PROGRESS IN OBESITY

ON

Boo

PROGRESS IN OBESITY RESEARCH: 9

Editors

Geraldo Medeiros-Neto
Alfredo Halpern
Claude Bouchard

Proceedings of the 9th International Congress on Obesity
Sao Paulo, 2002

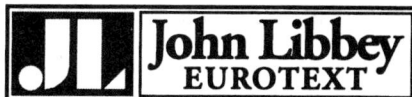

JL John Libbey EUROTEXT

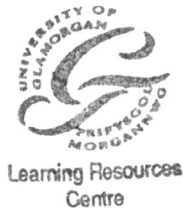

ISBN: 0-7420-0460-2
ISSN: 0962-7936

Editions John Libbey Eurotext
127, avenue de la République, 92120 Montrouge, France
Tél: 01 46 73 06 60
Email: contact@jle.com
Site internet: http://www.john-libbey-eurotext.fr

John Libbey Eurotext Limited
42–46 High Street, Esher, Surrey, KT10 9QY, United Kingdom

©2003

Table of Contents

Foreword

The International Association for the Study of Obesity approved in 1994 the proposal to hold its 2002 Congress in São Paulo at the invitation of the Brazilian Association for the Study of Obesity (ABESO). The 9th International Congress on Obesity was held in São Paulo from 24 to 29 August 2002. It was attended by about 3500 participants from 66 countries. This level of attendance is no doubt a reflection of the growing interest for adequate scientific foundations on the cause of the current obesity epidemic, its prevention and its treatment. The exciting advances made since the last ICO, held in Paris in 1998, played an important role in attracting the best and the brightest in the field to the São Paulo meeting despite the current financial difficulties and reluctance to travel in many countries of the world.

There were a total of about one thousand scientific presentations at the 9th ICO if one includes the traditional submitted free oral and poster papers. Among these, only authors of invited papers were asked to prepare a manuscript for this volume in the *Progress in Obesity Research* series. These papers were scheduled as plenary lectures, meet-the-professor sessions, debates, symposia or mini symposia. More than 220 papers are grouped in this publication under seven sections that coincide with the Programme Tracks used in the design of the Scientific Programme of the Congress. These Programme Tracks and corresponding sections are as follows:

Plenary lectures

1. Adipose tissue biology

2. Genetics of obesity

3. Prevention, behavioural aspects and childhood obesity

4. Epidemiology, health implications

5. Regulation of energy balance

6. Management and treatment

7. Continuing medical education

The authors were asked to write a short manuscript with strict limitations on the number of cited references. The purpose of the volume is not to be encyclopaedic but rather to provide a compendium of the key concepts and the essentials of the recent advances in obesity research. Despite the page limit imposed on the invited authors, we believe that this publication, like the previous volumes in this series, will constitute an excellent resource for those who are interested in understanding where research and professional practice stand today.

As Editors, we would like to express our gratitude to Anne Grauer and her associates at Paradigma for their help in the management of the collection of the manuscripts in a timely fashion. We would also like to thank the Publishers, John Libbey, for its effort to ensure that the *Progress in Obesity Research 9* was published as soon as possible after the Congress.

The Editors
Geraldo Medeiros-Neto, Alfredo Halpern and Claude Bouchard

PLENARY LECTURES

Progress in Obesity Research: 9. Edited by *Geraldo Medeiros-Neto, Alfredo Halpern and Claude Bouchard*
©2003 John Libbey Eurotext Ltd, pp. 3–9.

CHAPTER 1

Obesity research from genome to population: an integrative view

David B. Allison

Department of Biostatistics, Section on Statistical Genetics & Department of Nutrition Sciences, Clinical Nutrition Research Unit, University of Alabama at Birmingham, Ryals Public Health Building Room 327, 1665 University Boulevard, Birmingham, Alabama 35294-0022, USA
[e-mail: dallison@uab.edu]

It is a great honour to have the opportunity to share some thoughts on obesity research with my friends and colleagues on the occasion of receiving the Andre Mayer Award. Preparing these remarks was initially difficult. Putting one's own work into perspective and deciding why it is important is not an easy thing. To get some help, I turned to some of the writings of previous IASO award recipients. I found myself drawn back to a manuscript written by Dr. Jules Hirsch, a scientist I have long admired for his insight and eloquence, upon his acceptance of the 1986 Willendorf Award[1]. Dr. Hirsch opined that there were three types of researchers which he referred to as *moles, mutts* and *mappers*. Moles are scientists who pick a particular narrow research area in which to focus their efforts. Focus is the key word for these individuals. These scientists burrow ever deeper into a narrow area of research until they become the world's unquestioned expert on that very focused topic. Mutts are scientists that 'sniff around' turning over a rock here, a log there, occasionally discovering a new finding, but never staying on one topic for long. Mappers are the final category. Mappers are individuals who map out a whole new terrain. They see something new and open up new territories that large numbers of other investigators can then follow them into. Mappers, in the Kuhnian sense[2] might be said to be doing extraparadigmatic research. By definition, few of us can be mappers. If a mapper is somebody that many people follow, then not many people can be mappers or there will be no one to follow. I do not consider myself to have yet done any research that makes me worthy of being considered a mapper. I also know that I am unequivocally not a mole. I have not stuck with a single, narrowly-defined topic of research and plumbed ever deeper into that one endless series of narrowing concentric circles. Therefore I was left feeling as though I must be a mutt. And, while I like mutts rather well, it did not seem to me to be especially flattering to consider myself a mutt in this context (though I am confident others have occasionally considered me so in other contexts). I therefore began to wonder if there might not be some merit to considering some additional categories of obesity researchers.

In thinking about what a new category might be, I recalled the Arthurian legends. In T.H. White's *The Once and Future King*[3], Merlin teaches young Arthur a number of lessons by turning him into different animals. At one point, Merlin turns Arthur into a goose so that he may fly over England. As Arthur flies over England Merlin asks him 'What do you see?' Arthur replies that he sees the various kingdoms that comprise England below. Merlin points out that there are actually no boundaries between these kingdoms to be seen. Arthur literally sees that there are no such boundaries or rather, that all boundaries are simply human made, arbitrary lines. This important lesson allowed Arthur to try to move ahead and unify previously disparate kingdoms.

Just as land masses are often divided into arbitrary subunits, scientific inquiry is often divided up into arbitrary disciplines, topics, and subunits. To some extent, these disciplines, topics, and subdisciplines have utility by helping us arrange useful meetings, research centres, departments, and working groups. However, these divisions can sometimes impede the development of knowledge. My remaining remarks will talk about the researcher as bird. That is, the researcher as an individual who sometimes can see

3

past boundaries and thereby create new knowledge. I will illustrate this by beginning with a focus on genetic and environmental influences on body weight and fat.

Genes and environments

Animal breeders and livestock ranchers have known for centuries that animals can be selectively bred for numerous traits, including body weight and fatness. Pigs, cattle, chickens, quail, several aquatic species, and other species have been effectively selectively bred for traits related to body weight and composition[4]. In fact, average body fatness of pigs raised for human consumption has decreased dramatically in recent years, largely attributable to selective breeding for leanness. Most geneticists believe there is no stronger evidence for genetic influence on a trait than the ability to selectively breed for the trait. Thus, these data indicate the strong effect that genetic factors can have on fatness. Ironically, despite the fact that that this evidence of a genetic influence on fatness has been around for centuries, it was not until the early 1980's that the work of Albert Stunkard[5], clearly a 'bird' with a big picture view of things, published several seminal twin and adoption studies did people come to accept that there could be a genetic influence on adiposity in humans.

During the same time interval that fatness has radically decreased in pigs, fatness has radically increased in humans. Worldwide, our population is fatter now than it has ever been before[6] and this trend shows no sign of abating[7]. These joint observations, reduced adiposity in pigs due to selective breeding and increased adiposity in humans over a short period of time, clearly indicates the critical role of both genes and environments in explaining inter-individual variations in adiposity. The human gene pool is unlikely to have changed in important ways in a decade, and yet in the last decade BMI's of the American public and much of the world have steadily increased. What this points out is that a complete understanding of obesity cannot be obtained by studying either genetics or the environment, it can only be obtained by studying both genetics and the environment.

How heritable is BMI?

Heritability can be defined as the proportion of within population phenotypic variance that is due to within population genotypic variations. In humans, there are several types of studies that can be used to estimate the heritability of a trait. These include family and adoption studies, ordinary twin studies in which similarity of monozygotic twins is compared to the similarity of dizygotic twins, studies of monozygotic twins reared apart (i.e. twin separated at or shortly after birth), and studies of virtual twins (i.e. biologically unrelated individuals who are reared together as siblings and have the same or virtually the same date of birth). Numerous such studies have been conducted.

Family and adoption studies have generally estimated heritability to be in the range of 25–50 per cent[8]. Ordinary twin studies have generally estimated heritability to be in the range of 50–85 per cent[8]. This has led to some confusion in the field. Which is the correct answer? If one only has these two types of studies, it is difficult to tell. Each type of study is susceptible to different biases. In my experience, people often seem to be more acutely aware of and more likely to leap to point out the potential biases of the ordinary twin studies. The Achilles' heel of the ordinary twin study is the so-called 'equal environments assumption' which states that monozygotic twins that are treated no more similarly to their co-twins with respect to environmental factors that influence the trait under study than are dizygotic twins. If this assumption is violated, that is, if monozygotic twins are treated more similarly with respect to factors that influence their BMI's, then estimates of heritability from ordinary twin studies would be upwardly biased. In contrast, family and adoption studies are susceptible to different biases. I will not review them all here, but a detailed exposition can be found elsewhere[8]. In general, the important limitation in family and adoption studies is they are not particularly effective in capturing non-additive genetic variance. Non-additive genetic variance includes genes that act in a dominant or recessive fashion, genes that act epistatically, and genes that interact with other factors such as age. We have ample evidence from a variety of studies including molecular studies in mouse models that indicate that each of these sources of variation are present with respect to body weight and body fatness. Thus, it is at least equally plausible that family and adoption studies erroneously underestimate heritability as it is plausible that twin studies erroneously overestimate heritability.

The easiest way out of this question is to bring in new types of data. To this end, Allison *et al.* studied several sets of monozygotic twins reared apart (MZAs). Studies of MZAs are not subject to the same potential biases as are ordinary twin studies. Using these MZAs Allison *et al.* estimated the heritability of BMI to be roughly 70 per cent. This is almost exactly what is obtained with ordinary twin studies, suggesting that ordinary twin studies were yielding accurate estimates. More recently, Segal and

Allison[10] conducted a study of virtual twins. Like MZAs, these virtual twin studies are not dependent upon the equal environments assumption in the same way as ordinary twin studies are. Segal and Allison estimated the heritability of BMI to be roughly 65 per cent. They further estimated that the majority of genetic variance in BMI was non-additive variance. Moving across these different types of designs allows one to get a better handle on the true impact of genetic variation within our population.

What about the environment?

Many people seem to resist the idea that heritability of BMI could be as high as 70 per cent because they seem to think this implies that the environment is therefore of little importance. However, we can consider the environment in this context, and show that indeed it can be of profound importance. First, it is critical to point out that heritability, as stated previously, only refers to the proportion to *within population* variation that is due to within population genotypic variation. It says nothing about the extent to which differences in population distributions across time or geography are due to genetic or environmental factors. Secondly, although it may seem that 70 per cent of the variation within our population is due to genetic variations is large, 30 per cent can be seen to be a substantial amount by adapting an approach from Hewitt[11]. Let us assume that the heritability of BMI is roughly 70 per cent and that the standard deviation (SD) of adult BMI is approximately 5.8 units. This implies that BMI, ignoring an additive constant, is equal to

$$5.8 \left(\sqrt{0.7}\, G + \sqrt{1 - 0.7}\, E \right).$$

In this formula, G denotes a variable we cannot at this point explicitly quantify. G is the optimal composite of those innumerable genetic factors that effect BMI, most of which we do not yet know. However, if we did know all these factors and could add them all up with the proper scaling and weighting, the resulting quantity could be denoted G. Similarly, E represents the optimal composite of the innumerable environmental factors that influence one's body weight, many of which are also unknown. Having defined this formula, it is simple to work through the algebra to show that a 1 SD decrease in the environmental factors that increase BMI would reduce BMI by approximately 3.2 units. For a person that is 173 cm tall (approximately the mean height for a US adult) this would correspond to a loss of approximately 9.6 kg. It is noteworthy that the average person who shows up for an obesity treatment trial weighs roughly 100 kg and loses, with the best available drugs we have today plus some behaviour therapy, approximately 10 per cent of their body weight, or 10 kg. This means that a 1 SD decrease in the environmental factors that effect BMI could achieve the same results as the best available pharmaceuticals. A 1 SD decrease in environmental risk factors may seem large, but if one thinks back to 'Statistics 101' one will recall that with a normally distributed trait moving from roughly the 68th percentile to roughly the 50th percentile (i.e. the median) is a move of roughly 1 SD. Therefore, if we could help all individuals who tended to be at high environmental risk for obesity move just to the point of what is currently an average environmental risk for obesity, among those individuals we would expect to decrease their BMI by an amount equivalent to what we can achieve with the best available pharmaceuticals and is clearly clinically significant weight loss[12]. Thus even with a strong heritability such as 0.70, the environment is hardly impotent or ignorable.

Multivariate statistics, molecular genetics, and clinical observations

One of my first forays into obesity research was conducted with my friend and colleague, Dr. Stanley Heshka[13,14]. As part of my doctoral dissertation, Dr. Heshka and I used multivariate statistical methods (cluster analysis) to try to define homogenous subgroups of obese individuals from among what appeared to be broad heterogeneous samples. Clearly we were not the first to think about this approach. Many others, notably George Bray[15], had discussed classification of obesities for many years. But our approach was one of the first to bring multivariate statistical procedures to bear on the matter. It is interesting that today, more than 10 years later, cluster analysis and data mining have become the rage as scientists try to plow through massive databases in search of peculiar patterns[16]. Dr. Heshka and I found several interesting patterns and subtypes of obesity. We conjectured that these subtypes might be useful as the field progressed into genetic research by offering more homogenous phenotypes for geneticists to aim their sights on. Although the specific types we tentatively elaborated may not ultimately prove to be the most useful for genetic research, in more recent years the general idea that we may be in a position to better understand obesities from a genetic point of view by defining specific subtypes has proven useful. There have now been a number of individuals identified that appear to be obese because of single gene mutations. For review, see Rankinen *et al.*[17] These cases makes an interesting point. In virtually all cases, the individuals identified are not only obese but also have some relatively specific pattern of phenotypes or symptoms – a syndrome if you will. For example, individuals homozygous for inactivating mutations in a leptin gene have no functional leptin, become massively obese, have a highly fatty body composition, and, without exogenous leptin, cannot reach sexual maturity even into adulthood. In these regards, they recapitulate the syndrome displayed by the mutant ob/ob mice. In contrast, individuals with mutations in the leptin receptor gene, have virtually the same phenotypic syndrome except like db/db mice, they have markedly elevated levels of serum leptin. Individuals with POMC mutations are not only obese but have vivid red hair[18]. Individuals with certain PPARγ are not only obese, but have relatively low insulin[19]. These observations suggest that when looking for cases of obesity in which we may find single gene mutations, we may wish to look for not only obesity itself, but for obesity coupled with an unusual pattern of other phenotypic factors.

This idea was presaged long ago by Francis Bacon who, in the *Novum Organum*, wrote 'Errors of nature, sports and monsters correct the understanding in regard to ordinary things, and reveal general forms for whoever knows the ways of nature will more easily notice her deviations; and, on the other hand, whoever knows her deviations will more accurately describe her ways'. Bacon's words remind us to be on the lookout for interesting observations. Many of the most interesting observations are unlikely to be made only by somebody who stays in the mouse lab, nor by anyone who stays only in a clinic. But an individual who appreciates both aspects of study, who moves from mouse lab to clinic, and from mouse literature to human literature may be able to see additional things. For example, it is now well documented that mice that are made null for a 5HT2c receptor gene develop both obesity and a low threshold for seizures[20]. Interestingly, the clinical literature reveals a case of 'Hernandez syndrome' in a 16-year-old Brazilian girl who displayed psychomotor retardation, epilepsy, a bulbous nose, and obesity[21]. Is it possible that this girl had a mutation in the 5HT2c receptor gene? The tubby gene, when mutated to an inactivating form, leads to obesity, retinal degeneration, and cochlear degeneration[22]. Interestingly, North et al.[23] report a case of identical female twins with retinal degeneration, obesity, and mental retardation. Is it possible that these twins had mutations in the tubby gene? Only individuals who are willing to cross boundaries from clinical to mouse lab and literature will be in a position to answer these questions.

Studies in mortality

The relation between obesity and mortality rate has been of long standing interest and controversy to our field. This is also an area where new findings may be made by crossing boundaries. A somewhat surprising boundary exists between those who study epidemiology as an applied discipline and those who study statistical methodology. Although the field of epidemiology relies heavily on statistical analysis, many statistical practices in the field seem to become 'grandfathered in' as accepted knowledge and investigators do not cross over into the statistical literature to evaluate whether this presumed knowledge is veridical. An prominent example in the obesity field is the idea that one should control for potential confounding by pre-existing disease through the use of a technique which can be referred to as early mortality exclusion. The rationale is that people who die early in a follow-up are likely to have been diseased. Such individuals are also likely to have recently lost weight due to their disease. Because diseased individuals are likely to die earlier, this can create a spurious association between thinness and early mortality. Some authors opined that a reasonable way to control for this potential confounding would be to eliminate from the analysis any subject who died early in the follow-up period of a mortality study. Although intuitively appealing, and ultimately accepted as virtual dogma in the obesity field, my colleagues and I were surprised to find when we plowed into the statistical literature that there were no papers or books proving the merits of this technique. We therefore set about a series of studies, including mathematical proof, computer simulation, and meta-analysis, which we believe, demonstrate that this method is not a valid method for controlling for pre-existing disease[24,25,26]. There is no question that there are some circumstances that one can postulate under which eliminating early deaths will control for pre-existing disease. Nevertheless, there are many others one can postulate under which eliminating early deaths will not offer such control. Therefore, by stepping outside the boundaries of applied epidemiologic analysis and looking at the more basic statistical literature, we are able to see that an accepted technique in the obesity field could not be counted upon to achieve its objectives, and better techniques need to be sought.

Another example of the benefits of crossing boundaries between subfields within the overall field of obesity concerns the use of BMI in mortality analysis. It appears that a commonly accepted belief is that (a) BMI is highly correlated with per cent body fat and (b) therefore, when BMI is used in mortality analyses it will give us the same answer we would obtain if we used measured body fat instead of BMI. In contrast, I suggest that while (a) I agree that BMI is highly correlated with per cent body fat, (b) despite this, when used in mortality analyses, BMI may give markedly different answers then we would obtain with measured body fat, if fat mass and fat-free mass have opposite effects on mortality rate. I became interested in this question while working at the New York Obesity Research Centre and collaborating closely with Dr. Steven B. Heymsfield and other experts in the field of body composition. Though body composition methodology per se was not my primary field of investigation, being involved in it through my collaborations with Dr. Heymsfield and others allowed me to consider its use in mortality analyses. It appears that most epidemiologists do not have such exposure and, therefore, rarely question the merits of rough proxies like BMI in mortality analyses. In 1997,[27] my colleagues and I were able to show that the following conditions are entirely compatible. Specifically, it is entirely possible for BMI to have a linear increasing association with per cent body fat, for fat mass to have a linear increasing association with mortality rate, for fat-free mass to have a linear decreasing association with mortality rate, and for BMI to still have a U-shaped relationship with mortality rate. Therefore, although previous authors have tried to dismiss the elevation in mortality that is observed among thin people as artifactual and due to confounding by either smoking or pre-existing disease, we offered an additional explanation. Specifically, we suggested the possibility that this elevation of mortality among thin individuals might be due to low lean body mass. Several studies have now begun to investigate this with, admittedly crude, measures of body composition. Results are not entirely consistent, but some studies support the conjecture[28] and we are hopeful that additional studies will be forthcoming with more rigorously measured body composition.

The relationship between weight change and mortality rate has been even more confusing than the relationship between BMI and mortality rate. Although it would seem intuitive that, at least among obese people, weight reduction would lead to increased longevity and decreased mortality rate, this has not been observed to date. The majority of studies that examine undifferentiated weight change among obese people as a predictor of mortality rate show that it is associated with increased rather than decreased mortality rate (see Gregg and Williamson, this volume). Nevertheless, obesity is conceptually defined as an excess of body fat and is only operationally defined as an excess of body weight. We therefore examined two epidemiologic studies, the Framingham study and the Tecumseh study, to see whether there were apparently differential effects of body weight loss and body fat loss on mortality rate. In these studies, our measurement of change in body fat was limited to rather crude skinfold indicators. Nevertheless, we obtained remarkably similar results across these two studies. In each study we found that, conditional upon change in weight, fat loss resulted in a decreased mortality rate. In contrast, conditional upon change in fat, weight loss resulted in increased mortality rate. These data suggest that the composition of weight loss may be critical. It further suggests several important future research needs. First, epidemiologic investigators need to cross outside the strict boundaries of their field, which only relies on BMI and begin collaborating with investigators who have the expertise and ability to rigorously measure body composition such that greater insights can be obtained. Second, it suggests that individuals conducting clinical investigations of obesity treatments, especially of novel anti-obesity medications, would be wise to consider using body fat reduction as their primary end point rather than body weight reduction, as is now the norm. Several new drugs are available that hold the potential to preferentially reduce body fat (e.g. leptin, axokine, etc.) and these potential effects should be pursued.

Finally, I wish to point out an interesting 'hole' in the obesity literature that, in my opinion, is indicative of the need for crossing boundaries between disciplines and research strategies. Although we regularly prescribe weight loss for obese individuals and prescribe a number of anti-obesity medications for individuals with the expectation that such treatments will, among other things, hopefully prolong life, it is noteworthy that, to my knowledge, there has never been a single study in rodents showing that rodents allowed to become obese and remain obese until early middle adulthood and then subsequently reduced through caloric restriction or anti-obesity medications, live longer. Relative to the many studies done in rodents with sham-feeding, cannulas, injections, transgenic over-expression, knockouts, inducible knockins, tissue-specific transgenics, and so on, a study which simply exposes rodents to different diets or pharmaceuticals and records the date on which each animal dies is extraordinarily simple. Despite its simplicity, it has never been done. Why? I suspect that it has never been done because most people who think about weight loss and mortality rate are epidemiologists, most of whom would never think of doing a study in rodents. In contrast, most people who do studies in rodents are currently high-level physiologists, neuroscientists, and molecular geneticists who enjoy sophisticated technology and would never consider a study that is so simple as to merely count death rates. Nevertheless, in collaboration with colleagues at the New York Obesity Research Center, including Dr. Joseph Vasselli, we have obtained funding from the National Institutes of Health to conduct such a study. This study is a collaboration that could only be done by people who appreciate both statistical and population research, as well as the strengths of experimental manipulation and the use of model organisms. Data are not yet in, but we look forward to sharing results with the field in the not too distant future.

In conclusion, I am thankful for the opportunity to have shared some of my thoughts with you, and deeply honored by receipt of this award. I hope that the examples that I have presented have at least been interesting. Moreover, if there are a few among you who, like me, despaired of being a mutt, I hope you may appreciate the merits and the possibility of being a bird.

References

1. Hirsch J. The Willendorf Lecture: The Judgment of Solomon (I Kings 3: 16–28), *Recent Advances in Obesity Research: V*, Berry EM, Blondheim, SH, Eliahou HE, Shafrir, E (eds). London: John Libbey, 1986. pp. 1–4.

2. Kuhn T. *Structure of scientific revolutions.* Chicago: University of Chicago Press; 1962.

3. White, TH. *The once and future king.* New York: GP Putnam & Sons; 1958.

4. Allison DB, Pietrobelli A, Faith MS, Fontaine KR, Gropp E, Fernández JR. *Genetic influences on obesity.* In: R. Eckel, editors. New York: Elsevier (in press).

5. Stunkard AJ, Sorenson TIA, Hanis C, Teasdale TW, Chakraborty R, Schull WJ, Schulsinger F. An adoption study of human obesity. *N Eng J Med* 1986; 314: 193–8.

6. Allison DB, Saunders S. Obesity in North America: An overview. *Medical Clinics of North America*, 2000; 84: 305–32.

7. Lewis CE, Jacobs DR Jr, McCreath H, Kiefe CI, Schreiner PJ, Smith DE, Williams OD. Weight gain continues in the 1990s: 10-year trends in weight and overweight from the CARDIA study. Coronary Artery Risk Development in Young Adults. *Am J Epidemiol* 2000 Jun 15; 2000; 151(12): 1172–81.

8. Maes HHM, Neale MC, Eaves LJ. Genetic and environmental factors in relative body weight and human adiposity. *Behav Genet* 1997; 27: 325–51.

9. Allison DB, Kaprio J, Korkeila M, Koskenvuo M, Neale MC, Hayakawa, K. The heritability of BMI among an international sample of monozygotic twins reared apart. *Int J Obes* 1996; 20: 501–6.

10. Segal N, Allison DB. Twins and virtual twins: bases of relative body weight revisited. *Int J Obes* 2002; 26: 437–41.

11. Hewitt JK. The genetics of obesity: What have genetic studies told us about the environment. *Behav Genet* 1997; 27: 353–8.

12. Knowler WC, Barrett-Connor E, Fowler SE, Hamman RF, Lachin JM, Walker EA, Nathan DM. Reduction in the incidence of type 2 diabetes with lifestyle intervention or metformin. *N Engl J Med* 2002; 346(6): 393–403.

13. Allison DB, Heshka S. Toward an empirically derived typology of obese persons. *Int J Obes* 1991; 15(11): 741–54.

14. Allison DB, Heshka S. Toward an empirically derived typology of obese persons: derivation in a nonclinical sample. *Int J Eat Disord* 1993; 13(1): 93–108.

15. Bray GA. Definition, measurement, and classification of the syndromes of obesity. *Int J Obes* 1978; 2(2): 99–112.

16. Altman RB, Raychaudhuri S. Whole-genome expression analysis: challenges beyond clustering. *Curr Opin Struct Biol* 2001; 11(3): 340–7.

17. Rankinen T, Perusse L, Weisnagel SJ, Snyder EE, Chagnon YC, Bouchard C. The human obesity gene map: the 2001 update. *Obes Res* 2002; 10(3): 196–243.

18. Krude H, Biebermann H, Luck W, Horn R, Brabant G, Gruters A. Severe early-onset obesity, adrenal insufficiency and red hair pigmentation caused by POMC mutations in humans. *Nature Genet* 1998; 19: 155–7.

19. Ristow M, Muller-Wieland D, Pfeiffer A, Krone W, Kahn CR. Obesity associated with a mutation in a genetic regulator of adipocyte differentiation. *N Engl J Med* 1998; 339(14): 953–9.

20. Tecott LH, Sun LM, Akana SF, Strack AM, Lowenstein DH, Dallman MF, Julius D. Eating disorder and epilepsy in mice lacking 5-HT2c serotonin receptors. *Nature* 1995; 374: 542–6.

21. Melo DG, Acosta AX, de Pina-Neto JM. Syndrome of psychomotor retardation, bulbous nose, and epilepsy (Hernandez Syndrome): A Brazilian Case. *Clin Dysmorphology* 1999; 8: 301–3.

22. Coleman DL, Eicher EM. Fat (fat) and tubby (tub): two autosomal recessive mutations causing obesity syndromes in the mouse. *J Hered* 1990 Nov-Dec; 81(6): 424–7.

23. North KN, Fulton AB, Whiteman DA. Identical twins with Cohen syndrome. *Am J Med Genet* 1995; 58: 54–8.

24. Allison DB, Heo M, Flanders DW, Faith MS, Williamson DF. Examination of 'early mortality exclusion' as an approach to control for confounding by occult disease in epidemiologic studies of mortality risk factors. *Am J Epidemiol* 1997; 146(8): 672–80.

25. Allison DB, Heo M, Flanders DW, Faith MS, Carpenter KM, Williamson DF. Simulation study of the effects of excluding early mortality on risk factor-mortality analyses in the presence of confounding due to occult disease: the example of body mass index. *Annals Epidemiol* 1999; 9: 132–42.

26. Allison DB, Faith MS, Heo M, Townsend-Butterworth D, Williamson DF. Meta-analysis of the effect of excluding early deaths on the estimated relationship between body mass index and mortality. *Obes Res* 1999; 7(4): 342–54.

27. Allison DB, Faith MS, Heo M, Kotler DP .Hypothesis concerning the U-shaped relation between body mass index and mortality. *Am J Epidemiol.* 1997 Aug 15; 146(4): 339–49.

28. Allison DB, Zhu S, Plankey M, Faith MS, Heo M. Differential associations of body mass index and adiposity with all-cause mortality among men in the first and second National Health and Nutrition Examination Surveys (NHANES I & NHANES II) follow-up studies. *Int J Obes* 2002; 26; 410–6.

Progress in Obesity Research: 9. Edited by *Geraldo Medeiros-Neto, Alfredo Halpern and Claude Bouchard*
©2003 John Libbey Eurotext Ltd, pp. 10–14.

CHAPTER 2

Uncoupling proteins

Daniel Ricquier

Centre National de la Recherche Scientifique, UPR 9078 Institut de Recherche Necker-Enfants Malades,
156 Rue de Vaugirard 75730 Paris Cedex 15, France
[e-mail: ricquier@infobiogen.fr]

The balance between energy intake and energy expenditure controls body weight. Energy is expended on basal metabolism, exercise, and adaptative thermogenesis, which is a response to environmental changes such as cold exposure, excess food intake, or infection. Cold-induced thermogenesis in rodents has long been known to involve brown adipose tissue and a mitochondrial uncoupling protein (UCP renamed UCP1)[1–3]. The discovery in 1997 of new uncoupling proteins triggered re-examination of the molecular mechanisms of thermogenesis, their potential contribution to the pathogenesis of obesity, and above all their utility in the search for drugs to combat obesity[4–7].

Energy balance and thermogenesis

Thermogenesis is a characteristic of endothermic animals, which explains why their body temperature is spontaneously close to 37 °C even if exposed to low temperatures. Outside periods of reproduction or lactation, all the energy in a resting adult derives from food intake and is lost in the form of heat released during cellular metabolism and substrate oxidation. Cellular metabolism generates heat and substrate oxidation occurs in mitochondria where it is coupled to the reduction of NAD or FAD to NADH and FADH. The oxidation of reduced coenzymes by the mitochondrial electron transport chain is in turn coupled to the building of a proton gradient across the inner mitochondrial membrane. ATP synthesis by mitochondria is coupled to the return of these protons to the mitochondrial matrix through ATP synthase. Mitchell's theory predicts that the leaks of mitochondrial membrane protons not coupled to the phosphorylation of ADP increase the dissipation of energy in the form of heat. Whereas it was long thought that energy metabolism was fully coupled to ATP production, it is now known that a significant proportion of mitochondrial respiration is not coupled to ATP synthesis.

Brown adipose tissue and UCP1

Much nonshivering thermogenesis in small mammals is achieved in the brown adipose tissue (BAT), which is located near large blood vessels. BAT is found in all small mammals and in the newborn of larger mammals, such as humans[1–3]. BAT consists of brown adipocytes which are morphologically and functionally distinct from white adipocytes. Brown adipocytes contain numerous mitochondria characterized by a highly developed inner membrane. Activation of thermogenesis in BAT occuring in newborns, rodents exposed to cold, and in animals emerging from hibernation is commanded by the central nervous system and the orthosympathetic fibres innervating each brown adipocyte. The norepinephrine released by these fibres binds to adrenergic receptors on the surface of the brown adipocytes. The later steps of the activation of thermogenesis in brown adipocytes are production of cyclic AMP, activation of lipolysis, and oxidation of fatty acids by the numerous mitochondria. Released fatty acids stimulate brown adipocyte respiration and heat production. In line with Mitchell's chemiosmotic theory, if proton leakage is activated by a signal such as free fatty acids in the case of the mitochondria of brown adipocytes, the respiratory rate is enhanced. If, in addition the activated proton leakage is independent of ADP phosphorylation, respiration is uncoupled from ATP synthesis and oxidation energy is dissipated in the form of heat. The protein responsible for proton leakage within the inner mitochondrial membrane and for respiratory uncoupling was identified in 1976–1977, purified in 1982, and its cDNA was cloned in 1984 (see reviews[1-3]). It has an apparent molecular weight of 33,000 and was originally called uncoupling protein (UCP). Known as UCP1 since the discovery of UCP2 in 1997, it is abundant in the inner membrane of the mitochondria of brown adipocytes and is specific to these cells. The expression of UCP1 in yeasts or mammalian cell lines induces partial uncoupling of respiration[6]. The protonophoric activity of UCP1 has been reconstituted in liposomes where it can be inhibited by nucleotides and activated by free fatty acids. The mechanism of action of UCP1 is a matter of debate: some scientists believe that it is a proton transporter, whilst others assert that it returns anionic fatty acids to the intermembrane space, after they have crossed the membrane in protonated form. UCP1 and the ADP/ATP translocator are similar in structure and derive from the same ancestral gene, like several other members of the family of mitochondrial transporters sequenced since. The observation that $Ucp1^{-/-}$ mice are unable to maintain body temperature in the cold proved that the UCP1-induced uncoupling of respiration was responsible for cold-activated nonshivering thermogenesis of rodents[8].

The novel uncoupling proteins: UCP2 and UCP3

Given their specific role in thermogenesis, it has always seemed logical that brown adipocytes be equipped with an original mechanism, partial uncoupling of respiration, brought into play by a specific protein, UCP1, which induces proton leakage. In fact, an explanation had to be sought for the heat-generating mechanisms in cells other than brown adipocytes since all metabolic reactions produce heat. Moreover, it was known that mitochondrial respiration is always accompanied by heat production as it is imperfectly coupled to ADP phosphorylation in all types of cells. To explain this incomplete coupling of respiration and the energy loss mechanism, some authors have invoked slippage of the respiratory chains, while others refer to proton leaks. Brand and coll. have calculated that proton leaks from the inner membrane of mitochondria of hepatocytes and myocytes could explain 26 per cent of the liver's oxygen consumption and 5 per cent of the skeletal muscle's, i.e. about 20 per cent of the body's basal metabolism (see review[6]).

UCP2: an homologue of the brown fat UCP present in various tissues

Analysing a library of cDNAs of mouse skeletal muscle with a probe corresponding to the brown fat UCP cDNA, we and others isolated a clone corresponding to a protein with 59 per cent sequence identity with the UCP of brown fat[4-5]. This new UCP, called UCP2, was also identified in humans. In contrast with UCP1, the mRNA of UCP2 is present in almost all tissues and many cell types, such as spleen, thymus, digestive tract, brain, adipose tissue, muscle, heart, adipocytes, myocytes, and macrophages. Expressed in yeasts, murine UCP2 decreases the potential of the mitochondrial membrane, raises the respiration rate and reduces sensitivity to uncouplers: UCP2 therefore uncouples respiration and appeared to be a second mitochondrial uncoupling protein[4-7,9]. The UCP2 gene is located on chromosome 7 of the mouse and chromosome 11 of humans, near a region linked to hyperinsulism and obesity[4]. The expression of UCP2 mRNA was measured in obesity-prone and obesity-resistant mice given a lipid-rich diet: the obesity-resistant mice overexpressed UCP2 mRNA in their adipose tissue. These findings, together with the function of the protein and the chromosomal location of its gene, led to propose a role for UCP2 in diet-induced thermogenesis[4].

UCP3: another UCP homologue predominantly present in skeletal muscle

cDNAs corresponding to UCP3, a protein homologous to UCP1 and UCP2, were cloned soon after the discovery of UCP2[10-13]. The amino acid sequence of UCP3 is 72 per cent identical to that of UCP2 and 57 per cent identical to that of UCP1. UCP3 mRNA is predominantly expressed in the skeletal muscles of humans, mice and rats. In mice, UCP3 mRNA is also present in the brown adipose tissue as well as in the white adipose tissue and the heart. Recent work has shown that human and murine $UCP2$ and $UCP3$ genes are on the same chromosome and are separated by a few kilobases[10,14].

avUCP and stUCP: bird and plant UCPs

More recently, we isolated and characterized a chicken UCP cDNA termed avUCP[15]. This gene is only expressed in skeletal muscles of birds and ducks and is induced upon exposure to the cold. Therefore avUCP seems to be involved in regulatory thermogenesis. In other respects, funtional studies of isolated plant mitochondria suggested that plants contain mitochondrial uncoupling proteins. Following this observation, a cDNA from a new UCP was isolated from a potato bank[16]. The sequence of the corresponding protein, called stUCP, was 44 per cent identical to that of UCP1 and 47 per cent identical to

Methods	UCP1	UCP2	UCP3
Liposome	H^+leak	H^+leak	H^+leak
Yeast	H^+leak	H^+leak	H^+leak
Overexp. tg mice	uncoupling	n.d.	H^+leak or not increased oxidation
-/- mice	uncoupling	ATP effect or not ROS effect	uncoupling or not ROS effect
Normal Animals	thermogenesis	ROS control insulin secretion	ROS control ?

Fig. 1. Comparison of UCP1, UCP2 and UCP3 according to analytical methods used.

that of UCP2. The mRNA of stUCP is present in most plant organs. The most surprising result was that stUCP2 mRNA is strongly induced in the leaves of plants exposed to a temperature of 4 °C. Cold therefore induces stUCP as it induces UCP1 in the brown adipose tissue of animals. However, plant and animal UCPs may have different functions.

Roles and functions of UCP2 and UCP3: an unresolved question

Numerous questions remain unanswered, notably concerning the exact catalytic activity of each UCP, the nature of the endogenous ligands of UCP2 and UCP3, and the mechanisms of transcriptional control of the UCP2 and UCP3 genes. These proteins may simply translocate protons. The protons translocating activity of UCP1 is markedly activated by free fatty acids. Others proposed that the three UCPs were active as fatty acid cycler through the membrane[17–18]. According to this later hypothesis, protonated fatty acids cross the membrane and release a proton on the matricial side; then, the UCP facilitates the translocation of the anionic form of fatty acids. High loads of UCP2 or UCP3 can uncouple respiration in yeast or mammalian cell, but it is not certain whether the low physiological levels of these proteins may be sufficient to induce a net uncoupling of respiration *in vivo*. The divergent observations of the regulation of the activities of UCP2 or UCP3 by fatty acids or nucleotides will require further studies. Interestingly, Moore *et al.* recently proposed that UCP2 and UCP3 could export fatty acid anion under conditions of elevated fatty acid oxidation[19]. Expression studies of UCP2 in pancreatic cells agree with an uncoupling activity. Another important role for UCP2 and UCP3 may be related to the control of reactive oxygen species (this point is discussed below in the section of transgenic mice).

Bouchard *et al.* first reported a strong linkage between markers encompassing the UCP2/UCP3 locus and resting metabolic rate in humans[20]. Then, common polymorphisms were identified in human UCP2 and UCP3 genes. However conflicting data regarding the association of these polymorphisms to body mass index, morbid obesity, susceptibility to obesity, metabolic efficiency, fat oxidation, pathogenesis of juvenile or maturity onset obesity, insulin resistance, susceptibility to gain fat with age, basal metabolic rate were obtained[6,7]. More recently, another common variant in the promoter region of human UCP2 was described (G/A at position bp −866 relatively to the transcriptional start site); this variant is associated with decreased risk of obesity in middle-aged humans in a cohort of 790 individuals[21].

Mice overexpressing human UCP1[22] or UCP3[23] in skeletal muscle weigh less, have a decreased amount of adipose tissue, and an increased resting oxygen consumption. These data support a role for the UCPs in activating substrate oxidation and are in agreement with a respiration uncoupling activity of a high level of UCP3 and its potential role in treatment of obesity. Several other teams inactivated UCP2 or UCP3 by gene targeting[24–27]. In contrast to the marked decreased in fat content of mice overexpressing UCP3 (see above), the Ucp2$^{-/-}$ or the Ucp3$^{-/-}$ mice are not obese, have a normal body temperature and no change in oxygen consumption. These data challenge the expected role of the novel UCPs in energy metabolism. However, analysis of the Ucp2$^{-/-}$ mice identified two interesting roles of UCP2. Guided by the fact that UCP2 is expressed at high level in the immune system[4], Arsenijevic *et al.* found that the mutant mice were more resistant to infection by a parasite[26]. In fact, disruption of the Ucp2 gene provokes an elevation of ROS level that facilitates the killing of the pathogens. It is unknown whether such an effect results directly from a net change in respiration coupling in mitochondria or from a modification of the mitochondrial membrane potential that controls mitochondrial ROS production. These data support a role for UCP2 in limiting ROS level in cells. In other respects, Zhang *et al.*

observed that the Ucp2 $^{-/-}$ mice were hypoglycaemic and hyperinsulinaemic[27]. This is due to a higher insulin secretion in response to glucose by pancreatic islets. The authors explained this higher insulin secretion as a consequence of increased ATP levels in the absence of UCP2 uncoupling activity in islets of mutant mice. The negative effect of UCP2 on insulin secretion was also observed during experiments of overexpression of UCP2 in pancreatic islets.

UCP2 and UCP3, recent data, conclusions and perspectives

UCP1 has a well-demonstrated uncoupling activity and an essential role in maintenance of body temperature in small rodents exposed to the cold, but the exact biochemical and physiological roles of UCP2 and UCP3 remain to be further identified. Certain data support a true activity of these UCPs in respiration uncoupling[28], other data do not agree with a role for these UCPs in controlling body weight or adiposity. Interestingly, a strong association between UCP3 gene and obesity-related phenotypes was recently calculated using a new GA repeat microsatellite located in intervening sequence 6[29]. UCP2 and UCP3 appear to be genes limiting ROS level in cells and UCP2 as a gene controlling insulin secretion. The question of a direct regulation of UCP2 uncoupling activity by superoxide ion is presently debated[30-31]. Interestingly, the UCP2 gene is induced in apoptosis-sensitive lymphocytes after irradiation[32], in HeLa cells during oncosis[33], and in spinal cord of mice during experimental autoimmune encephalititis[34]. An open question is that of the exact amount of UCP2 and UCP3 in tissues since whatever is the exact intrinsic ability of these proteins to uncouple respiration from ATP synthesis, a certain amount of the proteins will be required to achieve a physiological uncoupling. In other respects, it should not be forgotten that a very small, but prolonged, change in level of coupling of mitochondrial respiration, i.e. change in efficiency of substrate oxidation, can significantly affect body adiposity.

Acknowledgements: The author is indebted to many colleagues in France and abroad and to the IASO Award Committee. Besides the outsanding contribution of F. Bouillaud, A-M. Cassard-Doulcier, C. Gelly, J-C. Kader, S. Klaus, C. Lévi-Meyrueis, B. Miroux, S. Raimbault and M-C. Alves-Guerra, L. Casteilla, E. Couplan, O. Champigny, C. Fleury, M-M. Gonzalez-Barroso, P. Hémon, M. Larose, G. Mory, C. Pecqueur, J-P. Revelli, S. Rousset, D. Vacher, F. Villarroya, the author acknowledges G. Ailhaud, J-M. Argiles, P. Arner, D. Arsenijevic, F. Assimacopoulos-Jeannet, J. Aubert, A. Basdevant, R. Bazin, C. Bouchard, L. Bukowiecki, M. Carruba, M. Cawthorne, Y. Chagnon, S. Cinti, S., K. Clément, S. Collins, B. Corkey, I. Cusin, C. Dani, Y. Deshayes, A. Doglio, C. Duchamp, L. Emorine, R. Falcou, C. Forest, P. Froguel, F. Fumeron, J-M. Garel, G. Garruti, J-P. Giacobino, L. Girardier, F. Goglia, M. Goubern, B. Guy-Grand, S. Krief, A. Hamann, G. Helmaier, J. Himms-Hagen, G. Hitman, B. Holloway, S. Inoue, B. Jeanrenaud, M. Klingenberg, A. Ktorza, D. Langin, M. Lafontan, M. Laloi, A. Lanni, C.S. Lin, F. Loönqvist, M-G. Mattei, B. Manning, M. Marzolo, F. Moreau, P. Muzzin, R. Nègrel, E. Nisoli, R.A. Norman, J. Nouguès, J-M. Oppert, L. Pénicaud, L. Pérusse, F. Picard, D. Richard, J. Seydoux, B. M. Spiegelman, E. Ravussin, Y. Reyne, E. Rial, F. Rohner-Jeanrenaud, S. Ross, D. Sanchis, M. Seldin, M. Stock, D. Strosberg, R. Surwit, M. Taouis, J. Thibault, R. Vettor, H. Vidal, K. Walder, C. Warden, J. Weissenbach, H. Wieneger, M. Yoshida. Our research is supported by Centre National de la Recherche Scientifique, Institut National de la Santé et de la Recherche Médicale, Association de Recherche sur le Cancer, Institut de Recherches International Servier, Human Frontier Science Programme Organization.

References

1. Nicholls DG, Locke RM. Thermogenic mechanisms in brown fat. *Physiol Rev* 1984; 64: 1–64.

2. Cannon B, Nedergaard J. The biochemistry of an inefficient tissue: brown adipose tissue. *Essays Biochem* 1985; 20: 110–64.

3. Himms-Hagen J, Ricquier D Brown adipose tissue. In: G. Bray, C. Bouchard and W. James, editors. *Handbook of obesity* pp. 415–41. New York, Basel, Hong Kong: Marcel Dekker, 1998.

4. Fleury C, Neverova S, Collins S, Raimbault S, Champigny O, Levi-Meyrueis *et al*. Uncoupling-protein-2: a novel gene linked to obesity and hyperinsulinemia. *Nature Genet* 1997; 15: 269–72.

5. Gimeno RE, Dembski M, Weng X, Deng NH, Shyjan AW, Gimeno CJ. Cloning and characterization of an uncoupling protein homolog: A potential molecular mediator of human thermogenesis. *Diabetes* 1997; 46: 900–6.

6. Ricquier D, Bouillaud F. The uncoupling protein homologues: UCP1, UCP2, UCP3, StUCP and AtUCP. *Biochem J* 2000 Jan 15; 345 Pt 2: 161–79. Review.

7. Boss O, Hagen T, Lowell BB Uncoupling Proteins 2 and 3. Potential regulators of mitochondrial energy metabolism. *Diabetes* 2000; 49: 143–56.

8. Enerback S, Jacobsson A, Simpson EM, Guerra C, Yamashita H, Harper YYE, Kozak LP. Mice lacking mitochondrial uncoupling protein are cold-sensitive but not obese. *Nature* 1997; 387: 90–4.

9. Rial E, Gonzalez-Barroso M, Fleury, Iturrizaga J, Jimenez-Jimenez J, Ricquier D, Goubern M, Bouillaud F. Retinoids activate proton transport by the uncoupling proteins UCP1 and UCP2. *EMBO J* 1999; 18: 5827–33.

10. Solanes G, Vidalpuig A, Grujic D, Flier JS, Lowell BB. The human uncoupling protein-3 gene – Genomic structure, chromosomal localization, and genetic basis for short and long form transcripts. *J Biol Chem* 1997; 272: 25433–36.

11. Boss O, Samec S, Paoloni-Giacobino A, Rossier C, Dulloo A, Seydoux J, Muzzin P, Giacobino JP. Uncoupling protein-3: a new member of the mitochondrial carrier family with tissue-specific expression. *FEBS Letters* 1997; 408: 39–42.

12. Vidal-Puig A, Solanes G, Grujic D, Flier J S, Lowell BB. UCP3: an uncoupling protein homologue expressed preferentially and abundantly in skeletal muscle and brown adipose tissue. *Biochem Biophys Res Commun* 1997; 235: 79–82.

13. Gong DW, He Y, Karas M, Reitman M. Uncoupling protein-3 is a mediator of thermogenesis regulated by thyroid hormone, beta3-adrenergic agonists, and leptin. *J Biol Chem* 1997; 272: 24129–32.

14. Pecqueur C, Cassard-Doulcier AM, Raimbault S, Miroux B, Fleury C, Gelly C *et al*. Functional organization of the human uncoupling protein-2 gene, and juxtaposition to the uncoupling protein-3 gene. *Biochem Biophys Res Commun* 1999; 255: 40–6.

15. Raimbault S, Dridi S, Denjean F, Lachuer J, Couplan E, Bouillaud F *et al*. An uncoupling protein homologue putatively involved in facultative muscle thermogenesis in birds. *Biochem J* 2001; 353: 441–4.

16. Laloi M, Klein M, Riesmeier JW, MullerRober B, Fleury C, Bouillaud F, Ricquier DA plant cold-induced uncoupling protein. *Nature* 1997; 389: 135–6.

17. Garlid KD, Jaburek M. The mechanism of proton transport mediated by mitochondrial uncoupling proteins. *FEBS Letters* 1998; 438: 10–4.

18. Jaburek M, Varecha M, Gimeno RE, Dembski M, Jezek P, Tartaglia LA, Garlid KD. Transport function and regulation of mitochondrial uncoupling proteins 2 and 3. *J Biol Chem* 1999; 274: 6003–7.

19. Moore GB, Himms-Hagen J, Harper ME, Clapham JC. Overexpression of UCP-3 in skeletal muscle of mice results in increased expression of mitochondrial thioesterase mRNA. *Biochem Biophys Res Comm* 2001; 283: 785–90.

20. Bouchard C, Pérusse L, Chagnon YC, Warden C, Ricquier D. Linkage between markers in the vicinity of the uncoupling protein 2 gene and resting metabolic rate in humans. *Hum Mol Genet* 1997; 6: 1887–9.

21. Esterbauer H, Schneitler C, Oberkofler H, Ebenbichler C, Paulweber B, Sandhofer F *et al*. A common polymorphism in the promoter of UCP2 is associated with decreased risk of obesity in middle-aged humans. *Nature Genet* 2001; 28: 178–83.

22. Li B, Nolte LA, Ju JS, Han DH, Coleman T, Holloszy JO, Semenkovich CF. Skeletal muscle respiratory uncoupling prevents diet-induced obesity and insulin resistance in mice. *Nature Med* 2000; 6: 1115–20.

23. Clapham JC, Arch JR, Chapman H, Haynes A, Lister C, Moore GB *et al*. Mice overexpressing human uncoupling protein-3 in skeletal muscle are hyperphagic and lean. *Nature* 2000; 406: 415–8.

24. Gong DW, Monemdjou S, Gavrilova O, Leon LR, Marcus-Samuels B,. Chou CJ *et al*. Lack of obesity and normal response to fasting and thyroid hormone in mice lacking uncoupling protein-3. *J Biol Chem* 2000; 275: 16251–7.

25. Vidal-Puig A J, Grujic D, Zhang CY, Hagen T, Boss O, Ido Y *et al*. Energy Metabolism in Uncoupling Protein 3 Gene Knockout Mice. *J Biol Chem* 2000; 275: 16258–66.

26. Arsenijevic D, Onuma H, Pecqueur C, Raimbault S, Manning B, Miroux B *et al*. Mice lacking uncoupling protein-2 survive to Toxoplasma gondii infection. A link with reactive oxygen species production and immunity. *Nature Genet* 2000; 26: 435–9.

27. Zhang C, Baffy G, Perret P, Krauss S, Peroni O, Grujic *et al*. Uncoupling protein-2 negatively regulates insulin secretion and is a major link between obesity, beta cell dysfunction, and type 2 diabetes. *Cell* 2001; 105: 745–55.

28. de Lange P, Lanni A, Beneduce L, Moreno M, Lombardi A. Silvestri E, Goglia F. Uncoupling protein-3 is a molecular determinant for the regulation of resting metabolic rate by thyroid hormone. *Endocrinology* 2001; 142: 3414–20.

29. Lanouette CM, Giacobino JP, Perusse L, Lacaille M, Yvon C, Chagnon M *et al*. Association between uncoupling protein 3 gene and obesity-related phenotypes in the Quebec Family Study. *Mol Med* 2001; 7: 433–41.

30. Echtay KS, Roussel D, St-Pierre J, Jekabsons MB, Cadenas S, Stuart JA *et al*. Superoxide activates mitochondrial uncoupling proteins. *Nature* 2002; 415: (6867): 96–9.

31. Couplan E, Gonzalez-Barroso MM, Alves-Guerra MC, Ricquier D, Goubern M, Bouillaud F. No evidence for a basal, retinoic or superoxide-induced uncoupling activity of the UCP2 present in spleen or lung mitochondria. *J Biol Chem* 2002; 277: 26268–75.

32. Voehrinher DW, Hirschberg DL, Xiao J, Lu Q, Roederer M, Lock CB *et al*. Gene microarray identification of redox and mitochondrial elements that control resistance or sensitivity to apoptosis. *Proc Natl Acad Sci USA* 2000; 97: 2680–5.

33. Mills EM, Xu D, Fergusson MM, Combs CA, Xu Y, Finkel T. Regulation of cellular oncosis by uncoupling protein 2. *J Biol Chem* 2002 Jul 26; 277(30): 27385–92.

34. Ibrahim SM, Mix E, Böttcher T, Koczan D, Gold R, Rolfs A, Thiesen, HJ. Gene expression profiling of the nervous system in murine experimental autoimmune encephalomyelitis. *Brain* 2001; 124: 1927–38.

Progress in Obesity Research: 9. Edited by *Geraldo Medeiros-Neto, Alfredo Halpern and Claude Bouchard*
©2003 John Libbey Eurotext Ltd, pp. 15–18.

CHAPTER 3

Transcriptional control of adipogenesis: interplay between C/EBPs and PPARγ in regulating adipocyte gene expression

Stephen R. Farmer

Department of Biochemistry, Boston University School of Medicine, 715 Albany Street, Boston, MA 02118, USA
[e-mail: farmer@biochem.bumc.bu.edu]

Introduction

During the last few years it has become increasing apparent that adipose tissue plays a central role in controlling energy balance in the organism[1]. Specifically, investigators have demonstrated that the adipocyte, in addition to facilitating the metabolism of glucose and lipids, secretes many proteins that regulate functions related to energy balance in other tissues including the brain, muscle and liver. These secreted proteins include many cytokines and hormones such as tumour necrosis factor alpha (TNFα), adiponectin and leptin. Understanding the molecular mechanisms regulating the expression of this large array of secreted proteins is presently an area of intense research in both basic and applied research. An approach to understanding these processes is to define the transcriptional events that regulate the differentiation of preadipocytes into mature adipocyte fat cells. This approach is particularly relevant since obesity is characterized by an increased adipose tissue mass that results from an expansion of the adipocyte population (i.e. differentiation of preadipocytes) as well as accumulation of triglycerides within already existing fat cells.

Regulation of adipogenesis: identification of a cascade of adipogenic transcription factors

Many of the studies, which have led to the identification of the transcriptional events regulating adipogenesis, have been performed in mouse mesenchymal cells in culture and in some cases confirmed in transgenic mice. The most frequently used model of adipogenesis in culture is the 3T3-L1 cell line of preadipocytes. Exposure of a confluent population of these cells to glucocorticoids (dexamethasone), isobutylmethylxanthine (MIX, a phosphodiesterase inhibitor which elevates intracellular cAMP levels), insulin and fetal bovine serum (FBS) induces differentiation. This process includes the re-entry of the quiescent, confluent preadipocytes into the cell cycle and passage through at least two rounds of cell division. This growth event is often referred to as clonal expansion and is considered to be a prerequisite for the subsequent transition into the terminal differentiation phase of adipogenesis. Coincident with clonal expansion, several transcription factors are expressed in a sequential manner, which are considered to initiate the cascade of adipogenic gene expression that leads to the formation of the mature fat cell phenotype[2]. One of the earliest events is the activation of expression of two members of the CCAAT/enhancer binding protein family[3], C/EBPβ and C/EBPδ, by mechanisms that involve glucocorticoids, cAMP and possibly the cAMP regulatory element binding protein, CREB[4]. An important role of both C/EBPβ and C/EBPδ appears to be activation of PPARγ[5,6], which is a member of the peroxisome proliferator-activated receptor family of nuclear hormone receptors. It is generally considered that PPARγ is the master regulator of adipogenesis[7,8]. In fact, ectopic expression of PPARγ in non-adipogenic fibroblasts under appropriate hormonal conditions induces their conversion into adipocytes[9]. This event involves the PPARγ-associated transcription of a series of target genes that encode proteins involved in several different biological processes. As expected, these include many enzymes and other proteins that regulate lipid and glucose metabolism in the mature fat cell such as the adipose-specific fatty acid binding protein (aP2)[10], fatty acid transport protein (FATP)[11], phosphoenolpyruvate kinase (PEPCK)[12] and the insulin-dependent glucose transporter (GLUT4)[13]. Induction of another key regulator of terminal adipogenesis, C/EBPα, appears to coincide with that of PPARγ , however the mechanisms responsible for this event are not as well defined as they are for the induction of PPARγ expression[7,14]. Once PPARγ and C/EBPα are expressed, they cooperate to ensure full expression of the mature adipocyte phenotype. This process includes a multitude of events including induction of additional transcription factors such as STAT 5A and B[15], suppression of growth-associated genes[2,16] as well as stimulation of insulin-dependent glucose transport[17,18].

Regulation of PPARγ expression and activity

PPARγ exists as two isoforms, γ1 and γ2, generated by alternative splicing of at least three different transcripts from the same gene[19,20]. Both isoforms share almost all the same exon sequences, except γ2 contains an additional 30 amino acids at the amino terminus[10,19]. The mouse and human PPARγ genes consist of greater than 100 kilobases, which contains at least nine exons[19,21]. Coding exons 1 to 6 are conserved between γ1 and γ2 and transcription of these is driven by two upstream promoters, P1 and P2. Transcription from the P1 promoter generates a large nuclear precursor mRNA that contains two additional untranslated γ1-specific exons, A1 and A2, that are spliced onto the 5' end of exons 1 to 6. The γ2 specific exon, B1, is transcribed from the P2 promoter and is also spliced onto the 5' end of exons 1 to 6 to generate an mRNA transcript in which both exon B1 and exons 1–6 are translated, giving rise to the longer γ2 isoform. The P1 promoter is at least 63 kilobases upstream of the P2 promoter and, consequently, it is very likely that each promoter contains specific regulatory DNA elements that direct transcription in a tissue-specific and differentiation-dependent manner. Transcription from the PPARγ gene has been detected in many different tissues in which the γ1 isoform is the predominant transcript[22]. In contrast, transcription from the P2 promoter is adipose tissue-selective, giving rise to abundant expression of the PPARγ2 isoform[10]. In fact, our recent studies (unpublished data) demonstrate that ectopic expression of C/EBPβ in non-adipogenic fibroblasts selectively activates the P2 promoter leading to abundant expression of PPARγ2. Exposure of these engineered cells to potent PPARγ ligands (see below) leads to conversion of these fibroblasts into adipocytes. The selective activation of the P2 promoter is consistent with other studies that have identified a C/EBP regulatory element within this region of the PPARγ gene[23].

As mentioned, the activity of PPARγ depends to a significant extent on its interaction with specific ligands that include various long chain polyunsaturated fatty acids (PUFAs) and their derivatives[24]. In fact, some members of the eicosinoid family of lipids (i.e. 15-deoxy-D12,14-prostaglandin J2 and 13S-HODE) have been shown to be high affinity ligands for PPARγ. Furthermore, there is a growing list of synthetic compounds currently being developed as drugs to sensitize individuals to insulin, which appear to act physiologically by regulating PPARγ activity in adipose tissue. Many of these drugs are also potent PPARγ ligands and are capable of inducing adipogenesis in various model systems including 3T3-L1 preadipocytes. For example, activation of PPARγ with the thiazolidinedione, troglitazone, induces many genes associated with the mature adipocyte phenotype and function[14].

It is generally accepted that natural PPARγ ligands exist in the differentiating preadipocyte, and that they play an important role in regulating PPARγ activity during adipogenesis. The mechanisms that regulate the production of these molecules, however, are unclear. Earlier studies by Spiegelman and collaborators demonstrated a role for ADD-1 (a member of the sterol regulatory element binding protein family, SREBP-1c) in stimulating PPARγ ligand production[25]. Our studies have also suggested a role for C/EBPβ since over-expression of a dominant negative isoform of C/EBPβ (LIP) renders 3T3-L1 preadipocytes dependent on an exogenous PPARγ-ligand for their differentiation into adipocytes[26].

Role of the MEK/ERK signaling pathway in regulating adipogenesis

In addition to these adipogenic transcription factors, it is quite apparent that signaling pathways play a role in coordinating the effects of the various adipogenic hormones in regulating adipogenesis. In our recent studies[27], we have questioned the role of the MEK/ERK signaling pathway in transmitting the effects of insulin and cAMP to the transcriptional machinery that regulates preadipocyte differentiation. Both insulin and cAMP have been shown to be required for the induction of adipogenesis in many mesenchymal cell lines including 3T3-L1 preadipocytes. The insulin receptor is a tyrosine kinase that can activate a series of signaling pathways including the Ras-MAPK pathway. The p42 (ERK2) and p44(ERK1) MAPKs are activated by phosphorylation on threonines and tyrosine residues by the dual specificity kinase MEK1, which induces their translocation into the nucleus where they activate or repress a variety of transcription factors involved in growth and differentiation. Our recent studies have shown that exposure of confluent, 3T3-L1 preadipocytes to the adipogenic inducers DEX, MIX and insulin induces MEK1 activity, which leads to the phosphorylation of both ERK 1 and ERK 2 during the initial 2–6 h of differentiation. In fact, it appears that insulin and MIX act in a synergistic manner to stimulate MEK1 activity. Inhibition of this activity by exposure of the cells to the MEK 1-specific inhibitor, U0126, prior to and during the first 24 h of differentiation significantly attenuates PPARγ and C/EBPβ gene expression. We were also able to demonstrate a direct relationship between MEK1 activity during the initial 6 h of differentiation and expression of the adipogenic genes. Incidentally, effectors that are potent inducers of the MEK/ERK signaling pathway such as FGF-2, when exposed to the cells for a limited period of time during this early phase of differentiation, were also capable of promoting adipogenesis. The MEK1 inhibitor had no effect on the ability of insulin and MIX to induce C/EBPβ expression suggesting the MEK/ERK signaling pathway is regulating adipogenesis at a step downstream of C/EBPβ. We questioned, therefore, whether activation of MEK/ERK activity potentiates the activity of C/EBPβ in inducing C/EBPα gene transcription. To address this question, we used a 3T3-L1 cell line, referred to as 4-2 cells, which contain a reporter gene composed of the C/EBPα minimal promoter regulating CAT expression in response to C/EBPβ activity. Exposure of 4-2 cells to DEX, MIX and insulin resulted in a burst of CAT activity at 36–60 h, which correlated with the expression of C/EBPβ during this early phase adipogenesis. Maximum stimulation of the MEK/ERK pathway by exposing the cells to FGF-2 along with the adipogenic hormones resulted in an even greater burst of activity. In fact, inhibition of this pathway by treating the cells with a MEK1 inhibitor, PD98059, significantly attenuated the induction of the C/EBPα minimal promoter by the various effectors as indicated by a PD98059-dependent decrease in CAT activity.

Concluding remarks

A therapeutic approach to treating obesity-related disorders is to develop drugs that modify adipose tissue function in obese individuals. This approach is validated by the successful use of two potent PPARγ ligands, rosiglitazone (Avandia™) and pioglitazone (Actos™), in controlling glucose homeostasis in humans[28]. As discussed above, PPARγ is a master regulator of adipogenesis and activation of its activity in adipocytes, by various ligands, alters expression of many proteins associated with energy balance including the insulin-dependent glucose transporter[13] and adiponectin[29]. Effectors that significantly modify PPARγ activity, therefore, are also targets for potential new therapeutics including signaling molecules (MEK/ERK) and additional transcription factors (C/EBPs).

Acknowledgement: This work was supported by National Institutes of Health Grant DK51586 and DK58825.

References

1. Bergman R N *et al.* Central role of the adipocyte in the metabolic syndrome. *J Investig Med* 2001; 49: 119–26.

2. Morrison R F, Farmer S R. Role of PPARγ in regulating a cascade expression of cyclin-dependent kinase inhibitors, p18(INK4c) and p21(Waf/Cip1), during adipogenesis. *J Biol Chem.* 1999: 274: 17088–97.

3. Cao Z, Umek RM, McKnight SL. Regulated expression of three C/EBP isoforms during adipose conversion of 3T3-L1 cells. *Genes Dev* 1991; 5: 1538–52.

4. Reusch J E, Colton L A, Klemm D J. CREB activation induces adipogenesis in 3T3-L1 cells. *Mol Cell Biol* 2000; 20: 1008–20.

5. Wu Z, Xie Y, Bucher N L R, Farmer S R. Conditional ectopic expression of C/EBPγ in NIH-3T3 cells induces PPARγ and stimulates adipogenesis. *Genes Dev.*1995; 9: 2350–63.

6. Wu Z, Bucher NLR, Farmer SR. Induction of peroxisome proliferator-activated receptor gamma during conversion of 3T3 fibroblasts into adipocytes is mediated by C/EBPβ, C/EBPδ and glucocorticoids. *Mol Cell Biol.* 1996; 16: 4128–36.

7. Rosen ED, Walkey CJ, PuigserverP, Spiegelman BM. Transcriptional regulation of adipogenesis. *Genes Dev* 2000; 14: 1293–307.

8. Rosen ED *et al.* C/EBPalpha induces adipogenesis through PPARgamma: a unified pathway. *Genes Dev* 2002; 16: 22–6.

9. Tontonoz P, Hu E, Spiegelman BM. Stimulation of adipogenesis in fibroblasts by PPARγ, a lipid-activated transcription factor. *Cell* 1994; 79: 1147–56.

10. Tontonoz P, Hu E, Graves R A, Budavari A I, Spiegelman BM. mPPARγ2: tissue-specific regulator of an adipocyte enhancer. *Genes Dev* 1994; 8: 1224–34.

11. Frohnert BI, Hui TY, Bernlohr DA. Identification of a functional peroxisome proliferator-responsive element in the murine fatty acid transport protein gene. *J Biol Chem* 1999; 274: 3970–7.

12. Tontonoz P, Hu E, Devine J, Beale EG, Spiegelman BM. PPAR gamma 2 regulates adipose expression of the phosphoenolpyruvate carboxykinase gene. *Mol Cell Biol* 1995; 15: 351–7.

13. Wu Z, Xie Y, Morrison RF, Bucher NLR, Farmer SR. PPARγ induces the insulin-dependent glucose transporter GLUT4 in the absence of C/EBPα during the conversion of 3T3 fibroblasts into adipocytes. *J Clin Invest* 1998; 101: 22–32.

14. Morrison RF, Farmer SR. Hormonal signaling and transcriptional control of adipocyte differentiation. *J Nutr* 2000; 130: 3116–21.

15. Stephens JM, Morrison RF, Wu Z, Farmer SR. PPARgamma ligand-dependent induction of STAT1, STAT5A, and STAT5B during adipogenesis. *Biochem Biophys Res Comm* 1999; 262: 216–22.

16. Altiok S, Xu M, Spiegelman BM. PPARgamma induces cell cycle withdrawal: inhibition of E2F/DP DNA-binding activity via down-regulation of PP2A. *Genes Dev* 1997; 11: 1987–98.

17. El-Jack AK, Hamm JK, Pilch PF, Farmer SR. Reconstitution of insulin-sensitive glucose transport in fibroblasts requires expression of both PPARγ and C/EBPα *J Biol Chem* 1999; 274: 7946–51.

18. Wu Z. *et al*. Cross-regulation of C/EBPα and PPARγ controls the transcriptional pathway of adipogenesis and insulin sensitivity. *Mol Cell* 1999; 3: 151–8.

19. Zhu Y. *et al*. Structural organization of mouse peroxisome proliferator-activated receptor γ(mPPARγ) gene: alternative promoter use and different splicing yield two mPPARγ isoforms. *Proc Natl Acad Sci USA* 1995; 92: 7921–5.

20. Fajas L, Fruchart JC, Auwerx J. PPARgamma3 mRNA: a distinct PPARgamma mRNA subtype transcribed from an independent promoter. *FEBS Letters* 1998; 438: 55–60.

21. Fajas L. *et al*. The organization, promoter analysis, and expression of the human PPARgamma gene. *J Biol Chem* 1997; 272: 18779–89.

22. Braissant O, Foufelle F, Scotto C, Dauca M, Wahli W. Differential expression of peroxisome proliferator-activated receptors (PPARs): distribution of PPAR-α, -β, and -γ in the adult rat. *Endocrinology* 1996; 137: 354–66.

23. Clarke SL, Robinson CE, Gimble, JM. CAAT/enhancer binding proteins directly modulate transcription from the peroxisome proliferator-activated receptor g2 promoter. *Biochem Biophys Res Commun* 1997; 240: 99–103.

24. Desvergne B, Wahli W. Peroxisome proliferator-activated receptors: nuclear control of metabolism. *Endocr Rev* 1999; 20: 649–88.

25. Kim JB, Wright HM, Wright M. Spiegelman BM. ADD1/SREBP1 activates PPAR gamma through the production of endogenous ligand. *Proc Natl Acad Sci USA* 1998; 95: 4333–7.

26. Hamm JK, Park BH, Farmer SR. A role for C/EBPbeta in regulating peroxisome proliferator-activated receptor gamma activity during adipogenesis in 3T3-L1 preadipocytes. *J Biol Chem* 2001; 276: 18464–71.

27. Prusty D, Park BH, Davis KE, Farmer SR. Activation of MEK/ERK signaling promotes adipogenesis by enhancing PPARgamma and C/EBPalpha gene expression during the differentiation of 3T3-L1 preadipocytes. *J Biol Chem* 2002; 20: 20.

28. Olefsky J M, Saltiel AR. PPAR gamma and the treatment of insulin resistance. *Trends Endocrinol Metab* 2000; 11: 362–8.

29. Combs TP et al.. Induction of adipocyte complement-related protein of 30 kilodaltons by PPARgamma agonists: a potential mechanism of insulin sensitization. *Endocrinology* 2002; 143: 998–1007.

CHAPTER 4

Evidence-based prevention

Shiriki Kumanyika

University of Pennsylvania School of Medicine, 8th Floor Blockley Hall, 423 Guardian Drive, Philadelphia, PA 19104,
USA
[e-mail: skumanyi@cceb.med.upenn.edu]

Introduction

Marked increases in the prevalence of obesity in adults have been documented throughout the world both in countries where the prevalence of obesity was already high and also in those where obesity has been relatively uncommon[1]. The seemingly limitless potential for obesity to prevail is reflected in the widely publicized obesity trends in the United States. Fifteen per cent of US adults were obese (defined as a body mass index [BMI] ≥ 30 kg/m^2) in 1980. In 1999 the per cent obese was nearly double, at 27 per cent, and subsequent reports suggest that the per cent obese has continued to rise[2,3]. With the emergence of this global epidemic, recognition of the need to put preventive strategies in place has increased, with a call for evidence as to what types of strategies may be effective[1,4]. However, compared to the vast resources devoted to obesity *treatment*[5], prevention has received relatively little attention. Strategies for obesity prevention require much more attention and a different paradigm.

Prevention arguments based on the situation in children are compelling. People recognize that what happens to children is a responsibility of the society at large, whereas with adults many will still view the problem more narrowly, as an issue of choice for individuals and, perhaps, their health care providers. Disturbing increases in obesity prevalence among children have been documented not only in western countries but also in countries such as Brazil, Costa Rica, Haiti, Japan, Egypt, Ghana, and Morocco[6]. These data show two to fourfold increases in obesity in pre-school and school-aged children in recent decades[6], and the possibility that these trends could continue unchecked is truly alarming. These trends thus portend an even greater population burden of adult obesity in the future. Moreover, obesity in childhood carries immediate deleterious and not necessarily reversible health and social consequences.

Definitions and causal pathways

To prevent obesity requires: (1) stabilizing the level of obesity in the population, (2) reducing obesity incidence, i.e. those whose BMI level increases to cross the threshold and, eventually, (3) reducing the number of obese people in the population[1]. Increases in the proportion of adults whose BMI levels are above the threshold that defines obesity (i.e. 30 kg/m^2, or the equivalent in children) are a direct function of the overall BMI distribution and directly correlated with the mean BMI level[7]. The ultimate goal is to achieve or maintain a population distribution centred on a mean of 21 to 23 kg/m^2.[1] This range is considered appropriate for limiting the proportion who are obese and to limit problems of underweight. We cannot forget that undernutrition is still a critical concern in certain population segments in countries where obesity is increasing overall.

What are the causes of widespread and increasing obesity in diverse societies, and what are the causes of the causes? Development of preventive strategies will require reflection on these pathways to identify potential points of leverage for removing or blocking the action of key factors, followed by research to demonstrate the ability to intervene successfully in these pathways. The proximal causes are self-evident: an excess of energy intake in relation to energy expenditure, leading to chronic, positive energy balance. Notwithstanding genetically-determined individual differences in susceptibility to weight

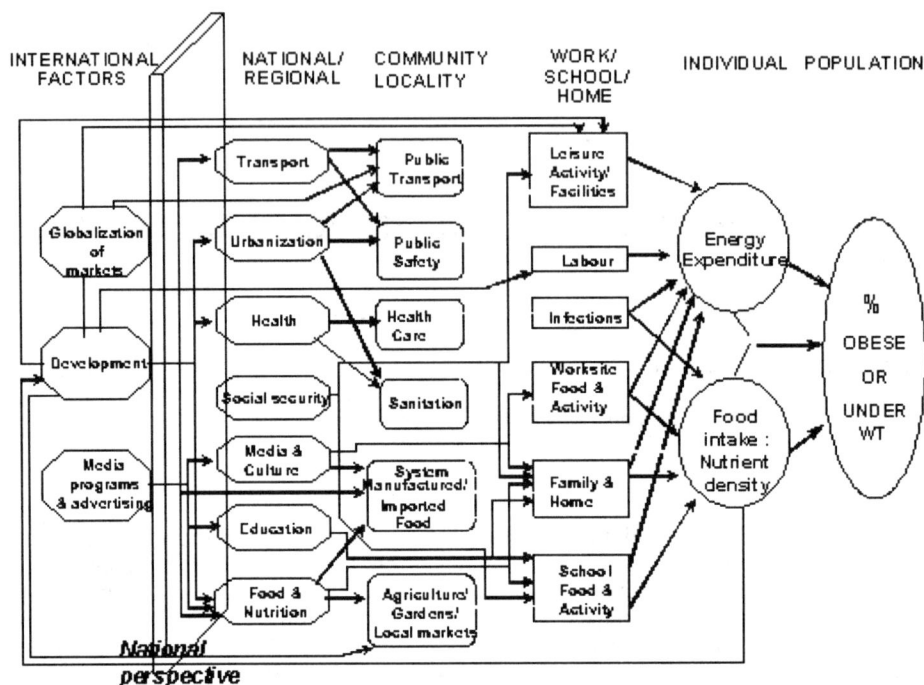

Fig. 1. Societal policies and processes influencing the population prevalence of obesity.

gain, most people are susceptible to becoming obese under the 'right' environmental circumstances, and these circumstances are increasingly present. In most cases, excess weight gain is quite gradual, perhaps even imperceptible on a day-to-day basis, although in some cultures perceptions about a body size that is healthy or unhealthy may allow obesity to occur and progress considerably without being viewed as problematic[4]. For example, particularly in low income communities, obese or overweight children who are active and socially well-adjusted may be perceived as simply more robust or healthy than their leaner peers[8].

Public education about the importance of weight control and how to achieve it is needed, but education alone is clearly insufficient. For example, in the United States, during the 1980s and 1990s, obesity prevalence doubled while the majority of adults were actively engaged in attempts to control their weight or lose weight[9]. However, societal trends leading to the unintentional or 'passive' overconsumption of food and to deprivation of opportunities to be physically active render many attempts at weight control either completely futile or only successful on a transient basis. Such trends include increased television viewing, reductions in physical education classes for school children, increasing dependence on automobiles, increased availability of food and marketing of very large portions of food, increased consumption of soft drinks, and more food eaten away from home[10].

The International Obesity Task Force framework for considering underlying causes of increases in obesity prevalence (Fig. 1) can be used to construct and deconstruct various possible prevention scenarios[4]. This framework depicts the vast array of macro-level and micro-level factors determining food intake and energy expenditure. These factors include global forces. Within countries there are influences at national, regional, community, and local levels. The behaviours of individuals are only partly a matter of personal choice. Individual choices are heavily influenced and limited by characteristics of the environment that are shaped by relatively remote forces[11,12].

Preventive strategies

There are different types of levels of preventive strategies[1]. In the most familiar classification, 'primary prevention' is defined as the reduction of risk to disease incidence, 'secondary prevention' as preventing disease progression, and 'tertiary prevention' as limiting the consequences of disease and preventing outcomes such as death or disability. 'Primordial prevention', prevention of the development of risk factors, is the stage before primary prevention. Other classifications are based on the segment of the population targeted and differentiate 'population approaches' that address the entire distribution, e.g. strategies to lower mean BMI, and 'high-risk' approaches, e.g. identifying and treating individuals or groups with high BMI levels. The categories of 'universal', 'selective' and 'targeted' prevention also refer to progressively more individualized approaches. A spectrum of prevention from distal to proximal factors has also been described, where distal or 'upstream' interventions focus on societal variables that will potentially impact on the entire population, e.g. changing policy and legislation related to taxes and food subsidies and the most proximal or 'downstream' approaches focus on improving the knowledge and skills of individuals. Population-oriented or environmental strategies are also termed public health strategies, in contrast to clinical strategies focusing on individuals. The term 'health promotion' emphasizes the importance of combining societal strategies with individually-oriented strategies, to increase the receptivity to and selection of favourable possibilities.

The enthusiasm for 'upstream' approaches and the understanding of what these approaches are and are not is quite limited among obesity researchers and health practitioners[13,14]. The model of obesity prevention as the treatment of preclinical obesity may seem comfortable and non-controversial. However, individually-oriented approaches alone cannot succeed in obesity prevention any more than tobacco control efforts could have succeeded without environmental and policy approaches[15]. Besides the paradigmatic issues, there are vested interests in industries, in the scientific community and in the population at large that support the status quo. These interests are well-served by arguments that obesity is determined at the individual level and should be approached primarily by case finding and treatment. Various stakeholders may have difficulty in accepting or may be unwilling to acknowledge the importance of making societal changes, often arguing that the problems are better resolved through the self-regulating aspects of the free-market system, that environmental pressures do not force autonomous individuals towards any particular set of choices, or – in the case of food advertising – that the right to advertise, even to very young children, is protected under the rights of free speech. Advances in the field of genetics are then discussed as possible 'preventive' tools, i.e. to screen and identify susceptible individuals.

Even where the need to approach the problem of obesity from a population perspective is recognized, those involved in developing and evaluating strategies are likely to be health professionals or scientists who feel ill-equipped to deal with policy and environmental issues such as price supports or transportation patterns[14], and whose thinking stays within the dominant biomedical paradigm in which clinical or treatment approaches are taken as the standard by which other interventions should be judged.

Differentiating prevention and treatment approaches

Articulating the differences between obesity prevention and obesity treatment is of paramount importance for avoiding the potentially destructive tendency to formulate and evaluate prevention strategies as a type of treatment. Heller and Page[16] have made the case well by identifying several dimensions on which clinical (i.e. treatment) and epidemiological (public health) approaches can be contrasted with respect to study design and statistical issues as well as implementation issues. Their excellent articulation of these critical paradigm issues can be summarized as follows. Whereas clinical approaches rely on refinements of randomized, controlled trials (RCTs), meta-analyses and systematic reviews, cost-effectiveness analyses and diagnostic tests for individuals, epidemiological approaches require the development of research approaches other than RCTs, the use of routinely collected data, and statistical approaches such as multi-level modeling that allow the simultaneous analysis of individual and contextual variables[16]. With respect to study design issues, it is especially unfortunate that efforts to educate clinicians about the rigors and internal validity of RCTs have been at the expense of categorizing other types of study designs (e.g. observational and quasi-experimental) as totally useless with this bias then carrying over to perceptions of what makes good evidence in the prevention domain. In addition, there still needs to be some approach available when there is as yet no evidence of any kind on the topic. In this sense, recourse to logic about causal pathways and common sense about actions that might help to reverse deleterious conditions in the physical or social environment is the counterpart of recourse to expert consensus or clinical judgment in a treatment situation.

Heller and Page[16] also make contrasts between the appropriate emphases in uses of clinical and epidemiological data for implementation. Clinical approaches are implemented by working towards improved access to information, clinical audits and clinical guidelines, and training of clinicians in critical appraisal of the scientific literature and seeking to make the 'best-case' scenarios from RCTs applicable to real life. Research on prevention must, by definition, be formulated for applicability to real life[17]. Improving access to information in epidemiological and preventive research means encouraging the routine collection of high quality data in natural settings across the health sector, calculating easy to understand population risk measures, and disseminating the results of model public health interventions[16]. Of particular importance on the public health side is not only that the data have direct relevance to policy and programmes but also that researchers learn the skill of making this data readily understandable to policy makers and to the public and educating them to use it.

The distinction between preventive and treatment approaches is somewhat blurred by the fact that high risk approaches, i.e. in which obesity prevention is defined as the identification and treatment of the subclinically obese, are indeed individually oriented and can be approached as 'treatments' where the goal is to stabilize weight rather than produce weight loss. This is a relevant but risky approach in that it can easily be seen to fail or, even if successful, be misinterpreted. For a number of methodological reasons, the likelihood of a statistically significant outcome is substantially less when the targeted outcome is prevention of weight gain than when the targeted outcome is substantial weight loss. Prevention studies are inherently less motivating because, for the participant in the intervention, the outcome is a *non*-event (no weight gain) rather than a readily observable event (weight loss). Hence, those individuals who are recruited to participate may have extremely high health motivations as well as knowledge and skill. The process of consenting individuals for such studies and then subsequently monitoring their behavioural and weight outcomes further adds to the potential for placebo effects and makes it both more difficult and less ethical to maintain a 'no-treatment' control. In fact, the behaviours of a sensitized group of individuals in a comparison group, as unconstrained by the intervention, may be more sensitive to any concurrent positive environmental changes. A complete litany of problems with the application of randomized trials in obesity prevention would include their low ecological relevance due to the distortion of reality that is inherent when taking internal validity as the most important criterion, various feasibility issues associated with randomization of both individuals and community units, and the inability to assess in field situations the critical process variable of individual energy balance.

Even when RCT approaches to obesity prevention result in a significant difference in the trajectory of weight change in the intervention vs. control groups, i.e. gradual weight gain versus maintenance at the same level, effects may be small and evident only over very long periods – periods that may outlast the funding for the study in question or the optimism of the investigator that an effect will indeed emerge. Moreover, because of the similarity in design to treatment studies, the small effects observed in prevention studies may be misconstrued as trivial individual-level effects when the correct interpretation is of a significant shift in the distribution of BMI in the population. RCTs of prevention have been successfully implemented in the area of sodium reduction and weight reduction for hypertension prevention to show the potential for small reductions in mean blood pressure levels that translate into substantial reductions in cardiovascular disease mortality[18]. Particularly for sodium reduction the intent was not to suggest direct dissemination of the extraordinary measures used to achieve the intervention effect. Rather, the demonstration of efficacy was intended to motivate changes in the food supply that would increase the ease and therefore the likelihood of sodium reduction in the general population.

Toward an obesity prevention paradigm

A paradigm shift to defining obesity prevention approaches as primarily population or environmentally oriented is needed: (1) to enhance understanding of the fundamental distinction between prevention and treatment and (2) to take advantage of the broader base of epidemiology and population sciences that is relevant to evidence for prevention. Such a paradigm shift would proceed with some critical *a priori* assumptions about causal pathways, for example, elaborating upon a general schema such as that shown in Fig. 1. Examples of a more refined logical framework that might be developed to analyse influences on energy intake and output in school or family settings are provided in a review by Dietz and Gortmaker[19] of childhood obesity prevention and treatment issues. Also relevant is the 'analysis grid for environments linked to obesity', or ANGELO, a tool proposed by Swinburn and colleagues[20] for analysing environmental factors and identifying possible places and ways to intervene.

Given the nature of the systems involved, it is clearly impossible to either anticipate all possible variations that may occur or to manipulate them in the manner of randomized trials. This is especially true for the macro-level forces that involve the production and manufacturing practices of huge multinational companies, economic policy, and mass media or for certain aspects of the physical environment. There are clearly many excellent strategic possibilities for intervention, but it is neither possible to intervene on them all at once nor to control the dynamics that are set into motion when the system is perturbed.

With respect to outcomes, environmental and population based approaches to obesity prevention are ultimately evaluated against the goal of stabilization of or shifting downward population mean BMI. However, just as the problem has evolved over decades, it may be decades before this goal can be achieved. In the short term one does have the ability to judge whether key indicators are tracking on the right course. Carefully chosen (e.g. for sensitivity and interpretability) process variables such as policy changes, accessibility of desirable options for food and physical activity as well as more proximal impacts on actual eating and physical activity behaviours are appropriate foci of evaluation[4]. Also, surveillance of environmental variables related to, although not directly targeted by, the intervention programme will be critical for identifying concurrent secular trends and interpreting the results of the intervention. Just as sophistication in the development of environmental interventions is growing, progress is also being made in the identification and refinement of a range of environmental and policy indicators[21,22].

The inherent difficulty of impacting upon the overall pathway with any given intervention, the inability to produce clear-cut or short-term effects on individuals exposed vs. not exposed to an intervention, and the need to take policy actions on the basis of common sense may combine to give preventive efforts a bad name, as unscientific or ineffective. This perspective is then taken up by those with vested interests in the status quo to argue that prevention doesn't work or that particular approaches are not justified and should not be supported. Advocates for prevention have a vested interest in identifying preventive approaches that do not work, but need to clearly establish the appropriate logic and methodology whereby this can be done. With respect to setting priorities, it will be most important to have strong evidence criteria and evidence when what is proposed goes against the dominant societal tendencies, because initiatives that are in line with dominant interests are likely to be less dependent on 'proving the case'.

The evidence at hand

Current evidence on obesity prevention consists of studies in children or adults where the outcome is BMI or weight[23–28] as well as studies of the impact of various interventions on physical activity[29] and eating behaviour variables[30]. Reviews and meta-analyses of changes in body weight[23–28] have focused on RCT designs and, not surprisingly given the foregoing discussion, have had mixed results and have overall been quite discouraging as to the potential for prevention. Studies in children have been more consistently promising than those in adults.

By contrast, recently published comprehensive, systematic reviews of the evidence for the effectiveness of interventions on physical activity[29] and on the intake of dietary fat and fruits and vegetables[30] have been very promising as to the potential for interventions to result in behavioural changes in the desired direction. In keeping with current conventions these reviews focused heavily on RCT-type studies, but the physical activity review in particular expanded the breadth of evidence to include other types of studies. For dietary behaviours the evidence tended to favour programmes among high risk populations and using behavioural modification strategies such as goal setting and small group discussions that have proven efficacious in treatment settings. For physical activity the promising interventions were more diverse and included informational, behavioural, and environmental approaches.

Summary and future directions

This brief review has focused on the mandate to put obesity prevention on a solid footing by first articulating a separate and appropriate paradigm and then following through with the compilation and dissemination of relevant evidence. The urgent need to act in this arena is evident from the current crisis of rapidly increasing obesity throughout the world and particularly among children who have the most to lose if effective prevention strategies cannot be developed and implemented. The needed strategies are a combination of environmentally-oriented, population based measures and individually-oriented approaches, with the former being the hardest to achieve. The beginnings of the needed paradigm shift are on the horizon but there is inadvertent competition from the movement for evidence-based medicine as well as deliberate resistance from diverse stakeholders who see many of the strategies recommended for prevention as a direct threat to their values and interests. Current evidence leaves much to be desired both with respect to study design and coverage of variables and pathways that must be a part of the ultimate equation for success. Accelerated efforts are needed.

References

1. World Health Organization. Obesity: preventing and managing the global epidemic. Report of a WHO Consultation. WHO Technical Report Series 894: Geneva 2000.

2. Centers for Disease Control and Prevention. National Center for Health Statistics. Prevalence of Overweight and Obesity Among Adults: United States, 1999; last reviewed 12/11/2000.Available from: URL: http://www.cdc.gov/nchs/products/pubs/pubd/hestats/obese/obs e99t2.htm (accessed on 29 May 2002).

3. Mokdad AH, Bowman BA, Ford ES, Vinicor F, Marks JS, Koplan JP. The continuing epidemics of obesity and diabetes in the United States. *JAMA* 2001; 286: 1195–200.

4. Kumanyika S, Jeffery RW, Morabia A, Ritenbaugh C and Antipatis VJ. Public Health Approaches to the Prevention of Obesity (PHAPO) Working Group of the International Obesity Task Force (IOTF). Obesity prevention: the case for action *Int J Obes Rel Metab Disord* 2002; 26: 425–36.

5. Natl Heart, Lung, Blood Inst Obes Educ Initiat. Clinical guidelines on the identification, evaluation, and treatment of overweight and obesity in adults. *Obes Res* 1998; 6 (Suppl 2): S51–S209.

6. Ebbeling CB, Pawlak DB, Ludwig DS. Childhood obesity. Public health crisis, common sense cure. *Lancet* 2002; 360: 473–82.

7. Rose G. Population distributions of risk and disease. *Nutr Metab Cardiovasc Dis* 1991; 1: 37–40.

8. Jain A, Sherman SN, Chamberlin DL, Carter Y, Powers SW, Whitaker RC. Why don't low-income mothers worry about their preschoolers being overweight? *Pediatrics* 2001; 107: 1138–1146.

9. Serdula MK, Mokdad AH, Williamson DF, Galuska DA, Mendlein JM, Heath GW. Prevalence of attempting weight loss and strategies for controlling weight. *JAMA* 1999; 13: 1353–1358.

10. French SA, Story M, Jeffery RW. Environmental influences on eating and physical activity. *Annu Rev Public Health* 2001; 22: 309–35.

11. Cockerham WC, Rûtten A, Abel T. Conceptualizing contemporary health lifestyles. Moving beyond Weber. *Sociol Q* 1997; 38: 321–42.

12. Nestle M, Jacobson MF. Halting the obesity epidemic. A public health policy approach. *Public Health Rep* 2000; 115: 12–24.

13. Kumanyika SK. Minisymposium on obesity: overview and some strategic considerations. *Annu Rev Public Health* 2001; 22: 293–308.

14. Antipatis VJ, Kumanyika SK, Jeffery RW, Morabia A, Ritenbaugh C. (1999)for the Public Health Approaches to the Prevention of Obesity (PHAPO) Working Group of the International Obesity Task Force. Confidence of health professionals in public health approaches to obesity prevention. *Int J Obes Rel Metab Disord* 23, 1004–1006.

15. Economos CD, Brownson RC, DeAngelis MA, Foerster SB, Foreman CT, Gregson J, Kumanyika SK, Pate RR.. What lessons have been learned from other attempts to guide social change? *Nutr Rev* 2001; 59: S40–S56.

16. Heller RF, Page J. A population perspective to evidence based medicine: evidence for population health. *J Epid Comm Health* 2002; 56: 45–7.

17. McGinnis J.M. Prevention research and its interface with policy. Defining the terms and challenges. *Prevent Med* 1994; 23: 618–9.

18. Trials of Hypertension Prevention Collaborative Research Group. Effects of weight loss and sodium reduction intervention on blood pressure and hypertension incidence in overweight persons with high-normal blood pressure. The Trials of Hypertension Prevention phase II. *Arch Internal Med* 1997; 157: 657–67.

19. Dietz WH, Gortmaker SL. Preventing obesity in children and adolescents. *Annu Rev Public Health* 2001; 22: 337–53.

20. Swinburn B, Egger G, Raza F. Dissecting obesogenic environments. The development and application of a framework for identifying and prioritizing environmental interventions for obesity. *Prevent Med* 1999; 29: 563–70.

21. Cheadle A, Sterling TD, Schmid TL, Fawcett SB. Promising community-level indicators for evaluating cardiovascular health promotion programs. *Health Educ Res* 2000; 15: 109–16.

22. Morland K, Wing S, Roux AD, Poole C. Neighborhood characteristics associated with the location of food stores and food service places. *Am J Prev Med* 2002; 22: 23–9.

23. Glenny AM, O'Meara S, Melville A, Sheldon TA, Wilson C. The treatment and prevention of obesity: a systematic review of the literature. *Int J Obes Rel Metab Disord.* 1997; 21: 715–37.

24. Resnicow K, Robinson TN. School-based cardiovascular disease prevention studies. Review and synthesis. *Ann Epidemiol* 1997; 7: S14–S31.

25. Story M. School-based approaches for preventing and treating obesity. *Int J Obes Rel Metab Disord* 1999; 2: S34–S51.

26. Hardeman W, Griffin S, Johnston M, Kinmonth AL, Wareham NJ. Interventions to prevent weight gain: a systematic review of psychological models and behaviour change methods. *Int J Obes Relat Metab Disord* 2000; 24(2): 131–43. Review.

27. Campbell K, Waters E, O'Meara S, Summerbell C. Interventions for preventing obesity in childhood. A systematic review. *Obes Rev* 2001; 2: 149–57.

28. Schmitz MK, Jeffery RW. Public health interventions for the prevention and treatment of obesity. *Medical Clinics of North America* 2000; 84: 491–512.

29. Kahn EM, Ramsey LT, Brownson RC, Heath GW, Howze EH, Powell KE, Stone EJ, Rajab MW, Corso P, and the Task Force on Community Preventive Services. The effectiveness of interventions to increase physical activity. *Am J Prev Med* 2002; 22 (Suppl 4),73–107.

30. Ammerman AS, Lindquist CH, Lohr KN, Hersey J. The efficacy of behavioural interventions to modify dietary fat and fruit and vegetable intake. A review of the evidence. *Prev Méd* 2002; 35: 25–41.

Progress in Obesity Research: 9. Edited by *Geraldo Medeiros-Neto, Alfredo Halpern and Claude Bouchard*
©2003 John Libbey Eurotext Ltd, pp. 26–28.

CHAPTER 5

The FLUORIDE hypothesis and DIOBESITY: How to prevent diabetes by preventing obesity

George A. Bray

Pennington Biomedical Research Center, Baton Rouge, LA 70808, USA
[e-mail: brayga@pbrc.edu]

Introduction

In the United States, body weight has increased slowly during most of the 20th century. Even before World War I, the life insurance industry had recognized that being overweight increased health risks. However, obesity palled in comparison to the search for new vitamins and the epidemic of heart disease that emerged as the old killers, tuberculosis and other infectious diseases, became treatable with antibiotics. Only at the end of the 20th century, when the rate of obesity accelerated, did people begin to take notice. When children and adolescents began to appear in endocrine clinics with obesity and diabetes, the problem began to take on a whole new dimension.

In this paper I will describe these two epidemics: the epidemic of obesity that precedes the epidemic of diabetes. I will describe some of the worldwide consequences of these epidemics. I will then briefly consider two treatment and preventive strategies that influence body weight. The first of these are the cognitive strategies – lifestyle, exercise and diet. The second alternative includes the procedures that adjust body fat 'automatically'. I have referred to these latter strategies for prevention and treatment as the 'fluoride hypothesis'. In this context, fluoride has two meanings. It refers to the molecule that when added to water or toothpaste reduces the incidence of dental caries. The second use is as an acronym for the types of messages that, like fluoride, would automatically adjust body fat. FLUORIDE in this context suggests that 'For Lowering Universal Obesity Rates, Implement Ideas that Don't Demand Effort'.

Epidemiology of obesity and diabetes

For the past 20 years, obesity has been increasing rapidly. By current definitions overweight, defined as a body mass index (BMI) of 25 to 30 kg/m^2, affects more than 60 per cent of adult Americans. A BMI > 30 kg/m^2 defines obesity and afflicts more than 30 per cent of adult Americans[1]. This epidemic of obesity is spreading throughout the world[2]. Of particular concern is the rising prevalence of obesity among children and adolescents, and its association with type 2 diabetes in adolescents.

There is also an epidemic of diabetes that now affects 6 per cent of Americans, with nearly an equal number undiagnosed. It is estimated that between 2000 and 2010 the number of diabetics worldwide will rise from 151 million to 221 million, a 45 per cent increase[3]. It is Asia and Africa that will bear the brunt of this increasing burden. Up to 50 per cent of adolescents with diabetes now have the type 2 form of this disease, in contrast with the near absence of type 2 in adolescents 10 years ago.

The causal relation of obesity to diabetes is suggested by the longitudinal studies in rhesus monkeys and Pima Indians. The first stage on the route to diabetes in a colony of rhesus monkeys is the appearance of obesity[4]. After obesity develops, glucose removal declines, insulin resistance appears and in animals whose beta cells are unable to cope with the extra demand for insulin, diabetes develops. Moreover, when weight gain is prevented for up to 10 years by restricting calories to keep weight stable, ɔ animals develop diabetes. Among the Pima Indians, there is a gradual increase in weight over the years prior to the onset of diabetes[5]. The likelihood of diabetes increases as insulin resistance becomes ever more severe.

Treatment and prevention

The standard approach to treatment is the use of lifestyle intervention, including diet and exercise. Use of these techniques has been shown to produce weight loss[6] and as a consequence, to decrease the need of antihypertensive medication or to slow the rate of conversion of impaired glucose tolerance to diabetes[7]. These techniques can be labeled as 'cognitive' strategies because they take a continuing effort on the part of the individual to make them work and to continue their effectiveness.

A number of recent studies have suggested that a significant component of body weight can be manipulated by settings that do not require the individual's participation. Breast feeding is the first example. In infants that are breast fed for more than 3 months, the risk of obesity at entry into school and in adolescence is significantly lower than infants who are breast fed less than 3 months[8]. This may be an example of 'infant imprinting'. Two other examples that fall into the category of fetal imprinting are the increased risk of obesity in offspring of diabetic mothers[9,10], and in the offspring of mothers who smoked during the individual's intrauterine period[11].

Other environmental agents also fall into this category. Smoking is well known to reduce weight, and smoking cessation is usually associated with weight gain. Nicotine is probably the actor in this case, since it will reduce food intake and increase thermogenesis in human beings. Dietary calcium intake is a dietary factor that works without 'attention'[12,13]. In epidemiological studies and in feeding trials, higher dietary calcium levels were associated with a reduced BMI.

A clinical trial with olestra illustrates the same principle. Olestra is an esterified form of sucrose that cooks and feels like 'fat' but that can't be digested by pancreatic lipase. When dietary fat is replaced by olestra, the diet has the same consistency and bulk, but has a reduced availability of fat. In a feeding trial, individuals whose diet had 25 per cent of its fat replaced by olestra lost significantly more weight than the group eating the control diet[14]. The precise explanation is not yet clear, but the implications are that changing the composition of the food supply might modify the human response to it.

Two medications also illustrate this point. The first group is of the 'atypical' antipsychotic drugs. Several of the more potent agents in this class are associated with weight gain. This can be as large as 10 per cent and is stable for as long as the drugs are continued. The other medication is metformin, which in a double-blind controlled trial produced a significant and consistent weight loss for more than 3 years without utilizing lifestyle or other cognitive techniques[7]. Along with the other events noted above, they suggest a new hypothesis to apply to the prevention of obesity.

The fluoride hypothesis

Fluoride is an element that can reduce the incidence of dental caries when added to the water supply. This effect does not require 'attention' or cognitive effort on the part of the individual. It is an automatic type of response. The alterations in body fat described above are similar to fluoride in that they don't require conscious intervention; rather, they are automatic or unconscious. The epidemic of dental caries could have been tackled by the cognitive strategies of increased brushing of the teeth and flossing. However, these cognitive approaches had not been successful, where the addition of fluoride to the water supply was so successful that it reduced the need for dentists and dental schools by nearly one-third.

The current epidemic of obesity may well reflect a defect in the feedback between energy expenditure and food intake, similar to the weakness of tooth enamel in the absence of fluoride. The report of 'toxins' that are found in adipose tissue suggests that the altered 'toxic' environment in which we live might have provided us with chemicals during the early stages of life that could have reprogrammed the 'fat' centres as does smoking or diabetes in the mother. I have labeled this hypothesis as the 'fluoride hypothesis' because it is analogous to what fluoride did for dental caries. It is also descriptive of one way to approach the current epidemic of obesity. 'For Lowering Universal Obesity Rates, Implement Ideas that Don't Demand Effort' describes this strategy.

If we were to use the fluoride hypothesis to tackle the current obesity epidemic, what approaches would we take? First, we would encourage more breast feeding. Second, we would discourage smoking during pregnancy, if not permanently. Third, we would evaluate the possibility of increasing calcium intake by clinical trials. Fourth, we would evaluate the nature of the changes in the food supply to look for other chemical entities that have appeared in the past 20 years that might act to 'imprint' the brain of newborn infants to alter their ability to couple the messages from food intake with their expenditure of energy. This is the message from the FLUORIDE hypothesis.

One interesting place to look might be in the food supply. A study by Van Dam *et al.* using data from the Health Professionals Follow-up Study showed that dietary fat was related to the incidence of diabetes, but not independent of body mass index[15]. This suggests that the dietary fat was affecting the incidence of diabetes by increasing body mass index. Of particular interest is the relation of processed meats to diabetes. Processed meats have a number of additives to provide a longer shelf life and reduce the risk of bacterial contamination. Could these 'preservatives', which are used in meats around the world, play a role in the relation of dietary fat to obesity and diabetes? It is only one idea suggested by the FLUORIDE hypothesis.

References

1. Flegal KM, Carroll MD, Kuczmarski RJ, Johnson CL. Overweight and obesity in the United States: prevalence and trends, 1960–1994. *Int J Obes Relat Metab Disord* 1998; 22: 39–47.

2. World Health Organization. Obesity: Preventing and Managing the Global Epidemic. Report of a WHO Consultation. Geneva: World Health Organization. WHO Technical Report Series 894, 2000.

3. King H, Aubert RE, Herman WH. Global burden of diabetes, 1995–2025: prevalence, numerical estimates, and projections. *Diabetes Care* 1998; 21: 1414–31.

4. Hansen BC, Jen KL, Pek SB, Wolfe RA. Fluctuations in basal plasma levels of pancreatic polypeptide in monkeys and humans. *Am J Physiol* 1985; 248: R739–47.

5. Ravussin E, Valencia ME, Esparza J *et al.* Effects of a traditional lifestyle on obesity in Pima Indians. *Diabetes Care* 1994; 17: 1067–74.

6. Wing RR. Behavioral approaches to the treatment of obesity. In: *Handbook of obesity*, GA Bray, C Bouchard, WPT James (eds), pp. 855–873. New York: Marcel Dekker, 1998.

7. Knowler WC, Barrett-Connor E, Fowler SE, Hamman RF, Lachin JM, Walker EA, Nathan DM; Diabetes Prevention Program Research Group. Reduction in the incidence of type 2 diabetes with lifestyle intervention or metformin. *N Engl J Med* 2002; 346: 393–403.

8. von Kries R, Koletzko B, Sauerwald T, von Mutius E, Barnert D, Grunert V, von Voss H. Breast feeding and obesity: cross sectional study. *BMJ* 1999; Jul 17; 319(7203): 147–50.

9. Silverman BL, Landsberg L, Metzger BE. Fetal hyperinsulinism in offspring of diabetic mothers. Association with the subsequent development of childhood obesity. *Ann NY Acad Sci* 1993; 699: 36–45.

10. Dabelea D, Hanson RL, Lindsay RS, Pettitt DJ, Imperatore G, Gabir MM, Roumain J, Bennett PH, Knowler WC. Intrauterine exposure to diabetes conveys risks for type 2 diabetes and obesity: a study of discordant sibships. *Diabetes* 2000; 49: 2208–11.

11. Power C, Jefferis BJ. Fetal environment and subsequent obesity: a study of maternal smoking. *Int J Epidemiol* 2002; Apr; 31(2): 413–9.

12. Zemel MB, Shi H, Greer B, Dirienzo D, Zemel PC. Regulation of adiposity by dietary calcium. *FASEB J* 2000; 14: 1132–8.

13. Davies KM, Heaney RP, Recker RR, Lappe JM, Barger-Lux MJ, Rafferty K, Hinders S. Calcium intake and body weight. *J Clin Endocrinol Metab* 2000; 85: 4635–4638.

14. Bray GA, Lovejoy JC, Most-Windhauser M, Smith SR, Volaufova J, Denkins Y, de Jonge L, Rood J, Lefevre M, Eldridge AL, Peters JC. A nine-month randomized clinical trial comparing a fat-substituted and fat-reduced diet in healthy obese men: The Ole Study. *Am J Clin Nutr* 2002.

15. van Dam RM, Willett WC, Rimm EB, Stampfer MJ, Hu FB. Dietary fat and meat intake in relation to risk of type 2 diabetes in men. *Diabetes Care* 2002; 25: 417–24.

Progress in Obesity Research: 9. Edited by *Geraldo Medeiros-Neto, Alfredo Halpern and Claude Bouchard*
©2003 John Libbey Eurotext Ltd, pp. 29–35.

CHAPTER 6

Obesity management: a priority in the primary and secondary prevention of cardiovascular disease

Jean-Pierre Després[1,2,3], Agnès Pascot[1], Isabelle Lemieux[1], Simone Lemieux[3], Benoît Lamarche[2,4], Charles Couillard[2,4] and Jean Bergeron[2]

[1]*Québec Heart Institute, Laval Hospital Research Center, Ste-Foy (Québec), Canada;* [2]*Lipid Research Center, CHUL Research Center, Ste-Foy (Québec), Canada;* [3]*Department of Food Sciences and Nutrition, Laval University, Ste-Foy (Québec), Canada;* [4]*Institute on Nutraceuticals and Nutritional Foods, Laval University, Ste-Foy (Québec), Canada*
[e-mail: jean-pierre.despres@crhl.ulaval.ca]

Introduction

The raising prevalence of obesity plays an important role in the epidemic of chronic complications such as type 2 diabetes, hypertension and cardiovascular disease[1]. However, as obesity is a heterogeneous condition, it is important to consider this notion in the evaluation of the risk associated with overweight/obesity. For instance, some very obese individuals are characterized by a normal blood pressure, a normal plasma lipoprotein-lipid profile and are euglycaemic despite a substantial excess of adipose tissue, whereas other subjects within a rather 'healthy' body weight range may sometimes have a substantially disturbed metabolic risk factor profile. The objective of this short paper is to provide evidence that visceral obesity is the obesity phenotype most likely associated with the highest risk of cardiovascular disease. Thus, until we appropriately manage this high-risk phenotype, the risk of chronic diseases will remain elevated among individuals characterized by this condition.

The contribution of obesity as the most common cause of chronic metabolic complications (including the metabolic syndrome) is not fully recognized

Obesity and type 2 diabetes have reached epidemic proportions in affluent societies and the increasing prevalence of these conditions is a source of concern[2-4]. For instance, obesity rates are projected to double over the next thirthy years[4,5] and, it has been projected that the worlwide number of type 2 diabetic patients will reach 270 millions in year 2025[6,7]. Among established coronary heart disease (CHD) risk factors, type 2 diabetes represents one of the most prevalent causes of CHD mortality and the majority of patients (65 to 80 per cent) diagnosed with type 2 diabetes will die from heart disease[8,9]. In this regard, Haffner and colleagues[10] published results of a prospective analysis documenting the high risk of myocardial infarction associated with type 2 diabetes. Over the 7-year follow-up period of the study, 3.5 per cent of nondiabetic asymptomatic individuals developed clinical ~s of CHD whereas this incidence reached 45 per cent among diabetic patients with established C¹ ~over, the incidence of myocardial infarction over the 7-year follow-up was 20.2 per cen' ~ patients initially asymptomatic for CHD, a value essentially similar to what was fou⸱ betic patients with already documented CHD (18.8 per cent)[10]. These results indic⸱ assessment standpoint, patients with type 2 diabetes without clinical signs of CH⸱ ered as patients with established CHD (secondary prevention). Therefore, from type 2 diabetes should be considered as a CHD risk equivalent[11].

Thus, the worldwide increase in the prevalence of obesity and of type 2 diab⸱ able challenge and a major burden for the health care system, emphasizi⸱

detection and management of these high-risk individuals. However, despite the fact that insulin resistance is a major risk factor for the later development of glucose intolerance and type 2 diabetes, cardiovascular disease may also develop even before the occurrence of hyperglycaemia or of type 2 diabetes. Thus, we have proposed that hyperglycaemia only represents the tip of an athero-thrombotic, inflammatory profile resulting from the presence of abdominal obesity and associated with a substantial increase in the risk of cardiovascular disease. Therefore, nondiabetic but overweight/obese patients with the features of the metabolic syndrome must be identified so that appropriate preventive measures are implemented in this subgroup of individuals at high risk for both type 2 diabetes and cardiovascular disease.

Visceral obesity: a high-risk phenotype

With the development of computed tomography and magnetic resonance imaging, it has become possible to distinguish the fat located in the abdominal cavity, the so-called intra-abdominal or visceral adipose tissue from the subcutaneous abdominal fat[12]. Using computed tomography, we have been able to show through several studies the important contribution of visceral adipose tissue to the metabolic complications of obesity despite the fact that this depot only represents a small proportion of the amount of total body fat[13-15].

We have used a very simple approach to sort out the respective contributions of visceral versus subcutaneous abdominal adipose tissue measured by computed tomography to the aetiology of the metabolic complications of obesity[13,14]. To achieve this goal, we have individually matched pairs of subjects for the same amount of total body fat but with either a low or high accumulation of visceral adipose tissue. In both men and women, we found that the subgroup of obese individuals with a high accumulation of visceral adipose tissue were characterized by the most severe metabolic disturbances, which included fasting hypertriglyceridaemia, reduced HDL-cholesterol concentration leading to a substantial increase in the total cholesterol/HDL-cholesterol ratio, glucose intolerance and hyperinsulinaemia resulting from *in vivo* insulin resistance, as well as a pro-thrombotic and inflammatory metabolic risk factor profile[13,14,16].

We also found that despite an apparent lack of difference in plasma LDL-cholesterol concentration, viscerally obese patients were characterized by an increased proportion of small, dense LDL particles, which were revealed by the presence of elevated apo B concentration as well as by a reduced size of the main LDL subpopulation assessed by polyacrylamide gradient gel electrophoresis[15]. Thus, the presence of an increased proportion of small, dense LDL particles cannot be appreciated by the measurement of LDL-cholesterol levels[17]. From a CHD assessment standpoint, the LDL-cholesterol concentration does not adequately reflect LDL quantity and quality in viscerally obese patients. However, fasting triglycerides, HDL-cholesterol and the cholesterol/HDL-cholesterol ratio have been found to be significant correlates of LDL particle size[17]. Recent data from our research group have also indicated that viscerally obese men with small LDL particles are also characterized by small HDL particles[18].

A fasting dyslipidaemic state is not the only metabolic alteration found in viscerally obese patients. There is also evidence that the expanded abdominal adipose tissue is an important site for the production of pro-thrombotic and inflammatory molecules[19-22]. For instance, plasma concentration of C-reactive protein (CRP), a marker of chronic inflammation which has been shown to predict the risk of myocardial infarction beyond classical risk factors[23], is markedly increased in viscerally obese patients[16]. It has also been demonstrated that waist girth, a simple anthropometric marker of abdominal obesity, was the best predictor of CRP levels[16]. Therefore, the cluster of metabolic abnormalities found among viscerally obese patients contributes to substantially increase the risk of an acute coronary syndrome due to the presence of an atherosclerotic, pro-thrombotic and inflammatory profile.

CHD risk in abdominally obese patients with the metabolic syndrome is not adequatelty estimated by traditional risk factors

Several papers from our laboratory have documented the metabolic complications associated with an excessive deposition of visceral adipose tissue. Overall, we found visceral abdominal obesity to be ociated, even in nondiabetic subjects, with all the features of the insulin resistance syndrome such rinsulinaemia, a greater glycaemic response to an oral glucose load, elevated triglyceride and ntrations, reduced HDL-cholesterol levels, an increased cholesterol/HDL-cholesterol ratio d proportion of small LDL particles[13-17]. These components of the insulin resistance

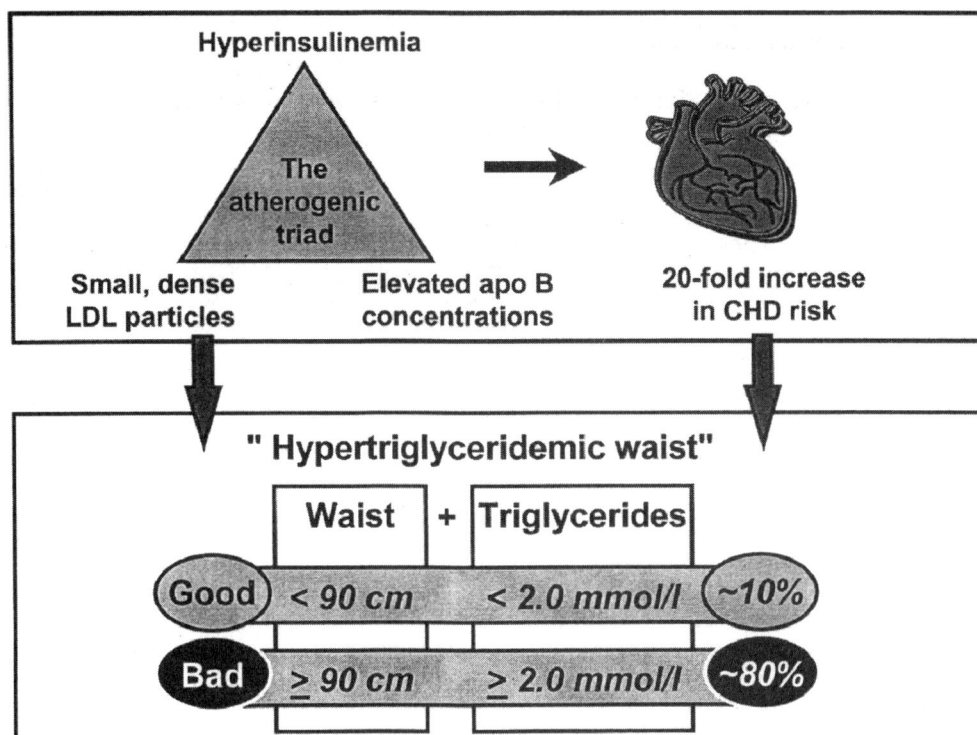

Fig. 1. Illustration of how 'hypertriglyceridaemic waist' could be used for the screening of high-risk patients characterized by the presence of the atherogenic metabolic triad (elevated apo B and insulin concentrations and small LDL particles) (adapted from Lemieux I *et al. Circulation* 2000; 102: 179–184).

syndrome have been shown in the cohort of middle-aged men of the Québec Cardiovascular Study to be associated with a substantial increase in the risk of CHD[24–26].

We were also interested to investigate whether our ability to discriminate individuals at high risk for CHD could be improved by simultaneously measuring three features of the metabolic syndrome (elevated apo B and insulin concentrations and small LDL particles) beyond what can be achieved using more traditional lipid risk factors (elevated triglyceride and LDL-cholesterol concentrations and reduced HDL-cholesterol levels) (Fig. 1)[27]. We found that being simultaneously characterized by the traditional lipid triad was associated with a 4.4-fold increase in the risk of CHD over the 5-year follow-up of our prospective study of middle-aged men[27]. However, the risk of CHD was increased by 20.8-fold among men simultaneously displaying the above features of the metabolic syndrome (hyperinsulinaemia, hyperapo B and small LDL size) and adjustment for the concomitant variation in the 'traditional' lipid triad failed to significantly alter this ratio, suggesting that this cluster of metabolic markers could improve our ability to identify individuals at high risk for CHD (Fig. 1)[27].

On the other hand, on the basis of the contribution of well known CHD risk factors, several guidelines recommend the use of the Framingham algorithm which considers age, total cholesterol, HDL-cholesterol, LDL-cholesterol, systolic and diastolic blood pressures, smoking and diabetic status in the CHD risk assessment[28]. A new notion introduced in the recently published NCEP-ATP III guidelines is the emphasis on the metabolic syndrome resulting from abdominal obesity[28]. Unfortunately, this highly prevalent atherogenic condition is not currently considered in the Framingham algorithm[29]. However, we have shown that asymptomatic men with an elevated waist girth (≥ 90 cm) and with moderate hypertriglyceridaemia (≥ 2.0 mmol/l) have a high likelihood (> 80 per cent) of being characterized by a triad of metabolic abnormalities (the atherogenic metabolic triad) which substantially increases their CHD risk even in the absence of elevated cholesterol and LDL-cholesterol or without traditional risk factors[30].

Although we observed in the Québec Cardiovascular Study that the Framingham algorithm adequately discriminates high-risk men characterized by traditional CHD risk factors, this algorithm was found to be misleading for a significant proportion of men with the metabolic syndrome and also at elevated risk for CHD, but not having the usual risk factors[31].

A simple clinical phenotype identifying the metabolic syndrome: 'hypertriglyceridaemic waist'

As most general physicians do not have access to insulin, apo B and LDL particle size measurements, we were interested in developing a simple algorithm which could be used in daily clinical practice to identify at low cost, high-risk individuals who would likely be carriers of this atherogenic metabolic triad[32]. On the basis of the very significant relationship between waist circumference and fasting insulin as well as apo B concentrations, we have used waist circumference as a surrogate anthropometric predictor for these two variables[32,33]. To predict the presence of small LDL particles, we and other groups had found that an elevated fasting triglyceride concentration was the best predictor of a reduced LDL particle size[15,34].

On the basis of these associations, we have used the combination of waist circumference and fasting triglyceride concentration to identify individuals characterized by this atherogenic metabolic triad (Fig. 1)[32]. A high proportion (more than 80 per cent) of men with simultaneous elevations in waist girth ($\geq$ 90 cm) and triglyceride levels ($\geq$ 2.0 mmol/l) were characterized by the atherogenic metabolic triad (Fig. 1)[32]. However, only 10 per cent of men with low triglycerides (< 2.0 mmol/l) and low waist girth (< 90 cm) had elevated apo B and insulin concentrations and small LDL particles[32]. Therefore, on the basis of the ability of this waist/triglyceride phenotype to predict this cluster of metabolic abnormalities, we have coined the term 'hypertriglyceridaemic waist' as a clinical phenotype defining a high-risk form of abdominal obesity.

Results published on the visceral obesity phenotype over the last 20 years have emphasized the importance of considering body fat distribution, especially visceral adipose tissue accumulation in the assessment of the obese patient. Nevertheless, it remains relevant for the clinician to measure weight and height and to calculate the body mass index (BMI) to position the patient in terms of relative weight. However, beyond the BMI, a waist circumference measurement will allow the physician to further characterize his/her patient for abdominal adipose tissue accumulation. In the presence of traditional risk factors such as hypertension, hypercholesterolaemia, smoking and type 2 diabetes, the presence of an elevated waist girth will substantially increase the risk of complications. However, the physician needs to keep in mind that even in the absence of these 'traditional' risk factors, the presence of the cluster of metabolic abnormalities of the insulin resistance syndrome will substantially increase the risk of CHD in the abdominally obese patient.

Need for weight loss – CHD prevention trials in high-risk overweight/obese patients

The best data available on the long-term benefits of moderate weight loss come from two landmark trials that were recently published: the Finnish Prevention of Diabetes study[35] and the American Diabetes Prevention Program[36]. Both trials recruited nondiabetic patients with impaired glucose tolerance who were randomized either to a lifestyle modification programme aiming at moderate weight loss (produced by a combination of increased physical activity and moderate reduction of caloric intake) or to a placebo group receiving usual medical care. In the American DPP, there was also another group who received metformin. Both trials were remarkably similar in showing that moderate weight loss induced by the lifestyle modification programme reduced the incidence of diabetes by 58 per cent. Furthermore, the American DPP showed that the risk of conversion from impaired glucose tolerance to diabetes was reduced to a greater extent (58 per cent) by lifestyle than by metformin (31 per cent). These landmark trials provide evidence that moderate weight loss produced by an improved diet and a more physically active lifestyle can decrease the risk of developing type 2 diabetes in a high-risk population with impaired glucose tolerance. In the Finnish DPP, a significant reduction in waist girth was also observed among patients with improved lifestyle[35].

A selective mobilization of visceral adipose tissue has also been reported with weight loss in viscerally obese patients[37] which could have a favourable impact not only on the dyslipidaemic profile and on indices of plasma glucose-insulin homeostasis, but such loss of visceral adipose tissue could also lead to significant reductions in plasma levels of thrombotic markers such as plasminogen activator inhibitor-1 as well as of inflammatory parameters such as cytokines and C-reactive protein concentrations[38]. These synchronized improvements in surrogate markers of atherosclerosis, thrombosis and inflammation could contribute to stabilize an unstable plaque possibly within only a few months of intervention, long before the normalization of body weight (Fig. 2). Obviously, this model is very speculative and

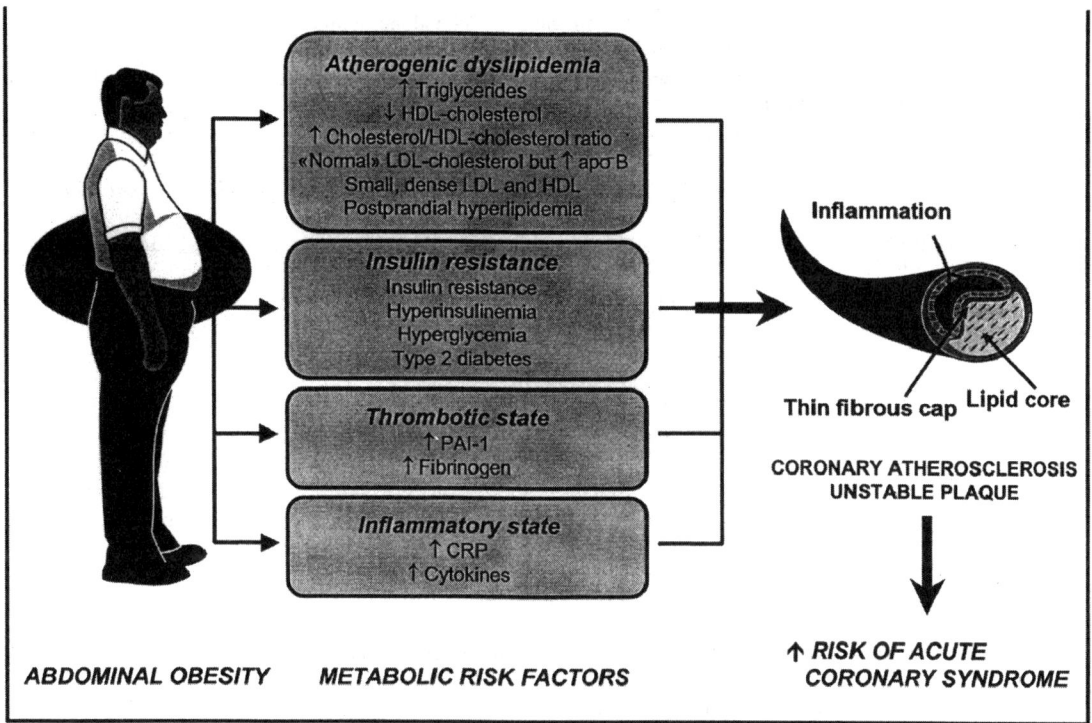

Fig. 2. Cluster of metabolic athero-thrombotic, pro-inflammatory disturbances resulting from visceral obesity, contributing not only to the progression of coronary atherosclerosis, but also increasing the risk of an acute coronary syndrome.

this possibility will have to be tested through randomized trials. Although two molecules (sibutramine and orlistat) are known to induce significant body weight loss[39,40], no study has been performed yet with these drugs in a high-risk population of patients characterized by visceral obesity and thus with the features of metabolic syndrome. However, on the basis of major metabolic improvements induced by moderate (5–10 per cent) weight loss, the relevance of an aggressive management of high-risk abdominally obese patients identified not only on the basis of body weight but also by waist circumference and fasting triglyceride measurements is emphasized.

Therefore, there has been a legitimate emphasis on the treatment of complications (by lifestyle interventions such as diet and exercise and/or pharmacotherapy) that are powerful risk factors for CHD such as hypertension, dyslipidaemia and diabetes. However, obesity has been ill-defined as a CHD risk factor, this situation being largely explained by its considerable heterogeneity as a phenotype. By being able to better identify a high-risk form of obesity, it is hoped that physicians will be encouraged to treat a common *cause* of the metabolic complications found in abdominally obese patients by focusing on waist circumference as another relevant therapeutic target.

Acknowledgements: This work was supported by the Canadian Institutes of Health Research (MT-14014) and the Canadian Diabetes Association. Jean-Pierre Després is chair professor of human nutrition and lipidology which is supported by Pfizer, Provigo and by the Foundation of the Québec Heart Institute. Benoît Lamarche is chair professor of Nutrition, Fonctional Foods and Cardiovascular Health from the Canada Research Chair programme. Simone Lemieux and Charles Couillard are research scholars from the Fonds de la Recherche en Santé du Québec. Jean Bergeron is a clinical research scholar from the Fonds de la Recherche en Santé du Québec.

References

1. Bray G, Bouchard C, James W. *Handbook of obesity*. USA: Marcel Dekker, Inc. 1998.

2. Mokdad AH, Ford ES, Bowman BA, Nelson DE, Engelgau, MM, Vinicor, F, *et al.* Diabetes trends in the US: 1990–1998. *Diabetes Care* 2000: 23, 1278–83.

3. World Health Organization. Preventing and managing the global epidemic. Geneva, Switerzerland: WHO Obesity Technical Report Series 894; 2000; 3–5 June.

4. Mokdad AH, Serdula MK, Dietz WH, Bowman BA, Marks JS, Koplan JP. The spread of the obesity epidemic in the United States, 1991–1998. *JAMA*. 1999; 282: 1519–22.

5. Kuczmarski RJ, Flegal KM, Campbell, SM, Johnson CL. Increasing prevalence of overweight among US adults. The National Health and Nutrition Examination Surveys, 1960 to 1991. *JAMA* 1994; 272: 205–11.

6. Zimmet PZ. Diabetes epidemiology as a tool to trigger diabetes research and care. *Diabetologia* 1999; 42: 499–518.

7. King H, Aubert RE, Herman WH. Global burden of diabetes, 1995–2025: prevalence, numerical estimates, and projections. *Diabetes Care* 1998; 21: 1414–31.

8. Grundy SM, Benjamin EJ, Burke GL, Chait A, Eckel RH, Howard BV, *et al.* Diabetes and cardiovascular disease. A statement for healthcare professionals from the American Heart Association. *Circulation* 1999; 100: 1134–46.

9. Kaukua J, Turpeinen A, Uusitupa M, Niskanen L. Clustering of cardiovascular risk factors in type 2 diabetes mellitus: prognostic significance and tracking. *Diabetes Obes Metabol* 2001; 3: 17–23.

10. Haffner SM, Lehto S, Ronnemaa T, Pyorala K, Laakso M. Mortality from coronary heart disease in subjects with type 2 diabetes and in nondiabetic subjects with and without prior myocardial infarction. *N Engl J Med* 1998; 339: 229–34.

11. Friesinger GC, Gavin JA. Diabetes and the cardiologists: a call to action. *J Am Col Cardiol* 2000; 35: 1130–33.

12. Ferland M, Després JP, Tremblay A, Pinault S, Nadeau A, Moorjani S *et al.* Assessment of adipose tissue distribution by computed axial tomography in obese women: association with body density and anthropometric measurements. *Br J Nutr* 1989; 61: 139–48.

13. Després JP, Moorjani S, Lupien PJ, Tremblay A, Nadeau A, Bouchard C. Regional distribution of body fat, plasma lipoproteins, and cardiovascular disease. *Arteriosclerosis* 1990; 10: 497–511.

14. Pouliot MC, Després JP, Nadeau A, Moorjani S, Prud'homme D, Lupien PJ *et al.* Visceral obesity in men. Associations with glucose tolerance, plasma insulin, and lipoprotein levels. *Diabetes* 1992; 41: 826–34.

15. Tchernof A, Lamarche B, Prud'homme D, Nadeau A, Moorjani S, Labrie F *et al.* The dense LDL phenotype. Association with plasma lipoprotein levels, visceral obesity, and hyperinsulinemia in men. *Diabetes Care* 1996; 19: 629–37.

16. Lemieux I, Pascot A, Prud'homme D, Alméras N, Bogaty P, Nadeau A, *et al.* Elevated C-reactive protein: another component of the atherothrombotic profile of abdominal obesity. *Arterioscler Thromb Vasc Biol* 2001; 21: 961–7.

17. Després JP. Health consequences of visceral obesity. *Ann Med* 2001; 33: 534–41.

18. Pascot A, Lemieux I, Prud'homme D, Tremblay A, Nadeau A, Couillard C, *et al.* Reduced HDL particle size as an additional feature of the atherogenic dyslipidemia of abdominal obesity. *J Lipid Res* 2001; 42: 2007–14.

19. Yudkin JS, Stehouwer CD, Emeis JJ, Coppack SW. C-reactive protein in healthy subjects: associations with obesity, insulin resistance, and endothelial dysfunction: a potential role for cytokines originating from adipose tissue? *Arterioscler Thromb Vasc Biol* 1999; 19: 972–8.

20. Juhan-Vague I, Alessi MC. PAI-1, obesity, insulin resistance and risk of cardiovascular events. *Thromb Haemost* 1997; 78: 656–60.

21. Juhan-Vague I, Morange P, Renucci JF, Alessi MC.): Fibrinogen, obesity and insulin resistance. *Blood Coagul Fibrinolysis* 1999 (10 Suppl 1): S25–8.

22. Garaulet M, Perex-Llamas F, Fuente T, Zamora S, Tebar FJ. Anthropometric, computed tomography and fat cell data in an obese population: relationship with insulin, leptin, tumor necrosis factor-alpha, sex hormone-binding globulin and sex hormones. *Eur J Endocrinol* 2000; 143: 657–66.

23. Libby P, Ridker PM, Maseri A. Inflammation and atherosclerosis. *Circulation* 2002; 105: 1135–43.

24. Després JP, Lamarche B, Mauriège P, Cantin B, Dagenais GR, Moorjani S *et al.* Hyperinsulinemia as an independent risk factor for ischemic heart disease. *N Engl J Med* 1996; 334: 952–7.

25. Lamarche B, Tchernof A, Moorjani S, Cantin B, Dagenais GR, Lupien PJ, *et al.* Small, dense low-density lipoprotein particles as a predictor of the risk of ischemic heart disease in men. Prospective results from the Québec Cardiovascular Study. *Circulation* 1997; 95: 69–75.

26. Lamarche B, Moorjani S, Lupien PJ, Cantin B, Bernard PM, Dagenais GR, *et al.* Apolipoprotein A-I and B levels and the risk of ischemic heart disease during a five-year follow-up of men in the Québec cardiovascular study. *Circulation* 1996; 94: 273–8.

27. Lamarche B, Tchernof A, Mauriège P, Cantin B, Dagenais GR, Lupien PJ, *et al.* Fasting insulin and apolipoprotein B levels and low-density lipoprotein particle size as risk factors for ischemic heart disease. *JAMA* 1998; 279: 1955–61.

28. Fodor JG, Frohlich JJ, Genest JJ, Jr., McPherson PR. Recommendations for the management and treatment of dyslipidemia. Report of the Working Group on Hypercholesterolemia and Other Dyslipidemias. *CMAJ* 2000; 162: 1441–7.

29. Wilson PW, D'Agostino RB, Levy D, Belanger AM, Silbershatz H. Kannel WB. Prediction of coronary heart disease using risk factor categories. *Circulation* 1998; 97: 1837–47.

30. Lamarche B, Tchernof A, Mauriège P, Cantin B, Dagenais GR, Lupien PJ, *et al.* Fasting insulin and apolipoprotein B levels and low-density lipoprotein particle size as risk factors for ischemic heart disease. *JAMA* 1998; 279: 1955–61.

31. Lemieux I, Lamarche B, St-Pierre A, Mauriège P, Dagenais GR, Després JP. Evidence from the Québec Cardiovascular Study that the Framingham risk chart may not detect a significant proportion of high risk men with the features of the insulin resistance syndrome. *Eur Heart J* 2001; 22: 630 (abstract).

32. Lemieux I, Pascot A, Couillard C, Lamarche B, Tchernof A, Alméras N *et al.* Hypertriglyceridemic waist. A marker of the atherogenic metabolic triad (hyperinsulinemia, hyperapolipoprotein B, small, dense LDL) in men? *Circulation* 2000; 102: 179–84.

33. Pouliot MC, Després JP, Lemieux S, Moorjani S, Bouchard C, Tremblay A *et al.* Waist circumference and abdominal sagittal diameter: best simple anthropometric indexes of abdominal visceral adipose tissue accumulation and related cardiovascular risk in men and women. *Am J Cardiol* 1994; 73: 460–8.

34. McNamara JR, Jenner JL, Li Z, Wilson PW, Schaefer EJ. Change in LDL particle size is associated with change in plasma triglyceride concentration. *Arterioscler Thromb* 1992; 12: 1284–90.

35. Tuomilehto J, Lindstrom J, Eriksson JG, Valle TT, Hamalainen H, Ilanne-Parikka P, *et al.* Prevention of type 2 diabetes mellitus by changes in lifestyle among subjects with impaired glucose tolerance. *N Engl J Med* 2001; 344: 1343–50.

36. Knowler WC, Barrett-Connor E., Fowler SE, Hamman RF, Lachin JM, Walker EA *et al.* Reduction in the incidence of type 2 diabetes with lifestyle intervention or metformin. *N Engl J Med* 2002; 346: 393–403.

37. Goodpaster,BH, Kelly DE, Wing RR, Meier A, Thaete FL. Effects of weight loss on regional fat distribution and insulin sensitivity in obesity. *Diabetes* 1999; 48: 839–47.

38. Després JP, Lemieux I, Prud'homme D. Treatment of obesity: need to focus on high risk abdominally obese patients. *BMJ* 2001; 322: 716–20.

39. Apfelbaum M, Vague P, Ziegler O, Hanotin C, Thomas F, Leutenegger E. Long-term maintenance of weight loss after a very-low-calorie diet: a randomized blinded trial of the efficacy and tolerability of sibutramine. *Am J Med* 1999; 106: 179–84.

40. Sjöström L, Rissanen A, Andersen T, Boldrin M, Golay A, Koppeschaar HP. Randomised placebo-controlled trial of orlistat for weight loss and prevention of weight regain in obese patients. European Multicentre Orlistat Study Group. *Lancet* 1998; 352: 167–72.

Progress in Obesity Research: 9. Edited by *Geraldo Medeiros-Neto, Alfredo Halpern and Claude Bouchard*
©2003 John Libbey Eurotext Ltd, pp. 36–39.

CHAPTER 7

Transcriptional profiling and gene discovery

Greg Collier[a,b], Andrea de Silva[a], Janette Tenne-Brown[a], Andrew Sanigorski[a],
David Segal[a], Lakshmi Kanthama and Ken Walder[a]

[a]*Metabolic Research Unit, School of Health Sciences, Deakin University, Geelong, Australia;*
[b]*Autogen Limited, Geelong, Australia*
[e-mail: barbedwa@deakin.edu.au]

DNA-based approaches for the discovery of genes that contribute to the development of type 2 diabetes have not been very successful despite substantial investment of time and money. The aetiology of a complex disease such as obesity or type 2 diabetes is not easily solved using current DNA-based approaches due to the multiple gene-gene and gene-environment interactions. Large numbers and/or variable combinations of small gene defects leading to the final disease state also complicate these analyses and make identification of important genes difficult. However, there are alternative strategies in the field of gene discovery such as RNA (gene expression) or proteomics-based approaches. Gene expression based technologies may prove to be a more rewarding approach to identify candidate genes, and in combination with appropriate animal models will be a powerful tool in understanding the underlying mechanisms of human polygenic diseases such as obesity and type 2 diabetes.

A number of RNA-based technologies are available to identify genes that are differentially expressed in various tissues. These include: differential display polymerase chain reaction (ddPCR); suppression subtractive hybridization (SSH); and cDNA microarrays. All of these techniques have been shown to be successful in identifying novel genes in a range of diseases. In our laboratory, differential gene expression profiling was used to identify tanis, a novel gene regulated by fasting and abnormally controlled in diabetic *Psammomys obesus*, a polygenic animal model of obesity and type 2 diabetes[1], and beacon, a novel gene involved in food intake and the control of body weight[2].

SSH is a powerful RNA-based technique that allows the comparison of two populations of mRNA and obtains clones of genes that are expressed in one population and not the other. The key advantage of this technique is its ability, via second-order hybridization kinetics, to exponentially amplify both rare and abundant differentially expressed transcripts while suppressing sequences that are common in both populations.

cDNA microarray experiments can provide gene expression data for thousands of genes and from large numbers of experimental samples. This technology is ideally suited to complex, multivariate analyses that generate detailed expression profiles, which in turn have the potential to increase our understanding of the underlying mechanisms associated with a disease. Current analysis techniques tend to focus on clustering algorithms that identify genes exhibiting similar expression patterns[3]. Recent advances in the analysis of microarray data have led to the construction of models to identify groups of genes involved in selected physiological processes[4]. Current progress in this field suggest that cDNA microarray technology will facilitate the identification of key genes and pathways involved in the pathogenesis of complex diseases such as obesity.

The power of these new technologies to detect differential gene expression is ideally suited to studies utilizing appropriate animal models of human disease. One such model, *Psammomys obesus* (Israeli Sand Rat) has been studied extensively in our laboratory[1,2,5–11]. *P. obesus* are gerbil-like rodents found in the desert areas of the Middle East and Northern Africa. They remain lean and free from diabetes in their native habitat, subsisting on a diet composed mainly of salt bush (*Atriplex halimus*)[12]. When taken into the laboratory, however, and allowed free access to standard rodent chow, varying degrees of obesity, insulin resistance and type 2 diabetes develop[5,13]. Adult *P. obesus* have a wide range of body weight and body fat content that forms a continuous distribution. It is the heterogeneous response to a relatively energy-dense diet that makes *P. obesus* more analogous to the pattern of human obesity and type 2 diabetes than homogenous single-gene animal models. A number of metabolic disturbances have been identified in obese, diabetic *P. obesus* relative to their lean littermates including hyperglycaaemia, insulin resistance, hyperphagia, obesity and dyslipidaemia[5–11].

The body weight distribution in *P. obesus* approximates a normal distribution and closely resembles that observed in human populations. Animals above the 75th percentile for body weight have increased body fat content and a greater risk of developing diabetes. Increased visceral fat content was also associated with elevated blood glucose and plasma insulin concentrations[11]. Cross-sectional analysis of the animal population of *P. obesus* reveals heterogenous distributions of blood glucose, plasma insulin and body weight[5,11]. It is this aspect of the development of diabetes and obesity in *P. obesus* which is of most importance, because these distributions are almost identical to the patterns observed in cross-sectional studies of human populations, including the inverted U-shaped relationship between blood glucose and insulin concentrations termed 'Starlings curve of the pancreas'[14,15]. Therefore, *P. obesus* represents an excellent animal model of obesity and type 2 diabetes that exhibits a phenotypic pattern closely resembling that observed in human population studies.

In our laboratory, the use of modern technologies to detect differential gene expression, in combination with an excellent animal model such as *P. obesus*, has resulted in the identification of novel genes important in the development of obesity and type 2 diabetes. Using ddPCR the beacon gene was identified as a transcript over-expressed in the hypothalamus of obese, diabetic *P. obesus*. Further studies in a larger group of animals demonstrated that the beacon gene was expressed in the hypothalamus in direct proportion to the body fat content[2]. Beacon is expressed ubiquitously throughout the body and encodes a small protein of 73 amino acids. The human beacon gene consists of 2194 nucleotides arranged into five exons and four introns and has been mapped to chromosome 19. The *P. obesus* beacon gene is composed of four exons, has a shorter 5'-untranslated region, and consequently lacks the first exon present in the human gene[2, Genebank Accession: AF318186]. Another novel gene, tanis, was overexpressed after fasting in the liver of obese, diabetic but not lean healthy *P. obesus*. The tanis gene comprises six exons on human chromosome 15q26.3 and encodes a 1155 nucleotide mRNA that produces a novel 189 amino acid protein with a single transmembrane region[1]. *In vitro* studies showed that tanis gene expression was suppressed by glucose in a range of cell lines. Yeast 2-hybrid and surface plasmon resonance studies showed that tanis interacts with serum amyloid a (SAA), an acute phase protein previously shown to be associated with type 2 diabetes[1].

However, candidate gene identification is only the first step in determining the gene's importance in the development of diabetes. It is necessary to determine the physiological function of the protein produced by the novel gene and to validate the potential of this protein as a therapeutic target. Recent years have seen the addition of various new tools to the existing classical biochemical techniques for understanding the role of proteins of unknown function. The research tools and strategies for functional studies that have been applied in our own and various other laboratories are outlined in Fig. 1 describing our technology platform used in these studies.

In our laboratory a research strategy is designed for each selected target based on the information obtained from bioinformatics and the physiological context in which the gene is discovered. The functional studies are directed to understand the function at a molecular level with isolated proteins, or at a cellular level by examining the altered biochemical or metabolic functions of cells as a consequence of inhibition or over-expression of the gene of interest. Where possible, we apply *in vivo* studies either by direct administration of the protein or by gene delivery into the animals using viral expression vectors.

It is helpful to have the purified protein available not only as a reagent for *in vivo* and *in vitro* experiments but also for raising antibodies. It is relatively more simple to genetically engineer bacterial strains and produce recombinant proteins than to isolate native proteins from tissue sources.

Monoclonal and polyclonal antibodies make valuable tools for several functional studies such as immuno-blotting, immuno-histochemistry and immuno-precipitation. Preparation of monoclonal antibodies is labour-intensive, but once the clones are established new stocks can be easily prepared. Work involved in producing polyclonal antibodies is less than for monoclonal antibodies and as they recognise multiple epitopes are in general more effective in recognizing antigens present in native or denatured conformations and for immuno-precipitation of antigens from dilute test samples.

A variety of eukaryotic plasmid and viral (retroviral or adenoviral) expression vectors can be employed to over-express genes of interest in insulin responsive cell lines such as differentiated 3T3-L1 (adipocyte), C2C12 or L6 (muscle), or HepG2 or H4IIE (hepatocyte) or min6 (pancreatic). As an alternative,

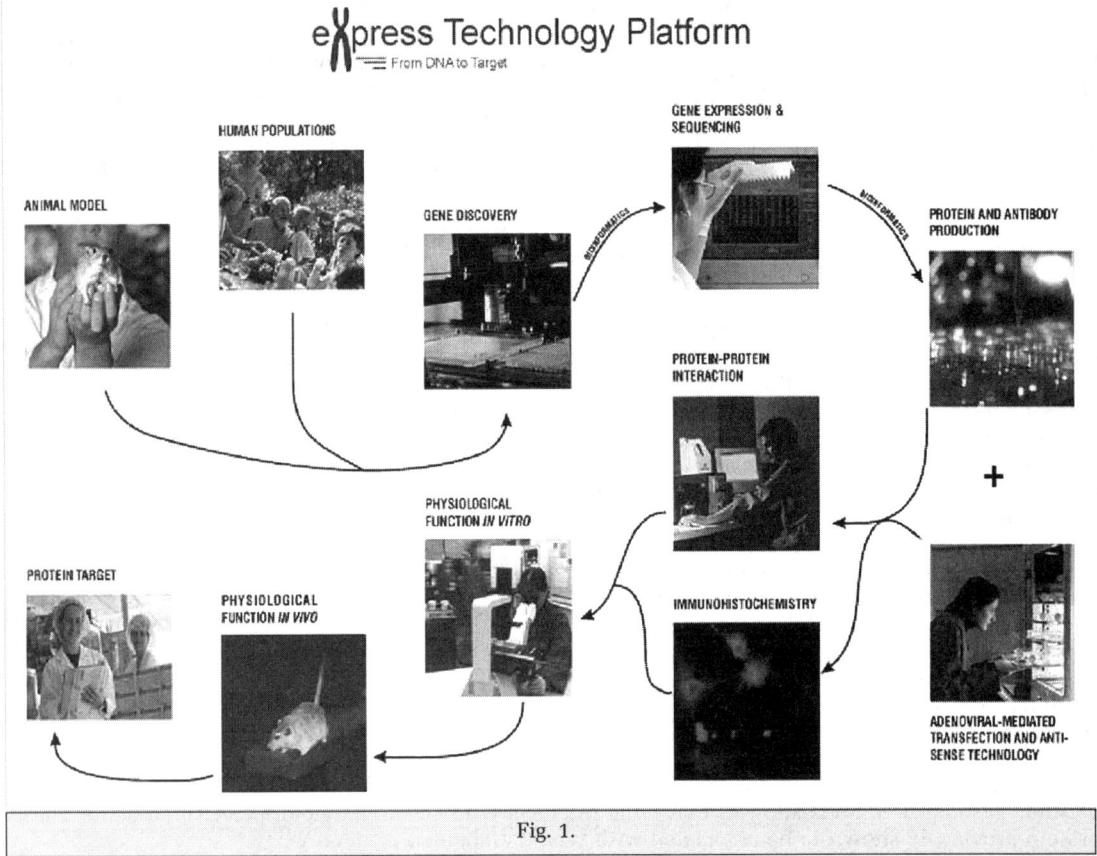

Fig. 1.

carefully designed antisense oligonucleotides or RNA interference vectors can be used to inhibit endogenous expression of genes of interest. Studies can be conducted in which the gene of interest is overexpressed or inhibited, and the cell's response to insulin, such as changes in glucose uptake, glycogen synthesis or lipogenesis is examined. This information can reveal the nature of metabolic pathways in which the gene of interest is involved. When the studies in cell culture models are completed our plan is to apply the same vectors or oligonucleotides that produce an effect for *in vivo* studies in live animals and validate the observed effects.

Almost all proteins fulfil their functional role via interaction with other proteins. Identification of interacting proteins and any knowledge of their functional properties can also provide clues for positioning the candidate protein in a defined signal transduction pathway. Protein-protein interactions can be identified using co-expression technologies such as the yeast 2-hybrid system[16–19], or biophysical techniques such as fluorescence and bioluminescence resonance energy transfer[20,21] or Biacore[22]. All of these techniques aim to identify interactions between two proteins.

We utilized the technologies described above to investigate the physiological function of two novel gene discoveries in our laboratory, beacon, an obesity gene, and tanis, a gene regulated by fasting. The physiological function of beacon in the regulation of energy balance was confirmed by direct admini-stration of the protein *in vivo* in *P. obesus*. Intracerebroventricular (ICV) administration of beacon for 7 days resulted in a dose-dependent increase in food intake and body weight gain, and resulted in a twofold increase in hypothalamic expression of NPY[2]. In addition, tanis expression was shown to be regulated by glucose, and the tanis protein interacts with SAA, an acute phase inflammatory protein[1]. The relationship between inflammation and diabetes has received intensive interest lately, as acute phase proteins including SAA and C-reactive protein have been shown to be good predictors of the development of diabetes and cardiovascular disease. These results suggest that tanis may be a new link between inflammation and diabetes which needs to be further investigated.

In summary, with the combination of an excellent animal model for the study of diabetes in *P. obesus*, and gene expression profiling technologies, we have discovered a number of novel genes, including beacon and tanis. Finally, it is hoped that with details of the pathway of beacon and tanis action defined, this information will be used for high throughput screening in the quest for a new therapeutic approach to obesity and diabetes.

References

1. Walder KL, Kantham J, McMillan *et al.* Tanis: A link between type 2 diabetes and inflammation? *Diabetes* 2002; 51: 1859–66.

2. Collier GRJ, McMillan K, Windmill *et al.* Beacon, a novel gene involved in the regulation of energy balance. *Diabetes* . 2000; 49: 1766–71.

3. Eisen Eisen MB, Spellman PT, Brown PO *et al.* Cluster analysis and display of genome wide expression patterns. *Proc Natl Acad Sci USA* 1998; 95: 14863–8.

4. Kim S, Dougherty ER, Chen Y. Multivariate measurement of gene expression relationships. Genomics 2000; 67: 201–9

5. Barnett M, Collier GR, Collier FM *et al.* A cross-sectional and short-term longitudinal characterization of NIDDM. In: Psammomys obesus. *Diabetologia* 1994; 37(7): 671–6.

6. Habito RC, Barnett M, Yamamoto A *et al.* Basal glucose turnover in Psammomys obesus: an animal model of Type 2 (non-insulin-dependent) diabetes mellitus. *Acta Diabetologica* 1995; 32(3): 187–92.

7. Collier GR, Walder K, Lewandowski P *et al.* Leptin and the development of obesity and diabetes. In Psammomys obesus. *Obes Res* 1997; 5: (5): 455–8.

8. Collier GR, de Silva A, Sanigorski A, Walder K, Yamamoto A, Zimmet P. Development of obesity and insulin resistance in the Israeli sand rat. In: Psammomys obesus. Does leptin play a role? *Ann NY Acad Sci* 1997; 827: 50–63 (review).

9. Walder K, Willet M, Zimmet P *et al.* Ob (obese) gene expression and leptin levels in Psammomys obesus. *Biochim Biophys Acta* 1997; 1354: 272–8.

10. Walder K, Lewandowski P, Morton G *et al.* Leptin resistance in a polygenic, hyperleptinemic animal model of obesity and NIDDM. In: Psammomys obesus. *Int J Obes* 1999; 2: 83–9.

11. Walder KR, Fahey RP, Morton GJ, Zimmet PZ, Collier GR. Characterization of obesity phenotypes. In: Psammomys obesus (Israeli sand rats). *Int J Exp Diab Res* 2000; 1(3): 177–84.

12. Shafrir E, Gutman A. Psammomys obesus of the Jerusalem colony: A model for nutritionally induced, non-insulin-dependent diabetes. *J Basic Clin Physiol Pharm* 1993; 4: 83–99.

13. Kalderon B, Gutman A, Levy E. Characterization of stages in the development of obesity-diabetes syndrome in sand rat (Psammomys obesus). *Diabetes* 1986; 35(6): 717–24.

14. Zimmet P, Whitehouse S, Kiss J. Ethnic variability in the plasma insulin response to oral glucose in Polynesian and Micronesian subjects. *Diabetes* 1979; 28: 624–8.

15. DeFronzo RA. The triumvirate B-cell, muscle and liver: A collusion responsible for NIDDM. *Diabetes* 1988; 37: 667–88.

16. Fields S, Song O. A novel genetic system to detect protein-protein interactions. *Nature* 1989; 340: 245–6.

17. Gyuris J, Golemis E, Chatkou H *et al.* Cdi 1, a human G1 and S phase protein phosphatase that associates with Cdk2. *Cell* 1993; 75: 791–803.

18. Durfee T, Becherern K, Chen PL. The retinoblastoma protein associates with the protein phosphatase type 1 catalytic subunit. *Genes Dev* 1993; 7: 555–69.

19. Vidal M, Brachmann RK, Fattaey A *et al.* Reverse two-hybrid and one-hybrid systems to detect dissociation of protein-protein and DNA-protein interactions. *Proc Natl Acad Sci* 1996; 93: 10315–20.

20. Damelin M, Silver P. Mapping interactions between nuclear transport factors in living cells reveals pathways through the nuclear pore complex. *Molecular Cell* 2000; 5: 133–40.

21. Angers S, Salahpour A, Joly E *et al.* Detection of B2 – adrenergic receptor dimerization in living cells using Bioluminescence resonance energy transfer (BRET). *Proc Natl Acad Sci* 2000; 97: 3684–9.

22. Nagata K, Handa H. *Real-time analysis of biomolecular interactions: applications of biocore.* Tokyo: Springer-Verlag; 2000.

Progress in Obesity Research: 9. Edited by *Geraldo Medeiros-Neto, Alfredo Halpern and Claude Bouchard*
©2003 John Libbey Eurotext Ltd, pp. 40–43.

CHAPTER 8

Can obese individuals be fit and how does it affect their health?

Steven N. Blair

President and CEO, Cooper Institute, 12330 Preston Road, Dallas, Texas 75230, USA
[e-mail: sblair@cooperinst.org]

Overweight and obesity are well established as health risks, and the prevalence of these conditions appears to be increasing rapidly in many countries around the world. There have been numerous calls to action to address the public health problem of overweight and obesity, from the World Health Organization and many national health authorities. The role of physical activity in relation to overweight or obesity and health status is mentioned in most reports and recommendations, but has not received appropriate emphasis. A fit and active way of life reduces the risk of substantial weight gain over time, is useful in weight loss programmes, appears to be crucial in maintaining weight loss, and provides health benefits to overweight and obese individuals. It is this last point that has largely been overlooked by those concerned with overweight and obesity, and is the subject of this report.

Influence of cardiorespiratory fitness on health outcomes

When Dr. Kenneth H. Cooper founded the Aerobics Center in 1970 he established The Cooper Clinic, a clinic devoted to the practice of preventive medicine, and The Cooper Institute, a non-profit research foundation. He had the vision to establish a data repository that included results of the preventive health examinations conducted at The Cooper Clinic and obtained the informed consent of the patients to be followed in a research study. The examination is a thorough one that includes a history and physical examination, and a wide range of clinical assessments – blood chemistries, blood pressure, anthropometry, pulmonary function, and a maximal exercise test on a treadmill. Data from the examinations are taken to The Cooper Institute and entered into a database that is the foundation of the Aerobics Center Longitudinal Study (ACLS). A schematic of the study is shown in Fig. 1.

Design of the Aerobics Center Longitudinal Study (ACLS)

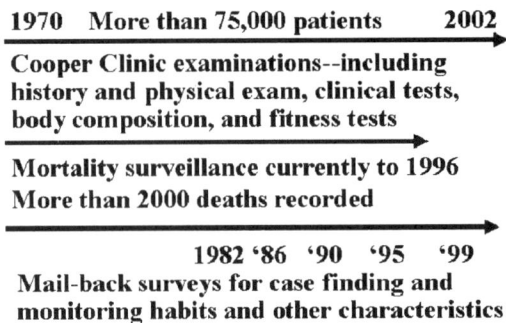

1970 **More than 75,000 patients**   2002

Cooper Clinic examinations--including history and physical exam, clinical tests, body composition, and fitness tests

Mortality surveillance currently to 1996 More than 2000 deaths recorded

                1982 '86 '90   '95   '99
Mail-back surveys for case finding and monitoring habits and other characteristics

Fig. 1. ©The Cooper Institute.

The overall purpose of the ACLS is to investigate the relation of physical activity, cardiorespiratory fitness, clinical variables, and other factors to future health outcomes. A major strength of the study is that all participants completed a maximal exercise test at baseline, and this provides an objective laboratory assessment of cardiorespiratory fitness. Cardiorespiratory fitness is an excellent marker for the physical activity pattern of the individual in the weeks and months prior to the treadmill test. In fact, I think that the treadmill test data provide a better indicator of a person's physical activity habits than can be obtained by self-reported physical questionnaires, which are crude and imprecise due to limitations of the method. Therefore, in the ACLS cardiorespiratory fitness is used as the exposure to evaluate the affect of sedentary habits on health outcomes. The treadmill test is a modified Balke protocol[1], which has been described in several earlier reports[2,3,4].

Time of the treadmill test is used to classify patients into low, moderate, and high categories of cardiorespiratory fitness. Distributions of treadmill times for women and men are created for age groups of 20–39 years, 40–49 years, 50–59 years, and 60+ years. The least fit 20 per cent in each age–sex group are assigned to the low fit category, the next 40 per cent of the distribution to the moderately fit category, and the most fit 40 per cent to the high fit category. Maximal treadmill times are converted to maximal METs based on published equations[5,6]. Maximal MET cutpoints for women and men for the three fitness categories in all age groups are shown in Tables 1 and 2.

Cardiorespiratory fitness and mortality

We have published several reports on the relation of cardiorespiratory fitness to cardiovascular disease (CVD) and all-cause mortality. The results have been consistent for women and for men, for healthy and unhealthy patients, and for middle-aged and older individuals. A representative example of these findings is shown in Fig. 2 for fitness and CVD mortality in women and men. These data are from a prospective study in 7,080 women and 25,340 men followed for approximately 8 years. There is a substantial difference in CVD mortality between the low and moderate fitness groups for both women and men, and a smaller difference in death rates between moderate and high fitness groups.

Cardiorespiratory fitness and mortality in overweight and obese individuals

We evaluated the relation of cardiorespiratory fitness to mortality in normal weight, overweight, and obese men for a satellite symposium of the 7th International Congress of Obesity in 1994. The results were somewhat surprising, with death rates in obese but fit men being substantially lower than the death rates in normal weight men who were unfit[7].

We have continued to investigate the interrelationships of fitness and fatness as predictors of mortality[8,9,10]. The results have remained consistent for men, and we have recently reported similar findings in ACLS women[11].

In one report we evaluated cardiorespiratory fitness and body composition as predictors of mortality[9]. In this study we used per cent body fat instead of BMI to classify study participants into lean, normal, and obese groups; and each of these fatness groups was further divided into unfit and fit (combined moderate and high fitness groups) categories. The study included 21,925 men examined at the Cooper Clinic and followed for an average of about 8 years, during which 428 men died. A summary of the results is presented in Fig. 3. In every fatness group, the unfit men had substantially higher death rates

Cardiorespiratory Fitness Categories, Men, ACLS

	Age Groups (years)			
	20-39	40-49	50-59	60+
Low fit	≤10.5	≤9.9	≤8.8	≤7.5
Mod fit	10.6-12.7	10.0-12.1	8.9-10.9	7.6-9.7
High fit	>12.7	>12.1	>10.9	>9.7

Table values are maximal METs attained during the exercise test

© Cooper Institute

Table 1.

Cardiorespiratory Fitness Categories, Women, ACLS

	Age Groups (years)			
	20-39	40-49	50-59	60+
Low fit	≤8.1	≤7.5	≤6.5	≤5.7
Mod fit	8.2-10.5	7.6-9.5	6.6-8.3	5.7-7.5
High fit	>10.5	>9.5	>8.3	>7.5

Table values are maximal METs attained during the exercise test

© Cooper Institute

Table 2.

CVD Deaths/10,000 PY

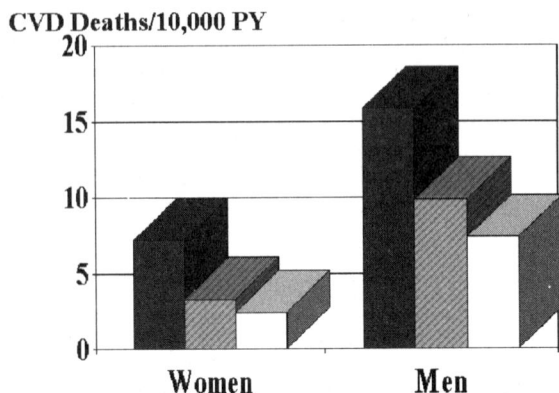

Adjusted for age, exam year, and other risk factors
Adapted from Blair SN et al. *JAMA* 1996; 276:205-10

Fig. 2. Cardiorespiratory fitness and cardiovascular disease mortality in women and men, ACLS. Fitness categories are – black bars = low fitness; striped bars = moderate fitness; and white bars = high fitness.

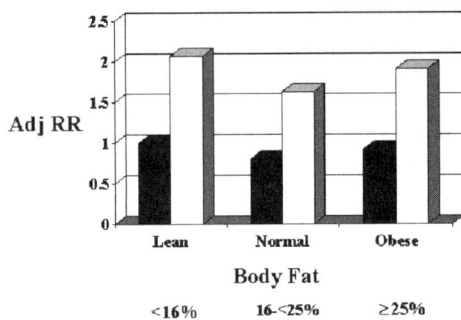

Lee CD et al. Am J Clin Nutr 1999.

Fig. 3. Adjusted relative risks for all-cause mortality for fit and unfit men in categories of per cent body fat. Relative risks for the fit men are the black bars and the unfit men are shown in the white bars. The relative risks are adjusted for age, examination year, smoking status, alcohol intake, and family history of cardiovascular disease.

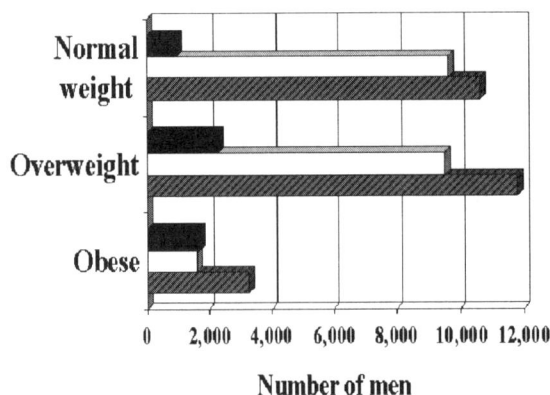

Wei M et al. *JAMA* 1999; 282:1547

Fig. 4. Number of men who were unfit (black bars) or fit (white bars) in normal weight (BMI 18.5 to 24.9), overweight (BMI 25.0 to 29.9), and obese (BMI ≥ 30.0) categories. The striped bars are the total number of men in the BMI category.

than the fit men, and there was no increased trend for mortality across fatness groups in the fit men. The unfit lean men were more than twice as likely to die during follow-up when compared with fit obese men. We found similar results in additional analyses performed only in non-smoking men and after exclusion of early mortality.

How many obese individuals are fit?

An important issue to consider in interpreting the results of analyses on fitness and fatness is whether or not many obese individuals are fit. Many believe that fatness is synonymous with being sedentary and unfit. We have examined this issue in the ACLS, and data on fit and unfit status of 25,714 men are shown in Fig. 4[10]. Nearly 90 per cent of the normal weight men are fit by ACLS standards, 80 per cent of the overweight are fit, and a surprising 49 per cent of the obese men are fit. We also find that a high proportion of obese women in the ACLS are fit, with 50 per cent of the women with a BMI of 30 meeting our fitness standard, and even in women with a BMI of 37 or more, approximately 20 per cent are fit[11].

Summary and conclusion

Low cardiorespiratory fitness is a strong predictor of CVD and all-cause mortality and moderate to high levels of fitness are protective. This relation holds in women and men; middle-aged and older individuals; healthy and unhealthy persons; and for those in normal weight, overweight, and obese categories. Data from the ACLS show death rates approximately twofold higher in normal weight individuals who are unfit, when compared with those who are obese but fit.

These findings should provide encouragement for overweight and obese individuals who exercise regularly, but still do not attain normal weight status. I do not advocate ignoring the health hazards and social stigma of overweight and obesity, which are numerous and well documented. I also do not mean to discourage individuals who strive to lose weight from giving up on that objective. However, the most important message from the research reviewed here is that being active and fit provides important health benefits for individuals of all shapes and sizes; and patients and health professionals should focus on being physically active.

Acknowledgement: The research reported here is supported in part by US National Institutes of Health grant from the National Institute on Aging – AG06495.

References

1. Balke B, Ware RW. An experimental study of physical fitness in Air Force personnel. *US Armed Forces Med J* 1959; 10: 675–88.

2. Blair SN, Kohl HW III, Paffenbarger RS Jr, Clark DG, Cooper KH, Gibbons LW. Physical fitness and all-cause mortality: a prospective study of healthy men and women. *JAMA* 1989; 262: 2395–201.

3. Kohl HW, Blair SN, Paffenbarger RS Jr, Macera CA, Kronenfeld JJ. A mail survey of physical activity habits as related to measured physical fitness. *Am J Epidemiol* 1988; 127: 1228–39.

4. Blair SN, Kohl HW, Barlow CE, Paffenbarger RS, Jr, Gibbons LW, Macera CA. Changes in physical fitness and all-cause mortality: prospective study of healthy and unhealthy men. *JAMA* 1995; 273: 1093–8.

5. Pollock ML, Bohannon RL, Cooper KH *et al.* A comparative analysis of four protocols for maximal treadmill stress testing. *Am Heart J* 1976; 92: 39–46.

6. Pollock ML, Foster C, Schmidt D, Hellman C, Linnerud AC, Ward A. Comparative analysis of physiologic responses to three different maximal graded exercise test protocols in healthy women. *Am Heart J* 1982; 103: 363–73.

7. Barlow CE, Kohl HW, III, Gibbons LW, Blair SN. Physical fitness, mortality and obesity. *Int J Obes* 1995; 19 (Suppl 4): S41–S44.

8. Lee CD, Jackson AS, Blair SN. US weight guidelines: Is it also important to consider cardiorespiratory fitness? *Int J Obes* 1998; 22: S2–S7.

9. Lee, CD, Blair, SN, Jackson, AS. Cardiorespiratory fitness, body composition, and all-cause and cardiovascular disease mortality in men. *Am J Clin Nutr* 1999; 69: 373–380.

10. Wei, M, Kampert, JB, Barlow, CE, Nichaman, MZ, Gibbons, LW, Paffenbarger, RS, Jr, Blair, SN. Relationship between low cardiorespiratory fitness and mortality in normal-weight, overweight, and obese men. *JAMA* 1999; 282: 1547–1553.

11. Farrell SW, Braun L, Barlow CE, Cheng YJ, Blair SN. The relation of body mass index, cardiorespiratory fitness, and all-cause mortality in women. *Obes Res* 2002; 10: 417–423.

Progress in Obesity Research: 9. Edited by *Geraldo Medeiros-Neto, Alfredo Halpern and Claude Bouchard*
©2003 John Libbey Eurotext Ltd, pp. 44–48.

CHAPTER 9

The costs of obesity

Ian D. Caterson

Human Nutrition Unit, School of Molecular & Microbial Biosciences, University of Sydney NSW 2006 Australia
[e-mail: I.Caterson@mmb.usyd.edu.au]

Introduction

Obesity is increasing in prevalence throughout the world and with this increase has come increased costs both to the individual and to health systems. In many countries there has been an increase in non-communicable diseases (particularly diabetes) consonant with the increase in obesity and this is causing health planners to look afresh at the costs of obesity. Health economists and politicians alike pretend to use such concrete dollar costs on which to base their predictions and plans for the health system and yet when it comes down to it there is a finite available sum for total health care. So to influence health care spending on obesity, an area, or disease, which has really not been funded in many health care systems, a strong case needs to be established. Calculating the cost of obesity in dollars alone has not been enough to change health care priorities yet, as every health area can produce evidence giving the cost of their area and so it has been difficult to produce change in the established funding models. What is necessary is an investigation of the costs of obesity, in monetary terms certainly, but this should be combined with other approaches and estimates (some of which will be discussed in this short paper) which shows how far reaching the effects of obesity are. It may be better to think and present the findings of such studies in terms of increasing funding for prevention of obesity (which may be a relatively small funding redistribution) rather seeking a major reallocation for treatment of established obesity per se (much of this cost is already included in the treatment of the many established chronic non-communicable diseases). Therefore novel factors need be included in any study of costs of obesity and the emphasis needs to be on a funding redistribution for the prevention of this disorder rather than on a major change in established treatment practices.

Alternate approaches

There is a standard approach used in many health economic analyses which determines the direct costs of obesity to the health care system. To this may be added the indirect costs (a cost which may vary from considerably depending on what is included) and intangible costs. It is this latter cost which is more nebulous currently but is one which needs refining and developing because it is this cost which will show how far reaching are the effects of obesity.

Other approaches include the calculation of disability adjusted life years (allowing obesity to be compared to other risk factors and diseases), the description of costs of environment changes necessitated by obesity (wider seats required in sports venues, fewer passengers able to be carried on a standard aircraft seating configuration, special facilities for the morbidly obese for example). Another such cost is the increasing difficulty of recruiting for the armed forces and other such organizations. As both the general population and this in the defence forces become more obese, either standards have to be relaxed, special programmes for weight loss and fitness instituted, machinery redesigned or a different mix of individuals recruited to enable all functions of the service to be fulfilled. In Singapore for example, all young men have to undertake a period of national service. Many were 'failing' the criteria for weight and it was necessary for an intensive programme for weight loss to be provided and for these overweight individuals to spend extra time (some 5 months) completing their national service[1]. While this has been presented as an example of how weight loss may be achieved, it may also

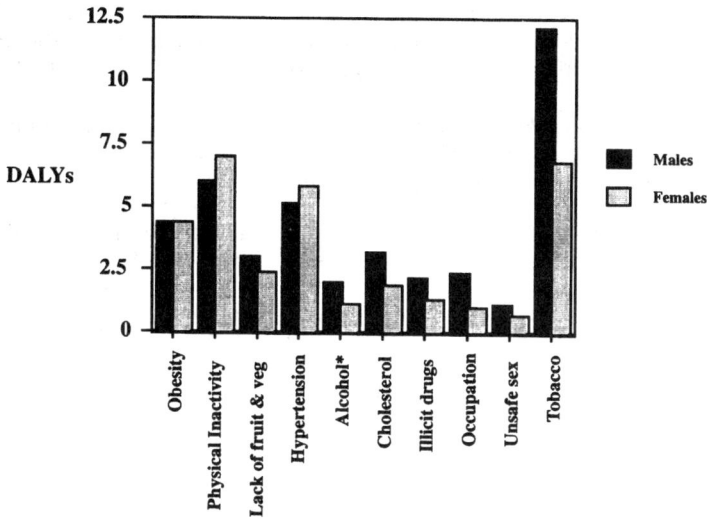

Fig. 1. Obesity as a risk factor, expressed as Diasability Adjusted Life Years (DALYs). Data obtained from Australian Institute of Health and Welfare[2]. *Alcohol is the sum of alcohol's harm and benefit.

be seen as added cost for the country (weight programme and extended service time) and the individual (extra time in national service with delayed entry into general workforce and chosen field).

While to some this may not seem to be a major problem or cost, it is such difficulties and costs repeated in many organizations and companies throughout modern society which will produce the greatest impetus to change and the prevention of obesity. There have been isolated reports of such types of change and the cost to an organization or the community, the documentation (and costs) of such environmental modification (and strengthening) is important. The need to change the environment (with a reduction in income or in efficiency of operation) will be a driving force in producing change in health care expenditure for obesity.

Other ways of looking at the economic costs of obesity include calculating years lost to disability (YLDs) or disability adjusted life years (DALYs), or quality adjusted life years. In Australia, Mathers et al., 1999[2] used such an approach as well as calculating the monetary cost in another publication (Mathers, 1999)[3]. They described 'risk factors' for the burden of disease in Australia and calculated these in disability adjusted life years (DALYs). The findings are given in Fig. 1. Whilst cigarette smoking was the major risk factor for men (some 12.5 DALYs), physical inactivity is the major risk factor for women. Obesity itself (after some adjustment because it was 'involved' in many of the other risk factors) caused some 4.2 DALYs in both men and women. It is interesting to note that the combination of obesity, physical inactivity and lack of fruit and vegetables (all involved in obesity really) make this lifestyle disorder complex the major risk factor in the burden of disease in Australia. This approach is worth emphasizing and similar analyses have been or are being performed in other places. This type of 'cost' makes an impact.

A further approach is to estimate the costs of disease treatment itself. For example Brown et al., 2001[4] have described the treatment costs of type 2 diabetes in this way contrasting diet treatment alone with drug treatment and the treatment of complications. The Philippines Association for the Study of Overweight and Obesity (PASOO – personal communication) have looked at the cost of treating obesity in their country. They have estimated the cost, including drug therapy to be of the order of US$1200 per year, of a similar order to the treatment of hypercholesterolaemia, but slightly more than than treatment of diabetes with sulphonylureas. Studies which compare the cost of obesity treatment, and the prevention of metabolic disease, with the cost of ongoing treatment of these diseases need to be performed.

Another way of examining the costs of obesity is by examining hospitalizations. In the US Navy where one might expect less obesity than in the general population, the cost of hospitalization due to obesity is $5million annually[5]. Obesity is also associated with a 36 per cent increase in outpatient and inpatient spending and a 77 per cent increase in medications, a greater cost than for smokers[6].

Standard approaches

Most such studies are prevalence studies in which the cost is determined in a defined time period. These are possible because the data collected by hospitals, health departments and authorities can be utilized. Another approach is an incidence based study, with the costs of new obesity and associated disease treatment in a cohort over a defined period being determined. Such studies are more difficult to perform as they usually require a special collection study. Most cost of obesity studies in the literature are prevalence studies.

There are three major costs of obesity given in such studies, though not all are reported in every study. Direct costs are those of the health care resources applied to both obesity and its associated conditions. Indirect costs are the reduction in the level of broader economic activity due to obesity. The wages and productivity lost due to sickness produced by obesity and the loss of productivity produced by the premature deaths due to obesity, are factors usually considered. There is no single way to calculate this cost and it is a more difficult calculation and more variable than the health care (or direct) costs. Most studies undertaken have used these two approaches in their calculations. Intangible or personal costs are the social and individual costs or losses associated with obesity. Some, such as the cost of commercial weight loss programmes, are relatively easy to estimate, but others are more difficult to ascertain and can be subject to the views of the particular health economist undertaking the study. For example, estimating the value of the reduced quality of life (QoL) produced by obesity requires both specific QoL measures and an estimate of the cost of a life year. Another variable is the grade of obesity. Estimation of the intangible cost has the greatest variability of these three cost types.

Reported costs of obesity

There are a large number of obesity cost or burden of illness studies and a number of recent studies from various countries are given in Table 1. There is a wide range of costs from a mere US$77 million in direct costs for New Zealand[7] where the prevalence of adult obesity is 19 per cent, to US$70 billion in the United States[8] with a prevalence of 25 per cent. In Australia the direct costs of obesity are estimated to be US$750 million (S. Crowley, personal communication) but the estimate has a wide range depending on what relative risk is employed. Differences in costs in the various countries may be due to different obesity prevalence, different absolute health costs in the treatment of obesity and its related diseases as well as differences in the methodology of performing the study. Some of these differences are the Body Mass Index (BMI) used to define obesity, the diseases included in the analysis and the relative risk factor employed. Overall the direct cost of obesity is between 2–5 per cent of the health care budget[9]. This cost may be greater in the United States[10]. Indirect costs are generally less than the direct health care costs but this cost was US$47.6 billion in the US in 1995[8].

Table 1. Reported economic costs of obesity

Year	Country	Direct cost	Indirect cost
1989	Netherlands[17]	DG 1 billion	
1990	USA[18]	US$45.8 billion	US$23 billion
1991	New Zealand[7]	NZ$135 million	
1990–91	UK[19]	GB£ 130 million	Included in cost
1992	France[20]	FF5.8billion	FF0.58 billion
1995	USA[8]	US$51.6 billion	US$47.6 billion
	USA[21]	US$70 billion	
1996	Australia	AU$0.84–1.4 billion	
1997	Canada[13]	C$0.83–3.4 billion	

These costs have been collated from various sources and the original references are cited. The Australian data is a personal communication from S. Crowley.

Several incidence studies which follow a representative cohort for some years have been performed. Thompson[11] estimated the lifetime costs of being at various BMI levels. For a BMI of 22.5 the lifetime cost of obesity was estimated to be US$19,300 in men and $18,600 in women. At a BMI of 37.5 the corresponding costs were US$35,2000 and $34,700. Then, lifetime costs could be extrapolated. In another study it was estimated that the cost of obesity would be 0.89–4.32 per cent of the US health care budget[12].

Recently, Segal and others prepared a report for the International Obesity Task Force. Using Australia studies with QoL measures and estimated value of life years lost due to obesity, they calculated that the intangible costs of obesity to the Australia population was of the order of US$5.5 billion. This report and the methodology used will be published by the IOTF.

Problems with study comparison

There are a number of factors which need to be taken into consideration when comparing reported costs. Firstly until recently different BMI cut-points for overweight and obesity were used. For example in a Canadian study[13] a BMI of 27 was used whereas many other studies use BMIs of 25 and/or 30. Seidell has reported costs of both overweight and obesity[9,14]. Three-quarters of the costs incurred were for the BMI range 25–30. One per cent of health care costs in the Netherlands were attributable to obesity and this contrasts with the 7 per cent of health care expenditure attributed in the US.

Secondly different obesity associated diseases are used in the analysis. Table 2 gives examples of the diseases included in studies. It is important to include musculoskeletal diseases (and many studies do not) as these disorders are a major cost in an ageing community. Similarly the costs of non-alcoholic steatohepatitis (NASH) need to be included, as this disorder may be the cause of 10 per cent of the cirrhosis in some societies. Cancer, endometrial cancer, postmenopausal breast cancer and bowel cancer are obesity related and need to be considered. To enable comparisons of obesity costs in the future it will be necessary to use a 'standard' list of diseases.

Table 2. Diseases utilized in cost of obesity studies and the range of relative risks (RR) employed

Frequency of use	Disease	Range of RR
Invariably	Type 2 diabetes	2.9–27.6
Frequently	Hypertension	2.51–4.3
	Coronary heart disease	1.72–3.5
	Gallbladder disease	1.85–10
	Cancer	1.16–1.5
Often	Dyslipidaemia	1.41–1.5
	Stroke	1.14–3.1
	Osteoarthritis	1.8
Occasionally	Gout	2.5
	Venous thrombosis	2.39

The use of conservative and higher RR enables allows the potential range of costs to be calculated.

A further problem is the calculation of the relative risk of any particular disease in a community or the availability of data (a large population-based study with both disease presence and BMI recorded) to allow this risk to be calculated. This relative risk is important because it allows the population attributable fraction (PAF) to be calculated. and this is used in the calculation of direct costs. The United States does have much of this data available, but other countries do not. Much of the US data is from Caucasian populations and may not be applicable to other ethnicities. There is also a wide variability in relative risk found and employed. Examples are given in Table 2. It may be better to use a conservative relative risk and a higher one and this will allow a range of obesity related costs to be calculated. For example, in Australia using this approach the range of direct costs of obesity is $830 million to $1.4 billion (S. Crowley, personal communication).

The risk of metabolic disease varies with the ethnicity of the population. For example it appears that Asian populations are at greater risk of diabetes, hypertension and dyslipidaemia[15]. Other groups may have greater risks for specific disorders. The Japanese population has a problem with hypertension which has a risk of 3.0 at a BMI of 24.9, the Chinese population has a greater risk of diabetes, non-alcoholic steatohepatitis (NASH) and of dyslipidaemia at BMI in the preobese range (BMI 25–29.9) than does the Caucasian population[16]. Until there are good relative risks determined for each population, those risks derived from Caucasian populations will continue to be used, with a probable under-estimation of the true costs of obesity in these populations and communities.

A further consideration is what cost centres to include in the calculation of direct costs. Usually included are personal health care, hospital care (both inpatient and outpatient services in public and private hospitals), medical services such as GP/primary care consultations, physicians' consultations, dietetic consultations and other allied health professionals' consultation, the cost of drugs and laboratory services. Other professional services can be included as can the cost of nursing home care. However this data may not be always available and there are many other possible inclusions such as the cost of prosthetic joint replacements. Each country and health system will have different ideas about what cost centres may be included and varying data available.

Other variable that is difficult to control is the basic cost of health care in various countries. In some, such as the US this may be very expensive whilst in others there are standard rates. Drug costs, availability and usage will vary as will availability and use of surgery for obesity. Such medical practice items will inflate or deflate obesity costs and so a truer comparison may be obtained by considering the direct cost of obesity as a percentage of total health care expenditure, but even this will not totally eliminate discrepancies and differences. Unless there is identical methodology, the use of appropriate relative risks and the cost is expressed per head of population, it will continue to be difficult to compare the cost of obesity in one country with the cost in another.

The calculation of indirect and intangible costs has even more inherent variability in what may be included and in the health economics methodology. A standard approach may be possible, but there needs to be a great deal of discussion and agreement before this will be possible.

References

1. Lee L, Kumar S, Leong LC. The impact of a five-month basic military training on the body weight and body fat of 197 moderately to severely obese Singaporean males aged 17 to 19 years. *Int J Obes* 1994; 18: 105–9.

2. Mathers C, Vos T, Stevenson C. The burden of disease and injury in Australia. Canberra: Australian Institute of Health and Welfare; 1999.

3. Mathers C, Penn R. Health system costs of cardiovascular diseases and diabetes in Australia 1993–94. Canberra: Australian Institute of Health and Welfare; 1999.

4. Brown JB, Nichols GA, Glauber HS, Bakst AW, Schaeffer M, Kelleher CC. Health care costs associated with escalation of drug treatment in type 2 diabetes mellitus. *Am J Health-Syst Pharm* 2001; 58: 151–7.

5. Bradham DD, South BR, Saunders HJ, Hauser MD, Pane KW, Dennis KE. Obesity-related hospitalization costs to the US Navy, 1993 to 1998. *Military Medicine* 2001; 166: 1–10.

6. Sturm R. DataWatch: The effects of obesity, smoking, and drinking on medical problems and costs. *Health Affairs* 2002; 21(2): 245–53.

7. Swinburn B, Ashton T, Gillespie J, Cox B, Menon A, Simmons D, Birbeck J. Health care costs of obesity in New Zealand. *Int J Obes* 1997; 21: 891–6.

8. Wolf AM, Colditz GA. Current estimates of the economic cost of obesity in the United States. *Obes Res* 1998; 6: 97–106.

9. Seidell JC. Societal and personal costs of obesity. *Exp Clin Endocrinol Diabetes* 1998; 106 (Suppl 2): 7–9.

10. Colditz G, Mariani A. The cost of obesity and sedentarism in the United States. In: *Physical activity and obesity*, Bouchard C (ed.), pp. 55–66. Champaign, IL: Human Kinetics; 2000.

11. Thompson D, Edelsberg J, Colditz G, Bird A, Oster G. Lifetime health and economic consequences of obesity. *Arch Int Med* 1999; 159: 2177–83.

12. Allison D, Zannolli R, Narayan K, Venkay M. The direct health care costs of obesity in the United States. *Am J Clin Nutr* 1999; 89: 1194–9.

13. Birmingham CL, Muller JL, Palepu A, Spinelli JJ, Anis AH The cost of obesity in Canada. *Canad Med Assoc J* 1999; 160: 503–6.

14. Seidell J. The impact of obesity on health status: some implications for health care costs. *Int J Obes* 1995; 19 (Suppl 6): S13–S16.

15. *The Asia-Pacific perspective: Redefining obesity and its treatment.* Zimmet P, Inoue S (eds). Hong Kong: WHO, IOTF, IASO; 2000.

16. Pan W-H. Epidemiology of obesity and dyslipidaemia. In: *Proc. Third World Congress of International Society for Apheresis.* Taipei, Taiwan; 2001.

17. Seidell JC. The impact of obesity on health status: some implications for health care costs. *Int J Obes* 1995; 19: S13–S16.

18. Wolf AM, Colditz GA. The cost of obesity: the US perspective. *Pharmacoeconomics* 1994; 5: 34–37.

19. West, R. Obesity. In: *Office of Health Economics monographs on current health issues.* Office of Health Economics. London: 1994. pp. 38–42.

20. Levy E, Levy P, LePen C, Basdevant. A. The economic cost of obesity: the French situation. *Int J Obes* 1995; 19: 788–92.

21. Colditz GA. Economic costs of obesity and inactivity. *Medicine and Science in Sports and Exercise* 1999 31: S663–S667.

Progress in Obesity Research: 9. Edited by *Geraldo Medeiros-Neto, Alfredo Halpern and Claude Bouchard*
©2003 John Libbey Eurotext Ltd, pp. 49–53.

CHAPTER 10

Subcutaneous and visceral adipose tissue: their relation to the metabolic syndrome

**Bernardo Léo Wajchenberg*, Antonio Carlos Lerário*,
Daniel Giannella-Neto* and Manoel de Souza Rocha****

Endocrine Service(Diabetes) and Radiology Division**, Hospital das Clínicas, Avenida Enéas Carvalho de Aguiar,
255, 05403-900 São Paulo SP,Brazil
[e-mail: bernarwaj@globo.com]*

Introduction

Many prospective studies have shown that excess of body fat in the upper part of the body (i.e. central or abdominal) is closely associated with glucose intolerance, hyperinsulinaemia, hypertriglyceridaemia and other features of the so-called metabolic syndrome,such as arterial hypertension, decreased levels of HDL and microalbuminuria[1,2]. In contrast, individuals with fat stored in gluteal-femoral or peripheral depots (lower body obesity) or female-type of fat distribution have a lower risk of morbidity from these metabolic disturbances. Imaging techniques, particularly computed tomography (CT), distinguished and allowed the measurements of the visceral (VAT) and abdominal subcutaneous components (SAT) of the upper-body fat. The VAT contained within the abdominal cavity, surrounding the internal organs, comprising the mesenteric and the greater and lesser omental depots, represent ~20 and 6 per cent of total body fat in men and women, respectively[3]. The SAT can be separated into a deep and superficial layers by the 'fascia superficialis', having been suggested by Smith *et al.*[4] as well as other investigators that deep SAT has a major influence on insulin sensitivity.In the lower body, all adipose depots are subcutaneous. Thus, increased VAT may be the most powerful risk factor related to the metabolic syndrome in central obesity,with further risk being added by the deep layer of SAT[5]. VAT and SAT are are morphologically *and* functionally different which may contribute to increased morbidity in visceral obesity. Thus, visceral cells have higher fatty acid turnover and lipolysis than subcutaneous cells and are also less responsive to the antilipolytic effect of insulin. The increased lipolysis is balanced by increased fatty acid transfer into these cells, permiting stability in cell size[5].Increased visceral fat cell free fatty acid flux could contribute to insulin resistance (IR) because these free fatty acids (FFAs) could be directed via portal venous system to the liver ('portal theory'), where they would induce changes in insulin signaling, promoting hepatic IR, leading to decreased inhibition of hepatic glucose output and reducing extraction of insulin, these effects contributing to hyperinsulinaemia. However, the increased release of FFAs from VAT leading to IR through effects on the liver, lacks supporting evidence *in vivo*, having been deduced indirectly rather than measured directly, the predominant source of FFAs probably being SAT[6]. Therefore, the observation of a link between accumulation of VAT and IR or the associated metabolic syndrome does not mean necessarily that the former causes the latter[7]. SAT and VAT are strongly correlated,the subcutaneous depot is generally considerably larger than the intra-abdominal and so has a great potential to contribute to IR through release of FFAs into the systemic circulation. However, total splanchnic blood supply increases postprandially as might the proportion of lipolysis from splanchnic (VAT) vs. subcutaneous fat (SAT), because of increased insulin and sympathetic activation after meals. Thus,the contribution of VAT to hepatic FFA uptake and systemic FFA appearance could be more substantial in the postprandial than in the fasting state[8].

VAT cells express a higher level of glucocorticoid receptors and have more lipoprotein lipase activation in response to glucocorticoids that subcutaneous adipocytes[5]. Thus, regional differences in processing and responses to glucocorticoids may be important in the genesis of inderdepot variation. Since leptin levels are correlated more closely with subcutaneous than with VAT and because leptin signals the state of fat stores to the brain, the VAT may be subject to less central nervous system regulation than peripheral. In addition to signaling the state of fat stores, leptin also has an insulin-sensitizing effect on muscle. Another secretory product by the adipocyte, adiponectin, is expressed predominantly in VAT and acts primarily on skeletal muscle in its fatty acid ß-oxidizing and insulin sensitizing effect[9]. Besides leptin and adiponectin, the list of secretory products of adipocytes includes, amongst others, with greater production by the visceral adipocytes, angiotensinogen, interleukin-6 and plasminogen activator inhibitor 1 (PAI-1) with well known peripheral actions. Besides the influences extrinsic to adipose cells, as above indicated, there are innate characteristics of that cells contributing to the distinct features of different fat depots: SAT preadipocytes have greater capacity for differentiation into lipid-storing adipocytes than those from visceral depots, being regulated in part by the nuclear hormone receptor peroxisome proliferator-activated receptor-γ (PPAR-γ).Activation of this receptor by synthetic ligands, such as thiazolidinediones (TZDs) or natural ligands, leads to stimulation of the differentiation pathway much greater in subcuta-neous than visceral human preadipocytes. Regional differences in preadipocyte apoptosis also occur. Tumour necrosis factor-α (TNF-α) regulates key components of fat metabolism and has a net effect to prevent obesity through inhibition of lipogenesis, increased lipolysis and inducing apoptosis of adipocytes (omental > subcutaneous)[10].

It seems increasingly likely that these special properties of VAT contribute to the morbidity associated with increased visceral fat mass. In effect, lean and obese individuals with most of their fat stored in VAT generally suffer greater adverse metabolic consequences than similarly normal weight or over-weight subjects with fat stored predominantly in subcutaneous depots[11]. Further confirmation that IR is related to VAT rather than SAT comes from results obtained in idential twins discordant for obesity[12], longitudinal studies[13] and intervention trials[14].

Material and methods

To investigate the relationship between abdominal fat distribution,by CT at the umbilicus and compo-nents of the metabolic syndrome, we have evaluated 55 women with normal oGTT, ages varying from 23 to 60 years and their ethnic groups: caucasian (50 per cent), mulatto (35 per cent) and black (15 per cent) correspondent to the population profile seen at The Hospital das Clinicas. The subjects were divided in three groups: 11 lean normal women (BMI: < 25 kg/m^2, two of them in the menopausal state, presenting visceral fat areas < 68 cm^2, correspondent to the mean + 2 SD for the normal females; 13 obese women with VAT ≤ 68 cm^2, four of them in menopause (30.7 per cent) and 31 obese individuals with VAT > 68 cm^2, and nine in menopause (29 per cent). The cutoff values, different for each gender, are considered to be related to increased cardiovascular risk[1].

All clinical and metabolic variables were tested for the adherence to normal distribution. Comparison between two groups was analysed employing Mann-Whitney test or Student t-test. Comparison be-tween the three groups was analysed with Kruskal-Wallis test or one-way analysis ot variance. Corre-lation between anthropometric, clinical and biochemical variables in a correlation matrix were analysed by Spearman test.Statistical significance was set to $P < 0.05$.All calculations were performed employing SigmaStat Statistical software for Windows version 2.03 (SPSS, Inc., Chicago, Illinois, USA).

Results and discussion

The clinical and metabolic characteristics of the study subjects are presented in Tables 1 and 2. Obese females with VAT within the normal range (≤ 68 cm^2) presented significantly higher BMI and WHR ($P < 0.05$), but not SAT, when compared to the normal lean females, suggesting that their higher BMI was more related to an increased peripheral fat masses. Systolic and diastolic blood pressures were also significantly higher in this group of obese individuals but still within the normal range (Table 1).Con-sidering the metabolic parameters (Table 2), the obese subjects with VAT ≤ 68 cm^2, despite presenting higher mean levels of fasting plasma glucose (FPG) and insulin (FI) as well as HOMA$_{IR}$ (Homeostasis model assessment for insulin resistance *in vivo*) they were not significantly different from those found in the lean control group, suggesting that the level of insulin resistance (IR) evaluated by the HOMA did not discriminate obese individuals with VAT within the normal range from the controls. Accord-ingly, when the glucose and insulin areas under the oGTT curves, above baseline, were taken into consideration, the higher mean insulin area, although non significant, correspondent to a similar mean glucose area in both groups of patients, are also suggestive for presence of IR in the obese subjects, although not significant by the statistical analyses. The only statistical significant difference between

Table 1. Clinical characteristics of the study subjects

	Lean	Obese	
	$VAT < 68 \text{ cm}^2$	$VAT \leq 68 \text{ cm}^2$	$VAT > 68 \text{ cm}^2$
No. of subjects	11	13	31
Age (years)	36.8 ± 2.5	37.8 ± 3.0	43.6 ± 2.0
BMI (kg/m^2)	22.1 ± 0.7*,**	35.1 ± 1.5	37.6 ± 1.2
WHR	0.77 ± 0.01*,**	0.93 ± 0.03***	0.91 ± 0.02
VAT (cm^2)	28.1 ± 5.5**	48.7 ± 4.0***	139.8 ± 12.4
SAT (cm^2)	128.4 ± 20.4**	304.1 ± 41.9***	458.6 ± 38.9
VAT/SAT	0.23 ± 0.02	0.18 ± 0.03	0.36 ± 0.05
Systolic BP	104.5 ± 3.6*,**	126.2 ± 5.6	137.4 ± 3.8
Diastolic BP	69.5 ± 2.7*,**	83.1 ± 3.1	92.3 ± 2.1

Values are mean ± SEM.
*Lean vs. obese VAT ≤ 68 cm^2; $P < 0.05$; **Lean vs. obese VAT > 68 cm^2; $P < 0.05$;
***Obese VAT ≤ 68 cm^2 vs. obese VAT > 68 cm^2; $P < 0.05$.

Table 2. Metabolic characteristics of the study subjects

	Lean	Obese	
	$VAT < 68 \text{ cm}^2$	$VAT \leq 68 \text{ cm}^2$	$VAT > 68 \text{ cm}^2$
Fasting plasma glucose (mg/dl)	84.5 ± 2.6**	95.4 ± 2.9	95.4 ± 2.4
Fasting 'true' insulin (μU/ml)	4.0 ± 0.9**	8.0 ± 1.3***	22.3 ± 4.0
HOMA$_{IR}$	0.84 ± 0.19**	1.87 ± 0.32***	5.40 ± 0.98
Glucose area under curve (oGTT) (mg/dl.min^{-1})	5205 ± 622	4729 ± 742	4699 ± 391
Insulin area under curve (oGTT) (μg/dl.min^{-1})	4890 ± 564**	7638 ± 1146	9311 ± 1053
Fasting FFA (μmol/l)	367 ± 51	434 ± 49	469 ± 40
%∇ FFA (oGTT) (% fasting FFA)	39.2 ± 3.3*,**	78.8 ± 3.1	72.4 ± 3.0
Triglycerides (mg/dl)	68.1 ± 6.4**	94.9 ± 8.0***	143.7 ± 12.1
Total cholesterol (mg/dl)	166.8 ± 10.8**	171.6 ± 7.6	201.0 ± 6.4
HDL-cholesterol (mg/dl)	51.1 ± 3.9	46.0 ± 3.8	44.9 ± 2.1
LDL-cholesterol (mg/dl)	102.1 ± 9.8**	105.8 ± 4.3	127.3 ± 5.8
Uric acid (mg/dl)	4.3 ± 0.1*,**	5.3 ± 0.2	5.4 ± 0.3

Values are mean ± SEM.
*Lean vs. obese VAT ≤ 68 cm^2; $P < 0.05$; **Lean vs. obese VAT > 68 cm^2; $P < 0.05$;
***Obese VAT ≤ 68 cm^2 vs. obese VAT > 68 cm^2; $P < 0.05$.

the two groups of subjects, regarding the metabolic parameters, besides serum uric acid (URA), was observed with the insulin-suppressed plasma FFA, at the end of the oral glucose tolerance test [FFA as percentage of fasting plasma FFA (per cent Δ FFA)], despite similar fasting FFA. Recently, Kelley *et al.*[15] studying type 2 diabetics, indicated that the strongest single correlate of IR in skeletal muscle was insulin-suppressed plasma FFA, suggesting that the severity of skeletal muscle insulin resistance in type 2 diabetes is closely related to the IR of suppressing lipolysis and that plasma FFA and VAT are key elements mediating the link between obesity and skeletal muscle IR in type 2 diabetes. From these findings[15] it can be suggested that in our obese females with VAT ≤ 68 cm^2, presenting higher mean values for SAT and VAT areas, although not significantly different from the control non-obese group, the insulin-suppressed plasma FFA was the most robust indicator for the presence of the state of IR. SAT, as a component of central obesity, could have a strong association with IR, retaining independent significance from VAT which is the major predictor of insulin sensitivity in majority of the reported studies (cited in[1]).In effect, there was a significant positive correlation among $HOMA_{IR}$ and VAT (r = 0.55, $P < 0.001$) and SAT (r = 0.38, $P < 0.05$) with data from all subjects being pooled. Our findings are consistent with the suggestion that VAT contributes more to IR than does SAT. Goodpaster and co-workers[16] have shown that both VAT and SAT were independently related to insulin sensitivity,the latter presenting a stronger association with IR evaluated by the euglycaemic clamp. However, it should be taken into consideration that in our measurements of SAT, as well as in the majority of other studies, it was not evaluated the deep SAT, which could be more relevant than total SAT to the metabolic variables[4].

SAT and VAT are themselves correlated,with correlation coefficients described from 0.72[17] to 0.92[7].In our subjects ,the correlation coefficient r between VAT and SAT, by pooling all data, was 0.43, which was highly significant ($P < 0.01$). SAT as VAT increased progressively from lean to the obese with highest VAT but only significantly in the latter group when compared either to the lean or to obese with VAT ≤ 68 cm^2 (Table 1). One approach to correct the VAT data for the SAT values would be to use the ratio VAT/SAT, a relative index of intraabdominal fat accumulation[18], also not discriminating the lean from the obese with VAT ≤ 68 cm^2 in relation to the $HOMA_{IR}$ and the insulin-suppressed FFA level.

When both groups of obese groups, with no significant differences in BMI and WHR, classified according to their VAT areas, were compared, those with significantly higher VAT, had also statistically greater SAT and VAT/SAT ratio, FI and $HOMA_{IR}$ suggesting decreased insulin sensitivity, associated with elevated mean levels of fasting serum lipids (except HDL-cholesterol) which however were not statistically different from those in the obese VAT ≤ 68 cm^2, except for the significantly higher triglycerides (TG). It is interesting to notice that the minimum value of FFA during oGTT, as percentage of fasting FFA (per cent Δ FFA), did not discriminate the two groups of obese subjects. These findings are at variance from those of Kelley et al.[15] probably related to the fact that insulin-suppressed plasma FFA was evaluated during euglycaemic clamping in their study while in our investigation it was obtained after an oral glucose load with its several variables. Thus,insulin-suppressed FFA, after an oGTT, could be considered as presenting specificity to indicate IR however not being sensitive enough for separating different levels of resistance in our obese subjects, evaluated by the HOMA.

Interestingly, SAT presented a strongest linear correlation with per cent Δ FFA (r = 0.50, $P < 0.01$) than VAT (r = 0.34, $P < 0.05$). These findings could suggest that subcutaneous adipocytes are more resistant to suppression of lipolysis (higher per cent Δ FFA) by insulin than adipocytes within omental and mesenteric fat, in accordance with the now classical concept that VAT present greater lipolytic activity than SAT[3].

The relationship between the components of the metabolic syndrome, obesity and fat distribution, as evaluated by Spearman rank order, indicated a significant correlation between VAT and the following: BMI (r = 0.66), systolic BP (r = 0.70), diastolic BP (r = 0.58), SAT (r = 0.59), VAT/SAT (r = 0.52), TG (r = 0.65), total cholesterol (r = 0.44), HDL-cholesterol (r = −0.34), LDL-cholesterol (r = 0.33), FI (0.59, $HOMA_{IR}$ (r = 0.68), per cent Δ FFA (r = 0.33) and insulin area (r = 0.41).On the other hand, there was a significant correlation between SAT and BMI (r = 0.68), WHR (0 = 0.35), systolic BP (r = 0.53) and diastolic BP (r = 0.46), total cholesterol (r = 0.32), LDL-cholesterol (0.32), FI (r = 0.43), $HOMA_{IR}$ (r = 0.66), per cent Δ FFA (r = 0.40) and insulin area (r = 0.44). The other parameters did not correlate significantly either with VAT or SAT. Thus, in our study, the VAT area presented a lower correlation than the correspondent SAT with the indices of adiposity, BMI and WHR, as expected considering the greater deposited fat size of the latter. However, the systolic and diastolic BP as well the serum lipids correlated more significantly with VAT than SAT except for per cent Δ FFA. Regarding glucose parameters, while fasting glucose correlated better with SAT, fasting insulin and $HOMA_{IR}$ did it with VAT.

References

1. Wajchenberg BL. Subcutaneous and visceral adipose tissue: Their relation to the metabolic syndrome. *Endocr Rev* 2000; 21: 697–738.

2. Alberti KG, Zimmet PZ. Definition, diagnosis and classification of diabetes mellitus and its complications. Part 1: diagnosis and classification of diabetes mellitus provisional report of a WHO consultation. *Diabet Med* 1998; July: 15 (7): 539–53.

3. Montague CT, O'Rahilly S. The perils of portliness. Causes and consequences of visceral adiposity. *Ann Rev Diabetes* 2001; 49: 1–8.

4. Smith SR, Lovejoy JC, Greenway F, Ryan D, deJonge L, de la Bretonne J, Volafova J, Bray GA. Contribution of total body fat, abdominal subcutaneous adipose tissue compartments, and visceral adipose tissue to the metabolic complications of obesity. *Metabolism* 2001; 50: 426–35.

5. Tchkonia T, Karagiannides I, Forse RA, Kirkland JL. Different fat depots are distinct mini-organs. *Current Opin Endocrinol Diabetes* 2001; 8: 227–34.

6. Guo Z. Hensrud DD, Johnson CM, Jensen MD. Regional postprandial fatty acid metabolism in different obesity phenotypes. *Diabetes* 1999; 48: 1586–92.

7. Frayn KN. Visceral fat and insulin resistance – causative or correlative? *Br J Nutr* 2000; 83 (Suppl 1): S71–S77.

8. Lewis GF, Carpentier A, Adeli K, Giacca A. Disordered fat storage and mobilization in the pathogenesis of insulin resistance and type 2 diabetes. *Endocr Rev* 2002; 23: 201–29.

9. Ito Y, Yamauchi T, Waki H, Kamon J, Uchida S, Kimura S, Kadowaki T. Direct effects of adiponectin on skeletal muscle. *Diabetes* 2002; 51 (Suppl 2): A 1868.

10. Sethi J, Hotamisligil GS. The role of TNF-α in adipocyte metabolism. *Semin Cell Dev Biol* 1999; 10: 19–29.

11. Ruderman N, Chisholm D, Pi-Sunyer X, Schneider S. The metabolically obese, normal-weight individual revisited. *Diabetes* 1998; 47: 699–713.

12. Rönnemaa T, Koskenvuo M, Marniemi J, Koivunen T, Sajantila A, Rissanen A *et al.* Glucose metabolism in identical twins discordant for obesity. The critical role of visceral fat. *J Clin Endocrinol Metab* 1997: 82: 383–7.

13. Lemieux S, Prud'homme D, Nadeau, A, Tremblay A, Bouchard, C, Desprès JP. Seven-year changes in body fat and visceral adipose tissue in women. *Diabetes Care* 1996; 19: 983–91.

14. Marks SJ, Moore NR, Clark MI, Strauss BJG, Hockaday TDR. Reduction of visceral adipose tissue and improvement of metabolic indices: effect of dexfenfluramine in NIDDM. *Obes Res* 1996; 4: 1–7.

15. Kelley DE, Williams KV, Price JC, McKolanis TM, Goodpaster BH, Thaete FL. Plasma fatty acids, adiposity,and varaiance of skeletal muscle insulin resistance in type 2 diabetes mellitus. *J Clin Endocrinol Metab* 2001; 86: 5412–9.

16. Goodpaster BH, Thaete FL, Simoneau J-A, Kelley DE. Sub-cutaneous abdominal fat and thigh muscle composition predict insulin sen-sitivity independently of visceral fat. *Diabetes* 1997; 46: 1579–85.

17. Abate B, Garg A, Peshock RM, Stray-Gundersen J Grundy SM. Relationships of generalized and regional adiposity to insulin sensitivity in men. *J Clin Invest* 1995; 96: 88–98.

18. Fujioka S, Matsuzawa Y, Tokunaga K, Tarui S. Contribution of intra-abdominal fat accumulation to the impairment of glucose and lipid metabolism in human obesity. *Metabolism* 1987; 36: 54–9.

Progress in Obesity Research: 9. Edited by *Geraldo Medeiros-Neto, Alfredo Halpern and Claude Bouchard*
©2003 John Libbey Eurotext Ltd, pp. 54–58.

CHAPTER 11

Influencing obesogenic environments to reduce obesity prevalence

Boyd Swinburn

School of Health Sciences, Deakin University, 221 Burwood Highway, Melbourne VIC 3125, Australia
[e-mail: swinburn@deakin.edu.au]

Introduction

The external environment has a powerful effect on the behaviour and therefore the health of individuals. The term 'obesogenic environments' is defined as 'the sum of influences that the surroundings, opportunities or conditions of life have on promoting obesity in individuals or populations'[1]. It is broader than just the physical environment and includes costs, laws, policies, social and cultural attitudes and values. At the other end of the spectrum, an environment that promotes leanness could be called 'leptogenic'.

The changing environments are probably the driving force behind the increasing obesity epidemic and therefore any prevention strategy must address those forces. The purpose of environmental change is 'to make the healthy choices the easy choices'. This is, of course, perfectly complementary to the role of individual and public education which is to promote and encourage people to make those healthy choices.

There are clear interactions on body weight between genes, behaviours and environments and these interactions appear more exaggerated compared with other continuous risk factors such as blood pressure and serum cholesterol[2]. As a population gets fatter, the frequency distribution curve for body mass index (BMI) shifts to the right and flattens out, but importantly, becomes skewed to the right. Assuming that the longitudinal progression of increasing BMI distribution follows the pattern seen in cross-sectional studies[2], a schema is shown in Fig. 1 for the change in BMI in two individuals as the environment becomes more obesogenic. Person A is genetically predisposed to be lean and remains so in both the leptogenic and obesogenic environments while taking the default behavioural choices offered in each environment. The small weight gain between the two environments is contrasted with Person B who is genetically predisposed to weight gain. By just taking the default behavioural choices offered by the two environments (such as walking or driving to work), he gains significantly more weight than Person A.

Strengths of an environment-centred approach

Table 1 lists some of the key strengths of an environmental/systems-based approach underpinning the obesity prevention efforts. Ideally, environmental interventions are part of a suite of strategies including social marketing, individual counseling and population education. However, an environment-centred approach (making healthy choices easier) brings with it a number of advantages particularly in relation to sustainability and reach. Obesity, like diabetes and coronary heart disease, has higher prevalence rates amongst the lower socio-economic status (SES) populations in high-income countries[3]. Low SES brings with it reduced lifestyle options and a lower uptake of health messages about behavioural changes for a healthy future. By influencing the 'default' choices in key environments, there is a much greater potential to affect overall diet and physical activity patterns in lower SES groups than by education strategies alone.

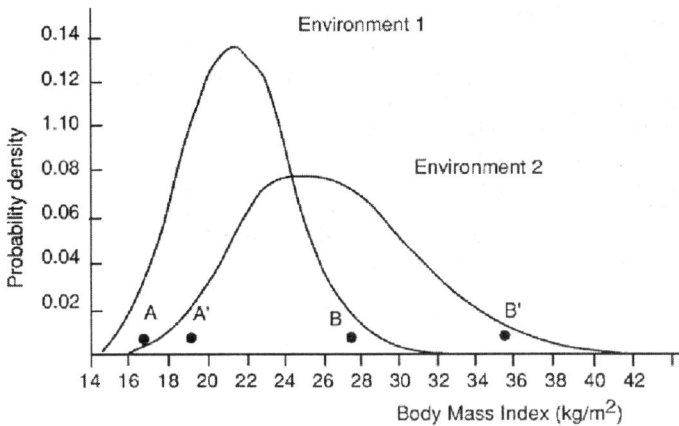

Fig. 1. Schema for gene-environment interactions for body mass index (BMI) assuming the adoption of default behaviour choices in each environment. The distribution curves for BMI are adapted from the two extreme populations from the Intersalt Study[2]. Environment 1 is considered 'leptogenic' and environment 2 is 'obesogenic'. Person A with a genetic predisposition to leanness gains a small amount of weight when moving to environment 2 (A'). Person B with a genetic predisposition to obesity gains a much larger amount of weight in the obesogenic environment (B') giving the distribution curve its characteristic skewed appearance.

Table 1. Strengths of an environment-centred approach to obesity prevention

Strength	Examples
Addresses underlying causes (i.e. potential for true prevention)	Parental fears for children's safety as the major reason for driving children to school – addressing the substance and perceptions related to the fears is likely to result in more active transport to school.
Becomes structural/systemic	Changing the physical environment for recreation, food laws, local government transport policies etc embeds the changes into the system.
Becomes the accepted norm	Regular availability of reduced fat milk, salad options, vegetable-based dishes etc helps to make them normative choices just as smokefree indoor environments helps to make non-smoking the norm.
Likely to be sustained	Systemic changes such as safe, attractive cycle networks or healthy school food menus which are backed by strong policies and traditions are more likely to sustain behaviours over the long term than media campaigns.
Influences the 'hard-to-reach'	Disadvantaged populations such those with low income or low educational attainment tend not to respond to health messages but they can still benefit from the fast food outlet which cooks lower fat French fries.
Less language dependent	Health messages and information are often aimed at a narrow population segment and are often not transmitted in the native tongue of ethnic minorities, but all can take advantage of public transport.
Can address inequities	Environmental interventions can not only reach populations with poor health outcomes but they can be differentially targeted to them such as improving bus services, school food programmes and active recreation amenities in poorer areas.
Usually cost effective	Environmental interventions (especially policy-based initiatives) are relatively inexpensive compared to individual-based approaches and media-based public education campaigns and even the expensive strategies (e.g. improving public transport) are often cost-effective in the long term.
Changes 'default' behaviour	Some food choices are highly influenced by price, labeling and availability and changing these factors shifts the 'default' food choices.
Minimizes message distortion	Education messages related to obesity (or foods which might promote weight loss) may be misconstrued or misapplied and this risk is minimized by a greater emphasis on providing and promoting healthy choices rather than preaching about unhealthy choices.

Strategies for obesity prevention

The action needed to reverse the current trends in obesity will have to be broad, serious and sustained to be successful. Action will be needed in multiple settings (for example schools, homes, neighbourhoods, workplace, food outlets) and backed up by supportive sector-based action (such as government policies and social marketing on nutrition and physical activity). One of theoretical models for grouping the influences on unhealthy weight gain is the classic epidemiological triad of host, vector, and environment[1,4]. This helps link obesity to previous population interventions that have successfully controlled other epidemics such as infectious diseases, smoking, coronary heart disease and injuries. The 'agent' in the Triad is the final pathway leading to weight gain and is defined as positive energy balance. The 'host' is the individual or population and education is the central strategy for host-based interventions. The 'vectors' of an overconsumption of total energy are predominantly energy-dense foods and drinks and large portion sizes[5-7]. High fat foods and high sugar drinks have been implicated as the energy-dense vectors for reductions in consumption[8,9]. The energy expenditure vectors are the mediators of reducing physical activity and promoting sedentary recreation and these are predominantly time/energy-saving machines such as cars and entertainment machines such as television. Many vector-based strategies involve technical/engineering solutions, for example, reducing the energy density of manufactured foods. An underlying principle in vector-based strategies is that targeting vectors related to high volume behaviours (such as reducing the fat content of French fries[10]) may only achieve small changes per individual but across the population, the changes can be significant.

The 'environment' incorporates not only the physical environment but also the economic, policy and socio-cultural environments. In general the environmental changes will need a strong lead from policy and/or social change. While the intervention strategies are different for each corner of the triad, they are all interconnected. The main lesson from other epidemics is that all three corners need to be addressed together to achieve success.

Dissecting 'obesogenic' environments

Within any setting (microenvironments such as homes) or sector (macroenviroments such as the food industry), one can pose a series of questions to 'scan' that environment for potential influences on eating and physical activity behaviours[1]:

- **Physical – What is available?** This includes not only the visible world of food and physical activity choices but also less tangible factors such as the availability of training opportunities, nutrition and exercise expertise, technological innovations, information and food labels.

- **Economic – What are the financial factors?** These refer to both the costs and incomes for consumers as well as the money spent on the promotion of healthy lifestyles by health departments, the advertising by fast food outlets and the government funding of roads, public transport, and recreation facilities.

- **Policy – What are the rules?** These refer to laws, regulations, policies (formal or informal), and institutional rules (including in the home) that impact on physical activity and eating behaviours.

- **Socio-cultural – What are the attitudes, perceptions, values and beliefs?** At a micro or setting level, these socio-cultural influences combine to give what is variously described as the 'culture' or 'ethos' of a school, home, workplace or neighborhood. At the macro-environmental level, the mass media are an important sector influencing the socio-cultural aspects of food and physical activity[11], particularly through the effects of advertising and marketing[12].

These questions form the basis of the ANGELO (Analysis Grid for Environments Linked to Obesity) framework that can be used with a group of stakeholders to identify and prioritize environmental strategies for intervention[1]. The prioritizing criteria include: Impact – what affect will changing the environmental factor have on behaviour? Relevance – is the environmental factor a big problem in our area? Changeability – is the environmental factor amenable to change?

Evidence that environments influence unhealthy weight gain

While the link between obesogenic environments and unhealthy weight gain seems intuitive, the evidence base for these links and their quantification is at an early stage. Most of the studies to date have been cross-sectional or case studies with some studies of quasi-experiments or natural experiments. Much more evidence is needed in this area, particularly on the impact of environmental interventions. The usual hierarchies of evidence strength will need to be adapted for environmental research where randomized controlled trials are rarely possible. For example, what is the evidence that home environments influence unhealthy weight gain in children? There have been very few studies in this area and none would qualify as grade 1 evidence[13], yet to state that the evidence is not strong enough to warrant including homes as a key environment for the prevention of unhealthy weight gain would be counter-intuitive. Similarly, the evidence that high volume television advertising of foods to young children influences their consumption of those foods is not available. There is a vast amount of data linking food promotions to sales but such information is rarely in the public domain. Does the huge advertising spend by the food industry directed at young children constitute evidence of effect? In the future, settings-based approaches to prevent unhealthy weight gain are likely to contain many components. For example, a school-based strategy could include curriculum programmes, nutrition and physical activity policies, parent education, changes to the school canteen, sports programmes and facilities, and safe walking and cycling routes to school. It may be possible to tease out the impact of some of the key interventions like the Planet Health project was able to do for reducing television viewing times[14], but this may become increasingly difficult to do as prevention programmes become more multidimensional and integrated into the school systems.

Environmental interventions in settings and sectors

There are multiple opportunities for incorporating environmental change into prevention programmes[15]. At a setting level, for example in neighbourhoods, childcare centres, workplaces and schools, environmental changes can be achieved through local action and the concerted efforts of a few individuals. To be successful, however, at a community level, several sectors need to be involved so that each reinforces the other. This is particularly important for school-based interventions where the home environment, the neighbourhood, the local sports and recreation clubs, and the local food outlets all contribute to the food and activity environments for children. It is too much to expect that a school-based programme can prevent unhealthy weight gain by itself.

Influencing environments at a sector level, such as strengthening regulations on food marketing to young children, achieving monitoring programmes for childhood obesity and its determinants, or getting manufacturers to reformulate food products, is very difficult. The major drivers of environmental change at this level will be a combination of enlightened government policies and public pressure for change. Commercial drivers continue to be instrumental in creating obesogenic environments, although there are some opportunities for those commercial drivers to help create more leptogenic environments. An example of this is supplying healthier food choices for health-conscious consumers. However, the conflicts between the commercial and public health agendas are too numerous for economic drivers from the commercial sector to be a leader in obesity prevention. Linking the health agenda to other agendas for change, such as reducing car traffic to reduce congestion and pollution, will strengthen efforts to influence the political decisions in government.

Conclusions

Building the evidence base around obesogenic environments is an urgent priority for obesity prevention. The ability to influence the key decision-makers about the need for an environment-centred approach will rest on the quality of that evidence as well as the public pressure for change. The opposition to changes that threaten commercial interests will be substantial and will also require a strong evidence base. However, actions to reduce the obesogenicity of our environments cannot await cast iron evidence because the epidemic is already upon us and because environmental change is usually slow. Building the evidence by intensively evaluating 'best guess' interventions as they are implemented is the prudent approach to take.

References

1. Swinburn B, Egger G, Raza F. Dissecting obesogenic environments: the development and application of a framework for identifying and prioritizing environmental interventions for obesity. *Prev Med* 1999; 29(6 Pt 1): 563–70.

2. Rose G. *The strategy of preventive medicine*. Oxford: Oxford University Press; 1993.

3. Stunkard AJ. Socioeconomic status and obesity. In: Cardew G (ed.) *The origins and consequences of obesity*, pp. 174–93. Chichester: Wiley; 1996.

4. Egger G, Swinburn B. An 'ecological' approach to the obesity pandemic. *BMJ* 1997; 315 (7106): 477–80.

5. Blundell JE, King NA. Overconsumption as a cause of weight gain: behavioural-physiological interactions in the control of food intake (appetite).Ciba Found Symp. 1996; 201: 138–54 (discussion 154–8, 188–93).

6. Prentice AM. Manipulation of dietary fat and energy density and subsequent effects on substrate flux and food intake. *Am J Clin Nutr* 1998; 67 (Suppl 3): S535–S541.

7. Rolls BJ, Engell D, Birch LL. Serving portion size influences 5-year-old but not 3-year-old children's food intakes. *J Am Diet Assoc* 2000; 100(2): 232–4.

8. Astrup A, Grunwald GK, Melanson EL, Saris WH, Hill JO. The role of low-fat diets in body weight control: a meta-analysis of *ad libitum* dietary intervention studies. *Int J Obes Relat Metab Disord* 2000; 24(12): 1545–52.

9. Ludwig DS, Peterson KE, Gortmaker SL. Relation between consumption of sugar-sweetened drinks and childhood obesity: a prospective, observational analysis. *Lancet* 2001; 357(9255): 505–8.

10. Morley-John J, Swinburn B, Metcalf P, Raza F, Wright H. Fat content of chips, quality of frying fat and deep-frying practices in New Zealand fast food outlets. *Aust NZ J Public Health* 2002; 26(2): 101–7.

11. MacLaren T. Messages for the masses: food and nutrition issues on television. *J Am Diet Assoc* 1997; 97(7): 733–4.

12. Serwer AE. McDonalds conquers the world. *Fortune* 1994; 130(8): 103–107.

13. Campbell K, Crawford D. Family food environments as determinants of preschool-aged children's eating behaviours: implications for obesity prevention policy: a review. *Aust J Nutr Diet* 2001; 58(1): 19–25.

14. Gortmaker SL, Peterson K, Wiecha J, Sobol AM, Dixit S, Fox MK, *et al*. Reducing obesity via a school-based interdisciplinary intervention among youth: Planet Health. *Arch Pediatr Adolesc Med* 1999; 153(4): 409–18.

15. French SA, Story M, Jeffery RW. Environmental influences on eating and physical activity. *Annu Rev Public Health* 2001; 22: 309–35.

Progress in Obesity Research: 9. Edited by *Geraldo Medeiros-Neto, Alfredo Halpern and Claude Bouchard*
©2003 John Libbey Eurotext Ltd, pp. 59–63.

CHAPTER 12

Neural pathways underlying food intake and energy homeostasis

Hans-Rudolf Berthoud

*Neurobiology of Nutrition Laboratory, Pennington Biomedical Research Center, Louisiana State University,
Baton Rouge, LA 70808, USA
[e-mail: berthohr@pbrc.edu]*

Introduction

Thrifty genes in a drastically changing environment are thought to be responsible for most of the obesity epidemic in affluent societies[1,2]. Availability of cheap calories from fat and sugar[3] combined with a sedentary lifestyle are overpowering a regulatory system that was designed to deal with a scarce supply of low calorie food, frequent famines, and high physical activity throughout the five million years of human evolution[4]. To survive in this harsh environment, genes were selected that: (1) produce heightened sensitivity to the perception of food cues, (2) allow large meals to be ingested when food was present, with weak negative feedback from satiety signals, (3) efficiently store temporary excess calories in fat depots, (4) produce mild insulin resistance to allow gluconeogenesis in times of famine, and (5) metabolize substrates for all energy needs economically and with minimal waste. In the new environment with high availability of carbohydrates and fat these genes have become a liability.

To tackle the obesity problem we have two options. We either change the environment, or we learn how the changed environment affects regulatory processes and come up with behavioural and pharmacological therapies. Human ingestive behaviour has changed drastically with industrialization. Market forces dictate highly palatable and calorically dense foods. Starting in early childhood the modern lifestyle brings exposure to a flood of powerful food cues. Because the nervous system is the main interface by which this environment influences regulatory processes, mechanisms of perception and cognition of food-related external stimuli may be key for finding successful therapies[4]. In this brief review I will describe the neural network of ingestive behaviour and energy homeostasis with emphasis on pathways linking extrahypothalamic structures involved in its cognitive aspects with hypothalamic and hindbrain areas involved in its metabolic aspects (see[5] for an in-depth review).

Ingestive behaviour involves more than swallowing food

Ingestive behaviour has been broken down into different phases using behavioural or neurological criteria. Most often an appetitive phase is distinguished from a consummatory phase. Watts[6] has provided a more detailed and accurate description of the cascade of events comprising ingestive behaviours.

In the initiation phase, the incentive value of a goal object (if present) and/or the internal state somehow make it possible for the organism to turn its attention to food. As mentioned above, food-related stimuli such as thought, sight and smell can be sufficient to arouse appetitive behaviour without any help from the internal state. On the other hand, in the absence of direct stimuli from food, the internal state is thought to selectively facilitate retrieval of memorial representations of food[7]. Neurologically, the initiation phase leads to a change in drive state, which allows appropriate motor program selection for the procurement phase.

In animals, the procurement phase can involve intense and prolonged foraging, as exemplified by the honeybee's waggle-dance, or the Canadian mountain goat engaging in a long and hazardous descent to find salt near a riverbank in the valley. Obviously, such behaviour is largely non-stereotypical and volitional and requires appropriate planning, memory, and reward mechanisms. Thus, it depends heavily on cortical cognitive, emotional and reward processing. Although many of these 'obstacles' to obtain food are no longer present for humans and animals in the modern environment, the relevant neural circuits that have been optimalized during millions of years of evolution are still functional, and may be an interesting substrate for behavioural and pharmacological intervention.

The consummation or consummatory phase begins when food is finally present and ingested. This phase involves stereotypic movements controlled by local circuits in the brainstem and spinal cord. It is also characterized by continuous sensing of the ingested foods and their constituent nutrients at the cephalic and gastrointestinal levels as well as the generation of associations between various sensory attributes[8]. During the course of a typical meal, humans also constantly compare the actual with the expected sensory attributes of each individual food component.

Finally, the mechanisms of satiation come into action, eventually leading to the termination of the meal. However, in a neurological sense, termination of the meal is not the end of an ingestive behaviour episode. Important information regarding the absorptive and post-absorptive consequences is gathered long after termination of a meal and stored in associative memories for future use. Furthermore, there is a certain behavioural sequence following a satiating meal, suggesting extensive cross talk between neurological systems controlling different behaviours. When naturally satiated, rats stop eating, groom and explore for a short time, and then rest or sleep.

Because most humans still ingest their daily food ration in only three discrete, scheduled meals, factors determining the size of these meals are of crucial importance for energy balance. Identification of mechanisms of satiation and meal termination has dominated research efforts, and a great number of putative satiety signals have been identified. However, satiety signals can be easily overridden by factors prevalent in the obesigenic environment, such as availability[9], variety[10], palatability[11,12], density[13], low cost[14], and social factors[15]. Most of these factors act directly on brain areas involved in hedonic and cognitive processing.

A hierarchy of neural pathways controlling energy homeostasis

The hypothalamic 'centre' hypothesis has dominated research on food intake during much of the last century. However, with the advent of neuronal tracing in the seventies, it became clear that the hypothalamus is well connected to most other areas of the brain and does not work in isolation. In particular it's strong reciprocal connections with certain areas in the caudal brainstem and spinal cord involved in oromotor, locomotor, and autonomic control[16–18], as well as prominent reciprocal connections with various cortico-limbic structures[19] suggested a much more distributed system.

Brainstem

The caudal medulla, perhaps together with the parabrachial complex in the pons, contains circuitry serving the three major components in energy homeostasis, food intake, energy assimilation, and energy expenditure[20].

Almost the entire alimentary canal, starting with the taste receptors in the oral cavity and ending with associated organs like pancreas and liver, is well represented in the dorsal vagal complex via sensory and motor fibres of the vagus and other cranial nerves[5,21]. This system is a major controller of the rate of assimilation of each of the three energy-providing macronutrients. The ventrolateral medulla contains major sympathetic pathways to organs such as the adrenal gland, liver, brown and white fat, and skeletal muscle involved in energy mobilization and expenditure[22]. The hindbrain also contains the sensory-motor control circuits for oromotor pattern generation[23], and together with the spinal cord, for locomotor pattern generation. In addition, absence of a blood brain barrier allows the area postrema and NTS easy access to circulating hormones and cytokines such as leptin, insulin, and amylin[24].

It was Grill and colleagues[25] that set out to demonstrate the intrinsic capacity of the brainstem to orchestrate ingestive behaviour. In a series of papers using the midbrain decerebrate rat and intraoral liquid food delivery as a model, an impressive catalog of integrative mechanisms complete within the brainstem was documented. The brainstem circuitry is capable to respond to short-term gastrointestinal signals but it cannot adjust intake to longer-term metabolic signals or to environmental signals requiring cognitive processing.

Hypothalamus

The recent progress in hypothalamic functional and chemical neuroanatomy has been discussed in several reviews[5,26,27] and is only briefly introduced here.

Strategically located in the midst of the mammalian neuraxis, the hypothalamus receives at least three distinct types of relevant information via direct or indirect neural connections as well as hormone receptors and substrate sensors bestowed on hypothalamic neurons. First, the medial and to a lesser extent the lateral hypothalamus receive a rich mix of information pertaining to the internal state of relative energy repletion/depletion through both neural inputs and hormone receptors. Second, the hypothalamus, particularly its lateral aspects, receives information from areas in the forebrain involved in the acquisition, storage, and retrieval of sensory representations of the external food space and internal food experience, as well as from the executive forebrain involved in behaviour selection and initiation. Third, specific hypothalamic nuclei receive information about the behavioural state, such as diurnal clock[28], physical activity-level, reproductive cycle, developmental stage, as well as imminent (e.g. fight and flight) and chronic (e.g. infection) stressors, that can potentially impact on short-term availability of fuels and long-term energy balance. In addition, rich intrahypothalamic connections facilitate further distribution of incoming information to various hypothalamic nuclei[29]. On the other hand, the hypothalamus has widespread neural projections to the same cortical areas it receives inputs[19], and many hypothalamic neurons are one synapse away from most endocrine systems and from both sympathetic and parasympathetic effector organs involved in the flux, storage, mobilization, and utilization of fuels.

Thus, the hypothalamus is crucial for deprivation-induced ingestion, the link between food intake and energy expenditure, and the modulation of brainstem reflex circuitry of ingestion. However, the hypothalamus does not contain the circuitry to adjust intake to many environmental signals affecting cognition, emotions, and reward expectancies.

Forebrain

Telencephalic structures are involved in the execution of mainly the initiation, procurement, and appetitive phases of ingestive behaviour and in associative learning before, during, and after the consummatory phase. One of the crucial factors for human evolution was the tremendous expansion of the cerebral cortex. It allowed what is usually referred to as higher neural functions, such as cognition, language, planning, consciousness and emotions, and as a consequence a completely new way to guarantee and satisfy nutritional needs. In neurological terms, the huge, flexible, and multidimensional computational capability of the cerebral cortex allows primates and even lower vertebrates to generate the most complex sensory representations of nutrients and the nutrient-related environment. A myriad of sensory information pertaining to the physical attributes of potential nutrients, their relationship to the environment (where and how to find), and their physico-chemical and neural interaction with the organism is collected through all senses and systematically refined and processed within specialized cortical areas.

Associative learning related to food intake is an important cognitive function. The organism presumably uses all of its senses to generate a large number of associations. Given the many sensory input channels with their qualitative, quantitative and temporal differences, even food items that are very similar produce a specific signature of sensory consequences in the broadest sense. Taste is just one, and may not be the most important, of the distinguishing features between two foods. Such associative learning enables the organism to use past experience for the management of daily nutritional requirements. By linking internal signals of metabolic repletion or depletion with external cues, it provides a mechanism to recognize the nutritive value of a food item before it is ingested.

The key areas of the cortex for ingestive behaviour control seem to be the visceral/taste, olfactory, and medial prefrontal areas as well as the hippocampal complex and the amygdala[5,30–32]. All of these areas are heavily interconnected. There is strong cortical input to hypothalamic nuclei involved in the control of food intake and energy balance[33]. Major inputs to the hypothalamus originate in the medial prefrontal, insular and olfactory cortices, the central and medial amygdala, and the entorhinal cortex and subiculum of the hippocampal complex. The lateral hypothalamus projects back to all of the cortical areas via direct orexin, melanin-concentrating hormone, and histaminergic projections[34], and indirectly, via the mesocortical dopamine system and the noradrenergic, serotonergic, and cholinergic 'arousal and attention' systems with various involvement of certain thalamic nuclei.

Another telencephalic area that has received the most attention is the nucleus accumbens. Together with the preforontal cortex and the amygdala, this nucleus seems to be involved in behaviour selection or suppression as dictated by motivation and optimization of pleasure and reward. Behavioural studies have come to the conclusion that humans and animals develop behavioural strategies to maximize the amount of pleasure to be derived[35]. Berridge has argued that reward contains distinguishable psychological and functional components, with different underlying neural substrates[36]. According to this theory, 'liking' is the pleasure derived from palatable food, and is associated with diffuse opioid and GABA/benzodiazepine systems distributed in the brainstem gustatory relay nuclei, the ventral striatum (and possibly other areas such as the amygdala, limbic cortex and hypothalamus), while 'wanting' represents the appetitive/incentive motivation component, associated with the meso-limbic and meso-cortical dopamine systems, including nucleus accumbens, medial prefrontal cortex, and possibly the amygdala.

How does the nucleus accumbens translate motivation into action? Food-related bits of information generated on-line in the association cortices or retrieved from storage in the hippocampal complex are continuously fed via glutamatergic projections into parallel loops to the nucleus accumbens shell and basolateral amygdala and back to the cortex via ventral pallidum and mediodorsal thalamus. Bits of information that achieve high motivational valence and arousal after an 'affective/emotional' filter in the amygdala and its effector responses, as well as the necessary level of 'wanting' after a 'pleasure' filter in the dopamine-gated nucleus accumbens shell, will become dominant through active suppression of undesirable bits of information. More and more behavioural motor programmes relevant to the dominant bits of information are then loaded into striatal motor pathways resulting in coordinated, goal-directed ingestive behaviour. The presence of projections from the accumbens shell to the lateral hypothalamus suggests an additional 'internal state filter' necessary for full expression of ingestive motor behaviour.

References

1. Neel JV. Diabetes mellitus: a 'thrifty' genotype rendered determined by progress? *Am J Hum Genet* 1962; 14: 353–363.

2. Ravussin E, Bogardus C. Energy balance and weight regulation: genetics versus environment. *Br J Nutr* 2000; 83 (Suppl 1): S17–20.

3. Drewnowski A. Nutrition transition and global dietary trends. *Nutrition* 2000; 16(7–8): 486–7.

4. Peters JC, Wyatt HR, Donahoo WT, Hill JO. From instinct to intellect: the challenge of maintaining healthy weight in the modern world. *Obes Rev* 2002; 3(2): 69–74.

5. Berthoud H-R. Multiple neural systems controlling food intake and body weight. *Neuroscience & Biobehavioral Rev* 2002; 26(4): 393–428.

6. Watts AG. Understanding the neural control of ingestive behaviors: helping to separate cause from effect with dehydration-associated anorexia. *Horm Behav* 2000; 37(4): 261–83.

7. Davidson TL. Pavlovian occasion setting: a link between physiological change and appetitive behavior. *Appetite* 2000; 35(3): 271–2.

8. Sclafani A. Psychobiology of food preferences. *Int J Obes Relat Metab Disord* 2001; 25 Suppl 5: S13–6.

9. Tordoff MG. Obesity by choice: the powerful influence of nutrient availability on nutrient intake. *Am J Physiol Regul Integr Comp Physiol* 2002; 282(5): R1536–9.

10. Treit D, Spetch ML, Deutsch JA. Variety in the flavor of food enhances eating in the rat: a controlled demonstration. *Physiol Behav* 1983; 30(2): 207–11.

11. Nasser J. Taste, food intake and obesity. *Obes Rev* 2001; 2(4): 213–8.

12. Sclafani A, Springer D. Dietary obesity in adult rats: similarities to hypothalamic and human obesity syndromes. *Physiol Behav* 1976; 17(3): 461–71.

13. Bell EA, Rolls BJ. Energy density of foods affects energy intake across multiple levels of fat content in lean and obese women. *Am J Clin Nutr* 2001; 73(6): 1010–8.

14. Morato S, Johnson DF, Collier G. Feeding patterns of rats when food-access cost is alternately low and high. *Physiol Behav* 1995; 57(1): 21–6.

15. De Castro J.M. Socio-cultural determinants of meal size and frequency. *Br J Nutr.* 1997; 77 (Suppl 1): S39–S54 (discussion S54–5).

16. Ricardo JA, Koh ET. Anatomical evidence of direct projections from the nucleus of the solitary tract to the hypothalamus, amygdala, and other forebrain structures in the rat. *Brain Res* 1978; 153(1): 1–26.

17. Sawchenko PE. Central connections of the sensory and motor nuclei of the vagus nerve. *J Auton Nerv Syst* 1983; 9(1): 13–26.

18. Ter Horst GJ, Copray JC, Liem RS, van Willigen JD. Projections from the rostral parvocellular reticular formation to pontine and medullary nuclei in the rat: involvement in autonomic regulation and orofacial motor control. *Neuroscience* 1991; 40(3): 735–58.

19. Saper CB. Hypothalamic connections with the cerebral cortex. *Prog Brain Res* 2000; 126: 39–48.

20. Grill HJ, Kaplan JM. The neuroanatomical axis for control of energy balance. *Front Neuroendocrinol* 2002; 23(1): 2–40.

21. Berthoud HR, Neuhuber WL. Functional and chemical anatomy of the afferent vagal system. *Auton Neurosci* 2000; 85(1–3): 1–17.

22. Morrison SF. Differential regulation of brown adipose and splanchnic sympathetic outflows in rat: roles of raphe and rostral ventrolateral medulla neurons. *Clin Exp Pharmacol Physiol* 2001; 28(1–2): 138–43.

23. Travers JB, Dinardo LA, Karimnamazi H. Motor and premotor mechanisms of licking. *Neurosci Biobehav Rev* 1997; 21(5): 631–47.

24. Grill HJ, Schwartz MW, Kaplan JM, Foxhall JS, Breininger J, Baskin DG. Evidence that the caudal brainstem is a target for the inhibitory effect of leptin on food intake. *Endocrinology* 2002; 143(1): 239–46.

25. Grill HJ, Kaplan JM. Caudal brainstem participates in the distributed neural control of feeding. In: Stricker EM (ed.) *Handbook of Behavioral Neurobiology*, pp. 125–149. New Jersey: Plenum Press; 1990.

26. Elmquist JK. Hypothalamic pathways underlying the endocrine, autonomic, and behavioral effects of leptin. *Physiol Behav* 2001; 74(4–5): 703–8.

27. Broberger C, Hokfelt T. Hypothalamic and vagal neuropeptide circuitries regulating food intake. *Physiol Behav* 2001; 74(4–5): 669–82.

28. Kalsbeek A, Fliers E, Franke AN, Wortel J, Buijs RM. Functional connections between the suprachiasmatic nucleus and the thyroid gland as revealed by lesioning and viral tracing techniques in the rat. *Endocrinology* 2000; 141(10): 3832–41.

29. Luiten PG, ter Horst GJ, Steffens AB. The hypothalamus, intrinsic connections and outflow pathways to the endocrine system in relation to the control of feeding and metabolism. *Prog Neurobiol* 1987; 28(1): 1–54.

30. Gautier JF, Chen K, Uecker A, Bandy D, Frost J, Salbe AD, *et al.* Regions of the human brain affected during a liquid-meal taste perception in the fasting state: a positron emission tomography study. *Am J Clin Nutr* 1999; 70(5): 806–10.

31. O'Doherty J, Rolls ET, Francis S, Bowtell R, McGlone F. Representation of pleasant and aversive taste in the human brain. *J Neurophysiol* 2001; 85(3): 1315–21.

32. Del Parigi A, Gautier JF, Chen K, Salbe AD, Ravussin E, Reiman E, *et al.* Neuroimaging and obesity: mapping the brain responses to hunger and satiation in humans using positron emission tomography. *Ann NY Acad Sci* 2002; 967: 389–97.

33. Simerly RB. Anatomical Substrates of Hypothalamic Integration. In: Paxinos G (ed), *The rat nervous system* (2nd edn), pp. 353–376. San Diego: Academic Press; 1995.

34. Bittencourt JC, Frigo L, Rissman RA, Casatti CA, Nahon JL, Bauer JA. The distribution of melanin-concentrating hormone in the monkey brain (Cebus apella). *Brain Res* 1998; 804(1): 140–3.

35. Balasko M, Cabanac M. Motivational conflict among water need, palatability, and cold discomfort in rats. *Physiol Behav* 1998; 65(1): 35–41.

36. Berridge KC. Food reward: brain substrates of wanting and liking. *Neurosci Biobehav Rev* 1996; 20(1): 1–25

TRACK I

ADIPOSE TISSUE BIOLOGY

Progress in Obesity Research: 9. Edited by *Geraldo Medeiros-Neto, Alfredo Halpern and Claude Bouchard*
©2003 John Libbey Eurotext Ltd, pp. 67–71.

CHAPTER 13

Methods for studying human adipose tissue *in vivo*

Keith N. Frayn

Oxford Centre for Diabetes, Endocrinology and Metabolism, Churchill Hospital, Oxford OX3 7LJ, UK
[email: keith.frayn@oxlip.ox.ac.uk]

Introduction: why study adipose tissue *in vivo*?

In a previous volume in this series I reviewed the reasons why it is necessary to conduct studies of adipose tissue metabolism *in vivo*[12]. In brief, adipose tissue is far more than just a collection of adipocytes each acting independently. It is a highly structured tissue whose activities are regulated by the autonomic nervous system, by the endocrine system and by a complex mixture of metabolites delivered in the blood and produced locally within the tissue. Furthermore, evidence of pulsatile leptin secretion suggests that adipocytes throughout the body may act in a synchronous manner[28,29]. Indeed, there are many aspects of adipose tissue function, such as blood flow and angiogenesis, that can only be studied *in vivo*. Understanding how adipose tissue operates and is regulated *in vivo* is a prime example of integrative physiology.

Since I reviewed methods for studying adipose tissue metabolism only four years ago, here my aims have been to (1) update that report, and (2) bring in aspects of adipose tissue other than metabolism that can be studied *in vivo*.

Imaging techniques: static

Adipose tissue is not homogeneous. Some adipose tissue depots, particularly central depots, are more highly associated with adverse complications (insulin resistance, cardiovascular disease risk factors) than are others. Whilst many studies have compared adipocytes from different depots *in vitro*, again we need ultimately to understand how these adipocytes function *in vivo* in their respective depots. One obvious example of where the *in vitro* perspective can be misleading is the following[13]. Several studies of adipocytes from different depots *in vitro* show that intra-abdominal adipocytes are characterized by high rates of lipolysis, which are not readily suppressed by insulin. In that case, it is not obvious why these adipocytes do not shrink and disappear: unless, of course, these high rates of lipolysis are matched at other times by equal rates of fatty acid uptake and storage. Fatty acid uptake, especially from lipoprotein-triacylglycerol, is not easily studied *in vitro*.

There have been some interesting recent developments in imaging of adipose tissue distribution *in vivo*. Computed tomography (CT) scans of intra-abdominal and subcutaneous adipose tissue have been used for many years to elucidate the depots that contribute most to the adverse effects of abdominal obesity[2]. More recently, CT and magnetic resonance imaging (MRI) have been used to study this in more detail. For instance, the subcutaneous abdominal adipose tissue is itself not homogeneous, and one study using CT suggests that only the deeper layers of the subcutaneous fat (below Scarpa's fascia) are associated with insulin resistance[25]. Using similar techniques, it was shown that deeper (sub-fascial) layers of thigh fat are associated with insulin resistance, whereas more superficial thigh fat is not[19]. At the same time, whole-body scans have been used to assess fat distribution, based on either MRI or the low-radiation dual-energy X-ray absorptiometry (DXA). Whole-body fat scans using MRI have shown that prediction of intra-abdominal fat from measurement of a single CT or MRI 'slice' is unreliable[42], and have highlighted the variability in body fat and its distribution[42].

Imaging techniques: dynamic

CT and MRI have also been used to follow changes in particular fat depots with physiological interventions. For instance, both subcutaneous abdominal and visceral fat are lost with weight loss, although only the latter correlates with the improvement in insulin sensitivity[18]. In contrast, there appears to be a selective loss of intra-abdominal adipose tissue with aerobic exercise training[41]. Changing from a diet rich in polyunsaturated fat to one rich in saturated fat produced an increase in subcutaneous abdominal fat[39], although, since this was only measured at a single level, this surprising result needs to be confirmed.

More dynamic measurements still can be made with the technique of positron emission tomography (PET), which has recently been applied to adipose tissue metabolism[43]. [18F]-2-fluoro-2-deoxy-D-glucose ([18F]FDG) was used to measure glucose uptake in adipose tissue in a study in which PET images were superimposed upon MR images to define regions of adipose tissue. At the same time, adipose tissue blood flow (ATBF) was measured using [15O]H$_2$O. Adipose tissue glucose uptake using [18F]FDG/PET correlated with glucose uptake measured using microdialysis (see below) in the same studies. Adipose tissue glucose uptake during insulin infusion was lower in obese subjects than in lean, and ATBF was also reduced in the obese ($P = 0.06$). This is an interesting development in methods for studying adipose tissue metabolism *in vivo*, although it must be remembered that PET is a specialized technique available in only a few centres, and there is not, as yet, a method for studying fatty acid and triacylglycerol metabolism in adipose tissue using PET.

Studies of adipose tissue metabolism and secretory functions

There has been an interesting development for studying fatty acid metabolism in rodents: the use of a fatty acid analogue, [9,10-3H]-(R)-2-bromopalmitate, to assess fatty acid uptake into tissues *in vivo*, in a similar manner to the use of 2-deoxy-D-glucose to study glucose uptake[33]. This technique can potentially be applied to all tissues and it might be thought that uptake of fatty acids (from the plasma non-esterified fatty acid fraction) is not a major metabolic pathway in adipose tissue *in vivo*. However, the technique has shown its usefulness in a study of the effects of the thiazolidinedione (TZD) antidiabetic agents on fatty acid 'trafficking' in tissues. These studies, in rats, suggested that a major effect of TZD treatment was to increase the capacity of adipose tissue to take up fatty acids[34].

In humans, two methods have continued to dominate this field: microdialysis[1] and arterio-venous difference measurements (both reviewed in[16]).

Microdialysis is a useful technique for assessing lipolysis by measurement of interstitial glycerol concentrations. Following the theme developed above of an increasing requirement to understand the metabolic differences between, and even within, adipose tissue depots, Enevoldsen *et al.*[9] have used ultrasonography to help them to place microdialysis probes into defined regions of human abdominal adipose tissue: superficial and deep layers (separated by Scarpa's fascia) and the depot inferior to the linea alba, in the round ligament, that they refer to as 'preperitoneal adipose tissue'. Measurements of lipolysis were made in the postabsorptive state, and during infusion of adrenaline. ATBF was also measured by ^{133}Xe washout (see below) in the same sub-depots. Contrary to expectations, these authors found that rates of lipolysis and blood flow were highest in the superficial layer. It is difficult as yet to reconcile these observations with the findings discussed above showing that the deeper layers are more strongly associated with insulin resistance, but this highlights the need to conduct metabolic studies of adipose tissue *in vivo*.

The use of arterio-venous difference methods for studying metabolism *in vivo* has a long history. It was applied specifically to human adipose tissue in 1989 with the development of a method for cannulating veins that drain subcutaneous abdominal adipose tissue[14,15]. This technique has continued to be informative and may be combined with stable isotopic tracer techniques to assess, for instance, the entrapment of lipoprotein-derived fatty acids in adipose tissue[10]. In addition, it has been combined with infusion of [3H]-noradrenaline to assess 'noradrenaline spillover' in adipose tissue, a measure of the sympathetic activation of the tissue[7,35]. Meal ingestion increases noradrenaline spillover in adipose tissue, and hence by implication sympathetic activation of adipose tissue[35]. Obese subjects had lower noradrenaline spillover in adipose tissue than lean[7].

As reviewed previously[12], arterio-venous difference measurements across specific adipose tissue depots have also been applied in other species including the tail of the fat-tailed sheep[17], the rat[27] and the dog[5].

Jensen and colleagues have used selective venous catheterization to provide further information on regional adipose tissue metabolism in humans[20,21,30]. Although they have not catheterized veins specifically draining adipose tissue depots, these authors have been able to assess regional contributions to lipolysis by using isotopic tracers to measure fatty acid production rates in different parts of the body. Infusion of a fatty acid tracer gives an estimate of the whole-body rate of fatty acid production; catheterization of the femoral or iliac vein gives the lower-body fatty acid production rate; catheterization of the hepatic vein gives the splanchnic fatty acid production rate; and the contribution of upper-body non-splanchnic (mainly superficial) depots to fatty acid production is assessed by difference. One of the consistent and striking findings to emerge from these elegant studies is that women with upper-body obesity have elevated whole-body fatty acid production rates compared with lower-body obese or lean women; but that the source of those excess fatty acids is primarily upper-body non-splanchnic adipose tissue, not visceral adipose tissue as has often been proposed[20]. Again, therefore, the findings of *in vitro* experiments (suggesting high rates of lipolysis in visceral adipocytes) have been contradicted when studies are performed *in vivo*.

Arterio-venous concentration differences have also been used to assess some of the secretory functions of adipose tissue. For instance, it was shown that adipose tissue is not a net producer of circulating tumour necrosis factor (TNF)-α *in vivo* in humans[32], although much attention has been paid to this cytokine as a possible signal between adipose and other tissues. On the other hand, both interleukin-6 and soluble TNF receptors are released into the circulation from human adipose tissue[31,32]. Human adipose tissue has also been shown to interconvert cortisone and cortisol *in vivo* using this technique[24]. Arterio-venous difference measurements have continued to be useful in elucidating the short-term control of leptin secretion in humans[8,11,26].

Adipose tissue blood flow (ATBF)

Adipose tissue is highly vascularized. An important theme to emerge from recent studies is that ATBF is regulated on a very short-term basis. ATBF increases after nutrient ingestion (even oral glucose)[4,36]. The increase is, in some people, several-fold within about 30 min, a much larger change than is seen in postprandial skeletal muscle blood flow (e.g. average 36 per cent increase after oral glucose[3]). Time-series and cross-correlation analysis suggests that this increase in blood flow is related to the plasma insulin peak[38]. Karpe *et al.* have now tested the effects of insulin on ATBF directly using the novel technique of 'microinfusion', in which agents can be delivered locally directly into the pool of ^{133}Xe injected into adipose tissue to measure washout (reflecting ATBF)[22]. Their conclusion is that insulin itself is not a direct vasodilator in human adipose tissue; instead, vasodilatation after oral glucose (or meals) is probably brought about by a local sympathetic activation in response to the insulin. This fits with an earlier observation that the increase in ATBF after a carbohydrate-rich meal is partially blocked by systemic propranolol infusion[37]. The role of the nitric oxide system, if any, in regulation of ATBF remains to be determined.

A further feature of the regulation of ATBF that has emerged clearly from recent studies is that not all people have the same responsiveness to nutrient ingestion. Obese subjects have a lower ATBF response to a meal than do lean[6,40]. This phenomenon of variability in ATBF responsiveness was analysed further in two independent groups of subjects[23]. Those whose ATBF response to a nutrient load was impaired were found to be characterized not primarily by a greater BMI than those with a good response, but more by measures of insulin resistance. In particular, a measurement of the ability of insulin to suppress non-esterified fatty acid concentrations was reduced in those with impaired ATBF regulation. This suggests that impaired ATBF regulation is associated with 'insulin resistance', particularly when measured in terms of adipose tissue insulin responsiveness[23].

Conclusion

Several of the findings reviewed have pointed to the need for an integrative, *in vivo* approach to studying adipose tissue metabolism and function. Adipose tissue, perhaps more than other tissues, is more than just a collection of its constituent cells, and findings from adipocytes *in vitro* cannot necessarily be extrapolated to the *in vivo* situation. Fortunately, there is a wide variety of methods available to study adipose tissue *in vivo*, where it truly belongs.

References

1. Arner P, Bolinder J, Eliasson A, Lundin A, Ungerstedt U. Microdialysis of adipose tissue and blood for *in vivo* lipolysis studies. *Am J Physiol* 1988; 255: E737–E742.

2. Ashwell M., Cole TJ, Dixon AK. Obesity: new insight into the anthropometric classification of fat distribution shown by computed tomography. *BMJ* 1985; 290: 1692–4.

3. Baron AD, Laakso M, Brechtel G, Hoit B, Watt C, Edelman SV. Reduced postprandial skeletal muscle blood flow contributes to glucose intolerance in human obesity. *J Clin Endocrinol Metab* 1990; 70: 1525–33.

4. Bülow J, Astrup A, Christensen NJ, Kastrup J. Blood flow in skin, subcutaneous adipose tissue and skeletal muscle in the forearm of normal man during an oral glucose load. *Acta Physiol Scand* 1987; 130: 657–61.

5. Bülow J, Madsen J. Influence of blood flow on fatty acid mobilization from lipolytically active adipose tissue. *Pflügers Archiv* 1981; 390: 169–74.

6. Coppack SW, Evans RD, Fisher RM, Frayn KN, Gibbons GF, Humphreys SM *et al.* Adipose tissue metabolism in obesity: lipase action *in vivo* before and after a mixed meal. *Metabolism* 1992; 1: 264–72.

7. Coppack SW, Horowitz JF, Paramore DS, Cryer PE, Royal HD, Klein S. Whole body, adipose tissue, and forearm norepinephrine kinetics in lean and obese women. *Am J Physiol* 1998; 75: E830–E834.

8. Coppack SW, Stanner S, Rawesh A, Goodrick S, Mohamed-Ali V. *In vivo* adipose tissue leptin production before and after a high carbohydrate meal. *Int J Obes* 1997; 1: S33.

9. Enevoldsen LH, Simonsen L, Stallknecht B, Galbo H, Bülow J. *In vivo* human lipolytic activity in preperitoneal and subdivisions of subcutaneous abdominal adipose tissue. *Am J Physiol Endocrinol Metab* 2001; 281: E1110–E1114.

10. Evans K, Burdge GC, Wootton SA, Clark ML, Frayn KN. Regulation of dietary fatty acid entrapment in subcutaneous adipose tissue and skeletal muscle. *Diabetes* 2002; 51: 2684–90.

11. Evans K, Clark ML, Frayn KN. Carbohydrate and fat have different effects on plasma leptin concentrations and adipose tissue leptin production. *Clin Sci* 2001; 100: 493–8.

12. Frayn KN. Methods for studying adipose tissue metabolism *in vivo*. In: *Progress in Obesity Research: 8*, Guy-Grand B, Ailhaud G (eds), pp.105–10. London: John Libbey 1999.

13. Frayn KN. Visceral fat and insulin resistance – causative or correlative? *Br J Nutr* 2000; 83 (Suppl 1): S71–S77.

14. Frayn KN, Coppack SW. Assessment of white adipose tissue metabolism by measurement of arteriovenous differences. *Methods Mol Biol* 2001; 155: 269–79.

15. Frayn KN, Coppack SW, Humphreys SM, Whyte PL. Metabolic characteristics of human adipose tissue *in vivo*. *Clin Sci* 1989; 76: 509–16.

16. Frayn KN, Macdonald IA. Assessment of substrate and energy metabolism *in vivo*. In: *Clinical research in diabetes and obesity*, Part 1: Methods, Assessment, and Metabolic Regulation. Draznin B, Rizza R (eds), pp.101–24. Totowa: NJ Humana Press; 1997.

17. Gooden JM, Campbell SL, van der Walt JG. Measurement of blood flow and lipolysis in the hindquarter tissues of the fat-tailed sheep *in vivo*. *Quart J Exp Physiol* 1986; 71: 537–47.

18. GoodpasterBH, Kelley DE, Wing RR, Meier A, Thaete FL. Effects of weight loss on regional fat distribution and insulin sensitivity in obesity. *Diabetes* 1999; 48: 839–47.

19. Goodpaster BH, Thaete FL, Kelley DE. Thigh adipose tissue distribution is associated with insulin resistance in obesity and in type 2 diabetes mellitus. *Am J Clin Nutr* 2000; 71: 885–92.

20. Guo Z, Hensrud DD, Johnson CM, Jensen MD. Regional postprandial fatty acid metabolism in different obesity phenotypes. *Diabetes* 1999; 48: 1586–92.

21. Jensen MD, Johnson CM. Contribution of leg and splanchnic free fatty acid (FFA) kinetics to postabsorptive FFA flux in men and women. *Metabolism* 1996; 45: 662–6.

22. Karpe F, Fielding BA, Ardilouze JL, Ilic V, Macdonald IA, Frayn KN. Effects of insulin on adipose tissue blood flow in man. *J Physiol* 2002; 540: 87–1093.

23. Karpe F, Fielding BA, Ilic V, Macdonald IA, Summers LKM, Frayn KN. Impaired postprandial adipose tissue blood flow response is related to aspects of insulin sensitivity. *Diabetes* 2002; 51: 2467–73.

24. Katz JR, Mohamed-Ali V, Wood PJ, Yudkin JS, Coppack SW. An *in vivo* study of the cortisol-cortisone shuttle in subcutaneous abdominal adipose tissue. *Clin Endocrinol* 1999; 50: 63–8.

25. Kelley DE, Thaete FL, Troost F, Huwe T, Goodpaster BH. Subdivisions of subcutaneous abdominal adipose tissue and insulin resistance. *Am J Physiol Endocrinol Metab* 2000; 278: E941–E948.

26. Klein S, Coppack SW, Mohamed-Ali V, Landt M. Adipose tissue leptin production and plasma leptin kinetics in humans. *Diabetes* 1996; 45: 984–7.

27. Kowalski TJ, Wu G, Watford M. Rat adipose tissue amino acid metabolism *in vivo* as assessed by microdialysis and arteriovenous techniques. *Am J Physiol* 1997; 273: E613–E622.

28. Licinio J, Mantzoros C, Negrao AB, Cizza G, Wong ML, Bongiorno PB *et al.* Human leptin levels are pulsatile and inversely related to pituitary-adrenal function. *Nature Med* 1997; 3: 575–9.

29. Licinio J, Negrao AB, Mantzoros C, Kaklamani V, Wong ML, Bongiorno PB. Synchronicity of frequently sampled, 24-h concentrations of circulating leptin, luteinizing hormone, and estradiol in healthy women. *Proc Natl Acad Sci USA* 1998; 95: 2541–6.

30. Martin ML, Jensen MD. Effects of body fat distribution on regional lipolysis in obesity. *J Clin Invest* 1991; 88: 609–13.

31. Mohamed-Ali V, Goodrick S, Bulmer K, Holly JM, Yudkin JS, Coppack SW. Production of soluble tumor necrosis factor receptors by human subcutaneous adipose tissue *in vivo*. *Am J Physiol* 1999; 277: E971–E975.

32. Mohamed-Ali V, Goodrick S, Rawesh A, Katz DR, Miles JM, Yudkin JS *et al.* Subcutaneous adipose tissue secretes interleukin-6 but not tumor necrosis-factor-α *in vivo. J Clin Endocrinol Metab* 1997; 82: 4196–200.

33. Oakes ND, Kjellstedt A, Forsberg GB, Clementz T, Camejo G, Furler SM *et al.* Development and initial evaluation of a novel method for assessing tissue-specific plasma free fatty acid utilization *in vivo* using (R)-2-bromopalmitate tracer. *J Lipid Res* 1999; 40: 1155–69.

34. Oakes ND, Thalén PG, Jacinto SM, Ljung B. Thiazolidinediones increase plasma-adipose tissue FFA exchange capacity and enhance insulin-mediated control of systemic FFA availability. *Diabetes* 2001; 50: 1158–65.

35. Patel JN, Eisenhofer G, Coppack SW, Miles JM. Norepinephrine spillover in forearm and subcutaneous adipose tissue before and after eating. *J Clin Endocrinol Metab* 1999; 84: 2815–19.

36. Samra JS, Frayn KN, Giddings JA, Clark ML, Macdonald IA. Modification and validation of a commercially available portable detector for measurement of adipose tissue blood flow. *Clin Physiol* 1995; 15: 241–8.

37. Simonsen L, Bülow J, Astrup A, Madsen J, Christensen NJ. Diet-induced changes in subcutaneous adipose tissue blood flow in man: effect of ß-adrenoceptor inhibition. *Acta Physiol Scand* 1990; 139: 341–6.

38. Summers LKM, Callow J, Samra JS, Macdonald IA, Matthews DR, Frayn KN. The effect on adipose tissue blood flow of isoenergetic mels containing different amounts and types of fat. *Int J Obes* 2001; 25: 1294–99.

39. Summers LKM, Fielding BA, Bradshaw HA, Ilic V, Beysen C, Clark ML. Substituting dietary saturated fat with polyunsaturated fat changes abdominal fat distribution and improves insulin sensitivity. *Diabetologia* 2002; 45: 369–77.

40. Summers LKM, Samra JS, Humphreys SM, Morris RJ, Frayn KN. Subcutaneous abdominal adipose tissue blood flow: variation within and between subjects and relationship to obesity. *Clin Sci* 1996; 91: 679–83.

41. Thomas EL, Brynes A, McCarthy J, Goldstone AP, Hajnal JV, Saeed N. Preferential loss of visceral fat following aerobic exercise, measured by magnetic resonance imaging. *Lipids* 2000; 35: 769–76.

42. Thomas EL, Saeed N, Hajnal JV, Brynes A, Goldstone AP, Frost G, Bell JD. Magnetic resonance imaging of total body fat. *J Appl Physiol* 1998; 85: 1778–85.

43. Virtanen KA, Peltoniemi P, Marjamäki P, Asola M, Strindberg L, Parkkola R *et al.* Human adipose tissue glucose uptake determined using [18F]-fluoro-deoxy-glucose ([18F]FDG) and PET in combination with microdialysis. *Diabetologia* 2001; 44: 2171–79.

Progress in Obesity Research: 9. Edited by *Geraldo Medeiros-Neto, Alfredo Halpern and Claude Bouchard*
©2003 John Libbey Eurotext Ltd, pp. 72–74.

CHAPTER 14

The study of gene expression in human adipose tissue

Hubert Vidal

INSERM U 449 and IFR 62, Faculté de Médecine RTH Laennec, Lyon, France
[e-mail: vidal@laennec.univ-lyon1.fr]

Introduction

Gene expression analysis is increasingly important in many fields of biological and molecular medicine research. Indeed, understanding the regulatory networks and mechanisms involved in the transcription of specific genes will most probably lead to the identification of genes relevant to new biological process, or implicated in disease. The dramatic increase in the prevalence of obesity urges us to better understand the molecular mechanisms underlying the different aspects of adipose tissue functions (such as adipocyte differentiation, the regulation of fatty acid storage and release, the production of adipocyte-derived products, etc.). Over the 15 last years, many important information and data regarding these processes have been obtained using adipose cell lines and rodent models of obesity. For the treatment of human obesity, it is now important to decipher these mechanisms in human adipose tissue directly. The investigation of the *in vivo* regulation of gene expression in human white adipose tissue relies on the ability to estimate the changes in specific mRNA levels in small fat biopsies that could be taken before and after an intervention (i.e. diet, exercise, drug treatment, etc.). Such study is limited by the size of the samples that could be taken and by the low yield in total RNA generally obtained from fat tissue that require highly sensitive methods to quantify specific mRNA molecules in order to estimate the expression levels of the genes of interest.

Preparation of RNA from human adipose tissue

The low stability of the mRNA molecules in crude tissue requires that the adipose tissue biopsies are taken under the least traumatic conditions and are rapidly frozen in liquid nitrogen. Using needle aspiration, 300 mg to 1.5 g of fat tissue can be routinely obtained at the level of umbilicus, under local anesthesia. The tissue should be removed rapidly (less than 5 min), washed with ice-cold saline buffer and immediately frozen. The tissue can be stored several months at −80 °C.

The high lipid content of fat tissue and the low amount of RNA in adipocytes result in difficulties to isolate total RNA using the classical methods based on guanidinium thiocyanate extraction followed by alcohol precipitation. In contrast, highly pure RNA preparations from low amount of adipose tissue can be obtained using commercially available kits that are based on the selective binding of RNA molecules on silica-gel supports. We have found that the RNeasy® minikit from Qiagen give highly reproducible results with very small amount (about 150 mg) of human adipose tissue[1,2]. However kits from other manufacturers can be satisfactorily used also.

After preparation, an important step is the quantification of the total RNA and the determination of its integrity. Spectrophotometer analysis is generally used. Integrity is verified on agarose gel stained with ethidium bromide, but the procedure requires rather large amount of material. The recently developed micro-electrophoresis instrument (Agilent 2100 Bioanalyser) is an alternative method to determine integrity and concentration of RNA preparations using extremely low amount of starting material (25 ng of RNA is sufficient).

The absorbance ratio (260/280 nm) is generally between 1.9 and 2.0 for total RNA preparations from human adipose tissue obtained with the RNeasy® minikit. The yield in total RNA is about 1.5 to 2 µg per 100 mg of tissue.

Quantification of specific mRNA using RT-PCR

The low yield in total RNA isolated from fat tissue requires a highly sensitive method to quantify specific mRNA molecules in order to estimate the expression levels of the genes of interest. A powerful method is the assay of mRNAs by quantitative RT-PCR. However, it should always keep in mind that RT-PCR are complex reactions, during which all the physical and chemical components are interdependent. The risk of contamination is also a major problem. In addition, the difficulty in obtaining accurate quantification of mRNA using PCR-based assays is mainly due to the exponential nature of the amplification process. Small variations in the amplification efficiency result in dramatic changes in product yields. To overcome these difficulties two approaches can be used: the quantification by competitive PCR and the direct measurement of the PCR products during the initial phase of the amplification process as performed in the real-time PCR.

Quantification of mRNA by RT-competitive PCR (RT-cPCR)

The competitive PCR involves the addition of known amount of either an exogenous synthetic RNA to the RT medium (competitive RT-PCR) or an exogenous DNA to the amplification mixture, after the RT step (RT-competitive PCR)[3,4]. The exogenous molecule (called competitor or internal standard) is co-amplified with the target in the same test tube, thereby standardizing the amplification process. During a competitive amplification, the ratio between the target and the competitor molecules remains constant during all the reaction. The amplification can thus be continued to the plateau phase of the reaction, resulting in the synthesis of PCR products that can be easily analysed[5]. The quantification of the ratio, at the end of the PCR, allows then the determination of the initial amount of target since the initial amount of competitor added in the tube is known.

However, for this quantitative PCR method to be accurate, the competitor and the target must be amplified with the same PCR efficiency[6]. The crucial issue of the RT-cPCR method is thus the design of the competitor DNA molecule. Because one of the determinant parameters of PCR efficiency is the hybridization of the primers to the templates, the target and competitor must be amplified using the same set of sense and antisense primers. In addition, the target and the competitor should generate distinguishable PCR products to allow the determination of their ratio at the end of the reaction. Different types of competitors have been reported in the literature. In most of the cases, they consist in a cDNA molecule with the same sequence as the target but with either a small deletion (less than 20 per cent of the total size), the addition of a small, but unrelated, sequence, or the modification of a restriction site[5].

Quantification of mRNA by real-time RT-PCR

Real-time (or kinetic) PCR methodologies relies on the direct recording during every cycles of a fluorescence signal generated by the accumulation of the PCR products. The principle of the quantification using real-time PCR is the determination of the threshold cycle (Ct), also called crossing point (Cp), that corresponds to the number of PCR cycles taken to reach a point in which the fluorescent signal is first recorded as statistically significant above background[7]. This point always occurs during the exponential phase of the amplification and thus is not affected by any reaction component that could become limitant at the plateau phase. The Ct (or Cp) value can be translated into quantitative result by reference to a standard curve amplified under the same conditions. Several suitable instrumentations are now competing on the market (i.e. from Applied Biosystems, Roche Diagnostics, Biorad, Stratagene, etc.). Several methodologies to produce a fluorescent signal that is proportional to the amount of the PCR product are also available. The simplest methods use fluorescent dyes (SYBR Green) that bind specifically to double-stranded DNA. Others rely on the hybridization of fluorescent-labeled probes to the correct amplicon (hybridization probes, hydrolysis or Taqman probes, molecular beacons, etc.). All these methods are described in detail in a recent review[8].

In our research group in the INSERM Unit 449 in Lyon, France, we have set up and validated RT-PCR assays for the quantification of a number of specific mRNAs in human adipose tissue and skeletal muscle. Using this methodology, we have investigated the regulation of gene expression during very low calorie diets in obese subjects[2,9] or the acute effects of insulin infusion in lean, obese and type 2 diabetic subjects[10,11]. More than 60 RT-PCR-based assays are running in our laboratory at the present time. Initially, we mainly developed RT-competitive PCR and found the method extremely reproducible

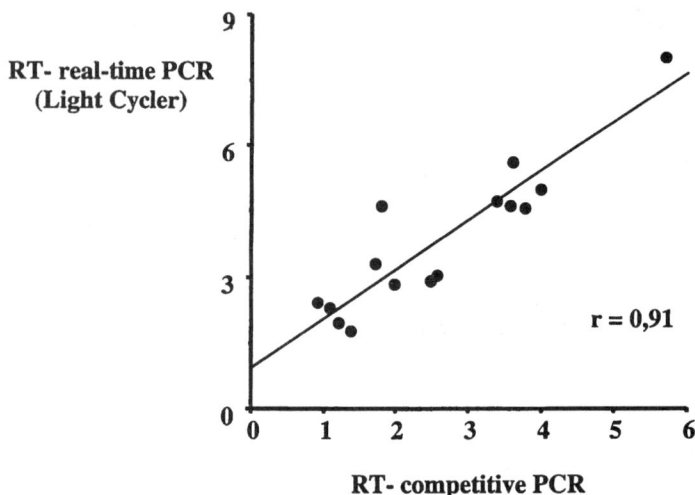

Fig. 1. Comparison of SREBP1c mRNA levels determined by RT- real-time PCR or by RT-competitive PCR.
Quantification of SREBP1c mRNA was performed with both methods in 15 different preparations of total RNA from human subcutaneous adipose tissue. The data are presented in amol/μg of total RNA.

(coefficient of variation lower than 10 per cent), allowing the precise quantification of low abundant transcripts[5]. We recently acquired a Light-Cycler (Roche Diagnostics) and found that real-time PCR give very similar results as competitive PCR. Figure 1 shows the data obtained for the quantification of the transcription factor SREBP1c in human adipose tissue biopsies using both methods. The main advantage of real-time PCR instruments is the fact that analysis does not require post-PCR manipulation, as it is the case for competitive PCR.

Analysis of gene expression and investigation of its regulation can therefore be performed in human fat tissue. The number of research groups using quantitative RT-PCR methodology in the field of obesity and nutrition research has rapidly increased during the last five years, as has the number and quality of publications dealing with the regulation of gene expression in human adipose tissue. Now, new methods to measure transcript abundance such as microarrays and DNA chips allow the parallel analysis of thousands of genes. Little work has yet been done using human adipose tissue, but an explosion of data can be expected in the near future.

References

1. Vidal H. Quantification of lipid-related mRNAs by RT-competitive PCR in human white adipose tissue biopsies. *Methods Mol Biol* 2001; 155: 83–8.

2. Vidal H, Auboeuf D, DeVos P, Staels B, Riou JP, Auwerx J, Laville M. The expression of ob gene is not acutely regulated by insulin and fasting in human abdominal subcutaneous adipose tissue. *J Clin Invest* 1996; 98: 251–5.

3. Ferré F. Quantitative or semi-quantitative PCR: reality versus myth. *PCR Methods Appl* 1992; 2: 1–9.

4. Gilliland G, Perrin S, Blanchard K, Bunn HF. Analysis of cytokine mRNA and DNA: detection and quantitation by competitive polymerase chain reaction. *Proc Natl Acad Sci USA* 1990; 87: 2725–9.

5. Auboeuf D, Vidal H. The use of the reverse transcription-competitive polymerase chain reaction to investigate the *in vivo* regulation of gene expression in small tissue samples. *Anal Biochem* 1997; 245: 141–8.

6. Raeymaekers L. A commentary on the practical applications of competitive PCR. *Genome Res* 1995; 5: 91–4.

7. Gibson UE, Heid CA, Williams PM. A novel method for real time quantitative RT-PCR. *Genome Res* 1996; 6: 995–1001.

8. Bustin SA. Absolute quantification of mRNA using real-time reverse transcription polymerase chain reaction assays. *J Mol Endocrinol* 2000; 25: 169–93.

9. Millet L, Vidal H, Andreelli F, Larrouy D, Riou JP, Ricquier D *et al.* Increased uncoupling protein-2 and -3 mRNA expression during fasting in obese and lean humans. *J Clin Invest* 1997; 100: 2665–70.

10. Rieusset J, Andreelli F, Auboeuf D, Roques M, Vallier P, Riou JP, Auwerx J *et al.* Insulin acutely regulates the expression of the peroxisome proliferator-activated receptor-γ in human adipocytes. *Diabetes* 1999; 48: 699–705.

11. Ducluzeau PH, Perretti N, Laville M, Andreelli F, Vega N, Riou JP *et al.* Regulation by insulin of gene expression in human skeletal muscle and adipose tissue: Evidence for specific defects in type 2 diabetes mellitus. *Diabetes* 2001; 50: 1134–42.

Progress in Obesity Research: 9. Edited by *Geraldo Medeiros-Neto, Alfredo Halpern and Claude Bouchard*
©2003 John Libbey Eurotext Ltd, pp. 75–79.

CHAPTER 15

Fatty acid transport: A physiological perspective

Azeddine Ibrahimi

Université Sidi Mohammed Ben Abdellah, Centre d'Etudes Universitaires de Taza, Taza, Morocco
[e-mail: Azeibrah@yahoo.com]

Introduction

Long-chain fatty acids (FA) are quantitatively the most important substrates for energy in humans and regulate a wide range of important biological processes[1]. On a more general level, FA have been implicated in the pathophysiology of obesity and diabetes, immune responses and atherosclerosis, cystic fibrosis and breast cancer[1]. This emphasizes their large potential role as general metabolic regulators and the importance of understanding the mechanisms mediating and regulating cellular uptake of FA.

The transport of FA across the cell plasma membrane may be viewed as the progression of three separate kinetic events: first, partitioning of unbound FA from the aqueous phase into the outer leaflet of the membrane; second, diffusion, or flip-flop, to the inner leaflet; and third dissociation of the FA from the inner leaflet to the cytoplasm. Studies of the transport of long-chain FA across model membranes indicate that flip-flop is the rate-limiting step[2]. For the uptake of physiologically important FA into giant unilamellar vesicles approaching cell size ($\geq$ 2000 Å) and lipid compositions, flip-flop times were shown to be between 1 and 10 s[2]. Given the unbound FA concentration in the blood and interstitium (5–11 nM), this intrinsic rate of transport may not be sufficient to meet the needs of tissues possessing a high metabolic capacity for FA such as adipose, liver or muscle tissues. Thus cells would need an efficient mechanism for recruiting FA to answer energy needs.

Studies by Abumrad *et al.* of FA permeation of adipocyte membranes[3] documented saturability of FA transfer under conditions where the FA was not metabolized and the sensitivity of the process to protein-modifying agents and to hormones[4]. The transport Km was observed to be in the low nanomolar range (7 nM), consistent with the expectation that the Km for protein-mediated transport should be within the physiological concentrations of unbound FA. FA transport was also shown to be partially inhibited by antibodies raised against FA transporters[5]. This notion led to the identification of three potential FA transport proteins named plasma membrane FA binding protein (FABPPM)[5,6] CD36[7,8] and a family of FA transport proteins (FATPs)[9,10]. We will focus in this review on the role of CD36 in FA transport.

CD36 (fatty acids translocase) as a facilitator of FA uptake

Studies by Harmon and Abumrad identified an 88 kDa membrane protein as a candidate FA carrier by covalent labeling with inhibitors of the FA-transport step[7]. The protein was isolated and then a full coding clone cDNA library was obtained based on its amino-terminal sequence. The clone coded for a protein with 85 per cent homology to human platelet CD36.

A considerable amount of data was obtained *in vitro*, supporting a role for CD36 in FA uptake. CD36 purified from adipose tissue reversibly bound FA with high affinity and specificity[11]. In Ob17PY fibroblasts, stable transfection of CD36 was associated with the appearance of a saturable, high affinity ($K_m \sim 4$ nM), and phloretin-sensitive component[12]. FA uptake increased and the magnitude of the increase generally correlated with the level of protein expression[12,13].

The expression pattern and regulation of CD36 level are consistent with its role in FA uptake. The distribution of CD36 favours tissues with a high metabolic capacity for FA such as adipose tissue, heart, and oxidative skeletal muscle[14,15]. Expression is also high in tissues exposed to large fluxes of FA such as microvascular endothelia, mammary secretory epithelia and enterocytes of the small intestine[16,17]. In muscle tissues, expression occurs with predominance in red oxidative fibres and is up-regulated with chronic muscle stimulation concomitant with an increase in the FA transport Vmax[15,18]. More direct and definitive data were obtained recently based on the availability of several models of altered CD36 expression (Table 1).

Table 1. Animal models with altered expression of CD36

Name	Genetic background	CD36 expression	Ref.
Rats			
SHR	CD36 –/–	No expression	20,21
SHR-ch4	CD36 +/+	Normal expression	20,21
SHR-TG19	CD36 +/+	Total overexpression*	22
Mice			
MCK-CD36	CD36 +/+	Overexpression in heart and muscle	19
CD36-null	CD36 –/–	No expression	23,26,27
GR-CD36	CD36 –/–	Rescued expression in heart and muscle	

*High expression in kidney and heart.

CD36 transgenic mice (MCK-CD36)

We generated transgenic mice with muscle-targeted CD36 over-expression by insertion of a CD36 cDNA under control of the muscle creatine kinase promoter[19]. The metabolic phenotype of these mice is consistent with greater peripheral FA utilization. These mice have less body fat and lower serum FA, triglyceride, and cholesterol. Blood glucose is increased, while insulin levels are higher in the fasted state. Most significantly the soleus muscle from these mice displays enhanced ability for FA oxidation in response to contraction[19].

SHR as a CD36-deficient rat model

In 1999, Aitman et al.[20] suggested, based on genetic linkage and microarray studies that CD36 deficiency underlies defects of FA metabolism and insulin responsiveness in the spontaneously hypertensive rat (SHR), a well studied model of human syndrome X. Aitman et al.[20] documented the complete absence of CD36 expression in the SHR. In later detailed studies Hajri et al.[21] demonstrated the loss of CD36 function in FA uptake in the SHR and its recovery in an SHR congenic strain, generated by Pravenec, Kurtz and colleagues[22] where a region of chromosome 4 containing the deletion variant of CD36 was replaced with the corresponding wild-type segment from the normotensive Brown Norway rat. FA uptake is significantly impaired in SHR heart, oxidative muscle, and adipose tissue while that of the glucose analog fluoro-2-deoxyglucose (FDG) is greatly increased[21]. These data confirmed that defective FA uptake is a primary factor behind some of the metabolic defects in the SHR. Transgenic expression of CD36 in SHR (SHR-TG19 rats) ameliorated insulin resistance and lowered serum fatty acids[22].

CD36 knockout models

CD36-null mice were generated by Febbraio et al.[23] and were shown to exhibit an increase in fasting serum FA, triglyceride, and cholesterol. Blood glucose and insulin levels were significantly decreased in the fasted state. Recently, a third mouse model was generated, which re-expresses CD36 in heart and skeletal muscle on the CD36-null background (Ibrahimi et al., unpublished observations). These mice, generated using the mouse muscle creatine kinase promoter, show rescue of the main abnormalities mentioned above.

Role of CD36 expression in adipocyte differentiation and obesity

In vitro studies with Ob1771 preadipocytes cells showed that CD36 mRNA is a marker of adipose differentiation[8]. CD36 mRNA and protein were induced by preadipocyte differentiation into adipocytes and induction is paralleled by an increase in the uptake of FA. The mRNA is also strongly induced by long-chain fatty acids in preadipocytes, similar to the mRNA of other genes coding for proteins involved in FA metabolism like acyl CoA synthetase and glycerolphosphate dehydrogenase[24].

In vivo, CD36-null mice have less body fat and their adipocytes lack the high affinity component of FA transport observed in wild type adipocytes expressing CD36[23]. Plasma from CD36-null mice showed low levels of leptin (Abumrad, personal communication). The decrease in leptin may be in part related to the fact that adipose tissue mass is lower in the CD36-null mice when compared to wild type mice. Another interesting finding is that food intake of the CD36-null mice is also significantly lower than that of wild type mice despite the lower leptin, suggesting that there may be increased sensitivity to leptin (Abumrad, personal communication). A recent report by Steinberg *et al.*[26] documented that chronic leptin treatment reduced CD36 mRNA. CD36 protein and FA uptake of muscle plasma membrane fractions were also reduced suggesting chronic regulation of CD36 level and FA uptake by leptin treatment. More studies are needed to investigate if leptin effects on body weight and on FA oxidation are modulated by expression levels of CD36 in muscle or adipose tissues.

Role of CD36 in muscle physiology and contractile activity

Muscle, especially that rich in red oxidative fibres has a high dependence on energy from FA oxidation. Coburn *et al.*[26] demonstrated that CD36-null mice have a greater than a 60 per cent reduction in FA uptake by heart and red muscle. As a result, CD36-null mice have a decreased ability to perform strenuous exercise (Ibrahimi *et al.*, unpublished data). In contrast, mice with CD36 overexpression perform better than wild type mice, which may reflect their enhanced ability for FA oxidation in response to contraction[19]. Bonen *et al.*[15,18] documented some of the molecular mechanisms involved in regulation of FA utilization by muscular activity. The acute regulation of FA uptake by muscle activity involves the translocation of CD36 from intracellular stores to the sarcolemma, analogous to the regulation of glucose uptake by membrane recruitment of GLUT-4[18].

Role of CD36 in insulin resistance and diabetes

More evidence for a role of CD36 in insulin responsiveness were obtained from studies with mice models[19,23,27]. These studies indicate that CD36 expression level strongly impacts muscle glucose utilization and insulin sensitivity. For example, transgenic mice overexpressing CD36 (6–8 months) show increases in plasma glucose and insulin levels[19]. On the other hand, CD36-null mice were hypoglycaemic[23], hypoinsulinaemic and more insulin sensitive than the wild type but they showed reduced tolerance to fructose induced insulin resistance[27]. Further studies should help document the role of FA utilization in insulin resistance and allow a better understanding of the molecular mechanisms involved.

Heart function

Under normal physiological conditions, optimal cardiac work is dependent on FA oxidation so as the heart must often respond to changes in the workload, FA metabolism must be regulated in such a manner as to allow a quick adaptation[28]. Studies with free fatty acid analogue 15-(*p*-iodophenyl)-3-(*R*,*S*)-methyl pentadecanoic acid (BMIPP) showed a defect in FA utilization and myocardial hypertrophy in CD36-null mice. They exhibited between 60–80 per cent reductions in BMIPP[27] uptake by heart tissue, which was similar in magnitude to that observed in CD36-deficient humans[29,30]. The effect of CD36 deficiency on FA transport in CD36-null mice and the SHR appears to lead to heart hypertrophy.

CD36 deficiency and myocardial hypertrophy in humans

The role of CD36 deficiency in the pathogenesis of cardiomyopathies in humans was investigated vigorously once evidence generated *in vitro* and later in laboratory animals documented the role of CD36 in FA utilization. Most of the studies were conducted in Japan where BMIPP is available commercially and used for clinical evaluation of cardiac FA metabolism by noninvasive imaging techniques. Patients with CD36 deficiency show reduced FA uptake in the heart[29], as visualized by scintigraphy using iodinated BMIPP. The deficiency may underlie some cases of cardiac hypertrophy[29,30] and incidence of CD36 deficiency in patients with heart diseases exceeds that in the general population[29]. These studies in humans document a strong association between CD36 deficiency, defective myocardial FA uptake and some forms of heart hypertrophy.

Conclusion

The identification of CD36 as a FA transporter has significantly contributed to the understanding of the regulation of FA uptake and utilization. A better knowledge of the metabolic role of CD36, and its physiological regulation by hormonal or nutritional factors, should contribute to the evaluation of the role played by lipid metabolism in the pathophysiological conditions such as obesity, insulin resistance and heart hypertrophy.

References

1. Abumrad NA, Harmon CM, Ibrahimi a. Membrane transport of long-chain fatty acids: evidence for a facilitated process. *J Lipid Res* 1998; 39: 2309–18.

2. Kleinfeld AM. Lipid phase fatty acid flip-flop, is it fast enough for cellular transport? *J Membr Biol* 2000; 175: 79–86.

3. Abumrad NA, Park JH, Park CR. Permeation of long-chain fatty acid into adipocytes. Kinetics, specificity, and evidence for involvement of a membrane protein. *J Biol Chem* 1984; 259: 8945–53.

4. Abumrad NA, Harmon CM, Barnela US *et al.* Insulin antagonism of catecholamine stimulation of fatty acid transport in the adipocyte. Studies on its mechanism of action. *J Biol Chem* 1988; 263: 14678–83.

5. Zhou SL, Stump D, Sorrentino D *et al.* Adipocyte differentiation of 3T3-L1 cells involves augmented expression of a 43-kDa plasma membrane fatty acid-binding protein. *J Biol Chem* 1992; 267: 14456–61.

6. Stremmel W, Lotz G, Strohmeyer G *et al.* Identification, isolation, and partial characterization of a fatty acid binding protein from rat jejunal microvillous membranes. *J Clin Invest* 1985; 75: 1068–76.

7. Harmon CM, Abumrad NA. Binding of sulphosuccinimidyl fatty acids to adipocyte membrane proteins: isolation and amino-terminal sequence of an 88-kD protein implicated in transport of long-chain fatty acids. *J Memb Biol* 1993; 133: 43–9.

8. Abumrad NA, el-Maghrabi MR, Amri EZ *et al.* Cloning of a rat adipocyte membrane protein implicated in binding or transport of long-chain fatty acids that is induced during preadipocyte differentiation. *J Biol Chem* 1993; 268: 17665–8.

9. Schaffer JE, Lodish HF. Expression cloning and characterization of a novel adipocyte long chain fatty acid transport protein. *Cell* 1994; 79: 427–36.

10. Hirsch D, Stahl A, Lodish HF. A family of fatty acid transporters conserved from mycobacterium to man. *Proc Natl Acad Sci USA* 1998; 95: 8625–9.

11. Baillie A, Coburn C, Abumrad N. Reversible binding of long-chain fatty acids to purified FAT, the adipose CD36 homolog. *J Memb Biol* 1996; 153.

12. Ibrahimi A, Sfeir Z, Magharaie H *et al.* Expression of the CD36 homolog in fibroblast cells: effects on fatty acid transport. *Proc Natl Acad Sci USA* 1996; 93: 2646–51.

13. Sfeir Z, Ibrahimi A, Amri E *et al.* CD36 antisense expression in 3T3-F442A preadipocytes. *Mol Cell Biochem* 1999; 192: 3–8.

14. Van Nieuwenhoven FA, Verstijnen CP, Abumrad NA *et al.* Putative membrane fatty acid translocase and cytoplasmic fatty acid-binding protein are co-expressed in rat heart and skeletal muscles. *Biochem Biophys Res Comm* 1995; 207: 747–52.

15. Bonen A, Dyck DJ, Ibrahimi A *et al.* Muscle contractile activity increases fatty acid metabolism and transport and FAT/CD36. *Am J Physiol* 1999; 276: E642–E649.

16. Greenwalt DE, Lipsky RH, Ockenhouse CF *et al.* Membrane glycoprotein CD36: a review of its roles in adherence, signal transduction, and transfusion medicine. *Blood* 1992; 80: 1105–15.

17. Poirier H, Degrace P, Niot I *et al.* Localization and regulation of the putative membrane fatty-acid transporter (FAT) in the small intestine. Comparison with fatty acid-binding proteins (FABP). *Eur J Biochem* 1996; 238: 368–73.

18. Bonen A, Luiken JJ, Arumugam Y *et al.* Acute regulation of fatty acid uptake involves the cellular redistribution of fatty acid translocase. *J Biol Chem* 2000; 275: 14501–8.

19. Ibrahimi A, Bonen A, Blinn WD *et al.* Muscle-specific overexpression of FAT/CD36 enhances fatty acid oxidation by contracting muscle, reduces plasma triglycerides and fatty acids, and increases plasma glucose and insulin. *J Biol Chem* 1999; 274: 26761–6.

20. Aitman TJ, Glazier AM, Wallace CA *et al.* Identification of Cd36 (Fat) as an insulin-resistance gene causing defective fatty acid and glucose metabolism in hypertensive rat. *Nature Genet* 1999; 21: 76–83.

21. Hajri T, Ibrahimi A, Coburn CT *et al.* Defective fatty acid uptake in the spontaneously hypertensive rat is a primary determinant of altered glucose metabolism, hyperinsulinemia, and myocardial hypertrophy. *J Biol Chem* 2001; 276: 23661–6.

22. Pravenec M, Landa V, Zidek V *et al.* Transgenic rescue of defective Cd36 ameliorates insulin resistance in spontaneously hypertensive rats. *Nature Genet* 2001; 27: 156–8.

23. Febbraio M, Abumrad NA, Hajjar DP *et al.* A null mutation in murine CD36 reveals an important role in fatty acid and lipoprotein metabolism. *J Biol Chem* 1999; 274: 19055–62.

24. Sfeir Z, Ibrahimi A, Amri E *et al.* Regulation of FAT/CD36 gene expression: further evidence in support of a role of the protein in fatty acid binding/transport. *Prostaglandins Leukot Essent Fatty Acids* 1997; 57: 17–21.

25. Steinberg GR, Dyck DJ, Calles-Escandon J *et al.* Chronic leptin administration decreases fatty acid uptake and fatty acid transporters in rat skeletal muscle. *J Biol Chem* 2002; 277: 8854–60.

26. Coburn CT, Knapp FF, Jr., Febbraio M *et al.* Defective uptake and utilization of long chain fatty acids in muscle and adipose tissues of CD36 knockout mice. *J Biol Chem* 2000; 275: 32523–9.

27. Hajri T, Han XX, Bonen A *et al.* Defective fatty acid uptake modulates insulin responsiveness and metabolic responses to diet in CD36-null mice. *J Clin Invest* 2002; 109: 1381–9.

28. Lopaschuk GD, Belke DD, Gamble J *et al.* Regulation of fatty acid oxidation in the mammalian heart in health and disease. *Biochim Biophys Acta* 1994; 1213: 263–76.

29. Hwang EH, Taki J, Yasue S *et al.* Absent myocardial iodine-123-BMIPP uptake and platelet/monocyte CD36 deficiency. *Nucl Med* 1998; 39: 1681–4.

30. Tanaka T, Nakata T, Oka T *et al.* Defect in human myocardial long-chain fatty acid uptake is caused by FAT/CD36 mutations. *J Lipid Res* 2001; 42: 751–9.

Progress in Obesity Research: 9. Edited by *Geraldo Medeiros-Neto, Alfredo Halpern and Claude Bouchard*
©2003 John Libbey Eurotext Ltd, pp. 80–82.

CHAPTER 16

Importance of adipocytokines in obesity-related diseases

Yuji Matsuzawa, Iichiro Shimomura, Shinji Kihara and Tohru Funahashi

Department of Internal Medicine and Molecular Science, Graduate School of Medicine, Osaka University, Osaka, Japan
[e-mail: matsuzawa-yuji@sumitomo-hp.or.jp]

The concept of adipocytokines and atherosclerosis

Adipose tissue has been long considered to be an organ only for storing excess energy as triglyceride, which itself is a very essential self-defence system for survival during starvation. In most of countries including many developing countries, people do not have to worry about lack of food as long as they are living without instability of a political situation and rather may easily gain excess adipose tissue by the tendency of overeating and physical inactivity, and recently obesity-related diseases have become the biggest problem all over the world. In order to elucidate the molecular mechanism of obesity-related diseases, we have investigated biological characteristic of adipose tissue analysing gene expression profile in visceral and subcutaneous fat. We initiated a systemic analysis of active genes by constructing a 3'-directed cDNA library, in which the mRNA population is faithfully reflected. Out of approximately 1000 independent clones, 60 per cent of the whole genes are already identified as 'known' human genes by searching in the non-EST division of the GenBank. The remaining 40 per cent of genes are novel and unidentified genes. We found unexpectedly high frequency of the genes encoding secretory proteins in adipose tissue most of which are important bioactive substances. The genes for plasmanogen activator inhibitor type 1 (PAI-1) and heparin binding EGF-like growth factor (HBEGF) are found to be highly expressed in adipose tissue. Especially, PAI-1 mRNA levels increased up to 10 times in visceral adipose tissue during development of obesity in ventromedial hypothalamic lesioned rats, while it remained unchanged in the subcutaneous adipose tissue. We also demonstrated that plasma levels of PAI-1 were significantly correlated with visceral adiposity determined by CT scan in human subjects. These data suggest that the secreted PAI-1 from accumulated visceral fat may contribute to the determination of plasma PAI-1 levels and, thus, may have an important role in the development of thrombotic disorders and atherosclerosis frequently found in obesity, especially visceral obesity[2].

The discovery of adiponectin and its clinical significance

As was mentioned above, 40 per cent of expressed genes in adipose tissue were unknown, in other words novel genes. The gene which expressed most abundantly and specifically in adipose tissue was also a novel gene. The molecule encoded by this gene, adipose most abundant gene transcript (apM-1) possesses a signal peptide, collagen-Re motif and globular domain and has the significant homology with collagen X, VIII and complement factor C1q[1]. We termed this matrix-like protein as adiponectin. We established the method for the determination of plasma adiponectin levels using enzyme-linked immunosorbent assay. Plasma levels of adiponectin in humans are substantially high, up to 5–10 pg/ml on average. Interestingly, plasma levels are negatively correlated with body mass index (BMI)[3], while leptin, another adipose tissue-specific secretory protein is known to increase with BMI. The negative correlation is stronger between adiponectin levels and visceral adiposity than between that and subcutaneous adiposity. Diabetic patients have lower adiponectin levels than control subjects. Diabetic patients with macroangiopathy have further lower levels of adiponectin[4]. The low level of adiponectin was also observed in diabetic subjects of Pima Indian.

From the observation in Pima Indian in collaboration with NIH group and in obese monkeys in collaboration with Barbara Hansen, we demonstrated that plasma levels of adiponectin are strongly correlated with insulin sensitivity[5,6,10]. These results suggest that the more important significance of adiponectin is that this protein shows lower levels in ischaemic heart disease[8]. Kaplan-Myer analysis in the subjects with renal insufficiency demonstrated that the subjects with hypoadiponectinaemia died of cardiac events more frequently during 4 years observation[7,9,11,12]. These data shows that hypoadiponectinaemia may be a novel and important risk factor of atherosclerotic diseases.

Cell biological functions of adiponectin

High concentration of adiponectin flows with blood stream inside of vascular walls. It is interesting to know whether adiponectin can enter into vascular walls. Immunohistochemical examination using antiadiponectin antibody demonstrated that there is no existence of adiponectin in the untreated normal vascular walls in rabbit. However markedly positive immunohistochemical stain was detected in the balloon-injured vascular walls. As adiponectin has been shown to have an ability to bind subendothelial collagen such as collagen V, VIII and X, endothelial injury may induce the entering of adiponectin into subendothelial space by binding to these collagens[13].

Atherosclerotic cellular changes consist of basically three cellular phenomena such as monocyte adhesion to endothelial cells by the expression of adhesion molecules, oxidized LDL uptake of macrophages through scavenger receptors and proliferation of migrated smooth muscle cells by the action of platelet-derived growth factors, PDGF or heparin binding EGF-like growth factor, HBEGF. Adiponectin has potentially inhibitory activities of these atherogenic cellular phenomena[13]. Physiological concentration of adiponectin was demonstrated to strongly inhibit the expression of adhesion molecules including ICAM-1, VCAM-1 and E-selectin. Adiponectin was shown to inhibit the TNF-α induced NF-k B activation through the inhibition of I-k B phospholyration, which might be a major molecular mechanism for the inhibition of monocyte adhesion to endothelial cells. Adiponectin also inhibits the expression of the scavenger receptor type A-1 of macrophages resulting markedly decreased uptake of oxidized LDL and inhibition of foam cell formation. In addition, adiponectin inhibits the proliferation and migration of smooth muscle cells. This inhibition was shown to be attributed to the binding competition to PDGF-BB receptor of adiponectin and the inhibition of signal transduction through EKP. From these vascular cellular functions, adiponectin may have a potential anti-atherogenicity. In human, many offensive factors are present including oxidized LDL, inflammatory stimuli and chemical substances which may induce vascular injuries. At that time, adiponectin secreted from adipose tissues may turn out to put off the fire of the vascular walls like firemen.

Genetic hypoadiponectinaemia and atherosclerosis

In order to know whether primary hypoadiponectinaemia causes metabolic disturbances including insulin resistance and atherosclerotic vascular changes we investigated the clinical profiles of the subjects with gene mutation of adiponectin which has been recently found. In the present we have found four types of misssence mutation in which I164 T mutation is the most frequent and accompanied with marked hypoadiponectinaemia. So far we found nine subjects with 1164T mutation and 8/9 are accompanied with hypertension or hyperlipidaemia and 9/9 are accompanied with impaired glucose metabolism including with IGT or DM. In addition, 6/9 already suffered of coronary artery disease[14]. These results suggest that genetic hypoadiponectinaemia may cause metabolic syndrome with a variety of metabolic and cardiovascular diseases.

In order to confirm this concept, we established the knockout mouse of adiponectin gene. The KO mice showed no specific phenotype, no high fat/high sucrose diet is loaded. However, high fat/high sucrose diet induced marked elevation of plasma glucose as well as plasma insulin levels in the KO mice. The KO mice also showed marked insulin resistance estimated by insulin tolerance test during high fat/high sucrose diet. The supplementation of adiponectin by adenovirus transfection clearly improved this insulin resistance. Increase of intimal smooth muscle cell proliferation also observed in the injured aorta in the KO mice which was rescued by the supplementation of adiponectin in adevirus tranfected KO mice[15,16].

These results together demonstrate that genetic hypoadiponectinaemia can be an important background for both insulin resistance and atherosclerotic vascular disease which may be corresponding so-called metabolic syndrome.

Conclusion

Obesity, especially visceral obesity causes the abnormalities of adipocyrokine secretion. The increase of TNF-α and PAI-1 secretion and the decreae of adiponectin secretion are typical cases which induce insulin resistance and more importantly may induce vascular changes directly. In the our recent studies on the genetic mutation of adiponectin gene in human sabjects and the KO mice clearly demonstrated that adiponectin may play a key role for metabolic syndrome.

References

1. Maeda K, Okubo K, Shimomura I, Funahashi T, Matsuzawa Y, Matsubara K. cDNA cloning and expression of a novel adipose specific collagen-like factor, apM1. *Biochem Biophys Res Comm* 1996; 221: 286–9.

2. Shimomura I, Funahashi T, Takahashi M, Maeda K, Kotani K, Nakamura T *et al.* Enhanced expression of PAI-1 in visceral fat: possible contributor to vascular disease in obesity. *Nature Med* 1996; 2: 800–3.

3. Arita Y, Kihara S, Ouchi N, Takahashi M, Maeda K, Miyagawa J *et al.* Paradoxical decrease of an adipose-specific protein, adiponectin, in obesity. *Biochem Biophys Res Commun* 1999; 257: 79–83.

4. Hotta K, Funahashi T, Arita Y, Takahashi M, Matsuda M, Okamoto Y *et al.* Plasma concentrations of a novel adipose-specific protein, adiponectin, in type 2 diabetic patients. *Arterioscler Thromb Vasc Biol* 2000; 20: 1595–9.

5. Hotta K, Funahashi T, Bodkin NL, Ortmeyer HK, Arita Y, Hansen BC, Matsuzawa Y. Circulating concentrations of the adipocyte protein adiponectin are decreased in parallel with reduced insulin sensitivity during the progression to type 2 diabetes in rhesus monkeys. *Diabetes* 2001; 50: 1126–33.

6. Lindsay RS, Funahashi T, Hanson RL, Matsuzawa Y, Tanaka S, Tataranni PA *et al.* Adiponectin and development of type 2 diabetes in the Pima Indian population. *Lancet* 2002; 360: 57–8.

7. Ouchi N, Kihara S, Arita Y, Maeda K, Kuriyama H, Okamoto Y *et al.* Novel modulator for endothelial adhesion molecules: adipocyte-derived plasma protein, adiponectin. *Circulation* 1999; 100: 2473–6.

8. Zoccali C, Mallamaci F, Tripepi G, Benedetto FA, Cutrupi S, Parlongo S Adiponectin, metabolic risk factors, and cardiovascular events among patients with end-stage renal disease. *J Am Soc Nephrol* 2002; 13: 134–41.

9. Ouchi N, Kihara S, Arita Y, Okamoto Y, Maeda K, Kuriyama *et al.* Adiponectin, an adipocyte-derived plasma protein, inhibits endothelial NF-kB signaling through a cAMP-dependent pathway. *Circulation* 2000; 102: 1296–301.

10. Stefan N, Vozarova B, Funahashi T, Matsuzawa Y, Weyer C, Lindsay RS. Plasma adiponectin concentration is associated with skeletal muscle insulin receptor tyrosine phosphorylation, and low plasma concentration precedes a decrease in whole-body insulin sensitivity in humans. *Diabetes* 2002; 51: 1884–8.

11. Ouchi N, Kihara S, Arita Y, Nishida M, Matsuyama A, Okamoto *et al.* Y Adipocyte-derived plasma protein, adiponectin, suppresses lipid accumulation and class A scavenger receptor expression in human monocyte-derived macrophages. *Circulation* 2001; 103: 1057–63.

12. Arita Y, Kihara S, Ouchi N, Maeda K, Kuriyama H, Okamoto Y *et al.* Adipocyte-derived plasma protein adiponectin acts as a platelet-derived growth factor-BB-binding protein and regulates growth factor-induced common postreceptor signal in vascular smooth muscle cell. *Circulation* 2002; 105: 2893–8.

13. Okamoto Y, Arita Y, Nishida M, Muraguchi M, Ouchi N, Takahashi M *et al.* An adipocyte-derived plasma protein, adiponectin, adheres to injured vascular walls. *Horm Metab Res* 2000; 32: 47–50.

14. Kondo H, Shimomura I, Matsukawa Y, Kumada M, Takahashi M, Matsuda M *et al.* Association of adiponectin mutation with type 2 diabetes: a candidate gene for the insulin resistance syndrome. *Diabetes* 2002; 51: 2325–8.

15. Maeda N, Shimomura I, Kishida K, Nishizawa H, Matsuda M, Nagaratani H *et al.* Diet-induced insulin resistance in mice lacking adiponectin / ACRP30. *Nature Med* 2002; 8: 731–7.

16. Matsuda M, Shimomura I, Sata M, Arita Y, Nishida M, Maeda N *et al.* Role of adiponectin in preventing vascular stenosis – the missing link of adipo-vascular axis. *J Biol Chem* 2002; 277: 37487–91.

Progress in Obesity Research: 9. Edited by *Geraldo Medeiros-Neto, Alfredo Halpern and Claude Bouchard*
©2003 John Libbey Eurotext Ltd, pp. 83–86.

CHAPTER 17

Paracrine and secretory functions of preadipose and adipose cells

Gérard Ailhaud

Centre de Biochimie (UMR6543CNRS), UNSA, Faculté des Sciences, Parc Valrose, 06108 Nice cedex 2, France
[e-mail: ailhaud@unice.fr]

Introduction

The lack of adipose tissue in lipoatrophic patients and fat-free mice is correlated with various disorders which include hepatic steatosis, dyslipidaemia, insulin-resistance and type 2 diabetes (NIDDM)[1]. The formation of adipose tissue is required to ensure physiological functions, i.e. glucose homeostasis, energy storage and reproductive functions. Unfortunately, excess of fat mass is also associated with most of the same metabolic disorders observed in lipoatrophy. The secretory properties of both adipocytes and precursor cells play an important role in these physiological and physipathological processes, underlying a cross-talk between adipose tissue and other organs as well as within the tissue itself.

Secreted factors from preadipocytes and adipogenesis

Extracellular factors secreted from preadipocytes and intracellular signaling pathways involved in early events of adipogenesis have been depicted over the last decade. Such studies have been made easier *in vitro* with the use of serum-free medium to culture adipose precursor cells and *in vivo* with the use of microdialysis technique. Preadipocytes are able to synthesize prostaglandin E_2, prostaglandin I_2 (prostacyclin) and trace levels of prostaglandin $F_{2\alpha}$ from arachidonic acid[2]. Antibodies added externally and directed against prostacyclin decrease by approximately 40 per cent but do not abolish the adipogenic effect of arachidonic acid whereas the two other prostaglandins do not show any adipogenic activity[3]. Thus prostacyclin is able after secretion to act as an autocrine/paracrine effector of adipogenesis. This adipogenic effect is also observed with adipose precursor cells from rat and human[4]. Prostacyclin and its stable analogue carbacyclin are able in clonal mouse preadipocytes to induce a rise in cAMP levels and an intracellular mobilization of calcium[4,5]. The critical role of prostacyclin as a locally-produced hormone raising cAMP and Ca^{2+} levels cannot be dissociated from the developmental stage of cells at which the effectors trigger transducing pathways. First, cAMP promotes the initiation of differentiation of 3T3-F442A preadipocytes but inhibits the late stage(s) of this process[6]. Second, the Ca^{2+}-calmodulin-sensitive protein kinase II, which is required for the differentiation of 3T3-L1 preadipocytes, exhibits at an early stage within a few hours two temporally distinct phases of activity after stimulation of adipogenesis[7,8]. It is likely that the time frame of exposure of clonal preadiopcytes to various effectors, i.e. the developmental stage at which the cells respond, explains the inhibitory or stimulatory effect previously reported.

Several additional observations demonstrate that prostacyclin is a potent adipogenic hormone: (1) it is active whithin a critical time-window during preadipocyte differentiation, consistent with the decrease in the expression of the cell surface IP receptor[4,9]; (2) through activation of its cell surface receptor, prostacyclin triggers the protein kinase A pathway and up-regulates the expression of the early transcription factors, C/EBPβ and C/EBPδ[10,11] which, in turn, up-regulate the expression of PPARγ2 critically required to terminate adipocyte differentiation[12-17]; (3) *in vivo*, after exposure of epididymal fat pad of rats by microdialysis to carbacyclin, there is an appearance within a few hours of lipid-containing cells expressing glycerol-3-phosphate dehydrogenase activity that demonstrates adipocyte formation[18]; (4)

carbacyclin is also a ligand of PPARδ[19], consistent with the activation of the genes encoding for the fatty acid translocase (FAT) and the adipocyte lipid-binding protein (ALBP) in PPARδ-overexpressing fibroblasts. Of note, PGD_2 and 15d-PGJ_2 are inactive[20].

Quite recently, the role of arachidonic acid in promoting mouse adipose tissue development early in life has been demonstrated. Prostacyclin through binding to the cell surface prostacyclin receptor IP-R and the activation of the cAMP-dependent pathway appears as a key player in mediating fat mass enlargement in response to polyunsaturated fatty acids of the n-6 series present in the diet during the pregnancy-suckling period (Massiéra *et al.*, unpublished data).

In addition to prostacyclin, preadipocytes secrete bioctive leukaemia inhibitory factor (LIF), and an antagonist of LIF receptor inhibits adipogenesis by approximately 60 per cent. Of interest, although this receptor remains expressed with differentiation, LIF production ceases in adipocytes. The capacity of lif-r$^{-/-}$ mouse embryonic stem cells to undergo adipogenesis is dramatically reduced. LIF addition stimulates adipocyte differentiation of preadipocytes and that of PPARγ agonist-treated mouse embryonic fibroblasts. As for the prostacyclin/IP-R system, expression of the early adipogenic transcription factors C/EPBβ and C/EBPδ is rapidly stimulated following exposure of preadipose cells to LIF. Selective inhibitors of mitogen-activated protein kinase kinase inhibit LIF-induced C/EBP gene expression and prevent adipocyte differentiation induced by LIF[21]. Studies of the mechanisms by which LIF and prostacyclin-induced signals are propagated to the nucleus have shown that both pathways share cAMP responsive element binding protein/activation transcription factor 1 (CREB/ATF-1) as common downstream effectors[11]. Invalidation of the *lif-r* gene is lethal, precluding any study of adipose tissue development. Not surprisingly, LIF-null mice are fully viable as LIF-R can be activated by other members of the interleukin-6 family. Taken together, it is clear that extensive redundancy is taking place to ensure differentiation of preadipocytes to adipocytes, in accordance with the need of adipose tissue formation. It is clear also that additional autocrine/paracrine effectors are secreted from preadipocytes, as shown recently for fibroblast growth factor 10 acting through its cognate cell surface receptor as the expession of C/EBPβ and development of white adipose tissue are markedly reduced in *fgf*10$^{-/-}$ mice[22].

Secreted factors from adipocytes and relationships with fat mass enlargement and metabolic disorders

Although leptin is a key factor secreted from adipocytes, a range of other protein factors are secreted. For the sake of clarity, a number of factors which regulate the expression of lipid and lipoprotein metabolism (lipoprotein lipase, cholesterol ester transfer protein, apolipoprotein E, acylation stimulating protein) can be distinguished from a number of secreted proteins that influence locally insulin resistance (tumour necrosis factor-α and interleukin-6) or influence systemically hemostasis (plasminogen-activator inhibitor factor-1) and possibly blood pressure (angiotensinogen, AGT). White adipose tissue (WAT) is a major extra-hepatic source of AGT due to adipocytes and WAT contains the components of the renin-angiotensin system which gives rise to angiotensin II (AngII) from AGT[23] whereas only glucocorticoids up-regulate AGT expression in adipocytes.

Hypertension is known as a frequent complication of obesity and although the mechanisms by which fat excess leads to hypertension have remained largely unknown, some reports suggest that increased adipose AGT production could contribute to the elevation of blood pressure in obese patients[25–27]. In order to gain insights into the relationships existing between adipose AGT, fat mass and blood pressure, we have recently generated transgenic mice which either over-express adipose AGT or in which AGT expression is restricted to adipose tissue. For that purpose the fat specific promoter of ALBP has been used to drive the targeted expression of rat agt cDNA in normotensive wild-type mice and in hypotensive AGT-null mice, respectively. Reexpression of AGT is confined to adipose tissue. AGT is secreted into the blood stream and leads to the restoration of normal blood pressure. In addition the fat mass, which was lowered in AGT null mice, is restored upon reexpression. Importantly, overexpression of AGT in adipose tissue leads to a series of consequences (i) adipocyte hypertrophy, (ii) fat mass enlargement, (iii) enhanced AGT levels from secretory fat tissue explants and enhanced AGT levels in blood, and (iv) increased blood pressure[28].

Quite recently has been developed another transgenic model in which 11-β-hydroxysteroid-dehydrogenase-type1 is overexpressed in adipose tissue[29]. Transgenic mice develop abdominal obesity and the main features of the metabolic syndrome. In particular, mesenteric AGT mRNA is increased, likely due to an increase in the activity of the glucocorticoid receptor subsequent to increased corticosterone levels *in situ*. Blood pressure measurements indicate that the animals are hypertensive. Taken together, these observations implicate adipose AGT in the regulation of blood pressure. In humans, when compared to lean subjects with body mass index (BMI) ~22, plasma AGT levels and blood pressure of obese patients with BMI ~33 are increased respectively by 15 per cent and 16 per cent[30], i.e. under conditions where adiposity is approximately doubled. These observations are entirely consistent with our findings in AGT overexpressing-mice compared with wild-type mice. Moreover AGT mRNA has been recently reported to be enhanced in adipose tissue of obese patients, likely due to adipocyte hypertrophy[30]. Therefore it is assumed that the contribution of adipose tissue to plasma AGT levels may become significant and lead to hypertension in many of the obese patients.

References

1. Moitra J, Mason MM, Olive M, Krylov D, Gavrilova O, Marcus-Samuel B *et al.* Life without white fat: a transgenic mouse. *Genes & Dev* 1998; 12: 3168–81.

2. Négrel R, Ailhaud G. Metabolism of arachidonic acid and prostaglandin synthesis in Ob17 preadipocyte cell line. *Biochem Biophys Res Commun* 1981; 98: 768–77.

3. Catalioto RM, Gaillard D, Maclouf J, Ailhaud G, Négrel R. Autocrine control of adipose cell differentiation by prostacyclin and PGF$_{2\alpha}$. *Biochim Biophys Acta* 1991; 1091: 364–9.

4. Vassaux G, Gaillard D, Ailhaud G, Négrel R. Prostacyclin is a specific effector of adipose cell differentiation: its dual role as a cAMP- and Ca^{2+}-elevating agent. *J Biol Chem* 1992; 267: 11092–7.

5. Vassaux G, Farahi Far D, Gaillard D, Ailhaud G, Négrel R. Inhibition of prostacyclin-induced calcium mobilization by phorbol esters in Ob1771 preadipocytes. *Prostaglandins* 1993; 46: 441–51.

6. Yarwood SJ, Kilgour E, Anderson NG. Cyclic AMP potentiates growth hormone-dependent differentiation of 3T3-F442A preadipocytes: possible involvement of the transcription factor CREB. *Mol Cell Endocrinol* 1998; 138: 41–50.

7. Wang HY, Goligorsky MS, Malbon CC. Temporal activation of Ca^{2+}-calmodium-sensitive protein kinase type II is obligate for adipogenesis. *J Biol Chem* 1997; 272: 1817–21.

8. Ntambi JM, Takova T. Role of Ca^{2+} in the early stages of murine adipocyte differentiation as evidenced by calcium mobilizing agents. *Differentiation* 1996; 60: 151–8.

9. Börglum JD, Pedersen SB, Ailhaud G, Négrel R, Richelsen B. Differential expression of prostaglandin receptor mRNAs during adipose cell differentiation. *Prostaglandins Other Lipid Mediat* 1999; 57: 305–17.

10. Aubert J, Saint-Marc P, Belmonte N, Dani C, Négrel R, Ailhaud G. Prostacyclin IP receptor up-regulates the early expression of C/EBPβ and C/EBPδ in preadipose cells. *Mol Cell Endocrinol* 2000; 160: 149–56.

11. Belmonte N, Phillips B, Massiéra F, Villageois P, Nichols J, Aubert J *et al.* Activation of extracellular signal-regulated kinases and CREB/ATF-1 mediate the expression of of C/EBPβ and C/EBPδ in preadipocytes. *Mol Endocrinol* 2001; 15: 2037–49.

12. Wu Z, Xie Y, Bucher NL, Farmer SR. Conditional ectopic expression of C/EBPβ in NIH-3T3 cells induces PPARγ and stimulates adipogenesis. *Genes Dev* 1995; 9: 2350–63.

13. Barak Y, Nelson MC, Ong ES, Jones YZ, Ruiz-Lozano P, Chien KR *et al.* PPARγ is required for placental, cardiac, and adipose tissue development. *Molecular Cell* 1999; 4: 585–95.

14. Kubota N, Terauchi Y, Mili H, Tamemoto H, Yamuachi T, Komeda K *et al.* PPARã mediates high-fat diet-induced adipocyte hypertrophy and insulin resistance. *Molecular Cell* 1999; 4: 597–609.

15. Rosen ED, Sarraf P, Troy AE, Bradwin G, Moore K, Milstone DS *et al.* PPARã is required for the differentiation of adipose tissue *in vivo* and *in vitro*. *Molecular Cell* 1999; 4: 611–7.

16. Ren D, Collingwood TN, Rebar EJ, Wolffe AP, Camp HS. PPARγ knockdown by engineered transcription factors: exogenous PPAR$_{γ2}$ but not PPAR$_{γ1}$ reactivates adipogenesis. *Genes Dev* 2002; 16: 27–32.

17. Rosen ED, Hsu CH, Wang X, Sakai S, Freeman MW, Gonzalez FJ, Spiegelman BM. C/EBPα induces adipogenesis through PPARγ: a unified pathway. *Genes Dev* 2002; 16: 22–6.

18. Saint-Marc P, Kozak LP, Ailhaud G, Darimont C, Négrel R. Angiotensin II as a trophic factor of white adipose tissue: stimulation of adipose cell formation. *Endocrinology* 2001; 142: 487–92.

19. Forman BM, Chen J, Evans RM. Hypolipidemic drugs, polyunsaturated fatty acids, and eicosanoids are ligands for peroxisome proliferator-activated receptors α and δ. *Proc Natl Acad Sci USA* 1997; 94: 4312–7.

20. Bastié C, Luquet S, Holst D, Jehl-Pietri C, Grimaldi P. Alterations of peroxisome proliferator-activated receptor δ activity affect fatty acid-controlled adipose differentiation. *J Biol Chem* 2000; 275: 38768–73.

21. Aubert J, Dessolin S, Belmonte N, Lo M, McKenzie FR, Staccini L *et al.* Leukemia Inhibitory Factor and its receptor promote adipocyte differentiation via the mitogen-activated protein kinase cascade. *J Biol Chem* 1999; 274: 24965–12.

22. Sakaue H, Kinishi M, Ogawa W, Asaki T, Mori T, Yamasaki M *et al.* Requqirement of fibroblast growth factor 10 in development of white adipose tissue. *Genes & Dev* 2002; 16: 908–12.

23. Engeli S, Négrel R, Sharma AM. Physiology and pathophysiology of the adipose tissue renin-angiotensin system. *Hypertension* 2000; 35: 1270–7.

24. Aubert J, Darimont C, Safonova I, Ailhaud G, Négrel R. Regulation by glucocorticoids of angiotensinogen gene expression and secretion in adipose cells. *Biochem J* 1997; 328: 701–6.

25. Cooper R, McFarlane AN, Bennett FI, Wilks R, Puras A, Tewskbury D *et al.* ACE, AGT, and obesity: a potential pathway leading to hypertension. *J Hum Hypertens* 1997; 11: 107–11.

26. Cooper R, Forrester T, Ogunbiyi O, Muffinda J. AGT levels and obesity in four black populations: ICSHIB Investigators. *J Hypertens* 1998; 16: 571–5.

27. Schorr U, Blaschke K, Turan S, Distler A, Sharma AM. Relationship between angiotensinogen, leptin and blood pressure levels in young normotensive men. J *Hypertens* 1998; 16: 1475–80.

28. Massiera F, Bloch-Faure M, Ceiler D, Murakami K, Fukamizu A, Gasc JM, Quignard-Boulange A, Negrel R, Ailhaud G, Seydoux J, Meneton P, Teboul M. Adipose angiotensinogen is involved in adipose tissue growth and blood pressure regulation. *FASEB J.* 2001; 15(14): 2727–9.

29. Masuzaki H, Paterson J, Shinyama H, Morton NM, Mullins JJ, Seckl JR. A transgenic model of visceral obesity and the metabolic syndrome. *Science.* 2001; 294(5549): 2166–70.

30. Van Harmelen V, Ariapart P, Hoffstedt J, Lundkvist I, Bringman S, Arner P Increased adipose angiotensinogen gene expression in human obesity. *Obes Res* 2000; 8: 337–41.

Progress in Obesity Research: 9. Edited by *Geraldo Medeiros-Neto, Alfredo Halpern and Claude Bouchard*
©2003 John Libbey Eurotext Ltd, pp. 87–95.

CHAPTER 18

Adipose tissue as an endocrine organ: regional differences in adipocyte endocrine function

James L. Kirkland*, Tamara Tchkonia, Nino Giorgadze and Tamar Pirtskhalava

*Departments of Medicine and Biochemistry, Boston University, 88 East Newton Street, F435, Boston, MA 02118, USA
[e-mail: kirkland@bu.edu]

Introduction

Adipose tissue is not only a site for lipid storage, but has equally important and very diverse endocrine functions. This has become increasingly apparent recently, particularly since the discovery of leptin[1]. Over the past couple of years, the list of hormones and autocrine/paracrine factors produced or processed by adipose tissue has grown extensively. Indeed, we have found over 80 secreted proteins in mass spectroscopic analyses of conditioned medium prepared from cultured human preadipocytes (unpublished observations). Together with published data about other factors released by fat tissue, the total number of such factors exceeds 120. Like certain endocrine organs, including the pituitary and adrenals, that produce different hormones in distinct regions within the organ, various fat depots exhibit distinct patterns of hormone production and processing. For example, abdominal subcutaneous fat releases more leptin than omental fat, and omental more plasminogen activator inhibitor-1 (PAI-1) and interleukin-6 (IL6) than subcutaneous fat[2–6]. Furthermore, the preadipocytes that account for anywhere from 15 to 50 per cent of cells in various fat depots have secretory profiles very different from those of fat cells. In this review, differentiation-dependent and regional differences in fat tissue endocrine function and responsible mechanisms will be emphasized, rather than effects of adipose-derived hormones on other organs, or effects of hormones produced by other organs on fat tissue.

Hormone and paracrine factor production

A hormone can be defined as a compound released systemically by an organ that has effects on distant organs. Adiponectin and resistin appear to meet this strict criterion. Other compounds with systemic effects that are released by fat tissue, such as leptin, angiotensin II (ANGII), IL-6, PAI-1, and serum amyloid A3 (SAA3), are hormone-like, as they are produced by other tissues in addition to fat. Fat tissue also processes a number of hormone precursors into active hormones, including angiotensinogen (AGT), membrane-bound tumour necrosis factor α (TNFα), glucocorticoids, and sex steroids. Most substances produced or processed by adipose tissue have local paracrine effects and direct autocrine effects on adipocytes, and a few have systemic effects. Examples of adipose tissue hormones and autocrine/paracrine factors, as well as differentiation-dependent and regional variations in their expression, appear in Table 1. A few of these will be considered here to illustrate general points about adipose tissue endocrine function.

The factor secreted by fat tissue that has received greatest attention (over 5000 papers since 1994) has been leptin. The primary role of leptin is to promote adaptation to energy deficiency, rather than to prevent fat accumulation. Leptin deficiency results in decreases in energy expenditure, satiety, insulin sensitivity, and fertility, as well as many other responses through effects on the brain, fat tissue, the thyroid, the immune system, bone, pancreas, intestine, kidney, and other tissues[7]. In addition to fat tissue, leptin is released by the stomach, placenta, and skeletal muscle. Leptin is a cytokine-like molecule, as are many of the proteins produced by adipose tissue, in keeping with the mesenchymal ancestry shared by adipocytes and monocytes/macrophages. Leptin release is regulated at the levels of transcription as well as posttranscriptionally[8]. Insulin, glucocorticoids, and acute TNFα treatment enhance leptin release, while β-adrenergic agonists and chronic TNFα exposure inhibit it[8–10]. Fat tissue not only releases leptin, but also soluble leptin receptors that bind leptin in blood, affecting its activity[11], adding another layer to the control exerted by fat tissue over effects of leptin on other tissues.

Interestingly, leptin administration results in more extensive loss of visceral than subcutaneous fat compared to control, pair-fed animals experiencing the same extent of weight loss[12]. This might suggest that the central nervous system contributes to control of regional fat distribution, through either neural or neuroendocrine outputs. Leptin may also have effects on visceral fat distinct from those on subcutaneous fat. Furthermore, since visceral fat turns over more rapidly and is more sensitive to lipolytic conditions than subcutaneous fat[13], reduction in food intake caused by leptin likely results in more rapid mobilization of fat from visceral depots.

Table 1. Examples of regional and differentiation-dependence of factors released by adipose tissue

Factor	Regional differences	Preadipocytes vs. fat cells
Leptin	Subcutaneous > visceral	Fat cells
Resistin	Abdominal > thigh	Fat cells
Adiponectin	?	Fat cells
Angiotensin II	Visceral > subcutaneous	Fat cells
PAI-1	Visceral > subcutaneous	Preadipocytes/fat cells
SAA3	?	Fat cells
Metallothionein	Brown > white fat	Similar in humans
IL-6	Visceral > subcutaneous	Preadipocytes (possibly fat cells)
TNFα	Variable	Preadipocytes and large fat cells
TGFβ	Similar	Fat cells
Adipsin	Similar	Fat cells
ASP (complement factor 3a)	Visceral > subcutaneous	Fat cells
Retinol binding protein	Similar	Fat cells
Basic FGF	Some isoforms subcutaneous, others visceral	Preadipocytes
Cholesterol ester transfer protein	Subcutaneous > visceral	Preadipocytes/fat cells
Hormones processed –		
Glucocorticoids/HSD-1	Visceral > subcutaneous	Preadipocytes/fat cells
Sex steroids/17β-HSD	Visceral > subcutaneous	Preadipocytes/fat cells
Sex steroids/aromatase	Subcutaneous > visceral	Preadipocytes

Leptin is not only produced by fat tissue with diverse effects on distant tissues, it has autocrine effects on fat cells. In addition to soluble leptin receptors, fat cells express the long form of the leptin receptor[14]. Expression of these receptors increases during adipogenesis[15]. Leptin promotes both preadipocyte replication and differentiation. Indeed, a theme repeated in the cases of most of the factors released by fat cells that affect other tissues is that these factors also have autocrine effects.

More leptin is produced by subcutaneous than visceral fat. This regional difference in leptin production is even evident in subcutaneous and omental preadipocytes isolated from the same subjects after being cultured under identical conditions, and in fat cells maintained in ceiling cultures[9,13]. Therefore, intrinsic mechanisms appear to contribute to distinct patterns of leptin production among cells from various fat depots (although interdepot differences in macrophage and mesothelial cell content occur, and these cell types could contaminate preadipocyte and ceiling cultures). Furthermore, increased fat cell size is associated with enhanced leptin release[16]. Since subcutaneous fat cells are generally larger than omental cells, this could contribute to regional differences in leptin production. A cycle can be envisaged than assures greater subcutaneous than visceral leptin production, since leptin promotes differentiation, leptin production increases with differentiation, and subcutaneous preadipocytes are more responsive than omental cells to agents that promote differentiation. Thiazolidinediones, which enhance activity of the adipogenic transcription factor, peroxisome proliferator activated receptor γ (PPARγ), inhibit leptin production through a direct inhibitory effect of PPARγ on the leptin promoter[17]. However, the other major adipogenic transcription factor, CCAAT/enhancer binding protein α (C/EBPα), stimulates leptin transcription. Although PPARγ expression is higher in differentiating subcutaneous than visceral preadipocytes, so is expression of C/EBPα[18], perhaps underlying both the increased leptin expression and larger fat cell size in subcutaneous fat. The finding that treating fat cells with rosiglitazone (a thiazolidinedione that binds to PPARγ, increasing its transactivating activity thereby inhibiting leptin production), equalizes subcutaneous and omental leptin expression[13], is in accord with this possibility. The precise mechanism responsible for initiating regional differences in leptin production remains to be determined.

Adiponectin (adipoQ, acrp30) fits the definition of a true hormone since its production appears to be limited to fat tissue[19]. Adiponectin is closely related to complement factor C1q, reflecting the shared mesenchymal ancestry of adipocytes and macrophages/monocytes. It acts on muscle to enhance fatty acid oxidation and on the liver to decrease glucose output. Overall, adiponectin results in enhanced insulin effects, reduced circulating free fatty acids, and weight loss without decreased food intake[19]. Reduced production of adiponectin by fat tissue is associated with insulin resistance. Insulin causes increased circulating adiponectin and β-agonists reduce adiponectin release[20]. More adiponectin is produced by fat cells than preadipocytes.

Release of resistin, like that of adiponectin, appears so far to be limited to fat tissue. Resistin impairs glucose tolerance and fat tissue glucose uptake[21]. It inhibits preadipocyte differentiation into fat cells. Obese rodents have increased serum resistin, but reduced fat tissue resistin mRNA, suggesting an important role of posttranscriptional regulation. Abdominal fat produces more of a human resistin homologue than subcutaneous fat from the thigh[22]. However, the closest human proteins to rodent resistin have only 60 per cent homology, and the relevance of resistin homologues to human fat biology remains to be clarified. This is an example of the considerable diversity in hormonal function encountered among species, and emphasizes the value of developing human fat model systems for the study of adipose tissue endocrine function and drug development.

Fat tissue expresses many of the elements of the renin-angiotensin system, including AGT, a renin-like activity, and angiotensin converting enzyme (ACE), resulting in generation of ANGII. ANGII activates production of certain prostaglandins in fat tissue, promotes lipogenesis, and increases IL-1βα, IL-6, PAI-1, and leptin release[23]. Transgenic mice overexpressing AGT in fat are obese[24]. In these animals, increased circulating ANGII and hypertension also occur, demonstrating that fat tissue ANGII can have systemic as well as local effects. Insulin and glucocorticoids promote release of AGT by fat cells[25]. Thus, fat tissue AGT production could be one link between insulin resistance and hypertension in obesity. While ANGII promotes lipogenesis and obesity, it interferes with preadipocyte differentiation[26], suggesting an effect of ANGII on preadipocytes distinct from that on differentiated adipocytes. This biphasic effect is not without precedent: cyclic AMP congeners promote preadipocyte differentiation, yet inhibit lipid accumulation by differentiated adipocytes.

AGT expression is greater in visceral than subcutaneous fat[27]. Since glucocorticoids stimulate AGT expression, higher visceral AGT may be a result of higher local glucocorticoid concentrations in visceral than subcutaneous fat (see below). Also, basal glucose uptake is higher in visceral than subcutaneous fat. Sp1, a transcription factor whose activity is enhanced by glycosylation, promotes AGT transcription[28]. Thus, increased glucose flux through the hexosamine biosythetic pathway resulting in protein glycosylation could contribute to increased visceral AGT expression.

PAI-1 is an anti-fibrinolytic protein that can contribute to hypercoagulability. Visceral fat produces more PAI-1 than subcutaneous fat[29,30], possibly contributing to the atherosclerosis associated with visceral obesity. As with AGT, insulin and glucocorticoids cause increased fat tissue PAI-1 expression[31]. ANGII itself increases fat cell PAI-1 expression[23] as does hyperglycaemia, possibly through activating the hexosamine biosynthetic pathway and Sp-1 glycosylation[32]. As with AGT, higher local glucocorticoid concentrations and glucose flux in visceral fat could contribute to the greater expression of PAI-1 in visceral fat. Most PAI-1 released by fat tissue comes from stromal cells, not fat cells[29]. Increased PAI-1 production by visceral fat is associated with increased abundance of stromal cells that stain for PAI-1, demonstrating the role that variations in fat tissue cellular composition among depots can play in the genesis of variations in secretory function[23].

Fat tissue releases IL-6[2] which, because it is relatively stable, enters the circulation and has systemic effects, including exacerbation of insulin resistance and hypertriglyceridaemia. Ninety per cent of the IL-6 in adipose tissue is generated by stromal-vascular cells, rather than fat cells[2]. β-agonists enhance production of IL-6 by fat tissue, but not macrophages. Thus, although fat cells have 'borrowed' IL-6 from macrophages, its regulation differs between these two cell types, a pattern evident in the cases of many other cytokines generated in adipose tissue. ANGII promotes IL-6 production[23], and more AGT is expressed by omental than subcutaneous fat[27], possibly contributing to the greater release of PAI-1 by omental than subcutaneous fat.

Fat cells produce many other hormone-like paracrine and autocrine factors, too numerous to consider in detail here. Broadly, these include cytokines (e.g. IL-6, IL-1β, TNFα), complement components (e.g. adiponectin, adipsin, acylation stimulating protein [ASP]), acute phase reactants (e.g. SAA3, metal-lothionein, Neu-related calcin), growth factors (e.g. insulin-like growth factor-1, basic fibroblast growth factor (FGF) subtypes, transforming growth factor β), factors involved in hemostasis (e.g. PAI-1), and other types of proteins (e.g. tissue inhibitors of metalloproteinases, retinol binding protein, bone-related peptides). Some of these factors have been well characterized (for example, TNFα). Others do not yet have functions in fat tissue that are fully understood. Additional autocrine/paracrine activities are known to exist, but the identities of the responsible compounds are as yet undetermined. For example, low molecular weight factors released by preadipocytes that inhibit preadipocyte replication exist[33], but their identities remain obscure.

Many of the paracrine and autocrine factors produced by adipose cells, as well as certain hormones such as ANGII, resemble those produced by the other mesenchymal cell types to which adipocytes are closely related. These include fibroblasts, myocytes, osteocytes, chondrocytes, renal mesangial cells, monocytes, and macrophages. In some cases, fat tissue has commandeered proteins produced by sister mesangial cell types to subserve a special, localized function in adipose tissue. The complement-related factors and ANGII are examples of this. For example, ASP produced by fat cells is complement factor 3a produced by monocytes, but in adipose tissue this complement factor induces lipid storage[34]. Some of the factors produced by adipose tissue that act in an autocrine or paracrine fashion can also act as hormones with systemic effects. Many, if not most, of these factors are produced to different extents in different fat depots. Some have greater effects on certain depots than others. For example, more ASP binds to subcutaneous than visceral fat cells[35]. Overall, visceral fat is more active in secreting these factors than subcutaneous fat tissue[36]. The larger size of the subcutaneous than visceral fat depot means that factors secreted by subcutaneous fat may have a greater systemic impact than those released by visceral fat. However, the venous drainage of certain visceral depots through the liver and other organs could amplify the impact of the large array of factors released by visceral fat.

Hormone processing

In addition to producing hormones and paracrine factors, fat tissue converts a number of inactive prohormones into locally active hormones. An example of this is conversion of ATG to active ANGII (see above). Glucocorticoid processing is another example. Inactive 11-keto steroids (such as cortisone in humans and 11-dehydrocorticosterone in rats) are converted into their active isoforms (cortisol and corticosterone, respectively) by 11β-hydroxysteroid dehydrogenase-1 (HSD-1). This enzyme is present in fat tissue and its activity is regulated by substrate availability, adipogenic transcription factors, and other mechanisms[37]. Adipogenic transcription factor activity, in turn, depends on the metabolic state of fat tissue. Activity of PPARγ, which downregulates HSD-1 expression, depends on the presence of ligands, including fatty acids. Thus, adipose tissue adds a layer of local metabolic control to the effects of systemic glucocorticoids.

More HSD-1 is expressed in human omental than subcutaneous adipose tissue[38]. Coupled with the higher abundance of glucocorticoid receptors in omental than subcutaneous fat[39], inactive circulating 11-keto steroids have a greater impact on visceral than subcutaneous fat tissue function. Increased visceral glucocorticoid receptor density may explain why uniform overexpression of HSD-1 in adipose tissue causes visceral obesity in transgenic mice[40]. Furthermore, HSD-1 can act as a dehydrogenase or an oxoreductase[37]. It is the latter activity that converts cortisone to cortisol. Oxoreductase activity of HSD-1 increases with differentiation and promotes further adipogenesis through enhanced cortisol generation. Possibly, the set-point for the switch between the dehydrogenase and oxoreductase activities of HSD-1 varies among fat depots.

Another example of adipose tissue fine-tuning of systemic hormonal signals is the processing of sex steroids. Type 3 17β-hydroxysteroid dehydrogenase (17β-HSD) catalyses conversion of androstenedione to testosterone. 17β-HSD activity is present in fat tissue[41]. In obese women, 17β-HSD mRNA levels are higher in visceral than subcutaneous fat relative to aromatase mRNA. If, in fact, significant amounts of testosterone are generated in visceral fat, these could act locally and reach the liver, possibly contributing to the metabolic syndrome, a possibility that remains to be tested.

Estrogens have pronounced effects on regional fat distribution, promoting an increase in the ratio of subcutaneous to visceral fat. Aromatase catalyses the synthesis of locally active estrogens from circulating C19 androgens. Aromatase expression is much higher in preadipocytes than fat cells[42]. Treatment of fat tissue with thiazolidinedione PPARγ ligands decreases aromatase expression, while TNFα enhances expression[43]. Aromatase expression is higher in subcutaneous than omental preadipocytes in both men and women[44]. Also in both men and women, cortisol induces aromatase expression in omental preadipocytes. However, while cortisol enhances subcutaneous preadipocyte aromatase expression in women, cortisol inhibits it in men. Since active estrogens can promote preadipocyte replication, these gender and regional differences in aromatase expression may predispose women to the development of subcutaneous obesity. The basis for these regional differences in preadipocyte aromatase expression is not yet entirely clear. Regional differences in aromatase expression may be coupled with regional differences in estrogen receptor (ER) responses to active estrogens. Human preadipocytes and fat cells express α and β type ER[45]. Interdepot and differentiation-dependent variation in feedback effects of estrogens on these receptors has been observed. Estrogens enhance expression of both ERα and β in subcutaneous and omental preadipocytes and enhance ERα expression in omental fat cells. However, in subcutaneous fat cells ERα (but not β) expression is inhibited by estrogens. This might explain why ERα knockout mice have an increased ratio of subcutaneous to visceral fat.

Regional differences in endocrine function

Regional differences in fat tissue production and processing of hormones and paracrine factors likely contribute to the metabolic syndrome and other consequences of visceral adiposity. Visceral lipectomy greatly improves insulin sensitivity and lipid profiles[46], demonstrating the distinct systemic impact of visceral fat. Furthermore, subcutaneous lipectomy, resulting in an increased ratio of visceral to subcutaneous fat, causes insulin resistance and elevated triglycerides[47]. What are the mechanisms that might constitute the basis for regional differences in endocrine function?

Regional differences in circulation, innervation, anatomic constraints, admixture of non-adipose cell types within fat depots, and other factors extrinsic to adipose cells could contribute to interdepot variation in responses, processing, and release of hormones. For example, omental fat tissue is more vascular than abdominal subcutaneous fat. Venous drainage of certain visceral fat depots is through the liver, which could potentiate effects of factors released by these depots on liver function.

Intrinsic differences in the characteristics of adipose cells themselves very likely also contribute. Even after many generations in identical cell culture conditions, and despite long term exposure to the same hormones, preadipocytes and fat cells from different fat depots retain distinct, depot-dependent characteristics[48]. For example, capacities to transfer fatty acids, express lipogenic enzymes, replicate, differentiate, and express the adipogenic transcription factors, C/EBPα and PPARγ, vary in cells from different fat depots after weeks or months in culture[18,49–51]. Epigenetic differences in fat cell DNA or other intrinsic processes could, through causing this regional variation in adipocyte transcription factor expression, impact expression of components of the pathways responsible for hormonal signaling, processing, and production (Fig. 1). For example, PPARγ activity inhibits HSD-1 expression. PPARγ expression is lower in omental than abdominal subcutaneous preadipocytes, even when these cells are isolated from the same subject, cultured under identical conditions in parallel, and exposed to supramaximal concentrations of a glucocorticoid that does not require activation by HSD-1[18]. HSD-1 activity is higher in omental than abdominal subcutaneous preadipocytes[38]. Thus, higher HSD-1 expression in omental cells could partly be a consequence of reduced PPARγ activity. A regionally-specific, fundamental mechanism intrinsic to adipose cells is likely to be upstream of regional differences in PPARγ expression, since the differences in PPARγ persist in cultured adipose cells. In concert with interdepot differences in circulation, innervation, and other factors extrinsic to adipose cells, it seems that fundamental, intrinsic, as yet unknown processes contribute to regional variation in the effects, processing, and release of hormones in adipose tissue.

Regional differences in fat tissue response to hormones can result in interdepot variation in hormone production. For example, regional variation in adipogenesis due to differences in HSD-1 activity would be predicted to contribute to variation in PPARγ activity in differentiating preadipocytes, in turn affecting HSD-1 and glucocorticoid levels. Similar cycles of events, likely with epigenetic or other intrinsic differences among depots as their starting point, could contribute to interdepot variation in estrogen receptor numbers, β-adrenergic signaling pathway components, ANGII generation, and other pathways that coordinate hormone responses in fat tissue.

ENDOCRINE INPUTS (pituitary, adrenal, pancreas, thyroid, gonads)

OTHER INPUTS (neural, metabolic, paracrine)

FUNDAMENTAL MECHANISMS INTRINSIC TO ADIPOSE CELLS

ADIPOSE TISSUE

HORMONE PRODUCTION (e.g. leptin, adiponectin)

HORMONE CONVERSION (e.g. sex steroids, glucocorticoids)

AUTOCRINE/ PARACRINE (e.g. IL-6, FGF, TNFα)

METABOLIC (e.g. FFA)

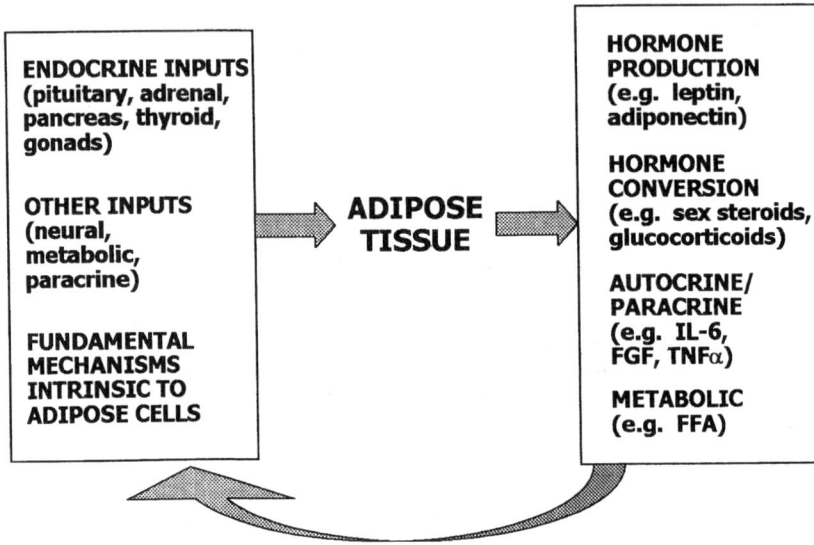

Fig. 1. Regulation and effects of adipose tissue endocrine function.

Not only are there general differences between visceral and subcutaneous fat, within these sites there are also differences. For example, mesenteric preadipocytes are more responsive to thiazolidinediones than omental cells[18]. Fat cells are also found in many tissues outside fat depots, including bone marrow and muscle. These cells can have distinct secretory profiles. For example, bone marrow fat cells produce factors that contribute to regulation of hematopoiesis and bone formation. Thus, adipose cells not only secrete factors that act on target tissues at a distance from fat depots, sometimes fat cells are in place within target tissues where they secrete regulatory factors.

Preadipocyte endocrine function differs from that of fat cells

Most of the factors released by fat tissue are produced in a differentiation-dependent manner. A larger than previously appreciated number of them are released to a greater extent by preadipocytes than fat cells. Anywhere from 15 to 50 per cent of the cells within fat tissue are preadipocytes, underscoring the relevance of preadipocyte characteristics to fat tissue function[52]. Preadipocyte responses to a number of hormones are distinct from those of fat tissue. For example, while preadipocytes have IGF-1 receptors that can be activated by high concentrations of insulin, they have few insulin receptors[53]. Preadipocytes have less G_i than fat cells, resulting in stimulation of cyclic AMP generation by adenosine and certain prostaglandins in preadipocytes, but inhibition in fat cells[54]. Stromal cells produce more IL-6 and certain FGF isoforms than fat cells[2,55], although differentiated preadipocytes can produce more IL-6 than undifferentiated cells[56]. Fat cells produce more leptin than preadipocytes. Preadipocyte processing of prohormones can be distinct from that in fat tissue. For example, aromatase is more highly expressed in preadipocytes than fat cells, while HSD-1 is more highly expressed in fat cells than preadipocytes. Since preadipocytes account for much of the cytokine and growth factor production by fat tissue, the variations in proportions of preadipocytes that occur among fat depots and with aging[52] likely contribute to regional differences in fat tissue endocrine function.

At least two preadipocyte subtypes exist[57]. One subtype is capable of extensive replication and differentiation, while the other is more limited. Both subtypes arise from the same parent cells. By transfecting human preadipocytes with a telomerase expression vector, stable strains originating from single preadipocytes can be generated[58]. When clones are derived from these strains, the two preadipocyte subtypes are still apparent, despite their identical ancestry. In preliminary studies, the proportions of these two subtypes vary among fat depots. Omental fat tissue contains many more of the slowly replicating, poorly differentiating preadipocytes. Perhaps it is this subtype that accounts for much of the production of those cytokines and growth factors that are released to a greater extent by omental than subcutaneous fat. Differences in function between these subtypes, such as capacities to release cytokines and growth factors, remain to be explored.

Conclusions

From the foregoing consideration of fat tissue endocrine function, the following basic patterns can be discerned. Adipose tissue shares a feature of the pituitary and adrenal glands as an endocrine organ: different regions within the adipose organ have distinct endocrine functions. Subcutaneous adipose tissue produces more leptin and coverts more estrogen precursors into active estrogen than does visceral fat. Visceral adipose tissue releases more IL-6 and PAI-1 and converts more cortisone to cortisol than does subcutaneous fat. Overall, visceral fat is a more active secretory tissue than subcutaneous fat[36,59].

Most factors released or processed by adipose tissue have predominantly local effects. Sometimes this is on fat tissue. In other situations, fat cells in other tissues produce factors that affect the function of those tissues, notably in bone marrow and muscle. Some factors released by fat tissue, including leptin, IL-6, PAI-1, acute phase reactants, and ANGII, have both significant local and systemic effects. Many of the hormones and autocrine/paracrine factors produced by adipocytes are 'borrowed' from other mesenchymal cell types and serve somewhat different functions in fat tissue.

Preadipocytes respond to, process, and produce hormones in ways distinct from fat cells. Indeed, preadipocytes are an important cell type in their own right: they are a major source of IL-6 and basic FGF and are the principal site of estrogen activation in fat tissue. Thus, varying ratios of preadipocytes to fat cells among depots would be predicted to affect fat tissue endocrine function in a regionally-distinct manner, a proposition that warrants further investigation. Furthermore, preadipocyte subtypes exist whose abundance varies among fat depots. Differences in the secretory profiles of these subtypes remain to be explored, as does the nature of the fat cells that develop from them. Variations among depots in content of macrophages and mesothelial cells may also contribute to regional variation in fat tissue endocrine function.

Adipose tissue can act as an endocrine way station, receiving hormonal signals and transducing their effects through local or systemic signals to other adipocytes as well as other tissues. Along the way, adipose tissue modulates these signals based on their metabolic state, sometimes in a depot-specific way, adding a level of control to effects or production of systemic hormonal signals.

Intrinsic differences in the characteristics of fat cells and preadipocytes are evident even in cells cultured under identical conditions for prolonged periods. Together with regional variation in circulation, innervation, presence of other cell types in fat depots, and other factors extrinsic to adipose cells, these intrinsic mechanisms contribute to regional differences in function. These intrinsic mechanisms act upstream of expression of the adipogenic transcription factors that control expression of the proteins that determine hormone production, processing, and effects on fat tissue, including receptors and post-receptor pathway components. Effectively, different fat depots are distinct endocrine mini-organs.

Abbreviations: plasminogen activator inhibitor-1 (PAI-1), interleukin (IL), angiotensin II (ANGII), serum amyloid A3 (SAA3), angiotensinogen (AGT), tumour necrosis factor α (TNFα), peroxisome proliferator-activated receptor γ (PPARγ), CCAAT/enhancer binding protein α (C/EBPα), angiotensin converting enzyme (ACE), fibroblast growth factor (FGF), acylation stimulating protein (ASP), 11β-hydroxysteroid dehydrogenase-1 (HSD-1), type 3 17β-hydroxysteroid dehydrogenase (17β-HSD), estrogen receptor (ER).

Acknowledgements: The authors are grateful to J. Armstrong for helpful discussions. This work was supported by NIH grants DK56891, AG/DK13925, and DK46200 (Adipocyte Core).

References

1. Zhang Y, Proenca R, Maffei M, Barone M, Leopold L, Friedman J. Positional cloning of the mouse obese gene and its human homologue. *Nature* 1994; 372: 425–32.

2. Fried SK, Bunkin DA, Greenberg AS. Omental and subcutaneous adipose tissues of obese subjects release interleukin-6: depot difference and regulation by glucocorticoid. *J Clin Endocrinol Metab* 1998; 83: 847–50.

3. Montague CT, Prins JB, Sanders L, Digby JE, O'Rahilly S. Depot- and sex-specific differences in human leptin mRNA expression: implications for the control of regional fat distribution. *Diabetes* 1997; 46(3): 342–7.

4. Harmelen V, Reynisdottir S, Eriksson P, Thorne A, Hoffstedt J, Lonnqvist F, Arner P. Leptin secretion from subcutaneous and visceral adipose tissue in women. *Diabetes* 1998; 47: 913–7.

5. Hube F, Lietz U, Igel M, Jensen PB, Tornqvist H, Joost HG, Haune H. Difference in leptin mRNA levels between omental and subcutaneous abdominal adipose tissue from obese humans. *Horm Metab Res* 1996; 28(12): 690–3.

6. Shimomura I, Funahashi T, Takahashi M, Maeda K, Kotani K, Nakamura T, *et al.* Enhanced expression of PAI-1 in visceral fat: Possible contributor to vascular disease in obesity. *Nature Med* 1996; 2(7): 800–3.

7. Friedman JM Halaas JL. Leptin and the regulation of body weight in mammals. *Nature* 1998; 95: 763–70.

8. Russell CD, Ricci MR, Brolin RE, Magill E, Fried SK. Regulation of leptin content of obese human adipose tissue. *Am J Physiol* 2001; 280: E399–E404.

9. Zhang HH, Kumar S, Barnett AH, Eggo MC. Intrinsic site-specific differences in the expression of leptin in adipocytes and its autocrine effects on glucose uptake. *J Clin Endocrinol Metab* 1999; 84: 2550–6.

10. Ricci MR, Fried SK. Isoproterenol decreases leptin expression in adipose tissue of obese humans. *Obes Res* 1999; 7: 233–40.

11. Brabant G, Nave H, Mayr B, Behrend M, van Harmelen V, Arner P. Secretion of freee and protein-bound leptin from subcutaneous adipose tissue of lean and obese women. *J Clin Endocrinol Metab* 2002; 87: 3966–70.

12. Barzilai N, Wang J, Massilon D, Vuguin P, Hawkins M, Rossetti L. Leptin selectively decreases visceral adiposity and enhances insulin action. *J Clin Invest* 1997; 100: 3105–10.

13. van Harmelen V, Dicker A, Ryden M, Hauner H, Lonnqvist F, Naslund E, Arner P. Increased lipolysis and decreased leptin production by human omental as compared with subcutaneous preadipocytes. *Diabetes* 2002; 51: 2029–36.

14. Bornstein SR, Abu-Asab M, Glasow A, Path G, Hauner H, Tsokos M *et al.* Immunohistochemical and ultrastructural localization of leptin and leptin receptor in human white adipose tissue and differentiating human adipose cells in primary culture. *Diabetes* 2000; 49: 532–8.

15. Machinal-Quelin F, Dieudonne MN, Leneveu MC, Pecuery R, Giudicelli Y. Proadipogenic effect of leptin on rat preadipocytes *in vitro*: activation of MAPK and STAT3 signaling pathways. *Am J Physiol* 2002; 282: C853–C863.

16. Zhang Y, Guo KY, Diaz PA, Heo M, Leibel RL. Determinants of leptin gene expression in fat depots of lean mice. *Am J Physiol* 2002; 282: R226–R234.

17. Hollenberg AN, Susulic VS, Madura JP, Zhang B, Moller DE, Tontonoz P *et al.* Functional antagonism between CCAAT/enhancer binding protein-α and peroxisome proliferator-activated receptor-γ on the leptin promoter. *J Biol Chem* 1997; 272(8): 5283–90.

18. Tchkonia T, Giorgadze N, Pirtshklava T, Tchoukalova Y, Karagiannides I, Forse RA *et al.* Fat depot origin affects adipogenesis in primary cultured and cloned human preadipocytes. *Am J Physiol* 2002; 282: R1286–R1296.

19. Berg AH, Combs TP, Scherer PE. ACRP30/adiponectin: an adipokine regulating glucose and lipid metabolism. *Trends Endocrinol Metab* 2002; 13: 84–9.

20. Delporte ML, Funahashi T, Takahashi M, Matsuzawa Y, Brichard SM. Pre- and post-translational negative effect of β-adrenoceptor agonists on adiponectin secretion: *in vitro* and *in vivo* studies. *Biochem J* 2002 (in press).

21. Steppan CM, Lazar MA. Resistin and obesity-associated insulin resistance. *Trends Endocrinol Metab* 2002; 13: 18–23.

22. McTernan CL, McTernan PG, Harte AL, Levick PL, Barnett AH, Kumar S. Resistin, central obesity, and type 2 diabetes. *Lancet* 2002; 359: 46–7.

23. Skurk T, Hauner H. Cytokine expression in cultured human adipocytes after ANG II stimulation. *Int J Obes Relat Metab Disord* 2002; 26 (Suppl 1): S120.

24. Massiera F, Bloch-Faure M, Ceiler D, Murakami K, Fukamizu A, Gasc JM *et al.* Adipose angiotensinogen is involved in adipose tissue growth and blood pressure regulation. *FASEB J* 2001; 15: 2727–9.

25. Aubert J, Safonova I, Negrel R, Ailhaud G. Insulin down-regulates angiotensinogen gene expression and angiotensinogen secretion in cultured adipose cells. *Biochem Biophys Res Commun* 1998; 250: 77–82.

26. Janke J, Engeli S, Gorzelniak K, Luft FC, Sharma AM. Mature adipocytes inhibit *in vitro* differentiation of human preadipocytes via angiotensin type 1 receptors. *Diabetes* 2002; 51: 1699–707.

27. Dusserre E, Moulin P, Vidal H. Differences in mRNA expression of the proteins secreted by the adipocytes in human subcutaneous and visceral adipose tissues. *Biochim Biophys Acta* 2000; 1500: 88–96.

28. Rohrwasser A, Zhang S, Dillon HF, Inoue I, Callaway CW, Hillas E. Contribution of Sp1 to initiation of transcription of angiotensinogen. *J Hum Genet* 2002; 47: 249–56.

29. Bastelica D, Morange P, Berthet B, Borghi H, Lacroix O, Grino M *et al.* Stromal cells are the main plasminogen activator-1-producing cells in human fat: evidence of differences between visceral and subcutaneous deposits. *Arterioscler Thromb Vasc Biol* 2002; 22: 173–8.

30. Halleux CM, Declerck PJ, Tran SL, Detry R, Brichard SM. Hormonal control of plasminogen activator inhibitor-1 gene expression and production by human adipose tissue: stimulation by glucocorticoids and inhibition by catecholamines. *J Clin Endocrinol Metab* 1999; 84: 4097–105.

31. Morange PE, Aubert J, Peiretti PF, Lijnen HR, Vague P, Verdier M *et al.* Glucocorticoids and insulin promote plasminogen activator inhibitor 1 production by human adipose tissue. *Diabetes* 1999; 48: 890–5.

32. Gabriely I, Yang XM, Callaway CW, Ma XH, Rossetti L, Barzilai N. Hyperglycemia induces PAI-1 gene expression in adipose tissue by activation of the hexosamine biosynthetic pathway. *Atherosclerosis* 2002; 160: 115–22.

33. Kirkland JL, Hollenberg CH. Inhibitors of preadipocyte replication: opportunities for the treatment of obesity. *Prog Mol Subcell Biol* 1998; 22: 177–95.

34. Sniderman AD, Maslowska M, Cianflone K. Of mice and men (and women) and the acylation-stimulating protein pathway. *Curr Opin Lipidol* 2000; 11: 291–6.

35. Saleh J, Christou N, Cianflone K. Regional specificity of ASP binding in human adipose tissue. *Am J Physiol* 1999; 276: E815–E821.

36. Matsuzawa Y. Importance of adipocytokines in obesity-related diseases. *Int J Obes Relat Metab Disord* 2002; 26 (Suppl 1): S63.

37. Bujalska IJ, Walker EA, Hewison M, Stewart PM. A switch in dehydrogenase to reductase activity of 11 beta-hydroxysteroid dehydrogenase type 1 upon differentiation of human omental adipose stromal cells. *J Clin Endocrinol Metab* 2002; 87: 1205–10.

38. Bujalska I, Kumar S, Stewart P. Does central obesity reflect 'Cushing's disease of the omentum'? *Lancet* 1997; 349: 1210–3.

39. Bronnegard M, Arner P, Hellstrom L, Akner G, Gustafsson JA. Glucocorticoid receptor messenger ribonucleic acid in different regions of human adipose tissue. *Endocrinology* 1990; 127: 1689–96.

40. Masuzaki H, Paterson J, Shinyama H, Mortin NM, Mullins JJ, Flier JS. A transgenic model of visceral obesity and the metabolic syndrome. *Science* 2001; 294: 2166–70.

41. Corbould AM, Bawden MJ, Lavranos TC, Rodgers RJ, Judd SJ. The effect of obesity on the ratio of type 3 17 beat-hydroxysteroid dehydrogenase mRNA to cytochrome P450 aromatase mRNA in subcutaneous abdominal and intra-abdominal adipose tissue of women. *Int J Obes Relat Metab Disord* 2002; 26: 165–75.

42. Clyne CD, Speed CJ, Zhou J, Simpson ER. Liver receptor homologue-1 (LRH-1) regulates expression of aromatase in preadipocytes. *J Biol Chem* 2002; 277: 20591–7.

43. Rubin GL, Duong JH, Clyne CD, Speed CJ, Murata Y, Gong C, Simpson ER. Ligands for the peroxisomal proliferator-activated receptor gamma and retinoid X receptor inhibit aromatase cytochrome P450 (CYP19) expression mediated by promoter II in human breast adipose. *Endocrinology* 2002; 143: 2863–71.

44. McTernan PG, Anderson LA, Anwar AJ, Eggo MC, Crocker J, Barnett AH. Glucocorticoid regulation of p450 aromatase activity in human adipose tissue: gender and site differences. *J Clin Endocrinol Metab* 2002; 87: 1327–36.

45. Anwar A, McTernan PG, Anderson LA, Askaa J, Moody CG, Barnett AH et al. Site-specific regulation of oestrogen receptor-alpha and -beta by oestradiol in human adipose tissue. *Diabetes Obes Metab* 2001; 3: 338–49.

46. Barzilai N, She L, Liu BQ, Vuguin P, Cohen P, Wang J, Rossetti L. Surgical removal of visceral fat reverses hepatic insulin resistance. *Diabetes* 1999; 48: 94–8.

47. Weber RV, Buckley MC, Fried SK, Kral JG. Subcutaneous lipectomy causes a metabolic syndrome in hamsters. *Am J Physiol* 2000; 279: R936–R943.

48. Tchkonia T, Karagiannides I, Forse RA, Kirkland JL. Different fat depots are distinct mini-organs. *Curr Opin Endocrinol Diabetes* 2001; 8: 227–34.

49. Caserta F, Tchkonia T, Civelek V, Prentki M, Brown NF, McGarry JD et al. Fat depot origin affects fatty acid handling in cultured rat and human preadipocytes. *Am J Physiol* 2001; 280: E238–E247.

50. Kirkland JL, Hollenberg CH, Gillon WS. Age, anatomic site, and the replication and differentiation of adipocyte precursors. *Am J Physiol* 1990; 258: C206–C210.

51. Wang H, Kirkland JL, Hollenberg CH. Varying capacities for replication of rat adipocyte precursor clones and adipose tissue growth. *J Clin Invest* 1989; 83: 1741–6.

52. Kirkland JL, Hollenberg CH, Kindler S, Gillon WS. Effects of age and anatomic site on preadipocyte number in rat fat depots. *J Gerontol* 1994; 49: B31-B35.

53. Smith PJ, Wise LS, Berkowitz R, Wan C, Rubin CS. Insulin-like growth factor-1 is an essential regulator of the differentiation of 3T3-L1 adipocytes. *J Biol Chem* 1988; 263: 9402–8.

54. Kirkland JL, Piñeyro MA, Lu Z, Gregerman RI. Hormone sensitive adenylyl cyclase in preadipocytes cultured from adipose tissue: comparison with 3T3-L1 cells and adipocytes. *J Cell Physiol* 1987; 133: 449–60.

55. Gabrielsson BG, Johansson JM, Jennische E, Jernas M, Itoh Y, Peltonen M. Depot-specific expression of fibroblast growth factors in human adipose tissue. *Obes Res* 2002; 10: 608–16.

56. Vicennati V, Vottero A, Friedman C, Papanicolaou DA. Hormonal regulation of interleukin-6 production in human adipocytes. *Int J Obes Relat Metab Disord* 2002; 26: 905–11.

57. Kirkland JL, Hollenberg CH, Gillon WS. Two preadipocyte subtypes cloned from human omental fat. *Obes Res* 1993; 1(2): 87–91.

58. Tchkonia T, DePonte M, Forse RA, Pirtskhalava T, Kirkland JL. Telomerase expression enhances differentiation of passaged human preadipocytes. *Obes Res* 2001; 9 (Suppl 3): S145.

59. Matsuzawa Y, Funahashi T, Nakamura T. Molecular mechanism of metabolic syndrome X: contribution of adipocytokines, adipocyte-derived bioactive substances. *Ann NY Acad Sci* 1999; 892: 146–54.

Progress in Obesity Research: 9. Edited by *Geraldo Medeiros-Neto, Alfredo Halpern and Claude Bouchard*
©2003 John Libbey Eurotext Ltd, pp. 96–100.

CHAPTER 19

Human adipocytes: differentiation and apoptosis

Martin Wabitsch, Pamela Fischer-Posovszky and Klaus-Michael Debatin

Research Laboratory, Pediatric Endocrinology, Department of Pediatrics, University of Ulm, 89075 Ulm, Germany
[e-mail: martin.wabitsch@medizin.uni-ulm.de]

Introduction

The energy content of the human body is under control of several regulatory systems. Changes of body energy content and changes of the size of adipose tissue, the major energy store of the body, are the result of the balance between energy intake and energy expenditure.

This review summarizes clinical observations with changes of adipose tissue mass and cellularity which are a basis for the identification of factors involved in adipose tissue growth. Data on the regulation of differentiation of human adipocytes *in vitro* are provided in relation to these observations. Finally, clinical and experimental evidence is shown that apoptosis of adipocytes in adipose tissue in man seems to be a relevant physiological mechanism involved in the regulation of human fat mass.

Changes of body fat stores during development

In a histological study of human fetuses it has been shown that between the 14th and 24th week of gestation the first fetal adipose tissue is visible. Morphologically, a local agglomeration of mesenchymal cells occurs resembling small tissue globules. Then capillaries grow into these globules and the first fat globules are present with cells characterized by a high content of triglycerides. During the further development cells get univacular lipid droplets. The typical fat globule which can be found in subcutaneous fat in the newborn have developped. The observation, that the first structure to be identified in a developing fat globule is a capillary, demonstrates the direct association between the development of fat cells and angiogenesis. In the last third of gestation the subcutaneous tissue of the fetus consists at nearly all locations of differentiated adipose tissue.

At birth, body fat content is around 13 per cent[1]. Until the end of the first year of live, the percentage of body fat content increases further to about 28 per cent in a normal weight infant. Normally, infants possess a considerable panniculus adiposus. One hundred years ago, Stratz described the different periods during infancy, childhood, and adolescents in which anthropometrical changes related to percentage adipose tissue occur[2]. The first increase of percentage body fat occuring until the end of the first year of life was called by Stratz 'first filling period'. This period is followed by a period called the 'first stretching period' during which the subcutaneous adipose tissue mass decreases and also the percentage of body fat decreases due to a relatively higher increase in lean body mass during growth. Later in development, these sinus-wave-like changes are repeated in a comparable way: body fat percentage increased between the 8th and 10th year of life, in an early period during puberty ('second filling period'). In boys a second 'stretching period' ('fat spurt') can be observed during the pubertal growth spurt. It has to be mentioned that this second stretching period during which at least a constancy of the amount of subcutaneous fat over several months can be observed is not detectable when following the development of body mass index probably due to the significant increase in lean mass especially muscel mass during this period. In girls the second filling period continues often during the following years and a further increase of body fat mass until adulthood occurs. The increase of body mass per se during growth and development can be devided in increase of fat free and increase of fat mass. The relation between these two increases is dependent of the biological age and shows changes in a sinus-wave-like manner. From this observation critical periods of adipose tissue development can be assumed. These periods of 'filling' and 'stretching' can be also readily demonstrated when the development of the sum of triceps and subscapular skinfold thicknesses during infancy childhood and adolescents is looked at.

Changes on cellular level related to changes in body fat

On the basis of their results derived from investigations of adipose tissue cellularity several authors (summarized in[3]) could identify two sensitive periods for adipose tissue development during childhood: one during the first year of life and another one just before puberty. Interestingly, these periods coincident with the first two filling periods described originally by Stratz. It seems that during the first year of life the increase in body fat content is mainly due to an increase in adipocyte volume. The further growth of adipose tissue especially in the second filling period is suggested to be mainly due to an increase in fat cell number without significant changes of fat cell volume.

On a cellular level, changes in adipose tissues size result from changes in adipocyte volume and adipocyte number. The volume of an adipocyte represents the balance between lipolysis and lipogenesis on the level of a specific cell. Changes in adipocyte number (increases or decreases) are the result of either a multiplication of preadipocytes and their subsequent differentiation into adipocytes resulting in an increase in fat mass or of dedifferentiation or apoptosis of existing adipocytes leading to a loss of adipose tissue mass. Although these cellular changes leading to a decrease in the number of adipocytes are theoretically possible there are not enough *in vivo* or *in vitro* data which could prove that the number of adipocytes really can be reduced in an individuum. More details about the regulation of adipocyte volume and number in man have been reviewed recently[4,5] and are summarized in the following paragraphs.

Preadipocytes in human adipose tissue

The existence of preadipocytes in postnatal life was originally suggested after demonstrating that cells of the stromal-vascular fraction of adipose tissue are able to incooperate [³H]-thymidin and that the radioactive labelled thymidin can be found lateron in mature adipocytes. The stromal-vascular fraction of the adipose tissue is a mixture of different cells like endothelian cells, blood cells, nerve cells, macrophages, and also preadipocytes.

Today, it is possible to isolate preadipocytes from adipose tissue of rodents and to study their proliferation and differentiation *in vitro*[6]. Earlier studies trying to characterize preadipocytes from human adipose tissue have not been very successfull since only a small part of the stromal-vascular fraction of human adipose tissue developped into mature adipocytes *in vitro*. After the establishment of a serum-free chemically defined culture system for human preadipocytes by the working group of Gerhard Ailhaud and our working group[7], it became possible to study more deeply the regulation of preadipocytes proliferation and adipose differentiation *in vitro*. It could be shown that almost all cells of the stromal-vascular fraction of human adipocyte tissue, which have been seeded in culture dishes accoording to an established method were preadipocytes, capable to differentiate into adipocytes after adequate stimulation. The newly differentiated human adipocytes can be cultured for several days in a monolayer and their metabolism can be further investigated[6].

In the undifferentiated stage, these preadipocytes possess multiple cytoplasmatic arms and are macroscopically not distinguishable from fibroblasts. During adipose differentiation the cells change their morphology. They get a round shape and their cytoplasm is going to be filled up slowly by multiple lipid droplets which increase in size. These morphological changes are the result of various biochemical processes during differentiation. At the end of their development the preadipocytes not only have acquired the phenotype of an adipocyte with an univacuolar lipid droplet but possess all biochemical characteristics of mature fat cells.

Age-dependency of differentiation of adipocyte precusror cells

When preadipocytes, derived from the subcutaneous adipose tissue of the abdominal wall, are cultured in a serum-free, adipogenic medium containing physiological concentrations of insulin, cortisol and triiodothyronin, it could be shown that in the case of young adults as donors up to 80 per cent of the preadipocytes are able to differentiate *in vitro* whereas in the case of 80 year old donors the differentiation capacity was around 20 per cent[7]. Nevertheless, these data show that also in old people adipose tissue contains preadipocytes which are able to differentiate after stimulation with physiological factors. Addition of serum to the culture medium or subsequent subculturing is accompanied with a rapid loss of the capacity of the cell to differentiate possibly due to antiadipogenic factors in serum[7]. In addition, we have data suggesting that the pool of adipocyte precursor cells in adipose tissue is decreasing with age. When the number of isolated precursor cells was calculated per 100 g adipose tissue prepared for their isolation, we obtain up to 40 million precursor cells when the tissue was obtained from young adults as compared to less than 10 million cells/100 g tissue when the tissue was obtained from subjects older than 50 years.

Proliferation and differentiation of preadipocytes from children at different ages

To our knowledge there is only one study in which proliferation and differentiation of preadipocytes derived from adipose tissue from children at different ages has been investigated[3]. The preadipocytes were isolated from adipose tissue according to an established protocol. The results of this study showed age-dependent differences in the proliferation activity and the differentiation capacity of these cells cultured under serum-containing conditions. In accordance with the cyclic development of fat-free body mass and body fat mass during growth it could be shown that in the first year of life and in a period just before puberty these cells showed a maximum in their proliferation capacity as well as in their differentiation capacity. These data support the concept that the development of adipose tissue during childhood occurs mainly through a formation of new fat cells during sensitive periods. These periods might also be sensitive periods for the development of obesity. Another interesting finding in this study has been the observation that in adipose tissue of children compared to the adipose tissue of adults a much higher percentage of small fat cells with a diameter below 25 micrometers can be found. This observation indicates a higher activity of formation of new fat cells during childhood which subsequently increase their volume. The data of these studies and more recent studies using serum-free culture conditions together show that the formation of new fat cells is depending on the age and occurs at high degree during childhood.

Hormonal factors regulating adipose differentiation in human adipose tissue

An adequate *in vitro* model for studying human adipocyte differentiation and metabolism has been described[6]. In the following part clinical observations are related to *in vitro* finding using the above mentioned model for studying human adipocyte differentiation and metabolism. Clinical observations demonstrate an important role of glucocorticoids, GH, insulin and thyroid hormones in the control of adipose tissue cellularity[5]. *In vitro* data have shown in addition that these hormones are important regulators of human adipocyte differentiation.

Hypothyroidism is associated with a decreased number of fat cells although adipose tissue mass might be increased in individuals. In cultures of human preadipocytes triiodthyronine is able to control proliferation dependend on the applied concentration. Physiological concentrations of T3 are able to decrease proliferation and stimulate differentiation in the presence of other adipogenic hormones.

GH-deficient children have slightly increased body fat stores. On the cellular level their adipose tissue consists of enlarged fat cells which are decreased in number compared to healthy patients of the same age[10]. Using cultured human preadipocytes it could be clearly shown that GH is able to stimulate the proliferation of preadipocytes by an induction of IGF-I expression and secretion. These cells are then ready to differentiate in the presence of adipogenic factors. In addition, GH itself has a significant metabolic effect inhibiting glucose uptake and lipogenesis (diabetogenic effect). GH shows a direct lipolytic effect in mature human adipocytes thus being able to decrease adipocyte volume[8].

Glucocorticoid excess in an individual leads to the phenotypic characteristics of Cushing syndrome with increased adipose tissue mass, especially in the abdominal region. On the cellular level using cultured human preadipocytes glucocorticoids are potent stimulators of adipocyte differentiation[7]. Their effect could be partly explained by increasing arachidonic acid availability and prostacyclin production[9].

Due to the structural similarity of the insulin receptor and the IGF-I receptor, both ligands, insulin and IGF-I are able to stimulate the one or the other receptor depending on the concentration used. Both receptors are expressed in undifferentiated human preadipocytes and in human adipocytes. Whereas IGF-I in physiological concentrations is able to stimulate the proliferation of human preadipocytes, insulin is leading to the same effect at supra-physiological concentrations possibly via the IGF-I receptor. In mature adipocytes insulin at physiological concentrations and IGF-I at supra-physiological concentrations is able to stimulate glucose uptake and lipogenesis as well as to inhibit lipolysis probably through the insulin receptor. Insulin in physiological concentrations is absolutely necessary for adipose differentiation of preadipocytes. IGF-I at supra-physiological concentrations can substitute for insulin (see also[10]). Since human preadipocytes and adipocytes secrete large amounts of IGF-1 and IGFBP-3[11] we suggest that these factors are involved in an auto-/paracrine regulation of adipocyte differentiation and metabolism.

Besides these examples of stimulating factors there are also several anti-adipogenic factors inhibiting the differentiation of human preadipocytes. Examples for these factors are TGFβ, TNFα, EGF and PDGF, which have been shown to inhibit differentiation of adipocyte precursor cells[5]. In one sense also GH belongs to these factors since its metabolic anti-insulin-like activity inhibits the phenotypical appearance of mature fat cells *in vitro*. There are certainly more yet unknown factors in human serum which are able to inhibit and therefore control adipose differentiation in man.

Human preadipocyte cell lines

Although findings on regulation of human adipose tissue obtained in primary human adipocyte precursor cells might be more relevant than findings obtained in rodent derived cells or clonal cell lines, their are certain disadvantages of this system (availablility of tissue, interindividual variations, limited number of cells from one patient). Recently we have described a human liposarcoma cell line and an adipocyte precursor cell strain obtained from an infant with Simpson-Golabi-Behmel syndrome (SGBS cells), both with high capacity for adipose differentiation[12,13]. The results obtained so far with the latter cells show that these cells might be an adequate model for studying human fat cell development and metabolism. Since their differentiation capacity remains high over more than 50 generations SGBS cells represent an almost unlimited source of human adipocyte precursor cells which can be used for further studies.

Clinical evidence of human adipocyte apoptosis

Apoptosis is physiological process occuring in several organs by which selected cells can be eliminated quickly and efficiently from the body. Recently, apoptosis of adipocytes could be demonstrated in adipose tissue of patients with tumour cachexia[14]. *In vitro* experiments have shown that TNFα can induce apoptosis of cultured human preadipocytes[15]. Apoptosis can be demonstrated in *in vitro* differentiated human adipocytes and in SGBS cells (publication in preparation). Besides tumour cachexia there are several other clinical findings which suggest that apoptosis of fat cells may occur in human adipose tissue. These are summarized in Table 1. Apoptosis of fat cells seem to be present especially in situations when a fast and extensive loss of fat mass occurs. In addition, it has been hypothetize that apoptosis of adipocyte is a physiological process which occurs in parallel to the differentiation of new adipocytes by which the number of fat cells in the body is kept within a certain regulated range[16,17].

Table 1. Clinical conditions providing evidence for fat cell apoptosis in man

Tumour cachexia
Extreme weight loss in obese individuals
Reduction of fat mass in old people
Loss of body fat in anorexia nervosa
Loss of adipose tissue in patients with acquired lipodystrophy (Lawrence syndrome, Barraquer-Simons syndrome)
HAART-associated lipodystrophy

Results from animal experiments support this modern concept of a continous turn-over of fat cells in adipose tissue. During starvation a reduction of DNA in white fat depots can be observed in rats[18]. Sprague-Dawley rats with streptozotocine-induced diabetes show a reductions of adipocytes which is reversed upon treatment with insulin[19]. Intrathecal applikationen of leptin in rats results in dramatic weight loss and an almost complete loss of adipose tissue due to apoptosis of fat cells[20]. Treatment of ob/ob mice with the central acting substances SKF 38393 and bromocriptin leads to weight loss and to apoptosis of adipocytes[30]. These data show that through yet unknown mechanisms the central nervous system is able to reduce the number of peripheral fat cells by apoptosis. Future studies have to prove the physiological importance of adipocyte apoptosis in man and identify possible regulators.

References

1. McLaren DS. A fresh look at some perinatal growth and nutritional standards. *World Rev Nutr Diet* 1987; 49: 87–120.

2. Stratz W. *der Körper des Kindes*. Stuttgart: Emke-Verlag; 1902. vol 1.

3. Hauner H, Wabitsch M, Pfeiffer EF. Proliferation and differentiation of adipocyte recursor cells from children at different ages; In: *Obesity in Europe 1988*; Björntorp P (eds). London: John Libbey; 1989. pp. 195–200.

4. Hauner H. Physiology of the fat cell, with emphasis on the role of growth hormone. *Acta Paediatr* 1991; 383 (Suppl): 47–51.

5. Ailhaud G, Hauner H. Development of white adipose tissue, In: *Handbook of obesity*, Bray *et al.* (eds) (2nd edn). 2002 (in press).

6. Hauner H, Skurk T, Wabitsch M. *Methods in molecular biology*. vol.155, pp. 239–43.

7. Hauner H, Entenmann G, Wabitsch M, Gaillard D, Ailhaud G, Negrel R, Pfeiffer EF. Promoting effect of glucocorticoids on the differentiation of human adipocyte precursor cells cultured in an chemically defined medium. *J Clin Invest* 1989; 84: 1663–70.

8. Wabitsch M, Braun S, Hauner H, Heinze E, Ilondo MM, Shymko R *et al*. Mitogenic and antiadipogenic properties of human growth hormone in human adipocyte precursor cells in primary culture. *Pediatr Res* 1996; 40: 450–6.

9. Gaillard D, Wabitsch M, Pipy B, Negrel R. Control of terminal differentiation of adipose precursor cells by glucocorticoids. *J Lipid Res* 1991; 32: 569–79.

10. Wabitsch M, Hauner H, Heinze E, Teller W. The Role of GH/IGF's in adipocyte differentiation. *Metabolism* 1995; 44 (Suppl): 45–9.

11. Wabitsch M, Heinze E, Debatin K-M, Blum WF. IGF-I and IGFBP-3-Expression in cultured human preadipocytes and adipocytes. *Horm Metab Res* 2000; 32: 555–9.

12. Wabitsch M, Brüderlein S, Melzner I, Braun M, Mechtersheimer G, Möller P. LiSa-2, a novel human liposarcoma cell line with a high capacity for terminal adipose differentiation. In: *Methods in molecular biology*. vol.155, 2000.

13. Wabitsch M, Brenner RE, Melzner I, Braun M, Möller P, Heinze E, Debatin K-M, Hauner H. Characterization of a human preadipocyte cell strain with high capacity for adipose differentiation. *Int J Obes* 2001; 25: 8–15.

14. Prins JB, Walker NI, Winterford CM, Cameron DP. Human adipocyte apoptosis occurs in malignancy. *Biochem Biophys Res Commun* 1994; 205: 625–30.

15. Prins JB, Niesler CU, Winterford CM *et al*. Tumor necrosis factors-α induces apoptosis of human adipose cells. *Diabetes* 1997; 46: 1939–44.

16. Prins JB, O'Rahilly SO. Regulation of adipose cell number in man. *Clin Sci* 1997; 92: 3–11.

17. Sorisky A, Magun R, Gagnon AM. Adipose cell apoptosis: death in the energy depot. *Int J Obes Relat Metab Disord* 2000; 4 (Suppl): S3–S7.

18. Miller AHJ, Faust IM, Goldberger AC, Hirsch J. effects of severe long-term food deprivation and refeeding on adipose tissue cells in rat. *Am J Physiol* 1983; 245: E74–E80.

19. Geloen A, Roy P, Bukowiecki LJ. Regression of white adipose tissue in diabetic rats. *Am J Physiol* 1989; E547–E553.

20. Qian H, Azain MJ, Compton MM *et al*. Brain Administration of leptin causes deletion of adipocytes by apoptosis. *Endocrinology* 1998; 139: 791–4.

21. Scislowski PW, Jetton TL. Dopamine receptor agonist treatment increases apoptosis and fatty acid oxidation of white adipose tissue in ob/ob mice. *Diabetes* 1999; 48 (Suppl): A266.

Progress in Obesity Research: 9. Edited by *Geraldo Medeiros-Neto, Alfredo Halpern and Claude Bouchard*
©2003 John Libbey Eurotext Ltd, pp. 101–104.

CHAPTER 20

Lysophosphatidic acid: a potential paracrine regulator of adipogenesis

Stéphane Gesta, Marie-Françoise Simon, Philippe Valet and Jean Sébastien Saulnier-Blache

INSERM U586, Rangueil Hospital, 31403 Toulouse, France
[e-mail: saulnier@toulouse.inserm.fr]

Introduction

The main function of adipose tissue is to store excess lipid energy. This function sits in specialized cells (adipocytes) issued from a specific programme of differentiation (adipogenesis) of precursor cells (preadipocytes). In young and adult mammals, preadipocytes and adipocytes are both present and closely linked to each other via local regulating factors[1]. Several bioactive mediators (tumour necrosis factor, angiotensinogen, leptin, fatty acids, monobutyrin, eicosanoids, lysophosphatidic acid, etc. ...) are released from adipocytes, some of them being able to regulate proliferation and differentiation of preadipocytes[2,3]. Our group has identified lysophosphatidic acid as one of the bioactive mediators released by adipocytes and potentially involved in the paracrine control of adipogenesis.

Lysophosphatidic acid (LPA) (1-acyl-sn-glycerol-3-phosphate) is a phospholipid known for years as a necessary intermediate of glycerolipid synthesis. More recently, LPA has emerged as a potent bioactive mediator able to regulate motility and proliferation of cultured cells by acting via specific G-protein coupled receptors. So far, three subtypes (LPA1, 2, and 3) of LPA receptors have been identified and cloned[4–6]. LPA1-R is strongly expressed in the central nervous system[7,8], and its invalidation in mouse leads to a significant reduction in the body size of neonates which is maintained in adults[9].

LPA has been detected (in an albumin-bound form) in several biological fluids such as serum, follicular fluids, ascites, lacrimal fluid, or extracellular fluid of adipose tissue. Extracellular release of LPA has initially been demonstrated from platelets during aggregation and more recently from some cancer cell lines, and from adipocytes[10,11].

According to the literature, the origin of cellular release of LPA remains controversial[10]. LPA can be synthesized extracellularly via phospholipase A2-[12] or lysophospholipase D-activities[13]. Alternatively, LPA could also be synthesized intracellularly by a glycerol-3-phosphate acyl-transferase[14] or monoacyl glycerol kinase[15]. Whether intracellular LPA can be externalized by passive or active diffusion remains a matter of debate.

In parallel, extracellular LPA can be hydrolysed and inactivated by a dephosphorylation-process catalysed by lipid phosphate phosphatases (LPP). Three genes encoding LPP isoenzymes (LPP-1, -2, and -3) have been identified in human and rodents[16] but their relative contribution in the catabolism of LPA is still unclear.

In 1998[11], our group has demonstrated that adipocytes are able to release LPA in their incubation medium, and that LPA is able to activate motility and proliferation of preadipocyte. Based on these observations we proposed that LPA might participate to the paracrine control of adipogenesis. Our investigations led us to analyse in more details the transduction pathways involved in the bioactivity of LPA in preadipocytes, and to determine the metabolic pathways responsible for the release of LPA by adipocytes. The objective of the present review is to summarize our main results, as well as to put into prospective our current view about the possible involvement of LPA in the development of adipose tissue.

Release of LPA by adipocytes

In 1998, Valet *et al.*[11] demonstrated that conditioned–media prepared from adipocytes (human and 3T3F442A) exposed to an α2-adrenergic challenge were able to activate motility (actino-myosine contraction) and proliferation of recipient 3T3F442A preadipocytes. These biological responses were completely abolished by treating the conditioned media with a lysophospholipase (phospholipase B). In parallel, LPA appeared as the only lysophospholipid sensitive to phospholipase B and able to activate preadipocyte motility and proliferation. LPA-like activity was also found in the extracellular fluid of human adipose tissue collected by microdialysis. Release of LPA by adipocytes was confirmed after identification of [^{32}P]LPA in the conditioned media of [^{32}P]-prelabeled adipocytes. In order to directly quantify the amount of LPA released by adipocytes, we developed a highly sensitive radioenzymatic assay based on the transformation of LPA into [^{14}C]phosphatidic acid using of a recombinant LPA-acyltransferase[17].

Influence of LPA on preadipocyte proliferation (role of the LPA1-receptor)

Transduction pathways of LPA signal were initially studied in 3T3F442A preadipocyte. LPA led to a rapid (within 15 min) and dose-dependent (EC50: 1–5 nM) activation of actino-myosin contraction, characterized by a spreading of preadipocyte onto their growing substrate (11). A longer (24–48 h) exposure to LPA led to a dose-dependent (EC50: 100–110 nM) increase in preadipocyte number associated with an increase in [^{3}H]thymidine incorporation. LPA was also found to activate proliferation of stroma-vascular cells (containing preadipocytes) isolated from normal mouse adipose tissue and maintained in primary culture (unpublished data). In 3T3F442A preadipocytes, LPA led to the tyrosyl-phosphorylation of the Mitogen Activated Protein Kinase (ERK1 and ERK2) and of the p125 Focal Adhesion Kinase (FAK). Whereas ERK activation was mediated by a pertussis-toxin-sensitive G-protein, FAK activation was pertussis-toxin insensitive but was dependent upon the activation of the small GTPase RhoA[18]. These results strongly suggested that LPA bioactivity in preadipocytes was receptor-mediated.

The most abundant LPA-receptor expressed in 3T3F442A preadipocytes is the LPA1-R subtype. This receptor is 10–50 more abundant than LPA2-R subtype. LPA3-R subtype is not expressed in 3T3F442A preadipocytes[19]. LPA1-R subtype mRNA expression was found to be strongly depressed when 3T3F442A preadipocytes are differentiated into adipocytes[19]. Similarly, in mouse adipose tissue, LPA1-R mRNA were more abundant in the stromal-vascular fraction than in adipocyte fraction (unpublished data). These observations strongly suggest that preadipocytes constitute the preferential target cells of LPA in the adipose tissue.

Permanent over-expression of an antisense RNA directed against LPA1-R subtype significantly attenuated the ability of LPA to activate both spreading and proliferation of 3T3F442A preadipocytes[19]. Similarly, stroma-vascular cells isolated from adipose tissue of LPA1-R knockout mice[9] are completely insensitive to LPA (unpublished data). All these results strongly suggest the predominant role of LPA1-R in bioactivity of LPA in preadipocytes.

Phenotype of LPA1-R knock-out mice

LPA1-R expression is elevated in the cerebral cortex and the olfactory bulb in mouse embryo. Targeted deletion of LPA1-R in mouse results in approximately 50 per cent neonatal lethality due to an impairment of suckling behaviour in neonatal pups. Survivors exhibit a reduced body size and reduced body weight[9]. Despite their growth alteration, LPA1-R knockout mice possesses similar, and sometime higher, amount of adipose tissue than wild type mice (unpublished data). In addition, LPA1-R knockout mice were completely insensitive to high fat diet-induced obesity, partly due to a reduction in food intake (unpublished data). Further analysis of LPA1-R knockout mice is now necessary to determine the specific contribution of preadipocyte LPA receptivity in alteration of adipose tissue development.

Metabolism of extracellular LPA in preadipocytes and adipocytes

Phospholipase A2-activity has previously been proposed to be at the origin of the release of LPA by platelets and ovarian cancer cells. In adipocytes, treatment with different phospholipase A2 inhibitors significantly reduced the release of eicosanoid, but not that of LPA (unpublished data). These results indicated the involvement of a phospholipase A2-independent metabolic pathway in the release of LPA by adipocytes.

We recently observed that, in parallel to LPA, culture media of adipocytes contained a LPA-synthesizing activity (LPA-SA). We identified this activity as a secreted lysophospholipase D (lysoPLD)-activity catalysing hydrolysis of lysophosphatidylcholine (LPC) (also secreted by adipocytes) into LPA[20]. Biochemical analysis revealed that lysoPLD-activity requires divalent ions (preferentially cobalt) for its activity, prefers acyl- rather than alkyl-LPC as substrate, is insensitive to primary alcohol (conversely to classical phospholipase D), and is strongly up-regulated during conversion of 3T3F442A preadipocytes into adipocytes[20]. We think that lysoPLD activity is mainly involved in release of LPA by adipocytes. Whereas lysoPLD activity has also been described in other biological fluids[10], the enzyme responsible for this activity remains unknown. We are in the process of purifying and cloning adipocyte lyso-PLD-activity[22].

In parallel to its synthesis, catabolic enzymes can inactivate LPA. By using radiolabled LPA as substrate we determined that more than 90 per cent of LPA hydrolysis results from its transformation into monoacyl glycerol phosphate[21]. This reaction is catalysed by lipid phosphate phosphohydrolases (LPP) located at the surface of preadipocyte and adipocyte plasma membrane. Three LPP subtypes (LPP-1, -2, and -3) are present in preadipocytes and adipocytes with the following rank order of expression of their mRNA: LPP-3 >> LPP1 > LPP2[21]. Inhibition of LPP activity with sodium orthovanadate significantly increases LPA release by adipocytes[21], indicating that these enzymes exert a constitutive negative influence on LPA release.

Perspectives

We have now clear evidences that LPA is released from adipocytes as the result of a fine-tuning of the balance between lysoPLD- and LPP-activities. In parallel, LPA is able to act on preadipocytes to regulate their growth via a specific receptor: the LPA1-receptor. Based upon these conclusions, LPA fulfills the criteria of a paracrine factor potentially involved in the regulation of adipogenesis.

So far, most of our investigations were performed *in vitro*, and further efforts will be necessary to determine whether LPA of the adipose tissue has an *in vivo* relevance. It will be necessary to identify the physiological and/or pathological situations (in animals and human) associated with modification of adipocyte-LPA release, and/or LPA1-receptor expression. It will also be necessary to complete the phenotype of LPA1-receptor knockout mice. Because this knockout is not tissue specific, we will have to discriminate between the effects directly due to alteration of preadipocyte LPA receptivity, and those due to the alteration of other organs involved in energy balance. In parallel, our results reveal that a fine tuning between lysoPLD- and LPP-activities conditions the amount of LPA released by adipocytes. Further efforts will be necessary to identify the factors (hormones, nutrients, pharmacological agents) able to control lysoPLD and/or LPP activities *in vivo*. Alternatively, transgenic alteration of lysoPLD and/or LPP expression will be an valuable approach to alter the amount of LPA in the adipose tissue and to determine the relevance of this bioactive phospholipid *in vivo*.

References

1. MacDougald OA, Mandrup S Adipogenesis: forces that tip the scales. *Trends Endocrinol Metab* 2002; 13: 5–11.

2. Négrel R. Paracrine/autocrine signals and adipogenesis. In: *Progress in Obesity Research: 8*. London: John Libbey, 1999.

3. Trayhurn P, Beattie JH Physiological role of adipose tissue: white adipose tissue as an endocrine and secretory organ. *Proc Nutr Soc* 2001; 60: 329–39.

4. Goetzl E, An S Diversity of cellular receptors and functions for the lysophospholipid growth factors lysophosphatidic acid and sphingosin 1-phosphate. *FASEB J* 12: 1589–98.

5. Chun J, Contos JJ. Munroe DA growing family of receptor genes for lysophosphatidic acid (LPA) and other lysophospholipids (LPs). *Cell Biochem Biophysics* 1999; 30: 213–42.

6. Hla T, Lee MJ, Ancellin N, Paik JH, Kluk MJ. Lysophospholipids – receptor revelations. *Science* 2001; 294: 1875–8.

7. Hecht JH, Weiner JA, Post SR, Chun J. Ventricular zone gene-1 (vzg-1) encodes a lysophosphatidic acid receptor expressed in neurogenic regions of the developing cerebral cortex. *J Cell Biol* 1996; 135: 1071–83.

8. Chun J. Lysophospholipid receptors: implications for neural signaling. *Crit Rev Neurobiol* 1999; 13: 151–68.

9. Contos JJ, Fukushima N, Weiner JA, Kaushal D, Chun J. Requirement for the lpA1 lysophosphatidic acid receptor gene in normal suckling behavior. *Proc Natl Acad Sci USA* 2000; 97: 13384–89.

10. Pages C, Simon MF, Valet P, Saulnier-Blache JS Lysophosphatidic acid synthesis and release. *Prostaglandins and other lipid mediators* 2001; 1: 1–10.

11. Valet P, Pages C, Jeanneton O, Daviaud D, Barbe P, Record M *et al*. Alpha2-adrenergic receptor-mediated release of lysophosphatidic acid by adipocytes. A paracrine signal for preadipocyte growth. *J Clin Invest* 1998; 101: 1431–8.

12. Fourcade O, Simon MF, Viodé C, Rugani N, Leballe F, Ragab A *et al.* Secretory phospholipase A2 generates the novel lipid mediator lysophosphatidic acid in membrane microvesicles shed from activated cells. *Cell* 1995; 80: 919–27.

13. Tokumura A, Harada K, Fukuzawa K, Tsukatani H. Involvement of lysophospholipase D in the production of lysophosphatidic acid in rat plasma. *Biochim Biophys Acta* 1986; 875: 31–8.

14. Haldar D, Vancura A. Glycerophosphate acyltransferase from liver. *Methods Enzymol* 1992; 209: 64–72.

15. Simpson C, Itabe H, Reynolds C, King W, Glomset J. Swiss 3T3 cells preferentially incorporate sn-2-arachidonoyl monoacylglycerol into sn-1-stearoyl-2-arachidonoyl phosphatidylinositol. *J Biol Chem* 1991; 266: 15902–9.

16. Waggoner DW, Xu J, Singh I, Jasinska R, Zhang QX, Brindley DN. Structural organization of mammalian lipid phosphate phosphatases: implications for signal transduction. *Biochim Biophys Acta* 1999; 1439: 299–316.

17. Saulnier-Blache JS, Girard A, Simon MF, Lafontan M, Valet P. A simple and highly sensitive radioenzymatic assay for lysophosphatidic acid quantification. *J Lipid Res* 2000; 41: 1947–51.

18. Pagès C, Girard A, Jeanneton O, Barbe P, Wolf C, Lafontan M *et al.* LPA as a paracrine mediator of adipocyte growth and function. *NY Acad Sci* 2000; 905: 159–64.

19. Pagès C, Daviaud D, An S, Krief S, Lafontan M, Valet P, Saulnier-Blache J. Endothelial Differentiation Gene-2 receptor is involved in lysophosphatidic acid-dependent control of 3T3F442A preadipocyte proliferation and spreading. *J Biol Chem* 2001; 276: 11599–605.

20. Gesta S, Simon M, Rey A, Sibrac D, Girard A, Lafontan M *et al.* Secretion of a lysophospholipase D activity by adipocytes: involvement in lysophosphatidic acid synthesis. *J Lipid Res* 2002; 43: 904–10.

21. Simon MF, Rey A, Castan-Laurel I, Gres S, Sibrac D, Valet P, Saulnier-Blache JS. Expression of ecto-lipid phosphate phosphohydrolases in 3T3F442A preadipocytes and adipocytes: involvement in the control of lysophosphatidic acid production. *J Biol Chem* 2002; 277: 23131–6.

22. Ferry G, Tellier E, Try A, Grés S, Naime I, Simon MF *et al.* Autotaxin is released from adipocytes, catalyses lysophosphatidic acid synthesis and activates preadipocyte proliferation. *J Biol Chem* 2003; 278: 18162-9.

Progress in Obesity Research: 9. Edited by *Geraldo Medeiros-Neto, Alfredo Halpern and Claude Bouchard*
©2003 John Libbey Eurotext Ltd, pp. 105–108.

CHAPTER 21

White adipose cell apoptosis

Alexander Sorisky and AnneMarie Gagnon

Department of Medicine and Biochemistry, Microbiology & Immunology, Ottawa Health Research Institute,
University of Ottawa, Ottawa, Canada
[e-mail: asorisky@ohri.ca]

Introduction to white adipose tissue – energy storage and much more

It was not long ago that adipose tissue was viewed as rather monotonous in its function, serving to store surplus energy as triacyglycerol, and to release it as free fatty acids (lipolysis) as a function of caloric demand. Over the past few years, adipocytes have been identified as a source of an exciting parade of bioactive factors that can influence metabolism and vascular biology[1]. In addition to an overflow of FFA into the circulation, altered secretion of these recently appreciated 'adipocytokines' in the setting of obesity may offer other mechanisms by which excess adipose tissue heightens the risk of type 2 diabetes and cardiovascular disease. For example, to mention a small subset, deficient adiponectin may increase insulin resistance by reducing fatty acid oxidation, increasing hepatic glucose production, and predisposing to vascular injury[2,3]. Over-production of tumour necrosis factor α (TNFα) may interfere with insulin signal transduction[4], and elevated plasminogen activator inhibitor 1 (PAI-1) may predispose to atherosclerosis[5].

Adipose tissue remodeling

Given that fat cells are an important source of cytokines/hormones/peptides, learning more about what regulates adipose tissue development and its remodeling during adult life is important. Adipose tissue mass is clearly influenced by adipocyte size[6]. However, there also appears to be a dynamic cellular turnover of adipose cells, consisting of the formation of adipocytes from fibroblast-like progenitor cells called preadipocytes, possible de-differentiation back to adipocytes, and apoptosis of preadipocytes and adipocytes[7]. This review will provide an update on adipose cell apoptosis.

Adipose tissue apoptosis in rodent models and humans

There are a variety of reports indicating that when rodents or humans are subjected to certain stresses, apoptosis can be detected in their adipose tissue. Reductions in adipose tissue cellularity (measured by tissue DNA content) have been described in rodents subjected to starvation or uncontrolled diabetes mellitus induced by streptozotocin, as recently reviewed[7]. Apoptosis, based on characteristic oligonucleosomal DNA laddering, has been documented in tissue explants from cachectic cancer patients[8]. A lipodystrophy syndrome associated with HIV infection and the use of protease inhibitor therapy results in remarkable atrophy of peripheral fat, and investigators have noted apoptosis, assessed by terminal deoxynucleotidyl transferase nick end labeling (TUNEL), in subcutaneous leg fat biopsies of such patients[9].

Other treatments have also been found to elicit adipose tissue apoptosis. When rats were administered intra-cerebroventricular leptin for 5 days (at doses that have no effect when given peripherally), apoptotic changes were seen in white adipose tissue, but not with pair-fed controls[10]. These included adipocyte loss, condensed chromatin in adipocytes, and a greater number of small adipocytes. High levels of peripheral leptin in rats have been generated by hepatic expression following adenoviral-leptin cDNA infusion, and though also leading to severe reductions in fat, did not change the DNA content of fat pads[11]. Decreases in fat also occurred following subcutaneous leptin administration, with no apoptosis detected[12].

Thiazolidinediones (TZD) are ligands and activators of peroxisome proliferator-activated receptor γ (PPARγ), a transcription factor expressed strongly in adipocytes that increases insulin sensitivity and activates adipogenesis[13]. When used as a treatment for type 2 diabetes mellitus, they cause a redistribution of adipose tissue in humans, with reductions in visceral intra-abdominal fat, and increases in subcutaneous fat[14]. TZD studies in obese Zucker rats have noted an actual reduction in adipocyte size, consistent with the established role of PPARγ in generating smaller newly differentiated adipocytes[15]. However, these rodent studies also demonstrated a selective apoptosis of enlarged hypertrophied adipocytes, contributing to the overall reduction in average adipocyte volume[15,16]. Recent work with obese Zucker rats have linked the TZD-induced large fat cell apoptosis with upregulation of galectin-12 mRNA in adipose tissue[17]. Galectin-12 belongs to the lectin family, proteins which bind carbohydrate residues on cell surface proteins, and some galectins are known to induce apoptosis in T cells.

Conjugated linoleic acid (CLA; conjugated dienoic derivatives of linoleic acid) supplementation to mice (1 % wt/wt with 10 per cent total fat diet) results in reduction of fat mass via apoptosis (within 5 days), possibly due to its ability to increase TNFα (see below)[18]. Upregulation of uncoupling protein 2 (UCP2) mRNA also occurred, and this was postulated to be linked to apoptosis via resulting decreased cellular ATP levels. Recently, it was reported that the reduction of fat in mice was specific to certain isomers of CLA; these authors also observed an increase in UCP2 mRNA, but TNFα mRNA decreased in their study[19].

Apoptosis induced in adipose cell culture models

Studies performed in this context have been aimed at a more mechanistic understanding of adipose cell apoptosis. One approach to induce apoptosis is growth factor deprivation (serum starvation). Growth factors may act to keep cells alive using a variety of signal transduction routes, including activation of phosphoinositide 3-kinase (PI3K) and its target, protein kinase B (PKB; also known as Akt). Using the 3T3-L1 preadipocyte cell line, two laboratories identified IGF-1 as a survival factor whose action was dependent on PI3K, but not mammalian target of rapamycin (mTOR) or p38 MAP kinase[20,21]. There were conflicting data about the requirement for p42/44 mitogen-activated protein kinase (MAPK) in this context. Another group has shown that constitutive activation of p38 MAPK actually induced cell death[22]. PI3K is able to generate two lipid products, PI(3,4,5)P3 and PI(3,4)P2, and also has the potential of acting as a serine protein kinase[23]. Exogenous PI(3,4,5)P3 was able to reduce apoptosis, and levels of activated caspase 3, in serum-deprived 3T3-L1 preadipocytes, either when added alone, or in the presence of IGF-1 when PI3K was pharmacologically inhibited. A similar pattern was observed with the ability of PI(3,4,5)P3 to induce PKB phosphorylation (indicative of activation), consistent with its proposed role in survival signaling. The transcription factor cAMP-response element-binding protein (CREB) influences 3T3-L1 adipocyte survival, by regulating the levels of PKB and potentially other proteins relevant to cell death[24].

Adipose cell culture models have also been used to explore apoptotic responses observed in vivo. For example, adipose tissue apoptosis in patients with HIV-associated lipodystrophy treated with protease inhibitors has prompted some investigators to examine the direct effect of these drugs on adipocyte apoptosis in culture[25].

With regards to adipose tissue remodeling via adipogenesis, an important question is whether there is a difference in susceptibility to apoptosis as a function of stage of differentiation. As 3T3-L1 preadipocytes differentiate into adipocytes, they acquire a resistance to apoptosis induced by growth factor deprivation[26,27]. This was documented by DNA laddering, Hoescht staining, and TUNEL. During differentiation, there was an upregulation in protein expression of two anti-apoptotic proteins, Bcl-2 and NAIP. It will be important to determine whether this occurs during human preadipocyte differentiation into adipocytes.

TNFα induces apoptosis in cultured human preadipocytes and in adipose tissue explants, and intra-abdominal omental preadipocytes are more susceptible compared to their subcutaneous counterparts[28,29]. Intracellular concentrations of ceramide rise upon TNFα stimulation, and a cell-permeable analogue of ceramide, C2-ceramide, causes apoptosis in rat preadipocyte cultures[30]. However, TNFα signaling is complex, and other signaling pathways are undoubtedly involved. Since higher amounts of TNFα are secreted by hypertrophied adipocytes in the obese state, it has been proposed that this cytokine may help curtail further adipose tissue accumulation via the induction of apoptosis[28].

Adipose tissue apoptosis: what are the implications?

A recent perspective, based on lean mouse models, distinguishes between reduced adipose tissue mass arising from a lack of normal adipocytes versus otherwise normal adipocytes that contain reduced amounts of triacylglycerol[31]. Although lean, the former results in insulin resistance and dyslipidaemia, similar to human congenital or acquired lipodystrophy. Clearly, an isolationist view of simply ablating large amounts of adipose tissue, without consideration of ongoing energy surplus and nutrient partioning/spillover, is not a viable therapeutic goal. In a similar vein, others have proposed that even in the case of an expanded adipose tissue mass, the inability to further increase storage capacity in the face of an unremitting positive energy balance may be the factor that results in ectopic fat accumulation in liver, muscle, and pancreatic β cells, contributing to the emergence of insulin resistance/type 2 diabetes mellitus in the obese[32,33].

We still know very little about *in vivo* rates, or the identity of environmental/genetic regulators, of adipose cell turnover within adipose tissue depots. Are there significant perturbations in the flux of these cells in individuals that are lipodystrophic, lean, obese, or obese and diabetic? Might cell turnover rates have an impact on overall adipose tissue lipogenesis and lipolysis, as well as adipocytokine secretion? Can the turnover of adipose cells be manipulated to remodel, but not ablate, adipose tissue to ameliorate insulin resistance? These are some of the questions that lie ahead in the field of adipose cell apoptosis.

References

1. Saltiel A. You are what you secrete. *Nature Med* 2001; 7: 887–8.

2. Berg AH *et al.* ACRP30/adiponectin: an adipocytokine regulating glucose and lipid metabolism. *Trends Endocrinol Metab* 2002; 13: 84–9.

3. Kubota N *et al.* Disruption of adiponectin causes insulin resistance and neointimal formation. *J Biol Chem* 2002; 277: 25863–6.

4. Hotamisligil GS *et al.* IRS-1-mediated inhibition of insulin receptor tyrosine kinase activity in TNF-alpha- and obesity-induced insulin resistance. *Science* 1996; 271: 665–8.

5. Juhan-Vague I, Alessi MC Regulation of fibrinolysis in the development of atherothrombosis: role of adipose tissue. *Thromb Haemost* 1999; 82: 832–6.

6. Hirsch J The search for new ways to treat obesity. *Proc Natl Acad Sci USA* 2002; 99: 9096–7.

7. Prins JB, O'Rahilly S Regulation of adipose cell number in man. *Clin Sci* 1997; 92: 3–11.

8. Prins JB *et al.* Human adipocyte apoptosis occurs in malignancy. *Biochem Biophys Res Commun* 1994; 205: 625–30.

9. Domingo P *et al.* Subcutaneous adipocyte apoptosis in HIV-1 protease inhibitor-associated lipodystrophy. *AIDS* 1999; 13: 2261–7.

10. Qian H *et al.* Brain administration of leptin causes deletion of adipocytes by apoptosis. *Endocrinology* 1998; 139: 791–4.

11. Zhou YT *et al.* Reversing adipocyte differentiation: implications for treatment of obesity. *Proc Natl Acad Sci USA* 1999; 96: 2391–5.

12. Sarmiento U *et al.* Morphologic and molecular changes induced by recombinant human leptin in the white and brown adipose tissues of C57BL/6 mice. *Lab Invest* 1997; 77: 243–56.

13. Rosen ED *et al.* Transcriptional regulation of adipogenesis. *Genes Dev* 2000; 14: 1293–307.

14. Kelly IE *et al.* Effects of a thiazolidinedione compound on body fat and fat distribution of patients with type 2 diabetes. *Diabetes Care* 1999; 22: 288–93.

15. Okuno A *et al.* Troglitazone increases the number of small adipocytes without change of white adipose tissue mass in obese Zucker rats. *J Clin Invest* 1998; 101: 1354–61.

16. Yamauchi T *et al.* The mechanisms by which both heterozygous peroxisome proliferator-activated receptor γ (PPARγ) deficiency and PPARγ agonist improve insulin sensitivity. *J Biol Chem* 2001; 276: 41245–54.

17. Hotta K *et al.* Galectin-12, as adipose-expressed galectin-like molecule possessing apoptosis-inducing activity. *J Biol Chem* 2001; 276: 34089–97.

18. Tsuboyama-Kasaoka N *et al.* Conjugated linoleic acid supplementation reduces adipose tissue by apoptosis and develops lipodystrophy in mice. *Diabetes* 2000; 49: 1534–42.

19. Roche HM *et al.* Isomer-dependent metabolic effects of conjugated linoleic acid. *Diabetes* 2002; 51: 2037–44.

20. Gagnon A *et al.* Phosphatidylinositol-3,4,5-trisphosphate is required for IGF-1-mediated survival of 3T3-L1 preadipocytes. *Endocrinology* 2001; 142: 205–12.

21. Niesler CU *et al.* IGF-1 inhibits apoptosis induced by serum withdrawal, but potentiates TNF-α-induced apoptosis, in 3T3-L1 preadipocytes. *J Endocrinol* 2000; 167: 165–74.

22. Engelman JA *et al.* Constitutively active mitogen-activated protein kinase 6 (MKK6) or salicylate induces spontaneous 3T3-L1 adipogenesis. *J Biol Chem* 1999; 274: 35630–8.

23. Cantley LC The phosphoinositide 3-kinase pathway. *Science* 2002; 296: 1655–7.

24. Reusch JEB, Klemm DJ. Inhibition of cAMP-response element-binding protein activity decreases protein kinase B/Akt expression in 3T3-L1 adipocytes and induces apoptosis. *J Biol Chem* 2002; 277: 1426–32.

25. Dowell P *et al.* Suppression of preadipocyte differentiation and promotion of adipocyte death by HIV protease inhibitors. *J Biol Chem* 2000; 275: 41325–32.

26. Magun R *et al.* The effect of adipocyte differentiation on the capacity of 3T3-L1 cells to undergo apoptosis in response to growth factor deprivation. *Int J Obes* 1998; 22: 567–71.

27. Magun R *et al.* Expression and regulation of neuronal apoptosis inhibitory protein during adipocyte differentiation. *Diabetes* 1998; 47: 1948–52.

28. Prins JB *et al.* Tumor necrosis factor-α induces apoptosis of human adipose cells. *Diabetes* 1997; 46: 1939–44.

29. Niesler CU *et al.* Human preadipocytes display a depot-specific susceptibility to apoptosis. *Diabetes* 1998; 47: 1365–8.

30. Kim HS *et al.* Induction of apoptosis by all-trans-retinoic acid and C2-ceramide treatment in rat stromal-vascular cultures. *Biochem Biophys Res Commun* 2000; 2000: 76–80.

31. Reitman ML Metabolic lessons from genetically lean mice. *Annu Rev Nutr* 2002; 22: 459–82.

32. Danforth E Jr. Failure of adipocyte differentiation causes type 2 diabetes mellitus? *Nature Genet* 2000; 26: 13.

33. Weyer C *et al.* Enlarged subcutaneous abdominal adipocyte size, but not obesity itself, predicts type 2 diabetes independent of insulin resistance. *Diabetolgia* 2000; 43: 1498–506.

CHAPTER 22

Brown fat cell apoptosis

Alessandra Bulbarelli[1], Annalisa Cardile[1], Michele O. Carruba[1,2] and Enzo Nisoli[1,2]

[1]*Center for Study and Research on Obesity, Department of Preclinical Sciences, LITA Vialba, L. Sacco Hospital, University of Milan, via G.B. Grassi, 74 – 20157 Milan, Italy and* [2]*Istituto Auxologico Italiano, via Spagnoletto 3, 20149, Milan, Italy*
[e-mail: enzo.nisoli@unimi.it]

Introduction

Anatomically an organ is defined as a series of tissues which jointly perform one or more interconnected functions. The 'adipose organ' is constituted by two different tissues: the white (WAT) and brown adipose tissues (BAT), which collaborate in apportioning the energy contained in lipids between thermogenesis and the other metabolic functions. Fat tissues are organized in discrete depots (subcutaneous or visceral depots) throughout the body, which are characterized by specific vascularization, innervation and cell pattern. In situations of thermogenic need the brown component becomes active and burns the energy provided essentially by the WAT. WAT is the principal site in the body for energy storage. It also helps to regulate energy homeostasis via the hormones it secretes, including leptin. The quantity of body fat varies widely in mammals, ranging from 2 per cent to > 50 per cent of body mass. This large variation in fat mass is determined by the individual's genetic background and by environmental factors, including diet and physical activity. Adipocytes also infiltrate many organs, such as skin, bone marrow and pancreas.

Typical pathologies of the adipose organ are obesity and lipoatrophy, which are characterized by increased or decreased fat stores, whose size is dependent on the number and volume of the adipocytes within them (Hauner[1]; Arner[2]). Adipocyte volume can increase or decrease through lipogenesis or lipolysis, respectively. Increase in adipocyte number can occur at any stage of life and is considered to result from one or more cycles of replication of preadipocytes (i.e. committed stem cells of mesenchymal origin) followed by their differentiation (Hauner[1]). Little is documented about the occurence or process of adipocyte loss, even if a number of recent reports suggest that adipocyte deletion occurs, and apoptosis is the cellular process involved.

Apoptosis

Apoptosis, or programmed cell death, is the process that removes surplus or harmful cells cleanly and specifically during animal development or ageing, in other words, is the highly conserved innate mechanism by which eukariotic cells commit suicide. For this reason apoptosis plays an essential role in the normal development of vertebrate. It is defined by a characteristic series of morphological and biochemical changes including membrane blebbing, external display of phosphatidylserine, cleavage of nuclear lamins and poly(ADP-ribose) polymerase, chomatine condensation, and DNA cleavage, culminating in fragmentation of the cell into apoptotic bodies (Evan[3]; Raff[4]; Yao and Cooper[5]).

The molecular mechanisms that regulate apoptosis are not yet completely understood. It is known that apoptosis can be induced by the transcriptional activation of genes, as well as by extracellular signals, delivered by cytotoxic cells, anti-cancer drugs and 'death-inducing' cytokines (death factors).

The mechanism by which apoptotic signals are transduced through the cell is well conserved among metazoan organisms (see Hengartner[6]). In mammalian cells, but not in nematodes, two families of proteins have been shown to play important roles in the regulation of cell death: members of the family of cysteine proteases related to the interleukin-1β converting enzyme (ICE), named caspases, and Bcl-2-related proteins.

Caspase enzymes

The best characterized signal transduction pathways that mediate apoptosis are the cell surface receptors of the tumour necrosis factor (TNF) family, including CD95 (Fas/Apo-1) and CD120a (p55 TNF-R1) (Tartaglia[7]; Wallach[8]). Engagement of Fas/TNF-R1 receptor by proteins like Fas or TNF-α (Nagata[9]) leads to formation of a protein complex known as the DISC (death-inducing signalling complex) (Medema[10]; Muzio[11]). This complex consists of Fas/TNF-R1, FADD (MORT1), and pro-caspase-8 (MACH/FLICE/Mhc5). Once pro-caspase-8 is recruited, it is processed and released from the complex in active form to activate the downstream 'effector' caspases (Medema[10]; Srinivasula[12]; Muzio[13]). The caspase family has been divided into different groups based upon sequence homology and substrate specificity: caspases 2, 3 and 7 as 'effector' of apoptosis and caspases 6, 8 and 9 as 'initiator'.

In particular, it has been shown that when procaspase-8 is processed to generate the active enzyme at the DISC, and it is released from the DISC cleaves and activates procaspase-3 (Kischkel[14]) with production of caspase-3. Caspase 3 has a short pro-domain and works as effector, by cleaving various intracellular substrates, eventually resulting in the morphological (i.e. well defined masses of condensed chromatin abutting the nuclear envelope, cell shrinkage, convolution of the nuclear and cellular outline and fragmentation of the cell to form membrane-bounded apoptotic bodies, which are phagocyted by adjacent cells) and biochemical changes (cleavage of the DNA between nucleosomes resulting in a ladder pattern on DNA gel electrophoresis) seen in cell undergoing apoptosis.

Bcl-2 family and related cytoplasmic proteins

The Bcl-2 family is composed of a number of gene that play a critical role in the control of mitochondrial integrity, since the loss of mitochondrial membrane potential is the ultimate determinant for apoptotic cell death. Some members of this family, such as Bax, Bid, Bak, and Bad, appear to promote apoptosis (Gross[15]). In contrast, the expression of other members, such as Bcl-2 and Ced 9, can prevent apoptosis by inhibiting adapters needed for activation of the caspases that dismantle the cell (Adams and Cory[16]; Boise and Thompson[17]).

Recently, Bcl-2 has been demonstrated to be involved in Fas-mediated apoptosis (Scaffidi[18]). Bcl-x, another member of the Bcl-2 family, has two alternatively spliced forms, the anti-apoptotic Bcl-xL and the apoptotic Bcl-xS (Min[19]). In particular, several studies suggest that Bcl-xL and Bcl-2 exert their antiapoptotic action upstream of the processing of certain caspases to their catalically active forms (Chinnaiyan[20]).

Mitochondria and apoptosis

Mitochondria are organelles with two well defined compartments: the matrix surrounded by the inner membrane (IM), and the intermembrane space surrounded by the outer membrane (OM). Apoptotic OM permeabilization involve the release of proteins which are normally confined to the intermembrane space of these organelles, including cytochrome c, certain procaspases, adenylate kinase 2 and apoptosis inducing factor.

Three phases of cell death can be distinguished: initiation, decision and degradation. During the first phase (initiation), cells accumulate effector molecules which directly act on mitochondria to determine the mitochondrial membrane permeabilization (MMP). The nature of these effectors depend on the death-inducing stimulus. During the second phase (decision), an MMP occurs, presumably through a limited set of mechanism, and seals the cell's fate. Finally the metabolic consequence of MMP as well as the leakage of proteins normally confined to mitochondria determines the catabolic features of cell death, with irreversible loss of vital cellular function and /or activation of nucleases and proteases (degradation).

It has been recently suggested that mitochondria are involved in apoptosis transduction signal. In particular, the pro-apoptotic members of the Bcl-2 family, which bear resemblance to channel-forming bacterial toxins, induce MMP when added to purified mitochondria as recombinant protein. This has been shown for Bax, Bak and Bid, and probably reflects the principal mechanism by which these proteins trigger cell death (Jürgensmeier[21], Pastorino[22]).

Accordingly, translocation of Bax from the cytosol (where it is present as a monomer) to mitochondrial membranes (where it forms a dimer or higher-order oligomers) has been reported in a wide array of apoptosis-inducing circumstances. The subcellular localization of Bad protein is regulated by kinase and phosphatases. Only non-phosphorylated Bad is able to interact and antagonize the anti-apoptotic

Bcl-2 or Bcl-XL on the outer membrane (OM). Bad can be phosphorylated on Ser 136 by Akt/PKB/RAC, or on Ser 112 by a mitochondrion anchored cAMP-dependent protein kinase A (Harada[23]). The OM-associated Raf 1 also stimulated the phosphorylation and inactivation of Bad.

Bid is another pro-apoptotic Bcl-2 family member that can traslocate to mitochondria. The cytosolic Bid is cleaved by Caspase-8, an apical caspase activated through ligation of TNF family death receptors. The truncated cleavage product (tBid) translocates to mitochondrial membranes. Bid$^{-/-}$ mice are resistant to hepatocyte apoptosis induced by antibody against CD95, emphasizing the importance of this pathway for CD95/Caspase-8 signalling in at least some tissues.

Taken into mind these notions, the present report would like to briefly review the first reports on the apoptotic mechanisms in brown and white fat cells, and the putative relevance of these mechanisms in physiological and pathophysiological conditions.

Brown adipose tissue

Apoptosis of cultured brown adipocytes

TNF-α has been recently shown to induce apoptosis of primary culture of rat brown adipocytes (Nisoli[24]). After 2 h of treatment 10 µg/ml cycloheximide (CHX), even if devoted of cytotoxicity *per se*, potentiates the TNF-α-induced apoptosis so that the addition of as little as 1 pM TNF-α led to nearly 50 per cent cytotoxicity. Transmission electron microscopy and measurements of the fragmentation of DNA into oligonucleosome-length fragments on gel electrophoresis confirmed that TNF-α plus CHX induced degeneration of brown adipocytes through an apoptotic pathway. In particular, transmission electron microscopy of TNF-α (10 pM) plus CHX (10 µg/ml) treated cells revealed compact patches of condensed nuclear chromatin. The cells were observed to be in various stages of degeneration, which is consistent with the asynchronism shown by phase-contrast microscopy. The cytoplasm was generally depleted of lipid droplets, and showed mitochondria and organelle breakdown.

These results were confirmed also by Porras[25] in rat fetal brown adipocytes in primary culture. Most of the fetal cells undergoing apoptosis after TNF-α treatment did not express PCNA, the δ subunit of DNA polymerase, that is maximally expressed during the S phase, suggesting an induction of apoptosis by TNF-α in non-proliferative cells. Interestingly, noradrenaline and insulin-like growth factor (IGF)-1 prevented TNF-α-induced apoptosis of brown adipocytes (Nisoli[24], Porras[25]).

In addition, serum deprivation of immortalized brown adipocyte cell line resulted in growth arrest in G0/G1 phases of the cell cycle and apoptosis (Navarro[26,27]). This was concurrent with a dramatic increase in the expression of the proapoptotic protein Bcl-XL, with a downregulation of Bcl-2 protein content and a loss of mitochondrial membrane potential. Both phosphatidylinositol (PI) 3-kinase and mitogen-activated protein kinase (MAPK) pathways are necessary for IGF-1 full survival effect under these experimental conditions (Navarro[26]).

Apoptosis of brown adipocytes as a physiological homeostatic process

Cold acclimation (4 °C), which is accompanied by heat production, increased the phosphorylation of MAPK (Erk1 and Erk2) in rat brown fat, and protected cells in the tissue from apoptosis (Lindquist and Rehnmark[28]). The cessation of the sympathetic stimulus, by transferring cold-adapted animals to termoneutral temperature (28 °C), caused an increase rate of apoptosis in the tissue. Thus, the regulation of cell survival is a process involved in the cold-induced hyperplasia of brown fat, as well as in eliminating redundant cells during the transition from the thermogenic to the non-thermogenic state.

Apoptosis of brown adipocytes as a pathophysiological process

Obesity in experimental models is ubiquitously associated with abnormalities in brown fat (Trayhurn[29], Himms-Hagen[30]). In adult obese animals the amount of thermogenically active BAT as well as the expression of β_3-adrenoceptors in brown adipocytes are substantially reduced potentially resulting in alterations of metabolic function and thermoregulation (Himms-Hagen and Desautels[31]; Muzzin[32]). The molecular basis of these obesity-related changes is poorly understood. Interestingly, in genetic models of obesity, the number of apoptotic cells in the brown fat is dramatically higher than that in control animals (Nisoli[24]). This may lead to reduction of the number of multilocular, thermogenically active brown fat cells and therefore cause BAT functional atrophy, which is characterized by defective thermoregulation in both genetic and dietary obesity. It is also worth noting that exposure of the obese rats to cold for some days, which increases BAT sympathetic activity, significantly decreased the number of apoptotic brown adipocytes in comparison with that observed in obese rats kept in an environment at room temperature (Nisoli[24]). Since it has been previously demonstrated that expression of TNF-α in adipose tissue is elevated in a variety of experimental obesity models and in obese humans (Hotamisligil[33]) these results may suggest that TNF-α -induced apoptosis is involved in pathogenetic processes that lead to or worsen obesity.

TNF-α and obesity-linked brown fat atrophy

As previously stated, obesity in experimental models is ubiquitously associated with abnormalities in BAT. In addition, since BAT is an important target for insulin action and other aspects of energy metabolism, its atrophy could further contribute to the abnormal metabolic profile in obesity. Recently, we have tested whether abnormal TNF-α production in obesity contributes to any of these abnormalities in BAT.

We first analysed the apoptosis of brown adipocytes in genetically obese (ob/ob) mice with targeted mutations either in p55, p75 or both TNF receptors. In these obese animals, signaling and function of TNF-α is partially or completely abolished (Uysal[34]). TUNEL staining was used for the *in situ* measurements of apoptotic cell number in BAT sections obtained from these animals. Our findings showed that there was significantly higher number of positive nuclei for DNA fragmentation in BAT of ob/ob animals (wild-type at TNF receptor loci) than in that of the lean control mice (65 ± 4 vs. 1 ± 0.5 per cent positive nuclei over total cell nuclei; $P < 0.005$). Apoptosis in TUNEL positive cells of BAT from genetically obese animals was further validated by several other techniques, including agarose gel electrophoresis and transmission electron microscopy. In contrast to the ob/ob animals, the number of apoptotic nuclei in the ob/ob mice lacking p55 (ob/ob-p55$^{-/-}$) or both TNF receptors (ob/ob-p55$^{-/-}$p75$^{-/-}$) were significantly lower and approached the ratios observed in the control lean mice (2 ± 0.3 and 4 ± 1 per cent positive nuclei, respectively; $P < 0.005$). In ob/ob mice lacking p75 TNF receptor (ob/ob-p75$^{-/-}$) the number of apoptotic cells (25 ± 3 per cent positive nuclei) was significantly higher than those seen in control lean animals as well as ob/ob-p55$^{-/-}$p75$^{-/-}$ mice, but lower than those seen in obese controls (ob/ob). It is known that in obese animals, the typical multilocular brown adipocytes (i.e. thermogenically active small fat cells with numerous small lipid droplets dispersed in the cytoplasmic space around a central nucleus) are substituted by unilocular adipocytes morphologically reminiscent of white adipocytes (i.e. large fat cells filled by a single lipid droplet that flattenes the nucleus to the cell membrane, and likely thermogenically inactive). Interestingly, the multilocular brown adipocytes in ob/ob mice lacking one or both TNF receptors were more abundant than in ob/ob mice (55.2, 70.2 and 86.1 per cent higher than ob/ob, in ob/ob-p75$^{-/}$, ob/ob-p55$^{-/-}$, and, ob/ob-p55$^{-/-}$p75$^{-/-}$, respectively). This pronounced multilocularity of adipocytes is likely to reflect active thermogenic metabolism of the cells. These findings demonstrate that the activity of TNF-α is the primary determinant of the BAT apoptosis and altered morphology of multilocular adipocytes seen in obesity since complete absence of TNF signaling confers essentially total protection from obesity-induced BAT apoptosis and the decline in the number of typical brown fat cells.

Since decreased β3-adrenoceptor expression and action in brown adipocytes are well-documented features of obesity, we examined the expression of β3-adrenoceptors in BAT of obese mice lacking TNF receptors. β3-adrenoceptor mRNA levels in ob/ob mice were significantly lower than the lean controls. Strikingly, in BAT of ob/ob-p55$^{-/-}$ p75$^{-/-}$ and ob/ob-p55$^{-/-}$ mice, the β3-adrenoceptor mRNA levels were much higher than those of ob/ob animals and comparable to those of lean mice. In contrast, the β3-adrenoceptor mRNA levels in BAT of ob/ob-p75$^{-/-}$ mice were low and comparable to those of ob/ob mice.

Noradrenaline-stimulation of β3-adrenoceptors induces BAT thermogenesis by activating an uncoupling mechanism to dissipate protons across the mitochondrial membrane. The mitochondrial uncoupling protein (UCP)-1 in the mitochondrial inner membrane of mammalian brown fat generates heat by uncoupling oxidative phosphorylation. This process protects against cold and regulates energy balance. Given the importance of UCP1 in the regulation of energy expenditure in rodents, we examined UCP1 expression in the BAT of obese mice lacking TNF receptors. Whilst the lack of p75 receptor alone did not change the UCP1 gene expression, the absence of p55 or both TNF receptors resulted in increased UCP1 mRNA levels compared to ob/ob mice. These data further support the evidence that the absence of TNF receptors increases the number of functionally active brown adipocytes.

To analyse the relevance of these changes *in vivo*, we assessed the effect of complete absence of TNF-α function on thermo-regulation in control and TNF receptor-deficient obese mice. The mice were exposed to cold (4 °C) for different periods of time and the rate and time of decline in core body temperature was used as a measure of sensitivity to cold and the thermo-adaptive capacity. These experiments demonstrated that the absence of both TNF receptors is accompanied by improved thermo-adaptation in ob/ob p55$^{-/-}$p75$^{-/-}$ mice compared to that of ob/ob mice with intact TNF-α function. These results suggest that TNF-α is at least partially responsible for altered BAT function in obese mice and lack of TNF receptors leads to significant improvement in thermo-adaptive capacity.

Nitric oxide and brown fat apoptosis

In addition, they may be consistent with a new approach to the treatment of obesity, that is the inhibition of brown fat apoptosis by modulating pharmacologically the effects of TNF-α and the molecular processes involved in the rescue of BAT apoptosis. It is interesting to note that noradrenaline, which antagonized the TNF-α-induced apoptosis is able to do so through the production of nitric oxide (NO), and consequent induction of heat shock protein (HSP)-70 (Nisoli[35]) and the induction of Bcl-2 gene expression in brown fat cells (Briscini[36]). Bcl-2 gene expression, at mRNA and protein level, is markedly reduced in BAT of genetically obese rodents (Briscini[36]). Both Bcl-2 and NO antagonize apoptosis of brown adipocytes, and their pharmacological modulation might reverse the obesity-linked brown fat atrophy.

Future perspectives in brown fat

Many questions remain unsolved in the apoptosis of brown fat. A direct involvement of this event in pathophysiological processes has to be firmly demonstrated, as well as the quantitative significance of apoptosis in the brown fat cell loss and BAT atrophy. Surely the study of expression and role of Fas and Fas-L in this tissue is relevant, and preliminary experiments show that this is the case. In addition, it will be important to understand any putative role of uncoupling proteins in the apoptotic processes in these cells. The capacity to uncouple the oxidative phosphorylation by UCP-1 may be relevant to face oxygen radicals accumulation in mitochondria, which is linked to cell damage. In general, brown adipocyte might be a good cell model to study the apoptotic processes.

White adipose tissue

Does apoptosis occur in WAT?

The relevance of apoptosis in white fat is extremely controversial. Even if Lindquist and Rehnmark[28] did not see any DNA fragmentation in rat white fat tissue, Prins[37,38] suggested that human white adipocytes differentiated in culture undergo apoptosis following growth factor deprivation, or mild heat injury, or TNF-α treatment. In control cultures, apoptotic indexes were betwen 0 and 2.3 per cent in all experiments. In the experimental systems, TNF-α induced apoptosis (assessed using morphological and biochemical criteria) in both preadipocytes and adipocytes, with indexes between 5 and 25 per cent.

Moreover, Prins[39] has reported that human white adipocyte apoptosis occurs *in vivo* and that the rates of adipocyte apoptosis appear higher in omental cells than in subcutaneous cells in patients with malignancy. The question of whether there might be a site-specific difference in the susceptibility of human preadipocytes to apoptosis was further studied in normal subjects without any medications known to affect adipose tissue mass, distribution, or metabolism, or severe systemic illness or known malignancy (Niesler[40]). Preadipocytes from the omental depot appeared to be more susceptible to apoptosis induced by both serum deprivation and the combined effect of TNF-α and serum deprivation.

The increment in apoptosis produced by TNF-α also appeared greater in omental than in subcutaneous cells. No difference in basal apoptosis between preadipocytes of the two depots was seen, although basal apoptotic indeces (< 1 per cent) were too low for precise quantification and comparison. These data strongly suggest an intrinsic difference between human preadipocytes from the two depots. Actually, levels of adipocyte expression of cellular inhibitor of apoptosis protein-2 (cIAP2) were reported to be higher in omental compared with subcutaneous adipocytes in normal weight to slightly obese individuals (Montague[41]). The cIAP 1 and 2 form a complex with the TRAFs 1 and 2, which are involved in the downstream signaling from TNF-α receptors. It has recently been demonstrated that when overexpressed in mammalian cells, cIAP2 activates NF-κB and suppresses TNF-α-induced cell death (Chu[42]). Therefore, a higher level of cIAP2 expression in the omental adipose depot may be related to the major susceptibility of this fat depot to TNF-α-induced apoptosis, in a sort of a counteregulatory mechanism to excessive apoptosis.

These findings may suggest that TNF-α, and possibly other related factors such as interleukin-6, are usually synthesized as controllers of adipocyte number and adipose mass: beyond a critical point these mechanisms are not able to face the increased fat mass and obesity develops.

Insights from adipogenic cell lines

Mouse fibroblast cell lines were established that could differentiate into adipocytes under certain tissue culture conditions, such as the addition of glucocorticoids, agents that increase cAMP, agonists of the IGF-1 receptor, and fetal bovine serum. Using these cell lines, in particular 3T3-L1 preadipocytes, it was found that following serum deprivation apoptosis occurred in preadipocytes, but not in differentiated adipocytes (Magun[43]). Consistent with the ability of the adipocytes to resist apoptosis, immunoblot analysis revealed that differentiated cell cultures expressed Bcl-2 at higher levels. In addition, the endonuclease DnaseI, which is believed to be responsible for the internucleosomal DNA cleavages that occur during apoptosis, was down-regulated during 3T3-L1 differentiation (Magun[43]). It should be noted that other factors may also potentially contribute to the resistance to apoptosis displayed by the differentiated adipocytes. Staiger and Loffler[44] reported that 3T3-L1 treated with corticosterone and cAMP-inducer IBMX in the absence of platelet-derived growth factor (PDGF) maintain confluence until day 2 and then showed a marked reduction in cell number. This was due to apoptosis as revealed by morphological features, vital dye exclusion and TUNEL sensitivity of dying cells.

Apoptosis of fat tissues: unanswered questions

As outlined above, recent years have witnessed an extraordinary increase in findings regarding the molecular control of apoptosis of fat tissues. These findings now lead to the next level of questions. Does apoptosis influence the homeostasis of white and brown adipose tissues? Do differences exist in the physiological relevance of apoptosis in the various fat depots? What are the physiological conditions that modulate apoptosis in fat tissues? Of particular interest is the relevance of feeding and/or fasting and dietary fats to serve as modulators of fat tissues apoptosis. Is this cellular event really involved in pathophysiological mechanisms, that can lead to obesity or lipoatrophy? And finally, can these studies contribute to development of new therapeutic strategies? Based upon recent progress, it is likely that answers to these questions will be forthcoming.

Since now it seems that apoptosis could be involved in at least two types of proposed therapies of fat tissue pathologies. Leptin, whose administration reduces food intake and increases energy expenditure, resulting in rapid loss of body fat depots in obese rodents and rare humans (Farooqi[45]), deletes white adipocytes by apoptosis when intracerebroventricularly infused in rats (Qian[46]). The apoptotic features were absent in control and pair-fed rats and in other tissues of leptin-treated animals. Finally, antibodies to rat adipocyte plasma membranes are able to destruct adipocytes, both *in vitro* and *in vivo*, by apoptotic and complement-mediated necrotic mechanisms (Flint[47]). The treated animals increased their lean tissue growth to compensate for lost fat. This approach could allow treatment to be targetted to localized sites, for example lipomas, without any risks associated with the need to deliver treatments systemically (Flint[48]). Thus, the fate of apoptosis in fat depots is waiting for novel playwriters.

References

1. Hauner H, Enternmann G, Wabitsch M, Gaillard D, Ailhaud G, Negrel R, Pfeiffer EF. Promoting effect of glucocorticoids on the differentiation of human adipocyte precursor cells cultured in a chemically defined medium. *J Clin Invest* 1989; 84: 1663–70.

2. Arner P. Control of lipolysis and its relevance to development of obesity in man. *Diabetes Metab Rev* 1988; 4: 507–15.

3. Evan GI, Wyllie AH, Gilbert CS, Littlewood TD, Land H, Brooks M *et al.* Induction of apoptosis in fibroblasts by c-myc protein. *Cell* 1992; 69: 119–28.

4. Raff M, Barres BA, Burne JF, Coles HS, Ishizaki Y, Jacobson MD. Programmed cell death and the control of cell survival: lessons from the nervous system. *Science* 1993; 267: 695–700.

5. Yao R, Cooper GM. Requirement for phosphatidylinositol-3 kinase in the prevention of apoptosis by nerve growth factor. *Science* 1995; 267: 2003–6.

6. Hengartner M. Death by crowd control. *Science* 1998; 281: 1298–9.

7. Tartaglia LA, Ayres TM, Wong GH, Goeddel DV. A novel domain within the 55 kd TNF receptor signals cell death. *Cell* 1993; 74: 845–53.

8. Wallach D, Kovalenko AV, Varfolomeev EE, Boldin MP. Death-inducing functions of ligands of the tumor necrosis factor family: a Sanhedrin verdict. *Curr Opin Immunol* 1998; 10: 279–88.

9. Nagata S Apoptosis by death factor. *Cell* 1997; 88: 355–65.

10. Medema JP, Scaffidi C, Kischkel FC, Shevchenko A, Mann M, Krammer PH, Peter ME. FLICE is activated by association with the CD95 death-inducing signaling complex (DISC). *EMBO J* 1997; 16: 2794–804.

11. Muzio M, Chinnaiyan AM, Kischkel FC, O'Rourke K, Shevchenko A, Ni J *et al.* FLICE, a novel FADD-homologous ICE/CED-3-like protease, is recruited to the CD95 (Fas/APO-1) death-inducing signaling complex. *Cell* 1996; 85: 817–27.

12. Srinivasula SM, Ahmad M, Fernandez-Alnemri T, Litwack G, Alnemri ES. Molecular ordering of the Fas-apoptotic pathway: the Fas/APO-1 protease Mch5 is a CrmA-inhibitable protease that activates multiple Ced-3/ICE-like cysteine proteases. *Proc Natl Acad Sci USA* 1996; 93: 14486–91.

13. Muzio M, Salvesen GS, Dixit VM FLICE induced apoptosis in a cell-free system. Cleavage of caspase zymogens. *J Biol Chem* 1997; 272: 2952–6.

14. Kischkel FC, Hellbardt S, Behrmann I, Germer M, Pawlita M, Krammer PH *et al.* Cytotoxicity-dependent APO-1 (Fas/CD95)-associated proteins form a death-inducing signaling complex (DISC) with the receptor. *EMBO J* 1995; 14: 5579–88.

15. Gross A, McDonnell JM, Korsmeyer SJ. BCL-2 family members and the mitochondria in apoptosis. *Genes Dev* 1999; 13: 1899–911.

16. Adams JM, Cory S. The Bcl-2 protein family: arbiters of cell survival. *Science* 1998; 281: 1322–6.

17. Boise LH, Thompson CB Bcl-x(L) can inhibit apoptosis in cells that have undergone Fas-induced protease activation. *Proc Natl Acad Sci USA* 1997; 94: 3759–64.

18. Scaffidi C, Fulda S, Srinivasan A, Friesen C, Li F, Tomaselli KJ *et al.* Two CD95 (APO-1/Fas) signaling pathways. *EMBO J* 1998; 17: 1675–87.

19. Minn AJ, Boise LH, Thompson CB. Bcl-x(S) antagonizes the protective effects of Bcl-x(L). *J Biol Chem* 1996; 271: 6306–312.

20. Chinnaiyan AM, Orth K, O'Rourke K, Duan H, Poirier GG, Dixit VM. Molecular ordering of the cell death pathway. Bcl-2 and Bcl-xL function upstream of the CED-3-like apoptotic proteases. *J Biol Chem* 1996; 271: 4573–6.

21. Jürgensmeier JM, Xie Z, Deveraux Q, Ellerby L, Bredesen D, Reed JC. Bax directly induces release of cytochrome c from isolated mitochondria. *Proc Natl Acad Sci USA* 1998; 95: 4997–5002.

22. Pastorino JG, Tafani M, Rothman RJ, Marcinkeviciute A, Hoek JB, Farber JL, Marcineviciute A. Functional consequences of the sustained or transient activation by Bax of the mitochondrial permeability transition pore. *J Biol Chem* 1999; 274: 31734–9.

23. Harada H, Becknell B, Wilm H, Mann M, Huang IJ, Taylor SS *et al.* Phosphorylation and inactivation of BAD by mitochondria-anchored protein kinase A. *Mol Cell* 1999; 3: 413–22.

24. Nisoli E, Briscini L, Tonello C, De Giuli-Morghen C, Carruba MO. Tumor necrosis factor-α induces apoptosis in rat brown adipocytes. *Cell Death & Differentiation* 1997; 4: 771–8.

25. Porras A, Alvarez AM, Valladares A, Benito M. TNF-α induces apoptosis in rat fetal brown adipocytes in primary culture. *FEBS Letters* 1997; 416: 324–8.

26. Navarro P, Valverde AM, Benito M, Lorenzo M. Insulin/IGF-I rescues immortalized brown adipocytes from apoptosis down-regulating Bcl-xS expression, in a PI 3-kinase- and Map kinase-dependent manner. *Exp Cell Res* 1998; 243: 213–21.

27. Navarro P, Valverde AM, Conejo R, Benito M, Lorenzo M. Inhibition of caspases rescues brown adipocytes from apoptosis downregulating BCL-XS and upregulating BCL-2 gene expression. *Exp Cell Res* 1999; 246: 301–7.

28. Lindquist JM, Rehnmark S. Ambient temperature regulation of apoptosis in brown adipose tissue. Erk1/2 promotes norepinephrine-dependent cell survival. *J Biol Chem* 1998; 273: 30147–56.

29. Trayhurn P. Brown adipose tissue and energy balance. In: *Brown adipose tissue* Trayhurn P, Nicholls DG (eds). London: Edward Arnold; 1986, pp. 299–338.

30. Himms-Hagen J. Brown adipose tissue thermogenesis and obesity. *Prog Lipid Res* 1989; 28: 67–115.

31. Himms-Hagen J, Desautels M. A mitochondrial defect in brown adipose tissue of obese (ob/ob) mouse: reduced binding of purine nucleotides and a failure to respond to cold by an increase in binding. *Biochem Biophys Res Commun* 1978; 83: 628–35.

32. Muzzin P, Revelli JP, Kuhne F, Gocayne JD, McCombie WR, Venter JC *et al.* An adipose tissue-specific β-adrenergic receptor. Molecular cloning and down-regulation in obesity. *J Biol Chem* 1991; 266: 24053–8.

33. Hotamisligil GS Mechanisms of TNF-α-induced insulin resistance. *Exp Clin Endocrinol Diabetes* 1999; 107: 119–25.

34. Uysal KT, Weisbrock SM, Marino MW, Hotamisligil GS. Protection from obesity-induced insulin resistance in mice lacking TNF-α function. *Nature* 1997; 389,: 610–4.

35. Nisoli E, Regianini L, Bulbarelli A, Briscini L, Bracale R, Carruba MO. Protective effects of noradrenaline against tumor necrosis factor-α-induced apoptosis in cultured rat brown adipocytes: role of nitric oxide-induced heat shock protein 70 expression. *Int J Obes* 2001; 25: 1421–30.

36. Briscini L, Tonello C, Dioni L, Carruba MO, Nisoli E. Bcl-2 and Bax are involved in the sympathetic protection of brown adipocytes from obesity-linked apoptosis. *FEBS Letters* 1998; 431: 80–4.

37. Prins JB, Walker NI, Winterford CM, Cameron DP. Apoptosis of human adipocytes *in vitro*. *Biochem Biophys Res Commun* 1994; 201: 500–7.

38. Prins JB, Walker NI, Winterford CM, Cameron DP. Human adipocyte apoptosis occurs in malignancy. *Biochem Biophys Res Commun* 1994; 205: 625–30.

39. Prins JB, Niesler CU, Winterford CM, Bright NA, Siddle K, O'Rahilly S *et al.* Tumor necrosis factor-α induces apoptosis of human adipose cells. *Diabetes* 1997; 46: 1939–44.

40. Niesler CU, Siddle K, Prins JB. Human preadipocytes display a depot-specific susceptibility to apoptosis. *Diabetes* 1998; 47: 1365–8.

41. Montague CT, Prins JB, Sanders L, Zhang J, Sewter CP, Digby J *et al.* Depot-related gene expression in human subcutaneous and omental adipocytes. *Diabetes* 1998; 47: 1384–91.

42. Chu ZL, McKinsey TA, Liu L, Gentry JJ, Malim MH, Ballard DW. Suppression of tumor necrosis factor-induced cell death by inhibitor of apoptosis c-IAP2 is under NF-κB control. *Proc Natl Acad Sci USA* 1997; 94: 10057–62.

43. Magun R, Boone DL, Tsang BK, Sorisky A. The effect of adipocyte differentiation on the capacity of 3T3-L1 cells to undergo apoptosis in response to growth factor deprivation. *Int J Obes* 1998; 22: 567–71.

44. Staiger H, Loffler G. The role of PDGF-dependent suppression of apoptosis in differentiating 3T3-L1 preadipocytes. *Eur J Cell Biol* 1998; 77: 220–7.

45. Farooqi IS, Jebb SA, Langmack G, Lawrence E, Cheetham CH, Prentice AM. Effects of recombinant leptin therapy in a child with congenital leptin deficiency. *N Engl J Med* 1999; 341: 879–84.

46. Qian H, Azain MJ, Compton MM, Hartzell DL, Hausman GJ, Baile CA. Brain administration of leptin causes deletion of adipocytes by apoptosis. *Endocrinology* 1998; 139: 791–4.

47. Flint DJ, Coggrave H, Futter CE, Gardner MJ, Clarke TJ. Stimulatory and cytotoxic effects of an antiserum to adipocyte plasma membranes on adipose tissue metabolism *in vitro* and *in vivo*. *Int J Obes* 1986; 10: 69–77.

48. Flint DJ Immunological manipulation of body composition. *Int J Obes* 1999; 23 (Suppl 5): S17.

Progress in Obesity Research: 9. Edited by *Geraldo Medeiros-Neto, Alfredo Halpern and Claude Bouchard*
©2003 John Libbey Eurotext Ltd, pp. 117–121.

CHAPTER 23

Regulation of human adipose tissue and skeletal muscle gene expression by thyroid hormone

Dominique Langin, Nathalie Viguerie, Pierre Barbe, Dominique Larrouy and Karine Clément

INSERM U586, Institut Louis Bugnard, CHU Rangueil, 31403 Toulouse Cedex 4 and Service de Médecine et Nutrition, Hôtel-Dieu, INSERM Avenir and EA 3502 Université Paris 6, France
[e-mail: langin@toulouse.inserm.fr]

Thyroid hormones control essential functions in development and metabolism. The major effects of thyroid hormones are mediated by modulation of gene transcription. Most of the characterized thyroid-response elements in target genes are positive cis-acting elements[1]. In the presence of triiodothyronine (T3), the thyroid hormone receptor undergoes a conformational change, which results in the replacement of a corepressor complex by a coactivator complex. The coactivator histone acetyl-transferase activity leads to an open transcriptionally active chromatin state. The recruitment of the receptor-associated protein complex may constitute a subsequent step in transcriptional activation by T3. In the absence of ligand, the heterodimer interacts with a corepressor complex with histone deacetylase activity. Histone deacetylation and DNA methylation both lead to transcriptional repression.

Adipose tissue and skeletal muscle are important targets of thyroid hormone action. A well-known effect of thyroid hormones is the alteration of the lipolytic response to catecholamines. In humans, hyperthyroidism enhances and hypothyroidism decreases lipolysis through different mechanisms. The induction of catecholamine-mediated lipolysis by thyroid hormones results from an increased β-adrenoceptor number and a decrease in phosphodiesterase activity[2,3]. Both regulations concur to an increase in cAMP level and hormone-sensitive lipase activity. Thyroid hormones are also major regulators of cellular respiration[4]. Hyperthyroidism and hypothyroidism are associated with increased and decreased mitochondrial respiration rates, respectively. Skeletal muscle accounts for most of the variation in metabolic rate between individuals[5]. Moreover, thyroid hormones are known to increase both skeletal muscle protein synthesis and degradation resulting in net protein breakdown[6].

Although thyroid hormones are key regulators of metabolism, few target genes had been identified and no large-scale studies had been performed in humans. In a series of studies, we have applied cDNA array and quantitative RT-PCR technologies to study the effect of thyroid hormone *in vivo* and *in vitro* on human adipose tissue and skeletal muscle[7–9]. Through the simultaneous investigation of thousands of genes, DNA arrays are ideally suited to unravel novel hormonal regulations.

Regulation of adipose tissue gene expression

To study the thyroid hormone regulation of gene expression in human adipocytes, we combined the use of cDNA arrays and primary culture of subcutaneous adipose tissue explants[8]. Culture of freshly isolated mature adipocytes is not appropriate because of decrease in gene expression over time and large differences in the viability of cells from different subjects. Primary cultures of human preadipocytes yield cells at different differentiation stages. It is therefore difficult to determine whether the observed hormonal regulation is due to an effect on differentiated adipocytes or on preadipocytes. Moreover, the differentiated cells do not recapitulate the full phenotype of mature adipocytes, i.e. large cells with unilocular lipid droplets and expression of late differentiation markers such as the α_2-adreno-ceptor (AR)[10]. We therefore chose to study hormonal regulation on adipose tissue explants. Explants partly maintain the *in vivo* structure of human adipose tissue that permits long-term culture with minimal change in gene expression. At the end of the treatment period, mature adipocytes are isolated. Gene expression is therefore measured on one single cell type.

Table 1. List of genes regulated by triiodothyronine *in vitro* in human adipocytes

Gene name	Biological process
G protein-coupled receptor RDC1	Signal transduction (putative)
G protein-coupled receptor kinase 4	G-protein linked receptor signalling pathway
Apolipoprotein D	Lipid metabolism
Squalene synthetase	Steroid biosynthesis
Lipopolysaccharide-binding protein	Cellular defence response
Lipopolysaccharide receptor	Apoptosis, inflammatory response, phagocytosis
Peptidyl-prolyl cis-trans isomerase	Apoptosis, protein folding
Hypoxia-inducible factor 2	Response to hypoxia
Neprilysin	Proteolysis and peptidolysis
Alcohol dehydrogenase 1A	Ethanol oxidation and metabolism
Cholinephosphate citidyltransferase 1	Phosphatidylcholine synthesis
Phosphoglycerate mutase 1	Glycolysis
Lymphocyte function-associated antigen 3	Cell-to-cell signalling
Inhibitory G protein α2 subunit	*G-protein linked receptor signalling pathway*
G protein β subunit-like protein 12	*Receptor for activated protein kinase C*
Sterol regulatory element binding protein 1	*Lipogenesis and adipogenesis*
Annexin 1	*Inflammatory response and signal transduction*
S100 calcium-binding protein A3	*Signal transduction*
α1,3-mannosyl-glycoprotein β1,2-N-acetylglucosaminyltransferase	*Protein glycosylation*

Up and downregulated genes are shown in plain and italicized fonts, respectively. Data are from reference[8].

Explant cultures were treated with 100 nM T3 for 24 h in serum-free medium. cDNA array experiments were carried out on subcutaneous adipose tissue preparations from several subjects. cDNA synthesis was performed using magnetic bead affinity enrichment of poly A^+ RNA and direct synthesis of cDNA probe using a primer mix corresponding to the genes represented on the cDNA array. Radioactive cDNA probe from either control or T3-treated cells were hybridized to Atlas Human cDNA expression arrays (Clontech) including 1176 cDNAs immobilized on a nylon membrane. The spots with low intensity were eliminated. Signal for each good quality spot was then normalized to housekeeping gene intensities. A threshold value of 1.3 for up or downregulation of significant genes was selected. This threshold value corresponds to variations that could confidently be confirmed using quantitative RT-PCR. The selection procedure yielded 13 genes that were upregulated and six genes that were downregulated (Table 1). The genes encoded proteins involved in signal transduction, lipid metabolism, apoptosis and inflammatory response. Interestingly, the transcription factor SREBP1-c was downregulated by T3. Studies in murine adipocyte cell lines have shown that SREBP1c influences positively adipogenesis and stimulates the expression of genes involved in lipogenesis[11]. Moreover, SREBP-1c may be a major mediator of insulin action on hepatic glucose and lipid metabolism gene expression[12]. The downregulation of SREBP-1c by T3 in mature adipocytes suggests that the transcription factor may be involved in the insulin-resistant state associated with hyperthyroidism. To confirm and extend the cDNA array data, we studied the expression of transcripts involved in adipose tissue lipolysis using quantitative RT-PCR. T3 increased *in vitro* the mRNA level of the lipolytic α_2-AR. Accordingly, hyperthyroidism is accompanied by an increase in α_2-AR number with no change in $\beta1$-AR level[13]. The activity of low K_m phosphodiesterase, an enzyme which hydrolyses cAMP into 5'AMP, is lower in hyperthyroid patients compared to euthyroid subjects[2]. The downregulation of phosphodiesterase activity contributes to an increase in fat cell cAMP levels and enhanced lipolysis. This activity is most likely attributable to PDE3B, which is a key cellular relay in the antilipolytic action of insulin. In human adipose tissue culture, T3 treatment led to a downregulation of PDE3B mRNA. The α_2-AR mediates through coupling to G_i proteins the antilipolytic effect of catecholamines[10]. The concomitant downregulation of α_2-AR and $G\alpha_{i2}$ mRNA levels may lead to a decreased antilipolytic potency of catecholamines. Together, these regulations favour an increase in intracellular cAMP levels and contribute to the enhanced lipolytic capacity of catecholamines during hyperthyroidism. T3 also induced an upregulation of uncoupling protein 2 mRNA expression. The increase is similar to the induction observed *in vivo* in human adipose tissue of subjects treated for 14 days with T3[7].

Regulation of skeletal muscle gene expression

To study the effect of thyroid hormone on skeletal muscle gene expression *in vivo*, healthy men were treated for 14 days with T3[7,9]. Biopsies of vastus lateralis skeletal muscle were performed at the beginning and the end of the treatment. Because the amount of total RNA obtained from skeletal muscle microbiopsies is limited, a two round amplification protocol that ensures high-fidelity mRNA amplification was used[14]. Fluorescently labeled cDNA probes were hybridized to 24,000 cDNA element microarrays (http: //genome-www4.stanford.edu/cgi-bin/sfgf/home.pl). Signals of bad quality or with low intensity were eliminated. Testing a large number of genes simultaneously requires one to implement a multiple comparison procedure, which guards against a large number of false positives. We therefore used Significant Analysis of Microarray, a non-parametric method that determines the expected proportion of false positives among all genes called significant[15]. On 18705 cDNAs, 449 were selected. Some selected genes were represented several times on the microarray. Consistent regulation among all replicates was used as a further selection step. A list of 381 upregulated and two downregulated genes was produced (Table 2). The upregulated genes showed a mean fold change above 1.4. To test the validity of the array experiments and statistical procedure, we performed real-time quantitative RT-PCR on six genes. For each gene, the data from quantitative RT-PCR confirmed the array data.

Table 2. Global changes of gene expression induced by thyroid hormone *in vivo* in human vastus lateralis skeletal muscle

Functional classes	Number	Functional classes	Number
Transcriptional control Transcription factors Coactivators/Corepressors Histone (de)acetylation	33	**Ribonucleoproteins and RNA metabolism** Pre-mRNA processing	16
Protein synthesis Ribosomal proteins Translation initiation factors	14	**Protein catabolism** Ubiquitin-proteasome pathway	20
Glucose and lipid metabolism Glycogen synthesis and glucose utilization	8	**Mitochondrial energy metabolism** Respiratory chain proteins Mitochondrial carriers Citric acid cycle	22
Signal transduction Protein phosphatases Protein kinases G proteins G protein-coupled receptors	36	**Cellular trafficking** Intracellular transport	13
Cytoskeleton	21	**Cellular immunity**	9
Miscellaneous	45	**Expressed sequence tags**	144

Data are from reference 9.

A global view of the changes shows that thyroid hormone specifically affects many genes that are related to the physiological effects of the hormone on protein and energy metabolism. The largest fraction of regulated genes was involved in the transcriptional and post-transcriptional control of protein synthesis. *In vivo*, multiple mechanisms can therefore account for the control of protein levels by T3. T3 increases the expression of numerous factors involved in transcriptional control, pre-mRNA processing and protein translation. Hence, protein synthesis may be promoted by thyroid hormone both directly through the direct effect of T3 on target gene promoters and indirectly through transcriptional control of proteins involved in transcriptional, post-transcriptional and translational mechanisms. Thyroid hormones are known to increase both skeletal muscle protein synthesis and degradation resulting in net protein breakdown[6]. Our data show a concomitant increase in mRNA expression of protein catabolism factors. Most changes affected the ubiquitin/proteasome pathway, which is part of the non-lysosomal degradation of intracellular proteins[16]. Another important group of genes upregulated by T3 encoded proteins of energy metabolism. These coregulations may contribute to the marked effect of T3 on skeletal muscle respiration[17].

Our study reveals that the transcriptional effect of T3 on skeletal muscle extends well beyond the classical metabolic effects of the hormone. Thirty-six signal transduction genes were upregulated. Through induction of receptor, G protein, protein kinase and protein phosphatase gene expression, thyroid hormone may exert its permissive effect on hormonal regulation of skeletal muscle metabolism. T3 may also influence cellular trafficking and tissue remodeling through increased expression of genes involved in protein transport and maturation, exchange between intracellular organelles and cytoskeleton assembly. Our data also identified 144 expressed sequence tags upregulated by T3, which correspond to novel putative target genes.

Thyroid hormones participate with insulin and catecholamines in the regulation of skeletal muscle metabolism. The antagonism to insulin action was illustrated by the mRNA increase of the p85α phosphatidylinositol 3-kinase regulatory subunit. Indeed, mice lacking p85α show increased insulin sensitivity[18]. Thyroid hormones enhance the effect of catecholamines. An induction of the β2-adrenergic receptor mRNA was observed consistent with the positive effects of T3 observed in human adipose tissue. As shown in hepatocytes, T3 upregulated enzymes involved in gluconeogenesis and glycogen metabolism[19,20]. Numerous genes of mitochondrial energy metabolism were upregulated, including several enzymes associated with the citric acid cycle. For the biogenesis of the respiratory apparatus, over 100 proteins are necessary[4]. Most of them are encoded in the nucleus with only 13 being encoded by the mitochondrial genome. Among the 50 independent mRNAs representing respiratory chain proteins on the microarray, 13 were upregulated during T3 treatment. The upregulated genes included several subunits of NADH: ubiquinone oxidoreductase (complex I) where proton translocation is coupled to electron transfer. Cytochrome c, a component of complex IV that donates electrons to the cytochrome oxidase complex, was markedly upregulated. We observed an increase of 2 cytochrome oxidase (complex IV) and 4 ATPsynthase (F1F0 ATPase or complex V) subunit mRNAs. The proteins of the respiratory chain need to be available in stoichiometric amounts for proper assembly in the inner mitochondrial membrane. T3 is a potent inducer of a subset of but not all nucleus-encoded respiratory chain genes[21]. This suggests that thyroid hormone yields an increase of the other components, indirectly through post-transcriptional mechanisms. The increase in genes encoding protein translation factors may participate in this mechanism. Moreover, T3 induced genes involved in mitochondrial protein translation such as the only known mitochondrial translation initiation factor MTIF2 and mitochondrial ribosomal proteins. Besides coupled respiration, thyroid hormones also increase uncoupled respiration and the leak of protons across the inner mitochondrial membrane. In humans, T3 treatment of young adults for 3 days promotes *in vivo* mitochondrial energy uncoupling in skeletal muscle[22]. T3 induced three putative candidates to explain the uncoupling effect: uncoupling protein 3 and adenine nucleotide translocases 1 and 2[23]. Genes of energy metabolism have recently been shown to be downregulated during caloric restriction in vastus lateralis muscle of male rhesus monkeys[24]. Caloric restriction is characterized by a decrease in plasma thyroid hormone level that leads to a decrease of the metabolic rate. Our data are therefore consistent with a role of thyroid hormone in caloric restriction-induced changes in energy metabolism gene expression.

Conclusions

To conclude, cDNA array data show that T3 regulates a large repertoire of genes in human adipose tissue and skeletal muscle. Sorting of regulated genes into functional classes in human tissues defined the molecular signatures that underlie the pleiotropic effect of thyroid hormone. In line with the known physiological effects of T3, induction of a large number of genes involved in protein turnover and metabolism was observed. The studies also reveal novel target cellular pathways. The impact on these pathways may help to understand the permissive effect of T3 on signal transduction cascades, intracellular transport and tissue remodeling. The studies also illustrate the value of a coupled use of DNA arrays with biopsies from human tissues to study *in vivo* and *in vitro* the physiological and pathological action of hormones.

References

1. Wu Y, Koenig RJ. Gene regulation by thyroid hormone. *Trends Endocrinol Metab* 2000; 11: 207–11.

2. Engfeldt P, Arner P, Bolinder J, Wennlund A, Östman J Phosphodiesterase activity in human adipose tissue in hyper- and hypothyroidism. *J Clin Endocrinol Metab* 1982; 4: 625–9.

3. Wahrenberg H, Engfeldt P, Arner P, Wennlund A, Ostman J. Adrenergic regulation of lipolysis in human adipocytes: findings in hyper- and hypothyroidism. *J Clin Endocrinol Metab* 1986; 63: 631–8.

4. Pillar TM, Seitz HJ. Thyroid hormone and gene expression in the regulation of mitochondrial respiratory function. *Eur J Endocrinol* 1997; 136: 231–9.

5. Zurlo F, Larson K, Bogardus C, Ravussin E. Skeletal muscle metabolism is a major determinant of resting energy expenditure. *J Clin Invest* 1990; 86; 1423–7.

6. Rooyackers OE, Sreekumaran Nair K. Hormonal regulation of human muscle protein metabolism. *Annu Rev Nutr* 1997; 17: 457–85.

7. Barbe P, Larrouy D, Boulanger C, Chevillotte E, Viguerie N, Thalamas C *et al.* Triiodothyronine-mediated up-regulation of UCP2 and UCP3 mRNA expression in human skeletal muscle without coordinated induction of mitochondrial respiratory chain genes. *FASEB J.* 2001; 15: 13–15.

8. Viguerie N, Millet L, Avizou S, Vidal H, Larrouy D, Langin D. Regulation of human adipocyte gene expression by thyroid hormone. *J Clin Endocrinol Metab* 2002; 87: 624–9.

9. Clément K, Viguerie N, Diehn M, Alizadeh A, Barbe P, Thalamas C *et al.* In vivo regulation of human skeletal muscle gene expression by thyroid hormone. *Genome Res* 2002; 12: 281–91.

10. Lafontan M, Berlan M. Fat cell α2-adrenoceptors: the regulation of fat cell function and lipolysis. *Endocr Rev* 1995; 16: 716–38.

11. Rosen ED, Walkey CJ, Puigserver P, Spiegelman BM. Transcriptional regulation of adipogenesis. *Genes Dev* 2000; 14: 1293–307.

12. Foretz M, Guichard C, Ferre P, Foufelle F. Sterol regulatory element binding protein-1c is a major mediator of insulin action on the hepatic expression of glucokinase and lipogenesis-related genes. *Proc Natl Acad Sci USA* 1999; 96: 12737–42.

13. Hellström L, Wahrenberg H, Reynisdottir S, Arner P. Catecholamine-induced adipocyte lipolysis in human hyperthyroidism. *J Clin Endocrinol Metab* 1997; 82: 159–66.

14. Wang E, Miller LD, Ohnmacht GA, Liu ET, Marincola FM. High-fidelity mRNA amplification for gene profiling. *Nature Biotechnol* 2000; 18: 457–9.

15. Tusher VG, Tibshirani R, Chu G. Significance analysis of microarrays applied to the ionizing radiation response. *Proc Natl Acad Sci USA* 2001; 98: 5116–21.

16. Tawa NE, Odessey R, Goldberg AL. Inhibitors of the proteasome reduce the accelerated proteolysis in atrophying rat skeletal muscles. *J Clin Invest* 1997; 100: 197–203.

17. Tata JR, Ernster L, Lindberg O, Arhenius E, Pedersen S, Hedman R. The action of thyroid hormones at the cellular level. *Biochem J* 1963; 86: 408–28.

18. Terauchi Y, Tsuji Y, Satoh S, Minoura H, Murakami K, Okuno A *et al.* Increased insulin sensitivity and hypoglycaemia in mice lacking the p85 alpha subunit of phosphoinositide 3-kinase. *Nature Genet* 1999; 21: 230–5.

19. Betley S, Peak M, Agius L. Triiodo-L-thyronine stimulates glycogen synthesis in rat hepatocyte cultures. *Mol Cell Biochem* 1993; 120: 151–8.

20. Swierczynski J, Mitchell DA, Reinhold DS, Salati LM, Stapleton SR, Klautky SA *et al.* Triiodothyronine-induced accumulations of malic enzyme, fatty acid synthase, acetyl-coenzyme A carboxylase, and their mRNAs are blocked by protein kinase inhibitors. Transcription is the affected step. *J Biol Chem* 1991; 266: 17459–66.

21. Wiesner RJ, Kurowski TT, Zak R. Regulation by thyroid hormone of nuclear and mitochondrial genes encoding subunits of cytochrome-c oxidase in rat liver and skeletal muscle. *Mol Endocrinol* 1992; 6: 1458–67.

22. Lebon V, Dufour S, Petersen KF, Ren J, Jucker BM, Slezak LA *et al.* Effect of triiodothyronine on mitochondrial energy coupling in human skeletal muscle. *J Clin Invest* 2001; 108: 733–7.

23. Skulachev VP. Anion carriers in fatty acid-mediated physiological uncoupling. *J Bioenergetics Biomembrane* 1999; 31: 431–45.

24. Kayo T, Allison DB, Weindruch R, Prolla TA. Influences of aging and caloric restriction on the transcriptional profile of skeletal muscle from rhesus monkeys. *Proc Natl Acad Sci USA* 2001; 98: 5093–8.

Progress in Obesity Research: 9. Edited by *Geraldo Medeiros-Neto, Alfredo Halpern and Claude Bouchard*
©2003 John Libbey Eurotext Ltd, pp. 122–126.

CHAPTER 24

Understanding of hormone signaling. DNA chips and beyond

Amilcar Flores-Morales and Gunnar Norstedt

Department of Molecular Medicine. Karolinska Institute. Stockholm 17176, Sweden
[e-mail: Amilcar.Flores@molmed.ki.se]

The postgenomic era has arrived in hormone research. The near completion of the of the human genome sequence will soon be followed by that of mouse and rat, the two most commonly used models in endocrine research[1-3]. These new developments promise to dramatically increase our understanding of both the genetic basis of endocrine disorders and the molecular mechanism behind the physiological actions of hormones. Whereas the traditional approach has put a focus on a narrow number of individual genes, including hormones, their receptors and signaling intermediaries, the genomic approach attempt to study the totality of genes in an organism. The significance of an increased understanding of the endocrine system requires little motivation. Endocrine related disorders including obesity and diabetes are among the most prevalent in the Western Society, therefore there is an urgent need to find novel means of diagnosis and treatment.

The knowledge on the function of most of the newly described genes is rudimentary as is our understanding of how non-coding regions in the genome regulate the expression of such genes. Computational approaches can use sequence homology analysis to predict domain structure and putative biochemical function of newly described genes[4,5]. This information can now be extracted for most of the genes in the genome but still experimental evidence must precede the assignment of genes to specific biological pathways. Since the understanding of endocrine regulation of tissue function makes up a significant fraction of our physiological knowledge, the annotations of genes in relation to hormone responsiveness should prove useful to place genes within biological pathways.

Biological experimentation is an area that is being revolutionized. New technologies are being developed in the areas of genomic, proteomics and cell biology that aim to speed up the discovery process[6]. The use of gene arrays for the parallel determination of the expression of tenths of thousands of genes in an easy to perform, commonly available assay makes this technology the most widely used source of genome scale experimental data in life sciences[7,8]. DNA microarrays are especially attractive in hormone research because the regulation of gene expression is a key mechanism whereby hormones exerts their physiological actions on targeted tissues. This is obvious in the case of steroid and thyroid hormones, whose receptors belong to the nuclear receptor family of transcription factors and are activated upon ligand binding[9]. Peptide hormones also regulate gene expression after activating complex cascades of intracellular signaling events upon binding to transmembrane receptors[10].

The possibility to acquire genome wide expression data impose new challenges to the endocrine researcher. Some are related to the efficient management and analysis of large volumes of data such as the construction of databases, the standardization of data description, creation of data exchange formats and other related tasks that are better solved by collaborating with software developers. Others are more pertinent to the biological researcher. This include, how to use our current knowledge and model systems to design experiments that make use of gene chips in order to obtain mechanistic information that goes beyond a mere phenomenological description of expression changes and are relevant to our biological problem.

The lack of standards for presenting and exchanging microarray data represents a serious shortcoming in this field, making it difficult to independently analyse and verify published microarray data and assemble large databases. The latter is essential since meta-analysis of large numbers of different

Table 1. Putative TRβ regulated in mice liver

| | | T3 treated | | Hypothyroid |
| | | T3+WT vs. WT | T3+TRβ (–/–) vs. TRβ (–/–) | |
ID[1]	Name	2 h	2 h	TRβ (–/–) vs. WT
RIAA32	alpha-2u globulin	3.46	0.52	8.56
RGIAX93	est	2.71	1.16	4.81
RGIAM95	nudix7	4.78	0.64	3.54
RNAC07	hepatic product spot 14	6.64	0.33	3.40
RGIAT71	squalene oxidase	5.48	2.10	3.17
RGIAJ68	glucose-6-phosphatase	2.23	0.65	3.14
RGIAE69	fatty-acid synthase	2.81	1.10	2.71
RGIAJ70	aquaporin 8	3.17	1.43	2.34
RGIAN56	malic enzyme	6.11	3.42	2.29
RGIAM83	GTPase activating protein rhoGAP	2.39	0.83	2.20
RGIAQ69	farnesyl pyrophosphate synthetase	2.87	1.24	2.19
RGIAN54	fatty acid synthase	3.39	1.11	2.13
RGIAM82	est	1.83	0.93	2.07
RGIAS25	podocalyxin	3.93	2.41	2.00
RGIAU16	cyclohydrolase	2.43	1.29	1.83
RGIAU48	N-ras p21 protein	1.79	1.15	1.68

transcript profiles by a variety of data mining algorithm would be a powerful way to extract valuable functional information about genes and their functional relationships beyond the scope originally intended when the expression measurements were taken[11,12]. To establish standards for expression data is however not an easy task. Expression data is rarely an absolute estimation of RNA content but usually presented as a relative change using a reference that is rarely standardized. Moreover, no standards exist to describe the multitude of possible biological experimentions that precedes the expression measurement. Certain steps are however taken to provide guidance in this matter. The members of the Microarray Database Expression group have proposed a set of guidelines to describe microarray data in a document called MIAME (Minimal Information about microarray experiments)[13]. MIAME intends to be a base to develop standards for microarray annotations. The lack of universal standards has not stopped the development of gene expression databases. Although, intended as public depository, databases such as Gene Expression Omnibus (GEO) at the National Center for Biotechnology Information, Bethesda, USA and ArrayExpress, at the European Bioinformatics Institute are not widely used[14,15]. Instead, the majority of datasets seems to be deposited within a university or local microarray facility. The importance of having DNA chips analysed in a consistent way and the data deposited in a relational database resides in providing quick and easy access to the data that greatly facilitate knowledge discovery. Questions, for example, can be asked to provide the expression changes of all members of nuclear receptor family along 20 different experimental paradigms. Answers to this type of queries will be literally one click away. More complex data mining including different kinds of cluster analysis and even basic statistical analysis are greatly facilitated by adequate data management[16–18].

The most common data mining tasks performed on microarray data aims to find subsets of genes that can be use to classify biological material, most commonly tumours[19,20], and find clusters of genes that have similar expression behaviour in multiple experiments[16,21]. It has been argued, that co-regulation along a variety of experiments may indicate that genes participate in common biological pathways. Therefore, this may be a way to functionally annotate genes or to discover new members in known pathways. While this may be true for some pathways, one can envisioned others where individual genes within the pathway could change in expression during time or where activation of certain genes require the previous activation of others (such cell cycle)[22]. Methodologies are emerging to unveil relationships that goes beyond simple co-regulation [23]. This include methods like the construction of gene networks[24–26] and multivariate analysis of expression relationships[27]. Often, an experimental design if carefully tailored will provide relevant mechanistic information with limited number of experiments.

In the field of endocrinology, it is an important to find out genes that are primary regulated by hormones. Primary regulated genes have a direct link to hormone-induced intracellular signals and can be characterized by the existence of the so called 'hormone response element' in their promoters. Gene products from such genes can in turn influence a number of other genes resulting in a physiological response. The hormone nuclear receptor family can be used as an example. We have recently show that genes that are primary targets of the isoform of thyroid hormone receptor can be extracted from the comparison of the effects of hypothyroidism and T3 treatment on gene expression in WT and TRβ[−/−] mice (Table 1)[28]. Such sets of co-regulated genes can be used to find transcription factors binding sites and promoter rules that can help to explain the organization of hormone regulated pathways. This is an especially hard task since the non-coding regions in the mammalian genome are large in comparison with the small size of transcription factor binding sites. This make finding functional sites by simple signature searching difficult since non functional sites are highly likely to appear in large number within the genome. Novel algorithms are appearing that can reduce this complexity by reducing the analysing the areas in the promoter that are evolutionary conserved between mouse and human[29].

As illustrated above, large-scale gene expression measurements can provide important novel hypothesis regarding mechanism of control of biological pathways. In most research labs the process of testing such hypothesis is performed using traditional approaches to study single gene function an in many cases is just limited to the confirmation using Northern Blot of RT-PCR of the results obtained using microarrays. This scenario is rapidly changing with new technologies available in the area of proteomics[30,31], molecular biology[32,33] and analytical chemistry[34,35] that allow genome wide evaluation of metabolites and protein levels, protein posttranslational modifications and protein-protein interactions. These technologies are costly and today they are available in few specialized laboratories. So far, most of the genome wide data published uses yeast as biological material. While findings in Saccharomyces cerevisiae can be explored to identify general architecture of intracellular pathways, experimental data needs to be acquired in endocrine relevant models in order to explain the complex action of hormones including issues such as multiplicity of actions and tissue specificity. Undoubtly, proteomics and metabolomics will be a powerful addition to expression data and the added layers of genome wide information will wider the rational basis from where novel hypothesis can be extracted. The process of testing such hypothesis is also rapidly changing with the development high throughput cellular assays for many biological pathways. Also important is our ability to overexpress genes or mutated variants using highly efficient transfection vectors[36,37]. Genes knockouts in mice, a most heralded technology considered the ultimate proof of a gene involvement in a physiological process is also being revolutionized and has been turn into a high throughput technique using random mutagenesis[38]. A very promising technology, within the purchase limits of must laboratories, make use of small interference RNA technology to knockout genes in cell cultures and can easily be converted into a high throughput assay[39,40]. It is evident that this the upcoming phase in biological research requires the assembly of many resources and a variety of different competences. The endocrinologist will have the challenge to integrate the information derive from a variety of sources and technologies and turn it into knowledge that contribute to the better understanding of the molecular basis of hormone actions.

The ultimate goal of endocrine research is to understand every detail and principle of the endocrine systems. This is essential to transform biological research from an empirical, phenomenological science that is today into an engineering discipline where the architecture and dynamics of the endocrine system is understood to a level that allow robust theoretical models to be build to simulate complex biological behaviour. These are the goals of the emerging discipline of System Biology[41]. The rapid accumulation of biological data at genomic scale will bring the necessary information to attempt this system level understanding, one that link physiological states of a system to molecular level mechanisms. This is not a trivial task but it is an urgent and important one since is increasingly evident that no individual is capable to comprehend in its totality even simple biological processes. The avalanche of new information brought in by an accelerated technological development will fill a purpose. However, the information has to be organized into abstract models, in order to be able to generate novel hypothesis that are truly relevant because they arise from the unbiased analysis of the current knowledge. Creating such models will require a very broad set of techniques to be deployed for each research area. Highly relevant is the creation of a computational framework and modeling and simulation theory applicable to biological systems[42]. To the experimental biologist this imposes higher demands than our current practice. A realistic attempt to build biological models requires large data sets that are comprehensive and systematically collected therefore require a communitarian rather than individual efforts.

Ideally, as many as possible features of the system should be measured simultaneously on a single sample. For dynamic modeling, fine grain time series are essential. Since this kind of data sets cannot be realistically generated for all possible cellular models, the establishments of standard experimental models that accurately reflect the *in vivo* behaviour and are widely use by the endocrine community is essential.

Hormonal systems are especially amenable to a systemic approach. First, a large body of information regarding both physiological effects and molecular mechanism of action are already available. Second is the existence of established models to generate the data required for biological modeling and to test and improve the validity of the derived hypothesis. Already several projects are ongoing with the objective of providing data and software for System Biology. For example, the Alliance for Cellular Signaling intends to perform a detailed exploration of the B-cell and the cardiomyocyte using genomic and proteomic tools [43]. More than 20 groups will contribute with data generated from the very same cellular models regarding the architecture of signaling networks in those cells. Organizing similar efforts for the study of hormone actions is an essential task of large value to increase our understanding of endocrine systems.

References

1. Venter JC *et al*. The sequence of the human genome. *Science* 2001; 291: 1304–51.

2. Lander ES *et al*. Initial sequencing and analysis of the human genome. *Nature* 2001; 409: 860–921.

3. Mural RJ *et al*. A comparison of whole-genome shotgun-derived mouse chromosome 16 and the human genome. *Science* 2002; 296: 1661–71.

4. Howard AD *et al*. Orphan G-protein-coupled receptors and natural ligand discovery. *Trends Pharmacol Sci* 2001; 22: 132–40.

5. Rock FL, Hardiman G, Timans JC, Kastelein RA, Bazan JF. A family of human receptors structurally related to Drosophila Toll. *Proc Natl Acad Sci USA* 1998; 95: 588–93.

6. Leo CP, Hsu SY, Hsueh AJ Hormonal genomics. *Endocr Rev* 2002; 23: 369–81.

7. Brown PO, Botstein D. Exploring the new world of the genome with DNA microarrays. *Nature Genet* 1999; 21: 33–7.

8. Lockhart DJ, Winzeler EA. Genomics, gene expression and DNA arrays. *Nature* 2000; 405: 827–36.

9. Willson TM, Moore JT. Minireview: genomics versus orphan nuclear receptors-a half-time report. *Mol Endocrinol* 2002; 16: 1135–44.

10. Flores-Morales A *et al*. Microarray analysis of the *in vivo* effects of hypophysectomy and growth hormone treatment on gene expression in the rat. *Endocrinology* 2001; 142: 3163–76.

11. Bussemaker HJ, Li H, Siggia ED. Regulatory element detection using correlation with expression. *Nature Genet* 2001; 27: 167–71.

12. Ge H, Liu Z, Church GM, Vidal M. Correlation between transcriptome and interactome mapping data from Saccharomyces cerevisiae. *Nature Genet* 2001; 29: 482–6.

13. Brazma A *et al*. Minimum information about a microarray experiment (MIAME)-toward standards for microarray data. *Nature Genet* 2001; 29: 365–71.

14. Edgar R, Domrachev M, Lash AE. Gene Expression Omnibus: NCBI gene expression and hybridization array data repository. *Nucleic Acids Res* 2002; 30: 207–10.

15. Kellam P. Microarray gene expression database: progress towards an international repository of gene expression data. *Genome Biol* 2001; 2(5): REPORTS4011.

16. Eisen MB, Spellman PT, Brown PO, Botstein D. Cluster analysis and display of genome-wide expression patterns. *Proc Natl Acad Sci USA* 1998; 95: 14863–8.

17. Nadon R, Shoemaker J. Statistical issues with microarrays: processing and analysis. *Trends Genet* 2002; 18: 265–71.

18. Kerr MK, Churchill GA. Statistical design and the analysis of gene expression microarray data. *Genet Res* 2001; 77: 123–8.

19. Beer DG *et al*. Gene-expression profiles predict survival of patients with lung adenocarcinoma. *Nature Med* 2002; 8: 816–24.

20. Hedenfalk I *et al*. Gene-expression profiles in hereditary breast cancer. *N Engl J Med* 2001; 344: 539–48.

21. Tavazoie S, Hughes JD, Campbell MJ, Cho RJ, Church GM. Systematic determination of genetic network architecture. *Nature Genet* 1999; 22: 281–5.

22. Qian J, Dolled-Filhart M, Lin J, Yu H, Gerstein M. Beyond synexpression relationships: local clustering of time-shifted and inverted gene expression profiles identifies new, biologically relevant interactions. *J Mol Biol* 2001; 314: 1053–66.

23. Zhou X, Kao MC, Wong WH. Transitive functional annotation by shortest-path analysis of gene expression data. *Proc Natl Acad Sci USA* 2002; 26: 26.
24. Winzeler EA *et al*. Functional characterization of the S. cerevisiae genome by gene deletion and parallel analysis. *Science* 1999; 285: 901–6.
25. Ross-Macdonald P *et al*. Large-scale analysis of the yeast genome by transposon tagging and gene disruption. *Nature* 1999; 402: 413–8.
26. Wagner A. Estimating coarse gene network structure from large-scale gene perturbation data. *Genome Res* 2002. 12: 309–15.
27. Kim S *et al*. Multivariate measurement of gene expression relationships. *Genomics* 2000; 67: 201–9.
28. Flores-Morales A *et al*. Patterns of liver gene expression governed by TRbeta. *Mol Endocrinol* 2002; 16: 1257–68.
29. Wasserman WW, Palumbo M, Thompson W, Fickett JW, Lawrence CE. Human-mouse genome comparisons to locate regulatory sites. *Nature Genet* 2000; 26: 225–8.
30. Zhou H, Ranish JA, Watts JD, Aebersold R. Quantitative proteome analysis by solid-phase isotope tagging and mass spectrometry. *Nat Biotechnol* 2002; 20: 512–5.
31. Templin MF *et al*. Protein microarray technology. *Trends Biotechnol* 2002; 20: 160–6.
32. Ito T *et al*. A comprehensive two-hybrid analysis to explore the yeast protein interactome. *Proc Natl Acad Sci USA* 2001; 98: 4569–74.
33. Ho Y *et al*. Systematic identification of protein complexes in Saccharomyces cerevisiae by mass spectrometry. *Nature* 2002; 415: 180–3.
34. Winssinger N, Ficarro S, Schultz PG, Harris JL. Profiling protein function with small molecule microarrays. *Proc Natl Acad Sci USA* 2002; 99: 11139–44.
35. Nicholson JK, Connelly J, Lindon JC, Holmes E. Metabonomics: a platform for studying drug toxicity and gene function. *Nat Rev Drug Discov* 2002; 1: 153–61.
36. Lesley SA. High-throughput proteomics: protein expression and purification in the postgenomic world. *Protein Expr Purif* 2001; 22: 159–64.
37. Koller D *et al*. A high-throughput alphavirus-based expression cloning system for mammalian cells. *Nat Biotechnol* 2001; 19: 851–5.
38. Brown SD, Balling R. Systematic approaches to mouse mutagenesis. *Curr Opin Genet Dev* 2001; 11: 268–73.
39. Paddison PJ, Caudy AA, Bernstein E, Hannon GJ, Conklin DS. Short hairpin RNAs (shRNAs) induce sequence-specific silencing in mammalian cells. *Genes Dev* 2002; 16: 948–58.
40. Lewis DL, Hagstrom JE, Loomis AG, Wolff JA, Herweijer H. Efficient delivery of siRNA for inhibition of gene expression in postnatal mice. *Nature Genet* 2002; 32: 107–8.
41. Kitano H. Systems biology: a brief overview. *Science* 2002; 295: 1662–4.
42. Loew LM, Schaff JC. The Virtual Cell: a software environment for computational cell biology. *Trends Biotechnol* 2001; 19: 401–6.
43. Systems biology's multiple maths. *Nature* 2000; 407: 819.

©2003 John Libbey Eurotext Ltd, pp. 127–130.

CHAPTER 25

Identification of genes which are differentially expressed in white and brown preadipocytes and analysis of their expression pattern during adipocyte differentiation

Stéphane Boeuf,[1] Martin Klingenspor,[2] Nicole L.W. van Hal,[3] Tatjana Schneider,[2] Jaap Keijer[3] and Susanne Klaus[1]

[1]*German Institute of Human Nutrition in Potsdam (DIfE), 14558 Bergholz-Rehbrücke, Germany;* [2]*Department of Biology, Philipps-University, 35043 Marburg, Germany;* [3]*RIKILT, Department of Safety and Health of Food, 6700 AE Wageningen, The Netherlands*
[e-mail: Klaus@www.dife.de]

Introduction

Adipose tissue is actively involved in energy homeostasis, playing a role not only in development of obesity but also insulin resistance and diabetes. In this respect, white (WAT) and brown adipose tissue (BAT) represent counter actors in energy partitioning, channeling lipid energy either to accumulation in WAT or to oxidation, i.e. dissipation in BAT[1]. Considerable progress has been made in elucidating the molecular mechanisms of adipocyte differentiation, which involves sequential activation of numerous transcription factors[2]. However, most of these studies focused on differentiation of white preadipocytes using established white preadipocyte cell lines[3] and very little is known about differentiation of brown preadipocytes. Today it is not known how and at which stage of development the differentiation of brown versus white fat is regulated. Brown and white adipocytes show distinct morphological and biochemical phenotypes *in vivo*[4]. When differentiated *in vitro*, brown adipocytes show a higher respiratory capacity than white adipocytes and express UCP1, a BAT specific protein which is considered to be a marker for brown adipocytes[5]. However, it is still not clear whether BAT and WAT derive from the same adipose precursor cells or arise independently from distinct mesenchymal stem cells.

We hypothesized that white and brown preadipocytes are already determined and thus represent distinct cell types. So far brown and white preadipocytes in culture cannot be discriminated either morphologically, biochemically or through marker genes. Starting from parallel primary cultures of white and brown preadipocytes we performed representational difference analysis (RDA), cloned around 250 cDNA fragments, and screened the expression of these cDNAs in cell culture and in tissue using DNA microarrays[6].

Methods

As a primary cell culture system we used the established and well characterized parallel culture of stromal vascular fraction from WAT and BAT of the Siberian dwarf hamster *Phodopus sungorus*[7]. Cells were grown to semi-confluency, total RNA was extracted and RDA performed as described[6]. The obtained cDNA fragments were cloned and spotted on glass slides together with approximately 50 control genes of established function in adipose tissue. Hybridization and analysis of microarrays was performed as described[6]. For evaluation of expression levels we used the double labeling method, comparing the expression of a given probe RNA with that of a reference RNA which consisted of pooled BAT and WAT samples. This way expression ratios probe/reference could be calculated and multiple hybridizations could be compared.

Results

Reproducibility of microarray hybridization

To check the Reproducibility of the microarray hybridization, each spot on the microarray was spotted in duplicate. Additionally, two separate hybridizations of the same probe RNA was performed. Duplicate spots showed very good correlation when plotted against each other. There was also a high reproducibility of the two hybridizations with less than 2 per cent of spots showing a more than twofold ratio difference. We thus considered differences in expression ratio of more than twofold as significant.

Comparison of white versus brown preadipocytes

Almost 30 per cent of the cloned cDNA fragments showed a ratio white preadipocytes to brown preadipocytes (W/B) or brown preadipocytes to white preadipocytes (B/W) higher than 2. These cDNA fragments were sequenced and matched to databases. In Table 1 are listed the genes with significant expression differences in white and brown preadipocytes: four show higher expression in white preadipocytes and eight higher expression in brown preadipocytes. Among the later is one so far completely unknown gene and one with no described function. Differential expression of these genes was confirmed by Northern blot (data not shown).

Table 1. Differentially expressed genes in white and brown preadipocytes

Function	ExpressionW/B	Accession	Gene
Complement	8.9	NM_008198	Complement factor B
	3.5	M29866	Complement vomponent C3
	3.9	NM_000063	Complement component C2
Metabolism	3.9	NM_004265	Delta 6 fatty acid desaturase (FADSD6)
Function	ExpressionW/B	Accession	Gene
Structure	2.9	NM_019143	Fibronectin
	2.3	NM_021895	Alpha actinin 4 (Actn4)
	2.1	AJ251198	Metargidin (MDC15 gene)
Transcription	2.4	NM_010882	Necdin
	2.2	NM_005336	Vigilin
	2.1	NM_015782	Small nuclear ribonucleoprotein polypeptide A (Snrpa)
Unknown	2.2	NM_006787	Hepatocellular carcinoma associated protein (HCAP)
	2.0	–	New (B26)

List of the difference products with a mean difference of expression level between white and brown preadipocytes higher than 2. The mean ratio of the expression levels from white preadipocytes compared to brown (expression W/B) or from brown preadipocytes compared to white (expression B/W) are shown for the white preadipocytes difference products and the brown preadipocytes difference products, respectively. Homologies to BLAST records were all higher than 80 per cent.

Expression pattern of difference products in cell culture

To obtain information about the expression of the spotted genes during differentiation of preadipocytes, the microarrays were hybridized with mRNA probes from confluent preadipocytes, preadipocytes entering differentiation, mature adipocytes and adipocytes treated with isoproterenol (see legend to Fig. 1 for details). In addition we hybridized the microarrays with mRNA from both BAT and WAT of several animals. Surprisingly, individual variation of gene expression was rather low in adipose tissue *in vivo* (data not shown). Figure 1A shows the expression pattern of delta 6 fatty acid desaturase

A

B

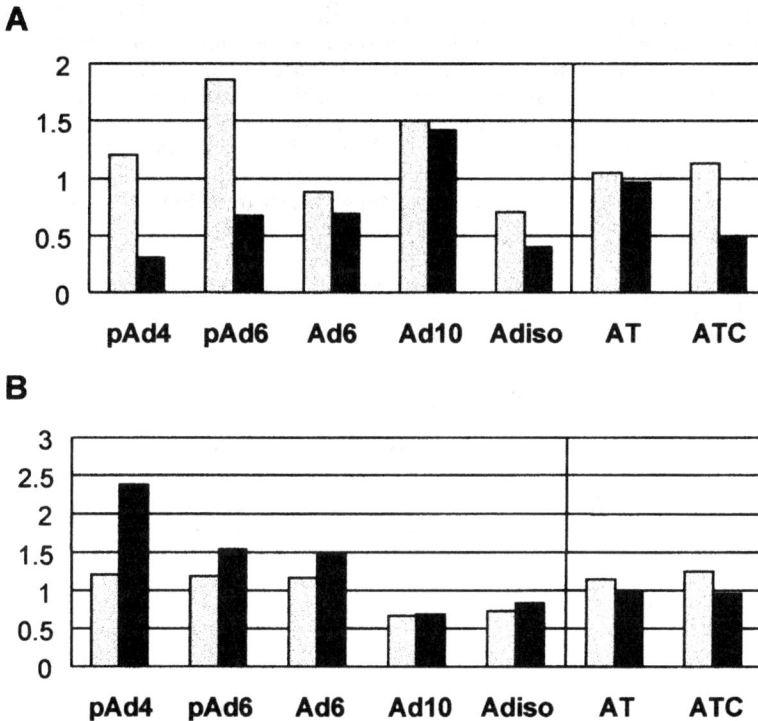

Fig. 1. Expression pattern of two genes with differential expression in white and brown preadipocytes. A Expression pattern of the new gene (B26) showing higher expression in brown preadipocytes. B Expression pattern of FADSD6 showing higher expression in brown preadipocytes. Light bars correspond to WAT, black bars to BAT.

pAd 4, Semi-confluent preadipocytes (day 4); pAd 6, Confluent preadipocytes (day 6); Ad 6, Preadipocytes beginning differentiation (day 6, treated with insulin); Ad 10, Mature adipocytes (day 10, treated with insulin); Ad iso, Adipocytes treated with isoproterenol (day 10, treated with insulin); AT, Pooled adipose tissue; ATC, Pooled adipose tissue from cold exposed animals.

(FADSD6), a gene with higher expression in white preadipocytes. In brown adipose cells, the expression level was higher in mature cells than in undifferentiated cells, whereas for white adipose cells there were high expression levels in both preadipocytes and in adipocytes. For both cells types, the expression was repressed by isoproterenol, i.e. ß-adrenergic stimulation. The complement factors show a very similar expression pattern (data not shown). Figure 1B shows the expression pattern of the new gene (B26): its expression in white preadipocytes did not change during differentiation, in BAT cultures however, its expression was high in preadipocytes and decreased during differentiation. There was no effect of ß-adrenergic treatment. The other clones identified with higher expression in brown preadipocytes (see Table 1) showed very similar expression patterns.

Discussion

Using a combination of a subtractive cDNA amplification (RDA) together with microarray screening we were able to identify genes with different expression levels in white and brown preadipocytes, many of which have so far not been implicated in adipocyte differentiation. The majority of differentially expressed genes surprisingly showed only two- to threefold difference in expression between white and brown preadipocytes. It seems that expression differences between white and brown preadipocytes are not as great as between preadipocytes and mature adipocytes. Our data suggest that there are rather subtle but relevant differences in expression levels of these genes.

A detailed discussion of the differentially expressed genes can be found in Boeuf *et al.*, 2001[6]. It is rather intriguing that the differentially expressed genes of one cell type (white or brown) all show very similar expression patterns, which are however different between the two cell types. It should also be noticed that the expression of many genes was rather different in BAT and WAT tissue compared to cell cultures. This could be due to the fact that adipose tissue consists of various cells different cell types beside adipocytes, and/or to different conditions *in vitro* versus *in vivo*.

In conclusion, we demonstrate that RDA in combination with DNA-microarray screening is a useful method for identification of genes with different expression levels in different cell populations or different physiological situations. We have identified several genes which show differential expression in white and brown preadipocyte as well as distinct patterns of expression during adipose conversion, among them one unknown gene. The function of these genes in adipogenesis remains to be investigated.

Acknowledgements: This study was supported by grants from the Deutsche Forschungsgemeinschaft (DFG) and by the European Commission (COST Action 918).

References

1. Klaus S. Brown adipocyte differentiation and function in energy metabolism. In: *Adipose tissues*, Klaus, S (ed.), pp. 82–96. Landes Bioscience, Medical Intelligence Unit. Austin: 2001.

2. Wu Z, Puigserver P, Spiegelman BM. Transcriptional activation of adipogenesis. *Curr Opin Cell Biol* 1999; 11: 689–94.

3. Ntambi JM, Young-Cheul K Adipocyte Differentiation and Gene Expression. *J Nutr* 2000; 130: 3122S–6S.

4. Cinti S. Morphology of the adipose organ. In: *Adipose tissues*, Klaus, S. (ed.),pp. 11–26. Landes Bioscience, Medical Intelligence Unit. Austin: 2001.

5. Klaus S, Ely M, Encke D, Heldmaier G. Functional assessment of white and brown adipocyte development and energy metabolism in cell culture. Dissociation of terminal differentiation and thermogenesis in brown adipocytes. *J Cell Sci* 1995; 08: 3171–80.

6. Boeuf S, Klingenspor M, van Hal N, Schneider T, Keijer J, Klaus S. Differential gene expression in white and brown preadipocytes. *Physiol Genomics* 2001; 7: 15–25.

7. Klaus S, Seivert A, Boeuf S. Effect of the beta-3-adrenergic agonist Cl316,243 on functional differentiation of white and brown adipocytes in primary cell culture. *Biochim Biophys Acta Mol Cell Res* 2001; 1539: 85–92.

Progress in Obesity Research: 9. Edited by *Geraldo Medeiros-Neto, Alfredo Halpern* and *Claude Bouchard*
©2003 John Libbey Eurotext Ltd, pp. 131–134.

CHAPTER 26

PPARγ: from cell proliferation to adipocyte differentiation

Lluis Fajas

Endocrinologie Moléculaire et Cellulaire des Cancers, INSERM U540, Montpellier, France
[e-mail: fajas@montp.inserm.fr]

Introduction

The peroxisome proliferator-activated receptor gamma (PPARγ) is a member of the nuclear receptor superfamily, which is activated by naturally occurring fatty acids or fatty acid derivatives. PPARγ heterodimerizes with retinoid X receptors (RXR) and regulates the transcription of numerous target genes after binding to specific response elements or PPREs, which are found in several genes involved in fat metabolism. Coordinate regulation of genes involved in fat uptake and storage by PPARγ underlies its effects on adipocyte differentiation.

Adipocyte differentiation is a highly regulated process taking place from birth throughout adult life. Adipose tissue is composed of adipocytes, which store energy in the form of triglycerides and release it as free fatty acids (for review see[1]). Excessive accumulation of adipose tissue leads to obesity whereas its absence is associated with lipodystrophic syndromes. PPARγ is highly expressed in the adipose tissue and is required for its development. During adipocyte differentiation, PPARγ regulates the expression of several adipose tissue specific genes. In fact, functional PPREs have been identified in several genes implicated in adipocyte differentiation. Good examples are aP2 2, phosphoenol pyruvate carboxykinase (PEPCK)[3], fatty acid transport protein-1 (FATP-1)[4], and lipoprotein lipase (LPL)[5], which are all regulated by PPARγ. The conclusive demonstration of the crucial role that PPARγ plays in adipogenesis comes from both, recent observations in PPARγ knock-out mice and the analysis of the mutations in the PPARγ gene in human subjects. PPARγ[−/−] mice are completely devoid of adipose tissue and PPARγ[+/−] mice are characterized by a decreased adipose tissue mass[6,7]. Injection of PPARγ[−/−] embryonic mice cells into wild-type blastocytes produces chimeric mice in which adipose tissue is composed exclusively with PPARγ[+/+] cells, demonstrating that PPARγ is necessary to ensure development of this tissue[8].

In humans, genetic studies have further contributed to determine the role of PPARγ in fat metabolism. Several mutations in the PPARγ gene have so far been described. A rare Pro115Gln mutation in the NH_2-terminal ligand-independent activation domain of PPARγ was found in four very obese subjects[9]. This mutation, which inhibits the phosphorylation at Ser112, resulted in a permanently active PPARγ and led to increased adipocyte differentiation and obesity[9]. Phosphorylation at Ser112 was proposed as a mechanism by which growth factors and insulin, through mitogen-activated protein kinase, decrease PPARγ activity and adipocyte differentiation[10,11]. Furthermore, a much more common Pro12Ala substitution in the PPARV2-specific exon B[12–15], resulting in a less active PPARγ form, is associated with a lower BMI. These results, together with the observations made on the Pro115Gln substitution, provide strong evidence for a role of PPARγ in the control of adipogenesis *in vivo*, such that a more active PPARγ (Pro115Gln) results in increased BMI[9], whereas the opposite is seen with a less active PPARγ (Pro12Ala)[13].

Three different mechanisms account for the regulation of PPARγ activity during adipogenesis (Fig. 1). First, transcription factors induced early in the differentiation process will trigger the expression of PPARγ. Second, several cofactors will modulate the activity of PPARγ. And finally, natural or synthetic

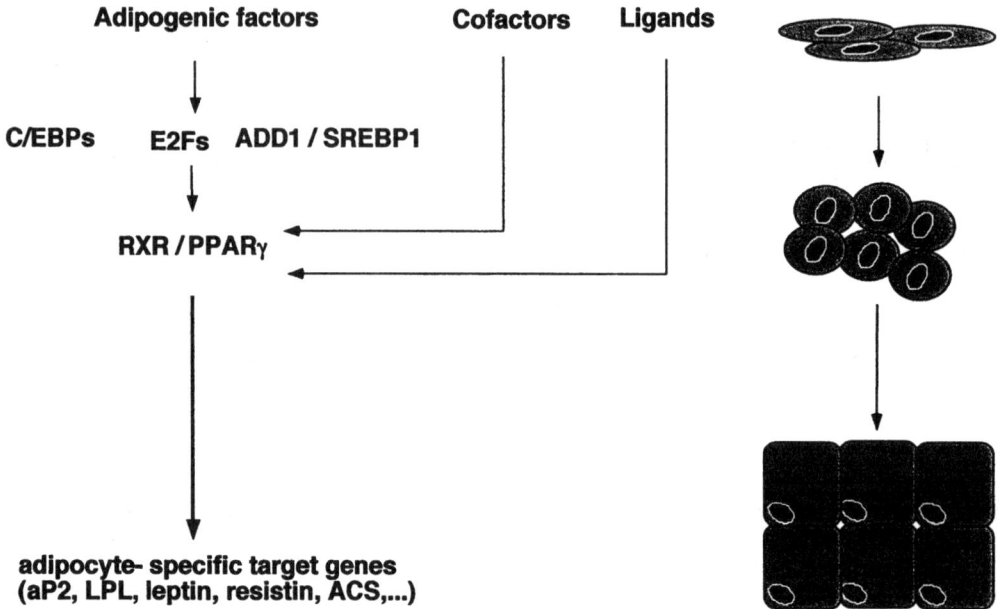

Fig. 1.

PPARγ ligands will also modulate its activity. The sum of all these mechanisms will determine the activity of PPARγ, and thus the degree of adipogenesis. I will discuss below each of these factors.

Transcription factors

Implication of the transcription factors C/EBPs, ADD-1/SREBP1, GATA, and others in the regulation of PPARγ is reviewed elsewhere[1].In this study I will focus on the participation of the E2F family of transcription factors in the regulation of PPARγ expression and its implication in the adipogenic process. In the first hours of adipocyte differentiation, an increase in the E2F activity has been observed[16] coincident with the required re-entry into cell cycle observed in hormonally induced preadipocytes. E2Fs are transcription factors which regulate the expression of genes involved in DNA synthesis (for review see[17–19]). Consequently, expression of these genes, such as cyclin D1, c-Myc, or cyclin E, is increased in the early stages of adipogenesis[20]. Interestingly, we have recently shown that E2F1 trigger the expression of PPARγ directly by binding to and transactivating the PPARγ1 promoter during the clonal expansion of the adipocyte differentiation process. Consistent with a positive role in adipogenesis, E2F1[-/-] mice have reduced fat mass and are protected against high fat diet induced obesity[21]. In contrast to E2F1, another member of the family, E2F4, which is considered as a repressor, represses the transcription of PPARγ, acting as a negative factor for adipogenesis. Consistent with this is the fact that E2F4[-/-] ES cells differentiate into adipocytes more easily than the wild type cells[21].

Cofactors

A functional class of proteins, called cofactors, was shown to play an important role in transcriptional control. Such cofactors also interact with nuclear receptors and they can either repress (corepressors) or enhance (coactivators) their transcriptional activities. An important number of cofactors interact with PPARγ. The CBP/p300 and the SRC family of cofactors, are reported to interact with PPARγ. CBP and p300 are two related and widely-expressed[22] cofactors. We have observed that CBP/p300 interacts with PPARγ. SRC-1 has been shown to interact in a yeast two-hybrid system with the PPARγ LBD[23]. Also other related members of the SRC family of cofactors such as Tif2/Grip1 and ACTR/RAC3/AIB/pCIP have been shown to interact with PPARγ in a manner similar to SRC-1. The PPAR binding protein (PBP)[24] (or TRAP 220 or DRIP 205) and PPAR gamma coactivator-1 (PGC-1)[25], were were also shown to be coactivators for PPARγ. SMRT is a corepressor, that inhibits retinoic acid receptor and thyroid hormone receptor-dependent transcription in absence of their respective ligands and it was suggested that SMRT may also be involved in down-modulating PPARγ-mediated gene transcription[26].

The retinoblastoma protein RB, which is a negative regulator of cell cycle, plays a dual role in adipocyte differentiation. During the clonal expansion phase RB plays a negative role by inhibiting re-entry into cell cycle following hormonal induction of preadipocytes. Consequently, RB has been found to be hyperphosphorylated, and thus inactive, in these early stages of adipogenesis[16]. In the later stages, RB positively regulates adipogenesis participating in the cell cycle exit required for terminal adipocyte differentiation. Consistent with this is the observation that pRB inactivation, by SV40 large T antigen, inhibits adipogenesis[27]. Moreover, pRB-deficient fibroblasts fail to differentiate into adipocytes when properly stimulated[28]. A second, positive role for RB in terminal adipocyte differentiation is the consequence of its stimulatory effect on the transactivation by the proadipogenic C/EBPs, which is mediated via a direct protein-protein interaction[28].

Since both PPARγ and RB are major regulators of cell proliferation and differentiation, a cross-talk between PPARγ and RB signaling might operate during adipocyte differentiation. We have shown that RB recruits histone deacetylase 3 (HDAC3) to PPARγ target promoters. Disruption of the PPARγ-RB-HDAC3 complex by phosphorylation of RB or inhibition of HDAC3 activity results in the activation of PPARγ translating in an increase in adipogenesis.

PPARγ ligands

Beside the sofar described natural and synthetic PPARγ ligands such as some prostaglandin derivatives and thiazolidinediones respectively, another PPARγ modulator, i.e. FMOC-L-Leucine (FMOC-L-Leu), was recently described in our laboratory[29]. FMOC-L-Leu has some similarity to the tyrosine-based PPARγ ligands, but unlike these last compounds have a rather weak affinity for PPARγ. Interestingly, two molecules of FMOC-L-Leu bind to the ligand binding domain of the receptor, as demonstrated by mass spectrometry of the PPARγ ligand binding domain and FMOC-L-Leu. This unique binding mode to PPARγ changes the cofactor preference of PPARγ, relative to classical agonist ligands, and resulted in distinct biological effects, characterized by strong insulin sensitization yet no weight gain.

Conclusions

Because of the central role that PPARγ plays in the differentiation of the adipocytes, we have studied its regulation in this process. We identified new transcription factors (E2Fs) which regulate PPARγ expression in the early stages of adipogenesis. Concerning its activity, we have shown that the RB-HDAC3 complex interact with PPARγ and represses its activity. We have also discovered that F-moc Leu, a new PPARγ partial agonist, recruits a specific set of cofactors to PPARγ resulting in a beneficial effect on glucose homeostasis without affecting body weight in mice.

References

1. Fajas L, Fruchart JC, Auwerx J. Transcriptional control of adipogenesis. *Curr Opinions Cell Biol* 1998; 10: 165–73.

2. Tontonoz P, Hu E, Graves RA, Budavari AI, Spiegelman BM. mPPARg2: tissue-specific regulator of an adipocyte enhancer. *Genes & Dev* 1994; 8: 1224–34.

3. Tontonoz P, Hu E, Devine J, Beale EG, Spiegelman BM. PPARg2 regulates adipose expression of the phosphoenolpyruvate carboxykinase gene. *Mol Cellular Biol* 1995; 15: 351–7.

4. Martin G, Schoonjans K, Lefebvre A, Staels B, Auwerx J. Coordinate regulation of the expression of the fatty acid transport protein (FATP) and acyl CoA synthetase genes by PPARα and PPARγ activators. *J Biol Chem* 1997; 272: 28210–7.

5. Schoonjans K, Peinado-Onsurbe J, Lefebvre AM, Heyman R, Briggs M, Deeb S, *et al.* PPAR1 and PPARγ activators direct a tissue-specific transcriptional response via a PPRE in the lipoprotein lipase gene. *EMBO J.* 1996; 15: 5336–48.

6. Kubota N, Terauchi Y, Miki H, Tamemoto H, Yamauchi T, Komeda K *et al.* PPARγ mediates high-fat diet-induced adipocyte hypertrophy and insulin resistance. *Mol Cell* 1999; 4: 597–609.

7. Miles PD, Barak Y, He W, Evans RM, Olefsky JM. Improved insulin-sensitivity in mice heterozygous for PPAR-gamma deficiency. *J Clin Invest* 2000; 105(3): 287–92.

8. Rosen ED, Sarraf P, Troy AE, Bradwin G, Moore K, Milstone DS *et al.* PPARgamma is required for the differentiation of adipose tissue *in vivo* and *in vitro. Mol Cell* 1999; 4: 611–7.

9. Ristow M, Muller-Wieland D, Pfeiffer A, Krone W, Kahn CR. Obesity associated with a mutation in a genetic regulator of adipocyte differentiation. *New Eng J Med* 1998; 339: 953–9.

10. Hu E, Kim JB, Sarraf P, Spiegelman BM. Inhibition of adipogenesis through MAP-kinase mediated phosphorylation of PPARγ. *Science* 1996; 274: 2100–3.

11. Camp HS, Tafuri SR. Regulation of peroxisome proliferator-activated receptor gamma activity by mitogen-activated protein kinase. *J Biol Chem* 1997; 272: 10811–6.

12. Yen CJ, Beamer BA, Negri C, Silver K, Brown KA, Yarnall DP *et al.* Molecular scanning of the human peroxisome proliferator activated receptor gamma gene in diabetic Caucasians: identification of a Pro12Ala PPARgamma 2 missense mutation. *Biochem Biophys Res Com* 1997; 241: 270–4.

13. Deeb S, Fajas L, Nemoto M, Laakso M, Fujimoto W, Auwerx J. A Pro 12 Ala substitution in the human peroxisome proliferator-activated receptor gamma2 is associated with decreased receptor activity, improved insulin sensitivity, and lowered body mass index. *Nature Genet* 1998; 20: 284–7.

14. Beamer BA, Yen CJ, Andersen RE, Muller D, Elahi D, Cheskin LJ *et al.* Association of the Pro12Ala variant in peroxisome proliferator-activated receptor gamma2 gene with obesity in two Caucasian populations. *Diabetes* 1998; 47: 1806–8.

15. Hara K, Okada T, Tobe K, Yasuda K, Mori Y, Kadowaki H *et al.* The Pro12Ala polymorphism in PPAR gamma2 may confer resistance to type 2 diabetes *Biochem Biophys Res Commun* 2000; 271(1): 212–216.

16. Richon V, Lyle RE, McGehee REJ. Regulation and expression of retinoblastoma proteins p107 and p130 during 3T3-L1 adipocyte differentiation. *J Biol Chem* 1997; 272: 10117–24.

17. Nevins JR. E2F: a link between the Rb tumor suppressor protein and viral oncoproteins. *Science* 1992; 258(5081): 424–9.

18. Helin K. Regulation of cell proliferation by the E2F transcription factors. *Curr Opin Genet Dev* 1998; 8(1): 28–35.

19. Sardet C, Le Cam L, Fabbrizio E, Vidal M. E2Fs and the retinoblastoma protein family. *Prog Gene Expression* 1997; 2: 1–62.

20. Reichert M, Eick D. Analysis of cell cycle arrest in adipocyte differentiation. *Oncogene* 1999; 18(2): 459–66.

21. Fajas L, Landsberg RL, Huss-Garcia Y, Sardet C, Lees JA, Auwerx J. E2Fs regulate adipogenesis. *Develop Cell* 2002; 3(1): 39–49.

22. Misiti S, Schomburg L, Yen PM, Chin WW. Expression and hormonal regulation of co-activator and corepressor genes. *Endocrinology* 1998; 139: 2493–500.

23. Zhu Y, Qi C, Calandra C, Rao MS, Reddy J. Cloning and identification of mouse steroid receptor coactivator-1 (mSRC-1), as a coactivator of peroxisome proliferator-activated receptor g. *Gene Expression* 1996; 6: 185–95.

24. Zhu Y, Qi C, Rao MS, Reddy JK. Isolation of and characterization of PBP, a protein that interacts with peroxisome proliferator activated receptor. *J Biol Chem* 1997; 272: 25500–06.

25. Puigserver P, Wu Z, Park CW, Graves R, Wright M, Spiegelman BM. A cold-inducible coactivator of nuclear receptors linked to adaptive thermogenesis. *Cell* 1998; 92: 829–39.

26. Lavinsky RM, Jepsen K, Heinzel T, Torchia J, Mullen TM, Schiff R *et al.* Diverse signalling pathways modulate nuclear receptor recruitment of N-CoR and SMRT complexes. *Proc Nat Acad Sci USA* 1998; 95: 2920–5.

27. Higgins C, Chatterjee S, Cherington V. The block of adipocyte differentiation by a C-terminally truncated, but not by full-length, simian virus 40 large tumor antigen is dependent on an intact retinoblastoma susceptibility protein family binding domain. *J Virol* 1996; 70: 745–52.

28. Chen PL, Riley DJ, Chen Y, Lee WH. Retinoblastoma protein positively regulates terminal adipocyte differentiation through direct interaction with C/EBPs. *Genes Dev* 1996; 10(21): 2794–804.

29. Rocchi S, Picard F, Vamecq J, Gelman L, Potier N, Zeyer D, *et al.* A unique PPARgamma ligand with potent insulin-sensitizing yet weak adipogenic activity. *Mol Cell* 2001; 8(4): 737–47.

Progress in Obesity Research: 9. Edited by *Geraldo Medeiros-Neto, Alfredo Halpern* and *Claude Bouchard*
©2003 John Libbey Eurotext Ltd, pp. 135–138.

CHAPTER 27

Mechanisms of βAR signaling in adipocytes and functional consequences on thermogenesis

Sheila Collins, Wenhong Cao, Jacques Robidoux and Kiefer W. Daniel

Departments of Psychiatry and Behavioral Sciences and Pharmacology and Cancer Biology,
Duke University Medical Center, Box 3557, Durham, NC 27710, USA
[e-mail: colli008@mc.duke.edu]

Long before the discovery of the β3AR and its recognition as a unique, adipocyte-specific receptor controlling lipolysis and thermogenesis, Rodbell and colleagues[1] made the observation that there was an unusual, biphasic stimulation of cAMP production in adipocytes in response to the β-adrenergic receptor agonist isoproterenol. Depending upon the concentration of GTP in the assay, isoproterenol could either stimulate or inhibit adenylyl cyclase activity in adipocyte plasma membranes. Murayama and Ui[2] showed that this inhibitory phase could be relieved by pretreatment of adipocytes with pertussis toxin (PTX).[1] This curious observation lay fallow until studied later in greater detail by Bégin-Heick[3–5]. However, it was not until the cloning and characterization of the β3AR gene and the development of selective β3AR agonists[6,7] that it was postulated that this novel adipocyte-specific βAR may be responsible for the biphasic adenylyl cyclase response in adipocytes[8]. We have previously noted that despite the relatively high level of expression of the β3AR in adipocytes, the efficiency of coupling of the β3AR to stimulation of adenylyl cyclase is low[9]. However, there has been no clear biochemical demonstration of physical coupling of the β3AR to Gi, other than comparative functional experiments in the presence or absence of PTX[10], nor has there been any indication of what additional second messenger pathway may be activated as a consequence of this putative coupling of β3AR to Gi.

Since the mid-1980s research in the field of G protein-coupled receptors has shown that they can mediate cellular growth or differentiation responses through the activation of MAP kinase cascades[11]. Receptors signaling via PTX-sensitive $G_{i/o}$ proteins, as well as PTX-insensitive $G_{q/11}$ proteins may activate the ERK1/2 MAP kinase cascade through a mechanism involving tyrosine protein phosphorylation and the activation of the low molecular weight G protein $p21^{ras}$[12–14]. Little is known about the potential role of βARs in the regulation of the MAP kinase pathway. Recently, our colleagues found that in fibroblasts the β2AR mediates Ras-dependent ERK1/2 activation through its ability to couple to a PTX-sensitive Gi protein[15]. β2AR coupling to Gi occurs as a result of PKA-dependent phosphorylation of the receptor, which effectively 'switches' receptor coupling from Gs to Gi proteins. In contrast, β2AR-mediated ERK1/2 activation in S49 lymphoma cells is an entirely Gs-dependent process[16]. In this system, PKA-mediated phosphorylation of the low molecular weight GTPase, Rap1, promotes Ras-independent ERK1/2 activation; this process was shown to be independent of β2AR interaction with $G_{i/o}$ proteins. Therefore, it is not yet clear whether there is a common mechanism by which βARs activate MAP kinase.

During the past few years we have probed the intracellular signaling cascades in adipocytes that are activated in response to βAR stimulation by catecholamines. This series of studies has led us to appreciate that there are several simultaneous and bifurcating pathways, each of which contributes to unique features of adipocytes metabolism. In the first set of studies we demonstrated that stimulation of the β3AR in adipocytes induces the direct activation of both Gs and Gi[17]. In these cells, Gs and Gi activation results in β3AR-mediated stimulation of both adenylyl cyclase and the activation of the ERK1/2 MAP kinase pathway, respectively. Unlike the β2AR signal in fibroblasts, β3AR activation of the ERK1/2 pathway is independent of cAMP and PKA. These data suggest that the promiscuous coupling of the β3AR in adipocytes permits the simultaneous transduction of two independent signaling pathways. Because GRK-mediated phosphorylation is necessary for β-arrestin binding, but the β3AR lacks sites for phosphorylation, we concluded that the β3AR must employ a novel mechanism of ERK activation. In this next series of studies we demonstrated that conserved proline-rich motifs in the third intracellular loop and carboxyl terminus of the β3AR directly recruit c-Src in a β3AR agonist- and PTX-sensitive manner[24]. This interaction occurs specifically through the SH3 domain of c-Src. Our findings establish a new mechanism whereby some GPCRs can acquire ligand-induced tyrosine kinase activity by means of direct recruitment of Src kinases. This property of the β3AR may be responsible, in part, for the unique physiological effects of selective β3AR agonists *in vivo*, such as their potency for stimulating lipolysis[18,19] and their ability to prevent or reverse obesity[6,20–23].

In the adipocyte, although the classic pattern of signal transduction through which βAR agonists exert their effects is increased cAMP production and activation of PKA, through the use of selective kinase inhibitors and cAMP mimetics, our recent results clearly show that cAMP and PKA activity are required for the subsequent activation of p38 MAPK by β3AR in adipocytes[25]. This pathway appears to be functional in both white and brown adipocytes. Because β3AR-selective agonists have thermogenic and anti-obesity effects, we also investigated the consequences of the p38 pathway on induction of the UCP1 gene in brown adipocytes. We show that p38 MAPK activity is absolutely required for the β-agonist-dependent increase in UCP1 mRNA and protein levels as well as transcriptional activation of the UCP1 promoter.

We did not focus extensively on the other members of the AR family in these studies but our data further suggest that all AR subtypes are capable of activating p38 MAPK in adipocytes because ISO, as well as provision of the adenylyl cyclase activator FSK or the cAMP mimetic dibutyryl cAMP, could elicit the same response. However, it is noteworthy that the amplitude of the stimulation of p38 MAPK by dibutyryl cAMP or FSK was smaller than that by CL or ISO. The reasons for this are not clear but appear to indicate the need for a signal that is specific to AR stimulation in addition to elevation of cAMP levels. One possibility could also be related to the isozymes of adenylyl cyclase that are expressed in adipocytes. We and others have shown that multiple adenylyl cyclase isoforms are expressed in white and brown adipocytes including the relatively abundant Type IX[32,33], which is insensitive to FSK[34,35].

Our results in both primary brown adipocytes and in transfected HIB-1B cells show that the cAMP-dependent increase in UCP1 expression through PKA and p38 MAPK targets the 2530/2310 enhancer region of the UCP1 promoter. This potent brown fat-specific enhancer was identified in the UCP1 gene as being responsible for tissue-specific and catecholamine-stimulated expression[26,27,29]. This region also contains a PPRE that appears critical for activity and when attached to a heterologous promoter also appeared to contribute to cAMP-responsiveness[28].

Since this most recent finding, we now have evidence that PPARγ-coactivator-1α is a key target of this β-adrenergic and p38 MAPK signaling. It requires the phosphorylation of PGC1α by p38 MAPK, and consequent increases in UCP1 gene transcription in animals and cell culture models.

The complexity of the signaling might insure that only when all of the relevant signaling molecules and the enzymes of signal transduction are present will there be appropriate gene expression for UCP1 (via p38 MAPK), or maximal lipolysis via the coordinated stimulation of HSL phosphorylation by both PKA and ERK1/2[30,31].

Abbreviations: β-AR: β-adrenergic receptor; MAPK: mitogen-activated protein kinase; PTX: pertussis toxin.

Acknowledgement: The author acknowledges grant funding NIH DK-57698 and NIH DK-54024.

References

1. Cooper DM, Schlegel W, Lin MC, Rodbell M. The fat cell adenylate cyclase system. Characterization and manipulation of its bimodal regulation by GTP. *J Biol Chem.* 1979; 254(18): 8927–31.

2. Murayama T, Ui M. Loss of the inhibitory function of the guanine nucleotide regulatory component of adenylate cyclase due to its ADP ribosylation by islet-activating protein, pertussis toxin, in adipocyte membranes. *J Biol Chem* 1983; 258(5): 3319–26.

3. Begin-Heick N. Absence of the inhibitory effect of guanine nucleotides on adenylate cyclase activity in white adipocyte membranes of the ob/ob mouse. Effect of the ob gene. *J Biol Chem.* 1985; 260(10): 6187–93.

4. Begin-Heick N. The response of adenylate cyclase to ACTH in adipocyte membranes of lean and obese mice. *Mol Cell Endocrinol* 1987; 53(1–2): 1–8.

5. Begin-Heick N. Quantification of the alpha and beta subunits of the transducing elements (Gs and Gi) of adenylate cyclase in adipocyte membranes from lean and obese (ob/ob) mice. *Biochem J* 1990; 15: 268(1): 83–9.

6. Arch Jr, Ainsworth AT, Cawthorne MA, Piercy V, Sennitt MV *et al.* Atypical beta-adrenoceptor on brown adipocytes as target for anti-obesity drugs. *Nature* 1984; 16: 309(5964): 163–5.

7. Bloom JD, Dutia MD, Johnson BD, Wissner A, Burns MG, Largis EE *et al.* Disodium (R,R)-5-[2-[[2-(3-chlorophenyl)-2-hydroxyethyl]-amino] propyl]-1,3-benzodioxole-2,2-dicarboxylate (CL 316,243). A potent beta-adrenergic agonist virtually specific for beta 3 receptors. A promising antidiabetic and antiobesity agent. *J Med Chem* 1992; 7: 35(16): 3081–4.

8. Begin-Heick, N. Beta 3-adrenergic activation of adenylyl cyclase in mouse white adipocytes: modulation by GTP and effect of obesity. *J Cell Biochem* 1995; 58(4): 464–73.

9. Collins S, Daniel KW, Rohlfs EM, Ramkumar V, Taylor IL, Gettys TW. Impaired expression and functional activity of the beta 3- and beta 1-adrenergic receptors in adipose tissue of congenitally obese (C57BL/6J ob/ob) mice. *Mol Endocrinol* 1994; 8(4): 518–27.

10. Chaudhry A, MacKenzie RG, Georgic LM, Granneman JG. *Cell Signal* 1994; 6: 457–65.

11. Van Biesen T, Luttrell LM, Hawes BE, Lefkowitz RJ. Mitogenic signaling via G protein-coupled receptors. *Endocr Rev* 1996; 17(6): 698–714.

12. Koch WJ, Hawes BE, Allen LF, Lefkowitz RJ. Direct evidence that Gi-coupled receptor stimulation of mitogen-activated protein kinase is mediated by G beta gamma activation of p21ras. *Proc Natl Acad Sci USA.* 1994; 91(26): 12706–10.

13. Van Biesen T, Hawes BE, Luttrell DK, Krueger KM, Touhara K, Porfiri E, Sakaue M, Luttrell LM, Lefkowitz RJ. Receptor-tyrosine-kinase- and G beta gamma-mediated MAP kinase activation by a common signalling pathway. *Nature* 1995; 376(6543): 781–4.

14. Crespo P, Xu N, Simonds WF, Gutkind JS. Ras-dependent activation of MAP kinase pathway mediated by G-protein beta gamma subunits. *Nature* 1994; 369(6479): 418–20.

15. Daaka Y, Luttrell LM, Lefkowitz RJ. Switching of the coupling of the beta2-adrenergic receptor to different G proteins by protein kinase A. *Nature.* 1997 Nov 6; 390(6655): 88–91. A *Nature* 1997; 390: 88–91.

16. Wan Y, Huang XY. Analysis of the Gs/mitogen-activated protein kinase pathway in mutant S49 cells.*J Biol Chem* 1998; 5; 273(23): 14533–7.

17. Soeder KJ, Snedden SK, Cao W, Della Rocca GJ, Daniel KW, Luttrell LM, Collins S. *J Biol Chem* 1999; 274: 12917–22.

18. Hollenga C, Brouwer F, Zaagsma J. Differences in functional cyclic AMP compartments mediating lipolysis by isoprenaline and BRL 37344 in four adipocyte types. *Eur J Pharmacol* 1991 6; 200(2–3): 325–30.

19. Hollenga C, Brouwer F, Zaagsma J. Relationship between lipolysis and cyclic AMP generation mediated by atypical beta-adrenoceptors in rat adipocytes. *Br J Pharmacol* 1991; 102(3): 577–80.

20. Largis EE, Burns MG, Muenkel HA *et al.* Antidiabetic and anti-obesity effects of a highly selective 3 adrenoreceptor agonist (CL 316,243). *Drug Development Res* 1994; 32: 69–76.

21. Himms-Hagen J, Cui J, Danforth E Jr, Taatjes DJ, Lang SS, Waters BL, Claus TH. Effect of CL-316,243, a thermogenic beta 3-agonist, on energy balance and brown and white adipose tissues in rats. *Am J Physiol* 1994 Apr; 266(4 Pt 2): R1371–82.

22. Himms-Hagen J, Cui J, Danforth E Jr, Taatjes DJ, Lang SS, Waters BL, Claus TH. Effect of CL-316,243, a thermogenic beta 3-agonist, on energy balance and brown and white adipose tissues in rats. *Am J Physiol.* 1994; 266(4 Pt 2): R1371–82.

23. Collins S, Daniel KW, Petro AE, Surwit RS. Strain-specific response to beta 3-adrenergic receptor agonist treatment of diet-induced obesity in mice. *Endocrinology* 1997; 138(1): 405–13.

24. Sasaki N, Uchida E, Niiyama M, Yoshida T, Saito M. J Vet Med Sci 1998; 60: 465–9.

25. Cao W, Luttrell LM, Medvedev AV, Pierce KL, Daniel KW, Dixon TM, Lefkowitz RJ, Collins S. Direct binding of activated c-Src to the beta 3-adrenergic receptor is required for MAP kinase activation. *J Biol Chem* 2000; 275(49): 38131–4.

26. Cao W, Medvedev AV, Daniel KW, Collins S. beta-Adrenergic activation of p38 MAP kinase in adipocytes: cAMP induction of the uncoupling protein 1 (UCP1) gene requires p38 MAP kinase. *J Biol Chem* 2001; 276(29): 27077–82.

27. Cassard-Doulcier AM, Gelly C, Fox N, Schrementi J, Raimbault S, Klaus S, Forest C, Bouillaud F, Ricquier D. Tissue-specific and beta-adrenergic regulation of the mitochondrial uncoupling protein gene: control by cis-acting elements in the 5'-flanking region. *Mol Endocrinol.* 1993; 7(4): 497–506.

28. Kozak UC, Kopecky J, Teisinger J, Enerback S, Boyer B, Kozak LP. An upstream enhancer regulating brown-fat-specific expression of the mitochondrial uncoupling protein gene. *Mol Cell Biol* 1994; 14(1): 59–67.

29. Sears IB, MacGinnitie MA, Kovacs LG, Graves RA. Differentiation-dependent expression of the brown adipocyte uncoupling protein gene: regulation by peroxisome proliferator-activated receptor gamma. *Mol Cell Biol* 1996; 16(7): 3410–9.

30. Cassard-Doulcier AM, Gelly C, Bouillaud F, Ricquier D. A 211-bp enhancer of the rat uncoupling protein-1 (UCP-1) gene controls specific and regulated expression in brown adipose tissue. *Biochem J* 1998; 15: 333(Pt 2): 243–6.

31. Greenberg AS, Shen WJ, Muliro K, Patel S, Souza SC, Roth RA, Kraemer FB. Stimulation of lipolysis and hormone-sensitive lipase via the extracellular signal-regulated kinase pathway. *J Biol Chem* 2001; 276(48): 45456–61.

32. Medvedev AV, Robidoux J, Bai X, Cao W, Floering LM, Daniel KW, Collins S. Regulation of the uncoupling protein-2 gene in INS-1 beta-cells by oleic acid. *J Biol Chem* 2002 J Biol Chem 2002; 277(45): 42639–44.

Progress in Obesity Research: 9. Edited by *Geraldo Medeiros-Neto, Alfredo Halpern and Claude Bouchard*
©2003 John Libbey Eurotext Ltd, pp. 139–144.

CHAPTER 28

Lipid mobilization and oxidation induced by alpha2-adrenergic receptor antagonists and natriuretic peptides

Max Lafontan, Michel Berlan, Daniel Rivière, François Crampes, Coralie Sengenes, Vladimir Stich*, Isabelle de Glisezinski, Isabelle Harant and Jean Galitzky

*Unité INSERM 586, Institut Louis Bugnard, CHU Rangueil, Université Paul Sabatier,31403 Toulouse cedex 4, France; and * Third Faculty of Medicine, Charles University, Prague, Czech Republic*
[e-mail: Max.Lafontan@toulouse.inserm.fr]

Introduction

Adipose tissue lipolysis, i.e. the catabolic process leading to the breakdown of fat cell triacylglycerols (TAG) into fatty acids and glycerol, delivers non-esterified fatty acids (NEFA) to circulation where NEFAs serve as the major circulating lipid fuel. When properly regulated, the process usually provides adjusted amounts of NEFAs to fat oxidizing tissues. The delineation of the molecular details of the lipolytic reaction and of the properties of the rate-limiting enzyme of lipolysis, hormone-sensitive lipase (HSL) has noticeably been improved during the last decade. In humans, alterations of hormone-sensitive lipase expression are associated with changes in lipolysis in various physiological and pathological states. Genetic studies have also shown that beta$_2$-adrenergic receptors and hormone-sensitive lipase genes may participate in the polygenic background of obesity[1]. Appropriate regulation of NEFA availability is important for human health. Circulating NEFA concentration is an independent risk factor for sudden death in middle-aged men[2]. Abnormalities of NEFA fluxes have been observed in some forms of obesities. Particularly, upper-body obesity results in several abnormalities of systemic NEFA availability that could contribute to the adverse health consequences usually described in this form of obesity.

The wide range of plasma NEFA availability is essentially related to adipose tissue lipolysis. The balance between hormones that stimulate (primarily catecholamines) and those that inhibit (insulin) HSL regulates adipose tissue lipolytic activity. Insulin role will not be considered in the present report. Studies performed on isolated fat cells from obese adults have demonstrated a reduced lipolytic sensitivity to catecholamines in subcutaneous abdominal adipose tissue. The lipolytic defects have been confirmed in *in vivo* studies[3-5]. Profound unresponsiveness of the subcutaneous adipose tissue to neurally-stimulated lipolysis has also been described in obese subjects[6]. Specific impairment in the capacity of beta$_2$-adrenergic receptors agonists to promote lipolysis, thermogenesis and lipid oxidation has been reported in middle-aged subjects and obese patients[7,8]. All the mechanistic aspects related to beta-adrenergic receptor alterations will not be considered here.

Alpha2-adrenergic receptors and the physiological regulation of lipolysis

Catecholamines are important stimulators of NEFA release under various conditions of stress and during exercise. Our group has devoted a number of studies to fat cell alpha$_2$-adrenergic receptors in humans[9]. *In vitro* assays on isolated human fat cells have delineated variations of human fat cell alpha$_2$-adrenergic receptors function and expression in various physiological and pathological situations. Activation of alpha$_2$-adrenergic receptors by epinephrine and norepinephrine impairs the beta-adrenergic component of catecholamine-induced lipolysis[10-13]. The strongest alpha$_2$-adrenergic effects

A

Number of $\beta_{1/2}$ and α_2-adrenergic receptors (per cell).

B

Increment in extracellular glycerol levels (μmol/l).

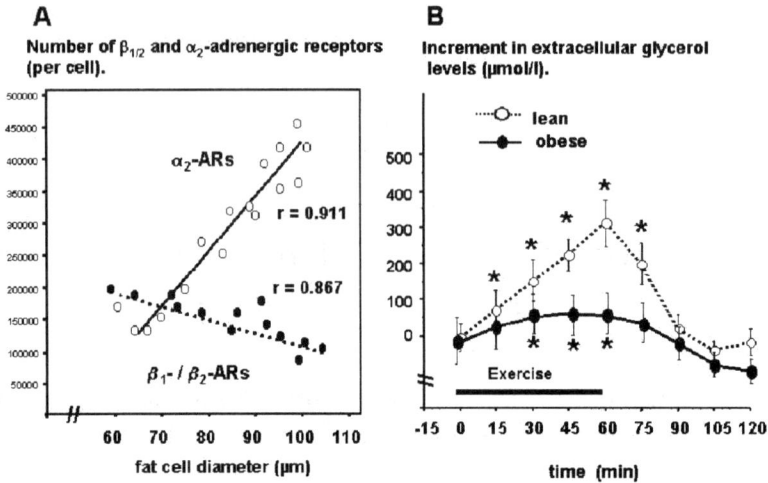

Fig. 1. Panel A: Relationships existing between beta1/beta2 and alpha2-adrenergic receptor expression and mean fat cell diameter in human fat cells originating from omental and subcutaneous fat deposits. Alpha2- and beta1-/beta2-adrenergic receptor number was determined using saturation binding studies on intact fat cells using [³H]RX821002 and [³H]CGP12177 respectively. Alpha2-adrenergic receptor expression was positively correlated to the increment of fat cell diameter while an inverse correlation was found for beta1-/beta2-adrenergic receptors. A similar relationship has also been observed in hamster white fat cells (see ref.[9]).

Panel B: Effect of exercise (1 h, 60-min and 50 per cent VO2max) on the extracellular glycerol concentrations measured by in situ microdialysis in the subcutaneous adipose tissue of lean and obese subjects. Exercise-induced lipid mobilization is impaired in subcutaneous adipose tissue of obese men. The blunting of lipid mobilization is suppressed by local administration of an alpha2-adrenergic receptor antagonist such as phentolamine (non selective alpha1/alpha2-antagonist) (see ref.[19]).

have been observed in the adipocytes from subcutaneous adipose tissue (SCAT) from men and women. In human SCAT fat cells where alpha2-adrenergic receptors outnumber beta-adrenergic receptors, the preferential recruitment of the alpha2-adrenergic receptors at the lowest catecholamine concentrations is leading to lipolysis inhibition[10]. Alpha2-adrenergic receptors are particularly expressed in SCAT adipocytes from obese subjects. There is a positive correlation between the level of expression of alpha2-adrenergic receptors (and a concomitant inverse relationship for the level of expression of beta1/beta2-adrenergic receptors) and fat cell hypertrophy (Fig. 1A). The recent in vivo results of the laboratory provide a response to an old question concerning the putative role of fat cell alpha2-adrenergic receptors in the physiological control of lipid mobilization.

Based on the utilization of in situ microdialysis technique, the results have allowed a better understanding of the relative contribution of the beta1-2/alpha2-adrenergic receptors in the control of lipolysis in vivo. Initial studies, performed in normal subjects, and based on the administration of an alpha2-agonist (clonidine) or catecholamines, directly in the microdialysis probe, have not been fully conclusive to attribute a physiological role to alpha2-adrenergic receptors[14,15]. Thus, exercise was selected as a prerequisite to promote a calibrated activation of sympathetic nervous system. Mild- or moderate-intensity exercise [25–65 per cent of maximal oxygen consumption (VO2max)] is associated with a 5–10 fold-increase in fat oxidation above resting amounts[16]. The catecholamine response to exercise increases lipolysis of adipose tissue TAG and presumably of intramuscular TAG in skeletal muscle. In addition to the well-identified contribution of beta-adrenergic receptors, it was shown that alpha2-adrenergic receptors are involved in the modulation of the lipolytic response initiated by acute bouts of exercise. The results have focused attention on the involvement of epinephrine in the control of lipid mobilization through activation of antilipolytic alpha2-adrenergic receptors in human subcutaneous adipose tissue during exercise[17,18]. It is noticeable that the alpha2-adrenergic effect was essentially observed when plasma epinephrine levels were increased.

Another study has shown that exercise-induced lipid mobilization is impaired in SCAT in obese men and the physiological stimulation of adipocyte alpha2-adrenergic receptors during exercise contributes to this impairment. The blunting of lipid mobilization was suppressed by local administration of an alpha$_2$-adrenergic receptor antagonist[19]. Striking interindividual differences were observed depending on the extent of fat deposits and the intensity of exercise. In heavily trained men, it was impossible to reveal any alpha$_2$-adrenergic effect in the reduced subcutaneous fat deposits of such subjects[20]. Moreover, sex-related differences in the lipid-mobilizing efficacy of physical exercise have been revealed in obese women[21]. Exercise-induced increments of plasma norepinephrine were found to be quite similar in both sexes. Striking differences were found in basal and exercise-induced increment in plasma epinephrine levels. Basal resting levels were lower in women than in men. Moreover the exercise-induced increment in epinephrine plasma levels was lower in obese or non-obese women than in men. It could be hypothesized, that activation of fat cell alpha$_2$-adrenergic receptors by exercise mainly occurs when epinephrine release occur, concomitantly with norepinephrine. Exercise-related activation of adrenal medulla and epinephrine release probably represents a negative stress for optimal lipid mobilization (epinephrine is known to have the highest affinity for alpha$_2$-adrenergic receptors). Thus, the functional studies, based on microdialysis investigation of local lipid mobilization in subcutaneous adipose tissue, suggest that, when looking for optimization of exercise-induced lipid mobilization it will be important to maximize positive stress (norepinephrine release) while minimizing negative stress (epinephrine release).

To attempt a modulation of exercise-induced lipid mobilization/utilization by alpha$_2$-antagonists, recent unpublished studies have been performed. It was possible to delineate oral doses of alpha$_2$-antagonists (yohimbine, idazoxan) that promote activation of SNS and increment of plasma norepinephrine levels without major cardiovascular events. Respiratory exchange ratio values, determined by indirect calorimetry, were decreased; a result suggesting that increased lipid oxidation could occur after alpha$_2$-antagonist administration. Thus, the alpha$_2$-antagonist-related increase in plasma NEFA levels, largely depending on exercise intensity, supplies NEFA to the exercising skeletal muscle. It remains to establish if there is some benefit to provide excess NEFA to the exercising muscle to improve muscle utilization (lipid oxidation). It will be important to settle if the lipolytic response matches skeletal muscle NEFA uptake and oxidation or if plasma NEFA delivery could exceed muscle uptake in such conditions. In the obese performing exercise, it seems that the omental and visceral fat deposits are sufficient to provide NEFA fuel to the exercising skeletal muscle. The peripheral component of the fat-mobilizing action of alpha$_2$-antagonist is supposed to concern fat deposits with adipocytes expressing high levels of alpha$_2$-adrenergic receptors. Is it truly safe to promote NEFA mobilization with an alpha$_2$-antagonist in the large mass of SCAT? High levels of alpha$_2$-adrenergic receptors in hypertrophied subcutaneous adipocytes are leading to limitation of lipolysis. When speculating about alpha$_2$-adrenergic receptors contribution in the adrenergic control of fat deposits, two opposite points of view could be put forward. If the resistance to lipid mobilization and fat loss is considered only, it could be suggested that alpha$_2$-adrenergic receptors stimulation is leading to adverse actions for mobilization of lipid stores. Nevertheless, if limitation of excessive lipolysis in large subcutaneous fat deposits is considered as being an healthy and beneficial action, limiting plasma NEFA excess, alpha$_2$-adrenergic receptors could contribute positively to the physiological adaptation taking place in hypertrophied adipocytes for limitation of their lipolytic activity. Increment of alpha$_2$-adrenergic receptors expression with fat cell hypertrophy has physiological relevance.

Natriuretic peptides – an emerging pathway in the control of lipolysis

A novel pathway for stimulation of lipolysis has recently been characterized in human fat cells[22]. Natriuretic peptides (NPs) i.e. atrial and brain natriuretic peptides (ANP and BNP), have been largely investigated in humans for their role in circulation homeostasis while the action of the C-type natriuretic peptide (CNP) is less known. In humans, natriuretic peptides are recognized to promote natriuresis, diuresis and vasodilatation together with inhibiting renin and aldosterone release. The signalling molecules for these hormones are natriuretic peptide receptor-A (NPR-A) and natriuretic peptide receptor-B (NPR-B) that are members of the cell surface family of guanylyl cyclase receptors, the enzymes that catalyse the synthesis of cyclic guanosine monophosphate (cGMP). Moreover, all NPs bind with relatively similar affinity to the natriuretic peptide clearance receptor C (NPR-C) which does not possess guanylyl cyclase activity and which is abundant in many tissues. NPR-C is considered to control local concentrations of NPs that are available to bind to NPR-A or B[23].

NPs (ANP, BNP and CNP) increased intracellular cGMP levels and stimulated lipolysis with a relative order of potency which was ANP > BNP > CNP; the effect of CNP being very weak. ANP-induced lipolysis could be mimicked using a cyclic cGMP analogue (bromo-cGMP) possessing plasma membrane permeation. The activation of a NPR-A receptor was required to trigger the lipolytic effect of NPs.

ANP-induced lipolysis was not modified by activation or inhibition of the adipocyte phosphodiesterase 3B or the inhibition of adenylyl cyclase. We have recently established the mechanism of the lipolytic pathway, i.e. the increase in cGMP contents is followed by an hormone-sensitive lipase phosphorylation mediated by the activation of cGMP-dependent protein kinase I (cGKI), the unique form cGK existing in human fat cells (Sengenes *et al.*, unpublished results). NPs exert a lipolytic effect through a cGMP-dependent action, which is completely different from the traditional intracellular pathways involved by catecholamine and insulin signalling. The lipolytic effect of NPs is not altered by insulin. To search for an ANP action *in vivo* and a putative influence of obesity on ANP responsiveness, we compared the lipolytic effects of human ANP (h-ANP) on isolated fat cells from SCAT from young, healthy lean and obese men. Moreover, the lipid mobilizing effects of an intravenous infusion of h-ANP was studied as well as various metabolic and cardiovascular parameters. Microdialysis probes were inserted into SCAT to measure modifications of the extracellular glycerol concentrations during h-ANP infusion. Spectral analysis of blood pressure and heart rate oscillations recorded using digital photoplethysmography were used to assess changes in autonomic nervous system activity. Human-ANP (h-ANP) induced a marked and similar increase in glycerol, NEFAs and a weak increase in plasma insulin levels in lean and obese. The effects of h-ANP infusion on the autonomic nervous system were similar in both groups. In SCAT, h-ANP infusion increased extracellular glycerol concentration and decreased local blood flow similarly in both groups. The increase in extracellular glycerol observed during h-ANP infusion was not modified when propranolol (non-selective beta-antagonist) was added in the microdialysis probe to prevent beta-adrenergic receptor activation[24]. These data show that ANP is a potent lipolytic hormone; its action is independent of the weak activation of the sympathetic nervous system promoted by h-ANP infusion. Moreover obesity did not modify the lipolytic and lipid mobilizing effect of ANP in young obese subjects. In a second study performed in obese women following a 28-day low-calorie diet, it was shown that the lipolytic and lipid mobilizing effects of ANP were significantly enhanced. It was postulated, based on previous studies in rats submitted to periods of fasting, that a reduction in NPR-C could lead to reduced uptake of ANP and thereby facilitate the expression of its lipolytic effect. Further studies are required to investigate whether NPs have a relevance regarding human physiology. Moreover, since plasma levels of NPs are considered as being predictors of heart failure, it could be of interest to analyse whether increased NPs production could influence the development of cachexia in patients with chronic heart failure or other diseases. The relevance of natriuretic peptides to the development of cachexia has recently been discussed[25].

Concluding remarks and perspectives

The knowledge of cellular events involved in the regulation and deregulation of lipolysis by catecholamines, lipolytic natriuretic peptides and antilipolytic agents have considerably been extended. Nevertheless, the exploration of the regulatory processes *in vivo* remains difficult. Adipose tissue is an organ with functional heterogeneity according to the anatomical location. Whole body and regional investigations of lipolytic processes have been improved by the concomitant development of *in situ* microdialysis, measurement of arterio-venous differences in abdominal subcutaneous adipose tissue and stable isotopes techniques. Because of its anatomical location, the direct assessment of the metabolic activity of intra-abdominal fat is not easily feasible in humans. It is probable that, in the near future, concomitant assessment of regional lipolysis in subcutaneous adipose tissue by *in situ* microdialysis and of the whole body lipolysis by stable labelled isotope kinetics will facilitate insight into the relative contribution of subcutaneous adipose tissues and other adipose tissues (presumably intra-abdominal and intra-muscular depots). The relationships existing between NEFA delivery by lipolysis, NEFA uptake and utilization by skeletal muscle during exercise merit deeper analyses.

Obese subjects seem to have an impaired utilization of NEFA in the muscle[26], and beta-adrenergic stimulation of lipolysis and fat oxidation have also been found to be impaired in the obese[8,27]. However, increase in plasma NEFA concentration leads to similar increases in lipid oxidation and energy expenditure in obese and lean men[28]. The accumulation of fat in obese subjects may therefore more likely be due to a defect in adipose tissue lipolysis than a defect in lipid oxidation. The subcutaneous deposits are usually more resistant to catecholamine-induced lipolysis due to the high level of expression of alpha$_2$-adrenergic receptors. However, depending on the patients, a possible deregulation of beta$_2$-adrenergic receptor function could be superimposed to the alpha$_2$-adrenergic effects. Management of beta-adrenergic responsiveness is not easy if the defect is related to beta$_2$-adrenergic receptor polymorphism leading to dysfunction. Nevertheless, physical training is known to improve beta-adrenergic responsiveness in subcutaneous adipose tissue[29,30]. There could be a rationale to propose pharmacotherapy based on the administration of alpha$_2$-adrenergic receptor antagonists to improve lipid mobilization/utilization. The recent results of the group have focused attention upon various factors which must be taken in account when exercise is prescribed to obese patients to optimise lipid mobilization in the various fat deposits. However, a number of metabolic and cardiovascular actions have not been studied so far and some limitations have been detected. For future investigations, sex-related and age-related differences will be important to take in account. Women are more capable than men of prompt and substantial increase in lipid mobilization in SCAT in response to moderate endurance exercise. Moreover, it is unknown if the differences persist or are worsened during ageing and fattening.

Concerning NPs-related questions, it is still necessary to provide additional physiological or pathological validation of ANP/BNP involvement in the regulation of lipid mobilization in situations related to physiological or altered pathological release of these hormones. Elevated levels of circulating NPs have been described in pathological states and are considered as valid indexes of disease severity. It is necessary to establish if they are contributing to disease in pro-cachectic situations such as chronic heart failure. Moreover it also remains to establish if this kind of new lipolytic agent (and related synthetic compounds), having beneficial actions on blood pressure and natriuresis, could offer some interest in the control of lipid mobilizing processes aiming at the improvement of lipid mobilization, energy expenditure and lipid oxidation.

References

1. Arner P. Catecholamine-induced lipolysis in obesity. *Int J Obes Metab Disord* 1999; 23 (Suppl 1): 10–13.

2. Jouven X, Charles MA, Desnos M, Ducimetière P Circulating non-esterified fatty acid level as a predictive risk factor for sudden death in population. *Circulation* 2001; 104: 756–61.

3. Bougnères P, Le Stunff C, Pecqueur C, Pinglier E, Adnot P, Ricquier D *In vivo* resistance of lipolysis to epinephrine. A new feature of childhood onset obesity. *J ClinInvest* 1997; 99: 2568–73.

4. Horowitz J F, Klein S Whole body and abdominal lipolytic sensitivity to epinephrine is suppressed in upper body obese women. *Am J Physiol* 2000; 278: E1144–E52.

5. Carel JC, Le Stunff C, Condamine L, Mallet E, Chaussain JL, Adnot P. Resistance to the lipolytic action of epinephrine: a new feature of protein Gs deficiency. *J Clin Endocr Metab* 1999; 84: 4127–31.

6. Dodt C, Lönnroth P, Fehm HL, Elam M. The subcutaneous lipolytic response to regional neural stimulation is reduced in obese women. *Diabetes* 2000; 49: 1875–9.

7. Enoksson S, Talbot M, Rife F, Tamborlane WV, Sherwin RS, Caprio S. Impaired *in vivo* stimulation of lipolysis in adipose tissue by selective β2-adrenergic agonist in obese adolescent girls. *Diabetes* 2000; 49: 2149–53.

8. Schiffelers SLH, Saris WHM, Boomsma F, Baak MA. Beta1- and Beta2-adrenoceptor-mediated thermogenesis and lipid utilization in obese and lean men. *J Clin Endocrinol Metab* 2001; 86: 2191–9.

9. Lafontan M, Berlan M. Fat cell α2-adrenoceptors: the regulation of fat cell function and lipolysis. *Endocrine Rev* 1995; 16: 716–38.

10. Mauriège P, Galitzky J, Berlan M, Lafontan M. Heterogeneous distribution of beta- and alpha2-adrenoceptor binding sites in human fat cells from various fat deposits: functional consequences. *Eur J Clin Invest* 1987; 17: 156–65.

11. Mauriège P, Després JP, Prud'homme D, Pouliot MC, Marcotte M, Tremblay A, Bouchard C. Regional variation in adipose tissue lipolysis in lean and obese men. *J Lipid Res* 1991; 32: 1625–33.

12. Mauriège P, Prud'homme D, Lemieux S, Tremblay A, Després JP. Regional differences in adipose tissue lipolysis from lean and obese women: existence of postreceptor alterations. *Am J Physiol* 1995; 269: E341–E50.

13. Mauriège P, Imbeault P, Langin D, Lacaille M, Alméras N, Tremblay A, Després JP. Regional and gender variations in adipose tissue lipolysis in response to weight loss. *J Lipid Res* 1999; 40: 1559–71.

14. Galitzky J, Lafontan M, Nordenström J, Arner P. Role of vascular alpha2-adrenoceptors in regulating lipid mobilization from human adipose tissue. *J Clin Invest* 1993; 91: 1997–2003.

15. Millet L, Barbe P, Lafontan M, Berlan M, Galitzky J. Catecholamine effects on lipolysis and blood flow in human abdominal and femoral adipose tissue. *J Appl Physiol* 1998; 85: 180–8.

16. Horowitz J, Klein S Lipid metabolism during endurance exercise. *Am J Clin Nutr* 2000; 72 (Suppl): 558S–563S.

17. Stich V, De Glisezinski I, Suljkovicova H, Crampes F, Galitzky J, Rivière D *et al.* Activation of antilipolytic α2-adrenergic receptors by epinephrine during exercise in human adipose tissue. *Am J Physiol* 1999; 277: R1076–83.

18. Stich V, De Glisezinski I, Berlan M, Bülow J, Galitzky J, Harant I, *et al.* Adipose tissue lipolysis is increased during a repeated bout of aerobic exercise. *J Appl Physiol* 2000; 88: 1277–283.

19. Stich V, De Glisezinski I, Crampes F, Hejnova J, Cottet-Emard JM, Galitzky J, *et al.* Activation of alpha(2)-adrenergic receptors impairs exercise-induced lipolysis in SCAT of obese subjects. *Am J Physiol Regul Integr Comp Physiol* 2000; 279(2): R499–504.

20. De Glisezinski I, Marion-Latard F, Crampes F, Berlan M, Hejnova J, Cottet-Emard JM *et al.* Lack of alpha2-adrenergic antilipolytic effect during exercise in subcutaneous adipose tissue of trained men. *J Appl Physiol* 2001; 91: 1760–5.

21. Stich V, Marion-Latard F, Hejnova J, Viguerie N, Lefort C, Suljkovicova H, *et al.* Hypocaloric diet reduces exercise-induced alpha2-adrenergic antilipolytic effect and alpha2-adrenergic receptor mRNA levels in adipose tissue of obese women. *J Clin Endocrinol Metab* 2002; 87: 1274–281.

22. Sengenes C, Berlan M, De Glisezinski I, Lafontan M, Galitzky J. Natriuretic peptides: a new lipolytic pathway in human adipocytes. *FASEB J* 2000; 14: 1345–51.

23. Potter LR, Hunter T. Guanylyl cyclase-linked natriuretic peptide receptors: structure and regulation. *J Biol Chem* 2001; 276: 6057–60.

24. Galitzky J, Sengenes C, Thalamas C, Marques MA, Senard JM, Lafontan M, Berlan M. The lipid mobilizing effect of atrial natriuretic peptide is unrelated to sympathetic nervous system activation or obesity in young men. *J Lipid Res* 2001; 42: 536–44.

25. Kalra PR, Tigas S. Regulation of lipolysis: natriuretic peptides and the development of cachexia. *Int J Cardiol* 2002; 85: 125–32.

26. Colberg SR, Simoneau JA, Thaete FL, Kelley DE. Skeletal muscle utilization of free fatty acids in women with visceral fat obesity. *J Clin Invest* 1995; 95: 1846–53.

27. Snitker S, Hellmer J, Boschmann M, Monroe MB, Ravussin E. Whole body fat oxidation is related to *in situ* adipose tissue lipolytic response to isoproterenol in males. *Am J Physiol* 1998; 275: E400–E4.

28. Schiffelers SLH, Saris WHM, Baak MA. The effects of an increased NEFA concentration on thermogenesis and substrate oxidation in obese and lean men. *Int J Obes* 2001; 25: 33–8.

29. De Glisezinski I, Crampes F, Harant I, Berlan M, Hejnova J, Langin D Endurance training changes in lipolytic responsiveness of obese adipose tissue. *Am J Physiol* 1998; 275: E951–E956.

30. Stich V, De Glisezinski I, Galitzky J, Hejnova J, Crampes F, Rivière D, Berlan M. Endurance training increases the β-adrenergic lipolytic response in subcutaneous adipose tissue in obese subjects. *Int J Obes* 1999; 23: 374–81.

Progress in Obesity Research: 9. Edited by *Geraldo Medeiros-Neto, Alfredo Halpern and Claude Bouchard*
©2003 John Libbey Eurotext Ltd, pp. 145–148.

CHAPTER 29

Selective PPARγ modulators for the treatment of diabetes and metabolic syndrome: new challenges and opportunities

Joel P. Berger

Department of Metabolic Disorders, Merck Research Laboratories, Rahway, NJ, USA
[e-mail: joel_berger@merck.com]

Introduction

The peroxisome proliferator-activated receptors (PPARs) form a subfamily within the nuclear receptor superfamily[1]. Three isoforms, encoded by separate genes, have been identified thus far: PPARγ, PPARα and PPARδ. The PPARs are ligand-dependent transcription factors that regulate target gene expression by binding to specific peroxisome proliferator response elements (PPREs) in enhancer sites of regulated genes (Fig. 1). Each receptor binds to its PPRE as a heterodimer with a retinoid X receptor (RXR). Upon binding an agonist, the conformation of a PPAR is altered and stabilized such that a binding cleft, made up in part of the C-terminal AF-2 domain, is created and recruitment of transcriptional coactivators occurs. Coactivators augment the ability of nuclear receptors to initiate the transcription process (2). Therefore, the result of the agonist-induced PPAR-coactivator interaction at the PPRE is an increase in gene transcription.

PPARγ is highly expressed in adipose tissue where it regulates numerous genes involved in lipid metabolism, adipogenesis and insulin signaling. Numerous fatty acids and their derivatives, including a variety of eicosanoids and prostaglandins, have been shown to serve as ligands of PPARγ[3]. Thus, this receptor may play a central role in sensing nutrient levels and modulating their metabolism. PPARγ is also expressed at lower levels in a broad range of cells and tissues including the heart, kidney, colon, vascular endothelial and smooth muscle cells, macrophages and bone cells. It appears to be able to affect a wide range of events in these tissues including atherosclerotic plaque formation and stability, inflammation, vascular tone, thrombosis, plasma volume levels and cardiac function and morphology.

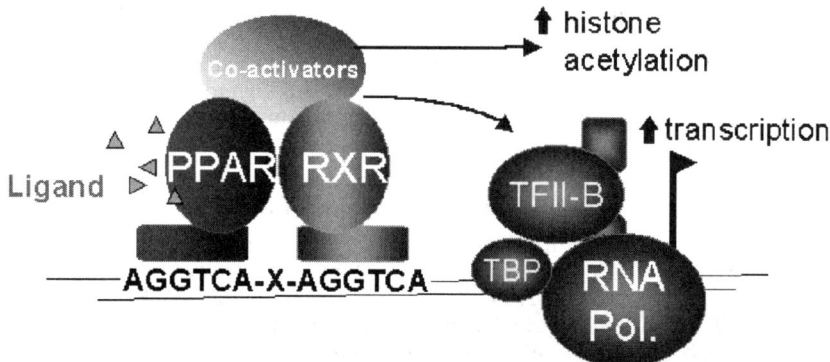

Fig. 1. Mechanism of transcriptional activation by PPAR.

rosiglitazone

nTZDpa

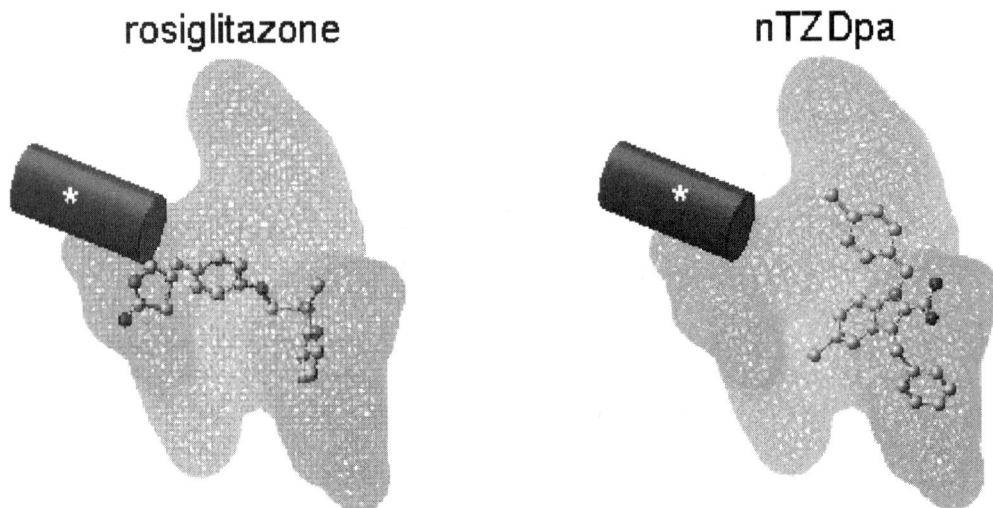

Fig. 2. Differential binding of rosiglitazone and nTZDpa to PPARγ ligand binding domain (red cylinder is helix 12; gold star is Tyr473).

PPARγ synthetic ligands

Thiazolidinediones (TZDs) were originally developed on the basis of their insulin-sensitizing effects in animal pharmacology studies. Subsequently, it was determined that TZDs are PPARγ ligands and agonists that demonstrate a definite correlation between their in vitro PPARγ activities and their in vivo insulin sensitizing actions[4-6]. Several TZDs, including rosiglitazone and pioglitazone, have insulin sensitizing and anti-diabetic activity in humans with type 2 diabetes and impaired glucose tolerance[7]. Farglitazar is a very potent non-TZD PPARγ-selective agonist that was recently shown to have anti-diabetic as well as lipid altering efficacy in humans[8]. In addition to these potent PPARγ ligands, a subset of non-steroidal anti-inflammatory drugs have displayed weak PPARγ activities[9].

Several unique PPARγ ligands have recently been described in the literature. A compound that partially activated PPARγ was shown to inhibit PPARγ agonist driven adipocyte differentiation in vitro[10]. A second PPARγ ligand antagonized the activation of the receptor by the PPARγ agonist rosiglitazone[11]. This compound was also shown to antagonize adipocyte differentiation in vitro. Another structurally unique compound, BADGE, was shown to have weak PPARγ antagonist activity and to also inhibit adipogenesis when studied under several in vitro conditions[12]. Unfortunately, no in vivo data was ever provided for any of these three novel PPARγ ligands. Moreover, these studies did not examine if the conformational state of PPARγ could be differentially affected by a partial agonist-antagonist nor did they address the hypothesis that partial agonism-antagonism of PPARγ might result in divergent patterns of gene expression. Recently, a newly characterized and relatively weak PPARγ agonist, FMOC-L-Leu, was described that displayed more modest in vitro adipogenic activity in comparison with 'classical' PPARγ agonists[13]. Surprisingly, FMOC-L-Leu did not antagonize, but actually augmented, the activity of PPARγ agonists in transactivation and gene expression studies thereby making its interaction with the receptor somewhat unclear. In vivo, this ligand was found to improve insulin sensitivity in rodent models of diabetes; however, no significant difference in weight gain was seen between animals treated with F-L-Leu or rosiglitazone.

A novel selective modulator of PPARγ

In competition binding assays, we found that the non-TZD compound nTZDpa (1-(p-chlorobenzyl)-5-chloro-3-phenylthiobenzyl-2-yl carboxylic acid) was a potent and selective PPARγ ligand and therefore did not differ significantly from previously described TZD and non-TZD PPARγ full agonists. However, in cell-based assays nTZDpa differed markedly from the aforementioned ligands in that it was only able to partially activate PPARγ. The physical basis for the activation of a nuclear receptor by its ligands appears to be the stabilization of the ligand: receptor complex into a limited number of conformations that can bind nuclear receptor coactivator proteins with increased affinity[14]. These complexes then interact with the cellular transcriptional machinery in a manner that increases the rate of transcription initiation. Both biochemical and structural biology techniques demonstrated that the unique binding of nTZDpa, not involving a direct interaction with Tyr473 in the AF-2 domain, produced PPARγ conformations of greater stability than the apo receptor, but of lesser stability than those generated by the classical full agonist rosiglitazone (Fig. 2). We have also observed that the binding of the partial agonist results in an apparently reduced affinity of PPARγ for transcriptional coactivators in comparison with full agonists. We conclude that nTZDpa acts as a partial agonist because, unlike full agonists, it does not stabilize PPARγ in the maximally active conformations that result in the highest affinity interactions with coactivators.

When 3T3-L1 adipocytes were treated with nTZDpa or several PPARγ full agonists and changes in mRNA expression were subsequently analysed using high-density oligonucleotide microarrays, clustering of the ligands according their gene expression patterns demonstrated that nTZDpa clustered well away from the full agonists. This separation was the result of two distinctive effects on gene expression by the partial agonist. First, nTZDpa did not alter the expression of as many genes as the full agonists. Second, nTZDpa often did not alter expression of the same genes to the same extent as the full agonists. These results demonstrate that the terms 'full agonist', 'partial agonist' and 'antagonist' are of limited value when used to describe the ability of ligands to alter gene expression. Wide-ranging gene profiling data now allow us to more fully describe the differential gene-regulating activities of nuclear receptor modulators.

High fat-fed C57BL/6J mice serve as a useful model of obesity and type 2 diabetes. Since they possess many of characteristics found in humans suffering from these maladies including hyperglycaemic, hyperinsulinaemic and hyperleptinaemic[15]. We observed that treatment of such animal with either a PPARγ TZD full agonist or nTZDpa significantly ameliorated these undesirable metabolic states, apparently by attenuating insulin resistance. Beyond these effects, however, the in vivo actions of these two PPARγ ligands showed important differences. While high fat-fed mice treated with the full agonist demonstrated robust weight gain, as a result of increased caloric intake and augmented feed efficiency, the nTZDpa-treated animals gained considerably less weight in large measure due to a significant diminution in feed efficiency. High fat feeding caused increases in several white adipose depots (epididymal, inguinal and retroperitoneal) as well as in intrascapular brown adipose tissue. The TZD increased subcutaneous (inguinal) fat with a concomitant reduction in visceral (retroperitoneal) fat as has previously been shown in human diabetics and rodent models[16,17]. In contrast, all four adipose depots were reduced in size following treatment of fat-fed mice with nTZDpa. These differences in adipose tissue weights were reflected in the changes seen in per cent body lipid. High fat-fed control mice as well as those treated with the PPARγ full agonist showed sizeable increases in whole body lipid content in comparison with lean mice while mice treated with nTZDpa had lower body lipid levels than mice in the two other high fat-fed groups. Conversely, while the high fat-fed control and full agonist-treated mice displayed decreased body protein vs. lean mice the nTZDpa-treated animals showed indistinguishable protein levels from the lean cohort.

In order to identify possible molecular mechanisms that might explain the similarities and differences between the in vivo actions of the PPARγ full agonist and nTZDpa, their effects on the regulation of a limited set of white adipose tissue genes was examined. Expression of genes encoding for biologically active proteins that are secreted by adipose tissue were regulated in a similar manner by both PPARγ effectors. Acrp30, an insulin sensitizing protein[18] which was downregulated in the diabetic mice, was upregulated by both ligands. TNFα, an insulin resistance causing cytokine[19] which was robustly upregulated in the insulin resistant mice, was normalized by treatment with either PPARγ ligand. Thus, altered expression of critical endocrine or paracrine factors in adipose tissue may be an important means by which the in vivo insulin sensitizing actions of PPARγ modulators is mediated. In contrast to their similar actions upon these effectors of insulin action, the PPARγ full agonist and nTZDpa had differential effects on the expression of a group of genes encoding for proteins involved in adipocyte lipid metabolism (FATP, CD36, LPL, aP2 and ACS) that were all downregulated in fat-fed mice. The PPARγ full agonist induced expression of these genes to normal or supernormal levels while nTZDpa either had no significant effect (aP2, CD36, FATP) or modestly downregulated (LPL, ACS) their expression. Such gene expression differences might be responsible for the divergent effects of the full agonist and nTZDpa on weight gain and adiposity.

Acknowledgement: I wish to thank the many biologists and chemists at Merck Reseach Laboratories as well as members of Dr. Richard Surwit's laboratory (Duke University Medical Center) who generated the results described in this manuscript.

References

1. Berger J, Moller DE. The mechanism of action of PPARs. *Ann Rev Med* 2002; 53: 409–35.

2. Xu L, Glass CK, Rosenfeld MG. Coactivator and corepressor complexes in nuclear receptor function. *Curr Opin Genet Dev* 1999; 9: 140–7.

3. Hihi AK, Michalik L, Wahli W. PPARs: transcriptional effectors of fatty acids and their derivatives. *Cell Mol Life Sci* 2002; 59: 790–8.

4. Lehmann JM, Moore LB, Smith-Oliver TA, Wilkison WO, Willson TM, Kliewer SA. An antidiabetic thiazolidinedione is a high affinity ligand for peroxisome proliferator-activated receptor γ. *J Biol Chem* 1995; 270: 12953–6.

5. Berger J, Bailey P, Biswas C, *et al.* Thiazolidinediones produce a conformational change in peroxisomal proliferator-activated receptor-γ: binding and activation correlate with antidiabetic actions in db/db mice. *Endocrinology* 1996; 137: 4189–95.

6. Willson TM, Cobb JE, Cowan DJ, *et al.* The structure-activity relationship between peroxisome proliferator-activated receptor gamma agonism and the antihyperglycemic activity of thiazolidinediones. *J Medicinal Chem* 1996; 39: 665–8.

7. Moller DE, Greene DA. Peroxisome proliferator-activated receptor (PPAR) gamma agonists for diabetes. *Adv Protein Chem* 2001; 56: 181–212.

8. Willson TM, Brown PJ, Sternbach DD, Henke BR. The PPARs: from orphan receptors to drug discovery. *J Med Chem* 2000; 43: 527–50.

9. Lehmann JM, Lenhard JM, Oliver BB, Ringold GM, Kliewer SA. Peroxisome proliferator-activated receptors alpha and gamma are activated by indomethacin and other non-steroidal anti-inflammatory drugs. *J Biol Chem* 1997; 272: 3406–10.

10. Oberfield JL, Collins JL, Holmes CP *et al.* A peroxisome proliferator-activated receptor gamma ligand inhibits adipocyte differentiation. *Proc Natl Acad Sci USA* 1999; 96: 6102–6.

11. Mukherjee R, Hoener PA, Jow L *et al.* A selective peroxisome proliferator-activated receptor-gamma (PPARgamma) modulator blocks adipocyte differentiation but stimulates glucose uptake in 3T3-L1 adipocytes. *Mol Endocrinol* 2000; 14: 1425–33.

12. Wright HM, Clish CB, Mikami T *et al.* A synthetic antagonist for the peroxisome proliferator-activated receptor gamma inhibits adipocyte differentiation. *J Biol Chem* 2000; 275: 1873–7.

13. Rocchi S, Picard F, Vamecq J *et al.* A unique PPARgamma ligand with potent insulin-sensitizing yet weak adipogenic activity. *Mol Cell* 2001; 8: 737–47.

14. McKenna NJ, O'Malley BW. From ligand to response: generating diversity in nuclear receptor coregulator function. *J Steroid Biochem Mol Biol* 2000; 74: 351–6.

15. Surwit RS, Kuhn CM, Cochrane C, McCubbin JA. Diet-induced type II diabetes in C57BL/6J mice. *Diabetes* 1988; 37: 1163–7.

16. Okuno A, Tamamoto H, Tobe K *et al.* Troglitazone increases the number of small adipocytes without the changes of white adipose tissue mass in obese Zucker rats. *J Clin Invest* 1998; 101: 1354–61.

17. Akazawa S, Sun F, Ito M, Kawasaki E, Eguchi K. Efficacy of troglitazone on body fat distribution in type 2 diabetes. *Diabetes Care* 2000; 23: 1067–71.

18. Combs TP, Berg AH, Obici S, Scherer PE, Rossetti L. Endogenous glucose production is inhibited by the adipose-derived protein Acrp30. *J Clin Invest* 2001; 108: 1875–81.

19. Hotamisligil GS, Shargill NS, Spiegelman BM. Adipose expression of tumor necrosis factor-alpha: direct role in obesity-linked insulin resistance. *Science* 1993; 259: 87–91.

20. Lebovitz HE. Differentiating members of the thiazolidinedione class: a focus on safety. *Diabetes Metab Res Rev* 2002; 18: S23–29.

21. Schoonjans K, Auwerx J. Thiazolidinediones: an update. *Lancet.* 2000; 355(9208): 1008–10.

Progress in Obesity Research: 9. Edited by *Geraldo Medeiros-Neto, Alfredo Halpern and Claude Bouchard*
©2003 John Libbey Eurotext Ltd, pp. 149–153.

CHAPTER 30

STAT 5A promotes adipogenesis in non-precursor cells

Z. Elizabeth Floyd and Jacqueline M. Stephens

Department of Biological Sciences, Louisiana State University, Baton Rouge, LA 70803, USA
[e-mail: jsteph1@lsu.edu]

Introduction

Obesity is a major risk factor for non-insulin-dependent diabetes and cardiovascular disease[1] and is the most common disorder in the industrial world. The disorder is characterized by excess adipose tissue resulting from an increase in adipocyte size and/or number[2]. Recent studies suggest that development of obesity may be linked to a breakdown in the regulatory mechanisms controlling adipocyte gene expression[3,4], and significant progress in understanding these mechanisms has been made by identifying the transcription factors involved in regulating gene expression during the formation and maintenance of adipocytes.

Three classes of transcription factors have been identified that directly affect adipogenesis. These include the nuclear hormone receptor, PPARγ, the basic-leucine zipper family members, C/EBPα, C/EBPβ, and C/EBPδ, and the basic-helix-loop-helix protein, SREBP1/ADD1[5,6]. C/EBPβand C/EBP are transiently expressed very early in adipocyte development, leading to the accumulation of PPARγand C/EBα[7]. Current models of adipogenesis propose that PPARγ is then responsible for the induction of C/EBPα, with both transcription factors being essential to the development and maintenance of adipocytes[6]. However, PPARγ can induce adipogenesis in the absence of C/EBPα[8], while C/EBPα requires the presence of PPARγ in order to induce adipogenesis[9]. These results position PPARγ as the central transcription factor in the development of adipocytes and suggest that PPARγ expression is controlled via C/EBP-dependent pathways.

However, other data demonstrate that PPARγ expression can be regulated in a C/EBP-independent manner. Adipose tissue from C/EBPβ and C/EBPδ knock-out mice express both PPARγ and C/EBPγ[10], indicating that induction of PPARγ expression is controlled by additional factors. Possible candidates include SREBP1/ADD1[11] and E2Fs[12], transcription factors that are induced during adipogenesis and participate in regulating PPARγ expression. Another group of proteins that may play a role in the regulation of PPARγ expression and adipogenesis is the STAT (Signal Transducers and Activators of Transcription) family of transcription factors[13,14].

STATs are a family of latent transcription factors that reside in the cytoplasm of resting cells. In response to various stimuli, STATs become tyrosine phosphorylated and translocate to the nucleus where they mediate transcriptional regulation. STATs can be rapidly activated to regulate gene expression and represent a relatively unexplored paradigm in the transcriptional regulation of fat cells[15]. A number of studies suggest that STAT 5 proteins may have important roles in fat cells. We have shown that the expression of STATs 5A and B proteins is highly induced during adipocyte differentiation and that the expression of STAT 5 proteins correlates with lipid accumulation and the expression of PPARγ and C/EBPγ[13,14,16]. STAT 5 antisense oligonucleotides have been shown to inhibit the growth hormone (GH)-dependent differentiation of 3T3-F442A preadipocytes[17] and the expression of a dominant negative STAT 5A in 3T3-L1 cells attenuates lipid accumulation[18]. Moreover, animal studies suggest that STATs 5A and 5B may function as important mediators of fat cell development. Transgenic knock-out animals lacking either the STAT 5A or 5B gene have reduced fat pad size, but mice lacking both STATs

5A and 5B have fat pads that are approximately *one-fifth* the size of wild type mice[19]. Other studies in these animals suggest that the lipolytic actions of growth hormone involve STAT 5 proteins[20].

STAT 5A and STAT 5B are highly related, but are encoded by two separate genes[21] and have been shown to have both essential and nonessential roles in cytokine responses[19]. Murine STAT 5A and 5B have 96 per cent sequence similarity and the major differences occur at the C-terminus, where the final eight residues are nonconserved between the two forms of STAT5 and STAT 5A is 12 residues longer that STAT 5B[21].

Our results clearly demonstrate that STAT 5A is sufficient to confer adipogenesis in fibroblast non-precursor cell lines. We observed that ectopic expression of STAT 5A alone, or in the presence of STAT 5B, is adipogenic in Balb/c cells as judged by cell morphology, marker gene expression, and lipid accumulation. Moreover, the adipogenesis of these cells occurs in the absence of thiazolidinediones. STAT 5B alone, unlike STAT 5A, is *not* adipogenic. However, the presence of STAT 5B enhances the adipogenic capabilities of STAT 5A.

Methods

Materials

Dulbecco's Modified Eagle's Media (DMEM) was purchased from Life Technologies. Bovine and fetal bovine serums (FBS) were obtained from Sigma and Life Technologies, respectively. Darglitizone was generously provided by Pfizer (Groton, CT).

Retroviral-mediated transfection in non-precursor cells

Retroviral-mediated stable expression of pBabe parental vector, pBabePPARγ2, pBabeSTAT5A, pBabeS-TAT5B and pBabeSTAT5A/B was generated in Balb/c cell lines. Recombinant retroviruses were produced as described[22,23].

Cell culture

Fibroblast cell lines ectopically expressing STAT5 genes were plated and grown to 2 days post confluence in DMEM with 10 per cent bovine serum. Medium was changed every 48 h. Cells were induced to differentiate by changing the medium to DMEM containing a standard induction cocktail of 10 per cent fetal bovine serum, 0.5 mM 3-isobutyl-1-methylxanthine, 1 µM dexamethasone, and 1.7 µM insulin (MDI). After 48 h this medium was replaced with DMEM supplemented with 10 per cent FBS, and cells were maintained in this medium. STAT5 stable cell lines were induced to differentiate in the presence or absence of 2.5 µM darglitizone. The Balb/c fibroblast cell line was obtained from the ATCC.

RNA analysis

Total RNA was isolated from cell monolayers with TriZOL (Invitrogen), according to the manufacturer's instructions with minor modifications. For Northern Blot analysis, 20 µg of total RNA was denatured in formamide and electrophoresed through a formaldehyde-agarose gel. The RNA was transferred to Zeta Probe-GT (Biorad), cross-linked, hybridized and washed as previously described[24]. Probes were labeled by random priming using the Klenow Fragment (Promega) and [γ^{32}P]dATP (Perkin Elmer, Life Sciences).

Results and discussion

In this study, we examined the adipogenic capabilities of STAT 5 proteins using ectopic expression in non-precursor fibroblast cell lines. To assess the role of STAT 5 in adipogenesis, we generated a series of stable cell lines that ectopically express STAT5 proteins in Balb/c non-precursor fibroblast cell lines. Cell lines containing the pBabe vector alone, pBabeSTAT5A, pBabeSTAT5B or the pBabeSTATs 5A and 5B (STAT5A/B) expression vectors in combination were then induced to differentiate at two days post confluence using the standard differentiation cocktail and adipogenesis was subsequently assayed by morphological and biochemical criteria. This approach has been very useful in examining other adipocyte transcription factors[9,25-27] since fibroblast cell lines do not normally undergo adipogenesis, even with the addition of the appropriate hormonal stimuli. This is significantly different than 3T3-L1 preadipocytes, which readily differentiate into adipocytes with the same hormonal stimuli[28].

As shown in Fig. 1A, ectopic expression of either STAT5A alone or STAT5A and STAT5B (STAT5A/B) in combination in Balb/c cells resulted in an adipocyte morphology as judged by Hoffman Optics. Using Northern blot analysis (Fig. 1B), we then assessed the adipogenesis of STAT5 Balb/c stable cell lines by examining the expression of PPARγ C/EBPγ, and aP2. While PPARγ and C/EBPγ are essential

A. Hoffman Modulation Contrast Optics

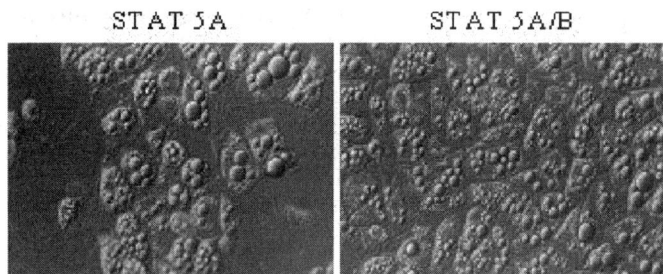

STAT 5A   STAT 5A/B

B. Northern Blot Analysis

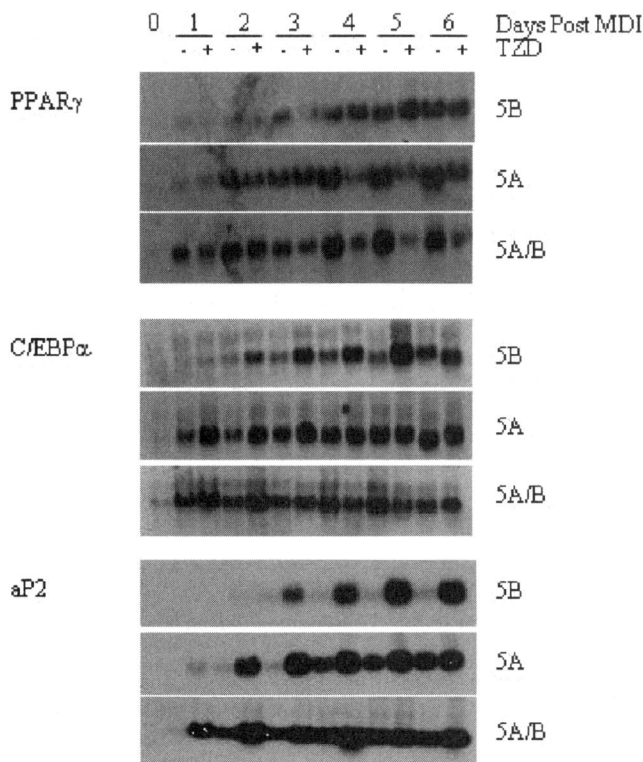

Fig. 1. STAT5A and STAT5A/B are adipogenic.
(A) Cell monolayers were photographed at 120 h after exposure to the MDI cocktail. The cells were maintained in the absence of thiazolidinediones.
(B) Total RNA was isolated at the indicated time points following induction of differentiation in the absence (-) or presence (+) of 2.5 μM darglitizone (TZD). Fifteen μM of total RNA was electrophoresed, transferred to nylon and subjected to Northern blot analysis for marker gene expression.

transcription factors in adipogenesis, aP2 is a fat-specific lipid binding protein expressed under the control of PPARγ[25]. Cells were induced to differentiate in the absence or presence of 2.5 mM darglitizone and total RNA was isolated at the indicated times. We observed an induction in PPARγ mRNA in STAT 5B cells at 3 days after the initiation of differentiation. Yet, the induction of PPARγ mRNA occurred at only 2 days after initiation of differentiation in STAT 5A cells and occurred within 1 day in STAT5A/B cells. A similar pattern was observed for the induction of C/EBPα mRNA. The induction of aP2 mRNA occurred in STAT 5B cells at day 3 and was expressed in a TZD-dependent manner. In STAT5A cells, aP2 mRNA was induced at day 2 in a TZD-dependent manner and in STAT 5A/B cells this mRNA was induced at day 1 in a similar manner. Interestingly, the expression of aP2 in STAT 5B cells was always dependent on the presence of TZD. Yet, in 5A cells or 5A/B cells, the expression of aP2 mRNA was *independent* of TZD in the later stages of adipogenesis, suggesting that these cells are capable of producing an endogenous PPARγ ligand.

STAT 5B, which only differs from STAT 5A by eight amino acids at the C-terminus, is not adipogenic but does enhance the adipogenic properties of STAT 5A. Our results indicate that STAT 5A is sufficient to induce adipogenesis in non-precursor cells in a process that is accompanied by an induction of PPARγ and C/EBPα.

Recent findings suggest that C/EBPα and PPARγ participate in a single pathway of fat cell development with PPARγ being the proximal effector of adipogenesis[9] We surmise that STAT 5 proteins participate in this identified pathway of fat cell development and hypothesize that

A. Induction of STAT5PY and PPARγ in 3T3-L1 Adipocytes

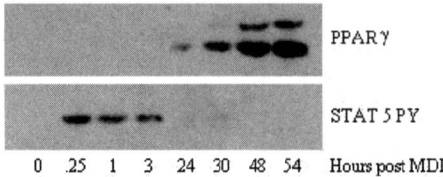

PPARγ

STAT5PY

0 .25 1 3 24 30 48 54   Hours post MDI

B. Schematic of STAT5A in Adipogenesis

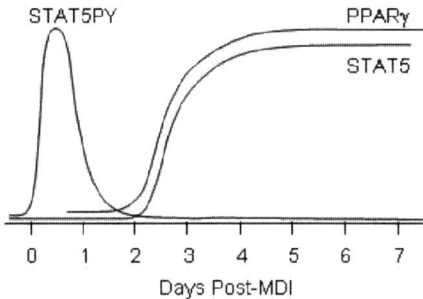

STAT5PY   PPARγ

STAT5

0   1   2   3   4   5   6   7
Days Post-MDI

Fig. 2. STAT5 activation precedes induction of PPARγ in adipogenesis.
(A) Whole cell extracts were harvested at the indicated time after induction of differentiation in 3T3-L1 preadipocytes. One hundred μg of each extract was analysed by SDS-PAGE, followed by transfer to nitrocellulose and detection using enhanced chemiluminescence (Pierce). (B) Schematic representation of the relationship between PPARγ expression and the induction of activated and total STAT5A during adipogenesis.

STAT 5A is an early effector of adipogenesis. This is supported by our data demonstrating that ectopic STAT 5A expression results in the induction of PPARγ expression in Balb/c fibroblasts as well as the early activation of STAT5 preceding the expression of PPARγ in 3T3-L1 adipocytes (Fig. 2A). The ability of STAT 5A to induce adipogenesis in non-precursor cells may be mediated by activated STAT5A directly regulating PPARγ expression at the early stages of adipogenesis (Fig. 2B). The increase in total STAT5A at the later stages of adipogenesis could, in turn, be analogous to the role played by E2F4 as a late suppressor of PPARγ[12]. In summary, our finding demonstrate that STAT 5A, alone or in the presence of STAT 5B is adipogenic in non-precursor cells, suggesting that STAT 5A and STAT 5B have non-redundant roles in adipogenesis. This is consistent with recent studies demonstrating that STAT 5 proteins are highly regulated in adipocytes[14,16], have the ability to influence adipogenesis[17,18] and that transgenic mice lacking either STAT 5 gene have a reduction in fat pad size[19].

Acknowledgements: We would like to thank Patricia Arbour-Reily and Kyle J. Waite for technical assistance.

References

1. Kersten S, Desvergne B, Wahli W. Roles of PPARs in health and disease. *Nature* 2000; 405(6785): 421–24.

2. Lazar MA. Becoming fat. *Genes Dev* 2002; 6(1): 1–5.

3. Flier JS. Diabetes. The missing link with obesity? *Nature* 2001; 409(6818): 292–3.

4. Saltiel AR, Kahn CR. Insulin signalling and the regulation of glucose and lipid metabolism. *Nature* 2001; 414(6865): 799–806.

5. Rangwala SM, Lazar MA. Transcriptional control of adipogenesis. *Annu Rev Nutr* 2000; 20: 535–59.

6. Rosen ED, Walkey CJ, Puigserver P, Spiegelman BM. Transcriptional regulation of adipogenesis. *Genes Dev* 2000; 14(11): 1293–307.

7. Darlington GJ, Ross SE, MacDougald OA. The role of C/EBP genes in adipocyte differentiation. *J Biol Chem* 1998; 273(46): 30057–60.

8. Wu Z, Rosen ED, Brun R, Hauser S, Adelmant G, Troy AE et al. Cross-regulation of C/EBP alpha and PPAR gamma controls the transcriptional pathway of adipogenesis and insulin sensitivity. *Mol Cell* 1999; 3(2): 151–158.

9. Rosen ED, Hsu CH, Wang X, Sakai S, Freeman MW, Gonzalez FJ, Spiegelman BM. C/EBPalpha induces adipogenesis through PPARgamma: a unified pathway. *Genes Dev* 2002; 16(1): 22–26.

10. Tanaka T, Yoshida N, Kishimoto T, Akira S. Defective adipocyte differentiation in mice lacking the C/EBPbeta and/or C/EBPdelta gene. *EMBO J* 1997; 16(24): 7432–43.

11. Fajas L, Schoonjans K, Gelman L, Kim JB, Najib J, Martin G et al. Regulation of peroxisome proliferator-activated receptor gamma expression by adipocyte differentiation and determination factor 1/sterol regulatory element

binding protein 1: implications for adipocyte differentiation and metabolism. *Mol Cell Biol* 1999; 19(8): 5495–5503.

12. Fajas L, Landsberg RL, Huss-Garcia Y, Sardet C, Lees JA, Auwerx J. E2Fs regulate adipocyte differentiation. *Dev Cell* 2002; 3(1): 39–49.

13. Stephens JM, Morrison RF, Wu Z, Farmer SR. PPARgamma ligand-dependent induction of STAT1, STAT5A, and STAT5B during adipogenesis. *Biochem Biophys Res Commun* 1999; 262(1): 216–22.

14. Stewart WC, Morrison RF, Young SL, Stephens JM. Regulation of signal transducers and activators of transcription (STATs) by effectors of adipogenesis: coordinate regulation of STATs 1, 5A, and 5B with peroxisome proliferator-activated receptor-gamma and C/AAAT enhancer binding protein-alpha. *Biochim Biophys Acta* 1999; 1452(2): 188–96.

15. Darnell JEJ. STATs and gene regulation. *Science* 1997; 277(5332): 1630–5.

16. Stephens JM, Morrison RF, Pilch PF. The expression and regulation of STATs during 3T3-L1 adipocyte differentiation. *J Biol Chem* 1996; 271(18): 10441–4.

17. Yarwood SJ, Sale EM, Sale GJ, Houslay MD, Kilgour E, Anderson NG. Growth hormone-dependent differentiation of 3T3-F442A preadipocytes requires Janus kinase/signal transducer and activator of transcription but not mitogen-activated protein kinase or p70 S6 kinase signaling. *J Biol Chem* 1999; 274(13): 8662–8.

18. Nanbu-Wakao R, Morikawa Y, Matsumura I, Masuho Y, Muramatsu MA, Senba E, Wakao H. Stimulation of 3T3-L1 Adipogenesis by Signal Transducer and Activator of Transcription 5. *Mol Endocrinol* 2002; 16(7): 1565–76.

19. Teglund S, McKay C, Schuetz E, van Deursen JM, Stravopodis D, Wang D *et al.* Stat5a and Stat5b proteins have essential and nonessential, or redundant, roles in cytokine responses. *Cell* 1998; 93(5): 841–50.

20. Fain JN, Ihle JH, Bahouth SW. Stimulation of lipolysis but not of leptin release by growth hormone is abolished in adipose tissue from Stat5a and b knockout mice. *Biochem Biophys Res Commun* 1999; 263(1): 201–5.

21. Liu X, Robinson GW, Gouilleux F, Groner B, Hennighausen L. Cloning and expression of Stat5 and an additional homologue (Stat5b) involved in prolactin signal transduction in mouse mammary tissue. *Proc Natl Acad Sci USA* 1995; 92(19): 8831–5.

22. Morgenstern JP, Land H. Advanced mammalian gene transfer: high titre retroviral vectors with multiple drug selection markers and a complementary helper-free packaging cell line. *Nucleic Acids Res* 1990; 18(12): 3587–96.

23. Pear WS, Nolan GP, Scott ML, Baltimore D. Production of high-titer helper-free retroviruses by transient transfection. *Proc Natl Acad Sci USA* 1993; 90(18): 8392–6.

24. Stephens JM, Pekala PH. Transcriptional repression of the C/EBP-alpha and GLUT4 genes in 3T3-L1 adipocytes by tumor necrosis factor-alpha. Regulations is coordinate and independent of protein synthesis. *J Biol Chem* 1992; 267(19): 13580–4.

25. Tontonoz P, Hu E, Spiegelman BM. Stimulation of adipogenesis in fibroblasts by PPAR gamma 2, a lipid-activated transcription factor. *Cell* 1994; 79(7): 1147–56.

26. Wu Z, Xie Y, Bucher NL, Farmer SR. Conditional ectopic expression of C/EBP beta in NIH-3T3 cells induces PPAR gamma and stimulates adipogenesis. *Genes Dev* 1995; 9(19): 2350–63.

27. Wu Z, Bucher NL, Farmer SR. Induction of peroxisome proliferator-activated receptor gamma during the conversion of 3T3 fibroblasts into adipocytes is mediated by C/EBPbeta, C/EBPdelta, and glucocorticoids. *Mol Cell Biol* 1996; 16(8): 4128–36.

28. Green H, Kehinde O. An established preadipose cell line and its differentiation in culture. II. Factors affecting the adipose conversion. *Cell* 1975; 5(1): 19–27.

Progress in Obesity Research: 9. Edited by *Geraldo Medeiros-Neto, Alfredo Halpern* and *Claude Bouchard*

CHAPTER 31

Sympathetic neurons and obesity related diseases – a role for FOXC2?

Sven Enerbäck

Medical Genetics, Department of Medical Biochemistry, Göteborg University, Box 440, SE 405 30 Göteborg, Sweden
[e-mail: sven.enerback@medgen.gu.se]

Direct innervation of WAT

In an early report by Mueller[1] a paraplegic patient in a cachectic state was reported to have selectively spared his adipose tissue on the denervated side. This is probably the first observation indicating a role for the nervous system in regulating the amount of adipose tissue. Since then many authors have used various techniques to surgically denervate adipose tissue. In early studies spinal cord lesions were used[1] the techniques have over the years become more sophisticated as selective axotomy of specific WAT depots was developed[2,3]. Unilaterally denervated WAT depots show an increase in size under normal conditions and resistance to starvation induced reduction, as compared with the intact contra-lateral side[4]. Even though altered rates of lipogenic and lipolytic activity in localized fad depots could be attributed to direct regulation by the sympathetic nervous system (SNS) and hence the variation observed in these experiments a consequence of the axotomy, altered blood flow and/or vessel permeability could also explain these findings. Direct electrical stimulation of nerves innervating specific WAT pads have been used to positively confirm the ablation studies. Several groups have shown that electrical stimulation of fat pad SNS efferent nerves leads to an increase in FFA release[5,6]. In some denervation experiments substances known to modulate SNS mediated signaling e.g. theophylline[7], β-adrenergic receptor blockers[6] have been administered into the fat pad's circulation, to examine the role of intracellular β-adrenergic pathways. These experiments support a view in which electrical activation of nerves leads to release of catecholamines that will activate intracellular lipolysis through a β-adrenergic pathway. As is the case for the denervation studies it is not possible to exclude a primary effect on the vasculature. Using fluorescent dyes Wirsén demonstrated for the first time catecholaminergic innervation of WAT and BAT[8]. Initially it was reported that only WAT vasculature was supplied by catecholaminergic innervation and not the adipocytes *per se*[9]. Using electron microscopy Slavin and Ballard could show that approximately 3 per cent of the adipocytes indeed received direct innervation of the SNS[10]. Injections of the retrograde fluorescent neural tracer fluorogold into epididymal or inguinal WAT fat pads revealed a more rostral position of neurons, in the sympathetic chain, that innervate the epididymal pad as compared with those innervating inguinal adipose tissue[11]. This interesting finding points out a possibility that different fat pads could be selectively regulated by the SNS. The question whether this diversity also is found in the brain was addressed using pseudorabies virus (PRV) as a transneuronal tract tracer. PRV is taken up by neurons and transported to higher CNS levels transsynaptically. Initial studies performed using PRV tracer failed to identify a specific WAT 'signature' in the CNS pattern of PRV positive cells[12]. Thus, no specific groups of cells in CNS seemed to be responsible for WAT SNS innervation. It rather appeared as if SNS innervation of WAT was part of a more general SNS outflow from the brain. However, in a more recent study from the same laboratory, analysing the pattern of PRV positive neurons that were immunocytochemically labeled to reveal their content of specifc neurotransmitters, the authors could identify a specific neurochemical identity of SNS outflow from brain to WAT[13]. This is potentially a very important finding since it points out that apart from circulating catecholamines, release of catecholamines by nerve endings in WAT could be specifically regulated at the CNS level.

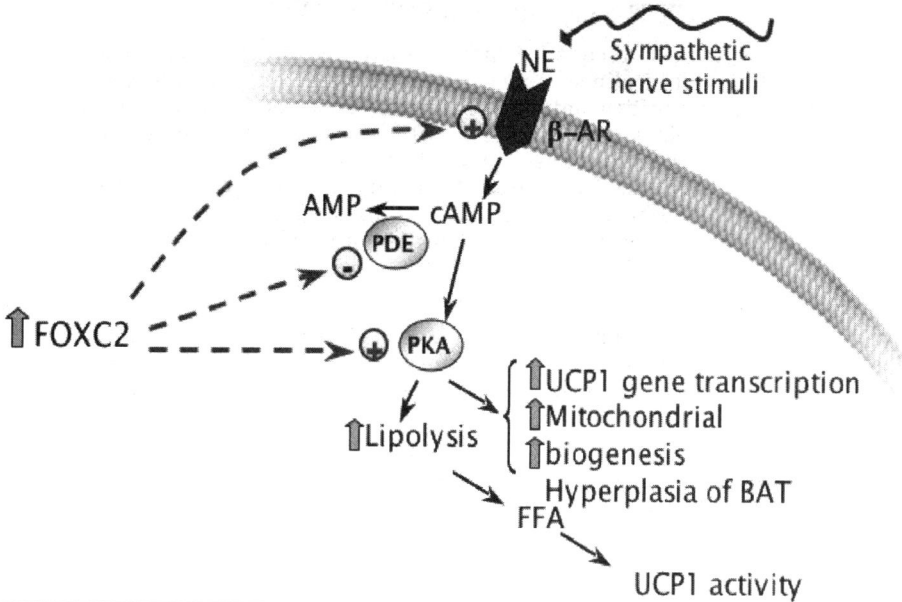

Fig. 1. FOXC2 induces increased sensitivity in the β-adrenergic pathway by acting at three different levels.

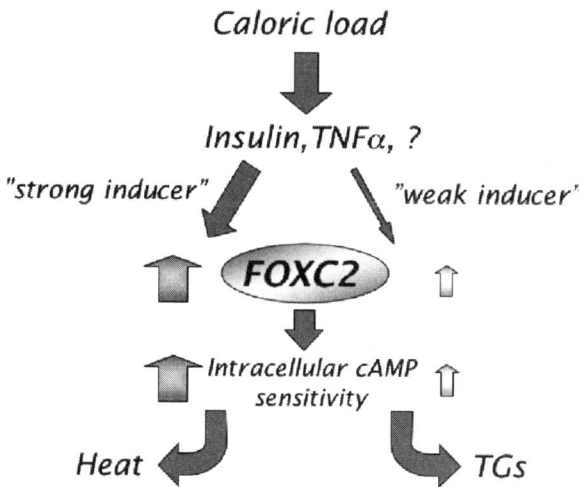

Fig. 2. FOXC2 as a regulator of metabolic efficency. According to this hypothesis a strong induction of FOXC2 in response to a caloric load leads to a metabolic situation in which a large portion of the ingested calories would be dissipated as heat, due to increased sensitivity of the β-adrenergic/PKA pathway, whereas a weaker induction induces conservation of the caloric load as triglycerides. [Reproduced with permission from *Cell*, copyright Elsevier Science.]

Physiological role of SNS in WAT

In general it is appreciated that the SNS plays an important role in regulating whole body adiposity, and that low sympathetic activity is associated with both experimental and clinical obesity. Adrenal medullary released epinephrine have been regarded as the major mediator of SNS effects. Recently, it has been shown, in a rodent model, that direct innervation of WAT plays an important role in regulating whole body adiposity[14]. Leptin can be regarded as a key afferent signal from WAT to the brain, by which the CNS receives, among other things, information regarding peripheral energy status. Catecholamines have been shown to decrease leptin expression both *in vitro* and *in vivo*[15]. In an elaborate feed back model Bray and York discuss the role of sympathetic modulation of leptin feed back to CNS as an important factor in regulating WAT metabolism[16]. This reinforces the possibility that one major role for catecholamines in WAT, apart from regulating lipolysis, could be to modulate leptin feed back to CNS.

155

FOXC2 a modulator of SNS in WAT?

In a recent publication we have studied mice that over-express the *forkhead* transcription factor FOXC2[17]. Such mice are lean and insulin sensitive. We propose that, on several levels, the β-adrenergic/PKA pathway is made more sensitive and that this leads to a metabolic situation characterized by: (i) induction of uncoupling protein 1 (ucp1) in WAT, (ii) increased mitochondrial function and biogenesis in WAT, and (iii) increased metabolism in WAT. The FOXC2-mediated changes in WAT is characterized by an increased level of cell surface located β-adrenergic receptors, decreased phosphodiesterase activity and altered PKA holoenzyme composition (Fig. 1). These changes all seem to enhance the catecholamine sensitivity of the adipocyte, and constitute a way by which FOXC2 can modulate SNS efferent signaling at the 'adipocyte-level'.

In this way FOXC2 would act as a regulator of the efficiency by which calories are converted to TGs (Fig. 2). The lean and insulin sensitive phenotype seen in mice over-expressing FOXC2 is due to a high sensitivity of adipocyte β-adrenergic pathways[17]. These findings raises the intriguing possibility that FOXC2 could act as an integrator molecule that transmit and convert external signals into appropriate metabolic responses in the adipocyte.

Acknowledgements: This work was made possible with support from The Swedish Medical Research Foundation, The Arne and IngaBritt Lundberg Foundation, The Juvenile Diabetes Foundation, The Wallenberg Foundation, Biovitrum Inc. and a Junior Individual Grant from The Swedish Foundation for Strategic Research to S.E.

References

1. Mansfeld G, Muller F. Der Einfluss der Nervensystem auf die Mobilisierung von Fett. *Arch Physiol* 1913; 152: 61–7.

2. Clement G. La mobilization des glycerides de reserve chez le rat. II. Influence du système nerveux sympathique. Etablissement d'un procédé de mesure de l'intensité de la mobilisation. *Arch Sci Physiol* 1950; 4: 13–29.

3. Cantu RC, Goodman HM. Effects of denervation and fasting on white adipose tissue. *Am J Physiol* 1967; 212: 207–12.

4. Beznak ABL, Hasch Z. The effect of sympathectomy on the fatty deposit in connective tissue. *QJ Exp Physiol* 1937; 27: 1–15.

5. Corell JW. Adipose tissue: ability to respond to nerve stimulation *in vitro*. *Science* 1963; 140: 387–8.

6. Rosell S. Release of free fatty acids from subcutaneous adipose tissue in dogs following sympathetic nerve stimulation. *Acta Physiol Scand* 1967; 67: 343–51.

7. Weiss B, Maickel RP. Sympathetic nervous control of adipose tissue lipolysis. *Int J Neuropharmacol* 1965; 7: 393–403.

8. Wirsén C. Adrenergic innervation of adipose tissue examined by fluorescence microscopy. *Nature* 1964; 202: 913.

9. Wirsén C. Studies in lipid mobilization with special reference to morphological and histochemical aspects. *Acta Physiol Scand* 1965; 65: 1–46.

10. Slavin BG, Ballard K. Morphological studies on the adrenergic innervation of white adipose tissue. *Anat Rec* 1978; 191: 377–90.

11. Youngstrom TG, Bartness TJ. Catecholaminergic innervation of white adipose tissue in the Siberian hamster. *Am J Physiol* 1995; 37: R744–R751.

12. Bamshad M, Aoki VT, Adkinson MG, Warren WS, Bartness TJ. Central nervous system origins of the sympathetic nervous system outflow to white adipose tissue. *Am J Physiol* 1998; 275: R291–R299.

13. Shi H, Bartness TJ. Neurochemical phenotype of sympathetic nervous system outflow from brain to white fat. *Brain Res Bull* 2001; 54: 375–85.

14. Demas GE, Bartness TJ. Direct innervation of white fat and adrenal medullary catecholamines mediate photoperiodic changes in body fat. *Am J Physiol* 2001; 281: R1499–R1505.

15. Fried SK, Ricci MR, Russel CD, Laferrere B. Regulation of leptin in humans. *J Nutr* 2000; 130: S3127–S3131.

16. Bray GA, York DA. The MONA LISA hypothesis in the time of leptin. *Recent Prog Horm Res* 1998; 53: 95–117.

17. Cederberg A, Gronning LM, Ahrén B, Taskén K, Carlsson P, Enerbäck S. FOXC2 is a winged helix gene that counteracts obesity, hypertriglyceridemia, and diet-induced insulin resistance. *Cell* 2001; 106: 563–73.

Progress in Obesity Research: 9. Edited by *Geraldo Medeiros-Neto, Alfredo Halpern and Claude Bouchard*
©2003 John Libbey Eurotext Ltd, pp. 157–160.

CHAPTER 32

Wnt signaling in regulation of adipogenesis

Kenneth A. Longo and Ormond A. MacDougald

Department of Molecular and Integrative Physiology, University of Michigan Medical School, Ann Arbor, Michigan 48109-0622, USA
[e-mail: macdouga@umich.edu]

The white adipocyte is the main site for storage and release of fatty acids in the body, and is a cornerstone in the regulation of metabolism and energy balance in humans. As such, a mechanistic understanding of the adipocyte has profound implications for the growing pandemic of obesity. Since the development of cell lines that have the potential to develop into adipocytes, much has been learned about the role of cell signaling pathways, transcription factors, and genes involved in carbohydrate and fatty acid metabolism during adipogenic conversion[1,2]. Conversion of 3T3-L1 preadipocytes to adipocytes *in vitro* requires 10 per cent fetal calf serum, methyl-isobutylxanthine, dexamethasone, and insulin. These components induce expression of adipogenic transcription factors C/EBPα and PPARγ, enzymes important for lipid synthesis and storage, proteins crucial for energy mobilization, and development of large intracellular triacylglycerol droplets[1–5]. Recent work from our laboratory has focused on the inhibition of these processes by Wnt signaling[2,6–8].

Wnt-1 was first identified as an insertion site for mouse mammary tumour virus in mammary carcinoma[9]. Since that time, a total of 23 vertebrate Wnts have been identified, with 19 in humans (http://www.stanford.edu/~rnusse/wntwindow.html). Wnts are secreted glycoproteins that associate with cell membranes. Wnts have profound effects on cell fate, including effects on differentiation, cell cycle and apoptosis[6,7,10–14].

Wnts interact with frizzled receptors, which are seven-transmembrane proteins that feature a cysteine-rich extracellular N-terminal region that is a candidate for the Wnt ligand binding domain[15]. Recently, the low density lipoprotein-related proteins (LRPs) have been demonstrated to enhance the interaction between Wnt and frizzled[16]. Mutations in the *Drosophila* LRP homologue *arrow* result in patterning defects that resemble *wingless* mutations in *Drosophila*, suggesting that both frizzled and LRP are required for Wnt signal transduction[16].

Wnt signaling can be regulated by a class of proteins called the secreted frizzled-related proteins. These proteins, with five known mammalian members, are homologous to the amino-terminal domain of frizzled receptors, which encode the Wnt ligand binding domain. As such, these proteins can bind Wnts, and block the ability of Wnt to signal through frizzled[17].

In the canonical Wnt pathway, Wnts interact with frizzled receptors to initiate a signal through the cytoplasmic protein dishevelled, to inhibit glycogen synthase kinase (GSK) -3 activity. Failure of GSK-3 to phosphorylate β-catenin leads to accumulation of β-catenin in the cytoplasm. β-catenin enters the nucleus and stimulates gene expression by binding members of the TCF/LEF family of transcription factors[18]. In the absence of Wnt ligand, dishevelled fails to inhibit GSK-3, which phosphorylates β-catenin and targets it to the proteasome complex for degradation[18]. Additionally, frizzleds can activate the jun N-terminal kinase pathway, and couple with G-proteins and activate other pathways, such as those that involve phospholipase C and intracellular calcium release[15,19].

Evidence that Wnt plays a role in adipogenesis was obtained with the 3T3-L1 preadipocyte line, which fails to differentiate into adipocytes in the presence of lithium, an inhibitor of GSK-3[7,20]. A more specific inhibitor of GSK-3, CHIR 99021, stabilizes β-catenin and also completely inhibits adipogenesis in 3T3-L1 cells[6]. The expression of C/EBPα and C/EBPα, considered the first wave of transcription factors expressed during the adipogenic programme, is unaffected by CHIR 99021. However, expression of C/EBPα and PPARγ, transcription factors that are necessary and sufficient for adipogenesis, is com-

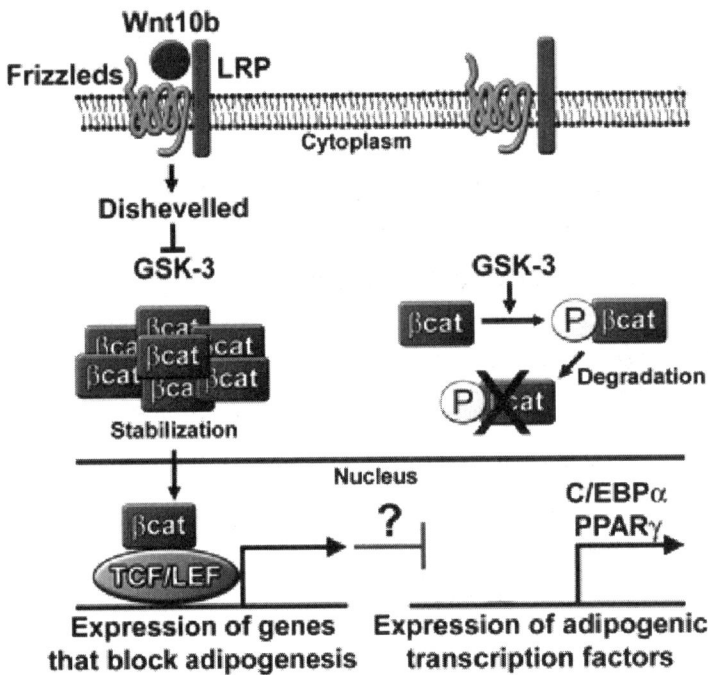

Fig. 1. Regulation of adipogenesis by Wnt signaling. Wnt10b acts through Frizzled receptors-1, -2, and/or -5 and coreceptors LRP5/6 to inhibit GSK-3. The reduced activity of GSK-3 results in hypophosphorylation and stabilization of β-catenin, which translocates to the nucleus and activates transcription through TCF/LEF transcription factors. Although the specific mechanism remains unknown, Wnt-induced changes in gene expression result in repression of the adipogenic transcription factors, C/EBPα and PPARγ. In the absence of Wnt signaling, GSK-3 phosphorylates β-catenin and targets it for ubiquitin-mediated turnover, thus releasing the repressive Wnt signal on adipogenic gene expression.

pletely blocked[6]. Although CHIR 99021 inhibits adipogenesis when added for any of the first three days after induction, it is not an effective inhibitor when applied after that time[6]. This suggests that inhibition of adipogenesis by Wnt occurs through the canonical pathway (Fig. 1).

Ectopic retroviral expression of Wnt-1 or a dominant-stable mutant of β-catenin both block adipogenesis[7]. As with CHIR 99021, Wnt-1 expression has no effect on C/EBPα or C/EBPγ, but completely inhibits expression of C/EBPα and PPARγ.[7] These data suggest that Wnt signaling blocks adipogenesis by inhibiting the ability of C/EBPα to induce these two key adipogenic transcription factors (Fig. 1). Consistent with Wnt-1 inhibiting adipogenesis through repression of C/EBPα and PPARγ , ectopic expression of these transcription factors rescues repressive effects of Wnt-1 on adipogenesis[7]. In contrast to 3T3-L1 cells, the 3T3-F442A cell line expresses undetectable levels of Wnt-10b mRNA, and undergoes spontaneous adipogenesis when injected into nude mice. However, these cells fail to differentiate *in vivo* when they ectopically express retroviral Wnt-1[7].

To determine whether adipogenesis is inhibited by endogenous Wnt signaling, the canonical pathway was blocked by ectopic expression of dominant negative TCF-4, which binds DNA but cannot activate transcription. 3T3-L1 preadipocytes in which Wnt signaling is repressed spontaneously differentiate into adipocytes *in vitro*, and *in vivo* when injected subcutaneously into nude mice[7]. These data provide compelling evidence that endogenous Wnt signaling represses adipogenesis, and this signal is mediated through the canonical Wnt pathway (Fig. 1).

A screen was performed to identify the endogenous Wnt that regulates adipogenesis. Differential RT-PCR using degenerate Wnt primers, and RNase protection assays, were used to narrow the field of potential candidates. Wnt-10b mRNA is expressed in 3T3-L1 preadipocytes, and declines upon induction of adipogenesis[7]. This pattern of expression is reflected *in vivo*, where Wnt-10b mRNA is expressed in the stromovascular fraction of white adipose tissue, but not in the adipocyte fraction[6]. When ectopically expressed in 3T3-L1 cells, Wnt-10b stabilizes β-catenin and blocks adipogenesis. The addition of secreted frizzled related protein-1 or -2 to 3T3-L1 cells causes spontaneous adipogenesis, suggesting that Wnt secretion by 3T3-L1 cells actively represses adipogenesis[6]. Collectively, these data indicate that Wnt-10b is expressed in 3T3-L1 cells, and acts through the canonical pathway to inhibit preadipocyte differentiation. Thus, an early event in the induction of adipogenesis is the rapid loss of Wnt-10b expression, which allows for subsequent expression of adipogenic genes[6,7].

To stimulate preadipocyte differentiation into adipocytes, 3T3-L1 cells are exposed to several inducers: fetal calf serum, methylisobutylxanthine, dexamethasone, and insulin. Additionally, a PPARγ agonist can also be used to stimulate adipogenesis. Application of these inducers to confluent 3T3-L1 preadipocytes initiates the cascade of genetic events that result in induction of proteins necessary for the adipocyte phenotype[1,2]. We explored the hypothesis that one or more of these agents might be responsible for the rapid decline of Wnt-10b mRNA, and hence alleviate inhibitory effects of Wnt-10b on adipogenesis. Upon treatment with inducers individually or in combination, only the phosphodiesterase inhibitor methyl-isobutylxanthine was sufficient to suppress Wnt-10b expression. Furthermore, the cAMP analog 8-bromo-cAMP and the adenylate cyclase activator forskolin both repressed Wnt-10b[6]. Taken together, these data indicate that elevated intracellular cAMP levels are responsible for the loss of Wnt-10b mRNA[6].

Another level of regulation of the Wnt signaling pathway occurs at the receptor level. Frizzled receptors -1, -2, and -5 are expressed in preadipocytes, and expression rapidly declines after induction of adipogenesis[6]. Although mRNA for the Wnt co-receptors LRP5 and LRP6 is unchanged during 3T3-L1 differentiation[6], these co-receptor mRNAs are present in stromovascular cells, but absent from adipocytes isolated from mouse white adipose tissue[6]. This decline in receptor and coreceptor expression during differentiation will render the preadipocyte refractory to autocrine or paracrine Wnt signals, and may be required for adipogenesis to occur.

Wnt inhibits adipogenesis through changes in gene transcription. To examine this mechanism, DNA microarrays were used to generate expression profiles for the differentiation of adipocytes *in vitro* (3T3-L1 preadipocytes to adipocytes) and *in vivo* (stromovascular cells and white adipocytes), as well as the effects of Wnt-1 signaling on gene expression in 3T3-L1 cells[8].

When expressed in 3T3-L1 cells induced to differentiate, Wnt-1 has a powerful repressive effect on expression of many cell cycle genes. Wnt-1 alters the activity of E2F4 and p130, in part by blockingthe repression of the cyclin dependent kinase inhibitors, p21 and p27[8], suggesting that Wnt-1 alters aspects of mitotic clonal expansion[8]. Wnt-1 also has dramatic effects on expression of genes involved in glycogen synthesis, the pentose phosphate shunt, glycolysis, oxidative phosphorylation, and lipogenesis[8]. As expected, the adipogenic transcription factors responsible for expression of many of these genes, C/EBPα, PPARγ, and SREBP1/ADD1, are repressed by Wnt-1.

Given the crucial role of Wnts in blocking adipogenesis *in vitro*, obvious questions have arisen about the role of Wnts, specifically Wnt-10b, *in vivo*. Wnt-10b mRNA is expressed in stromovascular cells, but is absent in adipocytes[6], suggesting that Wnt-10b is an endogenous regulator of white adipose tissue development. Currently, our laboratory is investigating the effects of Wnt-10b *in vivo* by using both knockout and transgenic animal models. The results of these studies should broaden our understanding of the role of Wnts in adipocyte biology, including pathologic conditions such as obesity and type 2 diabetes.

References

1. Green H, Meuth M. An established pre-adipose cell line and its differentiation in culture. *Cell* 1974; 3(2): 127–33.
2. MacDougald OA, Mandrup S. Adipogenesis: forces that tip the scales. *Trends Endocrinol Metab* 2002; 13(1): 5–11.
3. Rosen ED, Spiegelman BM. PPARgamma: a nuclear regulator of metabolism, differentiation, and cell growth. *J Biol Chem* 2001; 276(41): 37731–4.
4. Spiegelman BM, Flier JS. Obesity and the regulation of energy balance. *Cell* 2001; 104(4): 531–43.
5. Morrison RF, Farmer SR. Hormonal signaling and transcriptional control of adipocyte differentiation. *J Nutr* 2000; 130(12): S3116–S3121.
6. Bennett CN, Ross SE, Longo KA, Bajnok L, Hemati N, Johnson KW *et al.* Regulation of Wnt Signaling during Adipogenesis. *J Biol Chem* 2002; 277(34): 30998–1004.
7. Ross SE, Hemati N, Longo KA, Bennett CN, Lucas PC, Erickson RL *et al.* Inhibition of adipogenesis by Wnt signaling. *Science* 2000; 289(5481): 950–3.
8. Ross SE, Erickson RL, Gerin I, DeRose PM, Bajnok L, Longo KA *et al.* Microarray analyses during adipogenesis: understanding the effects of Wnt signaling on adipogenesis and the roles of liver X receptor alpha in adipocyte metabolism. *Mol Cell Biol* 2002; 22(16): 5989–99.
9. Nusse R, Varmus HE. Wnt genes. *Cell* 1992; 69(7): 1073–87.
10. Longo KA, Kennell JA, Ochocinska MJ, Ross SE, Wright WS, MacDougald OA. Wnt signaling protects 3T3-L1 preadipocytes from apoptosis through induction of insulin-like growth factors. *J Biol Chem* 2002; 1: 1.

11. Moon RT, Bowerman B, Boutros M, Perrimon N. The promise and perils of Wnt signaling through beta-catenin. *Science* 2002; 296(5573): 1644–6.

12. Hardt SE, Sadoshima J. Glycogen synthase kinase-3beta: a novel regulator of cardiac hypertrophy and development. *Circ Res* 2002; 90(10): 1055–63.

13. Peifer M, McEwen DG. The ballet of morphogenesis: unveiling the hidden choreographers. *Cell* 2002; 109(3): 271–4.

14. Van de Wetering M, de Lau W, Clevers H. WNT signaling and lymphocyte development. *Cell* 2002; 109 (Suppl): S13–S19.

15. Malbon CC, Wang H, Moon RT. Wnt signaling and heterotrimeric G-proteins: strange bedfellows or a classic romance? *Biochem Biophys Res Commun* 2001; 287(3): 589–93.

16. Bejsovec A. Wnt signaling: an embarrassment of receptors. *Curr Biol* 2000; 10(24): R919–R922.

17. Moon RT, Brown JD, Yang-Snyder JA, Miller JR. Structurally related receptors and Antagonists compete for secretes Wnt ligands. *Cell* 1997; 88: 725–728.

18. Akiyama T. Wnt/beta-catenin signaling. *Cytokine Growth Factor Rev* 2000; 11(4): 273–82.

19. Lisovsky M, Itoh K, Sokol SY. Frizzled receptors activate a novel JNK-dependent pathway that may lead to apoptosis. *Curr Biol* 2002; 12(1): 53–8.

20. Ross SE, Erickson RL, Hemati N, MacDougald OA. Glycogen synthase kinase 3 is an insulin-regulated C/EBPalpha kinase. *Mol Cell Biol* 1999; 19(12): 8433–41.

Progress in Obesity Research: 9. Edited by *Geraldo Medeiros-Neto, Alfredo Halpern and Claude Bouchard*
©2003 John Libbey Eurotext Ltd, pp. 161–164.

CHAPTER 33

Regional and gender differences in adipose tissue lipolysis

P. Mauriège

Division of Kinesiology, Laval University, Ste-Foy, Québec, Canada
[e-mail: pascale.mauriege@kin.msp.ulaval.ca]

Introduction

Since the pioneering clinical observations of Vague[1], it has become increasingly evident that men (or postmenopausal women) whose adipose tissue is predominantly located in the abdominal region are at greater risk of metabolic complications than premenopausal women who tend to accumulate fat preferentially in the gluteal and femoral depots[2–4]. In this regard, regional variation in adipose cell lipolysis has already been suggested as contributing to gender differences in body fat distribution[2–5].

Hormonal regulation of human adipose cell lipolysis

Briefly, hormone-sensitive lipase (HSL) is the rate-limiting enzyme in the hydrolysis of triglycerides stored in adipose tissue (AT)[5]. Among the various hormones which control lipid mobilization, catecholamines and insulin are the most potent regulators of *in vitro* adipose cell lipolysis, in adults[4,5]. The final response of adipocytes to catecholamines (antilipolytic or lipolytic effect) depends upon the functional balance between inhibitory α2- and stimulatory β-ARs whose activation modulates HSL activity, and thereby FFA and glycerol release[5]. Insulin interaction with its receptor activates the phosphatidyl-inositol kinase-3 (PIK-3)/phosphodiesterase-3 pathway which in turn decreases cAMP levels and lipolysis[4].

Regional and gender differences in adipose cell lipolysis

Regional and gender differences exist in the adipose cell lipolytic responsiveness to catecholamines and/or to insulin[2–4]. This functional heterogeneity is emphasized in some pathophysiological conditions such as *ageing and obesity on which special attention will be payed*[4]. In this regard, sc abdominal AT and omental depot (which is drained by the portal vein) have often been compared for both catecholamine and insulin actions[6–13]. Omental adipocytes displayed a greater lipolytic response to catecholamines than sc abdominal adipose cells in obese individuals, this effect being more pronounced in men than in women[6,8,10–12]. Minor regional differences in catecholamine-induced adipose cell lipolysis have also been found in lean men[7,12], although lean women were characterized by a higher lipolytic response to norepinephrine in sc abdominal (non-portal) than in omental (portal) adipose cells[7]. In contrast, the antilipolytic effect of insulin was lower in omental than in sc abdominal fat cells of obese male and female subjects[8–11,13] and of lean men[4 for review]. This observation was consistent with the greater insulin receptor (IR) affinity in sc abdominal than in omental adipocytes[4 for review]. As this regional variation may not entirely result from differences in the IR affinity, other events in the IR signalling cascade have been considered. In this regard, the blunted insulin-induced antilipolysis in omental adipocytes of both obese men and women[13], and thereby the increased FFA flux to the liver (an important risk factor in the metabolic complications related to obesity[2–4]) could be partly explained by reduced IR phosphorylation and signal transduction through an IR substrate-1 associated PIK-3 pathway.

Regional and gender differences in subcutaneous adipose cell lipolysis

Sc abdominal adipose cells were more responsive to catecholamine stimulation than femoral and gluteal adipocytes, irrespective of either the gender or the degree of obesity[14–18], mainly because of a greater β-AR density in the former adipocytes[4 for review]. Site differences in normal weight individuals were more marked in women than in men, a finding being mainly attributed to variations in the affinity properties of α2-ARs[16]. The influence of the level of body fatness on these regional variations has also been examined in men covering a wide range of fatness[17]. The marked antilipolytic effect of epinephrine in abdominal fat cells of obese subjects could be explained by an increased α2-adrenergic activity, whereas the exclusive lipolytic action of the hormone in abdominal adipocytes of lean individuals could be related to a weak α2-AR component. A similar study conducted on premenopausal women revealed that the greater antilipolytic response of abdominal and femoral adipocytes to epinephrine attests of a stronger α2-adrenergic inhibitory component in obese, as compared to lean individuals[18]. In addition to some alterations at receptor levels, post-receptor defects in catecholamine-induced lipolysis have also been found in sc adipocytes of obese subjects[4–5]. In this regard, Large et al.[19] have clearly shown that both HSL activity, protein content and mRNA level as well as the maximal abdominal adipose cell lipolytic response to post-adrenoceptor agents were decreased in upper-body obese men and women, as compared to non obese individuals, attesting thus of a reduced lipolytic capacity in obesity[19]. Sc abdominal adipose cells were also equally or more sensitive to the antilipolytic effect of this hormone than femoral and/or gluteal adipocytes, in obese individuals[9,21], a finding consistent with the enhanced IR affinity in the former cells[20]. The blunted insulin responsiveness observed in the femoral depot of both genders[22], and of lean women[18] has already been attributed to some alterations at a post-receptor level[22].

Regional and gender differences in visceral adipose cell lipolysis

Catecholamine-induced lipolysis was higher in portal (omental, mesenteric) than in non portal (retroperitoneal) adipocytes of lean men, while the reverse situation has been observed in lean women[7]. However, adipose cell lipolytic response to norepinephrine was as high in portal as in non portal depots in severely obese men and women[8]. On the other hand, insulin responsiveness was similar in both portal and non portal adipose cells of obese subjects[8]. Different catecholamine and insulin responsivenesses have also been observed in two visceral depots drained by the portal vein, in massively obese women[11]. Indeed, round ligament adipose cells displayed greater sensitivity and maximal antilipolytic response to insulin as well as higher α2-adrenergic antilipolytic component of epinephrine, when compared to omental adipocytes, suggesting that such distinct properties may represent a protective mechanism against the metabolic complications related to visceral obesity[2–4]. Similarly, omental adipose cells were more lipolytically responsive to norepinephrine than mesenteric adipocytes of severely obese women, but not in massively obese men[23]. Since metabolic complications of obesity are more commonly observed in men than in women[1–4], sex differences in visceral fat cell lipolysis may be thus of importance[23,24]. Indeed, although both responsiveness and sensitivity of omental adipose cells to insulin did not differ between genders, norepinephrine-induced lipolysis was higher in omental adipocytes of obese men, compared to obese women, mainly because of an increased β3-AR lipolytic sensitivity vs. a decreased α2-AR antilipolytic sensitivity[24], thus explaining the greater risk of coronary heart disease in men[1–4].

Influence of visceral obesity on subcutaneous adipose cell lipolysis

Although visceral adipocytes have a hyperlipolytic profile compared to sc fat cells[6–13], the relationship observed between visceral fat deposition and metabolic dysfunctions could also be partly attributed to enhanced lipolytic response of sc adipocytes[2–4]. However, most experiments published so far have generally compared subjects displaying a low visceral AT accumulation and small sc adipocytes with individuals showing a high intraabdominal fat deposition and large sc adipose cells. In this regard, subjects matched for similar age, body fatness and/or sc fat cell weight but displaying marked differences in visceral AT accumulation, were compared for regional adipose cell lipolysis. In this regard, Dowling et al.[25] have reported that both abdominal and gluteal adipose cells from upper-body obese (UBO) women were less sensitive to the antilipolytic effect of insulin, as compared to lower body obese (LBO) women. A similar study performed on overweight men[26] revealed a greater lipolysis in abdominal adipocytes of subjects displaying a high VAT accumulation, compared to those with a low VAT deposition.

162

Regional and gender differences in subcutaneous adipose cell lipolysis: influence of age

Ageing is also well known to be accompanied by body fat gain, and increased visceral AT accumulation, in both genders[2-4]. An enhanced adipose cell lipolytic response to catecholamines or insulin has commonly been observed in sc abdominal compared to gluteo-femoral regions of young men and women[6,9,11,14-18]. These site differences were, however, less pronounced in middle-aged men, because of a decreased fat cell lipolytic activity[22,31]. Discordant results have been reported with advancing age, in women, concerning the lack or the presence of regional variation in adipose cell lipolysis[22,27-30,32]. One reason for these conflicting data could be that subjects were not matched for total adiposity and regional fat distribution. The influence of body fat distribution on the adipose cell responsiveness to insulin has been shown in obese postmenopausal women matched for similar age and body fatness but displaying marked differences in visceral AT accumulation[28]. In the latter study, the maximal antilipolytic effect of insulin was similar in both abdominal and gluteal adipose cells, regardless of the subjects'visceral adiposity, at menopause. However, a similar matching procedure as that previously described[25,26,28] revealed that both UBO and LBO postmenopausal women were characterized by an increased lipolytic response of abdominal vs. gluteal adipose cells to epinephrine[29], mainly because of a lower $\alpha 2$-/β-AR ratio in the former adipocytes[30]. A study conducted on men confirmed that ageing was associated with a reduced adipose cell lipolytic capacity, via a decreased activation of the HSL complex, regardless of the region considered[31]. A comparison of pre- vs. postmenopausal women matched for body fatness, fat cell size and visceral AT accumulation, did not reveal significant change in regional adipose cell lipolysis[32].

Conclusion

As gender variation in body fat distribution is closely associated with sex steroids, it is tempting to speculate that such hormones are important factors in the regulation of sex- and site differences in adipose cell lipolysis. Further studies on the cellular actions of estrogens and androgens and the expression of the steroid converting enzymes would certainly help us to clarify the complex network of interactions among steroid hormones, regional adipose tissue distribution and lipolysis, and thereby obesity-related metabolic complications.

References

1. Vague, J.The degree of masculine differentiation of obesities: a factor determining predisposition to diabetes, atherosclerosis, gout and uric calculous disease. *Am J Clin Nutr* 1956; 4: 20–38.

2. Kissebah AH, Krakower GR. Regional adiposity and morbidity. *Physiol Rev* 1994; 74: 761–811.

3. Björntorp P. The regulation of adipose tissue distribution in humans. *Int J Obes* 1996; 20: 291–302.

4. Large V, Arner P. Regulation of lipolysis in humans. Pathophysiological modulation in obesity, diabetes and hyperlipidemia. *Diabetes & Metab* 1998; 24: 409–18.

5. Langin D, Lucas S, Lafontan M. Millenium fat cell lipolysis reveals unsuspected novel tracks. *Horm Metab Res* 2000; 32: 443–52.

6. Mauriège P, Galitzky J, Berlan M, Lafontan M. Heterogeneous distribution of beta- and alpha2-adrenoceptor binding sites in human fat cells from various deposits: functional consequences. *Eur J Clin Invest* 1987; 17: 156–65.

7. Rebuffé-Scrive M, Andersson B, Olbe L, Björntorp P. Metabolism of adipose tissue in intraabdominal depots of nonobese men and women. *Metabolism* 1989; 38: 453–8.

8. Rebuffé-Scrive M, Andersson B, Olbe L, Björntorp P. Metabolism of adipose tissue in intraabdominal depots of severely obese men and women. *Metabolism* 1990; 39: 1021–5.

9. Richelsen B, Pedersen SB, Moller-Pedersen T, Bak JF. Regional differences in triglyceride breakdown in human adipose tissue: effects of catecholamines, insulin and prostaglandin E$_2$. *Metabolism* 1991; 40: 990–6.

10. Marin P, Andersson B, Ottosson M, Olbe L, Chowdhury B, Kvist H *et al.* The morphology and metabolism of intraabdominal adipose tissue in men. *Metabolism* 1992; 4: 1242–8.

11. Mauriège P, Marette A, Atgié C, Bouchard C, Thériault G, Bukowiecki LJ, Marceau P *et al.* Regional variation in adipose tissue metabolism of severely obese women. *J Lipid Res* 1995; 36: 672–84.

12. Hoffstedt J, Arner P, Hellers G, Lönnqvist F. Variation in adrenergic regulation of lipolysis between omental and subcutaneous adipocytes from obese and non-obese men. *J Lipid Res* 1997; 38: 795–804.

13. Zierath JR, Livingston JN, Thörne A, Bolinder J, Reynisdottir S, Lönnqvist F, Arner P. Regional difference in insulin inhibition of NEFA release from human adipocytes: relation to insulin receptor phosphorylation and intracellular signalling through the insulin receptor substrate-1 pathway. *Diabetologia* 1998; 4: 1343–54.

14. Richelsen B. Increased alpha2- but similar beta-adrenergic receptor activities in subcutaneous gluteal adipocytes from females compared with males. Eur *J Clin Invest* 1986; 16: 302–9.

15. Leibel RL, Hirsch, J. Site- and sex-related differences in adrenoceptor status of human adipose tissue. *J Clin Endocrinol Metab* 1987; 64: 1205–10.

16. Wahrenberg H, Lönnqvist F, Arner P. Mechanisms underlying regional differences in lipolysis in human adipose tissue. *J Clin Invest* 1989; 84: 458–67.

17. Mauriège P, Després JP, Prud'homme D, Pouliot MC, Marcotte M, Tremblay A, Bouchard C. Regional variation in adipose tissue lipolysis in lean and obese men. *J Lipid Res* 1991; 32: 1625–33.

18. Mauriège P, Prud'homme D, Lemieux S, Tremblay A, Després JP. Regional differences in adipose tissue lipolysis from lean and obese women: existence of postreceptor alterations. *Am J Physiol* 1995; 269: E341–E350.

19. Large V, Reynisdottir S, Langin D, Fredby K, Klannemark M, Holm C, Arner P. Decreased expression and function of adipocyte hormone-sensitive lipase in subcutaneous fat cells of obese subjects. *J Lipid Res* 1999; 40: 2059–65.

20. Bolinder J, Engfeldt P, Ostman J, Arner P. Site differences in insulin receptor binding and insulin action in subcutaneous fat of obese females. *J Clin Endocrinol Metab* 1983; 57: 455–61.

21. Smith U, Hammersten J, Björntorp P, Kral JG. Regional differences and effects of weight reduction on human fat cell metabolism. Eur *J Clin Invest* 1979; 9: 327–32.

22. Rebuffé-Scrive M, Lönnroth P, Marin P, Wesslau C, Björntorp P, Smith U. Regional adipose tissue metabolism in men and postmenopausal women. *Int J Obes* 198; 711: 347–55.

23. Fried SK, Leibel RL, Edens NK, Kral JG. Lipolysis in intraabdominal adipose tissues of obese women and men. *Obes Res* 1993; 1: 443–8.

24. Lönnqvist F, Thörne A, Large V, Arner P. Sex differences in visceral fat lipolysis and metabolic complications of obesity. *Arterioscl Thromb Vasc* 1997; 17: 1472–80.

25. Dowling HJ, Fried SK, Pi-Sunyer FX. Insulin resistance in adipocytes of obese women: Effects of body fat distribution and race. *Metabolism* 1995; 44: 987–95.

26. Mauriège P, Brochu M, Prud'homme D, Tremblay A, Nadeau A, Lemieux S, Després JP. Is visceral adiposity a significant correlate of subcutaneous adipose cell lipolysis in men? *J Clin Endocrinol Metab* 1999; 84: 736–42.

27. Rebuffé-Scrive M, Eld J, Hafström LO, Björntorp P. Metabolism of mammary, abdominal and femoral adipocytes in women before and after menopause. *Metabolism* 1986; 35: 792–97.

28. Landin K, Lönnroth P, Krotkiewski M, Holm G, Smith U. Increased insulin resistance and fat cell lipolysis in obese but not lean women with a high waist/hip ratio. Eur *J Clin Invest* 1990; 20: 530–5.

29. Nicklas BJ, Rogus EM, Colman EG, Goldberg AP. Visceral adiposity, increased adipocyte lipolysis, and metabolic dysfunction in obese postmenopausal women. *Am J Physiol* 1996; 270: E72–E78.

30. Berman DM, Nicklas BJ, Rogus EM, Dennis KE, Goldberg AP. Regional differences in adrenoceptor binding and fat cell lipolysis in obese postmenopausal women. *Metabolism* 1998; 47; 467–73.

31. Imbeault P, Prud'homme D, Tremblay A, Després JP, Mauriège P. Adipose tissue metabolism in young and middle-aged men after control for total body fatness. *J Clin Endocrinol Metab* 2000; 85: 2455–62.

32. Mauriège P, Imbeault P, Prud'homme D, Tremblay A, Nadeau A, Després JP. Subcutaneous adipose tissue metabolism at menopause: importance of body fatness and regional fat distribution. *J Clin Endocrinol Metab* 2000; 85: 2446–54.

Progress in Obesity Research: 9. Edited by *Geraldo Medeiros-Neto, Alfredo Halpern and Claude Bouchard*
©2003 John Libbey Eurotext Ltd, pp. 165–170.

CHAPTER 34

Functional roles of perilipins and related lipid droplet-associated (PAT) proteins

Constantine Londos, Carole Sztalryd, John T. Tansey, Guoheng Xu, Xinyue Lu, Jai-Wei Gan and Alan R. Kimmel

National Institutes of Health, Bethesda, MD 10892-8028, USA
[e-mail: DeanL@intra.niddk.nih.gov]

Introduction

The triacylglycerols (TAG) stored in intracellular lipld storage droplets of adipocytes represent the major energy storage depots in animals. Energy, in the form of fatty acids, is released by lipolysis, a cAMP/protein kinase A-(PKA) mediated process in adipocytes. For many years, adipocyte lipolysis was thought to result primarily from PKA-mediated phosphorylation of hormone-sensitive lipase (HSL), the adipocyte enzyme thought to be responsible for lipolysis. This explanation seemed inadequate to us, because phosphorylation of HSL leads to only a twofold activation of catalytic activity *in vitro*, whereas *in vivo* activation of cellular PKA activity results in a 30- to 100-fold activation of cellular lipolytic activity in primary adipocytes. Two findings have radically altered our view of the lipolytic reaction. First, we found that HSL is a cytosolic enzyme in quiescent cells that rapidly translocates to the surface of the lipid droplet upon stimulation[1]. Initially, this was discovered by tracking HSL location in subcellular fractions of centrifuged homogenates of primary rat adipocytes. In unstimulated cells, HSL was found predominantly in the infranatant fraction below the floating fat cake, whereas in stimulated cells, the HSL was found associated with the floating fat cake, from which we concluded that the enzyme had migrated from the cytosol to the lipid droplet upon stimulation. Subsequently, this migration was confirmed by direct visualization of HSL in 3T3-LI adipocyte[2]. This delivery of the enzyme to its substrate seemed a more compelling basis for the magnitude of lipolytic activation than did catalytic activation. The second finding of note was our discovery of perilipin[3], a protein that coats the lipid droplet surface in adipocytes. This was a serendipitous finding of a heavily phosphorylated protein in the fat cake fraction of [P]loaded rat adipocytes[4], the same fraction to which HSL translocated upon stimulation. Since perilipin, like HSL, is polyphosphorylated by PKA, we hypothesized that peripilin is important in the lipolytic reaction, and we thus focused our efforts on perilipin function in lipolysis.

Type 2 diabetes mellitus is a major health problem in the Westen world, and one factor that correlates with type 2 diabetes mellitus is plasma fatty acid levels which are thought to arise from adipose tissue[5–7]. The role of adipose tissue is supported by studies showing that inhibition of adipocyte lipolysis by agonists of the adipocyte A1 adenosine receptor reverse diabetes in animal models[8,9]. Given the apparent central role of the adipocyte in propagating or exacerbating problems with diabetes mellitus, it is anticipated that an understanding of the molecular basis for the lipolytic reaction in adipocytes might lead to useful therapies for this disease.

We have applied two major approaches to assess perilipin function. First, we have expressed perilipin in cultured cell lines to determine if ectopic perilipins localize to lipid droplets and, if so, what are the effects of these proteins on the metabolism of neutral lipids within the droplets. Second, we have ablated the perilipin gene by homologous recombination in embryonic stem cells, which provided a source for adipocytes that lack perilipin.

As we review briefly below, the approaches noted above have yielded information on perilipin function.

165

Perilipin function

Previously, we found that a perilipin-related protein, ADRP, coats[10] the lipid droplets in most cells , whereas perilipin is expressed only in adipocytes and steroidogenic cells[11,12]. When we expressed perilipin A, the major splice variant of the perilipin gene, in fibroblastic cell lines (3T3-LI pre-adipocytes and CHO cells) the perilipin displaced the ADRP and the droplets acquired a coating of perilipin. These studies also indicated that perilipin exhibited a protective effect on intracellular triacylglycerols (TAG), since perilipin A expression in fibroblastic 3T3-LI pre-adipocytes led to a lengthening of the half-life of stored TAG by a factor of 4.5, from which we concluded that coating the intracellular lipid droplets lowered the access of the lipase(s) to the TAG within the core of the lipid droplets[13]. Further evidence for this protective function of perilipin was reported by Souza *et al.*[14] in a study on the lipolytic stimulation of 3T3-LI adipocytes by the cytokine TNFα. It was found that the cytokine reduced cellular perilipin, but that maintaining the perilipin using an adenovirus expression vector eliminated the TNF-α stimulated lipolysis. Perilipin A has six consensus sites for phosphorylation by PKA. Under the unstimulated condition, the introduction of perillpin A suppressed lipolysis of TAG within the lipid droplets, indicating that a major function of nonphosphorylated perilipin A is to protect neutral lipids from hydrolysis by endogenous lipases. The importance of this aspect of perilipin function is highlighted by the *perilipin* null animal, that exhibits a dearth of adipose tissue in all fat depots[15,16]. Lipolysis in CHO cells containing perilipin-coated droplets is inhibited by 90 per cent compared to hydrolysis in control cells with ADRPcoated lipid droplets[17]. Upon activation of PKA in CHO cells there is a sevenfold activation of lipolysis in the perilipin A cells, but not in control cells. Unlike adipocytes, which contain the PKA-regulated hormone-sensitive lipase, CHO cells contain no PKA-sensitive lipase. The PKA-mediated lipolytic response in CHO cells is mediated by phosphorylation of perilipin A alone, which appears to alter the lipid droplet surface to permit access of the endogenous lipase to the core TAG within lipid droplets. Thus, it is substrate access, and not the enzyme that is regulated by PKA. Further, this perilipin-mediated lipolytic activation, is abrogated by mutation of the serines within the three most N-terminal PKA phosphorylation sites within perilipin A[17]. An additional facet of this approach involved an exploration of the interplay between HSL and the perilipins. As noted above, upon stimulation of protein kinase (PKA) activity in adipocytes cytosolic HSL translocates to the surface of lipid droplets. We have introduced HSL tagged with GFP into CHO cells in which we also introduced perilipins. Upon PKA stimulation, HSL-GFP translocates from the cytosol to lipid droplets only in cells that also expressed perilipin A on their droplets. This does not occur in cells with ADPP on their droplets nor in cells expressing the perilipin in which the N-terminal PKA sites have been mutated (C. Sztalryd *et al.*, submitted). Thus, functional perilipin is required to induce HSL translocation. The importance of the HSL translocation reaction is highlighted in our studies on the perilipin null mice which show a loss of PKA-stimulated lipolysis (see below).

Animal studies

To assess the importance of perilipin in animal fat metabolism, we ablated the perilipin gene in mice using embryonic stem cell technology. The resulting animal was devoid of perilipin, and the adipocyte lipid droplets were now coated with ADRP[15]. This is a reversal of the perilipin process we described in differentiating murine adipocytes in culture, where the earliest lipid droplets are coated with ADRP. Shortly after the onset of perilipin expression, the lipid droplets acquire a coating of perilipin and the ADRP protein disappears, despite a rising level of ADRP MRNA expression[10]. We speculate that ADRP and perilipin compete for common space on the droplet surface and that when both proteins are present, perilipin binding prevails and ADRP is excluded. This speculation is boume out in our studies with fibroblasts, in which introduction of perilipin also reduces ADRP dramatically[17] . A major consequence of eliminating the perilipin gene in mice is a dramatic loss of adipose tissue, by nearly 60 per cent in both females and males (Fig. 1). Metabolic studies with isolated adipocytes reveal major functional consequences of the lack of perilipin. First, under carefully controlled conditions we had established previously[18] for managing isolated adipocytes, we found that basal lipolytic activity was elevated and, perhaps more importantly, there was a large loss in the ability to stimulate lipolysis with agents that elevated cAMP and activate PKA[15]. There was also a loss in the ability to elicit a lowering of the respiratory exchange ratio (RER) upon injection of a Beta-3-adrenergic receptor agonist, indicative of a loss in the lipolytic response in the *perilipin* null mice. In the normal animal, injection of the agonist led to a sharp decrease in the RER, which reflects the metabolism of fatty acids released from stimulated adipocytes. The fact that this did not occur in the *perilipin* null mice shows that as in the isolated adipocytes, the adipose cells fail to respond normally *in situ* to a lipolytic stimulus with an

Normal   Perilipin KO

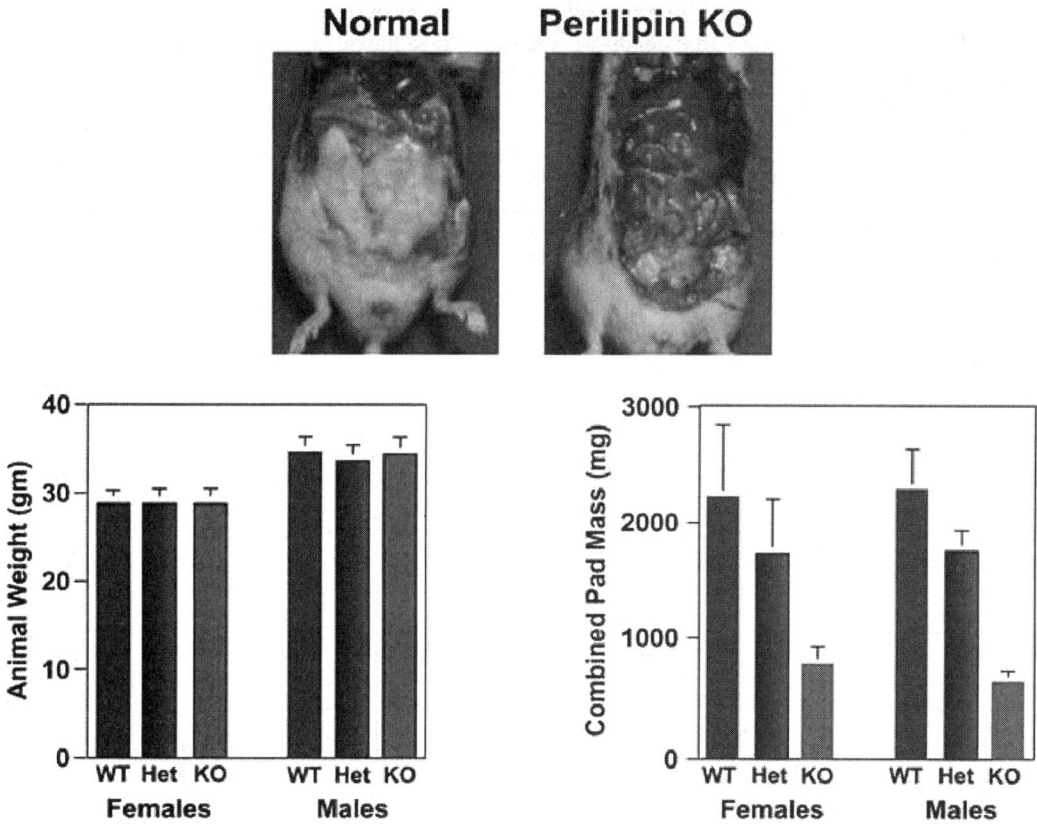

Fig. 1. Top panes are representative photographs of abdominal cavities of 22 week old wt (left) and *perilipin* null (right) mice. Lower bar graphs show (left) comparisons of animal weights of wt, heterozygote, and null mice. On lower right are comparisons of combined masses of reproductive, inguinal and retroperitoneal fat pads (adapted from Tansey *et al.*, ref.[15]).

outpouring of fatty acids. It appears that the elevated basal lipolysis in adipocytes of the perilipin null mouse has a greater impact on overall lipid metabolism than does the loss of stimulated lipolysis. The former would lead to a lessening of adipose lipids, where as the latter would lead to increase lipid storage. Since the animal clearly has a dramatic reduction in adipose lipid reserves, it appears that the elevated basal lipolysis is the predominant factor in determining the phenotype. Below, we discuss more recent mechanistic studies on the consequences of perilipin ablation on the activity of hormone-sensitive lipase in adipocytes. Oddly, despite their elevated basal lipolysis, the perilipin mouse did not exhibit elevated plasma free fatty acid concentrations, which may explain their failure to rapidly develop glucose intolerance. Rather, only a subset of the perilipin null mice showed glucose intolerance and apparent peripheral insulin resistance, and the animals that did so were only those that attained body weights of greater than 30 g. More recently we found that the perilipin null animals contain increased lipid depositions in their livers in the fed state, whereas the control animals exhibit hepatic lipid depositions only in the fasted state (C. Sztalryd, *J Cell Biol*, in press). Thus, the perilipin null mice appear to divert lipids from the adipose tissue to the liver. There were no differences in body weight between normal and *perilipin* null mice, and the latter exhibited a greater lean body mass and elevated metabolism, which may have contributed to the reduction in adipose mass. The null mice also contained increased plasma leptin concentrations, despite their lower adipose mass. In general, serum leptin value correlates with adipose mass. There was a much steeper relationship between plasma leptin and fat mass in the perilipin null mice than normal mice. The basis for this apparent increased leptin production in these animal remains unknown.

Perilipin and the action of HSL

We have found that the defect that leads to a failure to achieve hormone-stimulated lipolysis in adipocytes of the perilipin null mice lies downstream of the cell surface receptor beta-adrenergic receptor/G protein/adenylyl cyclase complex (Sztalryd *et al.*, submitted). Accordingly, we focused attention on the major event subsequent to cAMP generation and PKA activation in adipocytes, which is the interaction of HSL with the lipid droplets. To examine this translocation reaction, we developed lines of cultured cells from embryonic fibroblasts of normal and *perilipin* null animals, which could be differentiated into adipocytes. The cultured cells are more amenable to the examination of the HSL translocation than are the large primary adipocytes isolated from fat depots. Unsurprisingly, we found that HSL fails to translocate to lipid droplets upon stimulation of cells derived from perilipin null animals, whereas HSL translocated to lipid droplets in cell deri.ved from wild type animals. These results largely support our conclusions draw from CHO cell studies (above). The *perilipin* null mice serve to highlight two important functional roles of perilipin A. First, in the unstimulated state perilipin protects TAG within lipid droplets from hydrolysis and appears to be necessary for normal fat deposition. Second, in the stimulated state, perilipin A modifies the lipid droplet surface in such a manner that permits HSL to translocate to and attach to the droplet surface, where it hydrolyzes the core neutral lipids, primarily TAG.

An important question that arises relates to the mechanism by which phosphorylated perilipin facilitates HSL translocation. We reported previously that upon phosphorylation, perilipin disperses from large lipld droplets to numerous microdroplets . We further find that HSL occupies the space on larger droplets from which perilipin has departed. This does not preclude the possibility that HSL and perilipin directly interact, but such interaction may only be a very early event in HSL translocation, since as lipolysis progresses the two proteins are not co-localized (C. Sztalryd, *J Cell Biol*, in press).

In yet a another study, we have found that HSL translocation is not merely secondary to changes in the droplet surface. Rather, mutational analysis revealed that HSL must be PK-A phosphorylated in order to translocate. Like perilipin, HSL contains multiple sites for PKA phosphorylation, one (s563) known for many years and two (s659, s660) more recently discovered[21]. Single mutations of each of these serines to alanines does not eliminate HSL translocation, but double mutation of s659 and s660 to alanines abrogates HSL translocation. We conclude that phosphorylation of at least one of these two sites is required to induce HSL to translocate to the llpld droplet (C.-L. Su *et al.*, submitted).

Studies on ADR-P, TIP-47 and related proteins

Although the area of perilipin function is maturing, relatively little can be said about the function of perilipin-related proteins on lipid droplets. These include ADRP, TIP47 and the related proteins in *Drosophila melanogaster and Dictyostelium discoidium*[22,23], proteins that are encoded by members of an ancient gene family. ADRP is expressed in all cells, where it coats droplets in cells that do not express perilipin. In tissue scans, we found that ADRP was expressed in lung at a level second only to adipose tissue. Recently, in collaboration with John Torday (UCLA) we have pinpointed ADRP expression to pulmonary lipofibroblasts, cells with prominent lipid droplets that serve to remove lipid from the serum and apparently pass these lipids on to type 2 epithelial cells that synthesize and secrete surfactant. We find that type 2 epithelial cells can extract radiolabeled triolein from ADRP-coated lipid droplets isolated from cultured lipofibroblasts, and incorporate these fatty acids into radiolabled surfactant phospholipids[24]. Interestingly, antibodies against ADRP block the transfer of lipid into the type 2 cells, suggesting a role for ADRP in the lipofibroblast-to-type 2 cells transfer of lipids.

The issue of TIP-47 subcellular localization has been disputed. Initially, this protein was identified as a cargo factor in the trafficking of IGF-2 receptors[25]. Given its high homology to ADRP, two former members of this laboratory reported that TIP-47 localizes to lipid storage droplet[26]. Subsequently, this finding was disputed by the Pfeffer group at Stanford, who contended that the TIP-47 finding was an artifact, resulting from cross-reactivity of the TIP-47 antibody with ADRP[27]. More recently, using GFP-tagged TIP-47 plus anti-TIP-47 antibodies with no crossreactivity with ADRP, we demonstrated that TIP-47 does indeed localize to lipid droplets[28]. Like perilipin and ADRP, fusion constructs of the cDNAs for the related proteins of *Drosophila and Dictyostelium* to green floureseent protein localize exclusively to lipid droplets when expressed in the mammalian CHO cell line[28]. TIP-47 is the only product of this ancient family of genes that localizes to both lipid droplets and other cytoplasmic components. It may be reasonable to assume that these protein will be found to have roles in the metabolism of neutral lipids within the droplets that they coat.

Previously we found that a major mechanism for the regulation of perilipin expression was not at the transcriptional level but via protein stabilization upon binding to lipid droplets. More recently, we found that this post-translational mode of regulation applies also to ADRP. We have proposed that, in the absence of an available lipid droplet surface to which to bind, these proteins are synthesized and promptly degraded. We now find that both perilipin and ADRP are hydrolysed by a proteasomal process in the absence of lipid droplets to which to bind (G. Xu, submitted).

Concluding remarks

Before the discovery of perilipin, the molecular details of the reaction that governs lipolysis in adipocytes were unknown. Clearly, perilipin plays a critical role both in facilitating the deposition of TAG in adipose cells and in facilitating the action of HSL. Both the expression of perilipin in non-adipocytes and the knock-out of the perilipin gene have revealed important functional roles for perilipin. It will be interesting to examine animals that express only mutated forms of perilipin and the double mutant animal that expresses neither perilipin nor HSL. The sequence similarities between perilipin and ADRP led to the studies that also localized ADRP to lipid droplets. Whether or not the *ADRP* null animal will be as revealing as the *perilipin* null mouse remains to be determined. Of particular importance will be the fate of *ADRP* gene ablation on lipid metabolism in heart, skeletal muscle and liver. And, given our findings reviewed above on the possible role of ADRP in lung surfactant production, the *ADRP* null mice may reveal a fundamental role for this protein in animal lipid metabolism.

Acknowledgements: We should like to recognize the important contributions of our collaborators and co-workers in the research reviewed in this paper. These include, from Lund, Sweden, Drs. Cecilia Holm and Juan Antonio Contreras, from the NIH, Drs. Shinji Miura, Asma Amleh, Ms. Heidi Doward, and Ms. Jai-Wei Gan.

References

1. Egan JJ, Greenberg AS, Chang MK, Wek SA, Moos MC Jr, Londos C. Mechanism of hormone-stimulated lipolysis in adipocytes: translocation of hormone-sensitive lipase to the lipid storage droplet. *Proc Natl Acad Sci USA* 1992; 89: 8537–41.

2. Brasaemle DL, Levin DM, Adler-Wailes DC, Londos C. The lipolytic stimulation of 3T3-Ll adipocytes promotes the translocation of cytosolic hormone-sensitive lipase to the surfaces of lipid storage droplets. *Biochim Biophys Acta* 1999; 483: 251–62.

3. Greenberg AS, Egan JJ, Wek SA, Garty NB, Blanchette-Mackle EJ, Londos C. Perlllpin, a major hormonally regulated adipocyte-specific phosphoprotein associated with the periphery of lipid storage droplets. *J Biol Chem* 1991; 266: 11341–6.

4. Egan JJ, Greenberg AS, Chang MK, Londos C. Control of endogenous phosphorylation of the major CAMP-dependent protein kinase substrate in adipocytes by insulin and betaadrenergic stimulation. *J Biol Chem* 1990; 265: 18769–75.

5. Dresner A, Laurent D, Marcucci M, *et al.* Effects of free fatty acids on glucose transport and IRS-1-associated phosphatidylinositol 3-kinase activity. *J Clin Invest* 1999; 103: 253–259.

6. Roden M, Price TB, Perseghin G, Petersen KF, Rothman DL, Cline GW, Shulman GI. Mechanism of free fatty acid-induced insulin resistance in humans. *J Clin Invest* 1996; 97(12): 2859–65.

7. Bergman RN. New concepts in extracellular signaling for insulin action: the single gateway hypothesis. *Recent Prog Horm Res* 1997; 52: 359–85 (discussion 385–7)

8. Reaven GM, Chang H, Ho H, Jeng CY, Hoffman BB. Lowering of plasma glucose in diabetic rats by antilipolytic agents. *Am J Physiol* 1988; 254: E23–E30.

9. Bergman RN, Ader M. Free fatty acids and pathogenesis of type 2 diabetes mellitus. *Trends Endocrinol Metabl* 2000; 1: 351–6.

10. Brasaemle DL, Barber T, Wolins NE, Serrero G, Blanchette-Mackie EJ, Londos C. Adipose differentiation-related protein is an ubiquitously expressed lipid storage droplet associated protein. *J Lipid Res* 1997; 38: 2249–63.

11. Greenberg AS, Egan JJ, Wek SA, Moos MC Jr., Londos C, Kimmel AR. Isolation of cDNAs for perilipins A and B: sequence and expression of lipid droplet-associated proteins of adipocytes. *Proc Natl Acad Sci USA* 1993; 90: 12035–9.

12. Servetnick DA, Brasaemle DL, Gruia-Gray J, Kimmel AR, Wolff J, Londos C. Perilipins are associated with cholesteryl ester droplets in steroidogenic adrenal cortical and Leydig cells. *J Biol Chem* 1995; 270: 16970–3.

13. Brasaemle, DL, Rubin, B, Harten, I.A., Gruia-Gray, J.J., Kimmel, A.R., Londos, C. (2000) Perilipin A increases triacylglycerol storage by decreasing the rate of triacylglycerol hydrolysis. *J Biol Chem* 275, 38486-93.

14. Souza SC, de Vargas LM, Yamamoto MT, Lien P, Franciosa MD, Moss LG, Greenberg AS. Overexpression of perilipin A and B blocks the ability of tumor necrosis factor alpha to increase lipolysis in 3T3-LI adipocytes. *J Biol Chem* 1998; 273: 24665–9.

15. Tansey JT, Sztalryd C, Gruia-Gray J, Roush DL, Zee JV, Gavrilova O *et al*. Perilipin ablation results in a lean mouse with aberrant adipocyte lipolysis, enhanced leptin production, and resistance to diet-induced obesity. *Proc Natl Acad Sci USA* 2001; 98: 6494–9.

16. Martinez-Botas J, Anderson JB, Tessier D, Lapillone A, Chang BHJ, Quast MJ. Absence of perilipin results in leanness and reverses obesity in Lepr db/db mice. *Nature Genet* 2000; 26: 474–9.

17. Tansey, J.T. Huml, A.M., Vogt, R.,Davis, K., E. Jones, Jennifer. M., Fraser, K..A., Brasaemle, Dawn .L., Kimmel, Alan R., Londos, C. (2003) Functional Studies on Native and Mutated forms of Perilipins: A Role in Protein Kinase-A-activated lipolysis of triacylglycerols in CHO cells. *J Biol Chem* 2002; 278: 8401–6.

18. Honnor RC, Dhillon GS, Londos C. cAMP-dependent protein kinase and lipolysis in rat adipocytes. 1. Cell preparation, manipulation, and predictability in behavior. *J Biol Chem* 1985; 260: 15122–9.

19. Chen X, Iqbal N, Boden G. The effects of free fatty acids on gluconeogenesis and glycogenolysis in normal subjects. *J Clin Invest* 1999; 103: 365–72.

20. Londos C. Perilipins ADRP, and other proteins that associate with intracellular neutral lipid droplets in animal cells. *Semin Cell Dev Biol* 1999; 10: 51–8.

21. Anthonsen MW, Ronnstrand L, Wemstedt C, Degerman E, Holm C. Identification of novel phosphorylation sites in honnone- sensitive lipase that are phosphorylated in response to isoproterenol and govern activation properties *in vitro. J Biol Chem* 1998; 273: 215–21.

22. Miura S, Gan JW, Brzostowski J, Parisi MJ, Schultz CJ, Londos C *et al*. Functional conservation for lipid storage droplet association among perilipin-, ADRP-, and TEP 47-related proteins in mammals, drosophila, and dictylostellum. *J Biol Chem* 2002; 277: 32252–7.

23. Lu X, Gruia-Gray J, Copeland NG, Gilbert DJ, Jenkins NA, Londos C, Kimmel AR. The murine perilipin gene: the lipid droplet-associated perilipins derive from tissue-specific, MRNA splice variants and define a gene family of ancient origin. *Mamm Genome* 2001; 12: 741–9.

24. Schultz CJ, Torres E, Londos C, Torday JS. Possible role of adipocyte differentiation~related protein in lung surfactant phospholipid synthesis by epithelial type II cells. *Am J Physiol* 2002 (in press).

25. Diaz E, Pfeffer SR. TIP47: a cargo selection device for mannose Phosphate receptor trafficking. *Cell* 1998; 93: 433–43.

26. Wolins NE, Rubin B, Brasaemle DL. TIP47 associates with lipid droplets. *J Biol Chem* 2001; 276: 5101–8.

27. Barbero P, Buell E, Zulley S, Pfeffer SR. TIP47 is not a component of lipid droplets. *J Biol Chem* 2001.

28. Miura, S., Gan, J.-W., Parisi, M.J., Schultz, C.J., Oliver, B., Kimmel, A.R., Londos, C. (2002) Functional Conservation for Lipid Storage Droplet Proteins *Drosophila melanogaster* and *Dictyostelium discoidium*. *J Biol Chem* (2002) 277, 32252-7.

Progress in Obesity Research: 9. Edited by *Geraldo Medeiros-Neto, Alfredo Halpern and Claude Bouchard*
©2003 John Libbey Eurotext Ltd, pp. 171–175.

CHAPTER 35

Effect of exercise and calorie restriction on human adipose tissue lipolysis

Vladimir Stich[1], M. Berlan[2], M. Lafontan[2], N. Viguerie[2], J. Hejnova[1] and D. Langin[2]

[1]*Third Faculty of Medicine, Prague, Czech Republic;* [2]*INSERM U 317, Toulouse, France*
[e-mail: vladimír.stich@lf3.cuni.cz]

Obesity is associated with many metabolic disturbances. They imply a higher risk of developpement of diseases which worsen the health perspectives of obese patiens. The relevant disturbances are represented by insulin resistence, perturbations of energy metabolism (resting and postprandial) and deviations in fat metabolism represented by deviations in fat oxidation and in lipid mobilization, i.e. in adipose tissue lipolysis and skeletal muscle lipolysis. One of the main goals of therapy of obesity is a correction of these metabolic impairments: the correction may accompany the weight loss but it might occur in the absence of a major weight loss as well.

The main therapeutic interventions in obese patiens are represented by calorie restriction and exercise training. Their efect on adipose tissue lipolysis is the subject of this overview.

Adipose tissue lipolysis is the process which controls the breakdown of triacylglycerols (TAG) in adipose cells, i.e. the proces of hydrolysis of intracellular triacylglycerols giving rise to the formation of glycerol and non-esterified fatty acids (NEFA), released subsequently into the circulation. The released NEFA serve as energy substrate for the skeletal muscle. The plasma NEFA are not the only lipid-borne substrate for the muscle: the other sources being the intramuscular TAG and, possibly, TAG circulationg in blood. Their relative contribution to energy production varies in different physiological and pathological situations.

The adipose tissue lipolysis is, in combination with lipogenesis, the process which regulates the amount of triglycerides in the adipocyte and, thus, the adipose tissue mass. Furthermore, it controls the concentration of NEFA in the circulation and through this variable it is involved in the control of fat oxidation in the body, in the development of insulin resistence, and in the control of a number of processes in which the NEFA appear as important regulators (e.g. the effects of NEFA on expression of genes involved in the control of energy metabolism, as UCP 2,3, in relevant tissues, etc).

Adipose tissue lipolysis is a process is regulated mainly by catecholamines and insulin, although lipolytic effects of many other substances have been known since some time or have been reported recently (growth hormone, parathormone, leptin, tumour necrosis factor alpha, atrial natriuretic peptide etc.) with variable influences on lipolysis regulation. Catecholamines stimulate the lipolysis by activation of beta 1- and beta 2-adrenoreceptors (AR) (the role of beta 3-AR in the human white adipose tissue remaining questionable) and inhibit the lipolysis through activation of alpha2-AR[1]. Recently, the lipolytic effects of alpha1-agonists have been observed *in situ* – these findings, in authors' opinion, deserve further studies and verifications[2]. Adrenaline and noradrenaline stimulate and/or inhibit lipolysis depending on their relative affinity for adrenergic receptor subtypes, the relative number of fat cell β- and β₂-adrenergic receptors expressed in the fat cell and their coupling efficiency to heterotrimeric G proteins (Gs and Gi-protein, respectively) involved in the transduction of the signal to downstream elements of the lipolytic cascade (cAMP, protein-kinase A and the rate limiting enzyme of the lipolytic cascade hormone sensitive lipase). Insulin is a potent inhibitor of adipose tissue lipolysis.

Methods of measurement of adipose tissue lipolysis in humans.

(1) Whole body lipolysis is evaluated using measurement of turnover of substances labels with stable isotopes; (2) The regional lipolysis may be evaluated *in situ* in subcutaneous adipose tissue (SCAT)

using either microdialysis or arteriovenous cathetrization; (3) *In vitro* the rate of lipolysis is measured in isolated adipocytes in samples taken by needle biopsy from SCAT or, in rare experimental studies, by biopsy of visceral adipose tissue taken during the surgical interventions; (4) Alternatively, in the biopsy samples, the levels of mRNA for relevant proteins or the amount or activity of proteins are evaluated. When measuring the regional lipolysis the variations in respect to the region from which biopsy sample is taken must be taken into account.

Lipolysis in obese subjects

The regulation of lipolysis in adipose tissue was found to be disturbed in obese subjects in most studies. Using the simple measurementes of the response of plasma NEFA and glycerol to intravenous infusions of beta 1 and beta 2 agonists the lower increase of plasma glycerol and NEFA in response to beta 2 but not to beta 1 agonists in obese compared to lean subjects[3]. The increase in whole body lipolysis and in regional lipolysis in abdominal SCAT (evaluated using microdialysis) in response to intraveneous epinephrine infusion was found to be lower in obese patients[4]. In addition, a lower increase of adipose tissue blood flow in response to epinephrine was found in obese patients.[4]

In vitro studies give a deeper insight of possible mechanisms underlying the differences between obese and lean patiens. Epinephrine appears to be antilipolytic in lower concentrations in abdominal adipose tissue in obese subjects while it stimulates the lipolysis in lean ones[5]. The effect is region-dependent: the difference is not observable in femoral region. The antilipolytic effect of epinephrine in obese reflects the higher inhibitory action mediated by alpha2-AR. The stimulation mediated by beta-AR and beta 2-AR was also shown to be lower in upper body obese subjects[6]. The relationship between the excess fat mass and impairment of lipolysis is demonstrated by the negative correlation between BMI and beta-AR lipolytic sensitivity[6].

The relevance of the antilipolytic alpha2-mediated function of catecholamines can be demonstrated in physiologic conditions *in vivo*. Using microdialysis to measure lipolysis in abdominal SCAT during physical exercise it is observed that the blockade of alpha2-AR (by alpha2 inhibitor phentolamine) enhances the exercise-induced lipolysis: this effect is markedly more pronounced in obese subjects compared with lean[7].

Effect of calorie restriction and weight loss on the lipolytic profile of obese

Calorie restriction itself modifies the lipolysis regulation. The short term fasting induces an increase in whole body lipolysis in obese as well as in lean, the effect being lower in obese[8].

However, the fasting-induced enhancement of lipolysis is not observable in regional abdominal SCAT (assessed by arterio-venous catheterization) which suggests that SCAT – but not visceral adipose tissue – is resistant to this type of intervention in obese[8].

Very low calorie diets (VLCDs) modify the responsiveness of adipose tissue lipolysis in studies *in situ* and *in vitro*. An increase in basal and isoprenalin-stimulated lipolysis was found in several studies[9,10], accompanied with an increase of HSL activity[9]. Tle response of lipolysis regulation to VLCD appears to be genotype dependent[9]: in a group of monozygotic twins subjected to VLCD the high inter-pair variability is in contrast with the intra-pair ressemblance. The enhancing effect of this type of VLCD on beta adrenergic action was found *in situ* using microdialysis method[11]: the responses to isoprenalin and to beta 1- and beta 2- agonists was enhanced after the diet[11]. VLCD is accompanied by an increase in levels of mRNA of beta 2-AR in adipose tissue and borderline increase in mRNA of HSL[12].

The increase in beta2 mRNA is in agreement with a number of studies demonstrating the role of beta2 receptor in the adaptation of metabolism of AT to the dietary intervention[13,14] including those which show an association of polymorphism of beta-2 receptor with variations of lipolytic sensitivity and in fat mass, in general[13].

The above mentioned adaptations of the adrenergic lipolysis regulation seem to be in agreement with the idea of decisive role of the NEFA mobilization from adipose tissue for providing the energy substráte for the skeletal Muscle. However, the role of skeletal muscle lipolysis as an aditional source of fatty acids for fat oxidation during VLCD has been emphasized recently: VLCD did not modify the antilipolytic action of insulin in adipose tissue while this action was reduced in the skeletal muscle[15].

However, in addition to classical catecholamines and insulin additional mechanism which contribute to the adaptation of adipose tissue metabolism to the calorie restriction must be considred. Recently, a powerful lipolytic action of atrial natriuretic peptide (ANP) was shown. The lipolytic action of ANP is markedly enhanced in response to VLCD in isolated adipocytes *in vitro* and the enhancement of the lipolytic response to intravenous ANP infusion was demonstrated also *in situ*[16].

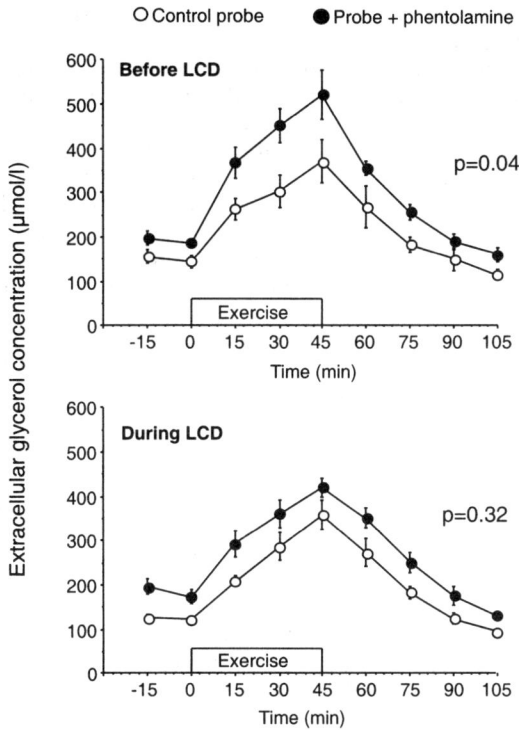

Fig. 1. Time-course of extracellular glycerol concentration in subcutaneous adipose tissue calculated from dialysate glycerol levels during the 45 min cycle-ergometer exercise before and after low-calorie-diet in obese women. The α2-adrenergic receptor antagonist phentolamine was ($\bullet$) or was not ($\circ$) added to the perfusion medium. Data are expressed as means $\pm$ SEM. $P < 0.05$ when compared to baseline value.

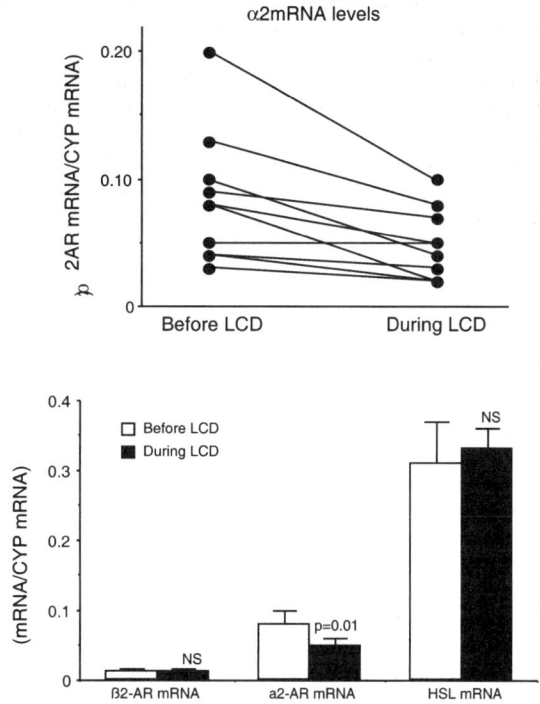

Fig. 2. Effect of low calorie diets.on α2-AR, β2 AR and hormone-sensitive lipase mRNA levels in subcutaneous adipose tissue of 10 obese women (lower panel). Evolution of individual values of α2-AR mRNA during the diet (upper panel). Amounts of mRNA were determined for each subject using RT-competitive PCR before and after the diet. Levels of mRNA were calculated as the ratio of mRNA level normalized to the house-keeping gene cyclophylin mRNA level.

The pattern of adaptation of lipolysis to the calorie restriction may be different after long-term moderate diets when exploration is performed in the state of weight maintenance.

In a study of 12 weeks' low calorie diet in obese women the upregulation of beta-2 AR mRNA was not observable while a marked reduction of alpha-2 mRNA occured[17]. This was associated with a reduction of alpha2 antilipolytic action *in situ* demonstrated during physical exercise.

The finding of the reduction of alpha2 mediated antilipolysis was observed also *in vitro* in a weight stable stage after 16 weeks' diet[18]. In the same study the regional and gender diferences in the adaptation of lipolysis to the diet were demonstrated. The reduction of alpha2 activity was evident in both abdominal and femoral region in women but only in abdominal region in men[18]. The gender and region related differences may be associated with the well-known preferential fat loss in abdominal region in both genders during the hypocaloric diets.

Physical activity and adipose tissue lipolysis

In contrast with calorie restriction the exercise training represents a certainly more physiological mode of therapeutic intervention in obesity. Adaptations of adipose tissue lipolysis are expectable in view of the training-induced increase in fat oxidation.

Numerous cross sectional studies have shown a higher catecholamine-stimulated lipolysis *in vitro* in trained subjects and demonstrated the sex-related[19] and adipose tissue region-related[20] differences in the adaptation. The training-induced adaptations occur in beta adrenergic pathway in both genders, while only women respond by adaptation (reduced efficiency) of alpha2 mediated pathway[20]. Moreover the latter adaptation in women occurs in abdominal tissue only.

Cross sectional comparison of *in situ* lipolysis using microdialysis has not found differences in the *in situ* epinephrine-stimulated glycerol release[21] which is not in agreement with the lower antilipolytic alpha 2-mediated action found in trained men[22].

Taking into account a number of biases of cross sectional training studies longitudinal follow- ups bring more relevant reflection of training-induced adaptations. Most of longitudinal studies have dealt with non obese subjects. The pioneering works of Depres *et al.*[23] have shown the increase in *in vitro* basal and epinephrine-stimulated lipolysis after 20 weeks' training, the effect being sex dependent, i.e. higher in men. In another study dealing with monozygotic overweight twin males the same authors[24] demonstrated the strong gene-training interaction in lipolysis adaptation to the training, i.e. strong intra-pair similarity of the change of lipolysis in response to the training.

In one of the few endurance training studies performed in obese men a 12 weeks' endurance training increased the *in vitro* lipolytic response to stimulation with beta and beta 1 agonists, and reduced the antilipolytic action mediated by alpha 2-AR and by insulin[25] and reduced the basl lipolysis and HSL activity. Adaptations occured on the post-receptor level as well. In a recent study of 12 weeks training in obese females, however, no changes in the epinephrine stimulated lipolysis at rest were found *in situ* (Stich *et al.*, *J Cell Biol*, in press data). Analysis of mRNA levels of the adrenoceptors in the adipose tissue did not show any training-induced changes in this study.

The lack of training-induced changes in adrenergic regulation of lipolysis in obese women might correspond to the lower training induced adaptation in women demonstrated in longitudunal follow up in non obese subjects[23].

Exercise training was shown to reduce insulin resistance of the skeletal muscle glucose uptake, the data on the effect of the training on the resistance to antilipolytic effect in adipose tissue are conflictiong. While a training-induced reduction of insulin supression of lipolysis was detected in SCAT *in vitro*[25] the *in vivo* investigations suggest a lack of any change of insulin antilipolytic action in SCAT and the increased sensitivity to insulin in visceral adipose tissue.

Most of the attention, in accordance with current clinical practice, was paid uptoday to the use of endurance training in therapy of oebsity. Taking into account the reported beneficial effects of strength training on various metabolic parameters the studies investigating the effect of strength training on adipose tissue characteristics are warranted.

Conclusions

Regulation of lipolysis in adipose tissue is disturbed in obese subjects. Calorie restriction as well as exercise training do affect the regulation of lipolysis. In most studies this effect goes in the direction towards correction of the abnormalities of regulation. The effect is, neverthless, variable depending not only on the mode of intervention (very low calorie diet vs. moderate low calorie diet vs. physical exercise) but also on genotype, gender, and adipose tissue region. More studies exploring interactions of these variables are needed in order to enable us to design more specifically the therapeutic intervention for each individual.

Acknowledgements: This work was supported by grant of the Czech Academy of Science 303/00/0649 and grant of the Czech Ministry of Health IGA 6836-3. The laboratories involved in the work participated in the FATLINK concerted action supported by the European Commission.

References

1. Lafontan M, Barbe P, Galitzky J *et al.* Adrenergic regulation of adipocyte metabolism. *Human Reprod* 1997; 12: 6–20.

2. Boschmann M, Krupp G, Luft FC, Klaus S, Jordan J. *In vivo* response to alpha(1)-adrenoreceptor stimulation in human white adipose tissue. *Obes Res* 2002; 10: 555–8.

3. Schiffelers SL, Saris WH, Boomsma F, van Baak MA. Beta(1)- and beta(2)-Adrenoceptor-mediated thermogenesis and lipid utilization in obese and lean men. *J Clin Endocrinol Metab* 2001; 86: 2191–9.

4. Horowitz JF, Klein S. Whole body and abdominal lipolytic sensitivity to epinephrine is suppressed in upper body obese women. *Am J Physiol Endocrinol Metab* 2000; 278: E1144–E1152.

5. Mauriège P, Després JP, Prud'homme D *et al.* Regional variation in adipose tissue lipolysis in lean and obese men. *J Lipid Res* 1991; 32: 1625–33.

6. Reynisdottir S, Wahrenberg H, Carlström K, Rössner S, Arner P. Catecholamine resistance in fat cells of women with upper body obesity due to decreased expression of beta2-adrenoceptors. *Diabetologia* 1994; 37: 428–35.

7.   Stich V, De Glisezinski I, Crampes F *et al.* Activation of alpha2-adrenergic receptors impairs exercise-induced lipolysis in SCAT of obese subjects. *Am J Physiol* 2000; 279: R499–R504.

8.   Horowitz JF, Coppack SW, Paramore D, Cryer PE, Zhao G, Klein S. Effect of short-term fasting on lipid kinetics in lean and obese women. *Am J Physiol* 1999; 276(2 Pt 1): E278–E284.

9.   Stich V, Harant I, De Glisezinski I, Crampes F, Berlan M, Kunesova M *et al.* Adipose tissue lipolysis and hormone-sensitive lipase expression during very-low-calorie diet in obese female identical twins. *J Clin Endocrinol Metab* 1997; 82: 739–44.

10. Hellstrom L, Reynisdottir S, Langin D, Rossner S, Arner P. Regulation of lipolysis in fat cells of obese women during long-term hypocaloric diet. *Int J Obes Relat Metab Disord* 1996; 20: 745–52.

11. Barbe P, Stich V, Galitzky J, Kunesova M, Hainer V, Lafontan M, Berlan M. *In vivo* increase in beta-adrenergic lipolytic response in subcutaneous adipose tissue of obese subjects submitted to a hypocaloric diet. *J Clin Endocrinol Metab* 1997; 82: 63–9.

12. Suljkovicoya H, Viguerie N, Kunesova M, Millet L, Avizou S, Hejnova J *et al.* Vyziva a metabolismus tukove tkane (Czech). *Cesk Fysiol* 2001; 50: 57–63.

13. Large V, Hellström L, Reynisdottir S, *et al.* Human beta2-adrenoceptor gene polymorphism are highly frequent in obesity and associated with altered adipocyte beta2-adrenoceptor function. *J Clin Invest* 1997; 100: 3005–13.

14. Lönnqvist F, Wahrenberg H, Hellstrom L, Reynisdottir S, Arner P. Lipolytic catecholamine resistance due to decreased ?2-adrenoceptor expression in fat cells. *J Clin Invest* 1992; 90: 2175–86.

15. Hagstrom-Toft E, Thorne A, Reynisdottir S, Moberg E, Rossner S, Bolinder J, Arner P. Evidence for a major role of skeletal muscle lipolysis in the regulation of lipid oxidation during caloric restriction *in vivo. Diabetes* 2001; 50: 1604–11.

16. Sengenes C, Stich V, Berlan M, Hejnova J, Lafontan M, Pariskova Z, Galitzky J. Increased lipolysis in adipose tissue and lipid mobilization to natriuretic peptides during low-calorie diet in obese women. *Int J Obes Relat Metab Disord* 2002; 26: 24–32.

17. Stich V, Marion-Latard F, Hejnova J, Viguerie N, Lefort C, Suljkovicova H *et al.* Hypocaloric diet reduces exercise-induced alpha 2-adrenergic antilipolytic effect and alpha 2-adrenergic receptor mRNA levels in adipose tissue of obese women. *J Clin Endocrinol Metab* 2002; 87: 1274–81.

18. Mauriège P, Imbeault P, Langin D *et al.* Regional and gender variations in adipose tissue lipolysis in response to weight loss. *J Lipid Res* 1999; 40: 1559–71.

19. Crampes F, Rivière D, Beauville M, Marceron M, Garrigues M. Lipolytic response of adipocytes to epinephrine in sedentary and exercice-trained subjects: sex-related differences. *Eur J Appl Physiol* 1989; 59: 249–55.

20. Mauriège P, Prudhomme D, Marcotte M, Yoshioka M, Tremblay A, Bouchard C *et al.* Regional differences in adipose tissue metabolism between sedentary and endurance-trained women. *Am J Physiol* 1997; 273: E497–E506.

21. Stallknecht B, Simonsen L, Bulow J, Vinten J, Galbo H. Effect of training on epinephrine-stimulated lipolysis determined by microdialysis in human adipose tissue. *Am J Physiol* 1995; 32: E1059–E1066.

22. De Glisezinski I, Marion-Latard F, Crampes F, Berlan M, Hejnova J, Cottet-Emard JM *et al.* Lack of alpha(2)-adrenergic antilipolytic effect during exercise in subcutaneous adipose tissue of trained men. *J Appl Physiol* 2001; 91: 1760–5.

23. Després JP, Bouchard C, Savard R, Tremblay A, Marcotte M, Theriault G. The effect of 20-week endurance training program on adipose tissue morphology and lipolysis in men and women. *Metab Clin Exp* 1984; 33: 235–9.

24. Després JP, Bouchard C, Savard R, Prud'homme D, Bukowiecki L, Theriault G. Adaptative changes to training in adipose tissue lipolysis are genotype dependent. *Int J Obes* 1984; 8: 87–95.

25. De Glisezinski I, Crampes F, Harant I, Berlan M, Hejnova J, Langin D *et al.* Endurance training changes in lipolytic responsiveness of obese adipose tissue. *Am J Physiol* 1998; 275(6 Pt 1): 951–6.

Progress in Obesity Research: 9. Edited by *Geraldo Medeiros-Neto, Alfredo Halpern and Claude Bouchard*
©2003 John Libbey Eurotext Ltd, pp. 176–179.

CHAPTER 36

Lipolysis in adipose tissue and skeletal muscle: what can be learned from stable isotope?

E.E. Blaak

Dept of Human Biology, Nutrition Research Centre, Maastricht, The Netherlands
[e-mail: E.Blaak@HB.Unimaas.nl]

Introduction

Whole body rate of production of glycerol is measured by using stable isotopes from the enrichment in blood glycerol when the stable isotope tracers ^{2}H- or ^{13}C labeled glycerol are used. Net production or utilization of glycerol by an organ or tissue is determined by multiplying the arterio-venous concentration difference of glycerol by a measure of blood flow. When blood glycerol is labeled the total uptake and/or release of glycerol by a tissue can be determined. Until recently, the whole body rate of appearance of glycerol (Ra) has been generally considered to be a good quantitative measure of whole body lipolysis[1-3]. The ratio of fatty acid to glycerol Ra has then been used as a quantitative index of intra-adipocyte fatty acid recycling, whereas the difference between fatty acid oxidation and three times glycerol Ra has been taken as measure of total fatty acid recycling.

Several assumptions underlie the use of glycerol Ra as measure of whole body lipolysis. Hydrolysis of triacylglycerol, both intracellular lipolysis as well as lipoprotein mediated triglyceride hydrolysis at the capillary endothelium, in muscle and adipose tissue leads to release of glycerol into the blood stream. Glycerol utilization has been assumed to occur mainly in liver and to some extent in kidney. Within the liver glycerol may be phosphorylated to glycerol-3-phosphate which may be reesterified to triacylglycerol in the fatty acid-triglyceride substrate cycle, whereas the remainder will enter the glycolytic/gluconeogenic metabolic pool. The glycerol carbon may then proceed to through glycolysis to pyruvate with resultant conversion to lactate or acetyl CoA, or it may be used by the gluconeogenic pathway to be released as glucose or stored as glycogen. The above described description is based on the precept that other tissues like muscle and adipose tissue[4,5] lack sufficient glycerolkinase activity to phosphorylate and metabolize glycerol any further. Tissues like adipose tissue and skeletal muscle which store considerable amount of triglyceride must then rely on glucose to provide glycerol-3-phosphate for fatty acid reesterification. There is accumulating evidence that extrahepatic glycerol kinase exists[6-10] and in this review evidence is presented that this enzyme plays a significant role in skeletal muscle. The presence of extrahepatic glycerolkinase activity may provide a new perspective on the relevance of glycerol to muscle and possibly adipose tissue metabolism, especially under conditions with elevated glycerol concentrations like fasting, obesity and type 2 diabetes mellitus.

Skeletal muscle glycerol metabolism

The first indications for a significant metabolism of glycerol in muscle came from studies of Elia and Kurpad[7], where it was found that the dilution of [^{2}H$_5$]-glycerol across skeletal muscle was greater than expected on basis of the arterio-venous glycerol concentration difference. Across the forearm, he found a 50 per cent loss of enriched glycerol. The finding of a significant uptake of glycerol by leg muscle, using tissue balance techniques in combination with stable isotope tracers of glycerol, was confirmed in studies of Coppack *et al.*[8], more recently. However, in the above studies, the infusion period was relatively short (1–3 h), opening the possibility that equilibration between labeled glycerol and the

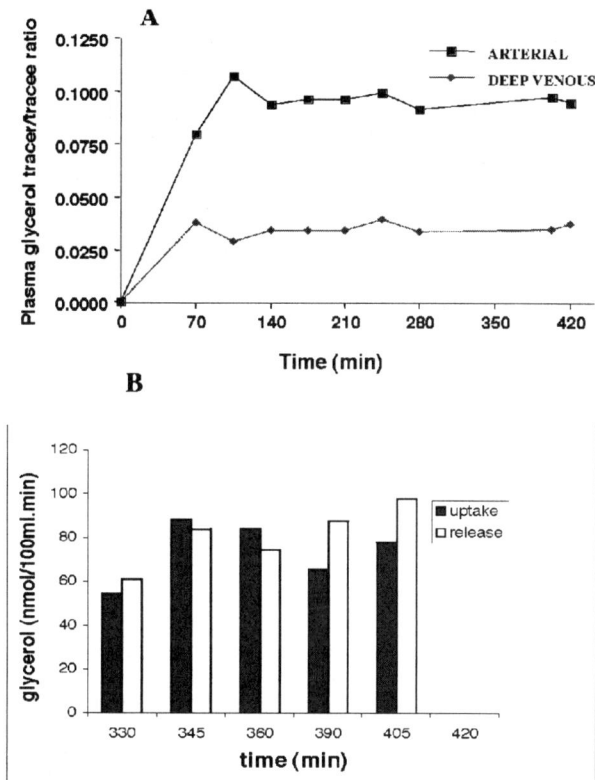

A

B

muscle glycerol pool is not complete during the relatively short infusion period. This might explain the disappearance of labeled glycerol into muscle glycerol pool. A second explanation is that there is indeed significant uptake of glycerol by skeletal muscle.

To investigate whether the duration of the infusion period may be of importance in determining skeletal muscle glycerol uptake and release, we investigated glycerol exchange and oxidation across muscle during a 7-h period of [²H₅]-glycerol infusion. In agreement with the data of Elia[7] and Coppack[8] preliminary data of our study (Blaak et al., 2002, unpublished observations) show that two-thirds of the label disappeared across muscle in the presence of an isotopic steady state (i.e arterial and deep venous glycerol tracer/tracee ratio remained constant during the 7-h period of infusion, Fig. 1A), indicating net uptake of glycerol by muscle (Fig. 1B). The fractional extraction of glycerol was 60 per cent, which is slightly higher than the 40–50 per cent found by Elia[7] and Coppack[8].

Beside muscle glycerol uptake during the 7-h period of [²H₅]-glycerol infusion we also determined glycerol oxidation by determining $^{13}CO_2$ exchange across muscle during an additional infusion of [U-^{13}C]-glycerol during the last 3 h of the protocol. Preliminary data in three subjects show no $^{13}CO_2$ production across muscle, indicating that glycerol oxidation in muscle is very low (Blaak et al., 2002, unpublished observations).

The extraction of glycerol by skeletal muscle, together with the finding of considerable uptake of glycerol by kidney (20 per cent, as calculated by Landau et al.[11]) indicate that there is considerable extrahepatic glycerol utilization and that liver is responsible for less than half of the postabsorptive glycerol utilization in contrast to previous assumptions[5]. Thus, these data indicate that muscle contains the enzymatic machinery to metabolize glycerol. There are two recent studies indicating functional glycerol kinase activity in muscle. Montell and coworkers[10] showed that glycerolkinase activity is present and functional in cultured human muscle cells, is inducible by insulin and enables the muscle cell to incorporate glycerol into lipids. Additionally, overexpression of glycerolkinase reveals that this enzyme is the rate limiting step in muscle glycerol metabolism and that elevated glycerol 3-P can also be diverted towards gluconeogenic-glycolyitic pathways.

Guo and Jensen[9] showed, using a stable isotope infusion of [^{14}C]- labeled glycerol, that muscle glycerol was incorporated into the intramuscular triacylglycerol (TAG) stores indicating that glycerol may be a significant and direct precursor for muscle TAG synthesis.

Adipose tissue glycerol metabolism

Adipose tissue is the largest store of triglyceride in the body, and therefore any functional glycerol kinase activity in this tissue would be correspondingly more significant. It has been generally assumed that glycerol-3-phosphate required for esterification in adipose tissue cannot be derived from glycerol to any significant extent, that glycerol kinase activity is extremely low and that essentially all adipose tissue glycerol is released without further metabolism. Based on the low activity of glycerol kinase in

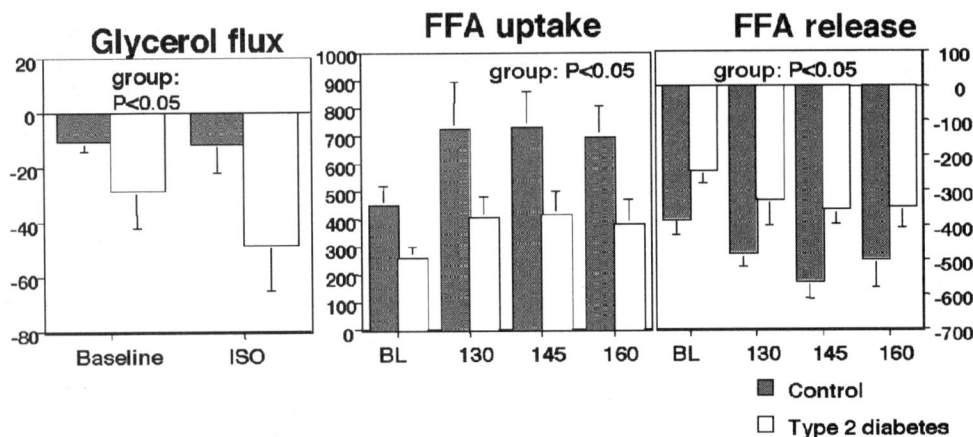

Fig. 2. Forearm muscle glycerol release and total FFA uptake and release (in nmol. 100 ml forearm tissue.min^{-1}) in type 2 diabetic subjects as compared to healthy controls during baseline conditions and during infusion of the non-selective ß-agonist isoprenaline (ISO); $n = 8$ in both groups, adapted from reference[16].

adipose tissue, glycerol utilization in this tissue has been estimated to be less than 1 per cent[12]. Klein *et al.*[13] and Coppack *et al.*[8] found no uptake of glycerol across adipose tissue. In contrast, Kurpad *et al.*[12] found uptake and dilution of [^{2}H$_5$] glycerol across abdominal subcutaneous adipose tissue. In these studies infusion was only 1 h, so that steady state may not have been achieved. In the study of Samra *et al.*[14] subjects fasted overnight were infused with [^{2}H$_5$]-glycerol for 7 h and arterial and adipose venous glycerol concentrations and enrichments were determined during the last 6 h. This study shows consistent uptake and dilution of [^{2}H$_5$]-glycerol across abdominal subcutaneous adipose tissue. The dilution of the labeled glycerol was consistently greater then expected from the measured net release of glycerol, indicative of significant uptake of glycerol by adipose tissue[14]. These data are consistent with some preliminary data of our group (Blaak *et al.*, 2002, unpublished observations) showing glycerol uptake by subcutaneous adipose tissue during a 7 h [^{2}H$_5$]-glycerol infusion. Fractional extraction of glycerol by adipose tissue in this study was on average 20 per cent.

Thus, although a significant glycerol utilization in adipose tissue has generally been assumed to be unlikely, the latter two studies indicate glycerol uptake in subcutaneous adipose tissue. There is an urgent need for further studies on adipose tissue to investigate if there is indeed significant glycerol uptake, phosphorylation and further glycerol metabolism in adipose tissue

Glycerol: a role in the increased triacylglycerol (TAG) storage in diabetic muscle?

Previous studies in our laboratory have shown a different handling of fatty acids in skeletal muscle of type 2 diabetic subjects as compared to control subjects using the forearm balance technique in combination with infusion of the fatty acid tracer [U-^{13}C]-palmitate. In type 2 diabetic muscle the oxidation of free fatty acids (FFA) extracted from plasma was diminished indicating an increased incorporation of FFA in the TAG stores[15]. Additionally, forearm glycerol release was increased and total forearm FFA release was impaired in these subjects, indicating a higher turnover of the TAG stores in the type 2 diabetic muscle[16] (Fig. 2). It is possible that glycerol can exert important influences on TAG storage under these circumstances since available evidence (see under muscle glycerol metabolism) suggests that glycerol can be metabolized in skeletal muscle and that glycerol through its conversion to glycerol-3-P by glycerolkinase may be an incorporated into muscle TAG. Importantly, recent studies have shown that intramuscular overstorage of TAG is closely correlated with muscle insulin resistance[17].

Implications of glycerol utilization by extrahepatic tissues

The indications of significant glycerol uptake and utilization by skeletal muscle suggest that glycerol release by muscle cannot be used to accurately reflect lipolysis in this tissue. Additionally, whole body glycerol turnover may not all be due to lipolysis, implying that the rate of glycerol appearance into blood may not be an accurate marker of systemic lipolysis.

With respect to adipose tissue metabolism, there are *in vivo* indications of significant adipose tissue glycerol uptake, although data are controversial. The former findings are preliminary in nature and require confirmation. Since adipose tissue is the largest store of TAG in the body, any significant glycerol utilization in adipose tissue may have an enormous impact on current thinking on adipose tissue metabolism, lipolysis and reesterification.

References

1. Boden G, Chem X, Desantis RA, Kendrick Z. Effect of insulin on fatty acid reesterification in healthy subjects. *Diabetes* 1993; 42: 1588–93.

2. Wolfe RR, Klein S, Carraro F, Weber JM. Role of triglyceride-fatty acid cycle in controlling fat metabolism in humans during and after exercise. *Am J Physiol.* 1990; 258(2 Pt 1): E382–W329.

3. Wolfe RR, Herndorn DN, Jahoor F, Miyoshi H, Wolfe M. Effect of severe burn injury on substrate cycling by glucose and fatty acids. *N Engl J Med* 1987; 317: 403–8.

4. Newsholme EA, Taylor K. Glycerol kinase activities from vertebrates and invertebrates. *Biochem J* 1969; 112: 465–74.

5. Lin ECC. Glycerol utilization and its regulation in mammals. *Annu Rev Biochem* 1977; 46: 765–95.

6. Frayn KN, Coppack SW, Humphreys SM. Glycerol and lactate uptake in the human forearm. *Metabolism* 1991; 40: 1317–19.

7. Elia M, Kahn K, Calder G, Kurpad A. Glycerol exchange across the human forearm assessed by a combination of tracer and arterio-venous exchange techniques. *Clin Sci* 1993; 84: 99–104.

8. Coppack SW, Persson M, Judd RL, Miles JM. Glycerol and nonesterified fatty acid metabolism in human muscle and adipose tissue *in vivo. Am J Physiol* 1999; 276(2 Pt 1): E233–E240.

9. Guo Z, Jensen MD. Blood glycerol is an important precursor for intramuscular triacylglycerol synthesis. *J Biol Chem* 1999; 274: 23702–6.

10. Montell E, Lerin C, Newgard CB, Gomez-Foix AM. Effects of modulation of glycerolkinase expression on lipid and carbohydrate metabolism in human muscle cells. *J Biol Chem* 2002; 277: 2682–6.

11. Landau BR, Wahren J, Previs SF, Ekberg K, Chandramouli V, Brunengraber H. Glycerol production and utilization in humans: sites and quantitation. *Am J Physiol* 1996; 271(6 Pt 1): E1110–E1117.

12. Kurpad A, Khan K, Calder AG, Coppack S, Frayn K, Macdonald I, Elia M. Effect of noradrenaline on glycerol turnover and lipolysis in the whole body and subcutaneous adipose tissue *in vivo. Clin Sci* 1994; 86: 177–84.

13. Klein S, Coppack S, Chinkes D, Villanueva-Meyer J. Regional transendothelial glycerol kinetics in humans. *FASEB Journal* 1996; 10: A520.

14. Samra JS, Clark ML, Humpreys SM, Bannister PA, Summers LKM, Macdonald IA, Frayn KN. Evidence for glycerol uptake by adipose tissue. *Proc Nutr Soc* 1999; 58: A164.

15. Blaak EE, Wagenmakers AJM. The fate of [U-13C]palmitate extracted by skeletal muscle in subjects with type 2 diabetes and control subjects. *Diabetes* 2002; 51: 784–9.

16. Blaak EE, Wagenmakers AJM, Glatz JFC, Wolffenbuttel BHR, Kemerink GJ, Langenberg CJM *et al.* Plasma free fatty acid utilization and fatty acid binding protein content are diminished in forearm skeletal muscle of type 2 diabetic subjects. *Am J Physiol* 2000; 279: E146–E154.

17. Perseghin G, Scifo P, De Cobelli F, Pagliato E, Battezzati A, Arcelloni C *et al.* Intramyocellular triglyceride content is a determinant of *in vivo* insulin resistance in humans. *Diabetes* 1999; 48(8): 1600–6.

Progress in Obesity Research: 9. Edited by *Geraldo Medeiros-Neto, Alfredo Halpern and Claude Bouchard*
©2003 John Libbey Eurotext Ltd, pp. 180–183.

CHAPTER 37

Adipocyte-derived NO: regulation and biological roles

Patrice Penfornis[1,2], Sonia Kapur[1,2], Frédéric Picard[1], Mylène Perreault[1,2], Yves Deshaies[1] and André Marette[1,2,3]

[1]*Department of Anatomy and Physiology;* [2]*Lipid Research Unit, Laval University Hospital Research Center, Québec, G1V 4G2; and* [3]*Institut des Nutraceutiques et des Aliments Fonctionnels, Laval University, Ste-Foy, Québec, G1K 7P4, Canada [e-mail: andre.marette@crchul.ulaval.ca]*

Introduction

The radical gas nitric oxide (NO) has been shown to participate in an ever-growing number of cellular processes. NO can be recognized as an intracellular second messenger, a local substance for regulation of neighboring cells, and a neurotransmitter. NO is synthetized from L-arginine by the enzyme nitric oxide synthase (NOS). There are at least three isotypes of NOS; the calcium-dependent endothelial cell NOS (eNOS) and neuronal type NOS (nNOS), and the so-called inducible, relatively calcium-independent NOS (iNOS). Unlike the other members of the NOS family, which are constitutive enzymes, iNOS cellular expression is limited under normal conditions. However, its expression is markedly stimulated by bacterial endotoxins or inflammatory cytokines in most cell types. When induced, this NOS isotype generates NO at a much higher rate and for longer periods of time than nNOS and eNOS enzymes[1]. It has been previously reported that white and brown adipose tissues express both iNOS and eNOS isoforms[2–6]. Expression of these enzymes in adipose tissue has also been confirmed in humans, both in health and diseased states[7–10]. However, the physio-pathological roles of NO in adipose tissues remains obscure. This short review focuses on recent work that has provided new insights on the regulation of NOS enzymes and NO production in white and brown fat and the emergence of key metabolic functions for this molecule in these tissues.

Expression of NOS enzymes in adipose tissues

Previous studies by us and others have shown that white and brown adipose tissues express two members of the NOS family, namely iNOS and eNOS (reviewed in[11,12]). Low but detectable expression of iNOS mRNA and protein can be found in adipose tissues of normal rats[3]. *In vivo* administration of bacterial LPS (a model of endotoxic shock) markedly increased iNOS expression in white and brown adipose tissues, raising iNOS enzymatic activity by 10–20-fold[3]. Importantly, the effect of LPS injection on adipose iNOS expression can be reproduced *in vitro* by chronically exposing cultured 3T3-L1 (white) and T37i (brown) adipocytes to cytokines and LPS[3,12]. Neither LPS alone nor individual cytokines were found to increase iNOS-mediated NO production in 3T3-L1 white adipocytes[3] and T37i brown adipocytes (Penfornis and Marette, unpublished data). These data suggest that iNOS induction in septic rats is mediated by a complex network of interactions between inflammatory cytokines and endotoxin at the level of the adipocyte.

Although eNOS can be detected in adipose tissue extracts, its presence within adipocytes has been called into question since eNOS cannot be detected in cultured 3T3-L1 adipocytes[3,12]. However, there is now evidence that eNOS can be detected in freshly isolated white adipocytes in both rats and humans[6,9,10]. This suggests that eNOS is expressed both in the vascular endothelial cells as well as in fat cells in adipose tissue, implicating hemodynamic and metabolic functions for this NOS isotype in this tissue.

Biological functions of NO in adipose tissues

NO is a pleiotropic molecule that likely plays multiple roles within adipose tissue including metabolic, hemodynamic, and immunologic. In this review, we will focus our attention on the metabolic function of NO with particular emphasis on the modulation of lipid and glucose metabolism in adipocytes and the potential for paracrine actions of the radical gas on neighboring muscle cells.

Role of NO in the regulation of lipolysis in adipose cells

One of the most important function of adipocytes is to store free fatty acids (FFA) in the form of triglycerides. Upon demand, lipolytic hormones and factors activate the breakdown of triglycerides into FFA and glycerol, a process controled by hormone sensitive lipase (HSL), the rate-limiting enzyme in the process known as lipolysis. Classical activators of lipolysis such as β-adrenergic agonists signal through activation of adenylyl cyclases and release of cyclic AMP. Cyclic AMP then induces activation of protein kinase A which in turns promotes phosphorylation and activation of HSL and its translocation on cellular lipid droplets.

Since adipocytes express NOS enzymes, it was of significant interest to test whether NO modulates lipolysis in fat cells. Gaudiot et al.[13] first reported that lipolysis was modulated by NO in isolated rat adipocytes. They found that NO donor drugs increase basal lipolysis despite the fact that authentic NO gas had no effect. On the other hand, NO donors and NO gas were also shown to inhibit isoproterenol-stimulated lipolysis, albeit via different mechanisms. However, caution must be exerted when examining the effect of NO donors or other exogenous NO generating systems since it was recently reported that NO attenuates the lipolytic effect of isoproterenol by an oxidation-linked inactivation of the β-adrenergic agonist[14]. In this regard, the use of specific inhibitors of NO synthesis may be more rewarding in attempting to uncover the role of NO in the control of lipolysis and other metabolic processes in fat cells. Andersson and colleagues, using a microdialysis technique, previously showed that N[G]-monomethyl L-arginine (L-NMMA), a specific NOS inhibitor, increases lipolysis independently of local blood flow changes in human adipose tissue[7]. This is in contrast with a more recent study showing that the NOS inhibitor diphenyliodonium (DPI) decreases both basal and dibutyryl cAMP-stimulated lipolysis, apparently by an antioxydant-related action[15]. Importantly, both L-NMMA and DPI inhibit eNOS and iNOS and it is therefore not possible to draw any conclusions as to the NOS isoform involved in the modulation of lipolysis in the above studies.

Cytokines and endotoxins induce iNOS expression in adipocytes but also increase lipolysis in adipose cells[16]. The possible relationship between iNOS induction and the lipolytic response to cytokines/LPS was investigated using the very selective and potent iNOS inhibitor 1400W[17]. Interestingly, 1400W further increased the lipolytic effects of cytokines/LPS on lipolysis, suggesting that NO is in fact a negative feedback regulator of cytokine-mediated lipolysis in adipose cells (Penfornis and Marette, unpublished data). Studies are currently underway to clarify the mechanism(s) by which NO modulates lipolysis and on the potential role of this regulatory pathway in the altered lipid metabolism found in obesity.

Role of NO in the modulation of LPL in adipose cells

NO has been previously reported to regulate lipoprotein metabolism in brown adipocytes. Uchida et al.[18] first reported that TNF-β-induced inhibition of lipoprotein lipase (LPL) activity was mediated by iNOS induction and NO production in brown adipocytes. Furthermore, we have recently confirmed that iNOS-mediated NO production down-regulates LPL activity in brown adipose tissue and skeletal muscle of LPS-challenged rats. Thus we found that LPS-induced LPL inhibition in skeletal muscle and brown fat was blocked by the specific iNOS inhibitor aminoguanidine (AGN) and was prevented in iNOS-deficient mice[19]. Surprisingly, although LPS also blunted LPL activity in white adipose tissue, this effect could not be restored by AGN treatment or by targeted disruption of the iNOS gene in mice, therefore suggesting that NO exerts a tissue-specific modulation of LPL activity in endotoxaemia. It may be speculated, however, that adipose-derived NO exerts some paracrine action on muscle LPL activity, thereby indirectly contributing to impaired lipoprotein catabolism and hypertriglyceridaemia in this model of septic shock.

Role of NO in the control of glucose metabolism

Insulin increases glucose disposal in skeletal muscle, heart and fat cells by a complex signaling cascade that eventually leads to the mobilization of GLUT4 glucose transporter proteins from intracellular storage vesicles to the cell surface membrane (see[20]). Overproduction of NO by iNOS induction has been previously shown to modulate glucose metabolism in rat skeletal muscle and cultured L6 myocytes[21,22]. In L6 myocytes, chronic treatment with cytokines and LPS caused a large increase in basal glucose transport but also completely inhibited the ability of insulin to stimulate glucose transport. Both effects were largely abrogated by the NOS inhibitor L-NAME[21]. In more recent studies, we have tested the potential role of NO in the regulation of glucose transport in white and brown adipocytes chronically exposed to cytokines and LPS[12]. Cytokines/LPS exposure markedly increased (3–4-fold) basal glucose transport in both 3T3-L1 white adipocytes and T37i brown fat cells. However, iNOS inhibition with 1400W failed to prevent the increase in basal glucose uptake in white adipocytes and only partially inhibited this effect in brown adipocytes. The cytokines/LPS mixture also markedly reduced insulin action on glucose uptake in both white and brown adipocytes but 1400W failed to reverse insulin resistance in both cell types.

In addition to its direct action to stimulate glucose transport in skeletal muscle, insulin also enhances tissue perfusion by vasodilatory mechanisms[23]. The stimulatory effect of insulin on blood flow has been reported to be dependent on eNOS[24,25]. This vascular action of insulin is believed to amplify the hormone action to enhance glucose uptake by increasing the delivery of glucose and insulin to the capillary bed. The implication of eNOS in insulin-mediated glucose disposal is supported by our previous observation that *in vivo* infusion of the NOS inhibitor L-NAME significantly reduced insulin-stimulated glucose uptake by muscles and adipose tissues[26]. A role for NO in modulating insulin-mediated glucose disposal is also supported by the finding that mice lacking eNOS develop insulin resistance[27]. Thus in summary, low physiological concentrations of NO may play a role in the stimulation of glucose utilization by insulin, but the available data strongly suggest that this is through the release of NO from eNOS and its effect on the tissues' vasculature rather than a direct action of NO on myocytes and adipose cells.

Role of NO in the pathogenesis of insulin resistance

As with any messenger molecule, there can be too little or too much of NO and pathological events ensue. Hence, most of the deleterious effects of NO on biological systems have been attributed to iNOS induction and chronic NO release (see[28] for a review). To evaluate the potential role of iNOS induction in the insulin resistance associated with obesity, we have recently tested whether iNOS is induced in muscle and adipose tissues of obese animals and if this was associated with the development of insulin resistance. We found that iNOS expression is markedly increased in muscle and adipose tissues of both genetic and dietary models of obesity[29]. To assess more directly the possible cause-effect relationship between iNOS induction and insulin resistance, we next subjected iNOS knockout mice and wild-type controls to a high-fat diet and measured insulin action *in vivo* and insulin signaling in muscle and fat. It was found that iNOS-deficient obese mice are protected from developing impairments of whole-body and skeletal muscle insulin-mediated glucose disposal when rendered obese by feeding a high-fat diet[29]. Surprisingly, insulin resistance in adipose tissue was not prevented in iNOS knockout mice fed the high-fat diet. This tissue-specific action of iNOS induction is in line with our *in vitro* studies showing that iNOS induction in cultured white and brown adipocytes does not lead to impaired insulin action on glucose transport in these cells[12]. Nevertheless, it may be possible that adipocyte-derived NO exerts some paracrine modulation of skeletal muscle insulin action. Indeed, NO is a low molecular weight, highly lipophilic molecule, and can diffuse rapidly to neighboring cells. It is therefore conceivable that iNOS induction and NO production by local adipose cells also contribute to muscle insulin resistance in obesity.

It will be interesting to test the hypothesis that iNOS is also responsible for the occurrence of dyslipidaemia in obesity. Interestingly, preliminary work suggests that mice with a targeted disruption of iNOS exhibited lower triglyceride levels when fed a high-fat diet as compared to wild-type counterparts (unpublished observations). This effect might be explained by the lack of negative modulation of muscle LPL activity in obese high-fat fed iNOS knockout mice as previously observed in endotoxin-challenged mice lacking iNOS.

Concluding remarks

It is now well recognized that adipose tissues are major sites of expression of NOS enzymes in both acute and chronic inflammatory settings including obesity. The functions of adipose NO are just beginning to be uncovered but there is already strong evidence for its modulatory effect on lipolysis, although the nature of this regulation remains to be clarified. More studies are also required to test the hypothesis that NO release by adipocytes can exert paracrine influences on skeletal muscle glucose and lipid metabolism, as is thought to be the case for other adipose-derived molecules including TNF-α, leptin and adiponectin.

Acknowledgements: The work presented in this review was supported by a grant from the Canadian Institutes for Health Research to A. Marette. P. Penfornis and M. Perreault were supported by a Doctoral studentship from the Canadian Institutes for Health Research.

References

1. Moncada S, Palmer RMJ, Higgs EA. Nitric oxide: physiology, pathophysiology and pharmacology. *Pharmacol Rev* 1991; 43: 109–42.

2. Giordano A, Tonello C, Bulbarelli A, Cozzi V, Cinti S, Carruba MO *et al.* Evidence for a functional nitric oxide synthase system in brown adipocyte nucleus. *FEBS Letters* 2002; 514(2–3): 135–40.

3. Kapur S, Marcotte B, Marette A. Mechanism of adipose tissue iNOS induction in endotoxemia. *Am J Physiol* 1999; 276(4 Pt l): E635–E641.

4. Nisoli E, Tonello C, Briscini L, Carruba MO. Inducible nitric oxide synthase in rat brown adipocytes: implications for blood flow to brown adipose tissue. *Endocrinology* 1997; 138(2): 676–82.

5. Ribiere C, Jaubert AM, Gaudiot N, Sabourault D, Marcus ML, Boucher JL *et al.* White adipose tissue nitric oxide synthase: a potential source for NO production. *Biochem Biophys Res Commun* 1996; 222(3): 706–12.

6. Ribiere C, Jaubert AM, Sabourault D, Lacasa D, Giudicelli Y. Insulin stimulates nitric oxide production in rat adipocytes. *Biochem Biophys Res Commun* 2002; 291(2): 394–9.

7. Andersson K, Gaudiot N, Ribiere C, Elizalde M, Giudicelli Y, Arner P. A nitric oxide-mediated mechanism regulates lipolysis in human adipose tissue *in vivo. Br J Pharmacol* 1999; 126(7): 1639–45.

8. Annane D, Sanquer S, Sebille V, Faye A, Djuranovic D, Raphael JC *et al.* Compartmentalised inducible nitric-oxide synthase activity in septic shock. *Lancet* 2000; 355(9210): 1143–8.

9. Elizalde M, Ryden M, van Harmelen V, Eneroth P, Gyllenhammar H, Holm C *et al.* Expression of nitric oxide synthases in subcutaneous adipose tissue of nonobese and obese humans. *J Lipid Res* 2000; 41(8): 1244–51.

10. Ryden M, Elizalde M, van Harmelen V, Ohlund A, Hoffstedt J, Bringman S *et al.* Increased expression of eNOS protein in omental versus subcutaneous adipose tissue in obese human subjects. *Int J Obes Relat Metab Disord* 2001; 25(6): 811–5.

11. Kapur S, Picard F, Perreault M, Deshaies Y, Marette A. Nitric oxide: a new player in the modulation of energy metabolism. *Int J Obes Relat Metab Disord* 2000; 24 (Suppl 4): S36–S40.

12. Pilon G, Penfornis P, Marette A. Nitric oxide production by adipocytes: a role in the pathogenesis of insulin resistance? *Horm Metab Res* 2000; 32(11–12): 480–4.

13. Gaudiot N, Jaubert AM, Charbonnier E, Sabourault D, Lacasa D, Giudicelli Y *et al.* Modulation of white adipose tissue lipolysis by nitric oxide. *J Biol Chem* 1998; 273(22): 13475–81.

14. Klatt P, Cacho J, Crespo MD, Herrera E, Ramos P. Nitric oxide inhibits isoproterenol-stimulated adipocyte lipolysis through oxidative inactivation of the beta-agonist. *Biochem J* 2000; 351(Pt 2): 485–93.

15. Gaudiot N, Ribiere C, Jaubert AM, Giudicelli Y. Endogenous nitric oxide is implicated in the regulation of lipolysis through antioxidant-related effect. *Am J Physiol Cell Physiol* 2000; 279(5): C1603–C1610.

16. Grunfeld C, Feingold KR. Regulation of lipid metabolism by cytokines during host defense. *Nutrition* 1996; 12 (Suppl 1): S24–S26.

17. Garvey EP, Oplinger JA, Furfine ES, Kiff RJ, Laszlo F, Whittle BJ *et al.* 1400W is a slow, tight binding, and highly selective inhibitor of inducible nitric-oxide synthase *in vitro* and *in vivo. J Biol Chem* 1997; 272(8): 4959–63.

18. Uchida Y, Tsukahara F, Ohba K, Ogawa A, Irie K, Fujii E *et al.* Nitric oxide mediates down regulation of lipoprotein lipase activity induced by tumor necrosis factor-alpha in brown adipocytes. *Eur J Pharmacol* 1997; 335(2–3): 235–43.

19. Picard F, Kapur S, Perreault M, Marette A, Deshaies Y. Nitric oxide mediates endotoxin-induced hypertriglyceridemia through its action on skeletal muscle lipoprotein lipase. *FASEB J* 2001; 15(10): 1828–30.

20. Watson RT, Pessin JE. Intracellular organization of insulin signaling and GLUT4 translocation. *Recent Prog Horm Res* 2001; 56: 175–93.

21. Bédard S, Marcotte B, Marette A. Cytokines modulate glucose transport in skeletal muscle by inducing the expression of inducible nitric oxide synthase. *Biochem J* 1997; 325(Pt 2): 487–93.

22. Kapur S, Bedard S, Marcotte B, Cote CH, Marette A. Expression of nitric oxide synthase in skeletal muscle: a novel role for nitric oxide as a modulator of insulin action. *Diabetes* 1997; 46(11): 1691–700.

23. Baron AD. The coupling of glucose metabolism and perfusion in human skeletal muscle. The potential role of endothelium-derived nitric oxide. *Diabetes* 1996; 45 (Suppl l): S105–S109.

24. Scherrer U, Randin D, Vollenweider P, Vollenweider L, Nicod P. Nitric oxide release accounts for insulin's vascular effects in humans. *J Clin Invest* 1994; 94: 2511–5.

25. Steinberg HO, Brechtel G, Johnson A, Fineberg N, Baron AD. Insulin-mediated skeletal muscle vasodilation is nitric oxide dependent. A novel action of insulin to increase nitric oxide release. *J Clin Invest* 1994; 94: 1172–9.

26. Roy D, Perreault M, Marette A. Insulin stimulation of glucose uptake in skeletal muscles and adipose tissues *in vivo* is NO dependent. *Am J Physiol* 1998; 274(4 Pt l): E692–E699.

27. Shankar RR, Wu Y, Shen HQ, Zhu JS, Baron AD. Mice with gene disruption of both endothelial and neuronal nitric oxide synthase exhibit insulin resistance. *Diabetes* 2000; 49(5): 684–7.

28. Nathan C. Inducible nitric oxide synthase: what difference does it make? *J Clin Invest* 1997; 100(10): 2417–23.

29. Perreault M, Marette A. Targeted disruption of inducible nitric oxide synthase protects against obesity-linked insulin resistance in muscle. *Nature Med* 2001; 7(10): 1138–43.

Progress in Obesity Research: 9. Edited by *Geraldo Medeiros-Neto, Alfredo Halpern and Claude Bouchard*
©2003 John Libbey Eurotext Ltd, pp. 184–188.

CHAPTER 38

Regulation of human adipocyte expression of secreted peptides

H. Hauner

Else-Kröner-Fresenius Centre for Nutritional Medicine, Technical University Munich, Ismaninger Str. 22, 81675 Munich
[e-mail: hans.hauner@wzw.tum.de

Introduction

Investigations on the physiological function of adipose tissue were long focussing on the uptake, storage and release of excess energy. In mammals, adipose tissue represents the most important depot for excess calories which are converted to and stored as triglycerides. This classical view of adipose tissue as a storage organ was challenged by surprising new findings during the last decade. Initiated by the observation of adipose expression of TNF-α[1] and further promoted by the discovery of leptin, a fat cell-specific hormone[2], a rapidly growing number of reports were recently published demonstrating that preadipocytes and adipocytes are also acting as endocrine cells which are able to produce and release a variety of factors which may generate signals acting at both the local as well as the systemic level.

Thus a new concept is arising which claims that fat cells maintain an intensive cross-talk with other cells and tissues. If the adipose tissue organ is part of an integrated network, it may become conceivable that disturbances at the fat cell level as found in the obese state may have fundamental consequences for the function of other tissue. Translated into human physiology this hypothesis could mean that an impaired secretory function of fat cells from obese subjects may directly cause or be involved in the pathogenesis of at least some of the well-known complications of obesity. Therefore, current efforts aiming to elucidate and to better understand the regulation of the secretory function of human fat cells may also have important preventive and therapeutic implications.

Although adipocytes produce and secrete prostaglandins, steroid hormones and possibly other non-protein low-molecular weight components that may be important in the complex cross-talk mentioned before, diverse peptides may play a central role in this network. The variety of proteins identified so far as products from fat cells can be classified into several groups as demonstrated in Table 1. Some of these factors act in an auto/paracrine fashion at the local level among them TNF-α and other cytokines, whereas others act more like classical hormones after being released into the circulation and communicate with distant organs among them leptin. Some of the secretory products, e.g. interleukin-6, may have both a local role as well as a systemic action. Some of these proteins have proinflammatory properties and could function as mediators of a chronic inflammatory process that may underly atherosclerosis and type 2 diabetes. In the following, two selected secretory products will be addressed in more detail. Both are known to be components of chronic inflammation.

Interleukin-6 (IL-6)

Among the many cytokines/chemokines produced by human adipocytes interleukin-6 (IL-6) appears to be of particular importance. Several recent studies have shown that adipocytes synthesize and release IL-6 into the circulation and that a close correlation exists between BMI and circulating IL-6 concentrations[3,4]. Furthermore, *in vitro* experiments revealed that omental fat cells secrete more IL-6 than subcutaneous adipocytes[5]. We recently reported that the expression and release of IL-6 is a differentiation-dependent phenomenon although preadipocytes are also able to produce large amounts of the cytokine. Such data are not easy to interpret as both culture conditions, e.g. the use of fetal bovine serum, and a variable contamination of the stromal cell fraction of human adipose tissue by monocytes/macrophages and other cell types may affect IL-6 production[6].

Table 1. Secretory proteins/peptides from human adipocytes with local and systemic action

Local action	Systemic action
TNF-α, TGF-β	IL-6, IL-8
IL-1β, IL-6	Leptin
Angiotensinogen	Angiotensinogen (?)
PAI-1 (?)	PAI-1
ASP, adipsin (?)	Adiponectin

Little is currently known about the regulation of IL-6 production in adipose tissue. Nevertheless, recent *in vitro* experiments demonstrated that catecholamines and other compounds known to increase intra-cellular cAMP rapidly increase both IL-6 expression and release[6]. These data are in agreement with previous observations that showed an elevation of IL-6 serum concentrations during stress, probably through a β-adrenergic receptor mechanism[7]. Therefore, it may be speculated that the dense sympathetic innervation of omental adipose tissue may contribute to the greater secretory capacity of adipocytes from this depot[5]. On the other hand, glucocorticoids were found to significantly reduce the adipose production of IL-6[6]. In further cell culture experiments performed by our group, it also turned out that Ang II is able to stimulate IL-6 release from cultured human fat cells in a dose- and time-dependent manner. This effect appears to be mainly mediated via the AT_1 receptor subtype, as specific blockers such as valsartan and candesartan were found to prevent this stimulatory action of Ang II almost completely. When the specific AT_2 receptor antagonist PD 123319 was used, there was no significant effect on IL-6 expression both at the mRNA and protein level. Further experiments demonstrated that Ang II may exert this action via the NFκB pathway as addition of Bay11-7082, a blocker of NFκB, was followed by a complete loss of the stimulatory action of Ang II on IL-6 secretion. In addition, Ang II was also found to stimulate the phosphorylation and nuclear translocation of the NFκB p65 subunit in human adipocytes in a time-dependent manner (manuscript in preparation).

Another question relates to the possible local action of IL-6. The specific receptor complex for IL-6 consisting of IL-6 receptor and gp 130 is clearly present on adipocytes as demonstrated by immunohistochemical studies, but so far we were able to show only minor actions of IL-6 at the local level. There was a rather weak lipolytic activity and a weak anti-adipogenic activity. In the presence of adipogenic factors, IL-6 was found to reduce the activity of glycerol-3-phosphate dehydrogenase, a marker enzyme of adipose differentiation, by approximately 30 per cent[6] indicating that IL-6 production could be involved in a negative feedback regulation that limits adipose tissue expansion. However, it should be emphasized that the catabolic effect of IL-6 was much weaker than that of TNF-α, another cytokine expressed by adipocytes[8]. In addition, there was no effect of IL-6 on basal and insulin-stimulated glucose transport in human adipocytes[6]. In contrast to other cytokines, IL-6 did not affect the production of plasminogen activator inhibitor-1 (PAI-1) in adipocytes.

Relevance of elevated circulating IL-6 concentrations in obesity

The question on the possible clinical significance of elevated IL-6 concentrations in human obesity is difficult to answer at present. Although IL-6 is a multi-functional protein that is produced by and acting in many tissues[9], there is little reliable information as to whether IL-6 contributes to the metabolic disturbances characteristic for obesity. In a recent study, there was an inverse association between adipose tissue IL-6 content and maximal *in vivo* insulin responsiveness measured during a hyperinsulinaemic euglycaemic clamp in obese subjects with and without type 2 diabetes[10]. Therefore, the authors claim that an increased IL-6 production by subcutaneous adipose tissue may contribute to the insulin-resistant state in human obesity. In addition, indirect evidence may support the notion that elevated IL-6 promotes chronic inflammation, e.g. by stimulating the production of C-reactive protein in hepatocytes[9]. IL-6 is also well known to have multiple endocrine actions, but it is only a matter of speculation whether the elevated IL-6 concentrations are also involved in the hormonal disturbances characteristic for obesity.

185

Angiotensin II

Ang II is the main biologically active product of angiotensinogen processing. It is now well established that human adipose cells express most components of the renin-angiotensin system[11–13]. There is also growing evidence that angiotensinogen expression is elevated in obesity and that omental fat cells produce more angiotensinogen than subcutaneous fat cells[14,15]. It is not clear at present whether Ang II is released into the circulation in relevant amounts and whether an increased release of this peptide is related to the increased incidence of hypertension in subjects with obesity. But there are some direct and indirect hints which may support this hypothesis[16].

Regulation of angiotensinogen expression

At present, there is limited information available on how angiotensinogen expression is regulated in adipocytes. Previous studies have shown that fasting is associated with a dramatic decrease in angiotensinogen expression, whereas refeeding results in an increased expression of angiotensinogen even above control levels[17]. Further experiments revealed that fatty acids and glucocorticoids increase angiotensinogen expression in clonal adipocyte cell lines[18,19], whereas conflicting results were reported concerning the role of insulin and sympathetic innervation[16]. In addition, most of these studies have been performed in rodent cell lines which are not fully representative for the situation in humans. Therefore, it remains to be determined how angiotensinogen expression is regulated in human adipose tissue.

Action of Ang II in adipose tissue

Apart from its vasoconstrictive action there is recent evidence that Ang II may have additional effects on metabolic pathways as well as on cytokine production and release. We recently studied the effect of angiotensin II on the expression of plasminogen activator inhibitor-1 (PAI-1) in human adipocytes. Ang II and its two metabolites Ang III and Ang IV were found to stimulate PAI-1 production via the AT_1 receptor subtype as specific antagonists abolished this effect[20].

We recently studied the effect of Ang II on the production and release of cytokines from human adipocytes. It turned out that Ang II promotes IL-6 synthesis and release from human adipocytes in primary culture. Preincubation with a specific AT_1 receptor antagonist substantially reduced the stimulatory action of Ang II arguing for an AT_1 receptor-mediated action. IL-8 is another proinflammatory cytokine which is produced in large amounts by adipocytes[21]. Incubation of human adipocytes with Ang II also resulted in a dose- and time-dependent stimulation of IL-8 release into the culture medium. Likewise, this effect was abolished by blockade of the AT_1 receptor. In contrast to its effect on IL-6 and IL-8, we could not demonstrate a similar effect of Ang II on the expression and release of IL-1β and TNF-α indicating that this peptide exerts a differential activation of cytokine expression using classical intracellular pathways. These data suggest that the beneficial effect of AT_1 receptor blockers on cardiovascular morbidity and mortality as recently demonstrated in a large intervention study[22] could also be due to such activities of these compounds. However, clinical studies are required to examine whether this *in vitro* finding in human adipocytes is of clinical importance.

Ang II has also direct effects on metabolic pathways in human preadipocytes and fat cells. It was originally shown by Jones *et al.* that Ang II promotes lipid accumulation in human adipocyte precursor cells. This group also demonstrated an increased expression of fatty acid synthetase, a key enzyme for lipogenesis[23]. In contrast, it was shown that Ang II reduces adipose differentiation in human adipocyte precursor cells[24,25], thereby indicating that this peptide may have different effects depending on the culture model and the experimental conditions. We recently observed a reduction of insulin-stimulated glucose uptake in *in vitro* differentiated fat cells. Subsequent experiments revealed that Ang II directly interferes with the insulin signalling pathway by reducing the extent of serine phosphorylation of proteinkinase B (Akt/PKB) which represents a key step in the intracellular signal transmission to the GLUT4 system. This finding suggests that changes in peptide expression in fat cells from obese subjects may be associated with the local development of insulin resistance.

Secretory function of human fat cells and muscular insulin resistance

Obesity is closely associated with insulin resistance and represents the major risk factor for the development of type 2 diabetes mellitus[26]. Insulin resistance is defined as a reduced glucose utilization upon insulin stimulation in muscle which is by far the most important organ for glucose disposal. Many studies in the past have convincingly shown that an excess of body fat is associated with muscular insulin resistance. A current upcoming hypothesis is that a negative cross-talk between excess body fat and skeletal muscle may impair insulin signalling and finally lead to muscle insulin resistance. To address this attractive hypothesis we recently established a co-culture system of human fat and skeletal muscle cells. In this model, insulin-induced tyrosine phosphorylation of insulin receptor substrate-1 (IRS-1) in the muscle cells was significantly reduced in the presence of fat cells or conditioned medium from fat cell cultures, whereas the expression of IRS-1 protein was unaltered. Troglitazone, an agonist of the nuclear transcription factor PPAR-γ, restored the insulin effect on IRS-1 phosphorylation in the co-culture model. Likewise, insulin-regulated activation of Akt/PKB, a serine kinase, in the human myocytes was significantly reduced after co-culture with adipocytes. Again, this inhibition was completely prevented by troglitazone. Further experiments clearly indicated that this effect was not due to TNF-α and resistin, respectively, two proteins released from adipose cells. These experiments suggest that secretory products from fat cells other than TNF-α and resistin induce insulin resistance in human skeletal muscle cells[27].

In additional experiments, we examined the effect of other possible mediators of insulin resistance from human fat cells. It turned out that Ang II has a weak negative effect on insulin signalling in human skeletal muscle cells with respect to IRS-1 tyrosine and Akt/PKB serine phosphorylation upon insulin stimulation. This effect was prevented by simultaneous addition of a specific AT_1 receptor antagonist. In contrast, addition of IL-6 at various concentrations had no clear effect on insulin signalling in human muscle cells. At present, there is good evidence that co-culture of human fat cells and muscle cells impairs insulin signalling in muscle cells due to secretory products from fat cells, but it is still unclear which factors are responsible for this inhibition. It is conceivable that the observed effect is the result of a mixed effect of inhibitory factors and we cannot exclude the possibility that some of these factors are still out of scope and need to be identified.

These experiments were carried out using fat cells only from healthy non-obese females. Therefore, it is completely unknown whether there is a difference between fat cells from lean and obese subjects and from diabetic vs. non-diabetic subjects. However, the current knowledge is in favour of the view that enlarged adipocytes may secrete more products which may induce insulin resistance. The only exception known so far is adiponectin whose synthesis and secretion is reduced in the obese state. However, low adiponectin serum concentrations appear to be associated with insulin resistance indicating that also reduced production of factors that protect from insulin resistance can cause metabolic disturbances[28]. As we are only at the beginning of a new understanding of the physiological role of adipose tissue, additional experiments are required to determine which adipocyte secretory factors could be responsible for the induction of insulin resistance in skeletal muscle and whether such information is also confirmed by clinical data.

In conclusion, recent studies clearly suggest that human fat cells secrete a variety of peptides that may be involved in the pathophysiology of the metabolic and cardiovascular complications of obesity. In particular, it is rather likely that secretory products are involved in the development of muscular insulin resistance which is a characteristic feature of human obesity. At present, it is rather unclear to which extent these *in vitro* observations are significant for the clinical situation. A better understanding of these processes and their regulation may be of crucial clinical importance as this may open new approaches to prevent or treat these adverse effects even if weight loss is not achieved or cannot be maintained.

Acknowledgements: The contributions by Th. Skurk, K. Röhrig and V. van Harmelen are gratefully acknowledged. I am also indebted to Prof. R. Olbrisch and Prof. B. Husemann for their help in obtaining adipose tissue samples.

References

1. Hotamisligil GS, Shargill NS, Spiegelman BM. Adipose expression of tumor necrosis factor-α: direct role in obesity-linked insulin resistance. *Science* 1993; 259: 87–91.

2. Zhang Y, Proenca R, Maffei M, Barone M, Leopold L, Friedman JM. Positional cloning of the mouse obese gene and its human homologue. *Nature* 1994; 372: 425–32.

3. Vgontzas AN, Papanicolaou DA, Bixler EO, Kales A, Tyson K, Chrousos GP. Elevation of plasma cytokines in disorders of excessive daytime sleepiness: role of sleep disturbance and obesity. *J Clin Endocrinol Metab* 1997; 8282: 1313–6.

4. Mohamed-Ali V, Goodrick S, Rawesh A, Katz DR, Miles JM, Yudkin JS *et al.* Subcutaneous adipose tissue releases interleukin-6, but not tumor necrosis factor-α, *in vivo*. *J Clin Endocrinol Metab* 1997; 82: 4196–200.

5. Fried SK, Bunkin BA, Greenberg AS. Omental and subcutaneous adipose tissues of obese subjects release interleukin-6: depot difference and regulation by glucocorticoids. *J Clin Endocrinol Metab* 1998; 83: 847–50.

6. Päth G, Bornstein SR, Gurniak S, Chrousos GP, Scherbaum WA, Hauner H. Human breast adipocytes express interleukin-6 (IL-6) and its receptor system: increased IL-6 production by β-adrenergic activation and effects of IL-6 on adipocyte function. *J Clin Endocrinol Metab* 2001; 86: 2281–8.

7. Soszynski D, Kozak W, Conn CA, Rudolph K, Kluger MJ. Beta-adrenoceptor antagonists suppress elevation in body temperature and increase in plasma IL-6 in rats exposed to open field. *Neuroendocrinology* 1996; 63: 459–67.

8. Hube F, Hauner H. The role of TNF-α in human adipose tissue: prevention of weight gain at the expense of insulin resistance? *Horm Metab Res* 1999; 31: 626–31.

9. Papanicolaou DA, Wilder RL, Manolagas SC, Chrousos GP. The pathophysiological roles of interleukin-6 in human disease. *Ann Intern Med* 1998; 128: 127–37.

10. Bastard JP, Maachi M, Van Nhieu JT, Jardel C, Bruckert E, Grimaldi A *et al.* Adipose tissue IL-6 content correlates to insulin activation of glucose uptake both *in vivo* and *in vitro*. *J Clin Endocrinol Metab* 2002; 87: 2084–9.

11. Karlsson C, Lindell K, Ottosson M, Sjöström L, Carlsson B, Carlsson LM. Human adipose tissue expresses angiotensinogen and the enzymes required for its conversion to angiotensin II. *J Clin Endocrinol Metab* 1998; 83: 3925–9.

12. Schling P, Mallow H, Trindl A, Löffler G. Evidence for a local renin-angiotensin system in primary cultured human preadipocytes. *Int J Obes* 1999; 23: 336–41.

13. Engeli S, Gorzelniak K, Kreutz R, Runkel N, Distler A, Sharma AM. Co-expression of renin-angiotensin system genes in human adipose tissue. *J Hypertens* 1999; 17: 555–60.

14. Van Harmelen V, Ariapart P, Hoffstedt J, Lundkvist I, Bringman S, Arner P. Increased adipose angiotensinogen gene expression in human adipose tissue. *Obes Res* 2000; 8: 337–41.

15. Van Harmelen V, Elizalde M, Ariapart P, Bergstedt-Lindqvist S, Reynisdottir S, Hoffstedt J *et al.* The association of human adipose angiotensinogen gene expression with abdominal fat distribution in obesity. *Int J Obes* 2000; 24: 673–8.

16. Engeli S, Negrel R, Sharma AM. Physiology and pathophysiology of the adipose tissue renin-angiotensin system. *Hypertension* 2000; 35: 1270–7.

17. Frederich RCJ, Kahn BB, Peach MJ, Flier JS. Tissue-specific nutritional regulation of angiotensinogen in adipose tissue. *Hypertension* 1992; 19: 339–44.

18. Safonova I, Aubert J, Negrel R, Ailhaud G. Regulation by fatty acids of angiotensinogen expression in preadipose cells. *Biochem J* 1997; 322: 235–9.

19. Aubert J, Darimont C, Safonova I, Ailhaud G, Negrel R. Regulation by glucocorticoids of AGT gene expression and secretion in adipose cells. *Biochem J* 1997; 328: 701–6.

20. Skurk T, Lee Y-M, Hauner H. Angiotensin II and its metabolites stimulate PAI-1 protein release from human adipocytes in primary culture. *Hypertension* 2001; 37: 1336–40.

21. Bruun JM, Pedersen SB, Richelsen B. Regulation of interleukin-8 production and gene expression in human adipose tissue *in vitro*. *J Clin Endocrinol Metab* 2001; 86: 1267–73.

22. Dahlöf B, Devereux RB, Kjeldsen SE, Julius S, Beevers G, de Faire U *et al.* Cardiovascular morbidity and mortality in the losartan intervention for endpoint reduction in hypertension study (LIFE): a randomized trial against atenolol. *Lancet* 2002; 359: 995–1003.

23. Jones BH, Standridge MK, Moustaid M. Angiotensin II increases lipogenesis in 3T3-L1 and human adipose cells. *Endocrinology* 1997; 138: 1512–9.

24. Schling P, Löffler G. Effects of angiotensin II on adipose conversion and expression of genes of the renin-angiotensin system in human preadipocytes. *Horm Metab Res* 2001; 33: 189–95.

25. Janke J, Engeli S, Gorzelniak K, Luft FC, Sharma AM. Mature adipocytes inhibit *in vitro* differentiation of human preadipocytes via angiotensin type 1 receptors. *Diabetes* 2002; 51: 1699–707.

26. Kahn BB, Flier JS. Obesity and insulin resistance. *J Clin Invest* 2000; 106: 473–81.

27. Dietze D, Koenen M, Röhrig K, Horikoshi H, Hauner H, Eckel J. Impairment of insulin signaling in human skeletal muscle cells by co-culture with human adipocytes. *Diabetes* 2002; 51: 2369–76.

28. Berg AH, Combs TP, Scherer PE. ACRP30/Adiponectin: an adipokine regulating glucose and lipid metabolism. *Trends Endocrinol Metab* 2002; 13: 84–9.

Progress in Obesity Research: 9. Edited by *Geraldo Medeiros-Neto, Alfredo Halpern and Claude Bouchard*
©2003 John Libbey Eurotext Ltd, pp. 189–192.

CHAPTER 39

Role of metallothioneins in adipose tissue: metallothionein as an *adipokine*

Paul Trayhurn[1] and John H. Beattie[2]

[1]*Liverpool Centre for Nutritional Genomics, Neuroendocrine & Obesity Biology Unit, Department of Medicine, University of Liverpool, University Clinical Departments, Liverpool L69 3GA, UK; and* [2]*Rowett Research Institute, Bucksburn, Aberdeen AB21 9SB, UK*
[E-mail: p.trayhurn@liverpool.ac.uk]

There has been a revolution in our understanding of the adipose organ in recent years, resulting from a major change in perspective on the physiological role of white adipose tissue. In addition to the core function in the storage of lipids and other roles such as thermal insulation (notably as blubber in marine mammals), it is now recognized that white adipose tissue is an endocrine organ. This followed the discovery in 1994 of the cytokine-like hormone, leptin[1]. Leptin has a wide range of biological effects, in addition to its key role as an adipocyte-derived signal in the regulation of energy balance[2].

Leptin is not the only hormone or protein factor secreted by white adipocytes. Indeed, there is a rapidly growing list of highly diverse proteins which are secreted[3–5] (Fig. 1), and these are increasingly known by the collective name *adipokines* or *adipocytokines* (adipokines is to be preferred since many of the proteins are *not* cytokines). The adipokines, together with lipid substances such as fatty acids, prostaglandins, cholesterol and retinol form what can be termed the '*secretome*' of the adipocyte – the totality of secretions from the cell. The adipokines include hormones such as adiponectin (also known as Acrp30, AdipoQ, ApM1 or GBP28), resistin and classical cytokines such as TNFα and interleukin-6. The full range of protein signals encompasses factors involved in vascular haemostasis (plasminogen activator inhibitor-1, tissue factor), blood pressure regulation (angiotensinogen), lipid metabolism (e.g. cholesteryl ester transfer protein, retinol binding protein) and the acute phase response (haptoglobin). In the first half of 2002 several putative new adipokines have been added to the list through the application of DNA microarrays and of proteomics[6,7].

In 1996 we reported that brown adipose tissue expresses a gene encoding a member of the metallothionein family of proteins[8]. Subsequent studies indicated that the metallothionein (MT) genes are also expressed in white adipose tissue, with MT itself being a secretory product of the white adipocyte[9]. In the present article we discuss the production and putative role of MT in adipose tissue.

What are the metallothioneins?

The MTs are a family of closely related proteins which currently number up to 12 member isoforms in human tissues. They are of low mol. wt. (approximately 6,000 *Mr*) with a very high cysteine content; indeed, one-third of the amino acids in the MTs are in the form of cysteine residues. Although these proteins were discovered some 30 years ago, there is no firm consensus as to their main biological function. They bind metals, and as such have a role in the homeostatic regulation of zinc concentrations and in the detoxification of non-essential heavy metals[10]. They can also function as antioxidants and may be involved in blood pressure regulation and in the protection against neurological disease[10]. There is additionally emerging evidence that the MTs could play a role in angiogenesis[11].

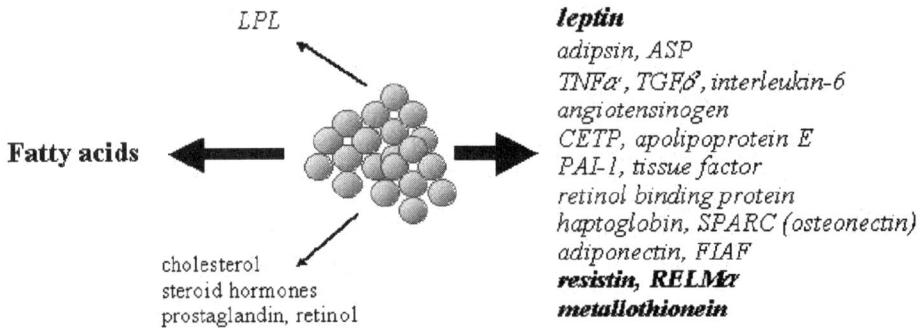

LPL

Fatty acids

cholesterol
steroid hormones
prostaglandin, retinol

leptin
adipsin, ASP
TNFα', TGFβ, interleukin-6
angiotensinogen
CETP, apolipoprotein E
PAI-1, tissue factor
retinol binding protein
haptoglobin, SPARC (osteonectin)
adiponectin, FIAF
resistin, RELMα
metallothionein

Fig. 1. The *secretome* of white adipocytes: the diagram shows a number of the adipokines and other secreted products from adipocytes. ASP, acylation-stimulating protein; CETP, cholesteryl ester transfer protein; FIAF, fasting-induced adipose factor; LPL, lipoprotein lipase; PAI-1, plasminogen activator inhibitor-1; RELMα, resistin-like molecule α; TGFβ, transforming growth factor β; TNFα, tumour necrosis factor α.

Metallothionein gene expression in adipose tissue

MT gene (MT-1) expression in rodent brown adipose tissue is markedly stimulated by exposure to cold[8,12], and the induction is more marked than that of UCP-1. The cold-induced expression of MT-1 in brown fat can be mimicked by the administration of noradrenaline, indicating that gene expression is stimulated through activation of the sympathetic innervation to the tissue[12]. This occurs via β-adrenoceptors (presumably the β3-subtype) since isoprenaline also stimulates MT-1 gene expression when injected into rodents[12]. The administration of metals such as zinc leads to a large increase in MT expression in liver and kidney, the traditional sites of the production of the protein, and this can also occur in brown adipose tissue – although the results are variable between rats and mice[8,12].

Subsequent studies have demonstrated that MT genes are expressed in white adipose tissue as well as in brown fat[9]. Expression occurs in each of the major white fat depots, both internal and subcutaneous, in mice and is associated with the mature adipocytes themselves rather than with the cells of the stromal-vascular fraction[9] (Fig. 2). Neither fasting nor the administration of zinc leads to any change in MT gene expression in white adipose tissue[9]. The lack of effect of zinc on expression is in marked contrast to the liver, where a major induction occurs. A small increase in MT mRNA level in epididymal white fat has been noted following the administration of a β3-adrenoceptor agonist, though not with noradrenaline[9].

Metallothionein secretion in cell culture

Expression of a gene does not, of course, mean that the encoded protein is secreted from a cell. We have therefore employed a rat primary cell culture system, in which fibroblastic preadipocytes are differentiated into mature adipocytes, to examine whether MT may be secreted from white adipose tissue. The MT-1 gene was found to be expressed in the adipocytes from the time at which differentiation was induced with a peak in mRNA level at two days post-induction – before the point at which expression of the late marker of adipocyte differentiation, adipsin, is evident[13]. Importantly, MT was found to be released into the culture medium by day two after the induction of differentiation, reaching

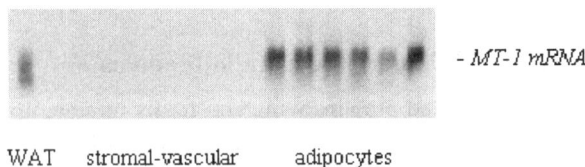

- *MT-1 mRNA*

WAT   stromal-vascular   adipocytes

Fig. 2. Metallothionein (MT-1) gene expression in mouse white adipocytes. A Northern blot was probed for MT-1 mRNA using a 28-mer antisense oligonucleotide (end-labelled with digoxigenin) with chemiluminescence-based detection. The blot shows epididymal white adipose tissue (WAT) and mature adipocytes and cells of the stromal-vascular fraction. Adapted from[4].

a peak from four to eight days post-induction[13]. In this system, release of MT continues throughout the culture period, albeit at a declining rate, with the peak in leptin secretion occurring later[13].

The addition of dexamethasone leads to a substantial increase in MT mRNA level in the adipocytes and to the release of the protein into the medium[13]. A stimulation of secretion has also been noted with insulin or leptin, but the effect is small such that these hormones are unlikely to play a significant role in the regulation of MT production in adipocytes[13]. Similarly, although forskolin and bromo-cAMP have a stimulatory effect, no response is observed with the addition of either noradrenaline or a selective β3-adrenoceptor agonist[13]. This suggests that catecholamines do not regulate MT production in white adipocytes, the stimulatory effect of high doses of the β3-adrenoceptor agonist observed *in vivo* reflecting an indirect rather than direct response[9].

The release of MT into the medium in cell culture appears to involve a specific secretory effect since measurements of lactate dehydrogenase indicate that it is not a reflection of general cell leakage. However, there is no obvious signal sequence in the MT protein, as would be expected with a classical secretion product.

Metallothionein expression in human adipose tissue

In recent studies we have explored whether the MT gene is expressed in human adipose tissue, in addition to rodents. It is not, of course, axiomatic that expression in laboratory animals means parallel expression in humans, as early studies on resistin have illustrated. Although the resistin gene is strongly expressed in adipose tissue from mice and rats[14,15], either no or extremely low expression was reported in the majority of subjects in initial studies on human tissue, even though highly sensitive RT-PCR procedures were employed to detect resistin mRNA[16,17].

MT gene expression is, however, readily evident in human subcutaneous adipose tissue; the presence of MT-2A mRNA, the MT-2A gene being the most commonly expressed member of the MT gene family in humans, is easily detected by Northern blotting[18]. Although expression occurs in mature adipocytes, in contrast to rodents expression is also evident in the cells of the stromal-vascular fraction. In a small sample of obese subjects the level of MT-2A mRNA in adipose tissue was significantly higher than in lean individuals, but no response to a two-week period of dietary restriction was noted[18].

These results indicate that MT gene expression occurs in human white adipocytes and is therefore not selective to rodent adipose tissue.

Metallothionein and obesity and diabetes

There is some evidence for links between MT and obesity and its associated disorders. Thus we have reported that one strain of MT knockout mice (MT-1 and MT-2 null) exhibited higher weight gain and moderate obesity as compared with a reference group of mice[19]. The MT-null animals had higher fat pad weights, increased level of *ob* mRNA in adipose tissue and substantially elevated plasma leptin concentrations[19]. It is, however, difficult at this stage to provide a clear mechanistic link between MT and energy balance, but the possibility that such a link exists is raised by these observations. Alternatively, mild obesity in MT-null mice could simply be a reflection of a rather distant secondary effect or the 'reprogramming' that can occur in transgenic animals.

A potential link between MT and the complications of diabetes comes from a recent report which has demonstrated that over-expression of MT in cardiomyocytes reduces the cardiomyopathy of the diabetic heart[20]. This important effect has been attributed to the antioxidant function of MT[20].

Coda

The key question with respect to the secretion of MT by white adipose tissue is the physiological significance of such a process. Given the strong expression of the protein on cold exposure in brown fat we originally suggested that MT may play an antioxidant role in protecting the cells from free radical damage generated by the very high rates of oxidation during thermogenesis[8]. In white adipose tissue, an antioxidant function is also conceivable in terms of a housekeeping role in preventing oxidation of the stored fatty acids. Similarly, secretion of the protein may protect fatty acids during their transport from the circulation to the fat cell. An alternative view is that MT may be involved in angiogenesis within adipose tissue – both brown and white forms – along with other adipokines such as leptin[21,22]. These possibilities need, however, to be tested and we are currently doing so through the use of MT knockout mice.

As noted above, MT is a low mol. wt cysteine-rich protein, and in this respect there are parallels with resistin and RELM-α (members of the RELM or FIZZ gene family) which share similar characteristics.

SPARC (or osteonectin) is a further high cysteine-containing protein which appears to be secreted from white adipocytes[23], although its mol. wt. is in excess of 50,000. Whether there is a meaningful connection between these proteins is unclear; nevertheless, it is of interest that a cell specialized for the storage of large amounts of lipid also secretes several proteins high in sulphur containing amino acids.

In summary, both brown and white adipose tissue produce the stress response and metal-binding protein MT, and in the case of white adipocytes the protein appears to be a member of the rapidly expanding range of adipocyte secretory proteins – the adipokines.

Acknowledgements: JHB is grateful to the Scottish Executive Environment and Rural Affairs Department for financial support.

References

1. Zhang YY, Proenca R, Maffei M, Barone M, Leopold L, Friedman JM. Positional cloning of the mouse obese gene and its human homolog. *Nature* 1994; 372: 425–32.

2. Trayhurn P, Hoggard N, Mercer JG, Rayner DV. Leptin: Fundamental aspects. *Int J Obes* 1999; 23: 22–8.

3. Mohamed-Ali V, Pinkney JH, Coppack SW. Adipose tissue as an endocrine and paracrine organ. *Int J Obes* 1998; 22: 1145–58.

4. Trayhurn P, Beattie JH. Physiological role of adipose tissue: White adipose tissue as an endocrine and secretory organ. *Proc Nutr Soc* 2001; 60: 329–39.

5. Frühbeck G, Gómez-Ambrosi J, Muruzabal FJ, Burrell MA. The adipocyte: A model for integration of endocrine and metabolic signaling in energy metabolism regulation. *Am J Physiol* 2001; 280: E827–E847.

6. Li J, Yu X, Pan W, Unger RH. Gene expression profile of rat adipose tissue at the onset of high-fat-diet obesity. *Am J Physiol* 2002; 282: E1334–E1341.

7. Kratchmarova I, Kalume DE, Blagoev B, Scherer PE, Podtelejnikov AV, Molina H *et al.* A proteomic approach for identification of secreted proteins during the differentiation of 3T3-L1 preadipocytes to adipocytes. *Mol Cell Proteomics* 2002; 1: 213–22.

8. Beattie JH, Black DJ, Wood AM, Trayhurn P. Cold-induced expression of the metallothionein-1 gene in brown adipose tissue of rats. *Am J Physiol* 1996; 270: R971–R977.

9. Trayhurn P, Duncan JS, Wood AM, Beattie JH. Metallothionein gene expression and secretion by white adipose tissue. *Am J Physiol* 2000; 279: R2329–R2335.

10. Lichtlen P, Schaffner W. The 'metal transcription factor' MTF-1: Biological facts and medical implications. *Swiss Med Weekly* 2001; 131: 647–52.

11. Giralt M, Penkowa M, Lago N, Molinero A, Hidalgo J. Metallothionein-1+2 protect the CNS after a focal brain injury. *Exp Neurol* 2002; 173: 114–28.

12. Beattie JH, Wood AM, Trayhurn P, Jasani J, Vincent A, McCormack G, West AK. Metallothionein is expressed in adipocytes of brown fat and is induced by catecholamines and zinc. *Am J Physiol* 2000; 278: R1082–R1089.

13. Trayhurn P, Duncan JS, Wood AM, Beattie JH. Regulation of metallothionein gene expression and secretion in rat adipocytes differentiated from preadipocytes in primary culture. *Horm Metab Res* 2000; 32: 542–7.

14. Steppan CM, Bailey ST, Bhat S, Brown EJ, Banerjee RR, Wright C *et al.* The hormone resistin links obesity to diabetes. *Nature* 2001; 409: 307–12.

15. Haugen F, Jorgensen A, Drevon CA, Trayhurn P. Inhibition by insulin of resistin gene expression in 3T3-L1 adipocytes. *FEBS Letters* 2001; 507: 105–8.

16. Nagaev I, Smith U. Insulin resistance and type 2 diabetes are not related to resistin expression in human fat cells or skeletal muscle. *Biochem Biophys Res Commun* 2001; 285: 561–4.

17. Savage DB, Sewter CP, Klenk ES, Segal DG, Vidal-Puig A, Considine RV, O'Rahilly S. Resistin/FIZZ3 expression in relation to obesity and peroxisome proliferator-activated receptor-gamma action in humans. *Diabetes* 2001; 50: 2199–202.

18. Do MS, Nam SY, Hong SE, Kim KW, Duncan JS, Beattie JH, Trayhurn P. Metallothionein gene expression in human adipose tissue from lean and obese subjects. *Horm Metab Res* 2002; 34: 348–51.

19. Beattie JH, Wood AM, Newman AM, Bremner I, Choo KHA, Michalska AE *et al.* Obesity and hyperleptinemia in metallothionein (-I and -II) null mice. *Proc Natl Acad Sci USA* 1998; 95: 358–63.

20. Liang Q, Carlson EC, Donthi RV, Kralik PM, Shen X, Epstein PN. Overexpression of metallothionein reduces diabetic cardiomyopathy. *Diabetes* 2002; 51: 174–81.

21. Sierra-Honigmann MR, Nath AK, Murakami C, GarciaCardena G, Papapetropoulos A, Sessa WC *et al.* Biological action of leptin as an angiogenic factor. *Science* 1998; 281: 1683–6.

22. Bouloumie A, Drexler HCA, Lafontan M, Busse R. Leptin, the product of *ob* gene, promotes angiogenesis. *Circulation Res* 1998; 83: 1059–66.

23. Tartare-Deckert S, Chavey C, Monthouel MN, Gautier N, Van Obberghen E. The matricellular protein SPARC/osteonectin as a newly identified factor up-regulated in obesity. *J Biol Chem* 2001; 276: 22231–7

Progress in Obesity Research: 9. Edited by *Geraldo Medeiros-Neto, Alfredo Halpern and Claude Bouchard*
©2003 John Libbey Eurotext Ltd, pp. 193–196.

CHAPTER 40

Hypoadiponectinaemia associates with insulin resistant syndrome

Iichiro Shimomura[1] and Yuji Matsuzawa[2]

[1]*Department of Medicine and Pathophysiology, Graduate School of Frontier Bioscience;* [2]*Department of Internal Medicine and Molecular Science, Graduate School of Medicine, Osaka University, 2-2 Yamadaoka, Suita, Osaka 565-0871, Japan*
[e-mail: ichi@fbs.osaka-u.ac.jp]

Introduction

The adipose tissue produces and secretes many bioactive substances, conceptualized as adipocytokines[1–4]. Dysregulated production of adipocytokines, such as tumour necrosis factor (TNF)-α, leptin, and plasminogen-activator inhibitor type 1 (PAI-1), is associated with the pathophysiology of obesity-related insulin resistance and thrombosis.
Adiponectin/ACRP30 is a novel adipocytokine, identified by our group through screening the adipose-specific genes in the human cDNA project[5]. Other groups independently cloned the mouse homologue of adiponectin as ACRP30[6] and AdipoQ[7], respectively. The protein contains the signal sequence and a collagen repeat domain at N-terminal, and the globular domain at C-terminal. Adiponectin/ACRP30 mRNA is exclusively expressed in adipose tissues in humans, monkeys, and mice.

Hypoadiponectinaemia in insulin resistant syndrome

Adiponectin/ACRP30 is abundantly present in plasma (range, 5–30 μg/ml)[8], but its adipose mRNA level and plasma levels decreased in obesity[7,8]. Plasma concentrations of adiponectin correlate inversely with body mass index (BMI). Interestingly, plasma concentrations of adiponectin were lower in the subject with type 2 diabetes and coronary artery disease even after adjustment for BMI[9,10]. During the course of development of diet-induced type 2 diabetes in rhesus monkey, reduction of plasma adiponectin occurs prior to the incidence of hyperinsulinaemia, which is used as a parameter of insulin resistance[11]. Hyperinsulinaemic euglycaemic clamp studies in human and monkey revealed that plasma concentrations of adiponectin significantly correlate with the degree of insulin sensitivity in whole body[11,12]. Moreover, adiponectin/ACRP30 treatment improved diabetes in mice[13–15]. These data suggested that adiponectin/ACRP30 is an insulin-sensitizing and anti-atherogenic hormone, and that reduced production of adiponectin/ACRP30 might relate to the pathophysiology of insulin resistance and atherosclerosis.

In vitro effects of adiponectin on insulin sensitivity and anti-atherogenesity

To confirm the hypothesis derived from the clinical studies, we conducted tissue-cultured experiments. For insulin sensitivity, adiponectin was capable of enhancing FATP-1 mRNA and activating IRS-1 associated PI3-kinase and glucose uptake in C2C12 myocytes[16]. FATP-1, fatty acid transport protein-1, facilitates fatty acid transport in muscle followed by fatty acid-catabolism via beta-oxidation. Quite interestingly, these enhancing effects of adiponectin on insulin sensitivity in myocytes were partially antagonized by TNFalpha, another adipocytokine[16].
For anti-atherogenesity, adiponectin suppressed TNFα-induced mRNA expression of adhesion molecules including VCAM-1, ICAM-1, and E-selectin in vascular endothelial cells, and monocyte attachment to endothelial cells[10,17]. Adiponectin also reduced lipid accumulation in human monocyte-derived macrophages through its suppressive effect on the expression of macrophage scavenger receptor[18].

Furthermore, recent analysis revealed that adiponctin suppressed the production of growth factors, such as PDGF, HB-EGF, bFGF and EGF, from activated endothelial cell, and inhibited these growth factors-induced proliferation and migration of smooth muscle cells[19,20].

These tissue cultured experiments strengthened the concept that adiponectin works as insulin sensitizing and anti-atherogenic hormone derived from adipose tissue.

Genetic hypoadiponectinaemia in human

We screened around 700 human subjects to identify the genetic mutations in the coding region of adiponectin gene. We identified four missense mutations (R112C, I164T, R221S, and H241P) in the globular domain[21]. Among these mutations, the frequency of I164T mutation (nine subjects) was highest. The subjects had significantly lower concentrations of plasma adiponectin, compared to wild type and other mutated subjects. The subjects carrying I164T mutation showed features of insulin resistant syndrome including impaired glucose tolerance (100 per cent), hyperlipidaemia (89 per cent), hypertension (100 per cent), and atherosclerotic disease (67 per cent). These findings suggested that primary hypoadiponectinaemia caused by genetic mutation of adiponectin gene, not by overcalorie, initiated insulin resistant syndrome in human. Recent genome-wide scan studies mapped a susceptibility locus for type 2 diabetes mellitus (DM) and the insulin resistant syndrome to chromosome 3q27, where the adiponectin gene is located[22,23]. Taken together, lower plasma concentration and/or reduced function of adiponectin are likely to induce insulin resistant syndrome in human.

Lessons from adiponectin knockout mice

Adiponectin knockout mice showed delayed clearance of plasma free fatty acid, low mRNA levels of muscle fatty acid transport protein (FATP)-1, high mRNA levels of adipose tumour necrosis factor (TNF)-α, and high plasma TNF-α concentrations[16]. The knockout mice exhibited severe diet-induced insulin resistance with reduced insulin receptor substrate (IRS)-1 associated phosphatidylinositol 3-kinase (PI3-kinase) in muscle. Adiponectin production by viral infection in knockout mice restored the reduction of FATP-1 mRNA, the increase of adipose TNF-α mRNA, and the diet-induced insulin resistance. Considering the opposite effects of adiponectin and TNFalpha to insulin sensitivity in cultured myocytes, the knockout mice studies demonstrated that low adiponectin and high TNF-α levels reduced muscle FATP-1 mRNA and IRS-1-mediated insulin signaling, resulting in severe diet-induced insulin resistance in the knockout mice. Further, we investigated *in vivo* role of adiponectin on the neointimal thickening after artery injury. Adiponectin knockout mice showed severe neointimal thickening and increased proliferation of vascular smooth muscle cells in mechanically injured arteries[20]. Adenovirus-mediated supplement of adiponectin attenuated neointimal proliferation. Together with the anti-atherogenic moieties of adiponectin in tissue cultures, the konockout mice analysis revealed that hypoadiponectinaemia itself can initiate the severer arterial wall response to vascular injury and the adiponectin supplement can reverse the phenomena.

In conclusion, the results from knockout mice studies strongly suggested that hypoadiponectinaemia is responsible for the development of type 2 diabetes, atherosclerotic changes, and vascular restenosis after angioplasty, in obese subjects, and that normalizing the plasma adiponectin should be a useful strategy to attack insulin resistance and vascular disease in obesity.

Therapeutic approach to hypoadiponectinaemia

Based on the results described above, there should be two therapeutic approach against the hypoadiponectinaemia-associated insulin resistant syndrome.

One is to aim at increasing plasma adiponectin levels, relative to those of plasma TNF-α. Previously, we reported the increasing effect of PPARgamma agonists on plasma adiponectin levels, through enhancing the expression of aidponectin mRNA in adipose cells[24]. Favourably, PPARgamma agonists also suppressed the TNFalpha production from adipose cells. Therefore, the effects of PPARgamma agonists on insulin resistant syndrome including type 2 diabetes and atheroscrelosis should be attributed, at least in part, to their increasing adiponectin and decreasing TNFalpha. The compounds like PPARgamma agonists will be screened simply by their activation on the transcription of adiponectin promoter using reporter analysis. More directly, another way is seeking for the drug to enhance the adiponectin secretion. Our recent analysis revealed that androgen specifically regulates the secretion of adiponectin without altering the mRNA and protein amounts of adiponecitn in adipocytes, suggesting the regulatory mechanism for adiponectin secretion[27]. To know the machinery how adiponectin

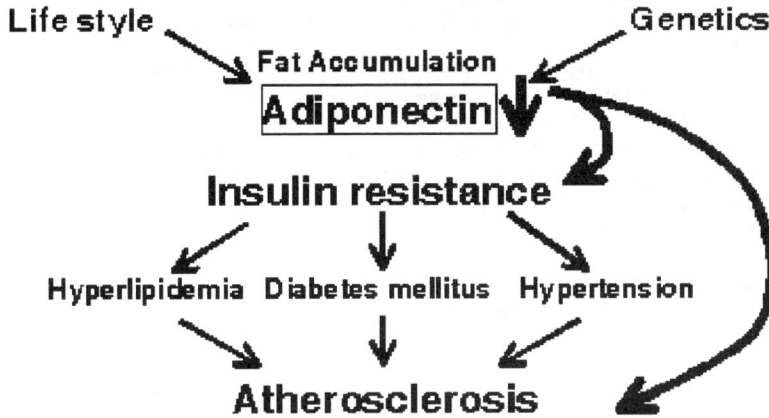

Fig. 1. Insulin resistant syndrome.

secretion is regulated should give a useful insight to develop the compound enhancing the secretion of adiponectin.

Another approach is create the agonist toward the adiponectin receptor. Obviously, we have to await the identification of the receptor. Now, numeral investigators in academics and companies are struggling for this mission.

Conclusion

The life style rampant in developed countries, more high fat-diet and less exercise, initiates hypoadiponectinaemia under the influence of genetic variation (Fig. 1). Once hypoadiponectinaemia is initiated, metabolic abnormalities and hypertension are driven by hypoadiponectinaemia-induced insulin resistance, and these abnormalities become causative for the development of athrosclerosis together with the direct atherogenic effect of hypoadiponectinaemia on artery. Hypoadiponectinaemia stands upstream in the pathophysiology of insulin resistant syndrome associated with obesity.

References

1. Shimomura I, Funahashi T, Takahashi M, Maeda K, Kotani K, Nakamura T *et al*. Enhanced expression of PAI-1 in visceral fat: possible contributor to vascular disease in obesity. *Nature Med* 1996; 2: 800–2.

2. Spiegelman BM, Flier JS. Adipogenesis and obesity: rounding out the big picture. *Cell* 1996; 87: 377–89.

3. Hotamisligil GS, Spiegelman BM. Tumor necrosis factor alpha: a key component of the obesity-diabetes link. *Diabetes* 1994; 43: 1271–8.

4. Friedman JM, Halaas JL. Leptin and the regulation of body weight in mammals. *Nature* 1998; 395: 763–70.

5. Maeda K, Okubo K, Shimomura I, Funahashi T, Matsuzawa Y, Matsubara K. cDNA cloning and expression of a novel adipose specific collagen-like factor, apM1 (Adipose most abundant gene transcript 1). *Biochem Biophys Res Commun*. 1996; 221: 286–9.

6. Scherer EP, Williams S, Fogliano M, Baldini G, Lodish HF. A novel serum protein similar to C1q, produced exclusively in adipocytes. *J Biol Chem* 1995; 270: 26746–9.

7. Hu E, Liang P, Spiegelman BM. AdipoQ is a novel adipose-specific gene dysregulated in obesity. *J Biol Chem* 1996; 271: 10697–703.

8. Arita Y, Kihara S, Ouchi N, Takahashi M, Maeda K, Miyagawa J *et al*. Paradoxical decrease of an adipose-specific protein, adiponectin, in obesity. *Biochem Biophys Res Commun* 1999; 257: 79–83.

9. Hotta K, Funahashi T, Arita Y, Takahashi M, Matsuda M, Okamoto Y *et al*. Plasma concentrations of a novel, adipose-specific protein, adiponectin, in type 2 diabetic patients. *Arterioscler Thromb Vasc Biol* 2000; 20: 1595–9.

10. Ouchi N, Kihara S, Arita Y, Maeda K, Kuriyama H, Okamoto Y *et al*. Novel modulator for endothelial adhesion molecules: adipocyte-derived plasma protein, adiponectin. *Circulation* 1999; 100: 2473–6.

11. Hotta K, Funahashi T, Bodkin NL, Ortmeyer HK, Arita Y, Hansen BC, Matsuzawa Y. Circulating concentrations of the adipocyte protein, adiponectin, are decreased in parallel with reduced insulin sensitivity during the progression to type-2 diabetes in rhesus monkeys. *Diabetes* 2001; 50: 1126–33.

12. Weyer C, Funahashi T, Tanaka S, Hotta K, Matsuzawa Y, Pratley RE, Tataranni PA. Hypoadiponectinemia in obesity and type 2 diabetes: close association with insulin resistance and hyperinsulinemia. *J Clin Endocrinol Metab* 2001; 86: 1930–5.

13. Fruebis J, Tsao TS, Javorschi S, Ebbets-Reed D, Erickson MR, Yen FT *et al*. Proteolytic cleavage product of 30-kDa adipocyte complement-related protein increases fatty acid oxidation in muscle and causes weight loss in mice. *Proc Natl Acad Sci USA* 2001; 98: 2005–10.

14. Yamauchi T, Kamon J, Waki H, Terauchi Y, Kubota N, Hara K *et al*. The fat-derived hormone adiponectin reverses insulin resistance associated with both lipoatrophy and obesity. *Nature Med* 2001; 7: 941–6.

15. Berg AH, Combs TP, Du X, Brownlee M, Scherer PE. The adipocyte-secreted protein Acrp30 enhances hepatic insulin action. *Nature Med* 2001; 7: 947–53.

16. Maeda N, Shimomura I, Kishida K, Nishizawa H, Matsuda M, Nagaretani H, *et al*. Diet-induced insulin resistance in mice lacking adiponectin/ACRP30. *Nature Med* 2002; 8: 731–7.

17. Ouchi N, Kihara S, Arita Y, Okamoto Y, Maeda K, Kuriyama H *et al*. Adiponectin, adipocyte-derived plasma protein, inhibits endothelial NF-βB signaling through cAMP-dependent pathway. *Circulation* 2000; 102: 1296–301.

18. Ouchi N, Kihara S, Arita Y, Nishida M, Matsuyama A, Okamoto Y *et al*. Adipocyte-derived plasma protein, adiponectin, suppresses lipid accumulation and class A scavenger receptor expression in human monocyte-derived macrophages. *Circulation* 2001; 103: 1057–63.

19. Arita Y, Kihara S, Ouchi N, Maeda K, Kuriyama H, Okamoto Y *et al*. Adipocyte-derived plasma protein adiponectin acts as a platelet-derived growth factor-BB-binding protein and regulates growth factor-induced common postreceptor signal in vascular smooth muscle cell. *Circulation* 2002; 105: 2893–8.

20. Matsuda M, Shimomura I, Sata M, Arita Y, Nishida M, Maeda N *et al*. Role of adiponectin in preventing vascular stenosis- the missing link of adipo-vascular axis. *J Biol Chem* 2002 (in press).

21. Kondo H, Shimomura I, Matsukawa Y, Kumada M, Takahashi M, Matsuda M *et al*. Association of adiponectin mutation with type 2 diabetes: a candidate gene for the insulin resistance syndrome. *Diabetes* 2002; 51: 2325–8.

22. Kissebah AH, Sonnenberg GE, Myklebust J, Goldstein M, Broman K, James RG *et al*. Quantitative trait loci on chromosomes 3 and 17 influence phenotypes of the metabolic syndrome. *Proc Natl Acad Sci USA* 2000; 97: 14478–83.

23. Vionnet N, Hani El-H, Dupont S, Gallina S, Francke S, Dotte S *et al*. Genomewide search for type 2 diabetes-susceptibility genes in French whites: evidence for a novel susceptibility locus for early-onset diabetes on chromosome 3q27-qter and independent replication of a type 2-diabetes locus on chromosome 1q21-q24. *Am J Hum Genet* 2000; 67: 1470–480

24. Nishizawa N, Shimomura I, Kishida K, Maeda N, Nagaretani H, Kuriyama H *et al*. Androgens downregulate plasma adiponectin, an insulin-sensitizing adipocyte-derived protein. *Diabetes* 2002 (in press).

Progress in Obesity Research: 9. Edited by *Geraldo Medeiros-Neto, Alfredo Halpern and Claude Bouchard*
©2003 John Libbey Eurotext Ltd, pp. 197–200.

CHAPTER 41

Chronic effects of insulin and glucocorticoids on the adipocyte: implications for the regulation of fat cell size in obesity

Susan K. Fried[1], Maria Trujillo[2], Yanxin Wang[2] and Andrew S. Greenberg[3]

[1]*Division of Gerontology, University of Maryland School of Medicine, Baltimore VA Medical Center, GRECC (BT/GR/18), 10 North Greene St., Baltimore, MD 21201, USA;* [2]*Department of Nutritional Science, Rutgers University, New Brunswick NJ 08901, USA;* [3]*HNRC, Tufts University, Boston, MA, USA*
[e-mail: sfried@rci.rutgers.edu]

Introduction

Hyperinsulinaemia is a hallmark of the obese state. While early in the development of obesity, adipocytes are highly sensitive and responsive to insulin, with enlargement of fat stores, adipocytes become progressively less sensitive to the ability of insulin to stimulate glucose transport and inhibit lipolysis. Fat cells tend to reach a maximal size at a point where the increased rate of fatty acid esterification is matched by higher rate of lipolysis. On a per cell basis, basal rates of glucose transport and metabolism are increased in enlarged adipocytes of the obese, compared to smaller adipocytes of lean individuals[1–3]. Thus, rates triglyceride turnover are elevated in enlarged adipocytes of the obese. The endocrine and paracrine determinants of the adaptation of fat cell metabolism to the obese state are only partly understood. In this chapter will review the evidence that chronic insulin and glucocorticoid levels play an important role in the modulation of adipocyte metabolic capacity. Additionally, depot-specific responses to chronic insulin and glucocorticoid appear to play an aetiologic role in the development of a visceral obesity.

Depot-specific effects of glucocorticoids

Fat cells from different depots vary in the rate of storage and turnover of triglyceride[4,5]. Visceral (omental and mesenteric fat cells) undergo enlargement in situations of cortisol excess, while peripheral adipose tissues are depleted. This phenomenon provides strong evidence that there are intrinsic differences in the metabolism of fat cells from different depots, or more specifically, altered responsiveness or sensitivity to cortisol. The ability of high concentrations of locally-produced cortisol to specifically increase visceral adipocyte was elegantly demonstrated by a recent study from Flier's group[6]. Overexpression of 11-beta-hydroxysteroid dehydrogenase in adipose tissue under the control of the aP2 promoter lead to the development of obesity with a specific increase in the size of mesenteric fat pads. It is interesting to note that this result contrasts with studies in which hypercortisolaemia is induced by adminstration of exogenous glucocorticoid or general stress, when catabolic effects and lower body weights are often observed[7,8]. This model therefore provides strong evidence that local metabolism of glucocorticoids is an important determinant of fat distribution.

Chronic hyperinsulinaemia and adipocyte metabolism

A number of components of the hormonal and paracrine milieu associated with obesity are thought to contribute to the alterations in adipocyte metabolism associated with the obese state. As judged by studies of adipose tissue or adipocytes in long-term culture *in vitro*, chronic hyperinsulinaemia

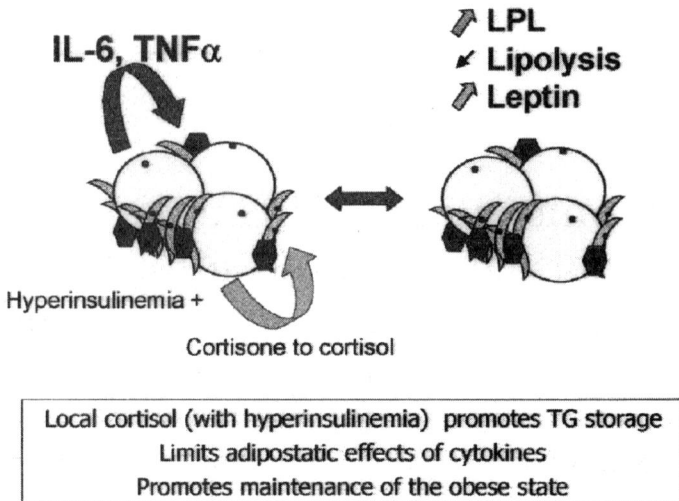

IL-6, TNFα

↗ LPL
↙ Lipolysis
↗ Leptin

Hyperinsulinemia +

Cortisone to cortisol

Local cortisol (with hyperinsulinemia) promotes TG storage
Limits adipostatic effects of cytokines
Promotes maintenance of the obese state

Fig. 1. Interactions of hormone and paracrine effects on fat cell size in obesity.

increases basal lipolytic rate, as measured by glycerol release. This effect is distinct from the acute antilipolytic effect of insulin[9,10]. The mechanism involves an increase in the expression of hormone sensitive lipase[10].

The effect chronic insulin to increase lipolysis may be mediated in part by insulin-induced increases in cytokine production. McTernan et al.[11] found that culture of isolated adipocytes with very high concentration of insulin increased tumour necrosis factor-α (TNF) secretion. Consistent with this observation, we find that prior culture of adipose tissue fragments from obese subjects for 7 days increases TNF release (unpublished observation). In 3T3-L1 adipocytes, chronic insulin also increases lipolysis. However, the time course of TNF and insulin stimulation of lipolysis differs. TNF, but not insulin, increases FA as well as glycerol release[12] because insulin also stimulated re-esterification.

Chronic culture with insulin also increases the production of interleukin-6 (IL6) by newly-differentia-tion human adipocytes in primary culture[13] and in cultured adipose tissue fragments (unpublished observation). We[14] and others[15] find that IL6 is lipolytic in human omental and subcutaneous adipose tissue. Thus, via a paracrine mechanism, IL6 may also contribute to the lipolytic action of insulin on adipose tissue.

Glucocorticoids and fat cell metabolism in obesity

Balancing the lipolytic effect of chronically high insulin levels, chronic exposure to cortisol may restrain basal lipolysis. Consistent with early report of Smith, Ottoson reported that culture of subcu-taneous human adipose tissue with cortisol (1 μM) in the presence of insulin (7 nM) decreased basal lipolysis and also decreased its' sensitivity to catecholamine stimulation[16]. Our laboratory finds that culture with 25 nM dexamethasone also decreases lipolysis during culture in the absence or presence of insulin (Wang, Greenberg and Fried, unpublished observation). Because studies of Ottosson, as well as our own, were carried out on tissue fragments, it cannot be determined whether the effects of glucocorticoids and insulin on lipolysis are directly on the adipocyte. The suppressive effect of gluco-corticoids on IL6 production[17] may also play a role. In contrast with these in vitro studies, the effects of hypercortisolaemia on lipolysis is controversial[18–20]. Adipocytes from patients with Cushings show impaired lipolytic responses to catecholamines[21]. The time of exposure, dose, and in vivo factors are likely to explain these discrepancies.

Glucocorticoids also promote triglyceride storage in adipocytes by increasing the activity of lipoprotein lipase (LPL), the enzyme that hydrolyses circulating triglycerides to fatty acids at the surface of the capillary endothelium[22]. In omental adipose tissue, culture with dexamethasone alone increases LPL activity and mRNA by about twofold, whereas in subcutaneous adipose tissue it has no effect. The increases responsiveness of omental adipose tissue to glucocorticoids is predicted by the higher con-centration of glucocorticoid receptors in this depot[23]. Surprisingly, however, we found that omental adipose tissue is less sensitive to the ability of dexamethasone to increase LPL activity in the presence of insulin (i.e. the dose-response curve was right-shifted)[22]. This finding suggested some desensitization of the glucocorticoid signaling system in omental adipose tissues. A possible explanation for this observation comes from new observations that human adipose tissue express 11-beta hydroxysteroid dehydrogenase. *In vivo*, this enzyme acts as reductase, converting inactive cortisone to cortisol[24]. The activity of HSD is higher in cultures of stromal cells derived from omental than subcutaneous abdominal adipose tissue[24], and our preliminary data show that higher omental HSD reductase activity in omental compared to subcutaneous adipose tissue cultured with insulin and dexamethasone. Thus, omental adipocytes may be exposed to chronically higher concentrations of cortisol. Since the maximal responsiveness of LPL to glucocorticoid is not decreased, local cortisol production in omental adipose tissue would be predicted to promote the expansion of fat cells in this depot.

Chronic effects of glucocorticoids and insulin on adipocyte glucose metabolism and insulin action

Addition of high concentrations of glucocorticoids to cultured adipocytes in the absence of insulin decreases glucose transport and induces insulin resistance[25]. However, in cultures of rat adipocytes, a permissive concentration of glucocorticoid is necessary for insulin to increase to increase the level of expression of the insulin-sensitive glucose transporter, GLUT4, gene[26]. This allows the cells to remain acutely responsive to the ability of insulin to increase glucose transport. Consistent with this observation in rat adipocytes, we find that culture of human adipose tissue with the combination of insulin and dexamethasone best maintains the ability of fat cells to respond to insulin with an increase in glucose metabolism[27]. Similar results were reported Cigolini and Smith[28], who also underlined the key importance of the insulin to glucocorticoid ratio in determining the metabolic effect of glucocorticosteroids, i.e. high doses can be catabolic while physiological doses promote fat deposition.

Insulin and glucocorticoid effects on adipose protein synthesis

Chronically high levels of insulin also produce a general increase in protein synthesis within adipose tissue, while dexamethasone has a suppressive effect[27]. This effect of insulin on general protein synthesis may contribute to the stimulatory effect of this hormone on the expression of many proteins. However, our recent studies show that relative rates of leptin biosynthesis are increased by prior culture with insulin for 24 h[29]. The insulin-induced increase in leptin synthesis appears to occurs without an increase in leptin mRNA levels, suggesting a translational effect. Bradley and Cheatham[30] also found that insulin increased leptin release independent of an increase in leptin RNA, although they did not directly measure relative rates of leptin synthesis in their experiments. In contrast to the effect of insulin on leptin synthesis, the effect of chronic insulin on LPL activity and relative rates of biosynthesis occur in parallel to an increase in LPL mRNA, i.e. a pre-translational effect[22]. Thus, it appears that chronic insulin may increase relative rates of synthesis of a subset of adipocyte genes. The mechanisms involved merit further investigation.

Acknowledgements: Our work was supported by NIH RO1 DK52398, and grants from Merck, Inc.

References

1. Hissin PJ, Foley JE, Wardzala LJ, Karnieli E, Simpson IA, Salans LB *et al.* Mechanism of insulin-resistant glucose transport activity in the enlarged adipose cell of the aged, obese rat. *J Clin Invest* 1982; 70(4): 780–90.

2. Digirolamo M, Howe MD, Esposito J, Thurman L, Owens JL. Metabolic patterns and insulin responsiveness of enlarging fat cells. *J Lipid Res* 1974; 15(4): 332–8.

3. Kashiwagi A, Verso MA, Andrews J, Vasquez B, Reaven G, Foley JE. *In vitro* insulin resistance of human adipocytes isolated from subjects with noninsulin-dependent diabetes mellitus. *J Clin Invest* 1983; 72(4): 1246–54.

4. Marin P, Oden B, Bjorntorp P. Assimilation and mobilization of triglycerides in subcutaneous abdominal and femoral adipose tissue *in vivo* in men: effects of androgens. *J Clin Endocrinol Metab* 1995; 80(1): 239–43.

5. Virtanen KA, Lonnroth P, Parkkola R, Peltoniemi P, Asola M, Viljanen T *et al.* Glucose uptake and perfusion in subcutaneous and visceral adipose tissue during insulin stimulation in nonobese and obese humans. *J Clin Endocrinol Metab* 2002; 87(8): 3902–10.

6. Masuzaki H, Paterson J, Shinyama H, Morton NM, Mullins JJ, Seckl JR *et al.* A transgenic model of viseral obesity and the metabolic syndrome. *Science* 2001; 294: 2166–70.

7. King BM, Zansler CA, Tatford AC, III, Neville KL, Sam H, Kass JM *et al.* Level of corticosterone replacement determines body weight gain in adrenalectomized rats with VMH lesions. *Physiol Behav* 1993; 54(6): 1187–90.

8. Rebuffé-Scrive M, Walsh UA, McEwen B, Rodin J. Effect of chronic stress and exogenous glucocorticoids on regional fat distribution and metabolism. *Physiol Behav* 1992; 52(3): 583–90.

9. Smith U, Jacobsson B. Studies of human adipose tissue in culture. II. Effects of insulin and of medium glucose on lipolysis and cell size. *Anat Rec* 1973; 176(2): 181–3.

10. Botion LM, Green A. Long-term regulation of lipolysis and hormone-sensitive lipase by insulin and glucose. *Diabetes* 1999; 48(9): 1691–7.

11. McTernan PG, Harte AL, Anderson LA, Green A, Smith SA, Holder JC *et al.* Insulin and rosiglitazone regulation of lipolysis and lipogenesis in human adipose tissue *in vitro*. *Diabetes* 2002; 51(5): 1493–8.

12. Rosenstock M, Greenberg AS, Rudich A. Distinct long-term regulation of glycerol and non-esterified fatty acid release by insulin and TNF-alpha in 3T3-L1 adipocytes. *Diabetologia* 2001; 44(1): 55–62.

13. Vicennati V, Vottero A, Friedman C, Papanicolaou DA. Hormonal regulation of interleukin-6 production in human adipocytes. *Int J Obes Relat Metab Disord* 2002; 26(7): 905–11.

14. Trujillo M, Sullivan S, Greenberg A, Fried SK. Interleukin-6 regulates human adipose tissue lipolysis and leptin production. *Diabetes* 2002.

15. Path G, Bornstein SR, Gurniak M, Chrousos GP, Scherbaum WA, Hauner H. Human breast adipocytes express interleukin-6 (IL-6) and its receptor system: increased IL-6 production by beta-adrenergic activation and effects of IL-6 on adipocyte function. *J Clin Endocrinol Metab* 2001; 86(5): 2281–8.

16. Ottosson M, Lonnroth P, Bjorntorp P, Eden S. Effects of cortisol and growth hormone on lipolysis in human adipose tissue. *J Clin Endocrinol Metab* 2000; 85(2): 799–803.

17. Fried SK, Bunkin DA, Greenberg AS. Omental and subcutaneous adipose tissues of obese subjects release interleukin-6: depot difference and regulation by glucocorticoid. *J Clin Endocrinol Metab* 1998; 83(3): 847–50.

18. Samra JS, Clark ML, Humphreys SM, Macdonald IA, Matthews DR, Frayn KN. Effects of morning rise in cortisol concentration on regulation of lipolysis in subcutaneous adipose tissue. *Am J Physiol* 1996; 271(6 Pt 1): E996–E1002.

19. Samra JS, Clark ML, Humphreys SM, Macdonald IA, Frayn KN. Regulation of lipid metabolism in adipose tissue during early starvation. *Am J Physiol* 1996; 271(3 Pt 1): E541–E546.

20. Djurhuus CB, Gravholt CH, Nielsen S, Mengel A, Christiansen JS, Schmitz OE *et al.* Effects of cortisol on lipolysis and regional interstitial glycerol levels in humans. *Am J Physiol Endocrinol Metab* 2002; 283(1): E172–E177.

21. Rebuffé-Scrive M, Krotkiewski M, Elfverson J, Bjorntorp P. Muscle and adipose tissue morphology and metabolism in Cushing's syndrome. *J Clin Endocrinol Metab* 1988; 67(6): 1122–8.

22. Fried SK, Russell CD, Grauso NL, Brolin RE. Lipoprotein lipase regulation by insulin and glucocorticoid in subcutaneous and omental adipose tissues of obese women and men. *J Clin Invest* 1993; 92(5): 2191–8.

23. Rebuffé-Scrive M, Lundholm K, Bjorntorp P. Glucocorticoid hormone binding to human adipose tissue. *Eur J Clin Invest* 1985; 15(5): 267–71.

24. Bujalska IJ, Kumar S, Stewart PM. Does central obesity reflect 'Cushing's disease of the omentum'? *Lancet* 1997; 349(9060): 1210–3.

25. Sakoda H, Ogihara T, Anai M, Funaki M, Inukai K, Katagiri H *et al.* Dexamethasone-induced insulin resistance in 3T3-L1 adipocytes is due to inhibition of glucose transport rather than insulin signal transduction. *Diabetes* 2000; 49(10): 1700–8.

26. Hajduch E, Hainault I, Meunier C, Jardel C, Hainque B, Guerre-Millo M *et al.* Regulation of glucose transporters in cultured rat adipocytes: synergistic effect of insulin and dexamethasone on GLUT4 gene expression through promoter activation. *Endocrinology* 1995; 136(11): 4782–9.

27. Appel B, Fried SK. Effects of insulin and dexamethasone on lipoprotein lipase in human adipose tissue. *Am J Physiol* 1992; 262(5 Pt 1): E695–E699.

28. Cigolini M, Smith U. Human adipose tissue in culture. VIII. Studies on the insulin-antagonistic effect of glucocorticoids. *Metabolism* 1979; 28(5): 502–10.

29. Wang Y, Greenberg A, Fried SK. Regulation of perilipin expression in obesity. *Diabetes* 2001.

30. Bradley RL, Cheatham B. Regulation of ob gene expression and leptin secretion by insulin and dexamethasone in rat adipocytes. *Diabetes* 1999; 48(2): 272–8.

Progress in Obesity Research: 9. Edited by *Geraldo Medeiros-Neto, Alfredo Halpern and Claude Bouchard*
©2003 John Libbey Eurotext Ltd, pp. 201–205.

CHAPTER 42

Anatomy of brown adipose tissue: the harlequin concept

Saverio Cinti, Raffaella Cancello, Maria Cristina Zingaretti, Enzo Ceresi, Rita De Matteis, Antonio Giordano, Jean Himms-Hagen and Daniel Ricquier

Institute of Normal Human Morphology, Faculty of Medicine, University of Ancona, Italy (SC,RC,MCZ,EC,RDeM,AG); Department of Biochemistry, Microbiology and Immunology, Faculty of Medicine, University of Ottawa, Canada (JHH); Centre de Recherche sur l'Endocrinologie Moléculaire et le Développement, Centre National de la Recherche Scientifique, Meudon, France (DR)
[e-mail: cinti@univpm.it]

Introduction

In all mammals (humans included) white and brown adipocytes are organized in a multidepot organ called the adipose organ. The adipose organ is composed of two main subcutaneous depots (anterior and posterior) and by several visceral depots. All depots are composed by two citotypes: white and brown adipocytes. The vascular tree is much more dense of capillaries in the areas composed by brown adipose tissue (BAT). The nerves contain different types of fibres of which the most represented at parenchymal level are the noradrenergic ones[1].

The morphology of white and brown adipocytes is quite different: lipids are organized in a unique droplet in white ('unilocular') and in many droplets in brown ('multilocular') adipocytes[1]. The main function of white adipocytes is to store highly energetic molecules in order to provide fuel (free fatty acids) to all other cells of the organism 24 h a day. White adipose tissue also secretes many other factors that affect the metabolism of the whole organism[2]. Brown adipocytes have a completely different functional role in the adipose organ: thermogenesis. This activity is mediated by a specific mitochondrial protein: UCP1[3]. The signals for brown adipocyte activation are cold and diet that induce activation of the sympathetic nervous system whose neurons of the sympathetic chain directly reach brown adipocytes in the adipose organ[4]. Noradrenaline activates ß3-adrenoceptors that induce the cascade of cell signalling to produce heat[5]. This activity of brown adipose tissue influences the eating behaviour and the energy balance, and transgenic mice lacking brown adipose tissue become obese[6]. Furthermore mice lacking all beta adrenergic receptors become massively obese under high fat diet in absence of any change of their eating behaviour and physical activity[7]. Of note, the mechanism responsible for this kind of obesity appears to be uncoupled from heat production because transgenic mice lacking UCP1 are cold sensitive but not obese[8]; on the other hand transgenic mice expressing UCP1 in white adipose tissue are resistant to obesity[9]. When brown adipose tissue is not adrenergically stimulated gradually converts into white adipose tissue[1]. The adipose organ is composed of subcutaneous and visceral depots all containing both white and brown adipocytes. The relative percentage of white and brown adipocytes in the organ is variable depending on strain, age, sex, environmental and nutritional conditions[10]. Genetically obese and diabetic rats as well as diet-induced obese rats have been successfully treated with ß3-adrenoceptor agonists and such treatment was accompanied by the appearance of brown adipose tissue in white depots[11]. We recently showed that white adipocytes can transdifferentiate into multilocular adipocytes in rats treated with the ß3-adrenoceptor agonist CL316,243[12].

Therefore, considering all together, and mainly these recently demonstrated phenomena of reciprocal transdifferentiation between white and brown adipocytes into the adipose organ, any functional characteristic of brown adipocytes physiology can be relevant for the whole functional activity of the adipose organ and consequently for the physiopathology of the obesity. Other proteins, called UCP2 and UCP3, with high homology to the UCP1, have been discovered. UCP2 and -3 are found in BAT as well as in many other mammalian tissues, but UCP1 is exclusively expressed in BAT[13-15]. Before the identification of UCP2 and UCP3 proteins, non-uniform staining of brown adipocytes has been reported by an immunohistochemical study with a rabbit antiserum against rat UCP, suggesting cellular heterogeneity of brown adipocytes in BAT[16]. To better understand this phenomenon, we studied by IHC the expression of UCP1 protein in animals exposed to different thermogenic stimuli using a polyclonal antibody specific for UCP1 that did not cross react with UCP2 and UCP3[17]. To verify if this non-homogeneous pattern of expression is due to a real non-homogeneous expression of the gene, we studied the *in situ* expression of the UCP1 mRNA in serial sections obtained from the same animals and we quantified the mitochondrial UCP1 expression at the ultrastructural level, by immunogold staining (IGS). Most of the results presented here have been recently published[18].

Materials and methods

Male 6-week-old Sprague–Dawley rats were acclimated to cold (4 °C for 20 h, acute stimulus; 4 °C for 2 weeks, chronic stimulus) and warm (28 °C for 2 weeks). The specific ß3-adrenoceptor pharmacological stimulus consisted of CL316,243 in saline solution (daily dose 1 mg/kg). Under anaesthesia rats were transcardially perfused with 4 per cent paraformaldehyde in 0.1 M phosphate buffer (PB), pH 7.4. Interscapular BAT, liver, kidney, spleen, skeletal muscle, and rat foetal liver were dissected, dehydrated, and paraffin-embedded. These tissues were used for tests of antibody specificity.

BAT sections were processed for immunohistochemistry (IHC) with ABC method using a polyclonal anti-rat UCP1 antibody raised in sheep diluted 1 : 12000[19] and, only for the acute cold stimulus group, with a polyclonal anti-rat inducible isoform of heme oxygenase 1 (HO1) anti-body raised in rabbit diluted 1 : 200 (Stress Gen Biotechnologies; Victoria, BC, Canada). Human BAT was processed for IHC with the same above mentioned anti-rat UCP1 antibody and with a monoclonal anti-human ß3-adrenoceptor antibody[20] diluted 1 : 1500. UCP1 specificity was tested at the same dilution on tissues expressing the highest levels of UCP2 (skeletal muscle, kidney, spleen, foetal liver)[13,14] and UCP3 (skeletal muscle)[15]. All the tissues resulted negative.

For electron microscopy tissue fragments were fixed in 2 per cent glutaraldehyde and 2 per cent paraformaldehyde in 0.1 M PB, pH 7.4, and postfixed in 1 per cent OsO4, dehydrated in ethanol, and embedded in an Epon–Araldite mixture, for the immoelectron microscopy grids were incubated with sheep anti-rat UCP1, diluted 1 : 400.

For morphometric analysis, 20 adjacent cells were randomly selected for each animal of the two groups, in total 60 cells for experimental group. Image analysis of electron micrographs was performed at a final magnification of 11,270 with a Kontron KS100 image analyser. Means were compared by two-way ANOVA.

For *in situ* hybridization (ISH) tests, animals were perfused in 4 per cent paraformaldehyde diluted in 1 x PBS; the same tissues indicated above (animal and tissue section) were dissected and paraffin-embedded. The probe (800-bp UCP1 cDNA fragment) was previously labelled by an RNA labelling kit. Transcription was performed for at least 2 h at 37 °C. See[18] for more details.

Results and discussion

The following results were obtained with specific anti-rat UCP1 and HO1 antibodies and rat UCP1 mRNA antisense riboprobes. No cross reactions with UCP2 (in liver, kidney, skeletal muscle, and foetal liver) and UCP3 (skeletal muscle) were observed by these techniques.

In BAT of cold exposed animals (acute cold-stressed) as well as in animals treated with the ß3-adrenoceptor agonist CL 316,243 electron microscopy revealed a uniform population of brown adipocytes with cytoplasm rich in well-developed mitochondria and few small lipid droplets (Fig. 1). UCP1 was expressed at the immunohistochemistry (IHC) level with different intensities of positivity in adjacent brown adipocytes. Adipocytes strongly positive, nearly completely negative, or weakly positive were clearly observed. This IHC pattern was previously defined as the 'harlequin effect' in a preliminary report by our team[21] (Fig. 2). The harlequin pattern was detectable in each lobule of each acute cold-stressed animal. UCP1 mRNA expression had a positivity pattern very similar to that of the protein IHC localization described above. Some cells also showed nuclear positivity, with or without cytoplasmic staining (Fig. 2). The same harlequin pattern was observed in brown adipose tissue of two patients suffering for phaeochromocytoma. Of note, the same brown adipose tissue of these patients showed an harlequin pattern of expression also for the ß3-adrenoceptors (Fig 2). Unfortunately, the antibodies used for the human tissues did not cross reacted with the murine antigens therefore the β3-adrenoceptor distribution at the parenchymal level in BAT of rats or mice was not studied, and we cannot exclude

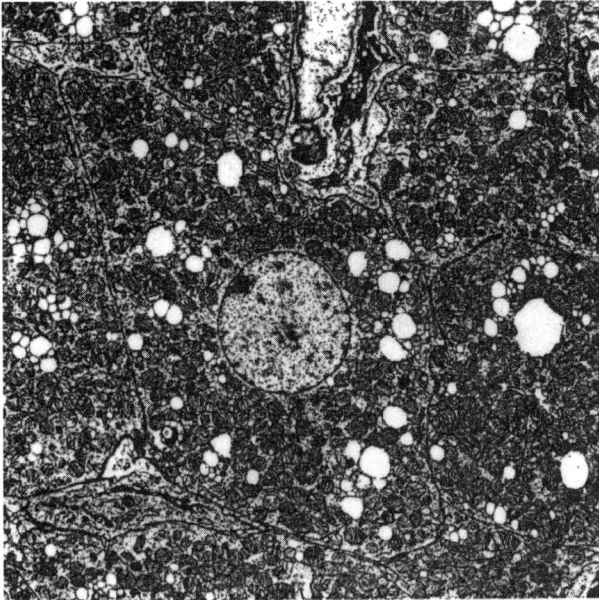

Fig. 1. Electron microscopy of brown adipose tissue of a rat treated with the ß₃ adrenoceptor agonist CL 316,243. The tissue ultrastructure was very similar to that of brown adipose tissue of acute cold exposed animals. Note the homogeneous aspect of the adipocytes. The cytoplasm is rich of well differentiated mitochondria and show several small lipid droplets (2000 x).

that a non-homogeneous distribution or down regulation of this receptor could be responsible, at least in part, for the phenomenon.

BAT of chronically cold-stressed animals was hypertrophic. UCP1 was weakly expressed at IHC level by all brown adipocytes of BAT, and only some lobules showed the harlequin effect. *In situ* hybridization revealed a UCP1 mRNA expression pattern similar to the IHC positivity.

After 7 days of CL316,243 treatment, the harlequin phenomenon was detectable in wide areas of BAT lobules, showing a pattern similar to that described for acute cold-stressed rats.

The environmental temperature of 28 °C is very close to thermoneutrality for rats. As a consequence, interscapular brown adipocyte morphology was greatly modified in these animals, mainly by a higher lipid accumulation at the cytoplasmic level. Mitochondria were numerous in all multilocular adipocytes but showed a lower density of cristae than those observed in cold or ß3-adrenoceptor-stimulated animals. UCP1 immunostaining, in BAT of these warm-acclimated rats, was weak and the harlequin phenomenon was not visible because strongly positive adipocytes were absent . UCP1 mRNA expression was not detectable.

Expression of UCP1 protein and mRNA was studied in serial sections only in BAT with a clear and diffuse harlequin pattern (i.e. acute cold-stressed and CL316,243-treated animals). Strongly immunoreactive cells stained positive for UCP1 protein and for the UCP1mRNA , but brown adipocytes strongly positive for UCP1 protein and negative for the UCP1 mRNA, as well as negative for both of them, were also found. Multilocular cells positive for the UCP1 mRNA and negative for UCP1 protein were not observed. UCP1 protein expression obtained with the IGS method was performed only in the experimental conditions in which the harlequin pattern was clear and diffuse in the tissue (acute cold and CL316,243) because only a restricted area of the tissue can be examined with this technique. Indeed, this technique aimed to compare the ultrastructure of adjacent adipocytes with different expression of UCP1. The numbers of UCP1/gold particles in mitochondria of brown adipocytes were significantly different in adjacent adipocytes. Comparison of the ultrastructure between cells with significantly different UCP1 expression showed no differences in mitochondrial numerical density and area.

An increase in UCP1 mRNA and protein in adrenergically stimulated BAT is well known[22–24]. Our data, showing the overlapping distribution pattern observed for UCP1 mRNA and protein, led us to postulate that the harlequin phenomenon could be the result of an alternative UCP1 gene activation and protein expression in neighbouring brown adipocytes. The most common finding in serial sections of cells positive for the protein and mRNA, or only for the protein, is in keeping with the longer lifespan of the protein and the tight correlation of UCP1 and its messenger production in BAT[25]. Furthermore, it has been shown that cold selectively destabilizes the mRNA for UCP1[24].

The absence of the harlequin phenomenon in non stimulated animals (warm-acclimated) shows a tight correlation with the very low level of activation of the UCP1 gene in brown adipocytes studied by the ISH technique. The distribution of parenchymal nerve fibres in IBAT of small mammals is dependent on the environmental temperature[26], and the norepinephrine concentration in this tissue is variable in different lobules[27].

However, the harlequin phenomenon is not due to these factors. In fact, it is also clearly evident in pharmacologically treated animals in which the adrenergic stimulus is independent of the distribution of nerve fibres. The reduction of the heterogeneous positivity pattern in chronic cold-stimulated

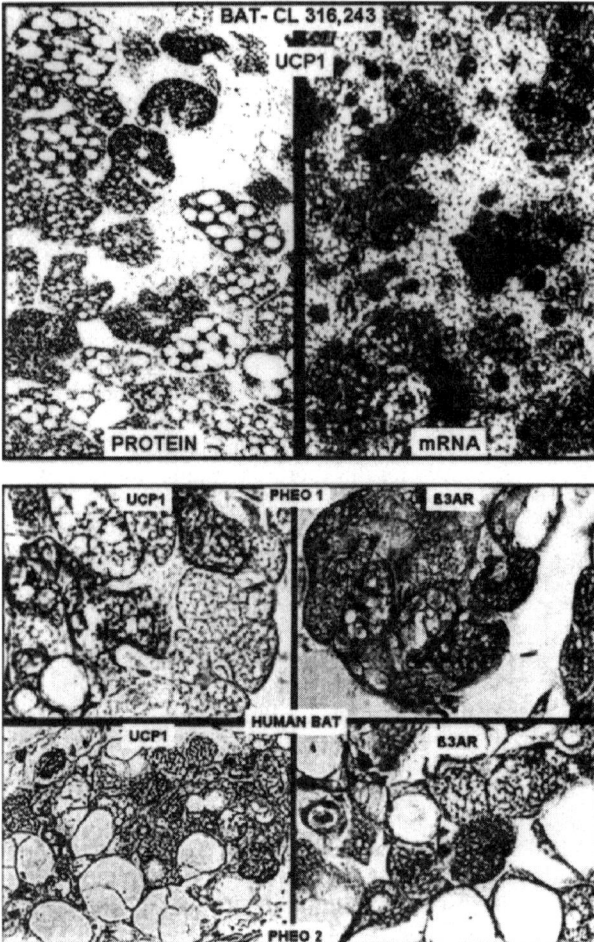

Fig. 2. Harlequin pattern. BAT-CL 316,243 UCP1: brown adipose tissue of a rat treated with the ß3 adrenoceptor agonist CL 316,243. On the left panel (protein) is shown the UCP1 immunoreactivity, in the right panel (mRNA) is shown the gene expression by *in situ* hybridization. Similar results were obtained in acute-cold treated animals (100x). The lower four panels show brown adipose tissue from two patients (pheo1 and pheo2) suffering for pheocromocytoma. In the left panels (UCP1) the immunoreactivity for UCP1 is shown. In the right panels the immunoreactivity for the ß3 adrenoceptor is shown.
In all panels is visible the different staining of neighbouring brown adipocytes (harlequin pattern) (100 x, lower left panel 20 x).

animals could be due to the hyperplasia of brown adipocytes that occurs in this condition[3] and suggests that an increased number of brown adipocytes would not require a maximal activation of each adipocyte. A possible relationship between cells highly positive for UCP1 and proximity to blood vessels can be excluded on the basis of the distribution of capillaries among brown adipocytes. In fact, every single cell is reached by at least one capillary in the brown adipose tissue[1].

When brown adipocytes are stimulated by norepinephrine, the rapid induction of UCP1 uncouples oxidative phosphorylation with a concomitant increase in metabolic rate and fat utilization. Increased free radical generation due to increased fatty acid oxidation, relative hypoxaemia, and heat production subjects brown adipocytes to metabolic stress. As a consequence, stimulated brown adipocytes produce different heat-shock proteins[22] and, specifically, the HO1 (also known as HSP32)[28]. HO1 expression increases in BAT of acute cold-stressed rats and, accordingly, norepinephrine up regulates its production in cultured brown adipocytes. Immunohistochemistry with anti-HO1 antibodies performed on brown fat of cold-exposed rats produces a harlequin pattern of staining very similar to that observed for UCP1 and UCP1 mRNA. Furthermore, the presence of brown adipocytes expressing both UCP1 and HO1 proteins in activated BAT suggests a simultaneous and/or induced activation of the two genes: HO1 protein and its by-products could be involved in the cell and tissue protection mechanisms triggered by heat produced by activated brown adipocytes. Of note, some nuclei of brown adipocytes also contain HO1, and their number increases after cold exposure[28].

Taken together, our observations suggest that the immunohistochemical 'harlequin' pattern is a true functional phenomenon. This alternative functional recruitment of noradrenergic-stimulated brown adipocytes could be a protective mechanism to avoid metabolic- and heat-production-dependent damage in activated cells, mainly under conditions of acute noradrenergic stress that probably require maximal heat production for each brown adipocyte.

References

1. Cinti S. *The adipose organ*. Milan: Kurtis, 1999.

2. Zhang YY, Proenca R, Maffei M, Barone M, Leopold L, Friedman JM. Positional cloning of the mouse obese gene and its human homologue. *Nature* 1994; 372: 425–32.

3. Himms–Hagen J, Ricquier D. Brown adipose tissue. *In handbook of obesity*, GA Bray, C Bouchard, WPT James (eds), pp. 415–41. New York: Marcel Dekker. 1998.

4. Girardier L, Seydoux J. Neural control of brown adipose tissue. In: *Brown adipose tissue*, P Trayhurn, DG Nicholls (eds), pp. 122–51. London: Edward Arnold, 1986.

5. Strosberg AD, Pietri-Rouxel F. Function and regulation of the beta 3-adrenoceptor. *Trends Pharmacol Sci* 1996; 17: 373–81.

6. Lowell BB, Susulic V, Hamann A *et al*. Development of obesity in transgenic mice after genetic ablation of brown adipose tissue. *Nature* 1993; 366: 740–2.

7. Bachman ES, Dhillon H, Zhang C-Y, Cinti S, Bianco AC, Kobilka BK, Lowell BB. βAR signaling required for diet-induced thermogenesis and obesity resistance. *Science* 2002; 297: 843–5.

8. Enerback S, Jacobsson A, Simpson EM, Guerra C, Yamashita H, Harper ME, Kozak LP. Mice lacking mitochondrial uncoupling protein are cold-sensitive but not obese. *Nature* 1997; 387: 90–4.

9. Kopecky J, Clarke J, Enerback B, Spiegelman B, Kozak LP. Ectopic expression of the mitochondrial uncoupling protein gene from the aP2 gene promoter prevents genetic obesity. *J Clin Inv* 1995; 96: 2914–23.

10. Cousin B, Cinti S, Morroni M *et al*. Occurrence of brown adipocytes in rat white adipose tissue: molecular and morphological characterization. *J Cell Sci* 1992; 103: 931–42.

11. Ghorbani M, Claus TH, Himms-Hagen J. Hypertrophy of brown adipocytes in brown and white adipose tissues and reversal of diet-induced obesity in rats treated with a β3-adrenoceptor agonist. *Biochem Pharmacol* 1997; 54: 121–31.

12. Himms-Hagen J, Melnyk A, Zingaretti MC, Ceresi E, Barbatelli G, Cinti S. Multilocular fat cells in WAT of CL-316243-trated rats derive directly from white adipocytes. *Am J Physiol Cell Physiol* 2000; 279: C670–C681.

13. Boss O, Samec S, Dulloo A, Seydoux J, Muzzin P, Giacobino JP. Tissue dependent upregulation of rat uncoupling protein-2 expression in response to fasting or cold. *FEBS Letters* 1997; 412: 111–4.

14. Fleury C, Neverova M, Collins S, Raimbault S, Champigny O, Levi Meyrueis C, *et al*. Uncoupling protein-2: a novel gene linked to obesity and hyperinsulinemia. *Nature Genet* 1997; 15: 269–72.

15. Vidal–Puig A, Solanes G, Grujic D, Flier JS, Lowell BB. UCP3, an uncoupling protein homologue expressed in skeletal muscle and brown adipose tissue. *Biochem Biophys Res Commun* 1997; 235: 79–82.

16. Cadrin M, Tolszczuk M, Guy J, Pelletier G, Freeman KB, Bukowiecki LJ. Immunohistochemical identification of the uncoupling protein in rat brown adipose tissue. *J Histochem Cytochem* 1985; 33: 150–4.

17. Pecqueur C, Alves–Guerra MC, Gelly C, Levi–Meyrueis C, Couplan E, Collins S *et al*. Uncoupling protein 2: *in vivo* distribution, induction upon oxidative stress and evidence for translational regulation. *J Biol Chem* 2000; 276: 8705–12.

18. Cinti S, Cancello R, Zingaretti MC, Ceresi E, De Matteis R, Giordano A *et al*. CL316,243 and cold stress induce heterogeneous expression of UCP1 mRNA and protein in rodent brown adipocytes. *J Histoch Cytochem* 2002; 50(1): 21–31.

19. Ricquier D, Barlet JP, Garel JM, Combes–George M, Dubois MP. An immunological study of the uncoupling protein of brown adipose tissue mitochondria. *Biochem J* 1983; 210: 859–66.

20. Chamberlain PD, Jennings KH, Paul F, Cordell J, Berry A, Holmes SD *et al*. The tissue distribution of the human ß3-adrenoceptor studies using a monoclonal antibody. *Int J Obes* 1999; 23: 1057–65.

21. Cinti S, De Matteis R, Zingaretti MC, Cancello R, Himms-Hagen J, Ricquier D. Harlequin secret: UCP-immunostained brown adipose tissue. *Int J Obes Relat Metab Disord* 1997; 21 (Suppl 2): S47.

22. Bouillaud F, Ricquier D, Mory G, Thibault J. Increased level of mRNA for the uncoupling protein in brown adipose tissue of rats during thermogenesis induced by cold exposure or norepi-nephrine infusion. *J Biol Chem* 1984; 25: 11583–6.

23. Ricquier D, Bouillaud F, Toumelin P, Mory G, Bazin R, Arch J, Penicaud L. Expression of uncoupling protein mRNA in thermogenic or weakly thermogenic brown adipose tissue. Evidence for a rapid beta-adrenoreceptor-mediated and transcrip-tionally regulated step during activation of thermogenesis. *J Biol Chem* 1986; 261: 13905–10.

24. Jacobsson A, Cannon B, Nedergaard J. Physiological activation of brown adipose tissue destabilizes thermogenin mRNA. *FEBS Letters* 1987; 224: 353–6.

25. Nedergaard J, Cannon B. Brown adipose tissue: development and function. In: *Fetal and neonatal physiology*, RA Polin, WW Fox (eds), pp. 478–89. London: WB Saunders; 1998.

26. De Matteis R, Ricquier D, Cinti S. TH-, NPY-, SP-, and CGRP-immunoreactive nerves in interscapular brown adipose tissue of adult rats acclimated at different temperatures: an immunohistochemical study. *J Neurocytol* 1998; 27: 877–86.

27. Foster DO, Depocas F, Zucker M. Heterogeneity of the sympathetic innervation of rat interscapular brown adipose tissue via intercostal nerves. *Can J Physiol Pharmacol* 1982; 60: 747–54.

28. Giordano A, Nisoli E, Tonello C, Cancello R, Carruba MO, Cinti S. Expression and distribution of heme oxygenase-1 and -2 in rat brown adipose tissue: the modulatory role of the noradren-ergic system. *FEBS Letters* 2000; 487: 171–5.

Progress in Obesity Research: 9. Edited by *Geraldo Medeiros-Neto, Alfredo Halpern and Claude Bouchard*
©2003 John Libbey Eurotext Ltd, pp. 206–210.

CHAPTER 43

Regulation of the UCP1 gene transcription: PPARα and RXR-dependent pathways define novel links between regulation of thermogenesis and lipid oxidation in brown adipocytes

Francesc Villarroya*, Pilar Yubero, M.José Barberà, Agatha Schlüter, Roser Iglesias and Marta Giralt

Department of Biochemistry and Molecular Biology. Universitat de Barcelona. Barcelona. Spain
[e-mail: gombau@porthos.bio.ub.es]

Introduction

The presence of UCP1 confers to brown adipose tissue its thermogenic capacity. After the discovery of UCP2 and UCP3, UCP1 remains as the only mitochondrial uncoupling protein unequivocally associated with adaptive thermogenesis in mammals. The physiological relevance of UCP1 in adult humans remains as a matter of debate due to the low amounts brown fat and UCP1 in adults. A weak UCP1 mRNA expression in white fat depots of adult humans and the association of polymorphisms of the human UCP1 gene with phenotypic features related to weight gain are recent findings to take into account in this debate[1].

The UCP1 gene is under a sensitive transcriptional regulation. It is now well established that sympathetic activity, which mediates thermogenic activation through norepinephrine interaction with β-adrenergic receptors in brown adipocytes, is a major inducer of UCP1 gene transcription in response to a cold environment or to overfeeding. However, the analysis of the transcriptional regulation of the UCP1 gene has revealed novel pathways of control which point to regulation of the thermogenic activity in response to fatty acid-related nutrients or metabolites and to a complex interaction with the noradrenergic pathway of regulation.

Functional structure of the 5' regulatory region of the UCP1 gene

The structure of the UCP1 gene in the mammalian species studied so far is similar. In rat, mouse and human the UCP1 gene is made of six exons and the introns position are essentially conserved[1]. The elements of transcriptional regulation of the UCP1 gene have been extensively studied for the rat and mouse genes and some data is available for the human gene. Transcriptional regulation of the rat UCP1 gene relies on the 5'-non-coding region. 4.5 kb upstream transcription initiation have been demonstrated to contain regulatory elements and transcription factors which control UCP1 gene transcription in response to signaling pathways that integrate cell-specificity, developmental and hormonal sensitivity of the gene[1].

Two major regulatory regions have been identified, a proximal one and an upstream enhancer of around 200pb. Transgenic mice bearing a construct containing the 211-bp enhancer region fused to 400 bp of the proximal promoter show specific transcription in brown fat and responsiveness to cold activation[2]. The proximal region of the rat or mouse UCP1 gene contains elements essential for basal promoter activity[2,3]. Moreover, it contains, close to the TATA box, a cAMP-responsive element (CRE) which is important for basal activity and norepineprine-mediated activation through protein kinase A.

Whereas CREB binds this element and mediates protein kinase A activation, c-Jun represses transcription by competing with CREB for binding this site[4]. This proximal site appears to mediate most of cAMP-dependent activation of the UCP1 gene although elements in the enhancer contribute to this effect. Upstream from the CRE, two sites mediate C/EBP-dependent regulation. C/EBPβ and C/EBPδ isoforms can bind and trans-activate the UCP1 promoter through these sites[5] and murine models 'knock-out' and 'knock-in' for C/EBPα have shown a major role for this family of transcription factors in development and differentiation-dependent expression of the UCP1 gene[6].

The upstream enhancer of the UCP1 gene is a complex region containing multiple regulatory elements, specially in response to members of the nuclear hormone receptors superfamily. Thus, at least three sites have been precisely characterized inside this enhancer region. An upstream PPAR-response element behaves as a responsive site to PPARα and to PPARγ[2] (see below). A second element consists in a retinoic acid-responsive site, able to mediate responsiveness to all-trans retinoic acid but of atypical structure as it contains RAR and RXR binding sites close to an AP1 site[9]. Finally, downstream elements in the enhancer behave as thyroid hormone response elements which could mediate the positive action of the T3 generated in brown adipocytes by deiodination of thyroxine[10]. Although less studied, major features of the transcriptional regulation of the human UCP1 gene as determined by transfection assays appear to be similar. There is also a distal enhancer region which provides responsiveness to cAMP and specially to retinoic acid[11].

PPARα-dependent activation of the UCP1 gene

A high expression of the peroxisome proliferator activated receptor α (PPARα) is characteristic feature of brown respect to white adipose tissue. This is consistent with the high capacity of lipid oxidation of brown fat and with the role of PPARα as a master transcription factor for the control of genes of lipid catabolism. Activators of PPARγ are fatty acids or hypolipidaemic drugs such as fibrates. PPARα activators induce UCP1 gene expression by activating the UCP1 gene promoter. through the PPAR-response element placed in the distal enhancer region of the UCP1 gene. The activation of the UCP1 gene by PPARα activators is enhanced by co-activators such as CBP and PPARγ-coactivator-1 (PGC-1)[8]. Acute treatment of rodents with PPARα activators induce the expression of the UCP1 gene but the extent of the effect is highly dependent on status of lipid metabolism able to provide endogenous PPARα ligand. For instance, lactating mice, in which brown adipose tissue is functionally atrophied and lipid oxidation is depressed, are highly sensitive to induce UCP1 gene expression in response to PPARα agonists[8,12]. Mice at 21 °C environment temperature, with a substantial extent of basal thermogenic and lipid oxidation activity, are much less sensitive.

Role of the PPARα-dependent pathway in thermogenic regulation

The action of norepinephrine on brown adipocytes cause a cAMP-dependent activation of hormone sensitive lipase which hydrolyses the stored triglycerides and release free fatty acids. These fatty acids, in addition to be the major substrate for thermogenesis and activators of UCP1 proton conductance activity, can act as activators of PPARα. Accordingly, cold exposure and β-adrenergic stimulation of brown adipose tissue results in activation of the PPARα pathway[13]. The upstream enhancer region of the UCP1 gene is responsive to norepineprine although it lacks a defined cAMP-responsive site. Several lines of evidence indicate that PPARα can mediate a role in this regulation and, for instance, when the PPAR-responsive element in the UCP1 is mutated, responsiveness of the UCP1 promoter is impaired[14]. Moreover, the PPARα-dependent pathway can integrate other adrenergic mediated signaling. In this sense, the co-activator PGC-1 is induced by adrenergic activation[15], it is a powerful activator of the PPARα-dependent induction of the UCP1 gene and it sensitizes the UCP1 promoter to the PPARα-ligand dependent stimulus[8]. Moreover, recent data have shown that the cAMP induction of the UCP1 gene enhancer requires p38 MAP kinase[16], a process in which PGC-1 may be involved[17] thus providing one more element for the interaction between cAMP and PPARα-mediated regulation. Finally, despite UCP1 mRNA expression is unaltered in PPARα-null mice in basal conditions, newborn mice devoid of PPARα show an impaired ability to induce UCP1 mRNA expression in response the thermic stress of birth (R. Iglesias and F. Villarroya, unpublished observations).

Phytanic acid, a novel activator of the UCP1 gene transcription, establishes a novel RXR-mediated pathway relating lipid metabolism and thermogenic activation

Phytanic acid (3,7,11,15-tetramethylhexadecanoic acid) is a phytol derivative, branched-chain fatty acid. The major sources of phytanic acid are dairy products or meat due to the high capacity of

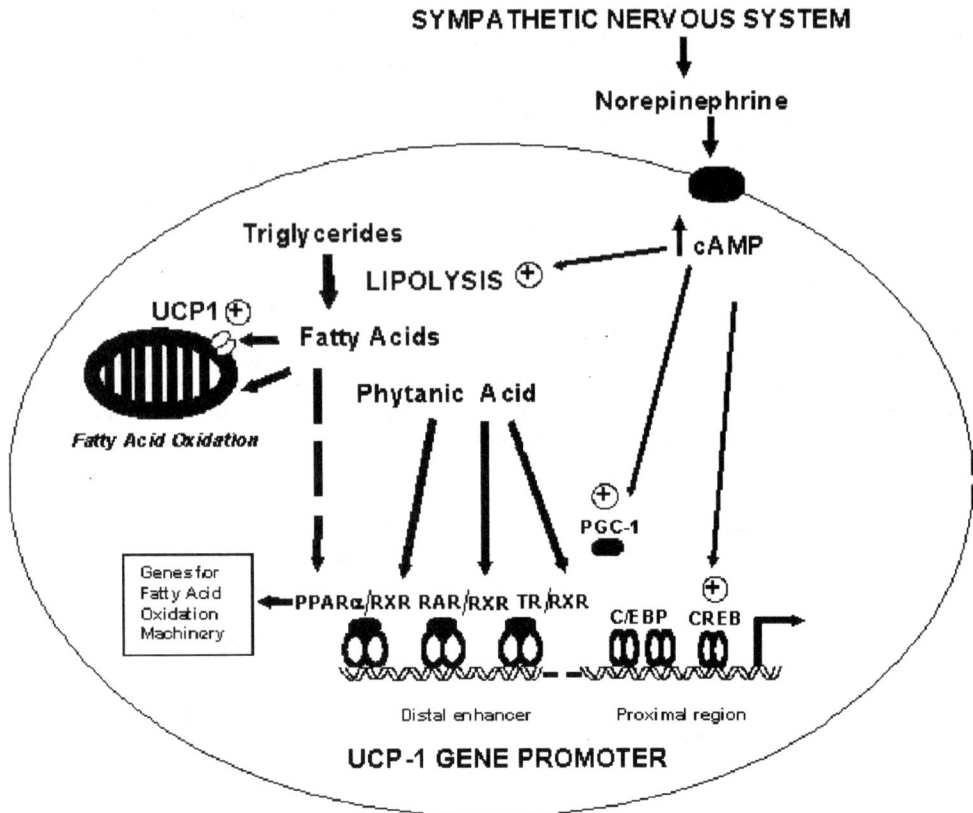

Fig. 1. Schematic representation of the action of phytanic acid and PPARα and RXR-dependent pathways of regulation of the UCP1 gene in the context of brown adipocyte thermogenic activation.

ruminants to breakdown chlorophyll and to oxidize its phytol side chain. Oxidation of phytanic acid in the body occurs in peroxisomes due to their machinery of α and β-oxidation including phytanoyl-CoA hydroxylase, a specific enzyme for the peroxisomal phytanic acid oxidation pathway[18].

Phytanic acid is a powerful activator of UCP1 gene expression[19]. It induces UCP1 gene transcription by activating three RXR-sensitive sites in the UCP1 enhancer region: the PPAR-responsive element, the retinoic acid responsive region and a thyroid responsive site (see Fig 1). All these sites bind heterodimers of nuclear hormone receptors with RXR, and phytanic acid acts additively upon these three regions. This is consistent with reports indicating that the RXR receptor can bind phytanic acid *in vitro*, with less affinity than 9-cis retinoic acid but in the range of physiological levels of phytanic acid[20]. The UCP1 gene enhancer region was known to be highly sensitive to the activation of the retinoic acid receptors RAR and RXR[21,22]. However, the physiological role of this regulatory pathway in relation to the biology of UCP1 gene expression is unknown. The action of phytanic acid, as a natural activator of RXR, can provide some answers to this issue. Circulating levels of phytanic acid in humans or rodents are in the micromolar range[18,23], close to the capacity to activate RXR, and circulating phytanic acid may influence UCP1 gene expression as a mechanism of sensing the nutritional status. However, a role of phytanic acid *in situ*, in relation to the specific thermogenic stimulus of brown fat, is also possible. Phytanic acid accumulates in brown adipose tissue fat depots as part of the stored triglycerides. When mice are suddenly exposed to a cold environment and thermogenesis is promoted, phytanic acid is released due to the activation of lipolysis, similarly to the other esterified fatty acids, and a transient appearance of high levels of free phytanic acid in the brown adipocyte is likely to occur[23]. The activation of RXR-binding sites in the UCP1 gene enhancer by phytanic acid may provide a further link between fatty acid oxidative pathways ands the requirement of enhanced UCP1 gene synthesis, in a sense similar to that reported above for the PPARα-dependent pathway.

Murine models in which to establish unequivocally the role of phytanic acid in UCP1 gene expression and brown fat thermogensis are scarce. However, mice with targeted disruption of the sterol carrier protein-2 show abnormally high levels of phytanic acid in blood, specially when fed diets rich in phytol. These mice remain lean despite becoming hyperphagic thus suggesting enhanced energy expenditure[24]. The involvement of high levels of UCP1 gene expression and brown fat activity in those mice should await further research.

Conclusions

Figure 1 shows an schematic drawing in which the novel PPARα and RXR-dependent pathways of regulation of the UCP1 gene transcription and the role of phytanic acid are integrated in the overall schema of functional regulation of the UCP1 gene. These mechanisms of regulation evidence the coordination of the regulation of UCP1 gene transcription with the overall process of lipid oxidation. Fatty acids were already known to act on brown fat thermogenesis at two levels: they provide the major fuel substrate and they activate the UCP1 proton conductance activity. Our present data point out to a third role of fatty acid derivatives as activators of UCP1 gene transcription in association with brown fat thermogenic activation.

Acknowledgements: Study supported by a grants from MECD, Spain (PM98-0188).

References

1. Ricquier D, Bouillaud F. The mitochondrial uncoupling protein: structural and genetic studies. Prog Nucleic Acid Res Mol Biol 1997; 56: 83–108.

2. Cassard-Doulcier AM, Gelly C, Fox N, Schrementi J, Raimbault S, Klaus S et al. Tissue-specific and beta-adrenergic regulation of the mitochondrial uncoupling protein gene: control by cis-acting elements in the 5'-flanking region. Mol Endocrinol 1993; 7: 497–506.

3. Kozak UC, Kopecky J, Teisinger J, Enerback S, Boyer B, Kozak LP. An upstream enhancer regulating brown-fat-specific expression of the mitochondrial uncoupling protein gene. Mol Cell Biol 1994; 14: 59–67.

4. Yubero P, Barberá MJ, Alvarez R, Viñas O, Mampel T, Iglesias R et al. Dominant negative regulation by c-Jun of transcription of the uncoupling protein-1 gene through a proximal cAMP-regulatory element: a mechanism for repressing basal and norepinephrine-induced expression of the gene before brown adipocyte differentiation. Mol Endocrinol 1998; 12: 1023–37.

5. Yubero P, Manchado C, Cassard-Doulcier AM, Mampel T, Viñas O, Iglesias R et al. CCAAT/enhancer binding proteins alpha and beta are transcriptional activators of the brown fat uncoupling protein gene promoter. Biochem Biophys Res Commun 1994; 198: 653–9.

6. Carmona MC, Iglesias R, Obregon MJ, Darlington GJ, Villarroya F, Giralt M. Mitochondrial biogenesis and thyroid status maturation in brown fat require CCAAT/enhancer-binding protein alpha. J Biol Chem 2002; 277: 21489–98.

7. Sears IB, MacGinnitie MA, Kovacs LG, Graves RA. Differentiation-dependent expression of the brown adipocyte uncoupling protein gene: regulation by peroxisome proliferator-activated receptor gamma. Mol Cell Biol 1996; 16: 3410–9.

8. Barberá MJ, Schlüter A, Pedraza N, Iglesias R, Villarroya F, Giralt M. Peroxisome proliferator-activated receptor alpha activates transcription of the brown fat uncoupling protein-1 gene. J Biol Chem 2001; 276: 1486–93.

9. Larose M, Cassard-Doulcier AM, Fleury C, Serra F, Champigny O, Bouillaud F, Ricquier D. Essential cis-acting elements in rat uncoupling protein gene are in an enhancer containing a complex retinoic acid response domain. J Biol Chem 1996; 271: 31533–42.

10. Rabelo R, Schifman A, Rubio A, Sheng X, Silva JE. Delineation of thyroid hormone-responsive sequences within a critical enhancer in the rat uncoupling protein gene. Endocrinology 1995; 136: 1003–13.

11. Gonzalez-Barroso M, Pecqueur C, Gelly C, Sanchis D, Alves-Guerra MC, Bouillaud F et al. Transcriptional activation of the human ucp1 gene in a rodent cell line. Synergism of retinoids, isoproterenol, and thiazolidinedione is mediated by a multipartite response element. J Biol Chem 2000; 275: 31722–32.

12. Pedraza N, Solanes G, Iglesias R, Vazquez M, Giralt M, Villarroya F. Differential regulation of expression of genes encoding uncoupling protein-2 and uncoupling protein-3 in brown adipose tissue during lactation in mice. Biochem J 2001; 355: 105–11.

13. Guardiola-Diaz HM, Rehnmark S, Usuda N, Albreksten T, Fetkamp D, Gustafsson JA, Alexson SE. Rat peroxisome proliferator-activated receptors and brown adipose tissue function during cold acclimatization. J Biol Chem 1999; 274: 23368–77.

14. Tai TA, Jennermann C, Brown KK, Oliver BB, MacGinnitie MA, Wilkison WO et al. Activation of the nuclear receptor peroxisome proliferator-activated receptor gamma promotes brown adipocyte differentiation. J Biol Chem 1996; 271: 29909–14.

15. Puigserver P, Wu Z, Park C, Graves R, Wright M, Spiegelman BM. A cold-inducible coactivator of nuclear receptors linked to adaptive thermogenesis. *Cell* 1998; 92: 829–39.

16. Cao W, Medvedev AV, Daniel KW, Collin S. beta-Adrenergic activation of p38 MAP kinase in adipocytes: cAMP induction of the uncoupling protein 1 (UCP1) gene requires p38 MAP kinase. *J Biol Chem* 2001; 276: 27077–82.

17. Puigserver P, Rhee J, Lin J, Wu Z, Yoon JC, Zhang CY *et al*. Cytokine stimulation of energy expenditure through p38 MAP kinase activation of PPARgamma coactivator1. *Mol Cell* 2001; 8: 971–82.

18. Verhoeven NM, Wanders RJ, Poll-The BT, Saudubray JM, Jakobs C. The metabolism of phytanic acid and pristanic acid in man: a review. *J Inherit Metab Dis* 1998; 21: 697–728.

19. Schlüter A, Barberá MJ, Iglesias R, Giralt M, Villarroya F. Phytanic acid, a novel activator of uncoupling protein-1 gene transcription and brown adipocyte differentiation. *Biochem J* 2002; 362: 61–9.

20. Lemotte PK, Keidel S, Apfel CM. Phytanic acid is a retinoid X receptor ligand. *Eur J Biochem* 1996; 236: 328–33.

21. Alvarez R, de Andrés J, Yubero P, Viñas O, Mampel T, Iglesias R *et al*. A novel regulatory pathway of brown fat thermogenesis. Retinoic acid is a transcriptional activator of the mitochondrial uncoupling protein gene. *J Biol Chem* 1995; 270: 5666–73.

22. Alvarez R, Checa ML, Brun S, Viñas O, Mampel T, Iglesias R *et al*. Both retinoic-acid-receptor and retinoid-X-receptor dependent signalling pathways mediate the induction of the brown-adipose tissue-uncoupling-protein-1 gene by retinoids. *Biochem J* 2000; 345: 91–7.

23. Schlüter A, Giralt M, Iglesias R, Villarroya F. Phytanic acid, but not pristanic acid, mediates the positive effects of phytol derivatives on brown adipocyte differentiation. *FEBS Letters* 2002; 517: 83–6.

24. Seedorf U, Raabe M, Ellinghaus P, Kannenberg F, Fobker M, Engel T *et al*. Defective peroxisomal catabolism of branched fatty acyl coenzyme A in mice lacking the sterol carrier protein-2/sterol carrier protein-x gene function. *Genes Dev* 1998; 12: 1189–201.

Progress in Obesity Research: 9. Edited by *Geraldo Medeiros-Neto, Alfredo Halpern and Claude Bouchard*
©2003 John Libbey Eurotext Ltd, pp. 211–213.

CHAPTER 44

Genetics of brown adipocyte development

Leslie P. Kozak*, Bingzhong Xue, Jong Rim, Ann Coulter and Robert Koza

Pennington Biomedical Research Center, 6400 Perkins Road, Baton Rouge, Louisiana 70808, USA
[e-mail: Kozaklp@pbrc.edu]

The two primary strategies for pharmacological intervention to reduce obesity are the development of agents that reduce food intake and those that enhance energy expenditure. This brief report will summarize the efforts to stimulate energy expenditure in our laboratory within the context of the many efforts by other laboratories around the world. At present the only established mechanism for reducing obesity by increasing energy expenditure in model organisms is through increased uncoupling of mitochondrial oxidative phosphorylation by the uncoupling proteins. Within the family of mitochondrial uncoupling proteins (UCPs,) which have been reproducibly investigated in detail, only the experiments with brown fat specific UCP1 have produced clear evidence that genetic and pharmacological manipulations to increase expression can result in reduced adiposity[1]. The genetic manipulations involve not only over-expression of transgenic mice, but also the targeted inactivation of genes that have led to unanticipated changes in transcription pathways that stimulate the brown adipocyte differentiation programme[2,3,4]. Over-expression of *Ucp3* has been achieved in the skeletal muscle of transgenic mice with a reduction in adiposity and an improvement in diet induced insulin resistance[5], but it is uncertain whether this is the result of a quasi-physiological increase in uncoupling or an increase in uncoupling that is toxic to the animal[6]. Evidence that excessive levels of uncoupling proteins can be toxic to the cell can occur even in brown adipocytes where it was found that the large increases in UCP1 in mice homozygous for a Ucp1 transgene driven by the constitutive aP2 promoter led to the death of brown adipocytes[1].

Paradoxically, most genetic manipulations or pharmacological treatments that reduce adiposity are accompanied more by an increase in UCP1 in ectopic sites rather than in interscapular brown adipocytes[7]. Based upon this observation in transgenic mice, we have speculated that the defined traditional brown fat depots, i.e. interscapular, thoracic and renal more effectively serve the regulation of body temperature while the regulation of body weight is served by those brown adipocytes diffusely distributed throughout traditional white fat depots. This interpretation is consistent with minimal effects of UCP1-deficiency on adiposity, in contrast to the cold sensitive phenotype of these animals[8]. Thus, it behoves us to focus attention on mechanisms for stimulating increases in brown adipocyte number in white fat depots. This focus is also important because of the concern that adult humans do not possess the traditional brown fat depots; rather, whatever is present in the human is diffusely localized.

Much molecular and cellular research has been done on the differentiation of the brown adipocyte and the regulation of *Ucp1* expression. Overviews of the pathways controlling expression of *Ucp1* have recently been described[7,9] and many of the same transcription and signaling pathways that act on the *Ucp1* gene are also involved in the induction of the brown adipocyte, particularly those associated with mitochondrial biogenesis. The major hormonal signal initiating the pathway is adrenergic signaling, principally through β1- and β3-adrenergic receptors. The stimulation of cAMP leads to a signaling pathway involving protein kinase A, p38 MAP kinase, Akt, and CREB[10,11]. This pathway or variations in it selects a repertoire of at least twelve transcription factors that have been shown to interact with the Ucp1 gene depending on the developmental age, physiological and hormonal responses required for diet or cold induced thermogenesis and whether the responding adipocyte is brown or white[7]. The outstanding questions associated with these mechanisms of energy expenditure that need to be answered if thermogenesis is to be a drug target for the treatment of obesity in humans are:

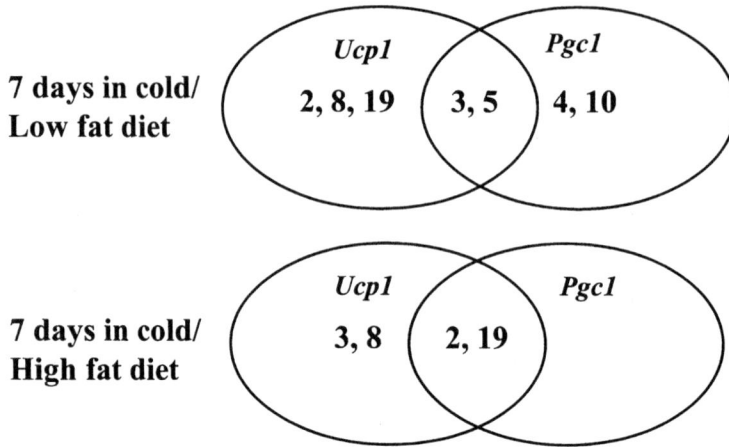

Fig. 1. Venn diagrams illustrating chromosomal locations of QTLs associated with the levels of *Ucp1* and *Pgc1* mRNA in the retroperitoneal fat depot of mice fed a low and high fat diet and exposed to the cold at 4 °C for 7 days.

1. How does the hypothalamus differentiate between dietary- and cold-induced thermogenesis?

2. If both cold exposure and diet stimulate the sympathetic nervous system, is there a qualitative or quantitative difference in signals acting on the adipocytes?

3. What is the mechanism for inducing increased numbers of brown adipocytes in white fat depots?

4. Can regulatory sites in the signaling or transcription pathway be identified that are independent of adrenergic signaling and therefore more selective for the stimulation of brown fat thermogenesis?

A genetic approach to aid in finding answers to the above questions became possible when it was discovered that inbred strains of mice varied phenotypically in the induction of brown adipocytes in traditional white fat depots[12]. These genetic studies have used quantitative trait locus (QTL) analysis to identify five genes, located on Chromosomes 2, 3, 5, 8 and 19 that control the levels of *Ucp1* mRNA in the retroperitoneal fat depot[13]. Remarkably none of these genes show variant expression in the interscapular brown fat depot. We have not analysed the QTLs in other white fat depots, but have data suggesting that some of the QTLs will also be controlling expression in these other depots. While pursuing the positional cloning of the QTLs for *Ucp1*, we have analysed the variation in expression of the *Pgc-1* (peroxisomal proliferator activated receptor coactivator) gene, because of the pivotal role played by *Pgc-1* in regulating genes associated with glucose and fat metabolism. The QTLs for *Pgc-1* overlap with those that control *Ucp1* and there is also no variation in the expression of *Pgc-1* in interscapular brown fat. This observation suggests that fundamental genetic differences exist between brown adipocytes that can be induced in white fat and those that exist in intrascapular fat.

A model that we are testing is based on the assumption that the adipocyte responding to adrenergic stimulation in the intrascapular fat depot of two month old mice is a fully differentiated brown adipocyte with all of the signaling and transcription pathways present and fully functional, whereas the adipocytes in the retroperitoneal fat must first proceed through a differentiation process similar to that of early development. How this occurs in adult white adipocytes independent of cell division is an additional interesting and important question? To determine whether this model can explain the difference in genetic variability in *Ucp1* expression between white and brown adipocytes, we have compared the early developmental pattern of expression of several transcriptional and signaling molecules associated with *Ucp1* expression in interscapular and retroperitoneal fat depots from B6 and A/J mice. No allelic difference in the expression of *Ucp1* or any other mRNA was found in intrascapular fat depots from mice between 18 days gestation and 4 months of age.

Interpreting the pattern of gene expression in retroperitoneal fat was more difficult. A large difference in the expression of *Ucp1* occurred between B6 and A/J mice that coincided with an early induction in expression that peaked at about 30 days of age and then declined to very low levels. *Pgc-1* expression also showed a developmental profile similar to *Ucp1*, although its expression remained elevated. At the peak of its expression the levels were about 30 per cent higher in A/J mice, which is much less than the four- to fivefold difference in expression observed in 2-month old mice exposed to the cold. The expression of ten other genes also showed a similar borderline difference. Only PPARα and the β3-adrenergic receptor showed large strain differences; however in the case of the β3-adrenergic receptor, it was the B6 strain that expressed higher levels. The data show that brown adipocytes in the retroperitoneal fat express allelic differences during early post-natal development when the bulk of development occurs for white fat depots. On the other hand, at no time could allelic differences be detected in the interscapular fat depot. This suggests that a fundamental difference in genetic program-ming of *Ucp1* expression exists between brown adipocytes in intrascapular fat and traditional white fat depots. With the exception of the QTL on Chromosome 8, which is located very close to the *Ucp1* structural gene, none of the other QTLs carry genes that have functions previously associated with *Ucp1* expression. The fact that the QTL on Chromosome 3 is a major locus controlling both *Ucp1* and *Pgc1* suggests very significant regulatory genes remain to be identified. Even more intriguing is the observa-tion that the significance of the QTL on Chromosome 3 for controlling *Pgc1* expression is completely lost when backcross progeny are fed a high fat diet from weaning until the two months of age when they are exposed to the cold. This suggests that Chromosome 3 is part of a pathway for stimulating energy expenditure through thermogenesis that is highly dependent on the fat composition of the diet. Although the QTL on Chromosome 3 appears particularly prominent with respect to diet-related expression of *Pgc-1* and *Ucp1*, the QTL data indicates that other genes are powerfully affected by the fat content of the diet as well. The nature of these macronutrient dietary effects on the QTLs associated with the regulation of both Ucp1 and Pgc-1 are illustrated on the Venn diagrams of Fig. 1.

References

1. Kozak LP, Harper ME. Mitochondrial uncoupling proteins in energy expenditure. *Annu Rev Nutr* 2000; 20: 339–63.

2. Cummings DE, Brandon EP, Planas JV, Motamed K, Idzerda RL, McKnight GS. Genetically lean mice result from targeted disruption of the RII beta subunit of protein kinase A [see comments]. *Nature* 1996; 382(6592): 622–6.

3. Cederberg A, Gronning LM, Ahren B, Tasken P, Carlsson P, Enerback S. FOXC2 is a winged helix gene that counteracts obesity, hypertriglceridemia, and diet-induced insulin resistance. *Cell* 2001; 106: 563–73.

4. Tsukiyama-Kohara K, Poulin F, Kohara M, DeMaria CT, Cheng A, Wu Z *et al.* Adipose tissue reduction in mice lacking the translational inhibitor 4E- BP1. *Nature Med* 2001; 7(10): 1128–32.

5. Clapham JC, Arch JR, Chapman H, Haynes A, Lister C, Moore GB *et al.* Mice overexpressing human uncoupling protein-3 in skeletal muscle are hyperphagic and lean. *Nature* 2000; 406(6794): 415–8.

6. Stuart JA, Harper JA, Brindle KM, Jekabsons MB, Brand MD. Physiological levels of mammalian uncoupling protein 2 do not uncouple yeast mitochondria. *J Biol Chem* 2001; 276(21): 18633–9.

7. Ricquier D, Kozak LP. Uncoupling proteins; In: *Handbook of obesity*, Bray GA, Bouchard C (eds), 2002 (in press).

8. Enerback S, Jacobsson A, Simpson EM, Guerra C, Yamashita H, Harper ME *et al.* Mice lacking mitochondrial uncoupling protein are cold-sensitive but not obese [see comments]. *Nature* 1997; 387(6628): 90–4.

9. Lowell BB, Spiegelman BM. Towards a molecular understanding of adaptive thermogenesis. *Nature* 2000; 404(6778): 652–60.

10. Cao W, Medvedev AV, Daniel KW, Collins S. beta -Adrenergic Activation of p38 MAP Kinase in Adipocytes. cAMP induction of the uncoupling protein 1 (UCP1) gene requires P38 MAP kinase. *J Biol Chem* 2001; 276(29): 27077–82.

11. Rim JS, Kozak LP. Regulatory motifs for CREB and Nfe2l2 transcription factors in the upstream enhancer of the mitochondrial uncoupling protein. *J Biol Chem* 2002.

12. Guerra C, Koza RA, Yamashita H, Walsh K, Kozak LP. Emergence of brown adipocytes in white fat in mice is under genetic control. Effects on body weight and adiposity. *J Clin Invest* 1998; 102(2): 412–20.

13. Koza RA, Hohmann SM, Guerra C, Rossmeisl M, Kozak LP. Synergistic gene interactions control the induction of the mitochondrial uncoupling protein (Ucp1) gene in white fat tissue. *J Biol Chem* 2000; 275(44): 34486–92.

Progress in Obesity Research: 9. Edited by *Geraldo Medeiros-Neto, Alfredo Halpern and Claude Bouchard*
©2003 John Libbey Eurotext Ltd, pp. 214–219.

CHAPTER 45

UCP1 expression in white adipose tissue and lipid metabolism

Jan Kopecký[1], Martin Rossmeisl[1], Pavel Flachs[1], Stanislav Kmoch[1], Kristina Bardová[1], Petr Brauner[1], Olga Matejková[1], Jana Šponarová[1], Tomáš Prazak[1], Michaela Thomason-Hughes[2] and Grahame Hardie[2]

[1]*Centre for Integrated Genomics, Institute of Physiology, Academy of Sciences of the Czech Republic, Vídeòská 1083, Prague 4, and Institute of Inherited Metabolic Diseases of the 1st Medical School, Charles University, Ke Karlovu 2, Prague 2, Czech Republic; and [2]Wellcome Trust Biocentre, University of Dundee, Dow Street, Dundee, DD1 5EH, UK*
[e-mail: kopecky@biomed.cas.cz]

Introduction

Many pieces of evidence suggest that metabolism of adipose tissue contributes to the control of body fat content. First, most of the candidate genes for obesity have important functions in adipocytes[1]. Second, mice that are prone or resistant to obesity were created by transgenic modification of adipose tissue (for review see ref.[2]). In these transgenic models, metabolic changes of white but not of brown adipose tissue are mostly responsible for the altered accretion of body fat, highlighting the importance of lipid metabolism in adipocytes of white fat. Evidently, treatment strategies for obesity and metabolic syndrome should include specific modifications of the metabolism of white adipose tissue.

Like in other tissues, mitochondria represent the main source of ATP even in white fat. Efficiency of ATP synthesis during oxidative phosphorylation and hence the rate of ATP synthesis depend on the proton leak of the inner mitochondrial membrane. Experiments of Brand and colleagues[3] suggest a general occurrence of proton leak in mitochondria *in vivo*. Several candidate genes for increasing the leak are expressed in adipocytes, namely the genes for uncoupling proteins (UCPs). In brown fat, UCP1, UCP2, UCP3 and UCP5 are expressed while in white fat only UCP2 and UCP5 genes are normally active[4,5]. Similarly to UCP1, also UCP2 and UCP3 probably enhance the proton leak, induce respiratory uncoupling, and decrease ATP synthesis[4,6]. That UCP1-mediated respiratory uncoupling in brown fat is involved in thermogenesis and in the control of energy balance is well known[4], while the physiological role of respiratory uncoupling and UCPs in white fat requires clarification. It may be hypothesized that uncoupling in white fat would increase energy expenditure and thermogenesis. However, the effect on energy balance may be relatively small because, e.g. in humans the contribution of white fat to resting metabolic rate is only about 5 per cent[7]. Alternatively, depression of ATP synthesis due to respiratory uncoupling in white fat, with consequent rise in ADP and AMP may result both in allosteric effects on the activities of key regulatory enzymes of sugar and lipid metabolism and in modulation of several intracellular regulatory pathways that reflect the intracellular energy status (see below). *In vitro* experiments suggest inhibition of fatty acid synthesis and enhanced glycolysis due to respiratory uncoupling in adipocytes[8]. Oxidation of FA in mitochondria is expected to increase, due to removal of the inhibition of FA transport to mitochondria by malonyl-CoA (the first committed intermediate in FA synthesis)[9] and also due to activation of mitochondrial biogenesis[10]. Lipolysis may be depressed[11].

Without complementary evidence from studies *in vivo*, the significance of the above findings on the links between energy and lipid metabolism in adipocytes would be limited. Therefore, the following paragraphs will focus on the relevant studies in humans and in experimental animals. The main focus will be on understanding the role of mitochondria and respiratory uncoupling in the control of lipid metabolism in adipocytes and in the mitigation of obesity.

Mitigation of obesity by ectopic UCP1 in white fat

The mechanism by which respiratory uncoupling may reduce accumulation of fat can be analysed in aP2-*Ucp1* transgenic mice in which the UCP1 gene is driven by the fat-specific aP2 promoter to achieve enhanced expression in both brown and white fat[12]. This transgenic mouse model was constructed well before the discoveries of UCP2 and UCP3 (see above). The animals are partially resistant to obesity related to age, induced by genetic background[12], or induced by feeding a high-fat-containing diet[13,14]. The resistance to obesity reflects lower accumulation of triacylglycerols in all fat depots, except for gonadal fat, which becomes relatively large[12-14]. Interestingly, reduction in total body weight becomes apparent when the animals are getting obese but not under standard conditions[12-14], similarly as in other models of obesity resistance induced by transgenic modification of adipose tissue or muscle metabolism. Transgenic UCP1 is present in both brown and white fat, while expression of the UCP1 endogene in brown fat is greatly reduced[12]. However, the obesity resistance results only from the transgenic modification of white fat[2]. The mechanism of brown fat atrophy in the transgenic mice is not clear[15].

Consequences of the expression of transgenic UCP1 in white fat, which induces the obesity resistance, has been studied in great detail. Transgenic UCP1 is contained in all the unilocular adipocytes[12]. Expression of the transgene differs in various fat depots, with gonadal fat showing a relatively low expression[16]. This may explain in part the lack of the effect of the transgene on the accumulation of lipids in gonadal fat (see above). However, even in the gonadal fat, transgenic UCP1 could decrease mitochondrial membrane potential in adipocytes[17] and elevate oxygen consumption twofold[14]. UCP1 also induces mitochondrial biogenesis in unilocular adipocytes, probably due to the up-regulation of the transcription factor NRF-1[18]. In adult mice, the total content of transgenic UCP1 in white fat does not exceed 2 per cent of the UCP1 in interscapular brown fat[12]. Apparently, only minute amounts of ectopic UCP1 in unilocular adipocytes of white fat can uncouple oxidative phosphorylation[17] and reduce accumulation of fat.

In agreement with the low oxidative capacity of white fat, the twofold increase of oxygen consumption brought about by transgenic UCP1 in this tissue (see above) results in only a marginal stimulation of the resting metabolic rate of mice[15]. The fact that UCP1 acts locally to reduce adiposity suggests that the reduction results not only from increased energy expenditure but also from a differential modification of lipid metabolism in various fat depots. Indeed, a strong diminution of FA synthesis was found in subcutaneous but not in gonadal fat of transgenic mice, reflecting the magnitude of UCP1 expression and the decrease of adiposity in different fat depots[16], as well as the drop in ATP/ADP ratio, that was observed only in the subcutaneous and not in the gonadal fat of transgenic mice[19]. The decrease of FA synthesis was accompanied by down-regulation of acetyl-CoA carboxylase, FA synthase 16 and peroxisomal proliferator-activated receptor β (our unpublished results) in white fat. The depression of FA synthesis by transgenic UCP1 was mediated by respiratory uncoupling, as confirmed by *in vitro* experiments[8,16]. Moreover, ectopic UCP1 in white fat affected also lipolysis and activity of lipoprotein lipase (LPL). Thus, the maximum lipolytic effect of noradrenaline was suppressed by 50 per cent in the subcutaneous but not in the gonadal fat of the transgenics. In parallel, UCP1 down-regulated the expression of hormone-sensitive lipase, lowered its activity, and altered the expression of G-proteins in adipocytes[19]. The activity of LPL was higher in the transgenic than in control mice while the stimulation of the activity by the transgene was significantly higher in animals fed high fat as compared with standard diet (our unpublished results). These results suggest that the uncoupling stimulates LPL-mediated clearance of triacylglycerols by adipose tissue. Accordingly, it was also found that plasma triacylglycerol levels were lower in transgenic than in control mice[13] and that the homozygous transgenic animals fed a high-fat diet had the lowest plasma triacylglycerol levels. Nonesterified FA in plasma were also depressed by the transgene (our unpublished results). The phenotype of aP2-*Ucp1* mice suggests that the main function of respiratory uncoupling and UCPs in white fat may be a modulation of lipogenesis, oxidation of substrates, lipolysis, and hormonal control of lipid metabolism.

AMP-activated protein kinase

The broad effect of the ectopic UCP1 on the metabolic properties of white adipose tissue is difficult to explain merely by respiratory uncoupling and it requires further clarification. In white fat, similarly as in other tissues, FA and carbohydrate metabolism is modulated by AMP-activated protein kinase (AMPK) which serves as a metabolic master switch[20]. In response to the fall in intracellular ATP/AMP ratio, AMPK becomes activated by phosphorylation of its β-subunit and the activated AMPK phosphorylates a number of enzymes involved in biosynthetic pathways, causing their inactivation and preventing further ATP utilization (for review see ref.[20]). In skeletal muscle, AMPK also up-regulates NRF-1 which induces mitochondrial biogenesis[21]. In adipocytes, AMPK is known to inhibit both lipolysis and lipogenesis by regulating directly the enzymes engaged in lipid metabolism[22]. In liver, the inhibitory effect of AMPK on lipogenesis is also indirect, being mediated by the transcription factor SREBP-1[23], which up-regulates the genes engaged in lipogenesis[24]. Thus, all the effects of transgenic UCP1 on biochemical characteristics of white fat of aP2-Ucp1 mice are in accordance with the activation of AMPK (see above). Indeed, it was observed that the UCP1-induced depression in ATP/ADP ratio in subcutaneous white fat of aP2-Ucp1 mice[19] was accompanied by reduction of the ATP/AMP ratio and that the aP2-Ucp1 transgene increased activity of AMPK in the subcutaneous but not in the gonadal fat (our unpublished results). Other studies indicated that the effect of leptin on lipid metabolism in muscle[25] was mediated by AMPK and that mutual links between AMPK activity and UCP3 expression existed in the muscle[26,27]. Therefore, AMPK may represent a link between respiratory uncoupling and lipid metabolism in white adipose tissue, and leptin signalling may involve respiratory uncoupling mediated by UCPs.

Biological significance of respiratory uncoupling in white fat

Substantial amount of evidence has accumulated indicating the involvement of mitochondrial UCPs in white fat in the control of adiposity. Even in adult humans, relatively low levels of the UCP1 transcript could be detected in various fat depots. In abdominal fat, UCP1 mRNA levels are negatively correlated with obesity[28] similarly to UCP2[29]. A common polymorphism in the promoter of the UCP2 gene is associated with decreased risk of obesity in middle-aged humans[30]. In humans, a negative correlation between heat production in adipocytes and body fat has also been found[7].

Table 1. Expression of UCPs, ATP/ADP ratio, and lipid metabolism in white fat under conditions associated with depression of adiposity

	aP2-Ucp1 mice	Leptin	Fasting	n-3 PUFAs	Bezafibrate	β-agonists
Expression of UCPs	↑UCP1[13]	↑UCP1[34] ↑UCP2[34]	↑UCP2[37]	↑UCP2[38] ↑UCP3[38]	↑UCP1[35] ↑UCP2[39] ↑UCP3[35,39]	↑UCP1[36] ↑UCP3[40]
ATP/ADP	↓ (n.p.)	?[25]	↓[41]	?	?	↓[41,42]
FA oxidation	↑[14]	↑[34]	↑ (n.p)	?	↑[39]	↑[43]
Lipogenesis	↓[16]	↓[34,44,45]	↓[46]	↓[47]	?	↓[48]
FA uptake	↑ (n.p.)	↑[34]	↓[49]	↑[50]	↑[39]	?

Data were obtained in mice, rats and humans. Leptin, the effects of peripheral administration of leptin; n-3 PUFAs, bezafibrate, and β-agonists (β-adrenoreceptor agonists), the effects of the respective compounds added to diet. Expression of various UCPs was characterized at the mRNA level. Some results refer to unpublished work performed in our group (n.p.). The effect on FA uptake by adipose tissues was mostly assessed through changes in the activity or expression of LPL.

It may be of practical importance to learn whether the efficiency of mitochondrial energy conversion and energy metabolism may affect adipocytes pharmacologically or by food, in order to counteract obesity. Therefore, it must be assessed whether such changes occur in adipocytes during treatment that affects adiposity, insulin resistance and other components of the metabolic syndrome. Several typical situations can be compared with the phenotype of aP2-Ucp1 mice, for instance administration of leptin, dietary n-3 polyunsaturated fatty acids (PUFAs), bezafibrate, and adrenoreceptor agonists, as well as the effect of fasting (Table 1 and ref.[31]). In all these situations, fat accumulation is reduced, signs of the metabolic syndrome are improved and metabolic features of adipocytes are changed in a similar way (Table 1). Thus, in most cases, expression of various UCPs is up-regulated, FA oxidation is increased, in situ lipogenesis is suppressed, and LPL-mediated clearance of triacylglycerols in white fat is augmented. Opposite changes in the activity of FA oxidation and lipogenesis probably reflect an inhibitory effect of malonyl-CoA on the transport of FA to mitochondrial matrix mediated by carnitine palmitoyl transferase-1[9]. Due to the low activity of the transferase in white fat, oxidation of FA is relatively slow and FA are directed toward esterification[32], unless the transferase is activated by leptin[33] or, possibly, by respiratory uncoupling. Furthermore, it is tempting to suggest that similar changes of lipid metabolism, occurring in white adipose tissue under the above situations leading to depressed accumulation of fat, involve up-regulation of mitochondrial UCPs and their effects on energy metabolism of adipocytes. Alteration of the energy status of adipocytes, as revealed by changes in the intracellular content of ATP and/or ATP/ADP and ATP/AMP ratios was not only detected in aP2-*Ucp1* mice, but also during fasting, or after administration of adrenergic compounds (Table 1). Moreover, the experiments in aP2-*Ucp1* mice (see above) strongly support the role of AMPK in adipocytes under conditions leading to depression of adiposity. The involvement of AMPK in the effect of leptin on lipid metabolism in skeletal muscle was found recently (see above). It remains to be clarified whether respiratory uncoupling and AMPK are involved in the changes of lipid metabolism in white fat under various circumstances that are associated with the depression of adiposity, besides the ectopic expression of UCP1 in white fat or the leptin treatment (see Table 1).

In spite of all the indirect evidence summarized above, the role of respiratory uncoupling in white fat cells in the control of lipid metabolism still remains to be definitively established. More studies focused on the energy metabolism in adipocytes, as well as on the links between UCPs and AMPK are necessary. Nevertheless, it is apparent that the energy status of fat cells has an important impact on various pathways of lipid metabolism that affect adiposity and mitigate obesity.

Acknowledgements: This work was supported by the Grant Agency of the Czech Republic (grant 303/02/1220) and the Ministry of Education of the Czech Republic (grant LN00A079).

Abbreviations: AMPK, AMP-activated protein kinase; aP2-*Ucp1* transgenic mouse, mouse with the expression of UCP1 from the fat-specific aP2 gene promoter; FA, fatty acids; LPL, lipoprotein lipase; PUFAs, polyunsaturated fatty acids; UCP, mitochondrial uncoupling protein.

References

1. Arner P. Obesity – a genetic disease of adipose tissue? *Br J Nutr* 2000; 83 (Suppl 1): S9–S16.

2. Kopecký J, Rossmeisl M, Flachs P, Bardová K, Brauner P. Mitochondrial uncoupling and lipid metabolism in adipocytes. *Biochem Soc Trans* 2001; 29: 791–7.

3. Brand MD, Brindle KM, Buckingham JA, Harper JA, Rolfe DF, Stuart JA. The significance and mechanism of mitochondrial proton conductance. *Int J Obes Relat Metab Disord* 1999; 23 (Suppl 6): S4–S11.

4. Ricquier D, Bouillaud F. The uncoupling protein homologues: UCP1, UCP2, UCP3, StUCP and AtUCP. *Biochem J* 2000; 345: 161–79.

5. Pecqueur C, Alves-Guerra MC, Gelly C, Lévi-Meyrueis C, Couplan E, Collins S *et al.* Uncoupling protein 2: *In vivo* distribution, induction upon oxidative stress and evidence for translational regulation. *J Biol Chem* 2001; 276: 8705–12.

6. Echtay KS, Winkler E, Frischmuth K, Klingenberg M. Uncoupling proteins 2 and 3 are highly active H^+ transporters and highly nucleotide sensitive when activated by coenzyme Q (ubiquinone). *Proc Natl Acad Sci USA* 2001; 98: 1416–21.

7. Bottcher H, Furst P. Decreased white fat cell thermogenesis in obese individuals. *Int J Obes* 1997; 21: 439–44.

8. Rognstad R, Katz J. The effect of 2,4-dinitrophenol on adipose-tissue metabolism. *Biochem J* 1969; 111: 431–44.

9. Saggerson ED, Carpenter CA. The effect of malonyl-CoA on overt and latent carnitine acyltransferase activities in rat liver and adipocyte mitochondria. *Biochem J* 1983; 210: 591–7.

10. Li B, Holloszy JO, Semenkovich CF. Respiratory uncoupling induces delta-aminolevulinate synthase expression through a nuclear respiratory factor-1-dependent mechanism in HeLa cells. *J Biol Chem* 1999; 274: 17534–40.

11. Fassina G, Dorigo P, Gaion RM. Equilibrium between metabolic pathways producing energy: A key factor in regulating lipolysis. *Pharm Res Commun* 1974; 6: 1–21.

12. Kopecký J, Clarke G, Enerbäck S, Spiegelman B, Kozak LP. Expression of the mitochondrial uncoupling protein gene from the aP2 gene promoter prevents genetic obesity. *J Clin Invest* 1995; 96: 2914–23.

13. Kopecký J, Hodný Z, Rossmeisl M, Syrový I, Kozak LP. Reduction of dietary obesity in the aP2-Ucp transgenic mice: Physiology and adipose tissue distribution. *Am J Physiol* 1996; 270: E768–E775.

14. Kopecký J, Rossmeisl M, Hodný Z, Syrový I, Horáková M, Kolarova P. Reduction of dietary obesity in the aP2-Ucp transgenic mice: Mechanism and adipose tissue morphology. *Am J Physiol* 1996; 270: E776–E786.

15. Štefl B, Janovská P, Hodný Z, Rossmeisl M, Horáková M, Syrový I *et al.* Brown fat is essential for cold-induced thermogenesis but not for obesity resistance in aP2-Ucp mice. *Am J Physiol* 1998; 274: E527–E533.

16. Rossmeisl M, Syrový I, Baumruk F, Flachs P, Janovská P, Kopecký J. Decreased fatty acid synthesis due to mitochondrial uncoupling in adipose tissue. *FASEB J* 2000; 14: 1793–800.

17. Baumruk F, Flachs P, Horáková M, Floryk D, Kopecký J. Transgenic UCP1 in white adipocytes modulates mitochondrial membrane potential. *FEBS Letters* 1999; 444: 206–10.

18. Rossmeisl M, Barbatelli G, Flachs P, Brauner P, Zingaretti MC, Marelli M et al. Expression of the uncoupling protein 1 from the aP2 gene promoter stimulates mitochondrial biogenesis in unilocular adipocytes in vivo. Eur J Biochem 2002; 269: 1–10.

19. Flachs P, Novotný J, Baumruk F, Bardová K, Bourová L, Mikšík I et al. Impaired noradrenaline-induced lipolysis in white fat of aP2-Ucp1 transgenic mice is associated with changes in G-protein levels. Biochem J 2002; 364: 369–76.

20. Winder WW, Hardie DG. AMP-activated protein kinase, a metabolic master switch: Possible roles in type 2 diabetes. Am J Physiol 1999; 277: 1–10.

21. Bergeron R, Ren JM, Cadman KS, Moore IK, Perret P, Pypaert M et al. Chronic activation of AMP kinase results in NRF-1 activation and mitochondrial biogenesis. Am J Physiol Endocrinol Metab 2001; 281: E1340–E1346.

22. Sullivan JE, Brocklehurst KJ, Marley AE, Carey F, Carling D, Beri RK. Inhibition of lipolysis and lipogenesis in isolated rat adipocytes with AICAR, a cell-permeable activator of AMP-activated protein kinase. FEBS Letters 1994; 353: 33–6.

23. Zhou G, Myers R, Li Y, Chen Y, Shen X, Fenyk-Melody J et al. Role of AMP-activated protein kinase in mechanism of metformin action. J Clin Invest 2001; 108: 1167–74.

24. Kim JB, Sarraf P, Wright M, Yao KM, Mueller E, Solanes G et al. Nutritional and insulin regulation of fatty acid synthetase and leptin gene expression through ADD1/SREBP1. J Clin Invest 1998; 101: 1–9.

25. Minokoshi Y, Kim YB, Peroni OD, Fryer LG, Muller C, Carling D, Kahn BB. Leptin stimulates fatty-acid oxidation by activating AMP-activated protein kinase. Nature 2002; 415: 339–43.

26. Pedersen SB, Lund, S, Buhl ES, Richelsen B. Insulin and contraction directly stimulate UCP2 and UCP3 mRNA expression in rat skeletal muscle in vitro. Biochem Biophys Res Commun 2001; 283: 19–25.

27. Zhou M, Lin BZ, Coughlin S, Vallega G, Pilch PF. UCP-3 expression in skeletal muscle: Effects of exercise, hypoxia, and AMP-activated protein kinase. Am J Physiol Endocrinol Metab 2000; 279: E622–E629.

28. Oberkofler H, Dallinger G, Liu YM, Hell E, Krempler F, Patsch W. Uncoupling protein gene: Quantification of expression levels in adipose tissues of obese and non-obese humans. J Lipid Res 1997; 38: 2125–33.

29. Oberkofler H, Liu YM, Esterbauer H, Hell E, Krempler F, Patsch W. Uncoupling protein-2 gene: Reduced mRNA expression in intraperitoneal adipose tissue of obese humans. Diabetologia 1998; 41: 940–6.

30. Esterbauer H, Schneitler C, Oberkofler H, Ebenbichler C, Paulweber B, Sandhofer F et al. A common polymorphism in the promoter of UCP2 is associated with decreased risk of obesity in middle-aged humans. Nature Genet 2001; 28: 178–83.

31. Yoshida T, Sakane N, Umekawa T, Kogure A, Kumamoto K, Kawada T et al. Nicotine induced uncoupling protein 1 in white adipose tissue of obese mice. Int J Obes 1999; 23: 570–5.

32. Martin BR, Denton RM. The intracellular localization of enzymes in white-adipose-tissue fat-cells and permeability properties of fat-cell mitochondria. Biochem J 1970; 117: 861–77.

33. Wang MY, Lee Y, Unger RH. Novel form of lipolysis induced by leptin. J Biol Chem 1999; 274: 17541–4.

34. Zhou YT, Wang ZW, Higa M, Newgard CB, Unger RH. Reversing adipocyte differentiation: Implications for treatment of obesity. Proc Natl Acad Sci USA 1999; 96: 2391–5.

35. Cabrero A, Llaverias G, Roglans N, Alegret M, Sanchez R, Adzet T et al. Uncoupling protein-3 mRNA levels are increased in white adipose tissue and skeletal muscle of bezafibrate-treated rats. Biochem Biophys Res Commun 1999; 260: 547–56.

36. Gong DW, He Y, Karas M, Reitman M. Uncoupling protein-3 is a mediator of thermogenesis regulated by thyroid hormone, beta3-adrenergic agonists, and leptin. J Biol Chem 1997; 272: 24129–32.

37. Millet L, Vidal H, Andreelli F, Larrouy D, Riou JP, Ricquier D et al. Increased uncoupling protein-2 and -3 mRNA expression during fasting in obese and lean humans. J Clin Invest 1997; 100: 2665–70.

38. Hun CS, Hasegawa K, Kawabata T, Kato M, Shimokawa T, Kagawa Y. Increased uncoupling protein2 mRNA in white adipose tissue, and decrease in leptin, visceral fat, blood glucose, and cholesterol in KK-Ay mice fed with eicosapentaenoic and docosahexaenoic acid in addition to linolenic acid. Biochem Biophys Res Commun 1999; 259: 85–90.

39. Cabrero A, Alegret M, Sanchez RM, Adzet T, Laguna JC, Vazquez M. Bezafibrate reduces mRNA levels of adipocyte markers and increases fatty acid oxidation in primary culture of adipocytes. Diabetes 2001; 50: 1883–90.

40. Yoshitomi H, Yamazaki K, Abe S, Tanaka I. Differential regulation of mouse uncoupling proteins among brown adipose tissue, white adipose tissue, and skeletal muscle in chronic beta 3 adrenergic receptor agonist treatment. Biochem Biophys Res Commun 1998; 253: 85–91.

41. Ho RJ, England R, Meng HC. Effect of glucose on lipolysis and energy metabolism in fat cells. Life Sci 1970; 9: 137–50.

42. Angel A, Desai KS, Halperin ML. Reduction in adipocyte ATP by lipolytic agents: Relation to intracellular free fatty acid accumulation. J Lipid Res 1971; 12: 203–13.

43. Himms-Hagen J, Melnyk A, Zingaretti MC, Ceresi E, Barbatelli G, Cinti S. Multilocular fat cells in WAT of CL-316243-treated rats derive directly from white adipocytes. *Am J Physiol Cell Physiol* 2000; 279: C670–C681.

44. Soukas A, Cohen P, Socci ND, Friedman JM. Leptin-specific patterns of gene expression in white adipose tissue. *Genes Dev* 2000; 14: 963–80.

45. Ceddia RB, William WN, Lima FB, Flandin P, Curi R, Giacobino JP. Leptin stimulates uncoupling protein-2 mRNA expression and Krebs cycle activity and inhibits lipid synthesis in isolated rat white adipocytes. *Eur J Biochem* 2000; 267: 5952–8.

46. Iritani N, Fukuda H, Tada K. Nutritional regulation of lipogenic enzyme gene expression in rat epididymal adipose tissue. *J Biochem* 1996; 120: 242–8.

47. Clarke SD. Polyunsaturated fatty acid regulation of gene transcription: a molecular mechanism to improve the metabolic syndrome. *J Nutr* 2001; 131: 1129–32.

48. Rodbell M. Metabolism of isolated fat cells. I. Effects of hormones on glucose metabolism and lipolysis. *J Biol Chem* 1964; 239: 375–80.

49. Kalderon B, Mayorek N, Berry E, Zevit N, Bar-Tana J. Fatty acid cycling in the fasting rat. *Am J Physiol Endocrinol Metab* 2000; 279: E221–E227.

50. Benhizia F, Hainault I, Serougne C, Lagrande D, Hajduch E, Guichard C et al. Effects of fish oil-lard diet on rat plasma lipoproteins, liver FAS, and lipolytic enzymes. *Am J Physiol* 1994; 267: E975–E982.

Progress in Obesity Research: 9. Edited by *Geraldo Medeiros-Neto, Alfredo Halpern and Claude Bouchard*
©2003 John Libbey Eurotext Ltd, pp. 220–222.

CHAPTER 46

Lessons from ß3- to ß1/ß2/ß3-adrenoceptor knockout mice

J.-P. Giacobino

Département de Biochimie médicale, Centre Médical universitaire, 1 rue Michel Servet, 1211 Geneva 4, Switzerland
[e-mail: Giacobino@medecine.unige.ch]

The ß-adrenoceptor family

Epinephrine and norepinephrine are the main effectors of the adrenal medulla and of the sympathetic nervous system. They mediate their effects through α- and ß-adrenoceptors. The ß-family consists of three subtypes: ß1-, ß2- and ß3-adrenoceptors. ß-adrenoceptors are involved in development, behaviour, heart function, smooth muscle tone and energy metabolism.

We are going to focus in this presentation on the role of ß-adrenoceptors in the control of energy metabolism.

In brown adipose tissue (BAT) the three ß-adrenoceptor subtypes coexist. The ß3-adrenoceptor however is largely predominant representing 70 per cent of the total ß population[1]. Cold exposure or overfeeding induces a stimulation of the BAT sympathetic nervous system. The norepinephrine released by sympathetic nerve endings induces, mainly via the ß3-adrenoceptor, an increase in lipolysis, intracellular FFA and UCP1 activity and expression which results in an increase in heat production. The extra heat production induced by overfeeding is called diet-induced thermogenesis (DIT) and that induced by cold exposure, cold-induced thermogenesis (CIT).

In white adipose tissue (WAT) the three ß-adrenoceptor subtypes also coexist, the ß3-adrenoceptor being predominant[1]. Fasting induces a stimulation of the sympathetic nervous system of the WAT and of the secretion of catecholamines by the adrenals. Catecholamines induce an increase in lipolysis and in FFA release into the blood.

Both adaptive thermogenesis and mobilization of FFA from the lipid stores should prevent the development of obesity.

Surprisingly, none of the ß-adrenoceptor knockout (KO) mice so far generated, i.e. ß1-KO, ß3-KO, ß2-KO, ß1/ß2-KO[2-5] became overtly obese or were cold sensitive. These weak metabolic phenotypes suggested a functional redundancy of the ß-adrenoceptor subtypes or compensations by pathways other than the ß-adrenoceptor system. To investigate these hypotheses, we generated various ß-adrenoceptor-KO mice.

I will present data on the four ßKO models which we are presently phenotyping in our laboratory. Most of the data are unpublished and the models that we are going to compare are still, for three of them, in a mixed genetic background. Our KO models are the following: ß3KO in a mixed background: C57BL/6J and 129Sv/ev (ß3KO)[3], ß3KO in a pure background: C57BL/6J (pure ß3KO), double ß1/ß2KO in a mixed background: C57BL/6J, 129Sv/J, FVB/N and DBA/2 kindly provided by Dr B.K. Kobilka[5] (DKO) and triple ß1/ß2/ß3KO in the same mixed background obtained by crossing our ß3KO model and the DKO mice of Dr. B.K. Kobilka (TKO).

'Obesity' in ß3KO to TKO mice

A study of the DKO mice revealed the following phenotype. In DKO mice as compared to their WT controls, body weight on a chow diet, cold resistance and UCP1 mRNA expression in BAT both at 24 °C or after 2–10 day of cold exposure were normal.

Therefore the β_1/β_2 adrenoceptors in WT mice do not seem to play a role in the control of energy metabolism. Does this mean that the β_3-adrenoceptor alone is in charge of the control of energy metabolism?

Our first comparison is that of body weights in β_3KO and TKO 5 months old male mice under standard conditions, i.e. on a chow diet. No change in body weight was observed in β_3KO[3] and pure β_3KO mice and a significant increase of 16 per cent in TKO as compared to WT mice.

Note that in 5-month-old male mice, 2 month on a high fat diet, Bachman et al.[6] report an increase in body weight of 54 per cent in TKO as compared to WT mice. It is noteworthy that all these changes occur without any increase in food intake.

These results show that in the absence of the β_3-adrenoceptor, β_1/β_2-adrenoceptors are recruited and participate in the control of energy balance, preventing an increase in body weight. If they are knocked out, body weight increases. Therefore, in the control of body weight, β_1/β_2-adrenoceptors act as fully competent jokers.

The second comparison deals with body composition in β_3KO and TKO mice under standard conditions. The percentage body fat is increased by a 33 per cent in β_3KO[3] and by 64 per cent in TKO mice. Therefore, in the control of body fat, β_1/β_2-adrenoceptors seem to act as partially competent jokers.

The higher adiposity of TKO as compared to WT mice despite similar food intake, reflects a higher food efficiency. This could be explained, by a defect in DIT. This hypothesis is supported by the abnormal morphological appearance of the brown adipocytes. Indeed, in TKO mice, brown adipocytes do not display their classical multilocular appearance and consist exclusively of unilocular cells. It is also supported by the data of Bachman et al.[6] who showed a decreased DIT in their model of TKO mice.

The TKO data support the hypothesis that ß-adrenoceptor signalling is required for DIT.

Cold resistance in ß₃KO to TKO mice

At 24 °C, the 'body temperature of pure β_3KO mice was not significantly different from that of wild type animals, During cold exposure, body temperature of pure β_3-KO mice was between 0.4 and 0.7 degree lower than that of wild type controls.

The colonic temperature of TKO mice kept at 24 °C, was 1.2 °C lower than that of the WT mice. Furthermore, TKO mice were clearly cold intolerant. Indeed, after a period of cold exposure varying between 1 and 24 h, colonic temperature in 10 out of 13 TKO mice slowly decreased and suddenly markedly dropped. TKO mice surviving cold exposure during 48 h had after this period of time a body temperature about 4 °C lower than that of WT mice and performed intense shivering, as assessed by visual inspection.

Therefore, in the control of cold resistance, β_1/β_2 adrenoceptors act as or partially competent jokers. The TKO data support the hypothesis that ß-adrenoceptor signalling is required for CIT.

In conclusion TKO induces a phenotype deviating more from normality than β_3KO as for as body weight, adiposity, BAT morphology and cold-sensitivity are concerned.

Unexpected phenotypes

The phenotyping of the β_3KO to TKO models also yield unexpected results. Let us consider three sets of such results.

Unexpected phenotype 1

In β_3KO mice on a chow diet, the percentage body fat is increased by 34 per cent and in β_3KO mice on a high fat diet by 47 per cent as compared to WT mice[3].

The correlation between circulating leptin level and adiposity is well documented in rodents[7]. We therefore expected an increase in leptin in β_3KO as compared to WT mice. However, despite the increase in adiposity, leptin levels were not found to be increased in β_3KO on both a low or a high fat diet vs. WT mice[3].

These results suggested that the β_3-adrenoceptors somehow control the set point linking body fat content and circulating leptin level. An ideal model to study this change in set point will be our TKO mice with their large excess of body fat mass.

Unexpected phenotype 2

It is well known that classical WAT depots are infiltrated by multilocular mitochondria-rich adipocytes expressing UCP1. The emergence of these ectopic cells is induced by cold acclimation. This phenomenon is called recruitment. We studied the effect of the ß₃KO on UCP1 expression in the BAT and in the WAT.

The ß₃KO did not change UCP1 mRNA expression in the BAT of mice either at 24 °C or exposed at 6 °C for 48 h. The results obtained in the WAT differed dramatically from those in the BAT. In the WAT of WT mice, the basal level of UCP1 mRNA at 24 °C, was found to be increased 2.6-fold by cold exposure. The effects of a lack of ß₃-adrenoceptor were striking. The UCP1 mRNA expression levels in WAT of ß₃KO mice were strongly depressed, being only 5 per cent and 3 per cent those measured in wild type mice kept at 24 °C or exposed to 6 °C, respectively. The same pattern of responses was observed at the level of UCP1 protein.

Therefore in the control of recruitment in the WAT, the ß3-adrenoceptor cannot be replaced.

Unexpected phenotype 3

Here, we deal with a different aspect of the metabolism i.e. lipolysis in WAT.

In TKO mice lipolysis was expected to be decreased as compared to WT mice. We measured circulating free fatty acids (FFA) and glycerol as an index of their capacity to mobilize lipids from fat stores. Unexpectedly, in the fed state, TKO mice displayed higher FFA (1.3-fold) and glycerol (1.5-fold) levels as compared to WT controls. A 16 h-fasting period increased circulating FFA and glycerol levels in both WT and mutant mice. Again, TKO mice displayed higher FFA (1.6-fold) and glycerol (1.4-fold) levels as compared to WT controls.

These results demonstrate that ß-adrenergic signalling is not essential in the control of lipolysis in both the fed and fasted state. The paradoxical increase of FFA in TKO mice may reflect an effect on peripheral fatty acid utilization. The observation that both FFA and glycerol levels follow the same trend rather supports the hypothesis of an increased lipolysis. The mechanism of this paradoxical effect deserves further study.

References

1. Giacobino JP. Beta 3-adrenoceptor: an update. *Eur J Endocrinol* 1995; 132: 377–85.

2. Rohrer DK, Desai KH *et al.* Targeted disruption of the mouse beta1-adrenergic receptor gene: developmental and cardiovascular effects. *Proc Natl Acad Sci USA* 1996; 93: 7375–80.

3. Revelli JP, Preitner F *et al.* Targeted gene disruption reveals a leptin-independent role for the mouse beta3-adrenoceptor in the regulation of body composition. *J Clin Invest* 1997; 100: 1098–106.

4. Chruscinski AJ, Rohrer DK *et al.* Targeted disruption of the beta2 adrenergic receptor gene. *J Biol Chem* 1999; 274: 16694–700.

5. Rohrer DK, Chruscinski A *et al.* Cardiovascular and metabolic alterations in mice lacking both beta1- and beta2-adrenergic receptors. *J Biol Chem* 1999; 274: 16701–8.

6. Bachman ES, Dhillon H *et al.* betaAR signaling required for diet-induced thermogenesis and obesity resistance. *Science* 2002; 297: 843–5.

7. Maffei M, Halaas J *et al.* Leptin levels in human and rodent: measurement of plasma leptin and ob RNA in obese and weight-reduced subjects. *Nature Med* 1995; 1: 1155–61.

Progress in Obesity Research: 9. Edited by *Geraldo Medeiros-Neto, Alfredo Halpern* and *Claude Bouchard*
©2003 John Libbey Eurotext Ltd, pp. 223–225.

CHAPTER 47

Pathophysiologic and therapeutic implication of leptin in obesity-related complications: Lessons from transgenic skinny mice

Yoshihiro Ogawa and Kazuwa Nakao

*Department of Medicine and Clinical Science, Kyoto University Graduate School of Medicine,
54 Shogoin Kawahara-cho Sakyo-ku, Kyoto 606-8507, Japan
[e-mail: ogawa@kuhp-kyoto-u.ac.jp]*

Introduction

Obesity increases a risk of cardiovascular and metabolic lifestyle-related diseases such as diabetes, hypertension, and hyperlipidaemia[1]. The adipose tissue has been regarded as a triglyceride storage organ, but recent advances in molecular and cell biology have revealed that the adipose tissue is involved in the regulation of a variety of homeostatic processes as an important endocrine organ that secretes many biologically active substances (collectively termed adipocytokines) such as tumour necrosis factor-α, free fatty acids, and so forth[1].

Leptin is such an adipocytokine that decreases food intake and increases energy expenditure, thereby representing one of the defense mechanisms against the development of overweight or obesity[2]. Since its discovery in late 1994, the potential usefulness of leptin for treatment of obesity and obesity-related complications has come before the footlight. Numerous studies, however, have demonstrated that plasma leptin concentrations are elevated in obese subjects in proportion to the degree of adiposity[3], suggesting the state of leptin resistance. It is also tempting to speculate, although paradoxically, that hyperleptinaemia may play a role in the pathogenesis of obesity-related complications. To pursue the impact of chronic hyperleptinaemia *in vivo*, we have recently created transgenic skinny mice with elevated plasma leptin concentrations comparable to those found in markedly obese subjects[4]. Here we discuss the pathophysiologic and therapeutic implication of leptin based on the studies with transgenic skinny mice.

Transgenic skinny mice overexpressing leptin (Fig. 1)

We constructed a fusion gene comprising the human serum amyloid P component promoter and mouse leptin cDNA coding sequences so that the hormone expression might be targeted to the liver[4]. Plasma leptin concentrations are elevated in transgenic mice according to the copy numbers of the transgene incorporated, and have reached up to approximately 50 ng/ml in transgenic mice with 30 copies of the transgene. Their food intake and body weight are approximately 70 per cent of those of nontransgenic littermates. They are apparently devoid of white and brown adipose tissue. We, therefore, call these animals transgenic 'skinny' mice. The animals have proved to be the useful model system to investigate the functional role of chronic hyperleptinaemia *in vivo*[4-9].

Glucose metabolism in transgenic skinny mice

Evidence has accumulated indicating that leptin is involved in the regulation of glucose metabolism, thus suggesting the pathophysiological role of leptin in insulin resistance and diabetes. Transgenic skinny mice exhibit normoglycaemia despite hypoinsulinaemia relative to nontransgenic littermates[4].

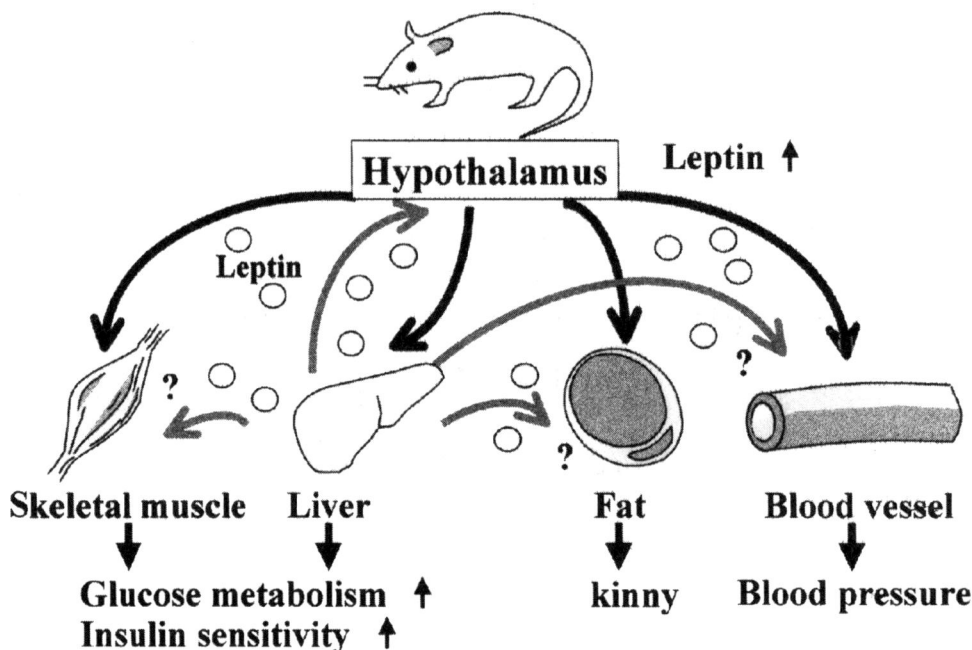

Fig. 1. Cardiovascular and metabolic phenotypes of transgenic skinny mice.

Glucose and insulin tolerance tests have revealed increased glucose metabolism and insulin sensitivity accompanied by increased insulin signaling in the skeletal muscle and liver. These findings suggest that leptin might be an antidiabetic factor.

Therapeutic implication of leptin in obesity-related diabetes

Weight reduction is one of the most powerful strategies for treatment of obesity and obesity-related complications such as obesity-related insulin-resistant diabetes and hypertension. However, molecular mechanisms responsible for it are poorly understood. Plasma leptin concentrations are reduced during caloric restriction or body weight loss, suggesting that leptin deficiency may play a role in the metabolic response to caloric restriction[10]. As a first step toward understanding the therapeutic implication of leptin in obesity-related insulin-resistant diabetes, we have crossed transgenic skinny mice (Tg/+) and KKAy (Ay/+) mice, a well-established model of late-onset obesity and type 2 diabetes[5]. The double transgenic mice (Tg/+: Ay/+ mice) are of normal weight with increased insulin sensitivity at younger ages. At older ages, however, they are phenotypically indistinguishable from Ay/+ mice; they both develop obesity, insulin-resistant diabetes, and blood pressure elevation similar to those in Ay/+ mice[5]. During caloric restriction, Ay/+ mice show hypoleptinaemia in parallel with body weight reduction. However, in response to caloric restriction, Tg/+: Ay/+ mice remain to be hyperleptinaemic despite body weight reduction, because of constitutive expression of the transgene in the liver. These observations suggest that Tg/+: Ay/+ mice are the unique experimental model to investigate the role of hypoleptinaemia during caloric restriction[5].

To obtain further insight into the therapeutic implication of leptin, we examined cardiovascular and metabolic responses of Tg/+: Ay/+ mice to caloric restriction. In response to caloric restriction, both Ay/+ and Tg/+: Ay/+ mice lose weight with the normalization of plasma glucose concentrations[5,6]. However, insulin resistance remains in Tg/+: Ay/+ mice in parallel with a decrease in plasma leptin concentrations. By contrast, insulin resistance is reversed in Tg/+ and Tg/+: Ay/+ mice after caloric restriction[5]. These observations suggest that weight reduction in combination with leptin supplementation is more efficacious than weight reduction alone for treatment of obesity-related insulin resistance and diabetes.

Pathophysiologic implication of leptin in obesity-related hypertension

Leptin is known to increase energy expenditure through the activation of sympathetic nervous system. Transgenic skinny mice show increased urinary catecholamine excretion relative to nontransgenic littermates, suggesting chronic sympathetic activation[6]. They exhibit 10~15 mmHg blood pressure elevation relative to nontransgenic littermates. Blood pressure elevation is normalized in transgenic skinny mice treated with α-adrenoceptor, β-adrenoceptor, and sympathetic ganglionic blockers that do not affect blood pressure in nontransgenic littermates. These findings suggest that chronic hyperleptinaemia can increase blood pressure through the sympathetic activation[6]. It has been proposed that insulin resistance or hyperinsulinaemia secondary to it may play a role in the pathogenesis of obesity-related hypertension[11]. Our data suggest that chronic hyperleptinaemia can cause blood pressure elevation through sympathetic activation without insulin resistance and hyperinsulinaemia. Thus, leptin may be involved in the pathogenesis of obesity-related hypertension via insulin-independent mechanisms.

We also examined blood pressure change in $Ay/+$ and $Tg/+: Ay/+$ mice during caloric restriction. Blood pressure elevation is reversed in $Ay/+$ mice after caloric restriction. By contrast, $Tg/+: Ay/+$ mice are still hypertensive after caloric restriction[6]. It is, therefore, likely that leptin deficiency may reverse the sympathetic activation, thus contributing to blood pressure reduction after caloric restriction.

Conclusion

Leptin is a major adipocytokine with multiple regulatory potentials and may play a role in obesity-related complications. Our transgenic skinny mice have provided new insight into the pathophysiologic and therapeutic implication of leptin in obesity-associated lifestyle-related diseases.

Acknowledgements: We thank Ms. Kitahata for secretarial assistance and Ms. M. Nagamoto and Ms. Inoue for technical assistance.

References

1. Spiegelman BM, Flier JS. Adipogenesis and obesity: rounding out the big problem. *Cell* 1996; 87: 377–89.

2. Friedman JM, Halaas JL. Leptin and the regulation of body weight in mammals *Nature* 1996; 395: 763–70.

3. Considine RV, Sinha MK, Heiman ML, Kriauciunas A, Stephens TW, Nyce MR *et al.* Serum immunoreactive-leptin concentrations in normal-weight and obese humans. *N Engl J Med* 1996; 334: 292–5.

4. Ogawa Y, Masuzaki H, Hosoda K, Aizawa-Abe M, Suga J, Suda M *et al.* Increased glucose metabolism and insulin sensitivity in transgenic skinny mice overexpressing leptin. *Diabetes* 1999; 48: 1822–9.

5. Masuzaki H, Ogawa Y, Aizawa-Abe M, Hosoda K, Suga J, Ebihara K *et al.* Glucose metabolism and insulin sensitivity in transgenic mice overexpressing leptin with lethal yellow agouti mutation: Usefulness of leptin for treatment of obesity-associated diabetes. *Diabetes* 1999; 48: 1615–22.

6. Aizawa-Abe M, Ogawa Y, Masuzaki H, Ebihara K, Satoh N, Iwai H *et al.* Pathophysiological role of leptin in obesity-related hypertension. *J Clin Invest* 2000; 105: 1243–52.

7. Yura S, Ogawa Y, Sagawa N, Masuzaki H, Itoh H, Ebihara K *et al.* Accelerated puberty and late-onset hypothalamic hypogonadism in female transgenic skinny mice overexpressing leptin. *J Clin Invest* 2000; 105: 749–55.

8. Matsuoka N, Ogawa Y, Masuzaki H, Ebihara K, Aizawa-Abe M, Satoh N *et al.* Decreased triglyceride-rich lipoproteins in transgenic skinny mice overexpressing leptin. *Am J Physiol* 2001; 280: E334–E339.

9. Ebihara K, Ogawa Y, Masuzaki H, Shintani M, Miyanaga F, Aizawa-Abe M *et al.* Transgenic overexpression of leptin rescues insulin resistance and diabetes in a mouse model of lipoatrophic diabetes. *Diabetes* 2001; 50: 1440–8.

10. Ahima RS, Prabakanan D, Mantzoros C, Qu D, Lowell B, Maratos-Flier E, Flier JS. Role of leptin in the neuroendocrine response to fasting. *Nature* 1996; 382: 250–2.

11. Landberg L, Krieger DR. Obesity, metabolism, and the sympathetic nervous system. Am J Hypertension 1989; 2: S125–S132.

TRACK II

GENETICS OF OBESITY

Progress in Obesity Research: 9. Edited by *Geraldo Medeiros-Neto, Alfredo Halpern and Claude Bouchard*
©2003 John Libbey Eurotext Ltd, pp. 229–233.

CHAPTER 48

Functional proteomics applied to obesity research

A. Donny Strosberg, Laurent Daviet and Catherine Borg-Capra

Research and Development, Hybrigenics SA, 3–5 Impasse Reille, Paris 75014, France
[e-mail: adstrosberg@hybrigenics.fr]

Introduction

Laboratory studies applied to Obesity research have, until recently, mostly been based on the use of molecular genetics. This was particularly evident in the remarkable analysis of the role of leptin in genetic models for murine obesity[1], later substantiated by the discovery of rare instances of human leptin mutations in children[2] and adults[3]. Mutational[4] or gene knock-out studies[5] for proteins such as the Beta 1, 2 and 3 adreno-receptors and several melanocortin receptors[6] also elegantly substantiated the role of such individual proteins in the homeostasis of fat metabolism.

There is little doubt however that obesity constitutes a multifactorial, multigenetic group of diseases that will require a systems approach to allow the development of appropriate, side effect-free therapeutic drugs. For such a broad approach, modern high-throughput technologies will need to be utilized. The first uses of genomics-derived tools have been promising but difficult to exploit: many genes were found to be associated with some forms of obesity, in many different patient groups.

A more mechanistic driven approach is clearly preferable to first unravel the pathways activated during differentiation of human adipocytes, then act on these pathways by specific and selective agents.

In this report we describe gene expression profiling and massive parallel protein interaction mapping applied to the human PAZ6 differentiated human adipocytes, and present here some of the results obtained with these technologies.

Methodology

Human PAZ6 cell line: Human brown pre-adipocytes were immortalized by microinjection of the genes encoding simian virus 40 T and t antigens under control of the human vimentin promoter[7].The resulting 'PAZ6' cells retain typical morphological characteristics after several months of culture and can be differentiated into adipocytes when treated with insulin, tri-iodothyronine, dexamethasone, IBMX and pioglitazone for 4 days following by 10 days with the same medium without IBMX.

In view of investigating the genes that are differentially expressed during differentiation of the PAZ6 cells, total mRNA from undifferentiated and 14-days-differentiated PAZ6 cells were extracted and analysed using the MPSS technology. In parallel, extracted mRNA was used for the construction of a cDNA library.

MPSS technology: Gene expression profiles were obtained using the massively parallel signature sequencing technology (MPSS), a novel sequencing approach developed by Brenner *et al.*[8] After constructing a microbead library of DNA templates by *in vitro* cloning, a planar array of a million template-containing microbeads was assembled in a flow cell. Sequences of the free ends of the cloned templates on each microbead were then simultaneously analysed using a fluorescence-based signature sequencing method that does not require DNA fragment separation. Signature sequence of 16–20 bases were obtained by repeated cycles of enzymatic cleavage, adaptor ligation and sequence interrogation by encoded hybridization probes.

Protein interaction mapping: The variant of yeast two-hybrid system developed by Fromont-Racine *et al.*[9], can be used to detect interactions between two known proteins or polypeptides and also to search

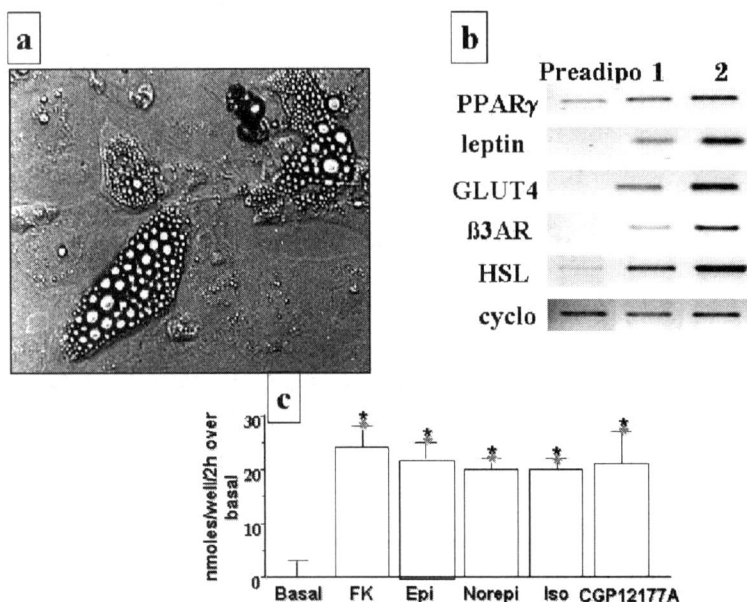

Fig. 1. (a) Morphological changes associated with differentiation of PAZ6 into fat-accumulating adipocytes; (b) Molecular markers in PAZ6 pre-adipocyte and adipocyte (1 and 2 weeks of differentiation): PPAR gamma, leptin, GLUT4, (ADRB3)(HSL) and cyclo; (c) Lipolysis in PAZ6 adipocytes. Lipolysis in PAZ6 cells was measured by glycerol released by incubation with 100 μM of various lipolytic agents: forskolin, epinephrine, norepinephrine, isoproterenol and ADRB3 agonists.

for unknown partners of a given protein. This high throughput yeast two hybrid assay was used to screen 43 proteins against a highly complex library encoded polypeptides constructed from total RNA extracted from differentiated PAZ6. All prey fragments were identified individually by sequence analysis and comparison with the genomic database via a dedicated integrated Laboratory Information Management System (the 'PIM Builder'). Protein interaction maps were built based on experimental data that yielded a heuristic value for each connection (the predicted Biological score, PBS). In addition, interactive domains were also identified.

PIM Rider analysis: To display and analyse the interaction data, we developed a software platform (The 'PIM Rider®'). The neighborhood of any protein within the protein interaction map was displayed with PBS scores for every connection.

A summary of information describing all interacting domains within a given protein can be displayed graphically. The PIM Rider also supplies a description of each gene with functional and genomic information, and includes links to significance bibliographic references and to relevant external data base.

Results

The PAZ6 immortalized human pre-adipocytes represent a unique model to study the physiology of human adipocytes. PAZ6 cells can be passaged in culture for several months without losing their morphological characteristics as well as their molecular markers.

These immortalized brown pre-adipocytes can readily be differentiated into adipocytes by treatment containing insulin, dexamethazone IBMX and pioglitazone. Morphological changes are associated with 14 days differentiation of PAZ6 (Fig. 1). These changes include the accumulation of multi-lobular fat droplets. Once differentiated, PAZ6 undergo lipolysis upon catecholamine stimulation.

PAZ6 cells express various markers found in or specific to human adipocytes including: PPAR gamma, leptin, glucose transporter (GLUT4), beta3 adreno-receptor, hormone sensitive lipase (HSL) all detected by PCR analysis (Fig. 1). An additional marker UCP1, specific to the brown adipocyte was also identified in the differentiated PAZ6 cells. Together, these characteristics confirm that PAZ6 are suitable immortalized human cells to investigate human adipocyte pathways implicated in the development of obesity.

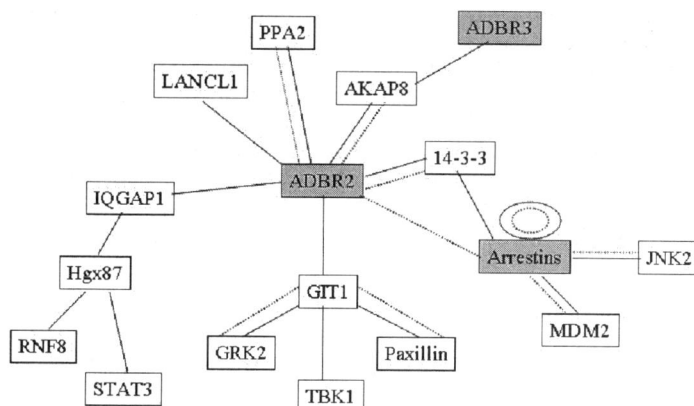

Fig. 2. A human adipocyte PIMRider screen shot displaying a portion of the protein interaction map around the ADRB2. Previously reported interactions are represented in dotted lines, whereas novel ones are illustrated in bold lines.

An increase in adipose tissue mass can be the result of the production of new fat cells through the process of adipogenesis. The characterization of novel genes that are highly expressed during adipose differentiation represents a privileged way to assess the mechanisms controlling adipogenesis and the maintenance of the mature adipocyte phenotype.

One attractive strategy for finding these novel genes involves examining differential gene expression. To this end, the MPSS technology was used at two different stages of PAZ6 cell development (pre-adipocytes and 14 days-differentiated adipocytes).

In total, 3,600 differentiated expressed genes were identified and could be grouped into four categories: (1) expressed in pre-adipocytes only (671 genes); (2) expressed in adipocytes only (990 genes); (3) up-regulated during differentiation (807 genes); and (4) down-regulated during differentiation (1148). Differentially expressed genes encode proteins involved in several main functions: adipogenesis, fatty acid oxidation, lipogenesis, mitochondrial respiration, protein secretion.

Some previously known up-regulated genes were identified. Among these, secreted proteins (SPARC/osteonectin, adipsin, leptin), transcription factors (STAT5, C/EBP gamma), enzymes (lipoprotein lipase, metalloproteinase 2, TIMP4,3, janus kinase) and others (CPTII, SOCS3, FABP). Several previously reported up-regulated genes were however not found. Among these, adreno-receptors ('ADRB'), leptin receptor, CD36, PPAR gamma, HSL, UCP and GLUT 4. This failure may be due to differences between primary cells and PAZ6 adipocytes, or to the fact that we are analysing human fat cells rather than the much more studied murine 3T3 L1 or F44A cell lines or last but not least to particular technical reasons. They are not due to reduced levels of expression, since very rare proteins were actually found to be expressed in the PAZ6 cells.

Newly up-regulated genes comprised receptors (several GPCRs: an orphan receptor, a cannabinoid receptor and the EDG2 receptor), secreted proteins (complement component, and frizzled-related proteins), transcription factors (zinc-finger proteins, forkhead transcription factors) and enzymes (kinases and metalloproteases).

Differential gene expression profile was complemented by protein-protein interaction information. To this end, eleven differentially expressed proteins were mapped for protein-protein interactions using a massively parallelized yeast-2 hybrid technology[10].

A separate specific goal was the identification of new interaction partners involved in intracellular signaling. A set of 32 proteins was selected. This set comprised (1) receptors, e.g. melatonin, the ADRB2, ADBR3, leptin receptor; (2) kinases, e.g. G-protein receptor kinases: GRK-2 and GRK3; (3) JAK2; (4) transcription factors, e.g: STAT 3; (5) suppressor of regulators of cytokine signaling such as SOCS family members, and (6) adaptor proteins, e.g: beta arrestin.

Differentially regulated proteins and proteins involved in intracellular signaling were assembled to build the human adipocyte PIM. This PIM was generated using protein-protein interaction information obtained for 43 proteins and 65 baits. Previously reported interactions were identified. This was the case for adaptor proteins and MAPKs such as beta arrestin and JNK 2 and JNK 3[11], adaptor proteins and E3 ubiquitin ligase like beta arrestin and mdm2[12], GPCR and adaptor protein such as beta 2 adrenergic receptor and AKAP[13], GPCR kinase and adaptor protein GTPase-activating protein like GRK2 and GIT[14], GPCR and phosphatase like ADRB2 and PP2A[15].

Interaction data were displayed and analysed using the PIMRider® technology that draws an automatic layout of the neighbourhood of a protein in a protein interaction map. As an example, Fig. 2 illustrates paths connecting signaling proteins in human PAZ6 adipocytes. Previously reported interactions are represented in dotted lines, whereas the novel ones are illustrated in bold lines.

The protein-protein interaction map enriches known signalling pathways and also reveals new biological pathways. For example, the GTPase activating protein GIT1 was reported to interact with GRK2 and Paxillin[14,16]. The protein interaction map reveals that GIT1 also directly interacts with the ADRB2, thus extending the signaling pathway of ADRB2 and further confirming a connection between small GTPases and ADRB2 signalling. The connection of beta-arrestin with mdm2, a protein involved in ubiquitination and with ADRB2 is consistent with a role of beta-arrestin in ADRB2 desensitization and degradation as suggested very recently[12]. A new structural link was also found between the 14-3-3 proteins and both beta-arrestin and ADRB2.

AKAP was reported earlier to interact with ADRB2; the new PIM reveals that the same AKAP protein may also connect with the ADRB3 suggesting that the AKAP proteins may similarly regulate ADRB3 function. Finally, with respect to the ADRB2 signaling pathway, two newly identified partners were identified: LANCL1 and IQGAP1.

Discussion

The first step in analysing differentiation-related pathways in human adipocytes is the establishment of a reliable and reproducible cellular system. The immortalized PAZ6 pre-adipocyte cell line was established several years ago by Zilberfarb *et al.*[7], and has since been validated by various laboratories in a number of publications which have demonstrated that these PAZ6 cells could indeed be differentiated into mature adipocytes which stably display most of the molecular markers and functionalities of human primary brown adipocytes[7,17].

These cells were thus deemed appropriate for creating protein interaction maps that would allow the elucidation of physiologic pathways involved in adipocyte differentiation. By applying the MPSS technology to the mRNAs prepared from differentiated PAZ6 adipocytes, we did not identify all of the molecular markers usually associated with mature adipocytes, but were gratified to find a number of molecular markers associated with adipocyte differentiation: leptin, and SPARC/osteonectin.

We then set out to use a number of the up-regulated genes as well as other marker genes described in the literature to develop protein interaction maps.

Sixty-five protein fragments were thus screened against a library containing independent clones. We analysed 3,600 interactions. These data, obtained with 43 proteins only represent a very small portion of the total human adipocyte interactome, if ones consider that a mature adipocyte probably expresses at least 10,000 proteins at any single time, that these vary in time, that these may not all be visualized in the yeast two-hybrid system used in this work. Only a relative small portion of these proteins (usually evaluated at 500) is probably selective for mature adipocytes.The data discussed here may thus be only a start of a much larger study.

The results reported so far appear to be reproducible and reliable. In fact we confirmed a number of interactions that had been published previously using similar or different proteomic or genetic association technologies.

Acknowledgements: We acknowledge the collaboration, in the initial steps of this work, of members of the CNRS UPR415 Unit (Tarik Issad and Vladimir Zilberfarb), of members of Lynx Inc (California) , and of Dr Simon Whiteside, then at Hybrigenics and now at Diversis in Cambridge, UK.

References

1. Friedman JM. Obesity in the new millennium. *Nature* 2000; 404: 632.

2. Montague CT, Farooqi IS, Whitehead JP, Soos MA, Rau H, Wareham NJ *et al.* Congenital leptin deficiency is associated with severe early-onset obesity in humans. *Nature* 1997; 387: 903–8.

3. Strobel A, Issad T, Camoin L, Ozata M, Strosberg AD. A leptin missense mutation associated with hypogonadism and morbid obesity. *Nature Genet* 1998; 18(3): 213–15.

4. Strosberg AD. *The β3-adrenoreceptor.* Taylor and Francis series in pharmaceutical sciences; 2000.

5. Bachman ES, Dhillon H, Zhang C-Y, Cinti S, Bianco AC, Kobilka BK *et al.* BetaAR signaling required for diet induced thermogenesis and obesity resistance. *Science* 2002; 297: 843–645.

6. Cone R. Haploinsufficiency of the melanocortin-4 receptor: part of a thrifty genotype? *J Clin Invest* 2000; 106(2): 185–7.

7. Zilberfarb V, Pietri-Rouxel F, Jockers R, Krief S, Delouis C, Isad T *et al.* Human immortalized brown adipocytes express functional beta3-adrenoceptor coupled to lipolysis. J *Cell Sci* 1997; 110(Pt7): 801–17.

8. Brenner S, Johnson M, Bridgham J, Golda G, Lloyd DH, Johnson D *et al.* Gene expression analysis by massively parallel signature sequencing (MPSS) on microbead arrays. *Nat Biotechnol* 2000; 18: 630–4.

9. Fromont-Racine M, Rain J-C, Legrain P. Towards a functional analysis of the yeast genome through exhaustive two-hybrid screens. *Nature Genet* 1997; 16: 277–82.

10. Rain J-C, Selig L, De Reuse H, Battaglia V, Reverdy C, Simon S *et al.* The protein-protein interaction map of Helicobacter pylori. *Nature* 2001; 409: 211–5.

11. McDonald, Chow CW, Miller WE, Laporte SA, Field ME, Lin FT *et al.* Beta arrestin 2: a receptor-regulated MAPK scaffold for the activation of JNK3. *Science* 2000; 290(5496): 1574–7.

12. Shenoy SK, McDonald PH, Kohout TA, Lefkowitz RS. Regulation of receptor fate by ubiquitination of activated beta 2-adrenergic receptor and beta arrestin. *Science* 2001; 294(5545): 1307–13.

13. Fraser ID, Cong M, Kim J, Rollins EN, Daaka Y, Lefkowitz RJ *et al.* Assembly of an A kinase-anchoring protein-beta(2)-adrenergic receptor complex facilitates receptor phosphorylation and signaling. *Curr Biol* 2000; 10(7): 409–12.

14. Premont RT, Claing A, Vitale N, Freeman JL, Pitcher JA, Patton WA *et al.* Related Articles, Domains, Nucleotide, Free in PMC, Protein beta2-Adrenergic receptor regulation by GIT1, a G protein-coupled receptor kinase-associated ADP ribosylation factor GTPase-activating protein. *Proc Natl Acad Sci USA* 1998 Nov 24; 95 (24): 14082–7.

15. Shih M, Lin F, Scott JD, Wang HY, Malbon CC. Dynamic complexes of beta2-adrenergic receptors with protein kinases and phosphatases and the role of gravin. *J Biol Chem* 1999; 274: 1588–95.

16. Zhao ZS, Manser E, Loo TH Lim L. Coupling of PAK-interacting exchange factor PIX to GIT1 promotes focal complex disassembly. *Mol Cell Biol* 2000; 20: 6354–63.

17. Oberkofler H, Esterbauer H, Linnemayr V, Strosberg AD, Krempler F, Patsch W. Peroxisome proliferator-activated receptor (PPAR) coactivator-1 recruitment regulates PPAR subtype specificity. *J Biol Chem* 2002; 277: 16750–7.

Progress in Obesity Research: 9. Edited by *Geraldo Medeiros-Neto, Alfredo Halpern and Claude Bouchard*
©2003 John Libbey Eurotext Ltd, pp. 234–236.

CHAPTER 49

Fine localization of genes influencing human obesity

R. Arlen Price

Center for Neurobiology and Behavior, University of Pennsylvania, Philadelphia, PA 19104, USA
[e-mail: arlen@bgl.psycha.upenn.edu]

Gene mapping studies

Rankinen and colleagues[7], in the annual obesity gene map update, report more than 250 genetic loci linked or associated with obesity in humans and animal models. These include 6 major genes from animal models (plus several knockouts), six major genes in humans, 25 genetic syndromes, 165 animal quantitative trait loci, 58 candidate genes with reported associations in humans, and 59 loci with at least one report of possible linkage. Considering all studies, every human chromosome has been implicated except the Y.

The linkage results come from some 44 separate publications, including 17 genome scans. Some of the scans involved reanalysis of the same cohort with different phenotypes. Scans not included in the annual review include several recent scans, some opportunistic analyses of height and weight in cohorts originally collected for other purposes. The number of loci (59+) is large, and some may well be false positives. However, 14 of the linkages have achieved at least minimal replication through an independent report of linkage to the same region. Most of these 'replications' are concentrated in only a few regions, including 1p31, 1q22, 2p22, 7q31, 10p12, 18q21, and 20q13. Of these regions, 10p12 and 2p22 appear to have the strongest and most consistent support. While much uncertainty remains, it is encouraging that the level of replication appears to be higher than for most other complex traits, e.g. NIDDM.

Regional gene mapping

Our recently published followup scan of three small regions of chromosome 10[6] illustrates some of the issues regarding the genome scans conducted thus far by others and by us. First, the sample sizes used have had low power to identify linkage to genes with small effects. (This weakness is not unique to our scan. Of the 10 scans recently reviewed by the PI[5], all but two of the samples included only about 500 individuals.) We did not detect the 10p peak on our first pass with 92 families. The earlier scan also missed a peak in chromosome region 7q31 in the 5' region of the leptin gene that we have identified in other studies using a finer map[4,8]. Second, support for linkage may be specific to a particular phenotype. In this case, the phenotype includes mild obesity occurring in families in which extreme obesity is also segregating. Third, the follow-up scan demonstrates the difficulty of replicating linkage results for complex traits having only modest gene effect sizes.

Another consideration is that most previous analyses have used only the simplest of genetic models. A few studies have considered two locus models acting either additively or interactively. However, no group has attempted a systematic screen for gene interactions. In addition, none have yet considered possible parent of origin effects associated with genomic imprinting. It will also be important to begin using sex specific phenotypes, e.g. by making opposite sex individuals phenotype unknown, and high resolution, sex specific recombination maps that have recently become available[3]. Given the relatively small gene effect sizes likely to be operative for obesity, more complex analyses may be essential for gene identification.

Regional linkage mapping has a long way to go before large-scale fine mapping efforts are justified. Because recombinations between markers and quantitative trait loci can only be inferred, the maximum resolution possible from linkage studies is about 1–2 per cent recombination (centamorgans, cM). The larger samples used in obesity linkage studies may have a resolution of 5–10 cM, while the average size obesity linkage study may have a resolution as poor as 20–30 cM. Clearly, more linkage studies are needed. Those studies will require much larger sample sizes and should utilize more realistic genetic models. Independent replication is also essential.

Fine mapping

Fine mapping will require methods other than linkage, particularly studies of genetic associations and/or linkage disequilibrium.

Associations between alleles arise because mutations occur on specific chromosome haplotypes or because equilibrium populations undergo bottlenecks or genetic drift, thereby increasing the associations among alleles in the preserved haplotypes. How long these associations are maintained depends on recombination, which in turn depends on physical distance. Initial disequilibrium for unlinked loci is decreased by half per generation, e.g. by more than 99.9 per cent within 10 generations, a little over two centuries. By comparison, 23,000 generations (about 460,000 years) would be required to reduce an association between tightly linked loci (about 30 kilobases, kb) by the same amount. Some early reports (Kruglyak 1999)[9] suggested that disequilibrium might only extend over much shorter distances of 3 to 30 kb. However, empirical studies indicate that the distances may be much larger, even in outbred populations. At the same time, there are gaps in disequilibrium over very short distances, perhaps due to gene conversion.

Rankinen *et al.*[7] summarized positive associations by over 180 studies to 58 candidate genes. Association studies have high error rates because cases and controls may differ in gene frequency due to chance or to population substructure. Recent studies[1] suggest that population substructure may be minimal provided samples are of at least moderate size (more than 500 individuals), ethnically homogeneous, and individuals with recent admixture are excluded. These findings are encouraging since large-scale case control studies provide a very powerful tool for fine mapping.

A recent advance in fine mapping is the detection of haplotype blocks with histories of very low recombination rates[2]. These blocks appear to have persisted in human evolution because of variability in recombination across the genome.

Case-control association studies can be very powerful but have created confusion because of small sample size and difficulty in replication. Large-scale studies having 500–1,000 cases and controls provide one of the most powerful tools available for fine mapping. Sample homogeneity is important, and in outbred populations recent admixture should be avoided. Sample heterogeneity can be tested and it may be possible to use genomic data to increase the matching of case and control groups.

Family based association methods are not subject to false positives due to population subdivision and may be the design of choice in some situations where heterogeneity is an issue. Preferential transmission of marker alleles from heterozygous parents in parent-offspring triads is not influenced by allele frequencies. However, triads are more difficult and expensive to collect than cases and controls and may be best used as an adjunct to case control designs, particularly for validation.

Summary and recommendations

Additional linkage studies are needed in order to improve the resolution of regional gene mapping. Larger samples and more realistic models will be needed. Models that should be considered include sex specific phenotypes, sex specific marker maps, gene-gene interactions, and parent of origin effects.

Case-control studies are powerful but underutilized. It is a useful design, but samples should be large and heterogeneity should be minimized.

Family-based studies are attractive because they are not influenced by sample structure. However, because of the additional effort and expense, they may be best used to validate and extend results from studies using cases and controls.

Acknowledgements: The preparation of this manuscript was supported by grants from the National Institutes of Health, R01DK44073, R01DK48950, and R01DK56210. Some unpublished results referred to in this paper were obtained through collaboration with Drs. Hongyu Zhao, Christopher Amos and Robert Nicholls. Drs. Wei-Dong Li and Chuanhui Dong, as well as Mr. Ding Li all made contributions to this work.

References

1. Ardlie KG, Lunetta KL, Seielstad M. Testing for population subdivision and association in four case-control studies. *Am J Hum Genet* 2002; 71: 304–11.

2. Gabriel SB, Shaffner SF, Nguyen H, Moore JM, Roy J, Blumenstiel B *et al*. The structure of haplotype blocks in the human genome. *Science* 2002; 296: 2225–9.

3. Kong A, Gubdjartsson DF, Sainz J, Jonsdottir GM, Budjonsson SA, Richardsson B *et al*. A high-resolution recombination map of the human genome. *Nature Genet* 2002; 31: 241–7.

4. Li W, Reed D, Lee J, Xu W, Kilker R, Sodam B *et al*. Sequence variants in the 5' flanking region of the leptin gene are associated with obesity in women. *Annals Hum Genet* 1999; 63: 227–34.

5. Price RA. Genetics and common obesities: Background, current status, strategies and future prospects. In: *Obesity: theory and therapy*, Chapter 4, Stunkard TWA (ed.). New York: Guilford Publications; 2002.

6. Price RA, Li WD, Bernstein A, Crystal A, Golding EM, Weisberg SJ *et al*. A locus affecting obesity in human chromosome region 10p12. *Diabetologia* 2001; 44: 363–6.

7. Rankinen T, Perusse L, Weisnagel SJ, Snyder EE, Chagnon YC, Bouchard C. The human obesity gene map: the 2001 update. *Obes Res* 2002; 10: 196–243.

8. Reed DR, Ding Y, Xu W, Cather C, Green ED, Price RA. Extreme obesity may be linked to markers flanking the human OB gene. *Diabetes* 1996; 45: 691–4.

9. Kruglyak L. Prospects for whole-genome linkage disequilibrium mapping of common disease genes. *Nature Genet* 1999; 22: 139–44.

Progress in Obesity Research: 9. Edited by *Geraldo Medeiros-Neto, Alfredo Halpern and Claude Bouchard*
©2003 John Libbey Eurotext Ltd, pp. 237–240.

CHAPTER 50

A cornucopia of study designs in the post genomics era: critical evaluation of methods using mouse models

Nancy A. Schonfeld-Warden[1] and Craig H. Warden[1,2]

[1]*Department of Pediatrics, UC Davis;* [2]*Rowe Program in Human Genetics and Section of Neurobiology, Physiology and Behavior, UC Davis, Davis CA 95616, USA*
[e-mail: chwarden@ucdavis.edu]

Genome progress summary

This review will discuss the impact of genome sequencing on study designs for obesity gene discovery in the 'post genomics' era. We will identify major methods for obesity gene discovery, including methods that existed before the genomics era that have benefited from completion of the genome sequencing projects, and we will also introduce study designs that are only now possible because this is the post genomics era. We focus on studies of obesity, but many of the methods we discuss work as well for any complex trait. We describe briefly the methods available for study designs, and we evaluate the strengths and weaknesses of each. We focus on the best methods to understand complex traits (where genes interact with other genes and with the environment), since such methods are likely to be relevant to understanding obesity. Finally, we focus on mouse models, since study designs in these models are greatly changed and improved in this post genomics era.

Introduction to post genomics study designs

Three general approaches are used widely to study phenotype effects of otherwise unknown genes. A simple but powerful study design is to use the new comprehensive gene lists to look for homologs of known obesity genes. This approach has been very productive, for instance aiding the identification of mitochondrial uncoupling protein 2 (UCP2) and agouti-related protein (AGRP)[1,2]. This fundamental genetic approach will retain its usefulness every time a new obesity gene is described.

Another approach to obesity gene discovery is to use assembled genome sequence as a guide to find genes with the same chromosomal positions as mapped obesity traits. Any lab that can map traits can use public (NCBI, ENSEMBL) and private (Celera) genome databases to identify positional candidate genes co-incident with such traits[3,4]. The assembled genome sequence is also an important tool for any approach that involves genome modification, such as gene-trap vectors and mutagenesis since the assembly itself facilitates identification of the mutated gene. Genome assemblies also now facilitate new tests of positional candidate genes, because we can now efficiently determine coding sequence for all of the many expressed genes co-incident with a mapped trait in normal and mutant mice.

The third approach is to use the new (almost) complete catalogs of genes to guide production of probes for mRNA expression profiles or to make collections of probes to detect gene x gene interactions with *in vitro* systems. Microarrays[5] produce 'expression profiles' that display relative amounts of thousands of different mRNAs in a tissue extract. These profiles show quantitative expression patterns of genes co-regulated over time or in health versus disease. For example, microarray analysis showed that leptin specifically represses mRNA levels for hepatic stearoyl-CoA desaturase (SCD-1). This led the investigators to produce SCD-1 knockout mice, which were lean and hypermetabolic[6].

However, expression profiles of mRNA levels are of limited usefulness because they provide information only about transcript levels. They do not yield information on translated proteins, post-translational modification, protein-protein interaction, gene-gene interaction, or cell biology/physiology[7].

Specific examples of post genomics study designs

We discussed above three widely used study designs that depend for success in part on the availability of the complete human and mouse genome sequences. Equally important to success is an appropriate animal model. With one exception[8,9], obesity genes were first identified in the laboratory mouse. All mouse genes (such as leptin) that are known to cause simple monogenic obesity syndromes have been cloned and these efforts have identified important mouse and homologous human obesity pathways[10]. However, many complex obesity genes and pathways remain undiscovered. Current methods to elucidate new obesity genes and pathways include those that identify natural alleles influencing obesity and methods to produce *in vivo* mutations of candidate obesity genes in mice that can be phenotyped.

Discovery of natural alleles influencing obesity

Many genes that influence fat accumulation exist within existing inbred strains of mice. The obesity effects of these genes may be hidden because they have relatively subtle effects or because any mouse strain carries genes that both promote and inhibit obesity. Common methods to identify these genes and observe their effects in mice include Quantitative Trait Locus (QTL) mapping and surveys of recombinant progeny of two inbred parental strains (congenic mice, recombinant inbred strains, recombinant congenic strains, and consomics[11,12]).

QTL mapping is a powerful method for defining the chromosomal positions of natural alleles that influence complex traits. Scores of obesity and related QTLs such as energy expenditure have been published[13]. The advantages of QTL mapping over other complex trait analytical methods are that it surveys natural alleles that may have been selected during evolution and it can be used to identify chromosomal loci that interact in any model including pure epistatic (no phenotype effects for either locus alone and effects only apparent for specific alleles of each locus together) or additive or dominant/recessive interactions.

The principal difficulty with QTL mapping is that it is slow to lead to identification of specific underlying genes. The primary reason for this is that QTLs are inherently large (10–20 cM) and thus include potentially hundreds of positional candidate genes and polymorphisms distinguishing any two strains used for QTL mapping. Thus, there will always be many candidate genes and polymorphisms in any QTL. This means that the gene(s) that underlie the QTL cannot be identified until the chromosomal region known to contain the QTL phenotype is narrowed. This problem has been solved by the production of congenic mouse strains, produced by crossing a 'donor' strain that carries a phenotype and hypothesized causative chromosomal region, with a phenotypically different 'background' strain. Repeated backcrossing and marker selection over 5–10 generations yield a congenic that differs from the background only in the donor chromosomal region of interest.

Mutations produced by human intervention

Methods for large-scale screens of mutagenized mouse genes for phenotype influences focus on phenotypes, specific genes, or all (any) genes.

Chemical mutagenesis

Random mutagenesis by ethane methylsulphonate (EMS) can alter function of any gene. Mutagenized male mice are bred to many females, and mice born to chemically mutagenized parents are trait-screened for dominant or recessive phenotypes[14]. The result is a high throughput screen system of mice collectively mutagenized for every gene. Dominant phenotype screens are easy because first-generation mice produced from mutagenized parents can be phenotyped since each mouse carries a finite number of mutations (perhaps 100). Recessive screens involve many F3 mice derived from each founder animal since only 25 per cent can be homozygous for any mutation.

The advantages of chemical mutagenesis are than many alleles can be generated for every gene and that positional cloning can isolate the genes underlying target phenotypes, since the mutations can be produced using inbred strains. Some of the disadvantages of chemical mutagenesis are that the phenotypes must be obvious and breedable (a problem for obesity models because most obese mice are infertile), and screens for epistasis and diet effects are not possible because a mutagenized animal probably would not have novel alleles of two different interacting obesity genes whose Mendelian inheritance can be confirmed by simple breeding tests.

Knockout mice

Knockout mice can be used to study the functions of specific genes *in vivo*, but the technology is too expensive (up to US$50,000 per knockout) for large-scale screens. Knockout production begins with homologous recombination to insert an inactivated allele of a specific gene into an embryonic stem cell line (ES), which can then be used to produce animals with the altered gene incorporated into the germ line. Some variants of the approach include tissue and time specific knockouts[15]. Generation of appropriate control mice for knockout experiments is tricky because all mice are genetic mixes and the admixture can affect obesity phenotypes profoundly.

Gene-traps

The gene-trap is a promoter less vector that depends on integration into a functioning gene for expression. They can be used to knock out or otherwise modify any gene expressed in ES cells[16]. In the mouse, the gene-trap process begins by integrating a gene-trap vector (with selectable markers) into ES cells. Clones that express an antibiotic resistance gene driven by the trapped gene's promoter are differentially selected and isolated. The DNA sequence from the mouse genomic DNA adjacent to the insertion site can be used to identify the 'trapped' gene. The result is libraries of ES cells with gene-traps in known and unknown genes, all usable for production of live animals.

Comparison and contrasts of study designs

Should any of the four gene discovery methods described above now be abandoned? For instance, in this era of animal model genetic manipulation, is gene discovery by QTL mapping obsolete? Or, do all the methods have advantages that make each useful, and shortcomings that limit them, so that all study designs are necessary in a comprehensive effort to understand the biological causes of human obesity? The unique and important advantage of QTL mapping over the other experimental approaches discussed above is that QTL mapping is the only method that can identify genes underlying gene x gene interactions. This is because QTL mapping experiments can screen thousands of allelic variants for phenotype effects in a single experiment, in fact all of the thousands of variants that differ between any two strains involved in a cross. QTL mapping experiments have already discovered many gene x gene interactions in obesity. Discovery of the underlying genes is essential for understanding mechanisms of obesity, especially human obesity which is very likely to involve gene x gene interactions.

QTL mapping takes much longer than other approaches to identify single underlying genes. In fact, it may not always be possible to use QTL mapping for this purpose because QTLs are too large to provide useful information about positional candidates. Thus, congenic strain production and phenotyping, which can take years, has been the next step for the isolation of QTL genes. The congenic regions of most congenic mouse strains include at least two and frequently hundreds of genes from the donor strains. However, once congenics have been established and shown to have a phenotype of interest, success at gene identification has become increasingly likely[17-20].

Advantages of chemical mutagenesis

Chemical mutagenesis is a powerful method for production of mice with altered phenotypes. These mice can be bred and used as tools for positional cloning to identify the mutated gene. The method clearly works and can be used to produce mice that should survey all genes for phenotype effects. Thus, chemical mutagenesis can identify genes whose individual single actions (monogenic effects) have detectable effects on complex traits[21].

Advantages of gene-trap experimental designs

It is easy to use gene sequence adjacent to a gene-trap vector to identify genes in ES cells that have gene-trap integration sites. This allows rapid selection and assembly of complete gene-trap libraries that could include thousands of ES cell lines each 'trapped' for one or more of each and every gene expressed by these cells. However, it is costly to transform mouse models with these cells, because the process involves blastocyst injection and implantation, with no guarantee of success. Nevertheless, the gene-trap's great advantage is that the chromosomal location of the mutant (knockout) gene is already known. Thus, it is usually easier and faster to use this type of model to identify obesity genes than it is to use chemically mutagenized mice, since a gene-trap mouse can identify a novel gene or allele by phenotype. Gene location can only be mapped in chemically mutagenized mice by crossing mouse lines, sometimes repeatedly over months and years.

Conclusions

Human obesity involves a complex interaction of many genes and pathways and is influenced by environment and natural genetic variation. Thus a complete understanding of obesity will involve identifying all genes and pathways that influence fat accumulation, understanding environment influences on these genes and pathways, and understanding allelic effects on gene: pathway: environment interactions. Although this work will take years, much of the task has been made infinitely easier by the completion of the human and mouse genome assemblies. Thus, 'post-genomics' investigators are free to focus on far more interesting topics such as characterizing gene function and on using this information to understand physiology and disease.

Acknowledgements: We thank Sean Barry for reviewing and editing the manuscript. This work was supported by NIH DK53993.

References

1. Fleury C, Neverova M, Collins S, Raimbault S, Champigny O, Levi-Meyrueis C *et al.* Uncoupling protein-2: a novel gene linked to obesity and hyperinsulinemia. *Nature Genet* 1997; 15: 269–72.

2. Ollmann MM, Wilson BD, Yang YK, Kerns JA, Chen Y, Gantz I *et al.* Antagonism of central melanocortin receptors *in vitro* and *in vivo* by agouti-related protein. *Science* 1997; 278: 135–8.

3. Hubbard T, Barker D, Birney E, Cameron G, Chen Y, Clark L *et al.* The Ensembl genome database project. *Nucleic Acids Res* 2002; 30: 38–41.

4. Kerlavage A, Bonazzi V, di Tommaso M, Lawrence C, Li P, Mayberry F *et al.* The celera discovery system. *Nucleic Acids Res* 2002; 30: 129–36.

5. Macgregor PF, Squire JA. Application of microarrays to the analysis of gene expression in cancer. *Clin Chem* 2002; 48: 1170–7.

6. Cohen P, Miyazaki M, Socci ND, Hagge-Greenberg A, Liedtke W, Soukas AA *et al.* Role for stearoyl-CoA desaturase-1 in leptin-mediated weight loss. *Science* 2002; 297: 240–3.

7. Daniel H. Genomics and proteomics: importance for the future of nutrition research. *Br J Nutr* 2002; 87 (Suppl 2): S305–S11.

8. Collier GR, McMillan JS, Windmill K, Walder K, Tenne-Brown J, de Silva A *et al.* Beacon: a novel gene involved in the regulation of energy balance. *Diabetes* 2000; 49: 1766–71.

9. Walder K, Kantham L, McMillan JS, Trevaskis J, Kerr L, De Silva A *et al.* Tanis: a link between type 2 diabetes and inflammation? *Diabetes* 2002; 51: 1859–66.

10. Fisler JS, Warden CH. Mapping of mouse obesity genes: A generic approach to a complex trait. *J Nutr* 1997; 127: S1909–S16.

11. Nadeau JH, Singer JB, Matin A, Lander ES. Analysing complex genetic traits with chromosome substitution strains. *Nature Genet* 2000; 24: 221–5.

12. Doerge RW. Mapping and analysis of quantitative trait loci in experimental populations. *Nat Rev Genet* 2002; 3: 43–52.

13. Rankinen T, Perusse L, Weisnagel SJ, Snyder EE, Chagnon YC, Bouchard C. The human obesity gene map: the 2001 update. *Obes Res* 2002; 10: 196–243.

14. Justice MJ. Capitalizing on large-scale mouse mutagenesis screens. *Nat Rev Genet* 2000; 1: 109–15.

15. Lewandoski M. Conditional control of gene expression in the mouse. *Nat Rev Genet* 2001; 2: 743–55.

16. Stanford WL, Cohn JB, Cordes SP. Gene-trap mutagenesis: past, present and beyond. *Nat Rev Genet* 2001; 2: 756–68.

17. Korstanje R, Paigen B. From QTL to gene: the harvest begins. *Nature Genet* 2002; 31: 235–6.

18. MacMurray AJ, Moralejo DH, Kwitek AE, Rutledge EA, Van Yserloo B, Gohlke P *et al.* Lymphopenia in the BB rat model of type 1 diabetes is due to a mutation in a novel immune-associated nucleotide (ian)-related gene. *Genome Res* 2002; 12: 1029–39.

19. Ma RZ, Gao J, Meeker ND, Fillmore PD, Tung KS, Watanabe T *et al.* Identification of Bphs, an autoimmune disease locus, as histamine receptor H1. *Science* 2002; 297: 620–3.

20. Mehrabian M, Allayee H, Wong J, Shih W, Wang XP, Shaposhnik Z *et al.* Identification of 5-lipoxygenase as a major gene contributing to atherosclerosis susceptibility in mice. *Circ Res* 2002; 91: 120–6.

21. Coghill EL, Hugill A, Parkinson N, Davison C, Glenister P, Clements S *et al.* A gene-driven approach to the identification of ENU mutants in the mouse. *Nature Genet* 2002; 30: 255–6.

Progress in Obesity Research: 9. Edited by *Geraldo Medeiros-Neto, Alfredo Halpern and Claude Bouchard*
©2003 John Libbey Eurotext Ltd, pp. 241–246.

CHAPTER 51

Large scale mouse mutagenesis programmes for identification of new obesity genes: pros and cons

Edward H. Leiter

The Jackson Laboratory, Bar Harbor, ME, 04609, USA
[e-mail: ehl@jax.org]

Introduction: statement defining the debate

The sequencing of the mouse genome has been completed and has provided a detailed genetic and physical map. Only between 1–2 per cent of this genome encodes the 30,000–40,000 expressed genes. The functions of only a fraction of these expressed genes have been identified. Hence, the effort to assign function to those genes that do produce proteins (functional genomics) is now where the major effort in mammalian genetics is being placed. This effort should lead to identification of many new moleculas (and novel drug targets) regulating somatic growth, adipogenesis, nutrient metabolism, and energy balance. The 'debate' presented in this essay focuses attention on the relative merits of generating new obesity-producing mutations by large-scale mutagenesis programmes versus in-depth analysis of known obesity-associated QTL. The argument for using chemical mutagenesis to generate dominant or recessive mutations inherited in a simple Mendelian trait (as opposed to 'chasing' QTL by sequencing numerous candidate genes and then validating the best candidate by testing *in vivo*) has been well made by Nadeau and Frankel[1]. Basically, the points these authors make are that dominant or recessive mutations with a discernible phenotype and inherited as a Mendelian trait in mice are readily identifiable in the current 'post-genome sequencing' era by physical mapping and positional cloning techniques.

In contrast to the relative case of identifying a null mutation in a gene produced in a chemical mutagenesis screen or by a spontaneous null mutation, establishing the physical identity of a QTL remains problematic ('the long and bumpy road') because these usually represent natural gene variants that have been differentially fixed among various inbred strains of mice. In many cases, they probably reflect mutations in regulatory sequences affecting mRNA levels or stability rather than exons encoding the protein structure. After a QTL has been delimited to a 2 cM or smaller region in a congenic stock, with retention of the altered phenotype (for example, altered fat depot weights), all the candidate genes in the arca must be evaluated, and then complex transgenic or knock-in technology must be employed for validation[1]. QTL analysis has indeed led to discovery of a few disease-associated genes in humans and rodents so that there is reason for optimism[2]. It is noteworthy that, in most of these cases of QTL gene discovery, a null allele from one strain (such as the intestinal phospholipase A2, *Pla2s*, resumed to be the *Mom* gene (modifier of *Min*, multiple intestinal neoplasias) was segregated against a functional allele. However, most QTL contributing to body mass and obesity probably have small additive or epistatic effects, so that isolation of only one in a congenic stock may well lead to loss of the phenotype used in its original identification. A recent review summarizes over 85 mouse QTL for body weight and more than 75 QTL for obesity[3]. This listing is by no means complete, and, to date, none have been identified definitively at the molecular level. The analysis of QTL on Chromosome 7 illustrate the problem.

Coincidence of multiple adiposity QTL on this chromosome following multiple interstram crosses have been reviewed[3]. Fine mapping of one of these suggests a novel ATPase with aminophospholipid translocase activity as a likely candidate gene[4,5]. However, knocking out the allele from one strain and knocking in the alternate allele by homologous recombination are the difficult steps that would have to be followed for validation of this gene as responsible for the QTL. Genome-wide mutagenesis, therefore, is an attractive alternative to 'QTL chasing' because of its potential to (theoretically) target every gene in the genome affecting a complex phenotype (e.g. obesity).

Large scale mouse 'muta' projects: what are are they and what do they involve?

Table 1 lists the major mouse mutagenesis centres and their web addresses. All centres treat parental male mice with the 'supermutagen' N-ethyl-N-nitrosurea (ENU). ENU primarily elicits A•T to T•A transversions and A•T to G•C transitions in spermatocytes, producing point mutations at a frequency of –1/1000 screened gametes. Mutations affecting fitness are often dominant embryonic lethals; non-lethal mutations with a visually discernible phenotype are much less prevalent. The mutations recovered include genes with splicing alterations, nonsense mutations, and missense mutations. Since mutagenized males (termed GO) are rendered transiently sterile by ENU treatment, they must be held for extended periods (typically 10–15 weeks) before they have recovered viable sperm count. This highlights one of the major requirements of any mutagenesis effort – the need for extensive vivarium facilities to hold mutagenized males and to generate and age their progeny. Excellent reviews of the various procedures used to screen progeny for dominant and recessive mutations have been published[6,7]. Dominant mutations can be uncovered in first generation (G1) progeny and confirmed in a second generation (G2). Recessive mutations require a three generation (G3) breeding scheme.

Table 1. Centres conducting high throughput mouse mutagenesis screens

UK Mouse Genome Centre, Harwell – ENU Mutagenesis Programme	http://www.mgu.har.mrc.ac.uk/mutabase/
ENU–Mouse Mutagenesis Screen in the German Human Genome Project	http://www.gsf.de/isg/groups/enu/
Neuroscience Mutagenesis Facility at the Jackson Laboratory	http://www.jax.orf/nmf/index.html
Mouse Heart, Lung, Blood and Sleep Disorders Center at the Jackson Laboratory	http://pga.jax.org
Baylor College of Medicine Mouse Genome Project	http://www.mouse-genome.bcm.tmc.edu/home.asp
Tennessee Mouse Genome Consortium	http://wtnmouse.org/
Mutagenesis at the McLaughlin Research Institute	http://www.montana.edu/wwwmri/enump.html
Centre for Modeling Human Disease at the Samuel Lunenfeld Research Institute	http://cmhd.mshri.on.ca/

ENU mutagenesis provides a chromosome unbiased (e.g. random) phenotype-driven genetic screen for mutations across the entire mouse genome. The key to successful mutation recovery in any of these programmes is the sophistication of the phenotyping protocols. The reader is referred to the webpages of the respective centres for details of the phenotypic screens employed and the success rate for recovery of heritable phenodeviants. Although not all centres are specifically seeking to uncover new obesity mutants, body weight is a parameter common to all screens. Table 2 below summarizes preliminary results concerning recovery of new obesity mutations and mice with diabetes-related phenotypes (impaired glucose tolerance, hyperglycaemia). In addition to mice with increased body fat, excessively lean mice are also generated in the mutagenesis programmes (not included in Table 2). Potential mutants ('putants') are first scored as phenodeviant if a specific phenotype such as body weight or body fat exceeds two standard deviations of what is considered as normative for the strain. Such 'putants' must be confirmed as bona fide mutants not only by a repetitive measurement for reproducibility of the trait in the proband, but also by recovery of more affected individuals in the same family, and demonstration of\ heritability into following generations. In the Neurosciences Mutagenesis Facility at The Jackson Laboratory, 20 individuals from each of 440 families established by mutagenized males are screened for phenodeviants. Identification of 'putants' requires careful analysis of the natural variation in the phenotype in question (for example, body weight).

Table 2. Heritable obesity (OB), diet-induced adiposity (AD), impaired glucose tolerance (IGT) or diabetes (DB) phenodeviants produced by genome-wide ENU mutagenesis

Programme	Strain	Screen	# Mice	# Phenodeviants
GGMC, Germany	C3HeB/FeJ	Dom. & recess.	40,000	7 OB*
Harwell, England	B6 x BALB/cJ	Dom. (behavioural)	25,000	2 OB*, 3 IGT
TJL (NMF)	B6	Dom. & recess.	8,800	1 OB
TJL (HLB)	B6	Dom. & recess.	4,000	23 AD*†, 2DB*

CGMC, German Gene Mutation Consortium; TJL, The Jackson Laboratoty; NMF, Neuroscience Mutagenesis Facility; HLB, Heart, Lung and Blood.
*'Putants', undergoing inheritance testing to confirm status as mutants; †Increase in per cent body fat without abnormally increased body weight during a 5 week period of feeding an atherogenic diet (1 per cent cholesterol, 0.5 per cent cholic acid, 15 per cent butter fat).

An excellent source for seeking normative data for various inbred strains is the Mouse Phenome Project website (http: //www.jax.org/phenome). Obviously, the domains included in a phenotyping screen determine the types of mutations recovered (behaviourial, metabolic, etc.). The phenotypic screens are labour-intensive, and the numbers of mice that can be processed through a complex phenotyping screen per week represent a bottleneck in most mutagenesis programmes. Most programmes seek to screen between 200–440 mutagenized genomes per year, with 20 progeny screened per G1 male, and 20 progeny per subsequent generation. This necessitates testing of approximately 85–160 mice per week (Karen Svenson, The Jackson Laboratory, personal communication). As noted in Table 2, the Heart, Lung, and Blood Mutagenesis programme at The Jackson Laboratory includes a 5-week period of feeding G3 mice an atherogenic diet containing 15 per cent fat (30 per cent calories). This G3 screen is generating heritable phenodeviants with increased per cent of body fat without an increase in body weight. If a mutation has been produced in a gene controlling adipogenic responses to elevated dietary fat, then establishing the heritability of this would require diet treatment of later generation mice. If 'putants' are discovered with juvenile obesity, they may prove difficult to breed, as evidenced by many of the spontaneously-occurring recessive obesity mutations which drastically curtail reproduction. In addition to the complexities of establishing the heritability of certain obesityrelevant genes that require environmental manipulations, another pitfall can be encountered in genome-based mutagenesis screens. It has been estimated that each generation of inbreeding results in homozygous fixation of at least three recessive mutations[8]. An elaborate phenotyping screen designed to identify 'putants' produced by mutagenesis may instead uncover one of these heretofore undiscovered mutant genes that will be widely distributed in individuals of the inbred strain. One such gene associated with epileptic seizure susceptibility was discovered through its prevalence in ENU-mutagenized B6 G1 males (Dr. Wayne Frankel, The Jackson Laboratory, personal communication).

Regional mutagenesis screens

One of the most commonly mutated obesity-producing genes in the mouse is that encoding the leptin receptor. Since the original report of the first mutation (*Leprdblj*) in 1966, at least seven other spontaneously-occurring and obesity-producing mutations in this gene have been uncovered over the ensuing 36 years, and two rat orthologs have been identified. Such an alleleic series represents a valuable tool for exploring structure/function relationships, but many of the mutant alleles are no longer available given the long period of time over which they have occurred. Mutagenesis now permits the investigator to generate such an allele series within a relatively short time frame. Such regional or allele-specific efforts usually take advantage of a linked coat colour mutation or other easily recognized phenotypic mutation (such as hairy ears). To illustrate, a stock of *LeVr*db_heterozygous 136 mice is available in which the misty (m) coat colour mutation is carried in close linkage to the mutant *Lepr*< !b allele. The coat colour phenotype of homozygous obese (m *Le*/m Lepr db)mice in this stock is greyish. If heterozygous GO males from this stock were mutagenized, mated to wild-type females, and obese mice with black coat colour recovered at G1, this would denote creation of a new (non-complementing) *Lepr* db mutation in the wild-type allele. However, since the obese mice would probably be infertile, this mutation could only be propagated by assisted reproduction techniques. Independent mutations at the *Lepr* locus occuring in primary spermatocytes and transmitted by GO males into reproductively-competent G1 mice with black lean phenotypes would have to be screened by test mating such G1 mice to m *Lepr* db/++ mice (also black, lean phenotypes). A non-complementing mutation in the *Lepr* locus would produce one-quarter black obese mice, with the two-thirds of the nonobese mice being carriers. Mutagenesis of germ-line competent embryonal stem cells *in vitro* is the most direct means for saturating a desired chromosome or chromosomal segment with mutations. The interested reader is referred to several excellent reviews that describe the various strategems in depth[6,7,9]. These strategems entail the use of homologous recombination to generate chromosome specific deletions[6] or inversions[10] in combination with transgenically-inserted coat colour or other visible transgenic markers ['balancer mutations'] or, alternatively, introduction of drug selection markers into a specific locus[11]. ES cell mutations are usually generated by irradiation (particularly deletions or inversions) or by treatment with another chemical point mutagen, ethylmethanesulphonate (EMS), *in vitro*. One 'chromosomal engineering' technique requires Cre/*LoxP* technology to produce an inversion in a chromosome of interest. Two *LoxP* sites are placed in the opposite orientation in ES cells so that the presence of the Cre recombinase in transgenic mice will produce an inverted chromosomal rearrangement. The targeted region is marked by a *Keratin 14* – a transgene so that the agouti phenotype produced by the dominant coat colour gene can mark the 'balancer chromosome' carrying the inversion. If C57BL/6 GO males are mutagenized and mated to females heterozygous for the agouti-marked 'balancer' chromosome, newly-generated homozygous recessive mutations can be identified in G3 homozygotes (those showing a non-agouti coat phenotype) Heterozygous carriers would show agouti coat colour. Agouti mice homozygous for the 'balancer' inversion would not survive.

Development of panels of chromosomally-engineered deletion stocks for chromosomespecific chemical mutagenesis both *in vitro* and *in vivo* is on-going in various laboratories. The interested reader is referred to several excellent reviews that describe the various at strategems in depth[6,7,9]. Region-specific screens using ES cells offer the advantage high mutagenesis frequencies, shortened breeding schemes, and isolation of mutations whose map position is known[6]. A bank of ES cells containing neo-Tk selection cassettes in all of the chromosomes has been developed at The Jackson Laboratory for chromosome-specific mutagenesis efforts (DELBank: http: //Iena jax.org/~jcs.html). Deletions in specific regions of each chromosome induced by ionizing radiation have been defined[12]. Availability of defined ES cell lines available in DELBank permit the investigator to use a point mutagen such as EMS (the latter much less hazardous than ENU to researchers working with mutagens *in vitro*) to mutate all or most genes in a defined chromosomal segment ('saturation mutagenesis')[12,13].

The other side of the search for mouse obesity genes – QTLs

Although both dominant and negative monogenic obesity genes have been described in rodents that produce juvenile onset obesity of the type that very likely will be produced in the large scale mutagenesis programmes, comparable loss-of-function mutations in the human orthologs to produce syndromic obesity are only rarely reported[14]. Human obesity and obesity-associated Type 2 diabetes (T2D) clearly show high heritability, but inheritance is not as a simple Mendelian trait. Most human obesity and most cases of type 2 diabetes, reflect complex interactions among networks of genes whose expression is influenced by age, sex, physical activity, and the nutritional environment[15]. Despite the formidable problems associated with QTL identification, this author would contend that knowledge of how QTL, in aggregate, produce a polygenic obesity syndrome will advance our understanding of the genetic basis of human obesities as much as complete loss of function mutations produced by mutagenesis or gene targeting efforts, but rarely observed in a natural population.

'Genetic architecture' is a term describing the full range of genetic effects on a phenotype. This architecture is not a fixed entity, but changes according to age and sex-mediated shifts in gene expression, as well as changes in the physical environment. Most common forms of obesity-induced T2D entail a complex interaction between multiple genes and the nutritional environment. It is conjectured that many of the genetic differences represented by QTLs identified in analysis of polygenic obesity sydromes in mice are not necessarily the consequence of mutations in the coding sequence of proteins, but rather in their regulatory sequences, rendering them hypo- or hyper-responsiveness to normal cellular signaling mechanisms. Quantitative trait locus (QTL) mapping has proven to be a powerful tool in dissecting the polygenic control of body size and fat depot development in mice (reviewed in[16–18]). Not surprisingly, QTL analysis has identified numerous loci controlling somatic growth and fat pad development in response to normal or high fat diets[16,17,19]. The New Zealand Obese (NZO) is an archetypal representative of a polygenic mouse obesity model. Leptin levels are initially normal, and signaling through the leptin receptor is also apparently normal[20]. However, this strain exhibits a defect in leptin transport across the blood-brain barrier[21]. Outcross of NZO with other inbred strains to identify locations of obesity and diabesity QTL have uncovered NZO-contributed QTL on

Chromosomes 1, 2, 5, 6, 7, 11, 12, 13 and 15[22–24] Genetic backcross analysis between NZO/HILt and either of two Swiss-derived inbred strains, NON/Lt or SJL/J, confirmed that diabesity in this polygenic obesity model represents a complex threshold phenomenon wherein the rate of early adiposity development establishes a diabetogenic level of insulin resistance[24,25]. Subsets of those NZO obesity QTL have been distributed into ten recombinant congenic strains (RCS) on the NON/Lt genetic background[26]. None of those RCS become as obese as the NZO parental strain, but all 10 RCS gain weight more rapidly then the NON/Lt parental strain. Each RCS, therefore, represents a different collection of NZO and NON interacting QTL that produce incremental levels of adiposity (and diabetogenic stress). Current gene expression microarray analysis of tissues from both parental strains, and the 10 RCS derived from them, should allow a molecular profiling as to how obesity (and diabesity) develops in response to the different combinations of QTLs.

Concluding remarks

What is particularly compelling about QTL analysis is the consistent finding that intercrosses between various inbred mouse strains often produce spontaneous development of obesity and diabesity in F1 or backcross generations[27–30]. Induction of obesity producing mutations in mice, without question, are key to discovery of new metabolic and endocrinologic regulatory pathways such as those in the leptin-leptin receptor pathway which led to identification of the 'adiposiat'[31]. At the same time, the deleterious interactions occuring among heterozygous combinations of different obesity QTL provide clear models for the 'epidemic' of obesity and T2D currently occurring in human societies living the modern 'Western lifestyle' of hyperalimentation accompanied by sedentary behaviours. Hence, knowledge gained by the discovery of the molecular nature of new targeted genes produced by either large scale mutagenesis programmes, or by selectively targeting candidate genes of interest, need to be accompanied by intensive analysis of QTL-induced obesity syndromes. Hopefully, convergence of these genetic initiatives will permit rational pharmacologic interventions based upon an individual's unique genome.

Acknowledgements: The author is indebted to Staff colleagues Drs. Tim O'Brien, Wayne Frankel, Jürgen Naggert, and Kevin Sebum, as well as Ms. Karen Svenson and Susan Carr, for sharing information and data regarding the mouse mutagenesis projects underway at The Jackson Laboratory. Dr. Neal Goodwin is also thanked for helpful discussions. The author was supported by NIH DK56853.

References

1. Nadeau JH, Frankel WN. The roads from phenotypic variation to gene discovery: mutagenesis versus QTLs. *Nature Genet* 2000; 25(4): 381–4.

2. Korstanje R, Paigen B. From QTL to gene: the harvest begins. *Nature Genet* 2002; 31: 235–6.

3. Brockmann GA, Bevova MR. Using mouse models to dissect the genetics of obesity. *Trends Genet* 2002; 18(7): 367–76.

4. Dhar M, Webb LS, Smith L, Hauser L, Johnson D, West DB. A novel ATPase on mouse chromosome 7 is a candidate gene for increased body fat. *Physiol Genomics* 2000; 4(1): 93–100.

5. Dhar M, Hauser L, Johnson D. An aminophospholipid translocase associated with body fat and type 2 diabetes phenotypes. *Obes Res* 2002; 10(7): 695–702.

6. O'Brien TP. *Mutagenesis and genetic screens in the mouse*, pp. 93–108. Boca Raton: CRC Press, 2001.

7. Justice ML. Capitalizing on large scale mouse mutagenesis screens. *Nature Reviews/Genetics* 2000; 1(2): 109–15.

8. Bailey D. How pure are inbred strains of mice. *Immunol Today* 1982; 3: 210–14.

9. You Y, Bergstrom R, Klemm M *et al.* Chromosomal deletion complexes in mice by radiation of embryonic stem cells. *Nature Genet* 1997; 15(3): 285–8.

10. Zheng B, Mills AA, Bradley A. Introducing defined chromosomal rearrangements into the mouse genome. *Methods* 2001; 24(1): 81–94.

11. Chen Y, Schimenti J, Magnuson T. Toward the yeastification of mouse genetics: chemical mutagenesis of embryonic stem cells. *Mamm Genome* 2000; 11(7): 598–602.

12. Goodwin NC, Ishida Y, Hartford S, *et al.* DelBank: a mouse ES-cell resource for generating deletions. *Nature Genet* 2001; 28(4): 310–1.

13. You Y, Browning VL, Schimenti JC. Generation of radiation-induced deletion complexes in the mouse genome using embryonic stem cells. *Methods* 1997; 13(4): 409–21.

14. Barsh GS, Farooqi IS, O'Rahilly S. Genetics of body-weight regulation. *Nature* 2000; 404: 644–51.

15. Elbein SC. Perspective: the search for genes for type 2 diabetes in the post-genome era. *Endocrinology* 2002; 143(6): 2012–8.

16. Mehrabian M, Wen PZ, Fisler J, Davis RC, Lusis AJ. Genetic loci controlling body fat, lipoprotein metabolism, and insulin levels in a multifactorial mouse model. *J Clin Invest* 1998; 101(11): 2485–96.

17. Pomp D. Genetic dissection of obesity in polygenic animal-models. *Behav Genet* 1997; 27(4): 285–306.

18. Kim JH, Nishina PM, Naggert JK. Genetic models for non insulin dependent diabetes mellitus in rodents. *J Basic Clin Physiol Pharmacol* 1998; 9(2–4): 325–45.

19. Cheverud JM, Routman EJ, Duarte FAM, van Swinderen B, Cothran K, Perel C. Quantitative trait loci for murine growth. *Genetics* 1996; 142: 1305–19.

20. Igel M, Becker W, Herberg L, Joost HG. Hyperleptinemia, leptin resistance, and polymorphic leptin receptor in the New Zealand obese mouse. *Endocrinology* 1997; 138(10): 4234–9.

21. Hileman SM, Pierroz DD, Masuzaki H *et al.* Characterizaton of short isoforms of the leptin receptor in rat cerebral microvessels and of brain uptake of leptin in mouse models of obesity. *Endocrinology* 2002; 143(3): 775–83.

22. Taylor BA, Wnek C, Schroeder D, Phillips SJ. Multiple obesity QTLs identified in an intercross between the NZO (New Zealand Obese) and the SM (small) mouse strains. *Mamm Genome* 2001; 12(2): 95–103.

23. Leiter EH, Reifsnyder PC, Flurkey K, Partke H-J, Junger E, Herberg L. Non-insulin dependent diabetes genes in mice: deleterious synergism by both parental genomes contributes to diabetogenic thresholds. *Diabetes* 1998; 47: 1287–95.

24. Reifsnyder PC, Churchill G, Leiter EH. Maternal environment and genotype interact to establish diabesity in mice. *Genome Res* 2000; 10(10): 1568–78.

25. Plum L, Kluge R, Giesen K, Altmuller J, Ortlepp JR, Joost HG. Type 2 diabetes-like hyperglycemia in a backcross model of NZO and SJL mice: characterization of a susceptibility locus on chromosome 4 and its relation with obesity. *Diabetes* 2000; 49(9): 1590–6.

26. Reifsnyder PC, Leiter EH. Deconstructing and reconstructing obesity-induced diabetes (diabesity) in mice. *Diabetes* 2002; 51(3): 825–32.

27. Cahill G, Jones E, Lauris V, Steinke J, Soeldner J. Studies on experimental diabetes in the Wellesley hybrid mouse. II. Serum insulin levels and response of peripheral tissues. *Diabetologia* 1967; 3: 171–4.

28. Leiter EH, Herberg L. The polygenetics of diabesity in mice. *Diabetes Rev* 1997; 5(2): 131–48.

29. Hattori M, Yamato E, Matsumoto E, *et al.* Occurrence of pretype I diabetes (pre-IDDM) and type II diabetes (NIDDM) in BC1 [(NOD x Mus spretus)F1 x NOD] mice. In: *Lessons from animal diabetes VI*; Shafrir E (eds), pp. 83–95. Boston: Birkhaüser, 1996.

30. Ranheim T, Dumke C, Schueler KL, Cartee GD, Attie AD. Interaction between BTBR and C57BL/6J genomes produces an insulin resistance syndrome in (BTBR x C57BL/6J) F1 mice. *Arterioscler Thromb Vasc Biol* 1997; 17(11): 3286–93.

31. Ioffe E, Moon B, Connolly E, Friedman JM. Abnormal regulation of the leptin gene in the pathogenesis of obesity. *Proc Natl Acad Sci USA* 1998; 95(20): 11852–7.

Progress in Obesity Research: 9. Edited by *Geraldo Medeiros-Neto, Alfredo Halpern* and *Claude Bouchard*
©2003 John Libbey Eurotext Ltd, pp. 247–249.

CHAPTER 52

The merits of the QTL approach in gene discovery in complex traits

Anthony G. Comuzzie

Department of Genetics, Southwest Foundation for Biomedical Research, San Antonio, Texas, USA
[e-mail: agcom@darwin.sfbr.org]

It has only been a little more than five years since the publication of the first genome scans focused on obesity-related phenotypes in humans (e.g. Comuzzie et al.[1]; Norman et al.[2], however, despite this relatively short time period (effectively the length of a single grant cycle) the insights that have been gained into the genetic influence on obesity-related phenotypes in humans is quit impressive. Contributing to this success has been the development of several important resources including (1) advances in analytical methods; (2) access to high-end computing resources; (3) access to economical (and reliable) high-throughput genotyping; and (4) improved definition of target phenotypes.

When selecting the most appropriate study design for genetic analyses it is necessary to consider the characteristics of the phenotypes to be studied. In the case of obesity we are dealing with a common, complex set of phenotypes with oligogenic architecture (i.e. several genes with a discernibly measurable effect expressed on a polygenic background) (Comuzzie[3]; Comuzzie et al.[4]). In addition, variation in these phenotypes is expressed in a continuous as opposed to a discrete pattern.

Genome scans versus the traditional candidate gene approach

Initial efforts to identify genes contributing to variation in complex diseases such as obesity, relied on the use of a candidate gene approach. This approach is based on the utilization of genes (often identified from knockout gene models in rodents) that are felt to be important contributors to the phenotypes of interest, unfortunately such an approach has not been that successful with regards to complex phenotypes in general, or with obesity-related phenotypes in particular.

As a result of the general pattern of mixed results produced by traditional candidate gene studies, a shift toward systematic genome-wide searches for the actual genes contributing to the observed variation in obesity-related phenotypes began (a pattern that was repeated across studies focusing on complex phenotypes in general). The principle distinction between the genome scanning efforts and those based on the 'traditional' candidate gene approach is the fact that no *a priori* assumptions concerning the potential importance of genes or chromosomal regions are made before starting the scan, but rather the variation across the entire genome is examined. In a genome scan, linkage analysis is conducted using a series of anonymous polymorphisms, scattered across the entire genome to identify quantitative trait loci (QTLs) affecting the phenotype of interest (Comuzzie[3]; Comuzzie et al.[4]). As a result, a genome scan is used to identify positional candidate genes, which then becomes the focus of more intensive follow-up analyses (e.g. combined linkage/disequilibrium analysis). A positional candidate gene differs from a 'traditional' candidate gene in that it is only considered as a candidate after the establishment of its proximity to a QTL that was identified via linkage analysis in a genome screen. Thus, the genome scan approach offers the potential of identifying new and/or previously unsuspected genes influencing the phenotype of interest. Under this approach a 'traditional' candidate gene, is not excluded from consideration since it only requires that such a gene reside in the region of the QTL linkage signal.

Current results of genome scans for obesity

Currently there is strong statistical support for approximately half a dozen QTLS influencing obesity-related phenotypes across a number of populations and ethnic groups. While some of these signals localize near genes that might have been considered *a priori* as candidate genes for obesity, several others offer evidence for previously unsuspected genes. As a result, there is an intriguing pattern of genetic contribution to obesity that has begun to emerge and which promises to greatly increase our understanding of the relationship between obesity and other chronic diseases such as coronary heart disease and type 2 diabetes.

To date significant linkage results for obesity-related phenotypes have been published from a relatively wide variety of human populations including Mexican Americans (Comuzzie et al.[1]), Native Americans (Norman et al.[2]; Norman et al.[5]); African American (Zhou et al.[6]); as well as several studies utilizing populations of western European origin [France (Hager et al.[7]; Vionnet et al.[8]); United States (Lee et al.[9]; Kissebah et al.[10]; Comuzzie et al.[11]); and Canada (Chagnon et al.[12])]. Even more important than the detection of significant linkage signals in any one of these studies, however, is the growing number of replications for a number of these human obesity QTLs across these various populations (Comuzzie et al.[4]). As a result there is now a clearly emerging pattern of approximately half a dozen genes with a substantial contribution to variation in obesity-related phenotypes in humans.

Replications

While the number of published genome scans focusing on human obesity is still relatively small, an interesting pattern is beginning to emerge with over half a dozen QTLS now appearing consistently across a variety of studies. Indeed, not only are these linkage signals supported by significant LOD scores, but many of these are in regions that contain very strong positional candidate genes for obesity-related phenotypes. The QTL on chromosome 2p first reported in Mexican Americans (Comuzzie et al.[2]) has now been replicated in a number of samples including French (Hager et al.[7]), African Americans (Rotimi et al.[13]), and Caucasians (Comuzzie et al.[11]). There is also strong evidence of replication for an obesity related QTL on the q arm of chromosome 3 across multiple studies including Caucasians (Kissebah et al.[10]; Vionnet et al.[8]), Native Americans (Walder et al.[14]); African Americans (Zhou et al.[6]), and South Pacific Islanders (Franke et al.[15]). There also appears to be a growing body of support within populations of western European origin for replication for an obesity QTL on 5cen-q (Hager et al.[7]; Comuzzie et al.[11]) and perhaps even tentative evidence in an African American sample as well (Zhou et al.[6]). Chromosome 10p also shows a pattern of replication for an obesity-related QTL across numerous studies and ethnic groups including Caucasians (Hager et al.[7]; Comuzzie et al.[11]; Hinney et al.[16]; Price et al.[17]) and South Pacific Islanders (Franke et al.[15]). Taken in total, this pattern of replications suggests that there are a group of genes with significant effects on the expression of obesity-related traits that appear to be present across populations, so that these linkage signals are not likely to reflect genetic effects unique to any particular ethnic group. Additionally, as the number of genome scans focusing on obesity continues to increase, and their results are published, there is every reason to believe that this pattern of replication will continue to be strengthened.

Conclusion

While obesity represents a complex biological phenomenon, the accumulating results from genetic analyses suggest that the task of dissecting out the relevant genetic contribution to its expression is not intractable. However, it has become increasingly clear that success in the efforts to identify specific genes affecting the expression of obesity is contingent upon the application of the most appropriate analytical tools for the job along with the collection of large informative data sets. Indeed, a striking, and fairly consistent, pattern of chromosomal regions with significant effects on obesity has begun to coalesce. There are already published replications for QTLs on chromosomes 2, 3, 5, 10 and 20 across several different populations and ethnic groups. Such a consistent pattern has important public health implications since it suggests that there are at least half a dozen or so obesity-related genes with common affects across populations.

While the results to date from genome scans are impressive, we still have important issues yet to address. The identification of QTLs is a critical first step in focusing our attention onto the most promising areas of the genome, but now we are faced with identifying the specific polymorphisms involved in the development of obesity. While such a task is not trival, there are promising new advances, both technical and analytical, which will make the sequencing and analysis of large spans of DNA in the region of these QTLs feasible. Indeed, given the findings from the genome scans which have accumulated since only the mid to late 1990s, combined with the continued development of technological and analytical advances, we are moving rapidly toward the ultimate goal of identifying the variations in specific genes influencing the expression of obesity and its associated phenotypes.

References

1. Comuzzie AG, Hixson JE, Almasy L, Mitchell BD, Mahaney MC, Dyer TD *et al.* A major quantitative trait locus determining serum leptin levels and fat mass is located on human chromosome 2. *Nature Genet* 1997; 15: 273–6.

2. Norman RA, Thompson DB, Foroud T, Garvey WT, Bennett PH, Bogardus C, Ravussin E. Genomewide search for genes influencing per cent body fat in Pima Indians: suggestive linkage at chromosome 11q21-q22. Pima Diabetes Gene Group. *Am J Hum Genet* 1997; 60: 166–73.

3. Comuzzie AG. The Genetic Contribution to Human Obesity: The Dissection of a Complex Phenotype. In F. Johnson and G. Foster (eds) *Obesity and human growth*, pp. 21–36. London: Smith-Gordon, 2001.

4. Comuzzie AG, Williams JT, Martin LJ, Blangero J. Searching for genes underlying normal variation in human adiposity. *J Molec Med* 2001; 79: 57–70.

5. Norman RA, Tataranni PA, Pratley R, Thompson DB, Hanson RL, Prochazka *et al.* Autosomal genomic scan for loci linked to obesity and energy metabolism in Pima Indians. *Am J Hum Genet* 1998; 62: 659–68.

6. Zhu X, Cooper RS, Luke A, Chen G, Wu X, Kan D *et al.* A genome-wide scan for obesity in African-Americans. *Diabetes* 2002; 51: 541–4.

7. Hager J, Dina C, Francke S, Dubois S, M Houari, Vatin V *et al.* A genome-wide scan for human obesity genes reveals a major susceptibility locus on chromosome 10. *Nature Genet* 1998; 20: 304–8.

8. Vionnet N, Hani EH, Dupont S, Gallina S, Francke S, Dotte S *et al.* Genomewide search for type 2 diabetes-susceptibility genes in French Whites: Evidence for a novel susceptibility locus for early-onset diabetes on chromosome 3q27-qter and independent replication of a type 2-diabeteslocus on chromosome 1q21-q24. *Am J Hum Genet* 2000; 67: 1470–80.

9. Lee JH, Reed DR, Li WD, Xu W, Joo EJ, Kilker RL *et al.* Genome scan for human obesity and linkage to markers in 20q13. *Am J Hum Genet* 1999; 64: 196–209.

10. Kissebah AH, Sonnenberg GE, Myklebust J, Goldstein M, Broman K, James RG *et al.* Quantitative trait loci on chromosomes 3 and 17 Influence phenotypes of the metabolic syndrome. *PNAS* 2000; 97: 14478–83.

11. Comuzzie AG, Funahashi T, Martin LJ, Sonnenberg G, Jacob H, Kwitek Black A *et al.* The genetic basis of plasma variation in adiponectin, a metabolic endophenotype for obesity and the metabolic syndrome. *J Clin Endocrinol Metab* 2001; 86: 4321–5.

12. Chagnon YC, Borecki IB, Perusse L, Roy S, Lacaille M, Chagnon M *et al.* Genome-wide search for genes related to the fat-free body mass in the Quebec family study. *Metabolism* 2000; 49: 203–7.

13. Rotimi CN, Comuzzie AG, Lowe WL, Luke A, Blangero J, Cooper RS. The quantitative trait locus on chromosome 2 for serum leptin levels is confirmed in African-Americans. *Diabetes* 1999; 48: 643–4.

14. Walder K, Hanson RL, Kobes S, Knowler WC, Ravussin E. An autosomal genomic scan for loci linked to plasma leptin concentration in Pima Indians. *Int J Obes Relat Metab Disord* 2000; 24: 559–65.

15. Francke S, Manraj M, Lacquemant C, Lecoeur C, Lepretre F, Passa P *et al.* A genome-wide scan for coronary heart disease suggests in: Indo- Mauritians a susceptibility locus on chromosome 16p13 and replicates linkage with the metabolic syndrome on 3q27. *Hum Mol Genet* 2001; 10: 2751–65.

16. Hinney A, Ziegler A, Oeffner F, Wedewardt C, Vogel M, Wulftange H *et al.* Independent confirmation of a major locus for obesity on chromosome 10. *J Clin Endocrinol Metab* 2000; 85: 2962–5.

17. Price RA, Li WD, Bernstein A, Crystal A, Golding EM, Weisberg SJ, Zuckerman WA. A locus affecting obesity in human chromosome region 10p12. *Diabetologia* 2001; 44: 363–6.

Progress in Obesity Research: 9. Edited by *Geraldo Medeiros-Neto, Alfredo Halpern and Claude Bouchard*

©2003 John Libbey Eurotext Ltd, pp. 250–259.

CHAPTER 53

Finding appropriate drug targets for obesity

Eric Ravussin

Pennington Biomedical Research Center, Baton Rouge, LA 70808-4124, USA
[e-mail: Ravusse@pbrc.edu]

Essential obesity in an 'obesigenic' environment

Although lifestyle and environmental influences on obesity are readily accepted, it is recognized that human obesity has an important genetic component as well. Obesity is characterized by a strong familial aggregation pattern and for most obese is clearly a polygenic condition. In the presence of a genetic predisposition to obesity, lifestyle and environmental conditions largely determine the severity of the disease. Within a population, the variability of the distribution of body mass index (or adiposity) in a given environment is mostly attributable to genes, whereas the average of the distributions is primarily determined by environmental conditions. An example can be derived from a population extremely susceptible to obesity and diabetes such as the Pima Indians. Pima Indians living in a 'restrictive' environment in the remote Mexican Sierra Madre mountains have a much lower prevalence of obesity and type 2 diabetes mellitus than Pima Indians living in Arizona[1] (who have the highest prevalence of type 2 diabetes in the world[2] and one of the highest prevalence of obesity[3]). When individuals from a population living in a 'restrictive' environment characterized by a traditional lifestyle evolve towards an 'obesigenic' environment, such as that found in industrialized countries, most individuals from this population will gain weight. However, those individuals with a high genetic predisposition for obesity will gain the most weight whereas those resistant to obesity will gain little weight.

Concept of 'essential obesity'

There has been considerable speculation concerning the reasons why the human genome could harbor so many genes predisposing to positive energy balance and obesity and so few to protective against weight gain. The most frequently stated theory is that of the 'thrifty genotype hypothesis'[4]. This hypothesis states that over mankind's history, individuals and populations have evolved in restrictive environments in which food was not very abundant and required much physical work to obtain. Hence, survival mechanisms have evolved to confer a protection against periods of food scarcity. Often-cited examples of such populations include the aboriginal populations of Australia, navigators of the Pacific Islands, and the Pima Indians of the United States, who were typically exposed to alternating periods of feast and famine. The 'thrifty genotype hypothesis' states that evolution in such a restrictive environment has progressively (or through genetic bottlenecks) selected for a 'thrifty genotype', conferring survival advantages in periods of famine, but resulting in liabilities in an affluent environment[5,6]. The hypothesis is not unreasonable, since the abundance of food and the lack of need for physical exercise to acquire food are fairly recent phenomena. One implication of the 'thrifty genotype hypothesis' is that it should not be surprising to observe that highly industrialized populations are now struggling with the problem of obesity due to rapid changes in environmental conditions. This has led to a second hypothesis which states that obesity in our present environment is an 'essential' condition, and only those with fewer obesity susceptibility genes are apt to resist our 'obesigenic' environment and remain normal weight without conscious effort[7]. Many individuals still overcome the development of obesity but at the cost of constant dietary restrain and regular self-imposed physical activity regimens. The common thread between these two hypotheses is that what was an asset in early mankind history has now rapidly become a liability.

Chase of obesity genes

Because of the apparent role of genes in the predisposition to obesity, a search for obesity susceptibility genes was initiated in different human populations during the 1990s. Variants in candidate genes (coding and promoter regions), positional candidate chromosomal regions, linkage studies in families, and association studies in affected vs. non-affected individuals have been used in the effort to identify genes[8,9]. The hope behind these studies was to identify new targets for the development of pharmacological agents.

Only a few single-gene mutations causally related to obesity have been detected in a small number of people. Mutations with strong effects were found in the leptin receptor gene[10], the leptin gene[11,12], the pro-opiomelanocortin gene[13], the prohormone convertase 1 gene[14], and the melanocortin MC4 receptor gene[15–18]. Several rare obesity-related Mendelian disorders are also known, and the loci for several of them have been mapped. The list of these syndromes is summarized in the latest annual human obesity gene map review[9] and include the Prader-Willi syndrome, different Bardet-Biedl syndromes, the Wilson-Turner syndrome and others.

To date, the results of at least six genome scans for human obesity related phenotypes have been reported; one in Mexican Americans[19], one in Pima Indians[20,21], one in French families[22], one in Americans with extreme obesity[23], one in French Canadian families from Quebec, and one in Amish families[24]. In these studies, the strongest linkages were observed on chromosomes 2P22-21, 10P12-3, 11Q22-24, and 20Q13. These different QTLs probably encode genes of importance for the susceptibility to obesity. The positional cloning of some of these QTLs is currently being pursued in several laboratories.

Numerous association studies have been conducted using DNA from case and control designs or comparing genotypes in samples characterized by heterogeneity in levels of adiposity. Association studies based on small sample size seem to be particularly vulnerable to false positive or false negative findings. Therefore, one should rely only on studies that have reasonable statistical power and on results that are replicated in different samples. At the present time, no strong definitive association with a mutation has been identified following these criteria. However genetic associations with levels of significance at $P < 0.001$ have been identified for variants in the following genes: the sodium potassium ATPase alpha$_2$ and beta$_1$ genes with respiratory quotient[25]; the promoter region of the pro-opiomelanocortin gene with plasma leptin concentration[26]; haplotype of variants in the UCP1 gene and β_3 receptor gene with weight loss[27]; β_2 adrenoreceptor gene with BMI[28]; UCP2 gene with BMI[29] or energy metabolism[30]; G protein β_3 subunit with BMI[31] and adenosine deaminase gene with BMI[32].

Since none of these associations has been proven to be the consequence of a mutation affecting the function or amount of a gene product, future genetic association studies need to be supported by cellular work identifying the functional consequences of the reported polymorphisms.

Pharmacological treatment of obesity

Weight gain results from a sustained imbalance between energy intake and energy expenditure favouring positive energy balance. However, this simple statement belies the complex, multi-factorial nature of obesity and the numerous biological and behavioural factors that can affect both sides of the energy balance equation[33–35]. In the context of a discussion on the implications of recent progress for potential drug targets for obesity, it is useful to consider the aetiology of the disease as a feedback model as proposed by Bray[36–38]. In such a model, afferent signals indicate to the central controllers in the brain, the state of the external and internal environments as they relate to food, metabolic rates and activity behaviour. In turn, these central controllers transduce these messages into efferent signals, governing the behavioural search for acquisition of food and modulating its subsequent deposition into energy storage compartments including adipose tissue, liver, and muscle. Finally, a component of the system regulates ingestion, digestion, absorption, transport, and storage of the ingested foods, as well as other related metabolic and behavioural functions. Each of these components of the system can be targeted for the development of drugs.

The beginning of modern obesity pharmacology as regards to obesity can be traced back a century ago, when the use of thyroid extract was first reported[36]. However, thyroid hormones had to be abandoned because of their adverse effects on the cardiovascular and skeletal muscle systems. In the 1920s it was observed that dinitrophenol, present in chemical dyes, caused weight loss in the workers that were exposed to it. The effect was due to an uncoupling of the phosphorylation of ATP from oxygen consumption, but it was quickly shown that treatment with dinitrophenol was associated with significant side effects, such as neuropathy and cataracts. Amphetamines were then introduced and found to be efficacious, but also to be addictive. Many drugs have been used to modulate food intake, mostly by their effect on monoamines, such as norepinephrine, serotonin and dopamine[38]. Serotonergic drugs such as fenfluramine and dexfenfluramine were developed and approved for use until it was discovered that dexfenfluramine alone or in combination was associated with valvular problems in some patients, after which it was withdrawn from the market.

There are only two obesity drugs left on the US and other markets at this time, namely sibutramine and orlistat. Sibutramine is a sympatheto-mimetic drug, which inhibits the central re-uptake of no-repinephrine, serotonin and to a lesser extent dopamine. Initially developed as an anti-depressant, it has been shown to decrease food intake in a dose-related fashion[39]. Sibutramine also seems to increase energy expenditure[40]. It is approved for long-term use, but is classified as a schedule 4 drug by the US Drug Enforcement Agency. Orlistat, an inhibitor of hepatic lipase, can be classified as a drug that alters metabolism by inhibiting the gastro-intestinal absorption of triglycerides. On a 30 per cent fat diet, orlistat produced a dose dependent increase in fecal fat loss and a similar dose related weight loss when used for a period of six months or more[41].

At least in the scientific community involved in obesity research, it is now well accepted that safe, efficacious drugs to treat obesity can and should be produced. Many pharmaceutical companies are now dedicating a large part of their Research and Development budget on 'obesity molecules'. However, one has to realize that drug development is a long process going from target identification and valida-tion to the launch of a medication on the market. After an obesity target is identified and validated, scientists have to develop *in vitro* and *in vivo* assays to screen and optimize a lead molecule that will eventually be administered to humans after extensive toxicology testing. This entire effort will take at least 3 years. After the initial first phase pharmacokinetic and safety studies (6 to 8 months), it takes at least another 18 months to perform the necessary proof of principle phase IB and phase II studies. Phase III studies for obesity compounds are required to last at least 2 years in a large number of patients. After collection of Phase III data, another year is necessary to prepare the entire data package required by regulatory agencies for drug registration. Summing all the above times, it becomes evident that the minimum duration for the development of a single anti obesity drug is 8–9 years. Such a stringent timeline is clearly without counting on unexpected events, which can stop or slow down the develop-ment of a given compound. Down time can be related to toxicology, formulation, bioavailability as well as manufacturing problems.

Potential targets for obesity drugs

Pharmaceutical agents may intervene at three different levels of the negative feedback model mentioned above. First, small molecules can reinforce the afferent signals from the periphery. Second, such molecules can target the central pathways involved in the regulation of food intake and energy expen-diture. Third, agents can increase directly peripheral energy expenditure and increase energy partition-ing towards muscle. Some of these targets have been reviewed elsewhere[42].

Afferent signals

The external environment and internal milieu provide signals that play a role in the control of feeding. External signals from sight, sound, smell, taste and touch all provide important elements in this feedback system. Gastrointestinal peptides have long been recognized as potential regulators of satiety. Cholecystokinine was one of the first peptides shown to reduce food intake[43]. Glucagon and glucagon-like peptide-1 (GLP-1) both reduce food intake in animals and humans[44]. Small molecules that may influence GLP-1 receptors (agonist activity), increase the release of GLP-1 from intestinal L cells, or increase the duration of action of GLP-1 could be candidates for drug therapies. Amylin seems to slow gastric emptying and decrease food intake in a direct and indirect manner[45]. Recently, it was shown that the infusion of the gut hormone PYY(3–36) significantly decreases appetite and reduces food intake in humans by 33 per cent over 24 h[46]. Enterostatin, the pentapeptide portion of pancreatic procolipase, reduces fat intake in some experimental models[47]. However, data in humans have not been conclusive. Nutrients such as glucose, pyruvate, lactate, and 3-hydroxybutyrate seem also to be afferent satiety signals. They all reduce food intake when injected into experimental animals.

Leptin, however, is the best-known and most studied afferent signal from adipose tissue and may be the most important hormone communicating information on body fat content to the central controllers of energy balance. Administration of leptin causes a decrease in food intake and an increase in energy expenditure[48,49]. These effects are driven by central regulatory mechanisms modulating orexigenic and anorectic neurons in the hypothalamus as well as activating the sympathetic nervous system in the brain stem. Clinical trials with leptin injections have shown that modest weight loss occurred at small doses but that local discomfort was registered at the injection site[50]. For these reasons and despite some promising results in patients with low leptin concentration and with lipodystrophy[51,52], it is unlikely that leptin itself will become an important obesity pharmacotherapy. However, the development of low molecular weight leptin receptor agonists remains an attractive and probably viable strategy. Such compounds would preferably be orally available and should cross the blood-brain barrier, thereby allowing a more potent stimulation of leptin receptors than a large protein, which is limited by saturable transport across the blood-brain barrier. Alternatively, sensitizers of the leptin pathway (allosteric enhancers) could be developed in the same way as insulin sensitizers.

CNS controllers

The central control systems for the regulation of food intake and energy expenditure are coordinated and controlled by neuronal systems converging on the ventral hypothalamus. It has been known for years that lesions in this region produce an increase or a decrease in weight, depending on the specific site of the lesion[37]. It is also known that monoamines, including norepinephrine, serotonin, dopamine and histamine modulate feeding[38,42]. Stimulation of the β_1 adrenoreceptor reduces food intake, whereas the stimulation of β_2 adrenoreceptors increases food intake in experimental animals. Receptors can be activated by agonist drugs, but also by releasing or inhibiting norepinephrine re-uptake in the vicinity of these receptors. Stimulation of dopamine receptors also reduces food intake probably by activation of the 5-HT2c-receptor[53]. Histamine receptors have also been identified as modulators of feeding and antagonists of the H3 receptor (an auto-receptor) could be targeted to increase the release of histamine in key central locations[54].

One of the most recent developments has been the identification of neuropeptides that play an important role in the regulation of both feeding and energy expenditure. These include neuropeptide Y, the pro-opiomelanocortin, the melanin-concentrating hormone (MCH), the agouti related protein and orexins. Neuropeptide Y is among the most potent stimulators of food intake. Antagonists to either the neuropeptide Y Y-1 or the neuropeptide Y Y-5 receptor are being explored as potential agents for the treatment of obesity[55]. Another attractive target is the melanocortin receptor system. Indeed, alpha-melanocyte stimulating hormone (α-MSH) caused a decrease in food intake. Furthermore, mice lacking pro-opiomelanocortin, the precursor of α-MSH, are obese[56]. Agonist and antagonist peptides of the melanocortin MC$_4$ receptor have been developed and cause the expected effect on feeding, i.e. decrease and increase, respectively. Finally, humans with functionally impaired melanocortin MC$_4$ receptors are obese[15-18]. The melanocortin receptor system therefore represents one of the major potential targets for the treatment of obesity. Agonists or allosteric enhancers of the melanocortin MC4 receptor may prove to be efficacious in humans as previously shown in rats and mice. Antagonists to the melanin-concentrating hormone (MCH) represent another potential approach for drug development. Knockout mice for the MCH gene are lean, suggesting that the peptide may have a physiological role in the control of food intake, energy expenditure and body fat stores[57]. Opioids also seem important in the regulation of feeding, and μ and κ receptors antagonists may be useful targets to decrease food intake[58]. Finally, antagonists of cannabinoid receptor 1 are potent inhibitors of food intake in animals[59,60] and are being tested as anti obesity agents in humans.

Efferent signals

The endocrine and autonomic systems are efferent control systems involved in the regulation of food intake and body fat stores. Since a low metabolic rate[61] and a low rate of fat oxidation[62] are risk factors for obesity, it is of interest to target molecular pathways involved in the regulation of energy expenditure and/or fat oxidation.

The ideal molecule to target energy metabolism at the periphery would be one that could both increase resting energy expenditure and fat oxidation. Several pharmaceutical companies are currently developing β_3 adrenoreceptor agonists for this purpose[63]. Further validation of the target was recently reported in transgenic animals[64]. The original uncoupling protein (UCP1) found in brown adipose tissue has a well-established role in temperature and body weight regulation in rodents[65]. Whether UCP1, UCP2, or UCP3 plays a role in the regulation of body weight in humans remains to be determined. Results from over expression of human uncoupling protein-3 in skeletal muscle of mice resulted in a lean mouse, suggesting that UCP3 may be a good target to increase metabolic rate[66].

Future pharmacological treatment

There are a number of features that would be desirable in a next generation obesity medication. The first is obviously safety as the history of the pharmacological treatment of obesity has been marked by several disasters[36]. This is particularly important because many people will seek pharmacological treatment for obesity, even if they have no clinical indication for drug therapy. Of course, an equally important feature for a new generation of drugs is efficacy. Future pharmacotherapy should be potent enough to induce a weight loss of at least 15 per cent of initial body weight on average. The mechanism of action will also be very important. Since almost all of the previous drugs were acting centrally and were associated with side effects, it would be preferable if some drugs of the next generation acted peripherally. Finally, since the pharmacological treatment of obesity requires lifelong therapy, the cost of such an agent should be affordable. If the cost of treating obesity exceeds the cost of treating its co-morbidities, then these new drugs are bound to fail on the market.

An important issue to keep in mind is the fact that the pharmacological treatment of the future will not cure obesity. Weight loss reaches a plateau after a few months of treatment as a result of many compensatory mechanisms having come into play and the re-equilibration of the energy balance. This reality has to be understood by both the patients and the health care providers if one wants to avoid the vicious cycles of frustration, which often occurs between parties when realistic expectations are not clearly established at the onset of the treatment[67].

Because of the above, combination therapy by targeting different mechanisms, is likely to be more efficacious. For instance, during the first phase of a weight loss programme, an appetite suppressant, in association with behavioural therapy, may be the most relevant approach. However, after two or three months of weight loss, an agent that increases energy expenditure and/or fat oxidation could be added to counteract the decrease in metabolic rate and sustain negative energy balance conditions. Together, an appetite suppressant and a stimulator of metabolic rate should be helpful in preventing some of the weight regain so commonly observed. Finally, further away in the future, the anticipated advances in human genomics and proteomics should make it possible to prescribe drugs designed to alleviate specific genetic 'deficiencies' identified by genotyping for mutations at relevant genes. These advances will allow the development of a treatment 'à la carte' approach.

In the pursuit of new pharmacological agents to target obesity via known or unknown mechanisms, pharmaceutical companies need to prioritize their efforts, taking into account the level of validation of targets. For the development of such a drug, one must show in pre-clinical models of obesity that the administration of the ligand to the targeted receptor or the modulators of enzymatic activity impacts food intake and/or energy expenditure. Second, the expression of the receptor and/or the ligand should be affected by changes in energy balance. Third, the histochemical/electrophysiological location of the target should preferably be present in tissues and areas previously described as being involved in the control of energy balance. Fourth, blockade or stimulation of peptide action by antibodies or antisense oligo-nucleotides should impact on energy balance. Finally, knockout or overexpression of the receptor or the ligand gene should impact energy balance and cause a change in body weight and adiposity.

There is presently an abundance of newly identified targets for potential development of pharmacological anti-obesity agents. For example, the creation of many new transgenic animals (gene knockout or overexpression) is providing an enormous wealth of relevant information. There are presently more than 75 genetically engineered mice presenting some perturbation of energy balance and/or fuel partitioning. The targeted genes encode for 25 receptors and transporters, 22 hormones and peptides, 14 metabolites, four signaling proteins, nine transcription factors/nuclear receptors and two structural genes. Information on the phenotypes of these transgenic animals has been reviewed in a book chapter by York[68].

The list of peptides affecting food intake and energy homeostasis is growing every month. The major orexigenic neuropeptides are: neuropeptide Y[55], melanin-concentrating hormone[57,69], orexin A and B[70–72], dynorphin[73], β-endorphin[74], and galanin[75]. On the other hand, many anorectic peptides have been discovered including αMSH[76], GLP-1[77], corticotropin releasing hormone (CRH)[78], urocortin[79], cocaine-amphetamine related transcript (CART)[80], neurotensin[81], neuromedin U[82], calcitonin[83], amylin[84], and enterostatin[47]. Some of these peptides not only impact food intake, but also energy expenditure in a reciprocal manner. All of the above targets have some degree of validation in pre-clinical models, or from gene knockout or gene overexpression studies. However, it should be noted that the melanocortin pathway, and especially the melanocortin MC_4 receptor, has the highest degree of validation, according to the criteria mentioned earlier. Agonists to the melanocortin MC_4 receptor may prove to be very potent in decreasing food intake and probably in increasing fat oxidation. However, proof of concept studies remain to be performed in humans with orally bioavailable melanocortin MC_4 receptor agonist molecules exhibiting an acceptable toxicology profile. It is important to note that, in general, it is easier for chemists to generate small molecules antagonizing a pathway, rather than stimulating a pathway. Therefore, molecules targeting 'orexigenic pathways' are likely to appear on the market before molecules targeting 'anorectic pathways'.

Table 1 presents some potential targets or pathways involved in an increase in energy expenditure and/or fat oxidation via central mechanisms or directly on peripheral tissues. At the present time, as mentioned earlier, the development of selective β3-adrenoreceptor agonists targeting the human receptor is receiving the most attention[63,64]. Previous compounds were generated against the rat receptor and have typically shown problems of bioavailability or lack of selectivity in humans. Leptin remains an attractive target because of the dual effect on food intake and energy metabolism. Whether or not small agonist molecule of the leptin receptor can be generated remains to be shown. Alternatively, molecules causing an allosteric enhancement of endogenous leptin action may be a viable strategy since obese patients already have high plasma and cerebrospinal fluid leptin concentrations.

Table 1. Potential targets (pathways) for increasing energy expenditure or fat oxidation or for inhibiting adipose tissue proliferation

Pathway	Activation (+) or Inhibition (−) to decrease obesity
Acetyl CoA carboxylase β (ACC2)	(−)
Adrenergic (β3)	(+)
Carnitine palmitoyltransferase 1 (MCPT1)	(+)
Diacylglycerol transferase (Dgat)	(−)
Stearoyl-CoA desaturase 1	(−)
Hmgic	(−)
Leptin (LEPR)	(+)
Peroxisome proliferator-activator receptor α (PPAR-α)	(+)
PPAR γ	(−)
PPAR γ coactivator1 (PGC1)	(+)
Sterol regulatory element binding protein (SREBP)	(−)
Thyroid hormones; (thyroid receptor β)	(+)
Uncoupling proteins (UCP)	(+)

Thyroid hormones have always represented an attractive target for stimulating energy expenditure. However, because of the well-known side effects on the cardiovascular system, molecules acting predominantly on the thyroid beta receptor in the muscle may be a potential means to increase energy expenditure[85] without unwanted effects. If uncoupling proteins can be activated only in desirable tissues, then they are likely to represent good targets for obesity[65]. Data from the knockout of the protein tyrosine phosphatase 1β indicate that inhibitors of this phosphotase may represent a viable way of increasing energy expenditure with a concomitant improvement of insulin sensitivity[86]. Among other potential obesity targets one can propose diacylglycerol acyltransferase (DGAT)[87], peroxisome proliferation-activated receptors (α and γ)[88-90] peroxisome proliferation-activated receptor gamma coactivator 1 (PGC1)[91,92], carnitine palmitoyltransferase[93], high-mobility group protein (HMGIC)[94], sterol regulatory element-binding protein (SREBP)[95,96] and stearoyl-CoA desaturase-1[97,98]. However, most of these pathways may need more validation before being considered true obesity targets. With our growing understanding of the biology of the human genome, it is very likely that new targets will be identified, validated and prioritized. A new generation of drugs with different mechanisms of action will be developed and used in combination therapy to treat the complex disease of obesity. Moreover, in the future, it is likely that the treatment of obesity will be characterized by growing individuality and sophistication. Regardless, it is certain that the coming years will see an explosion of research on target identification and target validation for the pharmacological treatment of obesity. However, given the epidemic nature of obesity at this time, only public health measures and drastic public policy changes can modify the 'obesigenic' environment[99]. Without major societal changes, it is almost certain that the obesity epidemic will continue to spread around the world in the present century. Pharmacology will mostly help obese individuals but populations' well being will be only helped by public health strategies.

References

1. Ravussin E, Valencia ME, Esparza J, Bennett PH, Schulz LO. Effects of a traditional lifestyle on obesity in Pima Indians. *Diabetes Care* 1994; 17: 1067–74.

2. Knowler WC, Pettitt DJ, Saad MF, Bennett PH. Diabetes mellitus in the Pima Indians: incidence, risk factors and pathogenesis. *Diabetes Metab Rev* 1990; 6: 1–27.

3. Knowler WC, Pettitt DJ, Saad MF, Charles MA, Nelson RG, Howard BV *et al*. Obesity in the Pima Indians: its magnitude and relationship with diabetes. *Am J Clin Nutr* 1991; 53: S1543–S51.

4. Neel JV. Diabetes mellitus: a 'thrifty' genotype rendered detrimental by progress? *Am J Hum Genet* 1962; 14: 353–63.

5. Neel JV. Diabetes mellitus: a 'thrifty' genotype rendered detrimental by 'progress'? 1962. *Bull World Health Organ* 1999; 77: 694–703 (discussion 692–693).

6. Neel JV. The 'thrifty genotype' in 1998. *Nutr Rev* 1999; 57: S2–S9.

7. Ravussin E, Bogardus C. A brief overview of human energy metabolism and its relationship to essential obesity. *Am J Clin Nutr* 1992; 55: S242–S245.

8. Barsh GS, Farooqi IS, O'Rahilly S. Genetics of body-weight regulation. *Nature* 2000; 404: 644–51.

9. Rankinen T, Perusse L, Weisnagel SJ, Snyder EE, Chagnon YC, Bouchard C. The human obesity gene map: the 2001 update. *Obes Res* 2002; 10: 196–243.

10. Clement K, Vaisse C, Lahlou N, Cabrol S, Pelloux V, Cassuto D *et al*. A mutation in the human leptin receptor gene causes obesity and pituitary dysfunction. *Nature* 1998; 392: 398–401.

11. Montague CT, Farooqi IS, Whitehead JP, Soos MA, Rau H, Wareham NJ *et al*. Congenital leptin deficiency is associated with severe early-onset obesity in humans. *Nature* 1997; 387: 903–8.

12. Strobel A, Issad T, Camoin L, Ozata M, Strosberg AD. A leptin missense mutation associated with hypogonadism and morbid obesity. *Nature Genet* 1998; 18: 213–5.

13. Krude H, Biebermann H, Luck W, Horn R, Brabant G, Gruters A. Severe early-onset obesity, adrenal insufficiency and red hair pigmentation caused by POMC mutations in humans. *Nature Genet* 1998; 19: 155–7.

14. Jackson RS, Creemers JW, Ohagi S, Raffin-Sanson ML, Sanders L, Montague CT *et al*. Obesity and impaired prohormone processing associated with mutations in the human prohormone convertase 1 gene. *Nature Genet* 1997; 16: 303–6.

15. Cone RD. Haploinsufficiency of the melanocortin-4 receptor: part of a thrifty genotype? *J Clin Invest* 2000; 106: 185–7.

16. Hinney A, Schmidt A, Nottebom K, Heibult O, Becker I, Ziegler A *et al*. Several mutations in the melanocortin-4 receptor gene including a nonsense and a frameshift mutation associated with dominantly inherited obesity in humans. *J Clin Endocrinol Metab* 1999; 84: 1483–6.

17. Vaisse C, Clement K, Guy-Grand B, Froguel P. A frameshift mutation in human MC4R is associated with a dominant form of obesity. *Nature Genet* 1998; 20: 113–4.

18. Yeo GS, Farooqi IS, Aminian S, Halsall DJ, Stanhope RG, O'Rahilly S. A frameshift mutation in MC4R associated with dominantly inherited human obesity. *Nature Genet* 1998; 20: 111–2.

19. Comuzzie AG, Hixson JE, Almasy L, Mitchell BD, Mahaney MC, Dyer TD *et al*. A major quantitative trait locus determining serum leptin levels and fat mass is located on human chromosome 2. *Nature Genet* 1997; 15: 273–6.

20. Norman RA, Tataranni PA, Pratley R, Thompson DB, Hanson RL, Prochazka M *et al*. Autosomal genomic scan for loci linked to obesity and energy metabolism in Pima Indians. *Am J Hum Genet* 1998; 62: 659–68.

21. Hanson RL, Ehm MG, Pettitt DJ, Prochazka M, Thompson DB, Timberlake D *et al*. An autosomal genomic scan for loci linked to type II diabetes mellitus and body-mass index in Pima Indians. *Am J Hum Genet* 1998; 63: 1130–8.

22. Hager J, Dina C, Francke S, Dubois S, Houari M, Vatin V *et al*. A genome-wide scan for human obesity genes reveals a major susceptibility locus on chromosome 10. *Nature Genet* 1998; 20: 304–8.

23. Lee JH, Reed DR, Li WD, Xu W, Joo EJ, Kilker RL *et al*. Genome scan for human obesity and linkage to markers in 20q13. *Am J Hum Genet* 1999; 64: 196–209.

24. Hsueh WC, Mitchell BD, Schneider JL, St Jean PL, Pollin TI, Ehm MG *et al*. Genome-wide scan of obesity in the Old Order Amish. *J Clin Endocrinol Metab* 2001; 86: 1199–205.

25. Katzmarzyk PT, Rankinen T, Perusse L, Deriaz O, Tremblay A, Borecki I *et al*. Linkage and association of the sodium potassium-adenosine triphosphatase alpha2 and beta1 genes with respiratory quotient and resting metabolic rate in the Quebec Family Study. *J Clin Endocrinol Metab* 1999; 84: 2093–7.

26. Hixson JE, Almasy L, Cole S, Birnbaum S, Mitchell BD, Mahaney MC *et al*. Normal variation in leptin levels in associated with polymorphisms in the proopiomelanocortin gene, POMC. *J Clin Endocrinol Metab* 1999; 84: 3187–91.

27. Kogure A, Yoshida T, Sakane N, Umekawa T, Takakura Y, Kondo M. Synergic effect of polymorphisms in uncoupling protein 1 and beta3-adrenergic receptor genes on weight loss in obese Japanese. *Diabetologia* 1998; 41: 1399.

28. Ishiyama-Shigemoto S, Yamada K, Yuan X, Ichikawa F, Nonaka K. Association of polymorphisms in the beta2-adrenergic receptor gene with obesity, hypertriglyceridaemia, and diabetes mellitus. *Diabetologia* 1999; 42: 98–101.

29. Cassell PG, Neverova M, Janmohamed S, Uwakwe N, Qureshi A, McCarthy MI *et al*. An uncoupling protein 2 gene variant is associated with a raised body mass index but not Type II diabetes. *Diabetologia* 1999; 42: 688–92.

30. Walder K, Norman RA, Hanson RL, Schrauwen P, Neverova M, Jenkinson CP *et al*. Association between uncoupling protein polymorphisms (UCP2-UCP3) and energy metabolism/obesity in Pima indians. *Hum Mol Genet* 1998; 7: 1431–5.

31. Siffert W, Forster P, Jockel KH, Mvere DA, Brinkmann B, Naber C *et al*. Worldwide ethnic distribution of the G protein beta3 subunit 825T allele and its association with obesity in Caucasian, Chinese, and Black African individuals. *J Am Soc Nephrol* 1999; 10: 1921–30.

32. Bottini E, Gloria-Bottini F. Adenosine deaminase and body mass index in non-insulin-dependent diabetes mellitus. *Metabolism* 1999; 48: 949–51.

33. Ravussin E, Swinburn BA. Metabolic predictors of obesity: cross-sectional versus longitudinal data. *Int J Obes Relat Metab Disord* 1993; 17 (Suppl 3): S28–S31 (discussion S41–S22).

34. Rosenbaum M, Leibel RL, Hirsch J. Obesity. *N Engl J Med* 1997; 337: 396–407.

35. Salbe AD, Ravussin E. The determinants of obesity. In: Bouchard C (ed.) *Physical activity and obesity*. Champaign, IL: Human Kinetics Publishers, 2000.

36. Bray GA. *Contemporary diagnosis and management of obesity*. Newton, PA: Handbooks in Health Care, 1998.

37. Bray GA. Obesity, a disorder of nutrient partitioning: the MONA LISA hypothesis. *J Nutr* 1991; 121: 1146–62.

38. Bray GA, Greenway FL. Current and potential drugs for treatment of obesity. *Endocr Rev* 1999; 20: 805–75.

39. Bray GA, Blackburn GL, Ferguson JM, Greenway FL, Jain AK, Mendel CM *et al*. Sibutramine produces dose-related weight loss. *Obes Res* 1999; 7: 189–98.

40. Danforth E Jr. Sibutramine and thermogenesis in humans. *Int J Obes Relat Metab Disord* 1999; 23: 1007–8.

41. Sjostrom L, Rissanen A, Andersen T, Boldrin M, Golay A, Koppeschaar HP *et al*. Randomised placebo-controlled trial of orlistat for weight loss and prevention of weight regain in obese patients. European Multicentre Orlistat Study Group. *Lancet* 1998; 352: 167–72.

42. Halford JC, Blundell JE. Pharmacology of appetite suppression. *Prog Drug Res* 2000; 54: 25–58.

43. Gutzwiller JP, Drewe J, Ketterer S, Hildebrand P, Krautheim A, Beglinger C. Interaction between CCK and a preload on reduction of food intake is mediated by CCK-A receptors in humans. *Am J Physiol Regul Integr Comp Physiol* 2000; 279: R189–R95.

44. Van Dijk G, Thiele TE. Glucagon-like peptide-1 (7-36) amide: a central regulator of satiety and interoceptive stress. *Neuropeptides* 1999; 33: 406–14.

45. Reidelberger RD, Kelsey L, Heimann D. Effects of amylin-related peptides on food intake, meal patterns, and gastric emptying in rats. *Am J Physiol Regul Integr Comp Physiol* 2002; 282: R1395–R404.

46. Batterham RL, Cowley MA, Small CJ, Herzog H, Cohen MA, Dakin CL *et al*. Gut hormone PYY(3-36) physiologically inhibits food intake. *Nature* 2002; 418: 650–4.

47. Erlanson-Albertsson C, York D. Enterostatin-a peptide regulating fat intake. *Obes Res* 1997; 5: 360–72.

48. Huang L, Li C. Leptin: a multifunctional hormone. *Cell Res* 2000; 10: 81–92.

49. Pelleymounter MA, Cullen MJ, Baker MB, Hecht R, Winters D, Boone T *et al*. Effects of the obese gene product on body weight regulation in ob/ob mice. *Science* 1995; 269: 540–3.

50. Heymsfield SB, Greenberg AS, Fujioka K, Dixon RM, Kushner R, Hunt T *et al*. Recombinant leptin for weight loss in obese and lean adults: a randomized, controlled, dose-escalation trial. *JAMA* 1999; 282: 1568–75.

51. Rosenbaum M, Murphy EM, Heymsfield SB, Matthews DE, Leibel RL. Low dose leptin administration reverses effects of sustained weight-reduction on energy expenditure and circulating concentrations of thyroid hormones. *J Clin Endocrinol Metab* 2002; 87: 2391–4.

52. Petersen KF, Oral EA, Dufour S, Befroy D, Ariyan C, Yu C *et al*. Leptin reverses insulin resistance and hepatic steatosis in patients with severe lipodystrophy. *J Clin Invest* 2002; 109: 1345–50.

53. Nonogaki K, Strack AM, Dallman MF, Tecott LH. Leptin-independent hyperphagia and type 2 diabetes in mice with a mutated serotonin 5-HT2C receptor gene. *Nature Med* 1998; 4: 1152–6.

54. Itoh E, Fujimiya M, Inui A. Thioperamide, a histamine H3 receptor antagonist, powerfully suppresses peptide YY-induced food intake in rats. *Biol Psychiatry* 1999; 45: 475–81.

55. Duhault J, Boulanger M, Chamorro S, Boutin JA, Della Zuana O, Douillet E *et al.* Food intake regulation in rodents: Y5 or Y1 NPY receptors or both? *Can J Physiol Pharmacol* 2000; 78: 173–85.

56. Yaswen L, Diehl N, Brennan MB, Hochgeschwender U. Obesity in the mouse model of pro-opiomelanocortin deficiency responds to peripheral melanocortin. *Nature Med* 1999; 5: 1066–70.

57. Shimada M, Tritos NA, Lowell BB, Flier JS, Maratos-Flier E. Mice lacking melanin-concentrating hormone are hypophagic and lean. *Nature* 1998; 396: 670–4.

58. Calo G, Guerrini R, Rizzi A, Salvadori S, Regoli D. Pharmacology of nociceptin and its receptor: a novel therapeutic target. *Br J Pharmacol* 2000; 129: 1261–83.

59. Rowland NE, Mukherjee M, Robertson K. Effects of the cannabinoid receptor antagonist SR 141716, alone and in combination with dexfenfluramine or naloxone, on food intake in rats. *Psychopharmacology* 2001; 159: 111–6.

60. Di Marzo V, Goparaju SK, Wang L, Liu J, Batkai S, Jarai Z *et al.* Leptin-regulated endocannabinoids are involved in maintaining food intake. *Nature* 2001; 410: 822–5.

61. Ravussin E, Lillioja S, Knowler WC, Christin L, Freymond D, Abbott WG *et al.* Reduced rate of energy expenditure as a risk factor for body-weight gain. *N Engl J Med* 1988; 318: 467–72.

62. Zurlo F, Lillioja S, Esposito-Del Puente A, Nyomba BL, Raz I, Saad MF *et al.* Low ratio of fat to carbohydrate oxidation as predictor of weight gain: study of 24-h RQ. *Am J Physiol* 1990; 259: E650–E7.

63. Weyer C, Gautier JF, Danforth E Jr. Development of beta 3-adrenoceptor agonists for the treatment of obesity and diabetes-an update. *Diabetes Metab* 1999; 25: 11–21.

64. Bachman ES, Dhillon H, Zhang CY, Cinti S, Bianco AC, Kobilka BK *et al.* betaAR signaling required for diet-induced thermogenesis and obesity resistance. *Science* 2002; 297: 843–5.

65. Ricquier D, Bouillaud F. The uncoupling protein homologues: UCP1, UCP2, UCP3, StUCP and AtUCP. *Biochem J* 2000; 345: Pt: 2: 161–79.

66. Clapham JC, Arch JR, Chapman H, Haynes A, Lister C, Moore GB *et al.* Mice overexpressing human uncoupling protein-3 in skeletal muscle are hyperphagic and lean. *Nature* 2000; 406: 415–8.

67. Garrow JS. Treatment of obesity. *Lancet* 1992; 340: 409–13.

68. York DA. Rodent models of obesity. In: *Handbook of obesity*, Bray GA, Bouchard C, James WP (eds). New York: Marcel Dekker, 2002 (in press).

69. Chambers J, Ames RS, Bergsma D, Muir A, Fitzgerald LR, Hervieu G *et al.* Melanin-concentrating hormone is the cognate ligand for the orphan G-protein-coupled receptor SLC-1. *Nature* 1999; 400: 261–5.

70. Edwards CM, Abusnana S, Sunter D, Murphy KG, Ghatei MA, Bloom SR. The effect of the orexins on food intake: comparison with neuropeptide Y, melanin-concentrating hormone and galanin. *J Endocrinol* 1999; 160: R7–R12.

71. Sakurai T, Amemiya A, Ishii M, Matsuzaki I, Chemelli RM, Tanaka H *et al.* Orexins and orexin receptors: a family of hypothalamic neuropeptides and G protein-coupled receptors that regulate feeding behavior. *Cell* 1998; 92: 573–85.

72. Yamanaka A, Sakurai T, Katsumoto T, Yanagisawa M, Goto K. Chronic intracerebroventricular administration of orexin-A to rats increases food intake in daytime, but has no effect on body weight. *Brain Res* 1999; 849: 248–52.

73. Lambert PD, Wilding JP, al-Dokhayel AA, Bohuon C, Comoy E, Gilbey SG *et al.* A role for neuropeptide-Y, dynorphin, and noradrenaline in the central control of food intake after food deprivation. *Endocrinology* 1993; 133: 29–32.

74. Grandison L, Guidotti A. Stimulation of food intake by muscimol and beta endorphin. *Neuropharmacology* 1977; 16: 533–66.

75. Kyrkouli SE, Stanley BG, Seirafi RD, Leibowitz SF. Stimulation of feeding by galanin: anatomical localization and behavioral specificity of this peptide's effects in the brain. *Peptides* 1990; 11: 995–1001.

76. Abbott CR, Rossi M, Kim M, AlAhmed SH, Taylor GM, Ghatei MA *et al.* Investigation of the melanocyte stimulating hormones on food intake. Lack of evidence to support a role for the melanocortin-3-receptor. *Brain Res* 2000; 869: 203–10.

77. Edwards CM, Abbott CR, Sunter D, Kim M, Dakin CL, Murphy KG *et al.* Cocaine-and amphetamine-regulated transcript, glucagon-like peptide-1 and corticotrophin releasing factor inhibit feeding via agouti-related protein independent pathways in the rat. *Brain Res* 2000; 866: 128–34.

78. Benoit SC, Thiele TE, Heinrichs SC, Rushing PA, Blake KA, Steeley RJ. Comparison of central administration of corticotropin-releasing hormone and urocortin on food intake, conditioned taste aversion, and c-Fos expression. *Peptides* 2000; 21: 345–51.

79. Bradbury MJ, McBurnie MI, Denton DA, Lee KF, Vale WW. Modulation of urocortin-induced hypophagia and weight loss by corticotropin-releasing factor receptor 1 deficiency in mice. *Endocrinology* 2000; 141: 2715–24.

80. Kristensen P, Judge ME, Thim L, Ribel U, Christjansen KN, Wulff BS *et al.* Hypothalamic CART is a new anorectic peptide regulated by leptin. *Nature* 1998; 393: 72–6.

81. Stanley BG, Hoebel BG, Leibowitz SF. Neurotensin: effects of hypothalamic and intravenous injections on eating and drinking in rats. *Peptides* 1983; 4: 493–500.

82. Howard AD, Wang R, Pong SS, Mellin TN, Strack A, Guan XM *et al.* Identification of receptors for neuromedin U and its role in feeding. *Nature* 2000; 406: 70–4.

83. Morley JE, Farr SA, Flood JF. Peripherally administered calcitonin gene-related peptide decreases food intake in mice. *Peptides* 1996; 17: 511–6.

84. Rushing PA, Lutz TA, Seeley RJ, Woods SC. Amylin and insulin interact to reduce food intake in rats. *Horm Metab Res* 2000; 32: 62–5.

85. Weiss RE, Murata Y, Cua K, Hayashi Y, Seo H, Refetoff S. Thyroid hormone action on liver, heart, and energy expenditure in thyroid hormone receptor beta-deficient mice. *Endocrinology* 1998; 139: 4945–52.

86. Elchebly M, Payette P, Michaliszyn E, Cromlish W, Collins S, Loy AL *et al.* Increased insulin sensitivity and obesity resistance in mice lacking the protein tyrosine phosphatase-1B gene. *Science* 1999; 283: 1544–8.

87. Smith SJ, Cases S, Jensen DR, Chen HC, Sande E, Tow B *et al.* Obesity resistance and multiple mechanisms of triglyceride synthesis in mice lacking Dgat. *Nature Genet* 2000; 25: 87–90.

88. Kubota N, Terauchi Y, Miki H, Tamemoto H, Yamauchi T, Komeda K *et al.* PPAR gamma mediates high-fat diet-induced adipocyte hypertrophy and insulin resistance. *Mol Cell* 1999; 4: 597–609.

89. Guerre-Millo M, Gervois P, Raspe E, Madsen L, Poulain P, Derudas B *et al.* Peroxisome proliferator-activated receptor alpha activators improve insulin sensitivity and reduce adiposity. *J Biol Chem* 2000; 275: 16638–42.

90. Willson TM, Brown PJ, Sternbach DD, Henke BR. The PPARs: from orphan receptors to drug discovery. *J Med Chem* 2000; 43: 527–50.

91. Lin J, Wu H, Tarr PT, Zhang CY, Wu Z, Boss O *et al.* Transcriptional co-activator PGC-1alpha drives the formation of slow-twitch muscle fibres. *Nature* 2002; 418: 797–801.

92. Wu Z, Puigserver P, Andersson U, Zhang C, Adelmant G, Mootha V *et al.* Mechanisms controlling mitochondrial biogenesis and respiration through the thermogenic coactivator PGC-1. *Cell* 1999; 98: 115–24.

93. Cohen I, Kohl C, McGarry JD, Girard J, Prip-Buus C. The N-terminal domain of rat liver carnitine palmitoyltransferase 1 mediates import into the outer mitochondrial membrane and is essential for activity and malonyl-CoA sensitivity. *J Biol Chem* 1998; 273: 29896–904.

94. Anand A, Chada K. *In vivo* modulation of Hmgic reduces obesity. *Nature Genet* 2000; 24: 377–80.

95. Boizard M, Le Liepvre X, Lemarchand P, Foufelle F, Ferre P, Dugail I. Obesity-related overexpression of fatty-acid synthase gene in adipose tissue involves sterol regulatory element-binding protein transcription factors. *J Biol Chem* 1998; 273: 29164–71.

96. Kakuma T, Lee Y, Higa M, Wang Z, Pan W, Shimomura I *et al.* Leptin, troglitazone, and the expression of sterol regulatory element binding proteins in liver and pancreatic islets. *Proc Natl Acad Sci USA* 2000; 97: 8536–41.

97. Ntambi JM, Miyazaki M, Stoehr JP, Lan H, Kendziorski CM, Yandell BS *et al.* Loss of stearoyl-CoA desaturase-1 function protects mice against adiposity. *Proc Natl Acad Sci USA* 2002; 99: 11482–6.

98. Cohen P, Miyazaki M, Socci ND, Hagge-Greenberg A, Liedtke W, Soukas AA *et al.* Role for stearoyl-CoA desaturase-1 in leptin-mediated weight loss. *Science* 2002; 297: 240–3.

99. Egger G, Swinburn B. An 'ecological' approach to the obesity pandemic. *BMJ* 1997; 315: 477–80.

Progress in Obesity Research: 9. Edited by *Geraldo Medeiros-Neto, Alfredo Halpern and Claude Bouchard*
©2003 John Libbey Eurotext Ltd, pp. 260–264.

CHAPTER 54

Delivering the next generation of anti-obesity therapies – challenges for pharmacogenomics, patients and the pharmaceutical industry

David J. Heal, Helen L. Rowley and Helen C. Jackson

RenaSci Consultancy Ltd, BioCity, Nottingham NG1 1GF, UK
[e-mail: david.heal@renasci.co.uk]

Introduction

With unrelenting momentum, the global pandemic of obesity has emerged as being the single major contributor to all-cause morbidity and mortality in Western industrialized nations. The World Health Organization has estimated that currently there are over 700 million overweight adults (BMI 25–30) and have predicted that by 2025 the number of obese adults (BMI > 30) will exceed 300 million. In most Western European countries, the prevalence of obesity ranges from 10–25 per cent in the adult population, but in the USA, Eastern and Mediterranean Europe, this figure can be much higher (30–40 per cent). A more sedentary pattern of work and leisure coupled with plentiful access to cheap, calorie-dense and highly palatable food is undoubtedly the major factor in creating this situation. Moreover, the export of our 'junk food culture' has led to the emergence of this problem in territories where the rates of obesity had previously been very low, e.g. the Far East including India, China and Japan. In a manner analogous to the globalization of obesity, the prevalence of this disorder is also increasing amongst children and initial results from the 1999 National Health and Nutrition Examination Survey (NHANES) using measured heights and weights indicated that an estimated 13 per cent of children aged 6–11 years and 14 per cent of adolescents aged 12–19 years were overweight in the USA at that time. Once again, the problem is not confined to the USA and it has been estimated that there are approximately 22 million children under 5 years of age who are obese.

Obesity impairs quality of life and is associated with increased morbidity and mortality resulting in an estimated ~400,000 deaths in the USA yearly. Morbidities associated with this chronic disease include hypertension, heart disease, type 2 diabetes mellitus, dyslipidaemia, stroke, gallbladder disease, aggravated osteoarthritis, sleep apnoea and breast, prostate, endometrial and colon cancers. The financial burden of obesity is heavy at both the individual and governmental level. It has been calculated that up to 6–8 per cent of the total healthcare budgets of Western industrialized nations is spent in treating overweight and obese patients. As an example, an estimated $51.6 billion or 5.7 per cent of the US healthcare budget was spent in treating this disorder and a further $47.6 billion was lost in indirect costs (lost wages through disability or illness and curtailed future earnings because of death). Added to this was a further ~$100 billion which was the cost of treating the co-morbid diseases resulting directly from obesity.

Past and present drugs for the treatment of obesity

The drugs which have been and are being used for the treatment of obesity are shown in Table 1. From all perspectives, i.e. patients', physicians' and governments', the treatment of obesity using pharmacotherapy has had a very chequered history. d-Amphetamine and methamphetamine were the first drugs to be introduced for the treatment of obesity in the 1940s. These 'appetite suppressants' were of

Table 1. Drugs used for the treatment of obesity

Drug	Tradename	Mode of action
Sibutramine	Meridia Reductil	Serotonin and noradrenaline reuptake inhibitor (SNRI)
Orlistat	Xenical	Peripheral lipase inhibitor
Fenfluramine[1]	Ponderax Pondimin	Serotonin and noradrenaline releasing agent
d-Fenfluramine[1]	Redux	Serotonin and noradrenaline releasing agent
d-Amphetamine [2] dl-Amphetamine	Durophet	Non-selective monoamine releasing agents
Methamphetamine[2]	Desoxyn	Non-selective monoamine releasing agent
Phentermine[2]	Ionamin Duromine	Non-selective monoamine releasing agent
Benzphetamine[2]	Didrex	Monoamine releaser (?)
Phendimetrazine[2]	Bontril	Monoamine releaser (?)
Mazindol[2]	Sanorex Teronac	Noradrenaline and dopamine reuptake inhibitor
Diethylpropion[2]	Tenuate Apisate	Sympathomimetic

[1]Product withdrawn globally; [2]Product withdrawn in Europe.

Table 2. Various approaches in discovery/development for novel anti-obesity drugs

Discovery/development	Compound	Mode of action	Company
Phase III (suspended)	Topiramate	Unknown	Johnson and Johnson
Phase III	Rimonabant	Cannabinoid (CB1) antagonist	Sanofi-Synthelabo
Phase III	CTNF (Ax15) Axokine	Ciliary neurotrophic factor	Regeneron
Phase III	Bupropion	Dopamine reuptake inhibitor	GSK
Phase II	P57	Hoodia-gordonii extract	Phytopharm/Pfizer
Phase II	Metraleptin	Leptin agonist	Amgen
Phase II	AOD 9604	Human growth hormone fragment	Metabolic
Phase II	ATL 962	Pancreatic lipase inhibitor	Alizyme
Phase II	BVT 933	$5-HT_{2C}$ agonist	Biovitrum
Phase II	RF 1051	Human steroidal hormone fragment	SuperGen
Phase II/I	SR 58611 SB 418790	β_3-Adrenoceptor agonist β_3-Adrenoceptor agonist	Sanofi-Synthelabo GSK
Phase I	GI 181771	CCK-A agonist	GSK
Preclinical	CP 671906-01 J 115814	NPY1 antagonist NPY1 antagonist	Neurogen/Pfizer Banyu
Preclinical	GI 264879A GW 569180A CGP 71683A L 152804	NPY5 antagonist NPY5 antagonist NPY5 antagonist NPY5 antagonist	GSK GSK Novartis Merck
Preclinical	Ro 27-3225 ME 10142	MC4 agonist MC4 agonist	Roche Melacure
Preclinical	SNAP 7941 T 22696	MCH1 antagonist MCH1 antagonist	Synaptic Takeda

limited therapeutic value because of the rapid development of tolerance to their actions resulting in short-term prescribing with rapid relapse at the end of treatment. The issue of poor efficacy was compounded by the emergence of a much more serious problem, i.e. their psychostimulant properties caused them to be diverted from clinical use into recreational drug abuse. This has resulted in an almost total suspension of their employment in tackling obesity. The search for a 'second generation' of drug candidates with equivalent or better efficacy than the amphetamines, but a much reduced potential for psychostimulant abuse, resulted in the discovery and development of drugs including phentermine, fenfluramine (and its active isomer, d-fenfluramine), diethylpropion and mazindol. In Europe, these 'second generation' drugs were extensively prescribed, but serious side-effect issues, particularly primary pulmonary hypertension (PPH) as reported by Abenhaim et al. (1996)[1] restricted the duration of treatment with these drugs and cautioned against combination drug therapy. In the USA, Weintraub et al. (1992)[2] reported that a combination of the depressant serotonergic drug, fenfluramine, with the activating sympathomimetic, phentermine, produced profound and prolonged weight loss in obese subjects; not only that, but this led to the hypothesis that the behavioural effects of these two agents effectively cancelled themselves out leading to the hypothesis that greater efficacy could be achieved with lower doses of each compound and with a reduced propensity for side-effects. This finding led to an upsurge in the aggressive pharmacological treatment of obesity. When this situation was fuelled by the introduction of the 'novel' serotonergic anti-obesity drug, d-fenfluramine, in 1996, the road to celebrity status for Redux® was already being mapped out. Like many previous glittering careers, this one was destined to end in failure and recrimination. Initially, it was the serious problems of PPH[1] and potential neurotoxicity[3] which critics claimed were largely ignored. However, it was multiple reports of a high proportion of cardiac valvulopathy in patients receiving the fenfluramines, either alone or in combination with phentermine (fen/phen)[4] which prompted the worldwide withdrawal of fenfluramine and d-fenfluramine and initiated a flurry of law suites against the manufacturers and anyone else who could be implicated in the debacle. In the European Union, which has traditionally taken a cautious stance on drug therapy for obesity, the regulatory authorities went much further by insisting on the withdrawal of all 'first and second generation' anti-obesity drugs on the basis of a poor or unproven risk-benefit ratio. The fallout from this has been enormous, especially in the USA where the confidence of physicians and patients in the pharmacotherapy of obesity has been seriously dented; it is likely that this situation will take several years to resolve fully. The late 1990s also saw the introduction of two new anti-obesity drugs with markedly different modes of action, i.e. sibutramine and orlistat. Sibutramine is a centrally-acting monoamine reuptake inhibitor that was initially developed as an antidepressant. Sibutramine's anti-obesity action appears to derive from its ability to reduce food intake by enhancing post-ingestive satiety, and perhaps also, its ability to prevent the reflex decrease in metabolic rate that accompanies reduced calorie intake. Animal studies have indicated that both effects can be explained by sibutramine's ability to block the reuptake of serotonin and noradrenaline in the brain[5]. The clinical use of sibutramine has not been associated with incidences of PPH or cardiac valvulopathy and there is no evidence that this drug has abuse liability in man. However, this drug does cause the cardiovascular side-effects (tachycardia and increased blood pressure) which require careful monitoring and also limit the dose that can be used in patients. Orlistat is a peripheral lipase inhibitor that prevents the absorption from the gut of approximately 30 per cent of calories consumed as fat. This drug has to be taken three times daily before meals and is effective when used in conjunction with a low fat diet. However, orlistat produces gastrointestinal disturbances which limit the dose that can be employed and these side-effects can be severe if orlistat is taken prior to the consumption of a high fat meal.

Expectations of physicians and patients

Current drug therapy produces weight loss of sufficient magnitude to produce clinical benefit, but the reductions in most instances do not meet the expectations of physicians and certainly not of their patients. In most clinical studies, the mean weight loss achieved with drug therapy is between 5 and 10 per cent, but the majority of patients and a significant number of physicians would like to see weight reductions of the order of 15–25 per cent or more. With current therapies, many patients are still obese after the weight loss has plateaued and most are still overweight. Furthermore, a significant proportion of patients do not achieve or sustain > 5 per cent weight loss that is generally accepted as being of clinical benefit. The poor safety record of anti-obesity drugs as a therapeutic class, i.e. first, diversion and abuse associated with the amphetamines, and latterly, PPH, cardiac valvulopathy and potential neurotoxicity with the fenfluramines, has created a climate of caution amongst physicians and regulatory agencies, especially as obesity is still not universally accepted as being a disease requiring pharmacological intervention. It is likely that novel drugs seeking regulatory approval and widespread acceptance by physicians will need to demonstrate improved clinical efficacy compared with existing therapies together with benign side-effect and adverse-event profiles.

Meeting the challenges

Responders versus non-responders

One key factor that arises from trials and general clinical experience is that no pharmacological intervention is universally effective and anti-obesity drugs are no exception to this rule. As an example, Bray *et al.* (1999)[6] demonstrated an excellent dose response relationship for weight loss over 6 months on sibutramine. However, at 10 and 15 mg daily, mean weight loss was respectively 6.1 per cent and 7.4 per cent for the completers, but using the more conservative 'last observation carried forward' analysis, these figures dropped to 4.7 per cent and 5.8 per cent. Although in this trial only 4 per cent of sibutramine discontinuations were ascribed directly to a lack of efficacy, it is generally accepted that for most anti-obesity drugs the figure is likely to be 10–25 per cent. In an ideal situation, patients not benefiting from therapy should not be exposed to the risk of drug treatment. Therefore, it is important that we achieve a greater understanding of why some patients are responders, but others are not. In this regard, genetic profiling of patients has potentially an important future role to play in defining which subpopulations of patients will achieve the greatest benefit from a particular drug intervention.

Drug combination therapy

One simple strategy to achieve greater clinical efficacy is to combine drug therapies with complimentary modes of action – this was the rationale for 'fen/phen'. However, as the pharmacology of neither drug was well understood, the reality turned out to be very different from the hypothesis. First, d-fenfluramine is not a 5-HT reuptake inhibitor[5], it acts solely through 5-HT release *in vivo*[7]. Second, its actions are not specific to 5-HT because it also releases noradrenaline[8]. Phentermine is also not a monoamine reuptake inhibitor, but is in fact a powerful releaser of noradrenaline, 5-HT and dopamine in the brain[7-9]. This drug is equipotent with d-amphetamine as a dopamine releaser and is a powerful psychostimulant at the doses required to reduce food intake[9]. Consistent with this finding, phentermine generalizes to cocaine in drug discrimination experiments (in house data) and is a positive reinforcer in primates trained to self-administer low doses of cocaine (Woolverton and Heal, in preparation). Thus, fenfluramine and phentermine each potentiates the action of the other on 5-HT and noradrenaline, and in addition, phentermine adds a powerful dopaminergic psychostimulant component. This profile is totally at odds with the previously accepted view that in the fen/phen combination fenfluramine specifically potentiated serotonergic function, whilst phentermine specifically potentiated noradrenergic function. Cardiac valvulopathy prompted the global withdrawal of the fenfluramines, and in turn, a keen desire to discover the mechanism responsible for this serious adverse event. Whilst much research has been focussed on the agonist actions of d-fenfluramine and d-norfenfluramine at 5-HT$_{2B}$ receptors on mitral valves, our approach has been to elucidate the role that 5-HT release from platelets and other peripheral tissues could play in activating this receptor population. Using microdialysis *in vitro* to measure platelet 5-HT release, we observed a profound dose-dependent effect of d-fenfluramine and d-norfenfluramine[10]. However, phentermine did not evoke 5-HT release from platelets, nor did it potentiate the release evoked by d-fenfluramine[10]. Since 5-HT is a powerful full agonist at 5-HT$_{2B}$ receptors, these findings provide an additional plausible mechanism to explain why the fenfluramines cause valvulopathy, but phentermine does not. Other combinations for obesity, including phentermine with the SSRI, fluoxetine (Phen/Pro) are being suggested as viable alternatives to fen/phen, but experience would indicate that assumptions about the pharmacology of drugs, especially in combination, are unwise and caution should be exercised before using patients as human guinea pigs.

New drug targets

In a review of this length, it is impossible to provide a comprehensive review of the 20 to 30 new approaches being pursued in the search for novel anti-obesity drugs which have reached the development stage of clinical candidate status and beyond (Table 2). Johnson and Johnson's topiramate has recently been suspended in Phase III for causing unacceptable CNS side-effects. Other late phase drugs include Sanofi-Synthelabo's CB1 antagonist, rimonabant, and Regeneron's CTNF drug. There is still interest in previously 'hot targets' like NPY, leptin and β$_3$-adrenoceptor agonists, but so far, there has been no unequivocal evidence to demonstrate clinical success with these particular approaches. Hypothalamic peptide targets, including MCH antagonists and MC4 agonists, are still being followed by many companies and recent animal data suggest that these approaches may yield some interesting new clinical candidates. There has also been a lot of interest in developing 5-HT$_{2C}$ agonists (to mimic d-fenfluramine's pharmacological actions); in this area Biovitrum's BVT-933 appears to be the clear leader at the present time. Overall, the decoding of the human genome and the successful application of technologies to de-orphanise receptors have provided a plethora of new targets which could herald the discovery of the next generation of anti-obesity drugs. Since the regulation of food intake and energy expenditure is fundamental to survival, the real challenge will be to identify those metabolic systems which cannot be overridden by the body's 'failsafe' homeostatic mechanisms. It is only by manipulating these fundamental regulators that there is an opportunity to deliver new drugs with significantly better efficacy than existing products. However, efficacy is not all that is required; new drugs will also need to deliver this enhanced performance with a benign profile of side-effects and minimal adverse advents.

Conclusions

The challenge thrown down by the increasingly global epidemic of obesity is one that cannot be met by any single technology or group in society. It is clear that patients, physicians, governments and researchers will each need to contribute substantially in order to regain the initiative in tackling the problem. Whilst new drug therapies are urgently required and much effort is being expended in achieving this objective, it is also clear that drugs alone cannot provide a panacea for obesity. It is probable that new drugs will deliver their optimum performance only in the situation where patients and physicians are committed to the objective of substantial, maintained weight-loss. The prospect of a new drug that will deliver major weight-loss without the requirement for a profound lifestyle change by the patient may be a pharmacological 'El Dorado' that is best left undiscovered.

References

1. Abenhaim L, Moride Y, Brenot F, Rich S, Benichou J, Kurz X et al. Appetite-suppressant drugs and the risk of primary pulmonary hypertension. N Eng J Med 1996; 335: 609–16.

2. Weintraub M, Sundaresan PR, Cox C. Long-term weight control study. VI. Individual participant response patterns. Clin Pharmacol Ther 1992; 51(5): 619–33.

3. McCann U, Hatzidimitriou G, Ridenour A, Fischer C, Yuan J, Katz J, et al. Dexfenfluramine and serotonin neurotoxicity: further preclinical evidence that clinical caution is indicated. J Pharmacol Exp Ther 1994; 269: 792–8.

4. Connolly HM, Crary JL, McGoon MD, Hensrud DD, Edwards BS, Edwards WD, et al. Valvular heart disease associated with fenfluramine-phentermine. N Eng J Med 1997; 337: 581–8.

5. Heal DJ, Aspley S, Prow MR, Jackson HC, Martin KF, Cheetham SC. Sibutramine: a novel anti-obesity drug. A review of the pharmacological evidence to differentiate it from d-aphetamine and d-fenfluramine. Int J Obes 1998; 22 (Suppl 1): S18–S28.

6. Bray GA, Blackburn GL, Ferguson JM, Greenway FL, Jain AK., Mendel CM et al. Sibutramine produces dose-related weight loss. Obes Res 1999; 7: 189–98.

7. Prow MR, Lancashire B, Aspley S, Heal DJ, Kilpatrick IC. Additive effects on rat brain 5HT release of combining phentermine with dexfenfluramine. Int J Obes 2001; 25: 1450–3.

8. Viggers J, Cheetham SC, Lancashire B, Prow M, Aspley S, Wortley KE et al. d-Fenfluramine and phentermine both enhance central noradrenergic function via release – contrast with reuptake inhibition by sibutramine. Int J Obes 1999; 23 (Suppl 5): P225.

9. Rowley HL, Butler SA, Prow MR, Dykes SG, Aspley S, Kilpatrick IC, Heal DJ. Comparison of the effects of sibutramine and other weight-modifying drugs on extracellular dopamine in the nucleus accumbens of freely moving rats. Synapse 2000; 38: 167–76.

10. Lane EL, Prow MR, Aspley S, Kilpatrick IC, Heal DJ. d-Fenfluramine releases 5-HT from whole blood of rats as measured by in vitro microdialysis. Br J Pharmacol 2000; 129: 155P.

Progress in Obesity Research: 9. Edited by *Geraldo Medeiros-Neto, Alfredo Halpern* and *Claude Bouchard*

©2003 John Libbey Eurotext Ltd, pp. 265–268.

CHAPTER 55

Molecular genetic basis of partial lipodystrophy: insights into requirements for adipocyte function

Richard C. Trembath

Professor of Medical Genetics, Division of Medical Genetics, Depts of Medicine and Genetics, Adrian Building, University of Leicester, University Road, Leicester LE1 7RH, UK
[e-mail: rtrembat@hgmp.mrc.ac.uk]

Introduction

The lipodystrophies are a heterogeneous group of disorders characterized by a regional or generalized absence of subcutaneous adipose tissue. At least 500 patients with various lipodystrophies have been reported in literature over the last 100 years[1]. Fat loss may be limited, resulting in well demarcated indentations of the subcutaneous structures (localized lipodystrophy) or extensive as seen in the congenital generalized form CGL, when the condition is also associated with significant metabolic disturbance including hypertriglycerideamia, diabetes mellitus and fatty infiltration of the liver. Recent progress through molecular genetic studies has led to a more logical classification of the lipodystrophies (see Table 1), and offers insight to critical molecular pathways in adipocyte function.

This review pays particular attention to recent progress in the molecular genetic basis of partial lipodystrophy an important natural model of the normal metabolic functions of subcutaneous fat. For completeness, brief mention is made of additional conditions characterized by varying degrees of lipoatrophy.

Table 1. Classification of lipodystrophies

Familial lipodystrophies	Acquired lipodystrophies
Congenital generalized lipodystrophy (Berardinelli-Seip syndrome)	Acquired generalized lipodystrophy (Lawrence syndrome)
Familial partial lipodystrophy (Dunnigan variety)	Acquired partial lipodystrophy (Barraquer-Simons syndrome)
Familial partial lipodystrophy (Köbberling variety)	Lipodystrophy in human immunodeficiency virus-infected patients
Familial partial lipodystrophy (mandibuloacral dysplasia variety)	Localized lipodystrophies
Familial lipodystrophies, other varieties	

Congenital generalized lipoatrophy

Congenital generalized lipoatrophy (Berardinelli-Seip syndrome OMIN 269700), is an autosomal recessive disorder leading to a near total absence of adipose tissue in subcutaneous, inter-abdominal and intra-thoracic sites. In contrast, normal amounts of fat maybe observed in the retro-orbital space, but also in the palms and soles, scalp and perineal regions. Additional features include acanthosis nigricans, acromegalic facies, hyper-androgenism in women and severe insulin resistance with impaired glucose tolerance and diabetes developing during teenage years. Most affected individuals develop significant hyper triglycerideamia, but with normal HDL-cholesterol levels.

Molecular genetics

Two genes have recently been reported to underlie CGL, with evidence of locus heterogeneity. BSCL1 on chromosome 9q34 was initially mapped using a number of consanguineous families. A positional candidate gene analysis identified mutations within the *AGPAT2* gene encoding 1-acylglycerol-3-phosphate O-acyltranserase 2, an enzyme that catalyses the acylation of licophosphatidic acid to form phosphotidic acid, a key intermediate in the biosynthesis of triacylglycerol and glycerophospholipids. *AGPAT2* transcripts are found to be highly expressed in adipose tissue, however, the mechanisms by which mutation in this enzyme leads to lipodystrophy remain unclear[2]. BSCL2 was also identified after a genome wide screen of consanguineous families with CGL. BSCL2 was localized to chromosome 11q13 and is a novel gene with significant homology to the murine guanine-nucleotide binding protein (G protein) gammer 3-linked gene (*Gng3lg*). Protein product of BSCL2 has been named serpin and limited studies to date indicate the transcript is predominantly expressed in brain and testes, including hypothalamic structures[3].

Partial lipodystrophy (PLD) (Dunnigan-Köbberling syndrome OMIN 151660)

Dunnigan (1974)[4] and Köbberling (1975)[5] independently described a familial disorder, partial lipodystrophy, which is characterized by the regional absence of subcutaneous adipose tissue. Although initially thought to be an x-linked dominant condition, analysis of further pedigrees reveal an autosomal dominant mode of transmission[6]. Anthropometric evaluation and cross-sectional imaging demonstrated the presence of fat in intra-abdominal and thoracic cavities and also within the subcutaneous tissues of the head and neck, but its complete absence from subcutaneous sites of the trunk and limbs. Skeletal muscle hypertrophy is present together with acanthosis nigricans, hirsutism and menstrual abnormalities and polycystic ovaries in females. The phenotype is more readily recognized in women with significant under reporting of the disorder in males, who maybe less severely affected by the metabolic complications of PLD. Intriguingly subcutaneous fat is present at birth with gradual loss occurring at or around puberty. Metabolically, most patients develop diabetes or impaired glucose tolerance after the age of 20, with characteristic high serum triglyceride yet below serum HGL cholesterol levels[6]. The Köbberling variant described in a small number of families, places emphasis on the loss of adipose tissue restricted to the extremities. It remains unclear whether this variant is a distinct entity or an allelic disorder with the Dunnigan phenotype.

Molecular genetics

Following a genome wide scan in affected multigenerational families, the gene for PLD was localized to the long arm of chromosome at 1q21. Discrete mutations within the LMNA gene encoding for the nuclear envelope protein Lamin A/C, have been identified in a number of PLD families[7–10]. Molecular implications of these findings are discussed below. A small number of patients have been described with a PLD phenotype characterized by loss of fat in due to heterozygous mutation in peroxisome proliferator-activated receptor-gamma, a transcription factor critical in apidocyte differention and glucose and lipid metabolism.

Familial partial lipodystrophy (mandibuloacral dysplasia variety OMIN 248370)

Mandibuloacral Dysplasia is an autosomal recessive disorder characterized by short stature, high pitched voice, mandibulohypoplasia, together with ectodermal defects, alipecia and nail dysplasia. Homozygous LMNA mutations have recently been identified in several in-bred families[11].

Acquired generalized lipodystrophy (Lawrence syndrome)

Lawrence syndrome is characterized by generalized absence of fat, insulin resistant diabetes mellitus, absence of ketosis, elevated basal metabolic rate and a severe hyperlipidaemia typically with hepotomegly. The disorder has its onset during late childhood or adolescence, a critical feature distinguishing it from familial CGL.

Acquired partial lipodystrophy (Barraquer-Simons syndromes)

Women are affected at least three times more frequently than men, with an onset typically before the age of 15 years. Fat loss classically involves the face, spreading to the neck, shoulders and upper extremities, yet often with excess fat in the hips and lower extremities. Approximately one third of patients develop a mesangio-capillary glomerulonephritis, typically more than 10 years after the onset of lipodystrophy. The molecular basis of the acquired lipodystrophy remains unclear[12], but increasing evidence of associated autoimmune disorders indicates that they represent an immunological-mediated processes. A rapidly growing literature on both the frequency and mechanisms leading to HIV associated lipodystrophy, a complication not confined to use of protease inhibitors, suggests that yet further insights into adipocyte function will soon emerge.

Nuclear infrastructure and laminopathies

The nuclear lamina is a network of polymeric filaments within the nucleus that consists of lamin proteins and associated lamin binding proteins [13]. Lamins are members of the intermediate filament family of proteins and have been classified by sequence into A and B types. The *LMNA* gene located at chromosome 1q 21 encodes for the major transcripts Lamin A and C which are ubiquitously expressed in differentiated cells and form small N-terminal head long coiled-coil rod and globular C-terminal tail domains[14-16]. Pairs of lamins interact in parallel via their coiled coil regions to form dimers. The lamina is thought to maintain nuclear structure and integrity and contribute to the regulation of chromatin organization.

Recently no fewer than five distinct phenotypes have been shown to arise from mutation of the LMNA gene, each targeted to different tissue types, whilst additional mutant alleles appear to lead to overlap syndromes. Dilated cardiomyopathy with conduction system disease (CMD1A)[17] and Emery-Dreifuss muscular dystrophy (EDMD-AD)[18], a progressive muscle wasting disorder with cardiac conduction defects, are both disorders of striated muscle. More recent detailed assessment has revealed evidence of lipodystrophy in some EDMD-AD patients with LMNA mutations[1]. In contrast, subjects with PLD appear to have hypertrophy of striated muscle and normal cardiac structures. Most recently, homozygous LMNA mutations have been reported in the rare disorders, axonal neuropathy (Charcot-Marie-Tooth disorder type 2)[19] (and mandibuloacral dysplasia[11], thereby expanding the phenotypic range seen in laminopathies. Lamin A/C is not essential for development, as the mouse LMNA knock-out displays both features of EMDM and has marked absence of subcutaneous white fat[20].

The molecular mechanisms by which defects of the nuclear envelope structure give rise to these various disorders remain unclear, being only in part reflected by the distribution of LMNA mutations within the gene, for example in EDMD, lesions appear distributed throughout the coding sequence, whilst in CMD1A, the mutations are mainly clustered within the coiled-coil domain, with the potential to disrupt the dimerization or lamin polymerization[21-23].

The crystal structure of the C-terminal domain of lamin A has been resolved and reveals the tightly clustered PLD amino-acid substitutions, lie on one face of the protein. Using the yeast two-hybrid screen[24], a number of lamin interacting proteins have been identified including the adipocyte differentiation factor, sterol response element binding protein 1 (SREBP1)[25-28]. These and related studies[29-31] raise the interesting possibility that at least some of the cell specific defects seen in the laminopathies reflect interference in critical protein-protein interactions . It is clear that further study of this interesting group of patients will continue to shed further light on the complex molecular pathways active in adipocytes and perhaps unexpectedly has contributed to the excitement amongst a broad range of biologists, with the identification of a range of human disorders due to defects in the nuclear envelope.

References

1. Garg A, Speckman RA, Bowcock AM. Multisystem dystrophy syndrome due to novel missense mutations in the amino-terminal head and alpha-helical rod domains of the lamin A/C gene. *Am J Med* 2002; 112(7): 549–55.

2. Agarwal AK, Arioglu E, de Almeida S, Akkoc N, Taylor SI *et al.* AGPAT2 is mutated in congenital generalized lipodystrophy linked to chromosome 9q34. *Nature Genet* 2002; 31: 21–3.

3. Magre J, Delepine M, Khallouf E, Gedde-Dahl T Jr, van Maldergem L, Sobel E *et al.* BSCL Working Group. Identification of the gene altered in Berardinelli-Seip congenital lipodystrophy on chromosome 11q13. *Nature Genet* 2001; 28(4): 365–70.

4. Dunnigan MG, Cochrane MA, Kelly A, Scott JW. Familial lipoatrophic diabetes with dominant transmission. A new syndrome. *Quart J Med* 1974; 43: 33–48.

5. Köbberling J, Willms B, Kattermann R, Creutzfeldt W. Lipodystrophy of the extremities. A dominantly inherited syndrome associated with lipatrophic diabetes. *Humangenetik* 1975; 29: 111–20.

6. Jackson SNJ, Howlett TA, McNally PG, O'Rahilly S, Trembath RC. Dunnigan–Kobberling syndrome: an autosomal dominant form of partial lipodystrophy. *Quart J Med* 1997; 90: 27–36.

7. Cao H, Hegele RA. Nuclear lamin A/C R482Q mutation in Canadian kindreds with Dunnigan-type familial partial lipodystrophy. *Hum Mol Genet* 2000; 9: 109–12.

8. Shackleton S, Lloyd DJ, Jackson SNJ, Evans R, Niermeijer MF, Singh BM et al. LMNA, encoding lamin A/C, is mutated in partial lipodystrophy. *Nature Genet* 2000; 24: 153–6.

9. Speckman RA, Garg A, Du F, Bennett L, Veile R, Arioglu E et al. Mutational and haplotype analyses of families with familial partial lipodystrophy (Dunnigan variety) reveal recurrent missense mutations in the globular C-terminal domain of lamin A/C. *Am J Hum Genet* 2000; 66: 1192–8.

10. Hegele RA. Molecular basis of partial lipodystrophy and prospects for therapy. *Trends Mol Med* 2001; 7: 121–6.

11. Novelli G, Muchir A, Sangiuolo F, Helbling-Leclerc A, D'Apice MR, Massart C et al. Mandibuloacral dysplasia is caused by a mutation in LMNA-encoding lamin A/C. *Am J Hum Genet* 2002; 71(2): 426–31.

12. Vigouroux C, Magre J, Vantyghem MC, Bourut C, Lascols O, Shackleton S et al. Lamin A/C gene: sex-determined expression of mutations in Dunnigan-type familial partial lipodystrophy and absence of coding mutations in congenital and acquired generalized lipoatrophy. *Diabetes* 2000; 49: 1958–62.

13. Stuurman N, Heins S, Aebi U. Nuclear lamins: their structure, assembly, and interactions. *J Struct Biol* 1998; 122: 42–66.

14. Fisher DZ, Chaudhary N, Blobel G. cDNA sequencing of nuclear lamin-a and lamin-C reveals primary and secondary structural homology to intermediate filament proteins. *Proc Natl Acad Sci USA* 1986; 83: 6450–4.

15. McKeon FD, Kirschner MW, Caput D. Homologies in both primary and secondary structure between nuclear envelope and intermediate filament proteins. *Nature* 1986; 319: 463–8.

16. Dhe-Paganon S, Werner ED, Chi YI, Shoelson SE. Structure of the globular tail of nuclear lamin. *J Biol Chem* 2002; 277(20): 17381–4.

17. Fatkin D, MacRae C, Sasaki T, Wolff MR, Porcu M, Frenneaux M et al. Missense mutations in the rod domain of the lamin A/C gene as causes of dilated cardiomyopathy and conduction-system disease. *N Engl J Med* 1999; 341: 1715–24.

18. Bonne G, DiBarletta MR, Varnous S, Becane HM, Hammouda EH, Merlini L et al. Mutations in the gene encoding lamin A/C cause autosomal dominant Emery–Dreifuss muscular dystrophy. *Nature Genet* 1999; 21: 285–8.

19. De Sandre-Giovannoli A, Chaouch M, Kozlov S, Vallat JM, Tazir M, Kassouri N et al. Homozygous defects in LMNA, encoding lamin A/C nuclear-envelope proteins, cause autosomal recessive axonal neuropathy in human (Charcot-Marie-Tooth disorder type 2) and mouse. *Am J Hum Genet* 2002; 70: 726–36.

20. Sullivan T, Escalante-Alcalde D, Bhatt H, Anver M, Bhat N, Nagashima K et al. Loss of A-type lamin expression compromises nuclear envelope integrity leading to muscular dystrophy. *J Cell Biol* 1999; 147: 913–9.

21. Hutchison CJ, Alvarez-Reyes M, Vaughan OA. Lamins in disease: why do ubiquitously expressed nuclear envelope proteins give rise to tissue-specific disease phenotypes? *J Cell Sci* 2001; 114: 9–19.

22. Wilson KL, Zastrow MS, Lee KK. Lamins and disease: insights into nuclear infrastructure. *Cell* 2001; 104: 647–50.

23. Vaughan OA, Alvarez-Reyes M, Bridger JM, Broers JLV, Ramaekers FCS, Wehnert M et al. Both emerin and lamin C depend on lamin A for localization at the nuclear envelope. *J Cell Sci* 2001; 114: 2577–90.

24. Lloyd DJ, Trembath RC, Shackleton S. A novel interaction between lamin A and SREBP1: implications for partial lipodystrophy and other laminopathies. *Hum Mol Genet* 2002; 11(7): 769–77.

25. Yokoyama C, Wang X, Briggs MR, Admon A, Wu J, Hua X et al. SREBP-1, a basic-helix–loop–helix–leucine zipper protein that controls transcription of the low density lipoprotein receptor gene. *Cell* 1993; 75: 187–97.

26. Tontonoz P, Kim JB, Graves RA, Spiegelman BM. ADD1: a novel helix–loop–helix transcription factor associated with adipocyte determination and differentiation. *Mol Cell Biol* 1993; 13: 4753–9.

27. Kim JB, Spiegelman BM. ADD1/SREBP1 promotes adipocyte differentiation and gene expression linked to fatty acid metabolism. *Genes Dev* 1996; 10: 1096–107.

28. Horton JD, Shimomura I, Brown MS, Hammer RE, Goldstein JL, Shimano H. Activation of cholesterol synthesis in preference to fatty acid synthesis in liver and adipose tissue of transgenic mice overproducing sterol regulatory element-binding protein-2. *J Clin Invest* 1998; 101: 2331–9.

29. Ostlund C, Bonne G, Schwartz K, Worman HJ. Properties of lamin A mutants found in Emery–Dreifuss muscular dystrophy, cardiomyopathy and Dunnigan-type partial lipodystrophy. *J Cell Sci* 2001; 114: 4435–45.

30. Raharjo WH, Enarson P, Sullivan T, Stewart C, Burke B. Nuclear envelope defects associated with LMNA mutations cause dilated cardiomyopathy and Emery–Dreifuss muscular dystrophy. *J Cell Sci* 2001; 114: 4447–57.

31. Vigouroux C, Auclair M, Dubosclard E, Pouchelet M, Capeau J, Courvalin J-C, Buendia B. Nuclear envelope disorganisation in fibroblasts from lipodystrophic patients with heterozygous R482Q/W mutations in the lamin A/C gene. *J Cell Sci* 2001; 114: 4459–68.

Progress in Obesity Research: 9. Edited by *Geraldo Medeiros-Neto, Alfredo Halpern and Claude Bouchard*
©2003 John Libbey Eurotext Ltd, pp. 269–271.

CHAPTER 56

Molecular genetic studies of porcine genes for obesity

Kwan-Suk Kim[1], Lloyd L. Anderson[1], James M. Reecy[1], Nguyet Thu Nguyen[1], Graham S. Plastow[2] and Max F. Rothschild[1]

[1]*Department of Animal Science, Iowa State University, Ames, IA 50011, USA;*
[2]*Sygen International, 2929 7th Street, Suite 130, Berkeley, CA 94710, USA*
[e-mail: kskim@iastate.edu]

Introduction

The physiological system governing energy storage in the form of fat might be the most fundamentally adaptive systems in humans and other animal species. These systems are now the target of extensive biomedical investigation to solve causes of human obesity. Experimental animals, mainly mice and rats, have been used for a number of obesity studies designed to identify genetic factors that regulate energy balance. Surgical, chemical, and dietary approaches have successfully revealed some physiological mechanisms leading to obesity. In addition, heritable forms of obesity in animals have been used as model organisms to identify genetic factors that may control human obesity. We have used the pig as a model to identify obesity-related genes for two reasons. First, the genetic components of human obesity may play important roles in regulation of pig performance traits such as fatness, growth rate, and feed intake. As pork is a principal source of animal protein and pork production is an important business in agriculture on a worldwide basis, this research can provide invaluable information for economically efficient lean pig production. More precisely, mapping of obesity-related genes on porcine chromosomes can be useful to breeding programmes for marker-assisted selection (MAS) of those performance traits. Second, numerous physiological similarities between pigs and humans suggest that the pig can be a useful model of human obesity (Houpt *et al.* 1979; Carey, 1997; Miller and Ullrey, 1987; Rapacz and Hasler-Rapacz, 1989)[7,13,15]. Furthermore, evolutionarily the pig genome is more closely related to human genome than small laboratory animal species. Thus, the identification of significant DNA polymorphisms in obesity-related genes in the pig genome might provide useful targets for the genetic study of human obesity.

Candidate gene studies in pigs

The number of genes or gene products that are known to control appetite or body weight is up to 130 and still increasing. Fifty-eight candidate genes were found to be significantly associated with obesity-related phenotypes in humans (Rankinen *et al.*, 2002)[14] and more than 10 of these have been studied in the pig in our laboratory.

One of the most significant discoveries was a polymorphism identified in the porcine *Melanocortin 4 receptor (MC4R)* gene (Kim *et al.*, 2000)[8]. This polymorphism revealed a missense mutation that replaces aspartic acid with asparagine at the amino acid position 298 of the MC4R protein. Interestingly, Asp298 is a well conserved amino acid within other MCR subtypes and in other species. This *MC4R* type was significantly associated with less backfat thickness, slower growth rate, and lower feed intake. In contrast, the Asn298 mutant was associated with increased backfat, higher feed intake, and faster growing pigs from several commercial populations. The strong association between the *MC4R* variants and fatness, growth rate, body weight, and feed intake probably result from the fact that the variant amino acid residues of the *MC4R* mutation cause a significant change of the MC4R function, and this hypothesis is under investigation.

Since similar MC4R mutations have been found in humans with morbid obesity (Rankinen *et al.*, 2002)[14], the pig MC4R mutation will be useful for studying the physiological relationship between melanocortin signaling and human obesity. New mutations from other porcine candidate genes are also under investigation and results from them may be useful to determine naturally occurring gene mutations that may be ultimately responsible for some of human obesity.

Quantitative trait loci (QTL) scanning in pigs

A significant number of QTL have been identified in the pig in recent years. Bidanel and Rothschild (2002)[3] recently reviewed all significant QTL studies performed with pigs. The first major QTL (named as *FAT1*) for fatness and growth was identified on chromosome 4 using a Wild Boar intercross (Anderson *et al.*, 1994)[1]. This *FAT1* region is homologous to parts of human chromosome 1 and 8. The latest comparative mapping results between humans and pigs indicate that the QTL is located in a region homologous to HSA1q (Berg *et al.*, 2002)[2].

Bidanel *et al.* (2001)[3] also conducted a QTL experiment with a Meishan x Large White F2 population and found several loci affecting important economic traits, such as growth rate and backfat thickness on chromosome 4 and 7. Wang *et al.* (1998)[16] directly searched for QTL on chromosomes 4 and 7 for performance traits in five Chinese x American breed cross families and identified QTL for average daily gain on chromosome 4 and QTL for backfat thickness on chromosome 7.

A recent QTL study conducted in our laboratory also identified a significant QTL for growth and fat content traits on the same region of pig chromosome 7 (Malek *et al.*, 2001)[10]. Further investigation using biological and positional candidate genes in that region revealed that polymorphisms in a candidate gene, *high mobility group A1* (*HMGA1*) were consistently associated with observed variation in the F2 pigs of the QTL population and other genetically diverse commercial populations (Kim *et al.*, 2002)[9]. The results obtained to date suggest that the *HMGA1* gene is a strong candidate for the QTL reported in pig chromosome 7. As the corresponding human and mouse chromosomal region is also known to be associated with obesity (Rankinen *et al.*, 2002), the *HMGA1* gene might be potentially important for human obesity and other model organisms. This result demonstrates that targeted comparative chromosomal studies that include pig genome may provide more information on the genetic control of human obesity.

Transcriptional profiling in pigs

Monitoring gene expression will be useful in elucidating molecular mechanisms in cells or tissues, and cDNA microarray can be a valuable tool for monitoring global gene expression difference in normal and obese individuals and in response to various environmental stimuli. Mathialagan *et al.* (2002)[11] investigated pig gene expression patterns using human microarrays. In pigs with high and low lean growth rates, phenotypic data and serum samples were collected at four different time points from weaning until slaughter, and seven tissues contributing to the regulation of metabolism and growth were collected for transcriptional profiling. Pooled RNA from each tissue from high lean and low lean groups were analysed on human microarrays. These microarrays identified 394 genes that maybe differentially expressed. The genomic location of these differentially expressed genes is being determined and the result will be useful for further identification of the candidate genes for studying the mechanism of growth and fat deposition in pigs as well as humans.

Conclusions

At present, limited genomic information and resources are available in pigs as compared to that of mice for being a model organism for complex genetic traits like obesity. However, several studies have demonstrated that studying the pig genome for genetic control of growth and fat deposition traits is valuable for its economic importance in the pork industry and potential application to human obesity (Ciobanu *et al.*, 2001; Kim *et al.*, 2000; Milan *et al.*, 2000)[6,9,12]. Comparative genome information between humans and pigs is well established; comparative map-based genetic study is possible for identifying responsible genes in the targeted QTL regions between humans and pigs (http: //www.toulouse.inra.fr/lgc/pig/compare/compare.htm).

The most difficult challenge remaining is the development of a dynamic system which can integrate the various research components such as genetic, genomic and physiological experiments for human medicine, and the pig can be a useful model to link these various research components for the development of an information system.

Acknowledgements: The authors are grateful to Jeannine Helm for technical assistance. Financial support provided by Sygen International and the Iowa Agriculture and Home Economics Experiment Station, Ames, IA is appreciated.

References

1. Andersson L, Haley CS, Ellegren H, Knott SA, Johansson M, Andersson K *et al.* Genetic mapping of quantitative trait loci for growth and fatness in pigs. *Science* 1994; 263: 1771–4.

2. Berg F, Archibald A, Anderson S, Andersson L, Moller M. Comparative genome analysis between pig chromosome 4 and human chromosome 1 and 8. Proceedings of the 28th International Conference on Animal Genetics. Gottingen; 2002.

3. Bidanel JP, Rothschild MF. Current status of quantitative trait locu mapping in pigs. *Pig News and Info* 2002; 23: 39–54.

4. Bidanel JP, Milan D, Iannuccelli N, Amigues Y, Boscher M, Bourgeois F *et al.* Detection of quantitative trait loci for growth and fatness in pigs. *Gen Sel Evol* 2001; 33: 289–309.

5. Carey GB. The swine as a model for studying exercise-induced changes in lipid metabolism. *Med Sci Sports Exerc* 1997; 29(11): 1437–43.

6. Ciobanu DC, Bastiaansen J, Malek M, Helm J, Woolard J, Plastow GS *et al.* Evidence for new alleles in the protein kinase AMP-activated, subunit gene associated with low glycogen content in pig skeletal muscle and improved meat quality. *Genetics* 2001; 159: 1151–62.

7. Houpt KA, Houpt TR, Pond WG. The pig as a model for the study of obesity and of control of food intake: a review. *Yale J Biol Med* 1979; 52: 307–29.

8. Kim KS, Larsen N, Short T, Plastow GS, Rothschild MF. A missense variant of the melanocortin 4 recptor gene is associated with fatness, growth and feed intake traits. *Mamm Genome* 2000; 11: 131–5.

9. Kim KS, Thomsen H, Bastiaansen J, Yuandan Z, Dekkers JCM, Plastow GS, Rothschild MF. Investigation of candidate genes for the growth and fatness QTL on pig chromosome 1, 7, and 13 in a Berkshire x Yorkshire family and commercial populations. Proceedings of the 28th International Conference on Animal Genetics, Gottingen; 2002.

10. Malek M, Dekkers JCM, Lee HK, Baas TJ, Rothschild MF. A molecular genome scan analysis to identify chromosomal region influencing economictraits in the pig. I. Growth and body composition. *Mamm Genome* 2001; 12: 630–6.

11. Mathialagan N, Dyer CJ, Leininger MT, Govinderajan K, Byatt JC, Buonomo FC, Spurlock M. Expression profiling of low and high lean pigs from weaning to finish. Proceedings of the Plant, Animal and Microbe Genomes X meeting. San Diego; 2002.

12. Milan D, Jeon TT, Looft C, Amarger V, Robic A, Thelander M *et al.* A mutation in PRKAG3 assoicated with excess glycogen content in pig skeletal muscle. *Science* 2000; 288: 1248–51.

13. Miller ER, Ullrey DE. The pig as a model for human nutrition. *Annu Rev Nutr* 1987; 7: 361.

14. Rankinen T, Perusse L, Weisnagel SJ, Snyder EE, Chagnon YC, Bouchard C. The human obesity gene map: the 2001 update. *Obes Res* 2002; 10: 196–243.

15. Rapacz J, Hasler-Rapacz J. Animal models: The pig. In: *Genetic factors in atherosclerosis: approaches and model systems*, Lusis AJ, Sparkes RS (eds), pp.139–69. 1989.

16. Wang L, Yu TP, Tuggle CK, Liu HG, Rothschild MF. A directed search for quantitative trait loci of chromosomes 4 and 7 in the pig. *J Anim Sci* 1998; 76: 2560–7.

Progress in Obesity Research: 9. Edited by *Geraldo Medeiros-Neto, Alfredo Halpern and Claude Bouchard*
©2003 John Libbey Eurotext Ltd, pp. 272–274.

CHAPTER 57

Muscle enhanced traits in sheep

N.E. Cockett[1], C.A. Bidwell[2], C. Charlier[3], M. Smit[1], K. Sergers[3], T.L. Shay[1], L. Karim[3], G.D. Snowder[4] and M. Georges[3]

[1]*Utah State University, Department of Animal, Dairy and Veterinary Sciences, Logan, UT 84322-4700, USA;*
[2]*Purdue University, Department of Animal Sciences, West Lafayette, IN 47907-1026, USA;* [3]*University of Liege,*
Department of Genetics, Liege, Belgium; [4]*USDA/ARS US Meat Animal Research Center, Clay Center, NE 68933, USA*
[e-mail: fanoelle@cc.usu.edu]

Introduction

Growth in a population of cells is an interaction between extracellular signals and intracellular programmes that increase cell numbers (hyperplasia) or increase cell size (hypertrophy). In skeletal muscle, hyperplasia is due to proliferation of mononucleated muscle progenitor cells called myoblasts. The myoblasts undergo terminal differentiation, exit the cell cycle, and fuse into new multinucleated myotubes or an existing muscle fibre. The multinucleated cell undergoes hypertrophy by the synthesis and accumulation of greater amounts of myofibrillar proteins and addition of new sarcomeres, causing the myofibres to grow in length and diameter.

Results and discussion

The *callipyge* gene is a mutation in sheep responsible for pronounced muscle hypertrophy, primarily in muscles of the pelvic limb (Koohmaraie[1]; Carpenter[2]). Interestingly, the hypertrophy is absent at birth and develops only after approximately three weeks of age; thus, there is no increased risk of dystocia for callipyge lambs and no differences in birth weights between callipyge and normal lambs (Jackson[3]). While no differences are found in weaning weight or postweaning average daily gain, feed efficiency is improved and feed intake is reduced in callipyge lambs (Jackson[3]). There is some negative influence of the gene on wool traits, with a decrease of 12.7 per cent in fleece weight and a decrease of 8.7 per cent in staple length in callipyge ewes, when compared to wool production in normal ewes (Jackson[3]).

Muscles from lambs expressing the callipyge phenotype enlarge to differing degrees, and not all muscles are affected (Koohmaraie[1]; Jackson[4]). The largest effect is found in the semimembranosus, with this muscle being 46 per cent larger in callipyge lamb carcasses than in normal lambs. Enlargement of the muscles is primarily due to myofibre hypertrophy. Carpenter[2] found larger average diameters of the fast twitch, oxidative and glycolytic (FOG) and fast twitch, glycolytic (FG) muscle fibres for callipyge muscles, but smaller average diameter for the callipyge slow twitch, oxidative (SO) fibres. Fibre content was decreased 33.3 per cent and 30.1 per cent for callipyge SO and FOG fibres, respectively, while content of FG fibres increased 35.7 per cent. Diameters of the three fibre types within the suprasinatus of callipyge and normal muscles did not differ. Increased muscle fibre diameter is evident in 5-week old (Lorenzen[5]) but not in 2-week-old lambs (Carpenter and Cockett[6]).

Callipyge animals are more desirable than normal animals for several carcass and meat characteristics (Koohmaraie[1]; Jackson[7]). Dressing percentage and ribeye area are dramatically increased (about 30 per cent) while all measures of fatness are decreased. Unfortunately, there is some concern with decreased tenderness of the loin (Kerth[8]; Koohmaraie[1]). This increased toughness seems to be limited to the callipyge loin and shoulder, with little or no effect on the leg. In consumer panel evaluations (Kerth[8]), 27.9 per cent more normal chops from the loin and 20.0 per cent more normal chops from the shoulder were rated acceptable for tenderness than the corresponding callipyge chops. However, percentage of leg chops that were rated accepted did not differ between callipyge and normal. Several postmortem tenderization methods are effective in improving the tenderness of callipyge lamb meat (Carpenter[9]). The *callipyge* locus has been mapped to the distal end of ovine chromosome 18 (Cockett[10]). Additional characterization of the locus has demonstrated a unique mode of inheritance termed 'polar overdominance' (Cockett[11]; Freking[12]), in which only heterozygous offspring inheriting the mutation from their sire express the phenotype. The three other genotypes are normal in appearance. Progeny data indicate that reactivation of the maternal *callipyge* allele occurs after passage through the male germ line, although this reactivation is not absolute (Cockett[11]).

Experiments directed towards understanding the functional basis of *callipyge* are ongoing. Using bovine YAC and BAC libraries and an ovine BAC library, physical contigs of bovine (Shay[13]) and ovine (Segers[14]) origin that contain the *callipyge* gene have been constructed. The contigs span a 900 kb interval flanked by *IDVGA30* and *OY3* microsatellites. The locus has been more precisely mapped to a 450 kb region, using breakpoint mapping and additional markers isolated from these contigs (Berghmans[15]). A 250 kb segment was subsequently sequenced; six genes were identified by comparison of the ovine sequence in this segment to orthologous human sequence from HSA14q (Charlier[16]). Two of the identified genes, *DLK1* and *GTL2*, have been previously described (Schmidt[17]), while the remaining genes, *DAT*, *PEG11*, *antiPEG11*, and *MEG8*, are novel. All six genes are strongly expressed in skeletal muscle and subject to parental imprinting in this tissue (Charlier[18]).

Northern blot analysis of muscle RNA demonstrates that expression of five of these genes (*DLK1, GTL2, PEG11, antiPEG11* and *MEG8*) are altered in a genotype- and muscle-specific manner (Bidwell[19]; Charlier[18]). These results suggest that the *callipyge* mutation modifies the activity of a common regulatory element, which could be either an enhancer (boosted by the callipyge mutation) or a silencer (inhibited by the callipyge mutation), in an age-dependent and muscle-specific manner. This altered regulatory element is then responsible for the enhanced expression of *DLK1*, *GTL2*, *PEG11*, *antiPEG11* and *MEG8*, and possibly other untested genes as well. It is likely that increased expression of one or more of these genes initiates the manifestation of the callipyge phenotype.

In another study (Smith[20]), 180 kb of the *callipyge* region was sequenced for phylogenetically related wild type and *CLPG* alleles. Over 300 polymorphisms were identified within the 180-kb sequence, but only one mutation was unique in animals possessing the *CLPG* allele. Genotypes of this marker displayed 100 per cent concordance in animals of known callipyge genotype. Additional experiments are ongoing to determine if this SNP is the causative *callipyge* mutation.

Characterization of another gene responsible for an increase in the rib eye muscle of lambs has been reported (Banks[21]). Effects of the *REM* locus are less dramatic than for *callipyge*, with an 11 per cent increase in muscle mass limited to the *longissimus*. The *REM* locus appears to act as a dominant gene and has only minor effects on meat tenderness (McEwan[22]). Using microsatellite markers from ovine chromosome 18, *REM* has been localized just distal to the *callipyge* position (McEwan[23]; Nicoll[24]; McEwan personal communication), suggesting that mutations in closely linked genes are responsible for the two hypertrophy phenotypes.

Conclusion

The control of myogenesis involves carefully orchestrated expression of specific genes. Reprogramming of this process by naturally occurring genetic mutations are responsible for muscle enhanced traits in farm animals, such as callipyge and rib eye muscling. Study of muscle hyperplasia and hypertrophy in livestock species will advance basic understanding of muscle formation.

References

1. Koohmaraie M, Shackelford SD, Wheeler TL, Lonergan SM, Doumit ME. A muscle hypertrophy condition in lamb (callipyge): characterization of effects on muscle growth and meat quality traits. *J Anim Sci* 1995; 73: 3596–607.

2. Carpenter CE, Rice OD, Cockett NE, Snowder GD. Histology and composition of muscles from normal and callipyge lambs. *J Anim Sci* 1996; 74: 388–93.

3. Jackson SP, Green RD, Miller MF. Phenotypic characterization of Rambouillet sheep expressing the callipyge gene: I. Inheritance of the condition and production characteristics. *J Anim Sci* 1997; 75: 14–21.

4. Jackson SP, Miller MF, Green RD. Phenotypic characterization of Rambouillet sheep expressing the callipyge gene: III. Muscle weights and muscle weight distribution. *J Anim Sci* 1997; 75: 133–9.

5. Lorenzen CL, Koohmaraie M, Shackelford SD, Jahoor F, Freetly HC, Wheeler TL *et al.* Protein kinetics in callipyge lambs. *J Anim Sci* 2000; 78: 78–87.

6. Carpenter CE, Cockett NE. Histology of longissimus muscle from 2-week-old and 8-week-old normal and callipyge lambs. Can *J Anim Sci* 2000; 80: 511–4.

7. Jackson SP, Miller MF, Green RD. Phenotypic characterization of Rambouillet sheep expressing the callipyge gene: II. Carcass characteristics and retail yield. *J Anim Sci* 1997; 75: 125–32.

8. Kerth CR, Jackson SP, Miller MF, Ramsey CB. Physiological and sensory characteristics of callipyge sheep. Texas Tech U Res Rep, Tech Rep No T-5-356, Lubbock: Texas Tech University, 1995, pp. 31–3.

9. Carpenter CE, Solomon MB, Snowder GD, Cockett NE, Busboom JR. Effects of electrical stimulation and conditioning, calcium chloride injection and aging on the acceptability of callipyge and normal lamb. *Sheep Goat Res J* 1997; 13: 127–34.

10. Cockett NE, Jackson SP, Shay TL, Nielsen D, Moore SS, Steele MR, *et al.* Chromosomal localization of the callipyge gene in sheep. *Proc Natl Acad Sci USA* 1994; 91: 3019–23.

11. Cockett NE, Jackson SP, Shay TL, Farnir F, Berghmans S, Snowder GD *et al.* Polar overdominance at the ovine callipyge locus. *Science* 1996; 273: 236–8.

12. Freking BA, Keele JW, Beattie CW, Kappes SM, Smith TPL, Sonstegard TS *et al.* Evaluation of the ovine callipyge locus: I. Relative chromosomal position and gene action. *J Anim Sci* 1998; 76: 2062–71.

13. Shay TL, Berghmans S, Segers K, Meyers S, Beever JE *et al.* Fine-mapping and construction of a bovine contig spanning the ovine callipyge locus. *Mamm Genome* 2001; 12: 141–9.

14. Segers K, Vaiman D, Berghmans S, Shay T, Beever J, Cockett N *et al.* Construction and characterization of an ovine BAC contig spanning the callipyge locus. *Anim Genet* 2000; 31: 352–9.

15. Berghmans S, Segers K, Shay T, Georges M, Cockett N, Charlier C. Breakpoint mapping positions the callipyge gene within a 450 kilobase chromosome segment containing the DLK and GTL2 genes. *Mamm Genome* 2001; 12: 183–5.

16. Charlier C, Segers K, Wagenaar D, Karim L, Berghmans S, Jaillon O *et al.* Human-ovine comparative sequencing of a 250kilobase imprinted domain encompassing the clpg gene and identification of novel imprinted transcripts: DLK1, GTL2, DAT, PERL, anitPERL and MEGC. *Genome Res* 2001; 11: 850–62.

17. Schmidt J, Matteson PG, Jones BK, Guan X-J, Tilghman SM. The Dlk1 and Gtl2 genes are linked and reciprocally imprinted. *Genes and Develop* 2000; 14: 1997–2002.

18. Charlier C, Segers K, Karim L, Shay T, Gyapay G, Cockett N, Georges M. The callipyge (CLPG) mutation enhances the expression of the co-regulated genes in cis without affecting their imprinting status. *Nature Genet* 2001; 27: 1–3.

19. Bidwell CA, Shay TL, Georges M, Beever JE, Berghmans S, Segers K *et al.* Differential expression of the GTL2 gene within the callipyge region of ovine chromosome 18. *Anim Genet* 2001; 32: 248–56.

20. Smith TP, Freking BA, Leymaster KA. Identification of an SNP associated with callipyge in sheep. Plant, Animal and Microbe Genomes X. San Diego; 2002. p. 224.

21. Banks R. The meat elite project: establishment and achievements of an elite meat sheep nucleus. *Proc Assoc Advance Anim Breed Genet* 1997; 12: 598–601.

22. McEwan JC, Broad TE, Jopson NB, Robertson TM, Glass BC, Burkin HB *et al.* Rib-eye muscling (REM) locus in sheep: Phenotypic effects and comparative genome localization., Minneapolis: Proceedings of the XXVIth International Conference on Animal Genetics; 2000, p. 25.

23. McEwan JC, Gerard EM, Jopson NB, Nicoll GB, Greer GJ, Dodds KG *et al.* Localization of a QTL for rib-eye muscling on OOV18. Auckland: Proceedings of the XXVIth International Conference on Animal Genetics; 1998, p. 101.

24. Nicoll GB, Burkin HR, Broad TE, Jopson NB, Greer GJ, Bain WE *et al.* Genetic linkage of microsatellite markers to the Carwell locus for rib-eye muscling in sheep. Proceedings of the VIth World Conference on Genetics Applied to Livestock Production, 1998; 26: 529.

Progress in Obesity Research: 9. Edited by *Geraldo Medeiros-Neto, Alfredo Halpern and Claude Bouchard*
©2003 John Libbey Eurotext Ltd, pp. 275–278.

CHAPTER 58

Genetic studies in *Psammomys obesus*

Ken Walder[a], David Segal[a], Jeremy Jowett[b], John Blangero[c], Paul Zimmet[b] and Greg Collier[ad]

[a]*Metabolic Research Unit, School of Health Sciences, Deakin University, Geelong, Australia;* [b]*International Diabetes Institute, Caulfield, Australia;* [c]*Autogen Center for Statistical Genomics, San Antonio, TX, USA;* [d]*Autogen Limited, Geelong, Australia*
[e-mail: barbedwa@deakin.edu.au]

Introduction

As the global epidemic of obesity and type 2 diabetes continues to escalate, the need for effective new treatment strategies increases. Despite great technological advances and huge investment of time and money to generate large amounts of genetic data, the rate of identification of genes contributing to the development of obesity and type 2 diabetes has been poor. This is partly due to the complexity of these disorders (exemplified by extensive genetic and allelic heterogeneity, and multiple gene-gene and gene-environment interactions) and inconsistencies in study design, subject ascertainment and data analysis methodologies across different populations that have hampered the identification of genomic regions replicably linked/associated with disease phenotypes. While genomic studies show great promise for the identification of disease-causing genes in obesity and type 2 diabetes, the difficulties encountered in fine mapping of causal variants have been great. The use of dense SNP maps across linked genomic regions to identify causal variants is perturbed by local variations in linkage disequilibrium, and the precise determination of what constitutes a causal variant can be very difficult.

Supplementing genomic data with appropriate gene expression profiles should greatly hasten the search for genes contributing to the development of obesity and type 2 diabetes. The advent of microarray technology has facilitated large scale comparisons of gene expression in diseased and healthy tissues. Genomic mapping of genes differentially expressed in key metabolic tissues (e.g. hypothalamus, muscle, liver, pancreas, adipose tissue) in obese and lean (or nGT and type 2 diabetic) subjects should provide new insights into genes involved in these disorders. However, there are limitations when conducting such studies in humans, for example the inability to obtain tissues (e.g. hypothalamus) collected under suitable conditions. Therefore appropriate animal models are required that accurately reflect the metabolic characteristics seen in obese/type 2 diabetic human subjects.

Psammomys obesus (the Israeli sand rat) is a unique, polygenic animal model of obesity and type 2 diabetes. In their natural desert habitat these animals remain lean and healthy on a low-energy diet of saltbush (*Atriplex halimus*)[1]. However, when housed in a laboratory setting and given *ad libitum* access to standard rodent laboratory chow, a proportion of the animals spontaneously develop a range of metabolic abnormalities including insulin resistance, obesity, type 2 diabetes and dyslipidaemia[1-8]. The distributions of body weight, glucose and insulin concentrations are continuous across the population of *P. obesus*, and closely approximate the distributions observed in human cross-sectional data (Fig. 1)[9,10].

We contend that targeted gene expression profiling studies in an appropriate animal model such as *P. obesus* and comparative genomic mapping of differentially expressed genes will facilitate the identification of genes contributing to the development of obesity and type 2 diabetes, highlighting new targets for the development of effective treatment strategies.

We extracted RNA and produced cDNA libraries derived from *P. obesus* hypothalamus, skeletal muscle and liver. Clones from each library were randomly picked, amplified by PCR, and the products purified and arrayed on chemically treated, optically flat microscope slides. The microarray specific for each *P.*

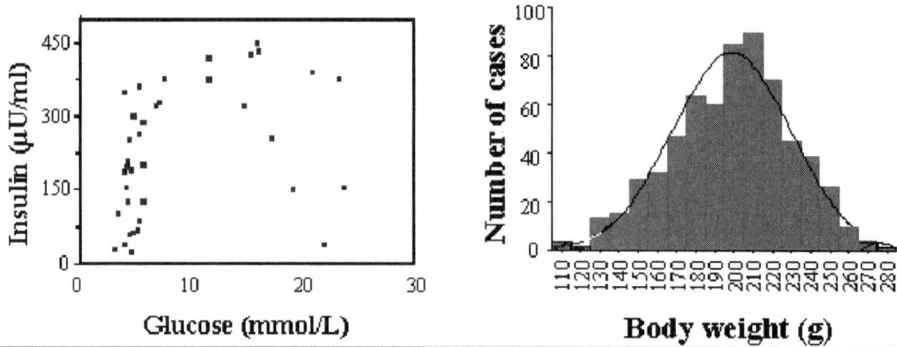

Fig. 1. Cross-sectional distributions of body weight, blood glucose and plasma insulin in 16-week-old *P. obesus*.

obesus tissue consists of ~12,000 elements plus several hundred control spots. We then conducted a range of experiments in lean, normal glucose tolerant and obese, type 2 diabetic *P. obesus*, including fasting (24 h), long term dietary energy restriction, exercise training etc. At defined stages during these experiments, tissues were collected and RNA extracted for microarray analysis. All RNA samples were indirectly labeled and competitively hybridized to *P. obesus* microarrays against standardized reference RNA samples specific for each tissue. After hybridization, microarrays were washed then scanned by laser fluorescence confocal microscopy and images extracted and analysed using commercial software programmes.

After conducting a number of such experiments in *P. obesus*, we have amassed an extensive warehouse of data containing more than 10 million datapoints for gene expression along with a range of phenotypic data such as body weight, percentage body fat, and circulating glucose and insulin concentrations. Mining this data has led to the identification of hundreds of genes with expression profiles implicating their involvement in obesity and/or type 2 diabetes. To limit the number of genes under investigation and focus further investigations on those genes most likely to contribute to the development of obesity and type 2 diabetes, we have undertaken extensive comparative genomic mapping of differentially expressed transcripts. Human homologues of genes differentially expressed in *P. obesus* were identified, and their genomic locations cross-referenced using our in-house database of chromosomal regions with evidence for linkage and/or association with obesity and diabetes phenotypes. An example of a genomic map showing the locations of a subset of genes differentially expressed in *P. obesus* is shown in Fig. 2. The genes were then ranked according to both their expression profiles and the strength of evidence for linkage with obesity/type 2 diabetes, and selected on the basis of this ranking for additional studies to confirm them as genuine targets for these diseases.

An example of the success of this approach is our recent discovery of beacon, a new candidate gene for obesity[11]. Beacon was first identified as a transcript with increased expression in the hypothalamus of obese, diabetic *P. obesus*. Sequencing revealed a 413bp mRNA with an open reading frame of 219bp encoding a novel 73 amino acid protein (predicted size 37.6 kDa). Taqman PCR was used to confirm elevated hypothalamic expression of beacon in obese *P. obesus*, and identified linear relationships between beacon gene expression and body weight and percentage body fat[11].

The human homologue of *P. obesus* beacon was identified on chromosome 19p13. Studies had previously shown linkage between this region of the genome and obesity-related phenotypes. A recent genome-wide linkage scan in 522 subjects from 99 families found evidence of linkage between this region and plasma leptin concentration, a proxy measure of body fat content ($P = 0.0009$)[12]. This suggests that variation at a gene in the region where beacon is located has a significant effect on body fat mass and circulating leptin levels. Furthermore, several animal obesity QTLs have been identified in mouse and rat genomes in regions syntenic with human chromosome 19p13 including Afpq6[13], Qlw9/Adip5[14] and Dmo5[15]. Collectively, there is a considerable body of evidence that a gene (or genes) located on chromosome 19p13 is involved in the regulation of energy balance and body fat mass. The combination of interesting initial expression data for beacon, along with its genomic location in a chromosomal region noted for linkage/association with obesity phenotypes, suggested that beacon was a candidate worthy of further investigation.

Beacon was found to be predominantly expressed in the retrochiasmatic nucleus of the hypothalamus, a region known to be involved in the regulation of food intake[11]. Hypothalamic beacon gene expression

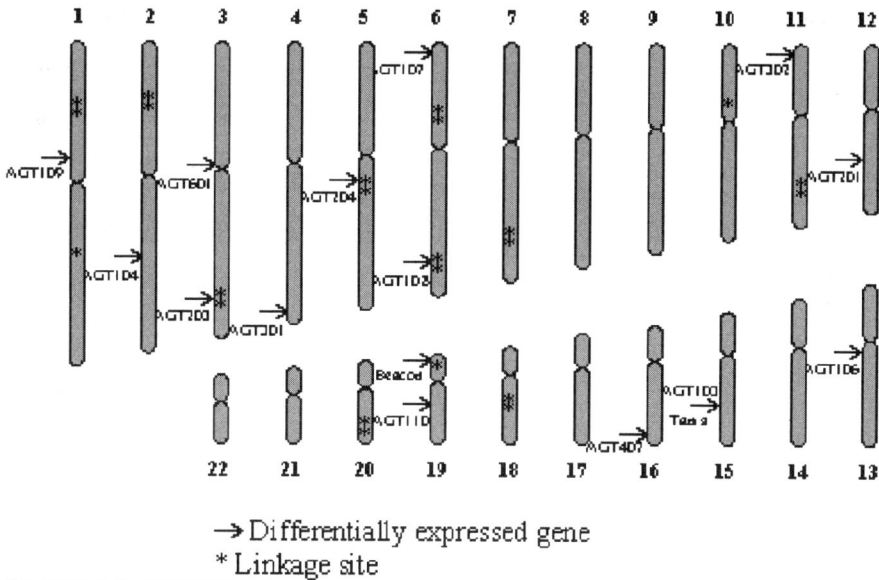

→ Differentially expressed gene
* Linkage site

Fig. 2. Genomic mapping of differentially expressed genes. Chromosomal regions showing evidence of linkage to obesity/type 2 diabetes are indicated by asterisks, while arrows denote the locations of human homologues of genes differentially expressed in *P. obesus*.

was elevated in *P. obesus* with a genetic predisposition for the development of obesity and diabetes before any increase in body weight, suggesting that overexpression of beacon may contribute to the development of obesity in these animals[16]. ICV administration of beacon to lean *P. obesus* significantly increased food intake and body weight gain, as well as increasing the hypothalamic gene expression of NPY, a known orexigenic neuropeptide[11]. Further studies demonstrated that the effects of beacon on body weight were due to accumulation of body fat, and no effects on energy expenditure or substrate partitioning were detected, suggesting that beacon acts to increase body fat accumulation through its effects on appetite[17].

Resequencing of the entire human beacon gene in 40 individuals identified four single nucleotide polymorphisms (SNPs): one in the 3'-untranslated region, exon 1 (non-coding), and introns 2 and 4. Minor allele frequencies ranged from 3–23 per cent These SNPs are currently being genotyped in a sample of 800 individuals and analysed for association with obesity-related phenotypes.

A number of studies are currently underway to determine the mechanism of action of beacon, including the generation of beacon-knockout mice, microarray analysis of cells treated with beacon, and investigation of proteins interacting with beacon through the use of yeast 2-hybrid screening and surface plasmon resonance analysis.

Collectively these data suggest that beacon is an exciting new obesity candidate gene, and further elucidation of the actions of beacon in the hypothalamus could lead to the development of more effective treatment strategies for obesity. Although the initial expression data for differential expression of beacon in the hypothalamus of *P. obesus* were not as extreme as some other transcripts, the combination of the expression data and the genomic location of beacon in a region known to be linked/associated with obesity phenotypes highlighted beacon as a potential new obesity candidate.

We have shown that an integrated approach using both expression profiling and genomic localization can lead to rapid identification of candidate genes for complex diseases such as obesity and type 2 diabetes. As technology continues to improve, we anticipate that the incorporation of proteomics data into such a model will further increase the power to discover genes. By combining data from the transcriptome and the genome, we have identified beacon as a promising new candidate gene for obesity.

References

1. Shafrir E, Gutman A. Psammomys obesus of the Jerusalem colony: A model for nutritionally induced, non-insulin-dependent diabetes. *J Basic Clin Physiol Pharm* 1993; 4: 83–99.

2. Barnett M, Collier GR, Collier FM *et al.* A cross-sectional and short-term longitudinal characterization of NIDDM in Psammomys obesus. *Diabetologia* 1994; 37: 671–6.

3. Collier GR, Walder K, Lewandowski P *et al.* Leptin and the development of obesity and diabetes in Psammomys obesus. *Obes Res* 1997; 5: (5)455–8.

4. Collier GR, de Silva A, Sanigorski A *et al.* Development of obesity and insulin resistance in the Israeli sand rat (Psammomys obesus). Does leptin play a role? *Ann NY Acad Sci* 1997; 20: 827: 50–63.

5. Walder K, Willet M, Zimmet P *et al.* Ob (obese) gene expression and leptin levels in Psammomys obesus. *Biochim Biophys Acta* 1997; 1354: 272–8.

6. Walder K, Lewandowski P, Morton G *et al.* Leptin resistance in a polygenic, hyperleptinemic animal model of obesity and NIDDM Psammomys obesus. *Int J Obes* 1999; 2: 83–9.

7. Walder KR, Fahey RP, Morton GJ *et al.* Characterization of obesity phenotypes in Psammomys obesus (Israeli sand rats). *Int J Exp Diab Res* 2000; 1: 177–84.

8. Kalderon B, Gutman A, Levy E. Characterization of stages in the development of obesity-diabetes syndrome in sand rat (Psammomys obesus). *Diabetes* 1996; 6: 717–24.

9. Zimmet P, Whitehouse S, Kiss J. Ethnic variability in the plasma insulin response to oral glucose in Polynesian and Micronesian subjects. *Diabetes* 1979; 28: 624–8.

10. DeFronzo RA. The triumvirate B-cell, muscle and liver: A collusion responsible for NIDDM. *Diabetes* 1988; 37: 667–88.

11. Collier GR, McMillan JS, Windmill K *et al.* Beacon: A novel gene involved in the regulation of energy balance. *Diabetes* 2000; 49: 1766–71.

12. Chagnon YC, Rice T, Perusse L *et al.* Genomic scan for genes affecting body composition before and after training in Caucasians from HERITAGE. *J Appl Physiol* 2000; 90: 1777–87.

13. Brockmann GA, Kratzsch J, Haley CS *et al.* Single QTL effects, epistasis, and pleiotropy account for two-thirds of the phenotypic F(2) variance in growth and obesity in DU6i x DBA/2 mice. *Genome Res* 2000; 10: 1941–57.

14. Cheverud JM, Vaughn TT, Pletscher LS *et al.* Genetic architecture of adiposity in the cross of LG/J and SM/J inbred mice. *Mamm Genome* 2001; 12: 3–12.

15. Watanabe T, Okuno S, Oga K *et al.* Genetic dissection of OLETF, a rat model for non-insulin-dependent diabetes mellitus: Quantitative trait locus analysis of (OLETF x BN) x OLETF. *Genomics* 1999; 58: 233–9.

16. Walder K, Ziv E, Kalman R *et al.* Elevated hypothalamic beacon gene expression in Psammomys obesus prone to develop obesity and type 2 diabetes. *Int J Obes* 2002; 26: 605–9.

17. Walder K, McMillan JS, Lee S *et al.* Effects of beacon administration on energy expenditure and substrate utilization in Psammomys obesus (Israeli sand rats). *Int J Obes* 2001; 25: 1281–5.

Progress in Obesity Research: 9. Edited by *Geraldo Medeiros-Neto, Alfredo Halpern and Claude Bouchard*
©2003 John Libbey Eurotext Ltd, pp. 279–284.

CHAPTER 59

A QTL regulating fasting insulin and adiposity on mouse chromosome 2

Aamir R. Zuberi

Pennington Biomedical Research Center, 6400 Perkins Road, Baton Rouge, LA 70810, USA
[e-mail: zuberia@pbrc.edu]

Introduction

Mouse chromosome 2 contains polymorphic genes regulating multiple metabolic phenotypes. To identify the genes regulating insulin homeostasis and adiposity on this chromosome, we are extending a research direction suggested by the data of Lembertas *et al.*[1] and of two publications from the Accili laboratory[2,3], and derived a new congenic mouse model in which to test the hypothesis that a polymorphic gene within the congenic segment regulates both circulating insulin concentrations and adiposity. The congenic B6.LPa mouse derives 99.98 per cent of its genome from the dietary obesity susceptible C57BL/6J (B6) genetic background strain except for a small 4.2–6.5 cM region of chromosome 2 derived from the dietary obesity resistant LP/J (LP) mouse. Male B6.LPa congenic mouse fed a low fat chow diet possess a 58 per cent lower fasting insulin concentration than age-matched B6 mice despite there being no significant differences in serum glucose levels. These mice also possess less adipose tissue and are leaner than B6 mice. Feeding mice a diet high in fat and sucrose can significantly increase the difference in adiposity between the strains. Although the fasting insulin concentrations of both B6.LPa and B6 mice become elevated in response to this diet, the insulin levels of B6.LPa mice remain significantly lower. The 10 Mb congenic interval contains many potential candidate genes but we are particularly intrigued by polymorphism in one novel gene, *Zfp106* with a potential role in insulin action and adiposity. This gene is expressed in insulin-responsive cells (except liver), is up-regulated in mice containing a targeted null allele of the insulin receptor (*insr*) gene, and appears to participate in the regulation of adipogenesis of 3T3-L1 cells. *Zfp106* also underlies a QTL regulating hyperinsulinemia in mice heterozygous for the targeted *insr* null mutation[3]. These data implicate *Zfp106* as a candidate for the QTL regulating circulating insulin concentrations regulatory phenotype and possibly for the adiposity QTL.

Background

Genetic linkage studies provide an effective tool to reveal the genetic components underlying susceptibility to obesity, diabetes, hyperinsulinaemia and other metabolic disorders. Although many studies have identified regions of the genome containing polymorphic genes regulating these metabolic phenotypes, until recently there has been limited progress in identifying the underlying genes. The availability of human and mouse genomic sequence identifying almost all of the genes in the genome in the Ensembl (www.ensembl.org) and Celera discovery system databases (www.celera.com), and the development of single nucleotide polymorphism (SNP) databases some of which identify genetic variation within genes (Celera SNP reference database), are valuable resources that will accelerate the identification of important genes encoding quantitative trait loci (QTL). Recently identified genes include *Cd36* as the gene underlying an insulin resistance QTL in the spontaneously hypertensive rat[4], and two mouse QTLs; *Pla2g2a* as the gene underlying *Mom1*[5], and *Mtap1* as the gene underlying *Moth1*, a modifier of hearing loss in the tubby mutant mouse[6]. Other QTL genes identified include the human CAPN10 diabetes susceptibility gene[7], a gene regulating milk yield in diary cattle[8], and a gene regulating flowering time in *Arabidopsis*[9].

Clearly, there is a multigenic component to the development of type 2 diabetes, hyperinsulinaemia and adiposity. QTL affecting adiposity, body weight, fed and fasting insulin and glucose are positioned throughout the mouse genome and have been recently reviewed[10]. With the possible exception of the *pfatp* ATPase, suggested as a candidate gene for a chromosome 7 adiposity QTL[11,12], the identities of the underlying genes remain uncertain; in part because of the challenging series of genetics and molecular approaches needed to confirm and fine-map the QTL. Typically, the QTL, initially identified from F2 or similar genetic crosses is confirmed by introgressing the trait-altering QTL region onto the genetic background of one of the parental strains to generate a congenic mouse, thereby, eliminating genetic variation between the congenic and background strain for all regions except the QTL of interest. A potential complication is that congenic strains containing large donor derived segments may contain more than one underlying gene influencing the same trait[13,14]. Once a QTL trait is assigned to a smaller genetic interval then additional higher resolution genetic mapping strategies, cDNA expression profiling and polymorphism screening coupled with candidate gene approaches represent effective strategies to identify the underlying gene.

Chromosome 2 and the genetic regulation of insulin concentration and adiposity

The insulin receptor deficient mouse

Pivotal studies by the Accili laboratory have determined that multiple genes, polymorphic between the B6 and 129 mouse strains, regulate the degree of hyperinsulinaemia in recombinant mice heterozygous for the targeted null allele of the insulin receptor (*insr*) gene[3]. One region of the genome exerting a major QTL effect maps to mouse chromosome 2. The complex biphasic distribution of the lod profile along this chromosome suggests the likelihood of at least two loci that modify the insulin phenotype, one mapping close to 25 cM and a second exerting a smaller effect mapping near 65 cM. The 1 lod interval for this second locus contains the murine *Zfp106* gene. In earlier studies, the Accili laboratory has shown that expression of this gene, initially designated *Sirm* (also known as *Sh3bp3* and *H3a*), is elevated in mice heterozygous or homozygous for the targeted *insr* gene[2]. Expression of *Sirm/Sh3bp3/H3a/Zfp106* is negatively regulated by insulin in wild-type *insr*+ cells. We previously speculated[15] and have since confirmed that *Sh3bp3* is an aberrantly spliced *Zfp106* transcript containing only exons 5 and 6 of the full-length gene. Importantly, two proline-rich regions in the exon 6-encoded domain of ZFP-106 associate with the SH3-domain containing protein, Grb-2 and the Src family tyrosine kinase, Fyn in an insulin dependent manner. The recruitment of Fyn and Grb-2 to ZFP-106 occurs in the absence of insulin[2]. ZFP-106 is also phosphorylated by the kinase activity of Fyn. Interestingly, Fyn is implicated in the adipocyte specific functions of insulin action[16,17]. As these interactions are destabilized by insulin, and *Zfp106* expression is downregulated by insulin, this suggests that ZFP-106 might function as a negative regulator of insulin action possibly affecting glucose uptake, one of the critical endpoints of insulin signaling.

We have determined the complete nucleotide sequence and intron-exon structure of *Zfp106*[15]; unpublished data). Furthermore, our studies reveal that the 90-kDa immunoreactive polypeptide observed by the Accili laboratory is the result of processing by a furin-like endoprotease of the predicted 200-kDa ZFP-106 precursor polypeptide at position 1030 of the full-length protein. The full-length 1888 amino acid protein contains three C2H2-type zinc finger domains and an extensive WD-40 repeat domain at the C-terminus, not present in the smaller 90 kDa SIRM subunit[15]. Although the highest RNA abundance of *Zfp106* is seen in skeletal and cardiac muscle, expression is also seen in other metabolically important and insulin-responsive tissues including the pancreas, adipocytes, and hypothalamus. Under normal conditions little or no expression is seen in liver, except in mice carrying at least one copy of the null *insr* allele[2]. *Zfp106* was initially cloned as a polymorphic gene encoding the important immunodominant H3a minor histocompatibility antigen that could facilitate tissue transplantation rejection[15]. Comparative sequencing of *Zfp106* reveals that the gene is highly polymorphic between B6 and the two closely related 129 and LP/J mouse strains. A total of 26 amino acid differences are observed between B6 and 129 (LP) that includes several non-conservative amino acid substitutions. A notable difference is that the 129 and LP-derived ZFP106 protein is three amino acids shorter than the B6 protein, as a consequence of a single 9-nucleotide deletion within one coding exon. The lack of polymorphism in ZFP-106 between 129 and LP is a consequence of the close genealogical relationship between these two strains 18, having derived from a common progenitor as recently as 1928.

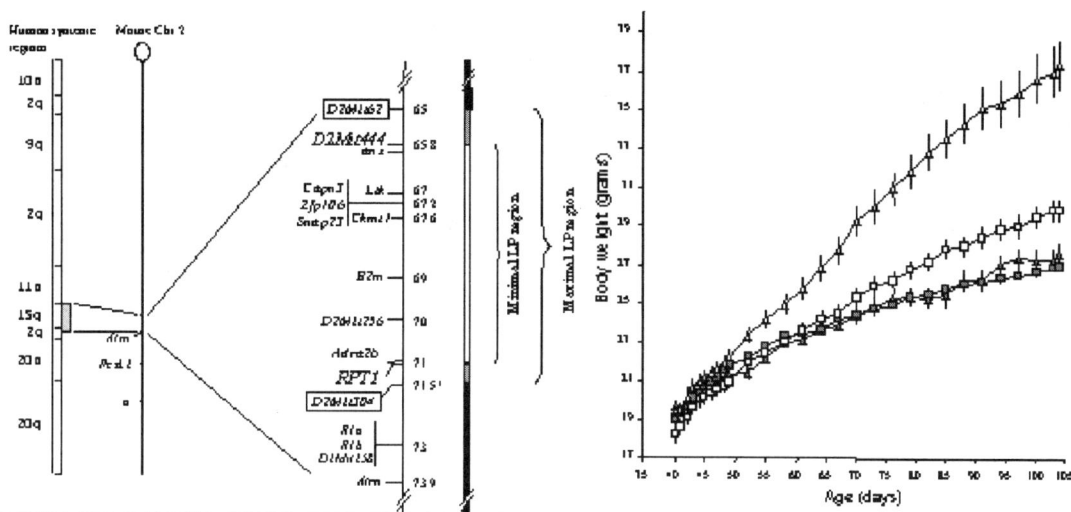

Fig. 1. Panel A (left). Extent of chromosome 2 LP-derived congenic DNA in the B6.LPa mouse. Syntenic relationships between relevant human chromosomes and mouse chromosome 2 are shown on the left, including the locations of the known obesity genes Atrn, Pcsk2 and agouti (a). The expanded region between D2Mit62 and Atrn provides a higher resolution of the minimal (white bar) and maximal extents of the LP-derived congenic segment. Black bars indicate B6 genomic DNA. The lightly shaded bars identify regions of uncertainty. Panel B (right). Body weight gain profiles of B6 (△) and B6.LPa (□) congenic mice fed either a HF diet (open symbols) or chow diet (closed symbols). Data are shown mean ± SE. Numbers of mice in each group are as follows: HF diet, B6 (n = 9), B6.LPa (n = 16); Chow diet, B6 (n = 9), B6.LPa (n = 12).

An adiposity QTL is positioned on mouse chromosome 2 in the vicinity of *Zfp106*

As part of an interesting study attempting to correlate human obesity QTL segregating in individuals of the Quebec Family Study and murine obesity QTLs mapping to the syntenic chromosomal regions, Lembertas *et al.* in 1997 determined that the B10.LP-*H3bH13b* mouse strain containing a large 33-cM LP/J derived chromosome 2 congenic interval on the C57BL/10 (B10) genetic background confers a reduction in body weight, adiposity and fasting insulin concentrations[1]. The differences in body weight and adiposity were significant despite the limited numbers of mice characterized. Despite the considerable benefits of having a congenic mouse strain manifesting a robust adiposity phenotype, a greater characterization of this mouse and fine-mapping of the underlying genes has not been reported, until now.

As part of a genetic strategy to identify polymorphic genes regulating adiposity and insulin homeostasis, we have extended the B10.LP-*H3bH13b* model and developed a novel subcongenic mouse line that carries a small 5.2–6.5 cM LP-donor region on the B6 genetic background. Characterization of this B6.LPa subcongenic strain (the donor LP segment was introgressed onto the more metabolically-defined B6 strain during strain construction) containing donor genomic DNA derived from the proximal end of the original 33-cM congenic interval confirms that a 10 Mb region of the genome is sufficient to confer reduced adiposity relative to the background strain and a resistance to dietary induced obesity in response to a high fat diet (Fig. 1). Interestingly, this subcongenic B6.LPa mouse strain also demonstrates a significant reduction in circulating fasting insulin concentrations on both chow and high fat diets relative to B6 mice. The polymorphic *Zfp106* gene maps within the congenic segment of the B6.LPa mouse, and continues to cosegregate with the phenotypes of interest, thereby remaining a viable candidate gene.

As *Zfp106* is also expressed in adipocytes, we characterized its role during adipogenesis of 3T3-L1 cells in more detail. Salvatore *et al.* reported that *Zfp106* RNA expression was observed in differentiated 3T3-L1 adipocytes but not in 3T3-L1 preadipocytes[2]. Our expression analysis reveals that *Zfp106* RNA abundance does not change during adipogenesis. Expression is seen in preadipocytes, mature adipocytes and daily at all intermediate stages. RNA abundance is, however, typically higher than observed *in vivo* in epididymal-derived adipocytes. During experiments attempting to perturb *Zfp106* expression in these cells, we have determined that over-expression of the full-length *Zfp106* cDNA in 3T3-L1

281

Table 1. Genetic studies identifying QTLs on mouse mid-chromosome 2

Parental strains	QTL	Phenotype	Ref.
AKR/J and C57L/J*	Obq3	Adiposity	21
NZO/H1J and SM/J*	Obq10	Adiposity	22
NZB/B1NJ and SM/J* B10.LP-*H3bH13b* (*D2Mit63-D2Mit227*)*	Mob5	Female body weight and adiposity Female adiposity and fasting insulin	1
C57BL/6 and CAST/Ei*	Mob6	Subcutaneous fat and minor body weight	19
Fat and Lean lines	Fob1	Adiposity	20
M16i and CAST/Ei	Pfat1	Adiposity and body weight	34
C57BL/6-*insr*[tm1Dac] and 129/Sv–*insr*[tm1Dac]*		Hyperinsulinaemia	3
DU6I and DBA/2		Serum IGF-1 levels (low lod score)	35
C3H/He and C57BL/6*		Intra peritoneal glucose tolerance test	36
SM/J and LG/J	Bgeq2	Early body weight	37
NOD.NOR (*D2Mit490-Pcna*)*	Idd13	Insulin dependent diabetes mellitus	28
BL and MH	Hlq2	Heat loss	38

Asterisk (*) indicates that the *Zfp106* allele in the B6.LPa congenic region is in linkage disequilibrium with the reported QTL. Two SNPs mapping to coding exons 6 and 12 were used to genotype *Zfp106* in the parental mouse strains. The fat and lean lines, M16i, DU6I, BL and MH strains were not genotyped.

preadipocytes inhibits adipogenesis. The mechanism whereby this phenotype is achieved is currently being investigated.

Thus, based on the reduction in circulating insulin concentrations (and possibly increased insulin sensitivity) and the altered adipocyte proliferative potential seen in the B6.LPa model, it is possible that both phenotypes could be attributable to polymorphism in the same gene. *Zfp106* remains a viable candidate for both phenotypes.

Several QTL overlap with a single region on mouse mid-chromosome 2 that includes the *Zfp106* gene. In addition to the chromosome 2 insulin regulating QTL reported by Kido *et al.*[3] and the adiposity QTL mapped to this region of the chromosome by Lembertas *et al.*[1], other recent reports suggest that this region of chromosome 2 may contain other QTL for adiposity, body weight, insulin, glucose tolerance, diabetes, IGF-1 and heat (Table 1). The 1 lod support interval for these related QTLs span the genetic position of *Zfp106* and in each case, with only a single exception between the SM/J and LG/J strains, we find that allelic variation in *Zfp106* is in linkage disequilibrium with the observed QTL.

As in Kido *et al.*[3], the biphasic distribution of lod scores along chromosome 2 in some crosses listed in Table 1 suggest the possibility of multiple genes underlying the QTL[19–22]. For example, the major QTL peaks of *Obq3* and *Obq10* map to proximal chromosome 2 but, in each case, the position of a smaller secondary lod peak is coincident with the *Zfp106* region[21,22].

Linkage and association studies in humans reveal polymorphic gene(s) regulating diabetes and energy expenditure map to regions syntenic with the mouse *Zfp106* gene.

The congenic region in B6.LPa mice on mouse chromosome 2 shares synteny with human chromosomes 15q15-q21 and 2p13-q13. Genetic variation in the calpain CAPN10 gene on human chromosome 2q37.3 underlies the NIDDM1 diabetes susceptibility locus[7,23] and NIDDM1 interacts synergistically with an unidentified gene positioned on human chromosome 15, close to the region syntenic with the murine B6.LPa congenic segment[24]. One other study[25] also reports a diabetes susceptibility locus mapping to chromosome 15q13-q21.

Lower levels of calpain CAPN3 gene expression have been correlated with increased adiposity, reduced carbohydrate oxidation and elevated circulating glucose and insulin concentrations[26]. Although similar to the effects of variation in CAPN10 on glucose regulation in Pima Indians[23], this observation is not supported by the phenotype of calpain 3-deficient mice[27]. Capn3 is positioned within the B6.LPa congenic region adjacent to the Zfp106 gene, and maps to the syntenic region on human chromosome 15q15-q21. Although differences in phenotype as a consequence of amino acid variation in proteins verses absence of the protein in targeted mice are possible – as has been demonstrated B2m and susceptibility to type 1 diabetes[28–30]; a role for CAPN3 in the regulation of adiposity and insulin must be viewed cautiously. Genetic variation in genes cosegregating with CAPN3 may also be consistent with the observations.

Other candidate genes within the B6.LPa congenic interval

The congenic region in B6.LPa mice maximally spans 6.5 cM from *D2Mit62* to *D2Mit304*. The latest Ensembl release (version 5.3a.1) of the B6 mouse genome sequence, places these flanking markers as 10 Mb apart on the physical map. One hundred and fifty genes are annotated within this interval, 56 of them being novel. Additional transcripts are suggested by Genescan profiling, cross-species sequence conservation with the syntenic regions of human chromosomes 15 and 2, and the mapping of genes and ESTs in multi-locus linkage crosses and radiation hybrid maps (www.informatics.jax.org). The actual number of genes within this interval is likely to increase as the annotation of the genome sequence continues and the 60 gaps in the contiguous sequence eliminated.

Genotyping of the B6.LPa congenic mouse excludes the known obesity genes *agouti*, *attractin* and the interleukin-1a and -1b genes, as candidates for the dietary obesity phenotype, but others remain. These include the ubiquitously expressed mitochondrial creatine kinase-1 gene (*Ckmt1*), tyrosine kinase genes *Ltk* and *Tyro3*, ryanodine receptor-3 (*Ryr3*), phospholipase Cβ2 (*Plcb2*), Calpain-3 (*Capn3*), Sorbitol dehydrogenase (*Sdh*), the neuroendocrine protein 7B2 required for peptide hormone processing (*Sgne1*), a cluster of Histidine decarboxylase genes (*Hdc*), and a number of genes involved in intracellular vesicle trafficking: Synaptosomal associated protein-23 (*Snap23*), Syntaxin-13 (*Syn13*), Microtubule associated protein-1 (*Mtap1*), and *Pallidin* (*Pldn*). The genes of the adrenergic receptor system have known effects on energy expenditure, obesity, and hypertension[31,32], and the adrenergic receptor, alpha-2B (*Adra2b*) gene is positioned within the congenic interval. Sequence variation within *Mtap1a* is associated with hearing loss in the tubby obese mouse[6] and may also regulate tubby retinal degeneration[33]. Our studies reveal a single amino acid polymorphism in the *Capn3* gene consisting of a conservative arginine to lysine substitution between B6 and LP at amino acid[66]. Only a single nucleotide difference was found between the B6 and LP alleles of *Snap23*, which is silent with respect to the encoded amino acid. Thus, at this level of analysis, these latter two genes are less likely candidates for the insulin and adiposity QTLs. Further fine-mapping of the gene(s) regulating the two traits and sequence comparisons of genes within the region using the Celera and Ensembl databases is the next step in extending these studies.

References

1. Lembertas AV, Perusse L, Chagnon YC, Fisler JS, Warden CH, Purcell-Huynh DA *et al.* Identification of an obesity quantitative trait locus on mouse chromosome 2 and evidence of linkage to body fat and insulin on the human homologous region 20q. *J Clin Invest* 1997; 100: 1240–47.

2. Salvatore P, Hanash CR, Kido Y, Imai Y, Accili D. Identification of sirm, a novel insulin-regulated SH3 binding protein that associates with Grb-2 and FYN *J Biol Chem* 1998; 273: 6989–97.

3. Kido Y, Philippe N, Schaffer AA, Accili D. Genetic modifiers of the insulin resistance phenotype in mice. *Diabetes* 2000; 49: 589–96.

4. Aitman T J, Glazier AM, Wallace CA, Cooper LD, Norsworthy PJ, Wahid FN *et al.* Identification of Cd36 (Fat) as an insulin-resistance gene causing defective fatty acid and glucose metabolism in hypertensive rats. *Nature Genet* 1999; 21: 76–83.

5. Gould KA, Dove WF. Analysis of the Mom1 modifier of intestinal neoplasia in mice. *Exp Lung Res* 1998; 24: 437–53.

6. Ikeda A, Zheng QY, Zuberi AR, Johnson KR, Naggert JK, Nishina PM. Microtubule-associated protein 1A is a modifier of tubby hearing (moth1). *Nature Genet* 2002; 30: 401–5.

7. Horikawa Y, Oda N, Cox NJ, Li X, Orho-Melander M, Hara M, *et al.* Genetic variation in the gene encoding calpain-10 is associated with type 2 diabetes mellitus. *Nature Genet* 2000; 26: 163–75.

8. Grisart B, Coppieters W, Farnir F, Karim L, Ford C, Berzi P, *et al.* Positional candidate cloning of a QTL in dairy cattle: identification of a missense mutation in the bovine DGAT1 gene with major effect on milk yield and composition. *Genome Res* 2002; 12: 222–31.

9. Din El-Assal S, Alonso-Blanco C, Peeters AJ, Raz V, Koornneef M. A QTL for flowering time in Arabidopsis reveals a novel allele of CRY2. *Nature Genet* 2001; 29: 435–40.

10. Brockmann GA, Bevova MR. Using mouse models to dissect the genetics of obesity. *Trends Genet* 2002; 18: 367–76.

11. Dhar M, Webb LS, Smith L, Hauser L, Johnson D, West DB. A novel ATPase on mouse chromosome 7 is a candidate gene for increased body fat. *Physiol Genomics* 2000; 4: 93–100.

12. Dhar M, Hauser L, Johnson D. An aminophospholipid translocase associated with body fat and type 2 diabetes phenotypes. *Obes Res* 2002; 10: 695–702.

13. Legare ME, Bartlett FS, Frankel WN. A major effect QTL determined by multiple genes in epileptic EL mice. *Genome Res* 2000; 10: 42–8.

14. Cormier RT, Bilger A, Lillich AJ, Halberg RB, Hong KH, Gould KA, *et al.* The Mom1AKR intestinal tumor resistance region consists of Pla2g2a and a locus distal to D4Mit64. *Oncogene* 2000; 19: 3182–92.

15. Zuberi AR, Christianson GJ, Mendoza LM, Shastri N, Roopenian DC. Positional cloning and molecular characterization of an immunodominant cytotoxic determinant of the mouse H3 minor histocompatibility complex. *Immunity* 1998; 9: 687–98.

16. Mastick CC, Brady MJ, Saltiel AR. Insulin stimulates the tyrosine phosphorylation of caveolin. *J Cell Biol* 1995; 129: 1523–31.

17. Mastick CC, Saltiel AR. Insulin-stimulated tyrosine phosphorylation of caveolin is specific for the differentiated adipocyte phenotype in 3T3-L1 cells. *J Biol Chem* 1997; 272: 20706–14.

18. Beck JA, Lloyd S, Hafezparast M, Lennon-Pierce M, Eppig JT, Festing MF, Fisher EM. Genealogies of mouse inbred strains. *Nature Genet* 2000; 24: 23–5.

19. Mehrabian M, Wen PZ, Fisler J, Davis RC, Lusis AJ. Genetic loci controlling body fat, lipoprotein metabolism, and insulin levels in a multifactorial mouse model. *J Clin Invest* 1998; 101: 2485–26.

20. Horvat S, Bunger L, Falconer VM, Mackay P, Law A, Bulfield G, Keightley PD. Mapping of obesity QTLs in a cross between mouse lines divergently selected on fat content. *Mamm Genome* 2000; 11: 2–7.

21. Taylor BA, Phillips SJ. Obesity QTLs on mouse chromosomes 2 and 17. *Genomics* 1997; 43: 249–57.

22. Taylor BA, Wnek C, Schroeder D, Phillips SJ. Multiple obesity QTLs identified in an intercross between the NZO (New Zealand obese) and the SM (small) mouse strains. *Mamm Genome* 2001; 12: 95–103.

23. Baier LJ, Permana PA, Yang X, Pratley RE, Hanson RL, Shen GQ, *et al.* A calpain-10 gene polymorphism is associated with reduced muscle mRNA levels and insulin resistance. *J Clin Invest* 2000; 106: R69–R73.

24. Cox NJ, Frigge M, Nicolae DL, Concannon P, Hanis CL, Bell GI, Kong A. Loci on chromosomes 2 (NIDDM1) and 15 interact to increase susceptibility to diabetes in Mexican Americans. *Nature Genet* 1999; 21: 213–5.

25. Mori Y, Otabe S, Dina C, Yasuda K, Populaire C, Lecoeur C, *et al.* Genome-wide search for type 2 diabetes in Japanese affected sib-pairs confirms susceptibility genes on 3q, 15q, and 20q and identifies two new candidate Loci on 7p and 11p. *Diabetes* 2002; 51: 1247–55.

26. Walder K, McMillan J, Lapsys N, Kriketos A, Trevaskis J, Civitarese A, *et al.* Calpain 3 gene expression in skeletal muscle is associated with body fat content and measures of insulin resistance. *Int J Obes* 2002; 26: 442–9.

27. Richard I, Roudaut C, Marchand S, Baghdiguian S, Herasse M, Stockholm D, *et al.* Loss of calpain 3 proteolytic activity leads to muscular dystrophy and to apoptosis-associated IkappaBalpha/nuclear factor kappaB pathway perturbation in mice. *J Cell Biol* 2000; 151: 1583–90.

28. Serreze DV, Bridgett M, Chapman HD, Chen E, Richard SD, Leiter EH. Subcongenic analysis of the Idd13 locus in NOD/Lt mice: evidence for several susceptibility genes including a possible diabetogenic role for beta 2-microglobulin. *J Immunol* 1998; 160: 1472–78.

29. Serreze DV, Leiter EH, Christianson GJ, Greiner D, Roopenian DC. Major histocompatibility complex class I-deficient NOD-B2mnull mice are diabetes and insulitis resistant. *Diabetes* 1994; 43: 505–9.

30. Hamilton-Williams EE, Serreze DV, Charlton B, Johnson EA, Marron MP, Mullbacher A, Slattery RM. Transgenic rescue implicates beta2-microglobulin as a diabetes susceptibility gene in nonobese diabetic (NOD) mice. *Proc Natl Acad Sci USA* 2001; 98: 11533–8.

31. Bray MS, Boerwinkle E. The role of beta(2)-adrenergic receptor variation in human hypertension. *Curr Hypertens Rep* 2000; 2: 39–43.

32. Hsueh WC, Cole SA, Shuldiner AR, Beamer BA, Blangero J, Hixson JE, *et al.* Interactions between variants in the beta3-adrenergic receptor and peroxisome proliferator-activated receptor-gamma2 genes and obesity. *Diabetes Care* 2001; 24: 672–7.

33. Ikeda A, Naggert JK, Nishina PM. Genetic modification of retinal degeneration in tubby mice. *Exp Eye Res* 2002; 74: 455–61.

34. Pomp D. Genetic dissection of obesity in polygenic animal models. *Behav Genet* 1997; 27: 285–306.

35. Brockmann GA, Kratzsch J, Haley CS, Renne U, Schwerin M, Karle S. Single QTL effects, epistasis, and pleiotropy account for two-thirds of the phenotypic F(2) variance of growth and obesity in DU6i x DBA/2 mice. *Genome Res* 2000; 10: 1941–57.

36. Kayo T, Fujita H, Nozaki J, E X, Koizumi A. Identification of two chromosomal loci determining glucose intolerance in a C57BL/6 mouse strain. *Comp Med* 2000; 50: 296–302.

37. Vaughn TT, Pletscher LS, Peripato A, King-Ellison K, Adams E, Erikson C, Cheverud JM. Mapping quantitative trait loci for murine growth: a closer look at genetic architecture. *Genet Res* 1999; 74: 313–22.

38. Moody DE, Pomp D, Nielsen MK, Van Vleck LD. Identification of quantitative trait loci influencing traits related to energy balance in selection and inbred lines of mice. *Genetics* 1999; 152: 699–711.

Progress in Obesity Research: 9. Edited by *Geraldo Medeiros-Neto, Alfredo Halpern and Claude Bouchard*
©2003 John Libbey Eurotext Ltd, pp. 285–287.

CHAPTER 60

Tissue-specific leptin receptor knockout studies of energy regulation

Streamson Chua, Jr., Julie McMinn, Thomas Ludwig[1], Ioannis Dragatsis[2], Paula Dietrich[2] and Barbara Kahn[3]

Department of Pediatrics and Institute of Human Nutrition, Columbia University, 1150 St. Nicholas Avenue, New York, NY 10032, USA; [1]Department of Anatomy and Cell Biology, Columbia University, 1150 St. Nicholas Avenue, New York, NY 10032, USA; [2]Department of Physiology, University of Tennessee, 894 Union, Nash Bldg, Memphis, TN 38163; [3]Division of Endocrinology, Diabetes and Metabolism, Beth Israel Deaconess Medical Center, 99 Brookline Avenue, Boston, MA 02215, USA
[e-mail: sc569@columbia.edu]

Introduction

The leptin-leptin receptor system is involved in multiple aspects of the regulation of energy balance[1]. Deficiencies of leptin and leptin receptor (*Lepr*) in rodents and humans lead to hyperphagia with early onset obesity and infertility. In addition, insulin resistance and cold intolerance are major features in rodent models of deficient leptin signalling[2]. It has been presumed that activation of leptin receptors on hypothalamic neurons mediates most of the actions of adipocyte-derived leptin[3]. However, the presence of leptin receptors in most peripheral tissues, such as bone and white adipose tissue, has suggested functions of leptin receptor that may or may not be related to energy balance. We have addressed this issue by examining the effects of genetic manipulations of leptin receptor expression on body composition, food intake, insulin sensitivity, and fertility.

Methods

Construction of novel *Lepr* alleles

We constructed the *Lepr-neo* allele based on a large EcoRI fragment from a BAC that contains most of the 3' region of *Lepr*. The construct contained coding exon 15, 16, 17 and 17'. Exon 17 is flanked by loxP sites and the upstream *loxP* site is followed by a *Pgk-npt* cassette flanked by *frt* sites. The construct was introduced into ES cells by electroporation and correctly targetted clones were identified by Southern blot analysis with an exon 14 probe after BamHI digestion. Two clones were used for injection into C57BL/6J blastocysts and one clone transmitted through the germline. Crosses with mice carrying an Actin-FLP transgene[4] generated the *Lepr-flox* allele. Crosses with mice carrying an Hsp70-CRE transgene[5] generated the *Lepr-d17* allele. Due to the numerous transgenes involved, these mice are maintained on a mixed C57BL/6J-129 background.

Tissue-specific deletion of *Lepr*

Mice heterozygous for the *Lepr-flox* allele were crossed with a brain-expressing CRE, CaMK2-CRE6 and an adipose tissue-expressing CRE7, aP2-CRE. Further crossing generated mice that were homozygous for *Lepr-flox* and carrying one of the CRE transgenes. Control mice, CRE-transgene-negative or *Lepr-flox*/+, were identified from siblings.

Phenotypic characterizations

Glucose and insulin were measured in tail blood in the fed and fasting states. Body weights were measured longitudinally at weekly intervals. Cold challenge tests were performed as previously described[3]. At sacrifice with carbon dioxide asphyxiation, carcasses were used for body composition analysis by DEXA. Tissues were also obtained for analysis of deletion of exon 17.

Table 1. Phenotypic characteristics of mice with various *Lepr* alleles and tissue-specific deletion of *Lepr*

Genotype	Body weight (g)	Glucose (mg/dl)	Insulin (ng/ml)	Fertility	Cold tolerance
+/+	28	133	0.9	+	+
Lepr-neo/neo	56.9*	392*	49.8*	–	–
Lepr-flox/flox	30.1	115	1.1	+	+
Lepr-d17/d17	53.1*	464*	18.7*	–	–
CaMK2-CRE Lepr-flox/flox	47.7^	158	97.6*	+	+/–
aP2-CRE Lepr-flox/flox	31.4	138	1.2	+	+

Values represent means of a group ($n = 4$–12) while + or – represents the presence or absence of the trait. *Represents a difference from wild type ($P < 0.05$, Wilcoxon ranked sign test) and ^ represents a difference from *Lepr–d17/d17*.

Results and discussion

Characterization of mice bearing three novel *Lepr* alleles

Mice homozygous for the three novel *Lepr* alleles (Fig. 1) – *Lepr-neo*, *Lepr-flox* and *Lepr-d17* – were characterized for various phenotypes characteristic of mice with leptin receptor mutations. Coding exon 17 encodes the membrane proximal region of LEPR and bears a motif required for JAK activation. Thus, the receptor encoded by *Lepr-d17* would be unable to activate the JAK-STAT pathway and we anticipated that *Lepr-d17* homozygous mice would show the characteristic obesity/diabetes syndrome of leptin receptor deficient mice. The body weights of *Lepr-d17* homozygotes are two- to threefold higher than control mice and this increased mass in primarily due to increased adipose tissue. Food intake measures indicated early onset hyperphagia. These mice are also insulin resistant with near normal blood glucose values and greatly elevated insulin concentrations. Test matings indicated that both sexes are infertile. Cold challenge tests also indicated defective BAT thermogenesis.

Surprisingly, *Lepr-neo* homozygous mice were phenotypically identical to LEPR-deficient mice, showing greatly increased fat mass, insulin resistance, cold intolerance and infertility. Examination of the expression of this allele indicated that the neo cassette interferes with proper splicing. This is not an uncommon observation since the neo cassette is known to have cryptic splice sites and can produce hypomorphic alleles.

The removal of the neo cassette with FLP recombinase generated the *Lepr-flox* allele. Mice homozgyous for *Lepr-flox* are phenotypically normal and are thus well suited for the analysis of effects of tissue-specific deletion of LEPR expression.

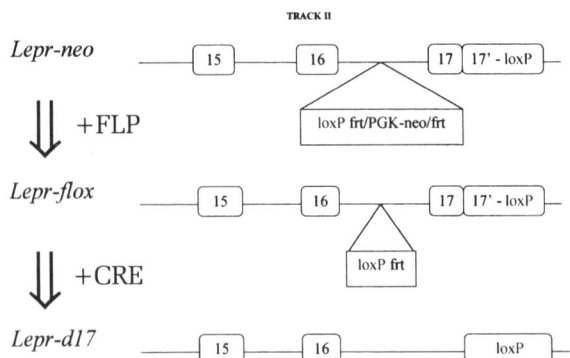

Fig. 1. Schematic representation of three *Lepr* alleles.

Deletion of *Lepr* in neurons and white fat

The effects of deleting *Lepr* specifically in two cell types was evaluated by tissue specific deletion of *Lepr* with transgenes expressing CRE in neurons (CaMK2-CRE) and white fat (aP2-CRE). We observed induction of obesity and insulin resistance by neuron-specific deletion of *Lepr*. In addition, measures of body composition indicated that all of the increased mass was due to accumulated fat. However, the degree of obesity was not as pronounced as in *Lepr-d17* homozygotes. Cold challenge tests indicated variability in individual mice with two of seven CaMK2-CRE *Lepr-flox* homozygotes showing cold intolerance. Furthermore, we did not see any effect on male infertility. We have not yet tested fertility in females. To examine this, we evaluated the degree of *Lepr* deletion in the brain and the hypothalamus. We observed variable degrees of deletion in individual mice and the range was from 70 per cent to 90 per cent deletion, based on semi-quantitative PCR. This estimate needs to consider that these measurements were on whole neural tissue, including glial components.

In contrast, the effect of deleting *Lepr* in white adipocytes was unremarkable. We were unable to distinguish any effect on body weight, food intake, or insulin sensitivity. Quantitative estimates of the degree of deletion suggested ~50–80 per cent deletion of *Lepr* in individual mice using DNA isolated from fat pads. The DNA would have contributions from the stroma vascular fraction, suggesting that a large number of adipocytes had deleted *Lepr*.

Summary

We have generated three new alleles of *Lepr* that are useful for testing of the phenotypic effects of spatial and temporal deletions of the leptin receptor gene. Two of the new alleles, *Lepr-neo* and *Lepr-d17*, are recessive alleles that produce the obesity/diabetes syndrome of leptin receptor deficiency. *Lepr-flox* is similar to the wild type allele since *Lepr-flox* homozygotes are identical to wild type mice. The *Lepr-neo* allele is a model wherein the effect of tissue-specific expression is activated by the action of FLP recombinase. This would be an interesting model to pursue over a *Lepr* transgene since the endogenous *Lepr-neo* alleles are converted to *Lepr-flox* alleles that are equivalent to wild type *Lepr* alleles. The *Lepr-flox* allele can be inactivated by the deletion of coding exon 17 via the action of CRE recombinase.

We have tested the phenotypic effects of neural- and adipocyte-specific deletions of *Lepr* in mice. Our studies indicate that even partial deletion of *Lepr* in neurons is sufficient to have an effect on food intake, body mass, and insulin sensitivity. However, male infertility and cold tolerance appear to require complete or near complete absence of LEPR function in the brain. The lack of an observable phenotype in mice lacking LEPR signalling in adipocytes suggests that LEPR signalling in adipocytes is not relevant to energy balance. However, quantification of the amount of coding exon 17 deletion in adipocytes indicated that we did not achieve 100 per cent excision. It is possible that near-complete coding exon 17 deletion is necessary to generate an observable phenotype. Moreover, it may be necessary to place these genetic manipulations on an inbred background to minimize heterogeneity. Taking all of these qualifications into consideration, the impact of LEPR signalling in white adipocytes on energy balance must be small whereas the LEPR signalling in the central nervous system plays a major role in energy balance.

Acknowledgements: This work was funded by grants DK57621 and DK26687.

References

1. Leibel RL, Chung WK, Chua SC Jr. The molecular genetics of rodent single gene obesities. *J Biol Chem* 1997; 272: 31937–40.

2. Chua SC Jr. Monogenic models of obesity. *Behav Genet* 1997; 27: 277–84.

3. Kowalski TJ, Liu SM, Leibel RL, Chua SC Jr. Transgenic complementation of leptin-receptor deficiency. I. Rescue of the obesity/diabetes phenotype of LEPR-null mice expressing a LEPR-B transgene. *Diabetes* 2001; 50: 425–35.

4. Dymecki SM. Flp recombinase promotes site-specific DNA recombination in embryonic stem cells and transgenic mice. *Proc Natl Acad Sci USA* 1996; 93: 6191–6.

5. Dietrich P, Dragatsis I, Xuan S, Zeitlin S, Efstratiadis A. Conditional mutagenesis in mice with heat shock promoter-driven cre transgenes. Mamm Genome 2000; 11: 196–205.

6. Dragatsis I, Zeitlin S. CaMKIIalpha-Cre transgene expression and recombination patterns in the mouse brain. Genesis 2000; 26: 133–5.

7. Abel ED, Peroni O, Kim JK, Kim YB, Boss O, Hadro E *et al.* Adipose-selective targeting of the GLUT4 gene impairs insulin action in muscle and liver. *Nature* 2001; 409: 729–33.

Progress in Obesity Research: 9. Edited by *Geraldo Medeiros-Neto, Alfredo Halpern and Claude Bouchard*
©2003 John Libbey Eurotext Ltd, pp. 288–292.

CHAPTER 61

Transgenic overexpression studies in obesity and diabetes

Fatima Bosch, Sylvie Franckhauser, Pedro Otaegui, Tura Ferre, Anna Pujol, Sergio Muñoz, Alex Mas, Antonio Hidalgo, Eduard Ayuso and Efren Riu

Department of Biochemistry and Molecular Biology, School of Veterinary Medicine and Center of Animal Biotechnology and Gene Therapy, Universitat Autónoma de Barcelona, 08193 Bellaterra, Spain
[e-mail: fatima.bosch@uab.es]

Introduction

Type 2 diabetes is among the most common metabolic disorders. It is characterized by decreased response of the liver and peripheral tissues to insulin (insulin resistance) and by insufficient compensatory insulin secretion[1-3]. When the β-cell no longer secretes enough insulin to compensate for the insulin resistance, fasting hyperglycaemia and overt diabetes develop[1,2]. In the western world there has been a marked increase in obesity, which is characterized by an alteration of the control of fat deposition and is frequently associated with dyslipidaemia, insulin resistance and type 2 diabetes[4,5]. Although skeletal muscle and adipose tissue contribute to the development of whole-body insulin resistance, liver dysfunction may also cause hyperglycaemia and insulin resistance[2,3].

Role of increased free fatty acid re-esterification by adipose tissue in the development of obesity and insulin resistance

Obesity is often associated with increased circulating levels of free fatty acids (FFA)[6]. Fatty acids released into the bloodstream result from the difference between hydrolysis of triglycerides in adipocytes during lipolysis and re-esterification of the FFA by fat cells through a futile cycle termed reesterification. FFA are esterified with glycerol 3-phosphate. In adipose tissue, glucose is considered to be the main precursor of glycerol 3-phosphate. When glucose supply is limited, as in starvation or low carbohydrate diet, glyceroneogenesis occurs in adipose tissue from pyruvate and aminoacids[7-9]. A regulatory step of this pathway is the conversion of oxaloacetate to phosphoenolpyruvate catalysed by phosphoenolpyruvate carboxykinase (PEPCK)[7].

We examined whether increased PEPCK activity in adipose tissue leads to higher glyceroneogenesis, and if so, whether this would increase lipid re-esterification and fat mass. To this end, transgenic mice overexpressing PEPCK specifically in adipose tissue were generated by using a chimeric gene in which PEPCK gene transcription was under the control of the constitutive and adipose-specific aP2 promoter[10,11]. We found that a primary metabolic alteration in adipose tissue, i.e. PEPCK overexpression, increased glyceroneogenesis, FFA re-esterification and lipid deposition[42]. This indicates direct involvement of PEPCK in the synthesis of glycerol 3-phosphate and shows the key role of glyceroneogenesis in FFA re-esterification and subsequent fat accumulation (Fig. 1). Furthermore, increased fat accumulation in BAT was also observed (Fig. 1), indicating that PEPCK is a key enzyme in this tissue. Our results are consistent with previous reports suggesting that PEPCK provides glycerol 3-phosphate during starvation, which maintains triglyceride synthesis by FFA re-esterification[12]. This may be considered as a negative feedback control on adipose tissue FFA output, which avoids the toxic effects of excess of circulating FFA[13,14]. Our results suggest that an increase in glycerol 3-phosphate concentration is sufficient to increase triglyceride synthesis. Furthermore, it raises the possibility that dysregulation of glyceroneogenesis might influence lipid deposition and therefore contribute to obesity. However, the role of increased PEPCK activity in fat tissue is unknown in human obesity.

Several spontaneous or genetically engineered animal models of hypertrophic obesity[15–17] result from alterations in energy intake or expenditure and are associated with insulin resistance. In contrast, aP2-PEPCK transgenic mice had similar food intake to controls. Moreover, these animals were normoglycaemic and normoinsulinaemic and did not show alterations in glucose or insulin tolerance tests. Skeletal muscle basal and insulin-stimulated glucose uptake and glycogen content were also unaffected, indicating that skeletal muscle of obese aP2-PEPCK transgenic mice remained insulin sensitive. Transgenic obese and control mice exhibited similar hepatic glucokinase activities and glycogen content, and both had normal serum trigly- ceride levels, indicating that triglyceride and glucose liver metabolism was not affected. Thus, obesity in homozygous aP2-PEPCK transgenic mice was due to a primary alteration in fat deposition since glucose homeostasis, whole-body and skeletal muscle insulin sensitivity, or liver glucose and triglycerides metabolism were not altered.

Obesity is generally associated with insulin resistance, thus favouring the development of diabetes. How enlarged adipose tissue mass affects insulin resistance is unclear, although several mechanisms have been proposed[5]. In humans, there is a positive correlation between the amount of visceral fat and the degree of insulin resistance[6]. The increased rate of lipolysis in this fat depot and the resulting increased plasma FFA level are believed to be responsible for the development of insulin resistance[6]. High circulating FFA may have deleterious effects on insulin uptake by the liver[18] and increase insulin secretion by the pancreatic B-cell[14], therefore leading to hyperinsulinaemia. Moreover, FFA increase gluconeogenesis in liver and inhibit insulin-stimulated glucose utilization in skeletal muscle[19,20]. Therefore, in obese aP2-PEPCK mice, the absence of insulin resistance may result from the low levels of circulating FFA due to enhanced re-esterification.

Prevention of insulin resistance and obesity by engineering the liver or the skeletal muscle to increase uptake glucose

Role of increased hepatic glucose uptake

The liver has a central role in glucose homeostasis. When plasma glucose is high the liver takes it up, and replenishes depleted glycogen stores. During starvation, the liver releases glucose to blood from glycogenolysis and gluconeogenesis. Although skeletal muscle and adipose tissue contribute to the development of whole-body insulin resistance, liver dysfunction may also cause hyperglycaemia and insulin resistance[2,3]. An excessive hepatic glucose output is tightly correlated with fasting hyperglycaemia in type 2 diabetes[2]. Transgenic mice overexpressing PEPCK, a key regulatory enzyme of gluconeogenesis, show increased chronic hepatic glucose production, hyperinsulinaemia, hyperglycaemia and insulin resistance[21]. Similarly, mice lacking insulin receptors in the liver display hyperglycaemia, hyperinsulinaemia, glucose intolerance and insulin resistance[3]. Furthermore, liver insulin resistance may result in increased B-cell insulin secretion and decreased hepatic insulin clearance, thus promoting the hyperinsulinaemia observed in type 2 diabetes[3,22]. The liver is also a key tissue for glucose uptake and storage, and may account for disposal of up to one third after an oral glucose load[2]. Therefore, the defect in hepatic glucose uptake observed in type 2 diabetes may have a role in the pathogenesis of insulin resistance and type 2 diabetes.

Engineering the liver to increase glucose uptake might prevent insulin resistance. Increased glucose utilization has been shown by increasing glucokinase (GK) gene expression, the main glucose phosphorylating enzyme in the liver[23–25]. An increase in glucose-6-phosphate stimulates transcription of genes of glycolytic and lipolytic enzymes and represses the expression of gluconeogenic genes[26,27]. The glucose response involves E-boxes within the glucose/carbohydrate regulatory elements located in the promoter of these genes[28]. c-Myc is a basic helix-loop-helix (bLHL)-leucine zipper transcription factor that interacts with E boxes with the sequence CACGTG[29,30]. We have shown that an increase in c-Myc protein in the liver of transgenic animals induces hepatic glycolysis, by increasing the expression of genes coding for enzymes that control the glycolytic pathway, in the absence of cell proliferation and transformation[31,32]. In addition, after an intraperitoneal glucose tolerance test, transgenic mice showed lower levels of blood glucose than controls, indicating that overexpression of c-Myc increased blood glucose disposal by the liver[31,32]. Furthermore, overexpression of c-Myc in streptozotocin-treated mice counteracts diabetic alterations through its ability to induce the expression of GK and thus hepatic glucose uptake and utilization, and to block the activation of gluconeogenesis and ketogenesis[32,43].

Transgenic mice overexpressing c-myc were also fed a high-fat diet to examine whether an increase in hepatic glucose disposal prevents obesity and insulin resistance. After feeding this diet, transgenic mice were lean and showed improved glucose disposal and normal levels of blood glucose and insulin, indicating that they had developed neither obesity nor insulin resistance[44]. In contrast, control mice

A)

Ventral view   **Epididymal fat**

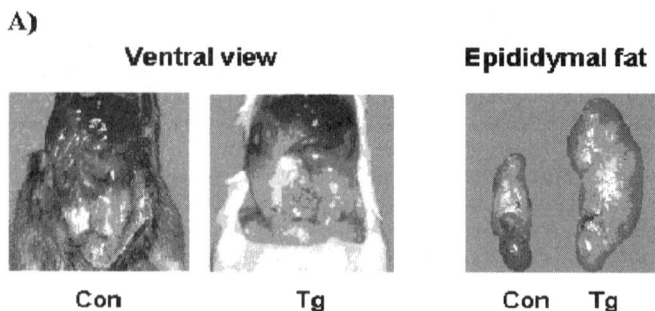

Con   Tg   Con   Tg

Fig. 1. (A) Ventral view showing increased adbominal fat in homozygous aP2/PEPCK transgenic mice compared to control mice. Homozygous transgenic mice presented also bigger epididymal fat pads. (B) Representative sections of epididymal WAT (top panel) and interscapular brown fat (bottom panel) from nontransgenic and heterozygous or homozygous transgenic mice stained with hematoxylin and eosin (x400).

B)

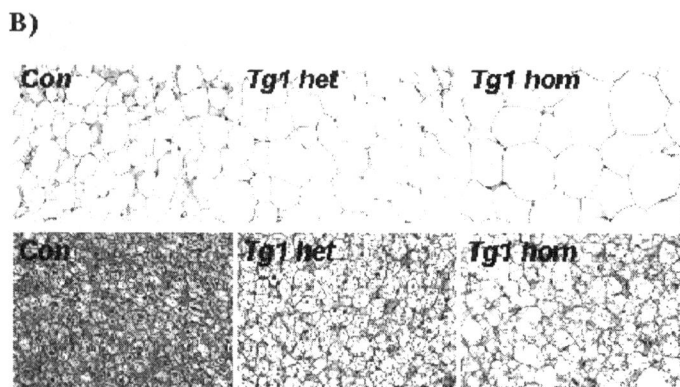

Con   Tg1 het   Tg1 hom

Con   Tg1 het   Tg1 hom

became obese, hyperglycaemic and hyperinsulinaemic. These findings in transgenic mice were parallel with normalization of hepatic GK and pyruvate kinase gene expression and enzyme activity, which led to normalization of intrahepatic glycogen content. In the liver of high fat-fed control mice, the expression of genes encoding proteins that control energy metabolism, such as sterol receptor element binding protein 1-c (SREBPI-c), peroxisome proliferator-activated-α (PPARα) and uncoupling protein-2 (UCP-2) was altered. In contrast, in the liver of high fat-fed transgenic mice the expression of these genes was normal. These results indicate that c-myc overexpression counteracted the obesity and insulin resistance induced by a high-fat diet by modulating the expression of genes that regulate hepatic metabolism. This transgenic model suggests that engineering the liver to increase glucose uptake and utilization, and/or block hepatic glucose production, may be a useful approach to prevent obesity, insulin resistance and type 2 diabetes.

Role of increased glucose phosphorylation by skeletal muscle

Skeletal muscle is the main tissue responsible for the insulin-stimulated disposal of a glucose load. Impaired glucose uptake by skeletal muscle is an early defect that is present in non-diabetic relatives of diabetic subjects[2]. Thus, skeletal muscle becomes a major site of insulin resistance in type 2 diabetes. Several reports suggest that glucose phosphorylation is a regulatory step in glucose utilization by skeletal muscle[33–35]. In type 2 diabetic patients, glucose transport in skeletal muscle in response to euglycaemic hyperinsulinaemia is impaired. However, glucose phosphorylation is impaired to an even greater extent, and as a result, the intracellular free glucose concentration increases[34]. This indicates that, while both glucose transport and phosphorylation are resistant to the action of insulin, impaired glucose phosphorylation is probably the key regulatory step for insulin action[34]. Furthermore, accumulation of intracellular free glucose was found after insulin treatment of both rat cardiac muscle[36] and isolated rat myocytes[37], which indicates that glucose phosphorylation is saturated. Accumulation of intracellular free glucose has also been observed in skeletal muscle of transgenic mice overexpressing GLUT1, showing that glucose phosphorylation is saturated as a result of increased glucose flux[38]. In skeletal muscle, conversion of glucose to glucose 6-phosphate is catalysed by hexokinases I and II (HKI and II)[39]. In an attempt to increase skeletal muscle glucose phosphorylation and to avoid the feed-back inhibition of HK activity by glucose 6-phosphate, the liver enzyme glucokinase (GK) was expressed in skeletal muscle of transgenic mice[40]. This resulted in increased glucose uptake and utilization by skeletal muscle and in increased glucose disposal after an intraperitoneal glucose load[40]. Similar results were obtained after adenovirus-mediated GK gene transfer to skeletal muscle of rats[41]. Furthermore, GK expression in the skeletal muscle reduces type 1 diabetic hyperglycaemia[40].

We have also examined whether GK gene expression in skeletal muscle of transgenic mice increases glucose phosphorylation and counteracts obesity and insulin resistance induced by a high-fat diet. Control mice fed this diet rapidly gained weight and became obese, while transgenic mice remained lean (P. Otaegui *et al.*, unpublished observations). Furthermore, high-fat fed control mice developed hyperglycaemia and hyperinsulinaemia, indicating that they were insulin resistant. In contrast, transgenic mice were normoglycaemic and showed a slight increase in serum insulin levels. In addition, transgenic mice improved whole-body glucose tolerance, normalization of insulin tolerance test and increased intramuscular concentrations of glucose 6-phosphate and glycogen. Furthermore, a parallel increase in uncoupling-protein 3 (UCP3) mRNA levels in skeletal muscle of GK-expressing transgenic mice was also observed. Also these data indicate that the increase in glucose phosphorylation by GK expression in skeletal muscle led to increased glucose utilization and energy expenditure that counteracted weight gain and mimicked a situation of insulin sensitivity. Therefore, our data suggest that the GK gene may be a good candidate to be expressed in skeletal muscle by using specific vectors, either viral or non-viral, for the gene therapy of type 2 diabetes. In this regard, preliminary studies demonstrated that electrotransfer of a GK chimeric gene to skeletal muscle led to GK gene expression and partially counteracted insulin resistance in animal models.

Thus, the results obtained in these transgenic models reinforce the key role of all these tissues, adipose tissue, liver and skeletal muscle, in the control of glucose and lipid homeostasis. They also provide evidence that as we understand more about the whole-body metabolic impact of altering key steps in major metabolic pathways, new interventions (pharmacological or gene therapy) to counteract insulin resistance and obesity may be designed.

Acknowledgements: Work in the author's laboratory has been supported by grants from European Union (QLRT-1999-00674) and CICYT (SAF99-0094) and Fondo Investigación Sanitaria (01/0427), Spain.

References

1. Polonsky KS, Sturis J, Bell GI. Non-insulin-dependent diabetes mellitus – A genetically programmed failure of the beta cell to compensate for insulin resistance. *N Engl J Med* 1996; 334: 777–83.

2. DeFronzo RA. Pathogenesis of type 2 diabetes: metabolic and molecular implications for identifying diabetes genes. *Diabetes Rev* 1997; 5: 177–269.

3. Michael MD, Kulkarni RN, Postic C, Previs SF, Shulman Gl, Magnuson MA, Kahn CR. Loss of insulin signaling in hepatocytes leads to severe insulin resistance and progressive hepatic dysfunction. *Mol Cell* 2000; 6: 87–97.

4. Montagne CT, O'Rahilly S. The perils of portliness. Causes and consequences of visceral adiposity. *Diabetes* 2000; 49: 883–8.

5. Kahn BB, Flier J. Obesity and insulin resistance. *J Clin Invest* 2000; 106: 473–81.

6. Jensen MD. Lipolysis: contribution from regional fat. *Annu Rev Nutr* 1997; 17: 127–39.

7. Ballard FJ, Hanson RW, Leveille GA. Phosphoenolpyruvate carboxykinase and the synthesis of glyceride-glycerol from pyruvate in adipose tissue. *J Biol Chem* 1967; 242: 2746–50.

8. Reshef L, Hanson RW, Ballard FJ. Glyceride-glycerol synthesis from pyruvate. *J Biol Chem* 1969; 244: 1994–2001.

9. Botion LM, Kettelhut IC, Migliorini RH. Increased adipose tissue glyceroneogenesis in rats adapted to a high protein, carbohydrate-free diet. *Horm Metab Res* 1995; 27: 310–3.

10. Yoo-Warren H, Monahan JE, Short J, Short H, Bruzel A, Wynshaw-Boris A, *et al.* Isolation and characterization of the gene coding for cytosolic phosphoenolpyruvate carboxykinase (GTP) from the rat. *Proc Natl Acad Sci USA* 1980; 80: 3656–60.

11. Graves RA, Tontonoz P, Platt KA, Ross SR, Spiegelman BM. Identification of a fat cell enhancer: analysis of requirements for adipose tissue-specific gene expression. *J Cell Biochem* 1992; 49: 219–24.

12. Hanson RW, Reshef L. Regulation of phosphoenolpyruvate carboxykinase (GTP) gene expression. *Annu Rev Biochem* 1997; 66: 581–11.

13. Unger RH. Lipotoxicity in the pathogenesis of obesity-dependent NIDDM. *Diabetes* 1995; 44: 863–70.

14. McGarry JD, Dobbins RL. Fatty acids, lipotoxicity and insulin secretion. *Diabetologia* 1999; 42: 128–38.

15. Chen D, Garg A. Monogenic disorders of obesity and body fat distribution. *J Lipid Res* 1999; 40: 1735–46.

16. Yen TY, Gill AM, Frigeri LG, Barsh GS, Wolff GL. Obesity, diabetes, and neoplasia in yellow A vy/- mice: ectopic expression of the agouti gene. *FASEB J* 1994; 8: 479–88.

291

17. Nonogaki K, Strack AM, Dallman MF, Tecott LM. Leptin-independent hyperphagia and type 2 diabetes in mice with a mutated serotonin 5-HT2c receptor gene. *Nature Med* 1998; 10: 1152–6.

18. Hennes MM, Shrago E, Kissebah AH. Receptor and postreceptor effects of free fatty acids (FFA) on hepatocyte insulin dynamics. *Int J Obes* 1990; 14: 831–41.

19. Saloranta C, Franssila-Kallunki A, Ekstrand A, Taskinene MR, Groop L. Modulation of hepatic glucose production by non-esterified fatty acids in type 2 (non-insulin-dependent) diabetes mellitus. *Diabetologia* 1991; 34: 409–15.

20. Boden G, Chen X, Ruiz J, White JV, Rossetti L. Mechanisms of fatty acid-induced inhibition of glucose uptake. *J Clin Invest* 1994; 93: 2438–46.

21. Valera A, Pujol A, Pelegrin M, Bosch F. Transgenic mice overexpressing phosphoenolpyruvate carboxykinase develop non-insulin-dependent diabetes mellitus. *Proc Natl Acad Sci USA* 1994; 91: 9151–4.

22. Duckworth WC, Bennett RG, Hamel FG. Insulin degradation: progress and potential. *Endocr Rev* 1998; 19: 608–24.

23. Ferre T, Riu E, Bosch F, Valera A. Evidence from transgenic mice that glucokinase is rate limiting for glucose utilization in the liver. *FASEB J* 1996; 10: 1213–18.

24. Ferre T, Pujol A, Riu E, Bosch F, Valera A. Correction of diabetic alterations by glucokinase. *Proc Natl Acad Sci USA* 1996; 93: 7225–30.

25. Hariharan N, Farrelly D, Hagan D, Hillyer D, Arbeeny C, Sabrah T et al. Expression of human hepatic glucokinase in transgenic mice liver results in decrease glucose levels and reduced body weight. *Diabetes* 1997; 46: 11–16.

26. Vaulont S, Vasseur-Cognet M, Kahn A. Glucose regulation of gene transcription. *J Biol Chem* 2000; 275: 31555–8.

27. Scott DK, O'Doherty RM, Stafford JM, Newgard CB, Granner DK. The repression of hormone-activated PEPCK gene expression by glucose is insulin-independent but requires glucose metabolism. *J Biol Chem* 1998; 273: 24145–51.

28. Girard J, Perdereau D, Foufelle F, Prip-Buus C, Ferre P. Regulation of lipogenic enzyme gene expression by nutrients and hormones. *FASEB J* 1994; 8: 36–42.

29. Liischer B, Eisenman RN. New light on Myc and Myb Partl. My *Genes Dev* 1990; 4: 2025–35.

30. Marcu KB, Bossone SA, Patel AJ. Myc function and regulation. *Annu Rev Biochem* 1992; 61: 809–60.

31. Valera A, Pujol A, Gregori X, Riu E, Visa J, Bosch F. Evidence from transgenic mice that myc regulates hepatic glycolysis. *FASEB J* 1995; 9: 1067–78.

32. Riu E, Bosch F, Valera A. Prevention of diabetic alterations in transgenic mice overexpressing Myc in the liver. *Proc Natl Acad Sci USA* 1996; 93: 2198–202.

33. Rothman D, Shulman R, Shulman G. 3 1 P nuclear magnetic resonance measurements of muscle glucose-6-phosphate. *J Clin Invest* 1992; 89: 1069–75.

34. Bonadonna RC, Del Prato S, Bonora E, Saccomani MP, Gulli G, Natali A et al. Roles of glucose transport and glucose phosphorylation in muscle insulin resistance of NIDDM. *Diabetes* 1996; 45: 915–25.

35. Pendergrass M, Koval J, Vogt C, Yki-Jarvinen H, Lozzo P, Pipek R et al. Insulin-induced hexokinase 11 expression is reduced in obesity and NIDDM. *Diabetes* 1998; 47: 387–94.

36. Cheung JY, Conover C, Regen DM, Whitfield CF, Morgan HE. Effect of insulin on kinetics of sugar transport in heart muscle. *Am J Physiol* 1978; 234: E70–E78.

37. Manchester J, Kong X, Nerbonne J, Lowry OH, Lawrence JC. Glucose transport and phosphorylation in single cardiac myocytes: rate-limiting steps in glucose metabolism. *Am J Physiol* 1994; 266: E326–E333.

38. Ren JM, Marshall BA, Gulve EA, Gao J, Johnson DW, Holloszy JO, Mueckler M. Evidence from transgenic mice that glucose transport is rate-limiting for glycogen deposition and glycolysis in skeletal muscle. *J Biol Chem* 1993; 268: 16113–5.

39. Printz RL, Magnuson MA, Granner DK. Mammalian glucokinase. *Annu Rev Nutr* 1993; 13: 463–96.

40. Otaegui PJ, Ferre T, Pujol A, Riu E, Jimenez R, Bosch F. Expression of glucokinase in skeletal muscle: a new approach to counteract diabetic hyperglycemia. *Hum Gene Ther* 11: 1543–52.

41. Jiménez-Chillarón JC, Newgard CB, Gómez-Foix AM. Increased glucose disposal induced by adenovirs mediated transfer of glucokinase to skeletal muscle *in vivo*. *FASEB J* 1999; 13: 2153–60.

42. Franckhauser S, Muñoz S, Pujol A, Casellas A, Riu E, Otaegui P, Su B, Bosch F. Increased fatty acid re-esterification by P-enolpyruvate carboxykinase overexpression in adipose tissue leads to obesity without insulin resistance. *Diabetes* 2002; 51: 624-30.

43. Riu E, Ferre T, Mas A, Hidalgo A, Franckhauser S and Bosch F. Overexpression of c-myc in diabetic mice restores altered expression of the transcription factor genes that regulate liver metabolism. *Biochem J* 2002; 368: 931-7.

44. Riu E, Ferre T, Hidalgo A, Mas A, Franckhauser S, Otaegui P and Bosch F. Overexpression of c-myc in the liver prevents obesity and insulin resistance. *FASEB J* 2003, in press.

Progress in Obesity Research: 9. Edited by *Geraldo Medeiros-Neto, Alfredo Halpern and Claude Bouchard*
©2003 John Libbey Eurotext Ltd, pp. 293–296.

CHAPTER 62

Role of genetic deficiency of fatty acid oxidation in metabolic syndrome/obesity

Philip A. Wood, David M. Kurtz, Keith B. Cox, Lara R. Nyman, Ada Elgavish, Doug A. Hamm, Barbara A. Gower and Tim R. Nagy

Department of Genetics and Nutrition Sciences, University of Alabama at Birmingham, USA
[e-mail: paw@uab.edu]

Introduction

Metabolic syndrome, also known as insulin resistance syndrome or syndrome X, is a common clinical entity characterized by a range of disorders tightly linked with insulin resistance and exacerbated by concurrent obesity[1]. In addition to insulin resistance (hyperinsulinaemia, decreased glucose tolerance, increased hepatic glucose output, fatty change in liver and muscle), these disorders include dyslipidaemia (increased VLDLs, increased small dense LDLs, and reduced HDLs), dysfunctional blood coagulation, and hypertension, frequently with cardiac hypertrophy. Many aspects of metabolic syndrome reflect a state of excess fatty acids and abnormally low fatty acid oxidation (FAO).

Through the work of many investigators, there is increasing evidence that aberrant fatty acid metabolism is a major factor in the development of insulin resistance, pancreatic β-cell dysfunction and eventually type 2 diabetes[2]. Furthermore, obesity is a major risk factor for the development of insulin resistance and metabolic syndrome. In his 2001 Banting lecture[2], the late Dr. J. Denis McGarry described evidence that strongly implicated dysfunctional fatty acid metabolism in the development of diabetes. McGarry, along with others, have demonstrated abnormal fatty acid oxidation in conditions of obesity and diabetes. Reaven[1] and others have shown strong evidence that diets rich in carbohydrates and low in unsaturated fat may be important in the development of metabolic syndrome or syndrome X. Other studies have shown a correlation between muscle triglyceride concentrations and excessive acyl-CoA with decreasing insulin sensitivity [2,3,4]. The build-up of excessive fatty acid substrates such as acyl-CoAs and diacylglycerols in cells, particularly in muscle and β-cells, may be a critical factor that induce cellular level dysfunction and insulin resistance.

We have used gene-targeting strategies to knockout several enzymes of mitochondrial fatty acid oxidation (FAO) in the mouse. These mutants have been reviewed recently [5,6], and include mice deficient in carnitine palmitoyltransferase-1a (liver isoform) (CPT-1a+/–, homozygous mice are lethal), long-chain acyl-CoA dehydrogenase (LCAD–/–) and very long-chain acyl-CoA dehydrogenase deficiency (VLCAD–/–). Using these mouse models of defective FAO, we posed the hypothesis that insulin resistance develops from an imbalance in fatty acid metabolism or a mismatch between fatty acid synthesis/intake and FAO. Thus, high calorie diets, characterized by high carbohydrates and low unsaturated fatty acids, may promote hyperinsulinaemia and excessive fatty acid synthesis resulting in obesity, insulin resistance and metabolic syndrome. Furthermore, this metabolic syndrome would be further exacerbated by inherited defects in FAO.

These mutants have a wide range of acute phenotypes[5–8] such as fasting intolerance, varying degrees of hypoglycaemia, and cold intolerance due to their inability to perform nonshivering thermogenesis[9]. These mice develop significantly elevated blood free fatty acids and fatty liver when fasted. We hypothesized that chronically elevated free fatty acids and concomitant intracellular accumulation of fatty acids, acyl-CoA and triglycerides would promote for the development of obesity, insulin resistance, and diabetes. Furthermore, we hypothesized that feeding a high-fat (HF) diet to LCAD–/– mice would exacerbate the development of insulin resistance and obesity. In this preliminary study, we analysed the physical and biochemical effects of feeding a HF diet or an isocaloric high carbohydrate (HC) diet to LCAD–/– and CPT1a+/– mice compared to age matched WT mice. Additionally, we evaluated body weights of mutants at older ages (LCAD–/–, VLCAD–/–) on a standard rodent diet to screen for those that may develop obesity as a function of their enzyme deficiency.

Materials and methods

Mice

Mice were either homozygous for null alleles at the long-chain acyl-CoA dehydrogenase locus (*Acadl* referred to as LCAD–/–)[8], very long-chain acyl-CoA dehydrogenase locus (*Acadvl* or VLCAD–/–)[9] or had C57BL/6NTac, 129S6/SvEvTac (B6,129) wild-type alleles (WT) at these two loci. An equivalent B6,129 background was maintained by using intercrosses within all three genotypes. In other experiments mice were heterozygous for a targeted mutation of liver isoform carnitine palmitoyltransferase-1a (*Cpt-1a* or CPT-1a+/–)(unpublished studies, Cox KB, Nyman LR, Wood PA) as CPT-1a–/– mice are nonviable. These mice were congenic on the 129S6 background as were the wild-type controls.

Mice were negative for murine pathogens based on serological assays for 10 different viruses, aerobic bacterial cultures of nasopharynx and cecum, examinations for endo- and ectoparasites, and histopathology of all major organs. All animal protocols were approved by the Institutional Animal Care and Use Committee of the University of Alabama at Birmingham.

Diets

Mice were fed either a standard rodent diet (10 per cent fat by calories-Teklad 7012) or custom diets formulated by Harlan-Teklad, Inc. (Madison, WI). The custom diets consisted of a high-fat (HF) diet (Teklad diet-TD 97268) contained 43 per cent fat (calorie per cent) by the addition of beef tallow as the major fat source and a high carbohydrate (HC) diet (Teklad diet-TD 97267) that was 14 per cent fat (calorie per cent) with starch making up the bulk of calories. Both diets were isocaloric and contained equal amounts of sucrose. The high fat diet was relatively high in saturated fat and cholesterol when compared to a standard rodent diet. Mice 17–19 days of age were weaned onto their respective diets.

Sample collection

Prior to sacrifice and sample collection, mice were fasted for 5 h. Blood was collected via intracardiac puncture under surgical anesthesia using CO_2 inhalation. Whole blood samples were allowed to coagulate on ice followed by immediate separation by centrifugation and sera collection. Sera was frozen at –80 °C until analysed.

Serum analyses

Triglycerides were measured in 10 μl of serum with the Ektachem DT II System (Johnson and Johnson Clinical Diagnostics). Insulin was measured by double-antibody radioimmunoassay in 30 μl serum (duplicate aliquots) with 'Sensitive Rat Insulin' reagents (Linco Research, Inc., St. Charles, MO). Assay sensitivity is approximately 0.066 ng/ml (30 μl sample size). Glucose was measured in 10 μl serum using an Ektachem DT II System (Johnson and Johnson Clinical Diagnostics).

Results and discussion

We found decreased blood glucose concentrations in all LCAD–/– mutant groups due to their inborn error of fatty acid oxidation. Severe hypoglycaemia is a common and highly significant clinical problem in children with these inherited enzyme deficiencies[5,6]. The surprising result was the significant hypertriglyceridaemia that occurred as a result of the HC diet rather than the HF diet. As shown in Fig. 1, the most severe hypertriglyceridaemia was found in the LCAD–/– males, while the lowest values were found in the LCAD+/+ females. The values in the groups on the high fat diet were similar regardless of sex or genotype. Insulin values in these same mice followed the blood glucose values for the most part (data not shown), i.e. the mutants had the lowest insulin values.

Furthermore, we found no evidence for increased bodyweight as compared to sex-matched controls for any of these mutants as shown in Fig. 2. The bodyweights shown are for LCAD–/–, WT, and VLCAD–/– mice fed a standard rodent diet with low-fat, but contained relatively unrefined carbohydrate sources such as ground corn, pulverized oats and wheat middlings. Although the VLCAD–/– mice were heavier, the differences compared to WT were not significant. In contrast, Strauss and colleagues[10] reported significant obesity in their independently derived VLCAD deficient mice. The CPT-1a+/– mutants were

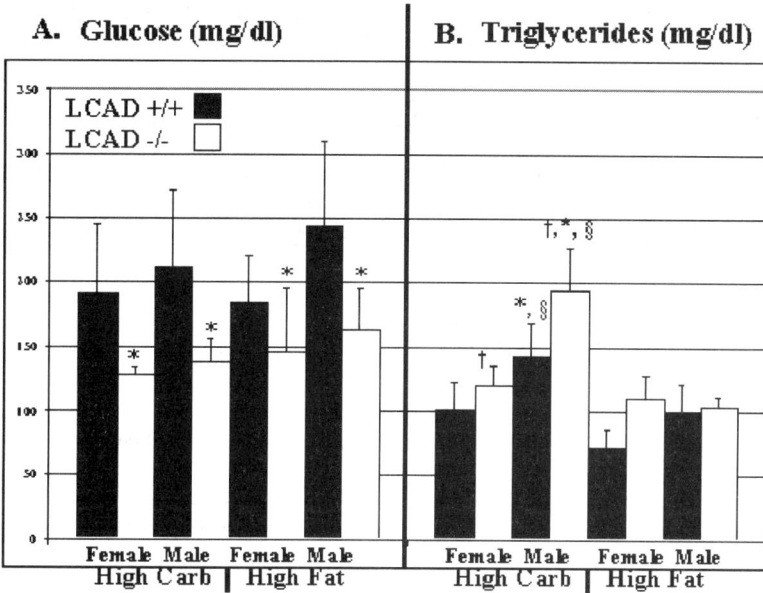

Fig. 1. (A) Blood glucose concentrations were significantly lower ($P < 0.001$) in all LCAD–/– groups regardless of diet or sex. (B) Blood triglyceride concentrations. *Both LCAD+/+ and –/– males on the high carbohydrate (HC) diet had significantly higher blood triglycerides ($P < 0.006$) than the females on the HC diet. †Both LCAD–/– males and females had significantly elevated triglycerides ($P <0.005$) as compared LCAD+/+ controls on the same diet. §Males on the high carbohydrate diet had significantly elevated triglycerides ($P < 0.001$) as

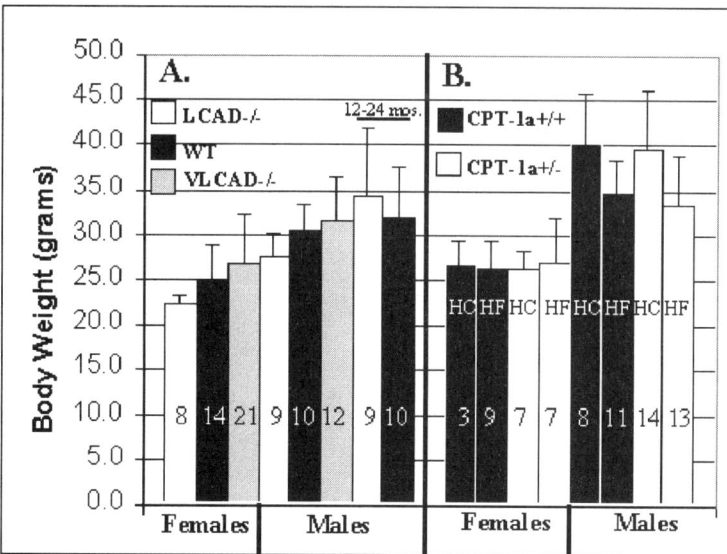

Fig. 2. (A) There were no significant differences in bodyweight found in mutant mice with LCAD deficiency, or VLCAD deficiency, as compared with their sex-matched wild-type (WT) controls. All mice were fed the standard rodent diet. All mice were of a C57BL/6Tac-129S6 mixed genetic background. Mice shown by the first 6 bars (left to right) were 5–8 months old and the last two bars of males were 12–24 months old. (B) The CPT-1a+/– mutants were congenic with WT on a 129S6 background and were fed either the high carbohydrate (HC) or high fat (HF) diets for 6 months. The mice were 7 months old when weighed. The number on the bar is equal to the number of mice analysed for that group.

fed the HF and HC diets for six months, but they likewise showed no evidence of differences in bodyweight as compared to their WT controls. There was a mild increase in bodyweight of males of both genotypes fed the HC diet as compared to the HF diet.

Overall, we found, like in metabolic syndrome, that a high carbohydrate diet, in contrast to an isocaloric high fat diet, promoted for development of hypertriglyceridaemia especially in LCAD–/– mice and this was independent of hyperglycaemia and hyperinsulinaemia. Furthermore, all three genetic defects in FAO failed to promote for increased bodyweight, regardless of diet or sex. Thus from these studies, we conclude that genetic defects in FAO may not play a major role in the development of obesity. Therefore, we speculate that defects in FAO may be important in facilitating metabolic conditions for elevated FFAs, elevated tissue triglycerides and HC diet induced hypertriglyceridaemia, but may not affect body mass.

Acknowledgements: These studies were supported by the following NIH grants RO1-RR02599 (PAW), T-32-RR07003 (to PAW for DMK, KBC), and UAB Clinical Nutrition Research Center P30 DK56336 (PAW, BAG, TRN).

References

1. Reaven G, Strom TK, Fox B. Syndrome X: *The silent killer, the new heart disease risk*. New York: Simon & Schuster, 2000.

2. McGarry JD. Dysregulation of fatty acid metabolism in the etiology of type 2 diabetes. *Diabetes* 2002; 51: 7–18.

3. Kelley DE, Mandarino LJ. Fuel selection in human skeletal muscle in insulin resistance. *Diabetes* 2000; 49: 677–83.

4. Shulman GI. Cellular mechanisms of insulin resistance. *J Clin Invest* 2000; 106: 171–6.

5. Wood PA. Defects in mitochondrial â-oxidation of fatty acids. *Curr Opin Lipidol* 1999; 10: 107–12.

6. Schuler AM, Wood PA. Mouse models for disorders of mitochondrial fatty acid β-oxidation. *ILAR J* 2002; 43: 57–65.

7. Cox KB, Hamm DA, Millington DS, Matern D, Vockley J, Rinaldo P *et al.* Gestational, pathologic, and biochemical differences between very long-chain acyl-CoA dehydrogenase deficiency and long-chain acyl-CoA dehydrogenase deficiency in the mouse. *Hum Mol Genet* 2001; 10: 2069–77.

8. Kurtz DM, Rinaldo P, Rhead WJ, Tian L, Millington DS, Vockley J *et al.* Targeted disruption of mouse long-chain acyl-CoA dehydrogenase reveals crucial roles for fatty acid oxidation. *Proc Natl Acad Sci USA* 1998; 95: 15592–7.

9. Guerra C, Koza RA, Walsh K, Kurtz DM, Wood PA, Kozak LP. Abnormal nonshivering thermogenesis in mice with inherited defects of fatty acid oxidation. *J Clin Invest* 1998; 102: 1724–31.

10. Exil V, Sims HF, Strauss AW. Obesity and tumors in the very long-chain acyl-CoA dehydrogenase deficient mice. *J Inherit Metab Dis* 2000; 23 (Suppl 1): 133.

Progress in Obesity Research: 9. Edited by *Geraldo Medeiros-Neto, Alfredo Halpern and Claude Bouchard*
©2003 John Libbey Eurotext Ltd, pp. 297–299.

CHAPTER 63

Human eating behaviour and obesity: laboratory phenotypes for genetics studies

Kathleen L. Keller[1], Clare Ridely[1], Angelo Pietrobelli[1,2] and Myles S. Faith[1]

[1]*NY Obesity Research Center, SD. Luke's-Roosevelt Hospital Center, Columbia University College of Physicians & Surgeons, New York, NY, USA;* [2]*Paediatric Unit, University of Verona Medical School, Verona, Italy*
[e-mail: kathleenkel@aol.com]

Introduction

There have been enormous advances into the genetics of obesity. Most human studies have used a variety of designs to investigate phenotypes of body composition, energy metabolism, and obesity-related risk factors (e.g. lipid and blood glucose levels, blood pressure). However, there have been few studies testing the genetic bases of human eating behaviours under controlled laboratory conditions. Studying human eating behaviour in the laboratory provides greater experimental control over extraneous 'noise' and bypasses the reporting biases associated with self-report methodology[1].

This brief review presents an overview of human studies addressing the genetics of laboratory-measured human eating behaviour. We include genetically 'uninformative' designs that compared obese and non-obese humans with respect to eating behaviour in the laboratory. These data are presented in order to illustrate the range of potential eating phenotypes for human genetic studies. The review also illustrates an ongoing evolution in the field from descriptive studies of obese/non-obese eating patterns to more refined studies of genetic/environmental influences on human eating behaviour.

Responsiveness to external cues

Historically, the study of the genetics of human eating behaviour can be linked to the seminal laboratory studies of Schachter and colleagues who posited that obese adults had eating patters characteristically similar to the ventromedial hypothalamus (VMH)-lesioned rat[2]. They proposed that obese humans were more 'innately' sensitive to external eating cues than non-obese humans, who were believed to be more sensitive to internal hunger/satiety cues. They designed a series of innovate studies to test this hypothesis in the laboratory (e.g. manipulating the intensive of lighting on experimental foods, the intensity with which subjects needed to work to obtain foods, etc.). Although the balance of data failed to support the internality-externality hypothesis, the importance of these studies with respect to their methodological rigor is noteworthy. These studies demonstrated that eating behaviour could be rigorously studied in the laboratory while being modeling after a viable animal model of obesity.

Rate of eating

From seminal animal studies[2] to Stunkard and Kaplan's[3] review of humans, rate-of-eating has been proposed to be a discriminating characteristic of the obese individual. Pioneering methods to measure rate of eating in humans were conducted by Jordan *et al.*[4] who measured the rate with which subjects consumed liquid meals. They showed that rate of sucking was associated with changes in reported hunger levels, but did not report on associations with weight status. Guss and Kissileff[5] subsequently developed the 'universal eating monitor' to measure rate of energy consumption over fixed time periods during *ad libitum* meals consumed in the laboratory. They demonstrated that the food intake curves of non-obese subjects, which were fit by quadratic curves, did not replicate among obese subjects. Despite its historical prominence, rate of eating in the laboratory has not been actively exploited for human genetics studies. The potential importance of this phenotype is suggested from infant studies showing that rate of sucking predicted increased weight as they developed[6].

Food choice selections

Genes might influence obesity through food selection. Stemming from behavioural economic theory and related animal studies[7], investigators have developed methods to test whether obese individuals exert more effort than non-obese individuals to gain access to high-fat/high-energy foods. These studies required subjects to work on computer tasks at different work intensity levels to earn access to obesity-promoting foods as opposed to healthier activities (e.g. access to nutritious foods and physical activity). Across a series of studies, Epstein and colleagues have demonstrated differences between obese and non-obese individuals with respect to food choices and have suggested that food (compared to other commodities) has a greater 'reinforcing value' for obese subjects[7]. Methods to assess the relative reinforcing value of food choices may yield new insights if used in the context of twin, adoption, and/or molecular studies.

Caloric compensation

'Caloric compensation' (CC) refers to the ability to adjust energy intake at a test meal proportional to energy previously consumed as a drink or snack[8]. Stemming from an extensive animal literature, procedures to test for CC in humans have tested the hypothesis that obese individuals are poorer at CC than non-obese individuals. Evidence dating back to Schachter's laboratory studies supports this hypothesis[2], as well metabolic ward studies showing that increasing body weight was associated with a greater coefficient of variation in energy intake[9]. However not all studies confirm this finding. Rolls et al.[10] failed to detect differences in CC ability strictly as a function of weight status in adults. They found that CC ability was more strongly determined by the macronutrient content of the preload (i.e. per cent fat vs. per cent carbohydrate), gender, and dietary restraint. These finding and other studies suggest that that CC ability may not reliably discriminate obese from non-obese individuals, and that other environmental and food characteristics (e.g. energy density[11]) need to be considered.

Building upon previous CC studies in adults, we conducted a laboratory study in order to test the heritability of energy intake[12]. We provided twins a multi-item buffet meal and computed total and macronutrient-specific intake by pre- and post-weighing food trays[12]. Results indicated that age- and sex-adjusted total caloric intake was significantly greater among monozygotic (MZ) (r = 0.80) than dizygotic (DZ) (r = 0.68) twins, consistent with the hypothesis of an additive genetic influence. Structural equation modeling estimated the heritability of food intake to be at 33 per cent, with 48 per cent and 19 per cent of the variance due to common and unique environmental effects respectively. Evidence for genetic influences on macronutrient intake was also established. We are currently following up this research in a paediatric twin sample[13]; preliminary results suggest a lack of a genetic influence on total energy intake but significant common and unique environmental influences[14].

Response to overfeeding

The study of gene-environment interactions may be critical for understanding human eating behaviour. Not all humans appear to have identical responses to energy and macronutrient intake, and certain genes may prevent certain individuals from excess weight gain during periods of overfeeding. The classical paper by Bouchard et al.[15] tested whether changes in body composition after exposure to overfeeding (i.e. 4.18 MJ/d energy surplus, 6 days a week over 100 days) were genetically influenced. Using 12 pairs of male MZ twins, they compared intra- and inter-pair differences in response to overfeeding. Data showed that variations in weight, fat mass, and fat-free mass changes were three times greater among than within pairs, suggesting a gene-environment interaction. Long-term under-feeding studies have also been carried out, and intra-pair resemblance has been observed for changes in body weight, fat mass, per cent body fat, body energy content, abdominal visceral fat, skinfolds, and respiratory exchange ratio during submaximal work[16].

Improvements in DNA collection methods may lead to the discovery of target genes that interact with diet to either predispose or protect against the development of obesity. One exemplary study published by the Bouchard group[17] found that metabolic responses to long-term overfeeding could were associated with particular polymorphisms at the Gln223Arg variant of the leptin receptor gene. This study illustrates the type of insights that can be achieved by bridging molecular analyses with human feeding protocols in the laboratory.

Conclusion

Historically, 'genetic' studies of human eating behaviour in the laboratory compared obese and non-obese individuals phenotypes based on animal models or theories. There does not appear to be one distinct phenotype that consistently discriminates the obese, perhaps suggesting the limitations of broad categorizations of obesity status for such studies. Although these studies were typically not designed to test for genetic influences per se, they nonetheless provided a foundation for more recent studies that have incorporated genetically informative designs (e.g. twin and overfeeding studies). A key issue for research is identifying those eating phenotypes that are most 'genetically loaded' and, hence, desirable for study. Genetics designs may provide new insights for human ingestive studies in several ways including the use of heritability studies to first determine those traits most genetically loaded and molecular studies to pinpoint specific genes influences those traits. The importance of animal obesity models cannot be overstated, was instrumental in Schachter's earliest work[2], and is expected to guide a new generation of feeding studies.

References

1. Schoeller DA, Fjeld CR. Human energy metabolism: What have we learned from the doubly labeled water method? *Annu Rev Nutr* 1991; 11: 355–73.

2. Schacheter S, Rodin J. Eds. *Obese humans and rats.* Publishers. Potomac: Lawrence Erlbaum Associates, 1994.

3. Stunkard AJ, Kaplan D. Eating in public places: a review of reports of the direct observation of eating behavior. *Int J Obes* 1977; 1: 89–101.

4. Jordan HA, Wieland WF, Zebley SP, Stellar E, Stunkard AJ. Direct measurement of food intake in man: A method for the objective study of eating behavior. Psychosomatic Med 28: 836–842. *Neuroscience Biobheh Rev* 1966; 24: 261–8.

5. Guss J, Kissileff HR. Microstructural analyses of human ingestive patterns: from description to mechanistic hypotheses, 2000.

6. Stunkard AJ, Berkowitz R, Stallings V *et al. Am J Clin Nut* 1999.

7. Epstein LH, Saelens BE. Behavioral economics of obesity: Fod intake and energy expenditure. In: *Reframing health behavior change with behavioral economics*, Bickel WK, Vuchinich RE (eds), pp. 293–311. Mahwah: Lawrence Erlbaum, 2000.

8. Kissileff HR. Satiating efficiency and a stategy for conducting food loading experiments. *Neuroscience Biobheh Rev* 1984; 8: 129–35.

9. Lissner L, Levitsky DA, Strupp BJ, Kalkwarf HJ, Roe DA. Dietary fat and the regulation of energy intake in human subjects. *Am J Clin Nutr* 1987; 46: 886–92.

10. Rolls BJ, Kim-Harris S, Fischman MW, Foltin RW, Moran TH, Stoner SA. Satiety after preloads with different amounts of fat and carbohydrate: implications for obesity. *Am J Clin Nutr* 1994; 60: 476–87.

11. Bell EA, Rolls BJ. Energy density of foods affects energy intake across multiple levels of fat content in lean and obese women. *Am J Clin Nutr* 2001; 73: 1010–8.

12. Faith MS, Rha SS, Neale MC, Allison DB. Evidence for genetic influences of human energy intake: results from a twin study using measured observations. *Behav Genetics* 1999; 29: 145–54.

13. Keller KL, Jozkowski K, Must S, Pietrobelli A, Faith MS. Caloric compensation ability in children: Associations with fat intake during *ad libitum* eating. *Int J Obes* (in press).

14. Faith MS, Keller KL, Pietrobelli A, Allison DB. Genetic and environmental influences on child energy intake. *Int J Obes* (in press).

15. Bouchard C, Tremblay A, Despres JP, Nadeau A, Lupien P, Theriault G *et al.* The response to long-term overfeeding in identical twins. *N Engl J Med* 1990; 322: 1477–82.

16. Tremblay A, Poehlman ET, Despres JP, Theriult G, Danforth E, Bouchard C. Endurance training with constant energy intake in identical twins: changes over time in energy expenditure and related hormones. *Metabolism*; 1997.

17. Ukkola O, Tremblay A, Despres J-P, Chagnon YC, Campfield LA, Bouchard C. Leptin receptor Gln223 Arg variant is associated with a cluster of metabolic abnormalities in response to long-term overfeeding. *J Internal Med* 2000; 248: 435–9.

Progress in Obesity Research: 9. Edited by *Geraldo Medeiros-Neto, Alfredo Halpern and Claude Bouchard*
©2003 John Libbey Eurotext Ltd, pp. 300–303.

CHAPTER 64

The genetics of physical activity level in humans

Tuomo Rankinen

Human Genomics Laboratory, Pennington Biomedical Research Center, Baton Rouge, LA 70808, USA
[e-mail: rankint@pbrc.edu]

Introduction

The beneficial effects of regular physical activity on primary and secondary prevention of several common chronic diseases have been well established and reduction of sedentarism is one of the corner stones of public health initiatives. The American Heart Association added physical inactivity on the list of major cardiovascular risk factors in 1992 and within a few years several federal agencies, such as the CDC, the Surgeon General and the NIH published their recommendations for physical activity to promote public health. The main challenge for implementation of these recommendations is the poor compliance to physical activity interventions. Since physical activity is a behavioural trait, research has mainly focused on finding psychological, social and environmental factors that contribute to levels of physical activity. Interest on the biological basis of physical activity has re-emerged recently[1,2] and advances in techniques of molecular genetic research have open new avenues to test these ideas. The purpose of this review is to summarize the data from genetic epidemiology studies, and to briefly discuss the potential candidate genes for physical activity.

Evidence from genetic epidemiology studies

Studies on the genetics of physical activity level are not extensive, but evidence from both twin and family studies suggest that genetic factors could be involved in the determination of physical activity level. Several twin studies have addressed the role of genetic factors in physical activity level and the findings from these studies are summarized in Table 1.

In a large cohort of mono- and dizygotic (MZ and DZ, respectively) male twin pairs over 18 years of age from the Finnish Twin Registry[3], information on intensity and duration of activity, years of participation in a given activity, physical activity on the job, and subjective opinion of the subject's own activity level was obtained from a questionnaire. A score of physical activity was generated from these variables using factor analysis, which was then used to compute correlations within MZ and DZ twin pairs. The results indicated an estimated heritability of 62 per cent for age-adjusted physical activity level. Heller *et al.* reported a significantly higher concordance within 94 pairs of MZ twins than within 106 pairs of DZ twins for participation in vigorous exercise in the past two weeks, and derived a heritability estimate of 39 per cent for this phenotype[4]. In another cohort of Finnish twins aged 16 years, leisure-time physical activity level outside the school was assessed using a questionnaire with two questions: one concerning the frequency and the other the intensity of the activities[5]. Based on these two questions the subjects were assigned to one of five classes of activity level. The results revealed greater intraclass correlations for MZ twins that for DZ twins for activity level (Table 1).

In the USA Vietnam Era Twin Registry (VETR) cohort, levels of moderate and vigorous activities were assessed using a mixed-mode mail and telephone survey in 3344 male twin pairs aged 33 to 51 years[6]. A clear pattern of familial clustering of both moderate and vigorous activities were observed, with the odds ratios for a twin to engage in physical activity when his co-twin also engaged in the same activity ranging from 1.25 (95 per cent; CI 1.21–1.30) to 4.60 (2.89–7.30). For the heritability analyses, only those twin pairs who saw each other at least once per month as adults were selected. Twin correlations for all activities were greater in MZ pairs (n = 1006) than in DZ pairs (n = 530). However, the heritability estimates were greater for vigorous activities such as jogging/running (0.53), racquet sports (0.48) and bicycling (0.58) than for moderate activities (from 0.12 to 0.40).

Table 1. Summary of the intraclass correlations from twin studies for physical activity level and physical activity-related phenotypes

Source	Physical activity trait	Age	Sex	Number of pairs		Correlation coefficients	
				MZ	DZ	MZ	DZ
Kaprio *et al.* (3)	Total physical activity	>18	M	1537	3507	0.57	0.26
Koopmans *et al.* (7)	Sports participation	18–22	M	249	241	0.89	0.60
			F	329	303	0.85	0.72
Aarnio *et al.* (5)	Leisure-time physical activity outside the school	16	M	147	191	0.72	0.45
		16	F	231	179	0.64	0.41
Lauderdale *et al.* (6)	Intermittent moderate activities	33–51	M	1006	530	0.38	0.12
	Jogging/running (> 10 miles/week)					0.53	0.07
	Strenuous racquet sports (> 5 h/week)					0.52	0.28
	Bicycling (> 50 miles/week)					0.58	0.14
	Swimming (> 2 miles/week)					0.39	0.35
Beunen and Thomis (8)	Sports participation	15	M	17	19	0.66	0.62
			F	17	19	0.98	0.71
Maia *et al.* (9)	Sports participation index	12–25	M	85	68	0.82	0.46
			F	118	85	0.90	0.53
	Leisure-time physical activity		M	85	68	0.69	0.22
			F	118	85	0.72	0.56
McGue *et al.* (10)	Self-rated ability on athletic competition	27–80	M	226	202	0.50[a]	0.26[a]
		27–86	F	452	345		
McGuire *et al.* (11)	Perceived athletic self-competence	10–18	M	45	49	0.58[a]	0.23[a]
		10–18	F	47	48		

a = Coefficients adjusted for sex.

Participation in sports activity may be influenced by genetic factors. In a study based on 1,294 families including both parents and 1,587 pairs of MZ and DZ twins, an estimated heritability of 45 per cent for sports participation was reported[7]. The remaining phenotypic variance was attributed to shared familial environment (44 per cent) and environmental factors unique to each individual (11 per cent). In the Leuven Longitudinal Twin Study, Beunen and Thomis reported that additive genetic factors explained 44 per cent and 83 per cent of the variation in sports participation index in 15-year-old girls and boys, respectively[8]. Similarly, Maia and coworkers detected greater heritabilities for sports participation index and leisure-time physical activity in Portuguese boys (63–68 per cent) than in girls (32–40 per cent)[9]. Moreover, psychological factors affecting sports participation may be characterized by a significant genetic component. In a cohort of 678 MZ and 547 DZ twin pairs, aged 27–86 years, an index of self-rated ability in athletic competition showed a genetic effect of 50.5 per cent while the remaining 49.5 per cent of the variance was due to nonshared environmental factors[10]. A very similar estimate of genetic effect was derived from data of 92 MZ twin pairs, 97 DZ twin pairs and 94 full sibling pairs, aged 10 to 18 years. The genetic effect for perceived athletic self-competence was 54 per cent whereas non-shared environmental factors contributed an additional 42 per cent of the variance[11].

Physical activity levels and patterns in children and their parents tend to be similar, but studies of familial aggregation of activity level and sports participation are relatively few. In 100 children, aged 4 to 7 years, and 99 mothers and 92 fathers from the Framingham Children's Study[12], data on habitual physical activity were obtained with an accelerometer for about 10 h per day for an average of 9 days in children and 8 days in fathers and mothers over the course of one year. Active fathers or active mothers were more likely to have active offspring than inactive fathers or mothers, with odds ratios of

3.5 and 2.0, respectively. When both parents were active, the children were 5.8 times more likely to be active as children of two inactive parents. These results are thus compatible with the notion that genetic or other factors transmitted across generations predispose a child to be active or inactive.

In the 1981 Canada Fitness Survey, a total of 18,073 individuals living in households across Canada completed a questionnaire on physical activity habits[13]. Detailed information on the frequency, duration and intensity of activities performed on a daily, weekly, monthly and yearly basis was used to estimate average daily energy expenditure for each individual. Familial correlations were 0.28, 0.12 and 0.21 for spouses (n = 1,024 pairs), parents and offspring (n = 1,622 pairs), and sibling pairs (n = 1,036), respectively. The lower correlations in parent-offspring and sibling pairs compared to spouses suggest only a small contribution of genetic factors in the familial aggregation of leisure-time energy expenditure.

In the Phase 1 of the Québec Family Study (QFS), path analysis procedures[14] were used to estimate the relative contribution of genetic and non-genetic factors to activity level. Two different indicators of physical activity, habitual physical activity and participation in moderate to vigorous physical activity, were obtained from a 3-day activity record completed by 1,610 members from 375 families encompassing nine types of relatives by descent or adoption. Most of the variation in the two indicators of habitual physical activity level was accounted for by non-transmissible environmental factors, with values reaching 71 per cent for habitual physical activity and 88 per cent for exercise participation. The transmission effect across generations was also significant. The estimate for habitual physical activity was 29 per cent, and it was entirely attributable to genetic factors. The corresponding estimate for participation in moderate to vigorous physical activity was 12 per cent, and it was accounted for by cultural transmission with no genetic effect. Since habitual physical activity was computed as the sum of all activities, and participation in moderate to vigorous activity included only more vigorous activities, low intensity activities were probably those characterized by the significant genetic effect. The results were thus interpreted as an indication of inherited differences in the propensity to be spontaneously active or inactive (14). Recently, Simonen and coworkers investigated familial aggregation of physical activity level in nuclear families from the Phase 2 of the QFS[15]. Maximal heritabilities derived from the maximum likelihood estimates of familial correlations reached 25 per cent, 16 per cent and 19 per cent for the degree of inactivity, time spent in moderate to strenuous physical activities, and total level of physical activity, respectively[15].

Evidence from molecular studies

Molecular evidence for a genetic contribution to the regulation of physical activity level comes from neurological disorders in which either hyper- or hypoactivity is one of the clinical features. The dopamine (DA) transporter (DAT) and the DA receptors have been implicated in this context. DAT is expressed on the plasma membrane of dopaminergic neurons where it regulates the reuptake of dopamine into presynaptic terminals. The DAT knockout (KO) mice are lacking the transporter and thus are accumulating DA in the extracellular space of dopaminergic neurons. A prominent feature of these animals is their marked hyperactivity. For example, the DAT-KO mice show about a 12-fold higher locomotor activity in a novel environment than the wild-type animals[16]. On the other hand, the D2 dopamine receptor (DRD2) deficient mice exhibit markedly lower activity levels, quantified as the initiation of movement, time spent in motion, and horizontal distance travelled, than their strain-matched wild-type controls[17]. In addition to the DRD2 genotype, the genetic background of the animals influences the locomotor activity. This suggests that genetic factors besides the DRD2 locus influences the activity level regulation in these mice. Whether genetic variation at the DAT and DRD2 loci has any effect on the physical activity level in humans is unclear. However, both linkage and association studies in humans have indicated that the DAT locus is involved in the attention-deficient hyperactivity disorder[18-20], which has hyperactivity as one of its clinical features.

Another example of the potential involvement of a gene in physical activity regulation comes from the fruit fly (Drosophila melanogaster). These insects exhibit two distinct activity patterns related to food-search behaviour; rovers move about 2-times longer distances while feeding than sitters. This activity pattern is genetically determined and is regulated by the *dg2* gene, which encodes a cGMP-dependent protein kinase (PKG)[21]. PKG activity is significantly higher in wild-type rovers than in wild-type and mutant sitters and the activation of the *dg2* gene reverts foraging behaviour from a sitter to a rover. The role of the *dg2* gene in the regulation of food-search behaviour was confirmed by overexpressing the dg2 gene in sitters, which resulted in a change of behaviour to the rover phenotype.

Summary

The studies summarized in this review indicate that several physical activity-related traits are influenced by genetic factors with maximal heritability estimates ranging from 20 to 60 per cent. The majority of the data available are based on genetic epidemiology studies, but results from animal studies suggest that single genes can markedly influence physical activity-related behaviour in experimental models suggesting that it will perhaps be possible to undertake in the future the genetic dissection at the molecular level of habitual physical activity as a behavioural phenotype in humans.

References

1. Rowland TW. The biological basis of physical activity. *Med Sci Sports Exerc* 1998; 30(3): 392–9.

2. Thorburn AW, Proietto J. Biological determinants of spontaneous physical activity. *Obes Rev* 2000; 1(2): 87–94.

3. Kaprio J, Koskenvuo M, Sarna S. Cigarette smoking, use of alcohol, and leisure-time physical activity among same-sexed adult male twins. *Prog Clin Biol Res* 1981; 69(Pt C): 37–46.

4. Heller RF, O'Connell DL, Roberts DC, Allen JR, Knapp JC, Steele PL *et al.* Lifestyle factors in monozygotic and dizygotic twins. *Genet Epidemiol* 1988; 5(5): 311–21.

5. Aarnio M, Winter T, Kujala UM, Kaprio J. Familial aggregation of leisure-time physical activity – a three generation study. *Int J Sports Med* 1997; 18(7): 549–56.

6. Lauderdale DS, Fabsitz R, Meyer JM, Sholinsky P, Ramakrishnan V, Goldberg J. Familial determinants of moderate and intense physical activity: a twin study. *Med Sci Sports Exerc* 1997; 29(8): 1062–8.

7. Koopmans JR, Van Doornen LJP, Boomsma DI. Smoking and sports participation. In: *Genetic factors in coronary heart disease*, Godlbourt U, De Faire U, Berge K (eds), pp. 217–235. Lancaster: Kluwer Academic; 1994.

8. Beunen G, Thomis M. Genetic determinants of sports participation and daily physical activity. *Int J Obes Relat Metab Disord* 1999; 23 (Suppl 3): S55–63.

9. Maia JA, Thomis M, Beunen G. Genetic factors in physical activity levels. A twin study. *Am J Prev Med* 2002; 23(2 Suppl 1): 87–91.

10. McGue M, Hirsch B, Lykken DT. Age and the self-perception of ability: a twin study analysis. *Psychol Aging* 1993; 8(1): 72–80.

11. McGuire S, Neiderhiser JM, Reiss D, Hetherington EM, Plomin R. Genetic and environmental influences on perceptions of self-worth and competence in adolescence: a study of twins, full siblings, and step-siblings. *Child Dev* 1994; 65(3): 785–99.

12. Moore LL, Lombardi DA, White MJ, Campbell JL, Oliveria SA, Ellison RC. Influence of parents' physical activity levels on activity levels of young children. *J Pediatr* 1991; 118(2): 215–9.

13. Perusse L, Leblanc C, Bouchard C. Familial resemblance in lifestyle components: results from the Canada Fitness Survey. *Can J Public Health* 1988; 79(3): 201–5.

14. Perusse L, Tremblay A, Leblanc C, Bouchard C. Genetic and environmental influences on level of habitual physical activity and exercise participation. *Am J Epidemiol* 1989; 129(5): 1012–22.

15. Simonen RL, Perusse L, Rankinen T, Rice T, Rao DC, Bouchard C. Familial aggregation of physical activity levels in the Quebec family study. *Med Sci Sports Exerc* 2002; 34(7): 1137–42.

16. Gainetdinov RR, Wetsel WC, Jones SR, Levin ED, Jaber M, Caron MG. Role of serotonin in the paradoxical calming effect of psychostimulants on hyperactivity. *Science* 1999; 283(5400): 397–401.

17. Kelly MA, Rubinstein M, Phillips TJ, Lessov CN, Burkhart-Kasch S, Zhang G *et al.* Locomotor activity in D2 dopamine receptor-deficient mice is determined by gene dosage, genetic background, and developmental adaptations. *J Neurosci* 1998; 18(9): 3470–9.

18. Gill M, Daly G, Heron S, Hawi Z, Fitzgerald M. Confirmation of association between attention deficit hyperactivity disorder and a dopamine transporter polymorphism. *Mol Psychiatry* 1997; 2(4): 311–3.

19. Cook EH, Jr., Stein MA, Krasowski MD, Cox NJ, Olkon DM, Kieffer JE *et al.* Association of attention-deficit disorder and the dopamine transporter gene. *Am J Hum Genet* 1995; 56(4): 993–8.

20. Waldman ID, Rowe DC, Abramowitz A, Kozel ST, Mohr JH, Sherman SL *et al.* Association and linkage of the dopamine transporter gene and attention-deficit hyperactivity disorder in children: heterogeneity owing to diagnostic subtype and severity. *Am J Hum Genet* 1998; 63(6): 1767–76.

21. Osborne KA, Robichon A, Burgess E, Butland S, Shaw RA, Coulthard A *et al.* Natural behaviour polymorphism due to a cGMP-dependent protein kinase of Drosophila. *Science* 1997; 277(5327): 834–6.

Progress in Obesity Research: 9. Edited by *Geraldo Medeiros-Neto, Alfredo Halpern and Claude Bouchard*
©2003 John Libbey Eurotext Ltd, pp. 304–306.

CHAPTER 65

The molecular basis of the mammalian sweet tooth

Danielle R. Reed, Xia Li, Alexander A. Bachmanov, Kirsten J. Mascioli and Gary K. Beauchamp

Monell Chemical Senses Center, Philadelphia PA 19104, USA
[e-mail: reed@monell.org]

The liking for sweet foods and drinks is considered to be a universal trait among many species of mammals and of humans, but in fact, there are differences among people and between species in the willingness to ingest sweeteners. Both types of differences, those between individuals and those between species, are greatest for artificial or high intensity sweeteners. However, since we are concerned here with the role that sweeteners play in obesity, we will restrict our discussion to naturally-occurring, nutritive sugars.

Three traits important in the characterization of the human response to sweet foodstuffs are: detection threshold, perceived intensity across a range of concentrations, and degree of liking. The relationship among these three traits is variable, and all three traits are rarely measured in the same subject. However, investigations in mice have shed some light on the relationship among these variables. Our research group has made a study over the last ten years of two inbred strains of mice, the C57BL/6J (B6) and the 129P3/J (129) strains. When sucrose is offered as a choice with water, B6 mice consume more sucrose at most concentrations, prefer sucrose at lower concentrations[2], and have increased peripheral nerve firing to sucrose concentrations compared with the 129 mice[9]. In other words, the more intense the sweet taste of sugar, the more mice like it.

Is the same true of humans? Several investigators have studied the response of humans to concentrated, naturally-occurring sugars and have divided people into two classes – those who increase their liking for sucrose as the concentration goes up and those that have an optimal 'middle of the road' concentration and then reduce their liking when the concentration is higher[22]. Such subjects find sucrose to be 'too sweet', i.e. is too intense and therefore unpleasant. Other people act like mice – more is better when it comes to sweetness.

The origins of these *individual differences* are not understood. However, some factors are known to reliably predict *group* differences in human sweet preference. There are racial and ethnic differences in sugar consumption that are independent of economic wealth. For instance, Japanese citizens consume half as much sugar compared with Swiss citizens[10]. Similarly, in the United States, populations of African descent prefer more highly sweetened foods than do those of European descent[21]. Children prefer more highly sweetened foods compared with adults[5]. Changes in metabolic state and meals are also associated with taste threshold for sugars; for instance, the lowering of blood glucose changes sucrose thresholds[6]. Similarly, ingestion of sweet foods and drinks decreases their subsequent pleasantness[4].

Individual differences in sweet preference in humans may be partially genetically determined. Several studies have examined the similarity in carbohydrate consumption among family members, demonstrating modest heritability, for a review see[19]. However, few studies specifically address the genetics of sweet preference, intensity ratings or threshold detection. One such study was conducted in twins, which reported little evidence of heritablity in sweet preference[7]. Even thought the initial forays to discover the genetic correlates of sucrose preference in humans were not encouraging , the compelling evidence in mice and rats led us to reexamine this issue.

In an ongoing study of the heritability of sucrose perception in humans, we are recruiting human families and comparing the degree of relatedness in the family members (e.g. grandparent–grandchild, parent–offspring) with their similarity in perception of sucrose intensity rating. Preliminary data analysis has shown that about 20 to 30 per cent of the phenotypic variance in sucrose intensity ratings can be explained by genetic relatedness. Therefore, we were encouraged to pursue this topic, and are now collecting this information from monozygotic and dizygotic twins. This work has been undertaken in collaboration with Drs. Nick Martin and Margie Wright (Australia) and Dr. Paul Breslin (Monell Chemical Senses Center).

In rodents, the preference for naturally occurring sweeteners is partially genetically determined, and this has led to substantial progress in understanding the molecular basis of sweet perception. In 1999, Hoon *et al.*[8], identified two receptors, T1R1 and T1R2*, which were thought to be taste receptors because they were expressed in taste receptor cells and, in the case of *Tas1r1*, because the gene was near the *Sac* locus. The *Sac* locus partially accounts for saccharin preference in mice, and the location of *Tas1r1* was consistent with a role for this receptor in the transduction of sweet taste perception. However, as we subsequently demonstrated, genetic mapping studies of sequence variants in *Tas1r1* excluded this gene as a candidate for the *Sac* locus[13]. Another member of the T1R family was soon discovered, *Tas1r3*, which probably corresponds to the *Sac* locus[1,12,15–17,20]. Support for this comes from congenic and transgenic mice experiments[1,17] and the behaviour of cells expressing this receptor in functional assays[13,17,18].

Proteins from the T1R family apparently interact at the surface of the taste receptor cell to produce functional receptors. Based on the cellular co-localization of T1R3 and T1R2 it appears that receptor dimerization is necessary for sweet compounds to properly interact with the receptor complex[14–17].

There are human orthologs of all of these genes (TAS1R1, TAS1R2 and TAS1R3), and we wondered whether DNA sequence variability existed in these receptors, and if so, whether this sequence variability could account for individual differences in the perception or liking for sweet solutions. Sequencing of these receptors in humans is ongoing, but at least one polymorphism has been identified in TAS1R3, which changes an alanine to a threonine in the extracellular portion of the molecule. Studies to discover additional sequence variability within these receptors and phenotype-genotype comparisons are ongoing.

Most discussion of the role of taste in the development and maintenance of obesity has been based upon the premise that obese people may have a higher preference or intake of sweets and therefore gain more weight. However, whether obese individuals have an increased liking for sweet foods has been contentious, complicated by the difficulties of accurately measuring food intake in humans. To circumvent the problem of report bias, a recent study found that although obese subjects do not report eating more sweet foods, they have more oral bacteria associated with sugar intake. This is a strategy that may outwit the report bias that plagues food intake research[3].

Rodent models have provided provocative data about the association of sucrose intake and obesity. In a recent report by Tordoff[23], rats offered one tubes of sucrose solution and five tubes of water became heavier and fatter than did those not offered sucrose solutions[23]. When rats were offered six tubes of sucrose and one tube of water they became even more obesity compared with other groups. The results of this study suggest that the more sources of sucrose offered, the more rats will eat, and the more weight they will gain. Little imagination is needed to extrapolate this experimental paradigm to current human circumstance of abundant and highly sweetened food and drink.

As mentioned above, metabolic state changes the preference for sweet solutions. One such phenomenon is the 'Cabananc effect'. Humans reduce their ratings of the pleasantness of sweet solutions after ingesting a large volume of sugar water relative to before ingesting sweetened water. The mechanisms for the decrease in pleasantness ratings are unknown. A recent study suggested that taste cells contain leptin receptors, and when the leptin receptors are not functioning adequately, as is the case in rats with mutations in the gene, then there is an increased avidity for sweet fluids[11]. Therefore, there may be a negative feedback loop such that increased body fat or food intake increases plasma leptin levels which in turn decrease the peripheral sensitivity to sweeteners. If the peripheral taste system is responsive to metabolic state, then this avenue of research may suggest potential new approach for obesity therapeutics.

The liking for sweet foods is but one piece of the puzzle of human obesity. The addition of prodigious amounts of pure sugar into the diet of man is a recent occurrence in the evolutionary time frame, one that coincides well with the development of obesity. Although nutritional advice changes frequently, the directive to reduce consumption of refined sugars has been one of the most stable nutritional

---

* The nomenclature is as follows: the structural gene for this receptor family is TAS1R, where TAS = taste, 1 = the first family discovered, and R = receptor. The proteins, in contrast to the genes, are referred to as T1RX. There are three protein members of this family identified to date, T1R1, T1R2 and T1R3. Gene symbols in humans are in UPPER CASE whereas symbols for mice are in lower case and are *italicized*.

recommendations. An aggressive research programme to understand individual differences in the preference for highly sweetened foods and drinks coupled with an investigation into the underlying mechanisms for these differences will pave the way to a better understanding of the treatment of obesity and other nutritional disorders.

Acknowledgements: This work was supported by National Institutes of Health grants R01DC00882 (GKB), R03DC03509, R01DC04188 and R01DK55853 (DRR), and R03DC03853 (AAB), and by a special grant from the Ambrose Monell Foundation. The assistance of R. Arlen Price in the early stages of this work is gratefully acknowledged. Michael G. Tordoff commented on a draft of this manuscript.

References

1. Bachmanov AA, Li X, Reed DR, Ohmen JD, Li S, Chen Z *et al*. Positional cloning of the mouse saccharin preference (Sac) locus. *Chem Senses* 2001; 26(7): 925–33.

2. Bachmanov AA, Tordoff MG, Beauchamp GK. Sweetener preference of C57BL/6ByJ and 129P3/J mice. *Chem Senses* 2001; 26(7): 905–13.

3. Barkeling B, Andersson I, Lindroos AK, Birkhed D, Rossner S. Intake of sweet foods and counts of cariogenic microorganisms in obese and normal-weight women. *Eur J Clin Nutr* 2001; 55(10): 850–855.

4. Cabanac M, Duclaux R. Specificity of internal signals in producing satiety for taste stimuli. *Nature* 1970; 227(261): 966–967.

5. Desor JA, Beauchamp GK. Longitudinal changes in sweet preferences in humans. *Physiol Behav* 1987; 39(5): 639–641.

6. Goetzi FR, Ahokas AJ, Payne JG. Occurrence in normal individuals of diurnal variations in acuity of the sense of taste for sucrose. *J Appl Physiol* 1950; 2: 619–26.

7. Greene LS, Desor JA, Maller O. Heredity and experience: their relative importance for the development of taste preference in man. *J Comp Physiol Psychol* 1975; 89(3): 279–284.

8. Hoon MA, Adler E, Lindemeier J, Battey JF, Ryba NJ, Zuker CS. Putative mammalian taste receptors: a class of taste-specific GPCRs with distinct topographic selectivity. *Cell* 1999; 96(4): 541–551.

9. Inoue M, McCaughey SA, Bachmanov AA, Beauchamp GK. Whole nerve chorda tympani responses to sweeteners in C57BL/6ByJ and 129P3/J mice. *Chem Senses* 2001; 26(7): 915–923.

10. Ishii H. Consumer perceptions of products containing sweeteners in Asian countries. *World Rev Nutr Diet* 1999; 85: 164–70.

11. Kawai K, Sugimcito K, Nakashima K, Miura H, Ninomiya Y. Leptin as a modulator of sweet taste sensitivities in mice. *Proc Natl Acad Sci USA* 2000; 97(20): 11044–11049.

12. Kitagawa M, Kusakabe Y, Miura H, Ninomiya Y, Hino A. Molecular genetic identification of a candidate receptor gene for sweet taste. *Biochem Biophys Res Commun* 2001; 283(1): 236–242.

13. Li X, lnoue M, Reed DR, Huque T, Puchaiski RB, Tordoff MG *et al*. High-resolution genetic mapping of the saccharin preference locus (*Sac*) and the putative sweet taste receptor (T1R1) gene (*Gpr70*) to mouse distal Chromosome 4. *Mamm Genome* 2001; 12(1): 13–16.

14. Li X, Staszewski L, Xu H, Durick K, Zoiier M, Adler E. Human receptors for sweet and umami taste. *Proc Natl Acad Sci* 2002; 99: 4692–6.

15. Max M, Shanker YG, Huang L, Rong M, Liu Z, Campagne F *et al*. *Tas1r3*, encoding a new candidate taste receptor, is allelic to the sweet responsiveness locus Sac. *Nature Genet* 2001; 28(1): 58–63.

16. Montmayeur JP, Liberies SD, Matsunami H, Buck LB. A candidate taste receptor gene near a sweet taste locus. *Nat Neurosci* 2001; 4(5): 492–498.

17. Nelson G, Chandrashekar J, Hoon MA, Feng L, Zhao G, Ryba NJ, Zuker CS. An amino-acid taste receptor. *Nature* 2002; 416(6877): 199–202.

18. Nelson G, Hoon MA, Chandrashekar J, Zhang Y, Ryba NJ, Zuker CS. Mammalian sweet taste receptors. *Cell* 2001; 106(3): 381–390.

19. Reed DR, Bachmanov AA, Beauchamp GK, Tordoff MG, Price RA. Heritable variation in food preferences and their contribution to obesity. *Behav Genet* 1997; 27(4)373–387.

20. Sainz E, Korley JN, Battey JF, Sullivan SL. Identification of a novel member of the TIR family of putative taste receptors. *J Neurochem* 2001; 77(3): 896–903.

21. Schiffman SS, Graham BG, Sattely-Miller EA, Peterson-Dancy M. Elevated and sustained desire for sweet taste in african-americans: a potential factor in the development of obesity. *Nutrition* 2000; 16(10): 886–893.

22. Thompson DA, Moskowitz HR, Campbell RG. Effects of body weight and food intake on pleasantness ratings for a sweet stimulus. *J Appl Physiol* 1976; 41(1): 77–83.

23. Tordoff MG. Obesity by choice: the powerful influence of nutrient vailability on nutrient intake. *Am J Physiol Regul Integr Comp Physiol* 2002; 282(5): R1536–1539.

Progress in Obesity Research: 9. Edited by *Geraldo Medeiros-Neto, Alfredo Halpern and Claude Bouchard*

CHAPTER 66

Genetics of eating disorders

Johannes Hebebrand and Anke Hinney

Clinical Research Group, Department of Child and Adolescent Psychiatry, Philipps-University of Marburg, Hans-Sachs-Str. 6, D-35033 Marburg, Germany
[e-mail: johannes.hebebrand@med.uni-marburg.de]

Twin and family studies

Anorexia nervosa and bulimia nervosa are complex diseases that are commonly defined by either the 'Diagnostic and Statistical Manual of Mental Disorders'-criteria (DSM, American Psychiatric Association, 1994) or the 'International Classification of Mental and Behavioural Disorders'-criteria (ICD-10, World Health Organization).

Evidence from family and twin studies suggests a genetic contribution to the aetiology of both anorexia and bulimia nervosa[3,10,22]. Holland *et al.*[16] showed proband-wise concordance rates for anorexia nervosa of 0.71 for monozygotic twins and 0.1 for dizygotic twins. Heritability estimates based on these rates ranged from 0.86 to 0.98[16]. Most twin studies have shown a higher concordance rate for monozygotic twins (approximately 0.44) than for dizygotic twins (approximately 0.13). Walters and Kendler[27] could not detect a genetic component to anorexia nervosa. They analysed a large epidemiological female twin sample (n = 2,163); only a small number of twins had retrospectively diagnosed anorexia nervosa; concordance rates were higher for dizygotic than for monozygotic twins. Interestingly, co-twins of twins with anorexia nervosa had significantly lower body mass index (BMI in kg/m^2) and higher depression rates than co-twins of unaffected twins.

Controlled family studies found an average 3 per cent lifetime risk of anorexia nervosa in first-degree relatives of patients compared to 0 per cent in about 1000 relatives of control subjects[6,21,26] equivalent to an approximate relative risk of at least 10. Anorexia nervosa was found to be rare in 1831 relatives of 504 patients with eating disorders, whereas full and partial syndromes aggregated in both anorexic and bulimic probands[26]. Relative risks were 11.3 and 12.3 for the full syndrome of anorexia nervosa in first-degree female relatives of patients with anorexia nervosa and bulimia nervosa, respectively[26], suggesting that specific genes can predispose to both eating disorders. The relative risks for bulimia nervosa were 4.2 and 4.4 for first-degree female relatives of patients with anorexia and bulimia nervosa, respectively. Overlapping of the genetic predisposition to both bulimia nervosa and depression was found in the Virginia twin study[28].

Candidate gene studies

The molecular genetic analysis of a complex phenotype basically involves two approaches: (i) association studies ('case-control-studies'), and (ii) linkage studies. Both approaches have been used in molecular genetic studies of eating disorders. The candidate gene approach relies on genetic, physiological, biochemical or pharmacological evidence to show the involvement of a specific gene in the phenotype under consideration. Candidate gene studies in eating disorders need to consider the following clinical considerations: (a) The prevalence of anorexia nervosa and bulimia nervosa is considerably higher in females (ratio 9: 1); (b) The manifestation periods for both anorexia nervosa and bulimia nervosa are predominantly in puberty and late adolescence, respectively; (c) Approximately 30 per cent of patients with anorexia nervosa later on develop bulimia nervosa, the opposite sequence is less frequent; (d) Obsessive compulsive behaviour is frequent in anorexia nervosa (Kaye *et al.*, 2000a; Kaye and Strober, 1999a).

In general terms, the narrower the pathways into the respective eating disorder, the fewer genes are likely to be involved. An example of such a narrow pathway into anorexia nervosa is the dysregulation of maintenance of a normal body weight upon weight loss, for whatever reason, during the critical age period. If, however, several different pathways can lead to the eating disorder, the greater the heterogeneity and the smaller the effect of a predisposing allele is likely to be.

Any neurochemical or neurobiological disturbance that persists upon recovery might be trait-related and implicated in the aetiology of the disorder. Studies pertaining to long-term follow-up patients with anorexia nervosa have shown that disturbances of monoaminergic pathways and weight regulation continue after recovery[5,9,19]. Based on results of these studies, genes involved in the serotonergic and dopaminergic systems and in weight regulation can be perceived as candidate genes. Because psychopathological features and extremely low body weight are inseparable in anorexia nervosa, this eating disorder can be considered as an extreme weight condition[10].

The role of variation in genes of the serotonergic system has been investigated extensively. This neurotransmitter system is regulated by tryptophan hydroxylase, the 5-HT transporter (SERT) and by several 5-HT receptors.Serotonin (5-hydroxytryptamine; 5-HT) is involved in a broad range of biological, physiological and behavioural functions[1,8]. Several lines of evidence implicate the serotonergic system in body weight regulation and more specifically in eating behaviour[1,8,24] and eating disorders[2,17]. In long-term weight-restored patients with anorexia nervosa or bulimia nervosa, 5-hydroxyindolacetic acid (5-HIAA) levels were elevated in cerebrospinal fluid in comparison with those of controls, suggesting that hyperserotonergic function is a trait marker in eating disorders[19]. The increased brain serotonin activity might pathophysiologically predispose to the development of eating disorders. In addition, increased serotonergic neurotransmission could account for characteristic psychopathological features such as perfectionism, rigidity and obsessiveness frequently associated with anorexia nervosa[18,20]. Despite this evidence for the involvement of the serotonergic system candidate gene studies including a meta-analysis for a 5-HT 2A receptor promoter polymorphism (−1438 A/G) have mostly been negative (Table 1).

The female predominance of anorexia nervosa, bulimia nervosa and extreme obesity[10] has led to the hypothesis that sex hormones might be involved in the development of weight extremes and in the aetiology of eating disorders. This is particularly so for anorexia nervosa where both the female predominance and the frequent onset around puberty point to a possible involvement of female sex hormones in the development of this eating disorder[29]. Estrogen levels increase dramatically with the onset of puberty in females. An exaggerated sensitivity of brain structures to the rising estrogen levels possibly mediated by estrogen receptors might represent a predisposition to the development of anorexia nervosa.

A systematic mutation screeing of the coding region of the *ESR2* revealed that the frequency of the 1082-G allele of a silent 1082 G/A polymorphism was increased in patients with anorexia nervosa compared to that of controls (obese and underweight) and of patients with bulimia nervosa. No evidence for an association between a second polymorphism (1730A/G) in the *ESR2* and anorexia nervosa was found[23]. In a second and not readily compatible study[4] the A-allele of the 1082 G/A polymorphism was more frequent in patients with anorexia nervosa (Table 1).

There has been a remarkable increase in the number of genetic studies pertaining to the regulation of body weight in the last few years. Principally, centrally expressed candidate genes appear more promising in eating disorders. Nevertheless, SNPs in peripherally expressed genes involved in weight regulation including genes for uncoupling protiens have been analysed in eating disorders (Table 1)[14]. Patients with anorexia nervosa have extremely low circulating leptin levels[9,10], thus signalling semi-starvation to the brain. Recently, it was shown that females with a past history of anorexia nervosa (followed-up 10 years after in-patient treatment) have a lower per cent body fat and a trend to lower serum leptin levels than the controls[5]. In other studies patients who had recovered from eating disorders also had reduced serum leptin levels after adjustment for BMI and/or fat mass, suggesting that relative hypoleptinaemia might be a trait marker in eating disorders. A mutation analysis of the coding region and part of the promoter region of the leptin gene in patients with anorexia nervosa has yielded negative results. Association studies based on other genes involved in weight regulation have also been negative (Table1).

Obesity has been identified as a risk factor for the development of BN. Accordingly, genotypes predisposing to obesity might be detected in patients with BN. A mutation screen in the melanocortin-4 receptor gene (*MC4R*) revealed that a single patient with both extreme obesity and BN had a haplo-insufficiency mutation in the *MC4R*. For the first time a genotype predisposing to obesity has been detected in an extremely obese patient with BN[12].

Table 1. Summary of association and transmission disequilibrium tests (TDT) pertaining to polymorphisms in different candidate genes in patients with anorexia nervosa (AN) or bulimia nervosa (BN)

Candidate gene[+]	Analysed polymorphism or genetic marker	P values for association tests (or TDT) of the rare allele to AN	P values for association tests (or TDT) of the rare allele to BN	References
Agouti related protein	526G>A (silent) is in linkage disequilibrium with Ala-67-Thr 605C>T (silent)	0.015	ND	Vink et al., 2001
β₃-adrenoceptor	Trp-64-Arg	NS	ND	
		NS (NS)	ND	Hinney et al., 1997b
Catechol-o-methyltransferase	Val-158-Met	(0.015)	ND	Frisch et al., 2001
Dopamine D4 receptor	13 bp deletion	NS	ND	Hinney et al., 1999c
	48 bp deletion	NS (NS)	ND	
Dopamine D3 receptor	BalI polymorphism in exon 1	NS	ND	Bruins-Slot et al., 1998
Estrogen β-receptor	1082G>A (silent)	0.04 for G-allele[a] sig. for A allele	NS	[a]Rosenkranz et al., 1998a
	1730A>G (silent)	NS	NS	[b]Eastwood et al., ????
Leptin	−1387G>A (promoter)	NS (NS)	NS[a]	[a]Hinney et al., 1998b
Melanocortin MC₄ receptor	Val-103-Ile	NS	NS	Hinney et al., 1999b
	Ile-251-Thr	NS	NS	
	Try-35-Stop		detected in a single obese patient	Hebebrand et al., 2002
Neuropeptid Y Y₁ receptor	PstI-polymorphism within the first intron	NS	ND	Rosenkranz et al., 1998b
Neuropeptid Y Y₅ receptor	1333G>A (silent)	NS	ND	Rosenkranz et al., 1998b
Pro-opiomelanocortin	Insertion of 9 bp between codon 73 and 74	NS	ND	Hinney et al., 1998a
5-HT₁ᵦreceptor	G861C polymorphism	ND	0.001 minimum lifetime BMI	Levitan et al., 2001
5-HT₁ᴅᵦreceptor	Phe-124-Cys	NS	ND	Hinney et al., 1999a

Table 1. *Continued.*

Candidate gene[+]	Analysed polymorphism or genetic marker	P values for association tests (or TDT) of the rare allele to AN	P values for association tests (or TDT) of the rare allele to BN	References
5-HT $_{2A}$receptor	−1438G>A (promoter)	0.02[a], NS[b,c,f,h,i], 0.005[d] 0.0001[e,g], 0.00014[k], (NS)[m]	NS[e,f,g], <0.01[i], 0.02[k]	[a]Collier et al., 1997; [b]Hinney et al., 1997c; [c]Campbell et al., 1998; [d]Sorbi et al., 1998; [e]Enoch et al. 1998; [f]Ziefler et al.,1999; [g]Nacmias et al., 1999; [h]Ando et al., 2001; [i]Nishiguchi et al., 2001; [k]Ricca et al., 2002; [m]Gorwood et al., 2002
	Thr-25-Asn	NS[bg]	NS[g]	
	102T>C (silent)	NS[g]	NS[g]	
	516C>T (silent)	NS[b]	NS[g]	
	His-452-Tyr	NS[bg]	NS[g]	
5-HT $_{2C}$receptor	Cys-23-Ser	NS[a,b,c]	NS[a,b]	[a]Nacmias et al., 1999; [b]Burnet et al., 1999; [c]Hinney et al., unpub. data
5-HT $_{7}$receptor	Pro-279-Leu	NS	ND	Hinney et al., 199a
Norepinephrine transporter gene promoter polymorphic region	4-bp deletion (S4) or insertion (L4) in AAGG4 repeat island	(TDT 87 Australian families; $P = 0.0052$)	ND	Urwin et al., 2002
Potassium channel hSKCa3	Coding CAG repeat	(0.0013 for longer alleles)	ND	Koronyo-Hamaoui et al., 2002
Serotonin transporter (SERT, 5-HTT)	44 bp Del/Ins (promoter)	NS[a,b,c] (NS)[a]	< 0.000[b]	[a]Hinney et al., 1997a; [b]Di Bella et al., 2000; [c]Sundramurthy et al., 2000; [d]Fumeron et al., 2001
Tryptophan hydroxylase	1095T>C (silent)	NS	ND	Han et al., 1999
Tumour necrosis factor alpha	3 promoter SNPs (−1031T>C; −863C>A; −857C>T	NS	ND	Ando et al., 2001
Uncoupling protein 2, 3	Flanking microsatellite markers	S for certain alleles[a], NS[b]		Campbell et al. Ho et al., 2002

[+]Genes in alphabetical order; AN, Anorexia nervosa; BN, Bilimia nervosa; TDT, Transmission disequilibrium test; S, Significant; NS, Not significant; ND, Not determined. For a complete reference list see Hinney, Remschmidt and Hedebrand, 2000. [a,b,c,etc.]refer to the references in the same row.

Genome wide linkage study

Despite considerable efforts, none of the candidate gene analyses has yielded unequivocal and clearly replicable evidence for the involvement of specific alleles in the aetiology of eating disorders. It has to kept in mind that molecular genetic studies pertaining to eating disorders have only recently been initiated on a larger scale. Furthermore, the candidate gene approach in anorexia nervosa is hampered by the fact that there is no clear cut evidence implicating a specific regulatory system.

In this situation a systematic genome-wide approach offers a viable alternative to detect genes involved in the aetiology of eating disorders. For anorexia nervosa, an international, multisite collaborative group (The Price Foundation Collaborative Group)[21] completed the collection of a large study group of patients with anorexia nervosa and affected relatives. All of the 196 ascertained index patients, mostly of Caucasian origin met DSM-IV criteria for anorexia nervosa; all 237 affected relatives met DSM-IV criteria for anorexia nervosa, bulimia nervosa, or eating disorders not otherwise specified. There were 229 relative pairs informative for linkage analysis; 64 per cent of the proband-relative pairs were anorexia nervosa-anorexia nervosa, 20 per cent were anorexia nervosa-bulimia nervosa, and 16 per cent were anorexia nervosa-eating disorders not otherwise specified.

The genome-wide linkage study of this study group, using 386 microsatellite markers, revealed a single multipoint nonparametric linkage score (NPL) above 1.5 on chromosome 4 (D4S2367). NPL > 1 were observed at an additional marker (D4S403) on chromosome 4 and on chromosomes 11 (D11S1392), 13 (D13S796) and 15 (D15S657), respectively. In a post hoc analysis only those 37 families were included in whom at least two individuals had the restricting type of anorexia nervosa. In this subgroup the highest NPL of 3.03 was obtained on chromosome 1p (D1S3721). In addition, all the regions which showed a NPL > 1 in the entire sample revealed NPL ≥ 1.5 in restricting subgroup. Interestingly, within the families that comprised this subgroup individuals affected with other eating disorders than the restricting subtype of anorexia nervosa also contributed to the positive NPL.

Conclusions and research directions

In forthcoming years we will hopefully gain a deeper insight into the genetic basis of eating disorders. Analysis of the genetic mechanisms underlying weight regulation is now progressing very rapidly. Results of this field of genetic research might prove valuable for the analysis of eating disorders. Both sets of results in both fields will be relevant for pharmacological research to identify new treatment strategies.

Acknowledgements: Our studies are funded by the Deutsche Forschungsgemeinschaft, the Bundesministerium für Bildung und Forschung and by the European Union (Framework V 'Factors in healthy eating').

References

Readers are invited to check Hinney, Remschmidt and Hebebrand (Eur J Pharmacology 410: 147–159; 2000) for a complete list of references.

1. Blundell JE, Lawton CL, Halford JC. Serotonin, eating behavior, and fat intake. *Obes Res* 1995; 3 (Suppl 4): S471–S476.
2. Brewerton TD, Jimerson DC. Studies of serotonin function in anorexia nervosa. *Psychiatry Res* 1996; 62: 31–42.
3. Bulik CM, Sullivan PF, Wade TD, Kendler KS. Twin studies of eating disdorders: a review. *Int J Eat Disord* 2000; 27: 1–20.
4. Eastwood H, Brown KM, Markovic D, Pieri LF. Variation in the ESR1 and ESR2 genes and genetic susceptibility to anorexia nervosa. *Mol Psychiatry* 2002; 7: 86–9.
5. Frey J, Hebebrand J, Muller B, Ziegler A, Blum WF, Remschmidt H *et al.* Reduced body fat in long-term followed-up female patients with anorexia nervosa. *J Psychiatr Res* 2000; 34: 83–8.
6. Gershon ES, Schreiber JL, Hamovit JR, Dibble ED, Kaye W, Nurnberger JI Jr *et al.* Clinical findings in patients with anorexia nervosa and affective illness in their relatives. *Am J Psychiatry* 1984; 141: 1419–22.
7. Price DE, Halmi KA, Fichter MM, Strober M, Woodside DB, Treasure JT *et al.* Evidence for a susceptibility gene for anorexia nervosa on chromosome 1. *Am J Hum Genet* 2002; 70: 787–92.
8. Halford JC, Blundell JE. Separate systems for serotonin and leptin in appetite control. *Ann Med* 2000; 32: 222–32.
9. Hebebrand J, Blum WF, Barth N, Coners H, Englaro P, Juul A *et al.* Leptin levels in patients with anorexia nervosa are reduced in the acute stage and elevated upon short-term weight restoration. *Mol Psychiatry* 1997; 2: 330–4.
10. Hebebrand J, Remschmidt H. Anorexia nervosa viewed as an extreme weight condition: genetic implications. *Hum Genet* 1995; 95: 1–11.

11. Hebebrand J, van der Heyden J, Devos R, Köpp W, Herpertz S, Remschmidt H, Herzog W. Plasma concentrations of obese protein in anorexia nervosa. *Lancet* 1995; 346: 1624–5.

12. Hebebrand J, Fichter M, Gerber G, Gorg T, Hermann H, Geller F *et al.* Genetic predisposition to obesity in bulimia nervosa: a mutation screen of the melanocortin-4 receptor gene. *Mol Psychiatry* 2002; 7: 647–51.

13. Hinney A, Remschmidt H, Hebebrand J. Candidate gene polymorphisms in eating disorders. *Eur J Pharmacol* 2000; 410: 147–59.

14. Hinney A, Lentes KU, Rosenkranz K, Barth N, Roth H, Ziegler A *et al.* Beta 3-adrenergic-receptor allele distributions in children, adolescents and young adults with obesity, underweight or anorexia nervosa. *Int J Obes Relat Metab Disord* 1997; 21: 224–30.

15. Hinney A, Schmidt A, Nottebom K, Heibült O, Becker I, Ziegler A *et al.* Several mutations in the melanocortin-4 receptor gene including a nonsense and a frameshift mutation associated with dominantly inherited obesity in humans. *J Clin Endocrinol Metab* 1999; 84: 1483–6.

16. Holland AJ, Sicotte N, Treasure J. Anorexia nervosa: evidence for a genetic basis. *J Psychosom Res* 1988; 32: 561–71.

17. Jimerson DC, Lesem MD, Kaye WH, Brewerton TD. Low serotonin and dopamine metabolite concentrations in cerebrospinal fluid from bulimic patients with frequent binge episodes. *Arch Gen Psychiatry* 1992; 49: 132–8.

18. Kaye W, Strober M. The neurobiology of eating disorders. In: *Neurobiological foundations of mental illness.* Charney DS, Nestler EJ, Bunney BS (eds), pp. 891–906. New York: Oxford University Press, 1999.

19. Kaye WH, Greeno CG, Moss H, Fernstrom J, Fernstrom M, Lilenfeld LR *et al.* Alterations in serotonin activity and psychiatric symptoms after recovery from bulimia nervosa. *Arch Gen Psychiatry* 1998; 55: 927–35.

20. Kaye WH, Klump KL, Frank GK, Strober M. Anorexia and bulimia nervosa. *Annu Rev Med* 2000; 51: 299–313.

21. Kaye WH, Lilenfeld LR, Berrettini WH, Strober M, Devlin B, Klump KL *et al.* A search for susceptibility loci for anorexia nervosa: methods and sample description. *Biol Psychiatry* 2000; 47: 794–803.

22. Kipman A, Gorwood P, Mouren-Simeoni MC, Ades J. Genetic factors in anorexia nervosa. *Eur Psychiatry* 1999; 14: 189–98.

23. Rosenkranz K, Hinney A, Ziegler A, Hermann H, Fichter M, Mayer H *et al.* Systematic mutation screening of the estrogen receptor beta gene in probands of different weight extremes: identification of several genetic variants. *J Clin Endocrinol Metab* 1998; 83: 4524–7.

24. Son JH, Baker H, Park DH, Joh TH. Drastic and selective hyperinnervation of central serotonergic neurons in a lethal neurodevelopmental mouse mutant, Anorexia (anx). Brain. *Res Mol Brain Res* 1994; 25: 129–34.

25. Strober M. Family-genetic studies of eating disorders. *J Clin Psychiatry* 1991; 52: 9–12.

26. Strober M, Freeman R, Lampert C, Diamond J, Kaye W. Controlled family study of anorexia nervosa and bulimia nervosa: evidence of shared liability and transmission of partial syndromes. *Am J Psychiatry* 2000; 157: 393–401.

27. Walters EE, Kendler KS. Anorexia nervosa and anorexic-like syndromes in a population-based female twin sample. *Am J Psychiatry* 1995; 152: 64–71.

28. Walters EE, Neale MC, Eaves LJ, Heath AC, Kessler RC, Kendler KS. Bulimia nervosa and major depression: a study of common genetic and environmental factors. *Psychol Med* 1992; 22: 617–22.

29. Young JK. Estrogen and the aetiology of anorexia nervosa. *Neurosci Biohav Rev* 1990; 15: 327–31.

Progress in Obesity Research: 9. Edited by *Geraldo Medeiros-Neto, Alfredo Halpern* and *Claude Bouchard*
©2003 John Libbey Eurotext Ltd, pp. 313–319.

CHAPTER 67

Mouse models for Prader-Willi and Angelman syndromes offer insights into novel obesity mechanisms

Robert D. Nicholls[1,2], Mihaela Stefan[1], Hong Ji[4], Yong Qi[3], R. Scott Frayo[5], Robert H. Wharton[6], Madhu S. Dhar[7], David E. Cummings[5], Mark I. Friedman[4] and Rexford S. Ahima[3]

[1]*Center for Neurobiology and Behavior, Department of Psychiatry,* [2]*Department of Genetics, and* [3]*Department of Medicine, University of Pennsylvania, Philadelphia, PA, USA;* [4]*Monell Chemical Senses Center, Philadelphia, PA, USA;* [5]*Department of Medicine, VA Puget Sound Health Care System, University of Washington, Seattle, WA, USA;* [6]*Spaulding Rehabilitation Hospital and Massachusetts General Hospital, Boston, MA;* [7]*University of Tennessee, Knoxville, TN, USA*
[e-mail: robertn@mail.med.upenn.edu]

Obesity in PWS and AS, and genetic basis of these disorders

Prader-Willi and Angelman syndromes (PWS and AS) are neurobehavioural and developmental syndromes that are associated with genetic defects of opposite parental origin in chromosome 15q11-q13. PWS infants have hypotonia and severe failure-to-thrive, with lack of the usual survival skills of an infant, including lack of cry and lack of contact with the mother[1]. Beginning from 1–3 years of age, there is onset of hyperphagia and severe obesity, an abnormal adipose tissue and muscle composition, short stature with growth hormone (GH) deficiency, hypogonadotropic hypogonadism, and mild-moderate mental retardation with behavioural disorders, including obsessive-compulsive disorder[2]. The hyperphagia in PWS is usually described as a failure to reach satiety and hence these individuals are constantly hungry. Without strict behavioural and dietary control, PWS individuals have severe mortality by the second or third decade of life due to cardiac or respiratory failure. Most morbidity in the syndrome occurs from complications of obesity, including kyphosis, sleep apnoea, lipolymphoedema, hypercholesterolaemia, impaired glucose tolerance, diabetes mellitus type 2, hypertriglyceridaemia, hypertension, and heart failure[3]. Occurring at a frequency of ~ 1/15,000 births, PWS is the most common form of genetic obesity and as such an understanding of this disorder should yield significant insights into the basis of obesity.

PWS is caused by loss of function of a unique set of at least ten genes from chromosome 15q11-q13 that normally only function when inherited from the father[4] (Figs. 1a, b). These defects include paternally derived 4 Mb deletions, maternal uniparental disomy (UPD) and paternally inherited imprinted defects[4]. The paternally expressed loci potentially involved in PWS include several intronless genes (*NDN, MAGEL2,* and *MKRN3/ZNF127*) as well as the complex *SNURF-SNRPN* polycistronic locus that encodes two proteins (SNURF, SmN) and at least 5 subfamilies of small nucleolar RNAs or snoRNAs (Figs. 1a, b), all nuclear in function and that may represent a mammalian operon[4–6]. It is also possible that additional genes will be identified in the PWS region as a consequence of the ongoing human and mouse genome sequencing projects, as several DNA sequence gaps remain within human 15q11-q13 and the homologous mouse chromosome 7C. Intriguingly, the ten known candidate genes in the PWS imprinted domain all appear to be regulatory in function and are likely to regulate several genetic pathways (Fig. 1c).

The basis of PWS is typically ascribed to hypothalamic deficiency, although peripheral metabolic deficiencies are also possible. The end result physiologically includes GH, IGF1 and IGFBP-3 deficien-

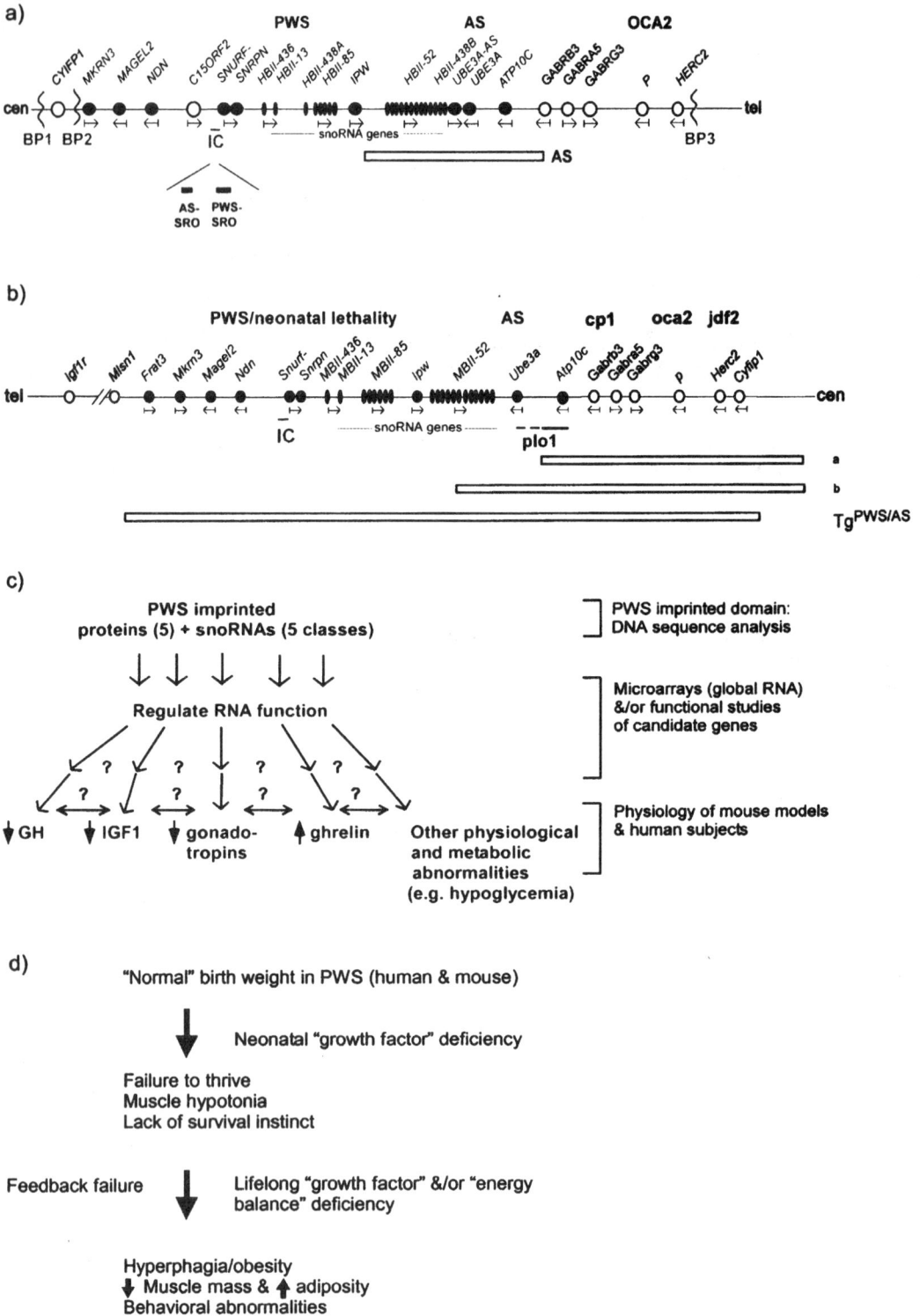

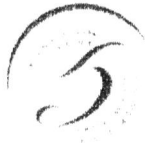

University of Glamorgan
Learning Resources Centre -
Glyntaff
Self Issue Receipt (GT1)

**Customer name: MR
OLUWATOBA ABIODUN**
Customer ID: ***********902

Title: Progress in obesity research: 9

ID: 7312580872
**Due: 23:59 Friday, 11 January
2013**

Total items: 1
11/12/2012 15:46

Thank you for using the Self-Service
system
Diolch yn fawr

cies[3], although the molecular basis for these hormonal changes is unknown and additional abnormalities may yet be discovered in PWS. For example, it has recently been found that the orexigenic hormone ghrelin has abnormal, very high levels in PWS[7]. Ghrelin is involved in increasing food intake and peripherally administered ghrelin increases body weight in both humans and animal models. Furthermore, ghrelin is the endogenous ligand for the growth hormone secretagogue receptor (GHS-R), and has adipogenic effects in addition to the orexigenic effects[8]. Therefore, it has been hypothesized that high ghrelin may drive the hyperphagia, abnormal body composition, and GH deficiency in PWS, the latter perhaps through an override inhibition[7]. Nevertheless, it remains possible that hyperghrelinaemia is a normal physiological response to PWS people constantly being hungry, and this or alternative mechanisms need to be distinguished by further clinical and mouse model studies before therapeutic approaches can be considered.

In contrast to PWS, AS patients have a severe neurological disease, associated with loss of function of imprinted, maternal-only expression of the *UBE3A* gene in the cerebellum and hippocampus of the brain. Defects leading to loss of functional *UBE3A* include maternally derived 4 Mb deletions, paternal UPD, maternally inherited imprinted defects, maternally inherited *UBE3A* single gene mutations, and an unknown fifth class[4,9]. The major clinical characteristics of AS include developmental delay, severe mental retardation with a lack of speech, movement ataxia, hyperactivity, seizures, aggressive behaviour, and excessive inappropriate laughter[4,9]. AS subjects in two molecular subclasses (UPD and imprinting defect) also have obesity, extending the phenotype, and these subjects have a body mass index (BMI) in the 80th–100th percentile for age[9]. The AS patients in the chromosome deletion class are less likely to have a high BMI[9], which may be due to the more severe movement disorder, hyperactivity, or other characteristics of this class compared to other classes.

Genetic mapping in the mouse based on overlapping deletions have suggested that a strong candidate gene for the obesity phenotype is *Atp10c*, which maps adjacent to *Ube3a* (Fig. 1b)[10]. In humans, *ATP10C* is imprinted with predominantly maternal expression in human brain and lymphocytes[11,12]. Although it is unproven as yet whether the mouse *Atp10c* gene shows imprinted, maternal-specific expression, given its association with maternally inherited increased body fat, it is likely to be imprinted; indeed, identification of tissues, cell types and/or developmental stages showing *Atp10c* imprinting may provide an important clue to the basis of obesity from loss of function of this gene.

Fig. 1(a). Genetic structure of the human chromosome 15q11-q13 imprinted domain involved in Prader-Willi and Angelman syndromes (PWS and AS). For AS, *UBE3A* structural gene mutations or IC mutations in imprinting defect patients occur ~ 500 kb apart. For PWS, IC mutations also occur. Symbols are: shaded circles, imprinted genes (all paternally expressed except for *UBE3A* and *ATP10C*, which are maternally expressed); open circles, non-imprinted genes; line arrows, transcriptional orientation of genes; zig-zag lines, PWS/AS common deletion breakpoints (BP) that occur in ~75 per cent of patients; open bar, 1 Mb deletion causing AS on maternal inheritance within a single Japanese family[28]; *HBII-85* and *HBII-52* snoRNAs are repeated 24 and 47 times[29]; OCA2, oculocutaneous albinism type II; SRO, shortest region of microdeletion overlap; *IPW* is identified[6] as *SNURF-SNRPN* exons 59-61. Three other genes located between BP1 and BP2 are not shown (Chai et al., submitted).

Fig. 1(b). Genetic structure of the mouse chromosome 7C imprinted domain homologous to PWS and AS genes, and deletion mapping to define the *p*-locus obesity (plo1) locus. Symbols are as for Fig. 1a; plo1, p-locus-associated obesity; cp1, cleft palate 1; jdf2, juvenile development and fertility[2]. Copies of the *MBII-85* and *MBII-52* snoRNAs are interspersed within 5' and 3' *Ipw* exons, which is presumably part of an extended *Snurf-Snrpn* transcript, as in human. The *Atp10c* gene has not yet been proven to be maternally expressed in any tissue in the mouse but is a strong candidate gene for maternally inherited obesity (i.e. plo1). The bars represent deletions, either transgene (Tg) insertion and deletion[17] (TgPWS/AS) or radiation-induced deletions that define plo1 [(a, b)][10] (R.D. Nicholls, M. Dhar, J.K. Greally, D.K. Johnson, unpublished data)]. The centromeric extent of the two radiation-induced deletions is not shown, and three other genes in the *Cyfip1* region (Chai et al., submitted) are not shown.

Fig. 1(c). Molecular basis for the Prader-Willi syndrome. Paternally-expressed imprinted genes in the PWS domain are hypothesized to function as nuclear regulatory molecules that control several genetic pathways (vertical arrows) leading to known human[3,4,7] and novel mouse (Stefan et al., unpublished data) endocrinological and physiological abnormalities in PWS. Horizontal arrows indicate potential interactions between pathways, while a '?' indicates unknown numbers of steps and members of hypothetical genetic pathways. At right are listed approaches that can be utilized to further elucidate each stage of the genetic pathways in PWS. $\downarrow$, decreased levels; $\uparrow$, increased levels.

Fig. 1(d). Metabolic feedback failure hypothesis in PWS. The absence of an unknown 'growth factor' in PWS is hypothesized to lead to neonatal failure-to-thrive in PWS in human and mice, and, as a consequence of a failure in metabolic feedback, to subsequent hyperphagia of children and adults.

Hypotheses for the metabolic and/or physiological basis of PWS

As yet, there is no known primary anatomical, biochemical or physiological abnormality in PWS. Identified physiological endpoints in PWS, as discussed above, can at the present time be considered to be secondary changes of unknown aetiology. Therefore, genetics holds the key to this disorder, and in particular to understanding and developing therapy for the overriding drive to eat and obesity that is of greatest concern for the PWS patient and family. While ten candidate genes in a 'PWS gene region' have been identified, no single gene has yet been directly linked to any clinical aspect of PWS. More importantly, the evidence to date suggests that these 'primary PWS genes' are involved in gene regulation, and hence that whole pathways of secondary and perhaps further downstream genes will be defective in PWS (Fig. 1c). These pathways may diverge, and perhaps interact, to produce the known (GH, IGF1 and gonadotropin deficiencies, and hyperghrelinaemia) and unknown physiological abnormalities in PWS.

Many imprinted loci regulate embryonic growth and this may underlie the evolutionary origin of imprinting for these genes (see ref.[13]). In a similar way, the evolutionary basis for imprinting in the PWS/AS domain may have come from phenotypic selection for a paternally-derived factor(s) involved in postnatal growth as a consequence of genetic conflict over maternal resources until the time of weaning[5,14]. The PWS neonatal phenotype is clearly consistent with this model. This view, along with the findings of normal birth weight of PWS babies and mouse pups, leads to the suggestion that maternal factors and/or the placenta may 'protect' the PWS embryo. Alternatively, the PWS genes may not be functional until after birth. We propose that the imprinted, paternally-derived 15q11-q13 gene(s) control expression of a factor(s) involved in postnatal growth that regulates neonatal feeding, muscle tone and other aspects of infant arousal, attention and maternal contact, and all are deficient in the PWS neonate (Fig. 1d). This 'growth factor' may be a primary metabolic molecule, of unknown identity. We propose that a normal feedback mechanism is absent in PWS, leading directly to the subsequent insatiable appetite, obesity, and abnormal body composition (Fig. 1d), and that may also relate to the behavioural problems of the PWS child and adult.

Mutations in the primary, imprinted PWS genes may not be associated with obesity and/or eating disorders in the general population, given that the PWS genes may also regulate behavioural and other phenotypes. Nevertheless, it is quite likely that genes along the unknown genetic pathways in PWS (Fig. 1c) – and that map to other chromosomal locations – will be found to show mutations or sequence variants that impact eating behaviour, energy regulation, and obesity. Consequently, the identification of all steps along the genetic pathways in PWS is essential and will provide numerous additional candidates for obesity genes. Furthermore, it is quite likely that inactivating mutations in *ATP10C* might be associated with obesity in the absence of a neurological condition, and these will show maternal inheritance only. To identify such cases, it is critical that genome scans for obesity-related phenotypes take into account parental transmission independently from fathers and mothers.

Mouse models of PWS and AS

The human PWS/AS region in chromosome 15q11-q13 is homologous to the central part of mouse chromosome 7, with conservation of gene content and imprinted features (Fig. 1b)[4]. Mouse models of PWS have been developed that have maternal UPD, an imprinting defect, or a paternally-derived chromosome deletion[15–17]. Similarly, mouse models of AS have paternal UPD, a maternally-derived chromosome deletion, or a 'knockout' of the *Ube3a* gene[17–19]. All three PWS mouse models have a close to normal birth weight and appearance, but share a very similar failure-to-thrive with early postnatal lethal phenotype, including hypotonia and respiration difficulties, which is equivalent to that of PWS infants. The deletion model resulted from a transgene insertion into mouse chromosome 7C, with a viable, fertile phenotype on maternal transmission allowing maintenance of the line (these animals are expected to have the mild neurobehavioural features of AS 'knockout' mouse models[19]), but transmission through males results in the mouse PWS phenotype[17].

Despite the failure of PWS mouse models to survive beyond ~1 week, access to critical tissues that may be abnormal in PWS – and which are not available from patients – will lead to significant insights into the pathophysiological basis of the disorder. Furthermore, half the offspring of each litter from paternal transmission of the deletion model have the PWS mouse phenotype and half are wildtype (WT), allowing direct comparisons to be made. We are presently performing detailed physiological, hormonal, metabolic, and blood chemistry experiments with PWS versus WT littermates, and have found widespread abnormalities beginning about 1 day postnatally (unpublished data). These studies are also examining hepatic energy status, since hepatic energy metabolism can have profound effects on feeding behaviour[20]. In addition, microarray studies to identify abnormally regulated genes in PWS mice are essential to identify candidate genes comprising the genetic pathways in PWS (Fig. 1c). Altered signaling among the hypothalamic arcuate nucleus neurons that co-produce the appetite-stimulating neuropeptide Y (NPY) and agouti related peptide (AgRP) or that produce the appetite inhibiting peptide α-melanocyte stimulating hormone (α-MSH) result in eating disorders[21,22]. Among the alterations in PWS of gene expression from secondary genetic and physiological pathways, this might include these hypothalamic genes encoding neuropeptides involved in eating behaviour. By mRNA *in situ* hybridization in brain slices from 3-day-old neonatal PWS mice, we found that *Agrp* mRNA was significantly reduced in PWS while mRNA expression of proopiomelanocortin (*Pomc*, the gene encoding α-MSH) was increased, compared to WT littermates, but *Npy* levels did not differ between PWS and WT mice[23]. These changes would be predicted to decrease appetite stimulating and augment appetite-inhibiting signals, and may contribute to a relative decrease in feeding (failure-to-thrive) of PWS mice[23]. Neither NPY nor AgRP have been found to be abnormal in a small number of PWS portmortum samples[24]. Therefore, since ghrelin activates NPY/AgRP neurons and inhibits α-MSH neurons[8], and since ghrelin is abnormally high in PWS subjects[7], the changes in neuropeptide gene expression are not as might be expected. Nevertheless, we need to determine the ghrelin levels in neonatal mice in order to fully examine this hypothesis, and, additionally, the status of hypothalamic expression of ghrelin[8] in PWS is unknown in both human and mouse.

It also remains unknown as to whether an adult mouse model will show additional features of PWS, such as hyperphagia and obesity. Generation of single gene mutations in the mouse, including primary PWS genes and those within PWS genetic pathways, transgene rescue studies, and/or clinical treatment of PWS neonatal mice will be necessary to determine this. Although mutations have been made in several PWS region candidate genes in the mouse, none have yet provided insight into the obesity phenotype of PWS[4].

As noted above, AS mouse models with a chromosome deletion are viable and fertile[17], but these become obese after 4–6 months of life when fed a low fat diet. AS mice with UPD also have a severe late-onset obesity[18]. Importantly, mice heterozygous for two *p*-locus deletions have significantly increased body fat (*p*-locus-associated obesity, or plo1) when the deletion is of maternal as compared to paternal inheritance (Fig. 1b)[10]. Based on deletion mapping, the only candidate gene within the plo1 region is the *Atp10c* gene encoding a P-type ATPase[10], which is proposed to function as a phospholipid translocase[25]. Mice with maternal deletions can have 1.5 to 2 times the body fat of those with the same deletion inherited paternally, with all adipose tissue depots equally affected. *Atp10c* is expressed at highest levels in white adipose tissue and testis[10]. To gain insight into the molecular basis of AS-associated obesity, we are performing detailed physiological and metabolic studies of AS deletion and both plo1 deletion mouse models, fed low (10 per cent) and 40 per cent high fat diets. Studies of *Atp10c* expression and tissue-specific imprinting are also ongoing, since these are necessary to identify the critical tissue(s) for body fat regulation by this gene.

Mechanism of genomic imprinting

Genomic imprinting plays a key role in the regulation of genes in the PWS and AS genomic region. Imprinting refers to a modification of DNA and chromatin proteins that occurs in the male and female germ cells, and is further regulated in the early preimplantation embryo[4,13] (Ohta *et al.*, submitted). These 'epigenetic' changes dependent on the sex of the parent-of-origin then result in differential expression of parental alleles during embryogenesis and subsequent development of the offspring. The establishment of imprints for the twelve known imprinted loci in the 2 Mb PWS/AS imprinted region (Fig. 1a,b), including all paternally and maternally expressed loci, are not independently regulated but are coordinately controlled in *cis* by a genetic element termed the imprinting centre (IC)[4]. Although a detailed discussion is beyond the scope of this chapter and can be found elsewhere[4] (Ohta *et al.*, submitted), a brief summary is of interest given that this mechanism controls at least two different pathways to abnormal body weight regulation in PWS and AS, respectively.

Defects in the imprinting process in PWS and AS patients, with mutations inherited paternally or maternally, respectively, provided the key to unlocking the mystery of how the imprint mechanism occurs. These mutations are microdeletions of 5 to > 100 kb that form the PWS-SRO and AS-SRO (Fig. 1a) and define the IC, leading to altered expression and DNA methylation patterns of all twelve imprinted genes in the PWS/AS region. The IC is located at the 5' end of the complex *SNURF-SNRPN* locus, and includes a series of duplicated, alternative upstream promoters, with at least two in human and ten in mouse (Ohta *et al.*, submitted). Two transcription factors that are putatively involved in somatic gene expression and in imprint establishment at each of these promoters have been identified.

Their activity at the upstream promoters during oogenesis and early preimplantation embryo development, or at the downstream *SNURF-SNRPN* promoter during spermatogenesis or later preimplantation embryo development correlates with the maternal or paternal imprint, respectively, suggesting that this controls the establishment of the imprints (Ohta *et al.*, submitted).

Concluding statements

Although a significant amount has been learnt about the homeostatic control of feeding behaviour, storage and utilization of fuels[26,27], there is much to learn and novel animal models for human disorders associated with obesity, such as PWS and AS as described here will play an important role in furthering our understanding. Future studies will identify the contribution of variation in genes within PWS genetic pathways as well as the *ATP10C* gene to human obesity and diabetes. These studies should aid the future development of rationale drug design or therapeutic approaches for obesity and diabetes-related phenotypes in PWS, AS, and the general population. In particular, PWS and AS mouse models will be invaluable for investigating potential therapeutic intervention approaches. Identification of the genetic pathways that control abnormal feeding behaviour in PWS, both a lack of feeding and survival skills in infants and the inability to stop eating in children and adults, as well as the basis of obesity in AS, can also be expected to shed significant light on genetic and physiological pathways involved in feeding behaviour and metabolism.

Note added in proof: The mouse *Atp10c* gene has been shown to be preferentially maternally expressed in several brain regions[30].

Acknowledgements: Work by the authors is funded from NIH grants HD36079 and HD31491 (RDN), DK53393 and DK45895 (MSD), DK53109 and DK36339 (MIF), a DERC pilot project under NIH P30-DK19525-26 (RDN and RSA), and the March of Dimes Birth Defects Foundation (RDN). We also acknowledge the wisdom of Dr. Richard Longnecker who established the PWS/AS transgenic mouse model in use in our laboratories.

References

1. Wharton RH, Levine K. Towards a new understanding of Prader-Willi syndrome: analysis and treatment recommendations. *The Gathered View* 1999; 8–12.

2. Cassidy SB. Prader-Willi syndrome. *J Med Genet* 1997; 34: 917–23.

3. Partsch C-J, Lammer C, Gillessen-Kaesbach G, Pankau R. Adult patients with Prader-Willi syndrome: clinical characteristics, life circumstances and growth hormone secretion. *Growth Hor IGF Res* 2000; (Suppl B): S81–S85.

4. Nicholls RD, Knepper JL. Genome organization, function and imprinting in Prader-Willi and Angelman syndromes. *Annu Rev Genomics Hum Genet* 2001; 2: 153–75.

5. Gray TA, Saitoh S, Nicholls RD. An imprinted, mammalian bicistronic transcript encodes two independent proteins. *Proc Natl Acad Sci USA* 1999; 96: 5616–21.

6. Runte M, Huttenhofer A, Gross S, Kiefmann M, Horsthemke B, Buiting K. The IC-SNURF-SNRPN transcript serves as a host for multiple small nucleolar RNA species and as an antisense RNA for UBE3A. *Hum Mol Genet* 2001; 10: 2687–700.

7. Cummings DE, Clement K, Purnell JQ, Vaisse C, Foster KE, Frayo RS *et al.* Elevated plasma ghrelin levels in Prader-Willi syndrome. *Nature Med* 2002; 8: 643–4.

8. Horvath TL, Diano S, Sotonyi P, Heiman M, Tschöp M. Minireview: Ghrelin and the regulation of energy balance – a hypothalamic perspective. *Endocrinology* 2001; 142: 4163–9.

9. Lossie AC, Whitney MM, Amidon D, Dong HJ, Chen P, Theriaque D *et al.* Distinct phenotypes distinguish the molecular classes of Angelman syndrome. *J Med Genet* 2001; 38: 834–45.

10. Dhar M, Webb LS, Smith L, Johnson D, West DB. A novel ATPase on mouse chromosome 7 is a candidate gene for increased body fat. Physiol. *Genomics* 2000; 4: 93–100.

11. Herzing LB, Kim SJ, Cook EH Jr, Ledbetter DH. The human aminophospholipid-transporting ATPase ATP10C maps adjacent to UBE3A and exhibits similar imprinted expression. *Am J Hum Genet* 2001; 68: 1501–5.

12. Meguro M, Kashiwagi A, Mitsuya K, Nakao M, Kondo I, Saitoh S *et al.* A novel maternally expressed gene, ATP10C, encodes a putative aminophospholipid translocase associated with Angelman syndrome. *Nature Genet* 2001; 28: 19–20.

13. Reik W, Walter J. Genomic imprinting: parental influence on the genome. *Nat Rev Genet* 2001; 2: 21–32.

14. Nicholls RD, Ohta T, Gray TA. Genetic abnormalities in Prader-Willi syndrome and lessons from mouse models. *Acta Paediatrica* 1999; 88 (Suppl. 433): 99–104.

15. Cattanach BM, Barr JA, Evans EP, Burtenshaw M, Beechey CV, Leff SE *et al.* A candidate mouse model for Prader-Willi syndrome which shows an absence of Snrpn expression. *Nature Genet* 1992; 2: 270–4.

318

16. Yang T, Adamson TE, Resnick JL, Leff S, Wevrick R, Francke U *et al.* A mouse model for Prader-Willi syndrome imprinting-centre mutations. *Nature Genet* 1998; 19: 25–31.

17. Gabriel JM, Merchant M, Ohta T, Ji Y, Caldwell RG, Ramsey MJ *et al.* A transgene insertion creating a heritable chromosome deletion mouse model of Prader-Willi and Angelman syndromes. *Proc Natl Acad Sci USA* 1999; 96: 9258–63.

18. Cattanach BM, Barr JA, Beechey CV, Martin J, Noebels J, Jones J. A candidate model for Angelman syndrome in the mouse. *Mamm Genome* 1997; 8: 472–8.

19. Jiang YH, Armstrong D, Albrecht U, Atkins CM, Noebels JL, Eichele G *et al.* Mutation of the Angelman ubiquitin ligase in mice causes increased cytoplasmic p53 and deficits of contextual learning and long-term potentiation. *Neuron* 1998; 21: 799–811.

20. Friedman MI. Fuel partitioning and food intake. *Am J Clin Nutr* 1998; 67: S513–S518.

21. Kalra SP, Dube MG, Pu S, Xu B, Horvath TL, Kalra PS. Interacting appetite-regulating pathways in the hypothalamic regulation of body weight. *Endocrin Rev* 1999; 20: 68–100.

22. Salton SRJ, Hahm S, Mizuno TM. Of mice and MEN: What transgenic models tell us about hypothalamic control of energy balance. *Neuron* 2000; 25: 265–8.

23. Ge Y-L, Ohta T, Driscoll DJ, Nicholls RD, Kalra S. Anorexigenic melanocortin signaling in the hypothalamus is augmented in association with failure-to-thrive in a transgenic mouse model for Prader-Willi syndrome. *Brain Res* 2002 Brain Res 2002; 957: 42–5.

24. Goldstone AP, Unmehopa UA, Bloom SR, Swaab DF. Hypothalamic NPY and agouti-related protein are increased in human illness but not Prader-Willi syndrome and other obese subjects. *J Clin Endocrinol Metab* 2002; 87: 927–37.

25. Halleck MS, Lawler JF Jr, Blackshaw S, Gao L, Nagarajan P, Hacker C *et al.* Differential expression of putative transbilayer amphipath transporters. *Physiol Genomics* 1999; 1: 139–50.

26. Ahima RS, Osei SY. Molecular regulation of eating behavior: new insights and prospects for therapeutic strategies. *Trends Mol Med* 2001; 7: 205–213.

27. Spiegelman BM, Flier JS. Obesity and the regulation of energy balance. *Cell* 2001; 104: 531–43.

28. Saitoh S, Kubota T, Ohta T, Jinno Y, Niikawa N, Sugimoto T *et al.* Familial Angelman syndrome caused by imprinted submicroscopic deletion encompassing GABAA receptor beta 3-subunit gene. *Lancet* 1992; 339: 366–7.

29. Cavaillé J, Buiting K, Kiefmann M, Lalande M, Brannan CI, Horsthemke B *et al.* Identification of brain-specific and imprinted small nucleolar RNA genes exhibiting an unusual genomic organization. *Proc Natl Acad Sci USA* 2000; 97: 14311–6.

30. Kashiwagi A, Meguro M, Hoshiya H, Haruta M, Ishino F, Shibihara T, Oshimura M. Predominant maternal expression of the mouse Atp10c in hippocampus and olfactory bulb. *J Hum Genet* 2003; 48: 194–8).

Progress in Obesity Research: 9. Edited by *Geraldo Medeiros-Neto, Alfredo Halpern and Claude Bouchard*
©2003 John Libbey Eurotext Ltd, pp. 320–323.

CHAPTER 68

Inherited lipodystrophic syndromes

Wendy K. Chung

Columbia University, USA
[e-mail: wkc15@columbia.edu]

Lipodystrophies are a diverse group of rare disorders that result in the selective loss of adipose tissue. The adipose tissue loss can be either generalized or regional and can be either inherited or acquired. Among the inherited lipodystrophies are the congenital generalized lipodystrophies also called Berardinelli-Seip syndrome and familial partial lipodystrophy including Dunnigan lipodystrophy and mandibuloacral dysplasia. Among the acquired forms of lipodystrophy are generalized lipodystrophy or Lawrence syndrome, partial lipodystrophy or Barraquer-Simons syndrome, localized lipodystrophy and HIV associated lipodystrophy. Regardless of the etiology, lipodystrophies are often associated with metabolic derangements of glucose metabolism that are more often associated with increased rather than decreased adiposity. The degree of insulin resistance and type 2 diabetes is often dependent upon the degree of adipose tissue loss.

Congenital generalized lipodystrophy (CGL)

Congenital generalized lipodystrophy is an autosomal recessive disorder associated with congenital complete absence of metabolically active adipose tissue found subcutaneously, intra-abdominally, intrathoracically, and within the bone marrow[16,25]. Mechanical adipose tissue in the palms, soles, scalp, orbits, perineum, and epidural space are maintained[11]. Affected individuals appear muscular, have hepatosplenomegaly, hypertrophic cardiomyopathy, and accelerated growth with acromegalic features including enlarged hands, feet, and mandible. Metabolic derangements include increased basal metabolic rate, hyperphagia, hypoleptinaemia, hypertriglyceridaemia that may result in eruptive xanthomas, acute pancreatitis and fatty liver infiltrate, low HDL, insulin resistance, and diabetes onset with puberty[11,15,16,25]. Females additionally often have polycystic ovaries and irregular menses.

CGL is a genetically heterogeneous disorder for which two genes have already been identified and for which at least a third as yet unidentified gene exists[23]. 1-acylglycerol-3-phosphate-O-acyltransferase 2 (*AGPAT2*) on 9q34 was the first of two genes identified in CLG[1] *AGPAT2* is the enzyme that catalyses acylation of lysophosphatidic acid to form phosphatidic acid, an intermediate in triglyceride synthesis. Without this enzyme, adipocytes are unable to synthesize triglycerides or produce the intracellular signaling molecules phosphatidylinositol, phosphatidylcholine, or phosphatidylethanolamine. Several mutations have been identified that are all predicted to result in loss of function of the enzyme[1].

A second gene for CGL was identified in subjects with classical features of CGL and associated with mental retardation in some affected individuals. Mutations in a novel gene of unknown function, *seipen*, were identified after linkage to 11q13 was established[18]. *Seipen* contains several hydrophobic regions suggestive of a transmembrane protein with homology with the murine guanine nucletide-ginding protein g3-linked gene (*Gng3lg*) that is expressed in the brain and testes. Based upon the pattern of expression and the associated metabolic derangements, *seipen* may represent a gene necessary for proper hypothalamic-pituitary function.

Familial partial lipodystrophy (FPLD)

FPLD is an autosomal dominantly inherited form of regional lipodystrophy with normal adipose tissue at birth that is gradually lost from the extremities and gluteal region with variable loss of truncal subcutaneous fat after puberty resulting in the appearance of increased muscularity[8,14]. Simultaneously, fat accumulates in the neck and face producing a Cushingoid appearance but without increased cortisol. Although both sexes are affected, the phenotype is more obvious in women producing an ascertainment bias that suggested x-linked inheritance with male lethality[17]. Associated metabolic abnormalities include hypertriglyceridaemia, low HDL, hypoleptinaemia, insulin resistance, type 2 diabetes, and in women polycystic ovaries and irregular menses[17]. The gene Lamin A/C (*LMNA*) was initially tested as a positional candidate gene after linkage on 1q21.2 was established and the gene had been implicated in Emery-Dreifuss muscular dystrophy that results in the selective loss of skeletal muscle fibres[3]. *LMNA* is a nuclear lamin that is alternatively spliced to produce both lamin A and C that differ in the C-termini[19]. Lamins A and C are intermediate filament proteins found in the nuclear envelop of terminally differentiated cells hypothesized to play role in DNA replication, chromatin organization, arrangement of nuclear pores, and anchoring nuclear membranes to direct traffic between the cytoplasm and nucleus. Lamins A and C have globular head and tail domains with a central rod domains. Hydrophobic residues in the rod domains promote dimerization, and dimers attach head to tail to form a meshwork inside the nuclear envelope. Interestingly, mutations in *LMNA* produce FPLD[5], Emery-Dreifuss muscular dystrophy (EMD2)[3], limb girdle muscular dystrophy with cardiac conduction abnormalities (LGMD1B), dilated cardiomyopathy (CMD1A)[4,10] and Charcot-Marie Tooth[7] depending on the location, type, and number of mutations. Mutations associated with FPLD generally localize to the surface of the globular C-terminus and often change charge. Recurrent mutations at amino acids 482 and 486 have been described and suggest that these amino acids are important for binding of transcription factors such as *SREBP-1*. Adipose tissue regional specificity may be the result of redundancy of other lamins expressed in each site. Recently, mutations in certain amino acids have also been associated with pleiotrophic effects including muscular dystrophy and/or myocardial dystrophy in addition to partial lipodystrophy[12]. Whether *LMNA* FPLD mutations are due to a loss or gain of function is not completely resolved; however, the phenotype of the *Lmna* knock out mouse consists only of a severe muscular dystrophy and cardiomyopathy without associated lipodystrophy[6] arguing that human *LMNA* mutations may be the result of unique gains of function.

Mandibuloacral dysplasia

Mandibuloacral dysplasia is an autosomal recessive form of familial partial lipodystrophy of the extremities associated with mandibular and clavicular hypoplasia, acral osteolysis, short stature, dental crowding, skin atrophy, alopecia and nail dysplasia[28]. Affected individual are homozygous for mutations in *LMNA* that are distinct from those associated with FPLD described above[21].

Mouse models of lipodystrophy

Although genetically aetiologically distinct from the human lipodystrophies, genetically manipulated mice provide useful models of lipodystrophy. Overexpression of *SREBP-1c* in adipose tissue under the control of aP2 produces disordered white and brown adipose tissue differentiation with some residual adipose tissue[27]. A dominant negative A-ZIP/F1 protein under the aP2 promoter inactivates the B-ZIP transcription factors including CEB/P and Jun resulting in the congenital absence of white and brown adipose tissue associated with severe metabolic derangements[20]. A third murine model with aP2 driven expression of diphtheria toxin A expression in white adipose tissue results in gradual loss of white adipose tissue until the age of 10 months[24]. All three models are associated with hypoleptinaemia, hypertriglyceridaemia, hepatic steatosis, insulin resistance, and diabetes that are proportional in degree to the amount of adipose tissue. The insulin resistance and diabetes associated with the lipodystrophies in mice can be reversed completely by transplantation of adipose tissue[13] or at least partially with treatment with leptin[9,26] although there may be other functions of adipose tissue besides leptin production that are necessary for normal glucose homeostatisis. Without the ability of white adipose tissue to store lipids, fat infiltrates the liver and muscle that may directly result in metabolic derangements.

Therapies for lipodystrophy

Leptin replacement in humans with lipodystrophies, similar to results in mice, produces normalization of hyperphagia, resting metabolic rate, hypertriglyceridaemia, insulin sensitivity and diabetes[22]. An alternative therapeutic option is thiazoladinediones that activate PPARγ to promote adipocyte differentiation and increase insulin sensitivity. Treatment with troglitazone produced a 3 per cent increase in fat associated with a decrease in RQ representing an increased oxidation of fats with concomitant normalization of insulin sensitivity and diabetes[2]. In the future, treatment with other safer thiazoladinediones in genetically at risk patients for FPLD prior to the onset of lipoatrophy may prevent metabolic derangements.

The new insight we have gained into the genetic aetiologies of inherited lipodystrophies should provide understanding of the central nervous system control of adipose tissue development, biochemical control of lipid storage, and the transcriptional controls of adipose tissue. These principles and the ability to therapeutically intervene with specific adipose derived proteins drugs to promote adipocyte differentiation can be also be applied to the more common acquired forms of lipodystrophy.

References

1. Agarwal AK, Garg A. A novel heterozygous mutation in peroxisome proliferator-activated receptor-gamma gene in a patient with familial partial lipodystrophy. *J Clin Endocrinol Metab* 2002; 87: 408–11.

2. Arioglu E, Duncan-Morin J, Sebring N, Rother KI, Gottlieb N, Lieberman J *et al.* Efficacy and safety of troglitazone in the treatment of lipodystrophy syndromes. *Ann Intern Med* 2000; 133: 263–74.

3. Bonne G, Di Barletta MR, Varnous S, Becane HM, Hammouda EH, Merlini L *et al.* Mutations in the gene encoding lamin A/C cause autosomal dominant Emery-Dreifuss muscular dystrophy. *Nature Genet* 1999; 21: 285–8.

4. Brodsky GL, Muntoni F, Miocic S, Sinagra G, Sewry C, Mestroni L. Lamin A/C gene mutation associated with dilated cardiomyopathy with variable skeletal muscle involvement. *Circulation* 2000; 101: 473–6.

5. Cao H, Hegele RA. Nuclear lamin A/C R482Q mutation in Canadian kindreds with Dunnigan- type familial partial lipodystrophy. *Hum Mol Genet* 2000; 9: 109–12.

6. Cutler DA, Sullivan T, Marcus-Samuels B, Stewart CL, Reitman ML. Characterization of adiposity and metabolism in Lmna-deficient mice. *Biochem Biophys Res Commun* 2002; 291: 522–7.

7. De Sandre-Giovannoli A, Chaouch M, Kozlov S, Vallat JM, Tazir M, Kassouri N *et al.* Homozygous defects in LMNA, encoding lamin A/C nuclear-envelope proteins, cause autosomal recessive axonal neuropathy in human (Charcot-Marie-Tooth disorder type 2) and mouse. *Am J Hum Genet* 2002; 70: 726–36.

8. Dunnigan MG, Cochrane MA, Kelly A, Scott JW. Familial lipoatrophic diabetes with dominant transmission. A new syndrome. *Q J Med* 1974; 43: 33–48.

9. Ebihara K, Ogawa Y, Masuzaki H, Shintani M, Miyanaga F, Aizawa-Abe M *et al.* Transgenic overexpression of leptin rescues insulin resistance and diabetes in a mouse model of lipoatrophic diabetes. *Diabetes* 2001; 50: 1440–8.

10. Fatkin D, MacRae C, Sasaki T, Wolff MR, Porcu M, Frenneaux M *et al.* Missense mutations in the rod domain of the lamin A/C gene as causes of dilated cardiomyopathy and conduction-system disease. *N Engl J Med* 1999; 341: 1715–24.

11. Garg A, Fleckenstein JL, Peshock RM, Grundy SM. Peculiar distribution of adipose tissue in patients with congenital generalized lipodystrophy. *J Clin Endocrinol Metab* 1992; 75: 358–61.

12. Garg A, Speckman RA, Bowcock AM. Multisystem dystrophy syndrome due to novel missense mutations in the amino-terminal head and alpha-helical rod domains of the lamin A/C gene. *Am J Med* 2002; 112: 549–55.

13. Gavrilova O, Marcus-Samuels B, Graham D, Kim JK, Shulman GI, Castle AL *et al.* Surgical implantation of adipose tissue reverses diabetes in lipoatrophic mice. *J Clin Invest* 2000; 105: 271–8.

14. Greene ML, Glueck CJ, Fujimoto WY, Seegmiller JE. Benign symmetric lipomatosis (Launois-Bensaude adenolipomatosis) with gout and hyperlipoproteinemia. *Am J Med* 1970; 48: 239–46.

15. Haque WA, Shimomura I, Matsuzawa Y, Garg A. Serum adiponectin and leptin levels in patients with lipodystrophies. *J Clin Endocrinol Metab* 2002; 87: 2395.

16. Seip M. Lipodystrophy and gigantism with associated endocrine manifestations. A new diencephalic syndrome? *Acta Paediatrica Scand* 1959; 48: 555–74.

17. Kobberling J, Dunnigan MG. Familial partial lipodystrophy: two types of an X linked dominant syndrome, lethal in the hemizygous state. *J Med Genet* 1986; 23: 120–7.

18. Magre J, Delepine M, Khallouf E, Gedde-Dahl T Jr, van Maldergem L, Sobel E *et al.* Identification of the gene altered in Berardinelli-Seip congenital lipodystrophy on chromosome 11q13. *Nature Genet* 2001; 28: 365–70.

19. McKeon FD, Kirschner MW, Caput D. Homologies in both primary and secondary structure between nuclear envelope and intermediate filament proteins. *Nature* 1986; 319: 463–8.

20. Moitra J, Mason MM, Olive M, Krylov D, Gavrilova O, Marcus-Samuels B *et al.* Life without white fat: a transgenic mouse. *Genes Dev* 1998; 12: 3168–81.

21. Novelli G, Muchir A, Sangiuolo F, Helbling-Leclerc A, D'Apice MR, Massart C *et al.* Mandibuloacral dysplasia is caused by a mutation in LMNA-encoding lamin A/C. *Am J Hum Genet* 2002; 71: 426–31.

22. Oral EA, Simha V, Ruiz E, Andewelt A, Premkumar A, Snell P *et al.* Leptin-replacement therapy for lipodystrophy. *N Engl J Med* 2002; 346: 570–8.

23. Rajab A, Heathcote K, Joshi S, Jeffery S, Patton M. Heterogeneity for congenital generalized lipodystrophy in seventeen patients from Oman. *Am J Med Genet* 2002; 110: 219–25.

24. Ross SR, Graves RA, Spiegelman BM. Targeted expression of a toxin gene to adipose tissue: transgenic mice resistant to obesity. *Genes Dev* 1993; 7: 1318–24.

25. Seip M, Trygstad O. Generalized lipodystrophy, congenital and acquired (lipoatrophy). *Acta Paediatrica* 1996; (Suppl)413: 2–28.

26. Shimomura I, Hammer RE, Ikemoto S, Brown MS, Goldstein JL. Leptin reverses insulin resistance and diabetes mellitus in mice with congenital lipodystrophy. *Nature* 1999; 401: 73–6.

27. Shimomura I, Hammer RE, Richardson JA, Ikemoto S, Bashmakov Y, Goldstein JL *et al.* Insulin resistance and diabetes mellitus in transgenic mice expressing nuclear SREBP-1c in adipose tissue: model for congenital generalized lipodystrophy. *Genes Dev* 1998; 12: 3182–94.

23. Young LW, Radebaugh JF, Rubin P, Sensenbrenner JA, Fiorelli G, McKusick VA. New syndrome manifested by mandibular hypoplasia, acroosteolysis, stiff joints and cutaneous atrophy (mandibuloacral dysplasia) in two unrelated boys. *Birth Defects Orig Artic Ser* 1971; 7: 291–7.

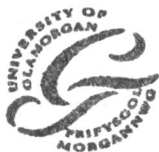

Progress in Obesity Research: 9. Edited by *Geraldo Medeiros-Neto, Alfredo Halpern and Claude Bouchard*
©2003 John Libbey Eurotext Ltd, pp. 324–327.

CHAPTER 69

Genetics of Bardet-Biedl syndrome: obesity and the Newfoundland population

William S. Davidson[1], Yanli Fan[1], Patrick S. Parfrey[2], Elizabeth Dicks[2], Susan Moore[2] and Jane S. Green[2]

[1]*Department of Molecular Biology and Biochemistry, Simon Fraser University, Burnaby, British Columbia, V5A 1S6, Canada; and* [2]*Faculty of Medicine, Memorial University of Newfoundland, St. John's, Newfoundland, A1B 3X9, Canada*
[e-mail: wdavidso@sfu.ca]

Clinical features

Bardet-Biedl syndrome (BBS) is characterized by dysmorphic extremities (post-axial polydactyly, syndactyly and brachydactyly), obesity, retinal dystrophy, hypogenitalism in males, and renal structural and functional abnormalities with secondary features that may include diabetes mellitus, endocrinological dysfunction, and learning difficulties[1,2]. Several syndromes share clinical features with BBS. Among these are Biemond syndrome, Alstrom syndrome, and McKusick Kaufmann syndrome (MKKS) but each is considered a different disorder (Table 1). It should be noted that MKKS differs from the other three syndromes with respect to the absence of obesity.

Genetic heterogeneity

BBS is genetically heterogeneous and has been mapped to six loci, each on a different chromosome: 11q13 (BBS1)[3], 16q21 (BBS2)[4] 3p12 (BBS3)[5] 15q22–23 (BBS4)[6] 2q31 (BBS5)[7] and 20p21 (BBS6)[8,9]. Evidence for a seventh BBS locus comes from the existence of families who can be excluded by haplotype analysis from BBS1-6[10]. Four BBS genes have been identified. The first of these was BBS6[8,9]. Homozygosity mapping in a consanguineous Newfoundland family, which had been excluded from BBS1-5, suggested that BBS6 mapped to 20p12[8]. Supporting evidence for this came from four other Newfoundland families and a critical region was defined which included the recently described gene for MKKS[11]. Given the overlapping clinical phenotype for the two syndromes and their concordant mapping position, the MKKS gene became a candidate for BBS6. Combinations of three mutations in the MKKS gene co-segregated with BBS6 in the five Newfoundland families confirming that MKKS and BBS6 were caused by mutations in the same gene. The MKKS/BBS6 protein is predicted to be a type 2 chaperonin. Members of this family of proteins are responsible for folding a wide range of proteins and it was anticipated that this would provide a clue for identifying candidate genes for BBS1-5. Unfortunately this has turned out not to be the case.

The genes for BBS2[12], BBS4[13], and BBS1[14] have subsequently been identified using standard positional cloning procedures. None of the predicted gene products of BBS2, BBS4 or BBS1 share any sequence similarity with chaperonins. The BBS4 protein is thought to function as an O-linked N-acetylglucosamine transferase[13]. However, although the BBS1 and BBS2 proteins display a region of weak similarity with one another, their predicted sequences did not provide any insight to their functions[12,14]. The gene associated with Alstrom syndrome (ALMS1) has also recently been identified[15,16]. Like the BBS1 and BBS2 proteins, the ALMS1 gene product does not share significant sequence similarity with any other proteins reported to date. It may be that the MKKS and BBS proteins, along with ALMS1, are part of a novel developmental pathway and disruptions to this pathway lead to overlapping phenotypes that vary depending on how effectively signals are transmitted along the pathway.

Table 1. Comparison of phenotypic traits among BBS and related syndromes

	BBS	Biemond	Alstrom	MKKS
MIM#	209900	210350	203800	236700
Obesity	X	X	X	–
Urogenital problems	X	X	–	X
Polydactyly	X	X	–	X
Eye problems	X	X	X	–
Kidney problems	X	X	–	–
Heart defects	–	–	–	X
Hearing loss	–	–	X	–

Pattern of inheritance

The pattern of segregation of BBS in families where consanguinity had been confirmed allowed the loci for BBS2-6 to be positioned on the genome using homozygosity mapping based on autosomal recessive inheritance[4-8]. Mapping of BBS1 was also based on the syndrome being inherited in this manner[3]. A survey of 92 pedigrees for which extensive genotype data were available, revealed that 14 per cent could be excluded from all of the six known BBS loci and for another 28 per cent it was impossible to assign a particular locus[10]. Although this has been taken as support for the presence of another, as yet unidentified locus (BBS7) another possibility has been presented that can account for this observation[17]. During a screen of BBS families for mutations in the BBS6 gene, it was found that several families harboured a single mutant BBS6 allele. One of these families was a consanguineous Newfoundland kindred. The affected and unaffected sibs shared the heterozygous state for the mutant BBS6 allele, but the affected also exhibited homozygosity by descent across the BBS2 locus. Sequence analysis of the BBS2 gene revealed a homozygous Y24X mutation in the affected individual. This observation prompted mutation analysis in the BBS2 and BBS6 genes in all families irrespective of haplotyping data. The results of this study showed that in some instances two mutations at a single BBS locus are not sufficient for the BBS phenotype to be manifested and it requires a third mutant allele at a second BBS locus for this to occur. Additional support for the triallelic inheritance model[17] came from a subsequent study that analysed the same cohort of families for mutations in the BBS4 gene[18]. It has been suggested that rather than calling this triallelic inheritance[17], it should be termed recessive inheritance with a modifier of penetrance[19].

Obesity in BBS

Obesity is the second most common manifestation of BBS after retinal dystrophy. It normally starts to be noticed in children between the ages of two and four and increases in severity with age. However, patients can reduce their weight with strict diet and exercise regimes. In adults, the obesity is usually restricted to the trunk and proximal limbs and less frequently to the face, but it has also been described as diffuse and non-specific in distribution during early life[20]. Definitions of obesity vary from study to study; however, 72 per cent of patients[2] were considered obese when the criterion was a BMI > 29 kg/m^2 and this figure rose to 88 per cent in another group of BBS patients[21] if the measure was a BMI > 28 kg/m^2. When obesity was defined as greater than the 90th percentile on the weight for height charts for Canadian men and women, 22 of 25 (88 per cent) Newfoundland BBS patients were considered obese and two of the three with normal weight had previously been obese[1]. Obesity was more pronounced in female Newfoundland BBS patients than their affected brothers[20]. The status of heterozygous carriers of a BBS mutant allele with respect to predisposition to obesity is unclear. Croft et al.[22] calculated the BMIs of 34 obligate BBS heterozygotes (parents of an affected individual) and suggested that BBS heterozygotes could account for approximately 3 per cent of all severely overweight white males in the USA. A more extensive study of BBS in British families found no excess of obesity among carrier parents; if anything, the average BMIs for both males and females were below those in the general population[2].

BBS in Newfoundland

BBS is a relatively rare syndrome (e.g. 1: 160,000 in Switzerland[23]); however, the incidence is much higher in some populations where consanguinity is more common due to social customs (e.g. 1: 13,500

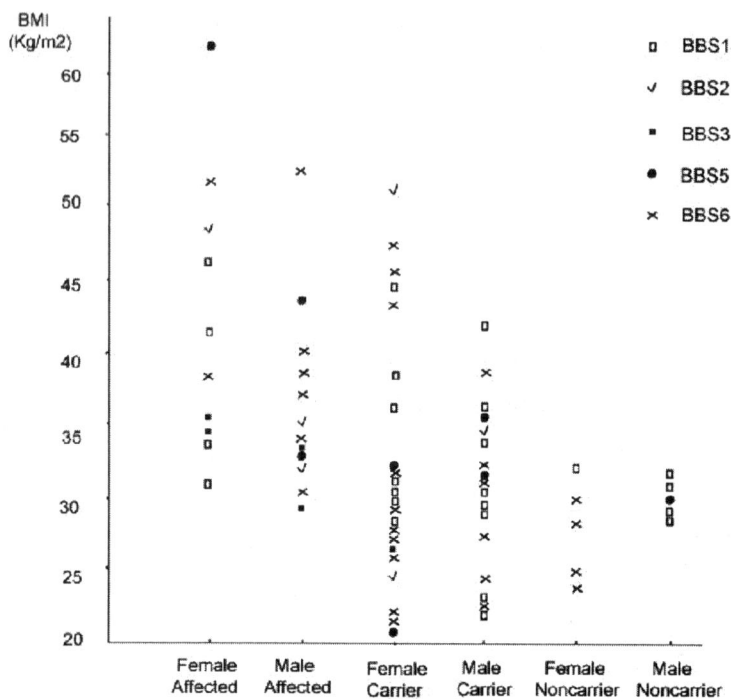

Fig. 1. Comparison of BMIs among members of Newfoundland BBS families according to sex and genotype at BBS loci.

among the Bedouin of Kuwait[24]) or as a result of founder effects (e.g. 1: 17,500 in Newfoundland[1]). Twenty-five BBS families have been identified in Newfoundland and they have been the subject of extensive clinical and genetic analyses. A surprising initial result from the genetic studies was that the high incidence of BBS in the Newfoundland population was not due to a single founder[25]. Extensive haplotype analysis and mutational analysis carried out on 17 of the families revealed that there are: six BBS1 families in which the affected individuals all carry the same mutation; one BBS2 family that is homozygous for the mutation; one BBS3 family; one BBS5 family; five BBS6 families in which three mutations segregate; one family which appears to be excluded from all known BBS loci; and two families which cannot be assigned unambiguously to any locus yet[26]. Therefore, this isolated island community contains a minimum of six BBS loci and a minimum of eight different BBS mutations.

As the high incidence of BBS in the Newfoundland population cannot be explained by a single founder event, we propose that the increase may be due to an underlying common modifier gene that is contributing through a mechanism such as triallelic inheritance[17] or else that during the course of colonization of Newfoundland there was selection for BBS heterozygotes[26]. Communities were founded around the coast of Newfoundland by small extended family groups in order to prosecute the inshore cod fishery. An enhanced ability to store fat may have provided a survival benefit in a cold, harsh environment where there was uncertainty about availability of food. In order to test this possibility we have begun to compare the phenotypes of affected individuals and their heterozygous and non-carrier relatives.

Our preliminary data for obesity (using BMI as an index) are shown in Fig. 1. These results reveal that there is no clustering of data with respect to BBS locus. A previous observation[20] that there is a tendency for female BBS patients to be more obese than affected males is supported. Male and female carriers of a mutant BBS gene tend to be more obese than their non-carrier counterparts. This study is being extended to include many more family members. In addition, obese individuals in the Newfoundland population who have no known genetic relationship to the BBS families will be examined to determine if they are carriers of mutations in the BBS genes whose structures are known.

Acknowledgements: We thank the Newfoundland BBS families who have been active participants in these studies. T. Young and M. Woods provided valuable discussions. This research was supported by the Canadian Institutes for Health Research, the Kidney Foundation of Canada, and the Janeway Foundation.

References

1. Green JS, Parfrey PS, Harnett JD, Farid NR, Cramer BC *et al.* The cardinal manifestations of Bardet-Biedl syndrome, a form of Laurence-Moon-Biedl syndrome. *N Eng J Med* 1989; 321: 1002–9.

2. Beales PL, Elcioglu N, Woolf AS, Parker D, Flinter FA. New criteria for improved diagnosis of Bardet-Biedl syndrome: results of a population survey. *J Med Genet* 1999; 36: 437–46.

3. Leppert M, Baird L, Anderson KL, Otterud B, Lupski JR *et al.* Bardet-Biedl syndrome is linked to DNA markers on chromosome 11q and is genetically heterogeneous. *Nature Genet* 1994; 7: 108–12.

4. Carmi R, Rokhlina T, Kwitek-Black AE, Elbedour K, Nishimura D *et al.* Use of a DNA pooling strategy to identify a human obesity syndrome locus on chromosome 15. *Hum Mol Genet* 1995; 4: 9–13.

5. Sheffield VC, Carmi R, Kwitek-Black AE, Rohklina T, Nishimura D *et al.* Identification of a Bardet-Biedl syndrome locus on chromosome 3 and evaluation of an efficient approach to homozygosity mapping. *Hum Mol Genet* 1994; 3: 1331–5.

6. Kwitek-Black AE, Carmi R, Duyk GM, Buetow KH, Elbedour K *et al.* Linkage of Bardet-Biedl syndrome to chromosome 16q and evidence for non-allelic genetic heterogeneity. *Nature Genet* 1993; 5: 392–6.

7. Young TL, Penney L, Woods MO, Parfrey PS, Green JS *et al.* A fifth locus for Bardet-Biedl syndrome maps to chromosome 2q31. *Am J Hum Genet* 64: 901–4.

8. Katsanis N, Beales PL, Woods MO, Lewis RA, Green JS *et al.* Mutations in MKKS cause obesity, retinal dystrophy and renal malformations associated with Bardet-Biedl syndrome. *Nature Genet* 2000; 26: 67–70.

9. Slavotinek AM, Stone EM, Mykytyn K, Heckenlively JR, Green JS *et al.* Mutations in MKKS cause Bardet-Biedl syndrome. *Nature Genet* 2000; 26: 15–16.

10. Beales PL, Katsanis N, Lewis RA, Ansley SJ, Elcioglu N *et al.* Genetic and mutational analyses of a large multiethnic Bardet-Biedl cohort reveal a minor involvement of BBS6 and delineate the critical intervals of other loci. *Am J Hum Genet* 2001; 68: 606–16.

11. Stone DL, Slavotinek A, Bouffard GG, Banerjee-Basu S, Baxevanis AD *et al.* Mutation of a gene encoding a putative chaperonin causes McKusick-Kaufman syndrome. *Nature Genet* 2000; 25: 79–82.

12. Nishimura DY, Searby CC, Carmi R, Elbedour K, Maldergem LV *et al.* Positioning cloning of a novel gene on chromosome 16q causing Bardet-Biedl syndrome (BBS2). *Hum Mol Genet* 2001; 10: 865–74.

13. Mykytyn K, Braun T, Carmi R, Haider NB, Searby CC *et al.* Identification of the gene that, when mutated, causes the human obesity syndrome BBS4. *Nature Genet* 2001; 28: 188–191.

14. Mykytyn K, Nishimura DY, Searby CC, Shastri M, Yen H *et al.* Identification of the gene (BBS1) most commonly involved in Bardet-Biedl syndrome, a complex human obesity syndrome. *Nature Genet* 2002; 31: 435–8.

15. Collin GB, Marshall JD, Ikeda A, So WV, Russell-Eggitt I *et al.* Mutations in ALMS1 cause obesity, type 2 diabetes and neurosensory degeneration in Alstrom syndrome. *Nature Genet* 2002; 31: 74–8.

16. Hearn T, Renforth GL, Spalluto C, Hanley NA, Piper K *et al.* Mutation of ALMS1, a large gene with a tandem repeat encoding 47 amino acids, causes Alstrom syndrome. *Nature Genet* 2002; 31: 79–83.

17. Katsanis N, Ansley SJ, Badano JL, Eichers ER, Lewis RA *et al.* Triallelic inheritance in Bardet-Biedl syndrome, a Mendelian recessive disorder. *Science* 2001; 293: 2256–9.

18. Katsanis N, Eichers ER, Ansley SJ, Lewis RA, Kayserili H *et al.* BBS4 is a minor contributor to Bardet-Biedl syndrome and may also participate in triallelic inheritance. *Am J Hum Genet* 2002; 71: 22–9.

19. Burghes AHM, Vaessin HEF, Chappelle A. The land between mendelian and multifactorial inheritance. *Science* 2001; 283: 2213–4.

20. O'Dea D, Parfrey PS, Harnett JD *et al.* The importance of renal impairment in the natural history of Bardet-Biedl syndrome. *Am J Kidney Dis* 1996; 27: 776–83.

21. Bruford EA, Riise R, Teague PW, Porter K, Thompson KL *et al.* Linkage mapping in 29 Bardet-Biedl syndrome families confirms loci in chromosomal regions 11q13, 15q22.3-q23, and 16q21. *Genomics* 1997; 41: 93–9.

22. Croft JB, Morrell D, Chase CL, Swift M. Obesity in heterozygous carriers of the gene for Bardet-Biedl syndrome. *Am J Med Genet* 1995; 12-5.

23. Klein D, Ammann F. The syndrome of Laurence-Moon-Bardet-Biedl and allied diseases in Switzerland. Clinical, genetic and epidemiological studies. *J Neuro Sci* 1969; 9: 479–513.

24. Farag TI, Teebi AS. High incidence of Bardet-Biedl syndrome among the Bedouin. *Clin Genet* 1989; 36: 463–5.

25. Woods MO, Young TL, Parfrey PS, Hefferton D, Green JS *et al.* Genetic heterogeneity of Bardet-Biedl syndrome in a distinct Canadian population: evidence for a fifth locus. *Genomics* 1999; 55: 2–9.

26. Parfrey PS, Davidson WS, Green JS. Clinical and genetic epidemiology of inherited renal disease in Newfoundland. *Kidney Int* 2002; 61: 1925–34.

327

Progress in Obesity Research: 9. Edited by *Geraldo Medeiros-Neto, Alfredo Halpern and Claude Bouchard*
©2003 John Libbey Eurotext Ltd, pp. 328–332.

CHAPTER 70

From monogenic to polygenic approach in the French population

Karine Clément and Arnaud Basdevant

*EA 3502, Paris 6 University, Department of Nutrition, Assistance Publique/Hôpitaux de Paris and INSERM 'Avenir'
Hôtel-Dieu. 75004 Paris, France
[e-mail: karine.clement@htd.ap-hop-paris.fr]*

Introduction

Obesity has become the highest-occurring nutritional disease[1]. In France, the current prevalence is 9.6 per cent in adults and 12–13 per cent in children. A recent INSERM (French institute for medical research) report anticipates a substantial increase in the prevalence of the disease in children in the coming decades and pleads for genetic/environment studies (*Obésité de l'enfant*, INSERM Ed., 2000). The inflation of energy stores (e.g. fat mass) results from the interaction of environmental and genetic factors[2]. The epidemic progression of obesity is a recent phenomenon which started in the last 30 years or so in Europe, a period too short to account for the selection of obesity genes in a large population. Except in rare situations[3–5] genetic causes are not responsible for the recent explosion of obesity but express themselves owing to external causes: increase in the food availability and/or physical inactivity are the two major contributors in a new social and economical context.

Adaptive responses to overfeeding drive mechanisms aimed at decreasing food intake and increasing energy output. These mechanisms involve a cross-talk between peripheral and central tissues which adequately respond to excess of energy input and storage by secreting specifc signals. Peripheral 'adiposity signals', such as insulin and leptin, are secreted in proportion to the energy stores. In the brain, a central controller system integrates these signals through various neuropeptides, either anabolic (e.g. peptides increasing food intake and/or decreasing energy expenditure) or catabolic. Then, peripheral effectors involved in energy storage (adipose tissue) or energy utilization (muscle, brown adipose tissue) respond to central or peripheral signal variations, in conjunction with hormones and circulating substrates[6,7]. Defective engagement of any of these elements may lead to abnormal control of food intake and/or energy expenditure. Obesity can be seen as an inappropriate adaptation of the systems involved in the control of energy balance to a context of overfeeding and/or inactivity. In order to dissect the molecular mechanisms leading to the development of obesity in the French population, we have been using genetic tools for more than 10 years.

Methods

Our group has contributed to this field by studying candidate genes of interest in cohorts of obese patients. Familial linkage and linkage disequilibrium approaches were used. They involved testing the association between obesity and a specific allele of a gene which appears to be a good candidate (e.g. a gene involved in the regulation of food intake and energy expenditure), either in a family study or in large cohorts of unrelated controls and patients. Individuals were characterized for genetic variations in candidate genes of obesity. We associated these genetic variations to given phenotypes related to common obesity. An alternative strategy, the genome wide scan, was used in this population in order to 'feed' the candidate gene approach with new genes. This strategy, attempts to mark genes purely by position and requires no presumption on the function of the genes.

These studies were conducted in severe obese phenotypes in sibpairs enriched in the same genetic background. The objective was to lower the genetic complexity and heterogeneity, thus to increase the power to detect the susceptibility genes. We have constituted banks of clinical data and DNA in large cohorts of morbidly obese patients (more than 2000 subjects and 500 families). These patients and their families have been characterized in the department of Nutrition in Hôtel-Dieu for parameters related to obesity (weight history, body composition, characteristics of food intake and physical activity) and features of insulin resistance. In severely obese populations, only a few individuals fell into rare or exceptional monogenic situation of obesity. The largest fraction presented with polygenic obesity, with multiple genes interacting with the environmental determinants.

Results and discussion

One family was identified with a leptin receptor mutation. This unique published case has completed the picture of rare monogenic situation due to mutation in genes encoding proteins that are strongly connected as part of the leptin loop and of the melanocortin pathway (one of the important catabolic circuits targeted by leptin in the hypothalamic cells). Indeed, mutations in the leptin and its receptor, in the pro-opiomelanocortin, pro-hormone convertase[1] and in the melanocortin receptor-4 genes were found in several populations[2]. In three sisters with the homozygous mutation in the leptin receptor, a truncation of the receptor abolishes leptin signaling, leading to a phenotype similar to that of individuals with leptin deficiency, although more severe. Homozygous carriers of a loss of function mutation in the leptin gene exhibit morbid obesity with onset in the first months of life, hypogonadotropic hypogonadisnn and central hypothyroidism[5]. Affected subjects continuously seek food and eat considerably more than their sibs. None of the heterozygous parents or sib are morbidly obese. The three sisters bearing the leptin receptor mutation also display a significant growth retardation due to impaired growth hormone secretion. Although, these situations of monogenic obesity are exceptional, they have contributed to validate the role of leptin axis not only in body weight regulation but also in the control of several endocrine functions. In addition, they represent unique models for human biology. For example, the mutation in the leptin receptor gene is a unique situation to study the role of leptin both at the central and peripheral levels. We have, for example, demonstrated that the full knock out of the leptin pathway in human is not responsible for compensatory hypersecretion of leptin. The high leptin concentrations found in the blood of affected patients were shown to be related to a decreased clearance of circulating leptin due to its trapping by a serum leptin-binding factor containing the truncated receptor.

The second group of monogenic forms of obesity is related to cases due to numerous mutations in the MC4R gene. Contrasting with the forms of monogenic obesity associated with multiple endocrine dysfunctions, mutations in the MC4R (the receptor of a MSH) cause non-syndromic obesity, dominantly and recessively inherited, with incomplete penetrance (in the families the mutation is not always associated with obesity) and variable expression (a similar mutation can yield various degrees of obesity)[3,9,10]. A trend toward a greater incidence of childhood obesity was found among the adult population we screened; however, by contrast with other studies in British population, no excessive hunger and food-seeking behaviour were evidenced by our studies. MC4R mutations represent a significant cause of obesity in morbidly obese children and adults (1 to 6 per cent). The MC4R gene was not only a good biological candidate. The fact that MC4R might be considered as a 'thrifty gene' (i.e. a gene whose product promotes energy efficiency) stems from several arguments repeatedly observed in different groups; cosegregation of phenotype and genotype among the families, population-based association (the mutations were found in obese groups, not in controls), functional consequences of the mutation. Its role was also validated in animal models (MC4RKO leads to obesity). Much efforts is still to be made to identify the mechanisms by which MC4R carriers develop an obese phenotype. The expression of the disease in mutation carriers is variable and the penetrance incomplete, emphasizing the role of environment as well as other genetic contributors. In addition, the described mutations have multiple functional consequences and their precise evaluation is still required.

In the most frequent forms of obesity, we faced several hypotheses[11]. One is the polygenic hypothesis where multiple genes with relatively small effects interact with numerous environmental factors – excess caloric intake and physical inactivity – and modulate the expression of obesity-related complex traits (modifier genes). One of the principal challenges of the molecular approach would be, however, to demonstrate that obesity is an oligogenic disease whose development can eventually be modulated by polygenic genes and by environmental influence. In the 'oligogenic' hypothesis, fewer genes with larger and measurable effects contribute to the phenotypic characteristics of obesities. Up to now, we have only been able to identify modifier genes such as minor contributors of morbid obesity-related features. We widely used the candidate gene approach and tested multiples genes based on their known or presumed biological role in energy homeostasis. Many plausible candidates were analysed for the presence of an association/linkage between genetic variant (SNPs, microsatellite markers) and several obesity-related phenotypes. Candidates were those whose product are involved:

(1)   In the control of food intake by the central and/or peripheral nervous system, such as leptin and leptin receptor, cholecystokinin and its receptors, glucagon like peptide 1, αMSH, neuropeptideY and receptors[112-116];

(2)   Energy expenditure (beta-adrenoceptors, UCPs), lipid metabolism including lipid oxidation, lipolysis, lipogenesis and more generally in adipose tissue metabolism, such as the lipoprotein lipase that provides fatty acids for the fat storage in adipose tissue and interacts with a coactivator apolipoprotein C2, the hormone-sensitive lipase, one of the enzymes determining whole-body fuel availability by catalysing the rate-limiting step of adipose tissue lipolysis, the peroxisome proliferator activated receptor, an important transcription factor activated by fatty acids that transactivates several genes involved in adipocyte metabolism and is critical for adipocyte differentiation;

(3)   In the modulation of insulin action and glucose metabolism in target tissues that may contribute to the excess of fat deposition and to the development of insulin resistance, associated with obesity. They included for example the sulphonylurea receptors, Isl-l, insulin receptor substrate 1, fatty acid-binding proteins etc.[12,24,25]

Constrasting with the MC4R gene situation, the supporting evidence of an implication of the tested genes were sometimes inconsistent or weak. The multiple association or linkage studies were sometimes validated by replication of data in unrelated individuals or families of different origin and sometimes discrepant[35].

The alternative approach to susceptibility gene discovery was the genome wide scan approach. Variations across the entire genome were analysed using polymorphic markers (380, average distance 9.25 cM,) in 264 sibling pairs. It provided statistical evidence for linkage for the existence of susceptibility genes in several regions including chromosomes 2p21 (lod-score 2.68), chromosome 10p11 (lod score 4.85) and on 5cen-q (lod-score 2.8). In addition, a few other markers showed increased allele sharing in the sibling pairs, although they did not meet enough criteria for linkage to a genome wide scan context. Some of them covered regions involved in obesity syndromes (like Bardet-Biedel, Prader-Willi or Cohen syndromes) or where a region showing positive linkage in other populations suggesting minor effects not detected by linkage or effects of other traits not studied in this population or others.

The suggestive linkage found in our population have been largely validated. At least two regions are reproducible in other populations with difference in ethnicity and probably in environmental factors. Genome wide scans for obesity genes carried out in Mexican and African American families also provided the chromosome 2p21 locus as a candidate that could explain a non-negligible part of the variance of leptin levels. The role of the chromosome 10 region in obesity was also confirmed in German young obese, in White Caucasiana in African American, and in the old order Amish[29-32]. Some concerns have been raised about the accuracy of the genome wide scan approach suggesting that evidence of linkage in multifactorial diseases can be confounded by the phenomenon of transmission ratio distortion that could result in non-Mendelian segregation of alleles from parents to their offspring. Using appropriate analysis in their cohort, the German group did not found any indication for the presence of sex of offspring transmission ratio distortion[29].

The next goal of this approach is to develop fine mapping strategies to identify the genes that underlie the related traits and further understand their role in body weight regulation. Chromosomal regions of linkage are refined using dense map of biallelic single-nucleotide polymorphisms (SNPs). DNA polymorphisms located away from the true functional variant can be associated with the disease or with the variation of an obesity associated trait. Relatively obvious candidate genes were sometimes located within the proximal region identified and their study help refining the maps. For example, the confidence interval surrounded the chromosome 2 region contains the POMC (Proopiomelanocortin) and UCN (Urocortin) loci. POMC and UCN are key neuropeptides synthesized by hypothalamic neurons that reduce food intake and body weight when given centrally. The stepwise process had involved to search for SNPs in those strong positional candidate. SNP markers are then systematically used for the detection of linkage disequilibrium mapping (LD mapping) in case and control cohorts, eventually completed by transmission disequilibrium test in the families. Linkage analysis confirmed the trend toward linkage between polymorphic markers around POMC and UCN and leptin and *BMI* but association studies revealed that the found mutations in *POMC* and UCN do not greatly contribute to the variance of obesity-related traits. We thus excluded a major role of these genes in our cohort.

A similar strategy was also used for the Lim domain homeobox gene, another positional candidate that maps to the 5q11q12 locus (a region enriched with candidate genes for obesity) linked to common obesity in French obese families[25]. Isl1 might play a role in body weight homeostasis via its transcriptional role on the preproglucagon gene (GCG). This gene encodes for the glucagon and glucagon-like peptides, GLP1 and GLP2, both potent inhibitors of food intake. In addition, glucagon and GLP proteins participate to glucose homeostasis. We performed association studies between obesity related phenotypes and several new variants 495 A>G (ATG = +1), −47A>G, and P168P (CCA > CCG) in obese and non-obese cohorts. No difference was observed between control and obese subjects showing that Isl1 doesn't contribute to the linkage at the 5q region. However in the obese group, the GG genotype of the −47 A>G variant was significantly less frequent in type 2 diabetic subjects and was associated with a decreased risk of being diabetic (OR = 0.41;). The −47A>G variant was also found associated with the body mass index in the morbidly obese group suggesting that isll itself or another nearby gene modulates the risk for T2DM in obese subjects and the severity of obesity. Other candidates located in those regions are under study.

In conclusion, extensive genetic screening in the French obese cohorts revealed the role of several candidates, with some of them being probably minor contributors, illustrating the complex heterogeneity and polygenic nature of obesities, even in its extreme form. They have indeed been related to the gravity of obesity (leptin), weight gain (B3AR, UCP1), metabolic complications such as diabetes (Isl1, sulphonylurea receptor), response to exercise (UCP3), biological parameters (leptin) etc. In contrast, many of other genes proposed as candidates in other populations were not validated in the French morbidly obese subjects[35].

Many efforts are now developed to demonstrate that obesity is also an oligogenic disease. The challenge is to identify the true aetiological gene variants, explaining the genome wide scan results. The future will tell us whether or not this approach is appropriate. Thanks to the increased availability of SNPs, human and mouse genomic sequence and maps, comparative and functional genomics, optimistic views suggest that many genes will be mapped in the next 10 years[36].

Acknowledgements: The authors thank senior researcher, post doctoral and PhD students, technicians, involved in the French connection for the genetic studies of obesities located at EA 3502, Paris 6 University, Hôtel-Dieu Hospital/Formation associée Claude Bemard, Contrat 'Avenir' Inserm, and CNRS UPRESA 8090 (Director Ph. Froguel). The studies presented here were supported by the Direction de la Recherche Clinique/Assistance Publique-Hopitaux de Paris and the Programme Hospitalier de Recherche Clinique (AOM 96088), Servier Research Institute (IRIS), the Fondation pour la Recherche Medicale and Groupe Lipide Nutrition.

References

1. Kopelman PG. Obesity as a medical problem. *Nature Genet* 2000; 404: 635–643.

2. Barsh GS, Farroqi IS, O'Rahilly S. Genetics of body weight regulation. *Nature Genet* 2000; 404: 644–651.

3. Vaisse C, Clement K, Durand E *et al.* Melanocortin-4 receptor mutations are a frequent and heterogeneous cause of morbid obesity. *J Clin Invest* 2000; 106: 253–62.

4. Farooqi IS, Yeo GS, Keogh JM *et al.* Dominant and recessive inheritance of morbid obesity associated with melanocortin 4 receptor deficiency. *J Clin Invest* 1998; 106: 271–79.

5. Clement K, Vaisse C, Lahlou N *et al.* A mutation in the human leptin receptor gene causes obesity and pituitary dysfunction. *Nature* 1998; 392: 398–401.

6. Kahn R. Triglycerides toggling the tummy. *Nature Genet* 2000; 25: 6–7.

7. Woods SC, Seeley RJ, Porte D *et al.* Signals that regulate food intake and energy homeostasis. *Science* 1998; 280: 1378–1383.

8. Lahlou N, Clement K, Carel JC, Vaisse C, Lotton C, Le Bihan Y *et al.* Soluble leptin receptor in serum of subjects with complete resistance to leptin: relation to fat mass. *Diabetes* 2000; 49: 1347–52.

9. Dubern B, Clément K, Pelloux V, Froguel P, Girardet JP, Guy-Grand B, Tounian P. Mutational analysis of melanocortin-4 receptor, agouti-related protein, and alpha-melanocyte-stimulating hormone genes in severely obese children. *J Pediatr* 2001; 139: 204–209.

10. Vaisse C, Clement K, Guy-Grand B, Froguel P. A frameshift mutation in the human melanocortin 4 receptor results in an autosomic dominant form of obesity. *Nature Genet* 1998; 20: 113–114.

11. Comuzzie AG, Williams JT, Martin LJ, J. Blangero. Searching for genes underlying normal variation in human adiposity. *J Mol Med* 2001; 79: 57–70.

12. Clement K, Dina C, Basdevant A, Chastang N, Pelloux V, Lahlou N, Berlan M, Langin D, Guy-Grand B, Froguel P. A sib-pair analysis study of 15 candidate genes in French families with morbid obesity: indication for linkage with islet 1 locus on chromosome 5 q. *Diabetes* 1999; 48: 398–402.

13. Clement K, Garner C, Hager J, Philippi A, Le Duc C, Carey A *et al*. Indication for linkage of the human OB gene region with extreme obesity. *Diabetes* 1996; 45: 687–690.

14. Rolland V, Clement K, Dugail I, Guy-Grand B, Basdevant A, Froguel P, Lavau M. Leptin receptor gene in a large cohort of massively obese subjects: no indication of the fa/fa rat mutation. Detection of an intronic variant with no association with obesity. *Obes Res* 1998; 6: 122–127.

15. Francke S, Clement K, Dina C, Inoue H, Behn P, Vatin V *et al*. Genetic studies of the leptin receptor gene in morbidly obese French Caucasian Families. *Hum Genet* 1997; 100: 491–496.

16. Roche C, Boutin P, Gyapay G, Basdevant A, Hager J, Guy-Grand B, Clement K, Froguel P. Genetic studies of neuropeptide Y receptors Y1 and Y5 regions in morbid obesity. *Diabetologia* 1997; 40: 671–675.

17. Clement K, Philippi A, Jury C, Pividal R, Hager J, Demenais F *et al*. Candidate gene approach of familial morbid obesity: linkage analysis of the glucocorticoid receptor gene. *Int J Obes* 1996; 20: 507–512.

18. Clement K, Hercberg S, Passinge B, Galan P, Varroud-Vial M, Shuldiner AR *et al*. The Pro115Gln and Pro12Ala PPAR gamma gene mutations in obesity and type 2 diabetes. *Int J Obes* 2000; 24: 391–3.

19. Clement K, Vaisse C, Manning BS, Basdevant A, Guy-Grand B, Ruiz J, Silver KD, Shuldiner AR, Froguel P, Strosberg AD. Genetic variation in the beta 3 adrenoreceptor and an increased capacity to gain weight in patients with morbid obesity. *New Engl J Med* 1995; 333: 452–454.

20. Clement K, Ruiz J, Cassard-Doulcier AM, Bouillaud F, Ricquier D, Basdevant A, Guy-Grand B, Froguel P. Additive effects of A->G (-3826) variant of the uncoupling protein gene and the Trp64Arg mutation of the beta-3 adrenergic receptor gene on gain weight in morbid obesity. *Int J Obes* 1996; 20: 1062–1066.

21. Otabe S, Clement K, Dubois S, Lepretre F, Pelloux V, Leibel R, Chung W, Boutin P, Guy-Grand B, Froguel P, Vasseur F. Mutation screening and association studies of the human UCP 3 gene in normoglycemic and diabetic morbidly obese patients. *Diabetes* 1999; 48: 206–208.

22. Otabe S, Clement K, Rich N, Warden C, Pecqueur C, Neverova M *et al*. Mutation screening of the human UCP2 gene in normoglycemic and NIDDM morbidily obese patients. *Diabetes* 1998; 47: 840–842.

23. Otabe S, Clement K, Dina C, Pelloux V, Guy-Grand B, Froguel P, Vasseur F. Genetic Variation in the 5' flanking region of the UCP3 gene is associated with body mass index in human in interaction with physical activity. *Diabetologia* 2000; 43: 245–9.

24. Hani E, Clement K, Velho G, Vionnet N, Hager J, Philippi A *et al*. Genetic studies of the Sulfonylurea Receptor gene locus in NIDDM and obesity among French Caucasians. *Diabetes* 1997; 46: 688–694.

25. Barat-Houari M, Clément K, Vatin V, Dina C, Le Gall G, Vasseur F *et al*. Positional candidate gene analysis of lim domain homeobox gene (Isl-1) on chromosome 5q11-q13 in French morbidly obese population shows indication for association with type 2 diabetes. *Diabetes* 2002; 51: 1640–1643.

26. Hager J, Dina C, Francke S, Dubois S, Houari M, Vatin V *et al*. A genome-wide scan for human obesity genes shows evidence for a major susceptibility locus on chromosome 10. *Nature Genet* 1998; 20: 304–338.

27. Comuzzie AG, Hixson JE, Almasy L *et al*. A major quantitative trait locus determining serum leptin levels and fat mass is located on human chromosome 2. *Nature Genet* 1997; 15(3): 273–276.

28. Rotimi CN, Comuzzie AG, Lowe WL *et al*. The quantitative trait locus on chromosome 2 for serum leptin levels is confirmed in African-Americans. *Diabetes* 1999; 48: 643–644.

29. Hinney A, Ziegler A, Oeffner F, Wedewardt C, Vogel M, Wulftange H *et al*. Independant confirmation of a major locus for obesity on chromosome 10. *J Clin Endocrinol Metab* 2000; 85(8): 2962–2965.

30. Rice T, Chagnon YC, Perusse L *et al*. A genomewide linkage scan for abdominal subcutaneous and visceral fat in black and white families: The HERITAGE family study. *Diabetes* 2002; 51(3): 848–855.

31. Hsueh WC, Mitchell BD, Schneider JL *et al*. Genome-wide scan of obesity in the old order Amish. *J Clin Endocrinol Metab* 2001; 86(3): 1199–1205.

32. Price RA, Li WD, Bernstein A, Crystal A, Golding EM *et al*. A locus affecting obesity in human chromosome region 10p12. *Diabetologia* 2001; 44: 363–366.

33. Delplanque J, Barat-Houari M, Dina C, Gallina P, Clement K, Guy-Grand B *et al*. Linkage and association studies between the proopiomelanocortin (POMC) gene and obesity in caucasian families. *Diabetologia* 2000; 43: 1554–7.

34. Delplanque J, Vasseur F, Durand E, Abderrahmani A, Dina C, Waeber G *et al*. Mutation screening of the urocortin gene: identification of new single nucleotide polymorphisms and association studies with obesity in French Caucasians. *J Clin Endocrinol Metab* 2002; 87: 867–9.

35. Rankinen T, Perusse L, Weisnagel SJ *et al*. The human obesity gene map: the 2001 update. *Obes Res* 2002; 10(3): 196–243.

36. Korstanje R, Paigen B. From QTL to gene. The harvest begin. *Nature Genet* 2002; 31: 235–236.

Progress in Obesity Research: 9. Edited by *Geraldo Medeiros-Neto, Alfredo Halpern and Claude Bouchard*
©2003 John Libbey Eurotext Ltd, pp. 333–337.

CHAPTER 71

Genome-wide scan studies of obesity-related phenotypes in the Quebec and HERITAGE Family Studies

Louis Pérusse[1], Yvon C. Chagnon[2] and Claude Bouchard[3]

[1]*Department of Preventive Medicine, Division of Kinesiology, PEPS, Laval University, Québec, Canada;*
[2]*Genetic and Molecular Psychiatry Unit, Laval University Robert Giffard Research Center, Québec, Canada;*
[3]*Human Genomics Laboratory, Pennington Biomedical Research Center Louisiana State University, Baton Rouge, USA*
[e-mail: louis.perusse@kin.msp.ulaval.ca]

Introduction

Genome-wide linkage studies are linkage studies performed with large number of polymorphic markers selected to cover the whole genome and tested for linkage with a variety of obesity phenotypes in order to detect Quantitative Trait Loci or QTLs. The obesity QTLs uncovered in such genome-wide scans lead to the identification of chromosomal regions, or in some cases of positional candidate genes, that can be further investigated for their role in the phenotype of interest. Several genome scans of obesity have been published since the first one reported in Pima Indians in 1997[1]. As of the time of the 9th International Congress on Obesity (ICO), about 25 genomic scans of obesity-related phenotypes, performed in 14 different populations, were published[2]. The Quebec Family Study (QFS) and the HERITAGE Family Study (HERITAGE) are two populations in which genome-wide scans of obesity have been performed. These two populations have the particularity of having phenotypes and markers that were measured and analysed using the same methodology. This offers a unique opportunity to compare results across populations and identify replications. This chapter will review the results of 4 genome-wide linkage studies reported in these two populations: one for fat free mass[3], one for body fat and body composition[4] and two for abdominal fat[5,6].

Description of the populations

The Quebec Family Study

The Quebec Family Study (QFS) is a prospective family study that was initiated in 1979. During Phase 1 of the study, and over a period of about four years, data were gathered on 1,630 subjects coming from 375 families of French descent living in the greater Quebec city area. These families were randomly ascertained with regards to obesity. During Phase 2 of the study, which began in 1992, 385 subjects from 105 Phase 1 families agreed to be measured for a second time after an average follow-up period of 12 years. Moreover, 263 subjects from 74 families with one or more obese members were recruited and 108 extended relatives from 46 Phase 1 families were incorporated into the study. Phase 3 of the study started in 1998 with 5-year follow-up measurements of families tested in Phase 2 and with recruitment of new obese families and/or sibships. As of August 2002, QFS included a total of 947 subjects from 223 families. A maximum of 530 sibpairs is available in QFS, including 111 male sibpairs, 182 female sibpairs and 235 opposite-sex sibpairs. The average BMI of the QFS subjects is 27.3 kg/m^2 and 27.7 kg/m^2 for males and females, respectively.

The HERITAGE Family Study

The HEart RIsk Factors Training And Genetics (HERITAGE) Family Study was designed to study the role of genetic factors in metabolic, cardiovascular and hormonal phenotypes before and in response to a standardized endurance-training programme[7]. The study includes 326 subjects from 127 Black families and 529 subjects from 101 Caucasian families consisting of the two parents and at least three biological offpring. The maximum number of sibpairs in Black families reached 148 (47 male sibpairs; 59 female sibpairs and 42 brother-sister pairs), while the corresponding number in Caucasian families was 415 (107 male sibpairs; 115 female sibpairs and 193 brother-sister pairs). The average BMI of the HERITAGE subjects is 26.6 kg/m^2 for both males and females. These subjects were submitted to a complete battery of tests before and after 20 weeks of endurance training on cycle ergometer. Details of the training programme can be found elsewhere[8]. Briefly, during the first two weeks, subjects trained at a heart rate corresponding to 55 per cent of their maximal oxygen consumption (VO$_2$ max) measured at baseline for 30 min. The duration and the intensity of the training sessions were gradually increased to reach 50 min at 75 per cent of the baseline VO$_2$ max for the last 6 weeks of the programme. The frequency of training was maintained at three times per week throughout the programme. A total of 742 subjects completed the training programme, 259 from Black families and 483 from White families. In subjects who completed the training, the response phenotypes were calculated as the difference between the pre- and post-training measures.

The phenotypes

Several variables related to obesity were measured in QFS and HERITAGE subjects. These include body mass index and subcutaneous fat assessed by the sum of eight skinfolds (SF8 = sum of biceps, triceps, thigh, calf, subscapular, suprailiac, abdominal and mid-axillary skinfolds) and leptin levels with (Lep-FM) and without (Lep) adjustment for fat mass in HERITAGE. Moreover, total body fat (FM), percentage body fat (%FAT) and fat free mass (FFM) were measured from body density measurements obtained by underwater weighing in both cohorts. Finally, total (ATF), visceral (AVF) and subcutaneous (ASF) abdominal adipose tissue areas were assessed by a CT scan obtained between the 4th and 5th lumbar vertebrae while subjects were in a supine position.

Linkage analyses

The phenotypes described above were adjusted for age and sex before being submitted to linkage analysis. In addition to the adjustment for age and sex, the response phenotypes were further adjusted for the baseline values. The genetic markers used for linkage analysis consisted of microsatellites mainly selected from the Marshfield panel 8a and the Genethon panel to cover the 22 autosomes. The panel of markers also includes polymorphisms in some candidate genes. For the QFS scan studies summarized here[3,5], the panel consists of 293 markers for an average map density of 11.9 cM. For HERITAGE studies, two panels of markers were used: one consisting of 344 markers with an average intermarker distance of 9.7 cM[4], and another consisting of 507 markers for an average map density of 7.0 cM[6]. The markers were tested for linkage with the adjusted phenotypes using the regression-based modified Haseman-Elston method[9] implemented in the SIBAPL2 software of SAGE[10] as well as a method based on variance components and implemented in the SEGPATH software[11]. Only significant linkage results, i.e. those with P values < 0.0023 or Lod scores ≥ 1.75 are reported.

Results

Fat free mass

Genome-wide linkage analyses of fat free mass were reported in QFS[3] and HERITAGE[4]. The study in QFS was based on 748 subjects from 194 families, while the one in HERITAGE was based on 522 subjects from 99 Caucasian families. The QTLs for fat free mass indentifed from these scans are summarized in Table 1. A total of five QTLs were found to influence FFM, four in QFS (1q44, 7p15.3, 15q26.2 and 16p32) and one in HERITAGE (18q12). One QTL affecting changes in FFM in response to training was also observed on 12q23.2. The strongest linkage was found on 15q26.3 (Lod = 3.56) with the insulin-like growth factor 1 receptor.

Body fatness

A genome-wide linkage analysis of phenotypes related to obesity was performed in 522 subjects from 99 HERITAGE Caucasian families[4]. The body fat phenotypes investigated included BMI, subcutaneous fat, FM, percentage fat and leptin levels (with and without adjustment for FM) in baseline and in response to training. The results are summarized in Table 2. A total of 11 QTLs were found to influence the various indicators of body fatness. These include five QTLs affecting specifically the changes of body fat in response to training (1q24.1, 1q31.1, 9q34.1, 11q21 and 18q21-q23) and three affecting specifically baseline phenotypes (8q24.1, 10q21-q22 and 14q11).

Table 1. Summary of QTLs affecting fat free mass in QFS and HERITAGE family studies*

Chromosome	Marker	Lod score	Cohort
1q44	D1S547	2.27	QFS
7p15.3	D7S1808	2.72	QFS
12q23.2	IGF1	2.30	HERITAGE
15q26.2	IGF1R	3.56	QFS
16p32	D16S748	2.10	QFS
18q12	D18S535	3.60	HERITAGE

*All QTLs are for fat free mass, except the one on 12q23.3, which is for changes in FFM in response to endurance training.
IGF1 = Insulin-like growth factor 1 (somatomedin C); IGF1R = Insulin-like growth factor 1 receptor.

Table 2. Summary of QTLs affecting body fatness in the HERITAGE family study

Chromosome	Marker	Phenotype	*P* value
1q24.1	ATP1A2	Δ%FAT	0.001
1q31.1	D1S1660	ΔFM, Δ%FAT	0.0006
5q14.1	D5S1725	BMI, ΔBMI, SF8	$0.002 < P < 0.0004$
8q24.1	D8S592	BMI, Lep	0.001
9q34.1	D9S282	ΔFM, Δ%FAT	$0.005 < P < 0.001$
10q21-q22	GATA121A08	Lep-FM	0.001
11q13	UCP3	FM, %FAT, ΔFM, Δ%FAT	$0.01 < P < 0.0009$
11q21	D11S2002	ΔFM, Δ%FAT	$0.01 < P < 0.0009$
14q11	D14S283	BMI, Lep, FM	$0.002 < P < 0.0006$
18q21-q23	D18S878	ΔFM, Δ%FAT	0.001
19p13.2	LDLR	SF8, Lep, ΔLep-FM, FM, %FAT	$0.01 < P < 0.0009$

%FAT = percentage body fat; FM = fat mass; SF8 = sum of eight skinfolds; Lep = leptin levels; Lep-FM = Leptin levels adjusted for fat mass; Δ = delta, i.e. changes between pre- and post-training values.
ATP1A2 = ATPase, Na^+/K^+ transporting, alpha 2 (+) polypeptide. UCP3 = Uncoupling protein 3 (mitochondrial, proton carrier). LDLR = Low density lipoprotein receptor.

Abdominal fat

Genome-wide linkage analyses of abdominal fat phenotypes were reported for both QFS[5] and HERITAGE[6] Family Studies. In QFS, the study was based on 521 adult subjects from 156 Caucasian families. In HERITAGE, linkage with abdominal fat was tested in 668 individuals from 99 White and 105 Black families. The linkages found for ATF, AVF and ASF, adjusted for total body fatness, are summarized in Table 3. A total of 18 QTLs were uncovered in the two populations: two for ATF (5q31.2, 7q36.2), two for AVF (2q22.1, 2q36.1) and the remainder for ASF. Only two QTLs, 4q31-q32 and 11p14.1, were replicated across the two populations.

Conclusions

The review of the genome scans of obesity performed in the QFS and HERITAGE family studies reveals that there are several regions potentially harboring genes influencing obesity in these two populations. The results reported so far have led to the identification of six QTLs for fat free mass, 11 QTLs for various indicators of body fatness and 18 QTLs for abdominal fat, independent of total body fatness. The large number of obesity QTLs uncovered in these two populations indicates that there are several genetic loci underlying the most common forms of human obesity.

Table 3.Summary of QTLs affecting abdominal fat areas measured by CT-scan in QFS and HERITAGE family studies

Chromosome	Marker	Phenotype[a]	Lod score	Cohort
1p11.2	D1S534	ASF	2.30	QFS
2p14	D2S1334	ASF_W	1.88	HERITAGE
2q22.1	D2S1399	AVF_W	2.33	HERITAGE
2q36.1	D2S434	AVF_W	2.49	HERITAGE
3p26.3	D3S2387	ASF_B	2.16	HERITAGE
3q29	D3S1311	ASF_B	2.45	HERITAGE
4p15.1	D4S2397	ASF	2.30	QFS
4q31-q32	D4S2431	ASF_B	2.34	HERITAGE
	D4S2417	ASF	1.76	QFS
5q31.2	D5S658	ATF_W	2.06	HERITAGE
		ASF_W	2.10	
7q31.1	D7S1875	ASF	1.97	QFS
7q36.2	D7S3070	ΔATF_B	2.53	HERITAGE
	NOS3	ΔATF_B	2.34	
9q22.1	D9S1122	ASF	2.37	QFS
11p14.1	GATA34E08	ASF_B	1.75	HERITAGE
		ASF	1.18	QFS
12q22-q24	IGF1	ASF	1.89	
	D12S2078	ASF	2.88	QFS
13q34	D13S285	ASF	1.92	QFS
14q24.1	D14S588	ASF_B	2.38	HERITAGE
17q21.1	D17S2180	ASF	2.24	QFS
22q11.23	D22S264	ASF_W	1.96	HERITAGE

[a]ASF = abdominal subcutaneous fat; ATF = total abdominal subcutaneous fat; AVF = Abdominal visceral fat. Δ = delta, i.e. changes between pre- and post-training values. Suffix B = is Blacks; Suffix W is Whites. IGF1 = Insulin-like growth factor 1 (somatomedin C). NOS3 = Nitric oxide synthase 3.

References

1. Norman RA, Thompson DB, Foroud T, Garvey WT, Bennett PH, Bogardus C, Ravussin E. Genome wide search for genes influencing per cent body fat in Pima Indians: suggestive linkage at chromosome 11q21-q22. *Am J Hum Genet* 1997; 60: 166–73.

2. Rankinen T, Pérusse L, Weisnagel SJ, Snyder EE, Chagnon YC, Bouchard C. The human obesity gene map: the 2001 update. *Obes Res* 2002; 10: 196–243.

3. Chagnon YC, Borecki IB, Pérusse L, Roy S, Lacaille M, Chagnon M *et al.* Genome-wide search for genes related to the fat-free body mass in the Quebec family study. *Metabolism* 2000; 49: 203–7.

4. Chagnon YC, Rice T, Pérusse L, Borecki IB, Ho-Kim MA, Lacaille M *et al.* Genomic scan for genes affecting body composition before and after training in Caucasians from HERITAGE. *J Appl Physiol* 2001; 90: 1777–87.

5. Pérusse L, Rice T, Chagnon YC, Després JP, Lemieux S, Roy S *et al.* A genome-wide scan for abdominal fat assessed by computed tomography in the Quebec Family Study. *Diabetes* 2001; 50: 614–21.

6. Rice T, Chagnon YC, Pérusse L, Borecki IB, Ukkola O, Rankinen T, *et al.* A genomewide linkage scan for abdominal subcutaneous and visceral fat in black and white families: The HERITAGE Family Study. *Diabetes* 2002; 51: 848–55.

7. Bouchard C, Leon AS, Rao DC, Skinner JS, Wilmore JH, Gagnon J. The HERITAGE Family Study. Aims, design, and measurement protocol. *Med Sci Sports Exerc* 1995; 27: 721–9.

8. Skinner JS, Wilmore KM, Krasnoff JB, Jaskolski A, Gagnon J, Province MA, *et al.* Adaptation to a standardized training program and changes in fitness in a large, heterogeneous population: the HERITAGE Family Study. *Med Sci Sports Exerc* 2000; 32: 157–61.

9. Elston RC, Buxbaum S, Jacobs KB, Olson JM. Haseman and Elston revisited. *Genet Epidemiol* 2000; 19: 1–17.

10. S.A.G.E. Statistical analysis for genetic epidemiology, release 4.0. Computer program package available from the Department of Epidemiology and Biostatistics, Rammelkamp Center for Education and research, Metro Health Campus, Case Western University. Cleveland, 2000.

11. Province MA, Rao DC. General purpose model and a computer program for combined segregation and path analysis (SEGPATH): automatically creating computer programs from symbolic language model specifications. *Genet Epidemiol* 1995; 12: 203–19.

Progress in Obesity Research: 9. Edited by *Geraldo Medeiros-Neto, Alfredo Halpern and Claude Bouchard*
©2003 John Libbey Eurotext Ltd, pp. 338–341.

CHAPTER 72

Genome scans for obesity – The USA studies

Kashif Munir[a], Braxton D. Mitchell[a] and Alan R. Shuldiner[a,b]

[a]*University of Maryland School of Medicine, Baltimore, MD, USA;* [b] *Geriatrics Research and Education Clinical Center, Baltimore Veterans Administration Medical Center, Baltimore, MD, USA*
[e-mail: ashuldin@medicine.umaryland.edu]

Introduction

Obesity is a complex phenotype determined by both genetic and environmental influences. It is estimated that up to 50 per cent or more of the variation in human obesity phenotypes is heritable[1]. Genome-wide scans have been successful in identifying genes for Mendelian diseases and are now being applied to complex diseases, including obesity. In genome scans, polymorphic short tandem repeat (STR) markers are genotyped at regular intervals throughout the genome in sibling pairs or larger family units. Linkage analysis is then performed to identify the chromosomal regions that affected (i.e. obese) family members share more commonly than would be expected by chance. Alternatively, quantitative trait linkage (QTL) analysis can be performed to determine if sharing of alleles at a given locus can account for the correlations among related individuals in obesity phenotypes (e.g. BMI, fat mass, plasma leptin levels). An advantage of genome-wide scans is that no prior assumptions about the potential importance of specific genes or regions of chromosomes are required; rather a systematic survey of the entire genome is made.

In recent years, an increasing number of genome scans for obesity and related phenotypes have been performed. Since complex traits like obesity are heterogeneous and polygenic by definition, statistical criteria for significant genome-wide linkage are likely to be too rigorous: few genome scans of obesity have resulted in linkages with LOD (log of the odds) scores meeting the genome-wide level of statistical significance of 3.3 proposed by Lander and Kruglyak[2]. Thus, replications of modest linkages across independent genome scans have become increasingly important in separating false positive linkages from linkages that are more likely to be true linkages. The successful positional cloning of obesity genes from linked regions, replicated or not, will ultimately determine the usefulness of genome-wide approaches.

This paper will review the complete genome scans performed in populations from the United States. A more complete review of genome scans both in humans and in animal models can be found elsewhere[3,4]. To date, the genome scans in the United States have been performed in four different ethnic groups: Caucasians, African Americans, Mexican-Americans and Native Americans (Pima Indians). Although all of these studies will be reviewed briefly, we will emphasize our studies in Amish Caucasians.

The Old Order Amish

The Old Order Amish who live in Lancaster County, Pennsylvania are a unique founder population. The Amish are rural-living and are characterized by their strict religious beliefs and distinct eschewal of technological innovation. They have a strong interest in ancestry and keep well-documented genealogies; nearly all of the Amish can trace their lineages back twelve to fourteen generations to a small number of founders who originated in Berne, Switzerland. The Amish Family Diabetes Study (AFDS)[5] was initiated in 1995 with the objective of identifying chromosomal regions and genes that predispose to type 2 diabetes and obesity. The AFDS now consists of over 1,400 subjects, most of whom have phenotypic measurements that include body mass index, body fat mass, blood pressure, plasma leptin, and glucose tolerance by 75-g oral glucose tolerance test. Most of these measures are significantly heritable in the Amish (e.g. h^2 for BMI = 0.42; leptin = 0.42; waist = 0.37; fasting glucose = 0.10; glucose at 120 min = 0.30)[5].

A genome-wide scan was conducted for obesity and related traits in the first 691 AFDS subjects, who comprise 28 large families and over 6,000 relationship pairs[6]. Three hundred and fifty-seven polymorphic STR markers were genotyped in these individuals (mean heterozygosity coefficient = 0.75; mean intermarker distance = 11 cM). Multipoint variance components linkage analysis revealed five chromosomal regions with evidence for linkage (i.e. LOD > 1.5) to one or more obesity-related traits (Table 1). The highest LOD score was that for BMI-adjusted leptin levels on chromosome 10p, near marker D10S220. This phenotype represents the residual variability of leptin after adjusting for BMI and may be regarded as a surrogate measure of leptin sensitivity for a given BMI. It is noteworthy that at least three prior studies have localized a very similar region of chromosome 10p12 as being linked to obesity[7–9]. The linkage to per cent body fat on chromosome 3p was less than 2 cM away from a linkage reported by Lee et al.[10] and Wu et al.[11] and the region on 7q was near linkages reported by others in Mexican-Americans[12], African Americans[11] and US Caucasians[11]. Intriguing positional candidate genes in these regions include PPAR-gamma (chromosome 3) and leptin (chromosome 7).

Table 1. Maximum LOD scores from multipoint linkage analysis of obesity-related traits in the Amish

Chromosome	Location (cM)	Nearest marker	Trait	LOD score (P value)
3	33	D3S3608	Per cent fat	1.61 (0.0032)
7	164	7S636	BMI-adjusted leptin	1.77 (0.0022)
10	71	10S220	BMI-adjusted leptin	2.73 (0.0002)
14	52	D14S276	Waist	1.80 (0.0020)
	86	D14S280	BMI-adjusted leptin	2.49 (0.0004)
16	1	D16S510	BMI	1.68 (0.0027)
	14	D16S407	Leptin	1.72 (0.0024)

In addition to the above-mentioned phenotypes, information regarding eating behaviour was obtained in AFDS subjects using the Three Factor Eating Behavior questionnaire devised by Stunkard and Messick[14]. The 51-item questionnaire assesses three aspects of eating behaviour: restraint, disinhibition and hunger. Restraint is defined as a cognitive avoidance of eating to control body weight. Disinhibition is loss of restraint resulting in overeating. Hunger measures the perceived need for food. All three eating behaviour traits were significantly and positively associated with body mass index (BMI)[15]. Interestingly, all three eating behaviours were significantly heritable even after adjusting for shared household (h^2 for restraint = 0.28; disinhibition = 0.40; hunger = 0.23; $P < 0.001$ for all)[15]. Genome-wide linkage analysis identified five chromosomal regions that were linked to eating behaviour traits (Table 2). There was suggestive evidence for linkage of restraint scores to chromosome 3 near marker D3S1304 with a LOD score of 2.5, the same region showing evidence for linkage to other obesity-related phenotypes[6,10,11] as well as on chromosome 6 near marker D6S276 with a maximum LOD score of 2.3. For disinhibition scores, the maximum LOD score of 1.6 occurred on chromosome 7 near marker D7S657 as well as on chromosome 16 near D16S752 with a LOD score of 1.4. Hunger scores showed a maximum LOD score of 1.4 on chromosome 3 near marker D3S1278. These studies, implicate for the first time, specific chromosomal regions (and putative genes) that regulate eating behaviour traits. Additional studies will be required to replicate these findings and ultimately to identify gene variants in the regions.

Table 2. Maximum LOD scores from multipoint linkage analysis of eating behaviour traits in the Amish

Chromosome	Location (cM)	Nearest marker	Trait	LOD score (P value)
3	19	D3S1304	Restraint	2.5 (0.0003)
	120	D3S1278	Hunger	1.4 (0.0053)
6	40	D6S276	Restraint	2.3 (0.0006)
7	105	D7S657	Disinhibition	1.6 (0.0033)
16	86	D16S752	Disinhibition	1.4 (0.0052)

Other US populations

A genome scan of 2209 Caucasian individuals from 507 families recruited from the TOPS (Take Off Pounds Sensibly, Inc.) membership revealed evidence for linkage of several obesity-related traits on chromosome 3q27 near marker D3S2427 (LOD scores = 3.30 for BMI, 2.40 for waist circumference, 3.54 for hip circumference and 3.17 for body weight). Plasma leptin levels showed the strongest evidence for linkage on chromosome 17p12 near marker D17S947 (LOD = 5.0). Possible candidate genes are the adiponectin gene (chromosome 3), and the PPAR-alpha gene (chromosome 17).

Deng et al.[17] studied 630 Caucasian subjects from 53 families and found a region on chromosome 2 near marker D2S347 with a maximum LOD score of 4.44 for BMI and 2.21 for body fat mass. There were additional QTLs for BMI on chromosome 1 near marker D1S468 (LOD = 2.09) and chromosome 4 near marker D4S1592 (LOD = 2.09). A potential candidate gene near the QTL on chromosome 1 includes the tumor necrosis factor-alpha receptor 2 gene.

In a genome scan of 513 predominantly US Caucasian members of 92 families with severe obesity, Lee et al.[10] found evidence of a QTL for BMI on chromosome 20q13. Affected sibling pair analysis yielded a LOD score of 3.17 near D20S476 in the same region. Possible candidate genes on chromosome 20q13 include the agouti-signaling protein (ASIP) gene and the CAAT/enhancer-binding protein beta.

A genome scan for QTLs influencing BMI was performed on Caucasian subjects in the National Heart, Lung, and Blood Institute Family Heart Study[11]. Over 4,000 subjects from two samples were studied. The strongest evidence for linkage was found on chromosome 7 at markers GATA43C11 and D7S1804 with a maximum LOD score of 4.9. This is the same region near the leptin gene that provided evidence of linkage to obesity-related traits in Mexican-Americans[12], African Americans[11], and the Amish[6,15].

A genome-wide scan for obesity and related traits was performed in Mexican-Americans participating in the San Antonio Family Heart Study[18]. QTLs influencing serum leptin levels and fat mass were found on chromosome 2p23. The maximum LOD score linked to serum leptin was 4.95 and for fat mass was 2.75, both near marker D2S1788. Possible candidate genes on chromosome 2 are the pro-opiomelano-cortin (POMC) gene and the glucokinase regulatory protein (GCKR) gene. Another suggestive area of linkage to leptin levels was observed on chromosome 8 near the beta-3-adrenergic receptor gene with a 2-point LOD score of 2.2. A subsequent genome scan of BMI was performed in these families, and a LOD score of 3.21 was observed on chromosome 8 in the region of the beta-3-adrenergic receptor gene[19].

In 618 African Americans from 202 families, the strongest evidence for linkage was found to percent body fat on chromosome 6 near marker D6S1959 (LOD = 2.7)[20]. For BMI, there was suggestive evidence of linkage on chromosome 5 near marker D5S817 (LOD = 1.9), and on chromosome 3 near marker D3S2477 (LOD = 1.8). The region on chromosome 3 has significant overlap with the previously described linkage by Kissebah et al.[16] in whites and may be considered a replication. This region contains the adiponectin gene.

The Pima Indian community of Arizona has been the subject of extensive efforts to identify genes influencing diabetes and obesity. BMI showed evidence for linkage on chromosome 11q near marker D11S4464 (LOD = 3.6), which was linked to diabetes as well[21]. Suggestive linkage to per cent body fat was found on chromosome 11 near marker D11S2366 (LOD = 2.1), and on chromosome 18 near marker D18S877 (LOD = 2.3)[22]. Possible candidate genes on chromosome 11 include the cluster of matrix metalloproteinase genes, which participate in the processing of tumor necrosis factor-alpha, and the gene for cytosolic glycerol-3-phosphate dehydrogenase, which plays an important role in lipid synthesis.

A combined analysis of genome scans using the interim results from the National Heart, Lung, and Blood Institute Family Blood Pressure Program was undertaken involving 6,849 individuals from four different ethnic groups (white, black, Mexican-American and Asian)[11]. The most significant linkage for BMI was found on chromosome 3 at marker D3S1764 (LOD = 3.45) for the GENOA network sample of blacks. Other suggestive areas of linkage for BMI were on chromosome 3 at marker D3S1259 (LOD = 2.03) for HyperGEN whites; chromosome 7 at marker D7S3051 (LOD = 2.66) for SAPPHIRe Asians; and at marker D7S2847 (LOD = 2.36) for HyperGEN blacks; chromosome 14 at marker D14S617 (LOD = 2.15) for HyperGEN blacks; chromosome 16 at marker GATA67G11 (LOD = 2.55) for GENOA whites; and chromosome 17 at marker D17S947 (LOD = 2.47) for GENOA whites. When the samples of the white populations were pooled, two regions showed suggestive linkage to BMI, chromosome 16 at marker GATA67G11 (LOD = 2.15), and chromosome 17 at marker D17S947 (LOD = 2.18). When samples of whites, blacks, and Mexican-Americans were combined, excluding Asians, there was evidence of linkage to BMI on chromosome 3 at marker D3S2427 (LOD = 3.40). This same region was observed to be linked to BMI by Kissebah et al. in whites[16].

340

Summary

Genome-wide scans for obesity phenotypes in multiple populations have led to the identification of several chromosomal regions that may harbour obesity susceptibility genes. As the number of scans has increased, several regions of replication have emerged, most notably on chromosomes 3, 7 and 10. The significance of these findings must await the eventual positional cloning of the putative obesity susceptibility genes in these regions.

References

1. Bouchard C, Perusse L, Rice T, Rao DC. The genetics of human obesity. In: *Handbook of obesity*, Bray BA, Bouchard C, James WPT (eds), pp. 157–90. New York: Marcel Dekker, 1998.

2. Lander E, Kruglyak L. Genetic dissection of complex traits: guidelines for interpreting and reporting linkage results. *Nat Genet* 1995; 11: 241–7.

3. Chagnon YC, Rankinen T, Snyder EE, Weisnagel SJ, Perusse L, Bouchard C. The human obesity map: the 2002 update. *Obes Res* 2003; 11: 313-367.

4. Comuzzie AG, Williams JT, Martin LJ, Blangero J. Searching for genes underlying normal variation in human adiposity. *J Mol Med* 2001; 79: 57–70.

5. Hsueh W-C, Mitchell BD, Aburomia R, Pollin T, Sakul H, Ehm MG *et al.* Diabetes in the Old Order Amish: Characterization and heritability analysis of the Amish Family Diabetes Study. *Diabetes Care* 2000; 23: 595–601.

6. Hsueh W-C, Mitchell BD, Schneider JL, St Jean PL, Pollin TI, Ehm MG *et al.* Genome-wide scan of obesity in the Old Order Amish. *J Clin Endocrinol Metab* 2001; 86: 1199–205.

7. Hager J, Dina C, Francke S, Dubois S, Houari M, Vatin V *et al.* A genome-wide scan for human obesity genes reveals a major susceptibility locus on chromosome 10. *Nat Genet* 1998; 20: 304–8.

8. Hinney A, Ziegler A, Oeffner F, Wedewardt C, Vogel M, Wulftange H *et al.* Independent confirmation of a major locus for obesity on chromosome 10. *J Clin Endocrinol Metab* 2000; 85: 2962–5.

9. Price RA, Li WD, Bernstein A, Crystal A, Golding EM, Weisberg SJ *et al.* A locus affecting obesity in human chromosome region 10p12. *Diabetologia* 2001; 44: 363–6.

10. Lee JH, Reed DR, Li WD, Xu W, Joo EJ, Kilker RL *et al.* Genome scan for human obesity and linkage to markers in 20q13. *Am J Hum Genet* 1999; 64: 196–209.

11. Wu X, Cooper RS, Borecki I, Hanis C, Bray M, Lewis CE *et al.* A combined analysis of genomewide linkage scans for body mass index from the National Heart, Lung, and Blood Institute Family Blood Pressure Program. *Am J Hum Genet* 2002; 70: 1247–56.

12. Duggirala R, Stern MP, Mitchell BD, Reinhart LJ, Shipman PA, Uresandi OC *et al.* Quantitative variation in obesity-related traits and insulin precursors linked to the OB gene region on human chromosome 7. *Am J Hum Genet* 1996; 59: 694–703.

13. Feitosa MF, Borecki IB, Rich SS, Arnett DK, Sholinsky P, Myers RH *et al.* Quantitative-trait loci influencing body-mass index reside on chromosomes 7 and 13: the National Heart, Lung, and Blood Institute Family Heart Study. *Am J Hum Genet* 2002; 70: 72–82.

14. Stunkard AJ, Messick S. The three-factor eating questionnaire to measure dietary restraint, disinhibition and hunger. *J Psychosom Res* 1985; 29: 71–83.

15. Steinle N, Hsueh W-C, Snitker S, Mitchell BD, Pollin TI, Sakul H *et al.* Eating behavior in the Old Order Amish: heritability analysis and a genome-wide linkage analysis. *Am J Clin Nutr* 2002; 75: 1098–106.

16. Kissebah AH, Sonnenberg GE, Myklebust J, Goldstein M, Broman K, James RG *et al.* Quantitative trait loci on chromosomes 3 and 17 influence phenotypes of the metabolic syndrome. *Proc Natl Acad Sci USA* 2000; 97: 14478–83.

17. Deng HW, Deng H, Liu YJ, Liu YZ, Xu FH, Shen H *et al.* A genomewide linkage scan for quantitative-trait loci for obesity phenotypes. *Am J Hum Genet* 2002; 70: 1138–51.

18. Comuzzie AG, Hixson JE, Almasy L, Mitchell BD, Mahaney MC, Dyer TD *et al.* A major quantitative trait locus determining serum leptin levels and fat mass is located on human chromosome 2. *Nat Genet* 1997; 15: 273–6.

19. Mitchell BD, Cole SA, Comuzzie AG, Almasy L, Blangero J, MacCluer JW *et al.* A quantitative trait locus influencing BMI maps to the region of the ß-3 adrenergic receptor. *Diabetes* 1999; 48: 1863–7.

20. Zhu X, Cooper RS, Luke A, Chen G, Wu X, Kan D *et al.* A genome-wide scan for obesity in African-Americans. *Diabetes* 2002; 51: 541–4.

21. Hanson RL, Ehm MG, Pettitt DJ, Prochazka M, Thompson DB, Timberlake D *et al.* An autosomal genomic scan for loci linked to type II diabetes mellitus and body-mass index in Pima Indians. *Am J Hum Genet* 1998; 63: 1130–8.

22. Norman RA, Thompson DB, Foroud T, Garvey WT, Bennett PH, Bogardus C *et al.* Genomewide search for genes influencing per cent body fat in Pima Indians: suggestive linkage at chromosome 11q21-q22. Pima Diabetes Gene Group. *Am J Hum Genet* 1997; 60: 166–73.

Progress in Obesity Research: 9. Edited by *Geraldo Medeiros-Neto, Alfredo Halpern and Claude Bouchard*
©2003 John Libbey Eurotext Ltd, pp. 342–347.

CHAPTER 73

Perils, pitfalls, and promise: expression profiling to diagnose obesity subtypes

Steven R. Smith, Andrey Ptitsyn and Hui Xie

Pennington Biomedical Research Center, 6400 Perkins Road, Baton Rouge, LA 70808, USA
[e-mail: smithsr@pbrc.edu]

Introduction

The current treatment recommendations for obesity are quite simple. All patients are essentially given the same advice: eat less, exercise more. In contrast, physicians and scientists realize that overweight and obese patients are unique. That is, patients respond by varying degrees to pharmacologic and other weight loss interventions. Unfortunately, our understanding of what characteristics will identify patients as 'responders' or 'non-responders' to a specific therapy is limited.

Interindividual variation in the response to therapy is in part due to differences in compliance with therapy[1], but degrees of response are also due to differences in the genetic and/or physiological makeup of an individual[2]. Greenway and Lefevre[2] showed that a polymorphism in the beta-3 adrenoreceptor gene was related to the weight loss during a combined pharmacologic and behaviour modification therapy. Nicklas *et al.* demonstrated that an uncommon polymorphism in the PPAR-γ gene was related to the ability of individuals to oxidize fat during weight loss[3]. For example, one-half of patients do not increase their resting energy expenditure more than 7 per cent when treated with a single dose of ephedra and caffeine (E + C)[4]. Importantly, this acute thermogenic response to caffeine predicts long-term weight loss success[5]. We know very little about why some patients respond and others do not, although these and other data strongly suggest a role of the sympathetic nervous system.

We are able to identify specific eating patterns such as the night eating syndrome and binge eating[6]. Recent advances also allow us to identify patients with cravings for certain types of foods[7]. Obese patients have also been grouped according to body fat patterning, i.e. central versus peripheral obesity. The latter classification is important to identify persons at highest risk for the metabolic complications of obesity[8–10]. The sequencing of the human genome provides a fantastic opportunity to advance our understanding of the responsiveness to adrenergic stimuli such as E + C[11,12]. Breast cancer, lymphoma, and prostate cancer can be separated into distinct phenotypic groups by simultaneously measuring the expression level for thousands of mRNAs[13–15]. This technique is known as cDNA 'microarray' technology. The data is then analysed using quantitative analysis of gene expression patterns, which together are called cluster analysis. The pattern of mRNAs present in an individual sample is known as an 'expression profile' which reflects the underlying pathophysiology of the tumour or disease[13]. When reduced in dimensionality, microarray data can be used to predict the prognosis of cancer patients and their response to chemotherapy[14]. Importantly, these techniques identify molecular pathways underlying specific tumour subtypes and identify surrogate markers, which predict the prognosis of cancer patients and their response to chemotherapy. Alizadeh *et al.* demonstrated that patients with B-cell lymphomas whose tumour mRNA clustered into the 'activated B-cell category' had a higher mortality and responded poorly to chemotherapy. The patients whose tumours clustered into the 'germinal centre' subtype had a much better response to chemotherapy and survived longer. An identical approach has also been applied to prostate and breast cancers.

Two important points must be considered regarding this experimental paradigm. First, *this technique does not rely upon a complete understanding of the underlying biology to advance our diagnostic and therapeutic acumen.* In other words, we do not necessarily need to understand the function of all of

Environment and genetics *converge* to regulate cellular function through coordinated regulation of large 'sets' of genes

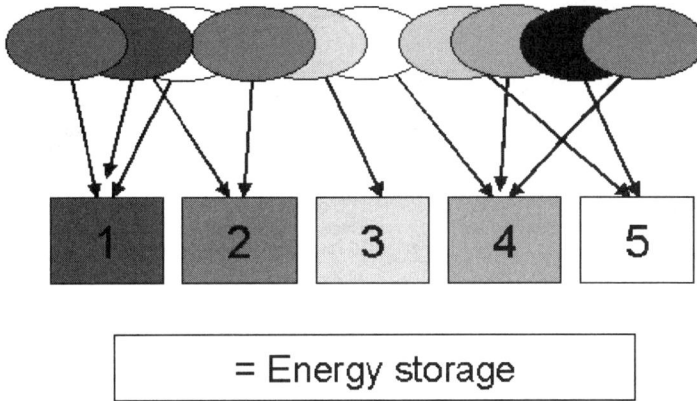

Fig. 1. Genes are regulated in groups or sets. These sets respond to the cellular environment and based on their genetic makeup. We do not need to know the upstream signals to use this information to classify patients into meaningful groups, nor do we need to know the function of the individual genes. Having some knowledge of the gene function or some *a priori* knowledge of the clinical classification allows us to use 'supervised' clustering techniques. More data is good.

the genes that make up the expression clusters to be able use the expression clusters to predict response to therapy . Second, all of these studies were able to advance our knowledge of tumour biology through identification of several dysregulated genes[16]. For example Dhanasekaran *et al.* demonstrated the novel gene 'hepsin' is related to survival of prostate cancer patients[17]. This gene had not been previously linked to prostate cancer and was discovered as a result of the combination of microarray and cluster analysis.

We are using a similar experimental design to separate obese patients into distinct groups based on their expression profiles ascertained by microarray analysis of skeletal muscle and adipose tissue mRNA. To take advantage of the post-genomic era[11,12] and harness the power of parallel data collection, we need robust statistical algorithms that reduce the dimensionality of the data.

'Having more data is good.'[18]

The reason that more data is good, is that we cannot, one gene at a time, move fast enough to test every biological hypothesis in a short period of time. Environment and genetics converge to regulate cellular function through coordinated regulation of large 'sets' of genes.

'... data sets produced in this way have emergent properties ... patterns and systematic features become apparent and we begin to build an integrated picture of the whole system.'[18]

We will follow the lead of the molecular oncologists who continue to push the technological envelope in order to improve patient care. In this paper, we will outline this approach.

An alternate approach is based on microarray technology. The microarray technique is fairly straight-forward in principle, but demanding with regards to the implementation, experimental design and quality control. Hundreds to thousands of DNA sequences are 'spotted' onto a single glass slide. One or two RNA samples are reverse transcribed generating cDNAs that are labeled with a unique fluorescent dye for each sample. The resulting cDNAs are then hybridized onto the slides containing the oligonucleotides representative of each gene. After washing, the slides are scanned with a laser. The intensity of the fluorescent signal is proportional to the amount of mRNA in the original sample.

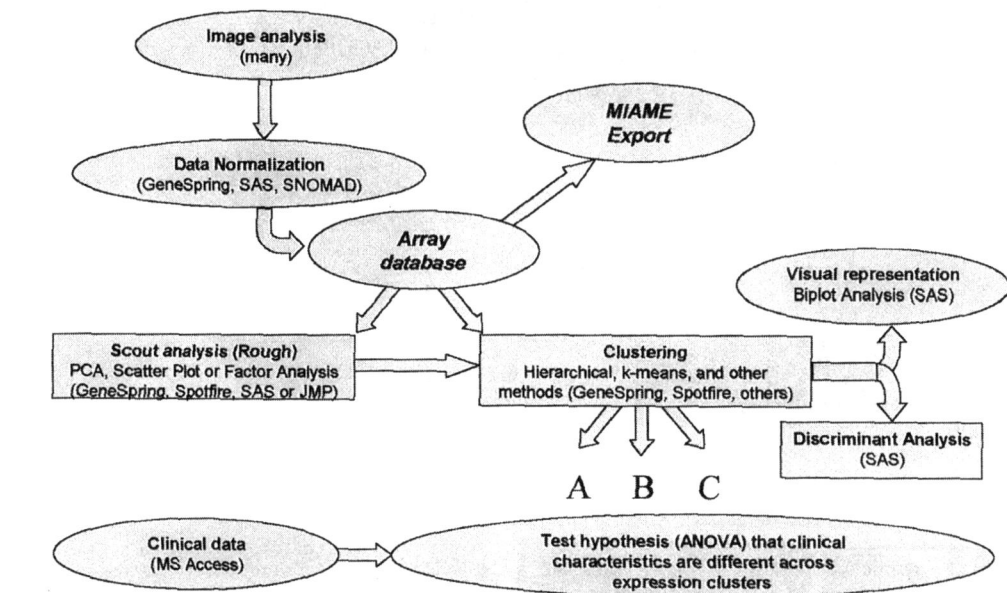

Fig. 2. An overview of the data flow and processing.
After an initial 'scout' principle components analysis, our approach is to allow the mRNA expression profile for each patient to agglomerate using hierarchical clustering and other clustering tools (in-development). The ultimate goal is to identify clusters that predict responsiveness to adrenergic therapy and other patient characteristics such as fat cell size, insulin resistance, fat distribution, etc.

Experimental design, data acquisition, and processing prior to analysis

We acknowledge the importance of robust experimental design and appropriate pre-processing of the microarray and clinical data[19,20]. The reader is referred to additional sources to review these topics[21,22].

Techniques to reduce the dimensionality of the data

There are many different types of statistical techniques that are used to reduce the multi-dimensional datasets into fewer (and hence understandable) dimensions. The number of statistical techniques applied to microarray data is on the rise with no signs of convergence in the field. For example, a recent survey of the literature recovered the following techniques: hierarchical clustering, K-means clustering, self-organizing maps/SOTA, singular value decomposition (a.k.a. principal components analysis), block clustering, gene 'shaving'/two-way clustering, associative memory neural network, relevance networks, shannon entropy, coupled two-way clustering, cluster-Rasch, TSVQ, supervised machine learning, support vector machine Roughly speaking, the techniques can be grouped into two categories: supervised and unsupervised.

'Unsupervised' clustering

As discussed by Ring and Ross unsupervised clustering '... allows the dominant gene-expression patterns in a dataset to drive the separation of clinical samples into groups on the basis of the overall similarity in expression pattern without allowing experimenter bias to influence the outcome'[23]. Of these methods, we will review two of the most popular and widely used: Hierarchical clustering and K-means clustering. The first used with microarray data was hierarchical clustering[24].

Hierarchical clustering

Hierarchical clustering reduces dimensionality based on the pair-wise distance between all genes in a set of experiments and subsequent agglomeration of clustered pairs into larger clusters, once again on the basis of distance. Hierarchical clustering is a 'bottom-up' method: each gene starts out in its own cluster and then is agglomerated to the closest pair of clusters at each stage producing a 'dendrogram'. This process continues until all the points are in one final cluster. The user then chooses the number of clusters that seems right and cuts the clustering tree at that point. One of the problems with this method is that there is no clear definition of the best level of the cluster.

K-means clustering

With this technique, the user must specify the number of starting points, k. Then a search algorithm goes out and finds k points in the data, called nodes. The routine goes through the rows and assigns each to the cluster that it is closest to. For each cluster, a new cluster centre is formed as the means (centroid) of the points currently in the cluster.

'Supervised' clustering

Regarding the classification of individuals into diagnostic categories, the best results are obtained with a training dataset, followed by a 'test' or confirmation data set. This technique relies upon *a priori* knowledge of gene behaviour or clinical classification[25,26]. These techniques will be useful at the later stages of our analysis after the subtypes are identified and diagnostic tests are developed for the clinic. Desirable features for any clustering method:

(1) *'Validation' and statistical analysis of the clustering model.* Statistical analysis of microarray data is just now moving to the forefront of the literature. The problems of having a large number of observations in a small population provide a daunting statistical problem. As mentioned above, a reduction in the multi-dimensional space helps, but knowing how good this process becomes quite difficult, but extremely important. Several techniques have been developed to address this need and numerous others are in-development. For example, the bootstrapping/ANOVA[27], FOM (figure of merit), and other techniques are appearing in the literature[28,29]. Again, It is important to remember that good statistical design is an important consideration and advance planning of the experiment is crucial.

(2) *Direct head-to-head comparison of multiple techniques is lacking.* The direct head-to-head comparison of these techniques is beneficial, but should not be considered a Darwinian survival of the fittest. Each statistical approach is likely to view the data from alternate viewpoints and may reveal patterns in the data not apparent from another perspective. The efforts of groups such as the microarray research coordination network (www.soph.uab.edu/mar) to provide standardized datasets in order to evaluate algorithms is applauded as an important component in the evolution of the field of microarray analysis.

An overview of our hypotheses and general approach

We are currently testing the hypotheses that the pattern of genes expressed in the skeletal muscle and adipose tissue from obese individuals will:

- **Identify distinct subtypes of obesity** that were previously undistinguishable;
- **Predict which patients will lose weight** during 6 months therapy with E+C; and
- **Correlate the subtypes identified** with the comorbidities of obesity.

The purpose of the final step in our analysis is to identify individual genes that are related to these three phenotypes of interest. It is important from a diagnostic standpoint to determine if a single gene might be representative of the entire cluster of genes from the primary analysis. If this were the case, a simple screening test might be developed to predict response. We will select genes based on the correlation coefficient of the relationship between the expression level on the microarray and the acute thermogenic response as described by Martin *et al.* using the PERMAX software package designed for this purpose[30]. Genes identified using this method will be confirmed using real-time RT-PCR on a PE7700 instrument (see[31] for a detailed description of the technique).

Perils and pitfalls

Although this process has been extremely valuable in understanding cancer, there are several pitfalls and perils when it comes to applying these techniques to obesity. As succinctly stated by Pritchard:

'Genetically diverse populations such as humans are likely to show even greater variability in gene expression than what we have observed among inbred mice. In addition, environmental

conditions cannot be carefully controlled in humans. These factors present challenges for microarray-based studies of human gene expression in vivo'[32].

An additional source of variability comes from the understanding that skeletal muscle biopsy samples are heterogeneous; containing blood vessels, neurons, adipocytes, and a range of fibre types. Similarly, adipose tissue biopsy samples are heterogeneous, containing adipocytes, blood vessels, neurons, mesenchymal stem cells, and fibroblasts/collagenous tissue.

This fact decreases the signal-to-noise ratio, unless variations in the proportions of these cell types are characteristic of the 'subtype' signal. Another major pitfall is if the brain/liver/islets are the master controllers of body weight and all other tissues follow. Again, reviewing Fig. 1 tells us that the sets of genes controlled by each of these factors in adipose tissue and skeletal muscle is influenced by the genetic makeup of the cell *and* the cellular environment (neural and endocrine inputs). Fortunately, we don't need to know to upstream signals to interpret their down stream effects, making this peril less concerning.

In summary, microarray expression data is useful for the 'molecular classification' of cancer and we believe that a careful application of this technology will lead to the identification of obesity subtypes. We believe that these molecular-diagnostic categories will lead to 'tailored obesity therapy' and an improved understanding of the obese patient.

Acknowledgements: I would like to acknowledge the support of the Bristol-Myers-Squibb Lipodystrophy initiative and the USDA that provide support for this work.

References

1. Guy-Grand B, Apfelbaum M, Crepaldi G, Gries A, Lefebvre P, Turner P. International trial of long-term dexfenfluramine in obesity. *Lancet* 1989; 2(8672): 1142–5.

2. Lefevre M, Greenway FL, Smith SR, Ryan DH, Bray GA, Morales S *et al.* Genetic Mutations That Predict Weight Loss In: An Obesity Treatment Program. *Int J Obes* 1998; 22 (Suppl 3): 61.

3. Nicklas BJ, van Rossum EF, Berman DM, Ryan AS, Dennis KE, Shuldiner AR. Genetic variation in the peroxisome proliferator-activated receptor- gamma2 gene (Pro12Ala) affects metabolic responses to weight loss and subsequent weight regain. *Diabetes* 2001; 50(9): 2172–6.

4. Liu YL, Toubro S, Astrup A, Stock MJ. Contribution of beta 3-adrenoceptor activation to ephedrine-induced thermogenesis in humans. *Int J Obes Relat Metab Disord* 1995; 19(9): 678–85.

5. Yoshida T, Sakane N, Umekawa T, Kondo M. Relationship between basal metabolic rate, thermogenic response to caffeine, and body weight loss following combined low calorie and exercise treatment in obese women. *Int J Obes Relat Metab Disord* 1994; 18(5): 345–50.

6. Stunkard A. Two eating disorders: binge eating disorder and the night eating syndrome. *Appetite* 2000; 34(3): 333–4.

7. Geiselman PJ, Anderson AM, Dowdy ML, West DB, Redmann SM, Smith SR. Reliability and validity of a macronutrient self-selection paradigm and a food preference questionnaire. *Physiol Behav* 1998; 63(5): 919–28.

8. Smith SR. The endocrinology of obesity. Endocrinology and Metabolism. Clinics of North America; 1996; 25: 921–42.

9. Smith SR. Regional Fat Distribution. In: *Nutrition genetic and obesity*, Bray GA, Ryan DH (eds), pp. 433–458. Baton Rouge: LSU Press, 1999.

10. Smith SR, Lovejoy JC, Greenway F, Ryan D, Dejonge L, De La Bretonne J *et al.* Contributions of total body fat, abdominal subcutaneous adipose tissue compartments, and visceral adipose tissue to the metabolic complications of obesity. *Metabolism* 2001; 50(4): 425–35.

11. Venter JC, Adams MD, Myers EW, Li PW, Mural RJ, Sutton GG *et al.* The sequence of the human genome. *Science* 2001; 291(5507): 1304–51.

12. Lander ES, Linton LM, Birren B, Nusbaum C, Zody MC, Baldwin J *et al.* Initial sequencing and analysis of the human genome. *Nature* 2001; 409(6822): 860–921.

13. West M, Blanchette C, Dressman H, Huang E, Ishida S, Spang R *et al.* Predicting the clinical status of human breast cancer by using gene expression profiles. *Proc Natl Acad Sci USA* 2001; 98(20): 11462–7.

14. Perou CM, Sorlie T, Eisen MB, van de Rijn M, Jeffrey SS, Rees CA *et al.* Molecular portraits of human breast tumours. *Nature* 2000; 406(6797): 747–52.

15. Sorlie T, Perou CM, Tibshirani R, Aas T, Geisler S, Johnsen H *et al.* Gene expression patterns of breast carcinomas distinguish tumor subclasses with clinical implications. *Proc Natl Acad Sci USA* 2001; 98(19): 10869–74.

16. Aitman TJ, Glazier AM, Wallace CA, Cooper LD, Norsworthy PJ, Wahid FN *et al.* Identification of Cd36 (Fat) as an insulin-resistance gene causing defective fatty acid and glucose metabolism in hypertensive rats [see comments]. *Nature Genet* 1999; 21(1): 76–83.

17. Dhanasekaran SM, Barrette TR, Ghosh D, Shah R, Varambally S, Kurachi K *et al.* Delineation of prognostic biomarkers in prostate cancer. *Nature* 2001; 412(6849): 822–6.

18. Brown PO, Botstein D. Exploring the new world of the genome with DNA microarrays. *Nature Genet* 1999; 21 (Suppl 1): 33–7.

19. Kerr MK, Churchill GA. Statistical design and the analysis of gene expression microarray data. Genet Res 2001; 77(2): 123–8.

20. Kerr MK, Martin M, Churchill GA. Analysis of variance for gene expression microarray data. J Comput Biol 2000; 7(6): 819–37.

21. Colantuoni C, Henry GW. SNOMAD – Standardization and NOrmalization of MicroArray Data.

22. Tinker NA. Data Pre-Processing Issues in Microarray Analysis. In: *A practical approach to microarray data analysis.* Amsterdam: Kluwer, 2002.

23. Ring BZ, Ross DT. Microarrays and molecular markers for tumor classification. Genome Biol 2002; 3(5): comment 2005.

24. Eisen MB, Spellman PT, Brown PO, Botstein D. Cluster analysis and display of genome-wide expression patterns. *Proc Natl Acad Sci USA* 1998; 95(25): 14863–8.

25. Yeang CH, Ramaswamy S, Tamayo P, Mukherjee S, Rifkin RM, Angelo M *et al.* Molecular classification of multiple tumor types. Bioinformatics 2001; 17 (Suppl 1): S316–S322.

26. Ramaswamy S, Tamayo P, Rifkin R, Mukherjee S, Yeang CH, Angelo M *et al.* Multiclass cancer diagnosis using tumor gene expression signatures. *Proc Natl Acad Sci USA* 2001; 98(26): 15149–54.

27. Kerr MK, Churchill GA. Bootstrapping cluster analysis: assessing the reliability of conclusions from microarray experiments. *Proc Natl Acad Sci USA* 2001; 98(16): 8961–5.

28. Yeung KY, Haynor D, Ruzzo W. Validating Clustering for Gene Expression Data: University of Washington. Report No. Technical Report UW-CSE-00-01-01; 2000

29. Herrero J, Valencia A, Dopazo J. A hierarchical unsupervised growing neural network for clustering gene expression patterns. Bioinformatics 2001; 17(2): 126–36.

30. Martin KJ, Graner E, Li Y, Price LM, Kritzman BM, Fournier MV *et al.* High-sensitivity array analysis of gene expression for the early detection of disseminated breast tumor cells in peripheral blood. *Proc Natl Acad Sci USA* 2001; 98(5): 2646–51.

31. Bustin SA. Absolute quantification of mRNA using real-time reverse transcription polymerase chain reaction assays. J *Mol Endocrinol* 2000; 25(2): 169–93.

32. Pritchard CC, Hsu L, Delrow J, Nelson PS. Project normal: defining normal variance in mouse gene expression. *Proc Natl Acad Sci USA* 2001; 98(23): 13266–71.

Progress in Obesity Research: 9. Edited by *Geraldo Medeiros-Neto, Alfredo Halpern and Claude Bouchard*
©2003 John Libbey Eurotext Ltd, pp. 348–351.

CHAPTER 74

Gene expression profiling of ageing and its retardation by caloric restriction

Tomas A. Prolla

Departments of Genetics and Medical Genetics, University of Wisconsin, 445 Henry Mall, Madison, WI, 53706, USA
[e-mail: taprolla@facstaff.wisc.edu]

Introduction

In order to gain a better understanding of general aspects of brain ageing, we are currently using DNA microarray analysis to study caloric restriction as a model system of ageing retardation in mammals[1,2,3]. These studies have shown the feasibility and utility of gene expression profiling to identify basic aspects of the ageing process. Caloric restriction (CR) retards the ageing process in laboratory rodents as characterized by a delayed occurrence or complete prevention of a broad spectrum of age-associated pathophysiological changes and a 30–50 per cent increase in maximum lifespan[4]. The maximum lifespan of fish, rotifers, spiders and other non-mammals is also extended by CR[4]. An active area of research in biological gerontology concerns the mechanisms by which CR retards the ageing process. There are five classes of interrelated and non-exclusive explanations for CR's mechanism: (i) decreases in oxidative stress; (ii) decreases in glycation or glycoxidation; (iii) decreases in body temperature and circulating thyroid hormone levels associated with a hypometabolic state; (iv) alterations in gene expression and protein degradation; and (v) neuroendocrine changes.

Animals and diets

Mice were purchased from Charles River Laboratories (Wilmington, MA) at 1.5 months of age. After receipt in Madison, the mice were housed singly in the specific pathogen-free Shared Aging Rodent Facility at the Madison Veterans Administration Geriatric Research, Education and Clinical Center, and provided a nonpurified diet (PLI 5001 [Purina Labs, St. Louis, MO]) and acidified water *ad libitum* for one week. The mice were then allocated into two groups and fed one of two nearly isocaloric (~4.1 kcal/g), semipurified diets. Each mouse in the control group was fed 84 kcal/week of the control diet (TD91349 [Teklad, Madison, WI]) which is ~5–20 per cent less than the range of individual *ad libitum* intakes. This dietary intake was used so that the control mice were not obese and retained motor activity up to the age of sacrifice. Each mouse subjected to CR was fed 62 kcal/week of the restricted diet (TD91351 [Teklad, Madison, WI]), resulting in a 26 per cent reduction of caloric intake. The latter diet was enriched in protein, vitamins and minerals such that CR and control mice were fed nearly identical amounts of these components. The fat component, corn oil, was at the same level (13.5 per cent) in both diets, leading to a 26 per cent reduction in fat intake for the calorie-restricted mice. The adult body weights of the mice averaged ~32 g for controls and ~23 g for those on CR. Mice were euthanized by rapid cervical dislocation, autopsied to exclude animals showing overt disease, and several tissues were collected and immediately flash-frozen in liquid nitrogen and then stored at –80 °C. All aspects of animal care were approved by the appropriate committees and conformed with institutional guidelines

Sample preparations and data collection

Total RNA was extracted from frozen tissue using TRIZOL reagent (Life Technologies) and a power homogenizer (Fisher Scientific) with the addition of chloroform for the phase separation before isopropyl alcohol precipitation of total RNA. Poly (A)$^+$ RNA was purified from the total RNA with oligo-dT linked Oligotex resin (Qiagen). One microgram of poly (A)$^+$ RNA was converted into double stranded cDNA (ds-cDNA) using SuperScript Choice System (Life Technologies) with an oligo dT primer containing a T7 RNA polymerase promoter region (Genset). After second strand synthesis, the reaction mixture was extracted with phenol/chloroform/isoamyl alcohol. Phase Lock Gel (5 Prime → 3 Prime, Inc.) was used to increase ds-cDNA recovery. The ds-cDNA was collected by ethanol precipitation. The pellet was resuspended in 3 μl of DEPC-treated water. *In vitro* transcription was performed using a T7 Megascript Kit (Ambion) with 1.5 μl of ds-cDNA template in the presence of a mixture of unlabeled ATP, CTP, GTP, and UTP and biotin-labeled CTP and UTP (bio-11-CTP and bio-16-UTP [Enzo]). Biotin-labeled cRNA was purified using a RNeasy affinity column (Qiagen). The amount of biotin-labeled cRNA was determined by measuring absorbance at 260 nm. Biotin-labeled cRNA was fragmented randomly to sizes ranging from 35 to 200 bases by incubating at 94 °C for 35 min in 40 mM Tris-acetate pH 8.1, 100 mM potassium acetate, and 30 mM magnesium acetate. The hybridization solutions contained 100 mM MES, 1 M [Na$^+$], 20 mM EDTA, and 0.01 per cent Tween 20. In addition, the hybridization solutions contained 50 pM oligonucleotide B2 (a biotin-labeled control oligonucleotide used for making grid alignments), 0.1 mg/ml herring sperm DNA, and 0.5 mg/ml acetylated BSA. The final concentration of fragmented cRNA was 0.05 μg/μl in the hybridization solutions. Hybridization solutions were heated to 99 °C for 5 min followed by 45 °C for 5 min prior to placing in the gene chips. Ten μg of cRNA was placed in the Affymetrix gene chip. Hybridizations were carried out at 45 °C for 16 h with mixing on a rotisserie at 60 rpm. Following hybridization, the hybridization solutions were removed, the Affyemetrix gene chips were installed in a fluidics system for washes and staining. The fluidics system (Affymetrix GeneChip Fluidics Station 400) performed two post hybridization washes (a non-stringent wash and a stringent wash), staining with streptavidin-phycoerythrin, and one post-stain wash. The gene chips were read at a resolution of 6 μm using a Hewlett Packard GeneArray Scanner. Data collected from two scanned images were used for the analysis. For methods on data analysis, please see our previous publications in the field[1-3].

The gene expression profile of ageing in the mouse brain

Of the 6347 genes surveyed, only 67 (1 per cent) displayed an increase greater than 1.7-fold in expression levels with ageing in the neocortex, whereas 63 (1 per cent) displayed an increase of more than 2.1-fold expression with ageing in the cerebellum (see www.wisc.edu/genetics/CATG/prolla/data/ageing/index.html for a full listing of genes). A subset of these genes was used for a comparison between oligonucleotide microarray data and TaqMan real time quantitative PCR assays, which demonstrated excellent overall agreement between the methods (Lee *et al.*, 2000). Of the upregulated genes, 20 per cent (14/67) and 27 per cent (17/63) could be assigned to an immune or inflammatory response in the neocortex and cerebellum, respectively (Table 1). Transcriptional alterations of several genes in this category were shared by the two brain regions, although fold-changes tended to be higher in the cerebellum. Interestingly, we saw a concerted induction of the complement cascade components C4, C1qA, C1qB and C1qC. Complement proteins are found in the senile plaques characteristic of Alzheimer's disease.

Table 1. Transcriptional evidence for an inflammatory response with aging in the mouse brain

Fold increase ↑ (SE)		Gene	CR prevention (%)	
Neocortex	**Cerebellum**		**N**	**C**
4.9 (0.2)	3.7 (0.3)	Complement C4	52	0
2.2 (0.2)	6.4 (0.9)	Lysozyme C	64	88
2.0 (0.2)	ND	CD40l receptor	58	–
1.9 (0.4)	4.7 (1.0)	Cyclophiin C-AP	100	0
1.9 (0.2)	3.9 (0.1)	Mps1	0	56
1.8 (0.1)	ND	C1q-B chain	100	–
1.8 (0.1)	4.1 (0.6)	C1q-C chain	75	56
1.7 (0.1)	4.4 (0.2)	C1q-A chain	100	80
1.7 (0.1)	ND	Cox-1	0	–

ND = not different with age.

Similar to previous data obtained from the gastrocnemius muscle[1], genes involved in a stress response (consistent with a state of oxidative stress and accumulation of damaged proteins) accounted for 24 per cent (16/67) and 13 per cent (8/63) of genes highly induced in the neocortex and cerebellum, respectively, of old animals (Table 1). These included the four cathepsins (lysosomal proteases) and the several heat-shock factors (e.g. Hsp40, Hsp27, Hsp59).

We also observed an induction of the early response genes junB and c-fos, which are co-induced in response to neocortical injury or hypoxic stress and GFAP, a marker of reactive astrocytosis induced in the ageing brain (Table 1). Taken as a whole, our observations support the concept that the ageing process in the brain is associated with a state of heightened immune reactivity and oxidative stress accompanied by the accumulation of altered or misfolded proteins. Therefore, a chronic state of oxidative stress appears to be a common transcriptional feature of ageing in both brain and skeletal muscle. Several transcripts which declined in expression encode nuclear genes involved in mitochondrial functions. These include NADP transhydrogenase, cytochrome-C-oxidase subunit VIII and the ATP synthetase-gamma and delta chains which are all either components of the mitochondrial electron transport system or support its function. This transcriptional profile suggests that mitochondrial function may be compromised in the aged brain, parallel to observations in skeletal muscle[1].

CR is associated with a transcriptional reprogramming in the brain

Of the largest age-associated changes in the neocortex (1.7-fold or more), 30 per cent (34/114) were prevented either completely or partially by CR. Remarkably, the effect of CR on age-associated alterations in gene expression was highly dependent on transcript class: CR influenced only 20 per cent (2/10) of the observed decreases in expression of genes involved in neuronal growth and plasticity, whereas it prevented 50 per cent (8/16) of the induction of stress response and 65 per cent (11/17) of immune response-related genes. A similar pattern was observed in the cerebellum. The effects of CR on immune and stress-related transcripts agree with studies suggesting reductions in both autoimmunity[4] and oxidative damage[5] occur in the brain of calorie-restricted mice.

As was observed in muscle, CR shifted the activity of several genes that were unaltered in expression with age (see www.wisc.edu/genetics/CATG/prolla/data/aging/index.html for a full listing of genes affected by caloric restriction in the neocortex). As compared to age-matched controls, CR induced the expression of 120 genes by 1.7-fold or more in the neocortex, which represent 1.9 per cent of the genes surveyed (Table 2). One of the largest classes of transcripts induced by CR was comprised of growth and neurotrophic factors (9 per cent). This class included the developmentally-regulated homeobox genes Hox2.5, Hoxb3 and Hoxa6, all of which may be involved in neural development, and the gene encoding neuroserpin, a factor that promotes neuronal plasticity. CR was associated with a reduction of 1.7-fold or greater in the expression of 84 genes in the neocortex. The largest functional class (11 per cent) consisted of genes involved in protein synthesis. Inflammatory-related transcripts downregulated by CR include the proinflammatory cytokine Mcp5. A state of lowered endogenous oxidative stress in CR mice is also suggested by reduced expression of the chaperone encoding genes Hsp27 and Cypa, and also the genes encoding the p65 and p100 subunits of NF-kB. Taken as a whole, these results suggest that metabolic alterations induced by CR may profoundly affect brain ageing.

Table 2. Transcriptional evidence for a stress response with ageing in the mouse brain

Fold increase ↑ (SE)		Gene	CR prevention (%)	
Neocortex	Cerebellum		N	C
2.4 (0.3)	3.8 (0.7)	GFAP	59	61
1.7 (0.3)	5.6 (2.6)	c-fos	100	59
1.7 (0.1)	4.7 (0.3)	Cathepsin S	56	62
1.8 (0.1)	2.6 (0.2)	Cathepsin D	64	38
1.9 (0.1)	2.1 (0.2)	Cathepsin Z	70	64
ND	2.9 (0.3)	Cathepsin H	–	55
1.8 (0.2)	3.1 (0.4)	HSP40 homolog 1	51	100
1.7 (0.2)	ND	HSP40 homolog 2	0	–
1.8 (0.3)	ND	Gadd153	0	–

ND = not different with age.

The gene expression profile of ageing and cr in rhesus monkey vastus lateralis muscle

We recently reported the effects of ageing and adult-onset CR on the gene expression profile of 7070 genes in the vastus lateralis muscle from rhesus monkeys[3]. The average lifespan of rhesus monkeys in our colony is ~27 years and the maximum lifespan is ~40 years. Gene expression analysis of old rhesus monkeys (mean age of 26 years) was compared to young animals (mean age of 8 years). Ageing resulted in a selective upregulation of transcripts involved in inflammation (a class not observed to be upregulated in the mouse gastrocnemius muscle) and oxidative stress, and a downregulation of genes involved in mitochondrial electron transport and oxidative phosphorylation. Middle-aged monkeys (mean age of 20 years) subjected to CR since early adulthood (mean age of 11 years) were studied to determine the gene expression profile induced by CR. CR resulted in an upregulation of cytoskeletal protein encoding genes, and also a decrease in the expression of genes involved in mitochondrial bioenergetics. Surprisingly, we did not observe any evidence for an inhibitory effect of adult-onset CR on age-related changes in gene expression. These results indicate that the induction of an oxidative stress-induced transcriptional response may be a common feature of ageing in skeletal muscle of rodents and primates, but the extent to which CR modifies these responses may be species-specific. However, critical differences in the experimental design of our mouse and monkey studies may explain the lack of efficacy of CR in retarding age-associated transcriptional changes in monkeys. Most notable are the early life onset of CR in the mouse study and the study of truly old calorie-restricted mice (vs. middle age calorie-restricted monkeys) in the mouse study.

Implications for ageing research

These data underscore the utility of high density oligonucleotide microarray gene expression analysis in the study of complex biological phenomena such as the ageing process and the response to CR. Further, gene chips are useful tools for evaluating the impact of nutritional interventions by providing a global, unbiased view of gene expression alterations. The promise of this approach derives from the ability to provide (eventually) a genome-wide screen within a single experimental setup. Proteomics is expected to offer similar opportunities. However, certain limitations are associated with data generated by microarrays. First, the observed collection of gene expression alterations in ageing whole tissues such as muscle and brain is complex, reflecting the presence of diverse cell types. Second, the ability of oligonucleotide microarrays to accurately measure mRNA levels for thousands of genes has predated the development of statistical tools to minimize the occurrence of false positives and false negatives. Additionally, changes in mRNA levels may not always result in a parallel alteration in protein levels. Nonetheless, the complete or partial prevention of the majority of the observed ageing alterations by CR in mouse muscle and the targeted prevention of stress response and inflammatory transcripts in the brain provide biological validation for this approach. Further, these data suggest that gene expression patterns can be used to assess the biological age of a tissue. Extension of our study to other organs should result in the identification of hundreds of tissue-specific biomarkers of ageing, facilitating the elucidation of ageing mechanisms and the development of interventions.

Acknowledgements: Supported by NIH grants P01 AG11915 (R.W.), R01 AG18922 (R.W.) and R01 CA78723 (T.A.P.). T.A.P. is a recipient of the Shaw Scientist (Milwaukee Foundation), Burroughs Wellcome Young Investigator, and Basil O'Connor (March of Dimes) awards.

References

1. Lee CK, Klopp RG, Weindruch R, Prolla TA. Gene expression profile of aging and its retardation by caloric restriction. *Science* 1999; 285: 1390–3.

2. Lee CK, Weindruch R, Prolla TA. Gene expression profile of the ageing brain. *Nature Genet* 2000; 25: 294–7.

3. Kayo T, Allison DB, Weindruch R, Prolla TA. Influences of aging and caloric restriction on the transcriptional profile of skeletal muscle from rhesus monkeys. *Proc Natl Acad Sci USA* 2001; 98: 5093–8.

4. Weindruch R, Walford RL. *The retardation of aging and disease by dietary restriction.* Springfield: CC Thomas; 1988.

5. Sohal RS, Agarwal S, Candas M, Forster MJ, Lal H. Effect of age and caloric restriction on DNA oxidative damage in different tissues of C56BL/6 mice. *Mech Ageing Dev* 1994; 76: 215–24.

Progress in Obesity Research: 9. Edited by *Geraldo Medeiros-Neto, Alfredo Halpern and Claude Bouchard*
©2003 John Libbey Eurotext Ltd, pp. 352–356.

CHAPTER 75

Mutation detection and association studies in experimental protocols: focus on ADRß3

Jeremy D. Walston

Associate Professor of Medicine, Johns Hopkins University School of Medicine, Baltimore, Maryland, USA
[e-mail: Jwalston@jhmi.edu]

Introduction

The beta-3 adrenoceptor (ADRß3) is a G-protein coupled, cell-membrane bound protein that is expressed in visceral adipose tissue, skeletal muscle, the GI tract, and the pancreas[4,5]. Stimulation of ADRß3 norepinephrine and epinephrine leads to an increase in intracellular concentration of cyclic AMP (cAMP), which in turn results in thermogenesis and lipolysis in fat and muscle tissue, and insulin release in the islet cells of the pancreas[4,5]. The Arg64 variant is located in the first intracellular loop of the receptor, an area thought important for G-protein interactions[1]. The variant is common in several populations, including Pima Indians (allele frequency 0.31), Japanese (0.20), Mexican Americans, (0.13), Caucasians from Baltimore, Maryland (0.08), and Samoans (0.06)[6].

First phase Arg64 ADRß3 association studies

The variant allele was first identified in an obese and diabetic Pima Indian cohort, where investigators found a significant association between the variant allele and accelerated onset of type 2 DM (5 years earlier) in those homozygous for the Arg64 allele compared to those homozygous for the Trp64 allele[1]. In addition, trends toward lower resting metabolic rate, increased BMI, and increased insulin resistance were associated with the Arg64 allele[1]. These findings supported the original hypothesis that the Arg64 variant receptor was functionally less efficient at thermogenesis and lipolysis, which in turn increased the chance of developing phenotypic traits related to obesity and type 2 DM. In order to better clarify the role of this gene variant in the development of these disorders, collaborative studies were developed that confirmed an association of the variant allele with earlier onset of type 2 DM (5 years in Arg64 heterozygotes compared to Trp64 homozygotes) and increased insulin resistance in a Finnish cohort, as well as an association of the Arg64 allele with increased BMI and rate of weight gain in French and Japanese cohorts[2,3,7]. Shortly thereafter, several other well performed studies were published that showed no association between the variant allele and BMI, weight gain, earlier onset of type 2 DM[4,8,9].

Meta-analyses

Two meta-analyses were performed and published in 1998 that attempted to summarize findings of the numerous smaller cohorts studied up until that time. The first meta-analysis by Allison *et al.* showed a statistically insignificant association between increased BMI and the Arg64 allele[10]. This study included over 7,000 subjects (5396 Trp/Trp, 2003 Trp/Arg heterozygotes or Arg/Arg homozygotes) from a number of ethnic groups and phenotype backgrounds. The mean BMI effect of this allele was found to be 0.19 kg/m^2 (CI 0.02–0.42, $P = 0.07$)[10]. Fujisawa *et al.* published a study in the same year from mixed ethnic and disease status populations using BMI measurements from 6789 Trp/Trp subjects and 2447 Trp/Arg heterozygous or Arg/Arg homozygous subjects (11), and identified a significant mean effect of the Arg allele on BMI of 0.30 (CI 0.13–0.47, $P < 0.05$). A third meta-analyses consisting only of Japanese subjects was published by Kurokawa *et al.* in 2001[12]. This study also demonstrated a significant Arg64 allele effect on BMI of 0.26 Kb/m^2 (CI 0.18–0.42, $P < 0.01$). These studies, along with the bulk of previously published studies, continued to support a modest role for the Arg64 allele in

BMI and other traits related to obesity and diabetes and are consistent with the magnitude of effect that investigators should expect in polygenic phenotypes[13].

Common design issues in candidate gene studies

Candidate gene associations studies have been criticized for a number of weaknesses that may contribute to the inconsistencies demonstrated in previous studies. First, type one errors (false positive results) may occur simply by chance alone; significant associations would be expected to occur in one of twenty association studies at a P value ≤ 0.05. Given that hundreds of analyses were undertaken that attempted to evaluate genotype-phenotype relationships, many positive results would be expected. Publication bias may also plays a role in increasing the acceptance of the effects of a candidate gene by the scientific community. Positive studies are far more likely to be submitted for publication and accepted for publication than negative association studies; this in turn may lead the scientific community to more readily accept the importance of a candidate gene.

Other design issues that need to be carefully considered in candidate gene analyses include those that result in type 2 or false negative errors. The Arg64 ADRß3 likely has only a modest effect on phenotypes such as BMI. Many if not most negative studies performed to date have been underpowered to detect such a modest effect. Ethnic background variability is a potential confounder and must be recognized in order to maximize the detection of single gene effects. Inconsistent phenotyping within and between cohorts also can result in both false positive and false negative results. Finally, obese, diabetic and insulin resistant states act as confounders on the ultimate gene effects. Because many of the cohorts studied to date have been selected from these diagnostic groups, the subtle gene effects or phenotypes may be undetectable in that physiologic milieu.

Next phase Arg64 ADRß3 association studies

In an attempt to overcome the potential confounders inherent in candidate gene analyses, a number of investigators designed prospective studies that attempted to better define the influence of the Arg64 allele on outcomes. In these protocols, investigators recruited by genotype, and designed protocols that controlled for the potential confounding variables of age, fat mass, BMI, and genetic or ethnic background.

Mitchell *et al.* used a sibling pair design, where the 45 Mexican-American sibling pairs were identical at a chromosome 2 obesity locus, but different at the Trp64Arg locus[14]. These investigators demonstrated a significant positive association with increased BMI, fat mass, and waist circumference and the Arg64 allele using this design. Garcia-Rubi *et al.* identified 14 Trp64Arg heterozygous, moderately obese, post menopausal Caucasian women, and matched them for age, race, post-menopausal status, intra-abdominal fat, BMI, and physical activity with 13 women with the Trp/Trp genotype[15]. The women were weight stabilized for one month, and underwent a hyperinsulinaemic, euglycaemic clamp. The results showed significantly lower glucose infusion rates (Trp/Arg, 241 ± 135 mg/min vs. Trp/Trp 379 ±172 mg/min, $P = 0.03$), and total glucose disposal (321 ± 111 mg/min vs. 441 ± 183 mg/min, $P = 0.05$). The results of this study have helped to further establish an Arg64 genotype effect, even in a heterozygous state, on glucose metabolism.

Walston *et al.* designed a study to recruit younger, non-diabetic and non-obese adults with the Arg/Arg genotype in order to maximize the ability to detect Arg64 effects on glucose metabolism. We first identified Arg64 homozygotes ($n = 20$), and then matched them by race, age, gender, BMI, and fat mass to Trp/Arg heterozygotes ($n = 23$) and Trp/Trp homozygotes ($n = 13$). All participants then underwent IV glucose tolerance testing after a 3 day high carbohydrate diet followed by an overnight fast. The mean acute insulin release in response to a glucose bolus (AIRg) was found to be significantly lower in those with the Arg/Arg genotypes (Trp/Trp 962 + 94 pmol/l vs. Trp/Arg 692 + 87 pmol/l vs. Arg/Arg 656 + 116 pmol/l, $P = 0.01$[16]. These results provided the first evidence that the Arg allele may impact insulin secretion, and suggests an additional physiologic basis for the finding of earlier onset of type 2 DM in previous population studies.

Resting metabolic rate (RMR) differences were found to differ modestly between Arg64 genotypes in previously designed association studies that included both obese and diabetic subjects from a wide age range[1,9,17]. Walston *et al.* studied the same younger, non-obese cohort described above to maximize the ability to detect RMR differences by genotype. The age, gender, ethnicity, fat mass, and BMI matched subjects underwent indirect calorimetry after a 12 hour fast and an overnight stay at a clinical research laboratory. The Arg64 homozygotes had a mean RMR that was 234 calories per day lower than the mean RMR of Trp64 homozygotes ($P \leq 0.01$)[18]. The results of these 'next phase' association studies, designed to control for several variables that may have confounded previous studies, have helped to

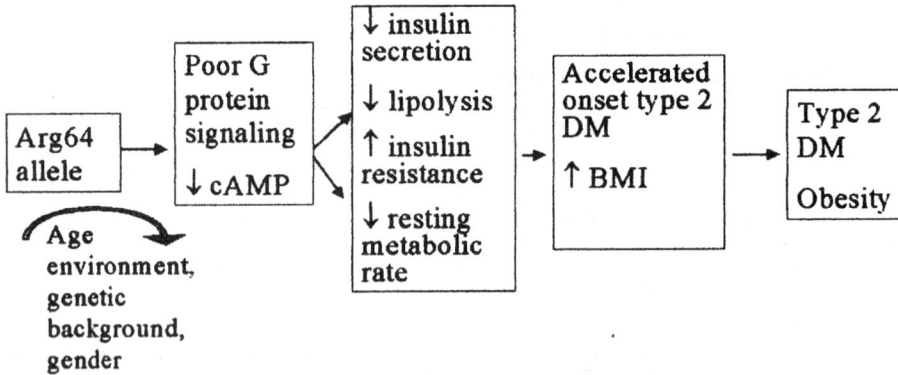

Fig. 1. Connecting Arg64 ADRß₃ Genotype to Phenotype. Initial association studies showed a relationship between genotype and distal outcomes (top arrow). Subsequently designed human studies have demonstrated important physiologic findings that have confirmed and extended the understanding of the Arg64 allele effects on phenotype (middle box).

further establish important Arg64 allele influenced phenotypes that connect this genotype to obesity and type 2 DM (Fig. 1).

Functional studies

Functional studies are also critical in further establishing the effect of gene variants on phenotype. A number of *in vitro* binding and signaling studies were undertaken shortly after the discovery of the ADRß₃ gene variant[19–22]. Most were performed by transfecting cells with either Trp64 or Arg64 ADRß₃ receptor producing plasmids and comparing binding and signaling properties between these receptors. All of these studies reported similar ligand binding properties between the Arg64 and Trp64 ADRß₃ receptors[19–22]. Three studies have identified markedly decreased G-protein signaling properties in the Arg64 transfected cells[20–22]. In two other functional studies, human omental fat samples, known to be rich in ADRß₃ were subjected to specific ADRß₃ agonists. Lipolytic response was found to be decreased by 25–50 per cent in Arg64 hetero- and homozygotes compared to Trp/Trp homozygotes[23,24]. Perfetti *et al.* demonstrated ADRß₃ receptor expression in ADRß₃ islets, and then showed that insulin producing cells transfected with Arg64 ADRß₃ receptors produced significantly less insulin than cells transfected with the Trp64 ADRß₃ receptor[5]. In fact, there was some evidence that the Arg64 receptor decreased the basal amount of insulin secretion. This study supported the findings of lower acute insulin release in Arg64 homozygotes, and provides further supportive evidence of the modest but real effect of the Arg64 ADRß₃ on phenotypes related to type 2 DM and obesity[16].

Gene-gene interactions

Because obesity and Type 2 DM are polygenic diseases, and because there are likely to be several genes of modest effect that contribute to phenotypes, several investigators have begun to study the combined effects of candidate genes. To date, there have been at least four studies of the combined effect of the Arg64 ADRß₃ allele on obesity and diabetes phenotypes. Hsueh *et al.* demonstrated a significant increase in BMI and insulin in those with the Arg64 allele and the Ala12 PPARgamma-2 variant allele in a cohort of 453 Mexican Americans[25]. Dionne *et al.* demonstrated significantly increased fat mass and per cent fat in those American Caucasians with the Glu9 α2b-ADR deletion and the Arg64 ADRß₃ allele (26). Finally, Mentuccia *et al.* have demonstrated increased BMI in those Caucasians with both the Ala982 type 2 deiodinase allele and the Arg64 ADRß₃ variant[27]. In all of these studies, the effect of the Arg64 allele alone was not sufficient to show a significant difference between genotypes; the combined effect of variant alleles was necessary to show the effect. These studies demonstrate additive or synergistic effects on phenotypes related to obesity, and type 2 DM, consistent with what is expected of genes of modest effects.

Discussion

Since the initial discovery of the Arg64 ADRß₃ allele in 1995 and its modest impact on phenotypes related to type 2 DM and obesity, many association studies have been designed to study the effects of

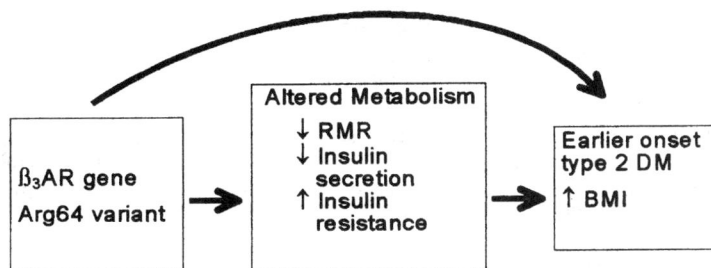

Fig. 2. Summary figure of causal pathway between Arg64 ADRß3 genotype and distal outcomes of type 2 DM and obesity. Functional and association studies have confirmed these relationships over the past several years. The critical potential confounders of age, environment, genetic background and gender likely influence this pathway at each step.

the allele in various ethnic groups[4]. Study design and interpretation issues, including publication bias, variable phenotyping, low power, and confounders of age, obesity, insulin resistance, and diabetic state have likely led to both false positive and false negative results. Several recent experimental protocols and meta-analyses were undertaken in order to overcome power issues and confounding variables and have helped to further establish a physiologic role for the Arg64 allele in insulin resistance and secretion and resting metabolic rate. Recent studies that evaluate the effect of allelic combinations have also helped to highlight the importance of this candidate gene in obesity and diabetes phenotypes. Functional studies have demonstrated the effect of the variant allele on decreased generation of cAMP, lower levels of lipolysis in human adipose cells, and lower levels of insulin secretion. The combined weight of these studies suggest a modest but real effect on the generation of cAMP, which in turn influences fat mass, insulin resistance, insulin secretion, lipolysis, and resting metabolic rate, which in turn may influence the development of both obesity and type 2 DM. Figure 2 summarizes these findings in a causal pathway. These findings are consistent with what investigators should expect in a polygenic disease where most genes will have a modest effect on phenotypic outcomes[13]. These studies and study design issues are highly relevant for other candidate gene studies, and indeed represent an important model for future approaches to candidate gene discovery efforts.

References

1. Walston J, Silver K, Bogardus C, Knowler WC, Celi FS, Austin S *et al.* Time of onset of non-insulin-dependent diabetes mellitus and genetic variation in the beta 3-adrenergic-receptor gene [See Comments]. *N Engl J Med* 1995; 333(6): 343–7.

2. Widen E, Lehto M, Kanninen T, Walston J, Shuldiner AR, Groop LC. Association of a polymorphism in the beta 3-adrenergic-receptor gene with features of the insulin resistance syndrome in Finns [See Comments]. *N Engl J Med* 1995; 333(6): 348–51.

3. Clement K, Vaisse C, Manning BS, Basdevant A, Guy-Grand B, Ruiz J *et al.* Genetic Variation in the beta 3-adrenergic receptor and an increased capacity to gain weight in patients with morbid obesity [See Comments]. *N Engl J Med* 1995; 333(6): 352–4.

4. Silver K, Shuldiner AR. Candidate genes for type II diabetes mellitus. LeRoith D and Olefskky J. *Diabetes mellitus: A fundamental and clinical text* (2nd edn), pp.709–19. Philadelphia: Lippincott, Williams & Wilkins, 2000.

5. Perfetti R, Hui H, Chamie K, Binder S, Seibert M, McLenithan J, Walston J. Pancreatic b-cells expressing the Arg64 variant of the beta-3-adrenergic receptor exhibit abnormal insulin secretary activity. J *Mol Endocrinol* 2001; 27(2): 133–44.

6. Silver K, Walston J, Wang Y, Dowse G, Zimmet P, Shuldiner AR. Molecular scanning for mutations in the beta 3-adrenergic receptor gene in nauruans with obesity and noninsulin-dependent diabetes mellitus. *J Clin Endocrinol Metab* 1996; 81(11): 4155–8.

7. Kadowaki H, Yasuda K, Iwamoto K, Otabe S, Shimokawa K, Silver K *et al.* A mutation in the beta 3-adrenergic receptor gene is associated with obesity and hyperinsulinemia in Japanese subjects. *Biochem Biophys Res Commun* 1995; 215(2): 555–60.

8. Elbein SC, Hoffman M, Barrett K, Wegner K, Miles C, Bachman K *et al*. Role of the beta 3-adrenergic receptor locus in obesity and noninsulin-dependent diabetes among members of Caucasian families with a diabetic sibling pair. *J Clin Endocrinol Metab* 1996; 81(12): 4422–7.

9. Gagnon J, Mauriege P, Roy S, Sjostrom D, Chagnon YC, Dionne FT *et al*. The Trp64Arg mutation of the beta3 adrenergic receptor gene has no effect on obesity phenotypes in the Quebec Family Study and Swedish Obese Subjects Cohorts. *J Clin Invest* 1996; 98(9): 2086–93.

10. Allison DB, Heo M, Faith MS, Pietrobelli A. Meta-Analysis of the Association of the Trp64Arg Polymorphism in the beta3 adrenergic receptor with body mass index. *Int J Obes Relat Metab Disord* 1998; 22(6): 559–66.

11. Fujisawa T, Ikegami H, Kawaguchi Y, Ogihara T. Meta-analysis of the association of Trp64Arg polymorphism of beta 3-adrenergic receptor gene with body mass index. *J Clin Endocrinol Metab* 1998; 83(7): 2441–4.

12. Kurokawa N, Nakai K, Kameo S, Liu ZM, Satoh H. Association of BMI with the beta3-adrenergic receptor gene polymorphism in Japanese: meta-analysis. *Obes Res* 2001; 9(12): 741–5.

13. Shuldiner AR, Sabra M. Trp64Arg beta3-adrenoceptor: when does a candidate gene become a disease-susceptibility gene? *Obes Res* 2001; 9(12): 806–9.

14. Mitchell BD, Blangero J, Comuzzie AG, Almasy LA, Shuldiner AR, Silver K *et al*. A paired sibling analysis of the beta-3 adrenergic receptor and obesity in Mexican Americans. *J Clin Invest* 1998; 101(3): 584–7.

15. Garcia-Rubi E, Starling RD, Tchernof A, Matthews DE, Walston JD, Shuldiner AR *et al*. Trp64Arg variant of the beta3-adrenoceptor and insulin resistance in obese postmenopausal women. *J Clin Endocrinol Metab* 1998; 83(11): 4002–5.

16. Walston J, Silver K, Hilfiker H, Andersen R, Seibert M, Beamer B *et al*. Insulin response to glucose is lower in individuals homozygous for the Arg64 variant of the beta-3-adrenergic receptor. *J Clin Endocrinol Metab* 2000.

17. Sipilainen R, Uusitupa M, Heikkinen S, Rissanen A, Laakso M. Polymorphism of the beta3-adrenergic receptor gene affects basal metabolic rate in obese Finns. *Diabetes* 1997; 46(1): 77–80.

18. Walston J, Andersen R, Seibert M, Hilfiker H, Beamer B, Blumenthal J, Poehlman E. Physiologic contributions of the Arg64 beta-3-adrenoceptor variant to the components of energy expenditure. *Obes Res* 2003; 11(4); 509–11.

19. Candelore MR, Deng L, Tota LM, Kelly LJ, Cascieri MA, Strader CD. Pharmacological characterization of a recently described human beta 3-adrenergic receptor mutant. *Endocrinology* 1996; 137(6): 2638–41.

20. Pietri-Rouxel F, St John Manning B, Gros J, Strosberg AD. The biochemical effect of the naturally occurring Trp64 – >Arg mutation on human beta3-adrenoceptor activity. *Eur J Biochem* 1997; 247(3): 1174–9.

21. Kimura K, Sasaki N, Asano A, Mizukami J, Kayahashi S, Kawada T *et al*. Mutated human beta3-adrenergic receptor (Trp64Arg) lowers the response to beta3-adrenergic agonists in transfected 3T3-L1 preadipocytes [In Process Citation]. *Horm Metab Res* 2000; 32(3): 91–6.

22. McLenithan J, Xu H, Pray J, Quon M, Shuldiner AR. W64R Is a naturally occurring dominant negative mutation in the beta-3-adrenergic receptor. *Diabetes* 2001; 50 (Suppl 2): 203–5.

23. Umekawa T, Yoshida T, Sakane N, Kogure A, Kondo M, Honjyo H. Trp64Arg mutation of beta3-adrenoceptor gene deteriorates lipolysis induced by beta3-adrenoceptor agonist in human omental adipocytes. *Diabetes* 1999; 48(1): 117–20.

24. Hoffstedt J, Poirier O, Thorne A, Lonnqvist F, Herrmann SM, Cambien F, Arner P. Polymorphism of the human beta3-adrenoceptor gene forms a well-conserved haplotype that is associated with moderate obesity and altered receptor function. *Diabetes* 1999; 48(1): 203–5.

25. Hsueh WC, Cole SA, Shuldiner AR, Beamer BA, Blangero J, Hixson JE *et al*. Interactions between variants in the beta3-adrenergic receptor and peroxisome proliferator-activated receptor-gamma2 genes and obesity. *Diabetes Care* 2001; 24(4): 672–7.

26. Dionne IJ, Turner AN, Tchernof A, Pollin TI, Avrithi D, Gray D *et al*. Identificaiton of an interactive effect of beta3-and alpha2b-adrenoceptor gene polymorphisms on fat mass in Caucasian women. *Diabetes* 2001; 50(1): 91–5.

27. Mentuccia D, Proietti-Pannunzi L, Tanner K, Bacci V, Pollin TI, Poehlman ET *et al*. Association between a novel variant of the human type 2 deiodinase gene Thr92Ala and insulin resistance: evidence of interaction with the Trp64Arg variant of the beta-3-adrenergic receptor. *Diabetes* 2002; 51(3): 880–3.

Progress in Obesity Research: 9. Edited by *Geraldo Medeiros-Neto, Alfredo Halpern and Claude Bouchard*
©2003 John Libbey Eurotext Ltd, pp. 357–362.

CHAPTER 76

Association studies in complex traits: single and multi-gene analyses of obesity and mental health diseases

Yvon C. Chagnon

Laval University Research Center Robert-Giffard, Genetic and Molecular Pshychiatry Unit, 2601 chemin de la Canardiere, room F-6459, Beauport (Quebec), G1J 2G3, Canada
[e-mail: yvon.chagnon@crulrg.ulaval.ca]

Introduction

Association studies are essential for the demonstration that a gene could be involved in the expression of a phenotype. However, its use in complex trait analysis such as the most common forms of obesity or mental health diseases is less evident. Most of the difficulties come from the multiple genes with individually low effects that are suspected to be involved in such traits together with their interactions between themselves and with environment. This short paper will review the main study designs and statistical tools available for association studies of complex traits. Examples of single-gene and multiple genes analysis will be given, whereas an example of a genomic approach for the determination of a gene effect will be shown. Finally, examples of candidate genes and quantitative trait loci (QTL) shared between two apparently distinct complex traits, obesity and schizophrenia, will be presented to illustrate plasticity and possible communality of genes effects.

Study designs for association tests

A recent review by Schulze and McMahon[1] give a comprehensive view of the association tests available and in which circumstances to use them. The main pitfall underlined by the authors is the stratification of the populations from where are taken the studied cohorts that could produce false positive results. Example of stratification is ethnicity with significant differences in gene frequencies observed between ethnic groups such as the complete inversion of the allele frequencies of a glutamine to arginine substitution at amino acid 223 (Q223R) of the leptin receptor (LEPR) gene between Pima Indians and Caucasian (see[2]). Other stratification factors are age for phenotypes showing significant different age of onset, sex or assortative mating. To control for such confounding factors, appropriate sampling and statistical analysis strategies have to be used. For example, the usually used case-control study design using chi square test to compare genotype or allele frequencies between both conditions need large number of homogeneous subjects according to age, sex, and ethnicity to be efficient. Comparison of frequencies is particularly demanding when gene-gene interaction is targeted. In a recent simulation, Gauderman[3] showed that for a gene-gene interaction of 1.5 raising the risk factor by 50 per cent in a recessive model where causative genotypes had a frequency of 40 per cent and 25 per cent in the population studied, and with 80 per cent power to detect the interaction, some 2,008 case-control pairs (~4,000 subjects) are needed. This number falls rapidly to 674 pairs for an interaction factor of 2.0, and to 270 pairs for a factor of 3.0. However, using a case-only study design that is not suitable for the evaluation of the single-gene effect but allow interaction analysis, these number fall to 947, 305 and 116 'subjects', not pairs, respectively. Another mostly family-based test, the transmission disequilibrium test or TDT, is now available that avoid most of the stratification problems. TDT hypothesized that alleles are transmitted randomly in absence of an association. The ideal unit of analysis is the triad formed by the two parents with one affected offspring. If only one parent genotype is available, TDT remains usable if marker analysed show multiple alleles and the affected child is heterozygous for this marker. TDT is also used for fine mapping as a test for association in presence of linkage. TDT test have been adapted to multiallelic markers (GTDT, ETDT), to sibships analysis (S-TDT, SDT), to parent reconstructed genotype when missing (RC-TDT), to chromosome X (X-TDT,XS-TDT,XRC-TDT), to extended pedigree (PDT), and quantitative trait (QTDT) (see[1]). Another possible association analysis for quantitative trait is covariance analysis where confounding factors such as age, sex, or ethnic origins for examples, and gene-gene and gene-environment interaction could be controlled for or estimated. We used thoroughly covariance analysis (GLM in SAS) in our candidate gene studies, initially on unrelated subjects, but more recently on all family subjects since an adjustment for familiality is now available (ProcMix in SAS). Following are some examples of our results in the Quebec Family Study (QFS) and in the HERITAGE Family Study.

Single-gene analysis: the leptin receptor (LEPR) gene

Table 1. Summary of association studies for the Q223R variant of LEPR. In results, the presence of the Q223 or R223 allele is higher (>) in higher BMI group or is associated with a greater (>) or lower (<) mean value of the phenotypes tested

Phenotypes	Populations	Tests	Results	References
BMI < 25 vs. > 25; %FAT	Caucasian m/f	CHI2; regression	Q223<; >4–5 per cent	[8]
Abdominal fat	Caucasian females	Anova	R233>	[7]
BMI; WC	Mixed (7C, 4B, 1H)	Meta-analysis	No	[24]
BMI; birth weight	India/Irish females	Anova	No	[25]
BMI; adiposity	Caucasian males 44–64 yr	Ancova	R223>	[4]
SBP/DBP	Caucasian males 50 yr	Ancova	Q223>	[6]
Leptin; TG; HDLC	Caucasian twin males	T-test (change)	R223>	[5]
BMI; TG; HDLC	Asiatic m/f 9–15 yr	Ancova	No	[26]
FFM	Caucasian males BMI<27	Ancova	Q223<	[2]
BMI>28 Vs <22; SF	Caucasian males 40–64 yr	CHI2; Anova	No	[10]
BMI, WHR	Caucasian m/f	Anova?	No	[27]
BMI>31 Vs lean	Caucasian males 18–26 yr	CHI2	No	[28]
BMI> 28 vs. <25	Asiatic m/f?	CHI2	No	[29]

m/f: males/females combined; 7C: 7 Caucasian samples; 4B: 4 Black samples; 1H: 1 Hispanic sample. WC: waist circumference; TG/HDLC: triglycerides/high density lipoprotein-cholesterol; SDP/DBP: systolic/diastolic blood pressure; FFM: fat free mass; SF: sum of skinfold; WHR: waist to hip ratio.

The leptin (LEP) gene and its receptor LEPR have been cloned in the mid-1990s from the spontaneously mutated mouse models Obese and Diabetes, respectively. In human, only two mutations have been found in LEP and one in LEPR inducing massive obesity and other metabolic perturbations. However, numerous polymorphisms have been reported for LEPR (see[2]), some of which showing associations with phenotypes of common obesity such as the body mass index (BMI) or fat mass (FM). Among them, the Q223R polymorphism had been the most extensively studied (Table 1). We have been the first group to report an association of LEPR and human body composition. For instance, we observed in QFS a weak association of the Q223 allele with a lower fat free mass but only in Caucasian males of BMI < 27 kg/m².[2] Later, we were able to evidence in HERITAGE, strong associations of the R223 allele with greater BMI and adiposity in middle-age Caucasian males[4], as with a lower change in leptin, triglycerides and high density lipoprotein-cholesterol in Caucasian twin males experiencing a restriction in calorie intake[5], and higher systolic and diastolic blood pressure in middle-age Caucasian males carrying the Q223 allele[6]. Finally, for Caucasian females, we observed a greater abdominal fat depot for those carrying the R223 allele[7]. The other positive result for this polymorphism were from Yiannakouris[8] that observed a lower frequency of the Q223 allele in Caucasians of both sexes of BMI > 25 kg/m² and a 4–5 per cent increase in per cent body fat, and in Pima Indians where an haplotype including the Q223R polymorphism showed a higher frequency in obese individuals[9]. Other studies reporting negative results differed from ours by the ethnic groups (India or Asiatic), statistical analysis (CHI2, Vs ANCOVA), grouping of subjects (age, sex, BMI, populations), and /or phenotypes analysed. For example, Gotoda[10] used a strategy very similar to our (ANCOVA on middle-age Caucasian males[4]), and the sum of skinfolds phenotype analysed in the Gotoda study showed also negative borderline result in our study ($P = 0.06$[4]).

Multiple genes analysis: gene-gene interaction

Few studies have targeted to evaluate gene-gene interaction. We have evaluated the interactions between β2- and β3-adrenergic receptors on abdominal fat in QFS [11]. Lipolysis is stimulated by ADRB3 activity whereas it is inhibit by ADRA2. Subjects ($n = 472$) were genotyped for the well-known ADRB3 Trp64Arg polymorphism, and for an ADRA2 6.7/6.3 KB Dra I restriction fragment length polymorphism (RFLP). Four groups of subjects were compared according if they carried one or both of the variant alleles (Arg64 and 6.3 KB, respectively) for total abdominal fat area (AFT; cm^2) determined by a computed tomography or CT scan. Carriers of the Arg64 and non-carrier of the 6.3 kb variant alleles showed a higher AFT then non-carriers of the Arg64 and carriers of the 6.3 kb ($\sim$410 Vs 370 cm^2; $P = 0.001$). These results let hypothesize that the ADRB3 Arg64 and ADRA2A 6.3 kb variant alleles are less efficient in their respective function of inducing or inhibiting lipolysis, respectively, since a higher amount of fat is observed in presence of Arg64 together with the absence of 6.3 kb. In another study, we have compared in QFS the interaction among the glucocorticoid receptor (GRL 2.3/4.5kb BclI RFLP), the lipoprotein lipase (LPL Ser447Ter), and ADRA2 (6.7/6.3 kb DraI RFLP) on subcutaneous fat evaluated using a sum of six skinfolds[12]. A more complex pattern of variation then above was observed where the strongest accumulation of subcutaneous fat was observed for individuals carrying simultaneously the variant alleles GRL 4.5 kb and ADRA2A 6.3 kb, and not carrying the LPL 447ter allele. This let suppose that the GRL 4.5 kb allele is less efficient to stimulate lipolysis directly and via the LPL for which it is already known that the 447ter allele has a higher lipolysis activity. However, this let suppose this time that the ADRA2A 6.3 KB allele is more efficient to inhibit lipolysis, which is in contradiction with the interpretation of the previous study. In any case, it is clear from this study that the combined analysis of multiple polymorphisms and genes will reach rapidly saturation because of the very large samples needed to get sufficient number of subjects per combined genotype groups. Equally, greater the number of genes and alleles involved in the comparison, greater will be the difficulty to have a comprehensive interpretation of the allele effects on the studied phenotypes. In summary, these results taken together underlined the importance of taking into account possible confounding factors such as ethnicity, age, sex, BMI in association studies to be able to uncover possible effect of a gene on a given phenotype.

Multiple genes analysis: genetic approach

The melanocortin receptor (MCR) system. The melanocortin system is central to food intake and body composition regulation (see[13]). We had analysed genetic polymorphisms of three melanocortin receptor (MC3R, MC4R, MC5R) genes, and of a gene encoding an antagonist of these receptors, the agouti-related peptide (AGRP) gene, in relation to body composition, food intake, and energy expenditure in QFS. In the first study[14], the variant alleles of a MC4R NcoI and of a MC5R PstI RFLPs were shown to associated, respectively, to a higher fatness ($0.004 < P < 0.002$) or a higher BMI ($P = 0.003$) but in females only, which contrast with associations of LEPR observed mainly in males. In contrast, the individuals homozygote for the variant allele of a +2138InsCAGACC polymorphism located 3' of MC3R maintained fatness at a constant level in normal weight (BMI < 25 kg/m^2; $0.0001 < P < 0.0003$) and overweight ($25 \leq$ BMI < 30 kg/m^2; $0.006 < P < 0.009$) subjects, which translated in a higher and lower adiposity, respectively in these two BMI classes[15]. This is not observed in obese subjects (BMI $\geq$ 30 kg/m^2) where, however, variant homozygotes showed a lower level of abdominal fat (–15 per cent; $P = 0.002$). In a comprehensive fashion, homozygote for the variant allele of the AGRP Ala67Thr polymorphism, which has shown to be associated with *Anorexia nervosa*, is associated with leanness in QFS, those subjects showing lower BMI, body weight, fat mass and fat free mass but with no obvious eating or energy expenditure disorder. These results illustrate how the different components of a same metabolic pathway could be involved in the regulation of a phenotype, here body composition, but in different ways some gene controlling general fatness (MC4R, MC5R), other body fat partitioning (MC3R), and other leanness (AGRP).

Multiple genes analysis: genomic approach. The uncoupling protein 3 (UCP3). We have studied a new microsatellite located in the intron 6 (GAIVS6) of UCP3 in relation to body composition and energy expenditure in QFS, and for their changes following 20 weeks endurance training in HERITAGE. Three main alleles named according to their apparent length in base pairs (bp) (238, 240 and 242 bp alleles) have been detected. We have observed significant greater changes in BMI and subcutaneous fat as estimated by the sum of eight skinfolds, among homozygote subjects for the 240 bp allele then those carrying the 238 bp allele, which themselves showed greater change then subjects carrying the 242 bp allele[16]. Moreover, we observed in QFS strongly significant higher BMI and adiposity in subjects homozygote for the 240 bp allele in contrast with those carrying the 238 bp allele that showed lower values[17]. The greater changes observed with the 240 bp allele in HERITAGE together with the greater fatness observed in QFS let us hypothesize that this allele provides a greater sensitivity to body composition changes according to genetic and environmental conditions faced by the subjects carrying this allele in two copies. However, despite the fact that the mean BMI or adiposity values for the carriers of the 238 bp allele was lower, some 238 bp carrier subjects were observed to be as obese as those homozygotes for the 240 bp allele, and homozygotes for the 240 bp allele as lean as those carrying the 238 bp allele. We interpreted this observation as the effect of a different genomic composition of individuals sharing the same UCP3 GAIVS6 genotype resulting in the expression or not of the associated phenotypes of leanness (238 bp allele) or obesity (240 bp allele). To evaluate these possible genomic differences, we have compared between subjects homozygote for the 238 bp allele, the overall gene expression in the skeletal muscle (*Vastus lateralis*) using Affymetrix microchips (6,800 genes and ESTs). Two groups of three obese subjects pooled together (mean BMI of 30.8 and 39.9 kg/m^2, respectively) vs. two groups of control subjects (mean BMI of 27.0 and 21.7 kg/m^2, respectively) were compared. The expression of between 1200 to 2000 genes were detected in the different four groups of subjects with some 25 genes showing a higher expression in obese individuals, and between 10 and 20 genes in controls. However, higher expression was replicated only for three genes in obese, and one gene in control. One of these three genes showing a nearly identical higher expression in obese was precisely UCP3, and it is striking that all subjects used in this gene expression experiment were selected according to a UCP3 genotype namely all were homozygote for the 238 bp allele. We interpreted these results as a relatively more homogenous genomic background of the subjects following their selection according to the UCP3 genotype allowing a more uniform expression of this gene among subjects analysed.

Obesity and mental health diseases: examples of common genes

Multiple genes interact together and with environment to express complex trait such as obesity. This is also true for other complex traits such as common mental health diseases including schizophrenia. Moreover, it appears very likely that the same genes and even mutations could be involved in more then one complex traits. For instance, numerous evidences emerge from the literature illustrating the possible genetic commonality between obesity and schizophrenia as illustrated in Table 2. Hence genes encoding receptors of the serotonin and dopamine systems, as genes related to the cholecystokinin system have been studied in relation to both obesity and schizophrenia. For example, serotonin is known to inhibit food intake and to be involved in behavioural and psychological processes. More particularly, the mouse knockout (KO) for the serotonin 2C receptor (5-HT$_{2C}$R) showed hyperphagia, become obese and has a lower ADRB3 activity. A polymorphism in 5-HT$_{2C}$R changing a cysteine for a serine at amino acid 23 (5-HT$_{2C}$R C23S) has been associated with weight loss, but also with a greater tardive dyskinisia (TD) following antipsychotic medication, whereas a change of a cytosine for a thymidine at nucleotide (nt) −759 in the promoter of 5-HT$_{2C}$R (5-HT$_{2C}$R −759C/T) has been associated with a lower weight gain under antipsychotics medication. Finally, a guanosine to adenine change at nt -1438 in the serotonin receptor 2A (5-HT$_{2A}$R −1438G/A) was associated with a lower energy intake (EI), BMI, waist to hip ratio (WHR), and abdominal depot (AD). The same hold true for the dopamine receptors that are involved in rewarding properties of food for its obesity aspect, and is blocked by antipsychotics for its schizophrenia aspect. It has been shown that the number of receptors of the dopamine receptor 2 (DRD2) is lower in obese subjects. Individuals carrying the C311 variant allele of the DRD2 S311C polymorphism had a greater BMI or lower 24 h energy expenditure (24hEE), whereas these individuals showed lower positive and negative symptoms in schizophrenia. In the other hand, individuals carrying a deletion of a cytosine at nt −141 of DRD2 (DRD2 −141C I/D) showed higher positive symptoms. As a last example of a candidate gene common to obesity and schizophrenia, the cholecystokinin (CCK) act as a satiety signal produced by the intestine, and is also candidate for schizophrenia because of its close co-localization with other neurotransmitters in the brain. Natural invalidation of the A receptor of CCK (CCKAR) in OLETF rat induced obesity and diabetes whereas the frequency of the −201G allele of the CCKAR −201A/G polymorphism was greater in schizophrenic patients. Similarly, frequencies of the variant alleles −36T and −215A, respectively from the CCK −36C/T, located in a sp1 transcription-regulating element of CCK gene, and CCKBR −215C/A polymorphisms were greater in schizophrenia. Same kind of evidences can be draw from genomic scan results for obesity and schizophrenia. For examples, a locus for schizophrenia has been reported on chromosome 9 at 9q34.1-q34.2 for schizophrenia[18], whereas we observed at the same location a possible locus for antipsychotics-induced obesity, and for BMI[19]. Similarly, we reported[20] as others, a locus for schizophrenia on chromosome 10 at 10p15.3-q11.2 as a locus for fat mass and BMI[19], whereas a locus for bipolar disorder[21] and for obesity[22,23] has also been reported in the same location. All these results support the hypothesis that same genes, and either same polymorphisms, could be involved in apparently different pathologies such as obesity and schizophrenia. The different combinations of gene polymorphisms and environment could produce the different phenotypes and pathologies.

Table 2. Examples of common genes and polymorphisms between obesity and schizophrenia (see text for abbreviations)

Genes	Obesity	Schizophrenia
Serotonin receptors	Inhibit food intake	Behavioural and psychological processes

	$5\text{-HT}_{2C}R$ C23S
	    Weight loss and <ADRB3
		$5\text{-HT}_{2C}R$ C23S
		    >TD (antipsychotics)

	$5\text{-HT}_{2C}R$ KO Hyperphagia and obesity	$5\text{-HT}_{2C}R$ -759C/T <weight gain (antipsychotics)
	$5\text{-HT}_{2A}R$-1438G/A <EI and <BMI-WHR,AD	
Dopamine receptors	Rewarding properties of food	Blocked by antipsychotics
	DRD2<# receptors	DRD2–141C I/D >+ symptoms
	DRD2 S311C >BMI and <24hEE	DRD2 S311C <+and- symptoms
Cholecystokinin	Satiety signal (intestine)	Co-localization neurotransmitters
	CCKAR KO OLETF rat Obesity/diabetes	CCKAR–201A/G >G
		CCK –36C/T (sp1) >T
		CCKBR –215C/A >A

Conclusion

In analysing the genetics of complex traits such as obesity and mental health diseases, flexibility is required in the study designs and in the interpretation of the results since complex traits are complex by definition, and probably more complex then we have imagined previously as examplified by the possible communality of genetic origin of apparently unrelated pathologies such as obesity and schizophrenia. New genomic tools such as gene expression microchips, PCR-based subtractive libraries, new efficient two-dimensional gels for protein expression, MALTI-DOF-based identification of proteins, and bioinformatic facilities will allow to attack these questions with a reasonable probability of success.

Acknowledgements: The author wants to acknowledge all collegues that have been involved in these works. The author also apologizes for references not reported in Table 2 due to space restrictions.

References

1. Schulze TG, McMahon FJ. Genetic association mapping at the crossroads: which test and why? Overview and practical guidelines. *Am J Med Genet* 2002; 114(1): 1–11.

2. Chagnon YC *et al.* Linkages and associations between the leptin receptor (LEPR) gene and human body composition in the Quebec Family Study. *Int J Obes Relat Metab Disord* 1999; 23(3): 278–86.

3. Gauderman WJ, Sample size requirements for association studies of gene-gene interaction. *Am J Epidemiol* 2002; 155(5): 478–84.

4. Chagnon YC *et al.* Associations between the leptin receptor gene and adiposity in middle- aged Caucasian males from the HERITAGE family study. *J Clin Endocrinol Metab* 2000; 85(1): 29–34.

5. Ukkola O *et al.* Leptin receptor Gln223Arg variant is associated with a cluster of metabolic abnormalities in response to long-term overfeeding. *J Intern Med* 2000; 248(5): p. 435–439.

6. Rosmond R *et al.* Hypertension in obesity and the leptin receptor gene locus. *J Clin Endocrinol Metab* 2000; 85(9): 3126–31.

7. Wauters M *et al.* Polymorphisms in the leptin receptor gene, body composition and fat distribution in overweight and obese women. *Int J Obes Relat Metab Disord* 2001; 25(5): 714–20.

8. Yiannakouris N *et al.* The Q223R polymorphism of the leptin receptor gene is significantly associated with obesity and predicts a small percentage of body weight and body composition variability. *J Clin Endocrinol Metab* 2001; 86(9): 4434–9.

9. Thompson DB *et al.* Structure and sequence variation at the human leptin receptor gene in lean and obese Pima Indians. *Hum Mol Genet* 1997; 6(5): 675–9.

10. Gotoda T *et al.* Leptin receptor gene variation and obesity: lack of association in a white British male population. *Hum Mol Genet* 1997; 6(6): 869–76.

11. Ukkola O *et al.* Interactions among the alpha2-, beta2-, and beta3-adrenergic receptor genes and obesity-related phenotypes in the Quebec Family Study. *Metabolism* 2000; 49(8): 1063–70.

12. Ukkola O *et al.* Interactions among the glucocorticoid receptor, lipoprotein lipase and adrenergic receptor genes and abdominal fat in the Quebec Family Study. *Int J Obes Relat Metab Disord* 2001; 25(9): 1332–9.

13. Chagnon YC Pérusse L, Bouchard C. The molecular and epidemiological genetics of obesity; In: *Handbook of Experimental pharmacology: obesity, pathology and therapy*, pp. 57–89. DLAT Heffner, 2000.

14. Chagnon YC *et al.* Linkage and association studies between the melanocortin receptors 4 and 5 genes and obesity-related phenotypes in the Quebec Family Study. *Mol Med* 1997; 3(10): 663–73.

15. Boucher N *et al.* A +2138InsCAGACC polymorphism of the melanocortin receptor 3 gene is associated in human with fat level and partitioning in interaction with body corpulence. *Mol Med* 2002; 8(3): 158–65.

16. Lanouette CM *et al.* Uncoupling protein 3 gene is associated with body composition changes with training in HERITAGE study. *J Appl Physiol* 2002; 92(3): 1111–8.

17. Lanouette CM *et al.* Association between uncoupling protein 3 gene and obesity-related phenotypes in the Quebec Family Study. *Mol Med* 2001; 7(7): 433–41.

18. Kaufmann CA *et al.* NIMH Genetics Initiative Millenium Schizophrenia Consortium: linkage analysis of African-American pedigrees. *Am J Med Genet* 1998; 81(4): 282–9.

19. Chagnon YC *et al.* Genomic scan for genes affecting body composition before and after training in Caucasians from HERITAGE. *J Appl Physiol* 2001; 90(5): 1777–87.

20. Maziade M *et al.* Chromosome 1q12-q22 linkage results in eastern Quebec families affected by schizophrenia. *Am J Med Genet* 2002; 114(1): 51–5.

21. Rice JP *et al.* Initial genome scan of the NIMH genetics initiative bipolar pedigrees: chromosomes 1, 6, 8, 10, and 12. *Am J Med Genet* 1997; 74(3): 247–53.

22. Hager J *et al.* A genome-wide scan for human obesity genes reveals a major susceptibility locus on chromosome 10. *Nature Genet* 1998; 20(3): 304–8.

23. Hinney A *et al.* Independent confirmation of a major locus for obesity on chromosome 10. *J Clin Endocrinol Metab* 2000; 85(8): p. 2962–5.

24. Heo M *et al.* Pooling analysis of genetic data: the association of leptin receptor (LEPR) polymorphisms with variables related to human adiposity. *Genetics* 2001; 159(3): 1163–78.

25. Rand L *et al.* Maternal leptin receptor gene variant Gln223Arg is not associated with variation in birth weight or maternal body mass index in UK and South Asian populations. *Int J Obes Relat Metab Disord* 2001; 25(5): p. 753–5.

26. Endo K *et al.* Association of Trp64Arg polymorphism of the beta3-adrenergic receptor gene and no association of Gln223Arg polymorphism of the leptin receptor gene in Japanese schoolchildren with obesity. *Int J Obes Relat Metab Disord* 2000; 24(4): 443–9.

27. Silver K *et al.* The Gln223Arg and Lys656Asn polymorphisms in the human leptin receptor do not associate with traits related to obesity. *Diabetes* 1997; 46(11): 1898–900.

28. Echwald SM *et al.* Amino acid variants in the human leptin receptor: lack of association to juvenile onset obesity. *Biochem Biophys Res Commun* 1997; 233(1): 248–52.

29. Matsuoka N *et al.* Human leptin receptor gene in obese Japanese subjects: evidence against either obesity-causing mutations or association of sequence variants with obesity. *Diabetologia* 1997; 40(10): 1204–10.

Progress in Obesity Research: 9. Edited by *Geraldo Medeiros-Neto, Alfredo Halpern and Claude Bouchard*
©2003 John Libbey Eurotext Ltd, pp. 363–365.

CHAPTER 77

Ghrelin

Olavi Ukkola

Department of Internal Medicine and Biocentre Oulu, University of Oulu, Finland
[e-mail: olavi.ukkola@oulu.fi]

Introduction

A novel gastrointestinal hormone, ghrelin, was identified from rat stomach by Kojima *et al.*[1] in 1999. Ghrelin is a 28 amino acid peptide hormone which has an unique feature: it is the first natural peptide with a hydroxyl group in the third serine residue acylated by n-octanoid acid[1]. Ghrelin is secreted mostly by stomach fundus[2] but also in small amounts by other tissues, like the pituitary[3], and the hypothalamus[1]. Ghrelin stimulates potently growth hormone (GH) release[1]. The n-octanoyl modification at Serine 3 residue is necessary for the GH-releasing potency of ghrelin[1] and the four first amino acids appears to constitute the active core of the molecule[4].

Ghrelin stimulates GH secretion

Ghrelin is involved in the regulation of pituitary GH secretion along with GH-releasing hormone (GHRH) and somatostatin. GH secretagogues (GHS's) are artificial compounds that release GH *in vitro*[5]. GHS's bind to their own receptors in the anterior pituitary but the endogenous ligand for these receptors had been unknown until the identification of ghrelin. This new gastrointestinal hormone revealed to be an endogenous ligand for the GHS receptor (GHS-R). The stimulatory effect of ghrelin on GH secretion is dose-dependent[6] and it has been shown in several studies[6,7]. Recently, a transgenic rat model, in which the expression of GHS-R protein was selectively attenuated, was generated[8]. Female rats had reduced GH secretion and plasma insulin-like growth factor-I levels suggesting that ghrelin might play a more important role in the regulation of GH secretion in female animals.

Ghrelin and the regulation of energy metabolism in rodent models

Tschöp *et al.*[9] found that peripheral daily administration of ghrelin caused weight gain by reducing fat utilization in rats and mice. In addition, continuous central ghrelin administration generated a dose-dependent increase in food intake and body weight. These findings were unexpected given the lipolytic effect of GH. However, the induction of positive energy balance by ghrelin was independent of its effect on GH secretion[9]. The stimulation of feeding in rodents has been confirmed in several other independent studies. Shintani *et al.*[10] observed that ghrelin reversed the leptin-induced inhibition of food intake and a decrease of hypothalamic neuropeptide Y (NPY) mRNA expression. The latter mechanism is thought to cause leptin's satiety effect. Therefore, ghrelin might be an endogenous leptin functional antagonist. Asakawa *et al.*[11] examined the effects of ghrelin on energy balance in association with leptin and vagal nerve activity in mice. They suggested that the orexigenic potency of ghrelin is caused by the activation of hypothalamic NPY and NPY1 receptor and the increase of gastric emptying. However, Kamegai *et al.*[12] presented for the first time evidence that the most important hypothalamic target of ghrelin might not be NPY but agouti related peptide. In rodents, serum ghrelin concentrations are increased by fasting and decreased by refeeding or oral glucose administration, but not by water ingestion[9].

Ghrelin and the regulation of energy metabolism in humans

Plasma ghrelin levels are influenced by acute[13] and chronic changes in nutritional state[14,15]. Recent data suggest a dramatic preprandial rise and postprandial fall in circulating ghrelin levels supporting the notion that ghrelin could be a physiological meal initiator[13]. Ghrelin enhances appetite and increases food intake in humans[16]. Interestingly, obese subjects have lower plasma ghrelin concentration than age-matched, lean controls[14]. Potential candidates for low ghrelin levels in obese individuals include chronic positive energy balance, leptin[10] and insulin. The effects of ghrelin on metabolism are exactly opposite to those of leptin. Weight loss increases circulating levels of ghrelin in human obesity supporting the notion that suppression of ghrelin in obesity is reversible[17]. Further evidence on the effects of ghrelin on body weight regulation was provided by Cumming et al.[18] who showed that gastric bypass was associated with markedly suppressed ghrelin levels, possibly contributing to the weight-reducing effect of the procedure. In contrast, the role of ghrelin in human obesity was challenged by the recent data[19] demonstrating that ghrelin was not related to the magnitude of body weight changes in either overfeeding or negative energy balance.

Ghrelin and glucose metabolism

Several studies[15,20-23] have provided evidence that ghrelin is involved in glucose and insulin metabolism. The effects of ghrelin on insulin metabolism may occur through its effects on energy metabolism. Indeed, fasting plasma ghrelin levels are negatively correlated with per cent body fat and fasting levels of insulin and leptin[14]. Central mechanisms controlling energy homeostasis including the activation of hypothalamic agouti related peptide or NPY neurones in the arcuate nucleus[24] may be involved in the interplay between hunger (ghrelin) and satiety (leptin, insulin) signals. In relation to meals, a secretion pattern of ghrelin reciprocal to that of insulin has been observed[13]. Food intake and glucose load have been shown to decrease plasma ghrelin levels[20] while insulin infusion decreased ghrelin levels in the study by Saad et al.[25]. These findings are in accordance with the theory that insulin may be an important regulator of plasma ghrelin levels in different states of nutrition. However, suppressive effect of parenteral administration of insulin on plasma ghrelin levels was not demonstrated in another study[21], and, on the contrary, Toshinai et al.[26] reported recently that the ghrelin mRNA level in the stomach increased after administration of insulin and leptin in mouse. Importantly, insulin and leptin have been shown to be independent determinants of fasting ghrelin concentrations[14]. Therefore, some additional mechanisms in addition to those related to adiposity, which could explain the interaction between ghrelin and insulin, must be considered. Ghrelin and its receptor are also expressed in pancreatic beta-cells[27]. However, studies about the effect of ghrelin on insulin secretion have been inconsistent in animal and human models and both stimulatory[22-23] and inhibitory[15] effects have been reported. Recently, ghrelin was reported to affect insulin signalling system in hepatoma cells[28].

Ghrelin polymorphisms in obesity

Ghrelin and preproghrelin sequences were determined in 96 unrelated female subjects with severe obesity and in 96 non-obese female controls of the Swedish Obese Subjects cohort[29]. A mutation at amino acid position 51 (Arg51Gln) of the preproghrelin sequence that corresponds to the last amino acid in mature ghrelin product was identified in six (all heterozygotes) obese subjects (6.3 per cent) but not among controls ($p<0.05$). The Arg51Gln mutation may alter the cleavage site of endoproteases and the length of the mature ghrelin product. Leu72Met polymorphism of the preproghrelin gene was detected in 15 obese and 12 control subjects. In conclusion, the data provided evidence that a low frequency sequence variations in the ghrelin gene could play a role in the aetiology of obesity. The further analysis did not confirm these findings although Arg51Gln mutation seemed to be associated with lower plasma ghrelin concentrations[30]. In addition, Met72 carrier status was protective against fat accumulation and associated metabolic co-morbidities[30].

Conclusions

Ghrelin is a gut-brain peptide that has somatotropic, orexigenic and adipogenic effects. Long-term administration of ghrelin agonist and antagonists will reveal, which of the two effects of ghrelin, adipogenic or somatotropic, dominates and determines the net influence on energy balance.

Acknowledgements: The author wishes to thank Dr. Claude Bouchard, Dr. Eric Ravussin and Monique Chagnon, ART, and all the staff in the Pennington Biomedical Research Center for their support and assistance in this project.

References

1. Kojima M, Hosoda H, Date Y, Nakazato M, Matsuo H, Kangawa K. Ghrelin is a growth-hormone-releasing acylated peptide from stomach. *Nature* 1999; 402: 656–60.

2. Date Y, Kojima M, Hosoda H, Sawaguchi A, Mondal MS, Suganamu T et al. Ghrelin, a novel growth hormone-releasing acylated peptide, is synthesized in a distinct endocrine cell type in the gastrointestinal tracts of rats and humans. *Endocrinology* 2000; 141: 4255–61.

3. Korbonits M, Bustin SA, Kojima M, Jordan S, Adams EF, Lowe DG et al. The Expression of the Growth Hormone Secretagogue Receptor Ligand Ghrelin in Normal and Abnormal Human Pituitary and Other Neuroendocrine Tumors. *J Clin Endocrinol Metab* 2001; 86: 881–7.

4. Bednarek MA, Feighner SD, Pong SS, McKee KK, Hreniuk DL, Silva MV *et al.* Structure-function studies on the new growth hormone-releasing peptide, ghrelin: minimal sequence of ghrelin necessary for activation of growth hormone secretagogue receptor 1a. *J Med Chem* 2000; 43: 4370–6.

5. Casanueva FF, Dieguez C. Growth hormone secretagogues: Physiological role and clinical utility. *Trends Endocrinol Metab* 1999; 10: 30–38.

6. Takaya K, Ariyasu H, Kanamoto N, Iwakura H, Yoshimoto A, Harada M *et al.* Ghrelin Strongly Stimulates Growth Hormone Release in Humans. *J Clin Endocrinol Metab* 2000; 85: 4908–11.

7. Arvat E, Di Vito L, Broglio F, Papotti M, Muccioli G, Dieguez C *et al.* Preliminary evidence that Ghrelin, the natural GH secretagogue (GHS)-receptor ligand, strongly stimulates GH secretion in humans. *J Endocrinol Invest* 2000; 23: 493–5.

8. Shuto Y, Shibasaki T, Otagiri A, Kuriyama H, Ohata H, Tamura H *et al.* Hypothalamic growth hormone secretagogue receptor regulates growth hormone secretion, feeding & adiposity. *J Clin Invest* 2002; 109: 1429–36.

9. Tschöp M, Smiley DL, Heiman ML. Ghrelin induces adiposity in rodents. *Nature* 2000; 407: 908–13.

10. Shintani M, Ogawa Y, Ebihara K, Aizawa-Abe M, Miynaga F, Takaya K *et al.* Ghrelin, an endogenous growth hormone secretagogue, is a novel orexigenic peptide that antagonizes leptin action through the activation of hypothalamic neuropeptide Y/Y1 receptor pathway. *Diabetes* 2001; 50: 227–32.

11. Asakawa A, Inui A, Kaga T, Yuzuriha H, Nagata T, Ueno N. Ghrelin is an appetite-stimulatory signal from stomach with structural resemblance to motilin. *Gastroenterology* 2001; 120: 337–45.

12. Kamegai J, Tamura H, Shimizu T, Ishii S, Sugihara H, Wakabayashi I. Central effect of ghrelin, an endogenous growth hormone secretagogue, on hypothalamic peptide gene expression. *Endocrinology* 2000; 141: 4797–800.

13. Cummings DE, Purnell JQ, Frayo RS, Schmidova K, Wisse BE, Weigle DS. A prandial rise in plasma ghrelin levels suggests a role in meal initiation in humans. *Diabetes* 2001; 50: 1714–9.

14. Tschöp M, Viswanath D, Weyer C, Tataranni PA, Ravussin E, Heiman ML. Circulating ghrelin levels are decreased in human obesity. *Diabetes* 2001; 50: 707–9.

15. Broglio F, Arvat E, Benso A, Gottero C, Muccioli G, Papotti M, *et al.* Ghrelin, a natural gh secretagogue produced by the stomach, induces hyperglycemia and reduces insulin secretion in humans. *J Clin Endocrinol Metab* 2001; 86: 5083.

16. Wren AM, Seal LJ, Cohen MA, Brynes AE, Frost GS, Murphy KG *et al.* Ghrelin enhances appetite and increases food intake in humans. *J Clin Endocrinol Metab* 2001; 86, 5992.

17. Hansen TK, Dall R, Hosoda H, Kojima M, Kangawa K, Christiansen JS, Jorgensen JO. Weight loss increases circulating levels of ghrelin in human obesity. *Clin Endocrinol* 2002; 56: 203–6.

18. Cummings DE, Weigle DS, Frayo RS, Breen PA, Ma MK, Dellinger EP, Purnell JQ. Plasma ghrelin levels after diet-induced weight loss or gastric bypass surgery. *N Engl J Med* 2002; 346: 1623–30.

19. Ravussin E, Tschöp M, Morales S, Bouchard C, Heiman ML. Plasma ghrelin concentration and energy balance: overfeeding and negative energy balance studies in twins. *J Clin Endocrinol Metab* 2001; 86: 4547.

20. Shiiya T, Nakazato M, Mizuta M, Date Y, Mondal MS, Tanaka M *et al.* Plasma ghrelin levels in lean and obese humans and the effect of glucose on ghrelin secretion. *J Clin Endocrinol Metab* 2002; 87: 240–4.

21. Caixas A, Bashore C, Nash W, Pi-Sunyer F, Laferrere B. Insulin, unlike food intake, does not suppress ghrelin in human subjects. *J Clin Endocrinol Metab* 2002; 87: 1902–6.

22. Lee HM, Wang G, Englander EW, Kojima M, Greeley GH Jr Ghrelin, a new gastrointestinal endocrine peptide that stimulates insulin secretion: enteric distribution, ontogeny, influence of endocrine, and dietary manipulations. *Endocrinology* 2002; 143: 185–90.

23. Date Y, Nakazato M, Hashiguchi S, Dezaki K, Mondal MS, Hosoda H *et al.* Ghrelin is present in pancreatic alpha-cells of humans and rats and stimulates insulin secretion. *Diabetes* 2002; 51: 124–9.

24. Williams G, Bing C, Cai XJ, Harrold JA, King PJ, Liu XH. The hypothalamus and the control of energy homeostasis: different circuits, different purposes. *Physiol Behav* 2001; 74: 683–701.

25. Saad MF, Bernaba B, Hwu CM, Jinagouda S, Fahmi S, Kogosov E, Boyadjian R. Insulin regulates plasma ghrelin concentration. *J Clin Endocrinol Metab* 2002; 87: 3997–4000.

26. Toshinai K, Mondal MS, Nakazato M, Date Y, Murakami N, Kojima M *et al.* Upregulation of Ghrelin expression in the stomach upon fasting, insulin-induced hypoglycemia, and leptin administration. *Biochem Biophys Res Commun* 2001; 281: 1220–5.

27. Wierup N, Svensson H, Mulder H, Sundler F. The ghrelin cell: a novel developmentally regulated islet cell in the human pancreas. *Regul Pept* 2002; 107: 63–9.

28. Murata M, Okimura Y, Iida K, Matsumoto M, Sowa H, Kaji H *et al.* Ghrelin modulates the downstream molecules of insulin signaling in hepatoma cells. *J Biol Chem* 2002; 277: 5667–74.

29. Ukkola O, Ravussin E, Jacobson P, Snyder EE, Chagnon M, Sjöström L, Bouchard C. Mutations in the Preproghrelin / Ghrelin Gene Associated with Obesity in Humans. *J Clin Endocrinol Metab* 2001; 86: 3996–9.

30. Ukkola O, Ravussin E, Jacobson P, Perusse L, Rankinen T, Tschop M *et al.* Role of ghrelin polymorphisms in obesity based on three different studies. *Obes Res* 2002; 10: 782–91.

Progress in Obesity Research: 9. Edited by *Geraldo Medeiros-Neto, Alfredo Halpern* and *Claude Bouchard*
©2003 John Libbey Eurotext Ltd, pp. 366–369.

CHAPTER 78

Methods to identify obesity and type 2 diabetes mellitus susceptibility genes in Pima Indians

Leslie Baier, Yunhua Li Muller, Peter Kovacs, Christopher Wiedrich, Kimberly Wiedrich, Jeffrey Sutherland, Pamela Thuillez, Michael Traurig and Clifton Bogardus

Phoenix Epidemiology and Clinical Research Branch, NIDDK, NIH, Phoenix Arizona, USA
[e-mail: lbaier@phx.niddk.nih.gov]

Introduction

The Pima Indians of Arizona have a high prevalence of obesity. In 1988, more than 80 per cent of Pima Indians between the ages of 20 and 55 years had a BMI > 27 kg/m[21] and the incidence of obesity has been steadily increasing. The Pima Indians also have the world's highest reported incidence and prevalence of T2DM[2]. Their diabetes is prototypic of this disease and is characterized by obesity, insulin resistance, insulin secretory dysfunction, and increased rates of endogenous glucose production[3]. Both obesity and T2DM in Pima Indians, as in other populations, have a substantial genetic basis[4]. Both diseases aggregate in families and both demonstrate a higher concordance rate among monozygotic twins as compared to dizygotic twins. Studies in monozygotic twins in non-Native American populations estimate that the heritability for BMI ranges from 0.60–0.80[5]. Studies of monogenic forms of T2DM led to the identification of several diabetes genes with major effects in rare families. These include genes that encode insulin, insulin receptor, glucokinase, three hepatic nuclear transcription factors (HNF-1a, -4a, 1b), and another transcription factor, IPF-1[6]. A few genes that can cause severe, rare forms of obesity, such as leptin and its receptor and the MC4 receptor, have also been characterized[7,8]. However, major genes that cause the most common forms or T2DM and obesity remain unknown. Moreover, none of the genes identified to date appear to have a major role in the pathogenesis of type 2 diabetes or obesity in Pima Indians.

In an effort to determine the genetic basis for obesity and T2DM in Pima Indians, we have undertaken a candidate gene approach as well as a genome scan approach. Candidate genes include genes that have a known physiologic role in glucose and/or lipid metabolism as well as genes that are associated with T2DM or BMI in other populations. To date, no variation in a physiologic candidate gene has been identified that has a major role in determining body mass index (BMI) or T2DM in Pima Indians.

We have recently completed a genomic scan in more than 1200 Pima Indians who had participated in a longitudinal study of diabetes[9]. Among 264 nuclear families containing 966 siblings, 516 highly informative autosomal markers, with a median distance between adjacent markers of 6.4 cM, were genotyped. Variance-components methods were used to test for linkage with an age-adjusted diabetes score and with BMI. In multipoint analyses, the strongest evidence for linkage with BMI (LOD = 3.6) was centred at marker D11S4464 on chromosome 11q (Fig. 1). This region also showed suggestive linkage to age-adjusted diabetes (LOD = 1.7). Bivariate linkage analysis for the combined phenotype 'diabesity' gave the strongest evidence for linkage (LOD = 5.2). The region of linkage is positioned at 11q23-24 (approximately 35 cM). Linkage of this region to T2DM in obese subjects has subsequently been replicated by the Diabetes Consortium, where the evidence for linkage comes from Mexican-American and Native American populations (Dr. Robert Hanson, personal communication). In addition, linkage to morbid obesity at marker D11S4464 has been demonstrated in males from multigenerational Utah Mormon pedigrees[10]. The aim of the current study is to identify obesity and/or diabetes susceptibility genes on 11q23-24 that gave rise to the linkage.

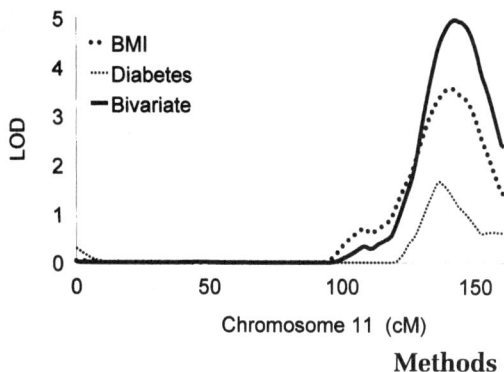

Fig. 1. Multipoint linkage results for chromosome 11 for BMI and for diabetes, adjusted for age and sex by a cumulative incidence method. The bivariate analysis tests the null hypothesis of no linkage with either phenotype (adapted from ref.[9]).

Methods

Linkage disequilibrium mapping of SNPs

Linkage disequilibrium analysis of SNPs is being used to narrow the chromosomal region along 11q23-24 harboring the susceptibility gene(s) for T2DM and BMI. Single nucleotide polymorphisms (SNPs) are being systematically identified and genotyped at 50 kB intervals across the 35 megabase region of linkage.

SNP identification/verification

Single nucleotide polymorphisms (SNPs) are systematically identified by searching public SNP databases and verifying the database SNP by sequencing 24 Pima Indian DNA samples. Alternatively, SNPs are identified *de novo* by directly sequencing segments of DNA in 24 DNA samples. For *de novo* sequencing, PCR primers are designed based on published sequence or sequence obtained by sequencing of bacterial artificial chromosome (BAC) ends that map to 11q23. PCR is typically performed with 100 ng of genomic DNA in buffer containing 1.5 mM MgCl$_2$, 0.25 mM dNTPs and 0.75U of AmpliTaq Gold (Perkin-Elmer) DNA polymerase. PCR conditions are typically 94 °C for 10 min followed by 33 cycles of 94 °C for 30 seconds, the optimal primer annealing temperature (55–60 °C) for 30 s, and 72 °C for 30 s, followed by a final extension at 72 °C for 10 min. Sequencing of the PCR product is done with both the forward and reverse PCR primers. DNA cycle sequencing is carried out using the Big Dye Terminator technology on a capillary DNA sequencer (Model 3700, Applied Biosystems, Inc). SNPs that have a minor allele frequency of 20 per cent or greater are considered 'informative' and are genotyped in 1229 Pima Indian DNA samples.

Individual genotyping of SNPs

Informative SNPs are genotyped in the Pima Indians used in our linkage study ($n = 1229$). Individual genotyping is done by either the Taqman allelic discrimination polymerase chain reaction technology, using a model 7700 ABI Prism instrument (PE Applied Biosystems) or the primer extension methodology of Pyosequencing, using a PSQ 96 system (Pyrosequencing, Inc.).

Positional candidate genes

Positional physiologic candidate genes are selected based on a perceivable function in a physiologic pathway relevant to T2DM and/or obesity. For each positional candidate gene, all exons, intron/exon boundaries, 5' and 3' untranslated regions and the putative promoter region are PCR amplified and sequenced, as above, in 24 Pima Indian DNA samples.

Results

To date we have sequenced 13 positional candidate genes that map to chromosome 11q23-24. These genes encode the serotonin receptor 3A, the dopamine receptor D2, four apolipoproteins (AIV, CIII, AI and AV), three transcription factors (PLZF, ZNF259 and PKNOX2), an opioid binding cell adhesion molecule (OPCML) and the THY-1, oxygen-regulated protein and glucose 6 phosphate transferase genes. SNPs were identified in all of these genes and were genotyped in DNA from 1229 Pima Indians. However, none of the nucleotide variants identified in these physiologic candidate genes accounted for the linkage to T2DM and BMI on chromosome 11q23-24[11,12].

Our goal for linkage disequilibrium mapping is to genotype an informative SNP every 50 kB across the 35 Mb region of linkage. This will require genotyping 700 informative SNPs. To date approximately 190 informative SNPs have been genotyped in 1229 Pima Indians. Of these 190 SNPs, approximately 160 were genotyped by the method of allelic discrimination and 30 were genotyped by the technique of Pyrosequencing. The physical map position of each SNP, based upon the human genome sequence

Association with BMI

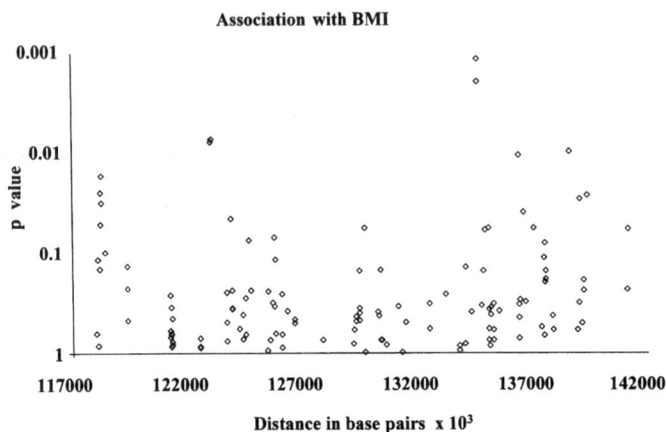

Fig. 2. Plot of 190 SNPs genotyped in 1229 individual DNA samples and analysed using an additive model for BMI. Data were adjusted for age and sex.

database (http: //www.ncbi.nlm.nih.gov), was plotted against the significance of the association of each SNP for both BMI and T2DM. SNPs that were significantly associated with BMI clustered in three distinct regions, at 119×10^6, 125×10^6 and 135×10^6 base pairs along chromosome 11 (Fig. 2). SNPs that were significantly associated with T2DM clustered around 137×10^6 base pairs (Fig. 3). We are currently filling in the gaps to complete a 50 kB map across the 35 Mb region.

Discussion

Positional cloning has had much success in the identification of genes and mutations for monogenic metabolic diseases. The same is not true for complex, polygenic diseases. In most cases, genome-wide linkage scans for complex diseases have identified large, poorly defined susceptibility regions. Subsequent linkage studies in either the same population or in a different population often fail to replicate the initial observations. Follow-up studies to identify the genetic variant(s) that gave rise to the linkage signal are laborious and expensive. Recently, however, linkage disequilibrium mapping of susceptibility regions has proven successful in identifying susceptibility genes for three complex disorders. The first example was the identification of the calpain 10 gene as a susceptibility gene for T2DM[13]. A genome scan in Mexican Americans in Starr County, Texas had identified linkage on chromosome 2q to T2DM[14]. The initial region of linkage encompassed a 12 cM region, and an interaction of the locus on chromosome 2 with a locus on chromosome 15 decreased the 1-LOD support interval from 12 cM to 7 cM. Linkage disequilibrium mapping was done by genotyping 133 SNPs, and haplotype analysis determined that SNP43, in combination with two other nearby SNPs, marked a heightened susceptibility to T2DM in Mexican Americans in Starr County, Texas. The combination of three SNPs in the calpain-10 gene also conveyed a risk in two northern European populations, whereas the single SNP43 was associated with increased insulin resistance in Pima Indians[15].

A second success of using linkage disequilibrium mapping to identify a susceptibility locus for a complex disease was the identification of variants in the NOD2 gene that conferred an increased risk for Crohn's disease[16]. In this study, linkage analysis identified a 20 million base pair region on chromosome 16 that appeared to harbor at least one risk gene. Subsequent mapping, using a database

Association with Diabetes

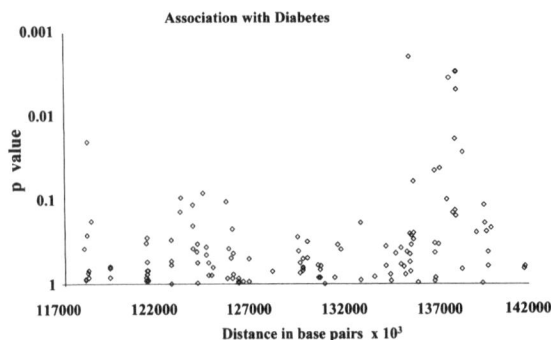

Fig. 3. Plot of 190 SNPs genotyped in 1229 individual DNA samples and analysed using an additive model for diabetes. Data were adjusted for age and sex.

search and non-SNP markers, narrowed the region to a 160,000 nucleotide span, and finally eleven SNPs were genotyped for linkage disequilibrium mapping. Interestingly, a subsequent study to replicate the use of microsatellite linkage and linkage disequilibrium mapping methods did not identify NOD2 as a Crohn's disease susceptibility gene, despite the presence of allelic association with NOD2 mutations[17].

Most recently, the ADAM33 gene was identified as a susceptibility gene for asthma and bronchial hyperresponsiveness by linkage disequilibrium mapping[18]. In this study, gene discovery efforts were centred on a 1-LOD-drop support interval for linkage to the bronchial hyperresponsiveness phenotype, which spanned 4.28 cM[18]. A total of 135 polymorphisms in 23 genes were analysed . Only SNPs within the ADAM33 gene were significantly associated with asthma using case-control, transmission disequilibrium and haplotype analysis.

The most marked difference between the three successful examples of using linkage disequilibrium mapping to identify a complex disease susceptibility locus and our study of chromosome 11q23-24 in Pima Indians is the interval initially obtained in the genome scan. The region of linkage on chromosome 2q to type 2 diabetes in Mexican Americans was narrowed to 7 cM, the region of linkage on chromosome 16 linked to Crohn's disease was narrowed to 160,000 base pairs, and the region of linkage on chromosome 20 was narrowed to approximately 4 cM prior to linkage disequlibrium mapping. Therefore, it is perhaps not surprising that in our 35 cM region, genotyping of approximately 190 SNPs has not yet clearly identified a susceptibility variant. It is likely that nearly double that number of SNPs must be systematically identified, mapped and genotyped before we are certain of the precise location of the variant gene(s).

References

1. Knowler WC *et al.* Obesity in the Pima Indians: its magnitude and relationship with diabetes. *Am J Clin Nutr* 1991; 53: S1543–S1551.

2. Knowler WC *et al.* Diabetes incidence and prevalence in Pima Indians: a 19-fold greater incidence than in Rochester, Minnesota. *Am J Epidemiology* 1978; 108: 497–505.

3. Bogardus C. Metabolic abnormalities in the development of non-insulin dependent diabetes mellitus. In: *Diabetes mellitus: a fundamental and clinical text*, D. LeRoith, S.I. Taylor, J.M. Olefsky (eds), pp. 459–67. Philadelphia: Lippincott-Raven, 1996.

4. Sakul H *et al.* Familiality of physical and metabolic characteristics that predict the development of non-insulin dependent diabetes mellitus in Pima Indians. *Am J Hum Genet* 1997; 60: 651–6.

5. Allison DB *et al.* The heritability of body mass index among an international sample of monozygotic twins reared apart. *Int J Obes Relat Metab Disord* 1996; 20: 501–6.

6. Elbein SC. The genetics of human non-insulin dependent (type 2) diabetes mellitus. *J Nutr* 1997; 127: S1891–S1896.

7. Montague CT *et al.* Congenital leptin deficiency is associated with severe early-onset obesity in humans. *Nature* 1997; 387: 903–8.

8. Vaisse C *et al.* A frameshift mutation in human MC4R is associated with a dominant form of obesity. *Nature Genet* 1998; 20: 113–4.

9. Hanson RL *et al.* An autosomal genomic scan for loci linked to type 2 diabetes mellitus and body mass index in Pima Indians: an obesity-diabetes locus at 11q23-25. *Am J Hum Genet* 1998; 63: 1130–8.

10. Stone S *et al.* A major predisposition locus for severe obesity at 4p15-p14. *Am J Hum Genet* 2002; 70: 1459–68.

11. Jenkinson CP *et al.* Association of dopamine D2 receptor polymorphisms Ser311Cys and Taq1A with obesity or type 2 diabetes mellitus in Pima Indians. *Int J Obes* 2000; 24: 1233–38.

12. Kovacs *et al.* Polymorphisms in the oxygen-regulated protein 150 gene (ORP150) are associated with insulin resistance in Pima Indians. *Diabetes* 2002; 51: 1618–21.

13. Horikawa Y *et al.* Genetic variation in the gene encoding calpain-10 is associated with type 2 diabetes mellitus. *Nature Genet* 2000; 26: 163–75.

14. Hanis CL *et al.* A genome-wide search for human non-insulin-dependent (type 2) diabetes genes reveals a major susceptibility locus in chromosome 2. *Nature Genet* 1996; 13: 161–6.

15. Baier LJ *et al.* A calpain-10 gene polymorphism is associated with reduced muscle mRNA levels and insulin resistance. *J Clin Invest* 2000; 106: R69–R73.

16. Hugot JP *et al.* Association of NOD2 leucine-rich repeat variants with susceptibility to Crohn's disease. *Nature* 2001; 411: 599–603.

17. Van Heel DA *et al.* Fine mapping of the IBD1 locuse did not identify Crohn-disease-associated NOD2 variants: implications for complex disease genetics. *Am J Med Genet* 2002; 111: 253–59.

18. Van Eerdewegh P *et al.* Association of the ADAM33 gene with asthma and bronchial hyperresponsiveness. *Nature* 418: 426–30.

Progress in Obesity Research: 9. Edited by *Geraldo Medeiros-Neto, Alfredo Halpern and Claude Bouchard*
©2003 John Libbey Eurotext Ltd, pp. 370–372.

CHAPTER 79

Association of the dopamine D2 receptor gene with obesity in native Brazilians

M.H. Hutz, V.S. Mattevi, S. Almeida, V.M. Zembrzuski and F.M. Salzano

Departamento de Genética, Instituto de Biociências, Universidade Federal do Rio Grande do Sul, Caixa Postal 15053, 91501-970 – Porto Alegre, RS, Brazil
[e-mail: mara.hutz@ufrgs.br]

Introduction

Obesity is a major predisposing factor for several chronic diseases including coronary heart disease, non-insulin dependent diabetes, hypertension, and hyperlipidaemia. It arises from complex interactions between genetics and environment which alter the delicate mechanism that regulates food intake and energy expenditure[1,2]. Genetic factors may account for as much as 70 per cent of the variability in human body weight[1]. The search for obesity genes requires a multifaceted approach that involves studies of potential candidate genes which can be chosen for their possible effects on body fat composition, anatomical distribution of fat, appetite regulation, and energy expenditure[2]. Several studies have suggested that there is variability in the efficiency with which humans store calories in the form of fat. However, evidences for the critical role of environmental factors in the development of obesity come from studies that showed that the incidence of obesity is rising in newly Westernized societies. An extreme example is found in the Pima population of the United States southwest, who are 25 kg heavier than Pima Indians living in Mexico[3,4]. The first group suffers from a syndrome of obesity and diabetes with a prevalence as high as 50 per cent, probably due to easy access to high-fat Western diet and reduction in physical activity[3].

The ingestion of food, like a variety of reinforcing substances such as alcohol and other drugs of abuse, can produce pleasure. Although, little is known about the reinforcing properties of these substances, there is general agreement that they are manifested in the dopaminergic reward pathways of the brain[5,6]. Evidence that the dopaminergic system may be implicated in appetite regulation is suggested by various drugs that interact with the dopamine D2 receptor (*DRD2*) and have ingestive side effects, in addition to their central neuroleptic effects. Dopaminergic agonists are powerful suppressors of appetite and weight gain, whereas antagonists enhance appetite[7]. Several genetic studies in human populations have shown an association of *DRD2* with obesity. Comings *et al.*[8], Noble *et al.*[9], and Spitz *et al.*[10] showed an association of the *DRD2 Taq*I A polymorphism with a higher body mass index (BMI) in Caucasians. Thomas *et al.*[11] reported an association of this *DRD2* polymorphism with increased skinfold thickness at the iliac and triceps in Chinese. In Pima Indians the *DRD2* Ser311Cys polymorphism was associated with a slightly higher BMI[12] and with reduced energy expenditure[13].

Native Brazilian populations constitute an excellent set of populations for investigating the interrelationship between obesity and genetics, because they have a relatively homogeneous genetic background with none or low levels of admixture with non-Indians, and their dietary habits and lifestyle also differ from those of Western societies. Epidemiological data, although poor, show a low frequency of cardiovascular diseases and few subjects with abnormal lipid or glucose levels. This situation seems to be changing in several populations, in particular in those groups that have engaged in intensive interaction with non-Indians and who have experienced a marked change in nutrition and lifestyle[14,15].

The major goal of this study was to evaluate the effect of the *DRD2 Taq*I A polymorphism on anthropometric parameters related to body mass and composition in Brazilian Amerindian subjects.

Subjects and methods

The Brazilian Indian samples consisted of 113 individuals from the Xavante, Zoró, Gavião, Suruí, and Kaingang tribes. The samples from the first four groups were collected in 1990, while the Kaingang samples were obtained in 2000. Linguistic, historical, demographic, genetic, and nutritional information about these populations had been reported previously[14–18]

The blood samples were collected with anticoagulant, refrigerated shortly afterwards, and transported in this condition to Porto Alegre. DNA was extracted from whole blood with standard procedures. The *Taq*I A locus was PCR amplified and genotyped as described[19].

Anthropometric data, including stature and weight were obtained from the adult population (21–74 years old) in all five groups, while skinfold thickness (triceps and subscapular) were gathered from Xavante, Zoró, Gavião and Suruí individuals only. The body mass index (BMI) was computed as weight in kilograms/stature in meters^2. Triceps and subscapular skinfold thickness was measured by means of a Lange caliper on the left side of the body as previously described[15]. Allele frequencies were estimated by gene counting. Standardization of the anthropometric data to account for sex and age differences was performed as described[15]. Differences between means for BMI and skinfold thickness were evaluated by analysis of variance (ANOVA). These analyses were performed with the SPSS V.8 statistical package.

Results and discussion

The mean BMI considering the five populations was 24.43 ± 3.86, with a range from 17 to 39. A BMI of 25 or higher, which could be classified as an indication of obesity, was observed in 39 per cent of the Indians investigated. The Kaingang have the highest proportion of overweight and obese individuals (45 per cent), whereas the lowest value was found in the Zoró (22 per cent). A BMI of 17, which is indicative of underweight was observed only in the Kaingang. In the other more isolated groups, the BMI ranged from 19 to 31.

Amerindians have the highest world prevalence of the *DRD2 Taq*I A *A1* allele (average of 12 Native American populations, 60 per cent), tested thus far[19,20]. No statistically significant differences in the frequency of *A1* carriers were observed when overweight plus obese individuals were compared with normal weight subjects ($P = 0.49$).

Table 1 shows mean BMI and mean skinfold thickness values by *DRD2* genotypes in the pooled five Native Brazilian populations. A highly significant association between BMI and the *Taq*I A polymorphism was observed ($P = 0.015$). Persons who were homozygous for the *A1* allele had on average a BMI 2.61 kg/m^2 higher than those with the *A2A2* genotype, while *A1A2* carriers show intermediate values. Skinfold thickness, was also associated with the *DRD2 Taq*I A polymorphism (Table 1). As in the previous analysis, higher values were observed in homozygous *A1A1* subjects, while carriers of the *A2A2* genotype have the lowest mean skinfold thickness ($P = 0.006$). The association between skinfold thickness and the *DRD2* gene had been previously investigated in Chinese[11] with significant results which are being replicated in the present study with Amerindians.

Table 1. Variation in anthropometric variables related to body mass and fat composition by *DRD2* genotypes in Native Brazilians

Genotype	BMI (kg/m^2)^1 Mean ± SD	Skinfold thickness (mm)^2 Mean ± SD
A1A1	25.55 ± 3.80	39.48 ± 10.35
A1A2	24.33 ± 3.96	31.87 ± 12.44
A2A2	22.93 ± 3.36	28.63 ± 6.94

^{1}ANOVA $P = 0.015$; ^{2}ANOVA $P = 0.006$.

The data from this study together with those from previous investigations[8–13]. suggest that the *DRD2* polymorphisms might influence obesity through the dopaminergic reward pathway. The consumption of food is essential for survival; the feeling of pleasure and satisfaction after the provision of nutrients strongly reinforces this action. Stimulation of this pathway may reduce the effectiveness of satiety factors, promoting overeating and leading to obesity[5,6]

The first candidate gene for obesity identified in Native Brazilians was the low-density-lipoprotein receptor (*LDLR*). In that study, performed in the same samples investigated herein, a haplotype derived from four restriction site polymorphisms was highly associated with BMI, skinfold thickness and the arm fat index[21].

Given the complex array of metabolic systems that are implicated in the development of obesity, it is not unexpected that genes involved in different metabolic processes like *LDLR* and *DRD2* have been associated with obesity in Native Brazilians. The probable small genetic effects determined by these genes could be overwhelmed by environment obesity factors in western societies.

Contemporary Brazilian Amerindian societies are experiencing drastic changes in their ways of living and diet. Santos and Coimbra[15] have verified, among the Suruí, that those individuals who have experienced the most intensive changes in diet and lifestyle are those with higher body mass and fat composition. A similar trend was also recently described for the Xavante communities[18]. It is important to understand the environmental changes responsible for this association and to relate them to a background of genetic predisposition, since individuals from these populations may develop an increased prevalence of metabolic diseases as their lifestyle becomes more westernized.

Acknowledgements: Thanks are due to the Fundação Nacional do Indío (FUNAI) for permission to study the Indians and for logistic assistance. The Indian leaders and the subjects of the investigation were adequately informed about the aims of the study and gave their approval, which is also acknowledged. We are very grateful to our colleagues Carlos E.A. Coimbra Jr and Ricardo V. Santos for the collection of blood and anthropometric data from four of the five Amerindian samples. Financial support was provided by Programa de Apoio a Núcleos de Excelência (PRONEX), Conselho Nacional de Desenvolvimento Científico e Tecnológico (CNPq), Financiadora de Estudos e Projetos (FINEP), and Fundação de Amparo à Pesquisa do Estado do Rio Grande do Sul (FAPERGS).

References

1. Barsh GS, Farooqi S, O'Rahilly S. Genetics of body-weight regulation. *Nature* 2000; 404: 644–51.

2. Kopelman PG. Obesity as a medical problem. *Nature* 2000; 404: 644–51.

3. Cone RD. Haploinsufficiency of the melanocortin-4 receptor: part of a thrifty genotype? *J Clin Invest* 2000; 106: 185–7.

4. Ravussin E. Metabolic differences and the development of obesity. *Metabolism* 1995; 9: 12–14.

5. Hoebel BG. Brain transmitters in food and drug reward. *Am J Clin Nutr* 1985; 42: 1133–50

6. Wise RA, Rompre PP. Brain dopamine and reward. *Annu Ver Psychol* 1989; 40: 191–225.

7. Doss FW. The effects of antypsichotic drugs on body weight. *J Clin Psychiat* 1979; 40: 528–30.

8. Comings DE, Flanagan SD, Dietz G, Muhleman D, Knell E, Gysin R. The dopamine D2 receptor (DRD2) as a major gene in obesity and height. *Biochem Med Metab Biol* 1993; 50: 176–85.

9. Noble EP, Noble RE, Richtie T, Syndulko K, Bohlman MC, Noble LA *et al.* D2 dopamine receptor gene and obesity. *Int J Eating Disord* 1994; 15: 205–17.

10. Spitz MR, Detry MA, Pillow PP, Hu Y, Amos CI, Hong WK, Wu X. Variant alleles of the dopamine receptor gene and obesity. *Nutr Res* 2000; 20: 371–80.

11. Thomas GN, Tomlinson B, Critchley JAJH. Modulation of blood pressure and obesity with the dopamine D2 receptor gene TaqI polymorphism. *Hypertension* 2000; 36: 177–82.

12. Jenkinson CP, Hanson R, Cray K, Wiedrich C, Knowler WC, Bogardus C, Baier L. Association of dopamine D2 receptor polymorphisms Ser311Cys and TaqI A with obesity or type 2 diabetes mellitus in Pima Indians. *Int J Obes* 2000; 24: 1233–8.

13. Tataranni PA, Baier L, Jenkinson CP, Harper I, Del Parigi A, Bogardus C. A Ser311Cys mutation in the human dopamine receptor D2 gene is associated with reduced energy expenditure. *Diabetes* 2001; 50: 901–4.

14. Salzano FM, Callegari-Jacques SM. *South American Indians: a case study in evolution.* Oxford: Clarendon Press; 1988.

15. Santos RV, Coimbra CEA Jr. Socioeconomic differentiation and body morphology in the Suruí of Southwestern Amazonia. *Curr Anthropol* 1996; 37: 851–6.

16. Salzano FM, Franco MHLP, Weimer TA, Callegari Jacques SM, Mestriner MA, Hutz *et al.* The Brazilian Xavante Indian revisited: new protein genetic studies. *Am J Phys Anthropol* 1997; 104: 23–34.

17. Salzano FM, Weimer TA, Franco MHLP, Callegari Jacques SM, Mestriner MA, Hutz MH *et al.* Protein genetic systems among the Tupi-Mondé Indians of the Brazilian Amazonia. *Am J Hum Biol* 1998; 10: 711–22.

18. Gugelmin SA, Santos RV. Human ecology and nutritional anthropometry of adult Xavante Indians in Mato Grosso, Brazil. *Cad Saúde Publica* 2001; 17: 313–22.

19. Hutz MH, Almeida S, Coimbra CEA Jr, Santos RV, Salzano FM. Haplotype and allele frequencies for three genes of the dopaminergic system in South American Indians. *Am J Hum Biol* 2000; 12: 638–45.

20. Kidd KK, Morar B, Castiglione CM, Zhao H, Pakstis AJ, Speed WC *et al.* A global survey haplotype frequencies and linkage disequilibrium at the DRD2 locus. *Hum Genet* 1998; 103: 211–27.

21. Mattevi VS, Coimbra CEA Jr, Santos RV, Salzano FM, Hutz MH. Association of the low-density-lipoprotein receptor gene with obesity in Native American populations. *Hum Genet* 2000; 106: 546–52.

Progress in Obesity Research: 9. Edited by *Geraldo Medeiros-Neto, Alfredo Halpern and Claude Bouchard*
©2003 John Libbey Eurotext Ltd, pp. 373–380.

CHAPTER 80

The search for obesity genes in isolated populations: Gullah-Speaking African Americans and the role of uncoupling protein 3 as a thrifty gene

W. Timothy Garvey*†, David C. McLean, Jr.* and Ida Spruill*

*Division of Endocrinology and Department of Medicine, Medical University of South Carolina, Charleston SC, 29425, USA; and †Ralph H. Johnson Veterans Affairs Medical Center, Charleston, SC 29403, USA
[e-mail: garveywt@musc.edu]

The Gullahs

Since the early 1700s, the barrier islands along the South Carolina Coast ('Sea Islands') and adjacent coastal communities have been inhabited by a unique African American population. Available anthropological, cultural, and historical data indicate that the Sea Islanders are descendants of people transported from the rice-growing areas of West Africa (i.e. Sierra Leone, Gambia, Senegal)[1]. Colonial plantation owners in the early 1700s sought out slaves from this region because of their rice growing expertise. The low country of South Carolina was ideally suited for rice cultivation, and plantation owners required tribes people from the 'grain coast' of West Africa (Mende, Temne, Kisi, etc.), with experience in this highly technical form of agriculture, to supply Europe with this leading cash crop. Linguistics also confirms the link with West Africa. Sea Island families speak the Gullah language, an English Creole very similar to the modern day language (Krio) spoken in Sierra Leone. Krio arose during the 1700s on the 'grain coast' of West Africa as English slave traders interacted with indigenous tribes, and was brought to the South Carolina Sea Islands as Africans were enslaved in this region. To this day, Gullah-speaking Sea Islanders have retained their African heritage, perhaps more than any other group of African Americans, and the cultural link with West Africa is reflected in regional cuisine, basketry, fish netting, folk medicine, music, and other cultural aspects. The Gullah-speaking African American population has multiple ideal characteristics for studying the genetic epidemiology of complex diseases.

Diseases

Polygenic diseases that afflict African Americans with a high degree of prevalence are also common on the Sea Islands, including, type 2 diabetes, obesity and hypertension. Due to genetic homogeneity and lifestyle, these diseases retain a high degree of familial segregation and relative genetic risk. For example, the relative risk (λ_s) for type 2 diabetes is 3.3, a figure that exceeds that in many other communities.

Culture and history preserves homogeneity

Our data to date indicate that the Gullahs are the most genetically homogeneous population of African descent in the United States[2–4], with estimated European Caucasian admixture of only 3.5 per cent (see below). Several factors have helped preserve the homogeneity of the Sea Islanders to the present day. First, unlike other regions of the Atlantic seaboard, numbers of Africans far exceeded that of Europeans in the South Carolina low country throughout the 1700s and early 1800s. Beginning in 1670, it is estimated that 40 per cent of Africans brought to the US as slaves entered through the port of Charleston, including more than 120,000 between 1716 and 1807, the primary era of legal slave trade into the US. Slaves entering at the port of Charleston originated from disparate sources, in particular, Senegal, Gambia, Sierra Leone, Ivory Coast, as well as the Congo and Angola[1,5]. However, Sierra Leone became a significant slave exportation site to the South Carolina low country as a result of regional expertise in rice agriculture. Many slaves imported through Charleston were brought to various inland areas, while slaves from rice-cultivating tribes on West Africa's grain coast were selectively retained on coastal plantations. Thus, the founding population for the Gullahs was relatively smaller and more geographically defined.

Second, the agricultural areas and estuary regions in the South Carolina low-country dedicated to rice cultivation were swampy low-lying areas rife with diseases such as yellow fever, malaria, and tuberculosis[1]. These areas were avoided by the Caucasian landowners who were content to live in Charleston or in manor houses, and, therefore, there was not much interaction (gene flow) between races. The slaves were largely supervised by African foremen and continued the collective farming practices that were successful in Africa. Third, geography also played a role since the Sea Islands were only accessible by boat, and bridges were not built to most of the islands until after World War II. The fourth factor was economics. After the Civil War, Gullah speaking African Americans continued to inhabit the Sea Islands, growing rice until the rice market deteriorated at the turn of the century, and then living on subsistence farming and fishing in subsequent decades. Because there was no industry or other opportunities for exploitation, there was no immigration of outsiders into these communities. This is changing in recent years with resort development and residential expansion. Finally, cultural identity and the Gullah language have acted to maintain genetic homogeneity.

Family structure

The population is comprised of relatively large, stable, multi-generation families. Family integrity is sustained by the strong cultural, religious, and family traditions of the Sea Islanders. Thus, it is common to find large families living for a long time in the same area. While there has been some emigration to northern American cities, there has been little immigration of African Americans born elsewhere into the Sea Islands. As a result of large stable families, family-based methods of statistical genetics analyses, such as traditional LOD scores, affected pedigree methods, and disequilibrium testing, can be effectively utilized in addition to sib-pair analyses and case control association studies. The availability of large families is countered by the very strong distrust of biomedical research which limits the participation of large pedigrees (see below).

Lifestyle

The Sea Islanders in general have relatively uniform rural lifestyle and dietary habits. The diet is very low in fibre content and rich in animal fats that are widely used in daily cooking (J. Haskill, D. Lackland, unpublished data). These attributes would predictably minimize individual co-variance resulting from environmental variables, and maximize the development of certain diseases, such as diabetes, obesity, arteriosclerosis, and cancer, in those individuals carrying susceptibility genes.

Population genetics

Table 1. Admixture estimates in African American populations[2,3]

Population	Admixture estimate (% ± SE)	Population	Admixture estimate (% ± SE)
Gullah Sea Islanders	3.5 ± 0.8	Pittsburgh	25.2 ± 2.7
Charlestone	9.8 ± 1.2	Baltimore	15.5 ± 2.6
Mississippi Delta	13.3 ± 1.9	New Orleans	22.5 ± 1.6
Chicago	18.8 ± 1.4	Jamaica	6.8 ± 1.3
New York	19.8 ± 2.1		

We have studied whether the population genetics of the Gullah correspond to the cultural and historic record with respect to the origins of the population. Our first series of studies used autosomal markers to assess European Caucasian admixture. These studies employed Ancestry Informative Markers (AIM) in collaboration with Dr. M. Shriver, which are autosomal polymorphisms showing large frequency differentials between major geographic or ethnic groups[2,3,6]. A panel of 10 AIMs were used to genotype DNA in multiple African American populations[2,3] and to estimate admixture proportions, as shown in Table 1.

The Gullahs by far have the lowest Caucasian admixture of any African American group ever studied[2,3], and the group with the second lowest admixture is the population of urban African Americans living in Charleston. Thus, the Sea Islanders constitute a unique African American population with low Caucasian admixture, a factor which enhances genetic epidemiology for complex disease genes.

We further employed mitochondrial DNA and Y chromosomal markers to study population origins and genetic distances between the Gullahs and Sierra Leone tribes4. For these studies, we selected current tribes in Sierra Leone to represent the primary parental population of the Gullahs and a generalized European Caucasian population from the US as the secondary parental population. The Sierra Leone sample includes individuals from eleven different tribal affiliations; the four most represented tribes in our sample were the Mende, Temne, Limba, and Creole tribes. These putative parental populations were studied relative to multiple North American diasporic populations including: the Sea Island Gullahs; urban African Americans living in Charleston, South Carolina; west coast African Americans living in Oakland, California; and Jamaicans.

We sampled seven mitochondrial DNA (mtDNA) polymorphisms and five Y-chromosomal DNA short tandem repeat (Y-STRs) polymorphisms, and constructed haplotypes to assess both maternal and paternal lineages, respectively[4]. mtDNA (specifically the hypervariable segments I and II of the D-loop) and Y-STRs share general features which makes each valuable for studying populations not long evolutionarily separated one from another. Specifically, both D-loop mtDNA and Y-STR: (i) are polymorphic with high mutation rates[7-12]; (ii) are non-recombining types of DNA[13,14] although rare exceptions have been noted for mtDNA[7,15]; (iii) have effective population sizes (Ne) reduced to 1/4 of autosomal loci and are thus more susceptible to both random genetic drift and bottlenecks[16]; and are inherited in essentially haploid fashion[16] although some cases of mtDNA heteroplasmy have been noted[7]. The primary differences in mtDNA and Y-STR are in their respective maternal[17] and paternal[16] inheritance patterns.

Genetic distance models based on analyses of the mtDNA and Y chromosome haplotypes (both D_A and Nei's standard genetic distance measurements) generally indicated that the closest relationships lie between the Sierra Leone and the Gullah samples. The Mende, Temne, Limba, and Creole tribes of Sierra Leone consistently grouped together. Closest to these tribes were the Gullah and Jamaican samples[4]. The genetic distances to the Sierra Leone tribes (and Gullahs) were progressively more remote when compared with the urban Charleston African American, followed by west coast African American, and finally the Caucasian samples. In addition, both mtDNA and Y-chromosome haplotypes exhibit low Caucasian admixture in a geographic core sub-sample of the Gullah, plus a sharp gradient of increasing Caucasian admixture through the larger Gullah community in the South Carolina low country, to urban African Americans living in Charleston, to west coast African Americans, consistent with autosomal admixture estimates[3]. Gullah and Jamaican samples exhibit extremely low maternal (mtDNA) with relatively higher paternal (Y-STR) Caucasian admixture levels, while the west coast African American sample reflects nearly equal mtDNA haplotype and Y-chromosome haplotype Caucasian admixture levels[4]. In conclusion, Gullah-speaking African Americans are more closely related to Sierra Leone tribes than are other African American populations, and exhibit by far the lowest degree of European Caucasian admixture. Thus, we believe that the Gullah-speaking African Americans offer a unique, relatively homogeneous population for genetic epidemiology.

Project sugar: ethical and social principles of community-based research

The unique characteristics of the Gullah population provide powerful rationale for an initiative to identify susceptibility genes for diabetes and obesity in African Americans. Investigators at the Medical University of South Carolina have commenced this study called Project Sugar with two principal goals, one of them scientific to complete a whole genome scan, and the other service-oriented to enhance patient outcomes for diabetes and obesity in the community. At the outset, Project Sugar together with community leaders established principles for the conduct of research in the Gullah community. Minority populations have unique biological, socio-demographic, economic, and cultural characteristics, and inadequate attention to those fundamental differences between and among minorities often lead to poor study participation by individuals from minority backgrounds. A palpable distrust for research has been widely acknowledged as a cause for minority under-representation in clinical trials, and this distrust presented the greatest challenge for achieving Project Sugar's scientific goals. The basis for this distrust is multifactorial[18], however, the Tuskegee Syphilis Experiment has contributed significantly. Therefore, Project Sugar could only be successful to the degree it merited the trust and participation of the community. Much of the success can be attributed to the practice of 'coordinated research', an approach that advocates providing coordinated tangible benefits to the community concomitant with data collection[19]. The goal is to build trust in communities that have been exploited by social and scientific research.

In adapting principles of coordinated research for Project Sugar, our efforts fell into three categories, **C P R** (Community identification, Plan for recruitment, Rewards to the community):

(i) Community identification. The goal is to identify the project with the community and the community with the project. All study personnel have a detailed understanding and respect for the Gullah history and culture, as an integral aspect of Project Sugar's study design. To vest the community in the project, community leaders and organizations were consulted up front and involved in the initial planning of the research project. Project Sugar hires staff who are living in Sea Island communities, and family recruitment and phenotyping is performed in the community in collaboration with trusted institutions such as public-health funded clinics, churches, and community centres. These community institutions are, thus, integrally involved in the conduct of the project as 'partners'. Importantly, the Project receives full oversight and guidance from a Citizens Advisory Board comprised of community leaders, scholars of African American culture, ministers, and patients with diabetes. This Board was empowered with decision making and charged with assuring that Project Sugar is conducted in the community's interest and in a culturally sensitive manner. The Board also serves as a forum for communication and intermediation with the community.

(ii) Recruitment plan. Project Sugar staff (i.e. RNs, LPNs, phlebotomists, assistants) have an understanding of health behaviours and needs as community residents. These staff not only conduct phenotyping studies, but also engage in health education in the community as well as one-on-one with patients and family members. Health education, referrals, and a small financial compensation is offered to study participants. Project Sugar participates in many community health fairs and wellness screenings where study volunteers are identified and recruited, or volunteers are referred form local clinics, churches, or community organizations. Studies (data collection, exam, blood drawing) are usually performed in local clinics providing health care to Sea Island residents, although home visits are also routine. Project Sugar advertises for volunteers in the minority owned print media, and the ads include a message of disease prevention. Most individuals are interested in prevention, because they have a parent, sibling or loved one who has already suffered from disease complications. Free screenings and education for all family members are always offered, and newsletters updating participants on Project Sugar, diabetes education, and diabetes news are mailed at intervals.

(iii) Tangible rewards to the community. Progress in meeting scientific goals must intimately be coupled with tangible and immediate benefits to the community. The Citizens Advisory Committee and community leaders decided what those benefits were to be, namely, health education, wellness screenings, and health care referrals. As a result, Project Sugar staff are extensively engaged in health education, and offer a variety of medical and social services and referrals. Study personnel attend community health fairs and health screenings on at least a weekly basis and offer free wellness and diabetes testing, as well as education and training for local health care professionals. Project Sugar maintains a Mobile health unit van equipped for education and health screening. These activities have helped vest the community in Project Sugar, and the investigator's budget has had to include funds for community outreach services/programmes in order to achieve the scientific objectives.

Uncoupling protein 3: a thrifty gene in African-derived populations?

Project Sugar is actively ascertaining a large number of pedigrees and sibships to support a whole genome scan for diabetes and obesity genes. We have also assessed a number of candidate genes including those encoding uncoupling proteins. Uncoupling protein 1 (UCP1) is a proton channel on the inner mitochondrial membrane in rodent brown fat that dissipates the proton gradient generated by mitochondrial respiration[20]. One possible mechanism for UCP action is that the transporter shuttles anionic free fatty acids (FFA) out of mitochondria where protons are added to them, and then they return to the mitochondrial matrix as neutral FFAs[21,22]. This uncouples respiration from oxidative phosphorylation and ATP synthesis and, thus, converts stored fuel into heat. Recently, two homologs, UCP2[23-25] and UCP3[25,26] have been found to be expressed in humans. UCP2 mRNA is expressed in multiple tissues in adults, and UCP3 expression is delimited to skeletal muscle, heart, and white fat. The expression of UCP2 and UCP3 in adult skeletal muscle indicates that these proteins have the potential to play an important role in energy balance[27]. However, current data suggest that these novel UCPs may not simply act to regulate thermogenesis but may have more complex metabolic roles. We have found that there is no correlation between muscle UCP2 or UCP3 protein levels and either resting energy expenditure or insulin-induced thermogenesis (analogous to thermic effect of food)[28,29]. Data from UCP2 and UCP3 knock-out mice also fail to show effects on thermogenesis or energy balance[30-33].

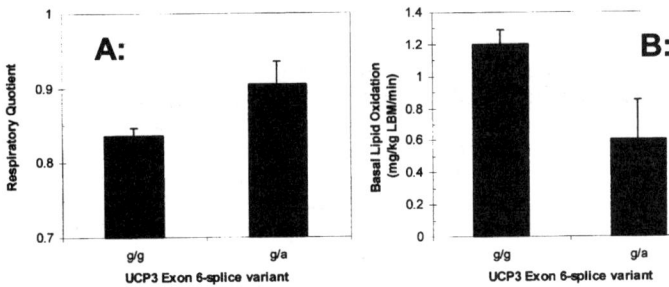

Fig. 1 (A and B).

In addition, starvation leads to enhanced expression of both UCP2 and UCP3 despite decreased thermogenesis in whole body and skeletal muscle[34–36]. These data are not consistent with a direct role for UCP2 or UCP3 in thermogenesis. However, many physiological states with increased muscle UCP expression do share in common higher circulating FFAs, suggesting a role for UCPs in lipid metabolism.

To determine whether UCP3 gene variation could contribute to human obesity, we assessed the nucleotide sequence of all six coding exons in 40 sequentially recruited subjects, comprising 20 Gullahs and 20 Caucasian Americans with obesity and diabetes[37]. This approach revealed one mutation and two polymorphisms in two Gullah probands. A G304A polymorphism in exon 3 was detected in one proband, resulting in a conservative amino acid substitution of a valine by an isoleucine (V102I). This polymorphism was found to have an allele frequency of ~18 per cent in both Gullah-speaking African Americans and the Mende tribe of Sierra Leone. Another proband (age 16, BMI 52, type 2 diabetes) was a compound heterozygote for the UCP3 gene. One allele contained a missense mutation (C427T) in exon 4 that introduced a premature stop codon at residue 143 (R143X). This mutation in effect truncates the C-terminal half of the protein containing three of the six UCP3 transmembrane domains. The other allele contained an intronic polymorphism in the splice-donor site for exon 6 (ggt-gat) resulting in loss of the splice junction, premature termination of the protein product, and deletion of the sixth transmembrane domain. The exon 6 splice donor-stop polymorphism was found to have an allele frequency of 10 per cent in both Gullah African Americans and the Mende tribe. The exon 6 splice donor and the V108I polymorphisms, as well as the R143X mutation, were exclusively observed in the African American and African populations, and were not detected in Caucasian Americans or Pima Native Americans.

To examine whether the two common polymorphisms (V102I and exon 6 splice donor) could contribute to obesity and type 2 diabetes, we performed case-control association and measured genotype analyses in Gullah-speaking African Americans. These studies included quantitative metabolic traits known to be involved in the pathogenesis of obesity, which were assessed as a function of genotype. We obtained largely negative data regarding the V102I polymorphism, however, the studies of the exon 6 splice donor polymorphism yielded interesting results[37]. Unrelated individuals with the exon 6 splice donor polymorphism were found to have a 50 per cent reduction in basal fat oxidation adjusted for lean body mass ($P = 0.0188$) and a marked elevation in the non-protein respiratory quotient ($P = 0.0079$), compared with wild type subjects (Figs. 1A and 1B). These metabolic alterations were not accompanied by any changes in resting energy expenditure adjusted for lean body mass. Thus, the exon 6 splice donor polymorphism appears to influence macronutrient fuel partitioning away from fat and in favour of carbohydrate to maintain the basal metabolic rate. We also examined whether the exon 6 splice donor polymorphism was associated with obesity, and we found no significant differences in BMI when comparing subgroups with and without the polymorphism in the population as a whole.

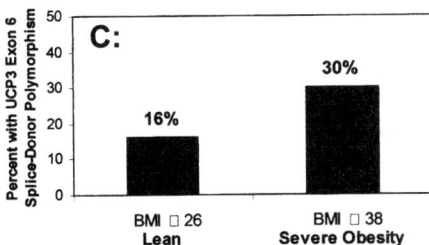

Fig. 1(C).

However, the Gullah-speaking African-American population is characterized by a high prevalence of obesity (mean BMI = 33 kg/m² among volunteers enrolled in Project Sugar), and we wondered whether this high prevalence could be masking the potential effect of a single obesity polygene on BMI. Closer examination of the data demonstrated that there was a progressive increase in allele frequency for the exon 6 splice donor polymorphism with increasing obesity when the population was analysed in discrete quartiles based on BMI. We then performed a truncated analysis in Fig. 1C, and observed that the frequency of the exon 6 splice donor polymorphism was nearly twice as great in the highest quartile with BMI = 38 (30 per cent) when compared with the leanest quartile with BMI = 26

(16 per cent). Thus, the effect of UCP3 gene variation on macronutrient fuel partitioning was associated with increased susceptibility for severe obesity.

An effect of the UCP3 exon 6 splice donor polymorphism to reduce fat oxidation would predictably promote fat storage and provide a mechanism by which UCP3 mutations could predispose to obesity. Indeed, increased RQ and low fat oxidation have previously been shown to be risk factors for future weight gain and the development of obesity[38,39]. We, therefore, propose that the UCP3 exon 6 splice donor polymorphism is functioning as a thrifty gene, as first purported by J. Neel in 1962[40]. Based on the identical allele frequency in Gullah, Jamaican, and Sierra Leone populations and the failure to detect the polymorphism in Caucasians and Native Americans, it would appear that the UCP3 polymorphism arose in the African continent and genotype frequencies have remained undisturbed in New World African-derived populations. Conceivably, this polymorphism could have arisen in west Africa (or elsewhere in sub-Saharan Africa) to alter UCP3 function in a manner that promotes fat storage during food abundance and increases survivability during famine. This 'thrifty' mechanism, however, may adversely lead to progressive obesity and diabetes in an alternative environment with chronic exposure to a high fat diet, as is the case for the Gullah-speaking African Americans.

The exon 6 splice donor polymorphism would interact with environment as an obesity susceptibility gene. In support of this point, we have identified another UCP mutation resulting in a non-conserved amino acid substitution (R70W) in a first generation Chinese American boy, age 15 years, with type 2 diabetes and BMI of 51 kg/m^2.[41] The mutation was inherited from his father who was lean (BMI 24) but also had type 2 diabetes. Dietary history revealed that the boy's father and mother adhered exclusively to a low-fat Old World diet consisting of rice, vegetables, and fish, while the boy consumed high-fat 'fast-foods' purchased daily from restaurants. Given the proposed involvement of UCP3 in macronutrient fuel partitioning, the exon 6 splice donor polymorphism could only predispose to fat accretion to the extent that individuals consume dietary fat. The difference in fat intake could account for the observed difference in body weight between father and son who were both heterozygotes for the R70W mutation. Along these same lines, Chung et al. did not observe any effect of the exon 6 splice donor polymorphism on BMI or energy expenditure in an African American population living in Maywood, Illinois, a suburb of Chicago[42]. This urban population displays much more Caucasian admixture and would be predicted to engage in more heterogeneous dietary practices compared with the genetically and culturally homogeneous Gullahs. Therefore, a rigorous study design controlling for environmental variables and genetic admixture is helpful for discerning effects of the UCP3 splice donor polymorphism on metabolism.

To study whether gene variation affects UCP3 functional activity, we expressed both wild type and polymorphic forms of UCP3 in Saccharomyces cerevisiae to determine their relative ability to disrupt proton gradients across the inner mitochondrial membrane[43]. In transformed yeast cells, UCP3 has previously been shown to uncouple mitochondrial respiration from ATP production, and this can be assessed by measuring the fluorescence of DiOC$_6$, a dye sensitive to the mitochondrial membrane potential[35]. Using this system, we demonstrated that both the R143X mutation found in the Gullah proband and the R70W mutation in the Chinese American boy impaired uncoupling properties of UCP3, while the V102I and exon 6 splice donor polymorphisms did not alter uncoupling capability, relative to the wild type protein[43]. However, UCPs do not appear to function as uncouplers in vivo in mammalian mitochondria, as evidenced by the absence of effect on thermogenesis in humans[28,29] and knock-out mice[30-33]. For these reasons, the study of uncoupling activity in transfected yeast may not be physiologically relevant to UCP action in humans, and not appropriate for assessing structure-function relationships for native gene variants.

Elevated circulating free fatty acids induce a significant increase in skeletal muscle UCP3 expression analogous to increased UCP3 expression observed during fasting[35,36,44]. Such induction of UCP3 may affect utilization of free fatty acids as fuel or help maintain the mitochondrial proton gradient necessary for oxidative ATP phosphorylation during fasting. Carriers of the exon 6 splice donor polymorphism had significantly reduced basal fat oxidation and elevated RQ, suggesting a predilection towards carbohydrate oxidation[37]. Consistent with this observation, we have found the increasing expression of UCP3 protein in skeletal muscle is associated with increased RQ and decreased rates of lipid oxidation[29]. The combined data strongly implicate a role for UCP3 in macronutrient fuel partitioning. The exon 6 splice polymorphism results in loss of the sixth transmembrane domain and the potential purine-nucleotide-binding domain (PNBD) at the carboxyl-terminus of the protein[37]. Binding of purines to PNBD is known to control coupling efficiency of UCP1 and to induce conformational changes[34]. Such loss of the PNBD and conformational shape in UCP3 could perhaps influence the functional role of UCP3 to regulate lipids as fuel substrates and affect the requirement of skeletal muscle tissue for lipids during food deprivation[45]. However, more rigorous structure-function analyses are necessary to determine the impact of gene variation on UCP3 function and to delineate the role of UCP3 in human metabolism.

In summary, these data establish the UCP3 exon 6 splice polymorphism as a susceptibility gene for severe obesity in African Americans, as a consequence of a reduction in basal fat oxidation and a high respiratory quotient. The observations implicate a role for UCP3 in macronutrient fuel partitioning[29,37] and indicate that UCP3 could function as a 'thrifty' gene[40] in African Americans. Hopefully, the ongoing study of Gullah-speaking African Americans, as well as other genetically and culturally homogeneous populations, will help further elucidate susceptibility genes for complex diseases.

Acknowledgements: The authors acknowledge the invaluable collaboration with Dr. Sahr Gevao at the University of Sierra Leone, Dr. Erol Y. Morrison at the University of the West Indies, and Owen S. Bernard of the Jamaican Diabetes Association. The work was supported by grants to WTG from the National Institutes of Health (DK-38765, DK-47461), the American Diabetes Association (GENNID), and the Department of Veteran Affairs Research Service. The work was also facilitated by a grant to MUSC from the W.M. Keck Foundation (Los Angeles, CA) in support of the Sea Island Family Project and Project Sugar. The General Clinical Research Center at the Medical University of South Carolina (RR0-0170) provided critical support for the project. The authors are indebted to all the staff and participating nurses in 'Project Sugar' for their field work on the Sea Islands of South Carolina and to participating Sea Island families.

References

1. Pollitzer WS. *The Gullah People and their African Heritage*, pp. 1–344. Athens: The University of Georgia Press; 1999.

2. Parra EJ, Marcini A, Akey J, Martinson J, Batzer MA, Cooper R *et al*. Estimating African American admixture proportions by use of population-specific alleles. *Am J Hum Genet* 1998; 63: 1839–51.

3. Parra EJ, Kittles RA, Argyropoulos G, Pfaff CL, Hiester K, Bonilla C *et al*. Ancestral proportions and admixture dynamics in geographically defined African Americans living in South Carolina. *Am J Phys Anthropol* 2001; 114: 18–29.

4. McLean DC, Page GP, Garvey WT. Mitochondrial DNA and Y-chromosome haplotypes of Gullah-speaking African Americans show closer genetic distance to Sierra Leoneans and lower Caucasian admixture than other new world African populations. *Am J Hum Genet* 2001; 69: A258.

5. Pollitzer WS. The relationship of the Gullah-speaking people of coastal South Carolina and Georgia to their African ancestors. *Historical Methods* 1993; 25: 53–67.

6. Shriver MD, Smith M, Jin L, Marcini A, Akey JM, Deka R, Ferrell RE. Forensic ethnic affiliation determination by use of population-specific allele DNA markers. *Am J Hum Genet* 1997; 60: 957–64.

7. Howell N, Kubacka I, Mackey DA. How rapidly does the human mitochondrial genome evolve? *Am J Hum Genet* 1996; 59: 501–9.

8. Sherry ST, Rogers AR, Harpending H, Soodyall H, Jenkins T, Stoneking M. Mismatch distributions of mtDNA reveal recent human population expansions. *Hum Biol* 1994; 66: 761–75.

9. Vigilant L, Stoneking M, Harpending H, Hawkes K, Wilson AC. African populations and the evolution of human mitochondrial DNA. *Science* 1991; 253: 1503–7.

10. Cooper G, Amos W, Hoffman D, Rubinsztein DC. Network analysis of human Y microsatellite haplotypes. *Hum Mol Genet* 1996; 5: 1759–66.

11. de Knijff P, Kayser M, Caglia A, Corach D, Fretwell N, Gehrig C *et al*. Chromosome Y microsatellites: population genetic and evolutionary aspects. *Int J Legal Med* 1997; 110: 134–49.

12. Ruiz Linares A, Nayar K, Goldstein DB, Hebert JM, Seielstad MT, Underhill PA *et al*. Geographic clustering of human Y-chromosome haplotypes. *Ann Hum Genet* 1996; 60: 401–8.

13. Hammer MF, Zegura SL The role of the Y chromosome in human evolutionary studies. *Evolutionary Anthropol* 1997; 5: 116–34.

14. Jobling MA, Tyler-Smith C. Fathers and sons: the Y chromosome and human evolution. *Trends Genet* 1995; 11: 449–56.

15. Awadalla P, Eyre-Walker A, Smith JM. Linkage disequilibrium and recombination in hominid mitochondrial DNA. *Science* 1999; 286: 2524–5.

16. Perez-Lezaun A, Calafell F, Seielstad M, Mateu E, Comas D, Bosch E, Bertranpetit J. Population genetics of Y-chromosome short tandem repeats in humans. *J Mol Evol* 1997; 45: 265–70.

17. Giles RE, Blanc H, Cann HM, Wallace DC. Maternal inheritance of human mitochondrial DNA. *Proc Natl Acad Sci USA* 1980; 77: 6715–9.

18. Gamble, V.N. Under the shadow of Tuskegee: African Americans and health care. *Am J Public Health* 1997; 87: 1773–8.

19. Jackson J, Slaughter S, Blake JH. The Sea Islands as a cultural resource. *The Black Scholar* 1974; 32–9.

20. Klaus S, Casteilla L, Bouillaud F, Ricquier D. The uncoupling protein UCP: a membraneous mitochondrial ion carrier exclusively expressed in brown adipose tissue. *Int J Biochem* 1991; 23: 791–801.

21. Jezek P, Orosz DE, Modriansky M, Garlid KD. Transport of anions and protons by the mitochondrial uncoupling protein and its regulation by nucleotides and fatty acids: a new look at an old hypothesis. *J Biol Chem* 1994; 269: 26184–90.

22. Skulachev VP. Fatty acid circuit as a physiological mechanism of uncoupling of oxidative phosphorylation. *FEBS Letters* 1991; 294: 158–62.

23. Fleury C, Neverova M, Collins S, Raimbault S, Champigny O, Levi-Meyrueis C et al. Uncoupling protein-2: a novel gene linked to obesity and hyperinsulinemia. *Nature Genet* 1997; 15: 269–72.

24. Gimeno RE, Dembski M, Weng X, Deng N, Shyjan AM, Gimeno CJ et al. Cloning and characterization of an uncoupling protein homolog: a potential molecular mediator of human thermogenesis. *Diabetes* 1997; 46: 900–6.

25. Boss O, Samec S, Paoloni-Giacobino A, Rossier C, Dulloo A, Seydoux J et al. Uncoupling protein-3: a new member of the mitochondrial carrier family with tissue-specific expression. *FEBS Letters* 1997; 408: 39–42.

26. Vidal-Puig A, Solanes G, Grujic D, Flier JS, Lowell BB. UCP3: an uncoupling protein homologue expressed preferentially and abundantly in skeletal muscle and brown adipose tissue. *Biochem Biophys Res Commun* 1997; 235: 79–82.

27. Ravussin E, Swinburn BA. Pathophysiology of obesity. *Lancet* 1992; 340: 404–8.

28. Bao S, Kennedy A, Wojciechowski B, Wallace P, Ganaway E, Garvey WT. Expression of mRNAs encoding uncoupling proteins in human skeletal muscle: effects of obesity and diabetes. *Diabetes* 1998; 47: 1935–40.

29. Willi SM, Maianu L, Kennedy A, Wojciechowski B, Bao S, Wallace P et al. The role of uncoupling proteins in metabolic fuel partitioning and human obesity. *Diabetes* 1998; 47: A13.

30. Arsenijevic D, Onuma H, Pecqueur C, Raimbault S, Manning BS, Miroux B et al. Disruption of the uncoupling protein-2 gene in mice reveals a role in immunity and reactive oxygen species production. *Nature Genet* 2000; 26: 435–9.

31. Zhang CY, Baffy G, Perret P, Krauss S, Peroni O, Grujic D et al. Uncoupling protein-2 negatively regulates insulin secretion and is a major link between obesity, beta cell dysfunction, and type 2 diabetes. *Cell* 2001; 105: 745–55.

32. Vidal-Puig AJ, Grujic D, Zhang CY, Hagen T, Boss O, Ido Y et al. Energy metabolism in uncoupling protein 3 gene knockout mice. *J Biol Chem* 2000; 275: 16258–66.

33. Gong DW, Monemdjou S, Gavrilova O, Leon LR, Marcus-Samuels B, Chou CJ et al. Lack of obesity and normal response to fasting and thyroid hormone in mice lacking uncoupling protein-3. *J Biol Chem* 2000; 275: 16251–7.

34. Boss O, Samec S, Dulloo A, Seydoux J, Muzzin P, Giacobino J-P. Tissue-dependent upregulation of rat uncoupling-2 expression in response to fasting or cold. *FEBS Letters* 1997; 412: 111–4.

35. Gong D-W, He Y, Karas M, Reitman M. Uncoupling protein-3 is a mediator of thermogenesis regulated by thyroid hormone, β3-adrenergic agonists, and leptin. *J Biol Chem* 1997; 272: 24129–32.

36. Millet L, Vidal H, Andreelli F, Larrouy D, Riou JP, Ricquier D et al. Increased uncoupling protein-2 and -3 mRNA expression during fasting in obese and lean humans. *J Clin Invest* 1997; 100: 2665–70.

37. Argyropoulos G, Brown AM, Willi SM, Zhu J-H, He Y, Reitman M et al. Effects of mutations in the human uncoupling protein 3 gene on the respiratory quotient and fat oxidation in severe obesity and type 2 diabetes mellitus. *J Clin Invest* 1998; 102: 1345–51.

38. Zurlo F, Lillioja S, Esposito-Del Puente A, Nyomba BL, Raz I, Saad MF et al. Low ratio of fat to carbohydrate oxidation as predictor of weight gain: study of 24-h RQ. *Am J Physiol* 1990; 259: E650–E657.

39. Ravussin E, Lillioja S, Knowler WC et al. Reduced rate of energy expenditure as a risk factor for body weight gain. *New Engl J Med* 1988; 318: 467–72.

40. Neel JV. Diabetes mellitus: a thrifty genotype rendered detrimental by progress. *Am J Hum Genet* 1962; 14: 353–62.

41. Brown AM, Willi SM, Argyropoulos G, Garvey WT. A novel missense mutation R70W in the human uncoupling protein 3 gene in a family with type 2 diabetes. *Hum Mutation* 1999; 13: 506–9.

42. Chung WK, Luke A, Cooper RS, Rotini C, Vidal-Puig A, Rosenbaum M et al. Genetic and physiologic analysis of the role of uncoupling protein 3 in human energy homeostasis. *Diabetes* 1999; 48: 1890–5.

43. Brown AM, Dolan JW, Willi SM, Garvey WT, Argyropoulos G. Endogenous mutations in human uncoupling protein 3 alter its functional properties. *FEBS Letters* 1999; 464: 189–93.

44. Weigle DS, Selfridge LE, Schwartz MW, Seeley RJ, Cummings DE, Havel PJ et al. Elevated free fatty acids induce uncoupling protein 3 expression in muscle. *Diabetes* 1998; 47: 298–302.

45. Samec S, Seydoux, J, Dulloo AG. Role of UCP homologues in skeletal muscles and brown adipose tissue: mediators of thermogenesis or regulators of lipids as fuel substrate. *FASEB J* 1998; 12: 715–24.

TRACK III

PREVENTION, BEHAVIOURAL ASPECTS AND CHILDHOOD OBESITY

©2003 John Libbey Eurotext Ltd, pp. 383–386.

CHAPTER 81

Is physical inactivity the cause or the consequence of obesity?

Liselotte Petersen and Thorkild I.A. Sørensen

Danish Epidemiology Science Centre at Institute of Preventive Medicine, Copenhagen University Hospital,
DK-1399 Copenhagen K, Denmark
[e-mail: tias@ipm.hosp.dk]

Introduction

The prevalence of obesity is rapidly increasing, and obesity has considerable adverse health effects. Since treatment often fails and since it is unfeasible to offer it in the magnitude requested, preventive measures are urgently needed[1].

Increased physical activity, and particularly avoidance of a sedentary lifestyle, is well established as a general health measure, because of the clear beneficial long-term effects on morbidity and mortality[2–4]. Numerous cross-sectional studies have shown an inverse association between leisure time physical activity (LTPA) and obesity[5,6], suggesting that physical inactivity may precede development of obesity. The task of interest for the present work is if physical activity also may provide long-term prevention of obesity in the general population, and which methodological points should be considered in the research of this question.

Methodology

Observational studies

Intervention studies, conducted as randomized controlled trials provide the optimal scientific evidence of effects, and in this sense they are superior to observational studies. Randomized controlled trials are feasible for short-term studies in selected populations, and they are typically used for weight loosing programmes among obese or volunteer experiments. As the interest here is the general population and the long-term effects, intervention studies addressing this question should be conducted as community trials. Regrettably such trials are hardly feasible and certainly expensive. Therefore, well conducted observational studies may provide the best evidence for the ability of physical activity to prevent obesity in a long-term perspective in the general population.

Interpretation of prospective studies

Some types of cross-sectional relations may generalize to prospective ones, for example in genetic epidemiology. Cross-sectional associations might be caused by a third factor, and even when an association is directly causal, the cross-sectional relation leaves open the question of direction. When developed, the outcome – here obesity – may alter the exposure – here physical activity.

Assessing possible causal relations is supported by the appropriate temporal sequence, here the appropriate sequence to support physical activity to prevent obesity is to measure physical activity among non-obese at one point in time and obesity at a later time point. Studies of concurrent changes in activity and BMI or obesity are essentially cross-sectional studies, since both outcome and exposure variables are measured at the same points in time, thereby the question of direction is still left open.

Study population, exposure and outcome

The general population is the focus, since a broad recommendation will be acceptable only when supported by studies in the general population.

Even though occupational physical activity also contributes to the energy expended, for the present research LTPA will be the exposure of interest, because only LTPA exhibits the inverse cross-sectional relation to obesity and LTPA is easier to modify and, therefore, better in accordance with the preventive aims.

As outcome measure one could consider changes in BMI or weight, but weight gain as such may not be relevant, since underweight people may benefit from gaining weight. Development of obesity is the measure to assess, thereby the question of prevention is distinguished from the possible effects of physical activity on obesity already developed.

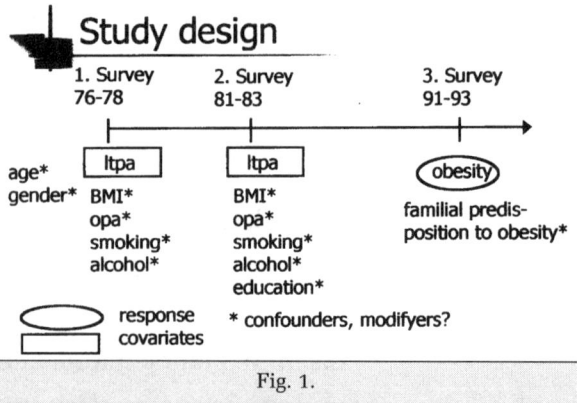

Fig. 1.

Confounding

Future weight changes and thereby development of obesity are dependent on current BMI and earlier changes in BMI[7], and the physical activity habits at and after baseline may depend on preceding changes in physical activity. Of particular importance is the tendency of extreme values of any feature that varies over time to become closer to the mean at next measurement – the socalled regression-to-the-mean phenomenon. The strong concurrent inverse relation between BMI and LTPA combined with the tracking of BMI and LTPA is the reason why baseline BMI, earlier changes in BMI and LTPA are possible confounders of the relation of interest.

Several other factors could be confounders, including occupational physical activity, gender, age, genetics, not least predisposition to obesity, and lifestyle, such as smoking status and alcohol consumption, and socio-economic status measured for example by education, employment or income. Finally, pre-existing diseases could influence obesity as well as physical activity level, and a supplementary analysis of disease-free subjects may reveal if diseases have confounded the results found.

Study example

In the Copenhagen City Heart Study, 5821 men and women, aged 25 to 83 years, were randomly selected within sex and age strata and examined at three surveys providing the opportunity to consider the first two as combined baseline, with information of both level and changes of risk factors, of possible modifiers and confounders as baseline information[8].

At the second survey, 5540 subjects were non-obese and thereby at risk of developing obesity (BMI $\geq$ 30 kg/m^2) before the third survey. Physical activity in leisure time was graded in four levels based on a questionnaire constructed by Saltin and Grimby[9] with minor modifications: (1) Physical inactivity: almost entirely sedentary (reading, TV, cinema) or light physical activity less than 2 hours per week; (2) Light physical activity: 2–4 h per week, e.g. walking, cycling, light gardening; (3) Moderate physical activity: more than 4 hours per week or more vigorous activity 2–4 h per week, e.g. brisk walking, fast cycling, heavy gardening, sports where you get sweaty or exhausted; (4) Highly vigorous physical activity: more than 4 h per week or regular heavy exercise or competitive sports several times per week. The questionnaire has been validated with respect to maximal oxygen uptake, which is increasing significantly from low to high level[10].

Using logistic regression, the odds ratios of developing obesity were estimated for men and women separately by level of LTPA at second survey. Analysis were, as argued for above, adjusted for baseline BMI and earlier changes in BMI and in LTPA. Further adjustments were made for age, smoking status, alcohol consumption, education, and familial predisposition to obesity.

Among women we found no significant association. Among men we found increasing risk of later obesity for those with high or medium activity compared to medium and low activity, with increasing significant trend from low through medium to high activity. No modifying or confounding effects of any of the variables were found on the effect of LTPA on later obesity. When excluding those with pre-existing diseases at 3rd survey, estimated odds ratios still suggest positive association between LTPA and becoming obese.

Referring to the above-mentioned methodological points, the study provides no evidence that LTPA prevents obesity in a free-living population in the long term.

Possible weaknesses in measures

One important question is if our inability to find the expected inverse relationship between physical activity and later obesity is due to the use of a too crude measure of physical activity without distinction between no and very low activity. However, in cross-sectional analyses, the measure of LTPA, as used here, is certainly strongly inversely correlated with concurrent BMI. Another question is whether the lack of a relationship is due to LTPA changes in the intervening time, but, as shown by Schnohr *et al.* in the same study population, LTPA, as measured here, at 1st and 2nd survey each has a strong predictive value with regard to long-term total mortality.[11]

Our results do not support that medium or high physical activity at baseline prevent obesity in the long term. This contradicts the intuitive ideas derived from the energy balance equation. The energy balance equation only tells us that physical activity can result in weight change if energy intake does not counterbalance the increased energy expenditure, which may occur in short-term studies, even in free-living subjects,[12] but possibly not in the long term. Furthermore, development of obesity corresponds to a very small positive energy balance, usually less than 1 per cent of the total energy turnover, and such a difference is too small to be estimated as a difference between measured energy intake and measured energy expenditure.

Comparison to other studies

The study of Williamson *et al.* of 3515 men and 5810 women aged 25 to 74 years of age, having baseline in 1971 to 75 and 10 years of follow-up[6]. Using weight gain in categories as outcome measure and adjusting for several confounders including baseline BMI, the association to LTPA at baseline and at follow-up was estimated. The analysis of 13 kilograms of gained weight showed no relation to baseline LTPA, but significantly increased risk of gain when ending up with low activity at follow-up compared to ending up with higher activity.

The study by Bild *et al.* of 1100 men and 1095 women aged 18 to 30 years of age, having baseline in 1985 and 2 years of follow-up[13]. Using weight loss of more than 5 per cent as outcome measure and adjusting for several confounders including baseline BMI, the association to LTPA at baseline (on a continuous scale) was estimated, that is odds ratios of weight loss for a person with a given level of LTPA compared to a person with lower LTPA. Among women no association were found, and for men, per 50 units increase in LTPA odds ratio of weight loss were significantly below one, which means that the more active the less chance of losing weight subsequently.

The study of Haapanen *et al.* of 2564 men and 2695 women aged 19 to 63 years of age, having baseline in 1980 and 10 years of follow-up[14]. Using weight gain of 5 kg or more and BMI of 26 or more as outcome measure and adjusting for several confounders, but not baseline BMI, the association to LTPA at baseline and at follow-up was estimated. The association to baseline LTPA was inconsistent, whereas the association to LTPA at follow-up showed increased odds of weight gain, when ending up at lower levels of LTPA.

The latter study does not adjust for baseline BMI. The study of Bild *et al.* suggests the opposite of preventing obesity by means of higher LTPA level. In the two others no association was found when taking into account the appropriate sequence of LTPA at baseline and subsequent weight change. They found strong association when considering LTPA at follow-up, the interpretation of which may be that preceding weight gain increases odds of a lower activity level.

Opposite causal direction

Consider the opposite causal direction, namely that obesity may lead to less activity. This would be in agreement with the cross-sectional relation as well as with the lack of preventive effect of LTPA on later development of obesity.

We have re-analysed data from the Copenhagen City Heart Study, and used low LTPA at third survey as outcome, adjusting for the relevant confounders and estimating the effects of BMI at an earlier point in time. We find that with increasing BMI at second survey the risk of low activity increases gradually with significant trends in both men and women.

Final discussion

We found an insignificant gender difference, suggesting no association between LTPA and later obesity in women and a weak positive association among men. On the other hand, our findings indicate that BMI is a strong determinant of later LTPA; the greater the BMI the greater the risk of being physically inactive 10 years later, also when adjustments were made for previous LTPA and possible confounders of the relation.

Earlier studies tend to interpret results as effects of LTPA on weight despite the lacking time sequence, but when requiring the appropriate time sequence to assess the causal direction, they do not disagree with our findings. Williamson *et al.* mention the possibility that weight gain effects activity level, but conclude the opposite.

When obesity has developed, the energy turnover increases and the energy requirement supporting a given physical activity increases as well[1]. In addition, it seems likely that a given level of physical activity elicits on average more discomfort, e.g. as musculoskeletal complaints, dyspnoe, exhaustion and sweating, the greater the overweight. This may reduce the motivation for physical activity and eventually reduce the actual physical activity.

Although our study does not exclude a short-term effect of LTPA on fat accumulation, our results do not support a long-term effect of physical activity on risk of later development of obesity. The cross-sectional inverse relation between obesity and LTPA seems too be due to the opposite causal direction, namely that obesity leads to less physical activity.

Conclusion

This study does not support that physical inactivity promotes development of obesity, but suggests that obesity may lead to physical inactivity.

Even though one would prefer randomized trials, the only feasible possibility for assessment of population-based long-term effects is observational studies. A study to support a recommendation of LTPA for obesity prevention should be conducted in the general non-obese population using obesity as outcome, or alternatively weight gain, either a high gain or a gain resulting in BMI above a high level. The study design should preferable adjust not only for baseline BMI, but also earlier changes in BMI and LTPA, which require measurements at three or more time points, and there should also be adjusted for other possible confounders. Last but not least, the interpretation of causal direction should be supported by the appropriate time sequence.

References

1. World Health Organistion. Obesity, preventing and managing the global epidemic. Report of a WHO Consultation on Obesity. WHO Technical Report Series (No. 894) Geneva 2000.

2. Paffenbarger RS, Hyde RT, Wing AL, Hsieh C. Physical activity, all-cause mortality, and longevity of college alumni. *N Eng J Med* 1986; 314(10): 605–13.

3. Hippe M, Vestbo J, Hein HO, Borch-Johnsen K, Jensen G, Sørensen TIA. Familial predisposition and suspectibility to the effect of other risk factors for myocardial infarction. *J Epidemiol Comm Health* 1999; 53: 269–76.

4. Andersen LB, Schnohr P, Schrol M, Hein HO. All-cause mortality associated with physical activity during leisure time, work, sport, and cycling to work. *Arch Intern Med* 2000; 160: 1621–28.

5. Fogelholm M, Kukkonen-Hajula K. Does Physical activity prevent Weight Gain – A systematic review. *Obes Rev* 2000; 1: 95–111.

6. Williamson DF, Madans J, Anda RF, Kleinman JC, Kahn HS, Byers T. 'Recreational physical activity and ten-year weight change in a US national cohort'. *Int J Obes* 1993; 17: 279–86.

7. Colditz GA, Willett WC, Stampfer MJ, London SJ, Segal MR, Speizer FE. *et al.* Patterns of weight change and their relation to diet in a cohort of healthy women. *Am J Clin Nutr* 1990; 51: 1100–1105.

8. Petersen L, Schnohr P, Sørensen TIA. Longitudinal study of the relation between physical activity and obesity in adults. Submitted.

9. Saltin B, Grimby G. Physiological analysis of middle-aged and old former athletes. Comparison with still active athletes of the same ages. *Circulation* 1968; 38: 1104–1115.

10. Saltin B. Physiological effects of physical conditioning. In: *Ischaemic heart disease. The strategy of postponement*, Hansen AT, Schnohr, Rose G (eds), pp. 104–115. Chicago: Year Book Medical Publishers and Copenhagen: FADL's Forlag, 1977.

11. Schnohr P, Scharling H, Jensen JS. Changes in physical activity and all-cause mortality in 7000 women and men. The Copenhagen City Heart Study. Submitted.

12. Stubbs RJ, Sepp A, Hughes DA, Johnstone AM, King N, Horgan G, Blundell JE. The effect of graded levels of exercise on energy intake and balance in free-living women. *Int J Obes* 2002; 26: 866–9.

13. Bild DE, Sholinsky P, Smith DE, Lewis CE, Hardin JM, Burke GL. Correlates and predictors of weight loss in young adults: the CARDIA study. *Int J Obes* 1996; 20: 47–55.

14. Haapanen N, Miilunpalo S, Pasanen M, Oja P, Vuori I. Association between leisure time physical activity and 10-year body mass change among working-aged men and women. *Int J Obes* 1997; 21: 288–96.

Progress in Obesity Research: 9. Edited by *Geraldo Medeiros-Neto, Alfredo Halpern and Claude Bouchard*
©2003 John Libbey Eurotext Ltd, pp. 387–391.

CHAPTER 82

Is there a place for dietary treatment of obesity given a 5-year 85 per cent relapse?

Teis Andersen

Hospital Direction, Roskilde County Hospital, University of Copenhagen, DK-4000 Roskilde, Denmark
[e-mail: rstan@ra.dk]

Introduction

Dietary treatment is the basic treatment for obesity. A huge number of different diets and a considerable number of adjuvant treatment components have been proposed – e.g. behavioural, pharmacological or surgical – in order to increase the efficacy of dietary treatment or to improve long-term outcome, or both. The vast number of such supportive treatment components has appeared because the efficacy – short-term and in particular long-term – has proved insufficient. Still dietary treatment is considered the basic treatment for obesity, implying that diet is the first-choice intervention. Given the large weight regain and the limited long-term success-rates it is reasonable to question whether dietary treatment for obesity is worthwhile at all. This review will discuss this issue, focusing on long-term observations in adults.

The importance of long-term outcome

In particular clinical situations weight loss can be considered relevant, even though successive long-term maintenance is not obtained. This may be the case for example in relation to female infertility and prior to elective surgery in order to reduce the risk of perioperative complications. In most situations, however, sustained weight loss is the aim. Although a final experimental proof of the effect of weight loss on mortality awaits the outcome of the Swedish SOS study, an abundance of evidence demonstrates that weight loss in obese patients reduces the prevalence and incidence of co-morbidities. Thus, the aim of lasting weight reduction relates to the intension not only to treat the overweight *per se* but also to improve the metabolic risk factors characterizing the obese. A transient weight loss will have only transient effect on the metabolic complications and probably no effect on mortality. Regain also calls for repeated weight loss attempts leading to a weight cycling which may be hazardous, especially when diets are nutritionally insufficient. Without any doubt the patients' goal is a lasting weight loss offering all the well-known psycho-social advantages.

Long-term results

What is then the potency of dietary treatment for obesity as to long-term maintenance of a significantly reduced weight? This review will deal with diets of any kind and will look also at the most typical supportive programmes and adjuvant treatments. 'Long-term maintenance' can be defined only arbitrarily as no lifetime studies exist. In a resent systematic review[1] no association was found between time of observation beyond 3 years (and up to 14 years) and success rate. In a meta-analysis[2] of US studies published between 1970 and 1999 the percentage maintained weight loss was 67 per cent, 44 per cent, 32 per cent, 28 per cent and 21 per cent after 1, 2, 3, 4 and 5 years of follow-up, respectively. The WHO report on obesity[3] recommends data on sustained weight loss be based on more than two years, preferably five years of observation. It might thus be concluded that 2 years of observation is too short and 3 years a more true cut-off point for evaluation of stable weight losses, although a continued weight regain and declining success rates thereafter cannot be ruled out. If not stated otherwise, observations will in this article be accepted as 'long-term' if based on at least three years of follow-up.

Other uncertainties appear when trying to evaluate the literature. The Ayyad review[1] identified from the chosen criteria for inclusion 17 papers reporting on 21 treatment groups and 3,030 patients, whereas the Anderson review[2] identified 16 papers with a follow-up of at least 3 years dealing with 24 patient groups and 1,926 patients starting treatment. Despite a limited overlap between the reports included in these comprehensive reviews, the total number of patients observed long-time and reported in the literature appears fairly small, in particular when considering the wide range of diets and regimens used. In addition, only about ¾ of the patients were available for follow-up, and a large fraction of the patients were followed-up by self-reported weights. Last but not least, the scientific quality of these publications was generally poor, and only three studies[1] had a relevant randomized design. No long-term study with allocation to either dietary treatment or no treatment was found. The consequent possibility that the long-term results of dietary treatment be underscored compared to the spontaneously increasing body weight has recently been supported by Kuller and coworkers[4] reporting a weight increase of 5.2 kg over 54 months in an untreated control group of peri-menopausal women. It has for long been a matter of dispute whether a marked energy restriction as obtained by very-low-calorie diets (VLCDs) lead to poorer long-term results than the use of more conventional diets offering more than 800 kcal (3.4 MJ) per day. The arguments against VLCD have been that excess loss of lean body mass would reduce basal metabolic rate and thus favour weight regain, and further that VLCD does not teach patients healthy food habits. The literature in general and a randomized controlled trial[5] (RCT) do not support this view. Ayyad[1] found only marginally higher success rates (18 per cent vs. 14 per cent) after conventional diet (CD) than after VLCD, whereas Anderson[2] reported better long-term outcomes after VLCD than after CD.

Another myth as to long-term outcomes of dietary treatment has been that rapid weight loss leads to poorer long-term results than a more slow weight loss. However, a RCT[6] (follow-up 2 years) has demonstrated that regain is not different in patients losing the same amount of weight in either 8 weeks (by VLCD) or in 17 weeks (by CD). Further, a large and rapid weight loss improved long-term outcome in a RCT[7], in which both assignment groups received behaviour modification (BM).

The composition of the diet as to energy providing nutrients has for decades attracted great attention among learned and unlearned. As described in the recent comprehensive review by Willet[8] the prescription of low-fat diets can bring about modest weight losses up to about 4 kg. Such weight losses are obviously the consequence of the energy deficit obtained and not of the change in macronutrient ratios. Thus, also long-term results will be totally dependent on the continued diet compliance. Swinburn[8] and co-workers recently illustrated this effect. A limited number of long-term RCTs on the effect of low-fat diets exists, but a part of these may have come out with biased results due to a lower attention paid to the control subjects. Generally, trials without this methodological flaw have not been able to demonstrate any sustained, clinically significant weight loss from low-fat diets[8,9]. This fact does not contradict that successful weight loss maintainers have been found to have a low intake of fat[2].

As patients' compliance with the prescribed diet is difficult to obtain and crucial for weight loss results, a number of adjuvant, supportive treatment components has been proposed. Their numerous modifications and their possible combinations do only allow the most important categories to be dealt with here.

It is a general experience that compliance and weight loss outcome are closely correlated with the intensity of the support programme, the frequency of the control visits and the enthusiasm of the care providers. This experience has been confirmed in long-term studies, in which a double success rate was characterizing study groups offered an active follow-up compared to passive assessment only[1]. Taking care of patients in groups – often named 'group therapy' – makes patient support more practicable and has also been found generally to be associated with better than average long-term results[1].

The term 'BM' is used for supportive programmes ranging from fairly simple advice about the patients' handling of various daily-life situations to structured, individualized psychological programmes. This variation may underlie the inconsistent findings as to effect of BM on long-term results[1]. Despite the widespread use of various BM programmes and their value short-term, use of BM cannot be said to be of proven value as to long-term benefit[10].

Physical activity is an intervention of its own right due to its direct influence on energy balance, and it has furthermore independent effects on metabolic complications of obesity. The latter fact makes physical activity advisable in obese subjects independent of weight loss attempts. Compliance seems to be the crucial factor for the benefit of physical activity on weight loss maintenance. Projects assuring a high level of physical activity generally come up with excellent weight maintenance[11]. Likewise, post-hoc analyses have shown a better weight loss maintenance in patients with a high exercise level[2] (2.7 years of follow-up). It can be argued that this relation may not exclusively be attributable to the exercise; it is probably also due to a high general motivation in this subgroup of patients and thus also to a good compliance with dietary recommendations. Nevertheless it seems safe to conclude that physical activity in theory and in practise supports weight maintenance when performed regularly and at a high level without being overcompensated by increased food intake. Vigorous motivational efforts are typically necessary. Simple counselling has only a dubious effect, which underlies the disappointing weight loss outcomes in community intervention studies[12].

However, evaluation of success rates depends on the goals set up. In a noteworthy controlled trial by Toumilehto and co-workers[13] the goal was not weight loss *per se* but prevention of manifest type 2 diabetes in overweight or obese subjects with impaired glucose tolerance. The intervention aimed at a reduced fat intake, an increase of fibre intake, and a higher exercise level. Despite a modest weight loss (group difference at one year 3.4 kg) a marked reduction in diabetes incidence was observed during further five years of follow-up. Thus, this study represents a goal-directed, combined intervention in subjects with high risk of metabolic complications, and it was successful despite a moderate dietary restriction focusing on fat intake. The target group and the outcomes were very much similar in the Diabetes Prevention Programme, in which, however, the diet was designed to obtain an initial 7 kg weight loss[14].

Drugs as adjuncts to dietary treatment have never been proved to improve long-term weight maintenance[15]. Orlistat – a pancreas lipase inhibitor – has been shown to reduce but not to eliminate regain in the year following treatment either with diet plus orlistat or diet plus placebo[16]. During the maintenance-year patients were prescribed an energy intake individually calculated to obtain energy balance and not a continued energy deficit that might have improved results. The proportion of patients successfully maintaining a weight loss of at least 5 per cent of their initial weight after either two years of orlistat treatment or two years of placebo was 1.5 times higher (57 per cent) in the former group.

Likewise, sibutramine – a norepinephrine and serotonine reuptake inhibitor – has been shown to improve the maintenance of a diet-induced weight loss during the succeeding 18 months leading to a regain 4 kg less than that observed in the placebo group[17]. This trial allowed a certain continued dietary energy deficit. The proportion of patients maintaining a weight loss of at least 5 per cent of their initial body weight was elevated by about 1.7 times (to about 70 per cent) in the sibutramine group compared to placebo.

Overall, orlistat and sibutramine are able to improve short-term maintenance of weight loss. Still, no investigation warrants a clinical use of these drugs for maintenance purposes for periods longer than one to two years.

The far best weight loss, weight maintenance and according control of co-morbidities have been obtained by surgical treatment[18]. Gastric procedures involving the stomach only (gastroplasty, gastric banding) are basically to be regarded as pure diet support interventions. Depending on the energy mal-absorption induced, gastric bypass surgery and bilio-pancreatic bypass surgery are to varying degrees also to be considered as support of a reducing diet. The physiological principles lying behind this outstanding efficacy will be returned to below.

Prediction of success and failure

It is a clinical experience that it is almost impossible from individual patient characteristics *before start of dietary treatment* to predict *long-term weight outcomes*. Although sparse[2], the literature on this particular issue confirms this impression. The literature is particularly limited as to prospectively planned studies of the issue. Gender, ethnicity, education, social class, marital status and number of children seem to be of no importance[2,19,20]. Higher age has inconsistently been found to be a positive predictor of weight maintenance[19]. As found in studies with shorter follow-up, some indication exists that initial degree of overweight is positively associated with the long-term weight loss, but reports are conflicting[19].

Barriers against maintenance – can they be overcome?

Several severe barriers against successful weight maintenance can be identified. They include decreased basal metabolic rate, decreased energy expenditure necessary for the same physical activity, a limited social drive to increase physical activity, habits as to physical activity, psychological and social factors related to food intake, easy food availability, and appetite.

Many of these barriers can be condensed into a need for raising the energy expenditure. Such change can be obtained only by pharmacological means or through increased physical activity. Centrally acting stimulating anorectics such as sibutramine have such effect[17], but side effects have so far limited the efficacy that can safely be obtained. Smoking, probably the most frequently used means against weigh gain and regain, also stimulates energy expenditure, but can for its detrimental health effects not be recommended. Thus, increase of physical activity seems to be a crucial issue, and successful long-term outcome of dietary treatment for obesity has repeatedly been shown to be linked to this factor. The diabetes prevention studies[13,14] previously dealt with were both successful in increasing the level of physical activity in their lifestyle intervention groups. Dieters successful as to long-term weight maintenance have in several studies[2,20,21] been found to be characterized by an elevated level of physical activity. As there is only a weak adaptive increase in resting energy expenditure in response to excess energy intake and insufficient environmental incitements in the modern society to increase physical activity, weight control has moved from an instinctual process to one that requires substantial cognitive effort[22]. Weight maintenance will be dependent also on a strong cognitive effort in relation to food intake. Accordingly, a continued dietary restraint as to energy and fat has been found to characterise weight loss maintainers[20,21].

It was previously stated that gastric surgery for obesity in principle was to be considered a technique to support dieting and maintenance of a lowered weight. The underlying physiological mechanism has not been known, but more than a decade ago it has been proposed that the gastric operations interfered with some type of messenger reducing appetite[23]. The hope for a 'pharmacological obesity operation' has recently been markedly increased by the detection of the hormone ghrelin, mainly secreted by the stomach and duodenum and implicated in mealtime hunger and long-term regulation of body weight. Ghrelin levels have been shown to increase after dietary weight loss and thus possibly add to an increased appetite and consequent maintenance problems. It is exciting that gastric bypass seems nearly to extinguish the ghrelin secretion[24]. It is probable that ghrelin thus represents the physiological explanation of the outstanding efficacy of gastric surgery as diet-supporting intervention. It can be hoped for that the principle of ghrelin antagonism in the future can be used pharmacologically for long-term weight loss maintenance.

Is there a place for dietary treatment – status, consequences and perspectives

It will hardly be an overstatement to postulate that frustration among caregivers and patients encompasses the field of dietary treatment for obesity due to poor long-term outcomes. If this frustration becomes the dominant force, patients will be pushed to, attracted to and kept in even less effective and probably harmful interventions, e.g. so-called 'alternative' treatments and smoking. The obligation for professionals is to use current knowledge as well as possible and to create new, useful knowledge.

First, a 15 per cent success rate as to weight loss maintenance is low but not negligible for a chronic disease. This rate can probably be raised by use of frequent, enthusiastic follow-up and in particular by better information on – and urge to – daily, considerable physical activity.

Another issue is proper selection of the patients on whom we spend the resources. Little is known about cost-effectiveness of various obesity treatments. It is obvious, however, that treatment efforts overall will be more cost-effective when a proper patient selection is performed. Because the metabolic risk profile demonstrably[13,14] can be improved long-term in patients at particular metabolic risk, and because these patients are likely to become the most expensive ones as to future health care, it would be advisable to focus on such high-risk patients. In a situation with few or none known predictors of a relevant and lasting treatment outcome, it might be proposed to use patients' readiness to perform daily physical activity at a reasonably increased level as a selection criterion for obesity treatment, as a maintained high level of physical activity seems to be a crucial factor for maintenance of weight loss. Genetic research may in the future make it possible more precisely to tailor the treatment to patient characteristics.

Dietary treatment supplemented with increased physical activity will without doubt remain central parts of obesity treatment. On the other hand it is obvious that adjuvant treatment modalities are necessary. Surgery for the morbidly obese has come up with the far best long-term results, whereas pharmacotherapy has not so far demonstrated to be the proper answer. It is to be hoped for that gastric surgery may uncover a useful principle for appetite control.

Further research – clinical as well as basic – is urgently needed. The clinical research should concentrate on strict RCTs. Resources should be made available so that long-term follow-up and scientific independency can be secured. As to basic research, particular hope can be attached to neuro-hormonal and genetic research.

Reference

1. Ayyad C, Andersen T. Long-term efficacy of dietary treatment of obesity: a systematic review of studies published between 1931 and 1999. *Obes Rev* 2000; 1: 113–19.

2. Anderson JW, Konz EC, Frederich RC,Wood CL. Long-term weight-loss maintenance: a meta-analysis of US studies. *Am J Clin Nutr* 2001; 74: 579–84.

3. World Health Organisation. Obesity – preventing and managing the global epidemic, p. 256. Geneva: World Health Organisation. 1998.

4. Kuller LH, Simkin-Silverman LR, Wing RR, Meilahn EN. Women's Healthy Lifestyle Project: A randomised clinical trial. Results at 54 months. *Circulation* 2001; 103: 32–7.

5. Wadden TA, Sternberg JA, Letizia KA, Stunkard AJ, Foster GD. Treatment of obesity by very low calorie diet, behaviour therapy and their combination: a five-year perspective. *Int J Obes* 1989; 13: 39–46.

6. Toubro S, Astrup A. Randomised comparison of diets for maintaining obese subjects' weight after major weight loss: *ad libitum*, low fat, high carbohydrate diet v fixed energy intake. *BMJ*1997; 314: 29–34.

7. Pekkarinen T, Mustajoki P. Comparison of behaviour therapy with and without very-low-energy diet in the treatment of morbid obesity. A 5-year outcome. *Arch Intern Med* 1997; 157: 1581–85.

8. Willett WC. Dietary fat plays a major role in obesity: no. *Obes Rev* 2002; 3: 59–68.

9. Swinburn BA, Metcalf PA, Ley SJ. Long-term (5 year) effects of reduced-fat diet intervention in individuals with glucose intolerance. *Diabetes Care* 2001; 24: 619–24.

10. Phelan S, Wadden TA. Combining behavioural and pharmacological treatments for obesity. *Obes Res* 2002; 10: 560–74.

11. Leermakers EA, Dunn AL, Blair SN. Exercise management of obesity. *Med Clin North Am* 2000; 84: 419–40.

12. Fogelholm M, Lathi-Koski M. Does physical activity prevent weight gain? Results from community interventions. *Obesity Matters* 2002; 3: 13–16.

13. Toumilehto J, Lindström J, Erisson JG, Valle TT, Hämäläinen H, Ilanne-Parikka P *et al.* Prevention of type 2 diabetes mellitus by changes in lifestyle among subjects with Impaired glucose tolerance. *N Engl J Med* 2001; 344: 1343–50.

14. Knowler WC, Barret-Connor E, Fowler SE, Hamman RF, Lachin JM, Walker EA, Nathan DM. Reduction in the incidence of type 2 diabetes with lifestyle intervention or metformin. *N Engl J Med* 2002; 346: 393–403.

15. Yanovski SZ, Yanovski JA. Obesity. *N Engl J Med* 2002; 346: 591–602.

16. Sjöström L, Rissanen A, Andersen T, Boldrin M, Golay A, Koppeschaar HPF, Krempf M. Randomised placebo-controlled trial of orlistat for weight loss and prevention of weight regain in obese patients. *Lancet* 1998; 352: 167–173.

17. James WPT, Astrup A, Finer N, Hilsted J, Kopelman P, Rössner S, Saris WHM, Van Gaal LF. Effect of sibutramine on weight maintenance after weight loss: a randomised trial. *Lancet* 2000; 356: 2119–125.

18. Livingston EH. Obesity and its surgical management. *Am J Surg* 2002; 184: 103–13.

19. Ogden J. The correlates of long-term weight loss: a group comparison study of obesity. *Int J Dis Relat Metab Dis* 2001; 24: 1018–25.

20. Crawford D, Jefferey RW, French SA. Can anyone successfully control their weight? Findings of a three year community-based study of men and women. *Int J Obes Relat Metab Dis* 2000; 24: 1007–1110.

21. McGuire MT, Wing RR, Klem ML, Hill JO. Behavioral strategies of individuals who have maintained long-term weight losses. *Obes Res* 1999; 7: 334–41.

22. Peters JC, Wyatt HR, Donahoo WT, Hill JO. From instinct to intellect: the challenge of maintaining healthy weight in the modern world. *Obes Rev* 2002; 3: 69–74.

23. Andersen T. Gastroplasty and very-low-calorie diet in the treatment of morbid obesity. *Dan Med Bull* 1990; 37: 359–370.

24. Cummings DE, Weigle DS, Frayo RS, Breen PA, Ma MK, Dellinger EP, Purnell JQ. Plasma ghrelin levels after diet-induced weight loss or gastric bypass surgery. *N Engl J Med* 2002; 346: 1623–30.

Progress in Obesity Research: 9. Edited by *Geraldo Medeiros-Neto, Alfredo Halpern and Claude Bouchard*
©2003 John Libbey Eurotext Ltd, pp. 392–396.

CHAPTER 83

How to measure energy intake in children and adults

Jeanne H.M. de Vries

Wageningen University, Department of Human Nutrition and Epidemiology, Bomenweg 2, 6703 HD Wageningen, The Netherlands
[e-mail: Jeanne.devries@wur.nl]

Introduction

Food consumption may be assessed for several purposes (Willett[1]). An important aim is to study the relationship between diet and disease in epidemiological studies. Assessment of food consumption is also important to monitor patients that are following dietary guidelines, or to measure the effect of dietary treatment in groups of patients according to evidence-based principles. In the treatment of patients, dietary assessment may be used for diagnosis, or counselling. Also, self-reporting of food intake could make patients more aware of their food habits, and motivate them to change their consumption, if necessary.

Diet is very complex and hard to measure. Several methods to assess intake have been developed, but no method is perfect (Bingham[2], Cameron[3]). They all suffer from measurement error, both systematic and random error. The scopes of error differ between the various methods, and between various populations; for example between lean and obese people, and between different age groups. Sources of error include underreporting of intake, incorrectly estimated portion sizes, and missing or inaccurate nutrient data in food composition tables. For all methods it is important that the measurement error or variability of the method is not too large relative to the actual variability in intake between subjects.

In obesity, the intakes of energy and macronutrients are especially of interest. Also, the consumption of specific food groups, for example snacks, is often assessed to evaluate intake with regard to a healthy food pattern. Therefore, this paper aims to present a brief overview of problems with respect to measuring the intake of energy and macronutrients, paying special attention to obese children and adults.

Methods

Dietary assessment methods can roughly be divided into methods assessing current diet, consisting of records and 24-h recalls, and methods assessing habitual diet, consisting of dietary histories and food frequency questionnaires. The intake data derived from these methods, combined with analytical data from food composition tables or chemical analysis, result in individual nutrient intakes. In addition to these methods, some biological indicators of dietary exposure have been developed, for example, protein in urine, and fatty acids in fat tissue (Willett[1], Kok[4]).

The mode of the report and the characteristics of the respondent, such as their age and culture, also determine the quality of the data collected by these methods (Carbone[5]). Modes of self-reporting include face-to-face interviews, telephone interviews, food diaries and records administered by computer or by tape. Not every mode is suitable for every study: the best mode of self-reporting depends on the research question and on the study population. For instance, if only a limited number of respondents in a population is literate, a diary is not a good choice, and in remote areas a face-to-face interview will not be a potential alternative. New, automated techniques could make some types of methods cheaper and more accessible. The use of computerized interviews might also lead to less socially desirable answering, resulting in better estimates of energy intake.

Measurement error

In selecting a method it is important to know what type of information is required: is this information about individual or group intake, food or food groups, all nutrients or only specific ones (Beaton[6]). For the required type of information, we have to deal with four types of error: random or systematic within-person error, and random or systematic between-person error. *Random within-person error* occurs for example when the method does not account for day-to-day variation of a person, when determining habitual consumption. It also occurs when types of foods or portion sizes are misestimated in a non-systematic way. Increasing the number of replicate measurements may blank out random within-person error. *Systematic within-person error* may be caused when a person under- or overestimates his food intake, for example if an important food is not included in a questionnaire. Repeated measurements do not decrease this type of error. *Random between person error* may be due to random and systematic within-person error, which is distributed randomly among individuals. As an overestimation by some individuals is counterbalanced by an underestimation by others, the estimated mean intake is consequently not biased. However, this type of error affects precision and widens the distribution artificially. Increasing the number of subjects or replicate measurements may improve precision, but not the validity of estimates for the percentage of undernourished subjects. *Systematic between-person error* is caused by systematic within-person error that is not randomly distributed among individuals, for example socially desirable answers given by groups of persons. As a consequence, the mean intake is not estimated correctly, nor is the percentage of undernourished persons.

Assessment of energy intake

There is a large variation in energy intake from day to day (Willett[1]). Therefore, one single recall or record does not represent a person's habitual energy intake. The number of days that is required to assess individual energy intake accurately depends on the within-person variability of intake, derived from information of at least 2 days. There is a simple formula (Beaton[7]) from which the required number of days may be calculated from the within-person variation.
This formula is $n = (Z^*CVw/D_0)^2$ where:

n = the number of days required,
$Z\_$ = normal deviate for the percentage of time the measured value should be within a specified limit,
CVw = the within-person coefficient of variation,
D_0 = the specified limit.

For example, if the CVw is 33 per cent: $n = (1.96 * 33\%/20\%)^2 = 10$ days. Thus, the number of days necessary to estimate a person's energy intake within 20 per cent will be 10 days. However, when subjects only should be classified according to their intake, fewer days will be sufficient. For example, for monitoring patients who lose body weight, assessing changes in energy intake is more interesting than determining absolute intakes.

Under- and over-reporting

To assess the validity of a method it is important to know whether there is a linear or a non-linear relationship between true and reported consumption (Fig. 1). In other words: whether there is differential or non-differential misclassification. If underreporting is linear to the level of intake serious bias in estimates of health risks can occur, but it will still be possible to rank subjects according to their energy intake or to assess changes in intake. On the other hand, if underreporting is non-linear to the level of intake, it will not be possible to rank subjects properly. In general, self-reports can validly identify associations between intake and disease or health. However, these methods cannot determine the actual level of consumption, which makes it difficult to set sensible limits for acceptable intake or to determine whether intakes meet recommended daily allowances (Beaton[6]).
It is difficult to determine whether self-reports underestimate or overestimate actual intake, because 'gold standards' to which assessment techniques can be validated are lacking. Energy requirements assessed by the doubly labelled water method (Schoeller[8]) are considered as a golden standard to assess energy intake. However, this method is expensive, and validation studies using this method are only performed in a limited number of subjects. As a consequence, often only so-called convergent validity can be determined by comparing one method with another. A high correlation between two methods does not necessarily mean that a method is valid, since errors of methods are often related, for example, when they both suffer from underreporting (Willett[1]).

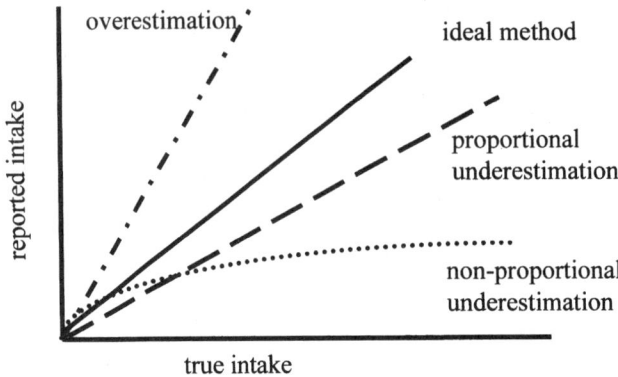

Fig. 1. Energy intake reporting: hypothetical curves of reported energy vs. true intake.

Underestimation of energy intake

Underestimation of energy intake is more common than overestimation. Schoeller[9] suggested that the reason of underreporting is that people report their intakes closer to perceived norms than to actual intakes. Thus, obese people tend to report their energy intake more towards that of lean people. The results of a large number of validation studies show that underreporting is on average about 20 per cent (Black[10]), with large differences between individuals and populations. Although results are not consistent, in general lean persons report their consumption better than obese (Lichtman[11]). We found an average underestimation of only 10 per cent by three-day records in 269 young lean and motivated subjects (de Vries[12]). However, underestimation by individuals might be much larger (Fig. 2; Siebelink *et al.*, 2003, unpublished). As the extent of underreporting is not necessarily the same for all subjects, it is not an option to correct estimated energy consumption by a specific factor as is done sometimes.

Underestimation of energy intake may be due to underreporting or undereating. Undereating could be tracked by measuring body weights during the period of reporting food intake.

Some foods and nutrients are more underreported than others (Goris[13], Heitmann[14]), but studies are not consistent in the types of foods and nutrients that are selectively underestimated. Some studies report underestimation of fat intake, others of carbohydrates, alcohol or specific foods such as snacks. It is also suggested that healthy foods, such as vegetables and fruit, are often overestimated.

When self-reports are repeated in the same subjects, underestimation increases (Goris[15]). This might be a problem, for example, when changes in intake are monitored. However, it is also shown that results improve when subjects are confronted with their own results of underestimation or when they are told that their intake is checked by another method (bogus pipeline).

In some cultures underreporting is greater than in others. This could be due to differences in food patterns between populations. It is assumed that regular patterns are easier to recall than patterns with a large variability. Also social acceptability could play a role: reporting could be more reliable in

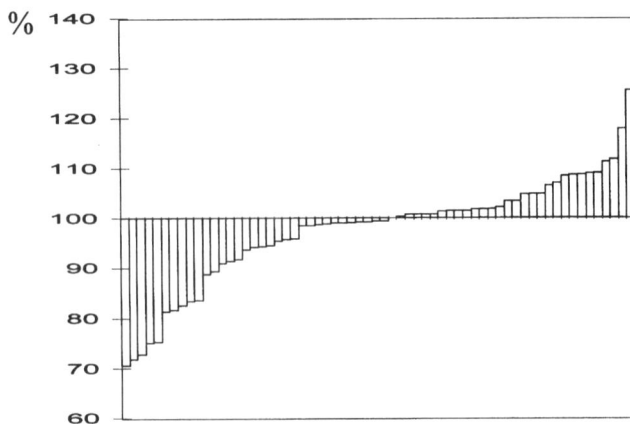

Fig. 2. Individual reported energy intake by a food frequency questionnaire as a percentage of actual energy intakes in 63 men.

populations where unhealthy food habits are more socially accepted. In the Seneca study, for example, a better relative validity of reporting of alcohol intake was found for the southern European centres than for the northern (van Staveren[16]).

Underestimation of portion sizes may be a reason of underestimation of energy intake (Young[17]). Underestimation may be very large, and occurs in all populations. However, portion sizes are also often overestimated. In addition, systematic bias in reporting portion sizes is mentioned, that is, small portions are overestimated, and large portions are underestimated. Estimations of portion sizes may be improved by the use of food models, weighing of portions, or training in estimating portions.

Measurement in children

Cognitive aspects influence the accuracy of dietary reporting in children. Compared to adults, children have limited cognitive ability to record or remember their diets, less knowledge of food and food preparation (Baranowski[18]), and more rapidly changing food patterns. Although adolescents have full cognitive ability and more knowledge about food than younger children do, other problems influence their self-reports, such as less structured food patterns and out-home eating. Also, the meaning of food changes to children as they get older: initially food satisfies hunger, but later on it becomes more a means of self-expression.

Reports by parents are not always reliable; especially they are not able to report a child's out-of-home eating (Livingstone[19]). In addition, as both parents work increasingly out-of-home, it will be more difficult to achieve accurate parental reports of children's eating. However, studies comparing parent's reports of their young children to estimates of expenditure determined by the doubly-labelled water method showed good agreement (Hill[20]).

It is thought that estimation of portion sizes is beyond the intellectual capacity of children. Although training may improve estimations, it has been shown that 35–50 per cent of the children's estimates did not correspond with parental reports (Livingstone[17]).

The ratio of the within variance of children is in general larger for older children than for younger children and adults. Therefore, more days are often needed to assess intake of older children. However, for specific populations or specific nutrients, within-person variation could be smaller, and number of reporting days could possibly be reduced. This could decrease the burden for patients and staff enormously. We compared fat intake assessed by three-day and four-day estimated food records in 167 children with cystic fibrosis (Spithoven *et al.*, unpublished. The within-person variation in their fat intake was 25 per cent, which is less than that of children reported by Willett[1]. Only 0.5 per cent of the children had deviations of more than 20 per cent in fat intake between estimates by three- and four-day records.

In a recent paper (Livingstone[17]), an overview of validation studies in children using energy requirements estimated by the doubly labelled water method was presented. It showed that underreporting increases with age, that obese children underreport more than their lean counterparts, and that underreporting by some dietary survey methods applied in specific age groups might perform better than others.

A method developed for adults does not necessary perform well in adolescents. We applied a food frequency questionnaire developed to assess the intake of energy, total fat, fatty acids and cholesterol in adults (Feunekes[21]) in 15-year-old adolescents (Droop[22]), and compared the results with those determined by a diet history. Although the adolescents reported the same food groups as the adults, and could be classified well according to their intake, they provided much higher estimates than adults did.

In choosing a method for children, practical aspects might also play a role. An easy method to apply in young children is a 24-h recall by telephone. We administered this method in 60 children of 5 and 6 years old (Aalbersberg *et al.*, 1999 unpublished). The interviews took on average 10 minutes. Eighty per cent of the parents were satisfied about this method, and preferred a telephone interview to a personal interview. In addition, energy intakes on group level agreed very well with energy requirements.

Improvements

It must be stressed that measurement error of methods could be reduced by practical improvements of methods, and the use of computers could make performances of methods easier. Major examples to deal with in surveys are incomplete time sampling, misestimation of portion size, and recall bias. The use of strictly standardized procedures for sampling, interviewer qualification and training, and quality control is needed in order to prevent or minimize errors. To assess portion sizes, a picture book or training in estimation of portion sizes is recommended.

Conclusions

To assess energy intake, several methods are available. The number of days needed depends on the method and the study population. Underreporting is common, especially in obesity. Therefore, it is recommended that other indicators of energy intake, such as body weight, height, and physical activity, are included. For children, the method chosen should be adapted to age and food patterns.

Reference

1. Willett W. *Nutritional epidemiology* (2nd edn). New York, Oxford: Oxford University Press; 1998.
2. Bingham SA. The dietary assessment of individuals; methods, accuracy, new techniques, and recommendations. *Nutr Abstr Rev* 1987; 57: 705–42.
3. Cameron ME, van Staveren WA. *Manual on methodology for food consumption studies*. Oxford: Oxford University Press; 1988.
4. Kok FJ, van 't Veer P. Overview of dietary markers of intake. In: *Biomarkers of dietary exposure*, FJ Kok, P van 't Veer (eds), pp. 27–36. London: Smith-Gordon, 1991.
5. Carbone ET, Campbell MK, Hones-Morreale L. Use of cognitive interview techniques in the development of nutrition surveys and interactive nutrition messages for low-income population. *J Am Diet Assoc* 2002; 102: 690–96.
6. Beaton GH. Approaches to analyses of dietary data: relationship between planned analyses and choice of methodology. *Am J Clin Nutr* 1994; 59 Suppl 253S–261S.
7. Beaton GH, Milner J, Corey P, McGuire V, Cousins M, Stewart E *et al.* Sources of variance in 24-hour dietary recall data: Implications for nutrition study design and interpretation. *Am J Clin Nutr* 1979; 32: 2546–49.
8. Schoeller DA. How accurate is self-reported dietary energy intake? *Nutr Rev* 1990; 48: 373–79.
9. Schoeller DA, Bandini LG, Dietz WH. Inaccuracies in self-reported intake identified by comparison with the doubly labelled water method. *Can J Physiol Pharmacol* 1990; 68: 941–49.
10. Black AE, Prentice AM, Goldberg GR, Jebb SA, Bingham SA, Livingstone MBE, Coward WA. Measurements of total energy expenditure provide insights into the validity of dietary measurements of energy intake. *J Am Diet Assoc* 1993; 93: 572–79.
11. Lichtman SW, Pisarska K, Berman ER, Pestone M, Dowling H, Offenbacher E *et al.* Discrepancy between self-reported and actual caloric intake and exercise in obese subjects. *N Engl J Med* 1992; 327: 1893–98.
12. De Vries JH, Zock PL, Mensink RP, Katan MB. Underestimation of energy intake by 3-d records compared with energy intake to maintain body weight in 269 non-obese adults. *Am J Clin Nutr* 1994; 60: 855–60.
13. Goris AH, Westerterp KRImproved reporting of habitual food intake after confrontation with earlier results on food reporting. *Br J Nutr* 2000; 83: 363–69.
14. Heitmann BL, Lissner L, Osler M. Do we eat less fat, or just report so? *Int J Obes Relat Metab Disord* 2000; 24: 435–42.
15. Goris AH, Meijer EP, Westerterp KR. Repeated measurement of habitual food intake increases underreporting and induces selective underreporting. *Br J Nutr* 2001; 85: 629–34.
16. Van Staveren WA, Burema J, Livingstone MBE. Evaluation of the dietary history method used in the SENECA study. *Eur J Clin Nutr* 1996; 50 Suppl 2: S47–S55.
17. Young LR, Nestle M. Portion sizes in dietary assessment: issues and policy implications. *Nutr Rev* 1995; 53: 149–58.
18. Baranowski T, Dome SB. A cognitive model of children's reporting of food intake. *Am J Clin Nutr* 1994; 59 Suppl 212S–217S.
19. Livingstone MBE, Robson PJ. Measurement of dietary intake in children. *Proc Nutr Soc* 2000; 59: 279–93.
20. Hill RJ, Davies PS. The validity of self-reported energy intake as determined using the doubly labelled water technique. *Br J Nutr* 2001; 85: 415–30.
21. Feunekes GIJ, van Staveren WA, de Vries JHM, Burema J, Hautvast JGAJ Relative and biomarker-based validity of a food frequency questionnaire estimating intake of fats and cholesterol. *Am J Clin Nutr* 1993; 58: 489–96.
22. Droop A, Feunekes GIJ, Ham E, Osendarp S, Burema J, van Staveren WA. Vetinneming van adolescenten. Validering van een voedselfrequentievragenlijst die de inneming van vet, vetzuren en cholesterol meet (in Dutch). *Tijdschr Soc Gezondheidsz* 1995; 73: 57–63.

Progress in Obesity Research: 9. Edited by *Geraldo Medeiros-Neto, Alfredo Halpern and Claude Bouchard*
©2003 John Libbey Eurotext Ltd, pp. 397–402.

CHAPTER 84

Is fat more fattening than carbohydrate?

Arne Astrup, Anne Raben, Anne Flint, Benjamin Buemann and Søren Toubro

Department of Human Nutrition, The Royal Veterinary and Agricultural University, Frederiksberg, Denmark
[e-mail: ast@kvl.dk]

The role of high fat diets for weight gain and obesity was assessed by the evidence based guidelines. Four meta-analyses of weight loss occurring on *ad libitum* low fat diets in intervention trials consistently demonstrate a highly significant weight loss of 3–4 kg in normal weight and overweight subjects. The analyses also found dose-response relationships so that the reduction in dietary energy from fat was positively associated with weight loss. Weight loss is also positively related to initial body weight, so a 10 per cent reduction in dietary fat is predicted to produce a 4–5 kg weight loss in an individual with a BMI of 30 kg/m². The non-fat component of the diet also should mainly consist of starchy, fibre-rich carbohydrates and protein. Whereas the glycaemic index of the carbohydrate may play a role for cardiovascular risk factors, there is so far little evidence to support that low glycaemic index foods facilitates weight control. By contrast, sugar in drinks is more likely to produce weight gain than solid sugar in foods. Although the evidence is weak alcoholic beverages seem to promote a positive energy balance, and wine may be more obesity promoting than beer. Protein is more satiating and thermogenic than carbohydrates, and one intervention study has shown that an *ad libitum* low-fat diet where carbohydrate was replaced by protein produced more weight loss after 6 months (8.1 vs. 5.9 kg).

Evidence based dietary guidelines

In order to prevent cardiovascular disease, cancer, obesity and type 2 diabetes it is recommended that dietary fat should be reduced from the 35–45 per cent of the total energy content, as is currently normal in most Western diets, to below 30 per cent. By contrast, a number of scientists claim that it is not the total fat content of the diet that counts, but that it is rather the type of fat eaten that is significant. They conclude that recommending a reduction in total dietary fat is misleading and unnecessary. Furthermore, it has been claimed that low fat diets may adversely affect cardiovascular risk factors[1].

We aim to use the evidence-based principle to assess the sufficiency of the existing documentation to substantiate whether one of the diets is superior to the other. Notably, meta-analysis of randomized controlled trials is recognized as being the strongest evidence, followed by experimental studies. Observational epidemiological studies are ranked at the bottom of the scale, with only opinions or clinical experience of respected authorities ranking lower.

The evidence linking dietary fat to energy balance and obesity

The possible link between dietary fat content and obesity must be exerted through an effect of dietary fat on energy balance. A positive energy balance can be facilitated, in theory, by a high fat diet through the promotion of overconsumption of energy, e.g. due to a lower satiating effect per Joule of a high fat vs. a low diet. Moreover, energy from fat could be more effectively absorbed from the intestine than carbohydrate and protein, and fat may also reduce energy expenditure, e.g. by a lower thermogenic effect of fat compared to carbohydrate and protein. It is likely that the effect on energy balance is predominantly exerted through an effect on intake, and the relation between dietary fat and body fat should therefore be studied under *ad libitum* conditions, where the studied individuals have free access to food. Consequently, studies where different diets are compared in isoenergetic amounts can only provide information about an effect on absorption and energy expenditure.

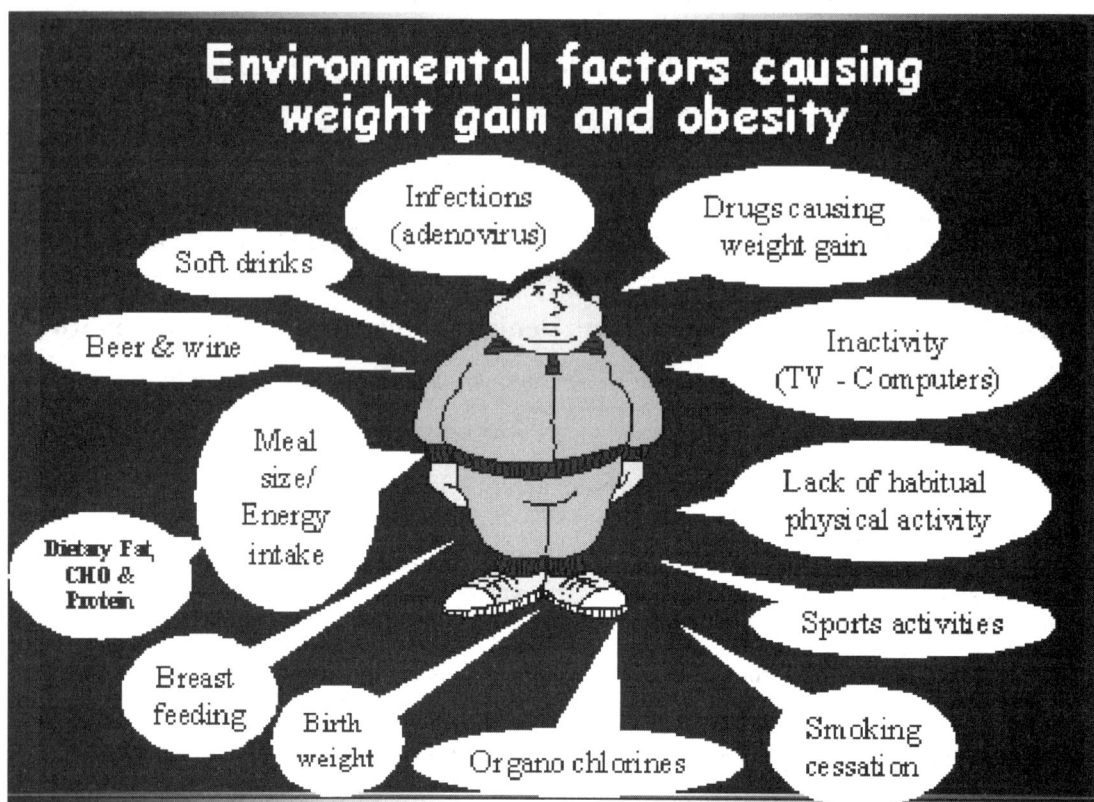

Fig. 1. Environmental factors contributing to weight gain and obesity. In the period from 1980 to 2002 in which population mean intakes of dietary fat has gone slightly down, the prevalence of overweight and obesity have continued to increase. This phenomenon has been called the 'American Paradox' and has been used as an arguments against any major role of dietary fat in the cause of the obesity epidemic. However, as shown in this cartoon many other risk factors of obesity have concomitantly changed so that the total risk has increased.

We are aware of four meta-analyses of controlled trials comparing low-fat diets with normal-fat diets as a control under *ad libitum* conditions.

In a systematic review and meta-analysis based on 28 intervention trials Bray and Popkin found that a reduction of 10 per cent in the proportion of energy from fat was associated with a reduction in weight of 16 g/d[2]. This corresponds to a weight loss of 2.9 kg over 6 months. We have conducted two more restrictive meta-analyses, including only studies with no intervention other than the *ad libitum* low-fat diet and a proper control[3-4]. The first analysis included a total of 1728 individuals, 1074 women and 654 men. Thirteen studies were randomized, controlled trials, 12 using a parallel design and one using a cross-over design. The control groups were either advised to continue their regular diet or to consume a diet with a fat content comparable to that of the background population. The low-fat interventions produced a weight loss of 2.4 kg more than in the control groups (95 per cent CI, 1.9–2.9; $P < 0.0001$) in the fixed effects analysis, and 2.5 kg more (1.5–3.5; $P < 0.0001$) in the random effects analysis. In a simple correlation analysis the major determinant of the weight loss difference was pre-treatment body weight ($r = 0.52$, $P < 0.05$). There was a dose-response relationship between the reduction in per cent dietary fat intake and weight loss after adjustment for pre-treatment body weight, ($r = 0.66$, $P < 0.005$). With no change in per cent dietary fat intake, no weight change occurred (intercept with 0: $P = 0.14$). The slope of the relation indicated that for every 1 per cent reduction in dietary fat a weight loss of 0.37 kg (0.15–0.60 kg/per cent) was achieved. Weight loss was not associated with the duration of the intervention.

Another meta-analysis, based on 37 dietary intervention studies, found weight loss in the intervention groups to be 2.79 kg larger than in the control groups, and there was a highly significant relation between reduction in dietary fat and weight loss[5]. For every 1 per cent decrease in energy from fat there was a 0.28 kg decrease in body weight.

Subsequently, we updated our initial meta-analysis and excluded trials in which the intervention group was instructed to increase physical activity in any way[5]. Two authors, independently of each other, selected the studies meeting the inclusion criteria and extracted data from 16 trials (duration of 2 ± 12 months) with 19 intervention groups, and enrolling a total of 1910 individuals. Fourteen of these studies were randomized. Weight loss was not the primary aim in 11 studies. Before the interventions the mean proportion of dietary energy from fat in the studies was 37.7 per cent in the low-fat groups, and 37.4 per cent in the control groups. The low-fat intervention produced a mean fat reduction of 10.2 per cent (8.1–12.3). Low-fat intervention groups showed a greater weight loss than control groups (3.2 kg, 1.9–4.5 kg; $P < 0.0001$), and a greater reduction in energy intake (1138 kJ/day, 564–1712 kJ/day, $P < 0.002$). A pre-treatment body weight 10 kg higher than the average was associated with a 2.6 kg greater difference in weight loss[5].

These four meta-analyses thus consistently show that a reduction in dietary fat without restriction of total energy intake causes reduction in caloric intake and weight loss in a dose-dependent fashion and may produce a modest, but clinically relevant, weight loss in overweight subjects.

Evidence from other lines of studies with lower evidence strength, such as experimental studies, consistently demonstrate that high-fat diets promote passive overconsumption of energy and increase the risk of weight gain and obesity (for review, see[6]). Observational studies, whether cross-sectional or longitudinal, also support that high dietary fat is positively associated with body weight and body fatness[7].

The non-fat component: carbohydrates and fibre

The importance of different types of carbohydrate on body weight has not been investigated as thoroughly as the role of the total fat content. A few recent studies have illuminated this area with regard to carbohydrate structure (e.g. simple/complex carbohydrates, sucrose/ starch). The largest and most recent one is the CARMEN multi-centre trial, which involved a total of 316 overweight subjects in five different countries[7]. In this study, the impact of 6 months' *ad libitum* intake of low-fat diets rich in either simple or complex carbohydrates on energy intake, body weight and risk factors was examined. The results showed that both low-fat diets reduced body weight by 1.6–2.4 kg compared with the normal-fat control diet, with no significant differences between simple and complex carbohydrates. The weight loss on both diets consisted mainly of fat mass. Furthermore, no detrimental effects on blood lipids were observed during either of the two carbohydrate diets. According to this study, the type of carbohydrate (simple sugars vs. complex carbohydrates) does not seem to have much importance for body weight regulation and risk factors as previously suggested.

The most probably reason for the observed weight loss on carbohydrate-rich diets is a spontaneous lower energy intake. Several mechanisms, probably all important, may be involved.

Firstly, the low energy density of carbohydrates is important. Thus one gram carbohydrate (17 kJ/g) provides less than half the calories of one gram fat (37 kJ/g). This fact means that a smaller amount of calories is consumed in a carbohydrate-rich meal than in a fat-rich meal of similar weight.

Secondly, but somewhat related, a starch- and fibre-rich diet often comprises surprisingly large volumes of foods. In one long-term study using such a diet, the large volume of foods was actually a problem for the volunteers to consume, especially for those with the highest energy requirements. The above two points together therefore mean that a much greater volume must be consumed in order to obtain a certain energy intake on a carbohydrate-rich diet. It is therefore plausible that energy intake decreases acutely and body weight decreases in the long term. This is a great advantage with regard to overweight. In developing countries the same effects may be hazardous and they are also a disadvantage for people engaging in elite sports, where a carbohydrate-rich diet is needed to optimize performance.

A third reason for a decreased energy intake is a slower gastric emptying rate on a fibre-rich diet. This effect, which may be related to an antral distention, is known to prolong feelings of fullness and satiety[6].

Fourthly, increased satiety due to increased plasma glucose (glucostatic theory) and liver glycogen concentrations (glycogenostatic theory) compared with a fat-rich diet may be important. The glucostatic theory has been supported by studies finding positive correlations between postprandial satiety and changes in plasma glucose and studies in rats and humans showing that meal initiation is preceded by a decrease in blood glucose concentration. Newer studies suggest that the glucose-induced plasma insulin increase is an important central satiety signal[8].

A fifth reason, which should also be considered, is the decreased energy availability of a high-fibre diet. Thus the ingestion of 64 g compared with 34 g dietary fibre/day for 10 weeks in lean healthy males, resulted in a reduction in protein utilization by 5.7 per cent and in fat utilization by 3.0 per cent. Total energy utilization decreased by 2.9 per cent equal to 400 kJ/day[9]. A theoretical calculation showed that if the fibre intake in a typical American diet was increased from 18 g/d to 36 g/d the amount of metabolizable energy would be reduced by 540 kJ/day.

Finally, carbohydrate-induced increases of satiating hormones (insulin, norepinephrine, GIP, GLP-1) may also play an important role.

Glycaemic index

The effects of a diet containing low or high GI foods on body weight have been very poorly investigated and the importance for energy balance is controversial[10–12]. In a systematic review of the different types of studies, Raben found that of the 31 studies that measured appetite sensations following low-Gi vs. high-GI meals, a low-GI meals produced greater satiety and reduced hunger in 15 studies, no difference was found in 14 studies, and in 2 studies the high-GI meals produced greatest satiety[11]. Similarly, among the 20 longer-term intervention studies identified, four studies found larger weight loss and 2 studies less weight loss on the low-GI diets, and 14 studies found no difference. Raben also points out that most of the studies are statistically underpowered to pick up clinically relevant differences in weight loss on the two types of diets.

A low-GI diet has in a majority of the published studies been found to produce favourable effects on risk markers of diabetes and cardiovascular diseases compared with a high-GI diet. Since most of the intervention studies have used diets aiming at energy balance or energy reduction the effects on body weight are, however, still unclear.

The non-fat component: soft drinks

It has been speculated that the removal of sucrose (carbohydrate) from the diet will increase the relative dietary fat content, which would then result in increased energy intake and body weight in the long term. A number of acute meal tests lasting from a few hours to 1–2 days have, however, produced conflicting results. In these studies sucrose have typically been exchanged for aspartame, saccharin and/or water and postprandial appetite sensations and/or *ad libitum* food intake have been monitored. Of more interest are therefore intervention studies lasting for weeks or months. The number of long term intervention studies (without caloric restriction) is scarce and have not lasted for more than 3 weeks. These intervention studies suggest, that an increased intake of artificial sweeteners decreases energy intake and body weight compared to sucrose. We investigated the effect of 10 week supplementation with either sucrose or artificial sweeteners on *ad libitum* food intake and body weight in two groups of overweight subjects[13]. About 80 per cent of the supplements were given as drinks and 28 per cent of the caloric intake came from sucrose in the sucrose group. Similar food items and volumes were given to the two groups. After 10 weeks, an increase in total energy intake (2.6 MJ/d), body weight (1.6 kg) and fat mass (1.3 kg) was seen in the sucrose group, whereas a decrease in the latter two (1.0 kg and 0.3 kg) was seen in the artificial sweetener group. One likely reason for the increased energy intake and body weight in the sucrose group is that about 70 per cent of the sucrose came from fluids. Calories from fluids have been shown to satisfy less than solid foods, and it is easier to overconsume energy when drinking compared with eating. That sucrose from fluids may be fattening was also suggested by a recent observational, prospective study in children, reporting that those with a high intake of sugar sweetened drinks were at an increased the risk of becoming overweight[14]. For overweight subjects it may therefore be preferential to choose drinks and foods containing artificial sweeteners rather than sucrose in order to prevent weight gain.

The non-fat component: protein

There is some concern that a high protein intake in infant formulas and during growth may increase the susceptibility to weight gain and obesity. However, a new study suggests that a high protein intake may be associated with a higher BMI due to a positive relationship with the size of the fat-free mass, not with body fat[15]. There is also a large body of experimental data to suggest that protein has a higher satiating power per calorie than carbohydrate and fat in adults. The impact on obesity and risk factors of replacing carbohydrate with protein in *ad libitum* low fat diets has been addressed in only one clinical trial. Two fat reduced diets (30 per cent of total energy), a high carbohydrate diet (protein 12 per cent of total energy) and a high-protein diet (protein 25 per cent of total energy) were compared in

65 obese patients[16]. Weight loss after 6 months was 5.1 kg in the high carbohydrate and 8.9 kg in the high protein groups, and more subjects lost >10 kg in the high protein group (35 per cent) than in the high carbohydrate group (9 per cent). The protein rich diet had no adverse effect on blood lipids, homocystein levels, renal function, or bone mineral density. Replacement of some dietary carbohydrate by protein in *ad libitum*, low fat diets may improve weight loss. More freedom to choose between protein rich and complex carbohydrate rich foods may encourage obese subjects to choose more lean meat and dairy products and hence improve adherence to low fat diets in weight reduction pro-grammes.

In conclusion, a dietary protein content up to 25 energy-% may be beneficial for weight regulation in adults (evidence category B). Protein allowances in diets for weight reduction and for diabetics of more than 20 energy- per cent should await confirmation of the positive results by more randomized trials.

Beer, wine and spirits

Even a moderate consumption of alcohol may constitute a significant part of the total energy intake. Studies using indirect calorimetry have shown that the thermogenic effect of a moderate alcohol intake corresponds to 18 to 28 per cent[17] of the energy it provides. The previous contention, based on studies with excessive intake in alcoholics[18], that alcohol is a non-nutritious substance which is totally dissipated as heat therefore appears to be a misconception and alcohol is now referred to as the forth macronutrient. But how does alcohol fit into a dietary regimen which aims for body weight control? There are several concerns to be raised. Alcohol may relieve the restrain on food intake resulting in a greater energy intake at the meals. Such an effect may be reflected by both a faster eating rate and an extended meal time when wine or beer are given as an appetizer compared to non-alcoholic drinks. In addition, alcohol may bypass the satiating impact from other macronutrients mediated by the different gastro-intestinal hormones. The response of gastro-intestinal hormones to alcohol is sparsely elucidated but pure alcohol has been reported not to elicit any CCK or gastrin release. However, inhibition of gastric emptying is probably a major factor for the role of these hormones in the termination of a meal and alcohol has been demonstrated also to retard gastric emptying when administered prior to the test meal by some undefined mechanisms[19]. A lack of or a blunted hormonal response to alcohol ingestion and absorption may mean that the energy in alcohol may not be compensated for in the same manner as is seen with the other macronutrients. Acute studies comparing *ad libitum* food intake when alcoholic beverages are consumed in fixed amounts with drinks containing isoenergetic amounts of other macronutrients have shown a higher energy intake with alcohol[20], while other experiments have failed to demonstrate such a difference. However, no or incomplete compensations for the energy in all sorts of beverages were detected in all these studies suggesting that appetite regulation responds insufficiently to energy in liquid form. Alcohol consumption may therefore promote a positive energy balance simply by being ingestion of liquid energy. A third concern is based on the capacity of alcohol to suppress the oxidation of other substrates. Alcohol is oxidized to acetate as instantly as possible in the liver, which in turn replaces fat as a substrate for peripheral oxidative metabolism.

In a study, 14 male subjects were instructed to drink 270 ml red wine at dinner during a 6-week period, but otherwise lived their normal daily life[21]. When compared to a control period, where the subjects refrained from drinking alcohol, no differences were found in body weight, body fat or energy intake assessed by a 3-day dietary record. Unfortunately, there are no other studies to support these results in other study groups and with other alcoholic beverages.

In conclusion, restrictions should be imposed on the intake of any energy dense beverage, alcoholic as well as non-alcoholic, if the aim is to achieve weight loss on a low fat diet. One may also have to consider that wine with its high energy density could be more risky to include in the daily life than light beer if body weight control is an important issue. Yet unpublished results from our lab are proposing that if red wine is provided *ad libitum* with an ordinary meal, total energy intake may be higher than if beer or soda is served. In the study, energy intake from the beverage was higher with wine and was not compensated for in the food intake.

Acknowledgements: Supported by grants from the Danish Medical Research Council and the Danish Food Technology and Nutrition Programme (FØTEK). Address reprint requests to A Astrup, FHE, Rolighedsvej 30, 1958 Frederiksberg C, Denmark.

Reference

1. Willett WC. Dietary fat plays a major role in obesity: no. *Obes Rev* 2002; 3: 59–68.

2. Bray GA, Popkin BM. Dietary fat intake does affect obesity. *Am J Clin Nutr* 1998; 68: 1157–1173.

3. Astrup A, Ryan L, Grunwald GK, Storgaard M, Saris W, Melanson E, Hill JO. The role of dietary fat in body fatness: evidence from a preliminary meta-analysis of *ad libitum* low fat dietary intervention studies. *Br J Nutr* 2000; 83 (Suppl 1): S25–32.

4. Astrup A, Grunwald GK, Melanson EL, Saris WHM, Hill JO. The role of low-fat diets in body weight control: a meta-analysis of *ad libitum* intervention studies. *Int J Obes* 2000; 24: 1545–52.

5. Yu-Poth S, Zhao G, Etherton T, Naglak M, Jonnalagadda, Kris-Etherton PM. Effects of the National Chelesterol Education Program's step I and step II dietary intervention programs on cardiovascular disease risk factors: a meta-analysis. *Am J Clin Nutr* 1999; 69: 632–46.

6. Astrup A, Buemann B, Flint A, Raben A. Low-fat diets and energy balance: how does the evidence stand in 2002? *Proc Nutr Soc* 2002; 61: 299–309.

7. Saris WHM, Astrup A, Prentice AM *et al*. Randomized controlled trial of changes in dietary carbohydrate/fat ratio and simple vs. complex carbohydrates on body weight and blood lipids. *Int J Obes* 2000; 24: 1310–18.

8. Verdich C, Toubro S, Buemann B, Lysgard Madsen J, Juul Holst J, Astrup A. The role of postprandial releases of insulin and incretin hormones in meal-induced satiety-effect of obesity and weight reduction. *Int J Obes Relat Metab Disord* 2001; 25: 1206–14.

9. Miles C. The metabolizable energy of diets differing in dietary fat and fiber measured in humans. *J Nutr* 1992; 122: 306–11.

10. Pawlak DB, Ebbeling CB, Ludwig DS. Should obese patients be counseled to follow a low-glycemic index diet? – Yes. *Obes Rev* 2002; 3: 235–43.

11. Raben A. Should obese patients be counseled to follow a low-glycemic index diet? – No. *Obes Rev* 2002; 3: 245–56.

12. Astrup A. The role of the glycemic index of foods in body weight regulation and obesity. Is more evidence needed? *Obes Rev* 2002; 3: 233.

13. Raben A, Vasilaras TH, Møller AC, Astrup A. Sucrose compared with artificial sweeteners: different effects on *ad libitum* food intake and body weight after 10 wk of supplementation in overweight subjects. *Am J Clin Nutr* 2002; 76: 721–93.

14. Ludwig DS, Peterson KE, Gortmaker SL. Relation between consumption of sugar-sweetened drinks and childhood obesity: a prospective, observational analysis. *Lancet* 2001; 357(9255): 505–8.

15. Hoppe C, Mølgaard C, Juul A, Michaelsen KF. Protein intake in infancy is related to body size but not to adiposity in 10-y old children. *Int J Obes Relat Metab Disord* 2001; S25: S64.

16. Skov AR, Toubro S, Rønn B, Holm L, Astrup A. Randomized trial on protein versus carbohydrate in *ad libitum* fat reduced diet for the treatment of obesity. *Int J Obes Relat Metab Disord* 1999; 23: 528–36.

17. Pirola RC, Lieber CS. The energy cost of the metabolism of drugs including ethanol. *Pharmacology* 1972; 7: 185–96.

18. Suter PM, Schutz Y, Jequier E. The effect of ethanol on fat storage in healthy subjects. *N Engl J Med* 1992; 326: 983–87.

19. Barboriak JJ, Meade RC. Effect of alcohol on gastric emptying in man. *Am J Clin Nutr* 1970; 23: 1151–53.

20. Westerterp-Plantenga MS, Verwegen CRT. The appetizing effect of an apéritif in overweight and normal-weight humans. *Am J Clin Nutr* 1999; 69: 205–12.

21. Cordain L, Bryan ED, Melby CL, Smith MJ. Influence of moderate daily wine consumption on body weight regulation and metabolism in healthy free-living males. *J Am Col Nutr* 1997; 16: 134–39.

Progress in Obesity Research: 9. Edited by *Geraldo Medeiros-Neto, Alfredo Halpern and Claude Bouchard*

CHAPTER 85

Do we have evidence that obesity prevention works?

T.P. Gill[1] and L. Lissner[2]

[1]*Centre for Public Health Nutrition, University of Sydney and the International Obesity TaskForce, Sydney, Australia;* [2]*Department of Primary Health Care, Sahlgrenska Academy at Göteborg University and Nordic School of Public Health, Sweden*
[e-mail: tim.gill@asso.org.au]

Introduction

Obesity rates are rising rapidly throughout the world and very few countries or communities have escaped this problem. Men, women and children are affected. Indeed, overweight, obesity and health problems associated with them are now so common and the rates have risen so quickly that many people question whether it is possible to prevent the problem[1,2]. According to the recent World Health Organization Consultation entitled 'Obesity: Preventing and Managing the Global Epidemic'[3], obesity prevention is one of the biggest challenges for the new millennium. Specifically, it was concluded that 'prevention of obesity should begin early in life and should involve the development and maintenance of lifelong healthy eating and physical activity patterns'. Moreover, prevention was described as 'not just the responsibility of individuals but also requiring structural changes in societies'. So is there any evidence that obesity prevention works or will work in the future? To answer that question it is important to first define what we mean by 'obesity prevention', how we define success and what do we require as evidence.

Prevention can occur on different levels. Traditionally prevention has been sub-classified into primary, secondary and tertiary interventions, an approach that has raised some ambiguity when applied to obesity prevention. For instance it is not clear how to classify prevention of adulthood obesity among obese children, or progression from overweight to obesity. As emphasized by the WHO Consultation, the current way of classifying preventive interventions is instead based on the level of intervention, and may be defined as universal/public health prevention (directed at all members of a community), selective prevention (directed at high-risk individuals and groups) and targeted prevention (directed at those with existing obesity or risk of obesity-related comorbidities).

When judging the evidence that obesity prevention is possible, it is necessary to consider the evidence at each of these levels of prevention. Within each type of intervention, it is then possible to apply different criteria of acceptable evidence. Clearly, it is not possible to apply usual standards of randomized controlled trials to broader levels of universal prevention, directed at all members of the community. On the other hand, targeted prevention programmes can and should apply such stringent standards whenever possible. The difficulties in evaluating the evidence from health promotion efforts is well recognized and has been summarized in the report of the WHO European Working group on Health Promotion Evaluation[4].

When assessing the success of an intervention it is also important to distinguish between the levels of intervention. The most common outcome measure usually applied to the evaluation of any obesity prevention programme is a significant reduction in the prevalence of obesity in the population. However, with such a strong secular increase in obesity an outright reduction in prevalence is highly unlikely and may be inappropriate even when interventions are intense and of long duration. Therefore the US Institute of Medicine proposed a range of appropriate outcomes for each level of obesity prevention[5]. Under their system appropriate policy and environmental changes, decreased rates of co-morbidities, prevention of weight gain in high risk individuals, improved lifestyle patterns as well as reduction in the mean population weight could be considered appropriate outcomes depending on the level of prevention.

The purpose of this dialogue is to evaluate the available evidence that obesity can be prevented. Dr. Gill will argue that we have evidence that prevention works, provided we are not clouded by narrow clinical view of obesity prevention and we have a public health perspective on what constitutes a successful intervention. However, Dr. Lissner will offer arguments that hard evidence is still lacking. They discuss evidence from community intervention trials, clinical trials, epidemiology and other indirect sources. These are summarized below.

Evidence from observational epidemiology

Although obesity prevalence is rising throughout the world there are certain countries and sections of society where rates have stabilized or reduced. For example between 1992 and 1998 the prevalence of childhood obesity dropped in Russia from 15.6 to 9.0 per cent[6]. In addition the rates of obesity in urban women in Brazil[7] and Japan[8] have also dropped in recent years. The mean BMI of a representative sample of middle-aged men and women in South West France has not increased over the past 15–20 years[9] and women from higher education grades in Finland showed far lower increases than the rest of the population, particularly in the 1970s to 1980s[10]. Similarly there are large variations in the level of obesity within similar countries in Europe with Norway and the Netherlands having much lower rates on obesity than Denmark and Sweden.

As mentioned previously, the wide evidence of the educational gradient in obesity is commonly given as a signal that educational programmes should work in halting the obesity epidemic. However, data from Finland[11] as well as Sweden[12,13] both suggest that the social gap is not continuing to get wider. Rather, obesity is affecting all social groups.

Observational epidemiologic studies can document the extent of the epidemic and can identify subgroups at risk who should be targeted for interventions. However this type of study cannot directly address whether prevention initiatives will work.

Intervention trials

Most of the available evidence, direct and indirect, on whether obesity prevention works, must come from intervention trials as opposed to observational studies. Thus, we have attempted to summarize the data from existing intervention studies below, separating into studies giving positive and negative results. This is not intended as a systematic review but as a balanced overview of available evidence on both sides of the debate.

Table 1 shows a list of trials that produced a positive impact on the weight status of the community. These examples have been drawn from all levels of obesity prevention and demonstrate a positive, although often small, effect of weight status. The strongest and most consistent evidence of the success of obesity prevention comes from targeted prevention trials, especially those studies that have addressed the progression to diabetes in persons identified as glucose intolerant. The four trials presented in the table have all produced significant reductions in diabetes rates by attention to exercise and diet with only small weight losses of around 3–4 kg on average. In addition, successful prevention of weight gain has been shown in community coronary heart disease prevention trials and school-based programmes.

Table 1. Evidence that prevention works

Study	Type of trial/level of prevention	Outcome	Reference
Pawtucket Heart Health programme	Community CHD prevention trial – Universal prevention Adults	Significant reduction in rate of increase of population mean BMI 1981–93	Carleton et al., 1995[14]
Mauritis NCD intervention programme	Community CHD prevention trial – Universal prevention Adults	Reduction in level of overweight and obesity in women from high in 1992 and stabilization in levels in men 1987–98	Zimmet et al., 2000[15]

Singapore Trim and Fit	School-based intervention – Universal prevention	Reduction in the level of obesity in children of over 2 per cent	Toh et al., 2002[16]
Keil study	School-based intervention – Universal prevention	Improvements in obesity-related behaviour and measures of adiposity (but not BMI) after 1 year	Muller et al., 2001[17]
Children's television reduction trial	School-based intervention – Universal prevention	Reduced body weight in children in intervention	Robinson, 1999[18]
Planet Health	School-based intervention – Universal prevention	Reduced adiposity in girls but not boys Improvements in obesity-related behaviours	Gortmaker et al., 1999[19]
Health-hunters	Intervention among offspring of the SOS trial participants – Selective prevention	Reduction in body weight in girls but not boys	Eiben, 2002[20]
Prevention trial for African American Women	Dietary intervention and group discussions in African American women and their daughters – Selective prevention	Improvements in fat intake but not body weight after 1 year	Stolley et al., 1997[21]
Diabetes Prevention trials Sweden 1991, China 1997, Finland 2000, USA 2001	Prevention of the progression to diabetes in adults with impaired GT – Targeted prevention	Reduction in body weight (1.8–6.0 per cent) Reduction in progression to diabetes (25–57 per cent)	Eiksson and Lingarde, 1991[22], Pan et al., 1997[23], Tuomilehto et al., 2001[24], Larkin, 2001[25]
Lifestyle Intervention trial	Intervention trial in adults with established CHD. Very low fat diet and exercise	Large weight loss and reduction in CVD risk	Ornish et al., 1998[26]
Epstein trials	Overweight children in family therapy – Targeted prevention	Reduced prevalence eof obesity after 10 years in family therapy groups	Epstein et al., 1994[27]
Flodmark trial	Family therapy intervention trail in 10–11-year-old very overweight children – Targeted prevention	Less progression of severe obesity in intervention group	Flodmark et al., 1993[28]

Table 2 lists a number of studies which suggest that evidence is lacking. The selected studies have been chosen on the basis of being large-scale public health interventions carried out in communities or schools. All of these studies could be considered to be aiming at universal prevention, although Pathways was conducted in a high-risk school population. It is very likely that other negative studies exist, both in the literature and particularly, in the 'never-published' category. Although the results of these trials were not statistically significant, in most cases the intervention community gained slightly less weight than the control community. One study is mentioned on both tables, because the authors reported a positive effect studying cross-sectional series of cohorts, but no difference when using longitudinal data comparing subjects who were present at all examinations[14]. Moreover, one of the 'negative' studies experienced a rather classic null finding, consisting of significant weight change in the intervention community, no such change in the control community, but no significant difference in changes or intervention effect[29]. Another negative study[30] reported no overall effect, but slightly more weight gain in the intervention area than the control area, possibly attributable to competition from smoking cessation efforts, a common situation in cardiovascular prevention campaigns. Most importantly when considering the studies together is the fact that most of the effort was placed on changing behaviour through knowledge, an approach which is no longer believed to be sufficient.

Finally, considering the two cited classroom interventions in children, educational efforts were strongly complemented with enhancing the physical education curriculum, and still there were no effects on anthropometric or direct indicators of body fatness in these ambitious, large-scale studies[31,32].

Table 2. Studies not providing evidence that prevention works

Study	Type of trial	Outcome	Reference
Minnesota Heart Health Programme (MHHP)	6-community CHD prevention	No overall effect of MHHP on BMI	Jeffery, 1995[33]
Stanford 5-city	Community CHD prevention	Similar rates of weight change in treatment and control cohorts	Farquhar, 1990[34]
Stanford 3 community	Community mass media CVD education	Marginal difference between two intervention areas and control community	Fortmann, 1981[35]
Pound of Prevention	Randomized (individual) trial consisting of no-contact control, education or education + incentives	No significant reduction in weight gain after 3 years with either intervention	Jeffery, 1999[36]
Pathways	School-based obesity intervention randomized to 41 schools	No significant 3-year difference in body fat or BMI. Reported differences in diet	Lohman et al., 2001[32]
CATCH	School-based randomized multicentre trial for CVD promotion in 96 schools	No significant effect on weight status after 2.5 years	Webber, 1996[31]
German Cardiovascular Prevention Study	Community intervention in six regions, one control region	3.5 year interim results: intervention +0.8 kg/m^2, reference +0.3 kg/m^2 (ns), decrease in smoking	Greiser, 1993[30]
Kilkenny Health Project	Community intervention, chronic disease reduction/universal	Both communities gained weight, only significant in control community, difference in difference not significant	Shelley et al., 1995[29]
Pawtucket	Community wide education	Effect not seen in cohort comparisons, only cross-sectionally, comparison city started out heavier	Carleton, 1995[14]
North Karelia Project	Community level health promotion	'Results not conclusive, but encouraging'	McAlister, 1982[37]

Other evidence

In addition to intervention trials that have addressed obesity or obesity-related behaviours there is a range of indirect evidence which either supports or opposes the proposition that obesity can be prevented.

Breastfeeding

There is some evidence that breastfeeding protects against the development of obesity in children who are breastfed for reasonable periods. Gilmann et al.[38] in a retrospective observational study found a significant odds ratio of 0.78 for adolescent overweight associated with breastfeeding. In contrast, Hediger et al.[39] using a similar design, found no reduced risk of being overweight associated with previous breastfeeding, but 'a reduced risk of being at risk'. Since these were both retrospective studies, the possibility of reporting error must be consdiered, as well as residual confounding by unmeasured factors that may relate both to breastfeeding and subsequent obesity.

Changes in dietary and exercise habits in children

It can be argued that poor diet and physical activity behaviours established in childhood and carried into adulthood are a major cause of chronic energy imbalance that leads to obesity and thus if appropriate behaviours can be established early in life it would make a major contribution to obesity prevention. However, certain potential fallacies of extrapolation must be considered.

Many intervention studies (set out above) which have failed to have a significant impact on body weight have still been able to demonstrate a positive influence on obesity-related behaviours such as fat intake, participation in physical activity or reduced levels of inactivity. A longitudinal study of fruit and vegetable consumption in children[40] showed that interventions can lead to improved behaviours over time and not just post intervention. Improvements in the intake of fruit and low fat snacks can be achieved by a simple manipulation of the price structure to make them more financially appealing[41].

Physical activity

Fogelholm[42] conducted a systematic review of the evidence from randomized trials and observational epidemiology that physical activity prevents weight gain. In the trials, mean weight regain was 0.28 kg/month with exercise and 0.33 kg/month without. The evidence from observational studies was mixed. It is concluded that 'the role of prescribed physical activity in prevention of weight gain remains modest'.

Past public health interventions

Other evidence that obesity can be prevented could be drawn from an examination of past public health programmes to tackle other chronic non-communicable diseases and risk factors such as CHD and smoking. All current obesity prevention initiatives have been short-term and addressed only a small number of contributing factors with little attention on environmental change. Much valuable evidence can be drawn from extensive community interventions such as the North Karelia project which took 10–20 years of sustained action over a variety of settings including education, policy change, fiscal interventions and improved health care to achieve meaningful improvements in health behaviours and CVD outcomes[43].

Discussion

There can be little doubt that obesity prevention offers the greatest hope for tackling the every increasing epidemic of obesity. However, the question remains as to whether we have sufficient evidence to indicate that obesity prevention works. As summarized in the concluding table, various arguments and counter-arguments have made in this debate.

Table 3. Summary of arguments pro and con

PRO	CON
A range of intervention studies show statistically significant effects on weight	Many of these effects are small and clinically insignificant Equally many studies show no effects and publication bias makes it likely that many more exist
Less educated sub-populations are at risk of obesity, so education related efforts should prevent obesity	Education-only interventions have been notoroiously ineffective, and the social gap is not obviously widening
Small changes demonstrated in the short term will produce important changes in the long-term	Fallacy of interpolation
We haven't always had the majority of the population being overweight, so prevention must be possible	In our current environment of ubiquitous food availability and predominant physical inactivity, there is no way to reverse the clock

Even unsuccessful inteventions (vis-à-vis weight) have observed promising changes in dietary and physical activity behaviours	Social desirability reporting biases may potentially invalidate much of this data
The strongest evidence that obesity can be prevented is in children	Lets get some more evidence that the improvements last until adulthood
Community level interventions cannot be judged by the standards of RCTs – other types of evidence more important (process-oriented etc)	Not normally viewed as acceptable level of evidence

In conclusion, despite the arguments pro and con summarized above, the discussants in this dialogue were able to agree on the following:

Do we have enough indirect evidence to support a *belief* in prevention?	Yes
Do we have *scientific* evidence that previous interventions have worked?	Some
Do we have evidence of *large* effects?	No
Do we have *enough consistent* evidence?	No
Do we have *sufficient evidence to act*?	Yes

Reference

1. Crawford D, Jeffery RW, French SA. Can anyone successfully control their weight? Findings of a three year community-based study of men and women. *Int J Obes* 2000; 24(9): 1107–10.

2. Foreyt J, Goodrick K. The ultimate triumph of obesity. *Lancet* 1995; 346(8968): 134–5.

3. World Health Organization (WHO). Obesity: Preventing and managing the global epidemic. Report of a WHO Consultation: WHO Technical Report Series 894 Geneva: World Health Organization, 2000.

4. World Health Organization (WHO). Health Promotion Evaluation: Recommendations to Polocymakers. Report of the WHO European Working Group on Health Promotion Evaluation. WHO Regional Office for Europe, Copenhagen,1999.

5. US Institute of Medicine. Reducing risks for mental disorders: Frontiers for preventative intervention research. Report of the Committee on Prevention of Medical Disorders. Div. Biobehavioural Sciences and Mental Disorders. Washington: National Academy Press, 1994.

6. Wang Y, Carlos Monteir C, and Popkin B. Trends of obesity and underweight in older children and adolescents in the United States, Brazil, China, and Russia. *Am J Clin Nutr* 2002; 75: 971–7.

7. Monteiro CA, D-A Benicio MH, Conde WL, Popkin BM. Shifting obesity trends in Brazil. *Eur J Clin Nutr* 2000; 54(4): 342–46.

8. Yoshiike N, Seino F, Tajima S, Aria Y, Kawano M, Furhata T, Inoue S. Twenty year changes in the prevalence of overweight in Japanese adults: The national nutrition survey 1976–95. *Obes Rev* 2002; 3: 183–90.

9. Marques-Vidal P., Ruidavets J-B, Cambou J-P, Ferrières J. Trends in overweight and obesity in middle-aged subjects from southwestern France, 1985–1997. *Int J Obes* 2002; 26: 732–34.

10. Lahti-Koski M, Vartiainen E, Mannisto S, Pietinen P Age, education and occupation as determinants of trends in body mass index in Finland from 1982 to 1997. *Int J Obes* 2000; 24(12): 1669–76.

11. Lahti-Koski M, Jousilahti P, Pietinen. Secular trends in body mass index by birth cohort in eastern Finland from 1972 to 1997. *Int J Obes* 2001; 25: 727–34.

12. Lissner L, Johansson SE, Rössner S, Qvist J, Wolk A. Social mapping of the obesity epidemic in Sweden. *Int J Obes* 2000; 24: 801–5.

13. Eiben G, Bengtsson C, Björkelund C, Dey D, Lissner L, Steen B. Obesity in 70-year old Swedes. Secular changes over a period of 30 years (abstract), Annual Meeting of the Swedish Medical AssociationGöteborg. Sweden; 2002.

14. Carleton RA, Lasater TM, Assaf AR, Feldman HA, McKinlay S. The Pawtucket Heart Health Program: Community Changes in Cardiovascular Risk factors and Projected Disease Risk. *Am J Pub Health* 1995; 5: 777–85.

15. Zimmet P. Diabetes and obesity worldwide – epidemics in full flight. Presented at the 60th Scientific Sessions of the American Diabetes Association; 10 June 2000; San Antonio, Texas.

16. Toh CM, Cutter J, Chew SK. School based intervention has reduced obesity in Singapore. *BMJ* 2002; 324: 7334–427.

17. Muller MJ, Asbeck I, Mast M, Langnase K, Grund A. Prevention of obesity-more than an intention. Concept and first results of the Kiel Obesity Prevention Study (KOPS). *Int J Obes* 2001; 25 (Suppl 1): S66–74.

18. Robinson TN. Reducing Children's Television Viewing to Prevent Obesity: A Randomized Controlled Trial. *JAMA* 1999; 282: 1561–67.

19. Gortmaker SL, Must A, Sobol AM, Peterson K, Colditz GA, Dietz WH. Television viewing as a cause of increasing obesity among children in the United States, 1986–1990. *Arch Pediatr Adolesc Med* 1996; 150(4): 356–62.

20. Eiben G, Lissner L. Health-Hunters (abstract, Swedish). Presented at the annual meeting of the Swedish Dietetic Association. Göteborg: Sweden; 2002.

21. Stolley MR, Fitzgibbon ML. Effects of an obesity prevention program on the eating behaviour of African American mothers and daughters. *Health Educ Behav* 1997; 24: 152–64.

22. Eriksson J, Forsen T, Tuomilehto J, Osmond C, Barker D. Size at birth, childhood growth and obesity in adult life. *Int J Obes* 2001; 25(5): 735–40.

23. Pan X-R, Lil G-W Hu Y-U *et al*. Effects of diet and exercise in preventing NIDDM in people with impaired glucose tolerance. *Diabetes Care* 1997; 20(4): 537–44.

24. Tuomilehto J, Lindstrom J, Eriksson JG, Valle TT, Hamalainen H, Ilanne_Parikka P *et al*. Prevention of type 2 diabetes mellitus by changes in lifestyle among subjects with impaired glucose tolerance. *N Engl J Med* 2001; 344(18): 1343–50.

25. Larkin M. Diet and exercise delay onset of type 2 diabetes, say US experts. *Lancet* 2001; 358: (Issue 9281) 563.

26. Ornish D, Scherwitz LW, Billings JH, Brown SE, Gould KL, Merritt TA, Sparler S, Armstrong WT, Ports TA, Kirkeeide RL, Hogeboom C, Brand RJ. Intensive lifestyle changes for reversal of coronary heart disease. *JAMA* 1998; 280(23): 2001–7.

27. Epstein LH, Valoski A, Wing RR, McCurley J. Ten-year outcomes of behavioral family-based treatment for childhood obesity. *Health Psychol* 1994; 13(5): 373–83.

28. Flodmark C-E, Ohlsson T, Ryden O, Sveger T. Prevention of progression to severe obesity in a groups of obese schoolchildren treated with family therapy. *Pediatrics* 1993; 91: 880–4.

29. Shelley E, Daly L, Collins C, Christie M, Conroy R, Gibney M *et al*. Cardiovascular risk factor changes in the Kilkenny Health Project. A community Health Promotion Programme. *Eur Heart J* 1995; 16: 752–60.

30. Greiser EM for German Cardiovascular Prevention Study Group. Risk factor Trends and Cardiovascular Mortality Risk after 3.5 years of Community-based Intervention in the German Cardiovascular Prevention Study. *Ann Epidemiol* 1993; 3 (Suppl): S13–S27.

31. Wang Y, Carlos Monteir C, Popkin B. Trends of obesity and underweight in older children and adolescents in the United States, Brazil, China, and Russia. *Am J Clin Nutr* 2002; 75: 971–7.

32. Lohman TG, Going S, Stweart D, Caballero B, Stevens J, Himes J *et al*. The effect of Pathways Obesity Prevention Study on Body Composition in Americna Children. *FASEB J* 2001; p.15 (abstract).

33. Jeffery RW, Gray CW, French SA, Hellerstedt WL, Murray D, Luepker RV, Blackburn H. Evaluation of weight reduction in a community intervention for cardiovascular disease risk: changes in body mass index in the minnesota Heart Health Program. *Int J Obes* 1995; 19: 30–9.

34. Farquhar JW, Fortmann SP, Flora JA, Taylor B, Haskell WL, Williams PT, Maccoby N, Wood PD. Effects of Coommnitywide Education on Cardiovascular Disearse Risk Factors. The Stanford Five-City Project. *JAMA* 1990; 264: 359–5.

35. Fortmann SP, Williams PT, Hulley SB, Haskell WL, Farquhar JW. Effect of health education on dietary beharior: the Stanford Three Community Study. *Am J Clin Nutr* 1981; 34: 2030–38.

36. Jeffery RW, French SA. Preventing Weight Gain in Adults: The Pound of Prevention Study. *Am J Public Health* 1999; 89: 747–51.

37. McAlister A, Puska P, Salonen JT, Tuomilehto J, Koskela K. Theory and Action for Health Promotion: Illustrations from the North Karelia Project. *Am J Public Health* 1982; 72: 43–50.

38. Gillman MW, Rifas-Shiman SL, Camargo CA, Berkey CS, Frazier AL, Rockett HRH, Field AE, Colditz GA. Risk of overweight among adolescents who were breastfed as infants. *JAMA* 2001; 285: 2461.67.

39. Hediger ML, Overpeck MD, Kuczmarski RJ, Ruan WJ. Association between infant breastfeeding and overweight in young children. *JAMA* 2001; 285: 2453–60.

40. Baranowski T, Mendlein J, Resicnow K, Frank E, Cullen, KW, Baranowski J. Physical activity and nutrition in children and youth: An overview of obesity prevention. *Prev Med* 2000; 31: s1–s10.

41. French SA, Story M, Jeffery RW. Environmental influences on eating and physical activity. *Ann Rev Public Health* 2001; 22: 309–35.

42. Fogelholm M, Kukkonen-Harjula K. Does physical activity prevent weight gain – a systematic review. *Obes Rev* 2000; 1: 95–111.

43. Puska P, Tuomilehto J, Nissinen A, Vartiainen E, editors. *The North Karelia Project: 20 years results and experiences.* Helsinki: National Public Health Institute, 1995.

Progress in Obesity Research: 9. Edited by *Geraldo Medeiros-Neto, Alfredo Halpern* and *Claude Bouchard*
©2003 John Libbey Eurotext Ltd, pp. 410–413.

CHAPTER 86

Smoking cessation in the development of obesity

Bruce B. Duncan

[1]*Graduate Studies Programme in Epidemiology, School of Medicine, Federal University of Rio Grande do Sul, Porto Alegre, RS, Brazil*
[e-mail: bbduncan@orion.ufrgs.br]

Risk of weight gain upon smoking cessation

Smokers are reported frequently[1,2], though not always[3], to have lower body mass indices than non-smokers. However, they pay a heavy price, in terms of weight gain, upon quitting. Data from US national representative samples are illustrative. Smoking quitters of 25 to 74 years of age, first examined the First National Health and Nutrition Examination Survey (NHANES I, 1971 to 1975) and then weighed a second time in the NHANES I Epidemiologic Follow-up Study (1982 to 1984), had adjusted weight gain attributable to the cessation of smoking of 2.8 kg (men) and 3.8 kg (women)[1]. The relative risk of major weight gain (greater than 13 kg) in those who quit smoking (as compared with those who continued to smoke) was 8.1 (95%CI, 4.4 to 14.9) in men and 5.8 (95%CI, 3.7 to 9.1) in women, and it remained high regardless of the duration of cessation. Blacks were at higher risk of major weight gain after quitting smoking. A similar analysis[4] was based on more recent (1988 through 1991) cross-sectional data of the Third National Health and Nutrition Examination Survey, which investigated 5247 adults 35 years of age or older. The investigators estimated 10 year weight gain comparing weight measured at the time of the exam with reported weight of 10 years earlier. The weight gain associated with the cessation of smoking (i.e. the difference in gain between smokers who quit and those who continued) was 4.4 kg for men and 5.0 kg for women. Smokers who had quit within the past 10 years had significantly greater adjusted odds to become overweight – 2.4 times those who had never smoked (95%CI 1.0 – 5.8) for men and 2.0 times for women (95%CI 1.0 – 3.9).

A 1998 systematic review found that, on average, sustained quitters gain about 5 to 6 kg in weight[5]. The risk of weight gain is highest during the 2 years immediately following smoking cessation, and declines thereafter.

Data of Klesges *et al.*[6] suggest that many studies may underestimate weight gain, to the extent that they utilized a single point estimate of cessation. They characterized 196 volunteers who participated in a smoking cessation programme as continuously smoking; continuously abstinent; or abstinent at one point, the 1-year follow-up visit, but not at others. Continuously abstinent participants gained 5.9 kg at 1 year, whereas those abstinent at 1 year but not consistently so throughout the study gained only 3.0 kg.

In this regard, one large and particularly well designed study[7], observing weight gain within the context of a randomized clinical trial of smoking cessation, demonstrated notably large gains. This report compared weight gain over a 5-year follow-up period in a cohort of 5,887 male and female smokers in the United States and Canada, aged 35–60 years, who were randomized to either smoking intervention or usual care. Among participants who achieved sustained quitting for 5 years, women gained, on average 5.2 kg the first year after quitting, and an additional 3.4 kg over the ensuing study years. Men gained a mean of 4.9 kg over the first year, and an additional 2.6 kg over the ensuing years. Over 5 years, 33 per cent of sustained quitters gained ≥ 10 kg compared with 6 per cent of continuing smokers. This study emphasizes also the extended nature of the phenomenon.

Physical exercise, older age, higher baseline body mass index, and lower rates of smoking attenuate the degree of weight gained after smoking cessation. Though ex-smokers may not, as a group, end up

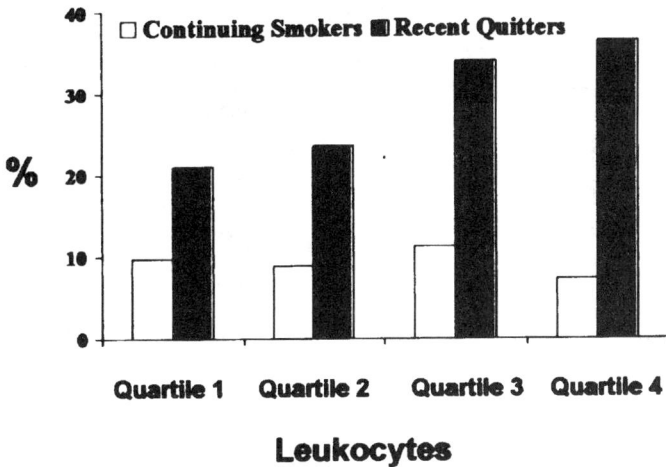

Fig. 1. Adjusted incidence of a large weight gain (per cent) in continuing smokers (white bars) and recent quitters (shaded bars) across quartiles of leukocyte count at baseline. Proportions estimated through logistic regression modeling adjusting to sample means for age, ethnicity, centre, gender and baseline weight, height, educational level, physical activity, cigarettes smoked per day and fasting insulin. Atherosclerosis Risk in Communities (ARIC) Study.

weighing more than never smokers, they do, as a group, in middle age, have a more central fat distribution[8].

The public health importance of smoking cessation as a contributing cause to the current obesity epidemic is little recognized. Flegal *et al.*, utilizing data from the third National Health and Nutrition Examination Survey[4] investigated the extent to which smoking cessation, in the presence of declining smoking prevalence, could be considered to contribute to the increasing prevalence of overweight. The proportion of US adults 35 to 74 years of age who were overweight increased by 9.6 per cent for men and 8.0 per cent for women from 1978 to 1990. Comparing this real distribution of weight gain with one based on hypothetical calculations which assumed that those who quit gained the same as continuing smokers, these authors estimated that about a quarter (2.3 of 9.6 percentage points) of the 10 year increase in the prevalence of overweight for men and about a sixth (1.3 of 8.0 percentage points) of the increase for women could be attributed to smoking cessation. Expressed in terms of the overall prevalence of obesity, the fraction of obesity attributable to smoking cessation over the previous decade would be 6.0 per cent for men and 3.2 per cent for women.

Of note is that sustained weight gain upon quitting is not reported universally. For example, a cross-sectional study analysing data from periodic health examinations for Japanese working men found little difference in the means of BMI between smoking quitters and current smokers 8–10 years after quitting[9]. For unknown reasons, many of the health risks of smoking appear less pronounced in Japan. Japan also has a lower prevalence of obesity than other countries with a similar level of affluence.

Further, this weight gain is not inevitable. For instance, in the setting of US military basic training, where access to food is limited and physical activity is emphasized, quitting smoking was not associated with weight gain[10].

Pathophysiology of weight gain upon cessation of smoking

Why smoking cessation should lead to weight gain is not clear. Nicotine has been cited by some as the culprit. Studies show an inverse association between weight gain and level of nicotine among those utilizing nicotine as an aid to quitting[11]. Nicotine raises levels of serotonin and dopamine in the lateral hypothalamic region, an area of the brain believed to be involved in the regulation of caloric ingestion[12]. Additionally, abstention from nicotine is associated with an increase in insulin[13], which, in turn, is associated with weight gain in adults[14]. More recently, smoking cessation has been shown to raise adipose tissue lipoprotein lipase (AT-LPL) activity[15]. Almost certainly, as signaling pathways for weight homeostasis become clearer over the next several years, additional mechanistic explanations for this smoking cessation effect will appear.

Possible importance of the presence of mild inflammation at quitting

A chronic, mild, systemic inflammatory state has been shown to precede and predict cardiovascular diseases and diabetes, as well as to be associated with the metabolic syndrome[16]. We have demonstrated in the ARIC Study, investigating weight change over a 3 year period of a biethnic cohort of 13017 middle-aged men and women, that elevated fibrinogen and leukocyte counts, as well as altera-

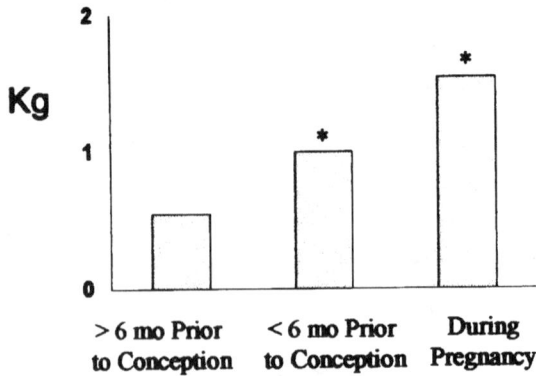

Fig. 2. Difference in weight gained during pregnancy, compared to that of never-smokers, for ex-smokers, in accordance with the moment of quitting smoking, adjusted through multiple linear regression for age, ethnicity, parity, clinical centre and pre-pregnancy body mass index. Brazilian Study of Gestational Diabetes, 1991–95. *$P < 0.05$ in comparison with non-smokers.

tion in several other markers of a chronic systemic inflammatory state, predict greater weight gain[17]. For example, study participants in the highest quartile of fibrinogen gained an estimated 0.23 kg/year more than those in the lowest quartile over 3 years of follow-up ($P < 0.001$).

We have recently extended this investigation, comparing gain in the individuals who continued to smoke with that in those who quit smoking during the 3 year follow-up. A large weight gain was defined as ≥ the 90th percentile of gains in the cohort. Figure 1 displays the adjusted percentage of individuals with large weight gains among continuing smokers and recent quitters, stratified by quartile of leukocyte count. As can be seen, there was relatively little difference in gain across leukocyte quartile in continuing smokers. In contrast, in quitters, the extent of the gain was directly proportional to baseline white cell count. This interaction between leukocyte count and quitting smoking, with respect to weight gain, was of borderline statistical significance ($P = 0.06$). However, the interaction, when the association was expressed in terms of the statistically more powerful endpoint of mean weight gain, was statistically significant ($P = 0.01$), as was a similar interaction between baseline fibrinogen level and smoking cessation ($P = 0.001$).

Smoking cessation and pregnancy

As pregnancy is a moment of important fat accumulation, often partially retained post-partum[18], we recently investigated the effect of quitting smoking on additional weight gain during pregnancy. We analysed data of 4000 pregnant women of greater ≥ 20 years of age, without known diabetes mellitus, interviewed between 20 and 28 weeks of pregnancy and then followed to delivery in general prenatal services in 6 Brazilian state capital cities between 1991 and 1995. We asked women about their pre-pregancy weight and their previous and current smoking history, and obtained data on their weights during pregnancy from chart review. At interview, 23 per cent were ex-smokers, and of these, 27.9 per cent had stopped during the pregnancy. Figure 2 displays the results for quitters. In multiply-adjusted analyses, those who had quit at least 6 months prior to pregancy gained 0.53 (95%CI 0.12–1.2) kg more than never smokers, those who quit during the 6 months immediately preceding pregnancy 1.0 (95%CI 0.31–1.7) kg more, and those who quit during pregnancy 1.5 (0.78–2.3) kg more. Additionally, continuing smokers gained 0.44 (IC95 per cent –0.11–0.98) kg more for every 10 cigarettes they reported decreasing during early pregnancy.

A possible extension of the effect of smoking cessation, of major potential public health importance, was recently reported by Montgomery and Eckbom[19,20], They investigated the effect of what might be interpreted as smoking cessation in the newborn. Utilizing data are from the British National Child Development Study (NCDS), based on an initial survey of births in March 1958, the authors characterized risk of obesity at ages 23 and 33 in the 11,359 offspring with available follow-up data. Maternal smoking status during pregnancy was characterized during the initial survey as non-, medium (1–9 cigarettes/day), heavy (> 10 cigarettes/day), and variable (a balance of medium and heavy) smoking. Height and weight of offspring were measured in follow-up examinations at ages 23 and 33. The adjusted odds ratios (and 95 per cent confidence intervals) for obesity at age 23 in offspring of smoking mothers, compared with offspring of non-smoking mothers, were 1.55 (0.97 to 2.47) 2.02 (1.07 to 3.82) and 2.56 (1.63 to 4.02) for medium, variable and heavy smoking in mothers, respectively. At age 33, these odds ratios had decreased somewhat, to 1.34 (1.07 to 1.69), 1.35 (0.95 to 1.92), and 1.38 (1.06 to 1.79), respectively, but still presented a statistically significant trend ($P = 0.003$).

In conclusion, smoking cessation is an important risk factor for weight gain in adulthood, and greater weight gain in pregnancy. Smokers having higher leukocyte counts and fibrinogen levels, perhaps indicating the presence of a chronic mild systemic inflammatory state, appear to be most susceptible to this gain. For women continuing to smoke during pregnancy, the risk of weight gain appears to be shifted to their offspring. The apparently ensuing increased weight gain in the offspring, likely due to withdrawal from smoking at a critical period, may provide an important mechanism by which smoking cessation can play a major role in the current epidemic of obesity.

References

1. Williamson DF, Madans J, Anda RF, Kleinman JC, Giovino GA, Byers T. Smoking cessation and severity of weight gain in a national cohort. *N Engl J Med* 1991; 324(11): 739–45.

2. Eisen SA, Lyons MJ, Goldberg J, True WR. The impact of cigarette and alcohol consumption on weight and obesity. An analysis of 1911 monozygotic male twin pairs. *Arch Intern Med* 1993; 153(21): 2457–63.

3. Klesges RC, Ward KD, Ray JW, Cutter G, Jacobs DR, Jr., Wagenknecht LE. The prospective relationships between smoking and weight in a young, biracial cohort: the Coronary Artery Risk Development in Young Adults Study. *J Consult Clin Psychol* 1998; 66(6): 987–93.

4. Flegal KM, Troiano RP, Pamuk ER, Kuczmarski RJ, Campbell SM. The influence of smoking cessation on the prevalence of overweight in the United States. *N Engl J Med* 1995; 333(18): 1165–70.

5. Froom P, Melamed S, Benbassat J. Smoking cessation and weight gain. *J Fam Pract* 1998; 46(6): 460–64.

6. Klesges RC, Winders SE, Meyers AW, Eck LH, Ward KD, Hultquist CM et al. How much weight gain occurs following smoking cessation? A comparison of weight gain using both continuous and point prevalence abstinence. *J Consult Clin Psychol* 1997; 65(2): 286–291.

7. O'Hara P, Connett JE, Lee WW, Nides M, Murray R, Wise R. Early and late weight gain following smoking cessation in the Lung Health Study. *Am J Epidemiol* 1998; 148(9): 821–830.

8. Duncan BB, Chambless LE, Schmidt MI, Szklo M, Folsom AR, Carpenter MA et al. Correlates of body fat distribution. Variation across categories of race, sex, and body mass in the atherosclerosis risk in communities study. The Atherosclerosis Risk in communities (ARIC) Study Investigators. *Ann Epidemiol* 1995; 5(3): 192–200.

9. Sakurai Y, Umeda T, Shinchi K, Honjo S, Wakabayashi K, Todoroki I et al. Relation of total and beverage-specific alcohol intake to body mass index and waist-to-hip ratio: a study of self-defense officials in Japan. *Eur J Epidemiol* 1997; 13(8): 893–98.

10. Talcott GW, Fiedler ER, Pascale RW, Klesges RC, Peterson AL, Johnson RS. Is weight gain after smoking cessation inevitable? *J Consult Clin Psychol* 1995; 63(2): 313–16.

11. Doherty K, Militello FS, Kinnunen T, Garvey AJ. Nicotine gum dose and weight gain after smoking cessation. *J Consult Clin Psychol* 1996; 64(4): 799–807.

12. Miyata G, Meguid MM, Fetissov SO, Torelli GF, Kim HJ. Nicotine's effect on hypothalamic neurotransmitters and appetite regulation. *Surgery* 1999; 126(2): 255–63.

13. Assali AR, Beigel Y, Schreibman R, Shafer Z, Fainaru M. Weight gain and insulin resistance during nicotine replacement therapy. *Clin Cardiol* 1999; 22(5): 357–60.

14. Folsom AR, Vitelli LL, Lewis CE, Schreiner PJ, Watson RL, Wagenknecht LE. Is fasting insulin concentration inversely associated with rate of weight gain? Contrasting findings from the CARDIA and ARIC study cohorts. *Int J Obes Relat Metab Disord* 1998; 22(1): 48–54.

15. Ferrara CM, Kumar M, Nicklas B, McCrone S, Goldberg AP. Weight gain and adipose tissue metabolism after smoking cessation in women. *Int J Obes Relat Metab Disord* 2001; 25(9): 1322–26.

16. Duncan BB, Schmidt MI. Chronic activation of the innate immune system may underlie the metabolic syndrome. *Sao Paulo Med J* 2001; 119(3): 122–27.

17. Duncan BB, Schmidt MI, Chambless LE, Folsom AR, Carpenter M, Heiss G. Fibrinogen, other putative markers of inflammation, and weight gain in middle-aged adults – the ARIC study. Atherosclerosis Risk in Communities. *Obes Res* 2000; 8(4): 279–86.

18. Kac G. Determinant factors of postpartum weight retention: a literature review. *Cad Saude Publica* 2001; 17(3): 455–466.

19. Montgomery SM, Ekbom A. Smoking during pregnancy and diabetes mellitus in a British longitudinal birth cohort. *BMJ* 2002; 324(7328): 26–7.

20. Montgomery SM. Re: Smoking out feeding's impact. *BMJ* 2002; 324: http: //bmj.com/cgi/eletters/324–7328/26.

Progress in Obesity Research: 9. Edited by *Geraldo Medeiros-Neto, Alfredo Halpern* and *Claude Bouchard*

©2003 John Libbey Eurotext Ltd, pp. 414–417.

CHAPTER 87

Environmental determinants of obesity: socioeconomic status, education and wealth

John P. Foreyt

Baylor College of Medicine, Houston, TX 77030, USA
[e-mail: jforeyt@bcm.tmc.edu]

Obesity is a major health hazard in most areas of the world. There are now more than 300 million obese individuals worldwide and more than 750 million overweight[1]. Data from the United States suggest that the entire population will be obese by the year 2230[2]. Obesity is associated with increased risks for morbidity and mortality, along with significant increases in health care costs for its comorbid conditions, especially type 2 diabetes and hypertension.

The aetiology of obesity is clearly multifactorial, although environmental forces appear to be the major determinant of the condition. This paper reviews socioeconomic status, education, and wealth as determinants of body weight.

The role of the environment

Obesity only recently has become a major health issue. It is still a relatively uncommon problem in non-industrial societies, although that fact appears to be changing quickly as societies shift to western lifestyles. Obesity is essentially absent in societies that exist as hunter-gatherers[3,4] (Table 1).

Table 1. Obesity is an environmental issue

- Obesity is a relatively recent public health concern

- Obesity is virtually nonexistent among hunter-gatherers

- Populations that transition to 'westernized lifestyles' experience significant and predictable increases in obesity and the 'diseases of civilization'

While obesity is increasing significantly in many societies, the reasons for the increase are not always apparent. The human gene pool has not changed in any real sense over the last 35,000 years, although the environment we live in has changed dramatically[5,6]. Obesity results primarily from a mismatch between our lifestyles and our genes. The western lifestyle is strongly associated with chronic and degenerative diseases[7]. The lifestyles of societies which still exist as hunter-gatherers suggest that in the distant past we had been significantly more active and our diets had been much less energy dense, with more fibre and less fat and calories than today[8]. Interestingly, the same genes that helped our ancestors survive are now a serious liability in a world with an abundance of food and little need to be active. Today, the main factors responsible for obesity are found in our environment. Our environment promotes the development of obesity through over-nutrition and under-activity. Socioeconomic status, education, and wealth play major roles in determining its development.

Socioeconomic status, education, and wealth

Socioeconomic status plays a major role in the development of obesity. In their classic review of 144 published studies of the relationship between socioeconomic status (SES) and obesity, Sobal and Stunkard[9] found a strong inverse relationship among women in developed societies, i.e. women of higher SES were significantly less obese than those of lower SES. However, the relationship was less clear for men and children in developed societies. They found an inconsistent relationship for both. Interestingly, there was a strong direct relationship between SES and obesity among women, men, and children in developing societies, i.e. the higher the SES, the higher the obesity in all three groups. The authors reviewed the social attitudes toward obesity and found the values congruent with the distribution of obesity by SES in both developed and developing societies. According to the authors, in developed societies, dietary restraint, increased physical activity, social mobility, and inheritance among higher SES women may mediate the attitudes about body weight that result in the inverse association between SES and the development of obesity. SES influences obesity through education, income, and occupation causing specific behavioural patterns which change energy intake, energy expenditure, and metabolic rate[10]. Likewise, obesity influences SES when its perception is influenced by prejudice, stigmatization and discrimination, significantly limiting access to higher SES[11] (Table 2).

Table 2. The relationship between socioeconomic status (SES) and obesity

- In developing countries, there tends to be a strong positive association between SES and obesity in women, men and children

- In developed countries, there tends to be a strong negative association between SES and obesity in women, although it is somewhat less consistent in men and children

This inverse relationship seen in developed countries is expected because food deprivation is rare although individuals in lower SES groups tend to eat less nutritious diets, which are lower in vegetables and fruits and are more energy-dense[10]. Many healthy food choices, including fish, lean meats, and fresh vegetables and fruits are oftentimes less available to individuals in lower SES groups[12]. The direct relationship seen in developing countries may be partly due to a perception that overweight is a positive attribute, an outward sign of affluence. Overweight oftentimes does not carry the same stigma as seen in developed countries among higher SES groups. For example, Reddy[13] examined the relationship between SES and body mass index (BMI) in 1,119 individuals from socio-economically diverse populations in southern Andhra Pradesh, India. Results showed a positive association between SES and BMI, qualitatively different from the negative association seen in developed countries. In contrast, Wardle, Waller and Jarvis[14] investigated socioeconomic predictors of obesity in more than 15,000 men and women in England. They found the opposite of Reddy, i.e. a negative association between SES and BMI, with the lowest obesity in the highest SES. Obesity risk in England was greater among both women and men with poorer economic circumstances and less education. They found that women and men who left school at an early age were more likely to be obese than those who stayed in school, with a graded effect across years of schooling. This finding was independent of other SES effects and was independent of age, ethnicity, and marital status. Studies in Sweden[15,16], Finland[17,18], Switzerland[19] and the United States[20,21] show similar results, i.e. a relationship between lack of education or lower SES and subsequent obesity. Because data on wealth are difficult to collect, SES, education, occupation or some composite measure is frequently used as surrogate for assessing income.

Data appear similar for children. For example, children in high SES groups are more likely to be obese in China and Russia, but children in low SES groups are more obese in the United States[22]. In the United States, the child's caretaker's SES, marital status, and social support predicted the child's risk of obesity. Lower SES, unmarried status of the caretaker, and lower expressive social support were associated with higher calorie intake and higher weight for height scores in the children[23]. In a study of the social and economic consequences of obesity in adolescents and young adults, Gortmaker and colleagues[24] found that women who had been overweight had completed fewer years of school, were less likely to be married, had lower household incomes, and had higher rates of household poverty than women who had not been overweight, independent of their baseline SES and aptitude test scores. Men who had been overweight were less likely to be married. The authors concluded that overweight during adolescence has important social and economic consequences and that discrimination against overweight individuals may explain their results.

Brazil appears to be somewhat of an exception to the data in developing countries but may be a sign of what is happening worldwide. Monteiro and colleagues[25] compared data collected in three comparable surveys in the two most populated Brazilian regions in 1975 ($n = 95{,}062$), 1989 ($n = 15{,}585$) and 1997 ($n = 10{,}680$). The earlier trends showed increasing obesity for all population groups (except men in rural areas). However, the most recent data suggested a more complex picture where increases in obesity were stronger in men than women, more rural than urban, and in poorer than richer families. Surprisingly, obesity was lower for women in higher SES groups, especially in urban areas. The authors concluded that this recent trend of a substantial reduction in the prevalence of obesity among upper SES urban women is unique in a developing country. They speculated that this declining obesity trend may be due to intense mass media aimed at combating sedentary lifestyle and encouraging healthier diets. This very interesting trend seen in Brazil may be a harbinger of a worldwide shift as developing countries continue to adopt western lifestyles. The richer, better educated individuals in these countries will become thinner, the poorer, less educated ones, fatter. The changing dietary patterns, the increasing life expectancy, and the shifts in SES and education will increasingly contribute to the problems of obesity and will have a major impact on the health and the health care resources of developing countries in the near future[26].

What can we do about it?

Our environment is the major cause of the increasing prevalence of obesity. Socioeconomic status, education, and wealth all play a significant role in determining our health, including our leanness or fatness. We are not going to return to hunter-gatherer lifestyles. The most promising targets to improve the health and well being of all of us are a focus on prevention of weight gain and on the development of strategies to promote healthy environmental changes[27]. Public health campaigns aimed at helping individuals reduce portion sizes, limit calories, and increase intake of healthy low-density foods, including vegetables and fruits, can help. The most important factor in weight loss is reduction of caloric intake and the emphasis should be on that fact. Working with food technologists and food manufacturers to develop appropriate food options could also be beneficial. Governments could provide subsidies for healthy foods.

Strategies for making the environment safer for increased physical activity, including attractive areas for walking, jogging and bicycling, needs to be a priority.

Because education is such a significant predictor of healthier weights, a focus on children and strong encouragement for them to stay in school should be a major priority.

References

1. International Obesity Task Force. Global burden of disease analyses: Body weights, prevalences of overweight and obesity and their impact on health. In: *World health reports*. Geneva: World Health Organization, WHO; 2002.

2. Foreyt JP, Goodrick GK The ultimate triumph of obesity. *Lancet* 1995; 346: 134–5.

3. World Health Organization (WHO). *Obesity: preventing and managing the global epidemic. Report of a WHO consultation on obesity*. Geneva: WHO; 1998.

4. Hewitt JK. The genetics of obesity: what have genetic studies told us about the environment. *Behav Genet* 1997; 27: 353–58.

5. Eaton SB, Konner M, Shostak M. Stone agers in the fast lane: chronic degenerative diseases in evolutionary perspective. *Am J Med* 1988; 84: 739–49.

6. Eaton SB, Konner M, Shostak M. *The paleolithic prescription*. New York: Harper & Row; 1988.

7. Popkin BM. The nutrition transition and its health implications in lower-income countries. *Public Health Nutr* 1998; 1: 5–21.

8. Burkitt DP, Eaton SB. Putting the wrong fuel in the tank. *Nutrition* 1989; 5: 189–91.

9. Sobal J, Stunkard AJ. Socioeconomic status and obesity: a review of the literature. *Psychol Bull* 1989; 105: 260–75.

10. Sobal J. Obesity and socioeconomic status: a framework for examining relationships between physical and social variables. *Med Anthropol* 1991; 13: 231–47.

11. Sri L. Sociodemographic characteristics and individual health behaviors. *S Med J* 1998; 91: 933–41.

12. Nestle M, Wing R, Birch L *et al*. Behavioral and social influences on food choice. *Nutr Rev* 1998; 56: S50–S74.

13. Reddy BN. Body mass index and its association with socioeconomic and behavioral variables among socioeconomically heterogeneous populations of Andhra Pradesh, India. *Human Biology* 1998; 70: 901–17.

14. Wardle J, Waller J, Jarvis MJ. Sex differences in the association of socioeconomic status with obesity. *Am J Public Health* 2002; 92: 1299–1304.

15. Kuskowska-Wolk A, Bergstrom R. Trends in body mass index and prevalence of obesity in Swedish women 1980–89. J *Epidemiol Comm Hlth* 1993; 47: 195–99.

16. Sundquist J, Johansson SE. The influence of socioeconomic status, ethnicity and lifestyle on body mass index in a longitudinal study. *Int J Epidemiol* 1998; 27: 57–63.

17. Rissanen AM, Heliovaara M, Knekt P, Reunanen A, Aromaa A. Determinents of weight gain and overweight in adult Finns. *Eur J Clin Nutr* 1991; 45: 419–30.

18. Laitinen J, Power C, Jarvelin MR. Family social class, maternal body mass index, childhood body mass index, and age at menarche as predictors of adult obesity. *Am J Clin Nutr* 2001; 74: 287–94.

19. Galobardes B, Morabia A, Bernstein MS. The differential effect of education and occupation on body mass and overweight in a sample of working people of the general population. *Annals Epidemiol* 2000; 10: 532–37.

20. Flegal KM, Harlan WR, Landis JR. Secular trends in body mass index and skinfold thickness with socioeconomic factors in young women. *Am J Clin Nutr* 1988; 48: 535–43.

21. Flegal KM, Harlan WR, Landis JR. Secular trends in body mass index and skinfold thickness with socioeconomic factors in young men. *Am J Clin Nutr* 1988; 48: 544–51.

22. Wang Y. Cross-national comparison of childhood obesity: the epidemic and the relationship between obesity and socioeconomic status. *Int J Epidemiol* 2001; 30: 1129–36.

23. Gerald LB, Anderson A, Johnson GD, Hoff C, Trimm RF. Social class, social support and obesity risk in children. *Child Care, Health & Development* 1994; 20: 145–63.

24. Gortmaker SL, Must A, Perrin JM, Sobol AM, Dietz WH. Social and economic consequences of overweight in adolescence and young adulthood. *NEJM* 1993; 329, 1008–12.

25. Monteiro CA, D'A Benicio MH, Conde WL, Popkin BM. Shifting obesity trends in Brazil. *Eur J Clin Nutr* 2000; 54: 342–6.

26. Popkin BM, Paeratakul S, Zhai F, Ge K. A review of dietary and environmental correlates of obesity with emphasis on developing countries. *Obes Res* 1995; 3 Suppl 2: 145s–153s.

27. Poston WSC, Foreyt JP. Obesity is an environmental issue. *Atherosclerosis* 1999; 146, 201–9.

Progress in Obesity Research: 9. Edited by *Geraldo Medeiros-Neto, Alfredo Halpern and Claude Bouchard*
©2003 John Libbey Eurotext Ltd, pp. 418–425.

CHAPTER 88

Interactions between energy intake and expenditure in the development and treatment of obesity

R. James Stubbs[1], Darren A. Hughes[1], Alexandra M. Johnstone[1], Graham W. Horgan[2], Neil King[3], Marinos Elia[4] and John E Blundell[3]

[1]*Rowett Research Institute, Greenburn Road, Bucksburn, Aberdeen AB21 9SB, UK;* [2]*Biomathematics and Statistics, Scotland, Rowett Research Institute, Greenburn Road, Bucksburn, Aberdeen AB21 9SB, UK;* [3]*BioPsychology Group, Psychology Department, Leeds University, Leeds LS2 9JT, UK;* [4]*Institute of Human Nutrition, Southampton General Hospital, Southampton, SO16 6YD*
[e-mail: j.stubbs@rri.sari.ac.uk]

Introduction

The effects that diet composition exerts on energy balance (EB) is becoming increasingly well documented[1]. Dietary macronutrients exert differential effects on energy intake (EI), both in the laboratory and in real life. Under normal conditions where fat contributes disproportionately to energy density (ED), protein, carbohydrate and fat exert hierarchical effects on satiety in the order protein >carbohydrate > fat. Alcohol appears to stimulate EI. In human appetite studies the main effect of controlling ED is to diminish the impact of differences in the satiating effects of fat and carbohydrate. ED exerts profound effects in constraining EI in short-to-medium term studies[2]. Subjects behave differently in longer-term interventions. In short-to-medium term laboratory studies, increases in ED (by various means) are more effective at increasing EI than at decreasing food intake. In longer term and cross-sectional studies conducted in naturalistic environments, increased ED appears to be more partially compensated to a greater extent.

Similarly, the effects of exercise on appetite and EB have become a little clearer in recent years. In the short-to-medium-term there is very poor coupling between exercise-induced changes in EE and EI. In the longer term it appears that greater compensation occurs. This appears to be the case either when a fit subject is training for an athletic event[3] or when obese subjects have lost weight using diet and /or exercise.

Thus while it appears that diet and/or exercise can exert profound effects on EB in the short-to-medium term, their appears to be greater compensation of EB in the longer term. This implies that some degree of cross talk is likely to occur between EI and EE in the development and treatment of obesity. What is the nature of this cross talk? Do sustained changes in EI or EE stimulate obligatory (passive) changes in other components of the EB equation (such as aspects of EE)? Do they also lead to facultative, active changes in EI and EE that restore EB? What is the relative importance of obligatory versus facultative changes in the components of EI and EE? Are perturbations of EB likely to produce similar changes in EI and EE? Do compensatory changes in the components of EI and EE respond symmetrically to positive and negative EB? In order to address these questions it is useful to structure the inquiry by examining interactions between EI and EE with reference to obesity development (weight gain) and obesity treatment (weight loss). There appear to be four main interactions to consider, two in relation to weight gain and two with respect to weight loss. In relation to weight gain it is valuable to ask: (1) Does sedentariness alter levels of EI or subsequent EE?, and (2) Do high levels of EI alter physical activity or exercise? In relation to weight loss the critical interactions are: (3) Do exercise-induced increases in EE drive EI upwards and undermine dietary approaches to weight management and (4) Do low levels of

EI elevate or decrease EE? Before addressing these specific issues it is valuable to consider the nature of EB control in humans.

The nature of EB control in humans

Feeding behaviour is governed by a redundant system that has numerous afferent inputs. Not all of these inputs are necessary for the system to function. Feeding behaviour can change in a number of measurable ways such as meal size, frequency, and the composition of foods selected, or the rate and manner in which foods are ingested. The system uses multiple sensory cues to learn about the consequences of ingesting certain foods. Mimicking the cues associated with certain foods can therefore, transiently at least, 'mislead' the system.

Energy balance control is sensitive to certain changes in the external and internal environment (e.g. temperature or pregnancy respectively) and to changes in the environmental supply of energy and nutrients. With respect to energy and nutrients, the sensitivity of the system (i.e. the capacity of the system to recognise changes in the environment) can often be greater than its responsiveness (i.e. its tendency to alter behaviour in order to maintain the constancy of the internal environment). Evolution has selected our physiology and behaviour to favour overconsumption rather than underconsumption[1]. This means that the system is more responsive to deficits in energy and nutrients than to increments. Being overweight is probably the result of largely 'normal' feeding responses when exposed to a western diet under modern sedentary conditions.

The system is interconnected with other biological systems that influence motivation and behaviour. Certain external and internal influences can greatly perturb the system in such a way that food (energy and nutrient) intake patterns become maladaptive. Other biobehavioural drives can override and distort the cues associated with feeding e.g during eating disorders.

There appears to be little evidence of regulatory signals that protect humans from slow, continuous weight gain under modern western conditions. Hence over half of the adult population of the western world are collectively overweight and obese[4]. Why this is so can be appreciated by considering the four interactions highlighted above.

Interaction 1: Does sedentariness alter levels of EI or subsequent EE?

Average daily energy expenditure (EE) appears to be less than was typical of the population several decades ago[5]. However, early estimates are imprecise since objective measures of free-living EE, using tracers, are a relatively recent phenomenon[6]. Nonetheless, it is generally accepted that western populations are more sedentary than they used to be. This is apparently because the estimated energy cost of common everyday activities and many work activities is believed to have declined in recent decades[5]. While people have on average, more leisure time than previously, it is often noted that may people spend less of it engaged in active pursuits[5]. The notion that the population is remarkably sedentary is supported by cross-sectional surveys of levels of activity amongst adults and children[7] and the fact that average levels of physical fitness are remarkably low in the population at large. Black *et al.* have estimated, from tracer studies, that the established limits of total daily EE range from 1.2–4.5 x BMR over periods of 2 weeks or more[8]. Intense, sustained activity tends to be a little lower for most people at ~2.3–2.9 x BMR[8]. The general (rather sedentary) population appear to be less variable with average TEE in the range 1.4–1.8 x BMR. This raises the important question: is there much scope to significantly effect EB by reducing physical activity within the normal range, given that modern lifestyles are apparently so sedentary?

There is very little *direct* evidence to link sedentariness to the development of a positive EB. Instead a number of intuitively obvious arguments and proxies of physical activity have been used in (largely) cross-sectional comparisons, to suggest that number of hours spent watching television, car ownership and the use of mobile phones are all factors lowering average physical activity in the population and predisposing us further to weight gain[9]. Despite the attractiveness of these arguments, it is remarkable that few studies have actually attempted to assess the impact on EB of imposing sedentary routines, within the normal range of activity, on healthy humans feeding *ad libitum*. The effects of inactivity on appetite and/or EI have been assessed in disease[10], in 6 degree head down tilt bedrest (as a model of zero gravity)[11] and as a consequence of life in space itself[12]. In addition, the effect of imposing a sedentary routine on healthy subjects has been examined in the short-term. For instance Murgatroyd *et al.* conducted 2-day treatments where subjects underwent active versus sedentary routines and consumed high vs. low fat diets, in a 2 x 2 design[13]. They noted that on a given diet subjects consumed the same level of energy regardless of the level of EE. Similarly Shepard *et al.* have noticed that when lean and obese subjects were placed in the calorimeter for a day, the decrease in activity associated with the sedentary environment of the calorimeter, generated a positive EB[14]. However, these assessments are very short and King *et al.* have noted that studies of this duration in general have produced no change in feeding behaviour, under a variety of conditions[15]. A recent study clamped total daily EE at ~1.4 and 1.8 x BMR, and examine the impact of this on motivation to eat and EI, for 7 consecutive days in 6 men, while continually resident in a whole body indirect calorimeter. EE amounted to 9.7 and 12.8 MJ/day, [F (1,5) = 53.67; P < 0.01 (sed = 0.41)], on the sedentary and active treatments, respectively. The corresponding values for EI were 13.5 and 14.4 MJ/d, [F (1,5) = 0.53; P = 0.463 (sed = 1.06)], respectively. By day 7, cumulative EB was 11.1 and 26.3 MJ, respectively. Most of the excess energy was stored as fat[16]. Importantly, there were no time trends in EI or EE over the 7 days of this study, indicating no tendency to compensate for an acute decrease in EE due to physical activity.

It is possible to detect decreases in EI as a response to a sustained decrease in EE. For instance in the unusual experimental model of 6 degree head down tilt bedrest, Ritz *et al.*[11] have shown that EI does significantly drop as a consequence of extreme sedentariness. Upon resumption of ambulatory activity EI begins to rise again. However the decrease in EI was not great and was insufficient to avoid a positive EB over a 6 week period of bedrest. The little evidence available relating to abrupt decreases in EE due to training cessation or injury suggests that acute decreases in EE, due to reduced activity lead to marked gain in body.

These insights are supported by a variety of observational studies. From the perspective of public health, there are a number of cross sectional studies that strongly suggest sedentariness is highly correlated with increased adiposity. For example, Martinez-Gonzalez *et al.* estimated the association of leisure-time sedentary and non-sedentary, self-reported activities on BMI and the prevalence of obesity in 15,239 subjects across the 15 member states of the European Union. They found that ...'obesity and a higher body weight are strongly associated with a sedentary lifestyle and a lack of physical activity in the adult population of the European Union'[7]. A number of studies suggest that the lifestyle correlates of a sedentary routine afford greater opportunity to overeat[17]. There is however little evidence that a sedentary routine promotes greater levels of EI *per se* (though it may afford opportunities for over-consumption), rather subjects appear to eat as they did during a prior period of greater EE and so EI overshoots EE leading to weight gain. These lines of evidence suggests that reduced EE due to activity is very weakly linked, through physiological signals, to EI and has little effect in reducing intake. Under these conditions it is likely that the rate of weight gain slows with time if energy requirements remain lowered. The extent to which this is due to passive or fixed changes in the components of EE or due to active cross talk between reduced activity and EI (or even components of EE) is at present unclear. There is more information on how these components of EB respond to energy deficits (See below).

The evidence thus suggests that the absence of strong cross-talk between reduced EE due to activity and *ad libitum* EI is responsible for the tendency to gain weight when activity is reduced, and food is available *ad libitum*. In modern society food is rarely not available *ad libitum*. It has recently been suggested that some people actively respond to overfeeding by increasing their ambulatory and positional movements. This has been termed the Non-Exercise Activity Thermogenesis (NEAT) phenomenon.

Interaction 2: Do high levels of energy intake alter subsequent EE?

Leibel *et al.*[18] examined the effects of altering body weight on EE and it's components (resting and nonresting EE, and the thermic effect of feeding) in 18 obese and 23 never-obese subjects. The subjects were studied at their usual body weight (UBW), after losing 10 to 20 per cent or gaining 10 per cent UBW by underfeeding or overfeeding, respectively. Maintenance of a body weight at a level 10 per cent or more below the UBW was associated with a mean (± SD) reduction in total EE of 25 ± 12.6 kJ/kgFFM/day in the subjects who had never been obese (P < 0.001) and 34 ± 21 kJ/kgFFM/day in the obese subjects (P < 0.001). This is equivalent to ~ 1.25 MJ/day and 2.1 MJ/day assuming a FFM (fat-free mass) of ~50 and ~63 kg in the lean and obese subjects respectively. Resting EE and non-resting EE each decreased 13 to 17 kJ/kgFFM/day in both groups of subjects (~0.65 and 1.2 MJ/day). Maintenance of body weight at a level 10 per cent above the usual weight was associated with an increase in total EE of 38 ± 29 kJ/kgFFM/day (~1.9 MJ/day) in the subjects who had never been obese (P < 0.001) and 33.6 ± 17 kJ/kgFFM/day (~2.4 MJ/day) in the obese subjects (P < 0.001). The thermic effect of feeding and non-resting EE increased by approximately 4 to 8 and 34 to 38 kJ/kgFFM/day, respectively, after weight gain. Clearly the greatest change in EE occurred through non-resting EE. The authors concluded that ... 'maintenance of a reduced or elevated body weight is associated with compensatory changes in EE, which oppose the maintenance of a body weight that is different from the usual weight'. It is important to distinguish here between fixed or obligatory changes in EE (see below), and active (compensatory) cross-talk between changes in EI and EE.

Subsequently Levine[19] published a study in which the physiological basis of variation in weight gain in response to overfeeding was investigated by measuring changes in energy storage and EE in 16 non-obese volunteers who were overfed by 4.2 MJ/day for 8 weeks[19]. DIT and BMR were not apparently related to fat gain. However fat gain was inversely related to *change* (increase) in NEAT (correlation coefficient = 0.77, $P < 0.001$), which ranged from 0–3 MJ/day. The authors reported that ~66 per cent of the increases in daily EE was due to increased NEAT. The results suggested that as humans overeat, activation of NEAT dissipates excess energy to preserve leanness, at least in some people. However, a potential problem with the data is that changes in EB were estimated as the fate of the 4.2 MJ/day in excess of requirements consumed by the 16 subjects over 8 weeks – assuming that all of the additional energy was consumed. Any non-compliance with this aggressive overfeeding regime in these 65 kg subjects would be registered as NEAT, since NEAT was estimated by difference. Average energy cost of weight gain in this study amounted to 4.2 x 56/4.7 = 50 MJ/kg. This is somewhat higher than literature values of 33 MJ/kg or below for subjects who were as lean as those in this study[20]. The possibility that subjects did not entirely comply with the overfeeding regime in this study cannot therefore be excluded. Other studies of overfeeding have not found so dramatic an effect of overfeeding on EE or its components[20,21]. This raises certain questions. Firstly, are changes in NEAT of 1–3 MJ/day feasible? Examining the difference in daily EE between two studies conducted by Stubbs *et al.* suggest so[23,24]. In two studies subjects consumed low, medium and high fat diets *ad libitum*, in one they were confined to a calorimeter in another they were semi-free living and ambulatory. The EE of the ambulatory subjects (with a similar height and weight as those in the chamber) was 2.8 MJ/day higher. Similarly in a calorimeter study which altered activity EE from 1.8 to 1.4 x BMR in lean men, daily EE was altered by ~ 3 MJ/day[16] Thus inter-individual variability in NEAT of 1–3 MJ/day is perfectly feasible. The degree of inter-individual variability in weight gain in response to overfeeding is not controversial. The critical question in our minds is 'Are there some people who specifically respond to overfeeding by increasing positional and postural activities by up to 1–3 MJ/day?' If so what are the mechanisms? Are there alternative or supplementary explanations?

It is known that during altered EB there are a number of small but significant changes in the components of EE. These include (i) Tissue dependent changes in sleeping and basal metabolic rate[25]; (ii) Changes in the energy cost of weight change alter as weight is gained or lost[20,26]; (iii) Exercise efficiency will alter as weight changes[27], (iv) As weight is gained or lost the energy cost of weight bearing activities will change[28], (v) During substantive overfeeding diet composition (fat vs. carbohydrate) will influence the energy cost of nutrient storage by ~ 15 per cent[29]. An important question is 'what is the aggregate effect of these changes on overall EB?' The responses (i–v) above are all 'obligatory' responses. The degree of inter-individual variability in these responses will define the scope within which various mechanisms of EB compensation can operate. The extent of inter-individual variability in these responses is not clear.

In addition to these obligatory changes, altered EB can stimulate active behavioural responses, which are presumably the consequence of cross-talk between EI and EE. Altered EB will lead to changes in the mode duration and intensity of physical activities, including postural and positional activities. In addition to changes in EE, the size, frequency and composition of ingestive events can also change. The relative importance of 'obligatory' versus facultative, behavioural responses as components of EB control, need to be defined.

Two interactions between EI and EE that are likely to predispose us to obesity development have been considered above. As regards interaction 1, there is little evidence that sedentariness alters levels of EI. This lack of cross-talk between altered EE and EI appears to promote a positive EB. Lifestyle studies also suggest that a sedentary routine actually offers the opportunity for over-consumption. Regarding interaction 2, (whether high levels of EI elevate or decrease EE), substantive changes in NEAT are feasible, but not clearly demonstrated. The jury is still out on this issue. The discussion of these two interactions between EI and EE highlights the need to focus research on measuring inter-individual variability in the several components of EI and EE. Which interactions between EI and EE are likely to help or hinder obesity treatment?

Interaction 3: Does exercise drive EI upwards and undermine dietary approaches to weight management?

Garrow has illustrated that the majority of subjects who lose weight through non-surgical treatment regain[30]. When comparing the effects of diet and exercise on weight regain some studies show little difference between diet and exercise[31]. There is a tendency for diet and exercise or exercise in the post-weight reduction period to increase the sustainability of weight loss[32]. There is little clear evidence however, that the increased EE due to exercise increases EI to the extent that it would undermine dieting to lose weight. This is probably because the increased EE due to exercise has a relatively weak impact on patterns of energy and nutrient intake in the short to medium term[33,15]. Furthermore, it has been shown that the more obese a person is, the harder, on average it is for them to increase EE through exercise due to their low VO₂max[34]. This means that in order to clearly examine the impact of sustained increases in EE due to exercise on obesity treatment a period of incremental training should be involved for very unfit subjects.

There is evidence that it takes considerable time for EI to adjust to elevations of EE. One direct intervention also supports this view. Lee *et al.* [35] studied the impact of five month basic military training on body weight, body fat and lean body mass in 197 Singapore males, classified as normal weight (BMI 24 to < 30), obese (BMI 30 to < 35) and very obese (BMI > 35). Two key features of this study are that training was incremental, allowing subjects to gradually become fitter, and food intake was *ad libitum*. Over the 5 months of training FFM did not change but subjects lost substantial amounts of weight and body fat. Subjects who were initially fatter lost more weight and more fat. This suggests that responses of intake to exercise-induced changes in EE may depend on how fat you are. In other words it is likely that fat mass is acting as an energy buffer and intake rises markedly when lean body mass is threatened by the exercise induced energy deficit. The importance of lean body mass changes in appetite control have been discussed by Stubbs and Elia (2000)[36]. If this is true then cross talk between elevated EE and EI is initially too weak and takes too long to activate, to seriously threaten dietary approaches to weight management. It appears that substantial fat loss is possible before intake begins to track a sustained elevation of EE.

Two studies have examined how much EE is required to sustain weight loss, i.e to prevent weight regain[32]. The estimate from the two studies are not dissimilar and suggest it takes around 40–47 kJ/kg/day of additional EE through physical activity, to prevent weight regain. This suggests that there are some powerful interactions trying to oppose the maintenance of weight loss, which raises a further question.

Interaction 4: Do low levels of EI elevate or decrease EE due to activity?

The issue of whether high levels of EI stimulate NEAT was discussed above. There is more evidence that low levels of EI do lower physical activity levels, at least in relatively lean men under conditions of acute[37] or prolonged[38] semi-starvation. Recent work by Johnstone (2002)[39] has examined the effect of three common forms of dietary restriction on physical activity patterns. Three studies were conducted in obese men (BMI 30–40, six subjects per group), (i) a total fast (to lose a nominal 5 per cent weight over 6 days); (ii) a very-low-calorie diet (VLCD, 2.5 MJ/day [8 g N/day] for 3 weeks); (iii) low-calorie diet (LCD, 5.2 MJ/day [8 g N/day] for 6 weeks), both to lose a nominal 10 per cent weight. Clearly, the energy deficit and rate of weight loss occurred in the order Fast > VLCD > LCD. At 5 per cent weight loss physical activity levels were 1.38, 1.71 and 1.84 x BMR respectively. All means were significantly different from each other ($P < 0.05$). These data suggest that in obese subjects the greater the rate of weight loss the greater the reduction in physical activity. These values amounted to a daily EE of around 11.5, 13.5 and 13.9 MJ/day. The difference in physical activity between the starvation and LCD amounted to 2.4 MJ/day. Thus there is evidence that an increased rate of weight loss through dietary restriction will produce a 'compensatory' decrease in physical activity. In this study the difference of intake between the fast and the LCD amounted to 5.0 MJ/day. The decrease in physical activity therefore compensated for 48 per cent of the difference in EI between the starvation and LCD regime.

It should be remembered that in addition to this active cross-talk between reduced EI and physical activity EE, there are the obligatory changes mentioned above. In these three studies for instance, BMR decreased by 0.5, 0.3 and 0.7 MJ/day at 5 per cent weight loss. The energy cost of weight change was also greater the slower the rate of weight loss due to the tissue composition of weight. The average (SD) energy cost of WL (MJ/kg), calculated from FM and FFM, was 23.2 (2), (28.1 deleting glycogen + water WL), 32.4 (2) and 36.0 (3), respectively ($P < 0.05$). At 5 per cent WL, the fraction of FM to total WL was 54 (68 per cent deleting glycogen + water WL), 70 and 82 per cent ($P < 0.05$), respectively. Much of the difference between (i) and (ii) plus (iii) is due to water loss. At 10 per cent WL, FM loss increased ($P < 0.05$) to 80 per cent and 91 per cent, in the VLCD and LCD groups[40]. These findings again point to the need to better quantify the aggregate effects of facultative (active) changes in behaviour *and* obligatory (or passive) changes in EB on overall predisposition to gain weight or succees at losing it. Indeed, it is important to be able to understand the relative contribution of obligatory changes in EB physiology versus active changes in behaviour as a means of compensating EB for perturbations of either EI or EE. It is also critically important to understand the relative contribution of different components of EI and EE to the overall compensation of EB. In this context Elia (unpublished) has recently re-examined the contribution of DIT, BMR and physical activity to the reduction in EE that occurred as a consequence of the 24 weeks semi-starvation to which Keys *et al.* subjected their subjects[39]. Daily EE fell by a remarkable 8.0 MJ/day over the 24 weeks. Of this 0.8 MJ/day was due to an estimated fall in DIT. BMR fell by 2.6 MJ/day. 65 per cent of this was tissue dependent and 35 per cent occurred over and above changes in lean tissue. The largest change in EE occurred due to a fall in physical activity (4.6 MJ/day). Of this 36 per cent was due to a decrease in the energy cost of activities and 64 per cent was due to a decrease in volitional physical activity. Thus the greatest single response to prolonged semi-starvation was a change in activity behaviour. As with other aspects of EB control, the change in EE alone was due to changes in several components, some of which were obligatory and some 'facultative' or 'adaptive'.

Measuring crosstalk between energy intake and expenditure

It is important to note that in recent years much attention has focussed on the role that diet composition plays in EB control in *ad libitum* feeding subjects. Far less attention has been paid to changes in EE in response to perturbed EB. Measuring the cross-talk between EI and EE *as a consequence* of perturbed EB is a conceptual step further. We are only beginning to simultaneously measure changes in all components of EB in response to altered EB, in order to assess the rate and extent of mechanisms of weight control. One preliminary study has given us an initial, albeit imperfect assessment of the rate and extent of compensation of EI and EE in response to perturbations of EB due to altered diet and exercise[41]. We assessed the effect of No-exercise, (NEX: control] and High exercise level [(Hex); (~4 MJ/day)] and two dietary manipulations [a high-fat (HF: 50 per cent of energy, 700 kJ/100 g) and low and high-fat (LF: 20 per cent of energy, 300 kJ/100 g)] on compensatory changes in EI and EE over 7 day periods. Nine lean men were each studied four times, in a 2 x 2 design. EI was directly quantified by weight of food consumed. EE was assessed by heart rate monitoring. Body weight was measured daily. Mean daily EE was 17.6 and 11.5 MJ/day ($P < 0.001$), on the pooled Hex and Nex treatments, respectively. EI was higher on HF diets (13.4 MJ/day pooled) compared to the LF diets (9.0 MJ/day) Regression analysis showed that these energy imbalances induced significant compensatory changes in EB over time of ~0.3–0.04 MJ/day ($P < 0.05$). These were due to changes in both EI and EE in the opposite direction to the perturbation in EB. These changes were significant, small but persistent, amounting to ~0.2 and ~0.35 MJ/day for EI and EE respectively. Compensation for a perturbation of EB of ~5 MJ/day would take 2–4 weeks and was more marked in relation to induced energy deficits that surfeits, provided compensation occurred at a linear rate. Compensation however tends not to occur at a linear rate as weight changes since weight gain or loss tends to plateau as weight change proceeds. While these estimates may be provisional and imperfect, they do suggest that (i) cross talk between changes in EI and EE does exist, (ii) this cross talk is stronger in relation to energy deficits than surfeits, and (iii) It takes weeks for significant compensatory changes in EB to occur in relation to a sustained perturbation of EB. In real life several of these influences are likely to be superimposed on each other, making the determinants of both EI and EE multifactorial. Interactions between the two will be similarly complex in both nature and their overall impact on EB, in the development and treatment of obesity.

References

1. Blundell JE, Stubbs RJ. Diet composition and the control of food intake in humans. In: *Handbook of obesity*, GE Bray, C Bouchard and WPT James (eds), pp. 243–72. New York, USA: Marcel Dekker; 1998.

2. Stubbs RJ, Johnstone AM, O'Reilly LM, Barton K, Reid C. The effect of covertly manipulating the energy density of mixed diets on *ad libitum* food intake in 'pseudo free-living' humans. *Int J Obes Relat Metab Disord.* 1998; 22(10): 980–7.

3. Blundell JE, King NA. Physical activity and regulation of food intake: current evidence. *Med Sci Sport Exer* 1999; 31 (11 Suppl): S573–S583.

4. World Health Organisation. Obesity: Preventing and Managing the Global Epidemic. Report of a WHO Consultation on Obesity; 3–5 June 1999; Geneva. (WHO/NUT/NCD/98.1).

5. *Allied Dunbar fitness survey activity and health research.* The Sports Council, London: UK; 1992.

6. Schoeller DA. Recent advances from application of doubly labeled water to measurement of human energy expenditure. *J Nutr* 1999; 129(10),1765–8.

7. Martinez-Gonzalez MA, Martinez JA, Hu FB, Gibney MJ, Kearney J. Physical inactivity, sedentary lifestyle and obesity in the European Union. *Int J Obes Relat Metab Disord* 1999; 23(11),1192–201.

8. Black AE, Coward WA, Cole TJ, Prentice AM. Human energy expenditure in affluent societies: an analysis of 574 doubly-labelled water measurements. *Eur J Clin Nutr* 1996; 50(2),72–92.

9. Prentice AM, Jebb SA. Obesity in Britain: gluttony or sloth? *BMJ*1995; 311(7002): 437–39.

10. Ritz P, Elia M. The effect of inactivity on dietary intake and energy homeostasis. *Proc Nutr Soc* 1999; 58(1),115–22.

11. Ritz P, Maillet A, Blanc S, Stubbs RJ. Observations in energy and macronutrient intake during prolonged bed-rest in a head-down tilt position. *Clin Nutr* 1999; 18: 203–7.

12. Lane HW, Gretebeck RJ, Schoeller DA., Davis-Street J, Socki RA, Gibson EK. Comparison of ground-based and space flight energy expenditure and water turnover in middle-aged healthy male US astronauts. *Am J Clin Nutr* 1997; 65(1): 4–12.

13. Murgatroyd PR, Goldberg GR, Leahy FE, Gilsenan MB, Prentice AM. Effects of inactivity and diet composition on human energy balance. *Int J Obes Relat Metab Disord* 1999; 23(12): 1269–75.

14. Shepard TY, Weil KM, Sharp TA, Grunwald GK, Bell ML, Hill JO, Eckel RH. Occasional physical inactivity combined with a high-fat diet may be important in the development and maintenance of obesity in human subjects. *Am J Clin Nutr* 2001; 73(4): 703–8.

15. King NA, Tremblay A, Blundell JE. Effects of exercise on appetite control: implications for energy balance. *Med Sci Sport Exer* 1997; 29: 1076–89.

16. Stubbs RJ, Johnstone AM, Hughes DA, Horgan G, King N. Blundell J. Effect of a decrease in physical activity on energy intake and balance. *Int J Obes* 2000 (in press).

17. Epstein LH, Paluch RA, Consalvi A, Riordan K, Scholl T. Effects of manipulating sedentary behavior on physical activity and food intake. *J Pediatr* 2002; 140(3): 334–9.

18. Leibel RL, Rosenbaum M, Hirsch J. Changes in energy expenditure resulting from altered body weight. *N Engl J Med* 1995; 332(10): 621–8.

19. Levine JA, Eberhardt NL, Jensen MD. Role of nonexercise activity thermogenesis in resistance to fat gain in humans. *Science* 1999; 283(5399): 212–4.

20. Forbes GB, Brown MR, Welle S, Lipinski BA. Deliberate overfeeding in women and men: energy cost and composition of the weight gain. *Br J Nutr* 1986; 56: 1–9.

21. Joosen AMCP, Bakker AHF, Westerterp KR. Metabolic response to short-term overfeeding. *Proc Nutr Soc* (in press).

22. Diaz EO, Prentice AM, Goldberg GR, Murgatroyd PR, Coward WA. Metabolic response to experimental overfeeding in lean and overweight healthy volunteers. *Am J Clin Nutr* 1992; 56(4): 641–55.

23. Stubbs RJ, Ritz P, Coward WA, Prentice AM. Covert manipulation of the ratio of dietary fat to carbohydrate and energy density: effect on food intake and energy balance in free-living men eating *ad libitum. Am J Clin Nutr* 1995; 62(2): 330–7.

24. Stubbs RJ, Harbron CG, Murgatroyd PR, Prentice AM. Covert manipulation of dietary fat and energy density: effect on substrate flux and food intake in men eating *ad libitum. Am J Clin Nutr* 1995; 62(2): 316–29.

25. Elia M. Energy expenditure in the whole body. In: *Energy metabolism: tissue determinants and cellular collaries*, JMT Kinney (ed.), pp.19–49. New York, USA: Raven Press; 1992.

26. Forbes GB, Kreipe RE, Lipinski B. Body composition and the energy cost of weight gain. *Hum Nutr: Clin Nutr* 1982; 36C: 485–87.

27. Shephard RJ, Lavallee H. *Physical fitness assessment – principles, practice and applications.* Springfield: CC Thomas; 1978.

28. Maldonado S, Mujika I, Padilla S. Influence of body mass and height on the energy cost of running in highly trained middle- and long-distance runners. *Int J Sports Med* 2002; 23(4): 268–72.

29. Horton TJ, Drougas H, Brachey A, Reed GW, Peters JC, Hill JO. Fat and carbohydrate overfeeding in humans: different effects on energy storage. *Am J Clin Nutr* 1995; 62(1): 19–29.

30. Garrow J. *Obesity and related diseases.* London: Churchill Livingston, 1988.

31. Saris WH. Physical inactivity and metabolic factors as predictors of weight gain. *Nutr Rev* 1996; 54(4 Pt 2): S110–5.

32. Saris WH. Does response of physical activity in the treatment of obesity – How much is enough to prevent unhealthy weight gain – Outcome of the first Mike Stock Conference. *Int J Obes* 2002; 26(S1): S108.

33. Blundell JE, King NA. Exercise, appetite control, and energy balance. *Nutrition* 2000; 16(7–8): 519–22.

34. Broeder CE, Burrhus KA, Svanevik LS, Wilmore JH. The effects of aerobic fitness on metabolic rate. *Am J Clin Nutr* 1992; 55: 795–801.

35. Lim CL, Lee LK. The effects of 20 weeks basic military training program on body composition, VO2max and aerobic fitness of obese recruits. *J Sport Med Phys Fit* 1994; 34(3): 271–8.

36. Stubbs RJ, Elia M. Macronutrients and Appetite Control with implications for the nutritional management of the malnourished. *Clin Nutr* 2001; 20 Suppl 1: 129–39.

37. Gibney ER. The physical, psychological and metabolic effects of nutritional depletion and subsequent repletion. PhD Thesis, Darwin College, University of Cambridge, UK; 2001.

38. Keys A, Brozek J, Henschel A, Mickelsen O, Taylor HL. *The biology of human starvation*. Minneapolis, USA: University of Minnesota Press, North Central Publishing; 1950.

39. Johnstone AM. Weight loss in human obesity. PhD Thesis, University of Aberdeen, UK; 2002.

40. Johnstone AM, Faber P, Gibney ER, Lobley GE, Horgan GW, Elia M, Stubbs RJ. Energy cost of weight loss in obese men. *Int J Obes* 2002; 26: S1–S98.

41. Johnstone AM, King N, Blundell JE, Farrelly H, Flemming M, Horgan G, Stubbs RJ. Effect of high fat V's low fat diets and exercise on hunger and appetite in lean men. *Int J Obes* 2001; 25(2): S18.

Progress in Obesity Research: 9. Edited by *Geraldo Medeiros-Neto, Alfredo Halpern and Claude Bouchard*
©2003 John Libbey Eurotext Ltd, pp. 426–430.

CHAPTER 89

What are the WHO recommendations for community based interventions?

W. Philip T. James

Chairman, International Obesity TaskForce, 231 North Gower Street, London NW1 2NS, UK
[e-mail: JeanHJames@aol.com]

The major conceptual development in community intervention came with the first cardiovascular analysis by the late Geoffrey Rose and Henry Blackburn who produced the 1982 Technical Report on cardiovascular disease[1] which was followed by reports on general preventive strategies[2] and children[3]. The broader perspective on adult chronic diseases came, however, in 1989 with the expert meeting in Geneva on diet, nutrition and the prevention of chronic diseases[4]. This WHO 797 report was published despite the opposition of the US government which had been intensely lobbied by sugar organizations keen to ensure that our report did not see the light of day. These developments reveal how public health initiatives are soon seen as political. The 797 report led to a prolonged battle by some elements of the food industry to limit the impact of the report but in practice it became a WHO best-seller. The 1997 obesity consultation itself[5] was seen as a threat by the sugar associated industrial groups who funded FAO to produce an earlier carbohydrate report supposedly exonerating sugars as conducive to either dental caries or excess weight gain.

In January 2002 the 797 report was re-evaluated by WHO and the draft placed on the WHO website for consultation. This re-evaluation reinforced the conclusions of the original Report and built on a newly released analysis by the International Agency on Research in Cancer[6] which dealt extensively with weight gain and physical inactivity and their association with the development of different cancers and our draft of a general WHO European report. The Pan American Health Organization has also recently produced a Latin American analysis linking poverty to a propensity to obesity[7] and Asian data had already stimulated WHO/IASO/IOTF to consider whether the acceptable or normal BMI range should be limited to an upper BMI value of 23 rather than 25[8] with lower waist circumference limits.

A coherent approach to preventive action

The children's report[3] set out a sequential scheme whereby a problem, e.g. obesity is identified, followed by the setting of national goals for limiting the problem, this being followed by a process of programme planning for preventive action. Mobilizing support for developing preventive action must include appropriate evaluation schemes. Evaluation is now not simply a way of justifying the programme but of analysing the appropriateness as well as the effectiveness of the selected action. The monitoring and evaluation of community action is becoming a critical tool which can justify early interventions in public health when the evidence for action is incomplete.

Specifying population rather than individual goals of global relevance

The Rose and Blackburn analysis of cardiovascular disease clearly set out the value of population rather than high risk strategies. They also specified both lower and upper dietary goals for the prevention of cardiovascular disease. Setting total fat goals of 15 per cent for the lower value and 30 per cent for the upper goal. We followed this in the 1990 chronic disease report[5] and Table 1 shows the values chosen. The lower total fat goal reflected intakes then known to apply to Japan, China and other developing countries with only modest evidence of childhood malnutrition, whereas the upper 30 per cent goal was a pragmatic goal to reduce total fat as a means for limiting saturated fatty acid (SFA) intake in the cardiovascular disease prone Western world. The upper 10 per cent goal for SFAs was an intermediate target, given the much lower Japanese and Mediterranean country intakes of SFAs and low heart disease rates. Similarly, the free sugar conclusions were based on the recognition that no free sugars were necessary for health and that Chinese, Japanese and traditional Mediterranean diets had negligible intakes.

Table 1. WHO 1990 population nutrient goals

	Limits for population average intakes	
	Lower	**Upper**
Total energy – see footnote*		
Total fat (% total energy)	15	30
Saturated fatty acids (% total energy)	0	10
Polyunsaturated F.As (% total energy)	3	7
Dietary cholesterol (mg/day)	0	300
Total carbohydrate (% total energy)	55	75
Complex carbohydrate (% total energy)	50	70
Dietary fibre (g/day)		
As non-starch polysaccharides (NSP)	16	24
As total dietary fibre	27	40
Free sugars (% total energy)	0	10
Protein (% total energy)	10	15
Salt (g/day)	–	6

*Energy intake needs to be sufficient to allow for normal childhood growth, for the needs of pregnancy and lactation, for work and desirable physical activities and to maintain appropriate body reserves of energy in children and adults. Adult populations on average should have a BMI of 20–22[5]. Note other important footnotes appear in the original.

The confusion of population goals

Very few doctors, given their focus on individual clinical cases, can cope with the concept of an average population goal. We set this out very clearly in the 1990 report[4]: to apply the population goal to almost all individuals, means that only 2–3 per cent should have intakes above 2 standard deviations beyond the mean and >10 per cent SFAs. This means that the population goal would in practice be only about 5 per cent SFA intake. Population goals are more applicable to families with men having greater food needs than women and children having needs proportionately smaller.

Specific obesity issues

The obesity report[5] considered two critical issues: the energy density of the diet and the amount of physical activity needed to maintain weight. We recognized that the data suggested that the fat content of the diet was the principal factor determining energy density and promoting excess weight gain. Thus Stubbs' work[9] on energy density where both fats and refined carbohydrates could confuse the appetite regulatory system, was linked with the Bray and Popkin global analysis[10] of the prevalence of overweight in relation to national dietary fat intakes. WHO then concluded that the optimum goal for preventing obesity might be 20–25 per cent fat with some data suggesting weight increases on fat intakes above 15 per cent[11].

The 2002 WHO analysis

The reanalysis of the importance of diet and physical inactivity involved the identification of those factors which promote or reduce the likelihood of a disease, these factors being classified as showing convincing, probably, possible or insufficient evidence. This classification evolved from that which we used for the World Cancer Research Fund report on diet and cancer[12]. With the current drive to assess evidence in the rigorous Cochrane Centre mode, there is a tendency to assume that unless one has a series of double-blind placebo controlled trials, then the evidence cannot be considered convincing. This is, of course, a ridiculous proposition when it comes to nutritional issues and simply shows the stereotyped thinking that takes over the medical profession, dominated as it is by individuals trained with a strong bias towards pharmacotherapy.

The background obesity document, developed by Swinburn's group, went one step further in tackling the basic causes of the societal behavioural patterns which lead to obesity. Thus the heavy marketing of energy-dense foods was considered as a probable cause for increasing the risk of obesity. Clearly there are no double-blind controlled trials in this domain, but unless one considers the socio-economic and other drivers for the environmental development of obesity, then one is simply not tackling the issue properly. We are, therefore, coming to recognise two arenas of evidence: the first based on the meticulous collection of data in epidemiological, metabolic and intervention studies, and the second dealing with the broader issues of societal change which are currently promoting so much ill-health.

One of the current issues is the optimum macronutrient content of the diet. Willett and colleagues' advocacy of high fat diets[13] is, on a global and evolutionary basis, remarkable since the billions living in Asia, Africa, Latin America and the Middle East have traditionally lived on low sugar, high carbo-hydrate, low fat intakes with 15 per cent of energy as fat. A 30 per cent fat diet is not low in fat: in practice, obesity emerges in florid form with all its comorbidities as fat intakes rise above 20 per cent. Now the free sugars, including the maltidextrins, were seen as probably promoting the development of obesity as well as dental caries. These conclusions were based on general data and clinical and physiological studies, e.g. meta-analyses of weight loss as fat intakes are reduced[14] and on new data on a double-blind controlled trial relating weight gain to sugar-rich soft drink consumption[15].

Physical activity and the optimum population BMI

Erlichman's major report and papers[16,17], for IOTF on the historical evolution of physical activity guidelines had been sent to the FAO meeting held in Rome in late 2001 and this also informed the WHO group meeting in Geneva in January. It was concluded that a physical activity level (PAL) of over 1.7, e.g. 1.8, was needed to maintain a healthy body weight in the current environment of high energy-dense foods, and this is equivalent to an hour's brisk walking a day rather than the classic 30 min walking a day for the prevention of cardiovascular diseases.

The other controversial problem for some was our original designation of a BMI of 21 to 23 as the average adult BMI for a population. There is no doubt that this low range is appropriate based on data from different parts of the world.

Preventive strategies

The two major intellectual developments in relation to preventive strategies came in the WHO 797 report and the obesity report which IOTF, with the major involvement of Tim Gill and his team within the IOTF office, had developed. One needs to distinguish between universal prevention directed at everyone in the community, selective prevention directed at high risk individuals and targeted preven-tion directed at those with existing problems of excess weight or diseases such as diabetes. A series of environmental strategies were set out including urban design and transport policies, laws and regula-tions relating to both food and activity, economic incentives for more appropriate community activity, changes in school curricular, in shifts in the criteria and taxes for food processing and catering, as well as in the area of health promotion and education. Subsidizing vegetables and fruit and providing companies with tax breaks for providing exercise and changing facilities for employees are other options. Nutritional standards and guidelines for public and private catering also need to change from the inept schemes used in most parts of the world. Food labelling and guidance is also currently locked into nutritionally inappropriate displays which simply satisfy food analysts and legal requirements without regard to how individuals can interpret these labels. The WHO 797 report showed how the WHO goals could be used to label foods as high, medium and low in fat, sugars etc. based on the total energy content of the food; this scheme then applies to individuals with remarkably different energy needs. Current advice on how much fat and energy to consume is in fundamental disagreement with the basic principles of individual needs.

One of the big problems is to shift the pervading view that prevention depends on education and individual advice. This is a tragic consequence of the dominance of Western thinking and the individu-alism found so prominently in the US. There is ample evidence, summarized by Jeffrey in this symposium, that effective community prevention cannot depend on individual health education. The ANGELO model developed by Egger and Swinburn[18] is now being used in a much broader way to assess the environmental strategies needed for preventing chronic diseases in general as well as obesity. We are using this approach for WHO Europe and have produced a major document which supports a diet action plan which over the next 5 years the Ministries of Health in the European region plan to implement with a new series of preventive programmes relating not only to dietary and physical activity changes, but also taking into account other issues such as food safety and sustainable agriculture.

The obesity report[5] reaffirmed the 1990 strategy of recognizing the distinct responsibilities of WHO, national governments, local Authorities, community or civil sector groups, as well as industry and the media in promoting change. We then proposed that each government should develop an inter-sectoral board relating to other government departments to promote environmental change. This was a mistake because the evidence now shows that ministry officials, and indeed Ministers, need to cope from day-to-day with the latest political demands; if they are put in charge of some new development, therefore, often nothing happens. Thus the 1992 World Nutrition Summit concerned with malnutrition led to the request for each country to develop a nutrition plan. Yet in our UN Commission on nutrition it became clear that more than a hundred governments had signed up to nutrition plans with presidential and prime ministerial signatures[19]. However, ten years later, these plans lie mouldering in filing cabinets in WHO and FAO with none of the other agencies or principal national academics knowing anything about them and with little evidence of any implementation. One must not rely on governments taking action to induce societal change.

The latest WHO developments

We are now engaged in a new WHO global analysis of the burden of disease relating to specific risk factors. BMI increases are emerging as exceptionally important since the associated risks of diabetes and cardiovascular disease are enormous. Weight gain and obesity have therefore now shot to the top of the world agenda in public health terms but the obesity community is in danger of not being ready to propose either preventive or therapeutic strategies. Too often we demand proof of every measure proposed. It is useful to be rigorous but, as recently proposed[20], it may be necessary to develop a common sense approach to obesity prevention. The remarkable escalation in childhood obesity and the emergence of adolescent type 2 diabetes confronts with a demand for rapid action without waiting for studies on the most efficacious methods needed for the prevention of these new scourges in 10 to 20 years' time. The evidence form major improvements in public health, e.g. in Finland for cardiovascular disease and Thailand for malnutrition, is that a co-ordinated programme of community-based action involving societal groups, the medical profession, local and central government and the drive from an independent academic but civil society based institution is crucial. The challenge now is whether we can learn from this experience when working to prevent obesity. Certainly WHO has now set a major challenge for the academic obesity community.

References

1. WHO. Prevention of Coronary Heart Disease. Technical Report Series 678, WHO, Geneva; 1982.

2. WHO. Community prevention and control of cardiovascular diseases. Technical Report Series No. 732, 1986.

3. WHO. Prevention in childhood and youth of adult cardiovascular diseases: time for action. Technical Report Series 792, 1990.

4. WHO. Diet, nutrition and the prevention of chronic diseases. Technical Report Series 797. WHO Geneva, 1990.

5. WHO 2000. Obesity: preventing and managing the global epidemic. WHO Technical Report Series No. 894. WHO, Geneva.

6. IARC. *Handbook of cancer prevention. Weight control and physical activity*. Vainio H, Bianchini F (eds), vol. 6. Lyon: France; IARC Publications; 2002.

7. Peña M, Bacallao J (eds). *Obesity and poverty*, pp. 41–49. Pan American Health Organization, Scientific Publication; 2000; 576.

8. WHO/IASO/IOTF The Asia-Pacific perspective: redefining obesity and its treatment. February 2000. Health Communications, Australia Pty Ltd. Available from: http://www.idi.org.au/obesity_report.htm.

9. Stubbs RJ, Johnstone AM, O'Reilly LM, Barton K, Reid C. The effect of covertly manipulating the energy density of mixed diets on *ad libitum* food intake in 'pseudo free-living' humans. *Int J Obes Relat Metab Disord* 1998; 22: 980–7.

10. Bray GA, Popkin BM. Dietary fat intake does affect obesity rate. *Am J Clin Nutr* 1998; 68: 1157–73.

11. Francois PJ, James WPT. An assessment of nutritional factors affecting the BMI of a population. *Eur J Clin Nutr* 1994; 48 Suppl 3: S110–S114.

12. World Cancer Research Fund/American Institute for Cancer Research (WCRF/AICR). Food, nutrition and the prevention of cancer: a global perspective. American Institute for Cancer Research: Washington DC, US; 1997.

13. Willett WC. Dietary fat plays a major role in obesity: no. *Obes Rev* 2002; 3(2): 59–68.

14. Astrup A, Grunwald GK, Melanson EL, Saris WH, Hill JO. The role of low-fat diets in body weight control: a meta-analysis of *ad libitum* dietary intervention studies. *Int J Obes Relat Metab Disord* 2000; 24(12): 1545–52.

15. Raben A, Vasilaras TH, Møller, Astrup A. Sucrose compared with artificial sweeteners: different effects on *ad libitum* food intake and body weight after 10 wk of supplementation in overweight subjects. *Am J Clin Nutr* 2002; 76 (in press).

16. Erlichman J, Kerbey AL, James WPT. Physical activity and its impact on health outcomes. Paper 1: the impact of physical activity on cardiovascular disease and all-cause mortality: an historical perspective. *Obes Rev* 2002; 3 (in press).

17. Erlichman J, Kerbey AL, James WPT. Physical activity and its impact on health outcomes. Paper 2: prevention of unhealthy weight gain and obesity by physical activity: an analysis of the evidence. *Obes Rev* 2002; 3 (in press).

18. Egger G, Swinburn B. An 'ecological' approach to the obesity pandemic. *BMJ* 1997; 315: 477–80.

19. James WPT, Norum K, Smitasiri S, Swaminathan MS, Tagwirye J, Uauy R, Ul Haq M. Ending Malnutrition by 2020: an Agenda for Change in the Millennium. Final Report to the ACC/SCN by the Commission on the Nutrition Challenges of the 21st Century. Supplement to the Food and Nutrition Bulletin.. UNU International Nutrition Foundation, USA. 2000 Sept/Oct.

20. Ebbeling CB, Pawlak DB, Ludwig DS. Childhood obesity: public-health crisis, common sense cure. *Lancet* 2002; 360.

Progress in Obesity Research: 9. Edited by *Geraldo Medeiros-Neto, Alfredo Halpern* and *Claude Bouchard*
©2003 John Libbey Eurotext Ltd, pp. 431–434.

CHAPTER 90

Community-based interventions and government policies for addressing the obesity epidemic

Robert W. Jeffery

Division of Epidemiology, University of Minnesota, School of Public Health, 1300 South Second Street, Suite 300, Minneapolis, Minnesota 55454-1015, USA
[e-mail: jeffery@epi.umn.edu]

Recent worldwide increases in the prevalence of obesity have been dramatic, and no more so anywhere in the world than in the United States. In the last 20 years, the average body weight of adults living in the US increased by 10 per cent and the population prevalence of obesity doubled. Nearly one in three adults in the US is now clinically obese[1]. Although obesity experts are not in consensus on the causes of recent trends in body weight, they are in agreement on two fundamental points: (1) the immediate causes of obesity are behavioural (i.e. people are eating more, being less physically active, or both), and (2) the causes of these behaviour changes are environmental rather than biological.

Unfortunately, population data on energy intake and physical activity in the US have not been very helpful in pinpointing behavioural causes of increasing obesity. Population surveys of individual food intake conducted between 1970 and the late 1990s have indicated relatively little change in per capita energy intake and in similar data on physical activity have shown little or no change as well. The apparent inability of current methods of diet and physical activity assessment to show which is contributing more to obesity has opened the field to widely divergent speculations about causes. Although this discussion is likely to continue, the present investigator believes that the arguments in favour of increased eating as the cause of increased obesity are better than those favouring decreased exercise. All energy intake comes from food, but only 30 to 40 per cent of energy expenditure is due to modifiable activity. Thus, equivalent changes in energy balance require a much smaller proportional change in eating than in activity.

A more empirical reason for favouring increased intake over decreased expenditure as the cause of the obesity epidemic in the US is food disappearance data. Although food disappearance data are certainly not equivalent to food intake, temporal trends in food supply have for the most part tracked the obesity epidemic. Prior to the onset of the obesity epidemic in about 1980, per capita food disappearance data were stable. After 1980, however, the per capita food disappearance began to increase and has continued to increase to the present. Overall, there has been about a 15 per cent increase in the annual per capita energy disappearance, which is roughly equivalent to what would be required to produce the observed changes in body weight.

Food supply data also provide interesting information about changes in diet composition. As per capita energy disappearance has risen, there has been an equally dramatic change in macronutrient composition. Increases have been much more dramatic in carbohydrates than in dietary fat. At the level of foods people eat, temporal trends have been even more complex. Beef and butter have decreased; chicken, fruits, vegetables, and sugar-free soft drinks have increased and so have cheese and caloric soft drinks. To date there have been no systematic attempts to empirically link specific food item availability to the obesity epidemic. However, food supply data clearly underscore the fact that in recent years the food environment in the US has evolved dynamically on a number of different dimensions.

Two other aspects of the changing food environment in the US deserve mention as well. Between about 1970 and the present, food has become more and more affordable, decreasing from 14 to 10 per cent of income. Accompanying this decrease in cost has been a dramatic shift toward eating away from home. The public health community has been particularly concerned about the trends in eating at 'fast food' restaurants. The fast food industry has been the most rapidly growing sector of the food distribution economy for 20 years and there is now increasing evidence that frequent eating at such establishments is associated with higher body weight[2].

Accompanying concerns about increased prevalence of eating away from home have also been concerns about the impact of food advertising on food choices. Advertising expenditures on food in the US are large, representing about $55 per year per capita. Advertising expenditures dwarf the expenditure by the US government on nutrition education of about $1.50 per year per capita. There is also evidence that the total amount of food advertising in the US has increased substantially over the last two decades; by one estimate, approximately doubling as a percentage of sales[3]. Recent evidence has also documented recent trends toward more and more food promotions based on quantity (i.e. larger portion sizes with little or no increase in price)[4].

Having made the case for food as a contributor to the obesity epidemic, it should be noted that there have also been a number of trends on the physical activity side of the energy balance equation that may also be making contributions to increasing body weights. These include the fact that reliance on motorized transportation to and from work has continued to increase throughout the period of the epidemic; the number of hours spent in passive entertainments, particularly TV viewing, has increased dramatically; and that time spent doing home chores has decreased while time spent in paid work has increased.

What can be done about the obesity epidemic?

During the 1980s and 1990s, three major health education projects aimed at population obesity were conducted at the University of Minnesota. The first, called the Healthy Worker Project (HWP), was a randomized trial of health education programmes delivered to adults in the general population through worksites[5]. Thirty-two worksites were recruited for the project that employed a total of approximately 20,000 people. Sixteen worksites were randomized to a treatment and 16 to a no-treatment control group. The treatment, delivered for 2 years, was comprised of face-to-face health education counseling in groups to interested individuals at their worksite.

The HWP was successful in recruiting over 2,000 individuals to weight loss programmes during the 2 years of the study who, on average, lost about 2 kg between their entry into the programmes and 6 months later. Unfortunately, however, the net benefits of providing these educational programmes over the entire 2 years was negligible. The difference in mean weight change between sites receiving the programmes and those not receiving the education programmes was only 0.1 BMI unit after 2 years.

The second health education project is the Minnesota Heart Health Program (MHHP)[6]. The MHHP was a 10-year research and demonstration project designed to evaluate the effectiveness of multicomponent interventions to reduce CVD incidence of mortality. The MHHP was not exclusively devoted to obesity. However, diet and exercise education provided as part of the project was very consistent with weight control messages. The MHHP involved six communities with a total population of about 500,000. The intervention was comprised of health education over a period of 7 years in multiple areas including individual risk factor screening and counseling, mass media, adult education classes, worksite interventions, interventions for children in schools, point-of-purchase education in restaurants and supermarkets, education of physicians about risk factor treatment, and others. MHHP was successful in reaching large numbers of people and positive changes in knowledge, attitudes, and in some self-reported behaviours related to obesity were observed. Nevertheless, over the 7 years of observation, we were unable to demonstrate that the health education programmes of the MHHP had a beneficial effect on body weight.

The third education project is the Pound of Prevention (POP) programme[7]. This project was a randomized trial evaluating the effectiveness of an educational programme for reducing rate of weight gain with age rather than weight loss. A diverse population of individuals was recruited to the study through public advertisement and randomized either to no treatment or to one of two education groups that received educational messages in monthly newsletters and periodic opportunities to participate in more active educational activities.

As in the previous two studies, participation in POP was good and changes in knowledge and behaviour were observed. However, this did not translate into changes in body weight over the 3 years of observation.

Partly in response to the lack of success in promoting weight control through public health education, the Minnesota research group began a series of studies in the early 1990s to look at factors other than health education in relation to obesity-related health behaviours. These researches have targeted both eating and exercise choices, although not yet body weight. The series of studies began with three pilot studies on eating choice that used a single subject ABA design in which food choices were observed first without intervention, second with intervention, and third without intervention again, all in the same setting. The first of these studies targeted healthy food choices (salad and fruit) in a cafeteria setting[8]. The study design involved 3 weeks of baseline observation of food choices, 3 weeks in which the price of targeted foods was reduced and the number of choices in each category was increased, and then a return to baseline conditions for 3 weeks. There was no education whatever in the study. The results were a threefold increase in fruit and salad purchases relative to baseline. A very similar study was done with adolescents in two schools and showed that children are also price-sensitive in fruit and vegetable purchases[9]. The third pilot study with the same design and results was done with low-fat snack items in vending machines[10].

These pilot studies led to a large-scale study that is to date the only large-scale outcome study of the effects of environmental interventions on food choice[11]. The study targeted low-fat vending snacks in 12 worksites and 12 schools, and evaluated both health education effects and price effects. Health education conditions were no education, labeling of low-fat products, and labeling products plus including signage in vending machines encouraging purchases of low-fat products. The price intervention was comprised of four conditions, equal prices for low and high-fat items, and 10, 25 and 50 per cent discounts for the lower fat items.

The effects of health education on food purchases in this study were statistically significant but small, an 8 per cent increase in the per cent of low-fat snack purchases. By contrast, the effects of price on low-fat snack purchases were strong, a 93 per cent increase in low-fat snack sales in the maximum price reduction condition with a graduated effect for lesser price subsidies.

Three studies similar to those done with food choice have also been done by University of Minnesota researchers on physical activity. In two we examined the effects of free memberships to exercise facilities as an incentive to increase physical activity participation. In both cases, reducing the price of access to high-quality community exercise facilities to zero did not increase use of those facilities. The other study examined ways to increase use of stairs rather than elevators in a public building. In a time-series design, we contrasted no intervention, signage encouraging stair rather than elevator use, and signage plus an art and music programme in the stairwells to make them more attractive. We found that the art and music programme increased usage by about 40 per cent, which was statistically significant.

Implications for public health policy

It is believed that on both theoretical and empirical grounds it should be possible to reduce population obesity through public health policy interventions. Environmental changes have caused population obesity and those changes for the most part are man made. Thus, in principle, we should be able to reverse them. Empirical work done on environmental change in health behaviours suggests a number of specific areas which public health policy interventions might target. For example, to achieve a goal of reducing body weight, the attractiveness and availability of food could be reduced by controlling the number of food outlets, controlling their number of hours of operation, or controlling other conditions of sale like portion sizes. Taxation policy could also be used to alter the price of foods, making either all foods less attractive or energy-dense foods less so in comparison to food with lower energy density. The education environment might also be controlled by limiting advertising of food products in order to lessen the impact of this as an inducement to overeat.

This having been said, however, meaningful change in the public health policy area in the US would be difficult. Obstacles to policy implementation include scientific ignorance about what behaviours or environmental conditions to target and political challenges due to the fact that effective policies would very likely have adverse effects on some people's lives and economic interests. Any public policy measures powerful enough to influence population obesity would almost certainly have disruptive influences on social and economic institutions whose consequence are hard to predict. Finally, and in some ways the most important, it is not clear if the general public in the US is ready for policy measures targeting eating and exercise behaviours.

The obesity epidemic has in many ways been a tremendous boon to obesity research. Much more money is now available to do all kinds of research in the area than was true 10 years ago. Even so, the research challenges posed by the obesity epidemic are considerable. There are conceptual challenges that we have yet come to grips with, particularly in regard to how to think about environmental determinants. We need more data on temporal trends in behaviours and environmental factors. Innovative experimental research that can help policy makers estimate the costs and potential effects of various public health policy measures on behaviour and body weight are also much needed.

Acknowledgements: This research was supported by grant number DK50456 from the National Institute of Diabetes and Digestive and Kidney Diseases.

Reference

1. French SA, Story M, Jeffery RW. Environmental influences on eating and physical activity. *Annu Rev Public Health* 2001; 22: 63–89.

2. Jeffery RW, French SA. Epidemic obesity in the United States: Are fast foods and television viewing contributing? *Am J Public Health* 1998; 88: 277–80.

3. Troy L. Report on 'Selected Operating Factors in per cent of Net Sales: Advertising'. In: *Almanac of business and industrial financial ratios*, L. Troy (ed.). Englewood Cliffs, NY: Prentice-Hall, 1978, 1985, 1990, 1993, 1998.

4. Young LR, Nestle M. The contribution of expanding portion sizes to the US obesity epidemic. *Am J Public Health* 2002; 92: 246–49.

5. Jeffery RW, Forster JL, French S, Kelder S, Lando H, McGovern P, Jacobs Jr DR, Baxter J. Healthy Worker Project: A worksite intervention for weight control and smoking cessation. *Am J Public Health* 1993; 83: 395–401.

6. Jeffery RW, Gray CW, French SA, Hellerstedt WL, Murray D, Luepker RV, Blackburn H. Evaluation of weight reduction in a community intervention for cardiovascular disease risk: Changes in body mass index in the Minnesota Heart Health Program. *Int J Obes* 1995; 19: 30–9.

7. Jeffery RW, French SA. Preventing weight gain in adults: The Pound of Prevention study. *Am J Public Health* 1999; 89: 747–51.

8. Jeffery RW, French SA, Raether C, Baxter JE. An environmental intervention to increase fruit and salad purchases in a cafeteria. *Prev Med* 1994; 23: 788–92.

9. French SA, Story M, Jeffery RW, Snyder P, Eisenberg M, Sidebottom A, Murray D. Pricing strategy to promote fruit and vegetable purchase in high school cafeterias. *J Am Diet Assoc.* 1997; 97: 1008–10.

10. French SA, Jeffery RW, Story M, Hannan P, Stat M, Snyder MP. Pricing strategy to promote low fat snack choices through vending machines. *Am J Public Health* 1997; 87: 849–51.

11. French SA, Jeffery RW, Story M, Breitlow KK, Baxter JS, Hannan P, Snyder MP. Pricing and promotion effects on low fat vending snack purchases: The CHIPS study. *Am J Public Health* 2001; 9: 112–7.

©2003 John Libbey Eurotext Ltd, pp. 435–438.

CHAPTER 91

Community based intervention and government policies: experience from Latin America

Walmir Coutinho

Catholic University of Rio de Janeiro, Department of Endocrinology, Av. Armando Lombardi, 800 Gr.238 - Barra da Tijuca, Rio de Janeiro-RJ, 22.640-000, Brazil
[e-mail: wcoutinho@openlink.com.br]

Obesity epidemic is rapidly escalating in most Latin-American countries, especially among lower income populations. Although several studies have provided alarming data about obesity epidemic in many Latin America countries, secular trends in the prevalence of obesity in Brazilian adults have been well documented with data from three nation-wide large-scale cross-sectional surveys undertaken in 1975, 1989 and 1997. About one third of the Brazilian population is presently considered overweight, whereas obesity prevalence is estimated to be approximately 10 per cent.

Nutrition transition seems to be the main explanation for the dramatic increase in obesity prevalence reported in the less developed (northeastern) region of Brazil and among lower income populations from the southeastern (more developed) region.

The shifts in employment structure and leisure time allocation led to increasingly sedentary lifestyle. Changes in food habits have been also very profound over the last decades, with important increases in fat intake being reported in all cities surveyed.

Surprising data emerged from the last survey, undertaken in 1997, when a remarkable decline in obesity prevalence was detected in the higher income group of southeastern women (from 13.2 per cent to 8.2 per cent).

Only in Scandinavian populations such declining trends had been previously described. Although much more information is still needed to allow an appropriate analysis, it seems reasonable to hypothesize that an intense mass media work focused on stimulating physical activity and better food habits has been effective in reaching at least the higher income women from the more developed parts of the country. Moreover, multivariate analysis of demographic, socioeconomic and anthropometric data indicate that, in transition societies, whereas income tends to be a risk factor for obesity, education tends to be protective.

The main public health implication arising from these findings seems to be the urgent need of specific education as the key element for the control of obesity epidemic.

The first steps

The main initiatives for the control of obesity epidemics in Latin America were developed trough collaborative work by the Ministry of Health, Brazilian Association for the Study of Obesity (ABESO) and local Governments.

A Latin American Consensus Meeting was promoted by Latin American Federation of Obesity Societies (FLASO) and ABESO in Rio de Janeiro in 1998, with the participation of Brazilian Ministry of Health. A Consensus document was published, suggesting several actions, such as regulation of consumer friendly food labeling, launching of healthy weight campaigns, promotion of healthy eating and physical activities in schools and work places and creation of facilities to stimulate the practice of physical activities in the streets.

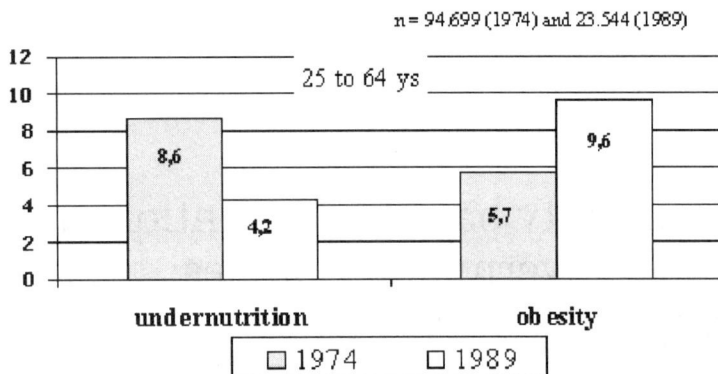

Fig. 1. Nutrition transition in Brazil. Monteiro *et al. Eur J Clin Nutr* 1995; 49: 105–13.

In 1999, the Ministry of Health instituted an official day for the fight against obesity (11 October) and the Brazilian Obesity Task Force (BOTF) was created. The first nationwide initiatives for obesity prevention were then designed, with the participation of many scientific societies, the food industry and consumers' associations.

Legislative and regulatory actions

All packaged foods in Brazil must list their content in calories, protein, carbohydrates and fats. The concept of 'nutritionally adequate serving sizes' was recently introduced, representing the usual consumption of the different foods and providing means of reinforcing unbalanced and erroneous eating patterns. The nutritional content of raw and unpacked foods will have to be informed at point of sale.

ABESO suggested that healthy foods should bear a green sign on the label and foods with high caloric density, high in saturated fat or sugar should be marked with a red sign.

To promote healthy eating in the schools, a new legislation was established in 2000, aiming to provide better school meals to elementary public school students (37 million children). The federal government, through monthly monetary transfers, funds the school meals programme. According to the new legislation, it is mandatory that a minimum of 70 per cent of the programme's annual budget of about US$500 million dollars is spent on fresh vegetables, fruits and minimally processed foods. Foods sold in public schools canteens will be probably regulated in the near future.

Information and communication activities

A Brazilian Food Guideline was created with the support of the Brazilian academic community. A new concept was introduced, the 'step-by-step route to healthy eating', proposing that people choose one of the 10 recommended steps and pursue it as a personal or family goal. A pre-tested self-assessment questionnaire, indicating the first step to be taken, was distributed to 10 million Brazilian adults in November 2001, during the national screening campaign for hypertension.

The messages stimulating the practice of physical activities will be delivered through the Ministry of Health's 'Agita Brazil' programme. To help consumers to take advantage of the seasonal variations in fruit and vegetable prices and make more valuable and healthier choices, a software program called 'Shop smart-the best buy' was produced and will be available at supermarkets.

To build the capacity of school teachers for nutrition promotion, healthy eating videos were introduced in the programme of a special TV channel created to train elementary school teachers. Four videos have been broadcast since April 1999, potentially reaching 37 million elementary school children.

Building the capacity of health workers to give advice on healthy eating was considered fundamental to guarantee sustainability for the whole strategy. Guidelines and manuals are being produced for 150,000 community health workers, who cover about 100 families each. Healthy eating and physical activity were included in the protocols used in health services to treat hypertensive and diabetic patients, and these protocols have already been provided to over 40,000 primary health care workers.

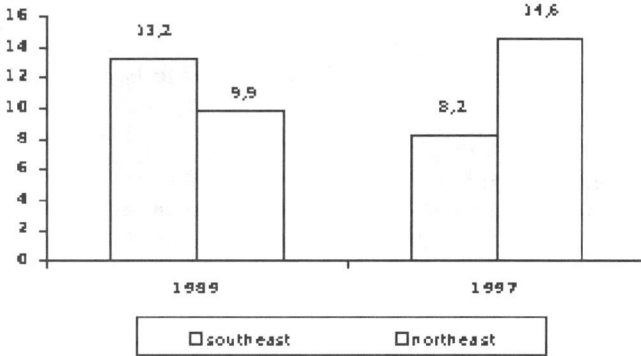

Fig. 2. Prevalence of obesity among women with the highest income in the Southeastern region. Monteiro and Conde, *Arq Bras Endocrinol Metab* 1999; 43(3).

ABESO programme for healthy weight education

Since 1999 a number of educational activities were planned and promoted by ABESO to develop healthy weight education in Brazil. More than 50 cities from all the regions of the country have already been covered with educational activities directed to physicians and other health professionals, aiming not only to optimize their ability in treating obese patients, but also to stimulate them to give advice on healthy eating and practicing of physical activity. Several types of scientific sessions have been used, such as interactive sessions, lectures and debates.

In 10 cities, the educational activities were also directed to the general public, with wide coverage by the media. Activities included workshops, 'food labs', lectures, festivals, anthropometric evaluation, and many other actions aiming to increase population's awareness about the risks of overweight and to encourage individuals to adhere to appropriate lifestyle changes.

During educational activities, many local initiative were initiated or supported, including several healthy weight promotion programmes in many cities all over the country.

Integrating approaches with other nutrition-related noncommunicable diseases

Brazilian Ministry of Health launched in 2001 a National screening campaign for diabetes and hypertension, aiming to identify new cases and refer them for treatment and to raise population awareness about these diseases. More than 20 million individuals aged 40 years or more have been already screened for diabetes, with elevated capillary glucose being detected in 2.9 million (14.66 per cent). Among 1,541,221 individuals who had their blood pressure checked, it was found elevated in 35 per cent of them.

The Ministry of Health is also using the data collected during the campaign to reorganize the components of the health care system involved with their treatment. In 2002, screening and management of obesity were also included in the scope of this campaign.

Community-based initiatives

At local government level, some initiatives have achieved remarkable results. In the city of Rio de Janeiro, a local plan was developed, aiming to improve health and to reduce inequalities, by promoting and supporting behaviour change. The action was focused to primary schools, heath centres, hospitals, working places and the community.

In schools, 530,000 healthy meals are provided everyday, at an annual cost of 27 million dollars. Nutrition education is being provided to teachers, students and workers involved with meal preparation, covering all 1,209 schools.

In all maternity hospitals, breast-feeding promotion is part of the programme. In health centres, healthy weight promotion was extended to 266,000 clients from the hypertension control programme and 58,000 clients from the diabetes control programme. Obesity management was instituted, including group approach and nutrition education.

At workplaces, the strategy was to work with the private sector, providing nutrition education, healthier meals and opportunities for physical activity to the municipal workers (180,000 people). At community level, many actions have been planned, like the 'healthy gastronomic festival'.

To promote physical activity, the 'Agita Rio' initiative is now to be launched, during the 7 April celebrations.

A very good example of legislation initiative, that can be easily reproduced in other cities, is the 'Healthy Street' law. It was passed in 1998 and allows the traffic to be interrupted during certain hours of the day or night and public security is provided so that people can exercise safely on the streets. Priority is given to the most deprived areas of the city, where security is poor and bicycle paths, sidewalks, sports facilities and pedestrian walkways are almost nonexistent.

Conclusions

Obesity is now recognized in Latin America as an overwhelming threat to the health of our population. Many achievements in healthy weight promotion in Brazil have been made possible by the collaborative efforts from the Federal Government, local governments, scientific societies and a number of other sectors of Brazilian society.

It is very important that Brazilian initiatives are replicated in other Latin American countries, and Latin American Obesity Task Force, affiliated to Latin American Federation of Obesity Societies has been working over the last two years trying to facilitate the collaboration between the Ministries of Health. It seems clear to us that any effort directed to the control of nutrition-related noncommunicable diseases, should involve, whenever possible, the Federal and local Governments, the Scientific and Academic societies and all relevant contributions we can recruit from many different sources, to fight sedentary life-style and to promote healthy eating habits. Regardless of all therapeutic resources, which urgently need to become available to our obese population, education and information seem to be the most cost-effective tools for the control of obesity epidemic and should be specially emphasized in developing countries.

References

1. Agencia Nacional de Vigilância Sanitária – regulations on nutrition labelling and serving sizes (RDC 39, 21 of March 2001 [On-line] Available from: URL: http://www.anvisa.gov.br [accessed 2 March 2002].

2. Brazil, Ministério da Saúde. Política Nacional de Alimentação e Nutrição / Secretaria de Políticas de Saúde – DFPD, Brasília, 2000. Brasil. [On-line] Available from: URL: http://www.saude.gov.br [Accessed 2 March 2002].

3. Brazil, Ministério da Saúde. Guias Alimentares para Crianças Menores de Dois Anos – Bases técnicas. Brasília: Brasil. 2001.

4. Coutinho W (Coordenador). Consenso Latino-Americano de Obesidade. Arquivos Brasileiros de Endocrinologia e Metabologia 1999.

5. Matsudo V, Matsudo S, Andrade D, Araujo T, Andrade E et al. A Promotion of physical activity in a developing country: the Agita Sao Paulo experience. Public Health Nutr (in press, 2002).

6. Monteiro CA, D'A Benicio MH, Conde WL, Popkin BM. 'Shifting Obesity Trends in Brazil'. Eur J Clin Nutr 2000; 54: 342–6.

Progress in Obesity Research: 9. Edited by *Geraldo Medeiros-Neto, Alfredo Halpern* and *Claude Bouchard*
©2003 John Libbey Eurotext Ltd, pp. 439–442.

CHAPTER 92

Success and failure in the maintenance of lost weight

Michael G. Perri

Department of Clinical and Health Psychology, University of Florida Health Science Center, PO Box 100165,
1600 SW Archer Road, Gainesville, FL 32610-0165, USA
[e-mail: mperri@hp.ufl.edu]

Introduction

Long-term studies of obesity treatment commonly paint a gloomy picture[1,2]. When weight-loss intervention ends, most patients gradually abandon changes in eating and exercise habits and regain weight[3]. On average, a return to baseline weight routinely occurs within 3 to 5 years of treatment[1–3]. If obese patients fail to maintain lost weight, the health benefits resulting from weight-loss treatments are likely to be negligible. Thus, improving the maintenance of lost weight represents a critical challenge in the management of obesity[4].

Some obese individuals experience long-term 'success' in weight management – a fact that is sometimes obscured by a simple examination of mean outcomes in follow-up studies. As many as 15–25 per cent of participants in lifestyle interventions successfully maintain 50 per cent or more of their initial weight losses 3 to 5 years after behavioural treatment[1]. Furthermore, clinical trials[3,4] have demonstrated that certain treatment strategies that may enhance the maintenance of lost weight. This paper provides an overview of factors associated with successful weight management with particular attention to promising strategies for improving long-term outcome in obesity treatment.

Contributors to the maintenance problem

Why is it so difficult for obese persons to sustain lost weight? A complex interaction of physiological, environmental, and psychological variables appears responsible for the weight-loss maintenance problem. Physiological factors, such as reduced metabolic rate resulting from sustained dieting, prime the obese person to regain lost weight[5,6]. Environmental factors, such as constant exposure to low cost, highly palatable, energy dense foods, combined with easy access to modern conveniences requiring low levels of energy expenditure, further dispose the individual to return to patterns of eating and physical inactivity that promote weight gain[7,8]. Furthermore, obese individuals view the degree of weight reduction commonly achieved in lifestyle and pharmacological treatments (i.e. 8–10 per cent) as 'disappointing'[9]. Consequently, they may not be sufficiently motivated to sustain what they view as insignificant weight change. Moreover, the most rewarding element of treatment, namely, weight loss, typically ends with the cessation of intervention. Consequently, many individuals perceive a high 'cost' associated with continued dietary control while experiencing no 'benefit' in terms of additional weight loss. Hence, they become dispirited, and small posttreatment weight gains commonly result in attributions of personal ineffectiveness, a sense of hopelessness, and an abandonment of the weight-control effort.

Findings from correlational studies

Despite the typical pattern of regain following an initial weight reduction, some individuals manage to succeed in sustaining clinically significant amounts of weight loss. Correlational studies[10–12] provide information about factors commonly associated with success (see Table 1). A high rate of attendances at treatment sessions and good initial adherence to intervention strategies (particularly self-monitoring) are positive predictors of favourable long-term outcome[10]. Similarly large initial weight losses are associated with greater amounts of weight loss maintained at follow-up[11], whereas the presence of binge eating coupled with depression is commonly associated with a poor outcome[12].

The National Weight Control Registry, an ongoing observational study[13] of individuals who have documented large weight losses, provides additional information about strategies associated with good long-term outcome. Successful maintainers typically consume a low-calorie, low-fat diet (approximately 1400 kcal/day with less than 25 per cent of energy from fats). Successful individuals are vigilant about their weight with 75 per cent reporting that they weigh themselves either daily or weekly. In addition, they are also committed to high levels of physical activity; 72 per cent report that expend more than 2000 kcal/week in exercise. Collectively, the Weight Loss Registry findings show that successful individuals demonstrate very active, ongoing efforts at weight control.

Findings from clinical trials

Over the past two decades, researchers have examined a wide array of strategies designed to improve long-term outcome in obesity treatment. Promising strategies include extended care programmes, the use of portion-controlled diets, home-based exercise regimens, and multi-component treatments (see Table 1).

Table 1. Factors associated with success in the management of obesity

Findings from correlational studies
High attendance at intervention sessions
Good 'early' adherence to treatment strategies
Absence of depression plus binge eating
Large initial weight loss
Long-term, continued intake of a low-fat, low-calorie diet
Long-term, continued self-monitoring of body weight
Long-term, continued completion of high levels of exercise
Findings from clinical trials
Continuing care through regular clinician-patient contacts following initial therapy
Prescribing a high frequency of moderate intensity, home-based aerobic exercise
Providing exercise equipment and prescribing exercise completion in short bouts
Providing portion controlled meals in combination with extended care
Combining pharmacotherapy, behaviour therapy, and portion-controlled diet

Extended care programmes

Improving the long-term effects of treatment involves finding ways to assist patients in sustaining key changes in the behaviours that regulate energy balance and weight loss. Perri and Corsica[3] recently reviewed the results of 13 studies in which behavioural weight-loss treatments were extended beyond six months through the use of weekly or biweekly treatment sessions. One year after the initiation of treatment, those groups that received behaviour therapy *with* extended contact successfully maintained 96.3 per cent of their initial losses. The inclusion of a control group (i.e. behavioural treatment without extended contact) in three of the studies permits a rough comparison of the groups with and without extended treatment. The groups *without* extended contact maintained 66.5 per cent of their initial weight reductions. Judging the effects of the extended-treatments by comparison with the standard-length groups suggests a beneficial impact for extended contact.

Portion controlled diets

Better long-term results might be obtained by directly altering the environment of obese individuals rather than relying on patients themselves to make all the required dietary changes. Accordingly, the provision of portion-controlled meals has been shown to improve weight-loss progress both during initial treatment and during the course of a 12-month maintenance period[14]. Moreover, the combination of monthly follow-up sessions with the provision of portion-controlled meals has shown good promise as a long-term maintenance strategy[15].

Exercise

Regular exercise produces many benefits for overweight individuals including increased energy expenditure and improvements in mood and self-concept. However, most controlled trials have failed to show that the combination of diet plus exercise produces greater maintenance of lost weight than diet alone[16]. The modest effects of exercise (particularly supervised group exercise) on long-term weight progress may be due to poor or inconsistent exercise adherence. Consequently, attention has turned to improving exercise adherence in obesity treatment. Promising approaches include: home-based exercise (rather than supervised group exercise)[17]; the provision of home exercise equipment combined with the use short rather than long bouts of exercise (e.g. four 10-min bouts vs. one 40-min bout)[18]; and prescriptions for aerobic exercise to be completed at a high frequency but moderate intensity[19].

Multi-component maintenance programmes

The ideal weight-loss maintenance programme would involve a matching of treatment methods to the specific needs of particular patients. However, an empirical database describing those procedures best suited to particular individuals is not yet available. Consequently, multi-component programmes have been developed with the expectation that some aspect of a multifaceted approach will benefit a particular individual. Empirically-tested, multi-component programmes have included ongoing professional contacts combined with training in problem-solving or relapse-prevention skills[20,21], social support[22,23], and high frequency exercise[23]. Most studies[20-23] have demonstrated that weight-loss treatments supplemented with multi-component maintenance programmes produce superior long-term results than treatments without maintenance programmes. However, continued contact may be the most important element in such programmes[4,23]. Recent findings[24,25] also suggest the benefits of multi-component programmes that combine behavioural and pharmacological approaches to the management of obesity.

References

1. Kramer FM, Jeffery RW, Forster JL, Snell MK. Long-term follow-up of behavioral treatment for obesity: Patterns of weight gain among men and women. *Int J Obes Relat Metab Disord* 1989; 13, 124–36.

2. Stalonas PM, Perri MG, Kerzner AB. Do behavioral treatments of obesity last? A five-year follow-up investigation. *Addict Behav* 1984; 9: 175–84.

3. Perri MG, Corsica JA. Improving the maintenance of weight lost inbehavioral treatment of obesity. In: *Obesity: theory and therapy* (3rd edn), TA Wadden, AJ Stunkard (eds), pp. 357–82. New York: Guilford, 2002.

4. Perri MG, Nezu AM, Viegener BJ. *Improving the long-term management of obesity: Theory, research, and clinical guidelines.* New York: John Wiley & Sons; 1992.

5. Leibel RL, Rosenbaum M, Hirsch J. Changes in energy expenditure resulting from altered body weight. *N Engl J Med* 1995; 332: 673–4.

6. Dulloo AG, Jacquet J. Adaptive reduction in basal metabolic rate in response to food deprivation in humans: a role for feedback signals from fat stores. *Am J Clin Nutr* 1998; 68: 599–606.

7. Poston WS, Foreyt JP. Obesity is an environmental issue. *Atherosclerosis* 1999; 146: 201–9.

8. Hill JO, Wyatt HR, Melanson EL. Genetic and environmental contributions to obesity. *Med Clin North Am* 2000; 84: 333–46.

9. Foster GD, Wadden TA, Vogt RA, Brewer G. What is a reasonable weight loss? Patients' expectations and evaluations of obesity treatment outcomes. *J Consult Clin Psychol* 1997; 65: 79–85.

10. Wadden TA, Letizia KA. Predictors of attrition and weight loss in patients treated by moderate and severe caloric restriction. In: *Treatment of the seriously obese patient*, TA Wadden, TB Van Itallie (eds), pp. 383–410. New York: Guilford Press; 1992.

11. Jeffery RW, Wing RR, Mayer RR. Are smaller weight losses or more achievable weight loss goals better in the long term for obese patients? *J Consult Clin Psychol* 1998; 66: 641–5.

12. Sherwood NE, Jeffery RW, Wing RR. Binge status as a predictor of weight loss treatment outcome. *Int J Obes Relat Metab Disord* 1999; 23: 485–93.

13. Wing RR, Hill JO. Successful weight loss maintenance. *Annu Rev Nutr* 2001; 21: 323–41.

14. Jeffery RW, Wing RR, Thorson C, Burton LR, Raether C, Harvey J, Mullen M. Strengthening behavioral interventions for weight loss: A randomized trial of food provision and monetary incentives. *J Consult Clin Psychol* 1993; 61: 1038–45.

15. Flechtner-Mors M, Ditschuneit HH, Johnson TD, Suchard MA, Adler G. Metabolic and weight loss effects of long-term dietary intervention in obese patients: four-year results. *Obes Res* 2000; 8: 399–402.

16. Wing RR. Physical activity in the treatment of the adulthood overweight and obesity: current evidence and research issues. *Med Sci Sports Exer* 1999; 31: S547–S552.

17. Perri MG, Martin AD, Leermakers EA, Sears SF, Notelovitz M. Effects of group- versus home-based exercise in the treatment of obesity. J *Consult Clin Psychol* 1997; 65: 278–85.

18. Jakicic JM, Winters C, Lang W, Wing RR. Effects of intermittent exercise and use of home exercise equipment on adherence, weight loss, and fitness in overweight women: a randomized trial. *JAMA* 1999; 282: 1554–60.

19. Perri MG, Anton SD, Durning PE, Ketterson TU, Sydeman SJ, Berlant NE, Kanasky WF Jr, Newton RL Jr, Limacher MC, Martin AD. Adherence to exercise prescriptions: Effects prescribing moderate versus higher levels of intensity and frequency. *Health Psychol* 2002; 21: 452–8.

20. Perri MG, Shapiro RM, Ludwig WW, Twentyman CT, McAdoo WG. Maintenance strategies for the treatment of obesity: An evaluation of relapse prevention training and posttreatment contact by mail and telephone. J *Consult Clin Psychol* 1984; 52: 404–13.

21. Perri MG, Nezu AM, McKelvey WF, Schein RL, Renjilian DA, Viegener BJ. Relapse prevention training and problem-solving therapy in the long-term management of obesity. J *Consult Clin Psychol* 2001; 69: 722–6.

22. Perri MG, McAdoo WG, Spevak PA, Newlin DB. Effect of a multicomponent maintenance program on long-term weight loss. J *Consult Clin Psychol* 1984; 52: 480–1.

23. Perri MG, McAllister DA, Gange JJ, Jordan RC, McAdoo WG, Nezu AM. Effects of four maintenance programs on the long-term management of obesity. J *Consult Clin Psychol* 1988; 56: 529–34.

24. Wadden TA, Berkowitz RI. Sarwer DB, Prus-Wisniewski R, Steinberg CM. Benefits of lifestyle modification in the pharmacologic treatment of obesity: a randomized trial. *Arch Int Med* 2001; 161: 218–227.

25. Phelan S, Wadden TA. Combining behavioral and pharmacological treatments for obesity. *Obes Res* 2002; 10: 560–74.

©2003 John Libbey Eurotext Ltd, pp. 443–446.

CHAPTER 93

Drug induced weight gain – psychoactive medications

Leif Breum

Department of Medicine, Endocrine Unit, Roskilde County Hospital Køge, University of Copenhagen, Hospital, DK-4600, Køge, Denmark
[e-mail: leif.breum@dadlnet.dk]

Introduction

Weight increase is a common, but often not recognized side-effect to many widely used psy-choactive medications. The weight gain may in susceptible individuals be substantial and result in obesity and associated co-morbidities. Both antipsychotic compounds, tricyclic anti-depressants, lithium and valproate are among those drugs often associated with persistent weight gain, which severely impedes compliance to an otherwise beneficial treatment. Since increase in appetite and weight gain often are seen as symptoms of improvement of the underlying psychiatric disease, the initial body weight is often markedly exceeded before the patients are offered dietary and exercise counselling. The mechanisms behind the weight gain and appetite changes are not fully understood. Many of the drugs interfere with central appetite-regulating neurotransmitters as such as serotonin, histamine and dopamine and might also affect appetite regulating neuropeptides and energy expenditure. Besides sedation, anticholinergic side-effects may also affect the energy balance by increasing the intake of energy containing beverages. There are only limited experiences with prevention strategies including anti-obesity drugs and much more research is needed.

Antidepressants

Body weight change is a frequent symptom of major depression due to alterations in appetite. Patients typically lose weight[1], although some do not[2]. Despite the introduction of specific serotonin reuptake inhibitors (SSRI) without weight gaining properties, tricyclic antidepressants remain the first choice of medication for the treatment of severe major depression. Amitriptyline[3,4] and imipramine[5-7] have most often been associated with increasing body weight during treatment and, within the tricyclic drug class, amitriptyline appears to promote weight gain to a much greater degree than others. It has not been possible to demonstrate a clear relationship between weight gain and clinical response[4,6] suggesting a more direct pharmacodynamic action independent of their effect on mood. Treatment with tricyclic compounds have been claimed not only to increase energy intake, but also to cause food specific cravings, particularly for 'sweets' or carbohydrates[3,5]. However, the desired 'carbohydrate" foods re-ported contained substantial amounts of fat (sometimes more than the CHO) and were all sweet tasting, like chocolate and pastry. More recent studies from Fernstrom, using more sophisticated and accurate tests for measuring food intake and food selection[6], have not been able to demonstrate marked changes in food preferences during a 4 months study[6]. The mechanism(s) by which antidepressants promote weight gain are not well understood and can reflect changes in energy balance produced by increases in caloric intake, reductions in energy expenditure, or both. In one of the few clinical studies per-formed, a consistent reduction of the resting metabolic rate was found in patients treated with tricyclic antidepressants[7]. Blockage of $5HT_{2C}$ receptors by TCA can increase appetite as demonstrated by the upregulation of these receptors in rat brain. Alternatively, dopamine (D2) receptors antagonism can also increase appetite (as demonstrated for antipsychotics, see below). Histamine H1 receptor antagonism may also be of importance. The SSRIs have proven to be effective in treatment of depression without a concomitant excessive weight gain. The lack of an appetite stimulating effect and possible enhance-ment of metabolic rate contribute to the weight stability properties observed. Although, some particular

SSRIs such as paroxetine occasionally produce significant weight gain[8], this class of serotonergic drugs may be an attractive treatment alternative in moderate ill patients in which drug-induced weight gain has been problematic.

Table 1. Psychoactive medication and obesity

Drug classes	Drugs which often induce weight gain	Drugs which seldom induce weight gain	Putative mechanisms for weight gain
Neuroleptics	Conventional antipsychotics	i.e. haloperidol, molindone	Increased appetite Carbohydrate (and fat) craving?
	High dose compounds such as chlorpromazepine	i.e. ziprasidone	Blockade of serotonin 5-HT$_{2C}$, histamine H$_1$ and dopamine receptors
Antidepressants	Tricyclic antidepressants such as amitryptyline, imipramine Lithium	SSRI drugs such as fluoxetine	Prenatal exposure (haloperidol) Breum et al. Int J Obes 1993;10: 609
	MAO inhibitors (older compounds)	Newer drugs such as meclobemide	Sedation Anticholinergic side effect
Mood stabilisers	Valproate, carbamazepine	i.e. topiramate	Increased insulin sensitivity (sulpiride) Changes in NPY?, leptin?, TNF-α?

Monoamine oxidase (MAO) inhibitors

Weight gain has been described in a relation to especially older MAO inhibitors, whereas this side-effect seems to be less prominent with the selective, reversible drugs such as meclobemide. These compounds may, therefore, represent an alternative treatment modality.

Lithium

Weight gain is often seen and affect between one-third to two-thirds of treated patients[9]. Weight gain appears to be dose-related, and this side-effect remains a leading reason for medication non-compliance[10]. Weight gain is more likely to occur in patients already overweight or with a genetic disposition, and seems more problematic in female patients[9]. The weight gain may amount up 10 kg during a 2- to 10-year period. Increased appetite, increased fluid intake, altered energy metabolism and endocrine changes, including medication-induced hypothyroidism have been proposed as possible mechanisms[9].

Antipsychotic medications

Weight gain as a side effect of antipsychotic treatment has been known for many years[11-13], but its importance in the clinical management of chronic schizophrenia has first recently been fully recognized following the development of new atypical neuroleptics with few or no extrapyramidal side-effects. Conventional antipsychotics such as phenothiazines have been shown to promote weight increase during the chronic treatment of schizophrenia. Placebo controlled trials have revealed that chlorpromazine, chlordiazepoxide and thioridazine cause a significant increase in weight[12,14]. Weight gain, albeit somewhat less extensive, has also been reported with low-dose agents such as haloperidol and fluphenazine[14,15]. It has been suggested that weight gain is not proportional to dose, since depot injections of varying dosages did not correlate with weight gain[14,16]. The weight gain occurs mostly during the first treatment months and can vary from 1 to 8 kg during several years to exorbitant weight increases within a short period of time. Numerous mechanisms have been proposed to explain this medication-induced weight gain. Increased appetite due to blockade of 5HT$_{2C}$ receptors as well as increased thirst due to anticholinergic effects resulting in increased fluid consumption have been suggested. Inactivity resulting from medication-related sedation may also be of importance. Among the novel atypical antipsychotics, clozapine is clearly associated with weight gain during treatment, and is along with olanzapine among the greatest weight gain promoters among the antipsychotics followed by risperidone and sertindole[15,17-19], while molindone and ziprasidone appears to have a weight neutral effect[15,20]. Both clozapine and olanzapine appear to increase leptin levels, but this may reflect body weight changes. The weight promoting mechanisms are, as for other psychoactive drugs, not fully understood. However, dopamine, 5HT$_{2C}$ and histamine binding properties seems to be of importance since a strong association have been demonstrated with compounds with high affinity for those receptors and weight gain[19]. Weight gain and obesity may also arise in children due to prenatal exposure to antipsychotic drugs such as haloperidol prescribed as an antiemetic drug to an otherwise healthy pregnant female[21]. It has been suggested, as for antidepressants, that weight gain during treatment is a positive sign of improvement[1] and necessary for a positive outcome. However, more recent data suggest that, in fact, weight gain is not necessary for achieving an effective therapeutic effect with improvement in symptoms[17]. It also important to notice that, at least for olanzapine, a dose reduction will not improve final outcome[18]. Novel antipsychotics such as clozapine and olanzapine have also been associated with an increased risk of diabetes and even ketoacidosis. In a recent study[22] the risk for developing diabetes was increased almost six times with olanzapine compared to placebo whereas no significant association was found with conventional drugs. It is still unclear wheter this risk is solely depending of the weight increase or by a more direct pharmacological action causing a decline in insulin sensitivity. Since weight gain occurs during the first treatment months, dietary advice, including avoidance of caloric beverages, regular weight control and exercise programmes must be initiated at the start of the treatment. In one of the few clinical studies, it has been shown that behavioural modification therapy could reduce the final weight increase with various antipsychotics, except for clozapine[19]. Studies with current anti-obesity drugs are not available except for a few short-term reports or abstracts pointing to a possible role for both orlistat and histamine H2 blockers, but this remains to be verified in larger long-term clinical studies.

Mood stabilizing drugs

Weight gain is a frequently described side-effect to valporate, a short chain fatty acid, widely used as treatment for mania and epilepsy[23]. In retrospective studies, valproate have been found to increase body weight by 4.0 to 7.5 kg in more than 60 per cent of the patients, but might often amount up to 20 kg resulting in discontinuation of the treatment. Unfortunately, it has been impossible to identify predictive markers separating weight gainers from weight-stable patients. The mechanisms are still widely unknown. Changes in thyroid hormones have been proposed as an contributing factor, but this was confirmed in later clinical studies[24]. Valproate is known to interfere with the GABA system, which might affect appetite regulation, but clinical human data are lacking. In one of the few physiological studies performed in patients treated with valproate[24], it was suggested that a reduced beta-oxidation of fatty acids could be of aetiologically importance since valproate is known to enhance the excretion of carnitine, which is an essential cofactor for the transport of fatty acids across the mitochondrial membrane. The impact of valproate on serum leptin and insulin levels have also been measured, but it seems to reflect the obese state rather than a specific effect of valproate treatment.

Animal studies are difficult to interpret since drug treatment decreases food intake and enhances energy expenditure in many species[25]. Weight gain is also a known side-effect of carbamazepine treatment of both epilepsy and mania. However, both the size of the problem as well as the number of studies is limited compared to valproate[26]. The mechanisms behind the weight gain are unknown, but since carbamazepin share some chemical properties with tricyclic antidepressants it could affect body weight regulation through the same 5HT and noradrenergic pathways increasing the appetite. During the last decade new drugs have been introduced into clinical practice. One of these drugs, vigabatrin, is normally better tolerated than the older compounds, but has recently been shown to be more frequently associated with weight gain than carbamazepine. In contrast to this finding, weight gain seems to be absent with newer compounds such as lamotrigin and topiramate, which could represent alternative treatment modalities[27].

Antianxiety drugs

Benzodiazepines have been shown to promote hyperphagia and weight gain in rodents due to an effect on the dopamine D2 receptors or gamma amino butyric acid neurones, although long-term experiments not have confirmed these findings. Data from the few clinical studies are inconsistent, but it is unlikely that these drugs cause significant weight gain in clinical practice.

Conclusions

Weight gain associated with tricyclic antidepressant, valproate and antipsychotic medications is problematic for many patients and often a reason for non-compliance. Dietary advice, avoidance of caloric beverages, regularly weight controls, and exercise programmes initiated at the start of the psychopharmacological treatment remain the fundament for prevention and treatment of drug-induced weight gain. Blood glucose and lipids should be measured at regular intervals. Specific pharmacological treatment with current anti-obesity drugs needs to be investigated further before any recommendations can be presented. If weight gain develops during treatment, reassessment of the indication for drug therapy or change of the psychopharmacological modality must be considered taken this serious side-effect into account.

References

1. Mezzich JE, Raab JS. Depressive symptomology across the Americas. *Arch Gen Psychiatry* 1980; 37: 818–823.

2. Stunkard AJ, Fernstrom MH, Price A, Frank E, Kupfer DJ. Direction of weight change in recurrent depression: A possible marker for subtypes of depression. *Arch Gen Psychiat* 1990; 47: 857–60.

3. Paykel ES, Meuller PS, DeLa Vergne PM. Amitriptyline, weight gain, and carbohydrate craving. *Br J Psychiat* 1973; 123: 501–7.

4. Fernstrom MH, Kupfer DJ. Antidepressant-induced weight gain: A comparison study of four medications. *Psychiat Res*1988; 26: 265–71.

5. Berken GH, Weinstein D, Stern WC. Weight gain: A side effect of tricyclic antidepressants. *J Affect Disord* 1984; 7: 133–8.

6. Fernstrom MH, Kupfer DJ. Imipramine treatment and preference for sweets. *Appetite* 1988; 10: 149–55.

7. Fernstrom MH, Spiker DG, Epstein LH, Kupfer DJ. Resting metabolic rate is reduced in patients treated with antidepressants. *Biol Psychiat* 1985; 688–92.

8. Sussman N, Ginsburg DL. Weight gain associated with SSRIs. *Primary Psychiatry* 1998; 5(1): 28–37.

9. Ackerman S, Nolan LJ. Bodyweight gain induced by psychotropic drugs: incidence, mechanisms, and management. *CNS Drugs* 1998; 9: 135–51.

10. John RE, McFarland BH Lithium use and discontinuation in a health maintenance organization. *Am J Psychiat* 1996; 153: 993–1000.

11. Mefford RB, Labrosse EH, Gawienowski AM, Williams, R. Influence of chlorpromazine on certain biochemical variables of chornic male schizophrenics. *J Nerv Ment Dis* 1958; 127: 167–79.

12. Planansky K, Heilizer F. Weight changes in relation to the characteristics of patients on chlorpromazine. *J Clin Exp Psychopathol* 1959; 20: 53–579.

13. Silverstone T, Smith G, Goodall E. Prevalence of obesity in patients receiving depot antipsychotics. *Br J Psychiat* 1988; 153: 214–217.

14. Ganguli R. Weight gain associated with antipsychotic drugs. *J Clin Psychiat* 1999; 60: S2: 20–24.

15. Allison DB, Mentore JL, Heo M, Chandler LP, Cappelleri JC, Infante MC, Weiden PJ. Antipsychotic-induced weight gain: a comprehensive research synthesis. *Am J Psychiatry* 1999; 156(11): 1686–96.

16. Johnson DA, Breen M. Weight changes with depot neuroleptic maintenance therapy. *Acta Psychiat Scand* 1979; 59: 525–8.

17. Leadbetter R, Shutty M, Pavalonis D *et al.* Clozapine-induced weight gain: prevalence and clinical relevance. *Am J Psychiat* 1992; 149: 68–72.

18. Kinon B, Basson B, Gilmore JA, Tollefson GD. Long-term olanzapine treatment: weight change and weight-related health factors in schizophrenia. *J Clin Psychiatry* 2001; 62(2): 92–100.

19. Wirshing DA, Wirshing WC, Kysar L, *et al.* Novel Antipsychotics: comparison of weight gain liabilities. *J Clin Psychiat* 1999; 60: 358–63.

20. Arato M, O'Connor R, Meltzer HY. On behalf of the ZEUS Study Group. A 1-year, double-blind, placebo-controlled trial of ziprasidone 40, 80 and 160 mg/day in chronic schizophrenia: the Ziprasidone Extended Use in schizo- phrenia (ZEUS) study. *Int Clin Psychopharmacol* 2002; 17(5): 207–15.

21. Breum L, Astrup AV, Quaade F. Increased appetite after prenatal haloperidol exposure – a case report. *Int J Obes* 1993; 10: 609.

22. Koro CE, Fedder DO, L'Italien GJ, Weiss SS, Magder LS, Kreyenbuhl J, Revicki DA, Buchanan RW. Assessment of independent effect of olanzapine and risperidone on risk of diabetes among patients with schizophrenia: population based nested case-control study. *BMJ* 2002; 3: 325(7358): 243.

23. Convanis A, Gupta K, Jeavons PM.Sodium valproate: Monotherapy and polytherapy. *Epilepsia* 1982; 23: 693–720.

24. Breum L, Astrup A, Gram L, Andersen T, Stokholm K H, Christensen N J, Werdelin L, Madsen J. Metabolic changes during treatment with valproate in humans: Implication for untoward weight gain. *Metabolism* 1992; 41: 666–70.

25. Horton R, Rothwell NJ, Stock MJ: Chronic inhibition of Gaba Transaminase results in activation of thermogenesis and brown fat in the rat. *Gen Pharm* 1988; 19: 403–5.

26. Mattson RH, Cramer JA, Collins JF. A comparison of valproate with carbamazepine for the treatment of complex partial seizures and secondarily generalized tonic-clonic seizures in adults. *N Engl J Med* 1992; 327: 765–71.

27. Yatham LN, Kusumakar V, Calabrese JR, Rao R, Scarrow G, Kroeker G. Third generation anticonvulsants in bipolar disorder: a review of efficacy and summary of clinical recommendations. *J Clin Psychiatry* 2002; 63(4): 275–83.

©2003 John Libbey Eurotext Ltd, pp. 447–450.

CHAPTER 94

Prescription medicines: modifiable contributor to obesity

Lawrence J. Cheskin

*Johns Hopkins Bloomberg School of Public Health, Johns Hopkins Weight Management Center,
2360 West Joppa Road, Suite 205, Lutherville, MD 21093, USA
[e-mail: Cheskin@jhmi.edu]*

Introduction

Given the striking increase in the prevalence of obesity worldwide over the past generation, and the difficulties typically encountered in treatment, any easily modified precipitants of weight gain we can identify would be most welcome. One such precipitant of weight gain may be prescription medications.

As obesity has increased in prevalence, there has also been a striking increase in the use of prescription medicines over the past generation. This increase in medication use is attributable to more widespread access to health care, increases in life expectancy, and more and more chronic health conditions becoming controllable through advances in pharmacotherapy.

While it would not be justified to conclude that the association of increased obesity rates and increased use of medications is causally linked, it is certainly possible that medications that are known to have a tendency to increase appetite or body weight account for or contribute to obesity in some individuals. Further, it is known that obese individuals are more likely to suffer such comorbidities as type 2 diabetes and hypertension, and thus are more likely to be prescribed medications that may contribute to weight gain.

Anecdotal experience at the Johns Hopkins Weight Management Center with patients reporting substantial weight gain temporally related to use of certain prescription medicines (see examples below) led to a more structured review of the phenomenon.

Case reports

Case A. A 42 year old health professional presented to the Johns Hopkins Weight Management Center for treatment of a 40 lb (18.2 kg) weight gain over the previous 18 months. She was of normal weight until beginning lithium carbonate and perpherazine for bipolar illness. Her psychiatrist felt that the lithium was essential, but changed the perphenazine to lozapine. With this change and a weight management programme she lost 35 lbs of the 40 gained.

Case B. A 36-year-old male supermarket pastry chef came to us for treatment of morbid obesity. He weighed 511 lb (232 kg) and was 68.5 in (1.74 m) tall, with a body mass index (BMI) of 76.7 kg/m². He had a 2½ year history of lower extremity pain, lymphedema, and recurrent cellulitis, treated with periodic courses of antibiotics and long-term prednisone therapy. He had gained 240 lb while taking prednisone. With discontinuance of prednisone, he stopped gaining weight and began to lose weight on a medical weight loss programme.

Methods

MEDLINE and the Micromedex Drug Information database (Micromedex, Englewood, Colorado, USA) were searched to identify and categorize prescription medications with side effects of weight gain or appetite increase. Possible alternative medications that are not known to cause these side effects are suggested for consideration when clinically appropriate. Mechanisms of weight gain are described when known, and guidelines for identification and management of medication-associated weight gain are offered.

Results

The findings are most readily described in tabular form. Each table contains a class of medication with member drugs that have been reported to be problematic, and possible alternative drugs that have not been reported to be problematic (Tables 1–5).

Table 1. Antihypertensives

Specific problem drugs	Alternative drugs
Nonselective b-blocker (propranolol)	Atenolol, metoprolol, labetalol, nadalol
One Ca-channel blocker (nisoldipine)	Diltiazem, nifedipine, verapamil, amlodipine
Most alpha-adrenergic blockers (prazocin, terazocin)	Doxazocine
Most centrally-acting agents (clonidine, methyldopa, guanethidine)	Guanfacine
ACE-inhibitors are not a problem	

Table 2. Antidiabetic agents

Specific problem drugs	Alternative drugs
Insulin	Once-daily insulin
Sulphonylureas (both 1st and 2nd generation)	Add metformin or acarbose
Insulin sensitizers including the thiazolidinediones are not problematic Metformin and acarbose may even help decrease weight	

Table 3. Psychoactive drugs

Specific problem drugs	Alternative drugs
Lithium carbonate	Valproate, carbamazepine
Most tricyclic antidepressants	Nortyptyline, SSRIs
MAOI phenylzine	Tranylcypromine, moclobemide
Clovoxamine	All other SSRIs
Antipsychotics: clozapine, chlorpromazine, thiothixene	Molindone, loxapine, ziprasadone

Table 4. Anticonvulsants

Specific problem drugs	Alternative drugs
Valproic acid, carbamazepine	Phenytoin, phenobarbital, topiramate

Table 5. Miscellaneous

Specific problem drugs	Alternative drugs
Clofibrate	Cholestyramine
Ketorolac	Other NSAIDs
Omeprazole	Other PPIs
Corticosteroids	Minimize dose, consider alternate day treatment

The most frequent mechanism of weight increase is an increase in appetite, such as is seen with certain psychoactive agents, anticonvulsants, antihypertensives, antihyperglycaemics, and hormonal agents. Other mechanisms include fluid retention, as may be seen with steroids, and increased metabolic efficiency, as may be seen when the hyperglycaemia of diabetes mellitus comes under control through use of insulin or other agents. In some cases, multiple mechanisms may coexist, such as in the example of steroids.

Sometimes, knowledge of the mechanisms of action of appetite-suppressing medications may help predict those medicines that can be expected to increase appetite. For example, beta-2 adrenergic agonists such as phentermine and diethylpropion are precribed as appetite suppressants, so it would be expected that centrally-active beta adrenergic *blockers* would be appetite stimulants, as indeed propranolol appears to be. On the other hand, several other, more selective beta blockers have not been reported to cause weight gain- it is likely that weight gain as a side effect would be seen most in those agents with particular avidity for central beta-2 receptors.

Discussion

Our knowledge of this area of weight control is derived largely from anecdotal reports and side effect profiles noted during clinical trials. Metaanalyses are beginning to appear[1,2], but much further work needs to be done. For example, there is little known about the frequency of noncompliance with medication prescriptions because of patients' perception of a medicine causing weight gain. Because of the lack of systematic searching for this side effect during clinical trials and clinical practice, it is likely that the lists compiled in this study are incomplete. In addition, idiosyncratic effects may be seen in individual patients such that the patient experiences weight gain that is not widely seen with a particular agent.

While it may be possible in some instances to do 'n of one' trials in specific patients by withdrawing the suspected drug to see whether the weight or appetite effect resolves, and even to reinstate the drug for further confirmation of the effect, this is unnecessary in most instances, since alternatives exist for most agents.

In some instances, weight gain may be viewed as a positive outcome, as when a depressed, underweight patient begins to respond to treatment and gains weight. This effect may be more clinical lore than fact, however[3]. Indeed, in the vast majority of patients with various conditions who experience weight gain or appetite increase, this is an undesirable and unexpected side effect of treatment. Weight gain in nonobese individuals may push them into the overweight or obese categories, while the already obese may experience the onset or exacerbation of obesity-related conditions.

Unfortunately, already obese individuals are most liable to being prescribed a medication that may cause weight gain because they have a higher risk of the diseases that are treated with medications. This may further exacerbate their comorbidities, setting up a potential 'vicious cycle' unless the problematic medicine is recognized and steps taken to provide alternatives as well as support for weight loss.

In at least one instance, there is evidence that the obese are more susceptible to medication induced weight gain for yet another reason – steroid agents are cleared less well and cortisol accumulates in higher concentrations in such target tissues as liver and visceral adipose tissue[4].

While the magnitude of the problem of medication-induced weight gain is essentially unknown, because of the number of drugs implicated and how commonly they are prescribed, it is likely to be substantial. Thus, it behooves practitioners to be aware of the possibility of weight gain related to medications. Guidelines are offered as follows:

1. Have a high index of suspicion and inquire specifically about appetite and weight effects when prescribing new medications or reviewing current medications in patients.

2. Be aware of the potential for weight effects in nonobese patients as they may be as concerned as obese individuals about weight gain.

3. Prevention is preferable to playing catch-up. Avoid problematic agents unless there is no acceptable alternative.

4. When patients are already taking a medication suspected as causing weight gain in that individual, stop the drug if possible, decrease the dose or frequency of administration if it is not possible to stop the agent, or provide an alternative agent not associated with weight gain.

5.   If none of the above changes in medication regimen are clinically feasible, provide the patient with support for dietary and other changes that may mitigate or counteract the problem.

6.   Be aware of medication-associated weight gain as a cause of noncompliance with prescribed regimens.

The health care provider who is knowledgeable about the mechanisms of medication-associated weight gain and specific agents commonly implicated can avoid most problems. Those problems that appear unexpectedly or are 'inherited' from previous care providers can usually be handled effectively by making appropriate medication substitutions or deletions as described above. Dealing knowledgeably and effectively with this underrecognized problem has the potential to contribute significantly to the fight against the rising tide of obesity among our patients, and is well worth the modest effort required.

References

1.   Allison DB, Mentore JL, Heo M, *et al.* Meta-analysis of the effects of anti-psychotic medication on weight gain. *Am J Psychiatry* 1999.

2.   Cheskin LJ, Bartlett SJ, Zayas R, Twilley CH, Allison DB, Contoreggi C Prescription Medications: A Modifiable Contributor to Obesity. *Southern Med J* 1999; 92: 898–904.

3.   Kupfer DJ, Copble PA, Rubinstein D Changes in weight during treatment for depression. *Psychosom Med* 1979; 41: 535–44.

4.   Andrew R, Phillips DI, Walker BR. Obesity and gender influence cortisol secretion and metabolism in man. *J Clin Endocrinol Metab* 1998; 83: 1806–9.

Progress in Obesity Research: 9. Edited by *Geraldo Medeiros-Neto, Alfredo Halpern and Claude Bouchard*

©2003 John Libbey Eurotext Ltd, pp. 451–455.

CHAPTER 95

The relationship between lifestyle and body composition from adolescence to adulthood:

Results of 23 years of follow-up in the Amsterdam Growth and Health Longitudinal Study (AGAHLS)

Han C.G. Kemper and Lando L.J. Koppes

Institute for Research in Extramural Medicine (EMGO Institute), VU University Medical Center (VUmc), Amsterdam, The Netherlands
[e-mail: hcg.kemper.emgo@med.vu.nl]

Introduction

Since the sixties there is a clear increase in the prevalence of overweightness (BMI > 25) and obesity (BMI > 30) not only in the US and Canada[1] but also in Europe. In the Netherlands the prevalence of obesity (BMI > 30) is estimated in 1997 as high as 7 per cent for adult men and as 11 per cent for adult women[2]. The increase is discernable in youth also[3]. Moreover there seems to be a clear relation between obesity and other biological risk indicators of cardiovascular diseases[4] such as hypertension, hypercholesterolaemia and type 2 diabetes. Obesity during childhood and adolescence is supposed to be an important determinant whether a subject will become obese as an adult[5,6]. It has been found that 40 per cent of children who were obese at age 7 years became obese adults, whereas more than 70 per cent of obese adolescents became obese adults.

Apart from genetic and environmental factors[7] also lifestyle factors are associated with the development of obesity in youth; important lifestyles in this respect are physical activity, dietary intake and early events in fetal and infantile growth. Food follows activity and the regulation of the energy balance and body weight seems to function better in situations were the demand of energy output is high and the energy intake is low. In modern western societies the situation is reversed (high energy intake and low energy output), leading to a gradual increase in body weight from childhood into adulthood. Most prevention programmes are focussed on healthy diets and a more physically active life because these two lifestyles are thought to be of major importance in the development of obesity. Therefore successful prevention of obesity may need to be started as early as in the growing years of the adolescence and should probably be focussed on dietary habits and habitual physical activity.

In this paper the results will be presented of a longitudinal study in a group of 13 year old healthy adolescent boys and girls, that are followed over a period of 23 years till age 36 years, about their pattern of dietary intake (DI) and physical activity (PA) on the one hand and the development of their body composition, measured as the body mass index (BMI) and the sum of four skinfolds (SFS) on the other hand. The data in this paper are collected as part of the Amsterdam Growth And Health Longitudinal Study (AGAHLS)[8,9].

The major goal of this paper is to determine the longitudinal relationship of two lifestyle factors (DI and PA) with two body composition measures BMI and SFS over 23 years of follow-up.

Methods

The Amsterdam Growth And Health Longitudinal Study (AGAHLS) used a multiple longitudinal design in which repeated measurements are in three birth cohorts (1962, 1963 and 1964) of males and females. The subjects were recruited as a whole sample from two secondary schools in Amsterdam and Purmerend (The Netherlands). Between 1976 and 2000 eight repeated measurements are completed: during the school period (13–16 years) four annual measurements, a fifth in 1985 (mean age 21 years), a sixth measurement in 1991 (mean age 27 years), a seventh measurement in 1996/1997 (mean age 32 years), and an eighth measurement in 2000 (mean age 36 years). Over the 15-year period the total drop-out rate was about 35 per cent. For the analyses in this study, data were used from 698 participants (331 men and 367 women) who on average attended 3.65 of the eight measurements.

The method to measure anthropometric and lifestyle factors have not changed over the 23 years of follow-up. All eight measurements were performed with identical procedures in all subjects. Anthropometric measurements of body height, body mass and four skinfolds (biceps, triceps, subscapular and crista iliac) were performed according standard procedures[10]. Body mass index (BMI), the ratio between body mass (kg) and body height squared (m^2), was used as an indirect measure of fat mass. The sum of four skinfolds (SFS) was used as a more direct measure of fat mass[11].

Two lifestyle factors have been monitored, dietary intake (DI), and physical activity (PA). DI was measured by a modification of the cross-check dietary history interview in a time frame of the last 3 months[12]. All subjects were interviewed by a dietitian to recall their usual intake of foods and drinks by reporting (a) the frequency (limited to at least twice a month), (b) the amounts (with models used to illustrate common portion sizes such as glasses, bowls, spoons and imitations of sizes of potatoes and fruits; a pair of scales to weigh sugar and butter addition), and (c) methods of preparation of the foods consumed. All consumed food items were transformed into nutrients in accordance with the Dutch Food and Nutrition Table[13]. As parameter of DI is chosen for the total energy intake (MJ/day).

Physical activity was measured with a standardized cross-check activity interview that was based on a questionnaire[14]. The interview was retrospective over the previous 3 months and covered the following areas: organized sports activities, unorganized sports activities (e.g. playing in the street), active transportation (e.g. bicycling), activities at home (gardening, playing with children), school (physical education) and at work (stair climbing). Only those physical activities were taken into account with a minimal duration of 5 min and an intensity level of four times basal metabolic rate (4 Mets). The physical activities were classified in three intensity levels: 4–7, 7–10, and >10 Mets, respectively[15]. The PA score was calculated as the average weekly time (minutes) spent, multiplied by the respective level of intensity. This weighted energy expenditure (Met·min/week) was used as the PA score of each subject for each year of measurement. In the last measurement period (2000) DI and PA were measured with a computerized version of the interviews (Bakker *et al.*, accepted for publication in *Eur J Clin Nutr*).

Longitudinal stability of both biological and lifestyle factors analysed using tracking analyses. In tracking analyses the initial value of a certain factor is regressed to the values of all later measurements of that factor, resulting in one standardized regression coefficient. This regression coefficient can be interpreted as a longitudinal correlation coefficient[16]. In the current analyses eight data points are used (at mean age 13, 14, 15, 16, 21, 27, 32 and 36 years, respectively). The stability coefficients were calculated with Generalized Estimating Equations (GEE), what has the major advantage that all available data are used[17].

Linear regression analyses were performed with GEE to study the relationship of DI and PA with BMI and SFS. To avoid that the longitudinal development of DI and PA confounded the relationship with SFS and BMI, z-scores of DI and PA were used. Analyses were performed both with actual values and with delta values (time *n* minus time *n* − 1), and corrections were made for gender and age. In the analyses PA was corrected for DI and vice versa.

In all analyses a probability level (*P*) of 5 per cent is used.

Results

In Table 1 mean and standard deviations are summarized of the male and female participants at the mean age of 36 years.

The differences between sexes are statistically significant in all anthropometric measures (*P* < 0.01). Males show significant higher DI and lower PA than females.

The longitudinal results of DI between age 13 and 36 years show an increase in energy intake in males from about 11.3 MJ per day at age 13 years to about 13.3 MJ per day at age 21 years, followed by a slight decrease to 12.5 MJ per day at age 36 years. In females the mean energy intake hardly changes between 13 and 36 years of age with mean values between 8.9 and 9.7 MJ per day. Males show significantly higher energy than females, at each year of measurement.

The longitudinal results of PA show a steep decrease in the energy expenditure in both sexes from age 13 to age 16: in boys from about 4700 Mets per week to about 3700 Mets per week and in girls from 3800 to 3200 Mets per week. During adolescence boys show a 20 per cent higher energy expenditure than girls. From age 21 to age 32 PA stabilizes at mean values between 2900 and 3600 MJ per week and there are no differences between males and females. At age 36 PA is increased in both sexes and the females show mean values of 5400 Mets per week compared to males with 4400 Mets per week.

Results of tracking analyses over the 23 years period indicate that DI and PA show relatively low stability with coefficients of, respectively 0.21 and 0.36 in men and of 0.41 and 0.44 in women. The stability of BMI and SFS is higher: 0.70 respectively 0.71 in men, and 0.70 respectively 0.75 in women.

Table 1. Mean and standard deviations (SD) of body height, body mass, sum of four skinfolds (SFS), body mass index (BMI), physical activity (PA) and dietary intake (DI) of the males and females at the mean age of 36 years

	Males n = 178	Females n = 200	P-value
Age (years)	36.0 (0.8)	36.1 (0.7)	n.s.
Body height (cm)	184 (6)	170 (6)	< 0.01
Body mass (kg)	83.8 (10.7)	67.9 (10.2)	< 0.01
SFS (mm)	47 (15)	55 (19)	< 0.01
BMI (kg/m²)	24.8 (2.7)	23.4 (3.3)	< 0.01
DI (MJ/day)	12.5 (3.1)	9.7 (2.1)	< 0.01
PA (kMET/week)	4.4 (2.7)	5.4 (3.7)	< 0.01

Significant differences between sexes ($P < 0.05$) are listed in the last column (n.s. = not significant).

Table 2. Regression coefficients (mean and 95 per cent CI) of actual and delta values of dietary intake (DI, MJ per day), and physical activity (PA, Mets·min/week) with sum of four skinfolds (SFS, mm) and Body mass index (BMI, kg/m2) of males and females over a period of 23 years between age 13 and 36 years

			Actual values		Change scores	
			b	95% CI	b	95% CI
PA	Men	SFS	−0.10	−0.19; −0.02	−0.06	−0.12; 0.00
		BMI	−0.18	−0.33; −0.03	−0.07	−0.17; 0.03
	Women	SFS	−0.04	−0.12; 0.05	−0.06	−0.14; 0.02
		BMI	0.06	−0.07; 0.19	−0.04	−0.14; 0.07
DI	Men	SFS	−0.10	−0.18; −0.03	−0.05	−0.12; 0.02
		BMI	0.10	−0.04; 0.24	0.06	−0.05; 0.17
	Women	SFS	−0.23	−0.33; −0.14	0.01	−0.09; 0.10
		BMI	−0.16	−0.30; −0.03	0.09	−0.03; 0.21

The longitudinal relationship of the actual values of PA with BMI and SFS (Table 2) resulted in significant ($P = 0.02$) negative regression coefficients in males but not in females. These regression coefficients should be interpreted as the following example: a one SD higher PA score is related to a 0.18 kg/m² BMI and a 0.10 cm smaller SFS. With DI however the regression coefficients with SFS are significant in males and females and with BMI only in females, but not in the expected direction: in males and females one SD lower DI was related with 0.10 cm and 0.23 cm higher SFS and in only females related with a 0.16 kg/m².

If the delta scores are used, an increase in PA is negatively related with SFS and BMI, but only significant for SFS in males. The regression of delta values of DI are not related with SFS and BMI.

Discussion

We found indeed that a higher SFS, BMI was related with a lower PA, but also with a lower DI. This unexpected result that a 23 years lower energy intake (per kg body mass) is significant related to a higher fat mass can be explained by two different reasons: (1) well-known is the phenomenon of underreporting of DI by the interview method: overweight and obese subjects are prone to 'forget' food stuffs or foodstuffs with a high energy density consumed in order to please the interviewer. Goris et al.[18] found in obese patients a percentage of underreporting of 30 per cent of foodstuffs with a high fat percentage; (2) repeated measurements, as in this longitudinal study can introduce negative testing effects as was found in the boys during adolescence[19]. That systematic differential underreporting could be the case is proved by the fact that analysis with delta values of DI with SFS and BMI resulted in coefficients that indicate positive trends.

During adolescence and young adulthood in the population of males and females from AGAHLS the PA, measured as the weighted energy expenditure (Mets·min/week) is decreasing rapidly but the DI, measured as the mean energy intake (MJ/day), is increasing in males during adolescence but not in females. DI and PA stabilize in both sexes between 21 and 36 years.

Fat mass, indirectly measured from BMI and SFS, is in both sexes gradually increasing in both males and females between 12 and 36 years. This development is resulting in an increasing prevalence rate of the percentage of subjects that are overweight (BMI > 25): in males: at age 13 less than 1 per cent is overweight but at 36 years 43 per cent of the males and 25 per cent of the females have a BMI > 25. These BMI values are almost comparable with recent data from the MORGEN study[20] in which in a random sample of the Dutch population the prevalence of risk indicators is monitored. The population from the AGAHLS longitudinal study can therefore be considered as representative for the whole Dutch population. Also other characteristics such as socio-economic status (SES) showed levels that are only slightly higher than the average Dutch population[8]. Although the prevalence of obesity is high, one must take into account that the majority of the males and females do show values of their fat mass that are in the normal range and are not showing any degree of obesity or overweight according the criteria of the World Health Organization[1].

The fat mass estimated BMI and SFS shows a relative high stability over the 23-year period. The stability coefficients of 0.70–0.75 are higher than other CVD risk indicators as diastolic blood pressure (0.34), systolic blood pressure (0.43) and equal to serum cholesterol (0.71)[17]. The high stability of fat mass is an important finding because this knowledge makes it possible to aim intervention towards this biological parameter early in adolescence.

The low stability coefficients of DI and PA demonstrate that these lifestyle parameters are less stable. Part of the low stability may be caused by the lack of reliability of the measurement method of these lifestyles by interview. However the reproducibility of both interview methods as estimated by inter-period correlations showed earlier that the zero interval of the slope of the regression line resulted in acceptable regression coefficients between 0.7 and 0.8[19].

The literature on the relation of both lifestyles PA and DI with body composition is scarce in this age group and gives a variety of results: cross sectional studies resulted in inverse relations[21–24]. One intervention study[25] shows no relation and a case-control study resulted in an inverse relation[26]. The reviews by Parizkova et al.[27] and Roberts et al.[28] and the meta-analysis of Ballor et al.[29] in general conclude that obesity in adolescents only can be altered by increasing PA and decreasing DI.

From the results it can be concluded that over the age period from 13–36 years BMI and SFS indicate a fairly good predictability; a high PA (actual and delta values) in males is related with a low SFS and BMI, but not in females. A high DI however is not related to a lower BMI and SFS. Therefore, promotion of physical activity in adolescence and young adult period seems to be effective in early prevention of obesity.

Acknowledgements: The AGAHLS is supported by multiple grants of the Dutch Prevention Fund, Dutch Heart Foundation, Dutch Ministry of Education, Culture and Science, Dutch Ministry of Well Being and Public Health, the Diary Foundation on Nutrition and Health and NOC/NSF. We like to thank all the men and women, who served as our longitudinal subjects since their early teenage years, for their cooperation in the repeated measurements of their growth, health and lifestyles over the past 23 years.

References

1. Seidell JC, Rissanen AM. In: *Handbook of obesity. Time trends in the worldwide prevalence of obesity* GA Bray, C Bouchard, WPT James (eds), pp. 79–91. New York: Marcel Dekker; 1998.

2. Volksgezondheid Toekomst Verkenning. De som der delen (in Dutch). Rijksinstituut voor Volksgezondheid en Milieu Elsevier/ Tijdstroom, Utrecht; 1997.

454

3. Gortmaker SL, Dietz WH, Sobol AM, Wehler CA. Increasing pediatric obesity in the United States. *Am J Dis Child* 1987; 141: 535–40.

4. Després J-P, Moorjani S, Lupien PJ, Tremblay A, Nadeau A, Bouchard C. Regional distribution of body fat, plasma lipoproteins, and cardiovascular disease. *Arteriosclerosis* 1990; 10: 497–511.

5. Kolata G. Obese children: a growing problem. *Science* 1986; 232: 20–1.

6. Guo SS, Roche AF, Chumlea WC, Gardner JD, Siervogel RM. The predictive value of childhood body mass index values for overweight at age 35 y. *Am J Clin Nutr* 1994; 59: 810–19.

7. Bray GA, Bouchard C, James WPT. *Handbook of obesity.* Marcel Dekker: New York; 1998.

8. Kemper HCG, editor. *Growth health and fitness of teenagers, longitudinal research in international perspective,* vol. 20. Medicine and Sport Science. Karger, Basel; 1985.

9. Kemper HCG (ed.) *The Amsterdam Growth Study, a longitudinal analysis of health, fitness, and lifestyle.* HK Sport Science Monograph. Human Kinetics: Champaign IL; 1995, vol. 6.

10. Weiner JS, Lourie JA. *Human biology, a guide to field methods. IBP Handbook no 9,* pp. 8–29. Oxford: Blackwell; 1969.

11. Durnin JVGA, Rahaman MM. The assessment of the amount of fat in human body measurements of skinfold thickness. *Br J Nutr* 1967; 21: 681–89.

12. Post GB. Nutrition in adolescence: A longitudinal study in dietary patterns from teenager to adult. [PhD Thesis], Agricultural University of Wageningen, De Vrieseborch, Haarlem, SO 1989,16.

13. Dutch Food and Nutrition Table (in Dutch) Zeist, Stichting, NEVO, Voorlichtingsburo voor de Voeding; 1985.

14. Verschuur, R. Daily physical activity and health: Longitudinal changes during the teenage period. [PhD Thesis]. University of Amsterdam, De Vrieseborch, Haarlem SO 12; 1987

15. Montoye HJ, Kemper HCG, Saris WHM, Washburn RA. Measuring physical activity and energy expenditure. *Human kinetics,* pp.123–83. Champaign IL, 1996.

16. Twisk JWR, Kemper HCG, Mechelen, W van, Post GB. Which lifestyle parameters discriminate high- from low-risk participants for coronary heart disease risk factors. Longitudinal analysis covering adolescence and young adulthood. *J Cardiovasc* 1997; Risk. 4: 393–400.

17. Twisk JWR, Kemper HCG, Mechelen W van, Post GB. Tracking of risk factors for coronary disease over a 14-period: A comparison between lifestyle and biologic risk factors with data from the Amsterdam Growth and Health Study. *Am J Epidemiol* 1997; 145(10): 889–98.

18. Goris AH, Westerterp-Plantinga MS, Westerterp KR. Undereating and underrecording of habitual food intake in obese men: selective underreporting of fat intake. *Am J Clin Nutr* 2000; 71(1): 130–34.

19. Kemper HCG, Mechelen W van, Post GB, Snel J, Twisk JWR, Lenthe FJ van, Welten DC. The Amsterdam Growth and Health Longitudinal Study, the past (1976–1996) and future (1997–?). Int J Sports Med 1997; 18: S141–S150.

20. Blokstra A, Seidell JC, Smit AH, Bueno de Mesquita HB,Verschuren WMM. Morgen Project (in Dutch). RIVM: Bilthoven, 1997.

21. Fripp RR, Hodgson JL, Kwiterovich PO, Werner JC, Schuler HG, Whitman V. Aerobic capacity, obesity and artherosclerotic risk factors in male adolescents. *Pediatrics* 1985; 75: 813.

22. Pena M, Baccallao J, Barta L, Amador M, Johnston FE. Fiber and exercise in the treatment of obese adolescents. *J Adolesc Health Care* 1989; 10: 30–4.

23. Bandini LG, Schoeller DA, Dietz WH. Energy expenditure in obese and non obese adolescents. *Pediatr Res* 1990; 27: 198–203.

24. Roberts SB, Young VR, Fuss P, Heyman MB, Fiatarone M, Dallal GE, Evans WJ. What are the dietary energy needs of elderly adults? *Int J Obes* 1992; 16: 969–76.

25. Blaak EE, Westerterp KR., Bar-Or O, Wouters LJM, Saris WHM. Total energy expenditure and spontaneous activity in relation to training in obese boys. *Am J Clin Nutr* 1992; 5(5): 777–782.

26. Moussa MAA, Skaik MB, Yaghy OY *et al.* Factors associated with obesity in school children. *Int J Obes* 1994; 18: 513–15.

27. Parizkova J. Physical training in weight reduction of obese adolescents. *Am J Clin Res* 1982; 34: 63–8.

28. Roberts SB. Abnormalities of energy expenditure and the development of obesity. *Obes Res* 1995; 3.

29. Ballor DL, Keessey RE. A meta-analysis of the factors affecting exercise-induced changes in body mass, fat mass and fat-free mass in males and females. *Int J Obes* 1991; 15: 717–26.

Progress in Obesity Research: 9. Edited by *Geraldo Medeiros-Neto, Alfredo Halpern and Claude Bouchard*
©2003 John Libbey Eurotext Ltd, pp. 456–461.

CHAPTER 96

The adiposity rebound and adult obesity

M.F. Rolland-Cachera[1], M. Deheeger[1] and F. Bellisle[2]

[1]*U557 INSERM, ISTNA – CNAM 2 rue Conté, 75003 Paris, France;* [2]*U341 INSERM Service Nutrition Hôtel Dieu, 75181 Paris, France*
[e-mail: cachera@cnam.fr]

Introduction

The treatment of constituted obesity is a very difficult and most often disappointing task. Preventing obesity could prove a more efficient approach. Then early markers of future body adiposity could be extremely useful for the paediatrician as guides for intervention. They are also useful tools for researchers to make progress in understanding the origin of obesity. Weight status at different ages are poor predictors of adult adiposity status and most obese adults were not obese as children. Less than 10 per cent of obese adults were overweight at age 7 years[1]. Other anthropometric parameters must be investigated. Age at adiposity rebound (AR), recorded on individual BMI growth curves, has been identified as an indicator predicting adult fatness. This indicator, may help identify the critical periods of adiposity development and the determinants of future obesity risks.

Adiposity development

Age at adiposity rebound

Adiposity development is generally assessed on the basis of weight and height measurements. As it is highly correlated with weight and body fat and weakly related to stature, the weight/height[2] Quételet or body mass index (BMI) has been selected to predict adiposity in children and BMI charts have been constructed for all ages throughout childhood[2] (Fig. 1).

The development of the BMI during growth parallels the development of more direct measures of body adiposity such as skinfolds. On the average, a rapid increase of the BMI occurs during the first year of life. The BMI subsequently declines and reaches a minimum by the age of 6 years, before beginning a sustained increase up to the end of growth. The point of minimal BMI value (the nadir of the BMI curve) is the start of the 'Adiposity rebound'[3].

Based on data published by Knittle et al.[4], we have suggested that the increase in BMI during the first year of life, followed by a decrease, corresponds to adipocyte size variations, while after the age of 6 years, the rise in BMI corresponds to a rise in adipocyte number. We then suggested that the age at AR may reflect the time when the steep increase in adipocyte number starts[3].

Assessment of the age at adiposity rebound

Different methods are used to assess age at AR. In some studies[3,5,6] BMI curves were drawn for each subject and timing of AR was assessed by visual inspection. This involves identifying an upward trend in the BMI after the nadir. In some cases, the descending phase of BMI is followed by a plateau. In this case, the age at AR corresponds to the start of the steep BMI increase (e.g. 8 years in case 4, Fig 1). In order to identify the upward trend in BMI, Dorosty et al.[6] specified that all consecutive measurements of the BMI after the nadir should show an increase, and required that any increase in the BMI after the nadir had to equal or exceed 0.1 kg/m[2]. Gasser[7] determined the AR from the velocity curve of the BMI. Age at AR corresponded to the point where the velocity curve became positive after a fall of BMI in infancy and early childhood.

Siervogel et al.[8], chose a polynomial model to describe the pattern of change in BMI. Age at minimum BMI was derived from this model. Other authors used the same approach[9–11].

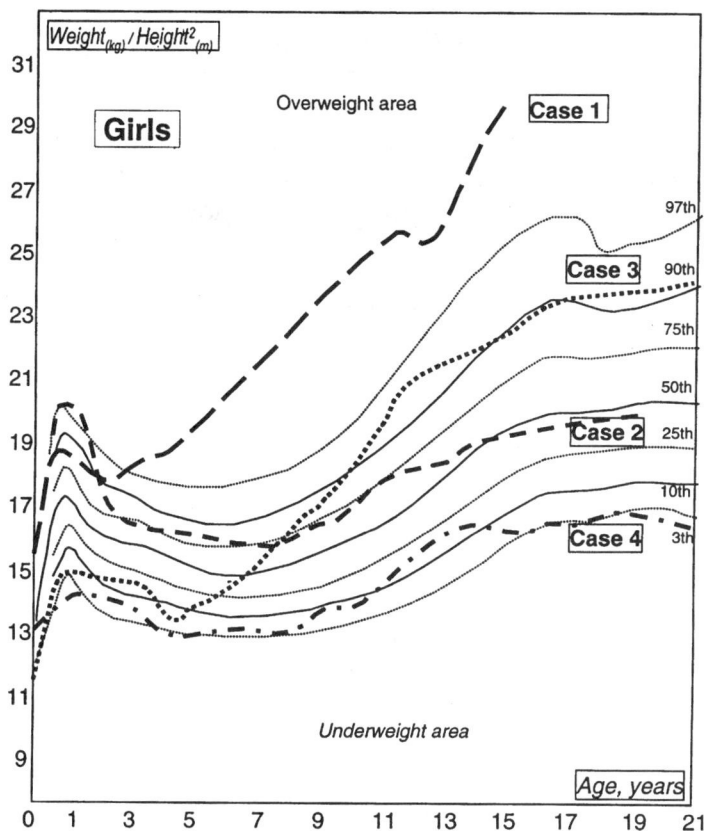

Fig. 1. Four examples of Body Mass Index development plotted against the French BMI reference charts (2): Case No. 1, fat child at one year, remained fat after an early adiposity rebound (2 years); case No. 2, fat child at one year, did not stay fat after a late adiposity rebound (8 years); case No. 3, lean child at one year, became fat after an early adiposity rebound (4.5 years); case No. 4, lean child at one year, remained lean after a late adiposity rebound (8 years).

Individual BMI pattern

Mean BMI during growth varies as described earlier, but individual BMI curves may have very different patterns[12] (Fig. 1). For example, a fat one-year-old child may become a normal weight adult after a late adiposity rebound (e.g. case 2), while a lean one-year-old child may become a fat adult after an early adiposity rebound (e.g. case 3). These individual BMI patterns explain why, before AR, the child's BMI predicts adult fatness only poorly. Case 3 in Fig. 1 (a thin child at 4 years becoming overweight after an early AR), points out that many cases of obesity which are diagnosed at adolescence actually have their origin much earlier in life.

Prediction of adult fatness

Several studies have investigated the associations between the age at adiposity rebound and the risk of adult adiposity. In the early 1980s, on the basis of the French sample of the International Growth Study, we established that age at AR was associated with BMI level at later ages[3]: the earlier the AR, the higher the BMI or the subscapular skinfold at the age of 21 years[12]. We also investigated the association between AR and bone age: an early AR was associated with advanced skeletal maturity[3]. This association, also reported by Williams et al.[10], is consistent with the accelerated growth observed in obese children[4]. Several authors reported the same association between an early adiposity rebound and increased risk of adult obesity[6–8,10,13,14].

In a longitudinal study conducted in Czech children aged from 1 month to 18 years, Prokopec and Bellisle[5] reported that in most cases (15 out of 18), overweight adults (BMI over 25 kg/m^2 at age of 18 years) had an early AR (before the age of 6 years) and all lean adults had late AR (after 6 years).

A retrospective study was conducted in adults by Whitaker et al.[9]. BMI curves were fitted for each subject between 1.5 and 16 years. Age and BMI level at AR were calculated from these curves. Adult obesity was associated with an early AR. After adjusting for parent BMI and BMI at AR, the odds ratio for adult obesity associated with early vs. late AR was 6.0 (95 per cent CI, 1.3–26.6). Based on the Fels longitudinal study, Guo et al.[11] examined BMI patterns from early childhood to 35–45 years. They showed that an early AR was related to adult overweight, more so in females than in males.

BMI pattern before the adiposity rebound

The association between age at AR and previous measurements was also investigated. While an early AR was associated with subsequent high adiposity, an opposite association was found between age at AR and BMI level in early life: an early adiposity rebound was associated with a lower BMI level at the age of one year[12]. This trend was recorded in boys and girls, but it reached significance only in girls. Similarly, Williams and Dickinson[15] found no association between age at AR and BMI at age 3 years in

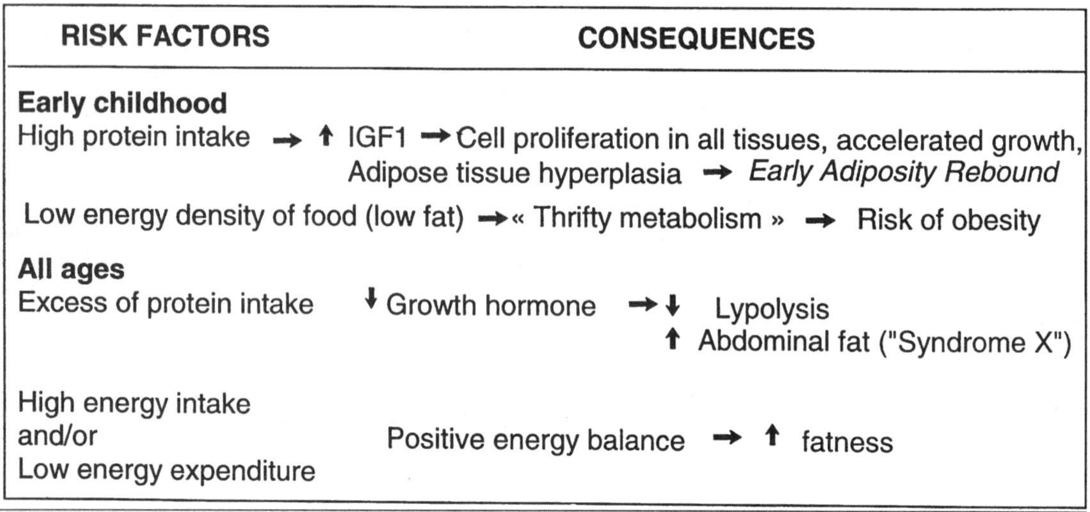

RISK FACTORS	CONSEQUENCES

Early childhood

High protein intake ➡ ⬆ IGF1 ➡ Cell proliferation in all tissues, accelerated growth, Adipose tissue hyperplasia ➡ *Early Adiposity Rebound*

Low energy density of food (low fat) ➡« Thrifty metabolism » ➡ Risk of obesity

All ages

Excess of protein intake   ⬇ Growth hormone ➡⬇ Lypolysis
⬆ Abdominal fat ("Syndrome X")

High energy intake
and/or   Positive energy balance ➡ ⬆ fatness
Low energy expenditure

Fig. 2. Hypothesis about the various origins of obesity.

boys and a lower BMI associated with an early adiposity rebound in girls. Dorosty *et al.*[6] found no association between the age at AR and BMI level before the AR.

In summary, while the age at AR is associated with high adult adiposity, it is not associated (or associated in an opposite direction) with adiposity in the first years of life.

BMI pattern in the obese

Mean age at AR in the French reference population[3] was 6.2 ± 1.6 years, varying from 3 to 9.5 years. Age at AR was also recorded in 62 obese children examined in a department of paediatric endocrinology. Mean age at AR was 3.2 ± 1.2 years. None of these obese children had an AR later than the age of 6 years. Two children had their AR at the age of 6 years (i.e. average) and more than half of them (55 per cent) had an AR at, or before, the age of 3 years[5]. Similar observation were reported elsewhere[16]. These observations, together with the data reported by Bellisle and Prokopec[5] showing that most obese subjects displayed an early AR contrast with the observation that most obese adults were not obese as children.

Age at adiposity rebound vs. BMI level by the age of 6 years

Some authors[7,10,13] noticed that the correlation between the BMI level of the child by the age at AR (6 or 7 years) and adult BMI was as good as or better than the correlation between age at AR and adult BMI. They concluded that recording the BMI by the age at AR was a more practical way of predicting adult BMI than assessing age at AR. Actually, different aspects must be considered.

A high BMI level at the age of 6 years is significantly associated with later high BMI, but also with previous high BMI levels. In the Zürich study[7], the correlation between BMI at 6 years and adult BMI was 0.60. It was of the same magnitude (r = 0.66) between the BMI at 6 years and the BMI at one year. By contrast, as described earlier, an early AR was associated with a high BMI at adult age, but with normal or even lower BMI level before the rebound. Consequently, as a rule, a fat child at age 6 years is likely to be always fat (such as case 1 in Fig. 1), while a child with an early AR may start with normal or even low adiposity in early life and develop fatness only from the time of AR (such as case 3 in Fig 1).

The inverse association described above between BMI level before and after AR was reported in various circumstances[17]. For example, comparing BMI curves from different countries, the median BMI level showed an opposite rank order before and after AR, i.e. a higher BMI by 2 years of age in Senegal as compared to the US, but after a late (8 years) and an early (5.3 years) AR respectively, a lower BMI level in Senegal as compared to the US.

The poor predictive value of adult obesity status based on childhood measurements, contrasts with studies showing that events in the critical period of fetal and/or early life can have lifetime health consequences. This idea was termed 'programming'[18]. Actually, determinants of adult weight status may have occurred in early childhood but their effect on weight may appear only several years later (e.g. in case 3, Fig. 1).

In summary, both markers (BMI by the age of 7 years and AR) predict adult fatness, but they correspond to different BMI patterns. These two markers are likely associated with different obesity promoting factors. They thus may give complementary information on the determinants of obesity development.

Factors associated with the age at adiposity rebound

Parental BMI

Three studies have examined the association between parental BMI and age at AR[6,9,15]. They all showed that parent obesity was associated with a younger age at AR.

Physical activity

Positive energy balance results from high intakes or low physical activity. Results of a longitudinal study showed that AR occurred earlier in children with a sedentary lifestyle[19].

Nutrition

Several studies have investigated the nutritional factors associated with age at AR. In a longitudinal study of nutrition and growth, nutritional intakes were assessed at the age of 2 years[20]. The association between nutritional intakes at the age of two years and age at AR were investigated. No association was found for energy, percentage of energy from fat or CHO and age at AR. A negative association was found between the percentage of protein intake and AR, i.e. the higher the percentage of protein consumed at the age of 2 years, the earlier the AR.

Dorosty *et al.*[6] conducted a prospective analysis in a cohort of children followed from birth to 5 years in the UK. They compared very early (before the age of 3.5 years), early (from 4 to 5 years) and later rebound (after 5 years). They found not evidence of associations between dietary protein or any other dietary variable recorded at the age of 18 months and timing of the adiposity rebound. They did not confirm the association between protein intake and age at AR. They also failed to reveal any association with either energy or fat intake. A study conducted in Italian children revealed an association between early high protein intake and increased BMI at the time of AR[21] while a study conducted in Australia[22] report a positive association between fat intake in infancy and body fatness at adolescence. These two last studies did not examine the association between nutritional intakes and the age at AR.

The results of the French study, suggesting a deleterious effect of excess protein intake, have underlined the inadequate nutrient balance of the infant diet in industrialized countries[23]. By the age of 1 year, the infant diet is characterized by a high intake of proteins ($\sim$ 4 g/kg body weight or 16 per cent of total energy) and a low intake of fat ($\sim$ 28 per cent). Protein intake represents about three to four times the protein needs. The nutrient imbalance is remarkable considering that human milk provides 6 per cent of energy as proteins and 54 per cent as fat. Paradoxically, the proportion of fat in the infant diet is low at a period of high energy needs. Subsequently, the percentage of energy provided by fat increases with age, whereas it should be high in early life and gradually decrease with age[17].

Protein intake and fatness development

Protein intake may alter fatness development in different ways.

Nutrient intake and hormonal status

We previously proposed that the characteristics of childhood obesity, i.e. increased stature and body mass (lean and fat)[4] were the consequence of high protein intakes. Changes in body composition could have occurred through changes in hormonal status[17,23]. High plasma insulin like growth fator-1 (IGF1) concentrations and reduced growth hormone (GH) secretion (spontaneous or in response to a wide variety of stimuli) are characteristic features of children with simple obesity[24]. As IGF1 promotes the differentiation of preadipocytes into adipocytes[25], a high protein intake may induce hyperplasia in adipose tissue. The early increase in adipocyte number reported in obese children[4] may be responsible for the early adiposity rebound recorded in the obese. In addition, high protein intake may, at any age, decrease GH levels, decreasing lipolysis and promoting the development and maintenance of high fat stores (Fig. 2).

Metabolic adaptation to a relative energy deficit in infancy

Energy intake in 1.5–2.5 year old English children declined from 1264 to 1045 kcal/day between 1967 and 1993[26]. The trend to decrease energy intake in the early period of life, also reported in other studies[17,27], can be the consequence of the low energy density of the low fat high protein diet currently consumed by infants of today[23]. The previously described BMI pattern associated with an early AR: low BMI level followed by high fatness can be the consequence of reduced energy balance in early life (Fig. 2). A relative energy deficit may programme 'thrifty metabolism', during the early phase of development. This adaptation may have adverse effects when, later in life, children will eat a more abundant high fat diet[17,27]. The low fat-energy diet consumed in early life may result from prevention strategies in industrialized countries and from poor living conditions in the developing world.

Conclusion

Because the weight status in infancy is a poor predictor of adult adiposity, prevention at the population level has been advocated[1]. However, identification of subjects at risk of obesity before adiposity reaches high levels, remains necessary. Age at AR seems to be a useful indicator to predict adult adiposity, for the paediatrician as a guide for intervention and for researchers to investigate the origins of obesity.

Most obese adults were not obese as they were a child[1]. By contrast most obese subjects displayed an early AR.

The early AR recorded in the obese suggests that determinants of obesity have operated early in life. Some hypotheses have been suggested, but no clear argument accounts for this phenomenon.

An early AR is associated with parental obesity. Nutritional intake may also affect the age at AR. More research on the circumstances associated with age at AR may help to identify the factors that promote obesity and may be useful in the prevention of obesity from an early stage of life.

References

1. Power C, Lake JK, Cole TJ. Measurements and long-term health risks of child and adolescent fatness. *Int J Obes* 1997; 21: 507–26.

2. Rolland-Cachera MF, Sempé M, Guilloud-Bataille M, Patois E, Péquignot-Guggenbuhl F, Fautrad V. Adiposity indices in children. *Am J Clin Nutr* 1982; 36: 178–84.

3. RollandCachera MF, Deheeger M, Bellisle F, Sempé M, Guilloud-Bataille M, Patois E. Adiposity rebound in children: a simple indicator for predicting obesity. *Am J Clin Nutr* 1984; 39: 29–35.

4. Knittle JL, Timmers K, Ginsberg-Fellner F, Brown RE, Katz DP. The growth of adipose tissue in children and adolescents. Cross sectional and longitudinal studies of adipose cell number and size. *J Clin Invest* 1979; 63: 239–46.

5. Prokopec M, Bellisle F. Adiposity in Czech children followed from one month of age to adulthood: analysis of individual BMI patterns. *Ann Hum Biol* 1993; 20: 51725.

6. Dorosty AR, Emmett PM, Cowin IS, Reilly JJ, and the ALSPAC Study team. Factors associated with early adiposity rebound. *Pediatrics* 2000; 105: 1115–8.

7. Gasser Th, Ziegler P, Seifert B, Molinari L, Lardo R, Prader A. Prediction of adult skinfolds and body mass from infancy through adolescence. *Ann Hum Biol* 1995, 22: 217–33.

8. Siervogel RM, Roche AF, Guo S, Mukherjee D, Chumlea WC. Patterns of change in weight/stature^2 from 2 to 18 years: findings from long-term serial data for children in the Fels longitudinal growth study. *Int J Obes* 1991; 15: 479–85.

9. Whitaker R, Pepe MS, Wright JA, Seidel KD, Dietz WH. Early adiposity rebound and the risk of adult obesity. *Pediatrics* 1998; 101: e5.

10. Williams S, Davie G, Lam F. Predicting BMI in young adults from childhood data using two approaches to modelling adiposity rebound. *Int J Obes* 1999; 23: 348–54.

11. Guo SS, Huang C, Maynard LM, Demerath E, Towne B, Chumlea WC, Siervogel RM. Body mass index during childhood, adolescence and young adulthood in relation to adult overweight and adiposity: the fels longitudinal study. *Int J Obes* 2000; 24: 1628–35.

12. Rolland-Cachera MF, Deheeger M, Avons P, Guilloud-Bataille M, Patois E, Sempé M. Tracking adiposity patterns from 1 month to adulthood. *Ann Hum Biol* 1987, 14: 219–22.

13. Freedman DS, Kettel Khan L, Serdula MK, Srinivan SR and Berenson GS. BMI rebound, childhood height and obesity among adults: the Bogalusa Heart study. *Int J Obes* 2001; 25: 543–9.

14. He Q, Karlberg J. Probability of adult overweight and risk change during the BMI rebound period. *Obes Res* 2002; 10: 135–40.

15. Williams S, Dickson N. Early growth, menarche and adiposity rebound. *Lancet* 2002; 359: 580–81.

16. Girardet JP, Tounian P, Le Bars MA, Boreux A. Obesité de l'enfant: intérêt des indicateurs cliniques d'évaluation. *Annales de Pédiatrie* 1993; 40: 297–303 (in French).

17. Rolland-Cachera MF. *Obesity among children and adolescents: the importance of early nutrition in Human Growth and Development,* Johnston FE, Zemel B, Eveleth PB (eds), pp. 245–58. London: Smith-Gordon; 1999.

18. Lucas A, Fewtrell MS, Cole TJ. Fetal origins of adult disease-the hypothesis revisited. *BMJ* 1999; 319: 245–9.

19. Deheeger M, Rolland-Cachera MF, Fontvieille AM. Physical Activity and body composition in 10-year-old French children: linkages with nutritional intake? *Int J Obes* 1997; 21: 372–9.

20. Rolland-Cachera MF, Deheeger M, Akrout M, Bellisle F. Influence of macronutrients on adiposity development: a follow up study of nutrition and growth from 10 months to 8 years of age. *Int J Obes* 1995; 19: 573–8.

21. Scaglioni S, Agostoni C, DeNotaris R, Radaelli G, Radice N, Valenti M, Giovannini M, Riva E. Early macronutrient intake and overweight at 5 years of age. *Int J Obes* 2000; 24: 777–81.

22. Magarey AM, Daniels LA, Boulton TJC and Cockington RA. Does fat intake predict adiposity in healthy children and adolescents aged 2–15? A longitudinal analysis. *Eur J Clin Nutr* 2001; 55: 471–81.

23. Rolland-Cachera MF, Deheeger M and Bellisle F. Increasing prevalence of obesity among 18-year-old males in Sweden: evidence for early determinants. *Acta Paediatrica* 1999; 88: 365–7.

24. Loche S, Cappa M, Borrelli A, Faedda A, Crino A, Cella SG, Corda R, Müller EE, Pintor C. Reduced growth hormone response to growth hormone-releasing hormone in children with simple obesity: evidence for somatomedin-C mediated inhibition *Clin Endocrinol* 1987; 27: 145–53.

25. Ailhaud G, Grimaldi P, Négrel R. A molecular view of adipose tissue. *Int J Obes* 1992, 16: 517–21.

26. Gregory JR, Collins DL, Davies PSW, Hughes JM, Clarke PC. *National diet and nutrition survey: Children aged 1.5 to 4.5 years,* p. 391. London: HMSO; 1995.

27. Rolland-Cachera MF, Deheeger M, Bellisle F. The Adiposity Rebound: its contribution to obesity in children and adults. In: *Obesity in childhood and adolescence,* Chunming Chen and WH Dietz (eds). Nestlé Nutrition Workshop Series, Pediatric Program 2001; 49: 99–118.

Progress in Obesity Research: 9. Edited by *Geraldo Medeiros-Neto, Alfredo Halpern* and *Claude Bouchard*
©2003 John Libbey Eurotext Ltd, pp. 462–467.

CHAPTER 97

Childhood obesity and adult risk of chronic disease: the Bogalusa heart study

G.S. Berenson, S.R. Srinivasan and W. Chen

Tulane Center for Cardiovascular Health, Tulane University Health Sciences Center, Departments of Epidemiology, Medicine, Pediatrics and Biochemistry, New Orleans, LA 70112, USA
[e-mail: berenson@tulane.edu]

Introduction

Cardiovascular (C-V) risk factors are detectable in childhood and are predictive of future risk for adult heart diseases. A number of epidemiologic studies have now established that risk factors in early life are associated with coronary artery disease (CAD) and essential hypertension[1–4]. It is also evident that early stages of diabetes mellitus begins in early life. The precise initiating factors of these diseases are still being investigated. Also, since the determinants of C-V risk begin early, it is prudent to begin prevention of adult C-V disease in childhood. Susceptibility to complex traits such as obesity, coronary atherosclerosis, essential hypertension and diabetes mellitus involve multiple genetic influences, but the development of these diseases are also greatly influenced by lifestyles and behaviours that occur over a long period of time. Unhealthy lifestyles like excess calories, a high-saturated fat and cholesterol diet, tobacco use, excess alcohol intake and physical inactivity interact with the intrinsic genetic makeup of an individual long before clinical events occur. What is now clear, C-V risk factors exist as a long-term burden on the C-V-renal system and that burden can be detected at an early age as predictive of disease later in life[5]. A major factor interrelated with risk is the increasing epidemic of obesity.

Population under study

The Bogalusa Heart Study is a comprehensive long-term study of infants, children, adolescents, and young adults in a stable, bi-racial (black-white), semi-rural community in Southeastern United States. The Study provides a database from birth to 38 years of age on some 16,000 subjects. Longitudinal observations have been made on approximately 3,500 individuals over a 20 to 25-year lifespan. Repeated and long-term observations provide an opportunity to study secular trends and predictability of future characteristics of adult C-V risk[4,5].

Secular trends

Obesity, in fact, is becoming a worldwide phenomenon associated with increasing CAD in developing countries. The increase of obesity has occurred in the general population of children and adults in the United States[6–8]. The increasing incidence of obesity in children is reflected in a similar trend in their parents[9]. During the decade of the 1970s to 1980s, an average increase of body weight of Bogalusa children was 2.5 kg, without an increase of height, Fig. 1. During the decade of the 1980s to 1990s the increase was 5 kg[7]. Although the explanation for this increase of body weight has been suggested to be due to greater inactivity from television watching[10], availability of inexpensive, energy-rich food has contributed to the increasing obesity[11]. This increase of obesity has important health implications, since there is already an indication that adult onset diabetes mellitus is increasing in the adult population in the United States and even occurring with a greater rate with adolescent age groups[12]. A tremendous amount of obesity occurs in young black females[13], in whom there is an even greater prevalence of diabetes.

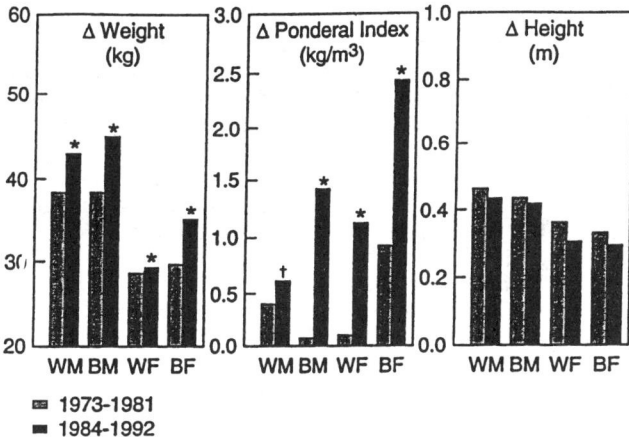

Fig. 1. Changes in anthropometric measurements of children aged 7–9 years over two 8-year periods, 1973–81 and 1984–92, in the Bogalusa Heart Study. Secular trends show significant increases in body weight and ponderal index (weight/height[3]) without significant change in height. ($P < 0.0001$; † $P < 0.05$) (Berenson[11]).

Tracking of risk factors

evels of risk factor variables in a child tend to remain (track) in a given rank relative to their peers ver time. The extent of tracking determines the predictability of future adult C-V risk. The fact that racking occurs strongly supports measuring risk factors in children. Risk factors track with varying degrees and as might be expected, the greatest tracking occurs for obesity measures, such as body weight and skinfolds[5,14,15]. Total cholesterol and LDL-cholesterol track almost as well. Lower levels of tracking occur for triglycerides, HDL-cholesterol and blood pressure. Systolic blood pressure tracks better than diastolic blood pressure, in part, due to limitations in measurements. The persistence of the risk factors over time becomes a burden that contributes to the development of adult heart diseases[16].

Genetics of obesity

Studies have shown consistently that 40–70 per cent of the variation in obesity-related traits, such as body mass index (BMI), skinfold thickness and fat mass, is heritable (17). Although more than 250 genes or chromosome regions have been associated or linked with cross-sectional measures of obesity[18], information is limited on genetic loci linked to long-term changes of BMI from childhood to adulthood. Using longitudinal measurements in sib-pairs who were enrolled in the Bogalusa Heart Study since childhood and followed over a 28-year period, a quadratic growth curve was developed to calculate longitudinal burden (area under the curve (AUC) divided by follow-up years) and longitudinal trends (incremental AUC above baseline and linear slope). In a variance-component multipoint linkage analysis, significant linkage to longitudinal measures of obesity was found in three chromosome regions of 5q23-q33 for incremental AUC (LOD = 3.8), 12q22-q24 for incremental AUC (LOD = 3.3) and slope (LOD = 4.3), and 18p11 for incremental AUC (LOD = 3.4), which harbour plausible obesity-related candidate genes of glucocorticoid receptor (GRL), adrenergic receptor (ADRβ2), insulin-like growth factor-I (IGF-I) and melanocortin-5 receptor (MC5R). These genes or loci close to them might affect the propensity to develop obesity from childhood[19].

Clustering of multiple risk factors

Obesity tends to occur in constellation with other risk factors. This aggregation or clustering of risk factors include adverse levels of blood pressure, lipids and lipoproteins, and variables of glucose homeostasis. The aggregation of risk factors occurs commonly in the adult population as in the insulin resistance syndrome, Syndrome X or the Deadly Quartet, characterized by visceral body fatness. Abdominal obesity is strongly associated with insulin resistance/hyperinsulinaemia and the attendant hypertension, dyslipidaemia and variety of factors that contribute to CAD, including prothrombotic and proinflammatory parameters. Since this metabolic cluster of risk factors begins in early life and is familial in nature, its occurrence produces a long-term burden that can have detrimental effects on the C-V system[20]. Figure 2, illustrates that obesity in early childhood precedes the hyperinsulinaemia[21]. The persistence of such multiple risk factors provides a density-exposure that enhances the development of C-V disease including progressive coronary atherosclerosis. These silent asymptomatic lesions herald the onset of morbidity from coronary heart disease.

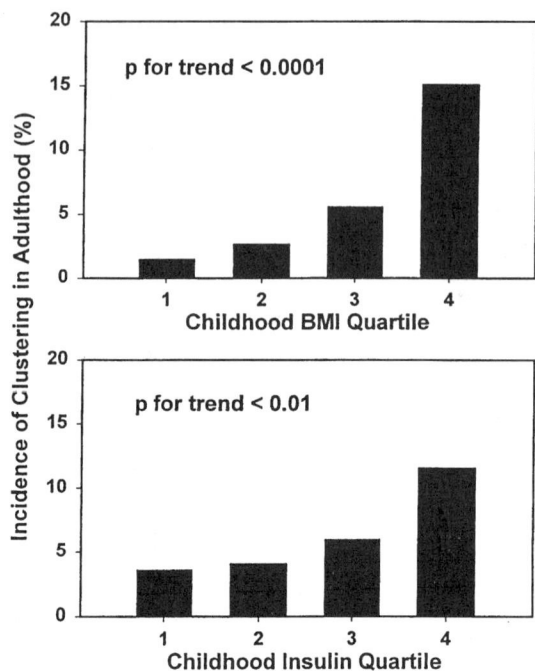

Fig. 2. Incidence of clustering of risk variables of syndrome X in adulthood by children BMI (A) and insulin (B) quartiles. The earliest childhood and latest adulthood measurements with a mean ± SD follow-up period of 11.6 ±3.4 years were used. Only those without clustering in childhood (n = 718) were included in the analysis. (Srinivasan[21]).

Anatomic observations

Anatomic studies provide the most impressive observations of the early natural history of hypertension and CAD. The early onset of essential hypertension and its effect on target organs are detectable by echocardiographic and Doppler studies. This non-invasive methodology provides evidence of early cardiac enlargement in children at the higher blood pressure levels (90th percentile)[22], levels which are much lower than considered abnormal by the clinical 140/90 or even lower by the JNC VI criteria used for adults. Generally at the level of 90th percentile and above underlying C-V changes are detected. In addition to cardiac enlargement, subtle changes of small renal arteries are altered related to blood pressure levels[23]. As noted above obesity and excess body fatness contributes to the adverse levels of lipids and blood pressure underlying these changes.

With regards to atherosclerosis, fatty streak lesions occur even in infants and young children in the aorta. Coronary lesions occur somewhat later in the second decade of life but show a marked increase in the young adult age[24]. Raised collagen-capped lesions appear with fatty streaks and 30 to 40 per cent of the vessel surfaces involved with the fibrous plaque type[25]. These lesions are progressive and although significant reduction of lumen size may not yet occur, they demonstrate the evidence of early CAD, ubiquitous in our population. Fatty streaks occur in 80 to 90 per cent of young individuals, both in the aorta and coronary vessels, while fibrous plaques progress to 60 to 70 per cent of lesions in coronary vessels by the third decade of life. Observations of Pathologic Determinants of Atherosclerosis in Youth (PDAY) study show these same findings[26]. Such observations indicate the widespread prevalence of atherosclerosis in our general population, as Silent Asymptomatic Disease[23-26].

Unique to the Bogalusa Heart Study is the opportunity to relate antemortem clinical risk factors to underlying atherosclerosis. Correlations of total LDL cholesterol are significantly related to the atherosclerotic involvement of the aorta, while lesions in the coronary vessels are associated more with multiple risk factors[27]. Obesity, higher blood pressure, VLDL cholesterol and lower HDL cholesterol are strongly correlated with the coronary lesions. As discussed above, multiple risk factors do occur in early life and their aggregation relates to changes in the coronary vessels. Of particular interest, the multiple risk factors are associated with an acceleration of coronary artery lesions. Using a multi-risk factor score, the presence of three or more risk factors greatly increases the severity of coronary atherosclerosis. These findings are in concert with the multi risk factor concept of Framingham in predicting of greater morbidity and mortality from a group of factors known to be associated with C-V risk. Recent studies in another vascular system also show that intima-media thickness in the common carotid and bifurcation segment relate strongly to increasing numbers of risk factors[28].

Effect of dietary intake

Although dietary intake is an important determinant of risk factors, a strong relationship of diet to risk factors within a given population consuming habitual high-fat, high-cholesterol and high-energy diet is difficult to establish. This is partly due to the difficulty of quantifying dietary intakes of individuals. In addition, for example, wide genetic variability in the response of serum cholesterol among individuals may undermine detecting the relationship between cholesterol intake and serum cholesterol levels.

Of note, alleles of aopE relate to variations of lipoprotein levels as well as lipoprotein response to diet[29]. Yet, cross-cultural, or multi-national studies, have detected relationships of diet and cultural factors to high or low levels of serum cholesterol and to clinical events related to C-V disease.

Dietary studies in children within this community do, however, show that a major portion, exceed even the first-level of moderation of diet recommended by the American Heart Association, i.e. of 30 per cent total fat and 10 per cent saturated fat. At these levels, some 60 per cent exceed the recommended cholesterol intake and some 80 per cent exceed dietary saturated fat[30]. Fortunately, secular trends in healthy dietary changes are occurring. Total fat has been reduced from 38 per cent of the diet to approximately 33 per cent in the population over the past two to three decades and cholesterol has been markedly reduced in the diet. The American Heart Association first-level recommended diet of 30 per cent fat, 10 per cent saturated fat is too liberal in terms of prevention. It has been noted regression of CAD does not occur in controls of many intervention clinical trials compared to drug effects, like statins. Still, the excess caloric intake related to inactivity remains as one of the main determinants of obesity[11].

An overview of findings on obesity in childhood

The adverse effects of obesity in childhood and its implications for adult heart disease are noted in the following:

1. The overall weight in children has increased in the Bogalusa Heart Study since beginning of observations in 1973–74, by an average increase of 5 kg. This has occurred without any striking increase in stature.

2. Obesity of children relates strongly to parental obesity.

3. A greater inactive lifestyle has contributed to an increase of body weight and fatness, i.e. television watching, computer games, and change in transportation.

4. Obesity in youth is highly predictive of obesity in adulthood.

5. Obesity and its interaction with other risk factors is associated with atherosclerotic coronary artery lesions in adolescents and young adults.

6. Obesity is related to higher insulin levels, serum total cholesterol, LDL-cholesterol, triglycerides and VLDL-cholesterol, and inversely with HDL-cholesterol. Obesity in childhood likely precedes the hyperinsulinaemia of adulthood. Further, higher blood pressure levels are associated with obesity, especially in white children.

7. Syndrome X and clustering of cardiovascular risk factors is associated with central fat deposition and the androgenic distribution of fat.

8. Genetic studies on the Bogalusa population show markers on five chromosomes are associated with BMI measured multiple times beginning in childhood.

Prevention

The importance of beginning primary prevention of obesity early in life has to be emphasized. Observations to establish effectiveness of primary prevention in the general population seems to be lacking. Incorporating dietary changes, increasing physical activity, and weight control reduction have enhanced the improvement of risk factors in a number of aggressive and controlled studies of small samples of individuals. Yet, this has not occurred in population-wide trends noted with obesity. Since the findings in the Bogalusa Heart Study point to the need to begin prevention in childhood, we developed a public health model, of a comprehensive health education programme (Health Ahead/Heart Smart) for elementary school children[31]. This programme addresses entire school environment, the classroom with extensive teacher's guides, the cafeteria, physical education, and even lifestyles of teachers and parents. In addition, teaching parents healthy lifestyles reinforces healthy influences on children[32].

These programmes recognize that lifestyles and behaviours that influence C-V risk factors are learned and begin early. Healthy lifestyles are encouraged to be adopted by both children and their parents, This concept is critical to modulating risk factors later in life. Prevention of cigarette smoking, increasing physical activity and marked reduction of saturated fat and cholesterol in the diet along with prevention of obesity are mandatory. Primary care physicians and paediatricians can play a major leadership role in the prevention of adult heart diseases, as they begin in childhood, by addressing the major problem of obesity through health education. Although there is controversy about screening for risk factor profiles at an early age[33], measurement of height, weight and waist measurements enabling following growth curves can be a basic part of health of children. Cardiologists and primary care physicians have a tremendous opportunity to guide prevention programmes for the young destined to be our next cardiac patients.

Acknowledgements: Grant Support: This research was supported by the National Heart, Lung and Blood Institute, Grant HL-38844, and NIH grant AG-16592. The authors wish to acknowledge the children and families in Bogalusa who made this research possible. The joint effort of the many individuals who have contributed to this study is gratefully acknowledged.

References

1. Lauer RM, Shekelle RB (eds). *Childhood prevention of atherosclerosis and hypertension*, p. 484. New York: Raven Press, 1980.

2. Berenson GS, McMahan CA, Voors AW, Webber LS, Srinivasan SR, Frank GC, Foster TA, Blonde CV. Cardiovascular risk factors in children – the early natural history of atherosclerosis and essential hypertension (editorial assistance: Andrews C, Hester HE). p. 450. New York: Oxford University Press, 1980.

3. Berenson GS (ed.). Causation of cardiovascular risk factors in children: perspectives on cardiovascular risk in early life, pp 408. New York: Raven Press, 1986.

. Webber LS, Wattigney WA, Srinivasan SR, Berenson GS (1995): Obesity studies in Bogalusa. *Am J Med Sci* 1995; 310(Suppl 1): S53–S61.

5. Berenson GS, Srinivasan SR, Hunter SM, Nicklas TA, Freedman DS, Shear CL, Webber LS. Risk factors in early life as predictors of adult heart disease: The Bogalusa Heart Study. *Am J Med Sci* 1989; 296: 141–51.

6. Mohdad AH, Serdula MK, Dietz WH, Bowman BA, Marks JS, Koplan JP. The spread of the obesity epidemic in the United States, 1991–1998. *JAMA* 1999; 282: 1519–22.

7. Gidding SS, Bao W, Srinivasan SR, Berenson GS. Effects of secular rends in obesity on coronary risk factors in children: The Bogalusa Heart Study. *J Pediatr* 1995; 127: 868–74.

8. Freedman DS, Srinivasan SR, Valdez RA, Williamson DF, Berenson GS. Secular increases in relative weight and adiposity among children over two decades: The Bogalusa Heart Study. *Pediatrics* 1997; 99: 420–6.

9. Bao W, Srinivasan SR, Valdez R, Greenlund KJ, Wattigney WA, Berenson GS. Longitudinal changes of cardiovascular risk from childhood to young adulthood in offspring of parents with coronary artery disease: The Bogalusa Heart Study. *JAMA* 1997; 278, 21; 1749–52.

10. Dietz WH Jr, Gortmaker SL. Do we fatten our children at the TV set? Obesity and television viewing in children and adolescents. *Pediatrics* 1985; 75: 807–12.

11. Berenson GS, Srinivasan SR, Nicklas TA. Atherosclerosis: A nutritional disease of childhood. *Am J Cardiol* 1998; 82: 22T–29T.

12. Srinivasan SR, Elkasabany A, Dalferes ER Jr, Bao W, Berenson GS. Characteristics of young offspring of type 2 diabetic parents in a biracial (black-white) community-based sample: The Bogalusa Heart Study. *Metabolism* 1998; 47: 998–1004.

13. Wattigney WA, Webber LS, Srinivasan SR, Berenson GS. The emergence of clinically abnormal levels of cardiovascular disease risk factor variables among young adults: The Bogalusa Heart Study. *Prev Med* 1995; 24: 612–26.

14. Bao W, Threefoot S, Srinivasan SR, Berenson GS. Essential hypertension predicted by tracking of elevated blood pressure from childhood to adulthood – The Bogalusa Heart Study. *Am J Hyperten* 1995; 8(7): 657–65.

15. Clarke WR, Schrott HG, Leaverton PE, Connor WE, Lauer RM. Tracking of blood lipids and blood pressure in school age children: The Muscatine Study. *Circulation* 1978; 58: 626–34.

16. Bao W, Srinivasan SR, Wattigney WA, Berenson GS. Persistence of multiple cardiovascular risk clustering related to Syndrome X from childhood to young adulthood. The Bogalusa Heart Study. *Arch Intern Med* 1994; 54: 1842–7.

17. Comuzzie AG, Allison DB. The search for human obesity genes. *Science* 1998; 280: 1374–7.

18. Perusse L, Chagnon YC, Weisnagel SJ, Rankinen T, Snyder E, Sands J, Bouchard C. The human obesity gene map: the 2000 update. *Obes Res* 2001; 9: 135–69.

19. Chen W, Li S, Srinivasan SR, Boerwinkle E, Berenson GS. A genome-wide scan for loci linked to 28-year longitudinal changes of body mass index from childhood to adulthood in white sibships: The Bogalusa Heart Study. Submitted to American Heart Association Meeting (2002).

20. Chen W, Srinivasan SR, Elkasabany A, Berenson GS. The association of cardiovascular risk factor clustering related to insulin resistance syndrome (Syndrome X) between young parents and their offspring: The Bogalusa Heart Study. *Atherosclerosis* 1999; 145: 197–205.

21. Srinivasan SR, Myers L, Berenson GS. Predictability of childhood adiposity and insulin for developing insulin resistance syndrome (Syndrome X) in young adulthood. *Diabetes* 2002; 51: 204–20.

22. Burke GL, Arcilla RA, Culpepper WS, Webber LS, Chiang RA, Berenson GS. Blood pressure and echocardiographic measures in children: The Bogalusa Heart Study. *Circulation* 1987; 75: 106–14.

23. Newman WP III, Freedman DS, Voors AW, Gard PD, Srinivasan SR, Cresanta JL, Williamson GS, Webber LS, Berenson GS. Relation of serum lipoprotein levels and systolic blood pressure to early atherosclerosis: The Bogalusa Heart Study. *N Engl J Med* 1986; 314: 138–44.

24. McGill HC Jr. Persistent problems in the pathogenesis of atherosclerosis. *Arteriosclerosis* 1984; 4: 443–54.

25. Berenson GS, Wattigney WA, Tracy RE, Newman WP III, Srinivasan SR, Webber LS, Dalferes ER, Jr, Strong JP. Atherosclerosis of the aorta and coronary arteries and cardiovascular risk factors in persons aged 6 to 30 years and studied at necropsy (The Bogalusa Heart Study). *Am J Cardiol* 1992; 70: 851–8.

26. McGill HC Jr, McMahan CA, Malcom RT, Oalmann MC, Strong JP. Effect of serum lipoproteins and smoking on atherosclerosis in young men and women. *Arterioscl Thromb Vasc Biol* 1997; 17: 95–106.

27. Berenson GS, Srinivasan SR, Bao W, Newman WP III, Tracy RE, Wattigney WA. Association between multiple cardiovascular risk factors and atherosclerosis in children and young adults. *N Engl J Med* 1998; 338, 23: 1650–6.

28. Urbina EM, Srinivasan SR, Tang R, Bond MG, Kieltyka L, Berenson GS. Impact of Multiple Coronary Risk Factors on the Intima-Media Thickness of Different Segments of Carotid Artery in Healthy Young Adults (The Bogalusa Heart Study). *Am J Cardiol* (in press)

29. Kesaniemi AY, Ehnholm C, Miettinen TA. Intestinal cholesterol absorption efficiency in man is related to apoprotein E phenotype. *J Clin Invest* 1987; 80: 578–81.

30. Nicklas TA. Dietary studies of children: the Bogalusa Heart Study Experience. *J Am Diet Assoc* 1995; 95: 1127–33.

31. Downey AM, Frank GC, Webber LS, Harsha DW, Virgilio SJ, Franklin FA, Berenson GS. Implementation of 'Heart Smart': A cardiovascular school health promotion program. *J Sch Health* 1987; 57(3): 98–104.

32. Johnson CC, Nicklas TA, Arbeit ML, Harsha DW, Mott DS, Hunter SM, Wattigney W, Berenson GS. Cardiovascular intervention for high-risk families: The Heart Smart Program. *Sou Med J* 1991; 84(11): 1305–12.

33. Berenson GS, Srinivasan SR, Webber LS. Cardiovascular risk factors in children - A challenge or a poor idea. *Nutr Metab Cardiovasc Dis* 1994; 4: 46–52.

Progress in Obesity Research: 9. Edited by *Geraldo Medeiros-Neto, Alfredo Halpern and Claude Bouchard*
©2003 John Libbey Eurotext Ltd, pp. 468–474.

CHAPTER 98

Alcohol, body mass index and body fat distribution in man

Yves Schutz

Institute of Physiology, Faculty of Medicine, University of Lausanne, Bugnon 7, CH-1005 Lausanne, Switzerland
[e-mail: yves.schutz@iphysiol.unil.ch]

Introduction

Nowadays, after almost one century of research, the controversy still exists as to whether pro-longed alcohol (ethanol = EtOH) consumption constitutes a risk factor for the developement of overweight and obesity in man.

The issue of the relationship between the amount of alcohol consumed and the level of body weight, BMI and body fat have plagued nutritionists (and alcohologists) for several decades. Many interesting reviews[1-4] debates[5-6], editorial and letters[7-8] have been published on this topic, but there is no real consensus in the literature on this issue. What proportion of the energy of the EtOH substrate can be extracted for use in the intermediary metabolism is the key question.

It's worth mentioning first some methodological points because these may constitute one critical factor susceptible to explain the continuing controversy in the literature.

The different approaches utilized to analyse the putative effects of alcohol on body weight have been the following:

(1)   Experimental studies of metabolic nature, investigating the full replacement or full addition of alcohol to food energy on the rate of heat production (energy expenditure) and substrate utilization of the other macronutrients co-ingested;

(2)   Psycho-behavioural investigations studying the effect of alcohol on the control of food intake mediated by a change in appetite; and

(3)   Epidemiological studies focusing on large human investigations in which an attempt was made to derive a relationship between alcohol intake and body weight in a large population.

A summary of the different factors influenced by alcohol consumption is shown in Fig. 1.

Effect of EtOH on body weight: metabolic inefficiency

Alcohol provides fuel energy to the body (29 kJ/g EtOH) but with a different metabolic efficiency as compared to other macronutrients: the postprandial thermogenesis of EtOH (increase in heat production after EtOH absorption) is much greater than that of mixed macronutrients, indicating that the net efficiency of energy utilization at high dosage of EtOH consumption is largely blunted. When full substitution of EtOH occurs (isocaloric replacement of carbohydrates/fat by EtOH), this theoretically results in a situation where the proportion of energy used by the body (= *net* Energy) is lower than with the other substrates. There is little doubt, nevertheless that the calories of alcohol do count despite what has been claimed, but the exact magnitude of this input may vary among individuals.

In chronic alcoholics, the net efficiency of energy utilization of EtOH is expected to be even lower than in social drinkers, due to the microsomal ethanol oxidizing system (MEOS) induction in the liver[9], so that an even lower fraction of EtOH energy is avalaible to the body for ATP production. It remain to be seen the level (and duration) of EtOH consumption required to induce the MEOS.

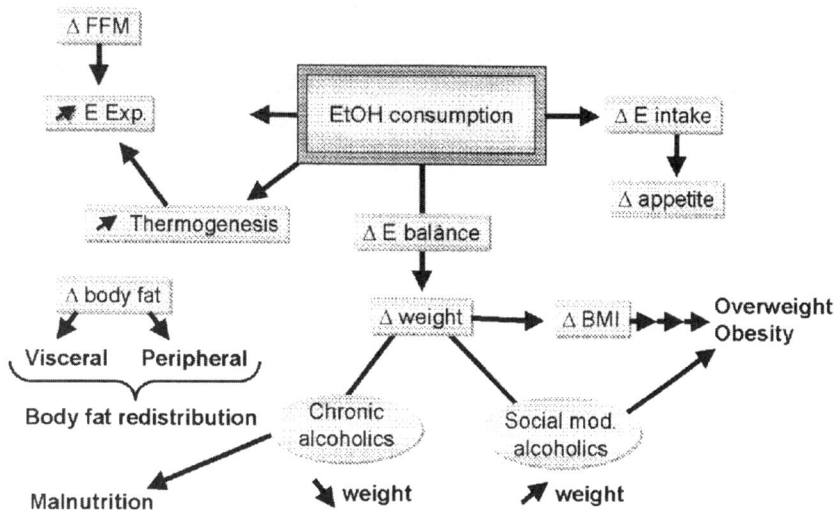

Fig. 1. Ethanol (EtOH) is susceptible to influence both energy intake (through a change in appetite) and energy expenditure (through increased thermogenesis as well as a change in FFM). The effect of EtOH on body weight and BMI seems to mostly depends upon the dosage of ethanol consumption, the type of consumption as well as the type of metabolization.

Another issue of interest is the demonstration that in alcoholic subjects the resting (basal) metabolic rate (measured without EtOH in the blood) was increased, as compared to matched controls, and this effect vanishes within a few days of abstinence[10]. This indicates that energy wastage in alcoholics occur, both in the postprandial phase (thermogenesis of EtOH) and the postabsorptive phase (resting energy expenditure).

The key issue in real life is whether moderate EtOH consumption (in non-alcoholics) favours body weight gain to the same extent as isoenergetic amount of macronutrient substrates. Since EtOH is a energetic substrate from which the body can extract about 3/4 of the gross energy value of EtOH[11], it seems unreasonable to compare EtOH energy added to a baseline diet with a control diet with no extra fuel added. Ideally, the effect of EtOH should be studied under three comparable situations:

(1) addition of EtOH vs. addition of other isocaloric macronutrients in 'overfeeding' conditions (i.e. positive energy balance);

(2) substitution of EtOH in eucaloric conditions (i.e. energy balance close to equilibrium); or

(3) combination of both situations (partly addition partly substitution).

EtOH is fully oxidized 'on line' in the body (in the liver primarily) and not stored as such, so that, in contrast to carbohydrates and lipids, no physiological feedback system exists for the control of food intake to response to a change in postprandial substrate storage. The effect of EtOH is mostly mediated by a decrease in utilization of other substrates (CHO and fat) rather than by an increase in fuel storage (sparing effect). The only exception is the process of lipogenesis from EtOH (see further).

Effect of addition vs. substitution of EtOH on body weight

General practitioners very often empirically observe that in plump (or obese) patients, who are social EtOH drinkers, the total suppression of alcohol leads to a decrease in body weight suggesting that ETOH is added to the diet. Therefore the total abstinence of alcohol in social drinkers, without voluntary calories replacemen from other drinks (i.e. sugar), can be considered as a complementary mean to obtain a better control of body weight, in particular when the adults get older.

Recently, Suter[12] claimed that there was a biphasic relationship between EtOH consumption and body weight (see Fig. 2). This indicates that at low alcohol intake, this substrate is generally added to the usual diet leading to positive energy balance and resulting in an increase in body weight up to a certain

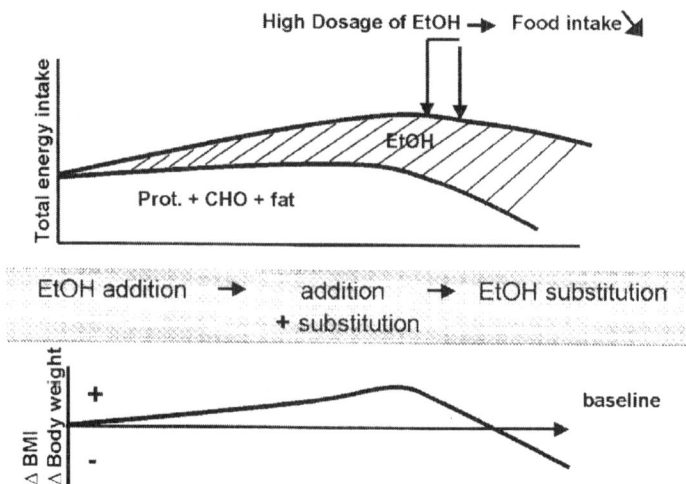

Fig. 2. Schematic hypothetical diagram showing the effect of prolonged alcohol consumption on body weight (adapted from Suter). At low to moderate level of consumption, ethanol engenders an increase of body weight through an increase in total energy intake (effect of ethanol addition) whereas at high alcohol consumption, total energy from food is curtailed and ethanol replaces energetic fuels (but with a blunted metabolic efficiency) so that the body weight tend to be lower as compared to the effect of ethanol substitution.

point. Then, the high dosage of EtOH (typically observed in alcoholics), results in a partial substitution of food energy by alcohol, diminishing nutrient intake.

The different pattern of food intake associated with alcohol consumption as well as behavioural factors such as a change in physical activity remain to be further studied.

The major nutritional factors involved in the effect of EtOH on body weight are the interaction between alcohol and the other macronutrients co-ingested, the proportion of 'addition' vs. 'substitution' of EtOH for food.

Whether obese men and women have a higher average consumption of EtOH than lean individuals remains to be investigated on the basis of a series of experimental studies in which as many confounding factors as possible are controlled.

To summarize, it can be hypothesize that small to moderate amount of EtOH consumption may lead to an increase in body weight because it is mostly taken in excess of habitual food (as 'apéritif[13]'), whereas elevated EtOH consumption may have divergent effect on body weight, since in chronic alcoholism the food intake is suppressed and leads to a progressive deterioration in nutritional status.

EtOH and fat metabolism

EtOH consumption has an effect on many lipidic sytems: chylomicrons, various lipids (sub)fractions in the blood, as well as fatty acids metabolism.

Briefly, alcohol increases the synthesis of triglycerides (net lipogenesis) in the liver, progressively leading to hepatic steathosis. It also stimulates the secretion of VLDL. These effect depends upon the dosage of EtOH and can be already observed in moderate EtOH consummers. Acute EtOH consumption inhibits lipid oxidation since it partially replaces fat as a source of calories but inhibition of other macronutrients is also observed[14].

This can theoretically result in a pervert and detrimental effect on body fat. In our classical metabolic study performed in a respiration chamber[15], fat oxidation suppression occurred not only when alcohol was added to the usual diet (hypercaloric conditions) but also when it was substituted (isocaloric conditions). Logically, when the body is exposed repeatedly to alcohol consumption, the metabolic situation is such that the lipid balance (and hence body fat) can be affected (see below), provided this effect is prolonged. All the effects described above depend upon the quantity of alcohol consumed, the chronicity of intake as well as hepatic metabolism.

Since obesity is defined as an excess body fat for size, one of the logical features to examine is the potential inflence of EtOH on overall fat balance (Fig. 3).

The physiological lipid balance of the body can be defined by the following equation:

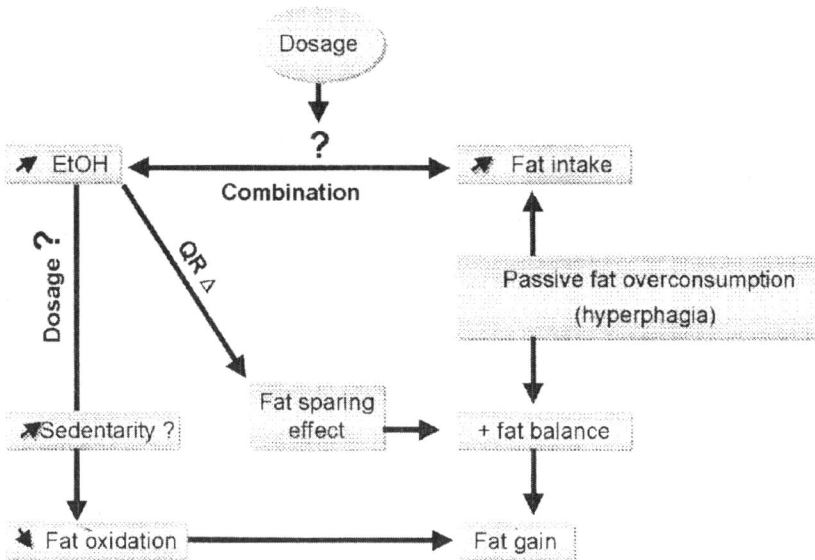

Fig. 3. Metabolic and behavioural effects of ethanol consumption leading to a change in fat balance and hence an effect on body fat. QR = respiratory quotient.

Fat balance = (exogenous fat intake + endogenous net fat synthesis) – (total fat oxidation)

where endogenous fat synthesis corresponds to the process of *de novo* lipogenesis from ethanol. Total fat oxidation represents the sum of exogenous + endogenous fat oxidations.

Using this straightforward physiological equation, it can be shown that ethanol consumption constitutes a potential risk factor for body weight (fat) gain, provided it can influence the different components of the fat balance equation. Three situations can be defined:

(1)   There is a passive overconsumption of exogenous fat when EtOH is co-ingested with food,

(2)   EtOH exerts a substantial inhibition of total fat oxidation, and

(3)   EtOH potentially influences endogenous fat synthesis by activating *de novo* lipogenesis[16].

More detailed analysis about these 3 possibilities have been thoroughly discussed[3].

Briefly co-ingestion of high fat with EtOH together with a blunting of fat oxidation rate would constitute a potent factor for increasing body fat, body weight and hence BMI.

One way to obviate this negative effect is to reequilibrate the energy balance by either decreasing fat intake or increasing fat oxidation through physical activity but this constitutes a somewhat theoretical situation with limited practical applications in a clinical setting.

Ethanol and body fat distribution

A few recent studies have been published on the issue, mostly of epidemiological nature[17-19], which will be briefly otlined. Recently, Buemann *et al.*[20] reviewed part of this topic and pointed out that cross-sectional epidemiological studies are more consistent than experimental studies in showing evidence that EtOH consumption, even at moderate levels, is associated with body fat distribution.

Dallongeville *et al.*[18] studied the influence of alcohol consumption and various beverages on waist girth and waist-to-hip ratio in a sample of men and women from France, a country where wine is the most commonly consumed alcoholic beverage. It was found that alcohol consumption was positively associated ($P < 0.0001$) with waist-to-hip ratio and waist girth, independently of BMI in women and in men.

The authors concluded that in French men and women, alcohol consumption is associated with greater android fat distribution independently of BMI. When genetic factors are kept constant, what would be the effect of increased OH consumption on body fat distribution? Marniemi *et al.*[19] have studied the

Alcohol ➚➚

↓

Hypothalamus arousal

| CRF ➚

Cortisol ➚ ────────────┐

↓   ↓

Fat redistribution   ➚ **Neoglucogenesis from endogenous protein (muscle)**

↓   ↓

➚ **Abdominal fat**   ➘ **fat-free mass**

⎵─────────────⎵

Δ body composition

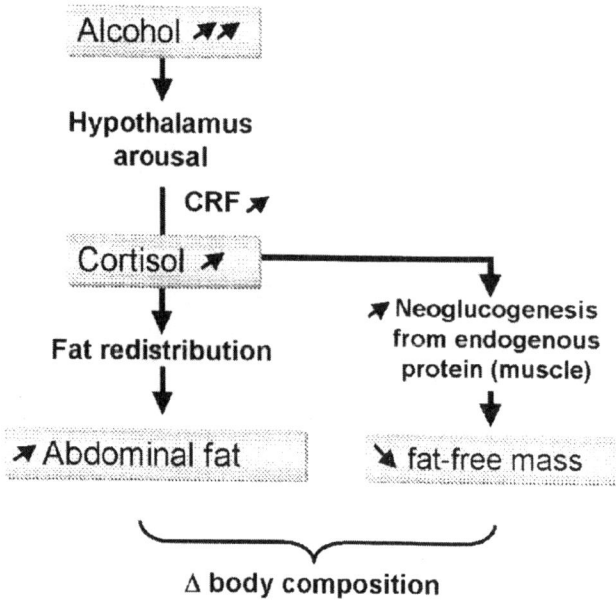

Fig. 4. Putative mechanism leading to visceral fat accumulation with high dosage of alcohol consumption. Increased neoglucogenesis through increased secretion of cortisol may lead to amino-acid mobilization from skeletal muscles, which may result in a decrease in muscle mass (fat-free mass) provoking, over the long term, a pseudo sarcopenic state.

association between psychosocial stress, obesity and body fat distribution in identical twins. The obese co-twins consumed almost 2.5 times as much alcohol, had higher daily urinary cortisol excretion and much higher visceral fat accumulation than their lean co-twins. However, this is only a very indirect evidence of an association between EtOH consumption and the visceral fat distribution because other nutritional factors may be involved.

In summary when adjustments are made for BMI and other confounding factors, EtOH consumption is generally correlated positively to waist-hip circumference, a proxy of abdominal (android) fat accumulation.

The mechanism behind increased abdominal fat consecutive to EtOH consumption is still debated. It is well known that hormonal factors (such as glucocorticoids and sexual hormones i.e. androgens) influence body fat distribution. Björntorp's group[21] made some hypotheses more than a decade ago, which are still relevant. The accumulation of intra-abdominal fat has been suggested to be the result of several factors acting in concert, one of which being alcohol and chronic stress. These factors cause the arousal of hypothalamic-pituitary-adrenal cortex axis. As shown in Fig. 4 the arousal of this axis increases the secretion of glucocorticoids (cortisol), resulting in body fat redistribution.

In parallel one can assume another effect of cortisol, which induces a stimulation of gluconeogenesis from amino acids, thus leading to an increase net breakdown of muscles tissues, whose magnitude remains to be determined. This is confirmed by an early study in which food energy was isocalorically replaced by EtOH, resulting in a small but persistent negative nitrogen balance[3].

The increased release of glucocorticoids may be dose-related and moderate levels of EtOH consumption may have much less effect on plasma cortisol[20]. Another factor which may play a role is the androgen level, which has been found to be associated to EtOH consumption in women (see Buemann et al.[20]). Let's recall that increased androgenic activity promotes abdominal fat accumulation in non-alcoholics non-obese premenopausal women. This is due to a rise in free testosterone and a depressed sex hormone-binding globulin (SHBG) which may be further compromised by a disturbance in hepatic function due to chronic alcohol consumption, the latter progressively leading to hepatic steathosis.

In summary, EtOH consumption seems to promote upper body fat accumulation. Whether or not this phenomenon of excessive relative fat accumulation in the abdominal area is also observed in alcoholics with a normal (or even low) BMI, remains to be further studied. Social (low to moderate) levels of alcohol consumption may have a significant effect over the long term. We should also keep in mind that in the ageing adult, visceral fat accumulation and BMI also increases with age without co-ingestion of EtOH!

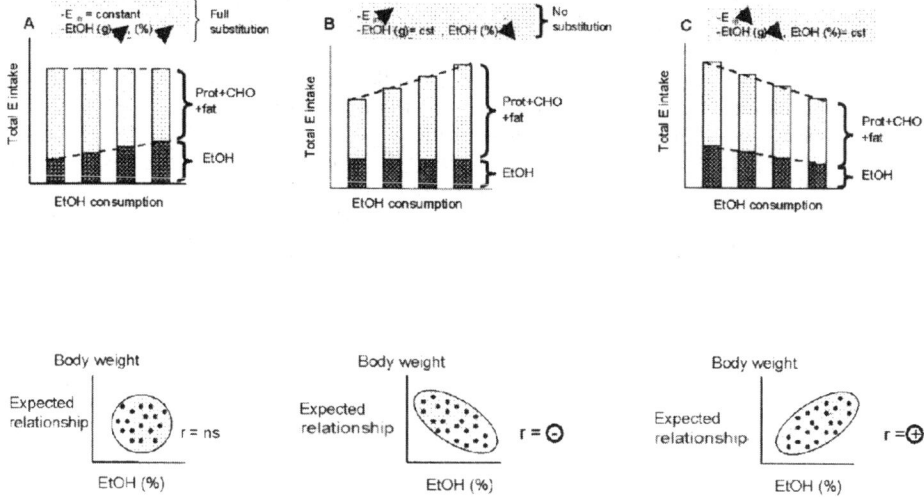

Fig. 5. Example of three theoretical profiles of ethanol consumption leading to spurious correlations with body weight. The uncertainty of the relationship between ethanol consumption (expressed either in absolute or relative terms), energy intake, and body weight is schematically shown. The hypothesis is made that total energy intake represents total energy requirement so that individuals with elevated body weights have (by definition) a higher energy requirement (and higher energy intake) than individuals with low body weights (assuming similar physical activity levels).

Epidemiological studies: the lack of consensus

Epidemiological studies have shown that when alcohol energy is additive to the usual diet, there is surprisingly no positive association between alcohol energy and body weight[22]. The lack of relationship between energy derived from alcohol and BMI has led to the suggestion that alcohol energy has a low metabolic efficiency (see above). As a result, surprisingly alcohol intake does not systematically increase body weight when this is judged on the basis of epidemiological studies. It is believed that at 'social dosage' EtOH supplements rather than displaces daily energy intake.

The lack of epidemiological evidence showing a clear relationship between daily alcohol consumption (expressed in energy units) and body weight is mostly true for men but not for women. Cross-sectional epidemiological surveys have shown that women who are moderate drinkers tend to have a lower (not higher) BMI than women not drinking[8].

The question is: does it seem reasonable to correlate the amount of alcohol consumed with body weight? Why not also analysing independently the relationship with other energetic macronutrients? How reasonable is it scientifically to correlate a substrate (alcohol) with body weight, the former contributing to (only) 10 per cent or less of total energy intake! What about the potential effect of the other energetic substrates contributing to the remaining 90 per cent?

In order to clarify the situation, a conceptual, schematic diagramme is presented (see Fig. 5) showing that almost any types of relationship can be developed between EtOH consumption and body weight and this is effectively what is found in the literature. This simplified demonstration is nevertheless based on many assumptions the main ones being that energy requirement is heavily dependent upon body weight. If variable degree of underreporting of EtOH would exist in function of BMI, this would constitute another bias than that examined here. In this demonstration, we mostly focus here on the expression of the results of EtOH consumption (total amount in gramme vs. per cent EtOH energy).

In the first theoretical example considered, the energy intake is assumed to be insensitive to the increase in EtOH consumption expressed either in absolute (g) or relative amount (%). There is full substitution. As a result, keeping confounding factors to a minimum, theoretically no relationship should be observed between the two variables.

In the second theoretical example, the amount of EtOH consumed would remain essentially constant irrespective of the total food intake. Therefore, the per cent EtOH energy in the diet decreases. There is no substitution at all ! As a result, a negative correlation is anticipated between EtOH and body weight, provided EtOH is expressed in relative amount (rather than in gramme).

473

In the third theoretical example, the amount of EtOH taken increase with total energy intake. As a result, one would expect a positive relationship between EtOH consumption (expressed in g) and body weight.

To summarize, this simplified visual demonstration indicates that, depending upon the different pattern of EtOH consumption in a population as well as the degree of replacement vs. substitution, the epidemiological studies could theoretically show either a positive relationship, no relationship, or a negative association. Physiologically there is no reason to think that the degree of substitution is perfect such as one calorie of EtOH would exactly replace one calorie of food substrate! As a result, part substitution and part replacement may co-exist but this situation has, as far as I am aware, not been studied experimentally yet!

Many questions remain for future research: Does alcohol influence appetite differently depending upon the EtOH dosage? This may explain the varying effect on body weight. Does liver metabolism play a role in this respect? Certainly yes. Does pleasure (of consuming attractive palatable alcoholic drinks) overcome the regulation? Is the EtOH molecule not very well sensed metabolically since it is ingested as a drink and not primarily stored? Does passive overconsumption occurs in a similar way as that described for exogenous fat or sugar drink?

All these questions may find an appropriate answer thanks to future research.

References

1. Prentice AM. Alcohol and obesity. *Int J Obes Relat Metab Disord* 1995; 19 Suppl: S44–50.

2. Westerterp PP, Prentice AM, Jéquier E. Alcohol and body weight. In: *Health issues related to alcohol consumption*, MacDonald I (ed.), pp. 103–23. Oxford: Blackwell Press, 1999.

3. Schutz Y. Role of substrate utilization and thermogenesis on body-weight control with particular reference to alcohol. *Proc Nutr Soc* 2000; 59: 511–17.

4. Muller MJ. Alcohol and body weight. *Z Gastroenterol* 1999; 37: 33–43.

5. Schutz Y. Alcohol calories count the same as other calories. *Int J Obes* 1995; 19 Suppl 2: 12–13.

6. Westertrep KR. Alcohol calories do not count the same as other calories. *Int J Obes* 1999; 19 Suppl 2: 14–15.

7. Jéquier E. Alcohol intake and body weight: a paradox. *Am J Clin Nutr* 1999; 69: 173–74.

8. McCarty MF. The alcohol paradox (letter) *Am J Clin Nutr* 1999; 70: 940–41.

9. Lieber CS. Perspectives: do alcohol calories count? *Am J Clin Nutr* 1991; 54: 976–82.

10. Levine JA, Harris MM, Morgan MY. Energy expenditure in chronic alcohol abuse. *Eur J Clin Invest* 2000; 30(9): 779–86.

11. Suter PM, Jéquier E, Schutz Y. Effect of ethanol on energy expenditure. *Am J Physiol* 1994; 266, R1204–R12.

12. Suter PM. Alkohol, Fettstoffwechsel und Körpergewicht. *Therapeutische Umschau* 2000; 57: 205–211 (German).

13. Westerterp-Plantenga MS, Verwegen CRT. The appetizing effect of an apéritif in overweight and normal-weight humans. *Am J Clin Nutr* 1999; 69: 205–12.

14. Shelmet JJ, Reichard GA, Skutches CL, Hoeldtke RD Owen OE, Boden G.: Ethanol causes acute inhibition of carbohydrate, fat, and protein oxidation and insulin resistance. *J Clin Invest* 1988; 81: 1137–45.

15. Suter PM, Jéquier E, Schutz Y. The effect of ethanol on fat storage in healthy subjects. *N Engl J Med* 1992; 326: 983–87.

16. Siler SQ, Neese RA, Hellerstein MK. De novo lipogenesis lipid kinetics, and whole-body lipid balances in humans after acute alcohol consumption. *Am J Clin Nutr* 1999; 70: 928–36.

17. Sakurai Y, Umeda T, Shinchi K, Honjo S, Wakabayashi K, Todoroki I. et al. Relation of total and beverage-specific alcohol intake to body mass index and waist-to-hip ratio: a study of self-defense officials in Japan. *Eur J Epidemiol* 1997; 8: 893–98.

18. Dallongeville J, Marecaux N, Ducimetiere P, Ferrieres J, Arveiler D, Bingham A et al. Influence of alcohol consumption and various beverages on waist girth and wais-to-hip ratio in a sample of French men and women. *Int J Obes Relat Metab Disord* 1998; 22: 1178–83.

19. Marniemi J, Kronholm E, Aunola S, Toikka T, Mattlar CE, Koskenvuo M, Ronnemaa T. Visceral fat and psychosocial stress in identical twins discordant for obesity. *J Intern Med* 2002; 251: 35–43.

20. Buemann B, Dyerberg J, Astrup A. Alcohol drinking and cardiac risk. *Nutr Res Rev* 2002; 15: 91–121.

21. Lapidus L, Bengtsson C, Hallstrom T, Bjorntorp P. Obesity, adipose tissue distribution and health in women – results from a population study in Gothenburg, Sweden. *Appetite.* 1989; 131: 25–35.

22. Colditz GA, Giovannuci E, Rimm EB et al. Alcohol intake in relation to diet and obesity in women and men. *Am J Clin Nutr* 1991; 54: 49–55.

Progress in Obesity Research: 9. Edited by *Geraldo Medeiros-Neto, Alfredo Halpern and Claude Bouchard*
©2003 John Libbey Eurotext Ltd, pp. 475–476.

CHAPTER 99

Alcohol, type of alcohol and waist circumference: results from the Copenhagen City Heart Study

Eva Soelberg Vadstrup, Liselotte Petersen, Thorkild I.A. Sørensen and Morten Grønbæk

Danish Epidemiology Science Centre at the Institute of Preventive Medicine, Copenhagen, Denmark; Centre for Alcohol Research, National Institute of Public Health, Copenhagen, Denmark
[e-mail: mg@niph.dk]

Introduction

A number of cross-sectional studies have assessed the relation between alcohol and high waist circumference. The results, however, are inconclusive. Some found a positive association[1-5], whereas others found a negative or no association between alcohol and abdominal adiposity in both men and women[6-10]. Only a few studies have examined the association between total alcohol consumption and obesity on a prospective basis. Some studies showed that men consuming alcohol had developed a higher body weight than did non-consumers, and women showed the opposite or no association[11,12]. These studies have considered neither type of alcohol nor waist circumference.

Methods

The present analysis concerns a sample of 6,886 subject, 2,916 men and 3,970 women, who attended both second and third examination at the Copenhagen City Heart Study and who contributed with complete information on the variables of interest. The subjects filled in a self-administered questionnaire concerning various health-related issues, including alcohol consumption, smoking habits, physical activity, school education, household income and deliveries. All statistical analyses were done by using SAS computer software[13]. Significance level of 5 per cent was used, and the estimated odds ratios were presented with 95 per cent confidence intervals (95 per cent CI).

Results

Men with a high alcohol intake had significantly increased risks of a high waist circumference, compared to the reference group (drinkers of 1–6 beverages per week). Thus, those with an intake of 14–27 beverages per week had an odds ratio of 1.50 (95 per cent CI 1.03–2.18) and those who had an intake of more than 28 beverages per week had an odds ratio of 1.65 (95 per cent CI 1.07–2.55)). A significant linear trend was found ($P = 0.019$). In women, the odds ratio for having a large waist circumference after 10 years was higher in women who ten years earlier drank 14–27 beverages per week and more than 28 beverages per week [1.20 (95 per cent CI 0.79–1.82) and 2.16 (95 per cent CI 0.86–5.14)], compared to the reference group. The trend was linear ($P = 0.008$). Men who drank 14–20 beers per week and more than 21 beers per week had higher odds ratios [1.15 (95 per cent CI 0.69–1.90) and 1.63 (95 per cent CI 0.99–2.67)] of having a large waist circumference after 10 years, compared with the reference group of drinkers of less than one beer per week. A significant linear trend was found ($P = 0.019$). For women, all groups had higher odds ratios of having a large waist circumference after 10 years, when compared with the reference group. Women who drank more than 14 beers per week had odds ratio 2.53 (95 per cent CI 0.92–6.34) of having a large waist circumference after 10 years (Fig. 1). The trend was linear ($P = 0.010$). Contrary to total alcohol and beer consumption, the odds ratios for having a large waist circumference after 10 years in men who drank 14–20 glasses of wine per week and more than 21 glasses of wine per week were lower [0.88 (95 per cent CI 0.39–1.94) and 0.49 (95 per cent CI 0.10–1.84)], than in the reference group. Women who drank more than 14 glasses of wine

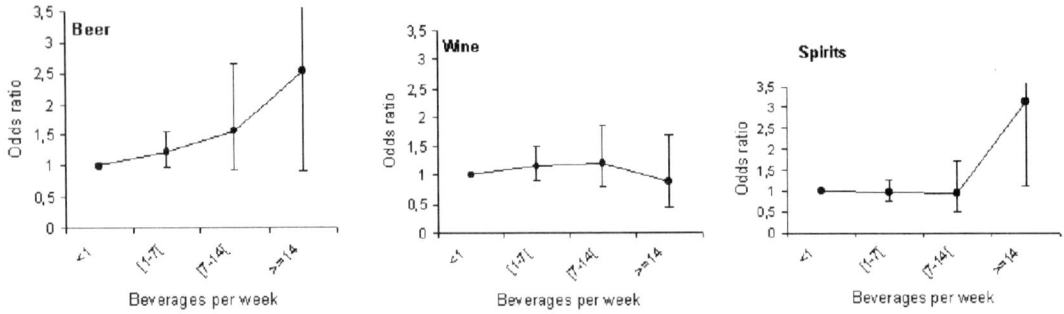

Fig. 1.

per week also had lower odds ratio 0.88 (95 per cent CI 0.44–1.69) of having a large waist circumference after 10 years than in the reference group (Fig. 1). No significant linear trend was found in either men or women ($P = 0.63$ and 0.88). Odds ratio for having a large waist circumference after 10 years in men who drank 7–13 glasses of spirits per week and 14–20 glasses per week was higher [1.37 (95 per cent CI 0.84–2.22) and 1.89 (95 per cent CI 0.81–4.36)] than in the reference group. Women had significantly higher odds ratio for having a large waist circumference after 10 years when drinking more than 14 glasses of spirits per week to 3.12 (95 per cent CI 1.12–8.52), compared to the reference group (Fig. 1). No significant linear trend was found in either men or women ($P = 0.28$ and 0.15).

In conclusion, a moderate to high consumption of alcohol and of beer and spirits is associated with later high waist circumference, whereas moderate to high wine consumption seems to have no effect. This may have implications for the interpretation of studies showing health benefits of wine.

References

1. Han TS, Bijnen FC, Lean ME, Seidell JC. Separate associations of waist and hip circumference with lifestyle factors. *Int J Epidemiol* 1998; 27(3): 422–30.

2. Laws A, Terry RB, Barrett-Connor E. Behavioral covariates of waist-to-hip ratio in Rancho Bernardo. *Am J Public Health* 1990; 80(11): 1358–62.

3. Marti B, Toumilehto J, Salomaa V, Kartovaara L, Korhonen HJ, Pietinen P. Body fat distribution in the Finnish population: environmental determinants and predictive power for cardiovascular risk factor levels. *J Epidemiol Community Health* 1991; 45(2): 131–7.

4. Dallongeville J, Marecaux N, Ducimetiere P, Ferrieres J, Arveiler D, Bingham A, Ruidavets JB, Simon C, Amouyel P. Influence of alcohol consumption and various beverage on waist girth and waist-to-hip ratio in a sample of French men and women. *Int J Obes Relat Metab Disord* 1998; 22(12): 1178–83.

5. Cigolini M, Targher G, Bergamo Andreis IA, Tonoli M, Filippi F, Muggeo M, De Sandre G. Moderate alcohol consumption and its relation to visceral fat and plasma androgens in healthy women. *Int J Obes Relat Metab Disord* 1996; 20(3): 206–12.

6. Kaye SA, Folsom AR, Prineas RJ, Potter JD, Gapstur SM. The association of body fat distribution with lifestyle and reproductive factors in a population study of postmenopausal women. *Int J Obes* 1990; 14(7): 583–91.

7. Keenan NL, Strogatz DS, James SA, Ammerman AS, Rice BL. Distribution and correlates of waist-to-hip ratio in black adults: the Pitt County Study. *Am J Epidemiol* 1992; 135(6): 678–84.

8. Haffner SM, Stern MP, Hazuda HP, Pugh J, Patterson JK, Malina R. Upper body and centralized adiposity in Mexican Americans and non-Hispanic whites: relationship to body mass index and other behavioral and demographic variables. *Int J Obes* 1986; 10(6): 493–502.

9. Slattery ML, McDonald A, Bild DE, Caan BJ, Hilner JE, Jacobs DR Jr., Liu K. Associations of body fat and its distribution with dietary intake, physical activity, alcohol, and smoking in blacks and whites. *Am J Clin Nutr* 1992; 55(5): 943–9.

10. Duncan BB, Chambless LE, Schmidt MI, Folsom AR, Szklo M, Crouse JR 3rd, Carpenter MA. Association of the waist-to-hip ratio is different with wine than with beer or hard liquor consumption. Atherosclerosis Risk in Communities Study Investigators. *Am J Epidemiol* 1995; 142(10): 1034–8.

11. Gordon T, Kannel WB. Drinking and its relation to smoking, BP, blood lipids, and uric acid. The Framingham study. *Arch Intern Med* 1983; 143(7): 1366–74.

12. Rissanen AM, Heliovaara M, Knekt P, Reunanen A, Aromaa A. Determinants of weight gain and overweight in adult Finns. *Eur J Clin Nutr* 1991; 45(9): 419–30.

13. SAS/STAT software: the GENMOD procedure, release 6.09. Cary, NC: SAS Institute; 1993.

Progress in Obesity Research: 9. Edited by *Geraldo Medeiros-Neto, Alfredo Halpern and Claude Bouchard*
©2003 John Libbey Eurotext Ltd, pp. 477–480.

CHAPTER 100

Effects of alcohol consumption on appetite

Margriet S. Westerterp-Plantenga

Department of Human Biology, University of Maastricht, The Netherlands
[e-mail: m.westerterp@hb.unimaas.nl]

Introduction

Low-level dietary exposure to ethanol via ingestion of fermenting fruit has probably characterized the predominantly frugivorous anthropoid lineage for about 40 million years. In contemporary human environments, excessive consumption of ethanol would then represent maladaptive development of ancestrally advantageous behaviours given *ad libitum* access to a compound otherwise found only within scarce nutritional substrates.

Evidence for alcohol preference in humans being regulated by the NPY system is given by a related polymorphism (Pro (7) substitution) in the signal peptide part of NPY, associated with a 34 per cent higher average alcohol consumption[12]. Several serotonin uptake blockers have been found to decrease alcohol intake[7], showing the rewarding effect of alcohol consumption. Evidence for the addictive effect appeared from the change in previously neutral stimuli associated with alcohol intake becoming conditioned cues that activate dopamine release and reward craving[8].

With respect to appetite and alcohol ingestion, relevant questions are whether appetite is influenced by alcohol consumption, whether the body recognizes alcohol-derived energy and regulates its intake as it does for the other macronutrients. These questions have been addressed in epidemiological, energy metabolism, and food intake studies.

Epidemiological studies of alcohol intake in relation to total energy intake have shown that in moderate alcohol consumers total energy intake increases when alcohol is introduced into the diet[1,4,5,11,14]. This suggests that alcohol derived energy is additive, and not recognized or regulated by the body; it does not replace energy from other substrates. Appetite seems to remain unchanged, and no compensatory decrease in the subsequent amount of food eaten was reported. This hypothesis was tested in several experimental studies.

Methods

The methods for investigating the effect of alcohol ingestion on appetite and food intake are either preload-test meal methods[10,13,20,22] or 24 h in house energy intake evaluations[6,18] or a combination[18,20]. All studies offered iso-volumetric drinks (330–392 ml) with 18–36 g alcohol vs. no alcohol as placebo. Not all studies applied an iso-energetic placebo. The studies were performed in men and women[20], only men[6,10,18,22], or only women[13].

We investigated the effects of a usual alcohol aperitif (34 g alcohol in 340 ml wine or beer) in comparison with iso-energetic (1 MJ) iso-volumetric (340 ml) fat-, protein-, and carbohydrate aperitifs (all fruit juices with similar tastes), and in comparison with an iso-volumetric water aperitif, on the short term appetite profile and subsequent energy intake in normal-weight and overweight men and women ($n = 52$)[20].

Lunch was offered 30 min after the aperitif was consumed, *ad lib*, from the universal eating monitor[20,21], and food intake during the rest of the day was recorded.

Poppit *et al.*[13] investigated the short-term effects of alcohol (31 g in gin, 392 ml) on hunger and energy intake in 20 partly dietary restrained, lean women. On four occasions subjects were given a randomized preload drink (alcohol, no alcohol, not iso-energetic carbohydrate, water), followed by visual analogue scales rating hunger and an *ad lib* test meal.

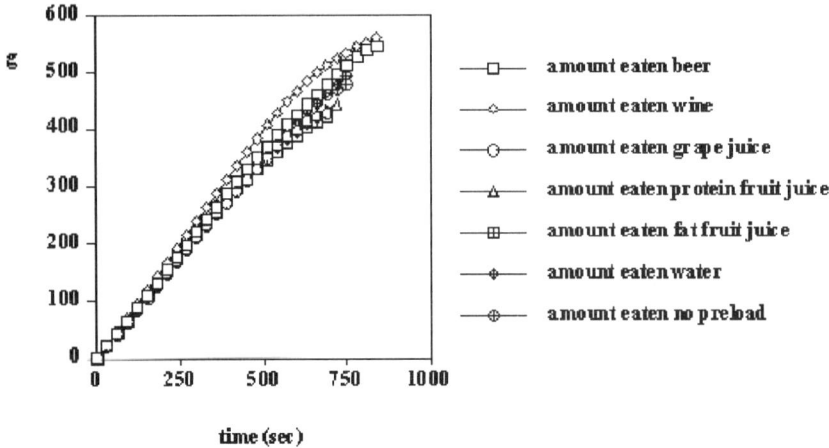

Fig. 1. Averaged cumulative amount ingested after the different preloads ($n = 52$) (SD range: ± 2 to ± 3 g ingested/min). The amount ingested after a beer or wine preload was significantly different from that after the other preloads, $P < 0.001$[20].

Yeomans et al.[22] evaluated the effects of alcohol (18 g, 330 ml) on appetite in 12 unrestrained and 10 restrained men during their lunch 20 min after consuming preloads consisting of water, an alcoholic fruit juice, and an iso-volumetric, iso-energetic non-alcoholic juice.

Hetherington et al.[10] investigated the effects of alcohol (24 g; 330 ml) on appetite and food intake in 26 males on three occasions. They compared two preload conditions, 30 min before lunch, offering 330 ml of a lager spiked with three units of alcohol (969 kJ), or 330 ml no-alcohol lager (264 kJ), or with a rest-condition. The test meal at lunch consisted of a buffet-style array of foods and chilled water.

Tremblay et al.[18] studied the effects of alcohol (25 g in beer, 341 ml vs. 341 ml iso-energetic de-alcoholized beer) and dietary fat on spontaneous energy and macronutrient intakes in eight male subjects who participated in a protocol including four randomly assigned 2 day sessions during which they ate ad libitum.

Foltin et al.[6] compared ethanol as an energy source in six young lean men, with dextrose containing beverages. On certain days, the subjects had to consume four beverages containing a total of 2.4 or 4.6 MJ, equivalent to 22 per cent and 42 per cent of usual energy intake. Each of four conditions (2.4 MJ ethanol (18 g, 330 ml) or dextrose); 4.6 MJ ethanol (36 g, 330 ml) or dextrose), consumed at four moments of time during the day, and a no-beverage control condition was examined for 2 days.

Results

We observed, in comparison to the iso-volumetric, iso-energetic fat, carbohydrate or protein appetizer, a higher energy intake after the aperitif (3.5 ± 0.3 MJ vs. 2.7 ± 0.2 MJ, $P < 0.001$), despite hedonic

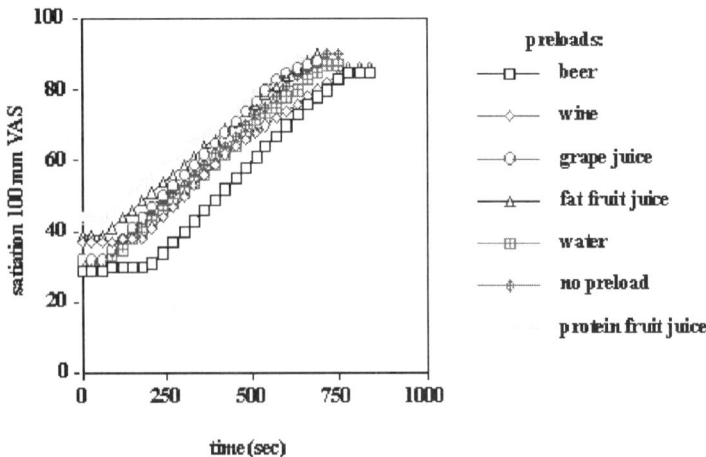

Fig. 2. Averaged visual analogue scale (VAS) satiety scores during the lunch meals after the different preloads ($n = 52$). (SD range: ± 3 to ± 12). The increase in satiety started later and the meal continued longer after maximum satiety with the beer and wine preloads than after the grape juice, cream fruit juice or protein fruit juice, $P < 0.01$[20].

ratings of the lunches being similar, in men as well as in women (Fig. 1)[20]. Eating rate was higher (44 ± 3 g/min vs. 38 ± 3 g/min, $P < 0.01$), meal duration longer (14 min vs. 12 min, $P < 0.01$), satiation started to increase later (3.5 min vs. 1.5 min, $P < 0.01$), and eating was prolonged after maximum satiation (2.5 min vs. 0.6 min, $P < 0.01$) (Fig. 2)[20]. Energy intake compensation during lunch, after the carbohydrate, protein or fat preload, compared to energy intake after the water preload, expressed as a percentage of the energy content of the preload, was on average 31 ± 4 per cent, while energy intake compensation after the alcohol preloads was on average –50 ± 8 per cent ($P < 0.01$)[20]. VAS ratings of light-headedness after the alcohol preloads and still 30 min after the subsequent meal, was larger than after the other preloads ($P < 0.001$)[20].

Energy intake during the rest of the day did not differ significantly among the different situations with energy containing preloads. Energy intake compensation (compared to energy intake after the water preload) after the energy containing preloads was then –40 ± 6 per cent for the alcohol preload (wine), –72 ± 9 per cent for the alcohol preload (beer), 32 ± 5 per cent for the carbohydrate preload, –6 ± 3 per cent for the fat preload, 67 ± 8 per cent for the protein preload, resulting in a higher 24 h energy intake on a day with alcohol preloads than on a day with water or no preloads ($P < 0.05$)[20].

Poppit *et al.*[13] reported no difference in hunger ratings nor in the amount of energy consumed during the test meal following any of the four preloads, in the women.

Yeomans *et al.*[22] reported that the unrestrained men ate significantly less after the juice preload, and ate most after the alcohol preload. In these men hunger increased more during the initial stages of the test meal after alcohol consumption. No effects were seen in the restrained men.

Hetherington *et al.*[10] reported that *ad libitum* intake at lunch was significantly higher following alcohol (7.3 ± 0.4 MJ) compared to both baseline (6.4 ± 0.3MJ) and the no-alcohol condition (6.5 ± 0.3 MJ), without differences in appetite ratings. Total energy intake, including energy from alcohol was enhanced in the alcohol condition by 30 per cent, suggesting that energy from alcohol is not compensated in the short-term and may even have a stimulatory effect on food intake.

Tremblay *et al.*[18] observed that alcohol had no inhibitory effect on food intake and its energy content was thus associated with an additional increase in 24 h energy intake. The enhancing effects of alcohol and dietary fat on daily energy intake were additive so that overfeeding was maximal (2.8 MJ/day) under a high fat + alcohol condition.

Foltin *et al.*[6] observed compensation for about 37 per cent of the energy contained in the beverages, such that total energy intake increased by 13 per cent under the 2.4 MJ conditions and 27 per cent under the 4.6 MJ conditions. There was no differential effect of ethanol content on energy intake, suggesting that effects of ethanol served in four separate quarter dosages, on intake of other foods can be accounted for by the energy content of ethanol, rather than by the pharmacological effects of ethanol.

Discussion

The appetizing effect of an alcohol aperitif compared to an iso-energetic (or not), iso-volumetric carbohydrate, protein or fat containing aperitif, all with similar hedonic values, was demonstrated in men and women as a larger meal size during the subsequent meal (20–30 min later)[10,20,22]. Poppit *et al.*[13] and Yeomans *et al.*[22] did not find a difference in energy intake after an alcohol and a carbohydrate preload, compared to after a water preload. The explanation for the difference in results cannot be the alcohol dosage, since stimulating appetite effects were found with dosages of 18–36 g alcohol, nor the comparison with a non iso-energetic preload, since Hetherington[10] reported increased intake after an alcohol preload even compared to a lower energy carbohydrate preload. Dietary restraint may have been a factor since Poppits' study[13] included dietary restrained women, and Yeomans[22] showed that in dietary restrained men intake and hunger was not altered by the alcohol preload compared to placebo. With respect to further possible energy intake compensation during the day, this was positive for successively protein, milkshake, and carbohydrate and negative for successively fat and alcohol[18,20]. However, the extend of energy intake compensation reported by Foltin *et al.*[6] was not specific for alcohol, but a general 37 per cent for the energy supplied by the beverages. The lack of a specific alcohol effect might be that the alcohol ingestion was spread over the day, in four drinks with 3½ h interval. The delayed fat oxidation not only lead to a lack of metabolic satiety, but also to a decrease in fat oxidation, e.g. by 73 per cent[15]. Moreover after 24 g alcohol ingestion, the fractional contribution of *de novo* lipogenesis rose from 2 ± 1 per cent to 30 ± 8 per cent[15].

Thus the overeating effect after an alcohol aperitif can only be prevented by taking a low dosage of alcohol each time[6] or by dietary restraint as was the case with Poppit[13] and with Yeomans[22]. Then also the increase of *de novo* lipogenesis will be limited, and body weight increase may be prevented. The other factor involved in the alcohol paradox may be habitual physical activity[19]. A positive relation was shown between habitual alcohol consumption and habitual physical activity, measured with a tri-axial accelerometer[19].

Thus, the suggested inverse relation between body mass index and alcohol intake at intakes ≤ 50 g/day in women[2,3,9] may be explained by dietary restraint[13,22], habitual physical activity[19] and spread alcohol consumption. At higher intakes of alcohol, light-headedness will play a role implying loss of control and of dietary restraint, resulting in increases in BMI[2,3,9].

In men, there is no such relation. Across a wide range of alcohol intake, men have similar BMIs[2,3,9]. This may be explained by the relationship between physical activity and alcohol intake[19]. It may be the habitually physically more active men, who drink.

References

1. Bebb HT, Houser H, Witschi JC, Littel AS, Fuller RK. Calorie and nutrient contribution of alcohol beverages to the usual diets of 155 adults. *Am J Clin Nutr* 1971; 24: 1042–52.

2. Colditz GA, Giovannucci E, Rimm EB, Stampfer MJ, Rosner B, Speizer FE, Gordis E, Willet WC. Alcohol intake in relation to diet and obesity in women and men. *Am J Clin Nutr* 1991: 54: 49–55.

3. Crouse JR, Grundy SM. Effects of alcohol on plasma lipo proteins and cholesterol and triglyceride metabolism in man. *J Lipid Res* 1984; 25: 486–96.

4. DeCastro JM, Orozco S. Moderate alcohol intake and spontaneous eating patterns of humans: evidence of unregulated supplementation. *Am J Clin Nutr* 1990; 62: 246–53.

5. Fisher M, Gorgon T. The relationship of drinking and smoking habits to diet: the lipid research clinics prevalence study. *Am J Clin Nutr* 1985; 41: 623–30.

6. Foltin RW, Kelly TH, Fischman MW. Ethanol as an energy source in humans: comparison with dextrose-containing beverages. *Appetite* 1993; 20: 95–110.

7. Gill K, Amit Z. Serotonin uptake blockers and voluntary alcohol consumption. A review of recent studies. *Recent Dev Alcohol* 1989; 7: 225–48.

8. Heinz A. Dopaminergic dysfunction in alcoholism and schizophrenia – psychopathological and behavioral correlates. *Eur Psychiatry* 2002; 17: 9–16.

9. Hellerstedt WL, Jeffery RW, Murray DM. The association between alcohol intake and adiposity in the general population, reviews and commentary. *Am J Epidemiol* 1990; 132: 594–611.

10. Hetherington MM, Cameron F, Wallis DJ, Pirie LM. Stimulation of appetite by alcohol. *Physiol Behav* 2001; 74: 283–89.

11. Jones BR, Barret-Conner E, Criqui MH, Holdbrook MJ. A community study of calorie and nutrient intake in drinkers and non-drinkers of alcohol. *Am J Clin Nutr* 1982; 35: 135–41.

12. Kauhunen J, Karvonen MK, Pesonen U, Koulu M, Tuomainen TP, Uusitupa MI, Salonen JT. Neuropeptide Y polymorphism and alcohol consumption in middle-aged men. *Am J Med Genet* 2000; 93: 117–21.

13. Poppit SD, Eckhardt JW, McGonagle J, Murgatroyd PR, Prentice AM. Short-term effects of alcohol consumption on appetite and energy intake. *Phys Behav* 1996; 60: 1063–70.

14. Rissanen A, Sarlio-Lahteenkorva S, Alfthan G, Gref CG, Keso L, Salaspuro M. Employed problem drinkers: a nutritional risk group? *Am J Clin Nutr* 1987; 45: 456–61.

15. Siler SQ, Neese RA, Hellerstein MK. De novo lipogenesis, lipid kinetics, and whole-body lipid balances in humans after acute alcohol consumption. *Am J Clin Nutr* 1999; 70: 928–36.

16. Sonko BJ, Prentice AM, Murgatroyd PR, Goldberg GR, van de Ven MLHM, Coward WA. Effect of alcohol on post-meal fat storage. *Am J Clin Nutr* 1994; 59: 619–25.

17. Suter PM, Schutz Y, Jequier E. The effect of ethanol on fat storage in healthy subjects. *N Engl J Med* 1992; 326: 983–87.

18. Tremblay A, Wouters E, Wenker M, St-Pierre S, Bouchard C, Despres JP. Alcohol and a high-fat diet: a combination favoring overfeeding. *Am J Clin Nutr* 1995; 62: 639–44.

19. Westerterp KR. Alcohol intake, physical activity and energy balance. *ICPFFI* XIII: 21; 2001.

20. Westerterp-Plantenga MS. Verwegen CRT. The appetizing effect of an aperitif in overweight and normal-weight humans. *Am J Clin Nutr* 1999; 69: 205–12.

21. Westerterp-Plantenga MS, Wouters L, ten Hoor F. Restrained eating, obesity, and cumulative food intake curves during four course meals. *Appetite* 1991; 16: 149–58.

22. Yeomans MR, Hails NJ, Nesic JS. Alcohol and the appetizer effect. *Behav Pharmacol* 1999; 10: 151–61.

Progress in Obesity Research: 9. Edited by *Geraldo Medeiros-Neto, Alfredo Halpern and Claude Bouchard*
©2003 John Libbey Eurotext Ltd, pp. 481–484.

CHAPTER 101

Alcohol and cardiovascular disease: the role of obesity as a possible confounder

S. Goya Wannamethee and A. Gerald Shaper

Dept of Primary Care and Population Science, Royal Free & University College Medical School, London NW3 2PF, UK
[e-mail: goya@pcps.ucl.ac.uk]

Introduction

In almost all epidemiological studies of alcohol and cardiovascular disease, non-drinking status is associated with increased risk of coronary heart disease compared with light or moderate alcohol intake, resulting in a J- or U-shaped curve[1-5]. Recent prospective studies suggest that this association is causal although the true magnitude of the effect is uncertain[6]. Plausible biological explanations include the effects of alcohol on lipid levels, haemostasis and platelet aggregation[2-5]. Alcohol consumption also increases energy balance which may enhance deposition of fat[7]. Obesity is a well established risk factor for CHD[8]. The epidemiological evidence relation to alcohol and body weight has been controversial[9]. In some studies light to moderate drinking has been shown to be associated with lower body mass index than observed in abstainers ('skinny drinkers') despite their higher total energy intakes, whereas in many studies heavy drinking is associated with increased risk of obesity[9]. In the majority of studies, BMI is included in multivariate adjustment and in virtually all these studies the inverse relationship associated with light to moderate drinking persists[2]. In this paper, we examine the role of obesity as a potential confounder in the alcohol-cardiovascular disease relationship. We present data on the relationship between alcohol intake and risk of major CHD events and cardiovascular mortality from a cohort of middle-aged British men followed for 21.8 years, stratified by body mass index.

Subjects and methods

The material presented in this paper comes from a prospective study of cardiovascular disease in 7735 men aged 40–59 years at entry recruited from the age-sex registers of one group general practice in each of 24 British towns and examined in 1978–80 (The British Regional Heart Study)[10]. The overall response rate was 78 per cent and men with pre-existing cardiovascular disease or on regular medical treatment were not excluded. Research nurses administered to each man a standard questionnaire (Q1) which included questions on frequency, quantity and type of alcohol consumption, smoking habits, physical activity and medical history.

Alcohol intake

At entry into the study the men were classified into five groups according to their estimated reported weekly intake: non-drinkers, occasional drinkers, light (1–15 units/week), moderate (16–42) and heavy (> 42 units/week)[11]. A UK unit is 8–10 g alcohol.

Body mass index

At screening weight and height were measured and body mass index (BMI) calculated as weight/height^2 was used as an index of relative weight. 'Obesity' was defined as BMI > = 28 kg/m^2, the upper fifth of the BMI distribution in all men.

Pre-existing disease

The men were asked whether a doctor had ever told them that they had angina or a heart attack, a stroke, diabetes or several other disorders. The WHO chest pain questionnaire for angina or possible myocardial infarction was administered to all men at screening and a three orthogonal lead electrocardiogram (ECG) was recorded at rest. Men with evidence of *CHD (undiagnosed)* were defined as those with no recall of a doctor diagnosis of CHD but who had a WHO (Rose) questionnaire response indicating angina or possible myocardial infarction or ECG evidence of definite or possible myocardial ischaemia or myocardial infarction.

Follow-up

All men were followed up for all cause mortality and for cardiovascular morbidity from the initial screening (Q1) and all deaths have been recorded to December 2000 (21.8 years from screening). Follow-up has been achieved in 99 per cent of the cohort. Analysis was restricted to men with no recall of a doctor diagnosis of CHD or stroke or diabetes ($n = 7171$) in whom there were 1143 major CHD events (502 non-fatal, 641 fatal) and 907 deaths from cardiovascular causes (641 CHD, 133 stroke, 133 other CVD).

Results and discussion

A non-linear relationship was seen between alcohol intake and age-adjusted rates for major CHD events and CVD mortality with the lowest rates in light and moderate drinkers (quadratic trend $P = 0.003$ and $P < 0.0001$ respectively). Table 1 shows the adjusted relative risks using occasional drinkers as the reference group, as non-drinkers are a small heterogenous group unsuitable for this purpose[12]. In this cohort alcohol intake showed a significant positive relationship with body mass index. The age-adjusted mean BMI for the five alcohol categories none, occasional, light, moderate and heavy were 25.4, 25.4, 25.3, 25.7 and 25.8 kg/m^2 ($P < 0.0001$ for trend). Additional adjustment for BMI made minor differences to the relationships (Table 1) and the quadratic trends remained significant ($P = 0.005$ and $P = 0.0002$ respectively).

Table 1. Alcohol intake and adjusted relative risk (RR) of major CHD events and CVD mortality in 7171 men with no recall of CHD, stroke or diabetes over 21.8 years mean follow-up

	N	Cases	Age-adjusted rates	Age-adjusted RR	Age + BMI adjusted RR	Adjusted* RR
CHD events (1143)						
None	400	76	10.1	1.05	1.06 (0.83, 1.37)	1.04 (0.80, 1.34)
Occasional	1707	300	9.6	1.00	1.00	1.00
Light	2363	348	7.6	0.79 (0.67, 0.92)	0.79 (0.68, 0.92)	0.87 (0.74, 1.01)
Moderate	1919	290	8.3	0.87 (0.74, 1.00)	0.85 (0.72, 1.00)	0.81 (0.69, 0.96)
Heavy	782	129	9.6	1.01 (0.82, 1.84)	0.97 (0.79, 1.20)	0.82 (0.67, 1.02)
Linear trend				n.s.	n.s.	$P = 0.006$
CVD mortality (907)						
None	400	65	7.9	1.11 (0.84, 1.46)	1.12 (1.11, 1.14)	1.08 (0.82, 1.43)
Occasional	1707	239	7.3	1.00	1.00	1.00
Light	2363	274	5.7	0.77 (0.65, 0.92)	0.78 (0.65, 0.92)	0.88 (0.74, 1.05)
Moderate	1919	220	6.1	0.84 (0.70, 1.00)	0.83 (0.69, 0.99)	0.79 (0.65, 0.95)
Heavy	782	109	7.9	1.12 (0.89, 1.41)	1.09 (0.87, 1.37)	0.89 (0.71, 1.13)
Linear trend				n.s.	n.s.	$P = 0.01$

*Adjusted for age, social class, smoking, physical activity, regular medication and pre-existing CHD (undiagnosed).
n.s. non-significant.

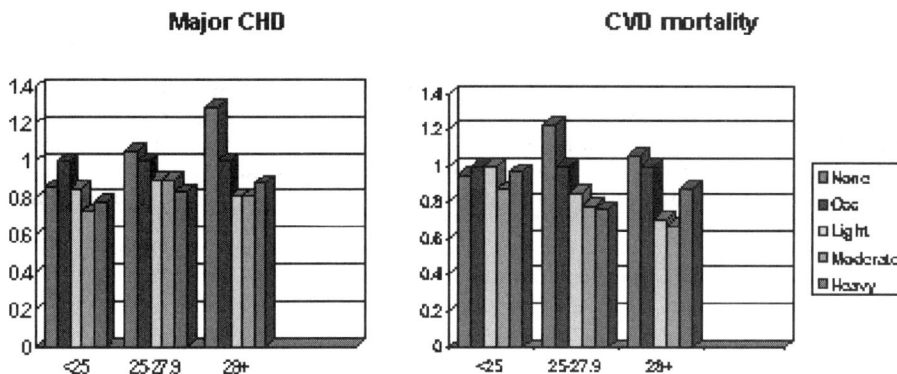

Fig. 1. Alcohol intake and adjusted (+) relative risk of major CHD events and CVD mortality by levels of BMI at baseline.*Adjusted for age, social class, smoking, physical activity, regular medication and pre-existing CHD (undiagnosed).

Further adjustment for other potential confounders, e.g. social class, smoking, physical activity, regular medication and pre-existing CHD (undiagnosed) attenuated the risk in heavy drinkers and all regular drinkers showed lower risk of major CHD events than occasional drinkers (Table 1). For cardiovascular mortality, risk decreased up to levels of moderate drinking beyond which risk started to increase.

Effects of obesity

We also examined the relationship between alcohol and major CHD events and CVD mortality stratified by initial BMI levels (< 25, $25-27.9$ and $28+$ kg/m^2). Major CHD events and CVD mortality rates increased with increasing BMI (age-adjusted rates/1000 person-years 7.2, 8.6 and 12.0 and 5.7, 6.2 and 9.3 respectively).

Obesity and CHD events

The inverse relationship between alcohol and major CHD events was seen within all BMI levels with all regular drinkers showing lower risk than occasional drinkers (Fig. 1). Among obese men non-drinkers showed a markedly increased risk compared to occasional drinkers. This is likely to be due to the particularly high prevalence of ill-health seen in this group of men. Non-drinkers overall tended to have a lower prevalence of diagnosed hypertension and measured systolic blood pressure than moderate and heavy drinkers and a similar prevalence of undiagnosed CHD and breathlessness to moderate and heavy drinkers. However, among the obese men, non-drinkers had by far the highest prevalence of diagnosed hypertension (27 per cent vs. 18–20 per cent in the other groups), the highest prevalence of breathlessness (21 per cent vs. 8–12 per cent in the other groups) and the highest prevalence of undiagnosed CHD (31 per cent vs. 26–28 per cent). It is likely than many of the obese non-drinkers have given up drinking due to obesity-related illnesses which is likely to inflate the risk seen in obese non-drinkers.

Obesity and cardiovascular mortality

For cardiovascular mortality, the lower risk associated with light and moderate drinking was more apparent in the heavier men. Among lean men (BMI < 25 kg/m^2) there was little difference in overall CVD mortality risk between the alcohol groups although moderate drinkers had the lowest risk. Cardiovascular mortality includes stroke mortality and the relationship between moderate alcohol intake and stroke is less consistent than that seen for CHD[13]. In the two heavier groups (>25 kg/m^2) a higher proportion of cardiovascular deaths were attributed to coronary heart disease than in lean men (74 per cent vs. 65 per cent) and this may explain the greater reduction in overall CVD mortality associated with moderate drinking in the heavier men rather than a true modifying effect of obesity. A test for interaction to assess whether the alcohol-CVD mortality relationship differed by BMI levels was not significant.

483

Caveats

We have not taken changes in alcohol intake during follow-up into account in this paper, but examination of changes in alcohol patterns over five years follow-up indicate that the majority of occasional drinkers tend to remain occasional drinkers and the majority of light drinkers tend to remain light drinkers[14]. Previous reports on alcohol and cardiovascular disease from this cohort taking account of changes in alcohol intake, show stable regular drinkers in particular stable light drinkers to have the lowest rates of cardiovascular disease[6,14]. The majority of heavy drinkers however, tend to reduce to light or moderate drinking status and some to non-drinking status during the course of follow-up[6,15]. The long term effect of heavy drinking on CVD risk based on one assessment in time is unlikely to represent the true effect and is likely to attenuate with longer follow-up[15]. This may explain the lack of adverse effect on overall CVD mortality in heavy drinkers using 21 year follow-up.

Conclusion

In this study of middle-aged men free of diagnosed CHD, stroke and diabetes, an inverse relationship was seen between alcohol and major CHD events and to a smaller extent with cardiovascular mortality after adjustment for potential confounders including BMI smoking, social class, physical activity and pre-existing disease. The inverse relationship with major CHD events was seen in both lean and heavier men. For cardiovascular mortality the lower risk associated with light to moderate drinking was more apparent in heavier men where CHD was more likely to be the cause of cardiovascular death. The relationship between alcohol and cardiovascular disease in men does not appear to be confounded by obesity.

References

1. Kannel WB, Ellison RC. Alcohol and coronary heart disease: the evidence for a protective effect. *Clin Chem Acta* 1996; 59–76.

2. Grobbee, EB Rimm, U Keil, Renaud S. Alcohol and the cardiovascular system. In: McDonald I (ed.) *Health issues related to alcohol consumption* (2nd edn), pp.125–180. ILSI Europe, Brussels; 1999.

3. Corrao G, Rubbiati L, Bagnardi V, Zambon A, Poikolainen K. Alcohol and coronary heart disease: a meta-analysis. *Addiction* 2000; 95: 1505–1523.

4. Goldberg DM, Soleas GJ, Levesque M. Moderate alcohol consumption: the gentle face of Janus. *Clin Biochem* 1999; 32: 505–18.

5. Rimm EB, Williams P, Fosher K, Criqui M, Stampfer MJ. A biologic basis for moderate alcohol consumption and lower coronary heart disease risk: a meta-analysis of effects on lipids and hemostatic factors. *BMJ* 1999; 319: 1523–28.

6. Shaper AG, Wannamethee SG. Epidemiological confounders in the relationship between alcohol and cardiovascular disease. In: R Paoletti (ed.). *Moderate alcohol consumption and cardiovascular disease*, pp.105–12. Kluwer Academic Publishers and Fondazione Giovanni Lorenzini; 2000.

7. Suter PM, Hasler E, Vetter W. Effects of alcohol on energy metabolism and body weight regulation: is alcohol a risk factor for obesity? *Nutr Rev* 1997; 55: 157–71.

8. Shaper AG, Wannamethee SG, Walker M. Body weight: implications for the prevention of coronary heart disease, stroke and diabetes mellitus in a cohort study of middle-aged men. *BMJ* 1997; 314: 1311–17.

9. Westerterp KR, Prentice AM, Jequier E. Alcohol and body weight. In: McDonald I (ed.) *Health issues related to alcohol consumption* (2nd edn), pp.103–123. ILSI Europe, Brussels; 1999.

10. Shaper AG, Pocock SJ, Walker M, Cohen NM, Wale CJ, Thomson AG. British Regional Heart Study: cardiovascular risk factors in middle-aged men in 24 towns. *BMJ* 1981; 282: 179–86.

11. Shaper AG, Wannamethee G, Walker M. Alcohol and mortality: explaining the U-shaped curve. *Lancet* 1988; ii: 1268–73.

12. Wannamethee SG, Shaper AG. Men who do not drink: a report from the British Regional Heart Study. *Int J Epidemiol* 1988; 17: 307–16.

13. Mazzaglia G, Britton AR, Altmann DR, Chenet L. Exploring the relationship between alcohol consumption and non-fatal or fatal stroke: a systematic review. *Addiction* 2001; 96: 1743–56.

14. Wannamethee SG, Shaper AG, Walker M. Taking up regular drinking in middle-age: effect on major coronary heart disease events and mortality. *Heart* 2002; 87: 32–6.

15. Wannamethee SG, Shaper AG, Walker M. Patterns of alcohol intake and risk of stroke in middle-aged British men. *Stroke* 1996; 27(6): 1033–9.

Progress in Obesity Research: 9. Edited by *Geraldo Medeiros-Neto, Alfredo Halpern and Claude Bouchard*
©2003 John Libbey Eurotext Ltd, pp. 485–488.

CHAPTER 102

Socioeconomic status and the obesity epidemic

Albert Stunkard and Kelly C. Allison

University of Pennsylvania, Philadelphia, PA 19104-3309, USA
[e-mail: stunkard@mail.med.upenn.edu; kca@mail.med.upenn.edu]

The epidemic of obesity that is sweeping the world has countless ill effects on current health and on health in the future. It has, however, one potential benefit, if we have the wit and energy to pursue it. It could lead us to a better understanding of the relationship between socioeconomic status (SES) and obesity, theoretically, and, ultimately, how to control obesity.

This was the optimistic view with which we began this report. It derives from the nature of our understanding of the relationship between SES and obesity. Since this relationship was first discovered in 1965[1], numerous papers have described its many aspects in all conceivable populations. The relationship that has been studied, however, has been primarily a static, descriptive one, exploring the associations of SES and obesity as they had existed at one point in time. The obesity epidemic should permit us to move from this study of associations at one point in time to the study of associations over time, from prevalence to prediction. Unfortunately, it has not. Accordingly, this report will describe what we know about the relationship of SES to lay a foundation for future studies that may make use of the information that can be gleaned from the epidemic. This task has been facilitated by a number of studies in different parts of the world that have assessed the relationship between SES and obesity, and also by the increase in the prevalence of obesity that has accompanied the epidemic.

A detailed review in 1989 revealed a very strong relationship between SES and obesity among women in all parts of the developed world and a similar, somewhat weaker, relationship between SES and obesity among men[2]. When we turn to the developing societies, the nature of the relationship between SES and obesity is quite different, almost the opposite of that found in the developed world.

We will summarize those findings by employing individual studies as the unit of analysis, counting the number of studies in the 1989 review that reported a particular pattern of SES-obesity relationships. This method controls for other factors that influence the prevalence of obesity, and focuses on the influence of SES. The method has the advantage of including a broad range of samples and the disadvantage of weighting large and small samples equally.

The 1989 review found that, among women in developed societies, 46 studies showed an inverse relationship between SES and obesity, seven studies showed no relationship and only one study showed a positive relationship. Among men in developed societies, the relationship was similar but weaker: 34 studies showed an inverse relationship, 15 showed no relationship and only nine showed a positive relationship. Children in developed societies showed relationships between SES and obesity similar to those of adults, but far weaker.

It should be noted that these relationships existed in developed societies with often affluent populations. Among developing societies, the relationship between SES and obesity, as we have noted, is the opposite of that in developed societies. Thus, in developing societies there was a strong positive relationship between SES and obesity. For both men and women, not a single study found an inverse relationship and 10 studies of women and 12 of men showed a direct relationship. Children in developing societies showed almost the same relationship between SES and obesity as did their parents. The number of studies of developing societies was limited, but the overwhelming strength of the relationship suggests that the results are valid.

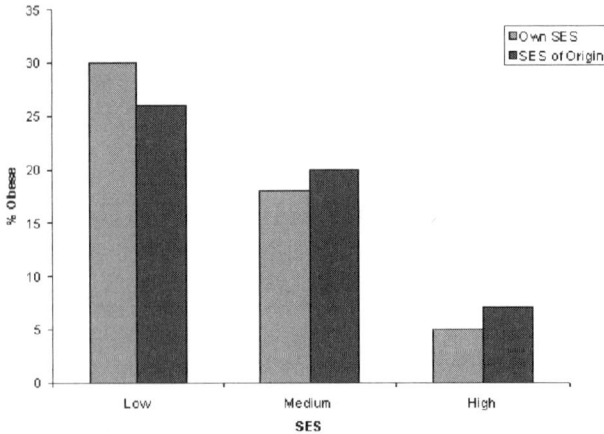

Fig. 1. Among persons in the lower SES, the prevalence of obesity was 30 per cent and it fell with increasing SES to a low of 5 per cent. The bars show the 'SES of origin', or the SES into which the person was born. People who fell in SES were more likely to be obese. People who rose in SES were less likely to be obese[1].

These finding pose the question that has eluded answer for the half century since it was first raised, 'What determines the relationship between SES and obesity?'

Understanding the relationship between SES and obesity, particularly in the developed world, has important theoretical and practical consequences. Among other things, such understanding would facilitate the development of public health measures that might, for example, reproduce the circumstances that make it possible for women of upper SES to control their obesity.

How are we to understand the relationship between SES and obesity? There are at least three possibilities: SES influences obesity, obesity influences SES and a common factor or factors influences both obesity and SES. There is evidence to support each of these possibilities.

A common factor is genetics. Genetics exerts a strong influence on the susceptibility to obesity. It is not as well known, but genetics may also influence SES[3]. Our growing understanding of genetics should help us to understand how its efforts may be reflected in its dual influence on both SES and obesity.

Turning to more established relationships, between SES and obesity and obesity and SES, the simplest explanation is that the relationship is bidirectional: each factor exerts an influence. The strongest support for this view may well be the analyses of the quasi-longitudinal Midtown Manhattan Study of 1660 persons in New York City, the first study to report a relationship between SES and obesity[1]. Figure 1 shows the strong inverse relationship between SES and obesity among women, which decreased from 30 per cent obesity in the lower SES to 5 per cent in the upper SES. The distinctive feature of this study, not since replicated, was information about the 'SES of origin', the SES into which the subjects had been born. This made it possible to assess the direction of causality between SES and obesity. Note that the SES of origin was almost the same as the subjects' own SES, suggesting that the SES into which one was born strongly determined one's own SES and one's obesity status. The few differences between own SES and SES of origin can be viewed as measures of social mobility. Among downwardly mobile women (whose present SES was lower than their SES of origin) the prevalence of obesity was 22 per cent, which was greater than that of women who remained in the SES of their origin (18 per cent) and far greater than that of those who were upwardly mobile (12 per cent).

Two large longitudinal studies in England could also be interpreted as showing that low childhood SES predicted the development of obesity in adult life[4,5]. The strongest evidence of the effect of parental SES on the BMI of their offspring came from the only study that controlled for parental BMI[3]. This adoption study in Denmark showed the familiar inverse relationship between SES and BMI of the adoptees. In addition, this study showed a correlation between the SES of both the adoptive and biological fathers and the BMI of the adoptees.

The evidence that SES influences obesity in no way contradicts the idea that obesity influences SES, and two studies have shown such a strong influence. In 1986, Sonne-Holm and Sorensen[6] showed that, over a period of 12.5 years, only 30 per cent of obese male Danish draftees rose above social class 2 (out of 7 social classes). By contrast, 51 per cent of a random sample of draftees did rise above level 2, a difference that the authors ascribed to the social handicap of obesity. More recently, Gortmaker et al.[7] provided further evidence of the deleterious effects of obesity on social functioning and social status. During a period of 7 years, obese adolescent girls were more likely than nonobese adolescent girls to complete fewer years of school, marry less often, have lower household income and higher levels of

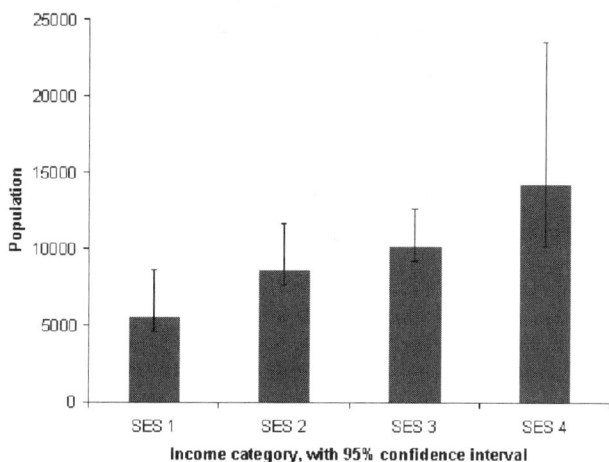

Fig. 2. The population per fast food outlet by measured SES. Note that there are 2.5 times more fast food outlets in the lower SES neighbourhoods than in the upper SES neighbourhoods[12].

household property. This effect of obesity was in striking contrast to the lack of effect on social functioning of a variety of other disabilities, including asthma, that showed no readily visible physical defects.

How does SES have an effect on body weight? The answer lies in gene by environment interactions. In any person genetic vulnerability and environmental challenges interact in such a way as to produce obesity or leanness. This interaction was demonstrated by a commingling analysis of the distribution of the BMI of identical twins. The distribution was compatible with the admixture of at least two component distributions, one for the overweight population and another for the remaining population[8]. The correlation between the BMI of twin pairs in the overweight population was far lower than that in the normal weight component. Greater genetic vulnerability interacted with stronger environmental influences to produce the overweight distribution. This analysis suggests that the obesity epidemic can be seen as an increased size of the overweight distribution, reflecting increasingly powerful environmental influences acting on genetically susceptible population[8,9].

This genetic susceptibility to environmental influences was well demonstrated by Bouchard's classic studies of overfeeding of identical twins[10]. The far higher correlation between twin pairs than the correlation among twin pairs indicated that it was genetic influences *among* twin pairs that determined their different responses to environmental challenge. This study, however, provided only a general description of the environmental influences on weight gain, no more than simply overfeeding by 1000 calories per day.

Environmental influences on body weight was provided by Heitman *et al.*[11] This study showed a differential effect of the fat content of diets upon genetic variation in weight gain. Thus, obese subjects with a familial predisposition to obesity showed a large increase in weight when the fat content of the diet exceeded a rather narrow threshold (3.9 mJ/day) and no increase in weight at a fat content of less than that. Subjects without a familial predisposition did not differ in weight gain with differing amounts of dietary fat.

The studies of Bouchard *et al.*[10] and Heitman *et al.*[11] demonstrate the varying vulnerability to weight gain, and presumably obesity, produced by gross environmental influences, such as feeding excess calories or large amounts of fat. We thus know in general how the environment influences obesity. But the control of obesity on a community-wide, or public health basis, will require greater specification of the environmental influences favouring obesity.

There had been reason to hope that the obesity epidemic might have made it apparent what these influences were. Unfortunately, such has not been the case. Despite this tantalizing opportunity, it has not been seized. We can only hope that this will be a major question to be answered: which institutions or organizations exert this influence in particular areas? Given the strong relationship between SES and obesity a potentially fruitful approach would be to assess the relative importance of these institutions or organizations at different levels of SES.

An imaginative study of just this type has been recently reported from Australia. Fast-food stores provide precisely the kind of highly palatable, high-fat, foods that fuel the epidemic of obesity. Reidpath *et al.*[12] examined the density of fast food stores in the community as a function of SES and found a striking relationship: a dose-response between SES and the density of fast-food outlets. People living in areas with the lowest SES had 2.5 times more exposure to these outlets than did people in the wealthiest SES areas. Thus, there was one fast-food store for every 5,600 persons in the lower SES areas compared to 1 store per 14,200 persons in the wealthiest SES areas.

This revealing study provides unequivocal support for the relationship between SES and the density of fast-food stores in the community. It may be that low SES encourages the introduction of fast food stores. But whatever led to their introduction, fast food stores contribute to the obesity epidemic and become clear targets in the effort to control obesity. Just what public health measures and government policies might reduce the frequency of fast food stores is not clear. This study makes clear the value of increasingly precise quantification of the influence of different institutions on the prevalence of obesity.

Fast-food stores are only one of the many influences fueling the obesity epidemic. The precision with which it was possible to relate their prevalence to areas defined by SES suggests that this type of study could provide useful information about these influences. Such a study in the magazine, *Men's Fitness* recently received considerable attention in the lay press when it proclaimed Philadelphia, the 'fattest city in America'[13]. Problems in the analysis of the study's data called into question its findings. But its methodology can serve as a model for future research. Its enumeration of obesity-promoting institutions in American cities provides a valuable inventory of critical environmental influences.

A first step in this future research could be to establish the frequency of obesity-promoting influences in areas defined, initially by SES level. Later analyses could move the dependent variable from SES to the geographical distribution of obesity, overweight and BMI. Mathematical models might relate obesity-promoting institutions to the prevalence of obesity in their geographical areas. In the process they might estimate which institutions provide the greatest contribution to the development of obesity and, ultimately, the costs and benefits of modifying these institutions.

It seems fit to end this talk by listing the attempts to modify the obesity-promoting institutions that afflict the lower SES. We can start with this inventory of institutions suggested by the *Men's Fitness* study: number of junk food stores, commuting time, alcohol consumption and number of bars, smoking prevalence, number of gymnasiums, number of sporting goods stores, per cent of population who exercise, fitness friendly climate, number of TV sets per capita, and access to healthcare.

References

1. Goldblatt PB, Moore ME, Stunkard AJ. Social factors in obesity. *JAMA* 1965; 152: 1039–42.

2. Sobal J, Stunkard AJ. Socioeconomic status and obesity: A review of the literature. *Psychol Bull.* 1989; 105: 260–75.

3. Teasdale TW, Sorensen TIA, Stunkard AJ. Genetic and early environmental components in sociodemographic influences on adult body fatness. *BMJ* 1990; 300: 1615–18.

4. Braddon FE, Rodgers SB, Wadsworth MD, Davies JM. Onset of obesity in a 36 year birth cohort study. *BMJ* 1986; 293: 299–303.

5. Power C, Moynihan C. Social class and changes in weight: height between childhood and early adulthood. *Int J Obes* 1988; 12: 445–53.

6. Sonne-Holm S, Sorensen TIA. Prospective study of attainment of social class of severely obese subjects in relation to parental social class, intelligence, and education. *BMJ* 1986; 292, 586–89.

7. Gortmaker SL, Must A, Perrin JM, Sobal AM, Dietz WH. Social and economic consequences of overweight in adolescence and young adulthood. *N Engl J Med* 1993; 329, 1008–12.

8. Price RA, Stunkard AJ. Commingling analysis of obesity in twins. *Human Hered* 1989; 30, 121–35.

9. Price RA, Ness R, Sorensen TIA. Changes in commingled body mass index distributions associated with secular trends in overweight among Danish young men. *Am J Epidem* 1991; 133, 501–10.

10. Bouchard C, Tremblay A, Despres JP, Nadeau A, Lupien PJ, Theriault G *et al.* The response to long-term overfeeding in identical twins. *N Engl J Med* 1990; 332, 1477–82.

11. Heitman BL, Lissner L, Sorensen TIA, Bengtsson C. Dietary fat intake and weight gain in women genetically predisposed for obesity. *Am J Clin Nutr* 1995; 61: 1213–17.

12. Reidpath DD, Burns C, Garrard J, Mahoney M, Townsend M. An ecological study of the relationship and environmental determinants of obesity. *Health & Place* 2002; 8,141–45.

13. Griffiths K. The fattest five. *Men's Fitness* 1999; 76–83.

Progress in Obesity Research: 9. Edited by *Geraldo Medeiros-Neto, Alfredo Halpern and Claude Bouchard*
©2003 John Libbey Eurotext Ltd, pp. 489–492.

CHAPTER 103

Behaviour and obesity: cause or consequence

David A. Levitsky

Division of Nutritional Sciences, Department of Psychology, Cornell University, Ithaca, NY 14853-6301, USA
[e-mail: dal4@cornell.edu]

Like the chicken and the egg, we have been considering the question of whether the behaviour of overeating causes obesity or does the biological state of obesity cause overeating? For the first half of this century, and earlier, obesity has been thought to be the consequence of overindulgent behaviour. Body weight was viewed as the algebraic summation of the energy consumed and energy expenditure. Because very few scientists believed that differences in energy expenditure contributed much to obesity, most researchers believed that obesity was caused simply by the behaviour of overeating.

This view radically shifted in the early 1960's due primarily to a couple of simple experiments and some profound thinking by Gordon Kennedy. He proposed that body weight (fat) was not a simple passive depot for differences in energy balance, but rather was part of a physiological process that actively regulated adipose tissue. The behaviour of eating was absolved as being the major cause of human obesity and was assigned to play a major role in correcting energetic errors to maintain the 'Set-Point' for fat stores at a constant value. As a result of this change in role for the behaviour of eating, the search for the major determinants that control body weight shifted from the exploration of the external stimuli that controlled the behaviour of eating to the search for the internal signals that transmitted information about state of the adipose tissue to the brain mechanisms that controlled eating behaviour. This approach to the study of behaviour and obesity received a major boost when leptin was suggested as the signal that transmitted information from adipose tissue to the brain[1].

Testing the hypothesis in humans: response to overfeeding and underfeeding

Although the Set-Point Theory has never been formally tested in humans as a viable theory of the regulation of body weight, I have been very interested in examining one of the critical components of the Set-Point Theory – the role of the control of food intake in the regulation of body weight. In animals, the classic demonstrations of the current view that the behaviour of eating is an integral part of the regulation of body weight is the overfeeding study. If rats are forced to gain weight, either by gastric intubation, repeated insulin injections, or feeding a high fat diet, then allowed to eat *ad libitum*, food intake is suppressed. Consequently, the animals loose the excess body weight and return to their pre-overfeeding weight. It was initially believed that the post-overfeeding anorexia was the only mechanism responsible for the recovery of body weight, but Almeida *et al.*[2] demonstrated that the reduction in food intake could account for only about half of the loss in body weight and that an increase in energy expenditure must occur that can explain the rest of the recovery of weight. Because almost no one had examined the recovery from overfeeding in humans and it appeared to be a classic test of the Set-Point Theory, Eva Obarzanek and I decided to explore it (Levitsky *et al.*, submitted). We examined a group of subjects in our 'Laboratory Restaurant' for two weeks during which time subjects consumed as much or as little food as they desired. However, during the study all their food they ate had to be dispensed through the Laboratory Restaurant because all food was carefully weighed before and after consumption. The subjects could take out snacks from the unit but they were pre-weighed and they had to return the container of uneaten food so that we could calculate the amount eaten. For the next 13 days, we had the subjects consume 130 per cent of the food they ate during the two week baseline. Following the period of overeating, the subjects returned to the free feeding situation and we again measured everything they ate.

As expected, all subjects gained weight during the period of overeating and then lost weight during the recovery. However, what was quite surprising was that the subjects lost the weight *without* reducing their food intake. In fact, daily food intake on the very first day of recovery returned precisely to baseline values, despite the fact that the subjects complained bitterly they couldn't eat another thing after completing the 13th day of overeating. Mean daily intake did not drop significantly below baseline line values at any time during the three weeks of recovery. Clearly, the role of the control of food intake was not as closely linked to the weight gain as the Set-Point Theory would suggest.The other classic demonstration that the control of food intake appears to be responsible for the regulation of body weight is the underfeeding study whereby following the restriction of food animals increase their daily food intake. Because of the unexpected results we obtained with overfeeding in humans, Lisa Jiaz and I investigated the degree to which humans responded to food deprivation with a precise increase in eating behaviour.

The study was conducted in the same Laboratory Restaurant as the overeeding study, but was done over a period of three, five-day weeks. During the first week, the subjects ate as much or as little as they wanted. As before they were served three meals and given the opportunity to take out snacks and all food intake was measured. On Monday of the second week, half of the subjects received the same food as was served the prior week but it was reduced to approximately 1200 kcal. The other half of the subjects received no food on Monday. From Tuesday until Friday, the subjects could again eat as much as they wanted. For the last week the conditions for the two groups were reversed.

To our surprise, daily food intake on Tuesday was not affected by either energy restriction or the total fast. Similarly, restricting food intake on Monday had no effect on the daily intake on any other day of the week. Thus, the eating behaviour of humans does not appear to be responsive to energy surfeits or energy deficit as would be predicted from the Set-Point Theory of the regulation of body weight.

Testing the hypothesis in humans: caloric compensation for changes in energy density

According to the Set-Point Theory of the regulation of body weight reducing the consumption of high fat is futile technique for losing body weight. Theoretically, a reduction in fat content of the diet should cause a reduction in adipose stores leading to an increase in food intake and a minimal loss in body weight. Anne Kendall-Casella and I[3] tested this prediction in a study in which we examined the effects of reducing the fat content of foods from a normal fat diet (34 per cent of calories as fat) to a lower fat version (25 per cent of calories as fat). As before, subjects ate only foods offered though the Laboratory Restaurant and all food that subjects ate was measured. The study lasted 22 weeks using a cross-over design so that every subject ate each diet for 11 weeks.

The results were very clear. Reducing the fat content of foods had no change in the volume of food consumed. Reducing the fat content of the foods from 34 per cent to 25 per cent resulted in an energy deficit of about 240 kcal per day which persisted for the 11 weeks of treatment. There was no indication that subjects would increase their intake of the lower fat foods to the that of the higher fat foods.

It has been argued that children, unlike adults, regulate energy intake more effectively than adults[4]. Thus, it is possible that adults do not demonstrate accurate caloric compensation for changes in their diet, but children do. To examine this question Gordana Mrdjenovic and I investigated the eating behaviour of children ages 5 to 11 who attended a summer camp at Cornell (in press). The intake of these children was measured daily for up to six weeks. The total variance of the intake for each meal was analysed for the effect of dietary composition at that meal and the composition of the foods served at the previous meal. The data showed that the amount of food a child consumed at a meal was inversely related to the energy density of the food suggesting that children do compensate for the energy content of the foods. However, we also observed that the amount of food served to the children was inversely related to the energy density of the diet. Indeed, of all the variables studied, the amount food served by the caregivers was by far the best predictor of how much food the child consumed. Moreover, when the amount of food served was used as a covariant, the energy consumed by the children at a meal was an increasing function of the energy density of the diet, similar to adults. Thus, in both adults and children, we have found no evidence that the control food intake responds to changes in the energy density of the diet in a way to maintain a constant energy intake. It appears that the greater the energy density of the diet, the greater the energy consumed. The outcome of such behaviour would be to produce a change in body weight that is directly related to the energy density of the diet. Body weight (fat stores) would then follow the change in the behaviour of eating, not the other way around as would be predicted from Set-Point Theory.

Amount Consumed (g)

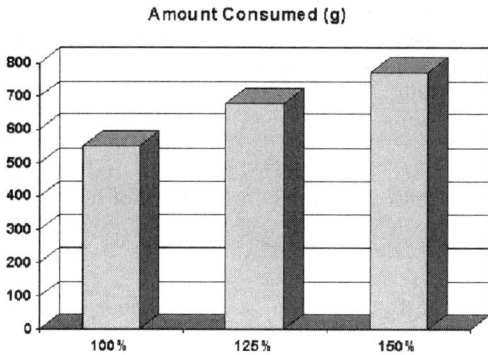

Fig. 1.

Testing the hypothesis in humans: changing portion size and skipping meals

The study of the eating behaviour of children demonstrated to us the powerful effect of serving size on food consumption and prompted us to look more closely at this effect. Trisha Yun and I examined the effect of experimentally altering the amount of food subjects are served on their plates on the amount of food they actually eat. Subjects were first brought into our Laboratory Restaurant and offered a buffet lunch in which they could determine their own portion size. The next week, the subjects returned for lunch, but this time the lunch was served to them. The subjects were divided into three groups. One group received 100 per cent of the amount they ate at the previous lunch, a second group was served 125 per cent, and a third group was served 150 per cent of the previous lunch. The subjects returned for lunch two more times where each subject received each of the three conditions in a counterbalanced order. The results are shown in Fig 1. The greater the amount of food the subjects were served, the more they ate. In fact, the amount of food they ate correlated very highly with the amount they were served ($r^2 = 0.99$).

If humans do not appear to respond to portion sizes with appropriate changes in their food intake, are they sensitive to the energetic effect of skipping meals? Amy Lanou and I examined the effect of skipping snacks on the amount of food humans consumed at meals. Subjects who routinely eat snacks and an equal number of subjects who don't eat snacks were recruited into a study of twenty-four hour food intake. For the first test, all subjects ate freely in the Laboratory Restaurant, taking whatever snacks they wished for twenty-four hours. The next week half the subjects were give a 250 kcal snack and asked to eat it between breakfast and lunch or between lunch and dinner. The other half of the subjects were told not to eat anything between meals. The conditions were reversed for the two groups on the following week. Eating a midmorning or midafternoon snack had absolutely no effect on the amount of food the subjects consumed at lunch or dinner. It appears that the more opportunities for the subjects to eat, the more they ate.

Sara Feldman and I performed a similar study to the snack study, but varied breakfast instead of snacks. We examined the effect in people who usually eat breakfast and those who don't. In one condition, everyone had to eat breakfast and in the other, no one ate breakfast. The amount of food consumed at lunch and dinner was measured. Skipping breakfast (620 kcal) increased the amount the subjects ate at lunch. However, the increase in lunch amounted to only 130 kcal over the amount the subject ate after eating breakfast. No effect of eating breakfast could be found at the midafternoon snack, dinner, or evening snack. The overall net energy effect was that skipping the breakfast meal resulted in nearly a 500 kcal reduction in energy.

Recently, Craig Halbmeier and I examined veracity of the weight gain popularly known as the Freshman 15 by weighing Freshman during their first week at Cornell and then again during the last week at Cornell. In addition, we asked them to answer a series of questions intended to examine what behaviours might have correlated with any change in weight. We observed the Freshman to gain 1.9 kg in their first 12 weeks at Cornell. Approximately, 25 per cent of the variance in the weight gain can be attributed to consuming 'junk food'. In addition eating multiple meals on weekends, evening snacks, lunch and dinner in dining halls, accounted for another 32 per cent of the variance. Clearly having increasing occasions to eat, correlates very highly with increased energy intake.

Conclusion to the chicken or the egg

The data presented above demonstrate quite convincingly that human eating behaviour does not appear to act to maintain body weight constant as suggested by the Set-Point Theory, but rather seems to determine body weight as suggested by the early researchers in this area. Indeed, human eating behaviour appears to be quite responsive to environmental stimuli such as the occasion to eat and portion size and not sensitive to changes in energy balance caused by over- and underfeeding.

If this conclusion is correct, then the most effective way to prevent or reverse the alarming increase in rates of overweight and obesity is to alter those stimuli that control eating behaviour. Such a task will not be easy because producing the changes necessary to alter human eating means confronting large segments of our population that have a vested interest in having humans eat as much as possible. Nevertheless, let me suggest various ways that we can make changes in our society that would reduce human food intake and offset the rise in overweight and obesity.

1. Subsidize low-fat foods

Despite the rhetoric from the many low-carbohydrate diet books, almost every laboratory study that has examined the effect of reducing fat intake has found that a reduction in the fat content of foods leads to an overall reduction in energy intake[5].

2. Limit the size of portions served in restaurants

One of the most consistent trends in the food industry is the increase in the number of meals, Americans eat outside the home. In addition, the sizes of portions served in restaurants and supermarkets has grown in the past 50 years. This is particularly true in fast food restaurants[6]. It is not unreasonable to limit the amount of food served at each meal to a value commensurate with body size. The difference between this reduced amount and what is now being served could still be given to the customer, but wrapped in 'doggie bags' to be used as another meal.

3. Remove vending machines

Although vending machines are a big business today, they provide the additional opportunities for people to snack. Their availability should be restricted.

4. Provide microwaves at work

Tax deductions could be used to increase the number of microwaves available at work. This would decrease the amount of food served at restaurants, but would also provide people an opportunity to bring the 'left-overs' from home. Foods prepared at home tend to be lower in fat and smaller in size than those purchased in restaurants[7].

5. Make the cost of health insurance contingent upon physical fitness

There is an increasing amount of data demonstrating that body weight per se may not be the critical variable in determining morbidity and mortality[8-11]. Rather the real culprit is a low level of physical activity and fitness. Physical fitness is a parameter that can be assessed and linking it to personal health insurance payments may be an effective means of motivating people to improve and maintain physical fitness.

References

1. Zhang Y, Proenca R, Maffei M, Barone M, Leopold L, Friedman JM. Positional cloning of the mouse obese gene and its human homologue. *Nature* 1994; 372: 425–32.

2. Almeida NG, Levitsky DA, Strupp B. Enhanced thermogenesis during recovery from diet-induced weight gain in the rat. *Am J Physiol* 1996; 271: R1380–7.

3. Kendall A, Levitsky DA, Strupp BJ, Lissner L. Weight loss on a low-fat diet: consequence of the imprecision of the control of food intake in humans. *Am J Clin Nutr* 1991; 53: 1124–29.

4. Birch LL, Deysher M. Caloric compensation and sensory specific satiety: evidence for self regulation of food intake by young children. *Appetite* 1986; 7: 323–31.

5. Levitsky DA. Macronutrient Intake and the Control of Body Weight. In: Coulston AM, Rock C, Monsen E (eds) *Nutrition and the prevention and treatment of disease*, pp. 499–516. San Diego: Academic Press; 2001.

6. Jeffery RW, French SA. Epidemic obesity in the United States: are fast foods and television viewing contributing? *Am J Public Health* 1998; 88: 277–80.

7. Young LR, Nestle M. The contribution of expanding portion sizes to the US obesity epidemic. *Am J Public Health* 2002; 92: 246–9.

8. Blair SN, Horton E, Leon AS, Lee IM, Drinkwater BL, Dishman RK *et al.* Physical activity, nutrition, and chronic disease. *Med Sci Sports Exerc* 1996; 28: 335–49.

9. Blair SN, Brodney S. Effects of physical inactivity and obesity on morbidity and mortality: current evidence and research issues. *Med Sci Sports Exerc* 1999; 31: S646–62.

10. Wei M, Kampert JB, Barlow CE, Nichaman MZ, Gibbons LW, Paffenbarger RS Jr, *et al.* Relationship between low cardiorespiratory fitness and mortality in normal-weight, overweight, and obese men. *JAMA* 1999; 282: 1547–53.

11. Lee CD, Blair SN, Jackson AS. Cardiorespiratory fitness, body composition, and all-cause and cardiovascular disease mortality in men. *Am J Clin Nutr* 1999; 69: 373–80.

Progress in Obesity Research: 9. Edited by *Geraldo Medeiros-Neto, Alfredo Halpern* and *Claude Bouchard*
©2003 John Libbey Eurotext Ltd, pp. 493–495.

CHAPTER 104

The society's view on obesity and the quality of life among the obese

Sirpa Sarlio-Lähteenkorva

Department of Public Health, P.O. Box 41, FIN-00014, University of Helsinki, Finland
[e-mail: sirpa.sarlio-lahteenkorva@helsinki.fi]

Ideal body size is culturally determined

Our ideas of 'ideal' body size are connected to cultural norms of beauty, normality and acceptable behaviour. Slim body is the most preferred body type in contemporary affluent societies, but this may not be true in all population groups and in other cultures. Access to food supplies, prevalence of obesity-related health problems, religious aspects and moral issues all have had an impact on attitudes toward obesity in different societies[1,2].

In their review on cross-cultural variation on ideal body type Brown and Konner (1987) show that in preindustrial societies overweight has been connected to various positive attributes such as prosperity, spiritual power, sexuality, maternity and nurturance. Ethnographic data on cross-cultural standards of female beauty show that plumpness, especially large or fat hips and legs, are (or have been) preferred by most societies where data on ideal standards are available. In Nigeria and some other parts of West Africa elite girls had even lived in special 'fattening huts' before marriage. Among Tarahumara's of North Mexico fat thighs are considered as the first requirement of beauty, a good-looking woman is called a 'beautiful thigh'[3].

In man obesity has been linked to positive attributes as well, including strength, prestige and spiritual power. The Bemba of South Africa believe that fatness demonstrates spiritual power in fending off the sorcery attacks. The corpulence of the seated Buddha symbolizes his divinity and otherworldliness. Japanese Sumo wrestlers have always intentionally builded large, fat bodies. Similar patterns of fattening young males wrestlers are found in Polynesia[3].

In these developing and preindustrial societies, however, obesity has usually been rare, and a direct relationship exists between socioeconomic status and obesity. It seems that when it is difficult to get access to food in sufficient quantities to become overweight, excess body weight is typically associated with high social status.

In modern societies people are constantly surrounded by food and most people have economic resources to eat as much as they like, so becoming obese is possible for the most. This affects prevalence of obesity, it's distribution in the population as well as ideas of ideal body shape. In modern societies, slenderness or even thinness has become a kind of status symbol, a marker of health, wealth and prosperity. Body can be seen as a kind of project or target, something that can be molded, shaped and reduced at will[4,5].

The pressures for thinness seem to be strongest in the most privileged groups of society, especially among females. Consequently, there is a strong inverse relationship between socioeconomic status and obesity among women in USA and most Western European societies. The data for men and children shows similar trends but, however, is inconsistent[6].

Discrimination and prejudice against obesity in modern societies

Pervasive stigmatization of obesity in modern societies has been documented in several studies. The degree of obesity is often directly related to the problems encountered in social and employment settings[7].

The background for prejudice and discrimination against obesity has been given many explanations. Religious and moral explanations emphasize that an early precedent for negative attitudes against obese was set when early Christian church included gluttony as one of the seven deadly sins. Originally emphasis was just in the overconsumption of food and drink, gluttony meant consuming more than needed and leaving others hungry. However, attitudes began to change in last century when gluttony was connected with fatness. At this period, criminologists experimented in using weight to index character. Later on, life insurance companies began to use weight to index mortality. Obesity was then increasingly seen as a visual evidence of gluttony, health problems or moral failure and judged unattractive[1].

Depreciating attitudes toward obesity continued to be a cultural norm and they can be reinforced by the currently popular assumptions that obesity is willfully incurred through 'bad' character, lack of willpower, laziness and emotional problems. Obese people are held responsible for their fatness[8]. Negative attitudes toward obesity may be learned very young. Even pre-school children aged below 6 years describe obese children with negative attributes[9]. Obese adolescent girls report more adverse social, educational and psychological correlates[10]. Clear and consistent stimatization, and in some cases discrimination, can be documented in three important areas of living: employment, health care, and education[7]. Obesity can thus be a major social liability.

Quality of life in obesity

Since obesity increases the risk of disability, morbidity and mortality[11], and is a largely unwanted condition is affluent societies, it can be expected that the quality of life is impaired among the obese. The concept 'Quality of life' is, however, difficult to define and operationalize. It is multidimensional, relative and theoretically it incorporates all aspects of life from macro societal and socio-demographic influences (e.g. income, educational attainment) to micro concerns such as individual's experiences and perception[12]. This poses inevitable challenges for measurement.

In research on health and health care, however, the focus usually has been on the impact of medical condition on functional health status and well-being, as perceived and reported by the patient. This so called health-related quality of life, HRQL, has been measured using either generic instruments or disease-specific instruments. Most common generic instrument is probably Medical Outcomes Study Short-Form Health Survey, SF-36 that measures HRQL among eight domains: physical functioning, role limitations owing to physical problems, body pain, general health perception, vitality, social functioning, mental health, and role limitations as a result of emotional problems[13]. Existing studies on obesity have mostly used generic measures, especially SF-36, although often combined with various study specific measures. There are also obesity-specific instruments such as impact of weight on quality of life questionnaire (IWQOL, IWQOL-lite), obesity-related well-being scale (ORWELL), obesity-related psychosocial problems (OP), obesity specific quality of life (OSQOL), etc. but the data on these specific measures is still quite limited[14].

Existing studies tend to demonstrate that obese persons experience significant impairments in their quality of life, with greater impairments associated with greater degrees of obesity. Moreover, obesity associated decrements on health-related quality of life tend to be most pronounced on physical domains of functioning such as general health, physical functioning, vitality, and bodily pain. Impairment in mental health, psychosocial domains or emotional well-being including life satisfaction is frequently reported, yet less pronounced than physical impairments. Several review articles on quality of life in obesity, especially HRQL has been published during past decade[13–16].

Relatively little is known about other domains of life. Moreover, although negative attitudes towards obesity[7] and inverse association between socioeconomic status and BMI in affluent societies[6] is well-known, macro societal and socio-demographic aspects of quality of life in obesity have received little attention. Even causal relationships between socioeconomic problems and obesity are still inadequately understood[17].

Prevalence of obesity is increasing worldwide and without effective prevention and management the medical complications of obesity threaten to overwhelm health services in the near future[11]. In order to tackle this problem and improve quality of life among the obese, we need to gain better understanding of the environmental and social determinants of weight gain. Above all, we need to learn more of the complex processes that hinder weight maintenance and impair quality of life among lower socioeconomic groups where obesity is most prevalent.

Weight loss and quality of life

Weight loss has been shown to improve quality of life in obese persons undergoing a variety of treatments[14,15]. However, significant and sustainable improvement in the health-related quality of life has been reported mostly among surgically treated morbidly obese patients with major weight loss. Although data on conventional treatment methods among milder forms of obesity suggest that even modest weight loss yields significant improvements, it is unknown whether these beneficial effects are sustained in the intermediate and long-term[13]. Indeed, since most weight loss results erode with time[11], studies reporting dramatic improvement in various areas of life after weight loss are perplexing.

If life really gets better after weight loss, why do most obese people fail to maintain their weight loss? It is possible that majority of obese people don't experience adequate and sustainable improvements in their quality of life to compensate for sacrifices they need to make in order to maintain their weight loss. Functional status or perceived health may improve but whether this leads to improvements in other domains of life remains an open question. Moreover, even positive changes such as greater acceptance in social relationships or promotions after weight loss may be problematic experiences since they tend to reveal hidden negative attitudes and discriminatory practices, often previously undiscovered by the individuals[18]. Indeed, one of the future challenges in obesity research is to develop methods that better capture complex processes that affect quality of life in weight changes.

References

1. Schwartz H. *Never satisfied. A cultural history of diets, fantasies and fat*. New York: The Free Press. Macmillan Inc; 1986.

2. de Darine I, Pollock NJ. *Social aspects of obesity*. Gordon and Breach Publishers; 1995.

3. Brown PJ, Konner M. Anthropological perspective on obesity. In: Wurtman RJ, Wurtman JJ (eds), *Human obesity*, pp. 29–46. New York; 1987.

4. Bordo S. *Unbearable weight. Feminism, Western culture and the body*. Berkley and Los Angeles: University of California Press; 1993.

5. Lupton D. *Food, the body and the self*. London: Sage publications; 1996.

6. Sobal J, Stunkard AJ. Socioeconomic status and obesity: a review of the literature. *Psychol Bull* 1989; 105, 260–75.

7. Puhl R, Brownell KD. Bias, discrimination, and obesity. *Obes Res* 2001; 9: 788–805.

8. Crocker J, Cornwell B, Major B. The stigma of overweight: affective consequences of attributional ambiguity. *J Pers Soc Psychol* 1993; 64: 60–70.

9. Turnbull JD, Heaslip S, McLeod HA. Pre-school children's attitudes to fat and normal male and female stimulus figures. *Int J Obes* 2000; 24: 1705–06.

10. Falkner NH, Neumark-Sztainer D, Story M, Jeffery RW, Beuhring T, Resnick MD. Social, educational, and psychological correlates of weight status in adolescents. *Obes Res* 2001; 9: 32–42.

11. WHO. Obesity: preventing and managing the global epidemic. Report of a WHO consultation on obesity. 3–5 June 1997; Geneva. World Health Organisation, 1998.

12. Bowling A. *Measuring health. A review of quality of life measurement scales*. Buckingham, UK: Open University Press; 1991.

13. Fontaine KR, Barofsky I. Obesity and health-realted quality of life. *Obes Rev* 2001; 2?173–82.

14. Kolotkin RL, Meter K, Williams GR. Quality of life in obesity. *Obes Rev* 2001; 2?219–29.

15. Kushner RF, Foster GD. Obesity and quality of life. *Nutrition* 2000; 16: 947–52.

16. Sarlio-Lähteenkorva S, Stunkard A, Rissanen A. Psychosocial factors and quality of life in obesity. *Int J Obes* 1995; 19 Suppl 6: S1–S5.

17. Stunkard AJ, Sörensen TIA. Obesity and socioeconomic status – a complex relation. *N Eng J Med* 1993; 329: 1036–37.

18. Sarlio-Lähteenkorva S. Weight loss and quality of life among obese people. *Social Indicators Res* 2001; 54: 329–54.

CHAPTER 105

Is there evidence for pregnancy as a cause for obesity?

Yvonne Linné

Obesity unit, Department of Medicine, M73 Huddinge University Hospital, Stockholm, Sweden
[e-mail: yvonne.linne@medhs.ki.se]

Introduction

Obesity among women is increasing rapidly all over the world[1,2], and more women in fertile age become overweight and obese. Weight development during adult life is characterized by a gradual increase in weight[1]. Body weight at one age is strongly correlated with body weight decades later, which suggests genetic influence on body weight[3]. However, the genotypical body weight development is depending upon environmental influences such as lifestyle[4,5], and various life events, e.g. illness[6], long-term medication[7] and pregnancy[8] can alter the genetically programmed weight gain trajectory.

Weight gain during pregnancy

Weight gain during pregnancy which is due to the foetus, placenta and expanded blood-volume has been calculated to be around 9.1 kg[9] the rest is an energy reserve for the mother to have to nourish her child.

The recommendations for weight gain during pregnancy have changed over time. In the 1950's the recommendation for weight gain during pregnancy was 7–8 kg to prevent makrosomia[10] and complicated deliveries. But when caesarean section become more common and alleviated the problem of weight, the recommendation become more liberal.

In the USA the Institute of medicine (IOM) has made recommendations according to pre-pregnancy weight and the recommendations are wide, spanning from 6.8 kg for overweight women to an upper limit of 18.0 kg for underweight women (Table 1).

Table 1. The recommended weight gain for women based on pre-pregnancy BMI according to the Institute of Medicine, USA[11]

Pre-pregnancy BMI	Recommended weight gain
Low pre-pregnancy weight (BMI under 19.8 kg/m^2)	12.5–18.0 kg
Normal pre-pregnancy weight (BMI 19.8–26.0 kg/m^2)	11.5–16.0 kg
High pre-pregnancy weight (BMI 26.0–29.0 kg/m^2)	7.0–11.5 kg
Very high pre-pregnancy weight (BMI over 29.0 kg/m^2)	6.8* kg

*Recommended minimum weight gain.

The IOM has also estimated that the cost of pregnancy is 1 kg/pregnancy but has also stated that more research needs to be done[11].

Weight retention after pregnancy

Overweight women world wide have reported that their weight problems started after pregnancy[8,12,13] and in a study at our unit 73 per cent of the female patients reported that their weight problems started

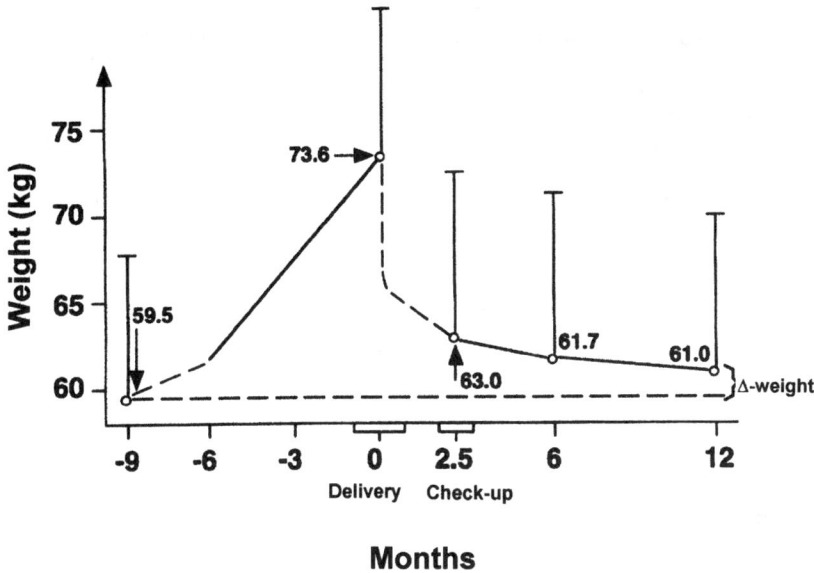

Months

Fig. 1. Weight development of 1423 Swedish women during pregnancy and up to 1 year after pregnancy.

with a pregnancy and that they gained more than 10 kg after their pregnancy. Demographic studies, however, have shown that women who have children weigh more than women without children and that weight increases with increasing parity[14–17].

Most studies report mean weight gains of 0.4–3.8 kg as a result of a pregnancy[17–20] with a range of women from 87 to 113,606 women. Figure 1 shows the weight development of 1423 Swedish women during pregnancy and up to 1 year after pregnancy. These studies have identified several factors that could be involved in the weight development after pregnancy. The strongest factor for retaining weight after pregnancy seems to be the weight gain during pregnancy[20–24]. High weight gain during pregnancy leads to high weight retention after pregnancy in a short time perspective. Smoking cessation, which fortunately often occurs when women learn of their pregnancy, will also make women retain more weight[25]. Changes in activity towards a more sedentary life style after pregnancy is also a risk factor[21,26,27] and socio-economic factors like low income are also associated with higher weight retention after pregnancy[21,28–30]. Some factors have been discussed as a way of controlling weight retention, such as breastfeeding[15,19,25,30]. However, there is no clear evidence that breastfeeding makes women lose more weight after pregnancy. But although the mean increase in weight after pregnancy is not that big, the wide range indicates substantial weight gain in a subset of women. Kappel *et al.* found in data from 2845 women that 25 per cent of white women and 40 per cent of the black women had gained more than 9 pounds at 8–10 weeks after delivery. Öhlin *et al.* found in 1432 women that before pregnancy 13 per cent where overweight and that number had increased to 21 per cent at one year[31].

So, for the average woman pregnancy does not cause obesity, but for a subgroup of women pregnancy is a risk factor of obesity. However, it has been hard with today's methods to identify witch women who is going to be obese.

But does pregnancy cause obesity in the long-term perspective?

The SPAWN (Stockholm Pregnancy And Women's Nutrition) study is a long-term follow-up study of women who delivered children in 1984–85 in Stockholm. The women where followed up to one year after pregnancy. Anthropometric measurements and questionnaire data were collected at 2.5, 6 and 12 months after delivery. The 1423 women who completed the whole study and filled out all questionnaires were asked to return 15 years later for a follow-up study. 563 women participated in the follow-up study SPAWN. To examine whether pregnancy had any impact on weight gain in these women, the sample was divided into two main groups, those who were normal weight before pregnancy and remained normal weight, and those who were normal weight before pregnancy and became overweight at 15 years of follow-up.

Women who become overweight had a higher pre-pregnant BMI (22.3 ± 1.5 kg/m^2 vs. 20.5 ± 1.6 kg/m^2, $P < 0.001$) but both groups were in the normal range of BMI (20–25). They gained more weight during pregnancy (16.3 ± 4.3 kg vs. 13.6 ± 3.7 kg, $P < 0.001$) and had retained more at 1 year of follow-up (normal weight 0.8 kg and overweight 3.1 kg). The women who became overweight also gained more from 1 year of follow-up until 15 years of follow-up (11.1 ± 6.5 kg vs. 4.5 ± 6.5 kg, $P < 0.001$). They had a higher BMI at 15 years of follow-up (27.5 ± 2.6 kg/m^2 vs. 22.5 ± 2.3 5 kg/m^2, $P < 0.001$). Age, number of children and other socio-economic factors did not differ between these two groups[32].

These data show that women who during 15 years increase from normal weight to overweight gain more weight during pregnancy, but they also gained more weight between one and 15 years of follow-up. Some of the weight gain, but not all, can be explained by their pregnancy.

Limitations on studies on pregnancy and weight gain

There are some limitations of studies of weight development after pregnancy.

1. Usually they use self-reported weight before pregnancy since most women contact the maternity clinic when they know they are pregnant. It is a well know phenomenon that women tend to underestimate their weight[33].

2. Few studies have representative control groups. To recruit a group of women that will not have children living in relationships and with the same socio-economical and educational level is obviously extremely difficult especially in the long-term perspective.

3. Interaction with other factors such as age, socio-economic variables are hard to rule out.

4. It is still unclear what is the optimal time period for a follow-up, at 6 months, 1 year or later?

Most studies have a follow-up time of one year. This is because if the follow-up time is shorter, women will not have been given enough time to lose their weight and if the follow-up time is longer there is a risk that the women become pregnant again.

References

1. Lissner L, Johansson SE, Qvist J, Rossner S, Wolk A. Social mapping of the obesity epidemic in Sweden. *Int J Obes Relat Metab Disord* 2000; 24: 801–5.

2. Statistics Office. *The health of adult Britain 1841–1994*. Vol. 1, pp. 112–13. London: The Stationery Office, 1997.

3. Arner P. Hunting for human obesity genes? Look in the adipose tissue! *Int J Obes Relat Metab Disord* 2000; 24 Suppl 4: S57–62.

4. DiPietro L. Physical activity, body weight, and adiposity: an epidemiologic perspective. *Exerc Sport Sci Rev* 1995; 23: 275–303.

5. JEBAT. Appetite controll and energy. *Nutr Res Rev* 1995; 8: 225–42.

6. WHO. Obesity: Preventing and managing the global epidemic. Report of a WHO Consultaton on Obesity, 3–5 June 1997; Geneva: WHO.

7. Fernstrom MH. Drugs that cause weight gain. *Obes Res* 1995; 3 Suppl 4: 435S–439S.

8. Rossner S. Pregnancy, weight cycling and weight gain in obesity. *Int J Obes Relat Metab Disord* 1992; 16: 145–7.

9. Hytten FE. Weight gain in pregnancy – 30 year of research. *S Afr Med J* 1981; 60: 15–9.

10. Dieckman WJ. *The toxemias of pregnancy* (2nd edn). St Louis Mo: The C.V. Mosby Co., 1952.

11. Institute of Medicine, Committee on Nutritional Status During Pregnancy, Weight Gain and Nutrient Supplemented. Washington DC: National Academy Press, 1990.

12. Mullins A. Overweight in pregnancy. *Lancet* 1960; i: 146–47.

13. Breadey P. Does pregnancy cause obesity? *Med J Aust* 1989; 151: 543–44.

14. Lowe G, JR G. Change in body weight associated with age and marital status. *BMJ* 1955; 1006–8.

15. Newcombe RG. Development of obesity in parous women. *J Epidemiol Community Health* 1982; 36: 306–9.

16. Brown JE, Kaye SA, Folsom AR. Parity-related weight change in women. *Int J Obes Relat Metab Disord* 1992; 16: 627–31.

17. Williamson DF, Madans J, Pamuk E, Flegal KM, Kendrick JS, Serdula MK. A prospective study of childbearing and 10-year weight gain in US white women 25 to 45 years of age. *Int J Obes Relat Metab Disord* 1994; 18: 561–9.

18. Schauberger C, Rooney B, Brimer L. Factors that influence weight loss in the puerperium. *Obstet Gynecol* 1992; 424–9.

19. Rookus MA, Rokebrand P, Burema J, Deurenberg P. The effect of pregnancy on the body mass index 9 months postpartum in 49 women. *Int J Obes* 1987; 11: 609–18.

20. Harris HE, Ellison GT, Holliday M, Lucassen E. The impact of pregnancy on the long-term weight gain of primiparous women in England. *Int J Obes Relat Metab Disord* 1997; 21: 747–55.

21. Walker LO. Predictors of weight gain at 6 and 18 months after childbirth: a pilot study. *J Obstet Gynecol Neonatal Nurse* 1996; 25: 39–48.

22. Crowell DT. Weight change in the postpartum period. A review of the literature. *J Nurse Midwifery* 1995; 40: 418–23.

23. Rossner S, Ohlin A. Pregnancy as a risk factor for obesity: lessons from the Stockholm Pregnancy and Weight Development Study. *Obes Res* 1995; 3 Suppl 2: 267s–275s.

24. Brewer MM, Bates MR, Vannoy LP. Postpartum changes in maternal weight and body fat depots in lactating vs. nonlactating women. *Am J Clin Nutr* 1989; 49: 259–65.

25. Ohlin A, Rossner S. Factors related to body weight changes during and after pregnancy: the Stockholm Pregnancy and Weight Development Study. *Obes Res* 1996; 4: 271–6.

26. Ohlin A, Rossner S. Trends in eating patterns, physical activity and socio-demographic factors in relation to postpartum body weight development. *Br J Nutr* 1994; 71: 457–70.

27. Harris HE, Ellison GT, Clement S. Do the psychosocial and behavioral changes that accompany motherhood influence the impact of pregnancy on long-term weight gain? *J Psychosom Obstet Gynaecol* 1999; 20: 65–79.

28. Harris HE, Ellison GT, Clement S. Relative importance of heritable characteristics and lifestyle in the development of maternal obesity. *J Epidemiol Community Health* 1999; 53: 66–74.

29. Parker JD, Abrams B. Differences in postpartum weight retention between black and white mothers. *Obstet Gynecol* 1993; 81: 768–74.

30. Potter S, Hannum S, McFarlin B, Essex-Sorlie D, Campbell E, Trupin S. Does infant feeding method influence maternal postpartum weight loss? *J Am Diet Assoc* 1991; 91: 441–6.

31. Ohlin A, Rossner S. Maternal body weight development after pregnancy. *Int J Obes* 1990; 14: 159–73.

32. Linné Y, Dye L, Barkeling B, Rössner S. Weight development over time in parous women- The SPAWN study – 15 years follow-up. 2002; Submitted.

33. Stewart A. The reliability and validty of self-repored weight and height. *J Chron Dis* 1982; 35: 295–309.

Progress in Obesity Research: 9. Edited by *Geraldo Medeiros-Neto, Alfredo Halpern and Claude Bouchard*
©2003 John Libbey Eurotext Ltd, pp. 500–503.

CHAPTER 106

Does breast-feeding protect the infant against obesity later in life

Kim Flcischer Michaelsen

Department of Human Nutrition, Royal Veterinary and Agricultural University, Rolighedsvej 30, DK-1958 Frederiksberg C, Denmark
[e-mail: kfm@kvl.dk]

Introduction

Many studies have examined whether breast-feeding has an effect on the development of obesity later in childhood, adolescence or young adulthood. Two reviews have evaluated the evidence. In 1999 Parsson *et al.* published an extensive review of childhood predictors of adult obesity[1], which also included a small review of infant feeding. The overall conclusion was that there was no consistent pattern. Most of the studies measured obesity as an outcome in children below 7 years. Also, it was mentioned that many of the studies did not control for appropriate confounders. More recently Butte published a more comprehensive review on the effect of breast-feeding on later obesity[2]. The review included 18 studies. She found that in most studies there was no effect of breast-feeding on later obesity. Only four studies showed an effect. She concluded that if there was an effect, it was probably weaker than genetic and other environmental factors.

After these two reviews were published several other studies have examined the association between breastfeeding and later obesity. In the following review the emphasis will be on these newer studies, but some of the more important older studies will also be mentioned.

How successful is the obese mother in breast-feeding?

Before examining the association between breast-feeding and obesity in the offspring, it is important to consider breast-feeding in obese mothers, since maternal obesity is regarded as one of the most important confounders of the association between breastfeeding and obesity in offspring. Both animal and human studies suggest that maternal obesity is associated with less successful breastfeeding[3]. In a study by Hilson *et al.*[4] initiation and duration of breast-feeding were examined in 810 white rural women from the US. Women who were overweight or obese were less successful in initiating breast-feeding when compared to normal weight women. Overweight and obese women who initiated breast-feeding were also more likely to discontinue it early. These effects were controlled for a number of factors that often co-vary with maternal obesity and breastfeeding.

There are several possible explanations why obese mothers are less successful in breast-feeding. It could be differences in the hormonal profiles between obese and normal weight mothers. It could also be because the infant has difficulties in suckling from the breast of the very obese mother. Another explanation could be residual confounding. While obesity is most prevalent among women with low educational and social status, in most societies women with a higher educational and social status breast-feed longer. Despite attempts to control for these factors, there might still be residual confounding.

The reduced initiation and duration of breast-feeding in obese mothers underline the importance of controlling for maternal obesity when examining the effect of breast-feeding on later obesity in the offspring. This was not done in many of the studies.

Studies examining breast-feeding and obesity in the off-spring

When reviewing the literature there are problems comparing the studies because the study designs differ considerably. Some studies compare no breastfeeding with any breastfeeding while others examine duration of breastfeeding but classify duration very differently. Some studies have used the duration of exclusive breastfeeding, while others have used the duration of any breastfeeding. Definition of overweight and obesity in childhood also differ but now there is agreement to use common cut-offs based on an international reference for BMI in childhood[5]. The degree to which the studies have controlled for potential confounders is also very different. This is especially a problem if there is no control for maternal obesity, and educational and socio-economic status of the parents. Another problem is the change over time in composition of infant formula, the alternative to breastfeeding. This is especially a problem in the studies with adult obesity as an outcome, since formula composition 30–50 years ago was very different from today's infant formula.

Childhood obesity

In a large study from Germany, von Kries *et al.*[6] examined more than 9,000 children at the age of 5–6 years. They found that the odds ratio of being overweight was 0.79 (95 per cent CI: 0.68–0.93), and for being obese 0.75 (0.57–0.98), if the child was breastfed. There was also a clear dose-response effect with duration of breastfeeding. The study was controlled for a number of potential confounders, but not for parental obesity. As a response to this study Wadsworth *et al.* analysed the effect of breastfeeding in a cohort of 3,731 infants born in 1945[7] and found no significant effect of breastfeeding on the prevalence of obesity at the age of six years.

In a more recent study from Germany the effect on obesity at the age of nine to10 years was examined in 2,108 children born in the mid-1980s[8]. After adjustment for confounders, breastfed infants were less likely to be obese (OR 0.66 (95 per cent CI: 0.52–0.87). Furthermore, there was a dose-response effect and parental weight was not controlled for.

In a study from Scotland by Armstrong *et al.* 32,200 children born in 1995 or 1996 were studied, but only up to the age of 39 to 42 months[9]. The odds ratio for developing obesity was 0.70 (CI 0.61–0.80). The study controlled for some potential confounders, but not for parental weight status.

In a cross sectional study of 2,685 US children aged three to five years, examined as part of the National Health and Nutrition Examination Survey (NHANES III), there was some protection of breastfeeding on being at risk of being overweight (BMI between the 85th and 94th percentile), but the pattern was inconsistent as the moderate effect on being overweight was not significant[10].

Obesity in adolescence

In a study from Canada 1,172 children were examined at the age of 12–18 years[11]. Breast-feeding protected against obesity and there was a dose-response effect with duration of breast-feeding. The study was controlled for sex, age, race, ethnicity, birth order, socio economic status, and family history of overweight and obesity. Family history of obesity was found to be a strong confounder.

A study from the US with more than 15,000 children aged nine to 14 years found that being only or mostly breastfed was associated with an odds-ratio of 0.78 (95 per cent CI: 0.66.0–91) of being overweight[12]. The confounders controlled for included the mother's BMI.

Adult obesity

Two small studies with individuals born in the mid 1940s have examined if there was an effect in adulthood. In a study from the US, Carney *et al.* examined 366 adults 20 to 30 years old[13]. There was no effect from breast-feeding, but only 18 per cent of the population was breast-fed for more than two weeks. In the other study by Marmott *et al.*, 172 adults were examined at the age of 32 years. Surprisingly, this study found that both weight, body mass index and skinfold was higher in the breast-fed individuals, but the study was not controlled for socio-economic status[14].

In a short report in a letter Poulton and Williams reported data from a cohort study in New Zealand, where about 1,000 individuals were followed from birth to 26 years[15]. Those breastfed for six months or more were less likely to be overweight at 26 years, but the association was weaker and non-significant when controlling for confounders including parental overweight.

We have studied the effect of breastfeeding on adult obesity in the Copenhagen Perinatal Cohort, which consists of 9,125 individuals born from 1959 to 1961[16]. The cohort is described in more detail in a recent paper in which we found that the duration of breast-feeding was positively associated in a dose-dependent manner with IQ in young adulthood[17]. In a sub sample of 2,601 males the following information was available: Duration of breast-feeding assessed by a questionnaire at 12 months and weight and length at draft board examination at 19 years. Breast-feeding did not protect against overweight (BMI > 25) or obesity (BMI > 30).

Possible causes

It is difficult to exclude that residual confounding could explain some of the positive findings even if most of the studies were controlled for parental education and social status. These two factors and several other family characteristics are strongly associated both to duration of breast-feeding and development of obesity later in life. The variables controlled for in the statistical analysis may not describe these effects fully. Another factor only controlled for in some studies is maternal cigarette smoking. Mothers who smoke are less likely to breast-feed and in the study by von Kries *et al.* maternal smoking during pregnancy increased the risk of the child being overweight and obese with more than 50 per cent in the final logistic regression model[6].

Despite these problems with the study design it is plausible that breast-feeding has an effect. If there is such an effect, there are several possible causes.

Human milk contains many bioactive factors including hormones, leptin and cytokines. It is possible that some of these factors could modulate the risk of developing obesity later in life. In one week old term infants the hormonal response, including insulin, to a meal was different in breastfed and formula fed infants[18]. Leptin is present in human milk and not in infant formula, but there seems to be no difference in serum leptin levels between breastfed and formula fed infants[19]. However, one study suggested that early feeding can programme leptin levels during adolescence[20].

Another reason could be differences in protein intake between breastfed and formula fed infants, as it has been suggested that a high protein intake in early life will increase the risk of obesity later during childhood[21]. Breastfed infants receive considerably less protein than formula fed infants. Typical values for protein content are human milk 8 g/l, infant formula 15 g/l and cow's milk 35 g/l. The epidemiological data supporting this hypothesis are, however, not strong. The most convincing study is by Scaglioni *et al.* who followed 147 Italian infants from one to five years[18]. The children who had a BMI above the 90 percentile at five years also had a higher protein intake at one year of age. Furthermore, breast-feeding tended to be shorter in the overweight children.

Parental care or interest is important for early feeding. It is possible that mothers who breast-feed are more caring and supportive on average during later childhood, which may have a protective effect against obesity. In a Danish study parental neglect in school-aged children was a very strong predictor for development of obesity in young adulthood[22].

It has also been suggested that breast-fed infants have a better satiety regulation. Breast milk composition and taste reflect the diet of the mother and changes considerably over time. This provides the infant with much more composite signals than the bottle-fed infant, and gives the infant a more active role. It is speculated that this could give a better satiety control later in life.

Conclusion

It is still not clear to what degree breast-feeding protects against obesity. Despite limitations in the study design the available studies make it plausible that there is an effect at least in some settings and during certain ages. None of the studies examining breastfeeding and adult obesity could find a significant effect. However, most of these studies are from early in the obesity epidemic, when the prevalence of obesity was not so high.

We need more large epidemiological studies with appropriate control for confounding, to determine the effect of breast-feeding on later obesity. We also need studies to explore the possible mechanisms by which breast-feeding may protect against obesity. Understanding these mechanisms could improve our understanding of the causes of obesity, and thereby be of value in both prevention and treatment of obesity.

Breast-feeding has many positive effects besides the possible effect on obesity[23]. These include protection against infections, which is most pronounced in populations with a high prevalence of infectious diseases. Furthermore, breast-feeding modulates the child's immune system and it has been shown that some immune related diseases are less prevalent among breast-fed infants. Breast-feeding is also likely to support the mental development of the infants[17,24]. Thus, there are many reasons why breastfeeding should be promoted. According to the new WHO recommendations infants should be breastfed exclusively for 6 months and thereafter continued with partial breastfeeding at least until the age of 12 months. Breastfeeding promotion programmes have shown to be effective and should also include the four goals of the 'Innocenti Declaration on the Protection, Promotion and Support of Breastfeeding' from a WHO/UNICEF meeting in 1990: (1) Appoint a national breastfeeding coordinator and committee, (2) Implement the Baby Friendly Hospital Initiative, (3) Implement the International Code of Marketing of Breast-Milk Substitutes, and (4) Implement legislation supporting breastfeeding rights of working mothers.

References

1. Parsons TJ, Power C, Logan S, Summerbell CD. Childhood predictor of adult obesity: a systematic review. *Int J Obes Relat Metab Disord* 1999; 23: S1–S107.

2. Butte NF. The role of breastfeeding in obesity. *Pediatr Clin North Am* 2001; 48: 189–98.

3. Rasmussen, KM., Hilson JA, Kjolhede CL. Obesity may impair lactogenesis II. *J Nutr* 2001; 131: 3009S–3011S.

4. Hilson JA, Rasmussen KM, Kjolhede CL. Maternal obesity and breast-feeding success in a rural population of white women. *Am J Clin Nutr* 1997; 66: 1371–78.

5. Cole TJ, Bellizzi MC, Flegal KM, Dietz WH. Establishing a standard definition for child overweight and obesity worldwide: international survey. *BMJ* 2000; 320: 1240–43.

6. von Kries R, Koletzko B, Sauerwald T, von Mutius E, Barnert D, Grunert V, von Voss H. Breast feeding and obesity: cross sectional study. *BMJ* 1999; 319: 147–50.

7. Wadsworth M, Marshall S, Hardy R, Paul A. Breast feeding and obesity. Relation may be accounted for by social factors. *BMJ* 1999; 319: 1576–1576.

8. Liese AD, Hirsch T, von Mutius E, Keil U, Leupold W, Weiland SK. Inverse association of overweight and breast feeding in 9 to 10-y-old children in Germany. *Int J Obes* 2001; 25: 1644–50.

9. Armstrong J, Reilly JJ. The Child Health Information Team Breastfeeding and lowering the risk of childhood obesity. *Lancet* 2002; 359: 2003–4.

10. Hediger ML, Overpeck MD, Kuczmarski RJ, June Ruan W. Association between infant breastfeeding and overweight in young children. *JAMA* 2001; 285: 2453–60.

11. Kramer MS. Do breast-feeding and delayed introduction of solid foods protect against subsequent obesity? *J Pediatr* 1981; 98: 883–7.

12. Gillman MW, Rifas-Shiman SL, Camargo CA, Berkey CS, Frazier AL, Rockett HRH *et al*. Risk of overweight among adolescents who were breastfed as infants. *JAMA* 2001; 285: 2461–67.

13. Charney E, Goodman HC, McBride M, Lyon B, Pratt R. Childhood antecedents of adult obesity. Do chubby infants become obese adults? *N Eng J Med* 1976; 295: 6–9.

14. Marmot MG, Page CM, Atkins E, Douglas JW. Effect of breast-feeding on plasma cholesterol and weight in young adults. *J Epidemiol Commun Health* 1980; 34: 164–7.

15. Poulton R, Williams S. Breastfeeding and risk of overweight. *JAMA* 2001; 286: 1449–49.

16. Michaelsen KF, Mortensen EL, Sørensen TIA, Schack-Nielsen L, Reinisch J M. Is duration of breastfeeding (BF) influencing the risk of obesity as adult? *Int J Obes* 2002; 26(1): S178 (abstract).

17. Mortensen EL, Michaelsen KF, Sanders SA, Reinisch JM. The association between duration of breastfeeding and adult intelligence. *JAMA* 2002; 287: 2365–71.

18. Lucas A, Sarson DL, Blackburn AM, Adrian TE, Aynsley-Green A, Bloom SR. Breast vs. bottle: endocrine responses are different with formula feeding. *Lancet* 1980; 14: 1268–69.

19. Lönnerdal B, Havel PJ. Serum leptin concentrations in infants: effects of diet, sex, and adiposity. *Am J Clin Nutr* 2000; 72: 484–9.

20. Singhal A, Farooqi IS, O'Rahilly S, Cole TJ, Fewtrell M, Lucas A. Early nutrition and leptin concentrations in later life. *Am J Clin Nutr* 2002; 75: 993–99.

21. Rolland-Cachera MF, Deheeger M, Akrout M, Bellisle F. Influence of macronutrients on adiposity development: a follow up study of nutrition and growth from 10 months to 8 years of age. *Int J Obes* 1995; 19: 573–78.

22. Lissau I, Sørensen TIA. Parental neglect during childhood and increased risk of obesity in young adulthood. *Lancet* 1994; 343: 324–27.

23. Heinig MJ, Dewey KG. Health advantages of breast-feeding for infants. *Nutr Res Rev* 1996; 9: 89–110.

24. Anderson JW, Johnstone BM, Remley DT. Breast-feeding and cognitive development: a meta-analysis. *Am J Clin Nutr* 1999; 70: 525–35.

Progress in Obesity Research: 9. Edited by *Geraldo Medeiros-Neto, Alfredo Halpern and Claude Bouchard*
©2003 John Libbey Eurotext Ltd, pp. 504–507.

CHAPTER 107

Small eaters or underreporters among obese?

Klaas R. Westerterp

Department of Human Biology, Maastricht University, The Netherlands
[e-mail: k.westerterp@hb.unimaas.nl]

Introduction

Food intake in humans in their own environment is one of the hardest parameters to measure. The assessment of food intake is prone to different types of error, depending on the method used. Most methods, like the food frequency questionnaire, dietary recall, dietary history and dietary record, rely on the reporting behaviour of the subject. Errors in food tables and coding errors are relatively small and are for all methods similar. Larger errors are due to the phenomenon that subjects give the wrong information. They report the perception of what they eat instead of the real consumption. For example, obese subjects often believe that their food intake is equal or even lower than the food intake of lean subjects and that their obesity is due to metabolic defects causing a low energy expenditure.

With the application of the doubly labeled water method for the measurement of total daily energy expenditure there is an accurate method for the validation of reported energy intake by subjects in free living situations. Three reviews reported on the accuracy of reported dietary energy intake using the doubly labeled water method as a reference. Schoeller[12] concluded that reported intakes tend to be lower than expenditure and thus are often underestimates of true habitual energy intake. It was speculated that individuals tend to report intakes that are closer to perceived norms than to actual intake. Black et al.[1] demonstrated good agreement between reported intake and measured expenditure when food intake was recorded by observers. They suggested that, ideally, all dietary studies should include independent measures of validity. Hill and Davies[9] identified factors involved in under-reporting including increased adiposity and/or body size, dieting and dietary restraint, gender, socioeconomic status, motivation, social expectations and the nature of the testing environment itself.

Here, the focus is on determinants of energy requirement, i.e. energy intake, determinants of discrepancies between reported intake and measured expenditure, and evidence for the existence of small eaters and large eaters.

Methods

Energy requirement was related to body size using the Maastricht data base of energy expenditure measurements with doubly labeled water. Exclusion criteria were age < 19, non-Caucasian, an intervention in energy intake, an intervention in physical activity including athletic performance, pregnancy, lactation and disease. Energy expenditure was measured over a two-week interval according to the Maastricht protocol as reported before[16], resulting in a figure for average daily metabolic rate (ADMR).

Determinants of discrepancies between reported intake and measured expenditure were evaluated from published studies including simultaneous measurement of reported intake and doubly labeled water assessed energy expenditure. Similarly, food intake in small eaters and large eaters was evaluated from published studies including simultaneous measurement of reported intake and doubly labeled water assessed energy expenditure.

Under reporting of habitual intake can be explained by under recording and under eating. Some studies discriminated between the two errors mentioned, by comparing reported food intake and water intake with energy expenditure and water loss. When subjects record food intake they record simultaneously water intake. In healthy individuals, water balance is preserved and is therefore an independent indicator for under recording. The recording precision of water intake is assumed to be representative for total food recording, as most foodstuffs contain water. Under-eating during food recording was monitored by measurement of body mass. Body mass changes over a food recording period are compared with normal body mass fluctuations.

Results

The Maastricht data base of energy expenditure measurements with doubly labeled water included 399 subjects meeting the formulated selection criteria. Subject characteristics are presented in Table 1. Energy requirement, as reflected in ADMR, showed a more than fourfold range from 4.1 to 18.4 MJ/day in women and from 5.0 to 21.5 MJ/day in men. In a stepwise multiple regression analysis, weight explained 48 per cent of the variance, followed by age (15 per cent), gender (7 per cent) and height (1 per cent). Energy requirement increases with weight, decreases with age, is higher in men than in women, and increases with height.

Table 1. Subject characteristics – mean ± sd (range)

	Women (*n* = 166)	Men (*n* = 233)
Age (years)	50 ± 25 (20–96)	49 ± 20 (19–96)
Height (m)	1.65 ± 0.07 (1.49–1.81)	1.77 ± 0.07 (1.60–1.97)
Body mass (kg)	70 ± 21 (38–164)	83 ± 20 (54–216)
ADMR (MJ/d)	9.8 ± 2.7 (4.1–18.4)	12.9 ± 3.1 (5.0–21.5)

Hill and Davies[9] recently reviewed studies using doubly labeled water in conjunction with self reported energy intake. Here, data included in the review are presented plus one study published afterwards[14]. Most studies showed a lower value for reported energy intake compared to measured total energy expenditure. Women did not show more or less under reporting than men. Values for normal-weight subjects were mostly in the range 0 to 25 per cent with a grand average of 16 per cent (Fig. 1). Values for obese subjects were more in the 25 to 50 per cent range with a grand average of 41 per cent, i.e. generally twice as high as in normal-weight subjects (Fig. 2).

The percentage under reporting, divided into under recording and a change in diet was observed in studies in lean women[3], obese men[4], elderly men and women[5], and depleted patients[6]. Both the obese men and lean women ate less, 26 per cent and 16 per cent, respectively, while recording food intake. The lean women, all dieticians, showed a high recording precision. The recording error observed in the obese men and in the elderly men and women, 12 per cent and 21 per cent, respectively, was probably

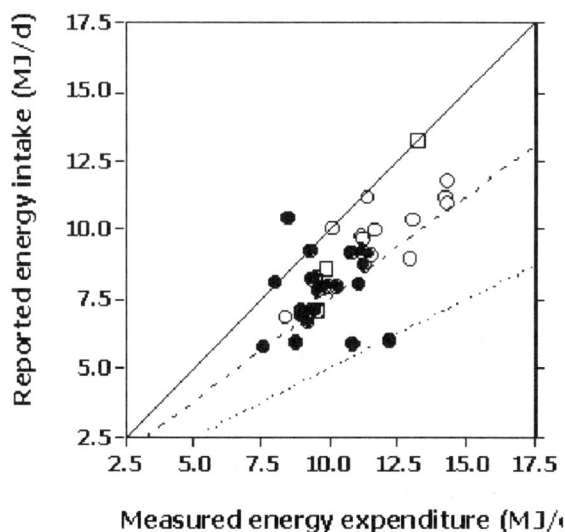

Fig. 1. Reported energy intake plotted against energy expenditure as measured with doubly labelled water of studies in normal weight (BMI 20–25 kg/m²) adult subjects – women: open dots (*n* = 482); men: closed dots (*n* = 226); gender mixed: squares (*n* = 46). The lines denote no under-reporting, 25 per cent under-reporting and 50 per cent under-reporting.

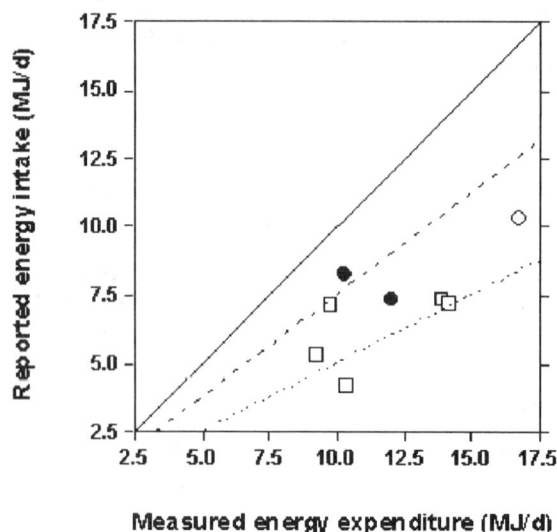

Fig. 2. Reported energy intake plotted against energy expenditure as measured with doubly labelled water of studies in obese subjects – women: open dots ($n = 17$); men: closed dots ($n = 30$); gender mixed: squares ($n = 85$). The lines denote no under-reporting, 25 per cent under-reporting and 50 per cent under-reporting

due to under estimation of food portion sizes and to not-recording of all foods consumed. Only the depleted patients reported their food intake accurately and they did not change their diet while recording food intake.

Clark *et al.*[2] compared self-reported food intake in 'large-' and 'small-eating' women with measured energy expenditure. Reported intake and measured expenditure in large- and small-eaters was, respectively, 10.5 MJ/day and 8.5 MJ/day, and 5.9 MJ/day and 11.3 MJ/day. Thus, large-eaters over reported 24 per cent and small-eaters under reported 48 per cent. In reality, the energy requirement of the small-eaters was higher than the energy requirement of the large-eaters.

Discussion

Energy requirement increases with increasing body size and thus obese subjects have to eat more than lean subjects to maintain the body size reached. We know this since the application of the doubly labeled water method to measure energy expenditure of subjects in free-living conditions. The current analysis shows body weight as the main determinant of daily energy expenditure. Body weight affects maintenance metabolism and activity induced energy expenditure. The effect of age on ADMR probably is through the change of body composition and physical activity with age. Increasing age is associated with lower activity levels and lower fat-free mass[15]. The higher ADMR in men compared to women with a similar body weight is mainly due to a gender difference in body composition. Women have a lower fat-free mass while activity levels are similar for women and men.

Misreporting of food intake has become clear since the application of doubly labeled water to measure energy expenditure as a reference method as well. Misreporting of food intake, mostly underreporting, is observed in many populations. People are likely to report intakes that are similar to the expectations for the population[12]. Obese subjects report an intake similar to or even lower than the intake of a non-obese subject. They show under recording and under eating while reporting food intake. The most likely reasons for under recording are probably under estimation of food portion sizes and to not-recording of all foods consumed. The portion size that is considered as normal by the obese is objectively considered as large[17]. If the portion sizes of foods are still calculated as 'normal' portion sizes by the dietician, an under reporting of food intake would be the result. Additionally, the recording of food intake by obese subjects might also be perceived as an opportunity to diet for these subjects[12].

Underreporting of food intake does not result from a systematical underestimation of portion sizes for all food items but seems to concern specific food items which are generally considered 'bad for health'[10]. The relation between nutrient intake and health parameters can be overestimated or hidden as a consequence of selective underreporting[11]. One example is the relation between fat intake and obesity entitled: 'the American paradox'. In the adult population the prevalence of overweight has increased since 1976 with 31 per cent and at the same time reported energy intake and percentage energy from fat has decreased. This might be due to a lower physical activity and a higher consumption of low-energy foods but underreporting has also increased since 1976[7]. Combining the results of studies showing selective underreporting of fat intake, the reported decrease in energy and fat intake in the US seems to be doubtful[4,8,13]. National health campaigns aimed at lowering fat intake might not be so successful as it is concluded from the results of national food consumption measurements showing a decline in reported fat intakes over several years.

In conclusion, habitual food intake in overweight individuals is higher than in gender, age and height matched normal-weight subjects, especially when they have a similar level of physical activity. Obese subjects under report food intake because of under recording and under eating during the observation interval. They selectively under report fat intake. There is no support for small eaters among the obese.

References

1. Black AE, Prentice AM, Goldberg GR, Jebb SA, Bingham SA, Livingstone MB, Coward WA. Measurements of total energy expenditure provide insights into the validity of dietary measurements of energy intake. *J Am Diet Assoc* 1993; 93: 572–79.

2. Clark D., Tomas F, Withers RT, Chandler C, Brinkman M, Phillips J, Berry M, Ballard FJ, Nestel P. Energy metabolism in free-living, 'large-eating' and 'small-eating' women: studies using $^2H_2^{18}O$. *Br J Nutr* 1994; 72: 21–31.

3. Goris AHC, Westerterp KR. Underreporting of habitual food intake is explained by undereating in highly motivated lean women. *J Nutr* 1999; 129: 878–82.

4. Goris AHC, Westerterp-Plantenga MS, Westerterp KR. Undereating and underrecording of habitual food intake in obese men: selective underreporting of fat intake. *Am J Clin Nutr* 2000; 71: 130–34.

5. Goris AHC, Meijer EP, Westerterp KR. Repeated measurement of habitual food intake increases under-reporting and induces selective under-reporting. *Br J Nutr* 2001; 85: 629–34.

6. Goris AHC, Vermeeren MAP, Wouters EFM, Schols AMWJ, Westerterp KR. Energy balance in depleted ambulatory patients with chronic obstructive pulmonary disease; the effect of physical activity and oral nutritional supplementation. *Br J Nutr* 2003; 89: 725–9.

7. Heini AF, Weinsier RL. Divergent trends in obesity and fat intake patterns: the American paradox. *Am J Med* 1997; 102: 259–64.

8. Heitmann B, Lissner L, Osler M. Do we eat less fat, or just report so? *Int J Obes* 2000; 24: 435–42.

9. Hill RJ, Davies PSW. The validity of self-reported energy intake as determined using the doubly labelled water technique. *Br J Nutr* 2001; 85: 415–30.

10. Lafay L, Mennen L, Basdevant A, Charles MA, Borys JM, Eschwege E. Romon M. Does energy intake underreporting involve all kinds of food or only specific food items? Results from the Fleurbaix Laventie Ville Sante (FLVS) study. *Int J Obes* 2000; 24: 1500–6.

11. Lissner L, Heitmann BL, Lindroos AK. Measuring intake in free-living human subjects: a question of bias. *Proc Nutr Soc* 1998; 57: 333–39.

12. Schoeller DA. How accurate is self-reported dietary intake? *Nutr Rev* 1990; 48: 373–379.

13. Tomoyasu N, Toth M. Poehlman E. Misreporting of total energy intake in older African Americans. *Int J Obes* 2000; 24: 20–6.

14. Weber JL, Reid PM, Greaves KA, DeLany JP, Stanford VA, Going SB *et al*. Validity of self-reported energy intake in lean and obese young women, using two nutrient databases, compared with total energy expenditure assessed by doubly labeled water. *Eur J Clin Nutr* 2001; 55: 940–50.

15. Westerterp KR, Meijer EP. Changes in physical activity patterns with age: a physiological perspective. *J Geront* 2001; 56A: 7–12.

16. Westerterp KR, Wouters L, Van Marken Lichtenbelt WD. The Maastricht protocol for the measurement of body composition and energy expenditure with labeled water. *Obes Res* 1995; 3: S1: 49–57.

17. Westerterp-Plantenga MS, Pasman WJ, Yedema MJW, Wijckmans-Duijsens NEG. Energy intake adaptation of food intake to extreme energy densities of food by obese and non-obese women. *Eur J Clin Nutr* 1996; 50: 401–7.

Progress in Obesity Research: 9. Edited by *Geraldo Medeiros-Neto, Alfredo Halpern and Claude Bouchard*
©2003 John Libbey Eurotext Ltd, pp. 508–518.

CHAPTER 108

Under-reporting in overweight subjects – is protein well reported?

S.D. Poppitt

Department of Medicine and Human Nutrition Unit, University of Auckland, Auckland, New Zealand
[e-mail: s.poppitt@auckland.ac.nz]

The problems of under-reporting

The inability to accurately report food intake is a major problem for nutrition trials attempting to assess the many and complex relationships between diet, health and disease. There is a convincing body of evidence that participants in trials fail to report significant portions of their diet and/or make short-term alterations to diet which invalidate attempts to assess habitual energy intake[1-6] and that this is commonly[7-10], although not always[11,12], worse in the obese and post-obese subject. A recent review of large national dietary surveys[13] has confirmed that under-reporting remains widespread[10,14-24], and data such as this has lead to the development of independent methods by which to validate intake of both energy and nutrients. Methods for independent estimates of energy intake (EI) include the measurement of energy expenditure (EE) by the doubly labelled water (DLW) technique, an expensive but well validated method[2,4,5,13,25] and the mathematical comparison between predicted EI (expressed as EI: BMR) and predicted EE (expressed as EE: BMR or physical activity level, PAL). This has generated cut-off values by which to evaluate reported EI as probable or unlikely estimates of actual EI [26,27]. Alternatively, energy adjustment as a method by which recall bias can be controlled is sometimes used[28,29], commonly assuming that measurement error is similar for all individuals and all macronutrients. Whether the adjustment of energy to compensate for under-reporting may distort disease risk ratios has been questioned[30-34] and recommendations for improved measurement methods rather than energy adjustment have been made[34].

Whilst the validation of energy is perhaps most crucial in diet surveys since under-reporting of food components is often related to general under-reporting of energy[35,36], the validation of individual nutrients is important for many trials. There remains considerable debate as to whether an estimate of energy under-reporting can be extrapolated to the individual macronutrients, fat, CHO protein or alcohol. There is little direct evidence that the under-reporting of macronutrients is proportional to either their percentage contribution to the diet or is equal across the diet, i.e. approximately 1/3 for each of the three food macronutrients (fat, CHO, protein). Despite this lack of evidence some epidemiological trials have assumed that, when expressed as a percentage of energy, macronutrient specific under-reporting is negligible and may be ignored even when energy reporting is grossly in error[35]. This has yet to be clarified.

Methods for the independent assessment of the macronutrients are considerably more problematic than for energy. As yet there are no widely used quantitative methods for assessment of CHO or fat intake in free-living populations, only a qualitative method for assessment of fatty acid composition of the diet through collection of venous blood and subsequent measurement of serum phospholipids, cholesterol esters and erythrocyte membranes, or adipose tissue samples. These are reasonably reliable methods that can determine habitual intake of dietary fat and/or changes made over a period of weeks or months in fat quality. They have been widely used in trials investigating the relationships between long-term intake of saturated and unsaturated fatty acids and diseases of middle age including cardiovascular disease and type 2 diabetes[37-43] They are also useful methods for assessing compliance in community based intervention trials since changes can be observed within a few weeks of dietary change.

Protein intake is considerably easier to validate since the assessment of urinary nitrogen (N) losses allow a quantitative estimate of N intake in individuals believed to be in N balance[44–46]. There are a number of assumptions associated with this method including (i) that the subjects are in N balance, (ii) urinary N losses are a constant proportion of total losses, and (iii) that a complete 24-h urine collection can be provided by the participant or in the absence of a full collection that, (iv) the use of ρ-aminobenzoic acid (PABA), as a marker of completeness of the urine collection, will allow retrospective calculation of the missing urinary N. This is discussed in more detail below. This paper addresses the question of whether under-reporting of protein intake is an important component in the under-reporting of energy intake in nutrition trials. It reviews recent work on biomarkers of protein intake and intervention trials which have measured the contribution of individual macronutrients to the missing energy component.

Biomarkers of total protein intake – the nitrogen balance method

When in N balance, total N intake should be equal to total N losses. This is the case for most adult participants of dietary surveys or intervention trials. Carefully conducted N balance studies have shown that losses occur through urinary (81 ± 5 per cent), faecal (13 ± 2 per cent), skin (4 ± 1 per cent), sweat, menstrual and other miscellaneous (< 1 per cent) routes[44], and that the percentage lost through each route is a constant fraction of total losses. This makes it possible to use a single marker, such as urinary losses, from which to calculate total N losses and hence evaluate N intake data:

$$\text{Predicted N}_{\text{intake}} \text{ (g/day)} = \text{Measured N}_{\text{losses (total)}} = \text{Measured N}_{\text{losses (urinary)}}/0.81$$

In subjects under-reporting N intake, urinary losses will tend to be greater than 81 ± 5 per cent of intake and in those over-reporting N intake, urinary losses will be less than 81 ± 5 per cent. An alternate method to allow for non-urinary N losses was proposed by Isaksson[47], who showed N losses from all other sources to be an average of 2.0 g N/day. Many trials use this method whereby,

$$\text{Predicted N}_{\text{intake}} \text{ (g/day)} = \text{Measured N}_{\text{losses (urinary)}} + 2 \text{ gN}$$

Ideally completeness of the 24-h urine collection must be verified using the PABACHEK method of Bingham and Cummings44. Subjects are asked to take three doses of 80 mg of PABA during the collection period, commonly with breakfast, lunch and dinner. PABA occurs in association with B vitamins in food, has no known toxicological or harmful effects and the metabolites are excreted in urine within 4–8 h post-dose. Percentage recovery of PABA provides a measure of collection of urine based on the assumption that PABA is excreted almost quantitatively and that a recovery of > 85 per cent represents a complete 24-h urine collection. A recent reanalysis has provided a method by which urine samples which contain < 85 per cent PABA can be mathematically adjusted to compensate for incomplete collection[48]. Using data from trials carried out on a total of 313 men and women in the UK and Sweden a linear equation was generated to calculate an adjusted N value for urines where PABA recoveries were 50–85 per cent:

$$\text{adjusted N (g)} = \text{excreted N} + [0.088 * (93 - \text{per cent PABA recovered})]$$

where 0.088 is a constant representing the slope of the PABA recovery and N excretion linear regression calculated from the validation trial of Johansson[48], and 93 per cent is the mean recovery of PABA in complete urine collections as calculated in the validation study of Bingham and Cummings[44]. There are no methods for adjustment of total N losses should the recovery of PABA fall below 50 per cent. The PABA analysis method has recently been updated from a colorimetric to HPLC method[49] which has eliminated problems such as the interference of a number of drug metabolites including paracetamol. The PABA recovery method is currently the only technique by which completeness of a 24-h urine sample can be quantified. It may be useful to note that although it appears extremely promising in the numerous relatively small validation studies that have been carried out over the last 20 years, it has yet to be fully validated in large scale trials to ensure factors such as age, gender, interaction with diet, and day to day biological variation do not invalidate the method. A recent publication by Kipnis and colleagues[50] however, in which the method was re-evaluated, has shown that whilst the ratio of urinary N to dietary N does not represent an exact biologic constant, effects of age, gender, source of protein intake and even person-specific bias have only minor and non-significant effects on the method. Their rigorous analysis concluded that 'these results suggest that urinary nitrogen level satisfies ... requirements for a reference instrument'[50].

Trials assessing protein reporting – dietary surveys

Many studies have attempted to investigate the extent of macronutrient specific under-reporting using the three compartment model of (i) total energy, (ii) protein energy, (iii) non-protein energy, and the simple equation of EI = [protein energy] + [non-protein energy] where non-protein energy comprises [fat + CHO energy] combined. No allowance is provided for alcohol energy. Independent assessment of energy reporting has commonly been provided by DLW and/or the physiological cut-off values of Goldberg[27] and Black[26] described above. Independent assessment of protein intake has been carried out using the N balance method of Bingham[44,51], using the factor for conversion of N to protein of between 5.8–6.5 (average 6.25), dependant upon the protein source. Any differential between reported energy and reported protein provides an estimate of the differential reporting of [fat + CHO] combined. Whilst this method cannot independently assess either fat or CHO, if energy is poorly reported but protein well reported it would seem reasonable to assume that it is within either the fat and/or the CHO component of the diet that the missing energy lies. This rather crude estimate of macronutrient under-reporting would of course be invalid should the reporting bias be due to undereating (dieting) rather than under-reporting of habitual diet *per se*.

Studies which investigated macronutrient specific under-reporting using these methods were identified from a computerized search of MEDLINE (National Library of Medicine, Bethesda, MD) and cross referencing (Table 1). Trials that have investigated bias in under-reporting without measurement of urinary N losses to validate protein intake have been excluded. Trials included both lean and obese individuals, and comments indicate when reporting was shown to be specifically related to BMI. No distinction was made between the reporting of men and women. For comparative purposes an arbitrary cut off for the definition of good reporting has been set at between 90–110 per cent of N validated intake. Forty studies were identified as using a variety of methods to assess intake, including 24-h recall, diet history, diet records, diet questionnaire (trial specific), food frequency questionnaire and weighed records. Many of the studies used more than one of these methods and a comparison of N (protein) intake with N losses was made for 67 dietary assessments. Overall protein reporting was excellent, with mean reported intake 100.4 ± 19 % (sd) of validated protein losses. Half of the studies reviewed (49 per cent) showed good reporting of protein, whilst the other half were divided between under-reporting (32 per cent) and over-reporting (19 per cent). When results from 10 trials using the weighed records 'gold standard' method were compared with N losses, 70 per cent show good and 30 per cent show poor protein reporting. Where validity of energy intake was assessed using DLW or a combination of estimated/measured BMR and an estimate of activity (PAL), the accuracy of reporting of non-protein [fat + CHO] energy has been calculated from the equation EI^{reported} = [protein energy]$_{reported}$ + [fat + CHO energy]$_{reported}$, as explained above (see Table 1). Alcohol intake was assumed to be zero for this model. In these 14 studies, energy reporting was 84 ± 9 per cent (sd) and protein reporting was 89 ± 10 per cent (sd) of validated intake. [Fat+CHO] reporting was calculated to be 83 ± 9 per cent (sd) of intake. In 12 of the 14 studies protein reporting was better than non-protein (fat + CHO) reporting. Where only the ratio of EI/BMR was published, [fat + CHO] reporting could not be calculated. Few studies which have attempted to validate protein intake using N losses have differentiated between lean and obese subjects, and no systematic evaluation has been made in this review.

Trials assessing protein reporting – controlled studies

There have also been trials that have attempted to measure the extent of nutrient under-reporting in the controlled conditions of a metabolic ward. In one such trial 33 lean and overweight women were asked to attend a metabolic facility in Cambridge, UK, ostensibly for measurement of body composition over a 2 day period[11]. During these 2 days participants were encouraged to eat freely from an extensive menu and, with no prior warning, were later asked to report their intake to a dietitian. Throughout the trial all foods eaten were carefully and covertly recorded to allow for comparison with the report provided by participants through 24-h recall. The trial showed that there was significant under-reporting of energy intake, that reported total CHO was significantly lower than measured, and that both protein and fat were well reported. (Fig. 1). Interestingly, it was apparent that much of this was driven by good reporting of main meals and poor reporting of between-meal snacks. A study in which restaurant clientele were questioned has also shown that food types less central to a meal, such as side dishes and condiments, tend to be badly reported when compared with entrees, main dishes and desserts[85]. Similar results were obtained in a study comparing sources of energy from meals versus

---

* 10 of the 67 assessments included correlations between N intake and losses but not per cent reporting. These were excluded from the summaries above.

Table 1. Studies in which 24-h urinary N losses have been used to assess the validity of dietary protein intake. Where DLW and/or predicted BMR has been used to assess the validity of dietary energy, an estimate of non-protein [fat + CHO] reporting is also shown

Author	Subjects	Diet assessment method	Energy expenditure method	N losses method	PA/BA	Dietary reporting
Steen et al., 1977[52]	M/F, 70 years (n = 370)	24-h R DH	Not assessed	24-h urine x 1	N	24-h R: poor protein reporting, 86% DH: good protein reporting, 95%
van Staveren et al., 1985[53]	M/F, 19–32 years (n = 44)	DH x 2	Not assessed	24-h urine x 2	N	DH: good protein reporting, 100%
Kahn, 1987[54]	M/F, 21+ years (n = 44)	24-h R	Not assessed	24-h urine x 1	N	24-h R: good protein reporting, 100%
Warwick et al., 1987[55]	M/F, young, lean (n = 37)	WR x 14d	Not assessed	24-h urine x 2	N	WR: good protein reporting, 91%
Hulten et al., 1990[56]	F, lean and obese 38–60 years (n = 154 205, 331)	DH-1968/9 DH-1974/5 DH-1980/1	Not assessed	24-h urine x 1	N	1968/9: good protein reporting, 97% 1974/5: good protein reporting, 105% 1980/1: protein over-reported, 120% worse reporting of protein in obese
Kunkel et al., 1991[57]	F, 40–92 years (n = 125)	DH DR x 7d	Not assessed	24-h urine x 1	N[1]	DR: protein over-reported, 112%
O'Donnell et al., 1991[58]	M/F, 18–65 years (n = 52)	DQ WR x 16d	Not assessed	24-h urine x 4	Y[2]	DQ:[3] protein reporting, r = 0.34** WR:[3] protein reporting, r = 0.56*** no data for% reporting provided
Johansson et al., 1992[59]	M/F, 27–61 years (n = 20)	24-h R x 16	Predicted BMR	24-h urine x 4	N	24-h R: poor protein reporting, 80% poor energy reporting, EI/BMR = 1.21
Petersen et al., 1992[60]	M/F, 20–31 years (n = 33)	DH DR x 4d	Not assessed	24-h urine x 1	Y	DH: good protein reporting, 107% DR: good protein reporting, 97%
Heitmann et al., 1993[7]	M/F, lean and obese, 35–65 years (n = 323)	D	Not assessed	24-h urine x 1	Y	DH: poor protein reporting, 85% worse reporting of protein in obese
Rothenberg, 1994[61]	M/F, 70 years (n = 76)	DR x4d FFQ	Predicted BMR	24-h urine x 1	N	DR: good protein reporting, 103%; energy reporting, EI/BMR = 1.27 FFQ: protein over-reported, 119%; energy reporting, EI/BMR = 1.64
Lindroos et al., 1993[62]	M/F, lean and obese, 21–61years (n = 64)	DR x 4d DQ	BMR measured[3]	24-h urine x 1	N	DR: poor protein reporting, 87%; poor energy reporting, 84%; calculate similar poor reporting of [fat +CHO], 84% DQ: protein over-reported, 111%; good energy reporting, 105%; calculate over-reporting of [fat +CHO], 104%

511

Table 1. *Continued.*

Author	Subjects	Diet assessment method	Energy expenditure method	N losses method	PA/BA	Dietary reporting
Bingham et al., 1995[45] Bingham and Day, 1997[63]	F, 50–65 years (n = 160)	24h-R x 2 DR x 7d FFQ x 4 WR x 16d (PETRA5)	Not assessed	24-h urine x 8	Y	24-h R: [3]poor protein reporting, r = 0.01–0.5 DR: [3]poor protein reporting, r = 0.6–0.7 FFQ: [3]poor protein reporting, r = 0.01–0.5 WR: [3]good protein reporting, 92%, r = 0.78–0.87
Black et al., 1995[9]	M/F, post-obese, 21–51years (n = 11)	DH x 2 WR x 10d + WR5 x 11d	DLW	24-h urine x 5	Y	WR: poor protein reporting, 77%; poor energy reporting, 76%; calculate similar poor reporting of [fat + CHO], 76%
Heitmann and Lissner, 1995[8]	M/F, 35–65 years (n = 323)	DH	Estimated from questionnaire	24-h urine x 1	Y	DH: poor protein reporting, 85%; poor energy reporting, 76%; calculate worse underreporting of [fat + CHO], 75%. worse reporting in obese
Kahn et al., 1995[64]	M/F, hyper-tensive, middle aged (n = 244)	24-h R	Not assessed	24-h urine x 1	N	24-h R: good protein reporting, 93%
Porrini et al., 1995[65]	M/F, young (n = 44)	FFQ WR x 7d	Not assessed	24-h urine x 3	N[1]	FFQ: good protein reporting, 100% WR: good protein reporting, 102%
Visser et al., 1995[66]	F, elderly (n = 12)	DH	24h EE measured[4] x 2	24-h urine x 4	N	DH: poor protein reporting, 90%; poor energy reporting, 88%; calculate similar poor reporting of [fat +CHO], 88%
Black et al., 1997[67]	M/F, 50–87 years (n = 45) and post obese (n = 11)	WR x 16d	BMR measured[4] DLW n = 45	24-h urine x 6	Y	WR: good protein reporting, 94%; poor energy reporting, 87%; calculate worse underreporting of [fat + CHO], 86%
Katsouyanni et al., 1997[68]	M/F, 25–67 years (n = 80)	24-h R x 12 FFQ x 2	Not assessed	24-h urine x 3	N	24-h R: protein reporting, 0.47 FFQ: protein reporting, 0.33
Moulin et al., 1997[69]	M/F, diabetics, 38–69years, (n = 15)	WR x 4d	Not assessed	24-h urine x 4	N	WR (high prot): good protein reporting, 105% WR (low prot): poor protein reporting, 87%
Ocke et al., 1997[70]	M/F, 20–70 years (n = 121)	24-h R x 12 FFQ	Predicted BMR	24-h urine x 4	Y	24-h R: poor protein reporting, 88% EI/BMR = not reported FFQ: good protein reporting, 91% EI/BMR: 1.46
Pisani et al., 1997[71]	M/F, middle aged (n = 197)	24-h R x 8–12 FFQ x 4	Predicted BMR	24-h urine x 4–6	N	24-h R: good protein reporting, r = 0.56; EI/BMR = 1.6; FFQ: poor protein reporting, r = 0.21; EI/BMR = 1.5

Table 1. Continued.

Author	Subjects	Diet assessment method	Energy expenditure method	N losses method	PA/BA	Dietary reporting
Riboli et al., 1997[72]	M/F, 50–69 years (n = 53)	DH FFQ WR x 18d	Not assessed	24-h urine x 6–8	N	DH: protein over-reported, 117% FFQ: protein over-reported, 117% WR: good protein reporting, 98%
Johansson et al., 1998[36]	F, lean and overweight, 20–50 years (n = 74)	FFQ WR x 4d	Predicted BMR	24-h urine x 1	Y	WR: poor protein reporting, 86% EI/BMR = 1.35
Klipstein-Grobusch et al., 1998[73]	M/F, middle aged/elderly (n = 80)	DR x 15d FFQ	Predicted BMR	24-h urine x 4	N	DR: good protein reporting, 107% EI/BMR = 1.44 FFQ: protein over-reported, 120% EI/BMR = 1.49
Kroke et al., 1999[74]	M/F, 35–67 years (n = 134)	24-h R x 12d FFQ	DLW n = 28 subset	24-h urine x 4	Y	24-h R: poor protein reporting, 72%; poor energy reporting, 74%; calculate similar poor reporting of [fat + CHO], 74% FFQ: poor protein reporting, 79% poor energy reporting, 80%; calculate similar poor reporting of [fat + CHO], 80%
Lindroos et al., 1999[12]	M/F, over-weight, 16–62 years (n = 29)	24-h R	24h EE measured[4]	24-h urine x 1	N	24-h R: poor protein reporting, 81%; good energy reporting, 99% (BUT under-reporting when compared to free-living EE); cannot assess [fat + CHO]
Luhmann et al., 1999[75]	M/F, 60+ years (n = 343)	DR x 3d	BMR measured[4]	24-h urine (n = 23)	N[1]	DR: good protein reporting, 100% EI/BMR = 1.6, worse energy reporting in obese
Black et al., 2000[13]	F, 50–65 years (n = 48)	DH WR x 16d[5]	DLW (subset n = 16)	24-h urine x 8	Y	DH: good protein reporting, 96%; good energy reporting, 95%; calculate similar good reporting of [fat + CHO], 95% WR: good protein reporting, 94%; poor energy reporting, 88%; calculate worse under-reporting of [fat +CHO], 87%
Daures et al., 2000[76]	M/F, middle aged (n = 87)	FFQ DR x 12d WR x 16d5	Predicted BMR	24-h urine x 4–8 (n = 40)	Y	FFQ: [3]protein reporting, r = 0.40 DR: [3]protein reporting, r = 0.43 WR: [3]protein reporting, r = 0.60 no data for% reporting provided
Heitmann et al., 2000[77]	M/F, 30–60years (n = 228, 122)	DH-1987/8 DH- 1993/4	Predicted BMR and activity questionnaire	24-h urine x 1	Y	1987/8: poor protein reporting, 85%; poor energy reporting, 76%; calculate worse under-reporting of [fat +CHO], 75% 1993/4: good protein reporting, 96%; poor energy reporting, 79%; calculate worse under-reporting of [fat + CHO], 76%

Table 1. *Continued.*

Author	Subjects	Diet assessment method	Energy expenditure method	N losses method	PA/ BA	Dietary reporting
Day et al., 2001[78]	M/F, 45–74 years (n = 123)	DR × 7d FFQ	Not assessed	24-h urine × 6	Y	DR: poor protein reporting, 88% FFQ: good protein reporting, 98%
Kipnis et al., 2001[50]	F, 50–65 years (n = 160)	FFQ WR × 16d[5]	Not assessed	24-h urine × 8	Y	Model suggests previous trials are underpowered and protein intake from FFQ is in error (no data on under-reporting provided)
MacIntyre et al., 2001[79]	M/F, 15–65 years (n = 74)	WR × 7d	Predicted BMR	24-h urine × 1 (n = 46)	Y	WR: Energy reporting was better than protein reporting. No data for% reporting provided
McKeown et al., 2001[80]	M/F, 45–74 years (n = 134)	DR × 14d FFQ × 2	Not reported	24-h urine × 6	Y	DR: good protein reporting, 104% FFQ: protein over-reported, 119%
Pedersen et al., 2001[81]	M/F, elderly (n = 34)	DH DR × 3d	Predicted BMR and activity questionnaire	24-h urine × 1	Y	DH: good protein reporting, 110%; poor energy reporting; assume worse [fat + CHO] under-reporting DR: good protein reporting, 110%; poor energy reporting; assume worse [fat + CHO] under-reporting
Sanchez-Castillo et al., 2001[82]	F, 20–45 years (n = 41)	WR × 7d	BMR measured[4]	24-h urine × 1	Y	WR: good protein reporting, 103% EI/BMR = 1.43
Schroder et al., 2001[83]	M/F, young/middle aged (n = 44)	24-h R × 3d FFQ DR × 3d	Not assessed	24-h urine × 6	N	24-h R: protein over-reported, 142% FFQ: protein over-reported, 187% DR: protein over-reported, 134%
Larsson et al., 2002[84]	M/F, 16–20 years (n = 32)	DH	DLW	24-h urine × 4	Y	DH: good agreement of N intake with losses (underestimate of 0.4 ± 1.9 g N/day); poor energy reporting, 87%; assume worse [fat + CHO] under-reporting

PABA, p-amino benzoic acid; M, male; F, female; BMR, basal metabolic rate; DLW, doubly labelled water; 24-h R, 24-h recall; DH, diet history; DR, diet record; DQ, diet questionnaire; FFQ, food frequency questionnaire; WR, weighed record; *P < 0.05, **P < 0.01, ***P < 0.001.
[1] 24-h creatinine excretion measured.
[2] PABA was used but recovery was so poor that the results were ignored and all 24-h urine collections were included in the final analysis.
[3] Pearsons correlation coefficient.
[4] Indirect calorimetry.
[5] Portable Electronic Tape Recorded Automatic (PETRA) scales, weight and a spoken description of each food are automatically recorded onto a cassette tape. Subjects are blinded to weight of food items.

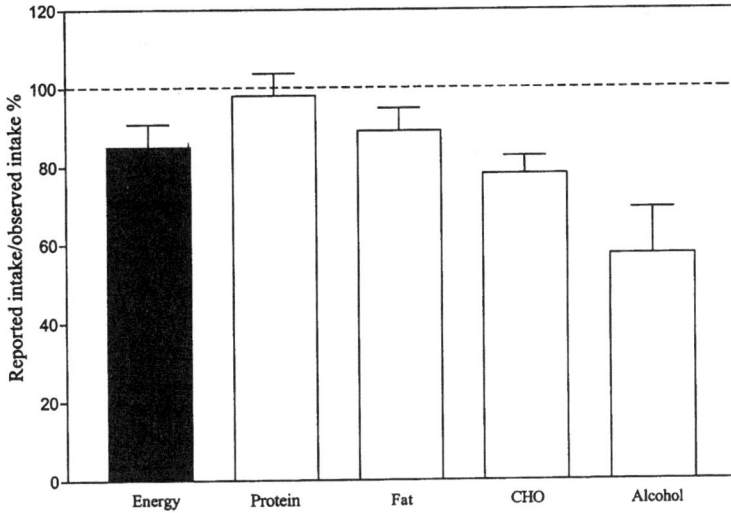

Fig. 1. Energy, protein, fat and CHO reporting in a group of 33 lean and obese women observed within a metabolic facility. Mean ± sem.

snacks both in a group of age stratified individuals[86] and in a study of obese men and women[8]. A recent trial by Goris and coworkers however showed no selective omission of snack foods, rather they showed worse reporting of lunch, dinner and evening snack foods when compared with breakfast and morning snacks[87].

Conclusions

There is some evidence from this review of diet survey studies that protein intake may be more reliably estimated than either energy or non-protein [fat + CHO] intake. The use of independent biomarkers by which to validate energy and macronutrient intakes is strongly recommended. Protein intake can be both easily and cheaply validated through 24-h urinary N collections, the completeness of which should be determined using the PABACHEK method.

References

1. Livingstone M et al. Accuracy of weighed dietary records in studies of diet and health. BMJ 1990; 300: 708–12.

2. Schoeller D, Bandini L, Dietz W. Inaccuracies in self reported intake identified by comparison with the doubly labelled water method. Can J Physiol Pharm 1990; 68: 941–49.

3. Bandini L, Schoeller D, Cyr H, Dietz W. A validation of reported energy intake in obese and non-obese adolescents. Am J Clin Nutr 1990; 52: 421–25.

4. Westerterp K, Verboeket-van-de-Venne W, Meijer G, tenHoor F. Self-reported intake as a measure for energy intake. A validation against doubly labelled water. Int J Obes 1991; 15: 3S.

5. Black A, Prentice A, Goldberg G. Measurements of total energy expenditure provide insights into the validity of dietary measurements of energy intake. J Am Diet Assoc 1993; 93: 572–79.

6. Black A. Physical activity levels (PAL) from a meta-analysis of doubly labeled water studies for validating energy intake as measured by dietary assessment. Nutr Rev 1996; 54: 170–74.

7. Heitmann B. The influence of fatness, weight change, slimming history and other lifestyle variables on diet reporting in adult Danish men and women aged 35–65 years. Int J Obes 1993; 17: 329–36.

8. Heitmann B, Lissner L. Dietary underreporting by obese individuals – is it specific or non-specific? BMJ 1995; 311: 986–89.

9. Black A, Jebb S, Runswick S, Poppitt S. The validation of energy and protein intakes by double-labeled water and 24-h urinary nitrogen excretion in post-obese subjects. J Hum Nutr Diet 1995; 8: 51–64.

10. Lafay L. et al. Determinants and nature of dietary underreporting in afree-living population: the Fleurbaix Laventie Ville-Sante (FLVS) Study. Int J Obes 1997; 27: 567–73.

11. Poppitt S, Swann D, Black A, Prentice A. Assessment of selective under-reporting of food intake by both obese and non-obese women in a metabolic facility. Int J Obes 1998; 22: 303–11.

12. Lindroos A, Lissner L, Sjostrom L. Does degree of obesity influence the validity of reported energy and protein intake? Results from the SOS Dietary Questionnaire. *Eur J Clin Nutr* 1999; 53: 375–78.

13. Black A, Welch A. Bingham S. Validation of dietary intakes measured by diet history against 24h urinary nitrogen excretion and energy expenditure measured by the doubly labelled water method in middle-aged women. *Br J Nutr* 2000; 83: 341–54.

14. Heywood P, Harvey P, Marks G. An evaluation of energy intake in the 1983 Australian National Dietary Survey of Adults. *Eur J Clin Nutr* 1993; 47: 604–6.

15. Klesges R, Eck L, Ray J. Who underreports dietary intake in dietary recall? Evidence from the second National Health and Nutrition Examination Survey. *J Consult Clin Psychol* 1995; 63: 438–44.

16. Ballard-Barbash R, Graubard I, Krebs-Smith S, Schatzkin A, Thompson F. Contribution of dieting to the inverse association between energy intake and body mass index. *Eur J Clin Nutr* 1996; 50: 98–106.

17. Fogelholm M, Mannisto S, Vartiainen E, Pietinen P. Determinants of energy balance and overweight in Finland 1982and 1992. *Int J Obes* 1996; 20; 1097–1104.

18. Briefel R, Sempos C, McDowell M, Chien S, Alaimo K. Dietary methods research in the third National Health and Nutrition Examination Survey: under-reporting of energy intake. *Am J Clin Nutr* 1997; 65: 1203S–1209S.

19. Price G, Paul A, Cole T, Wadsworth M. Characteristics of the low-energy reporters in alongitudinal national dietary survey. *Br J Nutr* 1997; 77: 833–51.

20. Pryor J, Vrijheid M, Nichols R, Kiggins M, Elliott P. Who are the 'low energy reporters' in the dietary and nutritional survey of British adults? *Int J Epidemiol* 1997; 26: 146–54.

21. Rothenberg E, Bosaeus I, Steen B. Evaluation of energy intake estimated by a diet history in three free-living 70 year old populations in Gothenberg, Sweden. *Eur J Clin Nutr* 1997; 51: 60–6.

22. Gnardellis C, Boulou C, Trichopolou A. Magnitude, determinants and impact of under-reporting of energy intake in a cohort study of Greece. *Public Health Nutr* 1998; 1: 131–37.

23. Braam L, Ocke M, Mesquita HB, Seidell J. Determinants of obesity-related underreporting of energy intake. *Am J Epidemiol* 1998; 147: 1081–86.

24. Voss S, Kroke A, Klipstein-Grobusch K, Boeing H. Is macronutrient composition of dietary intake data affected by underreporting. Results from the EPIC-Potsdam study. *Eur J Clin Nutr* 1998; 52: 119–126.

25. Lichtman S, Berman E, Pestone M. Discrepancy between self-reported and actual caloric intake and exercise in obese subjects. *N Engl J Med* 1992; 327: 1893–98.

26. Black A. *et al.* Critical evaluation of energy intake data using fundemantal principles of energy physiology: 2. Evaluating the results of published surveys. *Eur J Clin Nutr* 1991; 45: 583–99.

27. Goldberg G. *et al.* Critical evaluation of energy intake data using fundamental principles of energy physiology. 1. Derivation of cut-off values to identify under-recording. *Eur J Clin Nutr* 1991; 45: 569–81.

28. Willett W, Stampfer M. Implications for epidemiologic analyses. *Am J Epidemiol* 1986; 124: 17–27.

29. Trichopolous A. *et al.* Consumption of olive oil and specific food groups in relation to breast cancer risk in Greece. *J Nat Cancer Inst* 1995; 87: 110–16.

30. Flegal K. Energy underreporting: implications for the use of energy-adjusted nutrients in epidemiologic research. *Eur J Clin Nutr*, S17. s.d.

31. Evaluating epidemiologic evidence of the effects of food and nutrient exposures. *Am J Clin Nutr.* 1999 Jun; 69(6): 1339S–1344S. Review.

32. Flegal K, Larkin F. Partitioning macronutrient intake estimates from a food frequency questionnaire. *Am J Epidemiol* 1990; 131: 1046–58.

33. Brown C. *et al.* Energy adjustment methods for nutritional epidemiology: The effect of categorization. *Am J Epidemiol* 1994; 139: 323–38.

34. Wacholder S *et al.* Can energy adjustment separate the effects of energy from those of specific macronutrients? *Am J Epidemiol* 1995; 142: 225–6.

35. Bellach B, Kohlmeier L. Energy adjustment does not control for differential recall bias in nutritional epidemiology. *J Clin Epidemiol* 1998; 51: 393–98.

36. Willett W. *Nutritional epidemiology*. Oxford: Oxford University Press, 1998.

37. Johansson G, Akesson A, Berglund M, Vahter M. Validation with biological markers for food intake of a dietary assessment method used by Swedish women with three different dietary preferences. *Public Health Nutr* 1998; 1: 199–206.

38. Beynen A. A mathematical relationship between the fatty acid composition of the diet and that of adipose tissue in man. *Am J Clin Nutr* 1980; 81–5.

39. VanStaverenW. *et al.* Validity of the fatty acid composition of subcutaneous adipose tissue microbiopsies as an estimate of the diet of separate individuals. *Am J Epidemiol* 1986; 123: 455–63.

40. London S. *et al.* Fatty acid composition of subcutaneous adipose tissue and diet in postmenopausal US women. *Am J Clin Nutr* 1991; 54: 340–5

41. Hunter DJ, Rimm EB, Sacks FM, Stampfer MJ, Colditz GA, Litin LB, Willett WC. Comparison of measures of fatty acid intake by subcutaneous fat aspirate, food frequency questionnaire, and diet records in a free-living population of US men. *Am J Epidemiol* 1992; 135: 418–27.

42. Tjønneland A, Overvad K, Thorling E, Ewertz M. Adipose tissue fatty acids as biomarkers of dietary exposure in Danish men and women. *Am J Clin Nutr* 1993; 57: 629–33.

43. Sarkkinen E, Agren J, Ahola I, Ovaskinen M-L, Uusitupa M. Serum fatty acid composition of cholesterol esters, and erythrocyte and platelet membranes as indicators of long term adherence to fat-modified diets. *Am J Clin Nutr* 1994; 59: 364–70.

44. Ma J, Folsom AR, Eckfeldt JH, Lewis L, Chambless LE. Short- and long-term repeatability of fatty acid composition of human plasma phospholipids and cholesterol esters. The Atherosclerosis Risk in Communities (ARIC) Study Investigators. *Am J Clin Nutr*. 1995; 62(3): 572–8.

45. Bingham S, Cummings J. The use of 4-aminobenzoic acid as a marker to validate the completeness of 24 h urine collections in man. *Clin Sci* 1983; 64: 629–35.

46. Bingham S. *et al*. Validation of weighed records and other methods of dietary assessment using the 24h urine nitrogen technique and other biological markers. *Br J Nutr* 1995; 73: 531–50.

47. Bingham S. Urine nitrogen as an independent validatory measure of protein intake. *Br J Nutr* 1997; 77: 144–48.

48. Isaksson B. Urinary nitrogen output as a validity test in dietary surveys. *Am J Clin Nutr* 1980; 33: 4–5.

49. Johansson G, Bingham S, Vahtner M. A method to compensate for incomplete 24-hour urine collections in nutritional epidemiology studies. *Public Health Nutr* 1999; 2: 587–91.

50. Jakobsen J, Oveson L, Fagt S, Pedersen A. Para-aminobenzoic acid used as a marker for completeness of 24 hour urine: assessment of control limits for a specific HPLC method. *Eur J Clin Nutr* 1997; 51: 514–19.

51. Kipnis V. *et al*. Empirical evidence of correlated biases in dietary assessment instruments and its implications. *Am J Epidemiol* 2001; 153: 394–403.

52. Bingham S, Cummings J. Urine nitrogen as an independent validatory measure of dietary intake. *Am J Clin Nutr* 1985; 42: 1276–89.

53. Steen B, Isaksson B, Svanborg A. Intake of energy and nutrients and meal habits in 70-year-old males and females in Gothenburg, Sweden. A population study. *Acta Med Scand* 1977; 611: 39S–86S.

54. vanStaveren W, deBoer J, Burema J. Validity and reproducibility of a diet history method estimating the usual food intake during one month. *Am J Clin Nutr* 1985; 42: 554–9.

55. Kahn H. A step towards using urinary nitrogen as a tool for validating 24-hour dietary recall. *Eur J Epidemiol* 1987; 3: 308–11.

56. Warwick P, Williams L. Dietary intake of individuals interested in eating ahealthy diet: a validated study of intake before and after dietary advice. *Hum Nutr: Appl Nutr* 1987; 409–25.

57. Hulten B, Bengtsson C, Isaksson B. Some errors inherent in a longitudinal dietary survey revealed by the urine nitrogen test. *Eur J Clin Nutr* 1990; 44: 169–74.

58. Kunkel M, Beauchene R. Protein intake and urinary excretion of protein-derived metabolites in aging female vegetarians and nonvegetarians. *J Am Coll Nutr* 1991; 10: 308–14.

59. O'Donnell, M, Nelson M, Wise P, Walker D. A computerised diet questionnaire for use in diet health education.1. Development and validation. *Br J Nutr* 1991; 66: 3–15.

60. Johansson G, Callmer E, Gustafsson J. Validity of repeated measurements in a dietary intervention study. *Eur J Clin Nutr* 1992; 46: 717–28.

61. Petersen M, Haraldsdottir J, Hansen H, Jensen H, Sandstrom B. A new simplified dietary history method for measuring intake of energy and macronutrients. *Eur J Clin Nutr* 1992; 46: 551–59.

62. Rothenberg E. Validation of the food frequency questionnaire with the 4-day record method and analysis of 24-h urinary nitrogen. *Eur J Clin Nutr* 1994; 48: 725–35.

63. Lindroos A, Lissner L, Sjostrom L. Validity and reproducibility of a self administered dietary questionnaire in obese and non-obese subjects. *Eur J Clin Nutr* 1993; 47: 461–81.

64. Bingham S, Day N. Using biocheminal markers to assess the validity of prospective dietary assessment methods and the effect of energy adjustment. *Am J Clin Nutr* 1997; 65: 1130S–1137S.

65. Kahn H. *et al*. Validity of 24-hour dietary recall interviews conducted among volunteers in an adult working community. *Annals Epidemiol* 1995; 5: 484–9.

66. Porrini M, Gentile M, Fidanza F. Biochemical validation of a self-administered semi-quantitative food-frequency questionnaire. *Br J Nutr* 1995; 74: 323–3.

67. Visser M, deGroot L, Deurenberg P, vanStaveren W. Validation of dietary history method in a group of elderly women using measurements of total energy expenditure. *Br J Nutr* 1995; 74: 775–85.

68. Black A, Bingham S, Johansson G, Coward W. Validation of dietary intake of protein and energy against 24 hour urinary N and DLW energy expenditure in middle-aged women, retired men and post-obese subjects: comparisons with validation against presumed energy requirements. *Eur J Clin Nutr* 1997; 51: 405–13.

69. Katsouyanni K. *et al.* Reproducibility and relative validity of an extensive semi-quantitative food frequency questionnaire using dietary records and biochemical markers among Greek schoolteachers. *Int J Epidemiol* 1997; 26: S118–S127.

70. Moulin C. *et al.* Use of weighed diet records in the evaluation of diets with different protein contents in patients with type 2 diabetes. *Am J Clin Nutr* 1997; 67: 853–7.

71. Ocke M. *et al.* The Dutch EPIC food frequency questionnaire. II. Relative validity and reproducibility for nutrients. *Int J Epidemiol* 1997; 26: S49–58.

72. Pisani P. *et al.* Relative validity and reporducibility of a food frequency dietary questionnaire for use in the Italian EPIC Centre. *Int J Epidemiol* 1997; 26: S152–S160.

73. Riboli E, Elmstahl A, Saracci R, Gullberg B, Lindgarde F. The Malmo food study: validity of two dietary assessment methods for measuring nutrient intake. *Int J Epidemiol* 1997; 26: S161–S173.

74. Klipstein-Grobusch K. *et al.* Dietary assessment in the elderly: validation of a semiquantitative food frequency questionnaire. *Eur J Clin Nutr* 1998; 52: 588–96.

75. Kroke A. *et al.* Validation of a self-administered food frequency questionnaire administered in the European Prospective Investigation into Cancer and Nutrition (EPIC) Study: comparison of energy, protein and macronutrient intakes estimated with the doubly labelled water, urinary nitrogen and repeated 24-h dietary recall methods. *Am J Clin Nutr* 1999; 70: 439–47.

76. Luhrmann P, Herbert B, Gaster C, Neuhauser-Berthold M. Validation of a self-administered 3-day estimated dietary record for use in the elderly. *Eur J Nutr* 1999; 38: 235–40.

77. Daures J. *et al.* Validation of a food-frequency questionnaire using multiple-day records and biochemical markers: applications of the triads method. *J Epidemiol Biostatistics* 2000; 5: 109–15.

78. Heitmann B, Lissner L, Osler M. Do we eat less fat, or just report so? *Int J Obes* 2000; 24: 435–42.

79. Day N, McKeown N, Wong M, Welch A, Bingham, S. Epidemiological assessment of diet: a comparison of a 7-day diary with a food frequency questionnaire using urinary markers of nitrogen, potassium and sodium. *Int J Epidemiol* 2001; 30: 309–17.

80. MacIntyre U, Venter C, Vorster H, Steyn H. A combination of statistical methods for the analysis of the relative validation data of the quantitative food frequency questionnaire used in the THUSA study. Transition, Health and Urbanisation in South Africa. *Public Health Nutr* 2001; 4: 45–51.

81. McKeown N. *et al.* Use of biological markers to validate self-reported dietary intake in a random sample of the European Prospective Investigation into Cancer, United Kingdom Norfolk cohort. *Am J Clin Nutr* 2001; 74: 188–96.

82. Pedersen A, Fagt S, Ovesen L, Schroll M. Quality control including validation in dietary surveys of elderly subjects. The validation of a dietary history method (the SENECA-method) used in the 1914-population study in Glostrup of Danish men and women aged 80 years. *J Nutr Health & Aging* 2001; 5: 208–16.

83. Sanchez-Castillo C. *et al.* Are the proposed limits of energy intake: basal metabolic rate and dietary nitrogen: urinary nitrogen ratios suitable for validation of food intake? *Br J Nutr* 2001; 85: 725–31.

84. Schroder H. *et al.* Use of a three-day estimated food record, a 72-hour recall and a food-frequency questioonaire for dietary assessment in a Mediterranean Spanish population. *Clin Nutr* 2001; 20: 429–37.

85. Larsson C, Westerterp K, Johansson G. Validity of reported energy expenditure and enrgy and protein intakes in Swedish adolescent vegans and omnovores. *Am J Clin Nutr* 2002; 75: 268–74.

86. Beerman K, Dittus K. Sources of error associated with self-reports of food intake. *Nutr Rev* 1993; 13: 765–70.

87. Summerbell C, Moody R, Shanks J, Stock M, Geissler C. Sources of energy from meals vs. snacks in 220 people in four age groups. *Eur J Clin Nutr* 1995; 49: 33–41.

88. Goris A, Westerterp-Plantenga M, Westerterp K. Undereating and underrecording of habitual food intake in obese men: selective underreporting of fat intake. *Am J Clin Nutr* 2000; 71: 130–34.

Progress in Obesity Research: 9. Edited by *Geraldo Medeiros-Neto, Alfredo Halpern and Claude Bouchard*
©2003 John Libbey Eurotext Ltd, pp. 519–522.

CHAPTER 109

Reporting of fat and carbohydrate: the protein-energy-reporting method

Berit L. Heitmann

Research Unit for Dietary Studies, Danish Epidemiological Science Centre, Institute of Preventive Medicine, Copenhagen University Hospital, DK-1399 Copenhagen K, Denmark
[e-mail: blh@ipm.hosp.dk]

Introduction

Valid information on the habitual diet is difficult to obtain as all techniques rely on information supplied by the subjects themselves. Numerous papers have shown substantial underreporting of either dietary energy or protein using methods such as Doubly Labelled Water or 24-h urine nitrogen output as reference[1]. However, more recently it has been demonstrated that total underreported energy exceeds underreported energy from protein, e.g. only a fraction of the total calories underreported was energy from protein. As a consequence other macronutrients must have been underreported too, suggesting that foods rich in fat and/or carbohydrate are specifically underreported[2]. The present paper is concerned with this issue.

Estimating protein intake

A number of studies document that 24-h urinary nitrogen output can be used as a valid marker for protein intake at the population level, based on the fact, that most of the nitrogen derived from amino acids produced by protein catabolism, is excreted in urine. This is discussed elsewhere in these proceedings. In brief the principle behind this method relates to the fact that protein ingested in excess

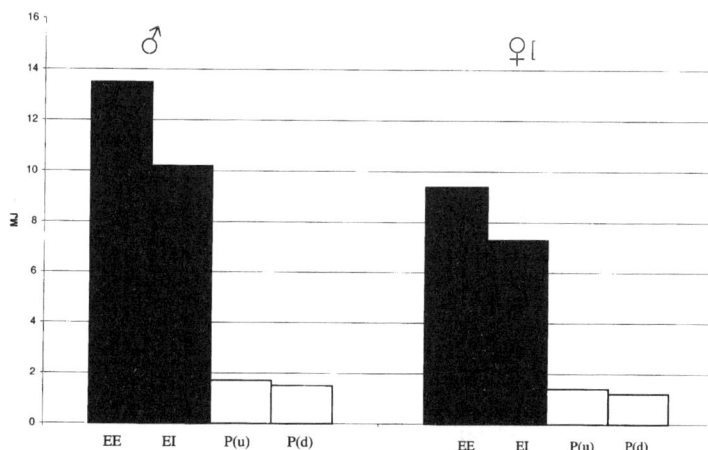

Fig. 1. Reported and measured intake (MJ) of total energy and energy from protein in men and women (from Heitmann & Lissner, 1995).
EE = Energy expenditure; EI = Energy intake (from diet);
P(u) = Energy from protein (calculated from urinary nitrogen); P(d) = Energy from protein (from diet).

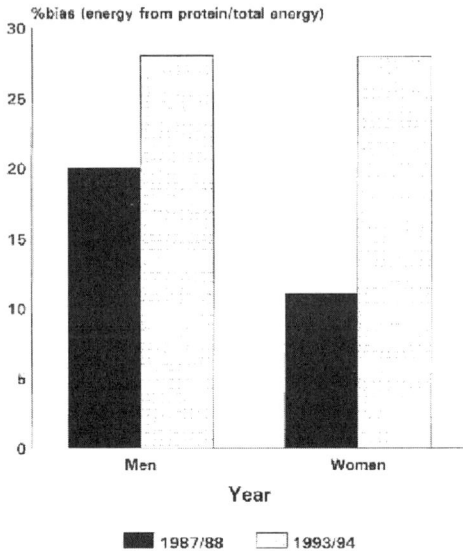

%bias (energy from protein/total energy)

Men   Woman

Year

■ 1987/88   □ 1993/94

Fig. 2. Degrees of underreported total energy relative to underreported energy from protein* from the surveys in 1987–88 and 1993–94 in Danish men and women (from Heitmann, Lissner & Osler, 2001).
* Protein intake (diet)/Protein intake (urine)
  Energy intake (diet)/Energy intake (24EE)

increase nitrogen excretion whereas when dietary protein is reduced, the amino acids are used more efficiently and less nitrogen is excreted[3,4].

Estimating total energy intake

Assuming energy balance, estimation of total energy intake can be made, both by the doubly labelled water method[5] and by the more simple estimates of 24-h energy expenditure (24EE) that are based on the calculation of multiples of physical activity level factors (PAL) and basal metabolic rate estimated from measures either of height and weight or of body composition[6]. The simple methods have shown good agreement with the doubly labelled water, albeit correct assessment of the PAL values is of great importance for the absolute agreement between the methods. These methods are discussed in more details elsewhere in these proceeding.

Underreporting of energy and protein

When diet intake is evaluated using methods that estimate total energy intake or protein intake, most studies find that habitual diet is generally underreported, and simultaneous use of both methods suggests that the same individuals are identified as underreporters by both methods[7]. Specifically the obese, but also subjects with a history of dieting, subject with a subjective weight problem, the so-called post-obese or other weight conscious subjects have been found to underreport their diet intake[1].

Reporting of fat and carbohydrate

There are no direct measures of fat or carbohydrate intakes although the fatty acids levels in blood, cell membranes and subcutaneous fat are possible indicators. However, the fatty acid profile more likely reflects the qualitative fatty acid intake than the absolute intake[8]. However, an indication that fat and/or carbohydrate may be underreported can be derived from a number of ways. For instance, a few studies have suggested selective underreporting of snacks, cakes, pastries, and confectionary types of food with a usually high fat and/or sugar content[9]. Alsoy results from different methods (food records, diet history interviews, quantative FFQs) have revealed differences in the densities from the macronutrients, even when energy intake was found to be similar using the different methods[10,11]. Such comparisons illustrate that bias in diet reporting of macronutrients may be method- and even population specific. Finally, more recently[12], Gorris et al. recorded both undereating and underrecording among 30 obese men keeping 7-day diet records. They defined underreporting as the difference between doubly labelled water estimated energy expenditure and energy intake computed from the food records. Undereating was calculated from the weight loss during the one-week observation. Underrecording was estimated from water losses assuming a similar accuracy of recording water intake and food intake. The data revealed a reverse relation between reported percentage of energy from fat and the percentage of

INTENSIFIED DIET CAMPAIGNS
Danish food agency, heart foundation, cancer society, and consumer agency

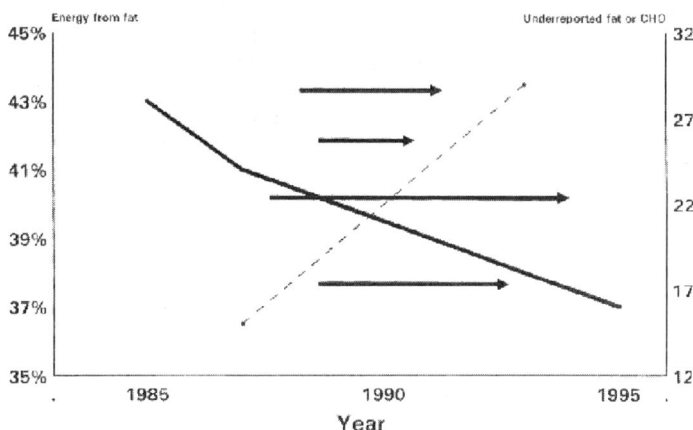

Fig. 3. The decrease in dietary energy from fat relative to bias in diet reporting and diet campaign activities in the period from 1985 to 1995 (data from the Danish food agency and Heitmann and Lissner, 1995 and Heitmann, Osler and Lissner 2000).

underreporting, suggesting a selective omission of fatty foods. A final approach has involved the comparison of underreported total energy in relation to underreported energy from protein, a so-called protein-energy reporting method[2]. The latter method will be discussed in the following.

The energy-protein-reporting method

The Energy-Protein-Reporting method uses discrepancies between reporting bias for total energy, and energy from protein to describe the size of underreported fat and/or carbohydrate.

The idea was developed[2] that underreporting of fat and/or carbohydrate could be quantified by estimating the absolute energy deficit from reported protein out of total underreported energy[2]. In the initial study, bias in dietary reporting of energy and protein intake was assessed by comparing data from a interview of dietary intake with data estimated from 24-h nitrogen output and estimated 24-h energy expenditure calculated from body composition and PAL. Completeness of 24-urine sample was monitored using the 4-aminobenzoic acid method. Basal energy expenditure was calculated according to a formulae developed by Garby et al.[13] based on fat-free mass and fat mass (derived from impedance). The physical activity level was assumed to be 1.55 in men and 1.56 in women for those who were unemployed or whose work was classified as sententry. 1.78 and 1.64 among those whose work was classified as light activity and 2.10 and 1.82 among those engaged in heavy and strengthened work or engaged actively in sports[14].

In total 322 subjects had complete information on diet intake and 24-h urine excretion and energy expenditure. In general estimates of total energy and total protein intake calculated from the dietary interview were lower than those calculated from the urine or energy expenditure analyses (all $P < 0.0001$). Estimate of percentage energy from protein calculated from the dietary interview was significantly higher than estimates based on urinary nitrogen (all $P < 0.0001$). Only 15 per cent and 28 per cent did not underreport total energy and protein respectively.

Figure 1 shows total energy and energy from protein estimated from reported dietary intake and calculated urinary nitrogen output/24-h energy expenditure in men and women. In both genders the difference between reported and estimated total energy was much larger than the difference for energy from protein.

A second study was performed 6 years later with similar information on total energy and protein intake from urinary nitrogen and estimates of 24-h energy expenditure[15]. This study showed an even larger underreporting of the fat and/or carbohydrate fraction of the diet (Fig. 2). The increase in reporting bias between the two surveys may offer one explanation for the apparent downward trend in reported fat intake seen in Denmark and possibly also other countries[15]. The results are in agreement with data from a Finnish study[16] and with food supply statistics also showing no increase in measured fat consumption[17].

In 1987–88 underreporting bias for fat and/or carbohydrate was more pronounced among the obese. In the second study performed in 1993–94 even the non-obese displayed substantial underreporting. The fraction of underreporting among obese is well described, whereas underreporting among lean and normal weight is less common. In Denmark several campaigns to reduce fat intake and intake of simple carbohydrates were launched in the late 1980s and in the beginning of the 1990s (Fig. 3). Assuming that the non-obese have no obvious social inclination to underreport their diet intake, the underreporting among the non-obese may suggest a possible increased awareness of diet intake related to intensified public health campaigns to reduce intake of fat and/or simple carbohydrates, that were not necessarily directed towards obesity prevention, but other conditions, such as cardiovascular disease and cancer.

Conclusion

Simultaneous use of methods that assess protein and energy intake has demonstrated that total energy is underreported more so than energy from protein suggesting that other macronutrients, e.g. fat and/or carbohydrate must be underreported too. Data from two studies performed six years apart suggest that the bias and underreporting is increasing, and that reporting bias was similar for the lean and the obese in the more recent data compared to the early study. It is possible that this fat/carbohydrate specific underreporting is responsible for the apparent trend of declining fat intake in Denmark. The findings have implications for our understanding of the health benefits of the apparent decline in dietary fat.

References

1. Heitmann BL. The influence of fatness, weight change, slimming history and other lifestyle variables on diet reporting in Danish men and women aged 35–65 years. *Int J Obes* 1993; 17: 329–36.

2. Heitmann BL, Lissner L. Dietary underreporting by obese individuals – is it specific or non-specific? *BMJ* 1995; 311: 986–9.

3. Isaksson B. Urinary nitrogen output as a validity test in dietary surveys. *Am J Clin Nutr* 1980; 33: 4–5.

4. Bingham SA, Cummings JH. Urine nitrogen as a independent validatory measure of dietary intake; a study of nitrogen balance in individuals consuming their normal diet. *Am J Clin Nutr* 1985; 42: 1276–89.

5. Schoeller DA, Racette SB. A review of field techniques for the assessment of energy expenditure. *J Nutr* 1990; 120 Suppl 11: 1492–5.

6. Black AE, Goldberg GR, Jebb SA, Livingstone MBE, Cole TJ, Prentice AM. Critical evaluation of energy intake data using fundamental principles of energy physiology: 2. Evaluating the results of published surveys. *Eur J Clin Nutr* 1991; 45: 583–99.

7. Bingham SA Validation of dietary assessment through biomarkers. In: *Biomarkers of dietary exposure*, Kok FJ, Vait Veer P (eds), pp. 41–52. London: Smith-Gordon; 1991.

8. Willett W. *Nutritional epidemiology* (2nd edn). Oxford University Press; 1998.

9. Poppitt SD, Swann D, Black AE, Prentice AM. Assessment of selective under-reporting of food intake by both obese and non-obese women in a metabolic facility. *Int J Obes* 1998; 22: 303–11.

10. Lissner L, Lindroos AK. Is dietary underreporting macronutrient-specific? *Eur J Clin Nutr* 1994; 48(6): 453–4.

11. Rutishauser IH. Is dietary underreporting macronutrient specific? *Eur J Clin Nutr* 1995; 49(3): 219–20.

12. Goris AHC, Westerterp-Plantenga MS, Westerterp KR. Undereating and underrecording of habitual food intake in obese men: selective underreporting of fat intake. *Eur J Clin Nutr* 2000; 71: 130–4.

13. Garby L, Garrow JS, Jørgensen B, Lammert O, Madsen K, Sørensen P, Webster J. Relation between energy expenditure and body composition in man; specific energy expenditure *in vivo* of the fat and fat-free tissue. *Eur J Clin Nutr* 1988; 42: 301–5.

14. Word Health Organisation. Measuring obesity-classification ad description of anthropometric data. Report on a Who consultation of the epidemiology of obesity. Warsaw 1987 Oct. 21–23; Copenhagen: WHO; 1989. (Nutrition Unit document, EUR/ICP/NUT 125).

15. Heitmann BL, Lissner L, Osler M. Do we eat less fat, or just report so? *Int J Obes* 2000; 24: 435–42.

16. Fogelhelm M, Mannisto S, Vartiainen E, Pietinen P. Determinants of energy balance and overweight in Finland 1982 and 1991. *Int J Obes Relat Metab Disord* 1996; 20(12): 1097–104.

17. *Statistisk Årbog 1995*. (Statistical Yearbook). Statistics Denmark; Copenhagen, 1995.

Progress in Obesity Research: 9. Edited by *Geraldo Medeiros-Neto, Alfredo Halpern and Claude Bouchard*
©2003 John Libbey Eurotext Ltd, pp. 523–526.

CHAPTER 110

Cognitive control of eating behaviour and long-term management of body weight in children and adults

Joachim Westenhoefer[1,2], Stephanie Fintelmann[3], Claudia Sievers[4], Jörg Spirik[2], Rainer Stachow[4], Astrid Stellfeldt[1,2], Uwe Tiedjen[4] and Bettina von Falck[1,2]

[1]*Hamburg University of Applied Sciences, Department of Nutrition and Home Economics, Hamburg, Germany;* [2]*HealthBehavior.de GmbH, Schwarzenbek, Germany;* [3]*Precon GmbH & Co KG, Bickenbach, Germany;* [4]*Fachklinik Sylt, Westerland, Germany*
[e-mail: joachim@westenhoefer.de]

Long-term results of obesity treatment are generally disappointing[1]. One of the reasons may be that the conscious and deliberate restriction of food intake, often denominated as dietary restraint or cognitive control of food intake, has been related to disordered eating patterns such as, for example, binge eating[2]. It has been shown however, that dietary restraint includes different aspects of behaviour that may have different consequences with regard to eating disorders and weight control. In particular, Westenhoefer and colleagues[3,4] have shown that flexible control of eating behaviour is associated with less disturbed eating patterns and better weight control, whereas rigid control of eating behaviour is associated with disordered eating patterns and poorer weight control. However, these findings were based on cross-sectional data or longitudinal data limited to one year. The present paper presents results extending these findings to periods of over three years.

Lean Habits Study

The Lean Habits Study is a prospective longitudinal study on the association between behaviour and long-term weight reduction. Since 1998 a cohort of over 8000 participants of the BCM Diet Programme has been recruited and is now followed up for three years.

The BCM Diet Programme is a treatment programme for overweight and obesity, which is offered by more than 1800 independent counselling practices in Germany and other European Countries. It aims at reducing body fat by a balanced diet rich in carbohydrates which is supplemented by a formula diet at the start of the programme. Counselling of the patients takes place in an open group format led primarily by physicians and includes behaviour modification techniques to induce a lasting change of diet and eating behaviour. Participants for the Lean Habits Study have been recruited at 400 counselling centres primarily in Germany.

Body weight has been measured as well as several behavioural factors assessed using a self-administered questionnaire at the beginning of the programme. For follow-up reassessments using the same measures take place after approximately 10 weeks and after one, two and three years.

For the present paper we investigated the influence of two sets of behavioural factors on successful weight reduction which was defined as a weight reduction of 5 per cent or more from baseline weight. Successful weight reduction was predicted by separate logistic regression analyses on two sets of behavioural variables. Set 1 consisted of flexible and rigid control of eating behaviour. These variables were assessed with short forms of the published scales[4]. Set 2 consisted of six questionnaire scales: meal rhythm (regular meal rhythm and meal frequency, avoidance of snacking and nibbling), food choice (avoidance of fatty foods, sweets or fatty snacks and preference of less fatty foods, vegetables and fruit), meal situations (sitting down, taking time and rest for eating, avoidance of other activities while eating), restricting quantity (of food eaten), physical activity (exercise and every day activities), coping with stress (e.g. subjective feeling of stress, conscious relaxation, eating behaviour and emotional stress). Successful weight reduction after one year was predicted from behaviour after 10 weeks, success after two years from behaviour after one year, and finally success after three years from behaviour after two years.

After one year, from the 8185 subjects who were included in the study for more than one year, 32.6 per cent had successfully reduced their weight by 5 per cent or more, 11.1 per cent had not sucessfully reduced their weight, and 56.4 per cent could not yet be reassessed. After two years, from the 7186 subjects included in the study for more than two years, 17.0 per cent had successfully reduced their weight, 11.1 per cent had not successfully reduced their weight, and 71.9 per cent could not yet be reassessed. After three years, from the 3472 subjects included in the study for more than three years, 12.4 per cent had successfully reduced their weight, 9.4 per cent were not successful in weight reduction, and 78.2 per cent could not yet be reassessed.

The logistic regression analyses (Table 1) of successful weight reduction on flexible and rigid control showed consistently that every additional score of flexible control significantly increased the likelihood of successful weight reduction (change of odds-ratio > 1) for one, two and three years. In addition, rigid control significantly decreased the likelihood of successful weight reduction (change of odds-ratio < 1) after one and two years.

Table 1. Results from the logistic regression analysis of successful weight reduction on behavioural factors

	Change in odds-ratio for successful weight reduction after		
	1 year	2 years	3 years
Logistic regression on			
flexible control	1.1*	1.3*	1.2*
rigid control	0.8*	0.8*	0.9
Logistic regression on			
meal rhythm	1.2*	1.2*	1.1
food choice	1.1*	1.2*	1.1
meal situations	1.1*	1.2*	1.2
restricting quantity	1.0	1.1	1.1
physical activity	1.0	1.0	1.1
coping with stress	1.1*	1.1*	1.1

*$P < 0.05$ for the corresponding regression coefficient.

Logistic regression analyses on the second set of behavioural variables (Table 1) showed, that the likelihood of successful weight reduction after one and two years was significantly increased by a regular meal rhythm, healthy food choices, appropriate meals situations and adequate coping with stress.

Weight maintenance in obese children and adolescents

In order to investigate the role of flexible and rigid control in the long-term weight management of children we conducted a follow-up study of obese children and adolescents who have undergone initial inpatient treatment for obesity in the Children and Adolescent Rehabilitation Hospital Sylt in Westerland, Germany. Included in the study were 307 boys and 355 girls, who participated between 1995 and 1998 in the obesity treatment. On initial treatment boys were on average 13.2 years old (range 8.7–18.0), girls 13.7 years (range 9.1–20.4). The average follow-up period was 43 ± 14 months (mean ± SD, range 22–68 months) after initial treatment. During follow-up assessment, weight and height was measured by the patients' physician and the patients completed a German children version of the Eating Inventory[5], including scales to assess flexible and rigid control. Relative body weight was evaluated using

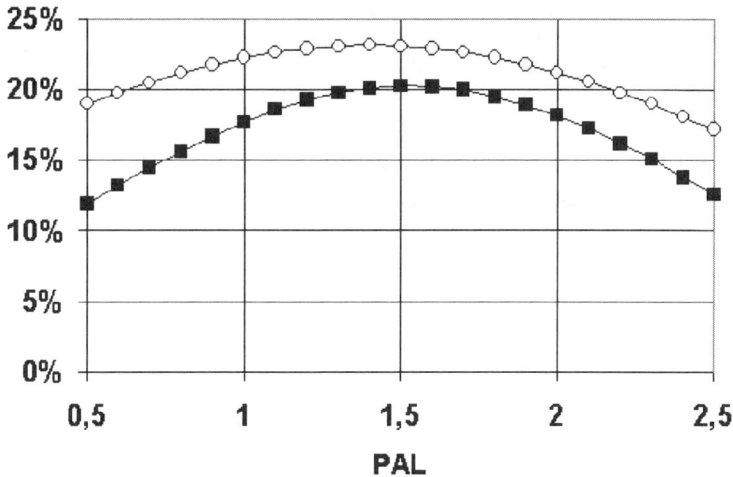

Fig. 1. Percentage of subjects with successful one-year weight reduction (women open circles; men: black squares) predicted by logistic regression analysis dependent on EI/BMR (adjusted for BMI and age).

the age and gender specific BMI standard deviation scores (BMI-SDS) computed by the LMS-method[6] in relation to the recently published German population norms[7].

Before initial treatment the 642 patients had a BMI-SDS of 2.1 ± 0.6 (mean ± SD) which was reduced to 1.9 ± 0.6 during treatment. At follow-up we were able to measure weight and height in 291 patients. Mean BMI-SDS at follow up was 1.8 ± 0.9. Children who maintained a BMI-SDS equal or below pre-treatment BMI-SDS were defined as successful weight maintainers ($n = 158$), children who had a BMI-SDS exceeding pre-treatment values were defined as unsuccessful ($n = 133$). When comparing successful weight maintainers and unsuccessful regainers, successful maintainers had significantly higher overall cognitive restraint scores and higher flexible control ($P < 0.05$), while they showed no difference in rigid control. Thus the importance of increased flexible control of eating behaviour for long-term weight control has been confirmed for children and adolescents.

Self-monitioring of eating behaviour and successful weight reduction

Self-monitoring of food intake is considered to be one of the key techniques of behaviour modification[8], which should be included in any basic obesity treatment[9]. Indeed, the ability to monitor food intake may be considered of central importance for adequate self-control of eating behaviour. Given this central importance of self-monitoring in the treatment of obesity, there is an apparent lack of knowledge about the consequences of inaccurate self-monitoring on the outcome of therapy. In order to investigate the consequences of inaccurate self-monitoring on attrition and successful weight reduction over one year we analysed the data of a rather large sample from a computer-assisted weight reduction programme.

The sample was selected from the participants of the Four-Seasons-Programme (Vier-Jahreszeiten-Kur), a computer-assisted weight reduction programme over 12 months[3,4]. For the present analysis we selected participants who kept dietary records for 5 to 14 days during initial assessment and who did not indicate a change of body weight while monitoring food intake. A total of 47,437 participants qualified for inclusion using these criteria. Self-reported energy intake EI was computed from the dietary records. In order to define possible over- or underreporting basal metabolic rate (BMR) was computed for each subject according to the Schofield-formulas based on sex, age and weight[10]. The ratio of self-reported energy intake to computed BMR (EI/BMR) was used to evaluate accurate self-monitoring and over- and underreporting. According to Black et al.[11] EI/BMR below 1.4 may be considered as indicative of underreporting, whereas EI/BMR above 2.0 are indicative for overreporting under normal conditions.

We used logistic regression analysis to predict successful weight reduction (5 per cent or more below baseline weight) after 1 year from EI/BMR ratios. As may be seen from Fig. 1, the highest rates of successful weight reduction are associated with EI/BMR ratios of 1.5 which are in the plausible biological range. However, subjects who severely underreport (EI/BMR < 1.0) or overreport (EI/BMR > 2.0) their intakes, are less likely to reduce their weight successfully after 1 year. A parallel analysis of the likelihood of staying in the programme for one year yielded very similar results (not shown). Thus, unrealistic self-monitoring of food intake and eating behaviour is associated with higher attrition from the weight management programme and poorer one year success in weight reduction.

Conclusions

Taken together the studies reported in the present paper show that certain behavioural factors are associated with successful long-term weight management. In particular, flexible control of eating behaviour has been shown to significantly increase the likelihood of successful weight reduction over periods of over three years, in adults as well as in children and adolescents. In contrast, rigid control of eating behaviour yields significantly poorer long-term weight control at least over periods of up to two years. In addition, a number of other behavioural factors, such as meal rhythm, meal situations and appropriate food choice are predictive of mediate term successful weight reduction. The results from the Four-Seasons-Programme show, that successful cognitive control of eating behaviour requires the ability to adequately perceive and monitor the own eating behaviour and food intake. Severe misperceptions and the misreporting of food intake have a negative impact on the participation in and outcomes of long-term weight management efforts. Thus increasing self-monitoring skills and flexible control of eating behaviour should be key requirements of future weight management attempts.

Reference

1. Ayyad C, Andersen T. Long-term efficacy of dietary treatment of obesity: a systematic review of studies published between 1931 and 1999. *Obes Rev* 2000; 1: 113–19.

2. Herman CP, Polivy J. Restrained eating. In: Stunkard A (ed.) *Obesity*, pp. 208–25. Philadelphia: Saunders; 1980.

3. Westenhoefer J. Dietary restraint and disinhibition: is restraint a homogeneous construct? *Appetite* 1991; 16: 45: 55.

4. Westenhoefer J, Stunkard AJ, Pudel V. Validation of the flexible and rigid control dimensions of dietary restraint. *Int J Eating Disord* 1999; 26: 53–64.

5. Stunkard AJ, Messick S. The three-factor eating questionnaire to measure dietary restraint, disinhibition and hunger. *J Psychosom Res* 1985; 29: 71–83.

6. Cole TJ. The LMS method for constructing normalized growth standards. *Eur J Clin Nutr* 1990; 44: 45–60.

7. Kromeyer-Hauschild K, Wabitsch M, Geller F, Ziegler A, Geiß HC, Hesse V *et al.* Perzentile für den Body Mass Index für das Kindes- und Jugendalter unter Heranziehung verschiedener deutscher Stichproben. Monatsschr. Kinderheilk. 2001; 149: 807–18.

8. Wing RR. Behavioral approaches to the treatment of obesity. In: Bray GA, Bouchard C, James WPT (eds) *Handbook of obesity*, pp. 855–73. New York: Marcel Dekker; 1998.

9. World Health Organisation Obesity. *Preventing and managing the global epidemic.* Geneva: WHO; 1998.

10. Schofield WN. Predicting basal metabolic rate, new standards and review of previous work. *Hum Nutr: Clin Nutr* 1985; 39 Suppl 1: 5–41.

11. Black AE, Coward WA, Cole TJ, Prentice AM. Human energy expenditure in affluent societies: an analysis of 574 doubly-labelled water measurements. *Eur J Clin Nutr* 1996; 50: 72–92.

Progress in Obesity Research: 9. Edited by *Geraldo Medeiros-Neto, Alfredo Halpern and Claude Bouchard*
©2003 John Libbey Eurotext Ltd, pp. 527–532.

CHAPTER 111

The relationship between low self-esteem and obesity

Andrew J. Hill

Academic Unit of Psychiatry and Behavioural Sciences, School of Medicine, University of Leeds, 15 Hyde Terrace, Leeds LS2 9LT, UK
[e-mail: a.j.hill@leeds.ac.uk]

Introduction

With the acceptance of an association with physical health problems, comes an increasing recognition that obesity has psychological consequences[1,2]. Obese adults are at increased risk of depression and binge eating disorder, especially if female. Most frequently observed is a relationship between obesity and low self-regard, in the form of body dissatisfaction, bodily shame, or low self-esteem. The purpose of this chapter is to ask some basic questions about the relationship between low self-esteem and obesity. First, what degree of association exists and by what is it moderated? Second, what is the likely direction of association and why is the association relatively weak? Third, how does obesity impact on different conceptualizations of self-esteem? Lastly, what are the treatment implications?

Obesity and global self-esteem

Low self-esteem and obesity do not invariably co-occur. Reviewing the literature on children and adolescents, French *et al.*[3] observed that only 13 of the 25 cross-sectional studies showed significantly lower self-esteem in obese youngsters. Adolescents aged 13–18 years showed the clearest effects, but little difference was apparent in children aged 7–12. Although in six of eight treatment studies weight loss programmes appeared to improve self-esteem, it was unclear whether these increases were related to enhanced weight loss. Moreover, even when detected, low self-esteem amounted to a modest impairment that rarely fell below the normal range.

These authors noted several features of the literature that contributed to the inconsistency in outcome. One was sample size, with nearly half of the studies reviewed including fewer than 100 participants. A second was the varying definitions of overweight and obesity adopted. And as important were inconsistencies in the type of self-esteem assessments.

To accommodate for these methodological issues, Miller and Downey[4] conducted a meta-analysis of all publications that included a global measure of self-esteem and the relevant statistics for testing the relationship between overweight or obesity and self-esteem. In all they found 91 effect sizes reported in 71 studies. The mean weighted correlation between overweight and global self-esteem was −0.18, equivalent to Cohen's d = −0.36 (95 per cent CI −0.33 to −0.40). Overall, this indicated a robust but small to moderate size relationship between overweight and self-esteem.

The large number of studies enabled Miller and Downey to examine the effect of several hypothesized moderating variables. Those with the greatest impact on effect size were weight dissatisfaction, gender, age, and socio-economic status (SES). Specifically, the correlations between overweight and global self-esteem were significantly higher in:

- Studies measuring weight dissatisfaction compared with actual weight (r = −0.34 vs. −0.12);

- Women than in men (−0.23 vs. −0.09);

- Young adults than in adolescents, than in children (−0.28 vs. −0.22 vs. −0.12);

- High SES than in low SES individuals (–0.31 vs. –0.16).

Interpreting associations

The preceding meta-analysis, while establishing that overweight and low global self-esteem are related, fails to answer two key questions. What is the direction of cause and effect, and why is the correlational relationship relatively weak?

In a review of the causes and consequences of low self-esteem, Emler[5] notes a range of different possibilities for explaining a correlational relationship between low self-esteem and a health outcome. In addition to it being either a direct or indirect causal influence, thereby making someone less able to implement behaviours necessary to slow weight gain, low self-esteem may act to mediate or moderate the effects of other environmental factors on obesity. In contrast, low self-esteem may itself be an effect or correlated outcome of being obese, an argument strongly supported by accounts of the stigmatization of obesity. Alternatively, and very likely in dynamic health situations, the relationship may represent a causal loop, such that low self-esteem and obesity both exert cause and effect on each other. Such causal loops are almost never closed, making them very difficult to break.

The complexity of the causal process in part explains why the correlational relationship is weak. Low self-esteem can have various effects on an obese person and their ability to alter behaviours relevant to energy balance. However, many factors contribute to the development and maintenance of obesity. Low self-esteem is probably a minor contributor, albeit one with the potential to interact with other risk factors. And weight is undoubtedly only one of several influences on an individual's sense of self-worth.

The alternative causal direction, of obesity leading to low self-esteem, has been the argument of choice. However, two further features of these measures are critical to understanding their weak inter-relationship. First, both are resistant to change. Obesity is notoriously difficult to reduce, and even when weight is lost much of it is regained. Self-esteem is also resistant to change since it is a higher order schema or internalized theory about the self. This deep knowledge structure is acquired early, often derived from emotionally significant experiences to which an individual has little conscious access[6]. Any threat to stability produces anxiety and is therefore avoided. It comes as a surprise to many that low self-esteem, like high self-esteem, is strongly defended.

Second, researchers have paid insufficient attention to the conceptualization of self-esteem and to how it is measured. Most psychologists and social scientists would agree that at its most basic, self-esteem represents a generalized feeling about the self that is more or less positive. This evaluation of global self-worth was the focus of the meta-analysis by Miller and Downey[4]. However, there are more elaborate conceptualizations, and two in particular offer interesting alternatives to the relationship between obesity and low self-esteem. These will be explored using the outcome of some our recent research with children and adolescents.

Domains of perceived competence

The representation of self-esteem as the ratio of a person's successes to their pretensions has been attributed to William James[6]. Fundamental to this idea is that self-esteem represents the personal evaluation of competence in areas that are deemed personally (and culturally) important. Someone with low self-esteem falls short of their ideals by perceiving themselves less competent in particular domains of skills or valued personal attributes. In addition, they may fail to discount the importance of domains in which they feel less competent. However, it is this discrepancy between competence and importance that defines overall self-worth.

Susan Harter has developed both this conceptualization and the associated assessments of perceived self-competence for several age groups[6]. She argues that for children domains of competence are set by parents (e.g. scholastic competence, behavioural conduct) and peers (physical appearance, social and athletic competences), and that these expand in number through adolescence into adulthood. The questionnaire assessments include several items from each domain, each item presenting respondents with two contrasting statements, for example in the domain of social competence, 'Some kids find it *hard* to make friends BUT other kids find it pretty *easy* to make friends.' The child has first to choose which description is most like them, and then rate their choice as either 'Sort of true for me' or 'Really true for me'. The result is a profile of competence in several domains, alongside an assessment of global self-worth, together with a measure of the perceived importance of each domain.

A few years ago, we reported that obese 9-year old girls scored significantly lower on physical appearance and athletic competence than their normal weight peers[7]. Importantly, their mean scores fell just below the mid-point of both these scales, indicating that on average, these obese girls judged themselves as more similar to the depictions of an unattractive and unathletic child. Although their rating of global self-worth was lower than that of normal weight girls, the difference just failed to reach statistical significance.

Girls aged 12, in their first year at senior school, show a similar impact of obesity (Murphy and Hill, in preparation). In this study there was a significant effect of obesity on overall self-esteem. The obese young adolescents had significantly lower athletic competence and global self-worth, and marginally lower physical appearance self-esteem. Interestingly, in neither the 12-year olds nor the 9-year olds was there an effect of obesity on domain importance. Neither age group of girls differed from their normal weight peers even on the domains (athletic and physical appearance) in which they considered themselves less competent. This suggests that obese girls were not responding to their reduced sense of competence by devaluing the importance of success in these domains.

A comparison of Junior and Senior school boys is also revealing in that it showed no relationship between obesity and low self-esteem on any aspect of perceived competence (Hill *et al.*, in preparation). Nor did being thin (BMI<15th percentile) have any consequence for self-esteem. For young and pre-adolescent British boys at least, body weight appears to have very little impact on self-evaluation.

The social basis of self-esteem

An alternative perspective on self-esteem derives from Charles Cooley's notion of the 'looking glass self'[5]. Here, self-esteem is primarily social in nature and is based on the judgments we imagine others to make of us. Those with low self-esteem perceive others to have little regard for them, and feel demeaned, neglected, or socially isolated. Especially influential are the behaviours and opinions of significant others such as parents, friends, and partners.

So what does this perspective hold for obesity? We have looked at peer popularity in several of the studies of obese children described above. In contrast with children's stereotyped perception of the social isolation of fat people[8], obese children do not rate themselves lower on Harter's scale of social competence than do their normal weight peers.

Indeed, this positive social view has some external credibility. We have used a peer nomination procedure to investigate children's popularity. This involves providing children with a same-sex class list and asking them to identify up to three others with whom they would most like to socialize inside and outside of class. The resulting popularity index shows that neither age group of obese girls or boys is disadvantaged in terms of peer choices. The one caveat is that a similar procedure to evaluate peer-rated attractiveness showed obese girls to be much less likely identified as attractive compared with their normal weight peers. Nine- and 12-year old normal weight girls received 4.6 and 2.6 attractiveness nominations compared with a mean of less than 1 nomination for either group of obese girls. And since attractiveness was the most important predictor of peer rated popularity[7], it may only be time before obese adolescent girls experience a decline in popularity.

Mark Leary has extended this social view to question the basic function of self-esteem[9]. His 'sociometer theory' proposes that the self-esteem system evolved as a monitor of social acceptance, it's motive being not to maintain self-esteem *per se*, but to avoid social devaluation and rejection. He argues that people are particularly sensitive to changes in relational evaluation, the degree to which others regard their relationship with the individual as valuable, important, or close. Accordingly, self-esteem is lowered by failure, criticism, or rejection and raised by success, praise and events associated with relational appreciation. Even the possibility of rejection can lower self-esteem. Low self-esteem is associated with believing oneself without the socially desirable attributes such as competence, likeability, or physical attractiveness. Overall, Leary considers that the relationship between low self-esteem and psychological problems has been overstated. Such problems (and by implication obesity) are not caused by low self-esteem but by a history of low relational evaluation, if not outright rejection. Accordingly, low self-esteem may parallel problems but is a co-effect rather than their cause.

Taking Leary's perspective on self-esteem as a gauge of social acceptance versus rejection, it is pertinent to look at circumstances where people have been socially rejected by being victimized because of their overweight. Some 40 per cent of US obese adults report having experienced weight-related mistreatment, over half of them from their spouse and two thirds from strangers[10]. The most frequently encountered stigmatizing situations included comments from children, people making negative personal assumptions, being stared at, and inappropriate comments from doctors[11]. Although encountered on average less than once per year they were not benign experiences. Stigmatization frequency was negatively correlated with measures of mental health, body dissatisfaction, and self-esteem and these

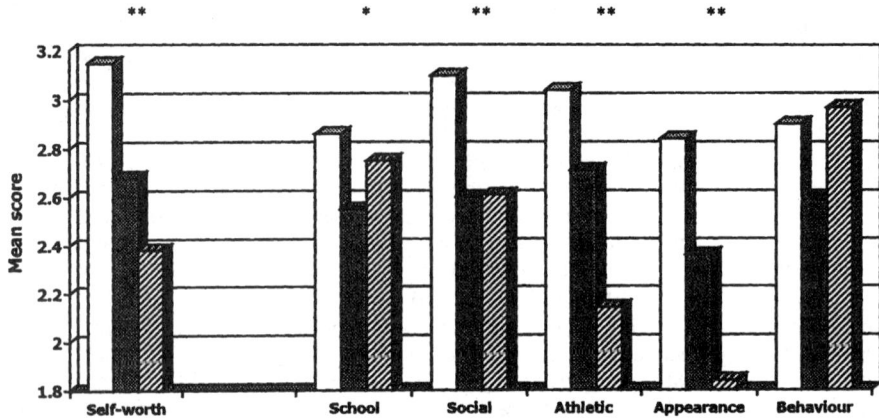

Fig. 1. Self-esteem in 12-year-old children not victimized (open columns), fat-teased boys (closed columns) and fat-teased girls (hatched columns). Significant effects of victimization, *P < 0.05, **P < 0.001.

associations were still present when BMI was included as a covariate. In other words, it was the frequency of these events that was important.

Children are part of this persecutory milieu. They stigmatise on the basis of appearance and in turn are stigmatized for overweight. We have looked at 'fat-teasing' in young adolescent children in the UK using questionnaire items inserted into Harter's Self-Perception Profile for Children[12]. In this study, 12 per cent of 12-year old girls and 16 per cent of boys described themselves as being teased or bullied for overweight. Although these victimized children were heavier than their non-victimized peers, less than half were either overweight or obese. Importantly, being fat-teased was associated with low body shape satisfaction and low self-esteem. As Fig. 1 shows, fat-teased girls and boys had significantly lower global self-worth, and lower perceived competence in all domains except behavioural conduct. Fat-teased girls in particular saw themselves as unattractive, unathletic and with low global self-worth. This portrayal was maintained when weight was added as a covariate, again showing the impact of victimization. However, victimization had no effect on the perceived importance of any of these domains. Once more, it would appear that these children were not modifying the importance of domains in which they judged themselves less competent.

The consequences of losing weight

If childhood (and adult) obesity does impact on self-esteem then treatments that lead to weight loss should be accompanied by self-esteem improvements, and the two outcomes related to each other. In the majority of intervention studies reviewed by French et al.[3] an increase in self-esteem was observed but without any association with body weight decrease.

In another of our studies we have looked at self-esteem in obese adolescents attending a residential, activity-based weight loss camp in the UK[13]. Fifty-seven obese adolescents (mean BMI = 32.6) attended the camp for an average of 4 weeks. They completed the Self-Perception Profile for Children at the start and end of their stay and were compared with an age-matched group of normal weight children. Over this period the campers lost 5.6 kg (SE ± 0.4), a highly significant decrease, reducing their mean BMI by 2.1 kg/m^2. In contrast, the comparison group showed a small but significant 0.4 kg/m^2 increase. Figure 2 summarizes the self-esteem of obese adolescents at both time periods. Overall, their scores were significantly lower than the comparison adolescents on every measure other than social acceptance. Significant group by time interactions showed that by the end of their stay the obese adolescents had increased their global self-worth, physical appearance and athletic competence. However, despite the improvement they still fell short of the positive self-perception of the comparison group and their self-perception remained as relatively unattractive and unathletic.

Several components of self-esteem were significantly and negatively correlated with BMI at the start of the camp (global self-worth r(93) = −0.44, P < 0.001; physical appearance r = −0.51, P < 0.001; athletic competence r = −0.30, P < 0.01). Most importantly, there was a significant correlation between the degree of BMI loss and the increase in global self-worth (r = 0.50, P < 0.001), physical appearance (r = 0.39, P < 0.001), and athletic competence (r = 0.28, P < 0.01). Restricting the analysis to campers

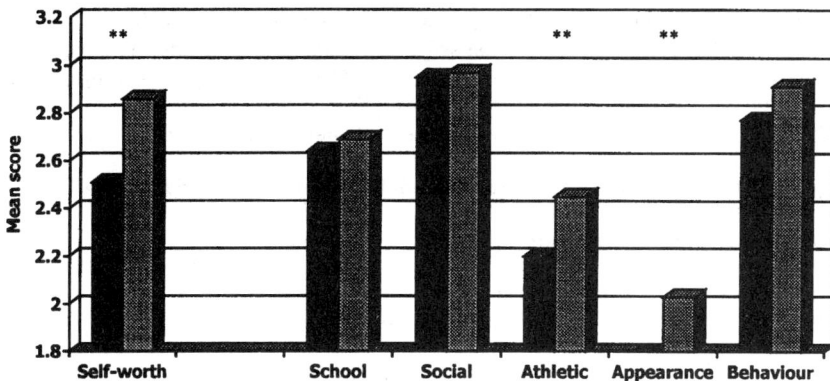

Fig. 2. Self-esteem in adolescents attending a summer weight-loss camp at the start (dark columns) and end (light columns) of their stay. Significant pre–post differences, **P < 0.001.

alone, only the relationship between BMI loss and increased global self-worth remained significant (r(55) = 0.43, P < 0.01). Finally, BMI was not associated with domain importance either at the start of the camp or in matching the degree of change. Indeed, in neither group of adolescents did domain importance change over the assessment period. The main psychological achievement of these weight-reducing obese adolescents therefore was to improve their current perception of physical attractiveness and athletic ability rather than re-negotiate the perceived importance of these attributes.

Conclusions

Low self-worth is not the only facet of self-esteem associated with obesity. For young adolescent girls at least, obesity is related to physical appearance dissatisfaction and poor athletic competence. Given the opportunity to lose weight these are the very areas that improve. Social acceptance is unaffected as long as the child is not victimized for their fatness.

Harter has suggested that low self-esteem adolescents may seek to improve their situation by discounting the importance of domains they perceive themselves to be low in competence[6]. No evidence for this was apparent in our research. Nor was there evidence of an alternative strategy: that of distorting perceived competence. Low physical appearance esteem concurrent with good social acceptance were validated by the obese girls' classmates.

It has also been observed that the perceived controllability of a stigma impacts on the attribution of prejudice and that obese college-age women are more likely to make internal attributions relating to their perceived personal inadequacy or lack of deservingness[14]. Many obese individuals are denied the use of self-esteem protective strategies such as externalizing blame since the clinical and public health climate for obesity reduction emphasizes individual eating and activity changes and the importance of will-power. The resultant self-blame may itself be part of the sustaining cycle of low self-esteem

A major challenge to providing effective treatment for child and adult obesity will be to enable a person to change weight-relevant behaviour in a state of high self-esteem and self-efficacy. Emler[5] notes that people with low self-esteem treat themselves badly and invite bad treatment by others. Health professionals working to achieve weight reduction must guard against acting on this invitation. A closer examination of the psychological defence processes that people use to maintain high self-esteem is well merited.

Acknowledgements: Thanks to Professor Ian Caterson, Human Nutrition Unit, Sydney University, for his assistance in the preparation of this chapter.

References

1. Friedman MA, Brownell KD. Psychological correlates of obesity: Moving to the next research generation. *Psychol Bull* 1995; 117: 3–20.

2. Hill AJ. Psychological aspects of obesity. *Psychiatry* 2002; 1: 28–32.

3. French SA, Story M, Perry CL. Self-esteem and obesity in children and adolescents: A literature review. *Obes Res* 1995; 3: 479–90.

4. Miller CT, Downey KT. A meta-analysis of heavyweight and self-esteem. *Pers Soc Psychol Rev* 1999; 3: 68–84.

5. Emler N. Self-esteem: *The costs and causes of low self-worth*. York: Joseph Rowntree Foundation; 2001.

6. Harter S. Causes and consequences of low self-esteem in children and adolescents. In: Baumeister RF (ed.) *Self-esteem: The puzzle of low self-regard*, pp. 87–116. New York. Plenum; 1993.

7. Phillips RG, Hill AJ. Fat, plain, but not friendless: Self-esteem and peer acceptance of obese pre-adolescent girls. *Int J Obes* 1998; 22: 287–93.

8. Hill AJ, Silver E. Fat, friendless and unhealthy: 9-year-old children's perception of body shape stereotypes. *Int J Obes* 1995; 19: 423–430.

9. Leary M. Making sense of self-esteem. *Curr Dir Psychol Sci* 1999; 8,32–5.

10. Falkner NH, French SA, Jeffery RW, Neumark-Sztainer D, Sherwood NE, Morton N. Mistreatment due to weight: Prevalence and sources of perceived mistreatment in women and men. *Obes Res* 1999; 7: 572–76.

11. Myers A, Rosen JC. Obesity stigmatisation and coping: Relation to mental health symptoms, body image, and self-esteem. *Int J Obes* 1999; 23: 221–30.

12. Hill AJ, Murphy JA. The psycho-social consequences of fat-teasing in young adolescent children. *Int J Obes* 2000; 24 Suppl 1: 161.

13. Walker LLM, Gately PJ, Bewick BM, Hill AJ. Children's weight loss camps: psychological benefit or jeopardy?. *Int J Obes* 2003; 27: 748–54.

14. Crocker J, Cornwell B, Major B. The stigma of overweight: Affective consequences of attributional ambiguity. *J Pers Soc Psychol* 1993; 64: 60–70.

Progress in Obesity Research: 9. Edited by *Geraldo Medeiros-Neto, Alfredo Halpern and Claude Bouchard*
©2003 John Libbey Eurotext Ltd, pp. 533–536.

CHAPTER 112

Menopausal turmoil: behaviour and obesity

Jorge Braguinsky

Ayacucho 1547 (1112) Buenos Aires, Argentina
[e-mail: jbraguin@ciudad.com.ar]

Introduction

Menopause is a powerful example of how a physiological phenomenon could be permeated by the influence of culture. During the very long history of men on Earth, menopause meant the disappearance of women from public life and their displacement to the rear of the house (symbolically: of life).

Moreover, her life expectancy (starting from menopause) was short so nobody, including herself, cared about how she looked then. But the 20th century changed the story. That century of revolutions included one which was dramatically important: the progressive achievement of women to new positions in society – in fact all positions were possible.

Menopause can be defined strictly as the permanent cessation of menstruation resulting from the loss of ovarian activity. The generally accepted clinical criterion to define the postmenopausal state is the absence of menses for at least 12 months. But menopause is not a single event. Instead, it is a series of changes that can start many years earlier and last into the 50s or even 60s. Sometimes menopause is considered an *estrogen deficiency disorder*. But menopause is a natural biological process, not just a medical problem. Nonetheless, many events are associated with this period, both physical and psychological.

Because *it is a cultural problem too*. If several generations ago not so many women lived beyond menopause, today many live as much as one third or more of their life after menopause.

Hormonal framework

With the menopause transition, estrogen levels decline progressively, while the ovaries continues to secrete some amount of androgens. Adrenal androgens such as DHEA, DHEAs, delta4 androstenedione, which can be converted to estogens in peripheral tissues, remain as the major source of estrogen in postmenopausal women (Table 1).

In contrast to the dramatic reduction in estradiol production, the decline in testosterone is smaller (–25 per cent) from 250 to 180 microns per day. Serum testosterone concentrations decline by 50 per cent after oophorectomy in postmenopausal women. It has been suggested that testosterone replacement can reverse the decline in sexual function and also improve psychological well-being[1].

Another important point is cortisol activity. The regulation of adipose tissue metabolism by steroid hormones is related to cortisol activity. Exceedingly high levels of cortisol, as in Cushing s Syndrome, lead to visceral fat accumulation. But cortisol levels are neither modified in a significant level by age nor by menopause.

Summing up, it is not so easy to discriminate the role of hormonal factors in the production of clinical and psychological factors that can appear in women in this period. We can come closer to the answer if we assume that the fluctuation levels of sex hormones and cortisol are possible causes of women's increased susceptibility to dysphoria. Table 2 is speculative, but helps.

It is possible that all the symptoms seen in women after 50s could be the result of the interplay of these hormones.

Hormonal production	
<u>Ovaries</u>	<u>Adrenal gland</u>
Estradiol, E_2 $\downarrow\downarrow$	Δ_4 Androstenedione $\downarrow$ AGE
Progesterone O	DHEA S $\downarrow$ AGE
Testosterone $\downarrow$ 25%	
Δ_4 Androstenedione $\downarrow$ > 50%	

Table 1.

MOOD		
$\downarrow\downarrow$ ESTRADIOL	$\downarrow\downarrow$ ANDROGENS	$\uparrow\uparrow$ CORTISOL
Climateric symptoms	Psychosocial asthenia	Depression
Being prone to depression		
	Loss of sexual desire	
Sometimes being recentful		

Table 2.

Obesity: role of hormones

Estradiol, E_2	$\rightarrow\rightarrow$	femoro-gluteal fat
Cortisol	$\rightarrow\rightarrow$	visceral fat
Androgens	$\rightarrow\rightarrow$	muscle

Table 3.

Mood, sexual disfunction and depressive sympotomes

Many studies (but not all) in the last years have found increased rates of depression in women aged 45 to 45 years, but the factors that influence these factors are not clearly understood. Recently Bossworth *et al.* assessed whether high rates of depressive symptoms were associated with menopausal status, climateric symptoms an use of replacement therapy. They found that 29 per cent of women reported a high level ($\geq$ 10) of depressive disorders.

Menopausal status was not associated with depressive symptoms

The prevalence of depressive disorders disorders has been consistently higher in women than in men, an these findings cross cultural, ethnic, socioeconmomic and geographical boundaries, Studd[3].

It has been suggested that not only do genetic and psychosocial factors account for this sexual disparity, but also biological and thus neuroendocrine factors, since the gender difference is seen only after the

General Characteristics of the Sample

	Premenopausal	Postmenopausal	p
N	21	39	
Age (y)	41.9 ± 8.0	60.9 ± 6.4	<0.0001
BMI (Kg/m²)	30.1 ± 5.5	29.0 ± 4.5	0.3937

Braguinsky, González, Katz, 2002

Table 1.

Premenopausal vs. Postmenopausal: How satisfied are you with love?
(QOLY, Quality of life Inventory, 1992.)

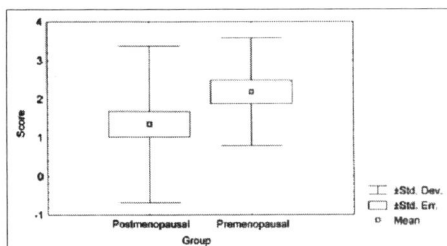

* Mann-Whitney Test p<0.05

Braguinsky, González, Katz 2

Table 3.

Premenopausal vs. Postmenopausal:
(Figure Rating Scale, 1991.)

**Correlation between Groups (pre / post menopausal)
and actual and ideal body figure (Spearman Correlation)**

	rS	t	p
Group & Actual Figure	0.21	1.643	0.106
Group & Ideal Figure	-0.68	-0.614	0.541

Correlation between actual and ideal body figure

	rS	t	p
Actual & Ideal	0.68	7.041	< 0.001

Braguinsky, González, Katz, 20

Table 5.

Premenopausal vs. Postmenopausal: Self - Esteem Score
(Rosenberg Self – Esteem Scale)

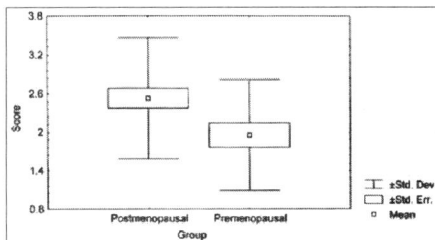

* Mann-Whitney Test p<0.05

Braguinsky, González, Katz 2

Table 2.

Premenopausal vs. Postmenopausal:
How confident are you about your capabilities
in doing everything to achieve love?
(QOLY, Quality of life Inventory, 1992.)

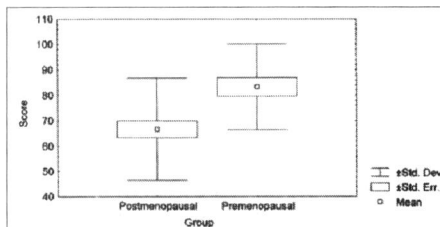

* Mann-Whitney Test p<0.05

Braguinsky, González, Katz 2

Table 4.

onset of puberty and persists until the age of 55. Controversy still exists with regard to whether there is an increased incidence of depression in the years surrounding menopause.

Our experience

I (JB) am the advisor to a very large lay association of obese people and we are studying this population. I will show here a small sample that can be useful for some final comments. The sample is composed of 60 women, 21 premenopausal and 39 postmenopausal.

Three tests were performed with all of them:

1. Rosenberg Self-Esteem Scale, Rosenberg 1965;

2. QOLY, quality of Life Inventory. Frisch, Cornell, Villanueva, Retzlaff, 1992;

3. Figure Rating Scale Thompson and Althabe, 1991.

Figure 1 shows that the differences in age in both groups are significant and the BMI are similar.
Figure 2 shows that the levels of self esteem appears as being higher in postmenopausal women. We think that it could be too speculative to try to give an explanation for this.
Figures 3 and 4, on the contrary, shows in the 2nd Study that premenopausal women are more satisfied with love and that premenopausal women are more confident about their capabilities in doing everything to achieve love.
Figure 5 shows that both groups have a good correlation between their actual and their ideal figure but there are no differences between the groups.
In spite of the fact that the number of patients in our sample is low, we think that the agreement of the results with those of most of the authors allows us to suppose that the most important factors involved in the production (or not) of mood perturbances including depression and dysthimia are social and cultural. In our sample the patients belong to a lay association with no professional direction, but for my advice.
They have weekly sessions or meetings and many assemblies, talks and conferences or lectures, and they are, usually, very successful in losing weight. They are very optimistic quite different from people that we can see in our offices, who seem to be more worried and guilty.
So it can be assumed that the environment that surrounds a menopausal woman, the way that society look at them, sharing or not, social tasks and games, and a very frequent and unveiled discussion of their obesities could be the main factors influencing mood, satisfaction, and sel-esteem in these women.

Obesity and menopause

A possible consequence of those hormonal shifts shown at the beginning is that menopause could also be a high-risk time for weight gain (with central distribution of fat) in women. Although the average women gains 2–5 pound during menopausal transition, some women are at risk of for greater weight gains. There is also a hormonal driven shift in body fat distribution from peripheral to abdominal at menopause, which may increase health risks in older women. In summary hormonal fluctuations across the female life span may explain the increased risks for obesity in women.
So, here again, the interplay between these hormones will determine not only the importance of the obesity but also the distribution of the adipose tissue that has been gained.

Reference

1. Shifren JL, Braunstein GD, Simon JA, Casson PR, Buster JE, Redmond GP *et al*. Transdermal testosterone treatment in women with impaired sexual function after oophorectomy. *N Engl J Med* 2000; 343: 682–8.

TRACK IV

EPIDEMIOLOGY, HEALTH IMPLICATIONS

Progress in Obesity Research: 9. Edited by *Geraldo Medeiros-Neto, Alfredo Halpern and Claude Bouchard*

©2003 John Libbey Eurotext Ltd, pp. 539–541.

CHAPTER 113

Estimating the health impact of obesity

Peter W.F. Wilson

Boston University School of Medicine, 715 Albany Street, Evans 204, Boston, MA 02118, USA
[e-mail: pwilson@bu.edu]

Introduction

Risk for a large number of health outcomes is increased in the presence of excessive adiposity. A variety of viewpoints can be undertaken, such as relative risk, population effects, and costs. The proportion of disease due to obesity has been estimated from several US studies. Cancers (breast, uterine, colon) tend to cluster at the lower end of the spectrum in the 10 per cent range, heart disease and hypertension are in the 15–20 per cent range, diabetes is in the 60 per cent range and sleep apnea is at the highest level, approaching 95 per cent[18].

Results[6,14]

The medical costs related to obesity provide a different account of the effects of obesity in adults. Oster and colleagues have estimated that hypertension (70million US$/year), coronary heart disease (85$ million US$/year) and type 2 diabetes mellitus (130million US$/year) cost US society the most in terms of dollars[12]. Other outcomes are important but the high cost of these diseases, coupled with the greatly increased risk observed in these persons underscores the importance of prevention and intervention for these outcomes.

It is possible to examine the relation between BMI level and various outcomes. For instance, the relation to excess adiposity for osteoarthritis, sleep apnea, and colon cancer is typically positive across all of the body mass index categories[4,7,19]. Care should be taken in the interpretation of some of these estimates as very low levels of adiposity are not necessarily indicative of good health. For instance, the BMI-mortality relation is U-shaped – persons at the lowest levels of BMI experience greater risk of death than persons at higher BMI levels[2]. Previous research has shown that cigarette smoking, underlying chronic diseases, and malignancy tend to account for the poor prognosis among persons at low BMI levels[5].

Discussion

Coronary heart disease and its underlying risk factors are highly related to excess adiposity. For instance, the prevalence of hypertension and mean lipid levels have been investigated for associations with higher levels of BMI in the Framingham Offspring cohort. The prevalence of hypertension (BP > 140/90 mm Hg or on therapy) was approximately 10 per cent at a BMI of 21 kg/m^2 and was greater in proportion to the BMI. At the obesity level (BMI > 30 kg/m^2) the prevalence of hypertension was approximately 40 per cent for middle-aged subjects[9].

Relations between BMI and lipids are more complex. With greater BMI lower mean levels of HDL-C and higher levels of VLDL-C and triglycerides have been observed . There is often no relation between LDL-C or total cholesterol and BMI.9 Earlier work in the Framingham Study showed that these greater VLDL and lower HDL levels in adults are largely due to weight gain between ages 20–50 years of age[1]. Lipoprotein patterns and their relation to obesity and weight change are more difficult to interpret in older persons after the age of 60 years of age as involuntary weight loss is common at that age.

The prevalence of diabetes is highly related to the BMI levels and weight gain in middle age is a key determinant of the later development of diabetes mellitus (figure Chan) and of risk factor clustering[3,16]. Conversely, sustained weight loss has been related to a decreased risk of subsequent type 2 diabetes mellitus in Framingham cohort participants. In comparisons to persons with a stable weight (less than

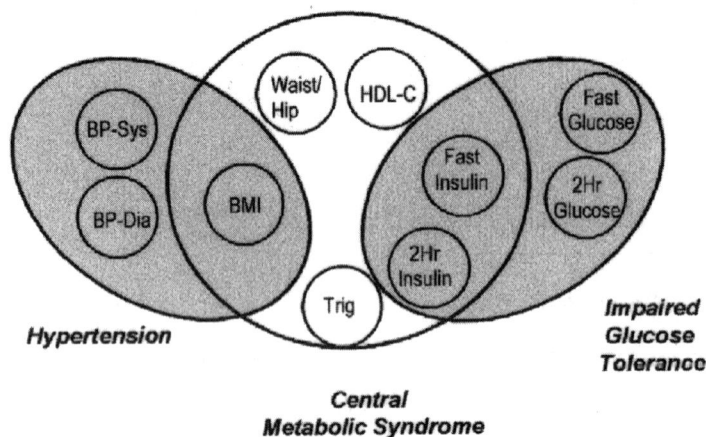

Fig. 1. Associations of risk factors considered for the metabolic syndrome. Results of principal components analysis from the Framingham Heart Study. After Meigs[10].

8 lb difference over 8 years), a loss of 8.1–15 lb conferred a 40 per cent lower risk of type 2 diabetes and a loss of more than 15 lb led to a 50 per cent lower risk of type 2 diabetes[11].

Obesity often co-exists with a variety of other risk factors that increase the risk for subsequent cardio-vascular disease or diabetes mellitus. This condition is characterized by risk factor clustering and hyperinsulinaemia. Population research has shown distinct clustering, especially for the variables in the central core of the metabolic syndrome (Fig. 1), as seen from the Framingham experience. The central factors are lipids (HDL-C and triglycerides), adiposity (BMI and waist or waist/hip), and insuli-naemia (fasting and post glucose challenge)[10]. In these correlational studies that used a technique called principal components analysis the systolic and diastolic blood pressure levels were not included in the central metabolic core. Similarly, the glucose variables from the glucose tolerance test were not in the central core, but the insulin levels were integral to the process. Such an approach is not definitive but does suggest that the metabolic syndrome, often called the insulin resistance syndrome, is not highly related to abnormal blood pressure levels or the presence of hypertension. Clinical research that uses glucose clamp data has provided different results and suggests that insulin resistance is consistently related to blood pressure[13].

Long-term follow up of Framingham participants for middle-aged and older Framingham participants has shown that higher BMI levels at a baseline exam are positively associated with the occurrence of later CHD in men and women (Fig. 2). The relations are also evident for the outcome stroke, although that the rates for that outcome are much lower and the events typically occur at a greater age[15]. Overall, the effects are cumulative and total CVD, representing the aggregate of coronary heart disease and stroke, is highly related to BMI level. The CVD effects are evident in both sexes, in younger (55–65 years) and older (66–74 years). Multivariate analyses of these outcomes typically shows that the effect of obesity on CVD risk is weakened greatly when risk factors such as HDL-C, hypertension, and

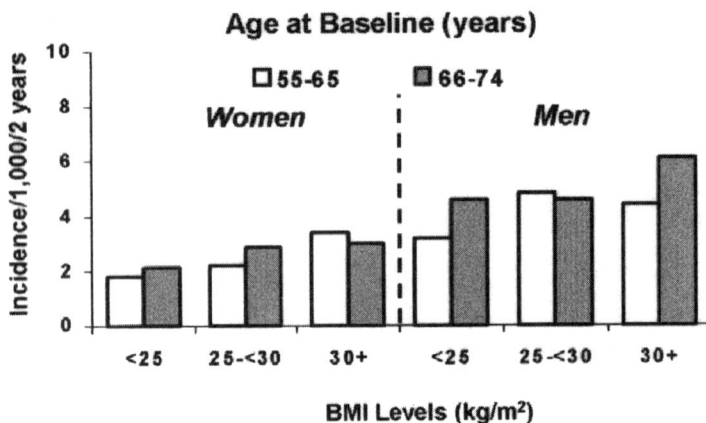

Fig. 2. 44-year experience of coronary heart disease risk in the Framingham cohort according to body mass index categories. Height and weight were obtained every 2 years and the 2 year incidence rates are shown. After Wilson[15].

diabetes are included in the prediction equations[17]. Recent research has shown that the congestive heart failure is also related to obesity and that direct effects can be attributed to this excess risk over and above the presence of hypertension or coronary artery disease. In the Framingham experience it was estimated that approximately 11 per cent of the cardiac failure event rate was attributable to a BMI > 30 kg/m^2.[8] This sort of result suggests that the primary causal factors are the lipids, blood pressure and diabetes itself and the obesity is a promoter of increased atherogenic risk through these factors and others.

Summary

A variety of outcomes have been related to adiposity. Most of the data from population studies have concentrated on using the body mass index as the measure of obesity for comparisons. As individuals with a BMI < 18.5 kg/m^2 often have chronic illnesses, this category is typically excluded from analyses and the referent group is typically in the 18.5–25 kg/m^2. With such an approach there are increased risks for many chronic disease outcomes. Especially important are the mild increases in relative risks for outcomes such as cardiovascular disease, hypertension, and diabetes at moderate degrees of adiposity. The increasing prevalence of persons in the overweight (BMI 25–30 kg/m^2) and the moderate relative risks for outcomes that are related to this category has led to greater population attributable risks for these outcomes.

References

1. Anderson KM, Wilson PWF, Garrison RJ, Castelli WP. Longitudinal and secular trends in lipoprotein cholesterol measurements in a general population sample: The Framingham Offspring Study. *Atherosclerosis* 1987; 68: 59–66.

2. Calle EE, Thun MJ, Petrelli JM, Rodriguez C,Heath CW Jr. Body-mass index and mortality in a prospective cohort of US adults. *N Eng J Med* 1999; 341: 1097–105.

3. Chan JM, Rimm EB, Colditz GA, Stampfer MJ, Willett WC. Obesity, fat distribution, and weight gain as risk factors for clinical diabetes in men. *Diabetes Care* 1994; 17: 961–9.

4. Felson DT, Zhang Y, Hannan MT, Naimark A, Weissman B, Aliabadi P, Levy D. Risk factors for incident radiographic knee osteoarthritis in the elderly: the Framingham Study.*Arthritis Rheum* 1997; 40: 728–33.

5. Garrison RJ, Castelli WP. Weight and thirty-year mortality of men in the Framingham Study. *Ann Intern Med* 1985; 103: 1006–9.

6. Gelber AC, Hochberg MC, Mead LA, Wang NY, Wigley FM, Klag MJ. Body mass index in young men and the risk of subsequent knee and hip osteoarthritis. *Am J Med* 1999; 107: 542–8.

7. Giovannucci E, Ascherio A, Rimm EB, Colditz GA, Stampfer MJ, Willett WC. Physical activity, obesity, and risk for colon cancer and adenoma in men. *Ann Intern Med* 1995; 122: 327–34.

8. Kenchaiah S, Evans JC, Levy D, Wilson PW, Benjamin EJ, Larson MG *et al.* Obesity and the risk of heart failure. *N Engl J Med* 2002; 347: 305–13.

9. Lamon-Fava S, Wilson PW, Schaefer EJ. Impact of body mass index on coronary heart disease risk factors in men and women. The Framingham Offspring Study. *Arterioscler Thromb Vasc Biol* 1996; 16: 1509–15.

10. Meigs JB, D'Agostino RB, Wilson PWF, Cupples LA, Nathan DM, Singer DE. Risk variable clustering in the insulin resistance syndrome. *Diabetes* 1997; 46: 1594–600.

11. Moore LL, Visioni AJ, Wilson PW, D'Agostino RB, Finkle WD, Ellison RC. Can sustained weight loss in overweight individuals reduce the risk of diabetes mellitus? *Epidemiology* 2000; 11: 269–73.

12. Oster G, Edelsberg J, O'Sullivan AK, Thompson D. The clinical and economic burden of obesity in a managed care setting. *Am J Managed Care* 2000; 6: 681–9.

13. Reaven GM. Insulin resistance and compensatory hyperinsulinemia: role in hypertension, dyslipidemia, and coronary heart disease. *Am Heart J* 1991; 121: 1283–88.

14. Suratt PM, Findley LJ. Driving with sleep apnea. *N Engl J Med* 1999; 340: 881–3.

15. Wilson PW, Kannel WB. Obesity, diabetes, and risk of cardiovascular disease in the elderly. *Am J Geriatr Cardiol* 2002; 11: 119–23.

16. Wilson PW, Kannel WB, Silbershatz H, D'Agostino RB. Clustering of metabolic factors and coronary heart disease. *Arch Intern Med* 1999; 159: 1104–9.

17. Wilson PWF, D'Agostino RB, Levy D, Belanger AM, Silbershatz H, Kannel WB. Prediction of coronary heart disease using risk factor categories. *Circulation* 1998; 97: 1837–47.

18. Wolf AM, Colditz GA. Current estimates of the economic cost of obesity in the United States. *Obes Res* 1998; 6: 97–106.

19. Young T, Shahar E, Nieto FJ, Redline S, Newman AB, Gottlieb DJ *et al.* Predictors of sleep-disordered breathing in community-dwelling adults: the Sleep Heart Health Study. *Arch Intern Med* 2002; 162: 893–900.

Progress in Obesity Research: 9. Edited by *Geraldo Medeiros-Neto, Alfredo Halpern and Claude Bouchard*
©2003 John Libbey Eurotext Ltd, pp. 542–546.

CHAPTER 114

Unraveling health implications of fatness and fitness

Ilkka Vuori

Tampere, Finland
[e-mail: ilkka.vuori@uta.fi]

Introduction

The world is experiencing a rapid change in the prevalence of diseases. The burden of infectious diseases is decreasing because of improved prevention and treatment, and that of chronic non-communicable diseases is increasing because of unfavourable behavioural and environmental changes such as tobacco use, unhealthy diet, physical inactivity, and pollution. The global burden of noncommunicable diseases was estimated to be 41 per cent in 1990, and it is expected to rise to 60 per cent in 2020[1]. The predicted development is not unavoidable, however. One strategy to combat chronic noncommunicable diseases, chosen e.g. by WHO, is to decrease the prevalence and severity of the most important risk factors that are common to many of these conditions. Fatness, i.e. overweight (body mass index, BMI 25.0–29.9 kg/m^2) and obesity (BMI 30.0 and over) and poor fitness as well as tobacco use are prime examples of these risk factors. The importance of fatness in this regard is well-known and begins to be understood and accepted among health professionals, policy makers and the general public. Fitness, however, is much less known and less appreciated risk factor of noncommunicable diseases. Fatness and fitness share much in common regarding their genesis, trends, effects on health and the mechanisms involved as well as strategies to prevent unhealthy weight gain and development of low fitness. Therefore, this paper examines especially the interrelationships of fatness and fitness and the implications of these relationships to prevention of noncommunicable diseases.

Prevalence, trends and health implications of fatness

Fatness has already reached epidemic proportions in many countries, both industrialized and those in economic transition. Fatness can affect all population groups, predominantly the lower socio-economic segments in affluent countries and the more well-off people in the poorer countries. Very alarmingly, fatness among children and adolescents is high in countries around the world. The trends indicate a rapid increase of fatness worldwide[1,2]. Fatness has strong impact on health, because it increases substantially the risk of many of the most common debilitating and lethal noncommunicable diseases and their precursors, e.g. coronary heart disease, stroke, Type 2 diabetes, hypertension, and several forms of cancer. Fatness increases also the risk of several conditions that decrease functional abilities and quality of life, and it leads commonly to negative psychosocial consequences[2,3]. Already the direct costs of fatness to health care are high, 2–6 per cent of total health care costs in many industrialized countries, and adding the indirect costs makes fatness a very expensive condition to national economies[1,3,4]. Taken together, the negative effects on health of fatness makes it one of the leading risk factors of the total burden of diseases especially in developed countries and also in developing countries with low mortality. However, even modest, about 10 per cent weight loss decreases significantly the risk of many obesity related diseases and improves quality of life[2–4].

Prevalence, trends, and health implications of fitness

Physical fitness is defined as 'a set of attributes that people have or achieve that relates to the ability to perform physical activity'. Many components of fitness are related to health status and can be influenced positively or negatively by physical activity. Health-related fitness is defined as a state characterized by (a) an ability to perform daily activities with vigour, and (b) demonstration of traits and capacities that are associated with low risk of premature development of hypokinetic diseases and conditions. Health-related fitness includes many components such as cardio-respiratory, metabolic, and morphological components, and each of these includes many subcomponents, e.g exercise capacity, heart and lung functions, and blood pressure in cardio-respiratory fitness, and glucose tolerance, insulin sensitivity, and lipid and lipoprotein metabolism in metabolic fitness[5]. All components of fitness are influenced strongly by hereditary factors[5]. However, they can also be influenced substantially by physical activity. Thus, fitness cannot be equated with physical activity, but physical activity is the strongest modifiable 'normal' factor that can influence fitness during ones lifetime.

The biological basis of health-related fitness or its components as predictors of health is theoretically sound, but its wide use for this purpose possesses several conceptual and practical problems. As a result, the predictive value of various components of fitness has not been studied for equally large number of health outcomes as is the case for fatness or physical activity. On the other hand, the predictive power of cardio-respiratory fitness has usually been stronger than that of physical activity in health outcomes that have been adequately studied in this respect. Thus, low levels of cardio-respiratory fitness has been shown to increase substantially and substantially more than low levels of physical activity the risk of, for example, all-cause mortality and development of cardiovascular diseases, coronary heart disease, and Type 2 diabetes[6,7]. The better predictive power of fitness as compared to physical activity is likely to be explained mainly by two factors: fitness is influenced more than activity by hereditary factors that are related also to the risk of several noncommunicable, particularly metabolic diseases, and fitness is usually assessed more accurately than activity.

The evidence of the relationships of physical activity and the risk of diseases and their precursors as well as of developing functional impairments has increased rapidly. Thorough reviews[2,8] of this evidence show that physical inactivity affects at least 20 of the most common and serious chronic disorders including coronary heart disease, stroke, congestive heart failure, hypertension, Type 2 diabetes, colon and breast cancer, gallstone formation, osteoporosis and related fractures, physical frailty, various types of cognitive dysfunction, and depression. The difference in risk between the sedentary and physically active populations is substantial, between 20 and 70 per cent in different conditions and different populations. Plausible biological mechanisms have been demonstrated or proposed for most of these relationships. Overweight and obesity increase the risk of most of these disorders. That means that in estimating the population attributable risk of either physical inactivity or obesity of these conditions the contribution of the other factor should be taken adequately into account.

The risk reduction is attained usually by moderate, frequent and continuous physical activity, but definite dose-response relationships have so far been assessed for only few diseases[9]. Currently physical activity for health, with the emphasis on prevention of cardiovascular diseases, is recommended as follows: People of all ages are advised to include a minimum of 30 min of physical activity of moderate intensity (such as brisk walking) on most, if not all, days of the week. Most people would attain greater health benefits by engaging in physical activity of more vigorous intensity or of longer duration. Cardio-respiratory endurance activity should be supplemented with strength-developing exercises at least twice per week for adults[10]. The scientific evidence for this recommendation comes mainly from studies on the relationships of physical activity and cardiovascular diseases and their precursors, and weight control has been of secondary importance in formulating the recommendation.

Assessment of population distribution of physical activity in general and in terms of sufficiency for health, and comparison of the results in different populations is hampered by lack of optimal, objective methods and insufficient standardization of the used methods. However, on the basis of available data it is obvious that the majority of population of most if not of all countries is not sufficiently physically active for health[2]. Because physical inactivity is so prevalent, the population attributable risk of physical inactivity is high for many diseases in many populations and even higher than that of some other 'major' risk factors[11].

The trends of physical activity indicate that physical activity related to work, transportation and domestic chores is decreasing globally, but the amount of leisure time physical activity shows variable changes during the past years in those few countries in which reliable data exist. The total amount of physical activity is, however, decreasing in most populations[2]. In terms of the risk of noncommunicable diseases this development is alarming.

Interrelationships between fatness, fitness, and physical activity

Is increased fatness caused by decreased physical activity?

The obesity epidemic could be caused by increased energy intake, decreased energy expenditure or by combination of them. Lack of data hampers exact analysis of the role of the two factors. However, it seems that during the development of the obesity epidemic the increase of energy intake has been modest at the most[12] or it may have even decreased[13]. No nationally representative data allow estimation of the average changes of energy expenditure, but decreased physical labour at work and in transport is obvious. Also in domestic chores opportunities to choose mechanized instead of physically active alternatives are numerous and realized by large numbers of people. These daily choices may lead to substantial decrease of energy expenditure during the course of weeks and months[12]. No data indicate that leisure time physical activity would have increased sufficiently to compensate for the highly probable decrease of energy expenditure in the other physical activity domains. In conclusion, it is very likely that decreased physical activity has contributed substantially to the obesity epidemic. An analysis of data from United States suggests that in that country about 40 per cent of the growth in weight over the last few decades may be due to expansion of food supply and about 60 per cent due to demand factors, notably fall in physical activity[14].

Is fatness likely to develop in unfit or physically inactive subjects?

Convincing evidence from laboratory, clinical, epidemiological and ecological studies indicates that low levels of habitual physical activity and low fitness increase substantially the risk of development of fatness[2,15]. Thorough analysis of the data suggests that maintenance of weight stability requires physical activity level (PAL, the ratio of total energy expenditure to the measured or estimated resting metabolic rate) of 1.8 or more in adults living in a Western society. This activity level corresponds to an additional 60–90 min of brisk walking daily in persons who normally undertake only modest exercise[2,3,15]. Complete sedentariness such as many hours of daily TV viewing has been shown to be an independent risk factor of weight gain in both children[16] and adults[17] through the very low energy expenditure and indirectly through increased consumption of snacks and drinks.

Is fatness a barrier to fitness and physical activity?

The limited number of studies that report physical activity level of a population by BMI strata show variable results, and fatness has not been found consistently to be a determinant of leisure time physical activity[18]. These findings are somewhat surprising, because fatness is known to decrease motivation and abilities for physical activity[19]. One reason for the variable findings, in addition to methodological issues, is that fatness is prevalent, and especially in affluent societies large numbers of overweight and obese individuals are trying to loose weight at any one time point, part of them by increasing their physical activity level[20,21]. Studies on adherence in various types of physical activity show generally high attrition rate among overweight and especially obese subjects[19]. Limiting factors that are specifically related to fatness include low fitness and low habituation to activity resulting in low exercise tolerance and development of musculo-skeletal symptoms, poor motor abilities leading to clumsiness and risk of injuries, and embarrassment and hygienic problems caused by fatness. Thus, fatness is a serious and common barrier for regular participation in physical activity. However, among large numbers of overweight and obese subjects it is a relative barrier as shown by their engagement in physical activity.

Are the negative health consequences of fatness caused partly by low fitness and insufficient physical activity?

Because low levels of physical activity and cardio-respiratory fitness contribute to the development and maintenance of fatness among a sizeable proportion of overweight and obese people it might be that part of the negative effects on health of fatness are in fact caused by low fitness and insufficient physical activity. This important issue has been examined especially by Blair and co-workers and summarized in a review article[6]. They present evidence from prospective epidemiological studies that there is an inverse gradient across fitness/physical activity categories in various strata of body habitus in the risk of all-cause mortality and coronary heart disease, hypertension, type 2 diabetes, ,and cancer morbidity or mortality, and the gradient is frequently steeper in the more obese subjects. Thus, the risk in fat and fit/active individuals is lower than that in fat and low-fit/sedentary subjects indicating that fitness and physical activity attenuate the risks associated with fatness. The evidence suggests that the magnitude of the attenuating effect of fitness/physical activity is in some health outcomes of the magnitude that the risk in fat but fit or active subjects is lower than that in non-fat and low-fit/sedentary individuals. This apparent protection of fitness and activity may extend to clearly obese men.

These findings are important but the evidence regarding the hypothesis of protective effect of fitness and physical activity against the consequences of fatness is still based on limited number of observational studies. The results of all these studies are not completely consistent and they are based mainly to a few cohorts of white middle-class men, and there is the possibility of self-selection to belong to the fit/physically active categories. On the other hand, the hypothesis is biologically plausible because good cardio-respiratory fitness and being physically active counteract the negative effects of fatness on most of the known metabolic risk factors of the fatness-related diseases[22]. Booth[8] stresses the pathophysiological role of insulin by stating that the human genotype requires sufficient use of muscles to maintain normal sensitivity to insulin. Physical inactivity would cause phenotypic expression of insulin resistance in skeletal muscle that would initiate whole body insulin resistance. This metabolic dysfunction manifests with different pathological phenomena based on the end organ involved, e.g. with the development of atherosclerosis, hypertension, visceral obesity, and Type 2 diabetes. Insulin resistance is one of the key elements also in the metabolic dysfunctions caused by obesity[22].

Practical implications

The strong multiple relationships between fatness, fitness, and physical activity have important implications. First, scientific evidence on these relationships and testing the 'Blair hypothesis' should be increased by conducting new analyses of suitable existing data sets and by including the research questions on fatness, fitness and physical activity as well as adequate measurements and parameters in appropriate new epidemiological studies and clinical trials. More knowledge is needed also of the optimal physical activity regimens to attain the metabolic benefits counteracting the effects of fatness. It is continuously warranted to recommend at least 30 min of moderate-intensity physical activity daily to attain a number of health benefits. However, current views suggest that about one hour of moderate-intensity activity is necessary for effective prevention of obesity and its deleterious consequences[2,3]. Vigorous intensity is likely to increase and add some benefits of physical activity as compared to the effects of moderate intensity activity, but the potential benefits have to be weighed against the decreased feasibility and safety of the activity[9].

Second, physical activity promotion should be one of the key components in the strategies and programmes aiming at prevention and control of obesity and related diseases. This work calls for development and testing of effective methods for individual counselling and community-wide promotion of physical activity. Even more importantly, physical activity should be seen as a fundamental human function that is continuously needed to maintain health and functional abilities in the same way as adequate nutrition. Consequently, all people should have opportunities for regular physical activity in their daily life. Sooner or later this challenge has to be taken seriously in order to prevent massive deterioration of health and functional abilities of the world population. The solutions are not easy because of the very strong societal structures and forces favouring sedentary ways of life. However, on the positive side there are numerous options to increase physical activity, and many of them are welcomed by large numbers of people of all ages and belonging to all social strata. The realization of the necessary opportunities requires deep-going changes in the attitudes, norms, and habits of the people, and functional and structural changes in the communities and in all settings of living.. These changes can be made only by developing and implementing multisectoral, integrated, and sustainable policies that enable the population at large to make continuously healthy choices in their daily life.

References

1. Kumanyika S, Jeffery RW, Morabia A, Ritenbaugh C,Antipatis VJ. Obesity prevention: the case for action. *Int J Obes* 2002; 26: 425–36.
2. International Agency for Research on Cancer: *IARC Handbooks of Cancer Prevention: Weight control and physical activity*, Vainio H, Bianchini F (eds), pp. 1–315 (vol 6). Lyon: IARC Press; 2001.
3. World Health Organization. Obesity: Preventing and managing the global epidemic. Report of a WHO consultation. Singapore: World Health Organ Tech Rep Ser; 2000; 894: i-xii, 1–253.
4. Oster G, Thompson D, Edelsberg J, Bird AP, Colditz A. Lifetime health and economic benefits of weight loss among obese persons. *Am J Public Health* 1999; 89: 1536–42.
5. Bouchard C, Malina RM, Pérusse L. *Genetics of fitness and physical performance*, pp. 1–398. Champaign: Human Kinetics; 1997.
6. Blair SN, Brodney S. Effects of physical activity and obesity on morbidity. *Med Sci Sport Exerc* 1999; 31: S646–S662.

7. Blair SN, Cheng Y, Holder JC. Is physical activity or physical fitness more important in defining health benefits? *Med Sci Sport Exerc* 2001; 33: S379–S399.

8. Booth FW, Chakravarthy MV, Gordon SE, Spangenburg EE. Waging war on physical inactivity: using modern molecular ammunition against an ancient enemy. *J Appl Physiol* 2002; 93: 3–30.

9. Kesäniemi YA, Danforth E, Jensen MD, Kopelman PG, Lefèbvre P, Reeder BA. Dose-response issues concerning physical activity and health: an evidence-based symposium. *Med Sci Sports Exerc* 2001; 33: S351–S358.

10. Department of Health and Human Services. *Physical Activity and Health: A report of the Surgeon General.* Atlanta: USDHSS, Centers for Disease Control and Prevention; 1996.

11. Haapanen-Niemi N, Vuori I, Pasanen M. Public health burden of coronary heart disease risk factors among middle-aged and elderly men. *Prev Med* 1999; 28: 343–8.

12. Blair SN, Nichaman MZ. The public health problem of increasing prevalence rates of obesity and what should be done about it. *Mayo Clin Proc* 2002; 77: 109–13.

13. Jebb SA, Moore MS. Contribution of a sedentary lifestyle and inactivity to the etiology of overweight and obesity: current evidence and research issues. *Med Sci Sports Exerc* 1999; 31: S534–S541.

14. Lakdawalla D, Philipson T. The growth of obesity and technological change: a theoretical and empirical examination. Working Paper 8946. National Bureau of Economic Research; 2002. URL: http://nber.org/papers/w8946

15. Erlichman J, Kerbey AL, James WPT. Physical activity and its impact on health outcomes. Paper 2: prevention of unhealthy weight gain and obesity by physical activity: an analysis of the evidence. *Obes Rev* 2002; 3 (in press).

16. Andersen RE, Crespo CJ, Bartlett SJ, Cheskin LJ, Pratt M. Relationship of physical activity and television watching with body weight and level of fatness among children. *JAMA* 1998; 279: 938–42.

17. Salmon J, Bauman A, Crawford D, Timperio A, Owen N. The association between television viewing and overweight among Australian adults participating in varying levels of leisure-time physical activity. *Int J Obes* 2000; 24: 600–6.

18. Sallis JF, Owen N. *Physical activity and behavioral medicine*, pp. 1–212. Thousand Oaks: Sage Publications; 1999.

19. Wilfley DE, Brownell KD. Physical activity and diet in weight loss. In: *Advances in exercise adherence* Dishman RK (ed.), pp. 361–393. Champaign: Human Kinetics; 1994.

20. Timperio A, Cameron-Smith D, Burns C, Salmon J, Crawford D. Physical activity beliefs and behaviours among adults attempting weight control. *Int J Obes* 2000; 24: 81–7.

21. Centers of Disease Control and Prevention. Prevalence of leisure-time physical activity among overweight adults – United States, 1998. *JAMA* 2000; 238: 2650–1.

22. Després JP, Lamarche B. Physical activity and the metabolic complications of obesity. In: *Physical activity and obesity*, Bouchard C (ed.), pp. 331–354. Champaign: Human Kinetics; 2000.

Progress in Obesity Research: 9. Edited by *Geraldo Medeiros-Neto, Alfredo Halpern* and *Claude Bouchard*
©2003 John Libbey Eurotext Ltd, pp. 547–553.

CHAPTER 115

We need ethnic-specific criteria for classification of BMI

Anoop Misra

Department of Medicine, All India Institute of Medical Sciences, New Delhi 110 029, India
[e-mail: anoopmisra@hotmail.com]

'Classifying an individual as lean, when in fact the individual is truly obese, may put this individual at risk for diseases associated with obesity and potentially delay possible beneficial therapy'
Smalley et al., Reassessment of body mass indices, 1990.

'Often the best predictor of future major disease is the presence of existing minor disease'
Geoffrey Rose, Sick individuals and sick populations, 2001.

Introduction

Obesity is an escalating global phenomenon. In some countries, nearly 30–50 per cent of the population is obese. It is of critical importance to have a correct method for the diagnosis of obesity. Imprecise methods would either over- or under diagnose obesity and would result in substantial shifts in its incidence and prevalence estimates. This would have far-reaching implications for the individuals, populations, and the health economics, both in developed as well as in the developing countries.

Body mass index (BMI) (ratio of height and weight, expressed as kg/m^2) is commonly used to define overweight and obesity based on the morbidity and mortality statistics from the Caucasian population. The lowest risks of developing type 2 diabetes mellitus, coronary heart disease (CHD) and hypertension has been reported between BMI values of 18.5 kg/m^2 and 25 kg/m^2.[1] A person with BMI > 25 kg/m^2 is defined as overweight and > 30 kg/m^2 is defined as obese[2]. These cut-offs for diagnosing overweight and obesity have been universally recommended. However, recent data suggest that, more appropriately, the criteria for the diagnosis of obesity should be modified considering the ethnicity of the individual.

A universal cut-off value of BMI could be applied to all ethnic groups if the composition of other body compartments (water, muscle, bone) remained constant in all individuals while body fat alone varied. In such a scenario, BMI would have a close and consistent correlation with the changes in the body fat. However, it is difficult to envisage such a situation since BMI would change in line with the changes in the proportion of any of the body compartments. This is clearly apparent in those with heavier muscle mass (e.g. professional wrestlers) as they would be defined as obese based on BMI, though their body fat may not be excessive. On the other hand, BMI value would not change appreciably if there is a proportional decrease in the muscle mass and increase in the body fat. Excess fat mass in such individuals may enhance their cardiovascular risk.

In the following brief review, evidence-based arguments will be presented to support ethnic-specific criteria for BMI. Authenticity of BMI cut-offs was considered by two criteria for the available studies; first, whether BMI cut-offs for overweight and obesity truly reflected excess adiposity, and, second, whether they corresponded to the excess cardiovascular morbidities.

Ethnic variations in the body composition

Fat-free mass (FFM)

Variations in the per cent body fat would occur if fat-free mass is altered due to ethnic differences in skeletal muscle, bone or non-skeletal skeletal muscle soft tissues. This is apparent upon comparison of body composition of blacks and whites[3]. Bone mineral content, bone mineral density (BMD), and skeletal muscle mass were reported to be significantly greater in black women as compared to whites[4]. Similarly, natives of Tonga had higher FFM, elbow breadth (indicative of larger skeletal size) and mid-arm muscle area as compared to Australian Caucasians[5]. On the contrary, smaller and 'slender' body frames are common in the Asian populations. Further, the Chinese males[6] and Asian Indians[7] were reported to have less lean mass as compared to Dutch Caucasians and Swedish males, respectively.

These data have important clinical implications. First, because of relative increase in the BMC and muscle mass, BMI value may increase though body fat may not be excessive. Misclassification of 12 per cent of black women as obese according to BMI criteria of obesity has been reported due to their greater muscle mass[8]. Second, errors in the estimation of fat mass by two-compartmental models may occur due to alterations in BMD and FFM[9].

Body fat

Table 1. Comparative statistics of BMI and per cent body fat in different ethnic groups

Author, year (ref)	Ethnic group (n)	BMI (kg/m^2)		per cent body fat	
		Men	Women	Men	Women
Wang et al., 1996 (14)	Whites (523)	25.2(3.3)	23.3(3.7)	19.6(6.7)	30.8(8.9)
	Blacks (180)	26.3(4.3)	28.5(5.9)	22.0(7.9)	38.2(9.6)
	Asians (267)[a]	23.3(2.9)	22.0(3.1)	21.3(6.4)	31.9(6.6)
	Puerto-Ricans (221)	27.4(4.7)	29.4(5.9)	24.8(8.3)	40.2(7.1)
Gallagher et al., 1996 (40)	Blacks (202)	25.8(3.3)	27.0(4.3)	21.7(7.9)	35.6(8.5)
	White (504)	25.2(3.1)	23.3(3.7)	21.2±7.8	30.3(8.6)
Luke et al., 1997 (22)	Nigerians (298)	21.7(3.9)	23.6(5.0)	11.4(7.5)	25.1(10.4)
	Jamaicans (240)	23.6(4.4)	27.0(6.0)	19.2(7.6)	35.3(8.4)
	US[b] (516)	27.0(5.7)	30.9(7.9)	27.1±7.8	42.2(7.9)
Gurrici et al., 1998 (12)	Indonesians (110)	24.3(3.3)	22.7(4.7)	28.3(6.2)	36.0(6.4)
	Dutch Caucasians (106)	26.2(3.6)	24.4(4.9)	26.5(7.6)	33.2(9.2)
Swinburn et al., 1999 (24)	Europeans (241)	25.6(3.5)	25.1(4.8)	20.7(8.0)	33.7(8.9)
	Maori (189)	30.5(5.0)	31.0(6.6)	27.8(8.1)	40.2(7.3)
	Samoans (185)	31.8(4.6)	33.3(6.3)	26.0(7.2)	40.8(6.8)
Yap et al., 2000 (10)	Chinese (108)	22.8(3.5)	22.1(4.8)	24.4(6.3)	33.3(6.3)
	Malays (76)	25.0(3.7)	24.5(4.8)	26.2(7.6)	35.8(6.4)
	Indians (107)	24.2(3.6)	24.9(5.2)	27.3(6.0)	35.8(5.6)
Dudeja et al., 2001 (17)	Asian Indians (86)	21.4(3.72)	23.3(5.49)	21.5(6.1)	34.9(4.2)
Ko et al., 2001 (11)	Hong Kong Chinese (5153)	23.4(3.3)	23.0(3.7)	21.4(5.9)	30.1(7.3)
He et al., 2001 (41)	Hong Kong Chinese (330)	23.0(3.8)	22.4(3.6)	23.0(7.0)	35.2(7.3)
Craig et al., 2001 (5)	Tongans (543)	30.3(0.3)*	32.6(0.4)	24.4(0.4)	40.5(0.4)
	Australians (393)	26.5(0.3)	25.8(0.4)	24.0(0.6)	37.0(0.5)

Data in mean (sd)
[a]Inclusive of subjects belonging to Japanese, Korean, Filipino and Chinese ethnicities, [b]Black immigrants in USA, [c]The majority of the subjects (98 per cent) was white. Adapted from Dudeja et al.[17]

Availability of newer techniques for the assessment of body composition has made it possible to study the variations in the body fat in a more precise manner. An overview of the data (Table 1) suggests that investigated ethnic groups could be broadly categorized into two categories; those having higher body fat at a relatively less BMI (e.g. Asians) and those with lesser amount of body fat at higher values of BMI (e.g. Tongans). The validity of BMI as a diagnostic marker for obesity would be compromised in both the situations. In such studies two reference markers have been considered; BMI cut-off values as defined from the data on Caucasians, and excess body fat as the standard for the diagnosis of obesity. However, since different methodologies have been employed to assess body composition in various studies, the comparisons of data are often difficult.

Relatively higher body fat for BMI

Asians: There is a mismatch of prevalence of obesity according to the current criteria and obesity-related co-morbidities in the Asian populations. The prevalence of obesity is nearly three times less in Asian ethnic groups as compared to Caucasians using the universal BMI cut-off (>30 kg/m^2), whereas the prevalence rates of the obesity-related diseases of the two populations are nearly similar.
A study on Asians in Singapore revealed high per cent body fat and lower BMI appropriate for body fat in Chinese, Malays and Asian Indians[10]. Ko *et al.*[11] reported that the prevalence of obesity (BMI $\geq$ 30 kg/m^2) in 5153 Hong Kong Chinese was only 3.4 per cent. However, prevalence of excess body fat was higher (26.9 per cent), comparable to the prevalence of obesity (BMI $\geq$ 30 kg/m^2) in Caucasians. Similar observations have been reported in the Indonesian population[12], and several Asian ethnic groups (Chinese, Japanese, Koreans and Filipinos) residing in New York, USA[13,14]. The observations by Deurenberg-Yap *et al.*[10] of high body fat at low BMI values in Asian Indians in Singapore have been supported by studies on Asian Indians residing in India[15] and immigrant Asian Indians in USA[16]. Dudeja *et al.*[17] used Receiver Operating Characteristic (ROC) curve analysis and reported misclassification of obesity in ~25 per cent men and ~70 per cent women in north India. Misclassification of obesity by BMI was also reported for Asian Indians with type 2 diabetes[18].
Several reasons could be responsible for the incongruous relationship between the BMI and body fat in the Asian populations. These include 'slender body frame', less lean mass, differences in the length of the lower extremities etc. Diet, physical activity, lifestyle, migration, genetic intermingling with people of other ethnic groups, and socio-economic strata, however, could influence the BMI and body fat relationship within an ethnic group. For example, body composition differences have been observed between Mainland Chinese and Hong Kong Chinese and subgroups of Indonesian population. Heterogeneity and migration of the Asian Indian population makes it likely the similar situation might also occur in them.
Though current BMI cut-offs have been based on the data on Caucasians, poor sensitivity and specificity of BMI for the diagnosis of obesity has also been shown in the Caucasian populations[19,20].

Relatively low body fat for BMI

Blacks: That blacks have more fat-free mass has been shown by several investigators. In addition, some evidence supports that they have relatively less body fat. A study on black women showed that they have higher value of BMI but similar amount of body fat as the Caucasian women[21]. Country-specific variations in BMI and body fat in the black population have also been reported. Luke *et al.*[22] compared anthropometry and body fat in 1054 black men and women from Nigeria, Jamaica and USA, using a standard protocol. Interestingly, the lowest values of BMI and body fat were observed in people from Nigeria, whereas blacks in USA had highest values of both the parameters. Further, although BMI correlated well to adiposity but it could not explain 25–39 per cent variance of body fat.
Polynesians: Rush *et al.*[23] showed that the BMI value of 30 for New Zealand Caucasians corresponded to BMI value of 34 for Polynesians at a comparable body fat. Mean values of BMI of Maori and Samoan Polynesians were reported to be higher by ~5–8 units than Europeans in New Zealand[24]. Based on the data, Swinburn *et al.*[24] proposed a higher BMI cut-off for diagnosing overweight and obesity in the Polynesian population (Table 2). Similarly, in the Tongan population, 90 per cent of the women $>$ 30 years of age were overweight, and 39 per cent women and 10 per cent men were obese using current BMI cut-offs[25]. When per cent body fat of Australian Caucasians at BMI cut-offs 25 and 30 were matched with Tongan population, the equivalent BMI values for Tongan men and women were much higher (Table 2).

Ratio of per cent body fat/BMI

This ratio gives estimate of per cent body fat per unit of BMI and should prove to be useful for inter-ethnic comparisons of body fat[17]. For example, per cent body fat/ BMI ratios for Tongans, Australians, Europeans, and Polynesian men and women range between 0.81–0.91 and 1.20–1.43, respectively. For Chinese, Malays and Asian Indians, however, the values are clearly higher, between 0.91–1.13 for men and between 1.31–1.57 for women. Of particular note, the highest value of the per cent body fat/BMI ratio among men was seen in Asian Indians.

Table 2. BMI cut-off values reported for various ethnic groups

Author, year (ref)	Ethnic group	Gender	Overweight (kg/m²)	Obesity (kg/m²)
Hortogagyi et al., 1994 (19)	Caucasians	Males[a] Females[c]		24.5[b] 22[b]
Wellens et al., 1996 (20)	Caucasian	Males[d] Females[e]		25[b] 23[b]
Gurrici et al., 1998 (12)	Indonesians[f]		–	27
Swinburn et al., 1999 (24)	Polynesians[g]		26–32	>32
Deurenberg-Yap et al., 2000 (10)	Chinese Malays Asian Indians		– – –	27 – 26
Ko et al., 2001 (11)	Hong Kong Chinese		23[b]	26[b]
He et al., 2001 (41)	Hong Kong Chinese	Males Females		24.6[h] 22.6[i]
Dudeja et al., 2001 (17)	Asian Indians	Males Females	21.5[b,j] 19[b,k]	–
Craig et al., 2001 (5)	Tongans	Males[l] Females[l]	27.5 28.8	35.8 35.1
Vikram et al., 2002 (18)	Asian Indians[m]	Males Females	22[b,j] 23[b,k]	– –

[a]Criteria for obesity, per cent body fat ≥ 25 per cent, BMI ≥ 28 kg/m²; [b]Receiver Operating Characteristic curve (ROC) analysis data; [c]Criteria for obesity, per cent body fat ≥ 30 per cent, BMI ≥ 27 kg/m²; [d]Cut-offs for ROC curve analysis, BMI–28 kg/m², and per cent body fat–25 per cent; [e]Cut-offs for ROC curve analysis, BMI–26 kg/m², and per cent body fat–33 per cent; [f]Data were compared to Dutch Caucasians; [g]Data were compared to New Zealand Caucasians; [h]Corresponding to 25 per cent body fat; [i]Corresponding to 35 per cent body fat; [j]25 per cent body fat as standard; [k]30 per cent body fat as standard; [l]Data were compared to Australian Caucasians; [m]Patients with type 2 diabetes.

Cardiovascular risk factor profile and its relation to BMI cut-offs and body fat

The true cut-off for defining obesity should correlate closely with the increased risk for adverse metabolic profile and cardiovascular morbidity and mortality. There is evidence that such a scenario occurs at lower BMI values in the Asian populations. Ko et al.[26] examined likelihood of having obesity-related morbidities in 1513 Hong Kong Chinese, and showed that the optimal BMI cut-offs to predict diabetes, hypertension and dyslipidaemia ranged between 23.0–24.3 kg/m² in both genders. In particular, the lowest cut-off value (~23 kg/m²) was observed for dyslipidaemia. Similar data were recorded recently for the Korean population[27]. Deurenberg-Yap et al.[28] also showed adverse metabolic profile at low BMI values in multi-ethnic population of Singapore. In the male population belonging to the BMI category 22–24 kg/m², ~24 per cent had hypercholesterolaemia, 33 per cent had hyper-triglyceridaemia, ~8 per cent had hypertension and ~5 per cent had diabetes mellitus. Furthermore, 54 per cent of the adult population had at least one risk factor even when BMI value was <25 kg/m².

In a recent study, cross-sectional data obtained from adults aged 30–65 years in China (n = 3,423), the Philippines (n = 1,929) and the USA (n = 7,957) were analysed by Bell et al.[29]. The odds ratio for prevalence of hypertension for Chinese men in the BMI range 23.0–24.9 kg/m² was 2.09 (95 per cent confidence intervals: 1.50–2.94), significantly more than the odds ratios seen in the Mexican-Americans, non-Hispanic whites and non-Hispanic blacks. Further, there was ~11 per cent increase in the prevalence of hypertension for Chinese men between BMI 23.0–24.9 kg/m², when compared to BMI between 18.5–22.9 kg/m², significantly higher than that observed for the other ethnic groups. Recent data of aboriginal Australians indicate increasing odds ratios for impaired glucose tolerance and diabetes from BMI value of 22 kg/m² onwards[30]. Similar to above data, our group has recorded higher odds ratios for various cardiovascular risk factors, particularly for hypertension and hypertriglyceridae-mia, in people with BMI < 25 kg/m² but having high per cent body fat (unpublished observations). More such data have been recently reported from India, Taiwan and China.

Overall, growing data suggest increase in the occurrence of cardiovascular risk factors at a 'non-obese' BMI range in Asian ethnic groups. These morbidities appear to be closely related to increase in the body fat.

'Non-obese people' with metabolic syndrome:

The observations of higher body fat and higher morbidities at a relatively lower BMI are conceptually supported and consolidated by studies on 'non-obese' subjects. Neil Ruderman introduced the concept 20 years back[31] of 'non-obese' people having predisposition for type 2 diabetes, dyslipidaemia, and premature atherosclerosis named as 'metabolically obese normal weight (MONW)' people. It is likely that MONW subjects have higher total body fat at a 'normal' value of BMI; hence, they are actually obese according to the excess adiposity. Indeed, Ruderman, recently emphasized that many of these people were 'mildly obese' and had BMI values in the upper range of normal, or had higher fat mass[32]. This concept was supported by studies of Hollenbeck and Reaven[33] where they showed that ~25 per cent of the healthy individuals were insulin resistant. Dvorack *et al.*[34] also reported high percentage body fat (31.8 ± 5.9 per cent) at a low mean BMI value (22.5 ± 2.0 kg/m^2) in normal weight non-obese women. Additionally these women had lower glucose disposal rate, hyperinsulinaemia, and dyslipidaemia.

Metabolic perturbations in such people could be due to an increase in the abdominal fat mass that may not affect overall adiposity[35,36]. For example, young Asian Indians having BMI in 'non-obese' range (23 ± 2 kg/m^2) had higher total abdominal and visceral fat and lower rate of glucose disposal as compared to the Caucasian subjects with comparable BMI values[37]. According to Banerji *et al.*[16], the majority (66 per cent) of 'non-obese' Asian Indians investigated by them was insulin resistant.

A cross-sectional study by Tanaka *et al.*[38] on normal weight (BMI between 18.5–25 kg/m^2) white population aged 17–60 years provide further supportive data. In this study, normal weight people were further divided by the quintiles of percentage body fat. Males in the upper quintile of per cent body fat (21.1–35.2 per cent) had higher odds ratio (3.15) for the risk factor variables that was significantly different from those in the first quintile of percentage body fat. In the normal weight group, subjects with at least one risk factor had significantly higher per cent body fat as compared to the subjects without any risk factors. Furthermore, overweight males (BMI between 25–30 kg/m^2) had odds ratio for risk factor variables similar to the normal weight subjects with high per cent body fat.

Taken together, the studies suggest that many 'non-obese' subjects are insulin resistant and have an adverse metabolic profile. These individuals have excess body fat and increased abdominal fat. This characteristic phenotype is frequently seen in the Asian populations[35].

Need for, and initiative towards establishing ethnic-specific BMI cut-offs

BMI cut-off values reported by various investigators are presented in Table 2. For all ethnic groups, except Polynesians and Tongans, the reported BMI cut-offs were lower than the currently accepted cut-offs. On the average, the values of the BMI reported for various ethnic groups differed by ~2–5 units as compared to the current cut-offs.

Prompted by increasing data, the World Health Organization (WHO) Expert Group suggested redefining the criteria for obesity in Asian population acknowledging the 'need for different standards that are culturally specific' in 2000 AD. In a monograph directed towards the populations of Asia-Pacific region, the proposed criterion for overweight was BMI 23–24.9 kg/m^2 and that for obesity was ≥ 25 kg/m^2.[39] The cut-off values for waist circumference were also lowered for the Asian populations. Supported by several recent studies, another WHO Expert Committee deliberated in Hong Kong in July 2002, and concluded that the individual countries should decide regarding the normal BMI categories for their populations, based on their morbidity and mortality data. The group reaffirmed that the optimum BMI range for the Asian population should be narrowed to 18.5–23 kg/m^2.

Overall, such modifications of BMI cut-offs appear to be scientifically justified and would result in more rational management of obesity and related co-morbidities. According to an estimate, lowering of BMI cut off value by ~3 units would increase the prevalence of obesity in any population by ~10–15 per cent. Accordingly, the expenditure on the health resources would increase.

References

1. Hoffmans MDAF, Kromhout D, Coulander C. The impact of body mass index of 78,612 18-year Dutch men on 32-year mortality of all causes. *J Clin Epidemiol* 1988; 41: 749–56.

2. World Health Organization. Obesity: preventing and managing the global epidemic. Report of a WHO consultation presented at: the World Health Organization. Geneva: World Health Organ Tech Rep Ser. 2000; 894: i-xii, 1–253.

3. Wagner DR, Heyward VH. Measures of body composition in blacks and whites: a comparative review. *Am J Clin Nutr* 2000; 71: 1392–402.

4. Ortiz O, Russell M, Daley TL *et al.* Differences in skeletal muscle and bone mineral mass between black and white females and their relevance to estimates of body composition. *Am J Clin Nutr* 1992; 55: 8–13.

5. Craig P, Halavatau V, Comino E, Caterson I. Differences in body composition between Tongans and Australians: time to rethink the healthy weight ranges? *Int J Obes Relat Metab Disord* 2001; 25: 1806–14.

6. Werkman A, Deurenberg-Yap M, Schmidt G, Deurenberg P. A Comparison between Composition and Density of the Fat-Free Mass of Young Adult Singaporean Chinese and Dutch Caucasians. *Ann Nutr Metab* 2000; 44: 235–42.

7. Chowdhury B, Lantz H, Sjostrom L. Computed tomography-determined body composition in relation to cardiovascular risk factors in Indian and matched Swedish males. *Metabolism* 1996; 45: 634–44.

8. Aloia JF, Vaswani A, Mikhail M, Flaster ER. Body composition by dual-energy X-ray absorptiometry in black compared with white women. *Osteoporos Int* 1999; 10: 114–9.

9. Schutte JE, Townsend EJ, Hugg J, Shoup RF, Malina RM, Blomqvist CG. Density of lean body mass is greater in blacks than in whites. *J Appl Physiol* 1984; 56: 1647–9.

10. Deurenberg-Yap M, Schmidt G, van Staveren WA, Deurenberg P. The paradox of low body mass index and high body fat percentage among Chinese, Malays and Indians in Singapore. *Int J Obes Relat Metab Disord* 2000; 24: 1011–7.

11. Ko GTC, Tang J, Chan JCN *et al.* Lower BMI cut-off value to define obesity in Hong Kong Chinese: an analysis based on body fat assessment by bioelectrical impedance. *Br J Nutr* 2001; 85: 239–42.

12. Gurrici S, Hartriyanti Y, Hautvast JG, Deurenberg P. Relationship between body fat and body mass index: differences between Indonesians and Dutch Caucasians. *Eur J Clin Nutr* 1998; 52: 779–83.

13. Wang J, Thornton JC, Russell M, Burastero S, Heymsfield S, Pierson RN Jr. Asians have lower body mass index (BMI) but higher per cent body fat than do whites: comparisons of anthropometric measurements. *Am J Clin Nutr* 1994; 60: 23–8.

14. Wang J, Thornton JC, Burastero S *et al.* Comparisons for body mass index and body fat per cent among Puerto Ricans, blacks, whites and Asians living in the New York City area. *Obes Res* 1996; 4: 377–84.

15. Misra A, Pandey RM, Devi JR, Sharma R, Vikram NK, Khanna N. High prevalence of diabetes, obesity and dyslipidaemia in urban slum population in northern India. *Int J Obes Relat Metab Disord* 2001; 25: 1722–9.

16. Banerji MA, Faridi N, Alturi R, Chaiken RL, Lebovitz HE. Body composition, visceral fat, leptin and insulin resistance in Asian Indian men. *J Clin Endocrinol Metab* 1999; 84: 137–44.

17. Dudeja V, Misra A, Pandey RM, Devina G, Kumar G, Vikram NK. BMI does not accurately predict overweight in Asian Indians in northern India. *Br J Nutr* 2001; 86: 105–12.

18. Vikram NK, Misra A, Pandey RM *et al.* Anthropometry and body composition in northern Asian Indian patients with type 2 diabetes: Receiver Operating Characteristics (ROC) Curve analysis of body mass index with percentage body fat as standard. *Diab Nutr Metab* 2003; 16: 32–40.

19. Hortobagyi T, Israel RG, O'Brien KF. Sensitivity and specificity of Quetelet index to assess obesity in men and women. *Eur J Clin Nutr* 1994; 48: 369–75.

20. Wellens RI, Roche AF, Khamis HJ, Jackson AS, Pollock ML, Siervogel RM. Relationship between the body mass index and body composition. *Obes Res* 1996; 4: 35–44.

21. Kleerekoper M, Nelson DA, Peterson EL, Wilson PS, Jacobsen G, Longcope C. Body composition and gonadal steroids in older white and black women. *J Clin Endocrinol Metab* 1994; 79: 775–9.

22. Luke A, Durazo-Arvizu R, Rotimi C *et al.* Relation between body mass index and body fat in black population samples from Nigeria, Jamaica, and the United States. *Am J Epidemiol* 1997; 145: 620–8.

23. Rush EC, Plank LD, Laulu MS, Robinson SM. Prediction of percentage body fat from anthropometric measurements: comparison of New Zealand European and Polynesian young women. *Am J Clin Nutr* 1997; 66: 2–7.

24. Swinburn BA, Ley SJ, Carmichael HE, Plank LD. Body size and composition in Polynesians. *Int J Obes Relat Metab Disord* 1999; 23: 1178–83.

25. Maclean E, Bach F, Badcock J. The 1996 national nutrition survey of Kingdom of Tonga: Summary report. South Pacific Commission; 1992 (technical paper no. 200).

26. Ko GTC, Chan JCN, Cockram CS, Woo J. Prediction of hypertension, diabetes, dyslipidemia or albuminuria using simple anthropometric indexes in Hong Kong Chinese. *Int J Obes* 1999; 23: 1136–1142.

27. Moon OR, Kim NS, Jang SM, Yoon TH, Kim SO. The relationship between body mass index and the prevalence of obesity-related diseases based on 1995 National Health Interview Survey in Korea. *Ob Rev* 2002; 3: 191–6.

28. Deurenberg-Yap M, Chew SK, Lin VF, Tan BY, van Staveren WA, Deurenberg P. Relationships between indices of obesity and its co-morbidities in multi-ethnic Singapore. *Int J Obes Relat Metab Disord* 2001; 25; 1554–62.

29. Bell AC, Adair LS, Popkin BM. Ethnic differences in the association between body mass index and hypertension. *Am J Epidemiol* 2002; 155: 346–53.

30. Daniel M, Rowlwy KG, McDermott R, O'Dea K. Diabetes and impaired glucose tolerance in Aboriginal Australians: prevalence and risk. *Diab Res Clin Pract* 2002; 57: 23–33.

31. Ruderman N, Schneider S, Berchtold SH. The 'metabolically obese' normal-weight individual. *Am J Clin Nutr* 1981; 34(8): 1617–21.

32. Ruderman N, Chisholm D, Pi-Sunyer X, Schneider S. The metabolically obese, normal-weight individual revisited. *Diabetes* 1998; 47: 699–713.

33. Hollenbeck CB, Reaven G. Variations in insulin-stimulated glucose uptake in healthy individuals with normal glucose tolerance. *J Clin Endocrinol Metab* 1987; 64: 1169–73.

34. Dvorak RV, DeNino WF, Ades PA, Poehlman ET. Phenotypic characteristics associated with insulin resistance in metabolically obese but normal-weight young women. *Diabetes* 1999; 48: 2210–4.

35. Misra A, Vikram NK. Clinical and pathophysiological consequences of abdominal adiposity and abdominal adipose tissue depots. *Nutrition* 2003; 19(5): 457–66.

36. Misra A, Athiko D, Sharma R, Pandey RM, Khanna N. Non-obese hyperlipidemic Asian northern Indian males have adverse anthropometric profile. *Nutr Metab Cardiovasc Dis* 2002; 12(4): 178–83..

37. Raji A, Seely EW, Arky RA, Simonson DC. Body fat distribution and insulin resistance in healthy Asian Indians and Caucasians. *J Clin Endocrinol Metab* 2001; 86: 5366–71.

38. Tanaka S, Togashi K, Rankinen T *et al.* Is adiposity at normal weight relevant for cardiovascular disease risk? *Int J Obes* 2002; 26: 176–83.

39. World Health Organisation. The Asia-Pacific Perspective. Redefining Obesity and its Treatment. International Diabetes Institute. Health Communications Australia Pty Ltd; 2000.

40. Gallagher D, Visser M, Sepulveda D, Pierson RN, Harris T, Heymsfield SB. How useful is body mass index for comparison of body fatness across age, sex, and ethnic groups? *Am J Epidemiol* 1996; 143: 228–39.

41. He M, Tan KC, Li ET, Kung AW. Body fat determination by dual energy X-ray absorptiometry and its relation to body mass index and waist circumference in Hong Kong Chinese. *Int J Obes Relat Metab Disord* 2001; 25: 748–52.

Progress in Obesity Research: 9. Edited by *Geraldo Medeiros-Neto, Alfredo Halpern and Claude Bouchard*
©2003 John Libbey Eurotext Ltd, pp. 554–557.

CHAPTER 116

BMI cutoffs for obesity should not vary by ethnic group

June Stevens

Departments of Nutrition and Epidemiology, School of Public Health, CB 7461, University of North Carolina, Chapel Hill, NC 27599, USA. [e-mail: June_Stevens@UNC.EDU

The World Health Organization (WHO)[1] has provided guidelines for the definition of overweight and obesity that use body mass index (BMI) as the criterion measure. Cutpoints of 25 kg/m^2 for overweight and 30 kg/m^2 for obesity have been rapidly adopted by many clinicians and researchers around the world. In February of 2000 a report was issued jointly by the Regional Office for the Western Pacific World Health Organization, the International Association for the Study of Obesity and the International Obesity Task Force which addressed the definitions of overweight and obesity in Asian populations[2]. The report states that, 'In Pacific Island populations e.g. Samoa, the recommended BMI standards should be higher than those recommended by WHO ..., whereas in certain other Asian populations such as Chinese and Japanese it is likely that they should be lower'.

The purpose of this paper is to present the arguments in favour of having a single set of BMI cutoffs for obesity (and overweight) for all ethnic groups. The arguments are presented in three main points: (1) BMI cutoff points for obesity should be based on risk rather than correlations with body fatness; (2) There is insufficient evidence on associations between BMI and mortality to support different cutpoints, i.e. lower cutpoints in Asians; (3) Defining cutoff points by ethnic groups, as opposed to other factors, is difficult to justify scientifically, socially and politically.

BMI cutoff points for obesity should be based on risk rather than correlations with body fatness

The WHO has defined obesity as 'a disease in which excess body fat has accumulated to an extent that health may be adversely affected'[1]. Recently several studies have confirmed that the degree of fatness varies among individuals with the same BMI and that there are significant differences by ethnic group. Deurenberg et al.[3] have shown that for the same level of fatness, African Americans have 1.3 kg/m^2 and Polynesians a 4.5 kg/m^2 higher BMI compared to Caucasians. In contrast, in Chinese, Ethiopians, Indonesians and Thais BMI's are 1.9, 4.6, 3.2 and 2.9 kg/m^2 lower than Caucasians respectively.

Though the ethnic differences in mean body fatness, for a given weight and height, are well established at this point in time, they have little impact on cutpoints for obesity if the differences in fatness do not explain differences in risk. Ultimately it is risk that is of concern to public health and clinical care. Were excess adiposity not associated with risk, it would be of only cosmetic interest. It happens that there is also diversity in the associations between adiposity and risk among ethnic groups. For instance, at the same BMI, on average African Americans have a lower per cent body fat compared to whites, yet at the same BMI they have a higher risk of diabetes and mortality. Therefore evidence that BMI is associated with different levels of adiposity in different ethnic groups does not form a firm basis for setting BMI cutpoints for obesity. Instead, associations of BMI with risk should be used as the basis of decision making.

Comparison of risk among ethnic groups must be done carefully with attention to the choice of an outcome and the measure of risk assessment. We compared associations with BMI in women from two different ethnic groups using four different outcomes (mortality, diabetes, hypertension and hypertriglyceridaemia) and three different risk estimates (absolute risk, relative risk and risk difference)[4]. We found that a higher, a lower, or a similar BMI cutpoint for obesity could be recommended for African American women relative to white women depending on the outcome and the measure of effect examined. In our examples, among African American women 'equivalent' BMI values to those in white women with a BMI of 30 ranged from absurdly low to absurdly high depending on the criteria used. As stated in our previous paper, 'There was essentially no BMI at which the incidence of death was as low in African American women as it was in white women with a BMI of 30, and there was no BMI at which the incidence of hypertriglyceridaemia was as high in African American women as it was in white women with a BMI of 30. Obviously factors other than body weight have powerful effects on these outcomes in African American and white women[4].'

Table 1. All-cause mortality by category of body mass index in Asians

Cohort	Body Mass Index (BMI) range risk estimates and 95 per cent confidence intervals						
MEN							
China[1]							
BMI categories	<18.5	18.5–<21.0	21.0–<23.5	23.5–<26.0	>26.0		
Rate ratios	1.16	1.06	1.00	1.02	1.04		
	(0.95–1.42)	(0.91–1.22)		(0.87–1.20)	(0.85–1.28)		
Japan[2]							
BMI categories	14.0–18.9	19.0–20.9	21.0–22.9	23.0–24.9	25.0–26.9	27.0–29.9	30.0–39.9
Rate ratios	2.26	1.57	1.33	1.00	1.14	1.38	1.97
	(1.66–3.08)	(1.25–1.98)	(1.09–1.63)		(0.90–1.45)	(1.03–1.83)	(1.27–3.06)
Hawaii[3]							
BMI categories	<19.6	19.6–21.3	21.4–24.8	24.9–29.2	29.3–32.5	>32.6	
Rate ratios	1.29	1.07	1.00	1.06	1.73	1.26	
	(1.09–1.52)	(0.92–1.24)		(0.99–1.26)	(1.30–2.29)	(0.76–2.08)	
Korea[4]							
BMI categories	18.0–19.9	20.0–21.9	22.0–23.9	24.0–25.9	26.0–27.9	28.0–29.9	>30.0
Rate ratios	1.17	1.06	1.0	0.96	0.98	0.97	1.47
	(1.11–1.24)	(1.01–1.11)		(0.91–1.01)	(0.92–1.04)	(0.86–1.09)	(1.21–1.77)
WOMEN							
Japan[2]							
BMI categories	14.0–18.9	19.0–20.9	21.0–22.9	23.0–24.9	25.0–26.9	27.0–29.9	30.0–39.9
Rate ratios	1.94	0.98	0.99	1.00	1.30	1.33	1.91
	(1.30–2.89)	(0.69–1.40)	(0.74–1.32)		(0.96–1.76)	(0.94–1.88)	(1.22–2.99)
Hawaii[3]							
BMI categories	<18.5	18.5–19.9	20.0–23.6	23.7–30.3	0.4–35.9		
Rate ratios	1.26	1.00	0.96	1.25	1.53		
	(0.98–1.61)		(0.79–1.17)	(1.02–1.53)	(1.06–2.22)		
MEN AND WOMEN							
China[5]							
BMI categories	<18.5	18.5–23.9	24–27.9	>28.0			
Rate ratios	1.21	1.00	0.91	1.12			
	(1.10–1.33)		(0.82–1.01)	(0.93–1.37)			

[1]Adapted from Yuan *et al.*[5]. Chinese men (*n* = 18,244) ages 45–64 years; self-reported height and weight; adjusted for age, smoking, alcohol and education;
[2]Adapted from Tsugane *et al.*[7] Japanese men (*n* = 19,500) and women (*n* = 21,315) ages 40–59 years; self-reported height and weight; adjusted for age, smoking alcohol and education;
[3]Adapted from Maskarinec *et al.*[8] Multi-ethnic men (*n* = 13,870) and women (13,808) ages > 30 years; self-reported height and weight; adjusted for age, smoking alcohol and education;
[4]Adapted from Song and Sung[10]. Korean men (*n* = 235,398) ages 40–64 years; measured height and weight; adjusted for age, smoking, income, alcohol and exercise;
[5]Adapted from Zhao *et al.*[6]. Chinese men (*n* = 15,723) and women (*n* = 14,837) ages 35–59 years.

It would be difficult to defend the use of any one disease over others to set standards for obesity. As an outcome for use in the establishment of weight standards, risk factors have little to offer. Risk factors do not, by themselves, cause a reduction in the quality or length of life. They are of importance because they are related to a 'hard outcome' (such as stroke, myocardial infarction or cancer) that does affect quality and length of life. Since the associations between risk factors and hard outcomes often vary by ethnic group, basing ethnic specific standards on risk factors (for example blood pressure or plasma cholesterol) has little appeal.

Table 2. Risk of diabetes in women from the Atherosclerosis in Communities Study (ARIC) cohort categorized by ethnicity, education or family history

Measure	Ethnicity			Education			Family history of diabetes mellitus		
	American White	African American	Δ	<High school	≥High school	Δ	No	Yes	Δ
Incidence per 1000 person-years									
Normal weight (BMI = 18.5–24.9)	3.1	6.2		5.9	3.2		6.2	2.8	
Obese (BMI ≥30)	18.1	23.2		23.5	19.3		26.0	18.2	
Risk ratio obese	5.8	3.8	2.0	4.0	6.1	2.1	4.2	6.5	2.3
Risk difference per 1000 person-years obese	15.0	17.0	2.0	17.6	16.1	1.5	19.8	15.4	4.4

Since the time of the Metropolitan Life Insurance Studies, mortality has been the outcome on which recommendations for weight for height were based. Mortality is unique, highly relevant, and easily and precisely measured. Mortality can be criticized as too extreme and too confounded by exposures other than body weight. An outcome that captures years of healthy, functional, high-quality life would be of great interest. Research in this area is needed, but it is unlikely that the scientific community will ever reach unanimity on how such an outcome should be defined and assessed.

As influential as the choice of the outcome used to set cutpoints, is the choice of the measure of effect, i.e. the type of calculated statistic used to draw conclusions. As stated in our previous paper[4], 'if the goal is to identify a level at which risk is elevated due to BMI, then some type of measure which considers differences in levels of baseline risk is needed. Both rate ratios and rate differences incorporate the level of risk at reference levels of BMI. However, we find the rate ratio the less attractive of the two measures of effect because equivalent multiplicative increases in risk can be associated with very different increases in the number of cases. The effect of obesity on the increase in the number of cases above that experienced by individuals at reference weight seems the most meaningful estimate for public health and policy decisions.' One such quantity is the rate or risk difference. Other types of estimates could also be of value.

Insufficient evidence on associations between BMI and mortality to support different cutpoints, i.e. lower cutpoints in Asians

Table 1 summarizes the data from several studies on the association between BMI and mortality. Support for the need to lower the cutoff points for overweight or obesity would come from studies showing that the risk of mortality was increased at a BMI below 25 or 30 compared to a lower reference level of BMI. For instance, if there were an increase in the risk of mortality at a BMI of 23–25 compared to a reference BMI of 18.5 to 22.9, this would give some indication that the current cutpoint of 25 for overweight was too high in that population. No such evidence is seen in any of the studies in Table 1. Careful examination of the table shows that statistically significant increases in mortality risk are not seen at a BMI lower than 25, and in general are present only at BMI levels above 30.

Additional evidence can be gleaned from a study by Maskarinec et al.[8] which examined the association in over 40,000 persons of Asian, Caucasian and Hawaiian ethnicity living in Hawaii. Models adjusted for age, education, and smoking showed very similar associations between BMI and mortality in the Asians studied as compared to the Caucasians and the Hawaiians. Similarly, in the Asia Pacific Cohort Studies Collaboration (APCSC) study of over 300,000 participants in 33 countries, there was no interaction by ethnicity between Asian and the Caucasian participants (the latter from Australia and New Zealand) for the associations of BMI with stroke ($P = 0.2$) or with ischaemic heart disease ($P = 0.4$)[9].

In sum, it appears that the currently recommended range of BMI levels (between 18.5 and 24.9) are consistent with the lowest risk of mortality in Asians. Further, studies that contrast the association of BMI with mortality or with other severe outcomes, such as stroke and ischaemic heart disease, provide no evidence that the association is different in Asians compared to Caucasians.

Defining cutoff points by ethnic groups, as opposed to other factors, is difficult to justify scientifically, socially and politically

In many epidemiologic studies ethnicity is measured by self-identification using one question and a check list. This variable is an indicator of a myriad of ill-defined environmental, cultural, social and familial factors. Usually geography or nationality is thought to contribute to ethnicity, but is not considered synonymous. In a multi-ethnic society such as the United States, it is likely that many individuals would have difficulty classifying themselves as belonging to only one ethnic group. Given the enormous stigma attached to obesity and the sensitivity of ethnic issues, it seems unlikely that formal policies setting different cutpoints for different ethnic groups in the United States would ever gain support. It is difficult to imagine different BMI cutoff points being used for different ethnic groups to determine things like insurance rates or the ability to serve in the military.

It can be questioned why the issue of having customized BMI cutpoints for obesity has focused on ethnicity. Using the same logic as that applied to ethnic groups, a case could be made for different BMI cutpoints for obesity for individuals of different educational levels or family medical history as well as other characteristics. Table 2 illustrates this point using data on the incidence of diabetes in women that was collected as part of the Atherosclerosis Risk in Communities (ARIC) Study. The risk of diabetes in obese as opposed to normal weight women is different by ethnicity whether measured by risk ratio or risk difference. However, there are also differences in the risk of diabetes in women with less than a high school education compared to those with more education, and the differences in the risk ratios and the risk differences are similar in magnitude to those seen for ethnicity. For family history of diabetes, differences in the risk ratios and the risk differences associated with obesity are also apparent. Similar types of analyses could be done for age and physical activity levels as well as other variables. Since a large part of ethnic variation can be accounted for by environmental and cultural factors that are subject to change, cutpoints specific to ethnic groups might have to be altered as their environment changed. For instance, an ethnic group that changed over time from being active to sedentary might also show a change in the associations between BMI and risk. Thus cutpoints based on risk estimates would need to be altered over time as behavioural variables changed, resulting in changes in the association between BMI and risk.

Conclusion

We have presented arguments in favour of promoting a single set of BMI cutoffs for obesity (and overweight) for all ethnic groups. Simplicity can be cited as a final, over arching reason to have a single BMI cutpoint for all populations. Using the same logic as that applied to BMI, a case could be made to have different cutpoints for different ethnic groups for other outcomes such as hypertension and diabetes, yet ethnic specific definitions have been avoided. Similarly, definitions of obesity should be kept simple. The BMI cutpoint for obesity provides, after all, only a crude indication of the status of an individual, and as such is appropriate in public health settings. Simplicity is well known to be a strong virtue of any health message to the public.

References

1. World Health Organization. Obesity: Preventing and Managing the Global Epidemic: Report of a WHO Consultation on Obesity. Geneva: World Health Organization Tech Rep Ser 2000; 894: i–xii, 1–253.

2. International Diabetes Institute. The Asia Pacific perspective: redefining obesity and its treatment. Geneva: WHO; 2000.

3. Deurenberg P, Yap M, van Staveren W. Body mass index and per cent body fat: a meta analysis among different ethnic groups. *Int J Obes* 1998; 22: 1164–71.

4. Stevens J, Juhaeri, Cai J, Jones DW. The effect of decision rules on the choice of a body mass index cutoff for obesity: examples from African American and white women. *Am J Clin Nutr* 2002; 75(6): 986–92.

5. Yuan JM, Ross R, Gao YT, Yu M. Body weight and mortality: a prospective evaluation in a cohort of middle-aged men in Shanghai, China. *Int J Epidemiol* 1998; 27: 824–32.

6. Zhao L, Zhou B, Wu Y, Li Y, Yang J. A prospective study on body mass index and mortality. *Chinese J Epid* 2002; 23: 24–7.

7. Tsugane S, Sasaki S, Tsubono Y. Under- and overweight impact on mortality among middle-aged Japanese men and women: a 10-y follow-up of JPHC study cohort I. *Int J Obes Relat Metab Disord.* 2002; 26(4): 529–37.

8. Maskarinec G, Meng L, Kolonel L. Alcohol intake, body weight, and mortality in a multiethnic prospective cohort. *Epidemiology* 1998; 9: 654–61.

9. Pan WH, Mhurchu C, Parag V, Zhang XH, Rodgers A. Body mass index and cardiovascular disease in Asian Pacific populations. *Am J Clin Nutr* 2002; 75: S408.

Progress in Obesity Research: 9. Edited by *Geraldo Medeiros-Neto, Alfredo Halpern* and *Claude Bouchard*
©2003 John Libbey Eurotext Ltd, pp. 558–560.

CHAPTER 117

Debate: Visceral obesity is just a marker of other factors which are responsible for the risks of obesity

Per Björntorp

Department of Heart and Lung Diseases, Sahlgren's Hospital, University of Göteborg, 41345 Göteborg, Sweden
[e-mail: Per Bjorntorp@hjl.gu.se]

The question to be discussed is the problem of whether visceral fat accumulation is responsible for the generation of risk factors leading to cardiovascular disease and diabetes type 2 or is just a marker of other factors responsible for disease generation.

Some years ago it was suggested that free fatty acids (FFA) from the visceral fat depot were affecting hepatic metabolism to cause increased synthesis of very low density lipoproteins, and hence in the next step, low density lipoproteins, both highly atherogenic. In addition FFA are known to stimulate hepatic gluconeogenesis, resulting in elevated circulating glucose. Finally, experiments with the perfused rat liver indicated that FFA were able to diminish hepatic clearance of insulin and therefore would be able to at least partly explain the prevailing hyperinsulinaemia. The background to this hypothesis was the findings of a very sensitive lipolytic process in visceral adipose tissue, combined with a blunted antilipolytic effect of insulin. Consequently it was hypothesized that elevated FFA concentrations in the portal vein, which drains visceral adipose tissue, were originating from enlarged visceral depots and then creating dyslipidaemia, hyperglycaemia and hyperinsulinaemia, all powerful risk factors for cardiovascular disease and diabetes[1].

A first question then arises, is excess exposure of the liver to FFA in the portal vein followed by these consequences. It seems reasonably well established that fatty acids are the rate limiting step for the synthesis of the lipoproteins mentioned. Furthermore, there seems to be good evidence for the gluconeogenic effects of FFA. The diminishing of hepatic clearance of insulin by FFA is found in experiments with the perfused rat liver and is well established in young rats. However, in older rats this is not that clear which might be due to the higher hepatic contents of triglycerides. The data from humans are scarce and uncertain.

Already when this hypothesis was published[1] it was suspected that there were central forces to driving both visceral fat accumulation and increasing lipid mobilization from adipose tissues, particularly from the sensitive visceral depot.

This hypothesis was based mainly on *in vitro* data. Small pieces of adipose tissue were incubated and release of glycerol measured in the basal condition and with stimulation by lipolytic agents. The results showed clearly that visceral fat mobilized more fat than subcutaneous adipose tissues. These data were then adjusted for the mass of visceral and other adipose tissues, and it was suggested that portal FFA probably were elevated in visceral obesity, and therefore could generate the risk factors mentioned above.

A major flaw of this interpretation is, however, that *in vitro* studies can not estimate the innervation and blood flow of the intact tissue. Both these factors are elevated in visceral fat in comparisons with other fat depots. The results obtained by calculations from *in vitro* data consequently were highly uncertain.

A problem with this whole area of research is that measurements in the portal vein in humans are almost impossible due to technical difficulties. Therefore other, more indirect techniques have to be used. One such technique is to infuse labeled fatty acids and estimate endogenous production by

Positive energy balance   Neuroendocrine and autonomic arousal

Obesity

Central obesity.
Elevated turn over
of visceral and
subq. fat

Free fatty acids

↓

Insulin resistance

↓

Diabetes, CVD

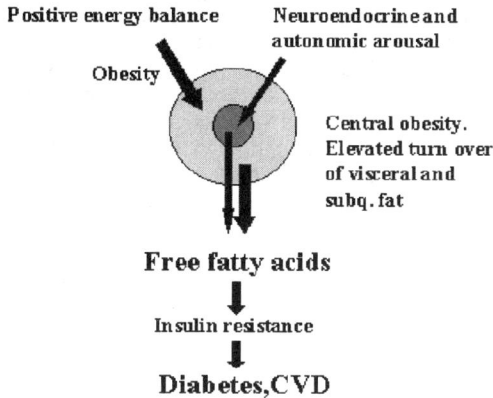

Fig. 1. The explanation to comorbidities in obesity. Obesity (large circle) is produced by positive energy balance. A neuroendocrine arousal is directing fat to central depots and increases lipid mobilization from the enlarged fat depots with elevated free fatty acids (FFA) and insulin resistance as consequences.

measuring the dilution of the label. When sampling FFA in the hepatic vein the concentration of the label is an estimate of the production of FFA from the visceral fat depot. It should, however, be remembered that there is also blood flow to the liver from the hepatic artery, that is, from systemic circulation. Therefore, the FFA production measured as dilution of labeled fatty acids in the hepatic vein is not only a result of visceral adipose tissue lipolysis, but also a measurement of lipolysis in other adipose tissue depots. Results from such studies suggest that lipolysis in general is elevated in abdominal obesity, that is both visceral and other depots have an increased contribution to elevated FFA in the portal vein[2]. Although these results open up the possibility that hepatic exposure for elevated levels of portal FFA may generate risk factors, it is not possible to conclude that this is a consequence of a large fraction of FFA from the visceral fat depot. In other words, this type of evidence does not show that visceral fat has any specific role in the generation of risk factors for prevalent disease.

There are also other approaches to this technically difficult problem. There are studies measuring the hepatic contents of lipid. Such studies show that in visceral obesity there are increased liver contents of triglyceride, presumably due to elevated exposure of the liver to FFA. There is also hyperinsulinaemia, proportional to the hepatic triglyceride contents. This picture then would be compatible with the hypothesis outlined above, and has been called the syndrome of 'fois gras', fatty liver[3]. However, again the important blood flow is not included, and the kinetics of the presumed events can not be evaluated. Another experimental approach to this problem utilizes the fact that adipose tissue triglycerides can be labeled by ingestion of a triglyceride load containing a small amount of labeled oleic acid[4]. By repeated biopsies the turnover of the depot fat can then be estimated and is found to be in the order 8, 6 and 3 months for femoral subcutaneous, abdominal subcutaneous and visceral fat. The turn over is probably dependent on FFA mobilization and therefore FFA flow in the portal vein and the systemic circulation can be estimated. Such calculations then result in an increased mobilization of FFA per unit mass of visceral fat in comparisons with other depots. However, due to the small total mass of visceral fat it is not likely that hepatic exposure of FFA from visceral fat would be of importance for the generation of risk factors.

Taken together at this point there is no definite evidence that increased FFA flow in the portal vein is responsible for the generation of risk factors for the development of cardiovascular disease and type 2 diabetes mellitus.

There are, however, other possibilities than FFA production from visceral fat. Recent experiments with mice, overexpressing ß-hydroxy steroid dehydrogenase 1 in adipose tissue show interesting results. This enzyme converts inactive glucocorticoids to active corticosterone and the genetic manipulation therefore results in oversecretion of the latter hormone. The results are insulin resistance and its consequences, an expected effect of corticosterone excess or, in humans, cortisol excess. The specific role of visceral fat for this event is, however, unclear[5].

Surgical removal of the omentum has been reported to be followed by an improvement of the symptoms characteristic of visceral obesity[6]. This would be compatible with a role for visceral fat in the pathogenesis of risk factors for disease. The results are, however, somewhat surprising because omental fat is a relatively minor part of intraabdominal fat, where usually mesenteric fat masses are greater, and these can not easily be removed by surgery. There are, however, remaining possibilities that omental fat has a specific secretory role producing factor(s) which are harmful.

The latter point seems to be the remaining possibility for a role of visceral fat. The mechanism that portal FFA are responsible is not totally refuted, but the evidence is incomplete. With the information available it seems rather unlikely that this is a pathogenetic pathway of importance. There is, however, strong evidence that systemic FFA concentrations are elevated in central obesity[7]. This is probably due

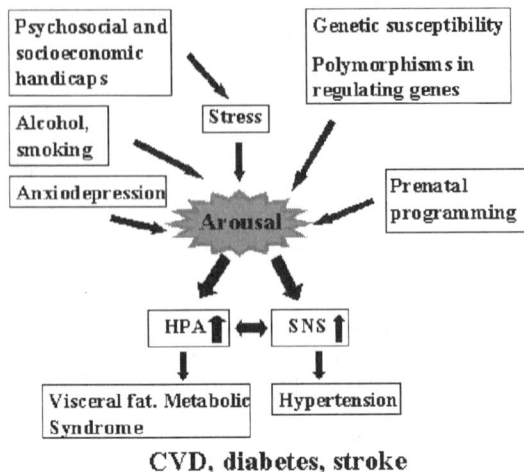

Psychosocial and socioeconomic handicaps

Genetic susceptibility

Polymorphisms in regulating genes

Alcohol, smoking

Stress

Anxiodepression

Arousal

Prenatal programming

HPA ↑ ⟷ SNS ↑

Visceral fat. Metabolic Syndrome

Hypertension

CVD, diabetes, stroke

Fig. 2. Background factors to the arousal syndrome responsible for the comorbidities of central obesity. Various environmental, genetic and perinatal programming factors cause a neuroendocrine and autonomic arousal with the consequences listed. Abreviations: HPA: Hypothalamic-pituitary adrenal axis. SNS: Central sympathetic nervous system. CVD: Cardiovascular disease (for details, see refs[8-10]).

to a combination of enlargement of adipose tissues in general and increased production of lipolytic agents, including elevated activity of the sympathetic nervous system in central obesity[8] (for schematic summary, see Fig.1).

In the discussion of various possibilities above it has been presumed that visceral fat has a specific role in risk factor generation, mainly via effects on the liver. A major problem with this reasoning is, however, that there is no explanation to the fact that excess fat is accumulated in visceral depots in the first place. Another type of hypothesis includes also this factor. This hypothesis has been described repeatedly recently[8-10]. In short, there is considerable evidence of a central arousal syndrome in visceral obesity. The resulting increased neuroendocrine-endocrine and autonomic nervous system activities are able to explain not only visceral fat accumulation but also the prevailing insulin resistance, due both to increased lipid mobilization in general and to the excess secretion of hormones known to create insulin resistance, such as cortisol. The advantage with this hypothesis is that it includes all observed abnormalities of central obesity and provides mechanistic explanations to these phenomena (for schematic summary, see Fig.2).

References

1. Björntorp P. 'Portal' adipose tissue as a generator of risk factors for cardiovascular disease and diabetes. *Arteriosclerosis* 1990; 10: 493–6.

2. Jensen MD, Haymond MW, Rizza RA, Cryer PE, Miles JM. Influence of body fat distribution on free fatty acid metabolism in obesity. *J Clin Invest* 1989; 83; 1168–73.

3. Björntorp P. Guest commentary: Liver triglycerides and metabolism. *Int J Obes* 1995; 19: 839–40.

4. Marin P, Lönn L, Andersson B, Odén O, Olbe L, Bengtsson BA., Björntorp P. Assimilation of triglycerides in subcutaneous and intraabdominal adipose tissues *in vivo* in men: Effects of testosterone. *J Clin Endocr Metab* 1996; 81: 1018–22.

5. Masuzaki H, Paterson J, Shinyama H, Morton NM, Mullins JJ, Seckl J, Flier JS. A transgenic model of visceral obesity and the metabolic syndrome. *Science* 2001; 294: 2166–70.

6. Thorne A, Lönnqvist F, Apelman J, Arner P. A pilot study of long-term effects of a novel obesity treatment: omentectomy in connection with adjustable gastric banding. *Int J Obes Relat Metab Disord* 2002; 26: 193–9.

7. Kissebah AH, Peiris AN. Biology of regional fat distribution: relationship to non-insulin-dependent diabetes mellitus. *Diabetes Metab Rer* 1989; 5: 83–109.

8. Björntorp P. The relationship between obesity and type 2 diabetes. In: *International textbook of diabetes mellitus*, Ferrannini E, Zimmet P, De Fronzo R, Keen H (eds). Chichester: Wiley.

9. Björntorp P. Visceral obesity: A 'Civilization Syndrome'. *Obes Res* 1993; 1: 206–22.

10. Björntorp P, Holm G, Rosmond R. Hypothalamic arousal, insulin resistance and type 2 diabetes mellitus. *Diabet Med* 1999; 16: 373–83.

CHAPTER 118

Obesity in the United States

Ali H. Mokdad

Centers for Disease Control and Prevention, Atlanta, GA 30333, USA
[e-mail: ahm1@cdc.gov]

Introduction

Obesity is a major cause of morbidity and mortality in the United States[1]. Each year, an estimated 300,000 US adults die of causes related to obesity[2]. Obesity also substantially increases morbidity and impairs quality of life[3–5]. Overall, the direct costs of obesity and physical inactivity account for approximately 9.4 per cent of US health care expenditures[6].

We used data from the Behavioral Risk Factor Surveillance System (BRFSS) to monitor obesity trends since 1991 and to examine changes in the prevalence of obesity among adults in the United States from 1991 to 2000. We also examined the prevalence of attempting to lose or maintain weight and the strategies used by Americans to lose or maintain weight.

Methods

The BRFSS is a cross-sectional telephone survey conducted by the state health departments with assistance from the Centers for Disease Control and Prevention. The BRFSS questionnaire consists primarily of questions about personal behaviours that increase risk for one or more of the 10 leading causes of death in the United States. The BRFSS uses a multistage cluster design based on random-digit dialing methods of sampling to select a representative sample from each state's noninstitutionalized civilian residents aged 18 years or older. Data collected from each state are pooled to produce nationally representative estimates. A detailed description of the survey methods is available elsewhere[7,8].

We used data on self-reported weight and height to calculate body mass index (BMI) as weight (kg)/height (m²). Participants were classified as obese if their BMI was greater than or equal to 30[9]. Extreme obesity (obesity class III) was classified as BMI greater than or equal to 40[9]. Self-reported weight and height were assessed by asking respondents, 'About how much do you weigh without shoes?' and 'About how tall are you without shoes?'

Participants were asked to report the type, duration, and frequency of the two leisure-time physical activities they had participated in most frequently in the past month. These questions were used to create a leisure-time physical activity score: (1) inactive, (2) irregularly active, (3) regular, not intense, and (4) regular, intense[10].

Respondents were asked 'Are you trying to lose weight?' Those who responded 'no' were asked 'Are you trying to maintain weight?' Respondents who answered 'yes' to either question were asked: (1) 'Are you trying to eat fewer calories or less fat to lose weight?'; (2) 'Are you using physical activity or exercise to lose weight or keep from gaining weight?'; and (3) 'In the past 12 months, has a doctor, nurse, or health professional given you advice about your weight?'

The 2000 BRFSS questionnaire included the fruit and vegetable (FV) module. We used these questions to classify participants into four groups of fruit and vegetable consumption: (1) less than once or not at all daily, (2) one to less than three times daily; (3) three to less than five times daily; and (4) five or more times daily. SAS and SUDAAN were used in the analyses and to account for the complex sampling design[11,12].

Table 1. Obesity prevalence among US adults, by selected characteristics, behavioural risk factor surveillance system, 1991 and 2000

	1991	2000	% difference
Total	12.0 (0.18)	19.8 (0.17)	65.0
Sex			
Male	11.7 (0.26)	20.2 (0.26)	72.6
Female	12.2 (0.24)	19.4 (0.21)	59.0
Age groups, year			
18–29	7.1 (0.29)	13.5 (0.33)	90.1
30–39	11.3 (0.34)	20.2 (0.36)	78.8
40–49	15.8 (0.48)	22.9 (0.41)	44.9
50–59	16.1 (0.58)	25.6 (0.47)	59.0
60–69	14.7 (0.52)	22.9 (0.50)	55.8
70+	11.4 (0.53)	15.5 (0.41)	36.0
Race			
White	11.3 (0.18)	18.5 (0.17)	63.7
Black	19.3 (0.68)	29.3 (0.59)	51.8
Hispanic	11.6 (0.76)	23.4 (0.77)	101.7
Other	7.3 (0.88)	12.0 (0.68)	64.4
Education levels			
Less than high school	16.5 (0.48)	26.1 (0.62)	58.2
High school	13.3 (0.30)	21.7 (0.30)	63.2
Some college	10.6 (0.36)	19.5 (0.31)	84.0
College +	8.0 (0.30)	15.2 (0.26)	90.0
Smoking status			
Never	12.0 (0.24)	19.9 (0.23)	65.8
Ex-smoker	14.0 (0.37)	22.7 (0.35)	62.1
Current	9.9 (0.32)	16.3 (0.35)	64.6

Results

A steady increase was observed in both sexes, all ages, all races, all education levels, and all smoking levels (Table 1). The prevalence of obesity increased by 65 per cent since 1991. A total of 38.8 million Americans were obese (19.6 million men and 19.2 million women).

Weight control practices varied by BMI. While most participants were trying to lose or maintain weight, 20.1 per cent of overweight participants and 13.5 per cent of obese participants were not trying to lose or maintain weight. About 27 per cent of Americans did not engage in any physical activity, and another 28.2 per cent were not regularly active. Only 24.4 per cent of Americans ate fruits and vegetables at least five times a day. Among obese participants who were trying to lose weight, only 42.8 per cent had been advised to lose weight by a health professional; 15.6 per cent of overweight participants had received such advice.

Comment

These data show that between 1991 and 2000, obesity increased in every state and across all age groups, races, educational levels, and smoking statuses. This rapid increase in obesity in all segments of the population and regions of the country implies that there have been broad sweeping changes in the society that are contributing to weight gain by fostering caloric imbalance.

Our estimates of the extent of the two epidemics of obesity and diabetes in the United States are conservative. In validation studies of self-reported weight and height, overweight subjects tend to underestimate their weight, and all participants tend to overestimate their height[13,14].

The strategies that Americans use to lose or maintain weight contribute to their failure to achieve their weight control objectives. We found that Americans have not increased their physical activity levels and their consumption of fruits and vegetables enough to control the obesity epidemic. Their physical activity patterns and their consumption of fruits and vegetables is still far below what will be needed to attain goals for healthy weight.

To control these dual epidemics, there is an urgent need to implement multi-component interventions for weight control, healthy eating, and physical activity. Health professionals should assess overweight and obesity, and recommend weight loss (using the combination of a low-calorie diet and increased physical activity) to overweight and obese patients, and weight maintenance to patients with normal weight. Workplaces must offer healthy food choices in their cafeterias and provide opportunities for employees to be physically active on site. Schools must offer more physical education that encourages lifelong physical activity. Urban policymakers must provide more sidewalks, bike paths, and other alternatives to cars. Parents need to reduce their children's TV and computer time and encourage active play. In general, restoring physical activity to our daily routines will be crucial.

References

1. Pi-Sunyer FX. Health implications of obesity. *Am J Clin Nutr* 1991; 53: S1595–S1603.

2. Allison D, Fontaine K, Manson J, Stevens J, VanItallie T. Annual deaths attributable to obesity in the United States. *JAMA* 1991; 282: 1530–8.

3. Must A, Spadano J, Coakley E, Field A, Colditz G, Dietz W. The disease burden associated with overweight and obesity. *JAMA* 1999; 282: 1523–9.

4. Fontaine K, Bartlett S. Estimating health-related quality of life in obese individuals. *Dis Manage Health Outcomes* 1998; 3: 61–70.

5. Ford ES, Moriarty DG, Zack MM, Mokdad AH, Chapman DP. Self-reported body mass index and health-related quality of life: Findings from the Behavioral Risk Factor Surveillance System. *Obes Res* 2001; 9(1): 21–31.

6. Colditz G. Economic costs of obesity and inactivity. *Med Sci Sports Exerc* 1999; 31(11): S663–7.

7. Nelson DE, Holtzman D, Waller M, Leutzinger CL, Condon K. Objectives and design of the Behavioral Risk Factor Surveillance System. Proceedings of the section on survey methods, American Statistical Association National Meeting. Dallas: TX; 1998. Remington PL, Smith MY, Williamson DF, Anda RF, Gentry EM, Hogelin CG. Design, characteristics, and usefulness of state-based behavioral risk factor surveillance: 1981–1987. *Public Health Rep* 1988; 103: 366–75.

8. National Institutes of Health National Heart, lung, and Blood Institute. Clinical guidelines on the identification, evaluation, and treatment of overweight and obesity in adults. The evidence report. NHLBI. *Obes Res*. 1998; 6 (Suppl 2): 51S–209S (Review).

9. Aspersen CJ, Pollard RA, Pratt SO. Scoring physical activity data with special consideration for elderly populations. In: Proceedings of the 21st National Meeting of the Public Health Conference on Records and Statistics: Data for an Aging Population, 13–15 July 1987. DHHHS, PHS, 88-1214. Hyattsville: National Center for Health Statistics; 1987.

10. SAS System version 8, SAS Institute Inc. Cary, NC. 2000.

11. Shah BV, Barnwell BG, Bieler GS. SUDAAN User's Manual, release 7.5. Research Triangle Park. NC: Research Triangle Institute; 2000.

12. Rowland ML. Self-reported weight and height. *Am J Clin Nutr* 1990: 52: 1125–33.

13. Palta M, Prineas RJ, Berman R, Hannan P. Comparison of self-reported and measured height and weight. *Am J Epidemiol* 1982; 115; 223–30.

©2003 John Libbey Eurotext Ltd, pp. 564–566.

CHAPTER 119

Women's obesity in the developing world is shifting toward the poor

Carlos A. Monteiro and Barry M. Popkin

Department of Nutrition and Center for Epidemiological Studies in Health and Nutrition, School of Public Health, University of Sao Paulo, Av. Dr. Arnaldo, 715, Sao Paulo, Brazil 01246-904; Carolina Population Center, University of North Carolina at Chapel Hill, University Square, CB# 8120, 123 W. Franklin St., Chapel Hill, NC 27516-3997, USA
[e-mail: carlosam@usp.br]

Introduction

There is abundant documentation on the large gap separating the poor from the rich in developing countries regarding the burden of disease as it concerns nutritional deficiencies, infections, and maternal and perinatal problems. For instance, in Brazil children with illiterate mothers are at least 10 times more likely to die before the age of 5 than are children whose mothers have a university education.[1] However, much less information is available on the social distribution of non-communicable diseases, including obesity, in the developing world.

An exhaustive review by Sobal and Stunkard[2] of the literature published between 1933 and 1988 on socioeconomic status (SES) and obesity found 130 studies conducted in developed populations and only 14 studies in developing populations. The review concluded that SES and obesity tended to be inversely related in developed populations (particularly among adult women) and directly related in developing populations. In nearly 90 per cent of the studies on developing populations, obesity was found to be more frequent among the higher SES groups; in nearly 10 per cent no association was detected and in none obesity was more frequent among the lower SES groups.

Results from cross-sectional studies conducted from 1987 to 1994 and published after the review made by Sobal and Stunkard have showed inverse or curvilinear associations between SES and women's obesity in middle-income developing countries as Chile, Brazil and Curaçao[3-6]. Besides that, in Brazil, the comparison of results from the most recent national survey conducted in 1997 with results from previous surveys conducted in 1975 and 1989 detected a progressive shifting in women' obesity from the higher to the lower income groups in the more developed south-eastern region and, in general, in urban areas[7,8].

A comprehensive study by Martorell *et al.*[9], based on reanalyses of data from 36 national surveys conducted between 1987 and 1996 on women of reproductive ages, added new valuable information on the social distribution of obesity in the developing world. In studying the association between the level of women's formal education (low and high) and obesity, Martorell found that, in very poor countries, obesity levels were greatly concentrated among higher income educated women while, in relatively more developed countries, obesity levels were more equally distributed in the general population.

Several emerging issues justify a reappraisal of the social distribution of adult female obesity in the developing world: (1) evidence that obesity is continuously increasing worldwide[10]; (2) an indication that this increase is occurring at a faster rate in the developing world[11,12]; and, most importantly, (3) the 17 new national surveys on women at reproductive ages conducted in developing countries between 1997 and 2000.

Methods

Most of data used in this article come from the Demographic Health Surveys (DHSs) files (downloaded from http://www.macroint.com/dhs/) or obtained directly from the State Statistical Offices that conducted these surveys. In our analyses, we included data from 32 DHSs conducted between 1992 and 2000. Eighteen of these surveys were conducted in Sub-Sahara African countries: Burkina Faso in 1992, Benin in 1996, Cameroon in 1998, Central African Republic in 1994, Cote d'Ivoire in 1994, Ghana in 1998, Kenya in 1998, Madagascar in 1997, Malawi in 1992, Mali in 1996, Namibia in 1992, Niger in 1998, Nigeria in 1999, Senegal in 1992, Tanzania in 1996, Uganda in 1995, Zambia in 1996, and Zimbabwe in 1994. Seven surveys were conducted in Latin American and Caribbean (LAC) countries: Bolivia in 1998, Brazil in 1996, Colombia in 2000, Dominican Republic in 1996, Guatemala in 1998, Haiti in 1994, and Peru in 2000. Three surveys were conducted in North African, Middle Eastern, and Central Eastern European countries: Egypt in 1995, Jordan in 1997, and Turkey in1998. Three surveys were conducted in Central Asian countries: Kazakhstan in 1999, Kyrgyzstan in 1997, and Uzbekistan in 1996. One survey was conducted in South Asia: India in 1999. For countries in which two or more DHSs were conducted between 1992 and 2000, we used only the most recent data. To increase the number of Asian countries in the study, we included in our analyses data from two surveys conducted in 1997 in China and Vietnam (The China Health and Nutrition Survey and the Vietnam Living Standard Measurement Survey).

We restricted our analyses to non-pregnant women aged 20 to 49 in all surveys. In the case of the DHSs, most women were mothers of children under five years of age.

We calculated for each country the overall prevalence of overweight women (BMI ≥ 25.0 kg/m^2) and the prevalence of overweight according to country-specific quartiles of women's years of formal education. We used sample weights so that all estimates are nationally representative (except for the China survey which represents eight provinces). To assess and test the direction of the association between SES and obesity in each country, we used age-adjusted odds ratios (with 95 per cent confidence intervals) for overweight in the higher education quartile (compared with the lower education quartile).

Results

Among the 18 Sub-Sahara African countries studied, the prevalence of overweight women was relatively low – averaging 14.2 per cent, and ranging from 4.6 per cent in Madagascar to 23.9 per cent in Nigeria. The prevalence of overweight women in these very low-income economies increased significantly with the level of formal education and the relative risk (age-adjusted odds ratio) of overweight among women in the higher education quartile (compared with women in the lower education quartile) – ranged from 1.88 (1.51–2.34) in Tanzania to 5.29 (4.06–6.90) in Niger.

The prevalence of overweight women was much higher in the seven LAC countries studied – averaging 41.1 per cent, and ranging from 12.1 per cent in Haiti to 53.9 per cent in Peru. A mixed picture characterizes the association between formal education and obesity in the LAC countries. Both in the very low-income economy of Haiti and in the low-income economy of Guatemala, the prevalence of overweight increased significantly with women's formal education and the relative risk of overweight in the higher quartile of education was of 3.29 (2.41–4.50) in Haiti and of 1.95 (1.60–2.38) in Guatemala. In the low-income economy of Bolivia and the middle-income economy of Peru, the prevalence of overweight was high and relatively stable throughout the four quartiles of formal education (approximately 50 per cent). In the middle-income economies of Colombia, the Dominican Republic, and Brazil, the prevalence of overweight decreased significantly with women's formal education and the relative protection against overweight among women in the higher education quartile (age-adjusted odds ratio) when compared with women in the lower education quartile was of 0.85 (0.71–1.03) in Colombia, 0.84 (0.74–0.96) in the Dominican Republic, and 0.80 (0.64–0.98) in Brazil.

The prevalence of overweight women was very high in the three Arab countries studied in North Africa, the Middle East and Central Eastern Europe: 53.4 per cent in Egypt, 55.3 per cent in Turkey, and 63.7 per cent in Jordan. In the low- to middle-income economy of Egypt, the prevalence of overweight increased significantly with formal education and the relative risk of overweight in the higher education quartile was of 2.45 (2.18–2.75). The prevalence of overweight decreased significantly with formal education in the middle-income economies of Turkey and Jordan and the relative protection against overweight in the higher education quartile was of 0.51 (0.41–0.63) and 0.71 (58–0.87), respectively.

The prevalence of overweight women was intermediate in the low-income economies of the three Central Asian countries studied: 26.1 per cent in Uzbekistan, 32.7 per cent in Kyrgyzstan, and 37.1 per cent in Kazakhstan. In Uzbekistan, the prevalence of overweight increased with women's formal education and the relative risk of overweight in the higher education quartile was of 1.23 (1.04–1.45). In Kyrgyzstan and Kazakhstan, the prevalence of overweight remained stable throughout the four education quartiles.

The prevalence of overweight women was relatively low in the countries studied in South, Southeast, and East Asia: 4.9 per cent in Vietnam, 11.5 per cent in India, and 18.5 per cent in China. The pattern of association between formal education and overweight, however, was very different in each country. In the very low-income economy of Vietnam, the prevalence of overweight increased slightly but significantly with formal education and the relative risk of overweight in the higher education quartile was of 1.45 (1.12–1.88). In the low-income economy of India, the prevalence of overweight increased enormously and significantly with formal education and the relative risk of overweight in the higher education quartile was of 7.80 (6.44–9.44). In the rapidly growing economy of China, the prevalence of overweight decreased significantly with formal education and the relative protection against overweight in the higher education quartile was of 0.74 (0.55–0.98).

Conclusions

Our analyses of data from national surveys collected in 34 developing countries between 1992 and 2000 demonstrated a direct association between SES and women's overweight in 70 per cent of the countries, no significant association in 12 per cent, and a significant inverse association in 18 per cent. If we were to exclude the poorly economically developed Sub-Sahara African countries, 37.5 per cent of countries would show a direct association, 25 per cent no association, and 37.5 per cent an inverse association between SES and overweight. The comparison of these findings with the results compiled by Sobal and Stunkard[2] (from surveys conducted between 1933 and 1987) and the findings from Martorell[8] (based on surveys conducted between 1987 and 1996) suggests that women's obesity in the developing world is increasingly shifting toward the poor. Furthermore, our study indicates that in the middle-income countries (and even in the low-income but rapidly growing economy of China) the burden of women's obesity is already concentrated in the lower SES groups. This may indicate that, in the absence of effective public actions, obesity can shift very rapidly toward the poor in most of the developing world.

References

1. UNICEF A infância brasileira nos anos 90. Brasília, DF Fundo das Nações Unidas para a Infância; 1998.

2. Sobal J, Stunkard AJ. Socioeconomic status and obesity: a review of the literature. *Psychol Bull* 1989; 105(2): 260–75.

3. Berrios CX, Jadue HL, Zenteno AJ, Ross AMI, Rodrigues HP. Prevalencias de factores de riesgo de enfermedaddes crónicas. Estudio en la población general de la Región Metropolitana. *Revista Medica de Chile* 1990; 118: 597–604.

4. Sichieri R, Coitinho DC, Leao MM, Recine E, Everhart JE. High temporal, geographical and income variation in body mass index among adults in Brazil. *Am J Public Health* 1994; 84: 793–8.

5. Monteiro CA, Mondini L, Souza ALM, Popkin BM. The nutrition transition in Brazil. *Eur J Clin Nutr* 1995: 4: 105–13.

6. Grol MEC, Eimers JM, Alberts JF, Bouter LM, Gerstenbluth I, Halabi Y, van Sondere E, van den Heubel WJA. Alarmingly high prevalence of obesity in Curaçao: data from an interview survey stratified for socioeconomic status. *Int J Obes* 1997; 21: 1002–9.

7. Monteiro CA, Conde WL. A tendência secular da obesidade Segundo estratos sociais: Nordeste e Sudeste do Brasil, 1975–1989–1997. *Arq Bras Endocrinol Metab* 1999; 43(3): 186–194.

8. Monteiro CA, Benicio MHD'A, Conde WL, Popkin BM. Shifting obesity trends in Brazil. *Eur J Clin Nutr* 2000; 54: 342–46.

9. Martorell R, Khan LK, Hughes ML, Grummer-Strawn LM. Obesity in women from developing countries. *Eur J Clin Nutr* 2000; 54: 247–52.

10. Word Health Organization. Obesity: preventing and managing the global epidemic. WHO Technical Report Series 894. Geneva: 2000.

11. Popkin BM. An overview on the nutrition transition and its health implications: the Bellagio meeting. *Public Health Nutr* 2002; 5: 93–103.

12. Popkin BM. The shift in stages of the nutrition transition in the developing world differs from past experiences! *Public Health Nutr* 2002; 5: 205–14.

Progress in Obesity Research: 9. Edited by *Geraldo Medeiros-Neto, Alfredo Halpern and Claude Bouchard*
©2003 John Libbey Eurotext Ltd, pp. 567–570.

CHAPTER 120

The shifts in diet, physical activity and obesity in the developing world appear to be speeding up!

Barry M. Popkin

Carolina Population Center, University of North Carolina Chapel Hill, University Square, CB# 8120, 123 W. Franklin St., Chapel Hill, NC 27516-3997, USA
[e-mail: popkin@unc.edu]

Introduction

This paper summarizes some issues and evidence that lead us to assert the experience (rapid onset of obesity and NR-NCD) may be unique. Understanding this topic is important for planning a strategy to prevent obesity and its complications in the developing world. Essentially the key assertions are:

- The speed of change appears unique due to the timing of the economic, technological, and social transformation now faced by lower and moderate income, transitional societies;

- The differences in the rates of change may be exacerbated by some biological relationships.

Assertion 1.
The shifts in dietary and activity patterns and body composition seem to be occurring more rapidly

The pace of the rapid nutrition transition shifts in diet and activity patterns from the period, termed the receding famine pattern, to one dominated by NR-NCDs seems to be accelerating in the lower and middle income transitional countries. We use nutrition rather than diet so that term NR-NCD's incorporate the effects of diet, physical activity, and body composition rather than solely focus on dietary patterns and their effects. This is based partially on incomplete information that seems to indicate that the prevalence of obesity and a number of NR-NCDs are increasing far much faster in the lower and middle income world than it has in the West. Another element is that the rapid changes in urban populations are much greater than that experienced a century or less ago in the West; yet another is the shift in occupation structure and the rapid introduction of the modern mass media. Underlying such changes is a general concern for rapid globalization as the root cause.

Clearly, there are quantitative and qualitative dimensions to these changes. On the one hand, changes toward a high density diet, reduced complex carbohydrates and other important elements, and inactivity may be proceeding faster than in the past. The shift from labour intensive occupations and leisure activities toward more capital-intensive, less strenuous work and leisure is also occurring faster. On the other hand, qualitative dimensions related to multidimensional aspects of the diet, activity, body composition, and disease shifts may exist. Social and economic stresses people face and feel as these changes occur might also be included.

At the start of the new Millennium, scholars often feel as if the pace and complexity of life, reflected in all aspects of work and play, are increasing exponentially; there are also unanticipated developments, new technologies, and the impact of a very modern, high-powered communications system. It is this sense of rapid change that makes it so important to understand what is happening and anticipate the way changes in patterns of diet, activity, and body composition are occurring. While the penetration and influence of modern communications, technology and economic systems – related to what is termed globalization – have been a dominant theme of the last few decades, there seem to be some unique issues that have led to a rapid increase of 'globalization and its impact'.

Placing the blame on globalization is, on the one hand, focusing on broad and vaguely measured set of forces; this ignores the need to be focused and specific which would allow us to develop potentially viable policy options. It is difficult to measure each element of this globalization equation and its impact. These processes certainly have been expanded, as indicated by enhanced free trade, a push toward reduction of trade barriers in the developing world, and the increasing penetration of international corporations into the commerce in each country (measured by share of GNP or manufacturing). Similarly, other economic issues related to enhanced value given to market forces and international capital markets are important. Equally, the increasing access to Western media, the removal of communication barriers enhanced by the World Wide Web, cable TV, mobile telephone systems, etc., is important. The accelerated introduction of Western technology into the manufacturing, basic sectors of agriculture, mining, and services is also a key element.

Another way to consider the types of changes the developing world is facing is to consider an urban squatter's life and a rural villager's life in China 20 years ago, and today. During the 1970s, food supply concerns still existed; there was no television; limited bus and mass transportation, little food trade, minimal processed food existed, and most rural and urban occupations were very labour intensive. Today, work and life activities have changed: small gas-powered tractors are available, modern industrial techniques are multiplying, offices are quite automated, soft drinks and many processed foods are found everywhere, TV's are found in about 89 per cent of households (at least a fifth of whom are linked to Hong Kong Star and western advertising and programming), younger children do not ride bicycles, and mass transit has become heavily used. Multiply such changes by similar ones occurring in much of Asia, North Africa, the Middle East, Latin America, and many areas (particularly cities) in sub-Saharan Africa and it is evident that the shift from a subsistence economy to a modern, industrialized one occurred in a span of 10–20 years; whereas, in Europe and other industrialized high income societies, this occurred over many decades or centuries.

To truly measure and examine these issues, we would need to compare changes in the 1980–2000 period, for countries that are low and middle income, with changes that occurred a half century earlier for the developing world. However, data on diet and activity patterns are not available and there is only minimal data on NR-NCDs and obesity.

Obesity trends

A recently published volume summarized many of the rapid shifts in obesity and overweight status in the regions of the developing world[1,2]. In China, we examined the shifts in body composition among adults aged 20–45 over an eight-year period[3]. As we have shown, not only did mean BMI increase, but the shape of the BMI distribution curve changed over the 8-year period[3]. From 1989 to 1997 the proportion of underweight men and women dropped considerably and the prevalence of both overweight and obesity increased greatly. In fact, the proportion of overweight or obese men more than doubled from 6.4.0 per cent to 14.5 per cent and the proportion of overweight or obese women increased 50 per cent from 11.5 per cent to 16.2 per cent.

In the Popkin 2002 paper we showed that the increase in the prevalence of overweight and obesity during the past several decades is much faster in the developing world. While in Europe and the US the annual percentage point increase in overweight plus obesity was about 0.3 to 0.5 percentage points of the total adult population per year, the same percentage point increase was double to fourfold that rate in a large number of developing countries.

Dietary changes: shift in the overall structure over time

The diets of the developing world are shifting equally rapidly. We do not have good data for most countries on total energy intake, but we do have reasonable data to examine shifts in the structure of the diet. Food balance data was used to examine the shift, over time, in the proportion of energy from fat[5]. We have shown dramatic increases in the energy density of the diet in China and other countries, large shifts toward increased edible oil intake, and increased sweetening of the diet by dramatic jumps in added sugar intake. The latter is based on unpublished research.

When we specifically examine the combined effect of these various shifts in the structure of rural and urban Chinese diets, we find an upward shift in the energy density of the foods consumed[4,5]. In this study, the kcal of energy intake from foods and alcohol per 100 grams of food in both urban and rural Chinese adult diets increased over 10 per cent (to 2.42) between 1989 and 1997. These are very rapid shifts in energy density. It is important to note that this value of 2.42 is not comparable with the normal measure of energy density of the diet. The normal method includes full measures of all beverages, while the Chinese Food Composition Table, from which this data was extracted, measures only a few beverages (milk, coconut juice, sugarcane juice, spirits, beer, wine, champagne, and brandy) and excludes many beverages, in particular tea and coffee. There are a number of clinical studies that varied the energy density of the diet in *ad libitum* studies. Each finds higher density increases, often only an increase as low as from 1 kcal/g to 1.3 kcal/g, can increase total energy intake[6,7]. For these reasons, energy density changes in China, and most likely in other developing countries, are critical components of dietary change to be monitored.

Physical activity shifts are equally rapid

There is much less data and analysis on the shifts, over time, in energy expenditures and physical activity patterns in general. Some published studies have demonstrated the remarkable shift in the structure of occupations, as well as in the activities performed in each occupation[8,9]. Using data from the China Health and Nutrition Survey (CHNS) results with adult physical activity patterns measured over the 1989–97 period to examine this topic, we have shown a remarkable downward shift for the proportion of adults, aged 20–45, whose daily activity profile categorizes them in a moderate category, compared to those in the light category over the last decade. In other work, we have shown that light and moderate activity profiles are linked with greater obesity[3,10].

Assertion 2.

Is the biology different? Or rather, do we have different social structures and body composition patterns that affect BMI-disease relationships? Or are there genetic variants that are important?

There are a number of different ways these questions could be answered in the affirmative. One is if the body composition and other unmeasured race – ethnic factors affect susceptibility to NR-NCDs. Another might be if previous disease patterns (e.g. the presence of malaria or other tropical diseases) led to disease patterns that predisposed the population to certain problems. One component of this might be the fetal insult syndrome developed and popularized by Barker[11].

There has been a growing body of research that shows the international standards, used to delineate who is overweight and obese, are not appropriate for many large subpopulations in the world. For instance, a BMI of 25 in an Asian adult appears to have a far greater adverse metabolic effect than in a Caucasian adult[12]. In fact, the World Health Organization (WHO) and the International Obesity Task Force (IOTF) formed a group of scientists and agencies in Asia to review this topic. This group held international meetings and has proposed a lower BMI cutoff for Asians of 23 for overweight and of 25 for obesity[13]. In one paper comparing China, the Philippines and US Hispanics, Blacks and whites, the odds of being hypertensive were higher for Chinese men and women compared the other subpopulation groups at lower BMI's in the 23–25 range[14]. Ethnic differences in the strength of the association between BMI and disease outcomes warrants further consideration.

What is not clear is how much of this difference between sub-populations BMI – diabetes or other BMI – morbidity relationships is a function of differences of body composition, metabolic or genetic factors, or social causes. Elsewhere we have shown that part of the apparent race – hypertension relationship may also be explained partially by socioeconomic status[14].

There is another pathway related to the role of previous health problems for which we have less understanding and no real documentation of its impact (e.g. malnutrition that caused a virus to mutate, parasitic infections that affected long-term absorption patterns, or a parasite that is linked with an unknown genotype – comparable to sickle cell anaemia and its evolutionary linkage with malaria). We have no basis for speculation about this potential pathway.

However, the final pathway – the effect of fetal and infant insults on subsequent metabolic function – is one that appears to be a critical area. If the rapid shifts toward positive energy imbalance are occurring concurrently with higher levels of low birth weight in a population, then this becomes a much more salient aspect of this argument. In the developing world, where intrauterine malnutrition rates are high and a high prevalence of nutrition insults during infancy exist, the work of Barker and many others portends important potential effects on the prevalence of NR-NCDs in the coming decades[11,15]. Not only is there an emerging consensus that fetal insults, in particular with regard to thin, low birth weight infants who subsequently face a shift in the stage of the transition and become overweight, are linked with increased risk of the NR-NCDs, but infancy may equally be a period of high

569

vulnerability. Studies by Hoffman *et al.*[16], suggest that fat metabolism of stunted infants is impaired to the extent that this could lead to increased obesity and other metabolic shifts. Other work on the role of stunting on obesity had suggested such an effect, but Hoffman's work suggests the mechanism, and fits with the correlational work[17].

Discussion

The shift toward the nutrition transition stage linked with a high level of NR-NCDs is finding most lower and middle income countries unprepared. The changes are occurring very rapidly and the costs, in terms of health, are great. Large populations are still undernourished and programmes and policies to address these new changes in a preventive way are not being developed. Further understanding of the causes and consequences of these shifts must be understood and far greater priority needs to be given to the area of prevention.

Acknowledgements: This study was supported in part by grants from the US National Institutes of Health (NIH) (R01-HD30880 and R01-HD38700). I thank Ms. Frances Dancy for her administrative assistance, Bill Shappell for editorial assistance.

References

1. Popkin BM. An overview on the nutrition transition and its health implications: the Bellagio meeting. *Publ Health Nutr* 2002; 5: 93–103.

2. Popkin BM, Doak C. The obesity epidemic is a worldwide phenomenon. *Nutr Rev* 1998; 56: 106–14.

3. Bell C, Ge K, Popkin BM. Weight gain and its predictors in Chinese Adults. *Int J Obes* 2001; 25: 1079–86.

4. Guo X, Mroz TA, Popkin BM, Zhai F. Structural changes in the impact of income on food consumption in China, 1989–93. *Econ Dev Cult* 2000; 48: 737–60.

5. Popkin BM, Lu B, Zhai F. Understanding the nutrition transition: Measuring rapid dietary: changes in transitional countries public health nutrition. *Publ Health Nutr* 2003; 5(6A): 947–53.

6. Drewnowski A. Energy density, palatability, and satiety: implications for weight control. *Nutr Rev* 1998; 56: 347–53.

7. Bell EA, Castellanos VH, Pelkman CL, Thorwart ML, Rolls BJ. Energy density of foods affects energy intake in normal-weight women. *Am J Clin Nutr* 1998; 67: 412–20.

8. Popkin BM. The nutrition transition and its health implications in lower income countries. *Publ Health Nutr* 1998; 1: 5–21.

9. Popkin BM. Urbanization, Lifestyle changes and the nutrition transition. *World Devel* 1999; 27: 1905–16.

10. Paeratakul S, Popkin BM, Ge K, Adair LS, Stevens J. Changes in diet and physical activity affect the body mass index of Chinese adults. *Int J Obes Relat Metab Disord* 1998; 22: 424–32.

11. Barker DJP. *Fetal origins of cardiovascular and lung disease.* New York: Marcel Dekker, 2001.

12. Deurenberg P, Yap M, Staveren WA. Body mass index and per cent body fat: a meta analysis among different ethnic groups. *Int J Obes* 1998; 22(12): 1164–71.

13. International Diabetes Institute. The Asia-Pacific Perspective: redefining obesity and its treatment. Health Communications Australia Pty Ltd; 2000.

14. Bell AC, Adair LS, Popkin BM. Ethnic differences in the association between body mass index and hypertension. *Am J Epidemiol* 2002; 155: 346–53.

15. Adair LS, Kuzawa CW, Borja J. Maternal energy stores and diet composition during pregnancy program adolescent blood pressure. *Circulation* 2001; 104: 1034–39.

16. Hoffman DJ, Roberts SB, Verreschi I, Martins PA, de Nascimento C, Tucker KL, Sawaya AL. Regulation of energy intake may be impaired in nutritionally stunted children from the shantytowns of São Paulo, Brazil. *J Nutr* 2000; 130(9): 2265–70.

17. Popkin BM, Richards MK, Monteiro C. Stunting is associated with overweight in children of four nations that are undergoing the nutrition transition. *J Nutr* 1996; 126: 3009–16.

Progress in Obesity Research: 9. Edited by *Geraldo Medeiros-Neto, Alfredo Halpern* and *Claude Bouchard*
©2003 John Libbey Eurotext Ltd, pp. 571–578.

CHAPTER 121

Prevalence and time trends of obesity in Europe

Jacob C. Seidell

Department of Nutrition and Health, Free University of Amsterdam and VU Medical Center Amsterdam; De Boelelaan 1085, 1081 HV Amsterdam, The Netherlands
[e-mail: seidell@bio.vu.nl]

Classification of obesity and fat distribution

The epidemiology of obesity has for many years been difficult to study because many countries had their own specific criteria for the classification of different degrees of overweight. Gradually, however during the 1990s, however, the body mass index (weight/height^2) became a universally accepted measure of the degree of overweight and now identical cut-points are recommended. The most recent classification of overweight in adults by the World Health Organization (WHO) is the following[1]:

Table 1

Classification	BMI (kg/m^2)	Associated health risks
Underweight	< 18.5	Low (but risk of other clinical problems increased)
Normal range	18.5–24.9	Average
Overweight (25.0 or higher)		
Pre-obese	25.0–29.9	Increased
Obese class I	30.0–34.9	Moderately increased
Obese class II	35.0–39.9	Severely increased
Obese class III	40 or higher	Very severely increased

In many community studies in affluent societies this scheme has been simplified and cut-off points of 25 and 30 kg/m^2 are used for descriptive purposes. Both the prevalence of very low BMI (< 18.5 kg/m^2) and very high BMI (40 kg/m^2 or higher) are usually low, in the order of 1–2 per cent or less. Researchers in Asian countries have already criticized these cut-points. The absolute health risks (particularly of type 2 diabetes mellitus) seem to be higher at any level of the body mass index in Chinese and South-Asian people, which is probably also true for Asians living elsewhere. There are some developments that indicate that the cut-points to designate obesity or overweight may be lowered by several units of body mass index (e.g. 23 kg/m^2 for overweight and 25 kg/m^2 for obesity in Asian populations. In countries such as China and India, with each over a billion inhabitants, small changes in the criteria for overweight or obesity potentially increases the world estimate of obesity by several hundred million (currently estimates are about 250 million worldwide).

Much research over the last decade has suggested that for an accurate classification of overweight and obesity with respect to the health risks one needs to focus in abdominal fat distribution. Traditionally this has been indicated by a relatively high waist-to-hip circumference ratio. Recently it has been proposed that the waist circumference alone may be a better and simpler measure of the health risks associated with abdominal fatness[2]. In 1998 the National Institutes of Health (National Heart, Lung and Blood Institute) adopted the BMI classification and combined this with waist cut-off points[3]. In this classification the combination of overweight (BMI between 25 and 30 kg/m^2) and moderate obesity (BMI between 30 and 35 kg/m^2) with a large waist circumference ($\geq$ 102 cm in men or $\geq$88 cm in women) is proposed to carry additional risk[3].

In this chapter I focus on the prevalence of overweight and obesity as indicated by the body mass index. The emphasis is on recent surveys and time-trends and data have been selected that are based on representative population surveys with measured weight and height.

The prevalence and time trends of obesity in adults in Europe

In many reviews it has been shown that obesity (defined as a body mass index of 30 kg/m^2 or higher) is a prevalent condition in most countries with established market economies[4,5]. There is a wide variation in the prevalence of obesity between and within these countries. It is quite easy to find places with at least twofold difference in the prevalence of obesity in one single country. In countries with established market economies, obesity is usually more frequent among those with relative low socio-economic status and the prevalence increases with age until about 60–70 years of age, after which the prevalence declines[6]. In most of these established market economies it has been shown that the prevalence is increasing over time[4,5]. Tables 1 and 2 show the increases in the prevalence of obesity in men and women aged 35–64 years in several centres participating in the WHO MONICA project[7]. It is clear that there is a rapid increase in the prevalence of obesity in most centres from countries in the European Union, particularly in men. The prevalence of obesity in men and women in European countries in the EU region (Table 2) is similar to a women/men prevalence ratio of 1.07 (range 0.56–1.29). In central and eastern European countries (Table 3) the prevalence is generally much higher in women than in men (average women/men prevalence ratio 2.03; range: 1.27–2.87).

In centres from countries in central and eastern Europe the prevalence of obesity in women may have stabilized or even slightly decreased but still those prevalences remain among the highest in Europe. A study by Molarius *et al.*[7] showed that the social class differences in the prevalence of obesity are increasing with time. Obesity becomes increasingly a lower class problem in Europe.

Table 2. Prevalence of obesity (age standardized per cent with BMI $\geq$ 30) in centres in EU countries participating in the first round of the MONICA study (May 1979 to February 1989) and the third round (June 1989 to November 1996) (adapted from Molarius *et al.*[7])

Country (centre) EU countries (+ Switzerland and Iceland)	Men		Women		Sex ratio 3rd round women/men
	1st	3rd round	1st	3rd round	
Belgium (Ghent)	9	20	11	11	1.10
Denmark (Glostrup)	11	13	10	12	0.92
Finland (north Karelia)	17	22	23	24	1.09
Finland (Kuopio)	18	24	20	25	1.04
Finland (Turku/Loimaa)	19	22	17	19	0.86
France (Toulouse)	9	13	11	10	0.77
France (Lille)	13	17	17	22	1.29
Germany (Augsburg, urban)	18	18	15	21	1.17
Germany (Augsburg, rural)	20	24	22	23	0.96
Iceland (Iceland)	12	17	14	18	1.06
Italy (area Brianza)	11	14	15	18	1.29
Italy (Friuli)	15	17	18	19	1.12
Spain (Catalonia)	10	16	23	25	1.56
Sweden (North)	11	14	14	14	1.00
Switzerland (Vaud/Fribourg)	12	16	12	9	0.56
Switzerland (Ticino)	19	13	14	16	1.23
United Kingdom (Belfast)	11	13	14	16	1.23
United Kingdom (Glasgow)	11	23	16	23	1.00
Mean	**13.7**	**17.0**	**16.4**	**18.8**	**1.07**

Table 3. Prevalence of obesity (age standardized per cent with BMI ≥ 30 kg/m²) of centres in countries in Central and Eastern Europe participating in the first round of the MONICA study (May 1979 to February 1989) and the third round (June 1989 to November 1996) (adapted from Molarius et al.[7])

Country (centre) Central and Eastern European countries	Men		Women		Sex ratio 3rd round women/men
	1st	3rd round	1st	3rd round	
Poland (Warsaw)	18	22	26	28	1.27
Poland (Tarnobrzeg)	13	15	32	37	2.47
Russia (Moscow)	14	8	33	21	2.63
Russia (Novosibirsk)	13	15	43	43	2.87
Czech Republic (rural CZE)	22	22	32	29	1.32
Yugoslavia (Novi Sad)	18	17	30	27	1.59
Mean	16.3	16.5	32.7	30.8	2.03

Table 4. Overweight (BMI 25–29.9 kg/m²) and obesity (BMI ≥ 30 kg/m²) levels in the Baltic States (adapted from Pomerleau et al.[8])

Country	Year of survey	Sample size	% overweight		% obese	
			Men	Women	Men	Women
Estonia	1997	1154	32.0	23.9	9.9	6.0
Latvia	1997	2292	41.0	33.0	9.5	17.4
Lithuania	1997	2096	41.9	32.7	11.4	18.3
Lithuania*	2000	2195	45.6	31.6	16.9	23.4
Kazakstan**	1995	3538	–	21.8	–	16.7
Uzbekistan**	1996	4077	–	16.3	–	5.4

*'Finbalt' study based on self-reported height and weight (Janina Petkeviciene, personal communication);
**Adapted from Martorell et al.[18].

There are only a few countries in Europe where the evaluation of long-term time-trends in obesity based on national survey data is feasible. Figure 1 shows the secular time trends of the prevalence of obesity in the Netherlands[8]. There data are based on self-reported height and weight and probably the true prevalence is about 2–4 per cent points high throughout the period. Other data based on measured heights and weights in three regions in the Netherlands have shown that the obesity prevalence in men and women aged 37–43 years was 9.3 per cent in women and 8.5 per cent in men which was considerably higher than the 6.2 per cent and women and 4.9 per cent in men in the period 1976–1980[9]. Figure 2 shows the time-trends in the UK. In the mid 1980s the prevalence of obesity in men was similar in these two countries but in the UK the increase in the prevalence has been much more dramatic than in the Netherlands[10].

Data from Eastern-Finland (Fig. 3) shows that the prevalence of obesity in men has dramatically increased over the last thirty years and has caught up with the much more stable high prevalence in women[11]. Data from German suggest that the prevalence of obesity in 1998 was about 24 per cent in women and 22 per cent in men in eastern Germany (the former DDR) and 21 per cent in women and 19 per cent in men in western Germany (the from BRD). These figures were slightly up from 1990–1992[12].

Table 4 shows the prevalence of obesity in some less well studied countries including some countries which previously were part of the Soviet Union[13]. In most of these surveys the prevalence in women was in the order of 15–20 per cent and this was considerably higher than the prevalences observed in men.

Figure 4 shows the women/men ratio of prevalence of obesity (BMI > 30 kg/m²) in 1997 in the United Kingdom, by age (older than 16). The prevalence is similar in 25–65 year old men and women but it is progressively higher with age in woman over the age of 65 years and it is also higher in women

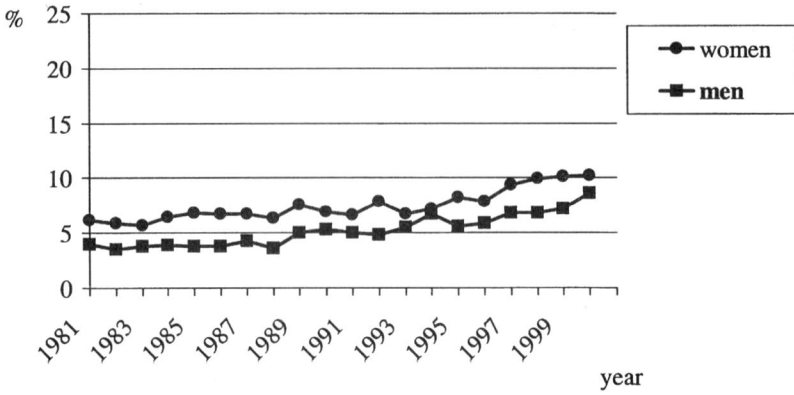

Fig. 1. Time-trends in the prevalence of obesity (BMI ≥ 30 kg/m^2) in the Netherlands (data from Statistics Netherlands (CBS)). Adapted from reference[8].

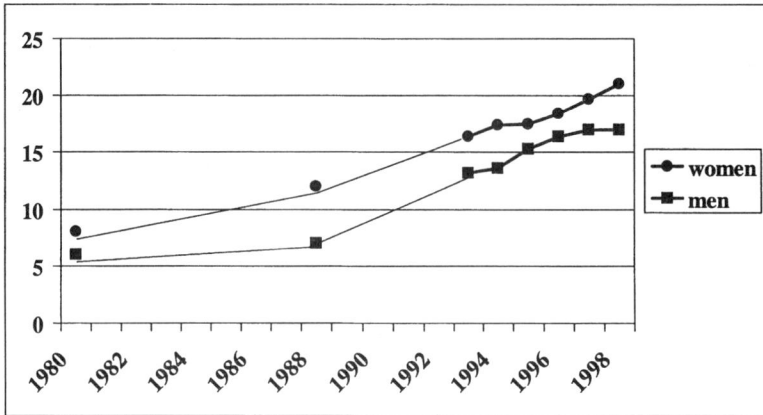

Fig. 2. Time trends in the prevalence of obesity (BMI ≥ 30 kg/m^2) in the UK (data from the Health Survey for England).

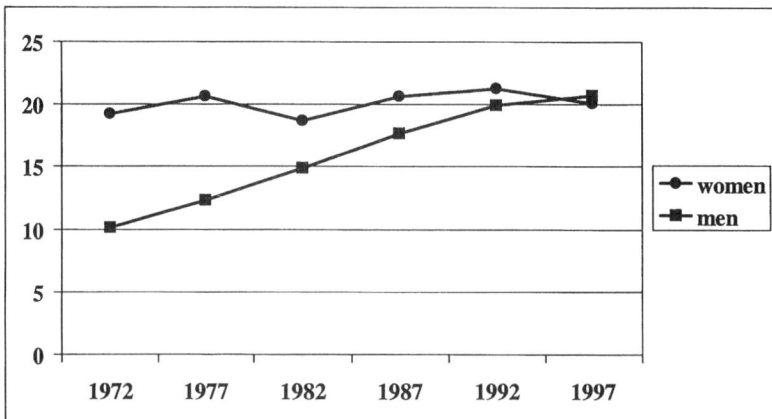

Fig. 3. Time trends in the prevalence of obesity (BMI ≥ 30 kg/m^2) in Finland (adapted from reference[11])

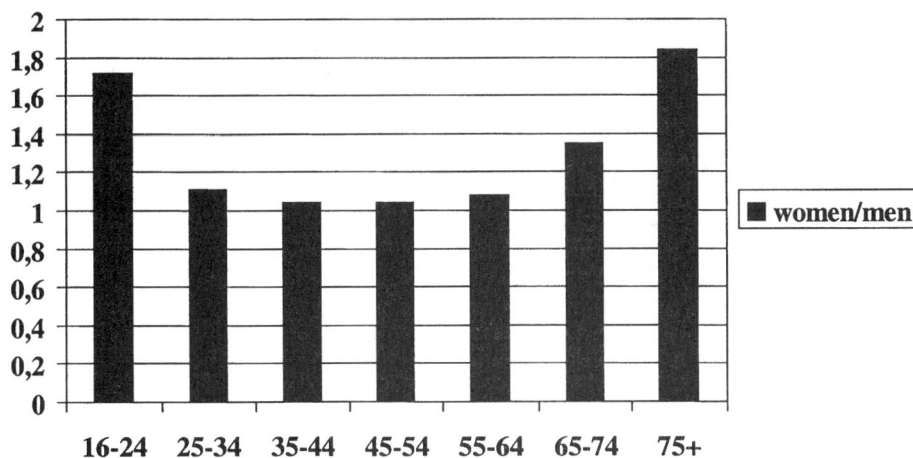

Fig. 4. The gender ratio (women/men) of the prevalence of obesity (BMI ≥ 30 kg/m²) by age in the Health Survey for England (ages 16+), 1997. Adapted from Seidell[9].

compared to men in the youngest age group (16–24 years). There are several possible explanations for the higher prevalence in women at older ages. It may be the result of a secular trend in which the prevalence of obesity has increased more in men from more recent birth cohorts than in women of the same age (as seen in the data from eastern Finland in Fig. 3). An alternative plausible explanation is a biological one. After menopause women may experience a greater increase in body fat mass compared to men as a result of the drop in estrogen levels.

A third explanation may be that obese men die more often prematurely than obese women do. The age-standardized absolute risk of some obesity related diseases such a coronary heart disease is higher among men than among women of the same age.

Explanations for the growing epidemic of obesity

Life-style changes

On an ecological level or population level these time trends are not too difficult to explain although exact quantification of different factors is almost impossible. On the one hand there is an increase in the average energy supply per capita. The World Health Report[14] has estimated that the average energy supply per capita and day in the world was 2,300 kcal in 1963; 2,440 kcal in 1971; 2,720 kcal in 1992 and it is estimated that in 2010 it will be 2,900 kcal. These increases are obviously not evenly distributed across the worlds' population and, sadly, many remain undernourished although in Asia (particularly China and India) and most of Latin America malnutrition is declining. The number of people with access to at least 2,700 kcal/day has increased from 0.145 billion in 1969–1971 to 1.8 billion in 1990–1992 and is estimated to grow to 2.7 billion in 2010. Even when corrected for the increase in the world's population this implies a more than tenfold increase in the number of people having access to high caloric diets. The globalization of agricultural production and food processing has not only affected the quantity of energy available per capita but also the energy density.

At the same time there are continuing changes in the physical demands of work and leisure time. Increasingly we are at leisure during working hours and we workout during leisure time. Mechanization of many types of work and changes in transportation are causing ever-increasing numbers of people to be sedentary for most of the time.

Increasing sedentary behaviour has been proposed to be one of the principal reasons for a further increase in the prevalence of obesity in countries with established market economies. Sedentary behaviour is poorly measured by the number of hours engaged in sports only. Large and important differences can be seen in the number of hours spent at sedentary jobs and in front of television or computer screens during leisure time. Transportation is almost certainly a factor as well. For example of short trips in the Netherlands 30 per cent are done by bicycle and 18 per cent by walking. In the UK these percentages are 8 per cent by cycling and 12 per cent walking and in the United States of America

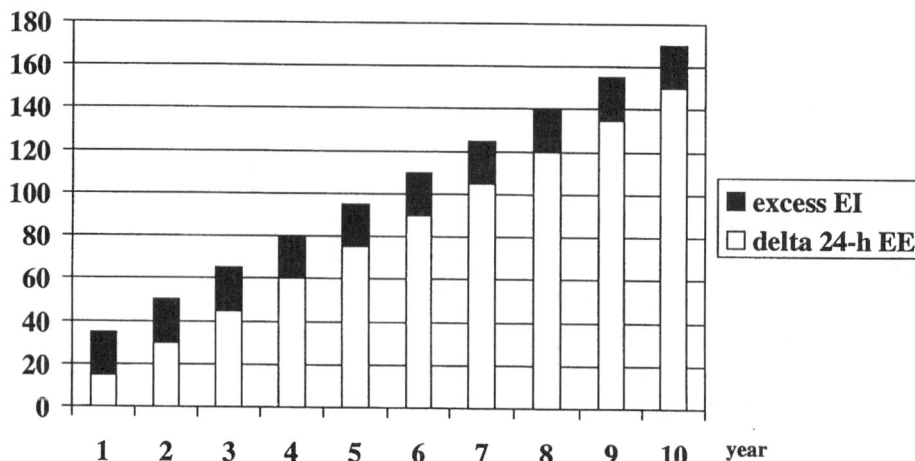

Fig. 5. Hypothetical calculations of the magnitude of a positive energy balance to gain 10 kilogram over 10 years. It is estimated that an excess enery intake (EI) of 20 kcal/day over a 1 year period leads to a weight gain of about 1 kg. One kilogram of weight gain is estimated to lead to about a 15 kcal/day increase in 24-h energy expenditure (EE) (derived data for women Prentice *et al.*, 1996[15]).

1 per cent by bicycle and 9 per cent by walking. These daily activities accumulated over a year can easily explain the small but persistent changes in energy balance needed to greatly increase the prevalence of obesity.

Figure 5 shows the disturbances in energy balance necessary to shift an individual's BMI from 23 to 26 kg/m². Energy intake in excess of energy expenditure only needs to be 20 kcal/day to produce about 1 kg weight gain over a year. This is in the order of 5 min of walking per day less or an additional can of beer per week. There are compensating increases in energy expenditure, however, which may range from 15 to 25 kcal/day/kg of weight gain in women and men respectively[15] so that the actual increase in energy intake or reduction in energy expenditure to achieve major weight change are much larger.

Data from eastern Finland suggests that the inverse relationship of BMI and physical activity in women increased over time suggesting that decline in physical activity has been of particular importance for maintaining the high prevalences of obesity in women[16].

Given the changes in lifestyles over the last decades in many parts of the world it is not surprising that people gain weight on the average although for many individuals this seems to remain a mystery. With small changes in average body weight the prevalence of obesity increases rapidly. For every unit increase in BMI there is an increase in the prevalence of obesity of five per cent points[1].

Social, economic and cultural determinants of the prevalence of obesity

There are many factors that affect energy balance and are determinants of obesity. The major determinants can be grouped into three groups[17]:

(a)   Biological influences and unalterable factors (e.g. age, sex, hormonal factors, and genetics);

(b)   Behavioural influences (which are the result of complex psychological factors, including habits, emotions, attitudes, beliefs, and cognitions developed through a background of learning history).

(c)   Environmental influences (physical, economic, and sociocultural environment).

Many behavioural and sociocultural factors that affect energy balance and obesity relate to eating habits and physical activity. Out of the many gender-related social determinants of obesity I briefly discuss the perception of overweight as a desirable or undesirable trait. The attitudes towards obesity vary greatly across social and ethnic groups and are related to the economic position of individuals and groups. In many affluent countries women experience social pressures to be thin. Katzmarzyk and Davis[18] studied the body weight and shape of Playboy centrefolds in the period 1978 to 1998 as an example of culturally 'ideal' women and noted that 70 per cent of them were underweight by WHO standards (BMI < 18.5 kg/m^2). They speculate that this phenomenon helps to explain the high levels of body dissatisfaction and disordered eating among women. It has been observed that these social pressures towards thinness are greater among women than among men and greater in women with high educational level compared to those with a low educational level. The prevalence of obesity is also sharply inversely associated with educational level. Black women in the US are more likely to be obese than white women, even when adjusted for socio-economic status, but they are less likely to perceive themselves as being overweight[19]. Such epidemiological data would suggest that the perception of overweight as an undesirable characteristic may play a role in the prevention of overweight particularly in young white women of high socio-economic background in affluent countries. This is undoubtedly an oversimplification but if true it does so against the potential cost of an increased risk of body dissatisfaction and perhaps disordered eating.

The perception of overweight among black women from disadvantaged communities in South Africa, where food insecurity is a continuous concern, is very different[20]. A qualitative in-depth survey of overweight women in these communities showed that the concept of an individual voluntarily regulating food intake when food was available was completely unacceptable. Increased body mass index was regarded as a token of well-being in that marital harmony was perceived to be reflected in increased body weight. Overweight children were regarded as reflecting health as it was associated with sufficient food supply and intake. According to a survey in a urban black population in the Cape Peninsula in South Africa more than half of the women above the age of 35 years were obese (BMI > 30 kg/m^2) whereas a considerable proportion of the children was undernourished[21]. The Cape Peninsula is an example of a population that has undergone rapid economic transition and which has moved from undernutrition to extreme overnutrition. Doak *et al.*[22] have similarly described the coexistence of overweight and underweight within households in Brazil, China and Russia with an underweight child coexisting with an overweight nonelderly adult being the predominant pair combination in all three countries. On an international level, Martorell *et al.*[23] have studied the prevalence of obesity in women aged 15–49 years in different regions of developing countries. The prevalence of obesity was estimated to be about 17 per cent in the Middle-East and North Africa, over 15 per cent in Central Eastern Europe/ Commonwealth of Independent States, about 6 per cent in Latin America and the Caribbean and less than 3 per cent in Sub Saharan Africa. There was a clear positive association between the gross national product (GNP) and the percentage of obesity up to a level of US$1500 GNP. With higher GNP's the relationship was no longer present. In these countries obesity was more prevalent in urban compared to rural areas and among people those with high educational level compared to those with low educational level. The relationship between obesity and the indicators of social class sharply diminished with an increase in the countries' GNP.

Such observations illustrate the complexities of the social determinants of obesity. In affluent countries the social pressures to thinness seem to be more intense in women than in men and in developing countries the pressures towards high body mass index seem also to be directed mainly to women. In affluent countries the preoccupation of diet is more common in those with high socio-economic status, whereas in developing countries a high body mass index is particularly appreciated in those with low socio-economic status. These social pressures may reflect many underlying issues among which food insecurity may be an important and often neglected element[24]. In societies where food security is never a problem obesity is common but not appreciated (particularly in women) whereas in food insecure societies obesity is uncommon in women but regarded as a desirable trait. In countries undergoing an economic transition and in immigrants from developing to developed countries the traditional perceptions of ideal body weight in women may be sustained. At the same time increases in food availability and decreases in energy expenditure promote weight gain. Such a mixture of attitudes and change of socio-economic conditions may, in part, be an explanation for the exceptionally rapid increase in the prevalence of obesity in particularly the women in such populations. Why the socio-cultural ideals vary more by socio-economic conditions among women than among men may be explained by the relative importance of energy reserves in women under conditions where the food supply is insecure. The energy reserves required for pregnancy and lactation may provide a biological basis for the cultural perception of an association between obesity and fertility. In situations where food is abundant throughout the year and no strenuous physical activity is required the cultural ideals about body shape seem to disappear.

These global issues apply also to Europe for several reasons. Firstly economic developments vary enormously across Europe and secondly because of the influx of immigrants from outside Europe which results in multicultural societies where a multitude of socio-cultural attitudes towards obesity and eating behaviour co-exist.

Conclusions

The prevalence of obesity is increasing at an alarming rate in many parts of the world. In white populations living in the west and north of Europe, Australia and the United States the prevalence of obesity is similarly high in men and women. In countries with relatively low gross national product such as those in central and eastern Europe, Asia, Latin-America and Africa the prevalence is 1.5 to 2 times higher among women than among men.

Within affluent societies the rates of obesity seem to be more common among women at older ages (65 years) and in groups with relatively low socio-economic status.

It can be tentatively concluded that obesity is particularly common in women living in relatively poor conditions.

References

1. World Health Organization. Obesity: preventing and managing the global epidemic. Technical Report Series, # 894, 2000.

2. Lean MEJ, Han TS, Seidell JC. Impairment of health and quality of life in men and women with a large waist. *Lancet* 1998; 351: 853–56.

3. NIH Clinical Guidelines on the Identification, evaluation, and treatment of overweight and obesity in adults: The Evidence Report. NIH, NHLBI 1998.

4. Seidell JC, Flegal KM. Assessing obesity: classification and epidemiology. *Br Med Bull* 1997; 53: 238–52.

5. Seidell JC, Rissanen A. World-wide prevalence of obesity and time-trends. In: *Handbook of obesity*, Bray GA, Bouchard C, James WTP (eds), pp. 79–91. New York: M Dekker Inc; 1997.

6. Seidell JC, Visscher TLS. Body weight and weight change and their health implications for the elderly. *Eur J Clin Nutr* 2000; 54(3): S33–S39.

7. Molarius A, Seidell JC, Sans S, Tuomilehto J, Kuulasmaa K. Educational level and relative body weight and changes in their associations over ten years – an international perspective from the WHO MONICA project. *Am J Public Health* 2000; 90: 1260–8.

8. Visscher TLS, Kromhout D, Seidell JC. Long-term and recent time trends in the prevalence of obesity among Dutch men and women. *Int J Obes* 2002; 26: 1218–24.

9. National Audit Office *Tackling obesity in England. Report by the comptroller and auditor general*; HC 220 Session 2000–2001. 2001 London Stationery Office.

10. Lahti-Koski M, Jousilahti P, Pietinen P. Secular trends in body mass index by birth cohort in eastern Finland from 1972 to 1997. *Int J Obes.* 2001; 25: 727–34.

11. Bergmann KE, Mensink GB. Anthropometric data and obesity. *Gesundheidswesen* 1999; 61: S115–S120.

12. Pomerleau J, Pudule I, Grinberga D, Kadziauskiene K, Abaravicius A, Bartkeviciute *et al.* Patterns of body weight in the Baltic republics. *Public Health Nutr* 2000; 3: 3–10.

13. Seidell JC. Obesity, insulin resistance and diabetes – a world-wide epidemic. *Br J Nutr* 2000; 1: S5–S8.

14. World Health Report. *Life in the 21st century – a vision for all*. World Health Report. Geneva; 1998.

15. Lahti K, Oski M, Pietinen P, Heliövaara M, Vartiainen E. Associations of body mass index and obesity with physical activity, food choices, alcohol intake, and smoking in the 1982–1997 FINRISK Studies. *Am J Clin Nutr* 2002; 75: 809–17.

16. Prentice AM, Black AE, Coward WA, Cole TJ. Energy expenditure in overweight and obese adults in affluent societies: an analysis of 319 doubly labelled water measurements. *Eur J Clin Nutr* 1996; 50: 93–7.

17. Egger G, Swinburn B. An ecological approach to the obesity pandemic. *BMJ* 1997; 315: 477–80.

18. Katzmarzyk P, Davis C. Thinness and body shape of Playboy centrefolds from 1978 to 1998. *Int J Obes* 2001; 25: 90–92.

19. Dawson DA. Ethnic differences in female overweight: data from the 1985 National Health Interview Survey. *Am J Public Health* 1988; 78: 1326–29.

20. Mvo Z, Dick J, Steyn K. Perceptions of overweight African women about acceptable body size of women and children. *Curationis* 1999; 22: 27–31.

21. Steyn K, Bourne L, Jooste P, Fourie JM, Rossouw K, Lombard C. Anthropometric profile of a black population of the Cape Peninsula in South Africa. *East Afr Med J* 1998; 75: 35–40.

22. Doak CM, Adair LS, Monteiro C, Popkin BM. Overweight and underweight coexist within households in Brazil, China and Russia. *J Nutr* 2000; 2965–71.

23. Martorell R, Kahn LK, Hughes ML, Grummer-Strawn LM. Obesity in women from developing countries. *Eur J Clin Nutr* 2000; 54: 247–52.

24. Olson CM. Nutrition and health outcomes associated with food insecurity and hunger. *J Nutr* 1999; 129(2): S521–S524.

Progress in Obesity Research: 9. Edited by *Geraldo Medeiros-Neto, Alfredo Halpern* and *Claude Bouchard*
©2003 John Libbey Eurotext Ltd, pp. 579–584.

CHAPTER 122

Cost-effectiveness of interventions for reducing body weight

Ping Zhang[1], Guijing Wang[2] and K.M.Venkat Narayan[1]

[1]*Division of Diabetes Translation,* [2]*Division of Nutrition and Physical Activity, Centers for Disease Control and Prevention, 4770 Buford Highway NE, Atlanta, GA 30341, USA*
[e-mail: paz2@cdc.gov]

Introduction

Economic analysis related to obesity has primarily focused on the consequences of obesity, i.e. the direct costs and the indirect costs associated with the disorder (cost of illness). The estimated direct and indirect costs demonstrate that obesity is a costly health problem, and the economic burden associated with the problem has been growing rapidly in the past several decades. In the United States, for example, the direct medical cost of obesity was estimated at $39.3 billion in 1986[1], increased to $45.8 billion in 1990[2], and to $52.64 billion in 1995, representing 5.7 per cent of the national health expenditures[3]. In Canada, the direct cost in 1997 was estimated at $1.8 billion, 2.4 per cent of the total health care expenditures[4]. In The Netherlands, the direct cost associated with overweight and obesity was about one billion Dutch guilders, which corresponds to about four per cent of total health care costs[5].

These findings are useful for educating and informing policy makers about the seriousness of the obesity problem in our society. The economic burden, however, does not represent the amount of money that society could save if the illness was eradicated. Rather, the economic burden equals the amount of money society could save only if the interventions used to treat the illness were unrealistically 100 per cent effective and cost free.

A primary consideration for policy makers is how to allocate the limited health care resources most effectively. Unfortunately, cost-of-illness estimates provide limited information in this regard. To determine how resources should be allocated among different programmes, accurate information is needed on the availability, costs, and effectiveness of treatment options. In many instance, high cost estimates of illnesses as documented by the cost-of-illness studies may merely reflect a lack of effective treatments. Thus, the high cost-of-illness estimates indicate that more research on finding effective treatments needs to be conducted before additional resources are invested in intervention programmes.

Health care resource allocation demands another type of economic analysis that is, the economic evaluation of different health interventions. The purpose of economic evaluation analysis is to determine the 'value' of health care resources invested in different health programmes. Cost-effectiveness analysis is the most common type of economic evaluation analysis used in health care field. This paper focuses on the cost-effectiveness of obesity interventions. In the following sections, we briefly describe the usefulness of cost-effectiveness analysis for health care decisions, and summarize specific cost-effectiveness studies of interventions for reducing body weight.

Using cost-effectiveness analysis for health care decisions

Cost-effectiveness analysis is an analytic tool in which costs and effects of a programme and at least one alternative are calculated and presented in a ratio of incremental cost to incremental effect[6]. The cost-effectiveness ratio (CER) of intervention A versus intervention B can be calculated by:

CER? incremental cost / incremental outcome

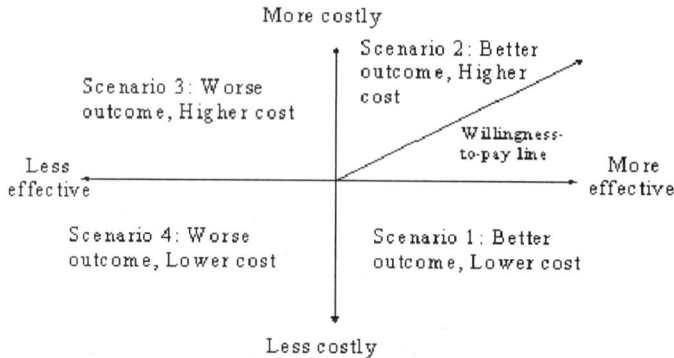

Fig. 1. A framework of using cost effectiveness analysis for allocating health care resources.

where incremental cost = cost of intervention B – cost of intervention A, and incremental outcome? health outcome of intervention B – health outcome of intervention A.

Health outcome can be measured in physical units such as number of pounds of body weight lost or number of life years gained. When the health outcome is measured by a quality-of-life adjusted measure, such as quality-adjusted life year (QALY), the cost-effectiveness analysis is referred to a cost-utility analysis. In addition, when the health outcome of intervention can be quantified in monetary terms, the cost-effectiveness analysis becomes a cost-benefit analysis. Because of the difficulties in converting health outcomes into a monetary value, cost-effectiveness analysis or cost-utility analysis is more often used.

Figure 1 illustrates the way in which the cost-effectiveness analysis can be used to aid our decisions on health care resources allocation[7]. In comparing intervention A with intervention B, four scenarios are possible in terms of effectiveness and cost. Scenario 1, better outcome at lower cost, is the most desirable of the four, but is probably the least often achieved in practice. Scenario 2, better outcome at higher cost, may be acceptable, depending on the extent to which the patient's outcome is improved and the increase in cost at which this is achieved. Scenario 3, worse outcome at higher cost, is the least desirable. Scenario 4, worse outcome at lower cost, may be acceptable depending on how much benefit is being forgone and whether and how the available resources are used.

Scenario 2 is the most common situation. This better-outcome and higher-cost quadrant can be further divided into two zones in terms of the acceptability of the higher costs. The willingness-to-pay (WTP) line (Fig. 1) represents how much a particular society is willing to pay for the intervention. Interventions with CERs above the WTP line are considered not acceptable by the society whereas interventions with CERs below the line are considered acceptable.

Cost-effectiveness of interventions for reducing body weight

We searched MEDLINE[8] and NHSEED[9] for articles published during the past 10 years (1993 to July 2002) on cost-effectiveness analysis of reducing body weight. We further scanned the reference lists of these articles to identify other related studies. We also identified unpublished studies from proceedings of professional meetings related to obesity. We used two criteria to determine which studies to include in our research. First, the studies had to be based on original data. Consequently, all review articles, book chapters, or editorial letters were excluded. Second, the studies had to be conducted according to the basic principles of CEA described by Udvarheyi[10] and others[6,11].

Four studies (three cost-utility analyses, and one cost-effectiveness analysis) met our inclusion criteria (Table 1)[12–15]. One study collected both effectiveness and cost data within the same clinical trial prospectively whereas the other three studies assembled data from published literature. The costs and health benefits were evaluated during periods ranging from 2 years to the end of the patients' lives. All studies adopted a health-care-system perspective although two of the studies also evaluated interventions from a societal perspective. A CEA from a societal perspective considers all costs (i.e. direct medical cost, direct nonmedical cost, and indirect cost) occurred as a result of an intervention while a CEA from a health-care-system perspective considers only the direct medical cost. Three kinds of interventions evaluated were lifestyle intervention, drug treatment, and surgical treatment. We con-

Table 1. The cost-effectiveness of interventions for reducing body weight (costs in year 2000, US$)

Reference	Study type	Intervention and population	Cost-effectiveness ratio	Comments on the study
DPP Research Group[12] (2002)	CUA	•Lifestyle intervention •Drug therapy (Metformin) •Persons with IGT, BMI m 24 •USA	•Lifestyle: $31,512/QALY •Metformin: $99,611/QALY	•Cost data were collected prospectively. •Was a large multi-centre study. •All costs (i.e. direct medical, direct non-medical, and indirect costs) were assessed. •Long-term health benefits were not included.
Lamotte et al.[13] (2002)	CEA	•Drug therapy (Orlistat) •Persons with diabetes, BMI m 28, with and without other CVD risk factors •Belgium	•No CVD risk factors: $18,451/LYG •Hypercholesterolaemia: US$6,821/LYG •Hypertension: $6,838/LYG •Hypercholesterolaemia and hypertension: US$3,196/LYG	•Effectiveness data were based on a 1-year clinical trial. •Health benefit was not discounted for the base case analysis. •Direct non-medical and indirect costs were not evaluated. •Validity of the Markov model used was not known. •Effect of intervention on patient's quality of life was not included. •Side effects of treatment were not included.
Foxcraft et al.[14] (1999)	CUA	•Drug therapy (Orlistat) •Persons with BMI m 30 •UK	$76,693/QALY	•Direct non-medical cost was not assessed. •Long-term benefits were not included. •Data on costs and quality of life were not collected prospectively.
Van Germet et al.[15] (1999)	CUA	•Vertical banded gastroplasty •Persons with BMI m 40 •Netherlands	–$4,139 to –$4,060 /QALY, depending on annual excess cost of obesity assumed	•Sample size was small. •Direct non-medical cost was not included. •Assumptions used for estimating the long-term health benefit and cost savings may be overoptimistic. •Sensitivity analysis was not performed. •Did not include cost of treating long-term complications.

BMI = body mass index, calculated as weight (kg)/height squared (m^2); CEA = cost-effectiveness analysis; CUA = cost-utility analysis; CVD = cardiovascular disease; IGT = impaired glucose tolerance; QALY = quality adjusted life year; and LYG = life year gained.

verted all costs to year 2000 US dollars by using consumer price indices if costs were reported in other years and by using exchange rates if costs were reported in foreign currency.

Cost-effectiveness of lifestyle intervention

The Diabetes Prevention Program (DPP) Research Group[12] assessed the cost-effectiveness of lifestyle intervention for preventing or delaying type 2 diabetes among persons with impaired glucose tolerance. The DPP was a large multi-centre clinical trial among 3,234 overweight or obese persons in the United States. The goals of the intervention were to achieve and maintain a weight reduction of at least 7 per cent of initial body weight through a healthy, low-calorie, low-fat diet and through physical activity of moderate intensity, such as brisk walking, for at least 150 min per week. A 16-lesson curriculum covering diet, exercise, and behaviour modification was designed specifically to help participants achieve these goals. The curriculum taught by case managers to participants on a one-to-one basis during the first 24 weeks after enrollment was flexible, culturally sensitive, and designed to meet the individual's unique needs. Subsequent individual sessions (usually monthly) and group sessions with the case managers reinforced the participants' behavioural changes. The placebo intervention in the DPP trial was a recommendation for lifestyle changes in the form of written information and an annual 20- to 30-minute individual session that emphasized the importance of a healthy lifestyle.

Compared with the placebo intervention over a 3-year period, the lifestyle intervention reduced participants' body weight by 5.5 kg and the incidence of type 2 diabetes by 58 per cent[16]. The lifestyle intervention cost US$2,269 more per participant from a health-care-system perspective and US$3,540 more from a societal perspective. In terms of the QALY gained, the lifestyle intervention cost US$31,512 from a health-care-system perspective and US$52,582 from a societal perspective.

Cost-effectiveness of drug therapies

The DPP trial also evaluated the use of medication Metformin for preventing or delaying type 2 diabetes[12]. Participants in the Metformin arm also received the same lifestyle recommendation as those in the placebo group. The Metformin intervention involved taking a dose of 850 mg daily during the first month of treatment. After one month, the dose was increased to 850 mg twice per day. Over a 3-year period, Metformin reduced participants' body weight by an average of 2.0 kg and the incidence of type 2 diabetes by 31 per cent[16]. Compared with the placebo intervention, the 3-year Metformin intervention cost US$2,191 more per participant from a health-care-system perspective and US$2,412 more per participant from a societal perspective. The cost per QALY gained with Metformin totaled US$99,611 from the perspective of a health-care-system and US$99,171 from a societal perspective.

A 2-year intervention that included Orlistat therapy of 12 mg three times per day plus a hypocaloric diet was compared with a 2-year hypocaloric diet alone over a period of 10 years[13]. The Orlistat therapy reduced a patient's body weight by 1.9 kg and improved the patient's HbA1c, blood pressure and cholesterol level in a 1-year clinical trial[17]. Translating this immediate health benefit into a long-term impact on mortality and on micro- and macro-vascular complications increased life expectancy over a period of 10 years as follows: 0.08 year for persons without other cardiovascular disease (CVD) risk factors, 0.204 year for persons with hypercholesterolaemia, 0.227 year for persons with hypertension, and 0.474 year for persons with both hypercholesterolaemia and hypertension. Over the 10-year period, the Orlistat therapy increased direct medical cost by US$1,485 for persons with no CVD risk factors, US$1,398 for persons with hypercholesterolaemia, US$1,549 for persons with hypertension and US$1,515 for persons with both hypercholesterolaemia and hypertension. In terms of cost per life year gained, the 2-year Orlistat treatment totaled US$18,451 for patients with no CVD risk factors, US$6,838 for patients with hypercholesterolaemia, US$6,821 for patients with hypertension, and US$3,196 for patients with both hypercholesterolaemia and hypertension.

The cost-effectiveness of Orlistat was also evaluated in a general obese population from the perspective of the National Health Service of the United Kingdom[14]. Currently, Orlistat can be prescribed for treating obese patients in conjunction with diet intervention for up to 2 years in the UK. The authors used published literature to estimate the health benefit of the drug therapy over 2 years based on the impact of a 10 per cent body weight loss on quality of life improvement. Compared with a diet intervention alone, the treatment of 100 obese persons with Orlistat resulted in a gain of 1.6 QALY with a cost of US$122,700. Thus, the drug therapy essentially cost US$76,693 per quality of life year gained.

Cost-effectiveness of surgical treatments

The health impact of vertical banded gastroplasty (VBG) surgery was evaluated based on the change in quality of life of 21 morbidly obese patients after 2 years following the surgery[15]. VBG surgery produced a body weight loss of 48.5 kg per patient at the end of year 2 post-surgery and improved the quality of life significantly. The surgery also lowered the per capita annual medical cost by US$783. Assuming that both health benefits and saving in medical costs would sustain, VBG surgery would extend a person's life by 3.6 years or by 12 years with an adjustment for improving the quality-of-life and would lower medical costs by US$1,226 until the patient reached age 65. VBG surgery also increased the probability of employment and reduced the number of work days absent, both would leading to an increase in earnings. Including this benefit, the surgical procedure would produce a cost savings ranging from US$48,707 to US$49,658 per person until the patient reached age 65.

Discussion and conclusions

The already high and ever increasing health and economic burdens of obesity suggest an urgent need for effective obesity prevention and treatment strategies. We examined the current evidence of cost-effectiveness of obesity treatment interventions. Unfortunately, comparisons of the cost-effectiveness of different interventions across the studies may not be appropriate for two reasons. First, different interventions were used for different clinical populations. Second, methodological differences exist for different studies, which may significantly affect the cost-effectiveness ratios. Nevertheless, the results of these studies demonstrate that interventions for reducing body weight across all three treatments could be good value for the health care investment. VBG for morbidly obese patients could both improve a patient's quality-of-life and lower medical costs[15] (i.e. the better-outcome and lower-cost quadrant – see Fig. 1). The CERs of all other interventions are in the better-outcome and higher-cost quadrant of Fig. 1, thus whether they should be adopted depends on where the WTP line is drawn. Without including long-term health benefits, lifestyle interventions for reducing body weight among persons with IGT cost approximately US$32,000 per QALY[12], which is comparable with the interventions that are commonly considered to be acceptable. A recent report, based on a simulation model, estimated that intensive glycaemic control for patients with newly diagnosed type 2 diabetes in the United States costs approximately US$41,000 per QALY gained over a lifetime[18]. Both hypertension screening and therapy for asymptomatic 20-year-old men would cost US$40,000 per QALY[19].

Results from those cost-effectiveness studies of reducing body weight could have major public health implications. First, the clinical and public health communities have been skeptical about interventions for reducing body weight, particularly lifestyle interventions, because of the lack of sustainable impact and the high cost[20]. The cost-effectiveness evidence, however, does not justify this skeptical perception. The cost-effectiveness ratios of the interventions evaluated are within the range commonly accepted by the society of developed nations. The DPP Research Group showed that lifestyle intervention could still be an attractive intervention for reducing body weight while the cost of the intervention was considered. Second, health insurance contracts routinely exclude obesity treatment[21]. According to the insurance industry, one reason for this exclusion is the lack of evidence of the cost-effectiveness of obesity treatments. Results of the cost-effectiveness studies demonstrate, however, that interventions for treating obesity are within the ranges of the cost-effectiveness of many treatments covered by health insurance for treating other illnesses.

The small number of cost-effectiveness studies on obesity treatment suggests that more economic evaluation research should be conducted. First, a major problem in synthesizing the literature is the high degree of differences among studies in their research perspective and their calculation of costs and benefits. These differences make the comparisons between the interventions impossible. In order to standardize the methods of cost-effectiveness studies, an expert panel of the US Public Health Services[6] has developed specific recommendations that should result in research findings that are more comparable. By addressing to these recommendations, the usefulness of cost-effectiveness studies would be greatly enhanced. Second, to conduct sound research on the cost-effectiveness of interventions, data on both effectiveness and cost should be collected systematically, especially alongside clinical trials. Although this requirement posts a challenge, researchers should view economic evaluation as a critical component of clinical trials. Finally, information is needed on the long-term effectiveness of obesity interventions. The longest clinical trial follow up among the four studies reviewed was 3 years (i.e. DPP study). The other three studies were based on clinical data of 2 years or less. Because many people regain weight after an intervention ends, the long-term effect of an intervention needs to be documented to ensure the true cost-effectiveness of the intervention. A longer-term follow up is also needed to correctly take into account the long-term effect of weight reduction on health outcomes.

References

1. Colditz GA. Economic costs of obesity. *Am J Clin Nutr* 1994; 55: S503–S507.

2. Wolf AM, Colditz GA. The cost of obesity, the US perspective. *Pharmaco Econ* 1994; 5(1): 34–7.

3. Wolf AM, Colditz GA. Current estimates of the economic cost of obesity in the United States. *Obes Res* 1998; 6: 97–106.

4. Birmingham CL, Muller JL, Palepu A, Spinelli JJ, Anis AH. The cost of obesity in Canada. *CMAJ* 1999; 160: 483–88.

5. Seidell JC, Deerenberg I. Obesity in Europe: prevalence and consequences for use of medical care. *Pharmaco Econ* 1994; 5(1): 38–44.

6. Gold MR, Siegel JE, Russell LB, Weinstein MC (eds). *Cost-effectiveness in health and medicine.* New York: Oxford University Press; 1996.

7. Laupacis A, Feeny D, Detsky A, Tugwell PX. How attractive does a new technology have to warrant adoption and utilization? Tentative guideline for using clinical and economic evaluations. *CMAJ* 1992; 146: 473–81.

8. National Library of Medicine. (2002). MEDLINE, available at www.nlm.nih.gov/databases/freemedl.html. Accessed on 8/20/2002.

9. National Health Service Economic Evaluation Database (NHSEED) (2002). Available at http://agatha.york.ac.uk/nhsdhp.htm. Accessed on 8/20/2002.

10. Udvarheyi S, Golditz GA, Rai A, Epstein AM. Cost-effectiveness and cost-benefit analysis in the medical literature: Are the methods being used correctly? *Ann Int Med* 1992; 116: 238–44.

11. Drummond MF, O'Brien B, Stoddart DL, Torrance GW. *Methods for the economic evaluation of health care programmes* (2nd edn). New York: Oxford University; 1997.

12. Diabetes Prevention Program (DPP) Research Group. The cost-effectiveness of DPP to delay or prevent type 2 diabetes. *Diabetes* 51 S2, A74. 62nd. San Francisco: Ann Meeting; 2002.

13. Lamotte M, Annemans L, Lefever A, Nechelput M, Masure J. A health economic model to assess the long-term effects and cost-effectiveness of Orlistat in obese type 2 diabetic patient. *Diabetes Care* 2002; 25: 303–8.

14. Foxcroft D, Ludders J. Orlistat for the treatment of obesity. Development and Evaluation Committee Report No. 101. Southampton: Wessex Institute for Health Research and Development 1999.

15. Van Germert WG, Adang EMM, Kop M, Vos G, Greve JWM, Soeters PB. A prospective cost-effectiveness analysis of vertical banded gastroplasty for the treatment of morbid obesity. *Obes Surg* 1999; 9: 484–491.

16. The Diabetes Prevention Program Research Group. Reduction in the incidence of type 2 diabetes with lifestyle modification or Metformin. *New Eng J Med* 2002; 346: 393–403.

17. Hollander PA, Elbein SC, Hirsch IB *et al.* Role of Orlistat in the treatment of obese patients with type 2 diabetes: A 1-year randomized double-blind study. *Diabetes Care* 1998; 21: 1288–94.

18. The CDC Diabetes Cost-Effectiveness Group. Cost-effectiveness of intensive glycemic control, intensified hypertension control, and serum cholesterol level reduction for type 2 diabetes. *JAMA* 2002; 287: 2542–51.

19. Chapman RH, Stone PW, Sandberg EA, Bell C, Neumann PJ. A comprehensive league table of cost-utility ratios and a sub-table of 'panel-worthy' studies. *Med Dec Mak* 2000; 20: 451–67.

20. Frank A. Utility and avoidance: medical professionals in the treatment of obesity. *JAMA* 1993; 269: 132–2133.

21. Martin LF, Robinson A, Moore BJ. Socioeconomic issues affecting the treatment of obesity in the new millennium. *Pharmaco Econ* 2000; 18: 335–53.

Progress in Obesity Research: 9. Edited by *Geraldo Medeiros-Neto, Alfredo Halpern* and *Claude Bouchard*
©2003 John Libbey Eurotext Ltd, pp. 585–590.

CHAPTER 123

Health system reform:
the obesity perspective

Leonie Segal

Health Economics Unit, CHPE, Monash University, Australia
[e-mail: Leonie.segal@buseco.monash.edu.au]

Role of obesity in health

Obesity is an established risk factor for CHD, stroke, hypertension, type 2 diabetes, osteoarthritis, colorectal and breast cancer and gall bladder disease. It is also a direct cause of loss of quality of life, through reduced capacity to fully engage in a range of social, family and work related activities and though negative societal attitudes. Obesity has a pervasive influence on survival and vulnerability to illness. Obesity is a current or emerging problem across Europe, North America, Australia and the Pacific, and much of Asia, South America and the former soviet economies.*

Considerable disease burden as measured by disability adjusted life years is attributed to obesity. A recent Australian study which measured disability adjusted life years, attributable to disease groups and risk factors[6], shows the burden of obesity to be greater than that of common diseases. It is responsible for more DALYs than diabetes, depression, musculoskeletal disorders, asthma or breast cancer, and similar to alcohol misuse (key results are summarized in Table 1).

Table 1. Attribution of disease burden: Australia, selected risk factors/diseases 1996

Risk factor	% total DALYs	Disease	% total DALYs
Smoking	9.8	Heart disease	11.9
Physical inactivity	6.6	Stroke	5.4
Alcohol	4.7	All musculoskeletal disorders	3.9
Obesity	4.3	Lung cancer	3.8
Inadequate intake fruit/vegetables	2.8	Depression	3.8
		Dementia	3.7
		Diabetes	3.2
		Asthma	2.6
		Breast cancer	2.6
		HIV AIDS	0.6

Source: Mathers *et al.*, 1999[6], Public Health Division, Depart. Human Services, Victoria, 1999.

The diseases that contribute most to excess morbidity and mortality from obesity are heart disease, type 2 diabetes and osteoarthritis (see Table 2 derived from Australian research).

* The role of risk factors in disease burden is dependent on stage of economic development. Malnutrition is the major cause of disease burden in sub-Saharan Africa and India, but not in established market economies (eme). While, physical inactivity is a source of disease burden in the eme, but not the developing world. (WHO 1998).

Table 2. DALYs attributable to obesity, Australia 1996

Attributable condition	DALYs	% of all Dalys attributed to obesity
Obesity	not calculated*	
Ischaemic heart disease	33,458	30.7
Type 2 diabetes mellitus	30,729	28.2
Osteoarthritis and back problems	18,919	17.4
Colorectal cancer	10,221	9.4
Ischaemic stroke and hypertension	9,787	8.9
Post-menopausal breast cancer	3,550	3.3
Gall bladder disease	1,023	0.9
Total	**109,040**	**100.0**

Source: Mathers *et al.* 1999[6].

Thus substantial benefits could be realized through reduction in rates of obesity. Furthermore, interventions designed to reduce obesity are likely to have a favourable impact on other risk factors such as physical inactivity and poor nutrition, potentially increasing the potential gains. However, it will not be possible to address this growing health problem without a responsive health system that will support the necessary redirection of resources to obesity prevention and management.

This paper is concerned with health system issues and the implications for obesity. The concept of the 'health system' is extremely broad. It encompasses (i) source of funds – how funds are generated to pay for health services, (ii) allocation of funds to populations; (iii) the regulatory framework, (iv) arrangements for paying providers, (v) accountability process; (vi) quality assurance mechanisms, and (vii) health services planning activities.

Health funding and delivery arrangements create incentives, which may either undermine or promote the capacity to address obesity. Financial incentives and direct public funding can be used to change the behaviours of health care providers and citizens to reduce the incidence and prevalence of obesity. Conversely, if incentives created by the health system are not understood and addressed, they could frustrate any solution to this problem. Any attempt to address the growing problem of obesity will require the application of resources. The major changes in behaviour that are required to address obesity can be expected to require a concerted system wide effort.

For instance, in Australia, a reduction in smoking between 1974 and 1995 (from 46 per cent to 27 per cent in males and from 31 per cent to 25 per cent in females) was supported by a massive public health campaign. This included legislation for smoke- free work places, recreational and eating venues, aggressive publicity campaigns highlighting the disease consequences of smoking, explicit warnings on cigarette packs (such as smoking kills), public funding of services to help smokers to quit, such as quit help lines and subsidy for nicotene replacement drugs together with high taxes on cigarettes.

Given that weight reduction is a far more complex issue than quitting smoking, and adoption of desirable eating habits and activity levels represents a challenging behaviour change task, substantial progress cannot be expected without a significant resource commitment, with relevant regulations to create an environment that supports healthy lifestyle choices.

Expenditure on prevention and management of obesity and attributable disease

It is almost certain that by far the majority of health sector resources allocated to obesity are directed to the treatment of attributable conditions, with very little spent on the prevention or management of obesity. Management largely occurs outside the 'health sector', through private weight loss agencies or the fitness industry. An estimate for Australia of health sector expenditure attributable to obesity is shown in Table 2[3]. Very few resources were allocated to prevention at less than US$25 million, with somewhat more for management of persons who are overweight or obese at less than US$60million, but over US$600 million for the management of attributable conditions – indicating an imbalance between prevention and management of obesity and treatment of attributable conditions.

Table 3. Estimated health sector expenditure on obesity prevention and management and treatment of attributable conditions, Australia 1996 ($US million)

Prevention of obesity	**15–25**
Management of obesity	**40–60**
Management of attributable conditions	**610**
CVD – hypertension, ischaemic heart disease, stroke	315
Osteoarthritis and back problems	182
Type 2 diabetes	108
Gallbladder disease	40
Cancers – colorectal, uterus, breast	33

Source: AIHW 2002[1], unpublished analysis by Segal, 2002.

There also appears to be a gross imbalance between expenditure and disease burden, given an attributable loss in quality of life and premature death, valued at just under US$6,000 million per year (see Fig. 1).

Fig. 1. Valuation of attributable loss in quality of life and premature deaths.

Estimates of the quality of life utility score (between 0 and 1, 1 representing best possible health and 0 death) were obtained from an Australian population survey using the AQoL (Assessment of Quality of Life utility instrument). Utility values were obtained for 2,934 persons. Mean utility score was found to be related to BMI: 0.85 for persons with a BMI 20–25, 0.82 for persons with a 25 < BMI < 30, 0.80 at a < 30 BMI < 35 and 0.76 for BMI > 30. The total annual value for the loss in quality was estimated at ~A$10,100 million per year, given a value of a life year of A$50,000 (~US$25,000), and applying known prevalence rates for overweight and obesity. In addition there were an estimated 31,000 premature deaths, due to obesity, a loss valued at A$1550. This suggests a total intangible cost of obesity for Australia in 1996 of ~A$11550 or just under US$6,000[11].

Availability of effective and cost-effective interventions

Contrary to popular opinion there is a substantial literature that illustrates the existence of effective approaches to reducing overweight (see for instance Segal, 2000, Chapter 7A2[12]). Studies demonstrate that small changes in weight can be clinically significant. Programmes which have only modest success rate can be highly cost-effective, given the potential benefits of weight reduction. For instance a media campaign that achieves sustained weight loss in only 0.1 per cent of overweigh/obese persons was found to be highly cost-effective (Segal et al., 1998)[9].

However, despite overwhelming evidence of the role of obesity as a major determinant of health and wellbeing and evidence that interventions to address obesity can be highly cost-effective, or even possibly cost saving (projected savings in downstream health care costs due to reduced morbidity less than initial programme costs), resources allocated to obesity prevention and control is invariably small. This finding is not uncommon. It is considered implausible that the optimal level of resources is now being allocated to obesity prevention and control.

Obesity seems to be viewed as a matter of personal choice and an area into which society does not intrude; even though the structure of modern society has set up the preconditions for obesity in the retail system, food production, urban design, product design, transport systems etc. that promote unhealthy food and activity choices. Arguably the failure to adequately resource obesity prevention and control represents a failure in heath funding and delivery arrangements. This is predicted from theoretical considerations, as discussed below.

Inefficiencies generated by health funding and delivery arrangements

Distortions in health funding and delivery arrangements arise in part from the nature of health and health care, and from governments responses, which may exacerbated rather than ameliorated the intrinsic aspects of market failure. Frequently, health funding arrangements promote a medical approach to health care. Health care systems tend to be reactive, responding to symptoms and disease with little capacity to promote wellbeing. These and other aspects of health funding and delivery arrangements will direct too few resources to obesity prevention and management, relative to the capacity of these services to contribute to health gain.

The distorted incentives responsible in large part for the misallocation of health resources arise through a range of common attributes such as:

(i)   *Programme based funding and multiple budgets* – common in many health delivery models which restrict the possibility of resource shifts between programmes and between health delivery settings, mode of intervention and stage of disease;

(ii) *Differential subsidies* – most societies subsidise access to health care to encourage use of health services by those in need. These subsidies however tend to support designated service types and delivery modalities, invariably favouring medical services, with allied health services or complementary practitioners often excluded from such arrangements.

(iii) *Multiple agencies* – in relation to obesity a wide range of agencies have a potential role, from both within the health sector and outside – such as transport, education, urban planning, retailing, building/work place design. This means that no one agency or funder has clearly defined responsibility for, or capacity to tackle obesity.

(iv) *Financial imperatives* – Agencies must be financially viable in the short term. This encourages a focus on service delivery to meet immediate and urgent needs, rather than a longer-term strategic response. The latter might suggest an investment in obesity control, where improved health outcomes should reduce costs downstream. However funding arrangements may make up-front investment, difficult if not impossible.

(v)   *Disempowerment of consumers* – consumers as patients and communities, generally lack the information to define and express their health needs. Under third-party payment, consumers also have no control over their health budget and have difficulty in participating effectively in determining the health services accessed at the individual or community level. In areas dominated by direct payment, consumers are actively seeking and paying for weight loss services, gym memberships etc. .., initiatives rarely embraced by the public system.

These distortions in the health sector can be classified as:

(1)   Supply side problems: which result in an inflexible and non-competitive supply system, with providers limited in the types of services that can be offered in meeting the health needs of individuals and the community;

(2)   Demand side attributes: reflecting disempowered consumers – as individuals and communities, which limit their capacity to determine their health needs, to establish the appropriate mix of services to meet those needs, to communicate those needs to providers and to redirect payments to elicit the required supply response[10].

Aspects of market failure tend to mean that the resourcing of programmes to address obesity will be inadequate. This is a concern, given the increasing prevalence of obesity, and the importance of obesity as a modifiable risk factor for common chronic diseases. Both demand and supply side issues need to be addressed if resources are to be allocated in a way that is efficient.

Health system reform – the performance of alternative capitated models

The health system structure has an influence on the health service mix and the resourcing of programmes to address obesity. Health system reform is for other reasons being actively pursued, largely in response to cost pressures, concerns about quality of care, about the health service mix and with health inequalities. A number of countries have introduced single budget-holding models, funded through risk adjusted capitation, as a central element of health system reform. Two contrasting models have been developed:

(1)   The competitive model where budget holders compete for enrollees; and

(2)   The non-competitive, where plan membership is by virtue of an objective attribute, such as residential location. The regional health authority is a common version of this model.

Under the *non-competitive model regional model*, a regional health authority has responsibility for the planning and purchasing of services for a defined population. The regional health budget is determined on the basis of a population based risk adjusted formula. This model is designed primarily to achieve equity between regions, but also to promote efficiency. Incentives for efficiency arise from low member turnover, combined with consolidated financial responsibility. This means that any downstream cost savings generated through investing in disease prevention through health promotion and best practice care will accrue to the regional health authority. Thus efficiency is promoted through the on-going responsibility for the health of a defined population. The non-competitive model supports the use of population based health services planning, and a long-term approach to care. The model requires a competent management, operating within an appropriate regulatory/policy framework and effective micro-management tools, such as the adoption of appropriate arrangements for paying providers and comprehensive quality assurance processes.

The capacity to develop a risk adjusted resource distribution formula that is robust at the regional or group level and promotes regional equity is confirmed by various examples (including the US Veterans Affairs model, DVA 2000, the NSW Area Health Authority model, NSW Health Dept 1999, and the UK resource distribution formula). Evidence also shows that the theoretical efficiency gains can be realized, provided there is a strong central agency policy role. This is demonstrated in the highly successful US Veterans Affairs model, an example of a non-competitive single fundholding model[5], where enhanced performance has been achieved through a range of quality assurance and management initiatives and a comprehensive approach to health service planning. Since the introduction of reforms, which commenced in the mid-1990s, there has been documented improvement in health outcomes and a reduction in the cost of care. This has been achieved through a redirection of resources to primary care and prevention and non-medical care (through for instance an expanded ambulatory care network and counseling centres), and away from in-patient care.

Under the competitive model, Health Plans compete for members and their risk adjusted capitated payments with the obligation to meet all their health care needs (with scope defined by the Fund). Efficiency is sought through the market mechanism of consumer choice. A range of regulatory arrangements may also be introduced to moderate undesirable elements of competition.

Equity can be addressed either through:

(i)   A universal model with funding via a central fund, and a centrally determined minimum care package, with equity and quality assurance supported by a strong central agency role. This model has been adopted, in part, in the Netherlands and Israel[8,14] (it has been referred to as 'managed competition').

(ii)   Support for selected 'needy' groups, such as those on low incomes and elderly, whose contributions are funded by the State. This approach has been adopted in the USA in the models of managed care, This model leaves many in need without access to care.

Concerns with the competitive model relate primarily to the capacity to develop robust risk adjusters, to reduce incentives for cream skimming – selective enrolment of persons with low expected expenditure relative to their capitated payment (see Morgan et al.[7]). Plans might thus seek to exclude obese persons. Efficiency may be compromised, as it may be easier to pursue cost control via risk selection rather than genuine efficiencies. There is no mechanism under the predominantly privately funded model for global cost control. Quality of care may be compromised, unless consumers can discriminate between Plans on the basis of quality. Under the competitive model, expected high turnover of membership, creates little incentive for primary prevention – where benefits accrue some years into the future and potentially reaped by another Fund. On the other hand Funds might offer preventative services, in an effort to attract healthier members.

The competitive model also offers opportunities for greater purchaser accountability to consumers and for innovative designs in payment and delivery systems, through dynamism from competitive pressures. Managed competition has theoretical appeal, supporting universality and opportunities for macro-level cost containment. It has particular appeal for those health systems operating within a sickness and social insurance system framework, supporting these funds to become pro-active third party purchasers in a market-driven environment, rather than remain simply as a premium collection agency for the central authorities.

However there are substantial conceptual and practical/technical problems associated with the competitive model. These relate in particular to (i) the development of robust risk-adjustment capitated payments; (ii) the capacity of consumers to discriminate amongst the offerings of health plans, (iii) the limited competition of both health plans and providers in rural and remote regions; (iv) the adequacy of quality assurance processes, especially where there is no strong central agency role, and (v) high transaction costs associated with a system of complex contractual arrangements between health schemes and providers. Finally the capacity of the competitive model to meet population-wide/public health needs and to support health promotion and other activities which yield benefits downstream has not been established. These concerns partly explain the relatively slow introduction of managed competition in European countries operating social insurance systems, overlaid by institutional resistance.

Whether policymakers are able to develop an appropriate regulatory framework which can distil the benefits of the market elements and support equity objectives whilst controlling sufficiently the potential adverse consequences is not known. Whether the benefits generated from capitated funding and competition amongst health schemes, outweigh the additional costs of operating a more complex system and the risk of unacceptable perverse impacts is an empirical issue, the answer to which cannot be readily discerned from the current health system reform experiments.

Population based health services planning and funds pooling – the regional based non-competitive model – is the subject of current debate in various countries including Australia[13]. The available evidence, while limited, suggests that there is some merit in the further exploration of this option. However, it is also clear that single fundholding with risk adjusted capitated payments is a permissive but not sufficient condition to promote efficiency and equity. Success also depends on an effective central agency able to promote competent management in the regions to undertake the health services planning and purchasing role and able to implement a sound quality assurance programme. And a central agency able to develop a robust capitation formula and core services entitlement.

Conclusion

Obesity is a serious health problem responsible for substantial loss in quality of life and life years. The response of the health system in terms of public resourcing of services to support those who are overweight is generally grossly inadequate, given the seriousness of the health problem, and the opportunities for improvement. The adoption of single fundholding models, particularly the non-competitive version, has the potential to redress this balance, provided such models are accompanied by a strong central agency role, to support an effective quality assurance process and accountability of health plan managers and a rigorous approach to health services planning.

References

1. AIHW Cost of illness data set 1995/96, Australian Institute of Health and Welfare, Canberra 2002.

2. AIHW Australia's Health, AIHW. Canberra 2000.

3. Department of Veterans Affairs, Veterans Helth Administration, VERA: Veterans equitable resource allocation: equity of funding and access to care across networks. Washington: DVA. 2000.

4. Glied S. *Handbook of health economics; managed care*, Culyer AJ, Newhouse JP (eds). Amsterdam; 2000 (Chapter 13).

5. Kizer K, Demakis J, Feussner J, Reinventing VA. Health Care. Systematizing quality improve-ment and quality innovation. *Medical Care* 2000; 38(6): 1–7 to 1–16.

6. Mathers C, Vos T, Stevenson C, Begg SJ. The burden of disease and injury in Australia. AIHW cat. no. PHE 17. Canberra: AIHW 1999.

7. Morgan R, De Vito CA, Persily N. The Medicare-HMO revolving door. The healthy go in and the sick go out. *N Engl J Med* 1997; 337(3): 169–75.

8. Schut F, van Doorslaer. Towards a reinforced agency role of health insurers in Belgium and the Netherlands. *Health Policy* 1999; 48: 47–67.

9. Segal L, Dalton A, Richardson J. Cost-effectiveness of the primary prevention of non-insulin dependent diabetes mellitus. *Health Promotion International* 1998; 13(3): 197–209.

10. Segal L. The importance of patient empowerment in health system reform. *Health Policy* 1998; 44: 31–44.

11. Segal L, McNeil H. Quality of Life and Obesity, CHPE Research report 17, Health Economics Unit, Monash University, 1999. Available from: URL: hhtp//chpe.monash.edu.au.

12. Segal L. Allocative efficiency in health: development of a priority setting model and application to NIDDM, doctoral thesis. Melbourne: Monash University; 2000.

13. Senate Community Affairs References Committee, Inquiry into Public hospital funding First report. Public hospital funding and options for reform. Canberra: Commonwealth of Australia; 2000.

14. Shmueli A, Chinitz D. Risk-adjusted capitation; the Israeli experience. *Eur J Public Health* 2001; 11(2): 182- 4.

15. Structural and Funding Policy Branch NSW Health Department, Resource Distribution Formula, Technical Paper, 1998/99 Revision. Sydney: NSW Health Department; 1999.

Progress in Obesity Research: 9. Edited by *Geraldo Medeiros-Neto, Alfredo Halpern* and *Claude Bouchard*
©2003 John Libbey Eurotext Ltd, pp. 591–595.

CHAPTER 124

What will society's response be to the obesity epidemic?

Louis F. Martin and William J. Raum

Louisiana State University Health Sciences Center, New Orleans, LA, USA
[e-mail: Lmarti1@lsuhsc.edu; wraum@lsuhsc.edu]

Introduction

Obesity is the second leading cause of morbidity and mortality in the United States (US)[1,2]. Although deaths and the total medical expenses associated with cigarette smoking[3,4] are still greater than those due to obesity, the incidence of obesity within the population is rising at an alarming rate[5]. These data have led both the US National Institutes of Health (NIH)[6] and the World Health Organization (WHO)[7] to identify obesity as the most important public health epidemic at the start of the 21st century. Obesity is associated with the development of numerous co-morbid medical conditions which cannot be effectively treated without treating the underlying obesity[8]. Obesity and its co-morbid medical problems account for over 5 per cent of the direct costs of medical care in the US[9].

Direct personal costs are high as well. The most obese segment of society faces discrimination that results in them obtaining fewer years of education, a lower household income, and less chance of being married than people of normal weight[10]. This level of discrimination causes a large portion of obese women (over 70 per cent) and obese men (over 20 per cent) to spend significant amounts of time and money in attempts to lose weight[11,12].

It is hard to accurately determine how much is spent per year on dieting because most estimates include the costs of low calorie carbonated beverages and snacks that might be purchased by those who are not dieting or are not overweight. The most reliable estimate of what the obese are willing to spend per year to lose weight may come from a Swedish study that specifically addressed the question of their willingness to pay (WTP) for an effective obesity treatment[13]. Over 3,000 Swedish adults between the ages of 37–60 years with a median monthly income (± SD) of US$1,300 ± 580 (in year 1998) responded providing a wide range that they were WTP, US$0–68,000. The mean cost they were WTP was US$3,300 and the median was US$2,600 or approximately 2 months pay. Over 50 per cent of the group were willing to assume a loan to obtain treatment. Those who were most willing to assume a loan were significantly heavier, had lower monthly incomes, and had more perceived health problems (but not documentation of increased disease burden) than those who were not willing to assume a loan to have treatment.

In spite of the documented health problems associated with obesity, the significant costs to society, and the willingness of the obese to spend money to lose weight, the societal response to the obesity epidemic has been minimal. As Segal[14] has documented, the governments of most developed nations spend much more of their health care funds on other less common diseases. Even though cost-effectiveness analysis (CEA)[15] have shown that obesity treatments are more effective than many other standard medical treatments, the majority of medical insurance contracts in the US contain exclusions for obesity treatments[16]. This occurs because the obese portion of most societies has not organized as an effective political lobbying group to demand that their medical problems obtain an appropriate share of government budgets. The lack of activism is thought to stem from the discrimination the obese have faced and their lack of self esteem[10,17].

Obstacles to identifying the costs associated with obesity

Governments respond to political pressure more easily than to data or logic. If obese citizens do not organize to effectively lobby and demand that governments spend a fair amount of their health resources on the problems of the obese, then the social order will not change.

Currently, there are multiple obstacles to identifying the true costs of effective obesity treatment. The coding and reimbursement system used by the US federal government and its medical insurance programmes discourages the reporting of obesity as a condition leading to therapeutic intervention through several mechanisms[16]. First, because many medical insurance plans do not pay for obesity treatment, if obesity is listed as a condition, the insurance payment is rejected. This discourages reporting of this condition even as a secondary, related medical problem. Secondly, the codes used to document obesity are antiquated. No height or weight data are required on any of the US administrative databases. The coding of diseases (the International Coding of Diseases, ICD) is owned by the WHO[16]. It does not separate obesity by body mass index as suggested by its own guidelines[7] and those of the NIH[6] into four or more classes-it uses only two. The ICD system has only four categories to define obesity conditions; it has a category for patients with a BMI > 40 kg/m^2, one for patients with a BMI > 30 kg/m^2, one for obesity associated with an underlying endocrine abnormality, and a new code that required years of lobbying to establish, to distinguish metabolic syndrome X. These entrenched administrative shortcoming[5] will be hard to reverse even when a will develops to reverse them.

As long as it is acceptable for the media and even physicians and government to discriminate against the obese[18,19], then it will be hard to effectively challenge the emerging obesity epidemic. The NIH and other research organizations must be encouraged to distribute government research funding in proportion to the costs of each disease to society[20]. Currently, although obesity is the second leading cause of death in America, only 1 per cent of the budget of the NIH are allocated to obesity research. Some of the reluctance to spend money on obesity treatments or research has been due to the perceived low level of success of most treatments and the multifactoral causes of obesity. Obesity is a chronic disease and most treatment does not produce a cure. Studies have shown that control does reduce morbidity. We do not ignore cancer because it is rarely curable. Why should we ignore obesity and what does it cost to do so?

Need to document the indirect costs of the obesity epidemic

There is vast body of knowledge that associates the development of obesity with increased health care costs and other societal expenses[5–9,16]. The increased costs of the medical problems of the obese all lead to indirect costs in the social security disability systems[21,22]. The standards used for the clothing industry, airlines, furniture fabrication, and even medical products are becoming obsolete as our societies become more obese.

In the US, Southwest Airlines announced this year that it wants people over 100 kg to buy two airline tickets to occupy two seats rather than one. The small size of airline seats relative to THE WEIGHT AND HEIGHT of society members is a subject of intense industrial debate. Consumer groups want the airlines to increase the space associated with each seat while the airlines resist this because of the desire to maintain profits. Because the comfort of all passengers are involved, in the near future political pressure will be applied from all, not just the obese.

The public school systems of the US and other developed countries are also facing a crisis[23]. The standard student desk with a half table (desk) connected to a seat has been a standard for over 50 years with sizes for elementary, middle school, and high school students. These standard sizes now accommodate less than 60 per cent of the students in many inner city schools with significant African American and/or Hispanic populations. School budgets do not have the flexibility to order bigger sizes, so many students are left in chairs without a desk top. Parents claim discrimination, worried that the lack of a desk top will decrease performance. The parents of obese children are already aware that their children face a heightened level of discrimination. They want the school's help to control their children's obesity. Instead, they often find the school administration contributing to their child's obesity by offering high fat, high calorie lunches and snack food in vending machines which earn school administrations extra income.[23].

Clothing and equipment standards for industry are becoming problematic. Hospitals, which provide uniforms for various staff members, provided four sizes for fifty years; small, medium, large, and extra large. Most hospitals have now had to add 2x, 3x and 4x to these four standard sizes and are still not accommodating all staff members. Hospitals also have to acquire super sized patients gowns, specially reinforced wheelchairs, stretchers, operating room tables, and other medical equipment items for over 10 per cent of their patients who weigh above the industrial standard of 150 kg. Many radiologic tables and other diagnostic services are not available to patients who weigh over 150 kg. This is becoming a malpractice issue in the US Office chairs, desks, and any weight or size limited piece of standard equipment in an office or especially in a governmental facility is a potential source of liability.

The problems outlined above are not static. Obesity levels are rising faster in adolescents and young adults[5-7] than in the older segments of the population. Definitions of 'standard size' are about to become obsolete. Businesses now complain about the rising costs of medical care. These businesses are about to be confronted with the more direct costs of having to change all of their equipment to fit the needs of more obese employees and clients.

Parallels to the societal response to smoking

One way to examine what society's response to the obesity epidemic may be to compare its response to the problems discovered to be secondary to cigarette use[3]. Until manufactured pre-rolled cigarettes became available at the turn of the 20th century, smoking was not considered a health hazard. Within 30 years of the introduction of pre-rolled, manufactured cigarettes, a surgeon in New Orleans, Alton Oschner, was able to document an association between cigarette consumption and lung cell metaplasia and cancer. In the US, the prepared food/fast food market started in the 1960s and matured in the late 1970s. High calorie, high fat food became readily available already prepared for consumption at prices almost equal to the raw ingredients. Calorie intake increased as automobile ownership expanded and manual labour tasks decreased in the home and at work. Within 30 years of these two events, long term epidemiologic studies show a clear association between the development of obesity and premature death[1,2].

The US Surgeon General declared smoking a major health risk in 1964[24]. Progressively, congress and local governments passed legislation restricting smoking in public places, increasing the taxes on cigarette consumption, and restricting cigarette advertising and access especially to minors. In 2001, the US Surgeon General published a 'Call to Action to Obesity'[25]. Public awareness of the problem is beginning to stir.

Public health officials, school administrators, and the public are becoming concerned about the increasing prevalence of obesity, especially in children. Much of the political pressure to contain smoking came from the public who was concerned about the ill effects of secondary smoke as they received passive consumption. Parents are now concerned that our society is causing their children to become obese before their children are old enough and mature enough to be actively concerned about what they eat – 'passive obesity'. Soft drink (sweetened carbonated beverages) companies and snack food manufacturers have paid public school systems to allow then to place dispensing machines in the schools[26]. Children purchase high calorie, high fat snacks on breaks and in place of more balanced meals distributed in the cafeteria which is often subsidized[23,27]. The schools claim they need this source of revenue to balance budgets that voters have reduced. The parents of school aged children have responded by sponsoring legislation to rid the schools of these dispensing machines and all 'junk' food (high calorie, high fat snacks)[26]. California has passed legislation to rid schools of junk food by 2004. Similar legislation is before other state legislative bodies. Several states have proposed placing a 2 cent per can tax on soft drinks[26]. California has proposed dedicating this tax to be used to restore physical education programmes in the less affluent school districts. California was the first state to reduce school taxes, especially property taxes, so that most physical education programmes had to be eliminated in the 1980s and 1990s. Elementary school children in California now average only 15 min a week of exercise in school[28]. In the 1960s, over 80 per cent of high school students had physical education while today less than 25 per cent have it[28].

Many state governments and individuals sued tobacco companies claiming that the companies had purposely tried to addict individuals by manipulating nicotine levels and not adequately informed the public of the dangers associated with smoking[29]. Some of these class action suits have required the tobacco companies to turn over billions of dollars to the states. Within the last year, obese individuals have begun suing fast food restaurants and soft drink manufacturers claiming they became obese because they consumed the companies high fat, high calorie products without realizing the consequences to their health and longevity of consuming their products[23]. Although it seems these suits have less merit than the ones against the tobacco companies, where nicotine was recognized as a drug, the suits still have a political impact.

The money that the states have received from the tobacco companies from their suits has usually been dedicated to improving health care of the indigent and for research and public education although, perversely, North Carolina has used the money to support farmers who grow tobacco[29]. The Shape Up America! Foundation has encouraged states to use some of these tobacco funds to help increase physical activity especially in children and the elderly. Two significant lobbying efforts involve developing parent groups to encourage children to walk to school and for cities to maintain good sidewalks and safe areas to walk. More activity along these lines is needed.

Cost effective treatment of obesity

Chapters in this book, *Progress in Obesity Research: 9*[14,15], outline how cost effective it is to treat obesity and suggest models that governments could use to be more effectively use their tax dollars to prevent obesity rather than treat the late consequences of a lifetime of being obese. Some of the resistance to using tax dollars to treat or prevent obesity has to do with the known difficulties of these approaches. Unlike smoking, food consumption cannot be eliminated. Diets have to be modified if people are to lose weight or obesity is to be prevented, but everyone still needs to eat to live. There seem to be inbred, genetic preferences that lead us to consume high fat foods, a survival instinct that is now destructive rather than protective. New obesity treatments have often failed or claimed fraudulent results. Obesity treatments that initially seemed successful have had untoward side effects. Amphetamines decreased appetite but were addictive[30]. Early surgical procedures which shortened the absorptive surface of the bowel successfully helped morbidly obese people return to almost normal, healthy weights but led to liver failure and death[31]. Fenfluramine treatment helped decrease weight but probably caused valvular heart damage in a small subsection of users[32]. Each of these failures causes a resistance to treatment that is at least an order of magnitude more then that generated by successful treatments.

The drive to find successful treatments and encourage prevention of obesity is still prevalent. Any effective drug treatment of obesity will produce significant profits for the company discovering the treatment. Researchers and public health officials have documented the rise of the obesity epidemic and its consequences like hurricane trackers watch the Caribbean during the summer hurricane season. The obesity epidemic, like a hurricane, is being ignored only at great risk to the unsuspecting general public. Pharmaceutical companies, commercial weight loss companies, self-help groups and surgeons have worked over four decades to improve obesity treatments[6,7]. Research has shown that intentional weight loss decreases the risk of early mortality from obesity[33], decreases the need to take medication for diabetes and hypertension, can reverse sleep apnea[34], depression and even decrease atherosclerotic plaque depth in diseased arteries[35].

Medical insurance companies in the US have no incentive to treat obesity, as their average client will change companies at least every three years and will not benefit from their clients long-term health improvement. Governments that provide health care for its citizens are aware that effective obesity treatments save money long term[16]. This is especially true for obese diabetics requiring multiple medications. It would also seem true of annual cost savings for any obese people hospitalized for co-morbid diseases associated with obesity. Obesity treatments can also be used to successfully delay premature retirement or decrease the number of sick days required per year. Research is especially needed to determine which morbidly obese children might be successfully treated.

In the 107th Congress, a bill was introduced in the US Senate entitled the 'Improved Nutrition and Physical Activity Act (IMPACT)' legislation. It is the first major piece of federal legislation aimed at finding ways to decrease obesity. Although it does not have the political support to become law in 2002, its very introduction increases the visability of the problem our nation is facing as our children become more obese. The bill had 11 sections but the majority of the proposed US$280 million in funding was to be directed at developing a Youth Media Campaign to prevent obesity, and to demonstration projects to treat or prevent obesity through community or school sponsored programmes. Funding was also to be allocated for training grants to recruit professionals to the field of obesity research and treatment, and for some specific types of research. Finding the political support to tackle a new problem that costs money is unusually rare, but possible. For example, over 20 years ago, Title X was introduced demanding equal funding for women's sports activities in public schools. In spite of enormous resistance from the male sports complex, it succeeded and the number of women in organized sport activities at all levels of public education dramatically increased[36]. Since the overall trend in society has been for a decrease of physical activity during the teen years[28], the impact of this legislation on the habits of our nation should not be underestimated.

References

1. Calle EE, Thun MJ, Petrelli JM *et al.* Body-mass index and mortality in a prospective cohort of US adults. *N Engl J Med* 1999; 341: 1097–105.

2. Allison DB, Fontaine KB, Manson JE *et al.* Annual deaths attributable to obesity in the United States. *JAMA.* 1999; 282: 1530–8.

3. Hodgson TR. Cigarette smoking and life time medical expenditures. *Milbank Q* 1992; 70: 81–125.

4. Center for Disease Control Prevention Cigarette smoking among adults United States 1991. *MMWR Morb Mortal Wkly Rev* 1993; 43: 230–3.

5. Mokdad AN, Serdula MK, Dietz WH *et al.* The spread of the obesity epidemic in the United States 1991–1998. *JAMA* 1999; 282: 1519–22.

6. National Hearth Lung and Blood Institute Clinical guidelines on the identification, evaluation, and treatment of overweight and obesity in adults; the evidence report. Washington: US Department of Health and Human Services; 1998.

7. World Health Organization. Obesity: preventing and managing the global epidemic. World Health Organization Technical Report Series. Geneva: WHO; 1998.

8. Jung RT. Obesity as a disease. *Br Med Bull* 1997; 53: 307–21.

9. Colditz GA.Economic costs of obesity. *Am J Clin Nutr* 1992; 55: S503–7.

10. Gortmaker SL, Must A, Perrin JM *et al.* Social and economic consequences of overweight un adolescence and young adulthood. *N Engl J Med* 1993; 329: 1008–12.

11. Horm J, Anderson K. Who in America is trying to lose weight? *Ann Intern Med* 1993; 119: 672–6.

12. Williamson DF, Serdula MK, Anda RF *et al.* Current weight loss attempts in adults. *Am J Public Health* 1992; 82: 1251–7.

13. Narbro K, Sjostrom L. Willingness to pay for obesity treatment. *Intl J Technology Assessment in Health Care* 2000; 16: 50–9.

14. Segal L. Health system reform: the obesity perspective. In: *Progress in Obesity Research: 9*, G Medeiros-Neto, A Halpern, C Bouchard (eds), pp. 585–90. Eastleigh, UK: John Libbey, 2003.

15. Zang P, Wang G, Narayan KMV. Cost-effectiveness of interventions for reducing body weight. In: *Progress in Obesity Research: 9*, Medeiros-Neto G, Halpern A, Bouchard C (eds), pp. 578–84. Eastleigh: John Libbey; 2003.

16. Martin LF, Robinson A, Moore BJ. Socioeconomic Issues Affecting the Treatment of Obesity in the New Millennium. *Pharmaco Economics* 2000; 18 (4): 335–53.

17. Martin LF. The biopsycho social characteristics of patients seeking treatment for obesity. *Obesity* 1999; 9: 235-43.

18. Coleman JA. Discrimination at large. *Newsweek* 1 August 1993; 1: 9.

19. Jindal B. Choice – sensitive health costs. *J La State Med Soc* 1997; 149: 62–7.

20. Gross CP, Anderson GF, Powe NR. The relationship between funding by the National Institutes of Health and the burden of disease. *N Engl J Med* 1999; 340: 1881–7.

21. Rissanen A, Heliovaara M, Knekt P *et al.* Risk of disability and mortality due to overweight in a Finnish population. *BMJ* 1990; 301: 835–7.

22. Narbo K, Jonsson W, Larwsson B *et al.* Economic consequences of sick leave and early retirement in obese Swedish women. *Int J Obes* 1996; 20: 895–903.

23. Tyre P. Fighting big fat. *Newsweek* 5 August 2002, pp. 38–40.

24. Terry LL. The Surgeon General's Report: Reducing the Health Consequences of Smoking. Washington: US Department of Health and Human Services, Public Health Service, Office of the Surgeon General; 1964.

25. Satcher D. The Surgeon General's call to action to prevent and decrease overweight and obesity. Rockville: US Department of Health and Human Services, Public Health Service, Office of the Surgeon General; 2001.

26. Tyre P. Drink up-and pay up. *Newsweek* 29 August 2002, p. 14.

27. Underwood A. How to flunk lunch. *Newsweek* 16 September 2002, p. 10.

28. Jackson DZ. When did phys ed become 'fizzed'? *The Times Picayune* 2 August 2002; B7.

29. Will G. States's tobacco policies take bizarre turns. *The Times Picayune* 26 September 2002; B7.

30. Bray GB. Pharmacologic therapy of obesity. *The management of eating disorders and obesity*, Goldstein DJ (eds), pp. 213–48. Totowa: Human Press; 1999.

31. Hocking MP, Duerson MC, O'Leary JP, Woodward ER. Jejunoileal bypass for morbid obesity. Late follow-up in 100 cases. *N Engl J Med* 1983; 308: 995–9.

32. Devereux RB. Appetite supressents and valvular heart disease. *N Engl J Med* 1998; 339: 765–7.

33. Williamson DR. Prospective study of intentional weight loss and mortality in never –smoking overweight US white women aged 40–64 years. *Am J Epidema* 1995; 141: 1128–41.

34. Pekarovics S, Raum WJ, Klein SR. Vertical banded gastroplasty versus gastric bypass: Weight loss and impact on comorbid conditions. *Obesity Surgery* 1998; 8: 169.

35. Buchwald H, Varco RL, Matts JP *et al.* Effect of partial ileal bypass surgery on mortality and morbidity from coronary heart disease in patients with hypercholesterolemia. *N Engl J Med* 1990; 323: 946–55.

36. Ramsey PG. The glory of competition, sports medicine docs talk about the world of sports. *UW Medicine* 2002; 25: 4.

Progress in Obesity Research: 9. Edited by *Geraldo Medeiros-Neto, Alfredo Halpern* and *Claude Bouchard*
©2003 John Libbey Eurotext Ltd, pp. 596–603.

CHAPTER 125

Obesity and musculoskeletal disorders

Tommy L.S. Visscher,[1,2,3] **Markku Heliövaara,**[2] **H. Susan J. Picavet,**[3]
Aila Rissanen[4] **and Jacob C Seidell**[1]

[1]*Department of Nutrition and Health, Faculty of Earth and Life Sciences, Free University, De Boelelaan 1085, 1081
HV, Amsterdam The Netherlands;* [2]*Department of Health and Disability, National Public Health Institute, Helsinki,
Finland;* [3]*Centre for Prevention and Health Services Research, National Institute for Public Health and the
Environment, Bilthoven, The Netherlands;* [4]*The Obesity Research Unit, Helsinki University Central Hospital, Helsinki,
Finland*
[e-mail: tommy.visscher@falw.vu.nl]

Obesity and musculoskeletal disorders

Obesity has a large public health impact, not only due to its relation with cardiovascular diseases and type 2 diabetes. Evidence is also accumulating for a relation between obesity and musculoskeletal disorders[1]. Besides the well documented relation between obesity and osteoarthirtis (OA), some studies have linked obesity to hyperuricaemia, gout, diffuse idiopathic spinal hyperostosis, low back pain, herniated intervertebral lumbar disc, neck pain, and shoulder joint pain.

It is important to study obesity in relation to musculoskeletal disorders, as musculoskeletal disorders are important determinants of work disability, impairment of everyday activities, pain, and impaired quality of life. This paper will discuss the body of evidence for associations between obesity and the risk of different musculoskeletal disorders and related disability.

Methods

A literature search was conducted to identify original and review articles on studies presenting results concerning the relation between obesity and one of the following musculoskeletal disorders: osteoarthritis, hyperuricaemia, gout, spinal hyperostosis, low back pain, herniated lumbar intervertebral disc, neck pain, and shoulder joint pain.

Both cross-sectional and longitudinal studies are considered. In cross-sectional studies one is uncertain what came first, obesity or the musculoskeletal disorder. Longitudinal studies are considered more suggestive for a causal relation between obesity and the musculoskeletal disorder than cross-sectional studies. When available, changes in body weight are described in relation to changes in outcome. Further, different endpoints are considered, including disease outcome, severity of disease symptoms and disease-related disabilities. For the purpose of this review, the terminology of 'excessive body weight' is used for different definitions of high body weight coming from different studies cited.

Knee osteoarthiritis

From the many musculoskeletal disorders that are potentially related to obesity, the strongest evidence is on the relation between obesity and knee osteoarthritis (OA). All of the several reviews written on this topic conclude that obesity is the most important modifiable risk factor for knee osteoarthritis[2-5]. Evidence is coming from both cross-sectional and longitudinal studies.

Many cross-sectional studies published since 1945 consistently conclude that obesity is associated with knee osteoarthritis. A dose-response relation between high body weight and knee OA could be taken to support a causal relation between excess body weight and knee OA. However, the relation could also be in opposite direction, as subjects with more severe knee OA will be less active and will thereby have a higher body weight. Supportive evidence for a causal relation between high BMI and knee OA, coming from a cross-sectional study, is the finding that patients with symptomatic and asymptomatic OA had similar BMI's[6].

The causal role between obesity and knee OA is confirmed in many longitudinal studies. Obesity or high BMI was related to radiographic knee OA[7-9] in both the patello-femoral and tibio-femoral joints[10], and to symptomatic knee OA[9,11]. A study that included both men and women, concluded that the relation between obesity and knee OA was stronger among men than among women[9]. Among patients with unilateral knee OA, excessive body weight was associated with OA in the contralateral knee[12]. A dose-response relation between body weight and knee OA was confirmed[12,13].

Baseline BMI at age 20–29 years baseline was more predictive for knee OA occurring in students who were followed for a median period of 36 years than was their BMI at ages 30–39 and BMI at age 40–49 years[14]. The authors concluded that a cumulative exposure of excessive body weight is related to a greater risk of knee OA. Another study concluded that past obesity during adulthood was related to knee OA in women, not in men[15].

While excessive body weight at baseline is related to the onset of knee osteoarthritis weight loss decreased the risk of osteoarthirtis[16], which is in our opinion the strongest evidence for emphasizing the need for weight gain prevention with regard to the prevention of osteoarthritis. The latter relation was found in women aged 60–66 years with a BMI ≥ 25 kg/m^2, not in women with BMI < 25 kg/m^2. One small randomized trial has been described (NIH) that reported a relation between an appetite suppressant related weight loss and with an improvement and signs of OA[17].

A relation between obesity and progression of knee OA has also been reported, although this relation was less strong with progression of OA than with incident OA[18]. Osteophyte scores became higher with higher BMI whereas differences in joint space narrowing and progression in Kellgren and Lawrence grade did not increase uniformly with obesity category[12]. Also, excessive body weight was related to knee OA leading and to prosthetic surgery[19] and to disability due to osteoarthritis[13].

The relation between excessive body weight and knee OA can be explained by increased pressure on the joints. This biomechanical explanation for the role of excessive body weight in OA is supported by the finding that excessive body weight was associated with severity in varus but not in valgus knees[20] and the finding that relative risks were higher for OA in the knee than in the hip[11,14]. Other factors that are likely to contribute to the risk of developing osteoarthritis are genetics, dietary intake, estrogen use and bone density (systemic factors) and muscle weakness and joint laxity (biomechanical factors).

Hip osteoarthiritis

The relation between obesity and hip OA has been described in several reviews[2-5]. While obesity is related to hip OA[2-5], the relation seems weaker than it is with knee OA[2-4]. Some studies do not report a relation between excess body weight and hip OA[4,5]. Excessive body weight is related to bilateral hip OA[2-4,18,21,22] and weaker[2] or not to unilateral hip OA[3]. Excessive body weight has been linked to incident symptomatic hip OA[2,23] and the relation between excess body weight and symptomatic hip OA seems stronger than its association with radiologic hip OA[4,24,25].

Three studies on body weight and hip OA with a longitudinal nature are reported.

One study assessed recalled body weight at age 30 or 40 years by method of interviewing in patients who received a hip prosthesis and compared these body weight to subjects from a general population. The mean body weight at age 30 or 40 years turned out to be higher in patients who received a hip prosthesis[26]. A second study identified 27 incident hip OA in women aged 20–89 years between 1990 and 1993. Body weight of these hip OA patients were available from 1989 onwards and the body weight closest to but before the date of hip OA was used for the analyses. These 27 women were matched to 27 women from the same study population, who were of the closest age and followed for the same period, but did not develop OA. Both body weight and body mass index were divided into tertiles. Crude odds ratios of hip OA for weight >70.0 kg was 11.9 with weight ≤ 60.4 kg as the reference. Crude odds ratios of hip OA for BMI > 27.8 kg/m^2 was 6.3 (95 per cent CI: 1.2–33.9) with BMI ≤ 23.9 kg/m^2 as the reference[11]. These high odds ratios are thus based on a longitudinal study design, but should be interpreted with some caution, since the mean length of time between body weight measurement and identification of OA was 4.5 months for cases and 10.3 months for controls. A third study with the baseline between 1948 and 1964 followed the incidence of hip OA among male students aged 20–29 at baseline. BMI was measured at age 20–29, 30–39, and at age 40–49 years. BMI tertiles were defined based on the BMI distribution at age 30–39 years. The incidence of hip OA was highest in the highest tertile of BMI at age 20–29, when measured at age 20–29 years and the incidence was lowest in the lowest tertile at age 30–39. A dose-response relation was not found for BMI tertiles at age 20–29 and 30–39[14]. BMI measured at age 40–49 was not related to the incidence of hip OA.

Regarding excess body weight and hip OA we conclude that excessive body weight is causally related to hip OA on basis of the following: (1) Most cross-sectional studies show a relation between excess bodyweight and hip OA; (2) Longitudinal analyses confirm a relation between BMI and hip OA, although data are scarce and relations are relatively weak; (3) The main plausible explanation for a causal relation between excessive body weight and *knee* OA, being high pressure on the joints, is likely to be true for the onset of *hip* OA, reflected by lower relative risks of excessive body weight for *hip* OA than for *knee* OA[11,14].

Hand osteoarthirtis

There seems to be evidence for a relation between excessive body weight and hand OA[2-5], but both cross-sectional and longitudinal studies provide conflicting results[2,5].

The relation between excess body weight and hand OA may be stronger in women than in men[27]. However, OA or disc degeneration with loss of joint space and joint destruction was noted in different hand joints in men in the highest quintiles of body mass index[28]. Body weight was higher in women with high osteophyte scores in the carpometacarpal joint, but no weight differences were seen between twin sisters with different osteophyte scores for the distal and proximal interphalangeal joints[10]. Another study found obesity modestly associated with carpometacarpal AO and distal interphalangeal OA[7].

As stated above, longitudinal studies showed mixed results. A relation of obesity with incidence and increasing grade of hand osteoarthritis was not found in a study on women aged 40 years and over[29]. In another longitudinal study, on women aged 20–89 years, excessive body weight was associated with incident hand OA, although no dose-response relation could be found and the mean length of time between body weight measurement and identification date of OA was only 4.5 months[11]. In a study with 23 years of follow-up, baseline excess body weight in men and women aged 50–74 years was related to the incidence of hand OA, with greater body weight leading to more severe hand OA[30].

Given that obesity is a risk factor for hand OA, mechanical pressure on the joints cannot be the explanation, suggesting that a metabolic intermediary (such as diabetes or lipid abnormalities) may account in part for this potent relationship, but no such intermediary has been found[3]. There is longitudinal evidence for a relation between obesity and hand OA, but the relation needs further investigation for an elucidative explanation.

Hyperuricaemia and gout

Gout is not a single disease. The term is used to describe a number of disorders in which crystals of monosodium urate monohydrate derived from hyperuricaemic body fluids give rise to inflammatory arthritis, tenosynovitis, bursitis or cellulites, tophaceous deposits, urolithiasis and renal diseases. Hyperuricaemia is a necessary but not a sufficient prerequisite for clinical manifestations of gout.

The relation between excessive body weight and gout has been presented in both cross-sectional and longitudinal studies[5]. A clear example of a cross-sectional study was a study performed in sumo-wrestlers. Sumo-wrestlers had much higher levels of serum uric-acid than age-matched men with lower weights[31]. Maoris, another example of population with large numbers of obese individuals, also have high prevalence of hyperuricaemia and gout[32]. A 6-year longitudinal study on Japanese middle-aged men, showed that obesity was among the predictors of the onset of hyperuricaemia, with an increasing incidence across the three BMI-categories[33]. Excessive weight seemed to be a risk factor for gout at lower levels of BMI in men than in women[34]. Not only BMI, but also the waist-thigh circumference ratio was clearly related to the onset of gout[35].

The potential importance of the duration of excessive body weight becomes clear from the finding that excessive body weight in childhood is a stronger risk factor for gout than excessive body weight in adulthood[36]. A recent review confirmed the importance of childhood obesity as risk factor for gout[37]. Both excessive weight and weight gain was related to onset of gout and development of the disease[38]. Hyperuricaemia is associated with cardiovascular diseases and insulin resistance[39-41]. This relation, in part, explains the common coexistence of hyperlipidaemia and glucose intolerance in patients with gout[39]. The co-existence of hyperuricaemia and gout[42] is illustrative for the role of obesity in the onset of gout. Obesity is associated with both the increase in the production of urate and a decrease in its excretion[43]. The accumulation of visceral fat is a probably stronger risk factor for increased uric acid concentration in serum and a decreased uric acid clearance than is overall fatness or the accumulation of subcutaneous fat[44]. The finding that obesity was also related to gout among hyperuraemic subjects[45], suggests that there are also other explanations for a relation between excessive weight and gout.

Low back pain

Low back pain can de defined as any reported pain occurring between the gluteal folds and the 12th rib[46]. Some authors include sciatica and cruralgia[46], others exclude pain due to pregnancy, menstruation, viral infection and cancer[47].

A relation between obesity and low back pain seems logical and obesity has been linked to an increased risk of low back pain and sciatica in a review dating from 1989. However, evidence for a relation between obesity and low back pain was weak[48]. According to a large systematic review of 56 journal articles reporting 65 epidemiologic studies dating from 1999, body weight should still be considered a possible weak risk factor for low back pain[49]. In a longitudinal study assessing excessive body weight in relation to low back pain episodes of different durations, a dose-response relation was only found for the relation between excessive body weight and long-term low back pain (> 30 days)[50]. For low back pain with a duration of 1–7, or 8–30 days, heavy overweight was less or not related, whereas moderate overweight was.

Further, increasing BMI has been linked to more frequent osteophytes at both dorsal and lumbar spine, although the relation was stronger at the dorsal spine[51]. In a study among middle-aged Dutch women, excessive body weight was linked to development of disc degeneration as detected by radiology[52].

It has been argued that some studies report a relation between obesity and low back pain, because of covariates that are associated with both obesity ands low back pain, such as low educational status, low occupational status, sedentary life-style and psychological distress[49]. In a Twin study, however, where these factors are generally similar within twins, obesity was still, although modestly, related to low back pain[50]. A recent longitudinal study concluded that excessive weight was not related to low back pain, when the relation was assessed in multi-variate models. However, only two categories of body mass index were compared: > 70th percentile vs. < 15th percentile[53].

Although the relation between obesity and the onset of low back pain is uncertain, obesity was clearly related to the onset of work disability due to low back pain[54]. That obesity is related to worsening of symptoms in low back patients is further suggested by the finding that a dose-response relation between excessive body weight and low back pain was only found for long-term low back pain (> 30 days)[50]. For low back pain episodes of shorter duration moderate overweight was associated to low back pain, whereas severe overweight was not or only weakly[50].

Obesity adds to intradiscal pressures as well as stresses in other spinal structures. However, no studies have been carried out to determine whether compressive overload of the disc arises from obesity as such, and whether any biological adaptation in the tissues of the disc follows the development of obesity[48]. The absent relation for severe overweight and short-term low back pain is compatible with the suggestion that subjects with severe overweight are relatively protected from high work-load, because of lack of strong physical conditions needed for heavy work. Higher odds ratios ratios of low back pain for large waist circumference than for high BMI, found in a cross-sectional study, suggest that an altered gait in subjects with a large waist circumference may have a causal role in the onset of low back pain[55].

Herniated lumbar intervertebral disc

Mean BMI was higher in Finns who needed an operation for lumbar disc herniation than the BMI in the general Finnish population[56]. Excessive body weight seemed important in the incidence of hospitalized lumbar disc lesions in holders of the US Army National Service Life Insurance policies[57]. The risk of herniated lumbar intervertebral disc was increased in categories of high BMI in men, but not in women, in a longitudinal study following a Finnish population sample[58]. A number of cross-sectional studies, however, failed to reveal such an association.

Diffuse idiopathic skeletal hyperostosis

Diffuse idiopathic skeletal hyperostosis (DISH) is a rheumatic disease characterized by a significant association with metabolic alterations, such as impaired lipidic profile[59].

The relation between excessive body weight and hyperostosis is found in longitudinal studies[59,60] and cross-sectional studies[72,73]. All studies are highly suggestive for a link with Syndrome X, but causal pathways are not yet clear. An increased serum level of growth hormone has been proposed to have a role.

Neck pain

Data on excessive body weight and neck pain are scarce. One longitudinal study reported a 1.4 to 1.5 increased risk for developing radiating neck pain (pain radiating to the upper extremity) in subjects with BMI above 26.0 kg/m^2 compared to those with BMI below 23.0 kg/m^2. A cross-sectional study suggested an association between excessive body weight and neck pain, defined as convincing history of severe, longstanding neck pain that had manifested symptoms during the previous month, a documented history of a previously diagnosed neck syndrome with convincing observable signs on physical examination, or mild or moderate neck pain with observable signs at the time of examination[61].

As direct high pressure on bones or tissues in the neck region cannot explain the relation between excessive body weight and neck pain, we hypothesise that the presence of abundant fat tissue complicates rotation movements of the neck.

Shoulder pain

A possible association between excessive body weight can be explained in a similar manner as the relation between excessive body weight and neck pain.

The association between excessive body weight was weak in a Finnish cross-sectional population based study, with an odds ratio being 1.3 (95 per cent CI: 0.8–2.0) for BMI of 35.0 kg/m^2 or more compared to BMI less than 25.0 kg/m^2. The relation was higher among employees of a large forestry company in Finland[62]. The relative risk of developing shoulder pain was 2.1 (95 per cent CI: 1.4–3.3) for BMI $\geq$ 29.0 kg/m^2 compared to BMI < 23.0 kg/m^2.

Our hypothesis that an abundant fat mass complicates rotation movements is confirmed by the finding of an association between excessive body weight and reduced shoulder flexion range[63].

Discussion

The studies described in this review suggest a link between excessive body weight to osteoarthritis in different joints, and to many other musculoskeletal disorders. Whereas the relation between excessive body weight and other musculoskeletal disorders than OA is not always clear, excessive body weight seems to be strongly related to the onset of severity of disease and disease-related disabilities. Exact estimations of relations could not yet be made within the scope of this review and is hampered by differences in study design, study populations, obesity indicators and different diagnosis criteria for the musculoskeletal disorders. However, it becomes clear that obesity is an important modifiable risk factor for musculoskeletal disorders and disability.

Osteoarthritis is the commonest single cause of disability[64] and the major reason for knee and hip replacements[65], as Cicuttini and Spector stated in their review[5]. Since the association between excessive body weight and knee OA is strong, monotonic, evident also in prospective studies, consistent between a multitude of studies, independent of other risk determinants, closer for bilateral than unilateral affection, concerning both symptomatic and non-symptomatic OA and biologically plausible, there seems to be no doubt about the major causal role of overweight in OA. Further, there is evidence that body weight is also important in patients who already developed OA. A lower body weight was associated with less severe symptoms in OA patients. In patients with OA obesity is related to the progression of knee OA symptoms[12,66] and as a consequence with attenuated balance[67] and future knee pain[68].

Low back pain is very common in western societies and a major cause of ill health and disability[48]. When a Dutch sample aged 25 years or more was asked whether one have had experienced at least one episode of low back pain during the past year 43.9 per cent answered positively. A total of 21.2 per cent reported chronic low back pain, i.e. back pain longer than 3 months[69]. Also for low back pain patients weight control deserves attention. Although a causal role of obesity in the onset of low back pain is unlikely, excessive body weight certainly predicts work disability due to back disorders[54].

Besides excessive body weight an increase in (work)load on the joints or tissues is likely to be a necessary factor, resulting in an interaction between excessive body weight and (work)load as some studies showed. *The failure to control* body weight is likely to be a crucial risk factor for a vicious circle of gaining weight, developing osteoarthritis, developing disability, becoming less physically active and thereby gaining weight resulting in more severe disease entity and/or worsening of symptoms and worsening of disabilities.

Both excessive body weight and musculoskeletal disorders are becoming more and more prevalent in western societies. Further, musculoskeletal disorders are highly disabling[70,71]. Due to the major causal role of excessive body weight in at least OA, gout and spinal hyperostosis, an increased attention for weight control programmes is warranted in the primary prevention of musculoskeletal disorders. In the secondary and tertiary prevention, the relation between excessive body weight and worsening of disease symptoms and onset of disabilities urge for a new paradigm for the treatment of OA in which the control of body weight gets high priority.

References

1. Visscher TLS, Seidell JC. The public health impact of obesity. *Annu Rev Public Health* 2001; 22: 355–75.

2. Silman AJ, Hochberg MC. *Epidemiologicy of the rheumatic diseases* (2nd edn). New York: Oxford University Press Inc; 2001.

3. Felson DT, Lawrence RC, Dieppe PA, Hirsch R, Helmick CG, Jordan JM *et al.* Osteoarthritis: new insights. Part 1: the disease and its risk factors. *Ann Intern Med* 2000; 133: 635–46.

4. Felson DT, Zhang Y. An update on the epidemiology of knee and hip osteoarthritis with a view to prevention. *Arthritis Rheum* 1998; 41: 1343–55.

5. Cicuttini M, Spector TD. *Obesity, arthritis, and gout.* New York: M Dekker 1997; 79–91.

6. Davis MA, Ettinger WH, Neuhaus JM. Obesity and osteoarthritis of the knee: evidence from the National Health and Nutrition Examination Survey (NHANES I). *Semin Arthritis Rheum* 1990; 20: 34–41.

7. Hart DJ, Spector TD. The relationship of obesity, fat distribution and osteoarthritis in women in the general population: the Chingford Study. *J Rheumatol* 1993; 20: 331–5.

8. Felson DT, Zhang Y, Hannan MT, Naimark A, Weissman B, Aliabadi P *et al.* Risk factors for incident radiographic knee osteoarthritis in the elderly: the Framingham Study. *Arthritis Rheum* 1997; 40: 728–33.

9. Felson DT, Anderson JJ, Naimark A, Walker AM, Meenan RF. Obesity and knee osteoarthritis. The Framingham Study. *Ann Intern Med* 1988; 109: 18–24.

10. Cicuttini FM, Baker JR, Spector TD. The association of obesity with osteoarthritis of the hand and knee in women: a twin study. *J Rheumatol* 1996; 23: 1221–6.

11. Oliveria SA, Felson DT, Cirillo PA, Reed JI, Walker AM. Body weight, body mass index, and incident symptomatic osteoarthritis of the hand, hip, and knee. *Epidemiology* 1999; 10: 161–6.

12. Spector TD, Hart DJ, Doyle DV. Incidence and progression of osteoarthritis in women with unilateral knee disease in the general population: the effect of obesity. *Ann Rheum Dis* 1994; 53: 565–8.

13. Manninen P, Riihimaki H, Heliovaara M, Makela P. Overweight, gender and knee osteoarthritis. *Int J Obes Relat Metab Disord* 1996; 20: 595–7.

14. Gelber AC, Hochberg MC, Mead LA, Wang NY, Wigley FM, Klag MJ. Body mass index in young men and the risk of subsequent knee and hip osteoarthritis. *Am J Med* 1999; 107: 542–8.

15. Noppa H, Andersson M, Bengtsson C, Bruce A, Isaksson B. Longitudinal studies of anthropometric data and body composition. The population study of women in Gotenberg, Sweden. *Am J Clin Nutr* 1980; 33: 155–62.

16. Felson DT, Zhang Y, Anthony JM, Naimark A, Anderson JJ. Weight loss reduces the risk for symptomatic knee osteoarthritis in women. The Framingham Study. *Ann Intern Med* 1992; 116: 535–9.

17. Williams RA, Foulsham BM. Weight reductaion in osteoarthritis using phentermine. *Practitioner* 1981; 225: 231–2.

18. Cooper C, Inskip H, Croft P, Campbell L, Smith G, McLaren M *et al.* Individual risk factors for hip osteoarthritis: obesity, hip injury, and physical activity. *Am J Epidemiol* 1998; 147: 516–22.

19. Sandmark H, Hogstedt C, Lewold S, Vingard E. Osteoarthrosis of the knee in men and women in association with overweight, smoking, and hormone therapy. *Ann Rheum Dis* 1999; 58: 151–5.

20. Sharma L, Lou C, Cahue S, Dunlop DD. The mechanism of the effect of obesity in knee osteoarthritis: the mediating role of malalignment. *Arthritis Rheum* 2000; 43: 568–75.

21. Tepper S, Hochberg MC. Factors associated with hip osteoarthritis: data from the First National Health and Nutrition Examination Survey (NHANES-I). *Am J Epidemiol* 1993; 137: 1081–8.

22. Heliövaara M, Mäkelä M, Impivaara O, Knekt P, Aromaa A, Sievers K. Association of overweight, trauma and workload with coxarthrosis. A health survey of 7, 217 persons. *Acta Orthop Scand* 1993; 64: 513–8.

23. Dennison EM, Arden NK, Kellingray S, Croft P, Coggon D, Cooper C. Hormone replacement therapy, other reproductive variables and symptomatic hip osteoarthritis in elderly white women: a case-control study. *Br J Rheumatol* 1998; 37: 1198–202.

24. Roach KE, Persky V, Miles T, Budiman-Mak E. Biomechanical aspects of occupation and osteoarthritis of the hip: a case-control study. *J Rheumatol* 1994; 21: 2334–40.

25. Kraus JF, D'Ambrosia RD, Smith EG, van Meter J, Borhani NO, Franti CE *et al.* An epidemiological study of severe osteoarthritis. *Orthopedics* 1978; 1: 37–42.

26. Olsen O, Vingard E, Koster M, Alfredsson L. Etiologic fractions for physical work load, sports and overweight in the occurrence of coxarthrosis. *Scand J Work Environ Health* 1994; 20: 184–8.

27. Acheson RM, Collart AB. New Haven survey of joint diseases. XVII. Relationship between some systemic characteristics and osteoarthrosis in a general population. *Ann Rheum Dis* 1975; 34: 379–87.

28. Van Saase JL, Vandenbroucke JP, van Romunde LK, Valkenburg HA. Osteoarthritis and obesity in the general population. A relationship calling for an explanation. *J Rheumatol* 1988; 15: 1152–8.

29. Hochberg MC, Lethbridge-Ceijku M, Wigley FM, Plato CC, Tobin JD. Factors predicting progression of hand osteoarthritis in males: data from the Baltimore Longitudinal study of Aging. *Arthritis Rheum* 1991; 34 (Suppl 9): S34.

30. Carman WJ, Sowers M, Hawthorne VM, Weissfeld LA. Obesity as a risk factor for osteoarthritis of the hand and wrist: a prospective study. *Am J Epidemiol* 1994; 139: 119–29.

31. Nishizawa T, Akaoka I, Nishida Y, Kawaguchi Y, Hayashi E. Some factors related to obesity in the Japanese sumo wrestler. *Am J Clin Nutr* 1976; 29: 1167–74.

32. Gibson T, Waterworth R, Hatfield P, Robinson G, Bremner K. Hyperuricaemia, gout and kidney function in New Zealand Maori men. *Br J Rheumatol* 1984; 23: 276–82.

33. Nakanishi N, Tatara K, Nakamura K, Suzuki K. Risk factors for the incidence of hyperuricaemia: a 6-year longitudinal study of middle-aged Japanese men. *Int J Epidemiol* 1999; 28: 888–93.

34. Seidell JC, Bakx KC, Dourenberg P, van den Hoogen HJ, Hautvast JG, Stijnen T. Overweight and chronic illness-a retrospective cohort study, with a follow-up of 6–17 years, in men and women of initially 20–50 years of age. *J Chronic Dis* 1986; 39: 585–93.

35. Seidell JC, Bakx JC, De Boer E, Deurenberg P, Hautvast JG. Fat distribution of overweight persons in relation to morbidity and subjective health. *Int J Obes* 1985; 9: 363–74.

36. Must A, Jacques PF, Dallal GE, Bajema CJ, Dietz WH. Long-term morbidity and mortality of overweight adolescents. A follow-up of the Harvard Growth Study of 1922 to 1935. *N Engl J Med* 1992; 327: 1350–5.

37. Maffeis C. Aetiology of overweight and obesity in children and adolescents. *Eur J Pediatr* 2000; 159(1): S35–44.

38. Roubenoff R. Gout and hyperuricemia. *Rheum Dis Clin North Am* 1990; 16: 539–50.

39. Wortmann RL. Gout and hyperuricemia. *Curr Opin Rheumatol* 2002; 14: 281–6.

40. Cigolini M, Targher G, Tonoli M, Manara F, Muggeo M, De Sandre G. Hyperuricaemia: relationships to body fat distribution and other components of the insulin resistance syndrome in 38-year-old healthy men and women. *Int J Obes Relat Metab Disord* 1995; 19: 92–6.

41. Vuorinen-Markkola H, Yki-Jarvinen H. Hyperuricemia and insulin resistance. *J Clin Endocrinol Metab* 1994; 78: 25–9.

42. Zavaroni I, Mazza S, Fantuzzi M, Dall'Aglio E, Bonora E, Delsignore R *et al*. Changes in insulin and lipid metabolism in males with asymptomatic hyperuricaemia. *J Intern Med* 1993; 234: 25–30.

43. Emmerson BT. The management of gout. *N Engl J Med* 1996; 334: 445–51.

44. Takahashi S, Yamamoto T, Tsutsumi Z, Moriwaki Y, Yamakita J, Higashino K. Close correlation between visceral fat accumulation and uric acid metabolism in healthy men. *Metabolism* 1997; 46: 1162–5.

45. Lin KC, Lin HY, Chou P. Community based epidemiological study on hyperuricemia and gout in Kin-Hu, Kinmen. *J Rheumatol* 2000; 27: 1045–50.

46. Anderson JA. Epidemiological aspects of back pain. *J Soc Occup Med* 1986; 36: 90–4.

47. McKinnon ME, Vickers MR, Ruddock VM, Townsend J, Meade TW. Community studies of the health service implications of low back pain. *Spine* 1997; 22: 2161–6.

48. Heliövaara M. Risk factors for low back pain and sciatica. *Ann Med* 1989; 21: 257–64.

49. Leboeuf-Y de C. Body weight and low back pain. A systematic literature review of 56 journal articles reporting on 65 epidemiologic studies. *Spine* 2000; 25: 226–37.

50. Leboeuf-Y de C, Kyvik KO, Bruun NH Low back pain and lifestyle. Part II-Obesity. Information from a population-based sample of 29,424 twin subjects. *Spine* 1999; 24(8): 779–83 (discussion 783–4).

51. O'Neill TW, McCloskey EV, Kanis JA, Bhalla AK, Reeve J, Reid DM *et al*. The distribution, determinants, and clinical correlates of vertebral osteophytosis: a population based survey. *J Rheumatol* 1999; 26: 842–8.

52. Symmons DP, van Hemert AM, Vandenbroucke JP, Valkenburg HA. A longitudinal study of back pain and radiological changes in the lumbar spines of middle aged women. II. Radiographic findings. *Ann Rheum Dis* 1991; 50: 162–6.

53. Power C, Frank J, Hertzman C, Schierhout G, Li L. Predictors of low back pain onset in a prospective British study. *Am J Public Health* 2001; 91: 1671–8.

54. Rissanen A, Heliövaara M, Knekt P, Reunanen A, Aromaa A, Maatela J. Risk of disability and mortality due to overweight in a Finnish population. *BMJ* 1990; 301: 835–7.

55. Han TS, Schouten JS, Lean ME, Seidell JC. The prevalence of low back pain and associations with body fatness, fat distribution and height. *Int J Obes* 1997; 21: 600–7.

56. Bostman OM. Prevalence of obesity among patients admitted for elective orthopaedic surgery. *Int J Obes Relat Metab Disord* 1994; 18: 709–13.

57. Hrubec Z, Nashold BS Jr. Epidemiology of lumbar disc lesions in the military in World War II. *Am J Epidemiol* 1975; 102: 367–76.

58. Heliövaara M. Body height, obesity, and risk of herniated lumbar intervertebral disc. *Spine* 1987; 12: 469–72.

59. Coaccioli S, Fatati G, Di Cato L, Marioli D, Patucchi E, Pizzuti C *et al.* Diffuse idiopathic skeletal hyperostosis in diabetes mellitus, impaired glucose tolerance and obesity. *Panminerva Med* 2000; 42: 247–51.

60. Julkunen H, Knekt P, Aromaa A. Spondylosis deformans and diffuse idiopathic skeletal hyperostosis (DISH) in Finland. *Scand J Rheumatol* 1981; 10: 193–203.

61. Mäkelä M, Heliövaara M, Sievers K, Impivaara O, Knekt P, Aromaa A. Prevalence, determinants, and consequences of chronic neck pain in Finland. *Am J Epidemiol* 1991; 134: 1356–67.

62. Miranda H, Viikari-Juntura E, Martikainen R, Takala EP, Riihimaki HA. prospective study of work related factors and physical exercise as predictors of shoulder pain. *Occup Environ Med* 2001; 58: 528–34.

63. Escalante A, Lichtenstein MJ, Hazuda HP. Determinants of shoulder and elbow flexion range: results from the San Antonio Longitudinal Study of Aging. *Arthritis Care Res* 1999; 12: 277–86.

64. Verbrugge LM. From sneezes to adieux: stages of health for American men and women. *Soc Sci Med* 1986; 22: 1195–212.

65. Bulstrode C. Keeping up with orthopaedic epidemics. *BMJ* (Clin Res Ed) 1987; 295: 514.

66. Cooper C, Snow S, McAlindon TE, Kellingray S, Stuart B, Coggon D *et al.* Risk factors for the incidence and progression of radiographic knee osteoarthritis. *Arthritis Rheum* 2000; 43: 995–1000.

67. Jadelis K, Miller ME, Ettinger WH Jr, Messier SP. Strength, balance, and the modifying effects of obesity and knee pain: results from the Observational Arthritis Study in Seniors (oasis). *J Am Geriatr Soc* 2001; 49: 884–91.

68. Schouten JSAG. The effect of body mass index and change in body weight on the progresion of knee osteoarthritis and knee pain. In: Schouten JSAG. *Osteoartrhitis of the knee*, pp. 165–76. The Netherlands: Thesis Eramsus Univeristy Medical Centre; 1991.

69. Picavet HS, Schouten JSAG. Musculoskeletal pain in the Netherlands: prevalences, consequences and risk groups, the DMC3-study. Submitted 2002.

70. Mäkelä M, Heliövaara M, Sievers K, Knekt P, Maatela J, Aromaa A. Musculoskeletal disorders as determinants of disability in Finns aged 30 years or more. *J Clin Epidimiol* 1993; 46: 549–59.

71. Croft PR, Macfarlane GJ, Papageorgiou AC, Thomas E, Silman AJ. Outcome of low back pain in general practice: a prospective study. *BMJ* 1998; 316: 1356–9.

72. Denko CW, Boja B, Moskowitz RW. Growth promoting peptides in osteoarthritis and diffuse idiopathic skeletal hyperostosis – insulin, insulin-like growth factor-I, growth hormone. *J Rheumatol* 1984; 21: 1725–30.

73. Littlejohn GO. Insulin and new formation in diffuse idiopathic skeletal hyperostosis. *Clin Rheumatol* 1985; 4: 294–300.

CHAPTER 126

The effects of obesity on asthma

John B. Dixon

Monash University Department of Surgery, Alfred Hospital, Melbourne, Victoria 3181, Australia
[e-mail: john.dixon@med.monash.edu.au]

Introduction

Over the last 20–30 year developed and developing communities have been in the grip of an obesity epidemic[1]. The prevalence of obesity (BMI > 30kg/m²) in the US was 16 per cent in 1976–80 and increased to 27 per cent by 1999. During the same period the incidence and prevalence of asthma has also increased substantially in both children and adults[2]. Between 1980 and 1994 the incidence of self reported asthma in US adults increased from 3.7 per cent to 5.4 per cent with an 80 per cent increase in women and 29 per cent in men[3].

Given the similar temporal changes observed in these two common conditions, an association may exist. The aim of this review was to assess the currently available literature in the English language from Medline regarding the relationship between obesity and asthma. Is there a positive relationship? What is the nature of the relationship? Is there evidence of causality? What are the implications for the management of asthma given our current knowledge?

Asthma

Asthma is a chronic inflammatory condition of the airways with many cells and cellular elements playing a role. Chronic inflammation leads to airway hyper-responsiveness leading to recurrent episodes of wheezing, coughing and breathlessness. The resulting airway obstruction is widespread, variable and often reversible.

Airway hyper-responsiveness (AHR) associated with asthma is measured using a dose response methacholine or histamine challenge to stimulate airway constriction. It is expressed as the percentage fall in forced expiratory volume in 1 s (FEV1)/concentration of methacholine.

Obesity and asthma in children and adolescence

Several cross-sectional studies have examined the relationship between BMI and asthma in children. A recent study of 5993 Australian primary school children with a mean age 9.7 years found a significant positive relationship between the prevalence of cough, wheeze, atopy and a diagnosis of asthma and BMI in girls but not in boys. However, this study failed to demonstrate increased airways hyper-responsiveness in these girls. Over 18,000 children in the UK were examined as part of the National Health and Growth Study. There was a positive association between wheeze and an asthma attack in the last year, and BMI but the relationship was attenuated in inner city boys[4]. Huang *et al.*, in a study of Taiwanese teenagers also found a sex difference with girls of higher BMI more likely to have a history of wheeze and asthma[5]. An increase in atopy and airways hyper-responsiveness was also demonstrated. Longitudinal studies have also found a positive association that is stronger in girls. The longitudinal Tucson Children's Respiratory Study examined 1246 US children and found there was no relationship between BMI in children at the age of 6 years and wheeze at any age[6]. However, girls who became overweight or obese between the ages of 6 and 11 years were seven times more likely to have developed new asthma symptoms by the ages of 11 to 13 years. Increased peak flow variability and bronchodilator responsiveness was also demonstrated. There was no similar effect in boys. The British Cohort Study 1970 reported very similar findings. BMI at age 10 years was not related to adult asthma but, by the age of 26 years, there was an increased incidence of self reported asthma especially in women[7]. In addition this study found that reported asthma was inversely related to birth weight, concluding that impaired fetal growth and adult fatness were risk factors for adult asthma.

An interesting study of cross-sectional trends from 8–9 year old Britons between 1982 and 1994 found no association between a diagnosis of asthma and asthma symptoms, and BMI in 1982, but a positive relationship in both boys and girls in 1994[8]. There was no BMI to year interaction found in this study leading to the conclusion that the association is recent and likely to be related to factors other than BMI, for example, lifestyle or dietary changes. It is worth noting that the selected age of the group may have been relevant with a possibility that early puberty changes may have confounded the results. The Tucson study found a significant difference between girls of age 6 and 11 years[6].

Obesity and asthma in adults

During the period from 1991–1995 there were 1596 new incident cases of physician diagnosed asthma with recent use of asthma medication reported in the US Nurses Health Study[9]. There was a positive association between asthma and BMI throughout the full range of BMI categories. Weight gain after the age of 18 years was associated with an increased risk of developing asthma over the next 4 years. The US CARDIA found that adult obesity and weight gain over 10 years was associated with newly diagnosed asthma in women but not in men[10]. The 1966-birth cohort study in Finland found that overweight or obesity at age 14 or 31 was associated with an increased risk of diagnosed asthma at age 31 years – again the association was stronger in women (Xu *et al.*, ATS abstract, 2000). These two latter studies found that the association was not explained by lower physical activity. A study of over 9000 adult subjects enrolled in the Canadian National Health Surveys reported that over a two-year period that the incidence of a new diagnosis of asthma was 1.6 per cent for men and 2.9 per cent for women[3]. High baseline BMI was a strong predictor in women but not men. A consistent problem associated with the above adult studies is the basis on which a diagnosis of asthma is made. None of these studies tested objective measures of asthma such as AHR.

Airway hyper-responsiveness was tested in a cross-sectional study of Australian adults[11]. Subjects were selected from three epidemiological studies in New South Wales between 1991 and 1997. In addition to symptoms or a diagnosis of asthma spirometry, skin testing for atopy and a methacholine airway challenge was performed. Subjects with a BMI greater than 35 kg/m² reported more wheezing, breathlessness, recent asthma and medication used for asthma. However there was no increased in atopy, bronchial obstruction as measured by FEV1/FVC or airways responsiveness. This study concluded that while obese subjects had symptoms highly suggestive of asthma an increased prevalence of 'true' asthma could not be supported. As part of the Veterans Administration Normative Aging Study of 1961 sixty-one men who developed airway hyper-responsiveness over a 4-year period were compared with matched controls[12]. The effects of initial BMI and change in BMI on the development of airway hyper-responsiveness were examined. The risk of developing AHR was lowest in the middle quintile of BMI (25.9–27.3) and increased for those in lower and higher quintiles. The odds ratio for developing AHR in highest quintile of BMI was 7.5 (95 per cent CI, 1.5–38). For men with an initial low BMI the increased risk of developing AHR was partly mediated by weight gain.

The effect of intentional weight loss on asthma

Several interventional studies have looked at the effect of weight loss surgery on asthma. We reported the effect of weight loss after Lap-Band® surgery[13]. Thirty-two consecutive patients who reported a history of physician diagnosed asthma were followed at least 1 year after surgery. The mean weight preoperatively was 125.2 ± 23 kg and at 1 year 89.3 ± 14 kg. A global asthma score was calculated to indicate the severity of asthma. The questionnaire included daily impact of asthma, effect on exercise, effect on sleep, hospitalization for asthma and all medications used. The mean preoperative modified Asthma Severity Score was 44.5 and at 1 year 14.3 ($P < 0.001$). All patients experienced an improvement in asthma with one third having resolution of all symptoms and requiring no asthma medication. Significantly fewer patients required daily preventative medication, none required oral steroids. No patient required admission to hospital for asthma during the 12 months after surgery whereas seven had been admitted to hospital, some on several occasions, for the treatment of asthma in the year prior to surgery. Similar improvements have also been reported with weight loss following gastric bypass surgery[14–16]. The only randomized study examined the effect of weight loss followed 19 patients losing weight with a very low calorie diet[17]. Subjects in the weight loss group experienced less dyspnoea, had improved FEV1 and used less breakthrough asthma medication. They also experienced fewer asthma exacebations and required less oral steroids. In a second study, performed by the same group from

Finland, 14 patients were found to have reduced diurnal and day to day peak expiratory flow variability, improved FEF 25-75, reduced airway resistance and improved functional residual capacity[18].

Causality: can obesity cause asthma?

Many aspects of the obesity – asthma relationship described above suggest causality. The increasing asthma prevalence with increasing BMI, together with the increase in risk of developing asthma with weight gain during puberty or later in life are suggestive of causality. The evidence although limited, that asthma improves with weight loss is strongly supportive. The above conditions fulfill the criteria of asthma, as defined as a clinical entity in the bulk of the studies, being a comorbidity of obesity. However, weakness lies in the strict definition of asthma. Few studies measured lung function and less bronchial responsiveness. Of those that did measure asthma more strictly with bronchial challenge, there were somewhat mixed results.

Some aspects of living with asthma may encourage the development of obesity. Asthma may limit physical activity leading to a more sedentary lifestyle. Treatment including both inhaled and oral steroids may predispose to weight gain. Given these theoretical possibilities longitudinal studies do not support a positive association.

Mechanisms for obesity – asthma link

Mechanical effects of obesity have predictable effects on lung function. Obesity is associated with reduced lung volumes, there is increased intra-abdominal pressure and splinting of the diaphragm, reduced chest wall compliance, increased small airways resistance, and increased blood volume and work of breathing[19,20]. Obesity is often associated with increased gastro-esophageal reflux, which may produce direct effects on the airway via microaspiration or indirect effects through neural reflexs[21]. Obesity is also associated with upper airway obstruction especially during sleep as indicated by snoring and obstructive sleep apnea and this may have adverse effects on lung function[22].

The following is a possible sequence for the development of increased airways resistance and responsiveness. Obesity is associated with a reduction in functional residual capacity and a reduced tidal volume with the tidal breaths taken closer to or around closing volume. This leads to a reduction in the middle part of the forced vital capacity (FVC) that is the forced expiratory flow between 25 per cent and 75 per cent (FEF 25–75) of FVC indicative of small airway narrowing[23]. It has been hypothesized that reduced small airway diameter leads to reduced small muscle stretching and latching leading to increased airway resistance and possibly responsiveness[24]. These effects would be seen to mimic, aggravate or cause asthma. It is important to emphasize that reduced lung volume may cause reduced airway caliber as a secondary effect and this could mimic asthma without accompanying airway inflammation or increased responsiveness.

Asthma and obesity are both increasing recognized as inflammatory conditions. Obesity with increased levels of inflammatory markers, leptin, TNF-alpha, IL-6 and IL-12, and asthma with increased levels of IL-4, IL-5 and TNF-alpha. There is the possibility of interaction between these pro-inflammatory cytokines whereby the inflammatory effect of obesity aggravates or triggers asthma[25].

Most studies indicate that the association between obesity and asthma is stronger in adolescent girls and women. Clearly sex hormone levels may be relevant with estrogen and its immune mediated effects a possible putative candidate.

There are also a number of possibilities for gene-environmental interactions leading to a recognizable association between asthma and obesity. The Barker hypothesis proposes that maternal nutrition during critical phases of pregnancy leads to intra-uterine gene programming. Abnormal maternal nutrition may predispose to an increased risk of disease later in life. Intra-uterine growth restriction is associated with increased risk of central obesity and asthma. Those with higher birth weight are also likely to go on to be larger children and adults and thus may also be at greater risk of developing asthma[7]. Higher fetal leptin levels are found in both underweight and overweight individuals. Our obesogenic environment with major changes in physical activity and dietary composition may also play a role in increasing the prevalence of both asthma and obesity. Obesity is also associated with significant body image, depression and psychosocial disturbance especially in younger women[26], these psychological factors may aggravate or trigger episodes of asthma.

Implications for the management of asthma

Symptoms of asthma are aggravated or caused by obesity and therefore weight reduction should be a key therapeutic goal in the management of the obese asthmatic. Advice regarding appropriate exercise, physical fitness, diet and behavioural changes to help treat and prevent further obesity are important. Oral steroids, which tend to encourage weight gain, should be avoided where possible and when necessary use kept to a minimum. To avoid the necessity for systemic steroids asthma preventative measures should be fully utilized. There remains the real possibility that some obese subjects that have been diagnosed with asthma do not have 'true asthma' and therefore asthma medication including steroids may be inappropriate. If an obese subject appears to have atypical asthma or is responding poorly to asthma therapy then early referral for diagnostic lung function is imperative.

Asthma, as defined loosely in many of the epidemiological studies, fulfills the criteria for being a true comorbidity of obesity. That is, the incidence increases with that of increasing obesity, the severity appears to increase with increasing obesity, weight gain increased the incidence and weight loss produces positive benefit with reduction or even resolution in asthma symptoms and reduction in the use of asthma medications[27]. It therefore may be argued that significant asthma in overweight and obese subjects lowers the threshold to weight loss interventions with the use of pharmacotherapy, very low calorie diets and obesity surgery at levels appropriate to those of subjects with significant obesity related comorbidity.

Table 1. Summary of important points

There is evidence of increased symptoms of asthma in obese adults and adolescents – the effect appears to be greater in females.
There is some evidence of increased airway hyper-responsiveness, atopy and airway obstruction in the obese.
Asthma symptoms may not always be asthma as we know it, i.e. associated with airways inflammation and hyper-responsiveness.
Weight loss is associated with reduced asthma symptoms, improved lung function and a reduction in medication used for asthma.
Asthma fulfills the criteria of being a comorbidity of obesity.
Weight reduction is an important part of the management of the obese asthmatic – thresholds should be lowered for the introduction of active obesity therapies.
If asthma is atypical or responds poorly to conventional therapy referral for diagnostic lung function study is imperative.

Conclusion

In conclusion the relationship between asthma and obesity needs further careful study. Strict criteria for a diagnosis of asthma, using objective lung function measures, need to be used to clarify the exact nature of asthma symptoms in obese subjects. Studying, in obese asthmatics, the effect of weight loss on lung function, preferably in randomized controlled trials, should provide valuable insights into the nature of the relationship. The effect of gender, sex hormones and inflammatory cytokines clearly needs further study. A summary of important points discussed in this chapter is listed in Table 1. In the meantime our current knowledge gives us some insight and assistance in managing our obese asthmatic patients.

References

1. World Health Organisation Obesity: Preventing and managing the global epidemic. World Health Organisation Technical Report Series. Geneva; 1998.

2. Alvey SD. Asthma emergency care: national guidelines summary. *Heart Lung* 2001; 30: 472–4.

3. Chen Y, Dales R, Tang M, Krewski D. Obesity may increase the incidence of asthma in women but not in men: longitudinal observations from the Canadian National Population Health Surveys. *Am J Epidemiol* 2002; 155: 191–7.

4. Figueroa-Munoz JI, Chinn S, Rona RJ. Association between obesity and asthma in 4–11 year old children in the UK. *Thorax* 2001; 56: 133–7.

5. Huang S, Shiao G, Chou P. Assoctation between body mass index and allergy in teenage girls in Taiwan. *Clin Exp Allergy* 1999; 29(3): 323–9.

6. Castro-Rodriguez JA, Holberg CJ, Morgan WJ, Wright AL, Martinez FD. Increased incidence of asthmalike symptoms in girls who become overweight or obese during the school years. *Am J Respir Crit Care Med* 2001; 163: 1344–9.

7. Shaheen S0, Sterne JA, Montgomery SM, Azima H. Birth weight, body mass index and asthma in young adults. *Thorax* 1999; 54: 3 96–402.

8. Chinn S, Rona RJ. Can the increase in body mass index explain the rising trend in asthma in children? *Thorax* 2001; 56: 845–50.

9. Camargo CA Jr, Weiss S T, Zhang S, Willett WC, Speizer FE. Prospective study of body mass index, weight change, and risk of adult- onset asthma in women. *Arch Intern Med* 1999; 159: 2582–8.

10. Beckett WS, Jacobs DR Jr, Yu X, Iribarren C, Williams 0D. Asthma is associated with weight gain in females but not males, independent of physical activity. *Am J Respir Crzt Care Med* 2001; 164: 2045–50.

11. Schachter LM, Salome CM, Peat JK, Woolcock AJ. Obesity is a risk for asthma and wheeze but not airway hyperresponsiveness. *Thorax* 2001; 56: 4–8.

12. Litonjua AA, Sparrow D,Celedon JC, DeMolles D, Weiss ST. Association of body mass index with the development of methacholine airway hyperresponsiveness in men: the normative Aging Study. *Thorax* 2002; 57: 581–5.

13. Dixon JB, Chapman L, O'Brien P. Marked improvement in asthma after LapBand surgery for morbid obesity. *Obes Surg* 1999; 9: 385–9.

14. Dhabuwala A, Cannan RJ, Stubbs RS. Improvement in co-morbidities following weight loss from gastric bypass surgery. *Obes Surg* 2000; 10: 428–35.

15. Murr MM, Siadati MR, Sarr MG. Results of Bariatric Surgery for Morbid Obesity in Patients Older than 50 Years. *Obes Surg* 1995; 5: 399–402.

16. Macgregor AM, Greenberg RA. Effect of Surgically Induced Weight Loss on Asthma in the Morbidly Obese. *Obes Surg* 1993; 3: 15–21.

17. Stenius-Aarniala B *et al.* Immediate and long term effects of weight reduction in obese people with asthma: randomised controlled study. *BMJ* 2000; 320: 827–32.

18. Hakala K, Stenius-Aarniala B, Sovijarvi A. Effects of weight loss on peak flow variability, airways obstruction, and lung volumes in obese patients with asthma. *Chest* 118, 2000; 1315–21.

19. Rorvik S, Bo G. Lung volumes and arterial blood gases in obesity. *Scand J Respir Dis* 1976; (95): 60–4.

20. Gibson GJ. Obesity, respiratory function and breathlessness. *Thorax* 2000; 55(1): S41–4.

21. Sontag S. Gastroesophageal Reflux and Asthma. *Am J Med* 1997; 103(3S): 84S–90.

22. Zerah-Lancner F *et al.* Pulmonary function in obese snorers with or without sleep apnea syndrome. *Am J Respir Crit Care Med* 1997; 156: 522–7.

23. Ho TF, Tay JS, Yip WC, Rajan U. Evaluation of lung function in Singapore obese children. *J Singapore Paediatr Soc* 1989; 31: 46–52.

24. Fredberg JJ *et al.* Airway smooth muscle, tidal stretches, and dynamically determined contractile states. *Am J Respir Crit Care Med* 1997; 156: 1752–9.

25. Tantisira KG, Weiss ST. Complex interactions in complex traits: obesity and asthma. *Thorax* 2001; 56 (Suppl 2): ii64–73.

26. Dixon JB, Dixon ME, O'Brien PE. Body image: appearance orientation and evaluation in the severely obese. Changes with weight loss. *Obes Surg* 2002; 12: 65–71.

27. Oria HE, Moorehead MK. Bariatric analysis and reporting out come system (BAROS). *Obes Surg* 1998; 8: 487–99.

Progress in Obesity Research: 9. Edited by *Geraldo Medeiros-Neto, Alfredo Halpern and Claude Bouchard*

CHAPTER 127

Quality of life: relationship to obesity

Ronette L. Kolotkin[1], Ross D. Crosby[2,3] and G. Rhys Williams[4]

[1]*Obesity and Quality of Life Consulting, Durham, NC, USA;* [2]*Neuropsychiatric Research Institute, Fargo, ND, USA;* [3]*University of North Dakota School of Medicine and Health Sciences, Fargo ND, USA;* [4]*Bristol-Myers Squibb, Princeton, NJ, USA*
[email: rkolotkin@yahoo.com]

In recent years there has been a great deal of interest in studying the impact of overweight and obesity on health-related quality of life (HRQOL)[1-6]. This paper examines (1) the relationship between BMI and quality of life, and (2) variables affecting the quality of life of persons with obesity.

The relationship between BMI and quality of life

Population studies

Population studies from Sweden[5], Australia[7], France[8] and the United States[9,10], demonstrate that as body mass index increases into the overweight and obese ranges, quality of life becomes more impaired. This impairment tends to occur primarily on the physical domains of quality of life as assessed by the SF-36[7-9,11], plus vitality[8,9]. Similarly, on the OSQOL, an obesity-specific quality of life instrument, quality of life impairment in the obese occurs primarily for physical state and vitality[8]. Those who have a BMI of 22–23 obtain optimal physical quality of life, and those with a BMI of 21 to 24 obtain optimal mental quality of life[7]. Underweight individuals as a group also demonstrate some quality of life impairment[5,7,12].

In a treatment-seeking sample, six out of eight scales of the SF-36 (physical scales plus vitality and social functioning) become more impaired with increasing obesity[13]. A similar relationship exists when quality of life is assessed using the IWQOL-Lite. As BMI increases, all scales show increasing impairment in quality of life[14,15].

Variables affecting quality of life in obese persons

Presence of co-morbid conditions

The presence of chronic illness in obese persons contributes greatly to impairment in the physical aspects of quality of life, but only slightly to impairment in the mental aspects of quality of life on the SF-36[11]. On the IWQOL-Lite, as the number of co-morbid conditions increases for obese persons, quality of life decreases on the physical function and sexual life domains[16].

Presence of pain

When SF-36 scores are compared for obese patients with and without pain, those with pain report greater quality of life impairment than those not reporting pain[17,18].

Presence of depression

The presence of depression is associated with greater quality of life impairment for obese subjects undergoing lap band surgery as compared to other obese patients undergoing this surgery[18].

Presence of binge eating disorder

Scores on the Binge Eating Scale are strongly associated with poor quality of life in obese outpatients[19]. Similarly, gastric bypass surgery patients with binge eating disorder show greater impairment as compared to other patients on four of the SF-36 scales (three of which are considered mental scales) plus the Mental Component Summary score[20]. On the IWQOL-Lite, patients with binge eating disorder have poorer quality of life on five of the six scales.

Treatment status

When obese treatment-seekers are compared to obese volunteers who are not seeking treatment, five scales of the SF-36 show greater impairment (the physical scales plus vitality)[21]. Similarly, obese people seeking a variety of weight loss treatments show significantly greater impairment on the IWQOL-Lite as compared to obese volunteers who are not seeking treatment[22].

Treatment intensity

The quality of life of obese persons seeking treatment differs according to the intensity of the treatment programme being sought. In one study, researchers found that within every BMI grouping, gastric bypass patients have the poorest quality of life (as assessed by the IWQOL-Lite), followed by day treatment patients, followed by those in weight programmes/studies, followed by clinical trials participants[22].

Gender

On the IWQOL-Lite sexual life and self-esteem scales, women have more impaired quality of life than men at every level of BMI[15]. Several other studies point to a greater impact of obesity on quality of life for women as compared to men[4,23–25].

Race

Findings on race and quality of life in obesity are inconsistent. On the IWQOL-Lite, Whites demonstrate significantly more impaired quality of life than African-Americans[22]. However, another study shows greater impairment for obese African-Americans than Whites[24], while another shows no difference between these racial groups[26].

Weight change

Numerous clinical reports and controlled research studies show that obese persons who lose weight (via surgical or non-surgical treatments) improve quality of life scores[27–33]. Even a modest sustained weight loss produces improvements in quality of life[34].

In the Nurses Health Study[9], a prospective study of health in women, weight change over a 4-year period (weight loss and weight gain) was associated with changes in the physical aspects of quality of life more than the mental aspects, as measured by the SF-36. In women who gain at least 9 kg over 4 years, all SF-36 scales become more impaired, particularly vitality, physical functioning, and bodily pain. For overweight and obese women, weight loss is associated with improved vitality, physical functioning, and bodily pain. For normal weight women, weight loss is associated with deterioration in these three scales.

Summary and conclusions

There is a consistent and strong relationship between quality of life variables and BMI, weight gain, and weight loss. Increasing BMI is associated with impaired quality of life (both generic and obesity-specific) in both population and treatment samples. On generic measures (and the OSQOL) the physical aspects of quality of life are more impaired than the mental aspects as BMI increases. On the IWQOL-Lite all scales show decreasing quality of life as BMI increases. Optimal quality of life scores are obtained for individuals with BMI's between 21 and 24, and underweight groups experience poor HRQOL equivalent to obese groups. Many factors affect the quality of life of obese persons, including the presence of co-morbid illness, pain, depression, and binge eating disorder. With further research we can discover the role played by other factors in the quality of life of obese persons. Since the elimination or cure of obesity is unlikely in the near future, providers may want to turn their attention to finding ways of enhancing and sustaining positive changes in the quality of life of obese persons.

References

1. Fontaine KR, Barofsky I. Obesity and health-related quality of life. *Obes Rev* 2001; 2: 173–82.
2. Kushner RF, Foster G. Obesity and quality of life. *Nutrition* 2000; 16: 947–52.
3. Kolotkin RL, Meter K, Williams GR. Quality of life and obesity. *Obes Rev* 2001; 2: 219–29.

4. Sullivan M, Karlsson J, Sjostrom L, Backman L, Bengtsson C, Bouchard C *et al.* Swedish obese subjects (SOS) – an intervention study of obesity. baseline evaluation of health and psychosocial functioning in the first 1743 subjects examined. *Int J Obes* 1993; 1743: 503–12.

5. Sullivan M, Karlsson J, Sjostrom L, Taft C. Why quality-of-life measures should be used in the treatment of patients with obesity. In: Bjorntorp P (ed.) *International textbook of obesity*, pp. 485–510. New York: John Wiley & Sons. 2001.

6. Fontaine KR, Bartlett SJ. Estimating health-related quality of life in obese individuals. *Dis Manage Health Outcomes* 1983; 3: 61–70.

7. Brown WJ, Dobson AJ, Mishra G. What is a healthy weight for middle aged women? *Int J Obes* 1998; 22: 520–28.

8. LePen C, Levy E, Loos F, Banzet M, Basdevant A. 'Specific' scale compared with 'generic' scale: a double measurement of the quality of life in a French community sample of obese subjects. *J Epidemiol Commun Hlth* 1998; 52: 445–50.

9. Fine JT, Colditz GA, Coakley EH, Moseley G, Manson JE, Willett WC, Kawachi I. A prospective study of weight change and health-related quality of life in women. *JAMA* 1999; 282: 2136–42.

10. Richards MM, Adams TD, Hunt SC. Functional status and emotional well-being, dietary intake, and physical activity of severely obese subjects. *J Am Diet Assoc* 2000; 100: 67–75.

11. Doll HA, Petersen SEK, Stewart-Brown SL. Obesity and physical and emotional well-being: Associations between body mass index, chronic illness, and the physical and mental components of the SF-36 questionnaire. *Obes Res* 2000; 8: 160–70.

12. Ford ES, Moriarty DG, Zack MM, Mokdad AH, Chapman DP. Self-reported body mass index and health-related quality of life: findings from the Behavioral Risk Factor Surveillance System. *Obes Res* 2001; 9: 21–31.

13. Fontaine KR, Cheskin LJ, Barofsky I. Health-related quality of life in obese persons seeking treatment. *J Fam Pract* 1996; 43: 265–70.

14. Kolotkin RL, Crosby RD. Psychometric evaluation of the Impact Of Weight On Quality Of Life-Lite Questionnaire (IWQOL-Lite) in a community sample. *Qual Life Res* 2002; 11: 157–71.

15. Kolotkin RL, Crosby RD, Kosloski KD, Williams GR. Development of a brief measure to assess quality of life in obesity. *Obes Res* 2001; 9: 102–11.

16. Kolotkin RL, Adams TD, Strong M, Pendleton R, Crosby RD. Health-related quality of life (HRQOL) in patients seeking gastric bypass surgery versus non-treatment-seeking controls. *Obes Surg* 2002; 12: 192.

17. Barofsky I, Fontaine KR, Cheskin LJ. Pain in the obese: impact on health-related quality-of-life. *Ann Behav Med* 1998; 408–10.

18. Dixon JB, Dixon ME, O'Brien PE. Quality of life after lap-band placement: influence of time, weight loss, and comorbidities. *Obes Res* 2001; 9: 713–21.

19. Marchesini G, Solaroli E, Baraldi L *et al.* Health-related quality of life in obesity: the role of eating behaviour. *Diabetes Nutr Metab* 2000; 13: 156–64.

20. De Zwaan M, Mitchell J, Howell L, Monson N, Swan-Kremeier L *et al.* Two measures of health related quality of life in morbid obesity: the role of binge eating, eating-specific and general psychopathology. *Obes Res* (in press).

21. Fontaine KR, Bartlett SJ, Barofsky I. Health-related quality of life among obese persons seeking and not currently seeking treatment. *Inter J Eat Dis* 2000; 27: 101–5.

22. Kolotkin RL, Crosby RD, Williams GR. Health-related quality of life varies among obese subgroups. *Obes Res* 2002; 10: 748–56.

23. Carpenter KM, Hasin DS, Allison DB, Faith MS. Relationships between obesity and DSM-IV major depressive disorder, suicide ideation, and suicide attempts: results from a general population study. *Am J Pub Health* 2000; 90: 251–7.

24. Katz D, McHorney C, Atkinson R. Impact of obesity on health-related quality of life in patients with chronic illness. *J Gen Int Med* 2000; 15: 789–96.

25. Mannucci E, Ricca V, Barciulli E, Di Bernardo M, Travaglini R, Cabras P, Rotella C. Quality of life and overweight: the obesity related well-being (Orwell97) questionnaire. *Add Behav* 1999; 24: 345–57.

26. Clarkson JR, Funkhouser ABS, Thornton JC, Yoshioka MRM, Mulvihill M, Pi-Sunyer X, Laferrere B. Quality of life in obese women. Effect of race, menopausal status and weight loss. *Obes Res* 2000; 8(1): S71.

27. Choban PS, Onyejekwe J, Burge JC, Flancbaum L. A health status assessment of the impact of weight loss following Roux-en-Y gastric bypass for clinically severe obesity. *J Am Coll Surg* 1999; 188: 491–7.

28. Karlsson J, Sjostrom L, Sullivan M. Swedish obese subjects (SOS) – an intervention study of obesity. Two-year follow-up of health-related quality of life (HRQOL) and eating behavior after gastric surgery for severe obesity. *Int J Obes* 1998; 22: 113–26.

29. Naslund I. Effects and Side-effects of obesity surgery in patients with BMI below or above 40 in the SOS (Swedish Obese Subjects) study. In: Guy-Grand B, Ailhaud G (eds) *Progress in Obesity Research: 8*, pp. 815–21. London: John Libbey; 1999.

30. Temple P, Travis B, Sachs L, Strasser S, Choban P, Flancbaum L. Functioning and well-being of patients before and after elective surgical procedures. *J Am Coll Surg* 1995; 181: 17–25.

31. Van Gemert WG, Adnang EM, Greve JW, Soeters PB. Quality of life assessment of morbidly obese patients: effect of weight-reducing surgery. *Am J Clin Nutr* 1998; 67(2): 197–201.

32. Rippe JM, Price JM, Hess SA, Kline G, DeMers KA, Damitz S *et al*. Improved psychological well being, quality of life, and health practices in moderately overweight women participating in a 12-week structured weight loss program. *Obes Res* 1998; 6: 208–18.

33. Kolotkin RL, Crosby RD, Williams GR, Hartley GG, Nicol S. The relationship between health-related quality of life and weight loss. *Obes Res* 2001; 9: 564–71.

34. Samsa GP, Kolotkin RL, Williams GR, Nguyen MR, Mendel C. Effect of moderate weight loss on health-related quality of life: an analysis of combined data from 4 randomized trials of sibutramine vs. placebo. *Am J Managed Care* 2001; 7: 875–83.

Progress in Obesity Research: 9. Edited by *Geraldo Medeiros-Neto, Alfredo Halpern and Claude Bouchard*
©2003 John Libbey Eurotext Ltd, pp. 613–617.

CHAPTER 128

Leptin and reproduction

Massimiliano Caprio, Elisa Fabbrini, Andrea M. Isidori, Antonio Aversa and Andrea Fabbri

Cattedra di Endocrinologia, Dipartimento di Medicina Interna, Universita' di Tor Vergata (MC, AA and AF) and Cattedra di Andrologia, Dipartimento di Fisiopatologia Medica, Università La Sapienza (MC, EF and AMI), 00100 Rome, Italy
[e-mail: massi71@hotmail.com]

Introduction

Leptin, from the Greek '????__' (thin), is a 16-kDa protein mainly produced by the adipose tissue[1], as well as by placenta, stomach and skeletal muscle[2]. The *ob* gene, consisting of three exons, encodes for leptin, whose tertiary structure resembles that of cytokines and lactogenic hormones. Leptin is cleaved from a 167 aminoacid precursor, circulates in the blood as a 146 aa mature protein[3], at concentrations paralleling the amount of fat reserves, and acts at the hypothalamic level as a satiety factor[1].

The identification and cloning of leptin receptor (Ob-R) in mice and humans have given new insights to the understanding of the complexity of actions and targets of leptin[4]. Ob-R belongs to the gp 130 family of cytokines receptors, it has a single membrane-spanning domain and exists in different isoforms (Ob-Ra, Ob-Rb, Ob-Rc, Ob-Rd, Ob-Re) which derive from alternative splicing of immature mRNA. All isoforms have an identical ligand binding domain but differ at the C-terminus. Only Ob-Rb contains a long intracellular domain and carries both protein motifs necessary for activation of the JAK-STAT pathway. Ob-Rb is mainly expressed in the hypothalamus; its expression is much lower in peripheral tissues, where the prevalent isoform is Ob-Ra. Ob-Ra has a short intracellular domain (< 30 aa) which contains only one out of two JAK binding domains and does not activate the JAK-STAT pathway[5]. Recent observations suggest that Ob-Ra performs signal transduction through MAP kinase[6].

The existence of an animal model with a homozygous mutation of the *ob* gene is a valuable tool for studying the biochemical messages between fat stores and the reproductive axis. The *ob/ob* mouse is infertile and has severe impairment of spermatogenesis, probably due to to an insufficient hypothalamic-pituitary drive and consequent low circulating gonadal steroids[1]. In *ob/ob* mice administration of leptin leads to weight gain of uterus and ovaries and seminal vesicles and testes in the female and male, respectively, and restores fertility in both genders[7,8]. Conversely, in the *ob/ob* mouse caloric restriction does not restore fertility, suggesting that obesity per se is not the cause of infertility in leptin deficiency, and that leptin is directly related to the modifications of reproductive capacity[7].

A mutation in the *db* gene, the gene encoding Ob-R, results in the synthesis of a truncated leptin receptor that is devoid of the intracellular domain[4]. The *db/db* mouse shows alterations of the reproductive function similar to those of the *ob/ob* mouse, but leptin treatment is unable either to modify the appetite of the animals or to restore fertility, since the defect is at the receptor level. *Ob* and *db* mutations have also been shown in humans, with similar phenotypic characteristics to those shown in mice[9–11].

Leptin and gonadal steroidogenesis

Leptin and ovary

Recent identification of Ob-R in several peripheral tissues, such as ovary, testis and adrenal gland[12–15], suggested that leptin may have a direct effect on downstream endocrine targets of the reproductive axis.

Several studies have been focused on the ovary, where the Ob-R expression is abundant. *In vitro* studies conducted on thecal and granulosa cells showed that leptin has a negative effect on ovarian steroid output, both in rodent and bovine models. In particular, it has been found that leptin inhibits insulin-induced progesterone and 17?-estradiol production by isolated bovine granulosa cells[14]; consistently with these findings, it has been shown that incubation of granulosa cells from fertile women with leptin, at concentrations between 10 and 100 ng/ml, significantly inhibits FSH- and IGF-I-stimulated estradiol production[15,16]. These observations indicate that leptin, at concentrations commonly found in obese women, has the potential to interfere with estradiol production by the dominant follicle *in vivo*, either directly, or through a reduction of the androgenic substrate derived by thecal cells. Also, excess of leptin may alter the ovarian response to local trophic stimuli, such as IGF-I, produced by the dominant follicle. If elevated leptin interferes with the development of the dominant follicle and reduces estradiol production, this phenomenon would lead to a lack of an adequate trigger for LH secretion and in turn anovulation. In agreement with this, recent studies showed that either *in vivo* administration of leptin in immature gonadotropin-primed rats or *in vitro* exposure of rat intact ovaries to leptin lead to a marked decline (3–4 times) in ovulation rate[17]. Taken together, these observations might in part explain the high incidence of reproductive dysfunction and the improvement of anovulation after weight loss in obese women[17].

Leptin and testis

The first identification of Ob-R in the testis is by Hoggard *et al.*[18] who detected mRNA for the common extracellular domain in murine spermatic cells and Leydig cells by *in situ* hybridization. Passage of leptin across the blood-testis barrier has also been investigated, showing that leptin enters the testis by a passive, non saturable process[19].

In recent studies we studied the expression of leptin receptor (Ob-R) in rat testes from gestational to adult age, in comparison with the pattern of expression of relaxin-like factor (RLF), a specific marker of Leydig cells differentiation status. Immunohistochemical analysis showed that in prenatal life Ob-R immunoreactivity was absent at early embryonic age (E14.5) and appeared at a late embryonic age (E19.5); in post-natal life, immunoreactivity was evident only after sexual maturation (35-, 60- and 90-days old), whereas it was absent in testes from sexually immature rats (7-, 14- and 21-days old). Immunoreaction was always confined to Leydig cells and no signal of Ob-R was detected within the tubules. The pattern of expression of Ob-R during testicular development was similar with that of RLF immunoreactivity, which was present in mature fetal as well as adult-type Leydig cells (Fig. 1). The pattern of expression of Ob-R in the testis was different from that observed in rat hypothalamus, where a marked Ob-R immunoreaction was evident both before and after sexual maturation. Ob-R was mainly localized in the arcuate nucleus and choroid plexus, with no significant difference in the intensity of Ob-R immunostaining before and after sexual maturation. These observations are in line with previous studies showing that Ob-R immunopositivity is present in paraventricular nucleus at late embryonic age, in the newborn and during the suckling period, even if at a weak level compared with the adult age[20]. Therefore it appears that different mechanisms control Ob-R expression in the testis and in the hypothalamus during development, probably through a tissue-specific different promoter[21] and/or a different local hormonal milieu. Semiquantitative RT-PCR results obtained on testes from rats of different ages were in line with the immunohistochemical data: Ob-R mRNA expression was significantly higher at late gestational (E19.5) vs. early gestational (E14.5) age. After birth (7- and 14-days old) Ob-R mRNA levels were similar with those found on day E14.5, showed a slight increase on day 21 and were much higher in mature testes, with a gradual increase from younger to older ages. Also, the developmental pattern of mRNA concentrations of the short (Ob-Ra) and long (Ob-Rb) isoforms of Ob-R was very similar to that of overall testicular Ob-R splice variants. These observations suggest that Ob-R expression is transcriptionally regulated, even if a post-transcriptional level of regulation cannot be excluded.

By using primary cultures of Leydig cells isolated from adult rats and a Leydig tumour cell line (MLTC-1), we demonstrated the expression of Ob-Rb (the long signaling isoform) in both these models by RT-PCR analysis. Upon binding with its receptor leptin was able to exert a rapid and dose-dependent inhibition of LH-stimulated testosterone production in mature adult Leydig cells in culture, enhancing the hCG-stimulated intracellular cAMP production[22]. Testosterone suppression was accompanied by a parallel reduction of androstenedione levels and a concomitant rise of the precursor metabolites 17-OH progesterone, progesterone and pregnenolone, compatibly with a leptin-induced lesion of 17-20 lyase activity, the enzyme that converts the 17??hydroxilated intermediates to androstenedione. Interestingly, and in analogy to what observed in primary rat Leydig cells, in MLTC-1 cells, a Leydig tumour cell line

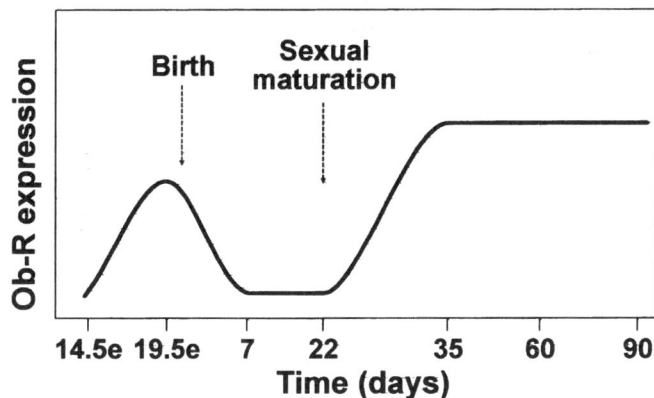

Fig. 1. Schematic representation of the developmental pattern of expression of leptin receptor (Ob-R) in rat Leydig cells. Before birth, Ob-R protein is not expressed at early embryonic age and becomes detectable at a later gestational age; after birth, it is again absent throughout the prepubertal period, and is switched on after sexual maturation. In addition, immature Leydig cells appear to be preserved by the deleterious effects of leptin on steroidogenesis observed in adult cells. It is conceivable that in rat Leydig cells leptin receptor is functional only after sexual maturation and, possibly, in the later phases of testicular embryogenesis.

not expressing the gene encoding for 17??hydroxilase/17-20 lyase and able to secrete only the precursor metabolites upstream 17?-hydroxilation (i.e. pregnenolone and progesterone), acute leptin tratment amplified hCG-induced intracellular cAMP without modifying steroid output[22]. These data further confirm that also MLTC cells express a functional leptin receptor, and that leptin actions occur downstream of progesterone synthesis. However, in Northern Blot studies leptin did not alter the accumulation of P450-17??mRNA from primary cultured rat Leydig cells, excluding that the rapid changes observed in hCG-induced steroidogenesis were mediated by a transcriptional regulation of P450-17??gene. A rapid post-translational regulation of 17-20 lyase enzimatic activity by leptin seems more likely. These observations indicate that leptin has the potential to modulate the paracrine network that controls gonadotropin-stimulated testicular steroidogenesis, similarly to what already observed in the ovary.

In line with the peculiar developmental pattern of expression of Ob-R in Leydig cells (Fig. 1), the inhibitory actions of leptin on hCG-induced testosterone production have been shown by our group also on late embryonic rat testicular cells in culture, where both immunohistochemical and RT-PCR studies showed the presence of Ob-R protein and trancript. On the other hand, leptin did not modify either hCG-stimulated testosterone or intracellular cAMP production by Leydig cells extracted by immature juvenile rats, where Ob-R immunostaining was negative and the relative abundance of Ob-R mRNA was low. Similar results were reported by other authors using slices of prepubertal testicular tissue incubated in the presence of hCG and leptin[23]. Taken together, these results indicate that leptin actions on Leydig cells are specific of late embryonic development and adult life and that in rat Leydig cells the Ob → Ob-R system is not functional before sexual maturation. We hypothesize that this system may protect Leydig cells from the possible deleterious effect of hyperleptinaemia on steroidogenesis in prepubertal age, ensuring a correct testis maturation and puberty.

Interestingly, the inhibitory effect of leptin on hCG-stimulated testosterone production appeared at concentrations within the range of circulating levels in obese men.

Several reports have addressed the association between leptin and circulating steroids in human males. Obese subjects, as a group, show elevated levels of leptin in blood and reduced androgen concentrations; also, it has been known for some time that the degree of androgen reduction is related to the amount of fat mass[24] and, recently, to leptin levels[25]. In addition, we found that the androgen response to hCG stimulation is impaired in obese men and multivariate analysis showed that leptin was the best hormonal predictor of the obesity-related reduction in androgen response to hCG stimulation[26]. In fact, in the moderate and massive obese men, the decreased testosterone (T) response to hCG was associated to a high net increase in 17?-progesterone (17-OH-P) levels. This led to elevated 17-OH-P/T molar ratios and increased percentage changes from baseline of 17-OH-P/T, which were 2 to 5 times higher than in controls (P < 0.05). The increases in 17-OH-P/T ratios, calculated at peak T values, were related to the amount of body fat and leptin (r = 0.45 at 48 h, P < 0.01)[26]. In line with the data obtained by *in vitro* studies on isolated rat Leydig cells, these findings indicate the presence of an enzymatic defect in the conversion of 17-OH-P to T, revealed by LH stimulation and related to the amount of fat mass and to circulating leptin levels. Taken together these observations indicate that leptin excess may have an important role in the development of reduced androgens output in male obesity.

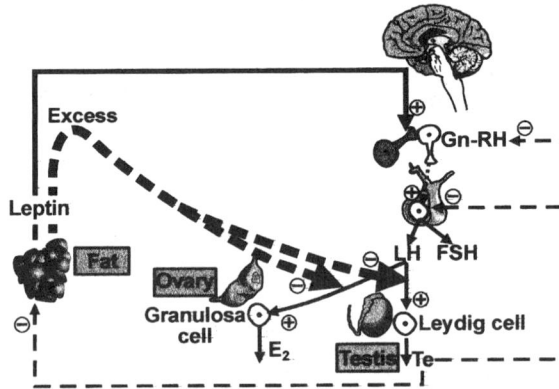

Fig. 2. Leptin and adipose tissue are systemic modulators of the HPG axis. Leptin acts at multiple levels of the reproductive axis, showing different effects on reproduction depending on its concentrations in the blood. The saturable system of leptin transport through the blood-brain barrier prevents that high levels of leptin reach hypothalamic receptors, where leptin exerts stimulatory actions on GnRH and in turn gonadotropin secretion. On the other hand excess of leptin has the potential to act on peripheral leptin receptors and to exert inhibitory actions on testicular and ovarian steroidogenesis. Testosterone in the long term acts on the adipose tissue inhibiting leptin synthesis and secretion, and closing the complex regulatory loop between leptin and the HPG axis. Solid lines = stimulatory actions; dashed lines = inhibitory actions.

Conclusions

The discovery of leptin, its receptors and mechanisms of action opens new and unexpected insights into the pathophysiology of reproduction. It is well established that leptin acts at various levels of the HPG axis, involving different tissues and multiple biochemical pathways. Its role on the reproductive function seems to be determined by different thresholds, depending on the site where leptin acts (Fig. 2) and on the tissue-specific expression of functional receptors. In fact, the different tissue-specific regulation of leptin receptor expression throughout development (Fig. 1) represents a further level of fine modulation of leptin actions at various anatomical levels, from embryonic life to adulthood, during the entire life-span.

It is possible that leptin has a dual effect on reproduction and that the major site of action may differ, depending on its circulating levels in the blood. The positive action of leptin at the hypothalamic-pituitary level may be critical as a trigger of puberty and play a predominant role during conditions with abnormally low plasma concentrations, such as in subjects with very low BMI (anorexic patients), or in patients with homozygous mutations of the *ob* gene. Conversely in obesity, leptin central receptors, able to signal extremely low ligand concentrations, are protected from hyperleptinaemia by the saturable transport system of the blood-brain barrier, while peripheral leptin receptors are directly exposed to high ligand concentrations, with consequent possible negative effects on gonadal steroidogenesis in both genders (Fig. 2). It can be hypothesized that a specific and narrow range of leptin concentrations is necessary to maintain a normal reproductive function, and that concentrations below or above these thresholds may interfere in opposing ways with the function of the HPG axis[27].

References

1. Zhang Y, Proenca R, Maffei M, Barone M, Leopold L, Friedman JM. Positional cloning of the mouse obese gene and its human homologue. *Nature* 1994; 372: 425–32.

2. Wang J, Liu R, Hawkins M, Barzilai N, Rossetti L. A nutrient-sensing pathway regulates leptin gene expression in muscle and fat. *Nature* 1998; 393: 684–8.

3. Sinha MK, Opentanova I, Ohannesian JP, Kolaczynski JW, Heiman ML *et al.* Evidence for free and bound leptin in human circulation. Studies in lean and obese subjects and during short-term fasting. *J Clin Invest* 1996; 98: 1277–82.

4. Tartaglia LA, Dembski M, Weng X, Deng N, Culpepper J, Devos R *et al.* Identification and expression cloning of a leptin receptor OB-R. *Cell* 1995; 83: 1263–71.

5. Tartaglia LA. The leptin receptor. *J Biol Chem* 1997; 272: 6093–96.

6. Bjorbaek C, Uotani S, da Silva B, Flier JS. Divergent signalling capacities of the long and short isoforms of the leptin receptor. *J Biol Chem* 1997; 272: 32686–95.

7. Chehab FF, Lim ME, Lu R. Correction of the sterility defect in homozygous obese female mice by treatment with human recombinant leptin. *Nature Genet* 1996; 12: 318–20.

8. Mounzih K, Lu R, Chehab FF. Leptin treatment rescues the sterility of genetically obese ob/ob males. *Endocrinology* 1997; 138: 1190–3.

9. Lingenfelter PA, Adler DA, Poslinski D, Thomas S, Elliott RW, Chapman VM *et al.* A leptin missense mutation associated with hypogonadism and morbid obesity. *Nature Genet* 1998; 18: 213–15.

10. Farooqi IS, Jebb SA, Langmack G, Lawrence E, Cheetham CH, Prentice AM *et al.* Effects of recombinant leptin therapy in a child with congenital leptin deficiency. *N Engl J Med* 1999; 341: 879–84.

11. Clement K, Vaisse C, Lahlou N, Cabrol S, Pelloux V, Cassuto D *et al.* A mutation in the human leptin receptor gene causes obesity and pituitary dysfunction. *Nature* 1998; 392: 398–401.

12. Zamorano PL, Mahesh VB, De Sevilla LM, Chorich LP, Bhat GK, Brann DW. Expression and localization of the leptin receptor in endocrine and neuroendocrine tissues of the rat. *Neuroendocrinology* 1997; 65: 223–8.

13. Glasow A, Haidan A, Hilbers U, Breidert M, Gillespie J, Scherbaum WA *et al.* Expression of Ob receptors in normal human adrenals: differential regulation of adrenocortical and adrenomedullary function by leptin. *J Clin Endocrinol Metab* 1998; 83: 4459–67.

14. Spicer JL, Francisco CC. The adipose obese gene product, leptin: evidence of a direct inhibitory role in ovarian function. *Endocrinology* 1997; 138: 3374–9.

15. Karlsson C, Lindell K, Svensson E, Bergh C, Lind P, Billig H *et al.* Expression of functional leptin receptors in the human ovary. *J Clin Endocrinol Metab* 1997; 82: 4144–8.

16. Agarwal SK, Vogel K, Weitsman SR, Magoffin DA. Leptin antagonizes the insulin-like growth factor-I augmentation of steroidogenesis in granulose and theca cells of the human ovary. *J Clin Endocrinol Metab* 1999; 84: 1071–6.

17. Duggal PS, Van Der Hoek KH, Milner CR, Ryan NK, Armstrong DT, Magoffin DA, Norman RJ. The *in vivo* and *in vitro* effects of exogenous leptin on ovulation in the rat. *Endocrinology* 2000; 141: 1971–6.

18. Hoggard N, Mercer JG, Rayner DV, Moar K, Trayhurn P, Williams LM. Localization of leptin receptor mRNA splice variants in murine peripheral tissues by RT-PCR and *in situ* hybridization. *Biochem Biophys Res Com* 1997; 232: 383–7.

19. Banks WA, McLay RN, Kastin AJ, Sarmiento U, Scully S. Passage of leptin across the blood-testis barrier. *Am J Physiol* 1999; 276: E1099–E1104.

20. Matsuda J, Yokota I, Tsuruo Y, Murakami T, Ishimura K, Shima K, Kuroda Y. Developmental changes in long-form leptin receptor expression and localization in rat brain. *Endocrinology* 1999; 140: 5233–38.

21. Mercer JG, Moar KM, Hoggard N, Strosberg AD, Froguel P, Bailleul B. B219/OB-R 5'-UTR and leptin receptor gene-related protein gene expression in mouse brain and placenta: tissue-specific leptin receptor promoter activity. *J Neuroendocrinol* 2000; 12: 649–55.

22. Caprio M, Isidori AM, Carta AR, Moretti C, Dufau ML, Fabbri A. Expression of functional leptin receptors in rodent Leydig cells. *Endocrinology* 1999; 140: 4939–47.

23. Tena-Sempere M, Pinella L, Gonzalez LC, Dieguez C, Casanueva FF, Aguilar E. Leptin inhibits testosterone secretion from adult rat testis *in vitro*. *J Endocrinol* 1999; 161: 211–8.

24. Zumoff B, Strain GW, Miller LK, Rosner W, Senie R, Seres DS, Rosenfeld RS. Plasma free and non-SHBG-bound testosterone are decreased in obese men in proportion of their degree of obesity. *J Clin Endocrinol Metab* 1990; 71: 929–31.

25. Vettor R, De Pergola G, Pagano C, Englaro P, Laudario E, Giorgino F *et al.* Gender differences in serum leptin in obese people: relationship with testosterone, body fat distribution and insulin sensitivity. *Eur J Clin Invest* 1997; 27: 1016–24.

26. Isidori AM, Caprio M, Strollo F, Moretti C, Frajese G, Isidori A, Fabbri A. Leptin and androgens in male obesity: evidence for leptin contribution to reduced androgens levels. *J Clin Endocrinol Metab* 1999; 84: 3673–80.

27. Caprio M, Fabbrini E, Isidori AM, Aversa A, Fabbri A. Leptin in reproduction. *Trends Endocrinol Metab* 2001; 12: 65–72.

28. Shepard DS Cost-effectiveness in Health and Medicine. Gold MR, Siegel JE, Russell LB, Weinstein MC, editors. New York: Oxford University Press. 1996. *J Ment Health Policy Econ* 1999; 2(2): 91–92.

29. Cartwright WS Methods for the economic evaluation of health care programmes, second edition. Drummond MF, O'Brien B, Stoddart GL, Torrance GW. Oxford: Oxford University Press, 1997. *J Ment Health Policy Econ* 1999; 2 (1): 43.

30. Mathers CD, Vos ET, Stevenson CE, Begg SJ. The burden of disease and injury in Australia. *Bull World Health Organ* 2001; 79(11): 1076–84.

Progress in Obesity Research: 9. Edited by *Geraldo Medeiros-Neto, Alfredo Halpern and Claude Bouchard*
©2003 John Libbey Eurotext Ltd, pp. 618–622.

CHAPTER 129

Unraveling the effects of lean body mass and fat mass on mortality

Angelo Pietrobelli[1,2] and Myles S. Faith[2]

[1]*Paediatric Unit, Verona University Medical School, Verona, (Italy);* [2]*Weight and Eating Disorders Program,
Unniversity of Pennsylvania School of Medicine, Philadelphia, PA, USA*
[e-mail: angpie@tin.it]

Introduction

The relationship between body composition components and mortality does not seem to be simple. On the one hand obesity is also associated with increased all-cause mortality rate and even small weight losses can be associated with short-term reduction in risk factors for disease[1,2]. There is strong evidence that weight loss in obese subjects improves risk factors for diabetes and cardiac vascular diseases. On the other hand, the majority of studies show that weight loss is associated with an increased mortality rate (Fig. 1)[3]. Such inconsistent findings in the literature may be attributable in part to body composition methods that could not disentangle fat- from lean body mass. Several studies suggest that better clarity may be achieved by modeling the independent effects of change in fat mass per se from change in total body mass[4]. The degree of health benefit may be dependent on the degree to which fat mass is lost and lean body mass is preserved[4-6].

The central aim of our paper is to discuss methods for body composition assessment that may provide new insights into the dynamic relationship between weight change and mortality rate.

Body composition assessment

As described in a classical paper published in the American Journal of Clinical Nutrition by Heymsfield's group in 1992 the composition of the human body can be divided in terms of an atomic model (i.e. oxygen, carbon, hydrogen, etc), a molecular model (i.e. water, lipid, protein, mineral and glycogen), a cellular model (i.e. cells, extracellular fluid, extracellular solid), or a tissue model (i.e. skeletal muscle, adipose tissue, visceral organs and residuals)[7]. Fat mass (FM) and fat free mass (FFM) are terms used frequently that refer to the classic two-component body composition model in which body is divided into fat and non fat tissue mass[7]. Measurement of body mass is extremely challenging, because we do not have direct measurements except for *in vivo* neutron activation analysis and chemical analysis of cadaver. There are various indirect methods for measuring fat and fat free mass, all of which have assumptions, and age-specific considerations. We note that age and growth influence the hydration and density of fat-free mass (Fig.2).

Hydrodensitometry

The hydrodensitometry system consists of a large tank of water (temperature of about 36 degrees Celsius) and a scale. The subject exhales maximally, submerges, and body weight is recorded to the scale. This is an estimate of weight underwater; the subject body weight is then measured outside the tank. Many researchers also measure residual lung volume during or following the underwater weighing procedures. The results are used to calculate body volume and body density (Db). Body density is then used to calculate the proportion of body weight as FM and FFM. The assumptions of this calculation are that the density of fat is constant (0.90 g/ml) and FFM is a homogeneous compartment with constant density 1.10 g/ml. In the classic two-component (2C) model of body composition, body weight is divided into FM and FFM[8]. The density of fat free mass is known to be influence by several

Weight loss ⟶ Short term reduction in
risk factors for disease

Obesity ⟶ Numerous morbidities

⟶ Increased all-cause
mortality

However

Weight loss ⟶ Increased mortality rate

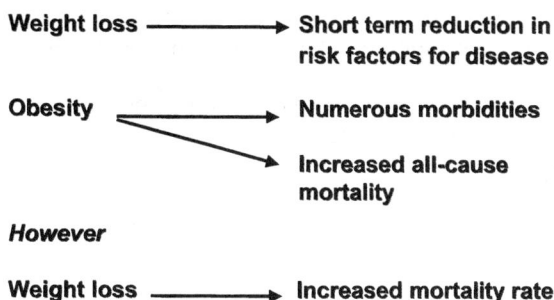

Fig. 1. The apparent paradox.

factors such as age, gender, ethnicity; there is limited information in children. Current limitation for applying densitometry to the general population includes practical problems (i.e. testing adherence is extremely difficult) and theoretic considerations. Recent developments used air rather than water displacement for measurements of volume and may be more practical for big samples. Recently we showed for the first time in a paediatric sample (48 children) a high correlation (r = 0.85) between body density by air displacement and hydrodensitometry. Among an adult sample (72 subjects) we found a high correlation (r^2 = 0.95) between body density by air displacement and hydrodensitometry[9].

Anthropometry

Estimation of fat mass from anthropometry involves development of prediction models in which anthropometric measures, in particular skinfolds, are related to body FM. Slaughter and colleagues developed body composition prediction equations from data on 310 paediatric subjects based on use of a multicompartimental model[10]. In the literature subscapular skinfold, triceps skinfold were use to estimate fat mass. Also triceps skinfold alone was use to estimate fat mass with prediction equation. Waist circumferences, a well-known measurements of body composition, is well correlated with cardiovascular risk disease in adults. We also found in children whose mean age was 8 years old that waist circumferences is a good predictor (r = 0.74) of overweight and/or obesity 4 years later when the subjects approached the puberty[11].

Bioimpedance

Bioimpedance (BIA) is a technique to use for assessing body composition in clinical and population-based studies. The technique is based on measurement of electrical resistance in the body to a tiny imperceptible current. This approach provides an estimate of total body water, which then be transformed into FFM. Essential considerations for obtaining valid data include the use of appropriate

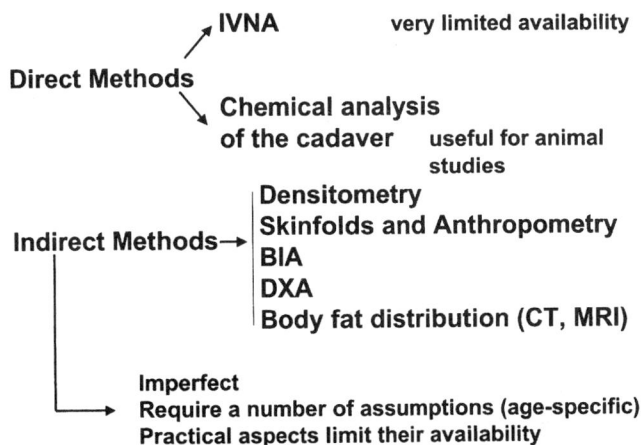

↗ **IVNA**   very limited availability

Direct Methods

↘ **Chemical analysis
of the cadaver**   useful for animal
studies

**Densitometry
Skinfolds and Anthropometry**
Indirect Methods→ **BIA**
DXA
Body fat distribution (CT, MRI)

Imperfect
⟶ **Require a number of assumptions (age-specific)**
Practical aspects limit their availability

Fig. 2. Methods used for body composition study.

equations (age and sex specific), standard measurement conditions and attention to subject-specific factors (i.e. position, time of the day, and room temperature among others)[12].

Dual energy X-ray absorptiometry

Recent advances in techniques to measure body composition have provided dual energy X-ray absorptiometry (DXA) for assessment of whole body as well as regional measurements of bone mass, lean mass and body fat. DXA quantifies the relative attenuation of the two main photon peaks as they pass through the body. They resolve body weight into bone mineral and lean and fat tissue masses[13].

Imaging

In adults, intraabdominal adipose tissue is related to cardiovascular risks. Recently *in vivo* imaging technique such as computed tomography (CT) and magnetic resonance imaging (MRI) have allowed more accurate measures of body fat distribution in adults. Goran and colleagues have conducted several studies in children using CT and MRI[14]. These two methods have a high degree of accuracy and reproducibility. However, they have disadvantages as cost, radiation exposure and limited to research setting[14].

Body mass index (BMI)and mortality

This review underscores the point that, in theory, there are several appealing possibilities, for human body composition measurements. However, in practice, especially in epidemiological studies, the filed has relied upon relatively very crude measurements of fat and fat mass. In the majority of the cases, BMI has been used. However, the relation between body weight/BMI and mortality remain controversial.

For the first time in 1999 Allison and colleagues did a study in order to tease apart the independent effects of weight loss and fat loss on all-cause mortality in two independent samples[4]. Specifically weight loss was hypothesized to be associated with an increasing all-cause mortality rate, whereas fat loss was hypothesized to be associated with a decreasing all-cause mortality rate. To test the hypothesis, we used data from two prospective longitudinal population-based cohort studies: The Tecumseh Community Health study and the Framingham Heart study. The Tecumseh study included over 1800 participants who were followed over 16 years. The Framingham Heart Study included over 2700 participants who were followed over 8 years. Fatness was measured by skinfold thickness (subscapular and triceps) in Tecumseh Study, and subscapular skinfold thickness in the Framingham Heart Study. Weight loss was calculated as weight at time 1 minus weight at time 2. Fat loss was calculated as the skinfolds taken at time 1 minus skinfolds at time 2. The results showed that weight loss was associated with *increased* mortality rate and fat loss with *decreased* mortality rate in the two independent samples. One standard deviation of weight loss (4.6 kg in Tecumseh and 6.7 kg in Framingham) increased the hazard rate 29 per cent and 39 per cent in the two samples respectively. Our hypotheses were supported in both data sets after adjusting for age, sex and smoking status across several sensitivity analyses. There is a clear trend toward increasing mortality rate with higher categories of weight loss and decreasing mortality rate with higher categories of fat loss[4].

A review of several studies presented in the literature illustrates the controversial relationship between weight and mortality. Williamson and colleagues performed a prospective analysis with a 12 years mortality follow up of 4,970 individuals with diabetes. Intentional weight loss was reported by 34 per cent of the cohort. After adjustment for initial BMI, sociodemographic factors, physical activity, intentional weight loss was associated with a 25 per cent reduction in mortality rate and a 28 per cent reduction in CDC and diabetes mortality[15]. They noted that intentional weight loss of 20–29 pounds was associated with the largest reduction in mortality (approximately 33 per cent)[15].

Farrell and colleagues followed 113,145 women and examined the relation of body mass index, cardio respiratory fitness, and all-cause mortality. They concluded that low cardio respiratory fitness is a strong predictor than BMI of all-cause mortality. They also suggested that clinicians should encourage overweight and obese to lose weight[16].

Very recently Allison and colleagues tested in 10,169 men the differential associations of BMI and adiposity with all cause mortality using the first and second National Health and Nutrition Examination Surveys. Subscapular and triceps skinfolds thickness were used as fat mass indicator whereas upper arm circumferences was used as a fat free mass indicator. They found that BMI had a U-shape relationship with mortality with nadir at 27 BMI. However, the relationship between FM and mortality was monotonic increasing and the relationship between FFM and mortality was monotonic decreasing[17]. The results support the hypothesis that the apparent deleterious effects of marked thinness may be due to the low fat and that marked leanness may have beneficial effects. Zhu and Allison using the same surveys tested the association of BMI and anthropometric indicators of fat mass and fat free mass with all cause mortality in women. The same body composition measurements were used, but different results were observed. Contrary to expectations, both FM and FFM had negative relationship with mortality. These different results may reflect sex differences in fat distribution. The authors speculated wheter fatness may have protective effects in women. However, they concluded that measurement issues might be responsible for the results. It is known that in women skinfold thickness is less reliable predictor of total fat than in men[18].

Lahmann and colleagues examined the association between different measure of adiposity and all cause mortality in a cohort of 10,902 men and 16,814 women. In both genders, linear and non-linear associations were observed with body fatness that could not detected with BMI. The authors also examined the association between body fat distribution and mortality. In both genders the rate of all-cause mortality were highest in subjects in the highest quintile of waist hip ratio[19].

Conclusion

Three conclusions emerge from this literature review:

(1)   An increased use of direct body fatness measurements and decreased reliance on BMI will promote better understanding of the U- or J-shaped obesity-mortality rate;

(2)   Weight change and fat change tend to be positively associated such that when individuals lose weight they also lose fat and vice versa;

(3)   Fat gain is associated with increased mortality rate.

It may be reasonable to interpret these results as indicating that FM loss is beneficial whereas lean body mass loss is deleterious and that the extent to which weight loss is beneficial or deleterious will depend of the composition of that weight loss.

These results underscore the importance of more precise body composition measurements for better understanding of mechanism of the effects of weight loss and fat loss in all-cause mortality. The data suggest also, that weight loss may be extend longevity if a sufficient proportion of the weight loss is lost as fat.

References

1.   Goldstein DJ. Beneficial effects of modest weight loss. *Int J Obes* 1992; 16: 397–415.

2.   Pi-Sunyer FX. A review of long term studies evaluating the efficacy of weight loss in ameliorating disorders associated with obesity. *Clin Ther* 1996; 18: 1006–35.

3.   Andres R, Muller DC, Sorkin JD. Long-term effects of change in body weight on all cause mortality: a review. *Ann Intern Med* 1993; 119: 737–43.

4.   Allison DB, Zannolli R, Faith MS, Heo M, Pietrobelli A, Van Itallie T B *et al*. Weight loss increases and fat loss decreases all-cause mortality rate: results from two independent cohort studies. *Int J Obes* 1999; 23: 603–11.

5.   Williamson D F, Pamuk E, Thun M, Flanders D, Byers T, Heath C. Prospective study of intentional weight loss and mortality in never-smoking overweight US white women aged 40–64 years. *Am J Epidemiol* 1995; 141: 1128–41.

6.   Williamson DF, Pamuk E, Thun M, Flanders D, Heath C, Byers T. Prospective study of intentional weight loss and mortality in overweight men aged 40–64 years. *Obes Res* 1997; 5 (Suppl 1): S94.

7.   Wang ZM, Pierson RN Jr, Heymsfield SB. The five level model: a new approach to organizing body composition research. *Am J Clin Nutr* 1992; 56: 19–28.

8.   Going SB. Densitometry. In: *Human body composition*, Roche AF, Heymsfield SB, Lohman TG (eds), pp. 3–24. Champagain: Human Kinetics, 1996.

9.   Nuñez C, Kovera AJ, Pietrobelli A, Heshka S, Horlick MH, Kehayias JJ *et al*. Body composition in children and adults by air displacement plethysmograph. *Eur J Clin Nutr* 1999; 53: 382–7.

10.   Slaughter MH, Lohman TG, Boileau RA, Horswill CA, Stillman RJ, van Loan MD, Bemben DA. Skinfold equations for estimation of body fatness in children and youth. *Hum Biol* 1988; 60: 709–23.

11.   Maffeis C, Grezzani A, Pietrobelli A, Provera S, Tatò L. Does waist circumference predict fat gain in children? *Obes Res* 2001; 25: 978–83.

12.   Heymsfield SB, Nuñez C, Pietrobelli A. Bioimpedance analysis: what are the next steps? *Nutr Clin Practice* 1997; 12: 201–3.

13. Pietrobelli A, Wang ZM, Formica C, Heymsfield SB. Dual energy X-ray absorptiometry: fat estimation error due to variation in soft tissue hydration. *Am J Physiol* 1998; 274: 808–16.

14. Goran MI. Measurement issue related to studies of childhood obesity. Assessment of body composition, body fat distribution, physical activity, and food intake. *Pediatrics* 1998; 1: 505–18.

15. Williamson DF, Thompson TJ, Thun M, Flanders D, Pamuk E, Byers T. Intentional weight loss and mortality among overweight individuals with diabetes. *Diabetes Care* 2000; 3: 1499–504.

16. Farrell SW, Braun L, Barlow CE, Cheng YJ, Blair SN. The relation of body mass index, cardiorespiratory fitness, and all-cause mortality in women. *Obes Res* 2002; 10: 417–23.

17. Allison DB, Zhu SK, Plankey M, Faith MS, Heo M. Differential association of body mass index and adiposity with all-cause mortality among men in the first and second National health and Nutrition Examination Surveys (NHANES I and NHANES II) follow up studies. *Int J Obes* 2002; 26: 410–6.

18. Zhu SK, Heo M, Plankey M, Faith MS, Allison DB. Association of body mass index and anthropometric indicators of fat mass and fat free mass with all cause mortality among women in the first and second National health and Nutrition Examination Surveys (NHANES I and NHANES II) follow up studies. *Ann Epidemiol* 2002; 286–93.

19. Lahman PH, Lissner L, Gullberg B, Berglund G. A prospective study of adiposity and all cause mortality: the Malmö diet and cancer study. *Obes Res* 2002; 10: 361–9.

Progress in Obesity Research: 9. Edited by *Geraldo Medeiros-Neto, Alfredo Halpern and Claude Bouchard*
©2003 John Libbey Eurotext Ltd, pp. 623–628.

CHAPTER 130

The impact of intentional weight loss on long-term health outcomes

Edward W. Gregg and David F. Williamson

Division of Diabetes Translation, National Center for Chronic Disease Prevention and Health Promotion, Centers for Disease Control and Prevention, Atlanta, GA 30341, USA
[e-mail: edg7@cdc.gov]

The prevalence of overweight and obesity continues to increase dramatically in the US and many other countries. During the last 20 years, the prevalence of overweight – BMI (kg/m^2) ≥ 25, includes obesity – increased from 47 per cent to 61 per cent and the prevalence of obesity *per se* (BMI ≥ 30) rose from 15 per cent to 27 per cent[1]. The greatest relative increases have been among the highest BMI categories (e.g. > 35) and the increases appear to have affected all age-ranges and several racial/ethnic groups in similar ways[2]. This epidemic is troubling because obesity is associated with many adverse health outcomes, including diabetes, gall bladder disease, coronary heart disease, osteoarthritis, and physical disability, and an increased risk of mortality, especially among younger adults[3].

Although obesity is clearly a growing problem with broad and profound health consequences, the effectiveness of weight loss as a public health response to this problem is unclear. On the one hand, short term weight loss has positive effects on several physiological parameters. For example, losing 5–12 per cent of one's weight using changes in lifestyle over 6–12 months may reduce systolic blood pressure by 3 to 10 mmHg, LDL cholesterol by 5 to 12 mg/dl, triglycerides by 10–20 mg/dl, and fasting glucose levels by 3 to 8 mg/dl; among persons with diabetes, weight loss reduces glycosylated hemoglobin levels by up to 2 percentage points[4–5].

On the other hand, there are several reasons to question whether losing weight in the short term will influence long-term disease outcomes. First, most people who try to lose weight end up regaining their weight. Even in the most effective circumstances, wherein weight loss is attempted in the form of consistent, multi-factorial, behavioural therapy over 6 months or more, one-third of peak weight loss is commonly regained over the subsequent year[6–7]. Second, even if weight loss is maintained over several years, it is unclear whether the initial rate of physiological benefit will continue for this longer period. In addition, we do not know whether the benefits obtained will be sufficient to reverse pre-existing pathology and thus influence long-term health outcomes. Third, numerous epidemiologic studies have found weight loss to be associated with increased, rather than decreased mortality risk, and have found an increased risk of such other outcomes as bone and muscle loss, osteoporotic fractures, and disability[8].

This literature is limited, however, by a lack of information on whether weight loss was intended. There is a potentially strong relationship between unintentional weight loss and underlying diseases such as cancer, depression, and end stage heart and lung disease, that may confound results even when researchers control for health status. Accordingly, we need to more specifically examine the long-term health effects of intentional weight loss.

In this review, we summarize the evidence from prospective cohort studies and controlled intervention trials that intentional weight loss is effective in reducing disease incidence and mortality.

Observational studies of intentional weight loss and mortality

In contrast to randomized controlled trials (RCTs), which examine interventions under ideal, recommended conditions, observational studies assess the impact of individual weight loss attempts under 'real world' conditions. Observational studies have typically assessed weight change and intent to lose weight using simple self-report questions at one time point, which is followed by a period of mortality ascertainment. Self-reported data indicate that most people who try to lose weight report cutting calories (73 per cent), exercising (50 per cent), or both cutting calories and exercise (37 per cent), but 31 per cent use one of several other methods, including skipping meals, attending special programmes, eating special products, taking diet pills, fasting, or purging, which may have varied success (Gregg, unpublished analyses from the 1991 US National Health Interview Survey). Thus, observational studies are designed to examine the impact of a broader set of behaviours than are RCTs.

Only a few observational cohort studies have examined the association between intentional weight loss and disease outcomes. A series of analyses that used data from the Cancer Prevention Study suggest that the association between intentional weight loss and mortality varies across different population subgroups and by cause of death[9-11]. Among a general population of overweight women aged 40–64 years, intentional weight loss was associated with 20 per cent reduced mortality among those with pre-existing conditions but not among healthy women[9]. The reduced mortality among women with health conditions was primarily due to a 30–40 per cent reduction in cancer mortality; there was only a weak (10 per cent), non-significant association with cardiovascular disease (CVD) mortality. In a separate analysis of persons with diabetes, intentional weight loss was associated with 25 per cent reduced all-cause mortality and a 28 per cent lower CVD mortality, with weight loss most protective (33 per cent reduction in all-cause mortality) among those reporting a 20–29 lb weight loss[10]. Among a general population of men, however, intentional weight loss was not associated with mortality regardless of pre-existing health status[11]. Unintentional weight loss in these analyses was either unrelated to mortality (men overall, women with pre-existing conditions) or associated with higher mortality (persons with diabetes, healthy women)[9-11].

Among women aged 55 to 69 with pre-existing health conditions enrolled in the Iowa Women's Health Study, there was an elevated mortality rate associated with intentional weight loss, but this finding was not statistically significant. Additionally, there was no association between intentional weight loss and mortality in the overall sample but unintentional weight loss was associated with increased mortality[12]. One other study (the Israeli Ischaemic Heart Disease Study) found higher mortality rates for persons who lost weight on a 'slimming diet' than for those who were not on a diet, but there was not adjustment for health status, smoking, behaviours, or obesity[13]. Thus, it is difficult to interpret their findings because of the lack of control for self-selection of sicker persons among the dieting group.

More recently, an analysis of 9-year mortality follow-up data of persons with diabetes from the 1989 National Health Interview Survey suggested that 'trying to lose weight' may be a more important predictor of mortality than actual weight loss[14]. Persons who were trying to lose weight had a 23 per cent lower mortality rate (HRR = 0.77, 95 per cent CI, 0.61–0.99) irrespective of weight change. Compared to persons reporting no weight loss and not trying to lose weight, persons who tried to lose weight but failed had a lower mortality rate (RR = 0.73, 0.55 to 0.96) while those who succeeded (i.e. intentional weight loss) had a non-significant reduction in mortality (RR = 0.82, 0.62–1.08). Persons with unintentional weight loss had a 58 per cent increased all-cause mortality rate.

Taken as a whole, observational studies have not consistently supported an association between intentional weight loss and mortality, and with the exception of the study conducted among persons with diabetes by Williamson et al.[10], there is no evidence for a dose-response association. These studies appear to refute the notion, however, that intentional weight loss is harmful[8]. At least three limitations should be considered when examining this literature. (1) the associations between weight loss and mortality reduction may be underestimated due to error in self-reported weight change; (2) the groups reporting intentional weight loss may be inflated by persons simultaneously undergoing unintentional weight loss related to underlying disease; if so, this would lead to an underestimate of the benefit of intentional weight loss; and finally; (3) there may be unexplored but important associations with disease incidence and quality of life outcomes that are not detected by studies of mortality.

Finally, it is important to distinguish the underlying purpose of observational studies and RCTs. Whereas RCTs are designed to test the true effectiveness of a defined intervention (for example, group-based lifestyle modification), observational studies examine the health outcomes associated with attempts to lose weight under everyday conditions; those studies may include a wide range of both recommended and non-recommended approaches. Quite possibly, the weight losses recorded in observational studies are less likely than weight losses recorded in RCTs to be followed by adequate maintenance of weight loss to effect disease outcomes.

Controlled trials: prevention and management of hypertension

Several RCTs conducted during the late 1980s and early 1990s examined the impact of lifestyle-based weight loss programmes on the development of clinically relevant hypertension[5]. These studies examined weight loss in combination with reduced sodium intake or nutritional supplements, making it difficult to interpret the independent effects of weight loss. However, these studies found that 2–4 year lifestyle-based weight loss programmes were feasible, that they could attain mean weight loss of 3–4 per cent, and that such effects could reduce medication needs in hypertensive patients.

More recent trials have tested the efficacy of long-term weight loss in the primary prevention of hypertension among high risk persons[15–17]. The Trials of Hypertension Prevention compared weight loss, decreased sodium intake, and use of other nutritional supplements (calcium, potassium, magnesium) to estimate their impact on blood pressure values and the incidence of hypertension among overweight persons aged 30–54 with high normal blood pressure[15]. The weight reduction group achieved a 4 per cent mean weight loss over 18 months, and of all the intervention conditions, weight loss had the greatest reduction in average blood pressure (2.9/2.3 mm/Hg) and incidence of hypertension (34 per cent lower than the control group).

In a follow-up 4-year multi-centre study, overweight persons randomized to lifestyle-based weight loss achieved a 4 per cent net weight loss over the first 6 months, accompanied by a mean blood pressure reduction of 2.7/3.7 mm/Hg[16]. After 3 years, their net weight loss was only 2 per cent and blood pressure reductions were modest (1.0/1.1 mm/Hg), but there was a significant 21 per cent reduction in incidence of hypertension. Additionally, the magnitude of risk reduction was directly associated with the success of the weight loss[17]. Compared to the control group, persons who maintained 4.5 kg (roughly 5 per cent) weight loss over 3 years had a 65 per cent lower hypertension incidence, and those who attained 4.5 kg after 6 months but relapsed to < 2.5 kg weight loss in the following 2.5 years had a 25 per cent risk reduction. There was no risk reduction for persons who were randomized to the intervention but failed to lose weight.

Controlled trials: diabetes prevention

A series of controlled trials testing whether lifestyle approaches can reduce diabetes incidence provide perhaps the strongest evidence to date for the value of lifestyle-based weight loss[18–21]. The first of these was conducted in Malmo, Sweden, where 260 men aged 47–49 with impaired glucose tolerance (IGT) were assigned (non-randomly) to a diet and exercise weight loss condition or to usual care[18]. After 6 years, men in the weight loss condition had maintained a 2.3 per cent weight loss (vs. a 0.5 per cent gain among control group) and a 63 per cent lower diabetes incidence. This study established the feasibility of long-term weight loss among persons with IGT, as well as an impressive magnitude of effect.

Using a randomized design in Da Qing, China, entire clinics of middle-aged (mean 45 years) persons with IGT were assigned to either diet (reduced fat and total intake), exercise, or diet plus exercise[19]. Participants in all three interventions had significant 29–32 per cent reductions in diabetes incidence, with no appreciable difference between groups. There were similar reductions in relative risk associated with the intervention among lean (BMI < 25) and overweight (BMI ≥ 25) persons. There was essentially no difference in weight change across the groups after 6 years, however, but the study did not report weight changes during earlier years of the study, which may have been more substantial and influenced diabetes risk.

More recently, the Finnish Diabetes Prevention Study examined the effects of a 2-year multidisciplinary intervention with goals of reducing body weight, lowering total and fat intake, and increasing physical activity and fibre intake among overweight, middle-aged adults with IGT[20]. The intervention achieved an average 2-year net weight loss of 3.8 per cent and a 58 per cent lower diabetes incidence, and it was estimated that 22 people with IGT needed to be treated with lifestyle intervention to prevent one case of diabetes per year. The study also found that the magnitude of reduction in diabetes incidence was associated with degree of weight loss, and with the number of study goals achieved.

One year later, the Diabetes Prevention Programme reported results from a similar type of intervention carried out in the US among a more ethnically diverse and more obese (mean BMI = 34, vs. 31 in the Finnish study) population, also with IGT[21]. Participants in the lifestyle intervention group had a achieved a mean net weight loss of 7 per cent, 6 per cent, and 4 per cent over 1, 2 and 4 years, respectively, and had a 58 per cent lower diabetes incidence rate than participants in the control group. It was estimated that seven people with IGT needed to be treated with lifestyle intervention to prevent one case of diabetes per year. Stratification by age, sex, ethnicity, or baseline BMI did not substantially alter the findings.

Taken as a whole, the four lifestyle intervention studies have encouraging implications for population-based prevention of diabetes and its complications[18-21]. In addition to showing an impressive magnitude of risk reduction (30–60 per cent across the trials), these studies demonstrated effectiveness across varied settings, cultures, and characteristics of patients. Key attributes of the most successful RCTs included intensive, extended contact in one-on-one or small group settings, combined steady reductions of total intake, fat intake < 30 per cent of total diet, and moderate intensity physical activity.

Controlled trials: weight loss and cardiovascular disease

Despite the consistent benefits of moderate weight loss on hypertension and diabetes, the effects of weight loss on CVD are less clear. Two studies have found a lowered risk of CVD to be associated with cardio-protective diets and weight loss[22-24]. Singh et al.[22] found that that among persons with heart disease, a vegetarian diet accompanied by 9 per cent weight loss over 6 months (vs. 3 per cent in a control condition) was associated with 40–50 per cent reductions in cardiac events, strokes, and mortality[22]. Similarly, Ornish et al. found that patients with heart disease randomized to an aggressive low fat/high fibre diet had an 8 per cent weight loss, and significant reductions in coronary stenosis over 5 years[23-24]. Although encouraging, these trials employed weight loss as an adjunct to an aggressive lipid lowering diet, making it unclear whether weight loss per se was responsible for the observed benefits. Other intervention studies have found that similar dietary approaches[25] or structured exercise[26] can influence atherosclerosis progression and CVD endpoints among persons with CHD without weight loss. In addition, no studies have examined the role of weight loss on primary prevention of CVD, although a long-term National Institutes of Health-funded clinical trial is underway in the US among persons with type 2 diabetes[27].

Obesity surgery studies

The most profound health benefits of weight loss have been observed in nonrandomized studies of obesity surgery conducted in the US and Sweden[28-30]. The Swedish Obese Subjects (SOS) Study is an ongoing trial of over 1800 men and women aged 37 to 60 (BMI > 34 for men and > 38 for women) who underwent bariatric surgery[29]. Compared to matched controls receiving conventional obesity treatment, the surgical patients had a net 22 per cent weight loss after 2 years, accompanied by a 98 per cent reduction in diabetes incidence and a 62 per cent reduction in hypertension incidence. There were also significant net reductions in dyspnea, walking-related chest pain, and psychiatric morbidity and significant improvements in mental well-being (anxiety, depression, mood)[29]. After 8 years, net weight loss was 17 per cent, and there was a 84 per cent reduction in diabetes incidence but no remaining difference in incidence of hypertension[30].

Summary and conclusions

Consistent evidence from RCTs now links multi-component lifestyle-based weight loss to moderate (20–30 per cent) reductions in hypertension incidence and substantial (30–60 per cent) decreases in diabetes incidence. Similar interventions appear to prevent CVD in persons with heart disease, but this evidence is less conclusive, and there is still no evidence for primary prevention of CVD with weight loss. Recent analyses from observational studies strongly suggest that intentional weight loss does not increase mortality. Whether intentional weight loss reduces mortality, however, remains unclear.

Many other questions remain about the potential benefits of weight loss. Benefits related to hypertension and diabetes have been demonstrated primarily among overweight persons with high-normal blood pressure, whereas diabetes prevention studies have observed benefits primarily among overweight/obese persons with IGT. Whether benefits can be generalized to the large segments of the population with normal glucose tolerance and lower body weight, or to older (i.e. > 65 years) persons remains unclear.

Perhaps the greatest challenge will be learning how to translate the findings related to lifestyle interventions into effective public health policy. The most successful RCTs employed intensive interventions aimed at long-term behaviour change, suggesting that a chronic disease model of care may be necessary to influence the risk of chronic disease. It is unclear whether health care systems in the US and other industrialized countries will adopt a chronic disease model of care for weight loss. At the same time, it remains unclear whether broad, less-focused, community and public health approaches to weight loss can achieve adequate impact on body weight to appreciably influence the risk of chronic disease

References

1. National Center for Health Statistics. Prevalence of overweight and obesity among adults. United States, 1999. [On-line] Available from: URL: http: //www.cdc.gov/nchs/products/pubs/pubd/hestats/obese/obse99.htm [Accessed 8/02/2002].

2. Mokdad AH, Serdula MK, Dietz WH, Bowman BA, Marks JS, Koplan JP. The spread of the obesity epidemic in the United States, 1991–1998. *JAMA* 1999; 282: 1519–22.

3. National Task Force on the Prevention and Treatment of obesity Overweight, obesity, and health risk. *Arch Intern Med* 2000; 160: 898–904.

4. Pi-Sunyer FX. A review of long-term studies evaluating the efficacy of weight loss in ameliorating disorders associated with obesity. *Clin Ther* 1996; 18: 1006–35.

5. Mertens IL, Van Gaal LF. Overweight, obesity, and blood pressure: the effects of modest weight reduction. *Obes Res* 2000; 8: 270–8.

6. Wing RR. Behavioral weight control. In: *Handbook of obesity treatment*, TA Wadden, AJ Stunkard (eds), p. 357. New York: The Guilford Press; 2002.

7. Perri MG, Corsica JA. Improving the maintenance of weight lost in behavioral treatment of obesity. In: *Handbook of obesity treatment*, TA Wadden, AJ Stunkard (eds), p. 357. New York: The Guilford Press; 2002.

8. Lee IM, Paffenbarger RS Jr. Is weight loss hazardous? *Nutr Rev* 1996; 54(4 pt 2): S116–S124 (review).

9. Williamson DF, Pamuk E, Thun M, Flanders D, Byers T, Heath C. Prospective study of intentional weight loss and mortality in never-smoking overweight US white women aged 40–64 years. *Am J Epidemiol* 1995; 141: 1128–41.

10. Williamson DF, Thompson TJ, Thun M, Flanders D, Pamuk E, Byers T. Intentional weight loss and mortality among overweight persons with diabetes. *Diabetes Care* 2000; 23: 1499–504.

11. Williamson DF, Pamuk E, Thun M, Flanders D, Byers T, Heath, C. Prospective study of intentional weight loss and mortality in overweight white men aged 40–64 years. *Am J Epidemiol* 1999; 149: 491–503.

12. French SA, Folsom AR, Jeffery RW, Williamson DF. Prospective study of intentionality of weight loss and mortality in older women: the Iowa Women's Health Study. *Am J Epidemiol* 1999; 149: 504–14.

13. Yaari S, Goldbourt U. Voluntary and involuntary weight loss: associations with long-term mortality in 9228 middle-aged and elderly men. *Am J Epidemiol* 1998; 148: 546–55

14. Gregg EW, Gerzoff RB, Thompson TT, Williamson DF. Trying to lose weight, losing weight, and 9-year mortality among overweight US diabetic adults. *Diabetes* 2002; 51(2): A226.

15. Trials of Hypertension Prevention Collaborative Research Group Effects of nonpharmacologic interventions on blood pressure of persons with high normal levels. *JAMA* 1992; 267: 1213–20.

16. The Trials of Hypertension Prevention Collaborative Research Group Effects of weight loss and sodium reduction intervention on blood pressure and hypertension incidence in overweight people with high-normal blood pressure. The Trials of Hypertension Prevention, phase III. *Arch Intern Med* 1997; 157: 657–67.

17. Stevens VJ, Obarzanek E, Cook NR, Lee IM, Appel LJ, Smith West D *et al*. For the Trials of Hypertension Prevention Research Group. Long-term weight loss and changes in blood pressure: results of the Trials of Hypertension Prevention, phase II. *Ann Intern Med* 2001; 134: 1–11.

18. Eriksson KF, Lindgärde F. Prevention of type 2 (non-insulin-dependent) diabetes mellitus by diet and physical exercise. The 6-year Malmo feasibility study. *Diabetologia* 1991; 34: 891–8

19. Pan XR, Li GW, Hu YH, Wang JX, Yang WY, An ZX *et al*. Effects of diet and exercise in preventing NIDDM in people with impaired glucose tolerance. The Da Qing IGT and Diabetes Study *Diabetes Care* 1997; 20: 537–44.

20. Tuomilehto J, Lindstrom J, Eriksson JG, Valle TT, Hamalainen H, Ilanne-Parikka P *et al*. Finnish Diabetes Prevention Study Group Prevention of type 2 diabetes mellitus by changes in lifestyle among subjects with impaired glucose tolerance. *N Engl J Med* 2001; 344(18): 1343–50.

21. Diabetes Prevention Program Research Group Reduction in the incidence of type 2 diabetes with lifestyle intervention or metformin. *N Engl J Med* 2002; 346: 393–403.

22. Singh RB, Rastogi SS, Verma R, Laxmi B, Singh R, Ghosh S *et al*. Randomised controlled trial of cardioprotective diet in patients with recent acute myocardial infarction: results of one-year follow-up. *BMJ* 1992; 304: 1015–19.

23. Ornish D, Brown SE, Scherwitz LW, Billings JH, Armstrong WT, Ports TA *et al*. Can lifestyle changes reverse coronary heart disease? The Lifestyle Heart Trial. *Lancet* 1990; 336: 129–33.

24. Ornish D, Scherwitz LW, Billings JH, Brown SE, Gould KL, Merritt TA *et al*. Intensive lifestyle changes for reversal of coronary heart disease. *JAMA* 1998; 280: 2001–7.

25. Watts GF, Lewis B, Brunt JNH, Lewis ES, Coltart DJ, Smith LDR *et al*. Effects of coronary artery disease of lipid-lowering diet, or diet plus cholestyramine, in the St Thomas Atherosclerosis Regression Study (STARS) *Lancet* 1992; 339: 563–9.

26. Schuler G, Hambrecht R, Schlierf G, Niebauer J, Hauer K, Neumann J *et al*. Regular physical exercise and low fat diet. Effects on progression of coronary artery disease. *Circulation* 1992; 86: 1–11.

27. Raczynski JM, Fujimoto WY, Kahn SE. For the Look Ahead Research Group. Early Recrutment results for the Look AHEAD Clinical Trial. *Diabetes* 51(2): A421.

28. MacDonald KG, Long SD, Swanson MS, Brown BM, Morris P, Dohm GL, Pories WJ. The gastric bypass operation reduces progression and mortality of non-insulin dependent diabetes mellitus. *J Gastrointestinal Surg* 1997; 1: 213–20.

29. Torgerson JS, Sjostrom L The Swedish Obese Subjects (SOS) study – rationale and results. *Int J Obes Relat Metab Disord* 2001; 25(1): S2–S4.

30. Sjostrom CD, Peltonen M, Wedel H, Sjostrom L. Differentiated long-term effects of intentional weight loss on diabetes and hypertension. *Hypertension* 2000; 36: 20–5.

Progress in Obesity Research: 9. Edited by *Geraldo Medeiros-Neto, Alfredo Halpern* and *Claude Bouchard*
©2003 John Libbey Eurotext Ltd, pp. 629–633.

CHAPTER 131

Epidemiology of adiposity in Africans in the Diaspora

Ike S. Okosun[1], K.M. Dinesh Chandra[2] and John M Boltri[3]

[1]*Department of Community Medicine, Mercer University School of Medicine, 1550 College St, Macon, GA 31207 USA;*
[2]*Department of Internal Medicine, Mercer University School of Medicine, 707 Pine St, Macon, GA 31201, USA;*
[3]*Department of Family Medicine, Mercer University School of Medicine, 1550 College Street, Macon, GA 31207, USA*
[e-mail: okosun_i@mercer.edu]

Introduction

In simple terms, obesity occurs as a result of energy imbalance when energy intake exceeds energy expenditure over a long period of time. Obesity is a marker for chronic diseases, of which cardiovascular diseases and cancers are major contributors to morbidity and mortality[1–3]. The two most common forms of adiposities are generalized and abdominal obesities. Body mass index (BMI), defined as weight in kilograms divided by the square of the height in meters, is a surrogate measure of generalized adiposity. A BMI of 30 or more is now widely accepted as the classification for generalized obesity[4]. Abdominal obesity is a more potent form of obesity that is highly correlated with visceral adiposity, generalized obesity and many cardiovascular diseases[5–6]. Waist circumference is a surrogate measure of abdominal obesity. Waist circumference values of ≥ 94 cm (~37 inches) in men and ≥ 80 cm (~32 inches) in women are the recommended abdominal obesity cut-points that are associated with obesity-related metabolic complications[4,7–8]. These complications include hyperinsulinaemia, glucose intolerance, hypertension, hypertriglyceridaemia, elevated levels of low-density lipoprotein (LDL-C), and low levels of high-density lipoprotein (HDL-C) cholesterol[9–12].

The prevalence of obesity and many of its associated metabolic complications are higher among peoples of West African origins (African Americans) in the United States compared with Whites[13–14]. The reason for this disparity is one of the most baffling questions in cardiovascular disease epidemiology. While various methodological attempts have been developed to explain Black–White differences for adiposity in the United States, many of these methods have been burdened with problems that have been difficult to resolve. Indeed, many studies that have been designed to explain the contributions of environmental factors in racial differences in obesity are fraught for their inability to clearly assess genetic contributions. An epidemiological investigation of Africans in the Diaspora offers an exceptional opportunity to study the role of nutritional transitions among contemporary populations sharing a common historical and genetic origin but under widely different environmental conditions.

Who are Africans in the Diaspora?

Africans in the Diaspora include over 11 million people who were transported from sub-Sahara Africa to provide labour in the New World colonies[15]. These Africans, who were brought into the Diaspora through the European slave trade, settled in North America, the Caribbean, Brazil and northern South America. Some Africans through recent voluntary migration are also found in the United States and the United Kingdom[15–16]. Other Africans occupy coastal regions of Central America including Argentina and other Andean countries[15]. Thus, Africans in the Diaspora occupy diverse socio-cultural environments that range from subsistence agriculture in sub-Saharan Africa, to urban and peri-urban small-market economies in the Caribbean, to industrialized societies in the United States and the United Kingdom[15]. Overall health and nutritional disparities between these populations reflects the economic and market conditions of these populations. An epidemiological investigation across these economic or social gradients (agriculture to industrial) allows historical understanding of diseases patterns. Because Africans in the Diaspora share a common ancestry and live under widely different environmental conditions, the basic assumption for using them in epidemiological understanding of diseases is that the genetic contribution to any variance in diseases is likely to be attenuated, thus, allowing study focus to be on the role of the environment.

Africans in Diaspora and nutritional transition

Sub-Sahara Africa is in the early stage of nutritional transition where malnutrition and undernutrition are the major causes of morbidity and mortality[17]. Many Caribbean nations represent the middle stage of nutritional transition where undernutrition and obesity coexist[18]. The United States and the United Kingdom represent the zenith of the nutritional transition, characterized by caloric excesses and diets that are high in fat and animal products. In the latter group, the effect of nutritional transition on health has been profound, and includes overweight, obesity and cardiovascular diseases[19-20].

Consequences of nutritional transitions are most ominous in populations undergoing social, cultural, and economic changes[21,22]. Indeed, Africans in the Diaspora have morbidity and mortality patterns that demonstrate the effect of socioeconomic and societal changes on a common substrate. These changes often termed 'westernization' are due to rapid urbanization and rise in socioeconomic status[23]. Westernization implies imitation of western lifestyle, including overindulgence in foods that are high in saturated fat, and sugar refined foods that are low in fibre, and an increase in smoking, sedentary lifestyle and urbanization. These factors, collectively known as 'civilization syndrome', often culminate in obesity[23].

What do we know from studying Africans in the Diaspora?

The best evidence of the effect of westernization on health comes from the International collaborative Study of Hypertension in Blacks (ICSHIB). Detailed accounts of ICSHIB sampling procedures have been published elsewhere[24-25]. Briefly, ICSHIB was a multi-site random sample of residential communities in West Africa (Nigeria and Cameroon), the Caribbean (Jamaica, St. Lucia and Barbados) and the United States. In Nigeria, a sampling method was designed to cover rural and urban sectors. The samples from Cameroon were mainly from civil servants from the capital city of Yaounde. The Caribbean samples were drawn from peri-urban areas of Spanish Town, Jamaica; Bridgetown Barbados; and Vieux Forte, St. Lucia. The United States sampling was carried out in Maywood, a suburban city west of Chicago, Illinois. Overall, the ICSHIB survey and data collection were carried out between 1991 and 1995 and covered a total of approximately 11,000 men and women 25–74 years of age.

In ICSHIB, measurement protocols were standardized across sites, and rigorous training techniques were implemented. Anthropometric measurements were obtained from participants without shoes and in light clothes. Weight was measured using electronic digital scales and recorded in pounds to the nearest 0.5 lb. Height was measured in meters to the nearest 0.1 cm against a vertical wall with a rigid headboard using an inelastic tape measure. Measurements of waist were made with a flexible tape for each subject to the nearest 0.1 cm. Waist measurement was made at the natural waist (narrowest part of the torso as seen from the front) or at midpoint between the bottom of the rib cage and 2 cm above the top of the iliac crest.

Anthropometrics across degree of westernization

Table 1 shows the mean values for the various anthropometric variables stratified by sex. The sites are listed in order of the degree of westernization, i.e. West Africa, Caribbean, and United States. In West Africa, Cameroon (samples drawn from civil servants representing a more affluent segment of the African population) is listed after Nigeria. Within the Caribbean, countries are listed in increasing order of gross national product (GNP). In 1990 per capital GNP for Jamaica, St. Lucia and Barbados were US$1103, US$1500 and US$5960, respectively[26]. In the absence of Cameroon data that represents a high socioeconomic group, a consistent gradient of increasing waist circumference (surrogate for abdominal obesity) is apparent. As expected a similar gradient was observed for weight and BMI. With the exception of Jamaica, men were heavier than women, however, women had a higher BMI than did men. A gradient of increasing values of weight, BMI and waist circumference was observed with increasing degree of westernization. A gradient of increasing values of weight, BMI and waist girth was observed from rural to urban in Nigerian men and women.

Table 1. Summary of the prevalence of adiposity in Africans in the Diaspora

Study site	Weight kg	Height cm	BMI kg/m^2	Waist cm	Prevalence of adiposity (%)	
					Generalized	Abdominal
MEN						
West Africa						
Nigeria	61.6 [10.8]	163.8 [9.5]	22.5 [4.6]	77.7 [9.1]	5.0	6.4
Rural	61.3 [10.6]	168.4 [7.4]	21.5 [3.4]	76.9 [8.2]	–	–
Urban	62.2 [11.8]	159.0 [9.1]	23.5 [5.4]	78.6 [9.9]	–	–
Cameroon	72.9 [13.0]	172.5 [7.2]	24.4 [4.2]	82.8 [11.1]	6.4	16.5
Caribbean						
Jamaica	70.3 [13.7]	172.1 [6.9]	23.7 [4.4]	80.8 [12.0]	7.2	14.3
St. Lucia	72.6 [11.4]	173.5 [7.4]	24.2 [3.7]	82.6 [9.5]	8.1	15.8
Barbados	76.4 [13.1]	170.0 [7.4]	25.9 [4.2]	86.0 [11.1]	10.3	21.4
United States	84.5 [18.0]	176.5 [7.3]	27.1 [5.5]	92.4 [14.0]	27.3	38.9
WOMEN						
West Africa						
Nigeria	58.0 [12.4]	157.8 [7.5]	22.9 [5.2]	75.7 [10.2]	11.0	26.3
Rural	57.2 [11.0]	158.3 [6.6]	22.8 [4.4]	73.9 [9.5]	–	–
Urban	59.8 [12.1]	156.9 [8.3]	23.0 [5.7]	78.0 [10.5]	–	–
Cameroon	72.9 [17.0]	161.2 [6.6]	28.1 [6.4]	84.8 [12.9]	15.8	62.8
Caribbean						
Jamaica	72.1 [17.4]	160.7 [6.4]	27.9 [6.4]	83.2 [12.7]	33.5	58.6
St. Lucia	72.3 [17.0]	162.8 [6.8]	27.3 [6.2]	85.5 [13.4]	28.9	62.1
Barbados	75.2 [20.9]	160.1 [6.3]	29.4 [6.3]	87.1 [12.6]	40.8	70.3
United States	82.4 [20.9]	163.4 [6.4]	30.8 [7.7]	91.4 [15.4]	49.0	76.4

Adapted from references[24,25] *Generalized obesity was defined as BMI >30 kg/m^2; Abdominal obesity was defined as waist circumference values of > 94 cm in men and > 80 cm in women.

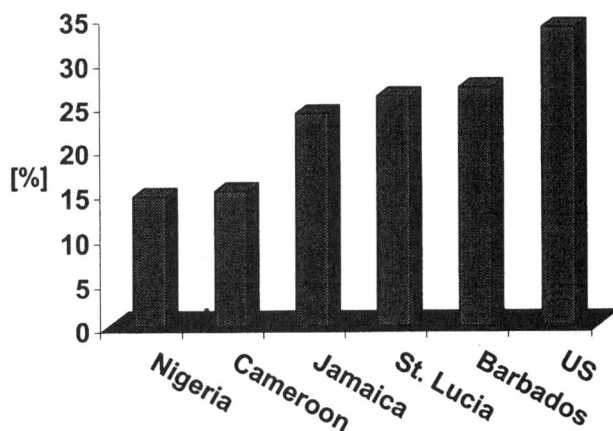

Fig. 1. Prevalence of hypertension in Africans in the Diaspora (adapted from reference[27]).

Adiposity across degree of westernization

Data from ICSHIB also provide a clear picture about the effect of westernization in adiposity. As shown from Table 1, there were gradients of increasing prevalences of generalized and abdominal adiposities from West Africa, to the Caribbean and to the United States. In men, the highest relative differences in prevalence values of generalized and abdominal obesities between Nigeria and United States were 22.3 per cent and 32.5 per cent, respectively. The corresponding values in women were 44 per cent and 50 per cent. Within the Caribbean, prevalences of generalized and abdominal adiposities were linear along per capita GNP. In these populations of Africans in the Diaspora, the prevalence of hypertension appears to be tightly linked to generalized and abdominal adiposities (Fig 1). A similar increasing prevalence of type 2 diabetes with increasing westernization was also observed using the population groups[27].

Adiposity and mortality

The positive association of obesity with increased mortality from cardiovascular diseases, including diabetes, cerebrovascular, and cardiovascular disease, and certain forms of cancer in many population groups is well known. However the relation between measures of adiposity and mortality has been a controversial topic. Some studies have noted no distinct relation[28]. Other studies have suggested that the relation is J-shaped, U-shaped, directly linear, or inversely linear between BMI and all-cause mortality[28]. Many of these studies are however limited by lack of data on the association between adiposity and mortality in Africans in the Diaspora. Many others have however observed that under-nutrition was a critically important nutritional variable for health among Africans outside industrialized nations[29,30]. Indeed, using data derived from an international collaborative study on chronic diseases in populations of the African Diaspora, Rotimi et al.[30] found that the prevalence of chronic energy deficiency was positively associated with increased risk of all-cause mortality in a cohort of adult Nigerians followed from 1992 to 1997.

Conclusion

The ICSHIB is a framework for understanding the effect of westernization in peoples with similar genetic background while residing in vastly different socio-cultural environments. As indicated by many studies, Africans in sub-Sahara countries, the source of Africans in Diaspora, have unnecessarily been overwhelmed with undernutrition, malnutrition and food scarcity. Infectious diseases such as malaria, tuberculosis and AIDS burden Africans in the less westernized nations, and no data exist on secular trends on obesity. There is no doubt that the adverse effects of lifestyle change due to increasing modernizations will lead to increase in obesity in the populations of the Africans in the Diaspora residing in Africa and the Caribbean. Also, because a large segment of these Africans reside in rural and underdeveloped areas, undernutrition and malnutrition will continue to be major public health problems.

Given the rapid rates of westernization in most developing nations, there is an urgent need to follow the lead of ICSHIB by developing large-scale longitudinal investigations to study the effect of these obesity phenotypes on morbidity and all-cause mortality. There is a need to link available obesity data to morbidity and mortality from various other studies and geographic locations in order to understand effect of westernization on a common substrate. Finally, while there is no doubt that westernization has a positive impact on overall health, there is a need to balance such impact against its negative effects. Public health awareness about good nutrition across populations of African descent may help in reducing the ill effects of westernization on overall health.

Acknowledgement: We thank Dr. Richard Cooper and ICSHIB investigators for the surveys.

References

1. Solomon CG, Manson JE. Related Articles Obesity and mortality: a review of the epidemiologic data. *Am J Clin Nutr* 1997; 66 (Suppl 4): S1044–S1050.

2. Cho E, Manson JE, Stampfer MJ, Solomon CG, Colditz GA, Speizer FE et al. A prospective study of obesity and risk of coronary heart disease among diabetic women. *Diabetes Care* 2002; 25: 1142–8.

3. Paeratakul S, Lovejoy JC, Ryan DH, Bray GA. The relation of gender, race and socioeconomic status to obesity and obesity comorbidities in a sample of US adults. *Int J Obes Relat Metab Disord* 2002; 26: 1205–10.

4. WHO/NUT/NCD/98.1 Obesity: preventing and managing the global epidemic. Report of a WHO consultation. World Health Organ Tech Rep Ser. 2000; 894: i-xii, 1–253.

5. Han TS, McNeill G, Baras P, Forester MA. Waist circumference predicts intra-abdominal fat better than waist: hip ratio in women. *Proc Nutr Soc* 1995; 54: 152A.

6. Lemieux S, Prud'homme D, Tremblay A, Bouchard C, Despres JP. Anthropometric correlates to changes in visceral adipose tissue over 7 years in women. *Int J Obes Relat Metab Disord* 1996; 7: 618–24.

7. Lean ME, Han TS, Morrison CE. Waist circumference as a measure for indicating need for weight management. *BMJ* 1995; 311: 158–61.

8. National Institute of Health/National Heart Lungs and Blood Clinical Guidelines on the Identification, Evaluation, and Treatment of Overweight and Obesity in Adults. The Evidence Report. *Obes Res* 1998; 6: S51–S209.

9. Haffner SM, Valdez RA, Hazed HP, Mitchell BD, Morales PA, Stern MP. Prospective analysis of the insulin-resistance syndrome (syndrome X). *Diabetes* 1992; 41: 715–22.

10. Gus M, Moreira LB, Pimentel M, Gleisener AL, Moraes RS, Fuchs FD. Association of various measurements of obesity and the prevalence of hypertension. *Arq Brás Cardiol* 1998; 2: 111–4.

11. Sattar N, Tan CE, Han TS, Forster L, Lean ME, Shepherd J, Packard CJ. Associations of indices of adiposity with atherogenic lipoprotein subfractions. *Int J Obes Relat Metab Disord* 1998; 5: 432–39.

12. Despres JP. Abdominal obesity as an important component of insulin-resistance syndrome. *Nutrition* 1993; 9: 452–9.

13. Mokdad AH, Serdula MK, Dietz WH, Bowman BA, Marks JS, Koplan JP. The spread of the obesity epidemic in the United States, 1991–1998. *JAMA* 1999; 27(282): 1519–22.

14. Harris M, Hadden W, Knowler W, Bennett PH. Prevalence of diabetes and impaired glucose tolerance in US populations aged 20–74. *Diabetes* 1987; 36: 523–34.

15. Curtin PD. *The Atlantic slave trade: a census.* Milwaukee WI: University of Wisconsin Press 1969.

16. Luke A, Cooper RS, Prewitt TE, Adeyemo AA, Forrester TE. Nutritional consequences of the African diaspora. *Annu Rev Nutr* 2001; 21: 47–71.

17. Drewnowski A, Popkin BM. The nutrition transition: new trends in the global diet. *Nutr Rev* 1997; 55: 31–43.

18. Hagley KE. Nutrition and health in the developing world: the Caribbean experience. *Proc Nutr Soc* 1993; 52: 183–7.

19. Flegal KM, Carroll MD, Kuczmarski RJ, Johnson CL. Overweight and obesity in the United States: prevalence and trends, 1960–1994. *Int J Obes Relat Metab Disord* 1998; 22: 39–47.

20. Burke JP, Williams K, Gaskill SP, Hazuda HP, Haffner SM, Stern MP. Rapid rise in the incidence of type 2 diabetes from 1987 to 1996: results from the San Antonio Heart Study. *Arch Intern Med* 1999; 159: 1450–6.

21. Sargeant LA, Bennett FI, Forrester TE, Cooper RS, Wilks RJ. Predicting incident of diabetes in Jamaica: the role of anthropometry. *Obes Res* 2002; 10: 792–8.

22. Alleyne SI, Morrison EY, Richards RR Some social factors related to control of diabetes mellitus in adult Jamaican patients. *Diabetes Care* 1979; 2: 401–8.

23. Trowell HC, Burkitt DP. *Westernizing Diseases: their emergence and prevention.* Harvard Press. Cambridge 1981.

24. Cooper R, Rotimi C, Ataman S, McGee D, Osotimehin B, Kadiri S *et al.* The prevalence of hypertension in seven populations of west African origin. *Am J Public* 1997; 87: 160–8.

25. Okosun IS, Forrester TE, Rotimi CN, Osotimehin BO, Cooper RS. Abdominal Obesity in Six Populations of West African Descent. Prevalence and Population Attributable Fraction of Hypertension. *J Obes Res* 1999; 7: 453–62.

26. Forrester T, Wilks R, Bennett F, McFarlane-Anderson N, McGee D, Cooper R, Fraser H. Obesity in the Caribbean. *Ciba Foundation Symposium* 1996; 201: 17–26.

27. Cooper RS, Rotimi CN, Kaufman JS, Owoaje EE, Fraser H, Forrester T *et al.* Prevalence of NIDDM among populations of the African diaspora. *Diabetes Care* 1997; 20: 343–8.

28. Baik I, Ascherio A, Rimm EB, Giovannucci E, Spiegelman D, Stampfer MJ, Willett WC. Adiposity and mortality in men. *Am J Epidemiol* 2000; 152: 264–71.

29. Martorell R, Khan LK, Hughes ML, Grummer-Strawn LM. Obesity in Latin American women and children. *J Nutr* 1998; 128: 1464–73.

30. Rotimi C, Okosun I, Johnson L, Owoaje E, Lawoyin T, Asuzu M *et al.* The distribution and mortality impact of chronic energy deficiency among adult Nigerian men and women. *Eur J Clin Nutr* 1999; 53: 734–9.

Progress in Obesity Research: 9. Edited by *Geraldo Medeiros-Neto, Alfredo Halpern and Claude Bouchard*
©2003 John Libbey Eurotext Ltd, pp. 634–638.

CHAPTER 132

Waist circumference, hip circumference and health outcomes

Kathryn M. Rexrode

Division of Preventive Medicine, Brigham and Women's Hospital, 900 Commonwealth Avenue, 3rd Floor, Boston, MA 02215, USA
[e-mail: krexrode@partners.org]

While waist/hip ratio (WHR) has been associated with multiple disease outcomes, as a ratio its interpretation is not direct. There are several advantages of circumference measurements. They are simple, requiring only an inexpensive tape measure. Their interpretation is direct and there is less measurement and calculation error than when a ratio is used. These advantages make them well suited for use in longitudinal studies as well as public health settings, if they are found to have significant disease associations. This paper will review the data from prospective studies on the separate associations of waist and hip circumference and disease outcomes, including diabetes, cardiovascular disease and mortality.

One difficulty in comparing results from different studies is that waist and hip circumference locations have been performed at different locations. Sites for the measurement of waist include at the level of the umbilicus[1-3], 2.5 cm above the umbilicus[4], at the right iliac crest[5] and midway between the lower rib and the iliac crest[6]. Some of these locations can be more easily performed without assistance than others. Hip circumferences have been measured at the largest measurement between the waist and thigh[1-3] the maximum buttocks measurement, and the widest trochanter measure[6].

Physiologically, enlarged waist circumference generally reflects increased fat deposition either in the subcutaneous or visceral layers. Using waist circumference residual scores after adjustment for BMI, larger than expected waist circumference was more closely associated with increased total body fat mass than fat-free mass[7]. In contrast, several different factors may influence hip circumference. Smaller hip circumference can be due to lower gluteal subcutaneous fat mass, decreased gluteal muscle or smaller pelvic bone width. Gender appears to modify the relationship between body circumferences and fat distribution. After adjusting for age and BMI, a large hip circumference residual was associated with decreased visceral fat in men but not women, and increased subcutaneous fat in both sexes[7]. Thus, WHR should not be interpreted as solely reflecting visceral fat. It also reflects regional fat distribution. In women, estrogen may help regulate preferential deposition of adipose in the hips, where fatty tissue has higher lipoprotein lipase activity and lower fatty acid turnover[8].

Waist circumference and risk of diabetes and hypertension

For diabetes, waist is a particularly strong risk factor. In the Nurses' Health Study (NHS), waist circumference had a stronger risk gradient for diabetes incidence than did BMI or WHR. Compared with the lowest quintile, women with a waist circumference ≥ 96.4 cm had an age-adjusted RR of 22.4 (95 per cent CI, 14.8–33.9); however, after controlling for BMI the risk was reduced to 6.2 (95 per cent CI, 3.5–11.0)[9]. In the Iowa Women's Health Study, waist circumference was also the single best measure of diabetes incidence, but the combination of WHR and BMI was the best predictor[10]. Results in men are slightly weaker. Men with a waist circumference ≥ 101.6 had an RR of 10.8 (95 per cent CI, 6.2–18.7) for diabetes, compared with the lowest waist quintile. Adjustment for BMI reduced the risk to 3.5 (95 per cent CI, 1.7–7.0)[11]. With regard to incident hypertension, women in the highest waist circumference tertile (> 91.4 cm) had an age-adjusted RR of 2.5 (95 per cent CI, 2.0–3.1) for developing hypertension

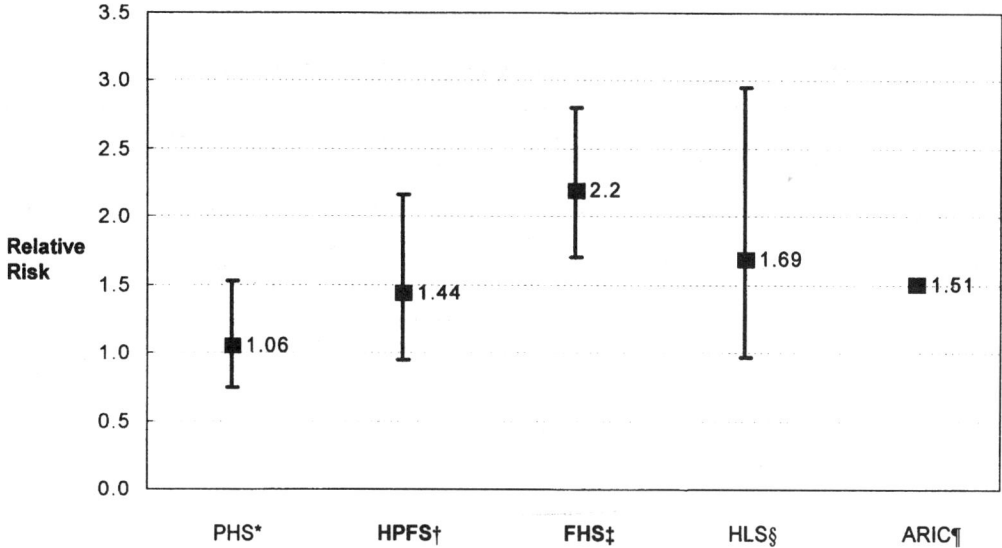

Fig. 1. Waist circumference and CVD in men.
*Physicians' Health Study(2) Multivariate including BMI. Quintiles;
†Health Professionals' Follow-up Study(3) Multivariate including BMI. Quintiles;
‡Framingham Heart Study(13) Age adjusted only, waist/height ratio.Quintiles;
§Health and Lifestyle Survey(22) Age and smoking adjusted. Quintiles;
¶Atherosclerosis Risk in Communities Study(14) Quintiles.

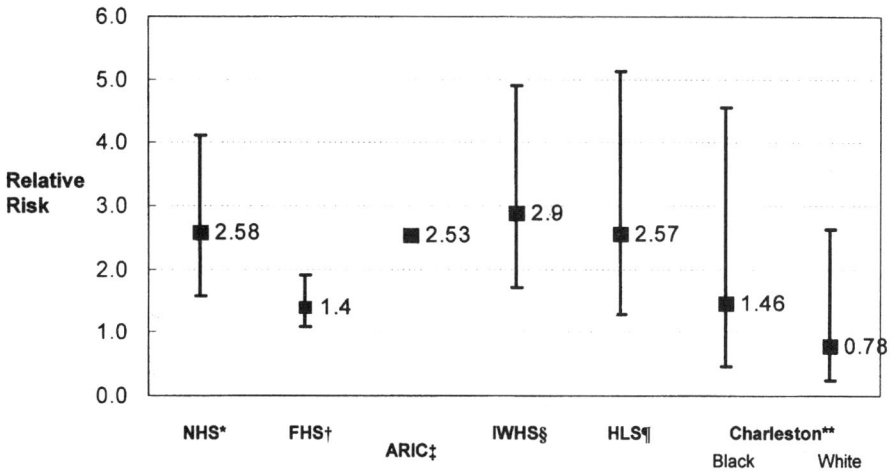

Fig. 2. Waist circumference and CVD in women
*Nurses' Health Study(1) Multivariate including BMI. Quintiles;
†Framingham Heart Study(13) Age adjusted only, waist/height ratio. Quintiles;
‡Atherosclerosis Risk in Communities(14) Quintiles;
§Iowa Women's Health Study(4) Age-adjusted only. Tertiles;
¶Health and Lifestyle Survey(22) Age and smoking adjusted. Quintiles;
**Charleston Heart Study(18) 85th vs. 15th percentiles.

during the subsequent two years[12]. Thus, waist circumference appears to be a particularly potent risk factor for the development of diabetes.

Waist circumference and risk of cardiovascular disease

As shown in Fig. 1, larger waist circumference has generally been associated with modestly increased risk of cardiovascular disease in men, though the risk estimates are generally weaker than for women. In the Physicians' Health Study, waist circumference was not significantly associated with increased risk of coronary heart disease, after adjustment for BMI. Men in the highest waist circumference quintile ($\geq$ 103.6) had an RR of 1.60 (95 per cent CI, 1.21–2.11) for coronary heart disease, but after adjustment for BMI the RR fell to 1.06 (95 per cent CI, 0.74–1.53)[2]. In the Health Professionals' Follow-up Study, men in the highest waist circumference quintile had a multivariate RR of 1.44 (95 per cent CI, 0.95–2.17) for coronary heart disease during three years of follow-up[3]. Men in the highest waist/height ratio quintile had a 2.2-fold age-adjusted increased risk of coronary heart disease mortality during 28 years of follow-up in the Framingham Heart Study[13]. Risk of heart disease was also increased 1.5-fold among men in the highest waist circumference quartile in the Atherosclerosis in Communities Study[14]. Thus, only the Framingham Heart Study found significantly elevated risks associated with coronary heart disease in men, but these were not adjusted for BMI.

As shown in Fig. 2, the associations between waist circumference and risk of coronary heart disease in women have been quite strong and consistent. In the Nurses' Health Study, women in the highest waist circumference quintile ($\geq$ 86.3 cm) had an RR of 2.58 (95 per cent CI, 1.58–4.22) for coronary heart disease, after adjusting for BMI and other cardiovascular risk factors[1]. In subgroup analyses, large waist circumference was a stronger risk factor for heart disease among women less than age 60 years of age (RR = 4.17) than those age 60 years or older (RR = 1.98). Risk gradients were strongest among normal weight women (BMI $\geq$ 25 kg/m^2) and those who did not use hormone replacement therapy[1]. Similarly, women in the highest waist circumference tertile (< 91.4 cm) had an age-adjusted RR of 2.9 (95 per cent CI, 1.7–4.9) for coronary heart disease mortality in the Iowa Women's Health Study[4]. In both the Nurses' Health Study and the Iowa Women's Health Study, WHR was a slightly stronger risk factor for coronary heart disease than was waist circumference. In the Atherosclerosis in Communities Study, women in the highest waist circumference quartile had a 2.5-fold increased risk of coronary heart disease during 6.2 years of follow-up[14]. The risk for extreme waist circumference quintiles was 1.4 (95 per cent CI, 1.1–1.9) in Framingham Heart Study[13].

Waist circumference has also been associated with risk of stoke, although the risks are somewhat more modest than those observed for coronary heart disease. In the Health Professionals' Follow-up Study, men in the highest waist circumference quintile had an RR of 1.52 (0.82–2.82) for stroke, whereas those in the highest WHR quintile had an RR for stroke of 2.3 (1.3–4.4)[15]. In the Framingham Heart Study, men in the highest waist circumference quintile had an RR of 2.0 (1.3–3.2) for stroke, while women in the highest quintile had an RR of 1.4 (1.0–2.2)[13]. In the Iowa Women's Health Study, women in the highest waist circumference tertile (> 91.4 cm) had an age-adjusted RR of 2.0 (95 per cent CI, 1.4–2.9) for stroke during the subsequent two years[12].

Waist circumference and mortality

Larger waist circumference has been weakly associated with all-cause mortality. In the Rotterdam Study, nonsmoking men with a waist circumference $\geq$ 101 cm had an age-adjusted hazard ratio of 1.6 (95 per cent CI, 0.8–3.4) for all cause mortality. Waist circumference was not associated with mortality among past or current male smokers. For women, waist circumference was not associated with all-cause mortality among any of the smoking groups[16]. In the Iowa Women's Health Study, WHR was the best predictor of total mortality but there was a modest association with waist circumference. Women in the highest waist circumference quintile had a multivariate RR of 1.2 (95 per cent CI, 1.1–0.4) for all-cause mortality over a twelve-year period. For cancer mortality, the risk associated with being in the highest waist circumference quintile was 1.2 (95 per cent CI, 0.96–1.4)[17]. In the Charleston Heart Study, waist circumference was more strongly associated with mortality in white than black women, but risk was higher for black than white men. Being in the 85th percentile of waist circumference was associated with a relative hazard of 1.75 (95 per cent CI, 0.87–3.51) for all cause mortality among white women, whereas for black women the hazard was 1.17 (95 per cent CI, 0.54–2.55)[18]. Among men in the Charleston Heart Study, black men with a waist circumference at the 85th percentile had a relative hazard for all-cause mortality of 1.96 (95 per cent CI, 0.97–3.95), while the association was null for white men[19].

Hip circumference and health outcomes

Since waist and hip are highly correlated (r = 0.76)[1], residual analysis is one method used to assess the independent effects of waist and hip on health outcomes. The residual of hip circumference after adjustment for BMI indicates the deviation from the expected hip circumference value at a given BMI. In a cross-sectional study, having larger than expected waist circumferences was associated with a 1.58 and 1.39 increased odds of hypertension among black men and women, respectively. The corresponding odds of hypertension in white men and women were 0.96 and 1.08[20]. In the Quebec Family Study, waist and hip circumference had independent and opposite effects on cardiovascular risk factors. Narrower than expected hips were directly related to HDL cholesterol and inversely associated with triglycerides, insulin and glucose in men. In women, hip residuals were negatively correlated only with triglycerides and insulin[7].

Hip circumference has less consistently been associated with health outcomes. In a cross-sectional study, men who had smaller than expected hip circumferences based on their BMI (lowest waist residual tertile) had a 3.7-fold increased risk of prevalent diabetes, while women had a 2.1-fold increased risk[21]. In men, smaller hips were associated with increased odds of diabetes, regardless of waist circumference, while for women the combination of smaller hips and larger waist was the most important risk factor[21]. In a prospective study in men, those in the highest height-adjusted hip circumference quintile had a sevenfold increased risk of diabetes incidence, but this became nonsignificant after adjustment for BMI[11].

One study has reported striking disease associations for hip circumference. In the Gothenburg Study, women in the highest quartile of hip circumference (> 103.5 cm) had reduced risks of myocardial infarction (RR 0.34, 95 per cent CI: 0.14–0.79), cardiovascular disease (RR 0.43, 95 per cent CI: 0.23–0.82) as well as total mortality (RR 0.59, 95 per cent CI, 0.35–0.99) during 24 years of follow-up, after controlling for BMI, waist, age and smoking[22]. In residual analyses, women with smaller than expected hip circumferences had significantly increased risks for total mortality as well as for myocardial infarction, cardiovascular disease and diabetes during follow-up[22]. However, other prospective studies have failed to find an association with crude hip circumference. Hip circumference quintiles were not associated with risk of coronary heart disease in women (*P* trend 0.78), after controlling for waist and height quintiles as well as other cardiovascular risk factors in the Nurses' Health Study. Women in the highest hip quintile had an RR of 0.81 (Rexrode, unpublished data). Larger hip circumference was also not associated with reduced risk of coronary heart disease in the Health Professionals' Follow-up Study. Men in the highest hip circumference quintile (≥ 108cm) had a multivariate RR of 0.93 (95 per cent CI, 0.62–1.38) for coronary heart disease, compared with those in the lowest quartile[3]. Additional prospective analyses on hip circumference using residuals would be helpful in assessing the independent associations of hip on disease outcomes.

In summary, waist and hip circumference are easily obtained anthropometric measurements that have significant associations with disease outcomes. The previously observed associations for WHR, may not just be due to the waist component, since hip circumference in some cases seems to add additional information about regional fat distribution that may contribute to disease risk. Waist and hip circumference should continue to be measured in epidemiologic studies. Optimal locations for measurement of circumference should be standardized, based on ease of measurement and disease prediction.

References

1. Rexrode KM, Carey VJ, Hennekens CH, Walters EE, Colditz GA, Stampfer MJ *et al.* Abdominal adiposity and coronary heart disease in women. *JAMA* 1998; 280(21): 1843–8.

2. Rexrode KM, Buring JE, Manson JE. Abdominal and total adiposity and risk of coronary heart disease in men. *Int J Obes Relat Metab Disord* 2001; 25(7): 1047–56.

3. Rimm EB, Stampfer MJ, Giovannucci E, Ascherio A, Spiegelman D, Colditz GA *et al.* Body size and fat distribution as predictors of coronary heart disease among middle-aged and older US men. *Am J Epidemiol* 1995; 141(12): 1117–27.

4. Prineas RJ, Folsom AR, Kaye AS. Central adiposity and increased risk of coronary artery disease mortality in older women. *Ann Epidemiol* 1993; 3(1): 35–41.

5. Lapidus L, Bengtsson C, Larsson B, Pennert K, Rybo E, Sjostrom L. Distribution of adipose tissue and risk of cardiovascular disease and death: a 12 year follow up of participants in the population study of women in Gothenburg, Sweden. *BMJ* 1984; 289(6454): 1257–61.

6. World Health Organization. Measuring obesity: classification and description of anthropometric data. World Health Organization. Copenhagen 1989.

7. Seidell JC, Perusse L, Despres JP, Bouchard C. Waist and hip circumferences have independent and opposite effects on cardiovascular disease risk factors: the Quebec Family Study. *Am J Clin Nutr* 2001; 74: 315–21.

8. Lindberg UB, Crona N, Silfverstolpe G, Bjorntorp P, Rebuffé-Scrive M. Regional adipose tissue metabolism in postmenopausal women after treatment with exogenous sex steroids. *Horm Metab Res* 1990; 22(6): 345–51.

9. Carey VJ, Walters EE, Colditz GA, Solomon CG, Willett WC, Rosner BA *et al.* Body fat distribution and risk of non-insulin-dependent diabetes mellitus in women. The Nurses' Health Study. *Am J Epidemiol* 1997; 145(7): 614–9.

10. Kaye SA, Folsom AR, Sprafka JM, Prineas RJ, Wallace RB. Increased incidence of diabetes mellitus in relation to abdominal adiposity in older women. *J Clin Epidemiol* 1991; 44(3): 329–34.

11. Chan JM, Rimm EB, Colditz GA, Stampfer MJ, Willett WC. Obesity, fat distribution, and weight gain as risk factors for clinical diabetes in men. *Diabetes Care* 1994; 17(9): 961–9.

12. Folsom AR, Prineas RJ, Kaye SA, Munger RG. Incidence of hypertension and stroke in relation to body fat distribution and other risk factors in older women. *Stroke* 1990; 21(5): 701–6.

13. Higgins M, Kannel W, Garrison R, Pinsky J, Stokes Jd. Hazards of obesity – the Framingham experience. *Acta Med Scand* Suppl 1988; 723: 23–36.

14. Folsom AR, Stevens J, Schreiner PJ, McGovern PG. Body mass index, waist/hip ratio, and coronary heart disease incidence in African Americans and whites. Atherosclerosis Risk in Communities Study Investigators. *Am J Epidemiol* 1998; 148(12): 1187–94.

15. Walker SP, Rimm EB, Ascherio A, Kawachi I, Stampfer MJ, Willett WC. Body size and fat distribution as predictors of stroke among US men. *Am J Epidemiol* 1996; 144(12): 1143–50.

16. Visscher TL, Seidell JC, Molarius A, van der Kuip D, Hofman A, Witteman JC. A comparison of body mass index, waist-hip ratio and waist circumference as predictors of all-cause mortality among the elderly: the Rotterdam study. *Int J Obes Relat Metab Disord* 2001; 25(11): 1730–5.

17. Folsom AR, Kushi LH, Anderson KE, Mink PJ, Olson JE, Hong CP *et al.* Associations of general and abdominal obesity with multiple health outcomes in older women: the Iowa Women's Health Study. *Arch Intern Med* 2000; 160(14): 2117–28.

18. Stevens J, Keil JE, Rust PF, Tyroler HA, Davis CE, Gazes PC. Body mass index and body girths as predictors of mortality in black and white women. *Arch Intern Med* 1992; 152(6): 1257–62.

19. Stevens J, Keil JE, Rust PF, Verdugo RR, Davis CE, Tyroler HA *et al.* Body mass index and body girths as predictors of mortality in black and white men. *Am J Epidemiol* 1992; 135(10): 1137–46.

20. Okosun IS, Choi S, Dent MM, Jobin T, Dever GE. Abdominal obesity defined as a larger than expected waist girth is associated with racial/ethnic differences in risk of hypertension. *J Hum Hypertens* 2001; 15(5): 307–12.

21. Seidell JC, Han TS, Feskens EJ, Lean ME. Narrow hips and broad waist circumferences independently contribute to increased risk of non-insulin-dependent diabetes mellitus. *J Intern Med* 1997; 242(5): 401–6.

22. Lissner L, Bjorkelund C, Heitmann BL, Seidell JC, Bengtsson C. Larger hip circumference independently predicts health and longevity in a Swedish female cohort. *Obes Res* 2001; 9(10): 644–6.

23. Cox BD, Whichelow MJ, Prevost AT. The development of cardiovascular disease in relation to anthropometric indices and hypertension in British adults. *Int J Obes Relat Metab Disord* 1998; 22(10): 966–73.

Progress in Obesity Research: 9. Edited by *Geraldo Medeiros-Neto, Alfredo Halpern and Claude Bouchard*
©2003 John Libbey Eurotext Ltd, pp. 639–643.

CHAPTER 133

Alternative anthropometric measures of risk: possible improvements on the waist-hip ratio

Henry S. Kahn

Division of Diabetes Translation, National Center for Chronic Disease Prevention and Health Promotion, US Centers for Disease Control and Prevention (CDC), Atlanta, Georgia 30341, USA
[e-mail: hkahn@cdc.gov]

The concept of a 'waist-hip ratio' (WHR) is now so common in the field of obesity epidemiology that one might fail to remember what this familiar phrase literally means. A WHR requires us to make two specific measurements. But how sure are we that 'waist' circumference is an optimal dimension for estimating 'upper-body' or 'central' mass? Do we know that 'hip' circumference is an optimal dimension for estimating 'lower-body' or 'peripheral' size? Is the hip circumference a useful reference against which to compare waist circumference?

Imagine that we had a fresh opportunity to select the anthropometric dimensions that best represent 'upper' and 'lower' tissue mass for epidemiological purposes while taking into account all that has been learned since WHR was first popularized in 1984[1,2]. Would we still choose WHR as a gauge of disease risk?

To approach this question, I will compare waist circumference with sagittal abdominal diameter (SAD), a measurement that was debated in 1994 at the 7th International Congress on Obesity[3,4]. I will also compare hip circumference with mid-thigh circumference (MTC). For each of these alternative measurements, I will examine the rationale that supports its use, the details of its definition, its emerging reported benefits, and its limitations. Then I will consider using these alternative dimensions in a ratio that might improve on the traditional WHR.

Sagittal abdominal diameter

Researchers in the US have measured SAD in standing subjects by applying a caliper at the level midway between the lower rib margin and the iliac crest[5] or, more recently, at the umbilicus. A French group applied a caliper at the inferior thoracic level[6] (personal communication from Dr. M-A Charles), although it is unclear if their participants were standing or supine. British researchers have also determined the 'minimum' SAD from side-view photographs of standing, unclothed women. No published biological rationale has been provided for SAD protocols in the standing posture.

Measuring SAD in the *supine* posture became more common after Kvist *et al.* reported that the volume of visceral adipose tissue (VAT) was strongly correlated with SAD measured at the L4-L5 level[7]. The subjects of this study had to be recumbent since the investigators used multi-scan, computerized-to-mographic (CT) methods to measure both VAT volume and SAD at several levels. For subjects in the supine posture, increased VAT volume tends to elevate the abdominal wall in the sagittal direction. Subcutaneous anterior or lateral abdominal adipose tissue, however, either compresses the abdomen or tends to flow out at the flanks[8]. For this reason variance in supine SAD might be expected to reflect primarily variance in the volume of VAT. To the extent that supine SAD includes subcutaneous fat, it would be primarily fat from the posterior subcutaneous truncal area. Thus, compared to a standing measurement supine SAD arguably incorporates a more specific estimate of the two adipose depots (visceral and posterior truncal subcutaneous) that are most closely associated with cardiovascular risk. Measured at the level of L4-L5, supine SAD explained about 82 per cent of the variance in VAT volume for both sexes. In comparison, supine SAD at the L3-L4 level explained about 80 per cent of the VAT variance, and waist circumference or WHR explained < 74 per cent of the variance in VAT volume[4,7].

While some investigators have continued to measure supine SAD from CT[9,10] or magnetic-resonance images[11], most researchers do not depend on these expensive technologies for measurement of SAD. Inexpensive bedside methods measure supine SAD as the distance from the examination table to a horizontal ruler placed on the subject's abdomen[12-14] or by employing various sliding-beam calipers (see Fig. 1) for the same purpose[15-22].

The low-technology, caliper measurements of supine SAD appear to be well correlated with VAT volume[18] (r = 0.92), a correlation as strong as Kvist's earlier observation using SAD measured from CT scans. Caliper-measured SAD is also reasonably well correlated with a variety of risk variables (e.g. lipid, insulin, C-peptide, glucose, and uric acid levels; blood pressure, intra-abdominal pressure; lung function; metabolic syndrome; combined risk scores). For these variables, the correlation coefficients for SAD rival or tend to exceed those found using waist circumference in cross-sectional studies[13,14,16,17,20,21]. The superiority of SAD to waist circumference in these cross-sectional studies may be only marginal, however, and might be clearer for male than female research subjects[11,13,14,16,21,22]. Among published cross-sectional studies that compared SAD with waist circumference, the advantages of SAD appear to be strongest when SAD was measured at the level of the iliac crests (i.e. L4-L5)[13,20,22] than at the level of the natural waist[17], at the umbilicus[14,16], or at the largest supine diameter[21]. Longitudinal studies of men have showed that changes in supine SAD were better correlated than changes in waist circumference with the men's changes in VAT volume[23], insulin sensitivity, fat mass, total cholesterol/HDL-cholesterol, and VO_{2max}.[15]

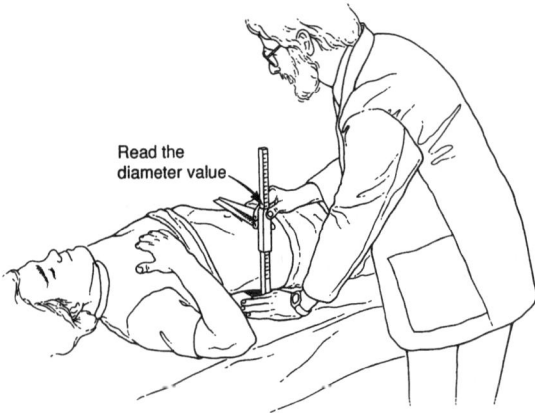

Fig. 1. A sliding-beam caliper for bedside measurement of the supine sagittal abdominal diameter (SAD).

Table 1. Anthropometric comparisons between incident cases of nonfatal coronary heart disease and neighbourhood controls, Atlanta, USA (from Kahn et al.[19])

	Means ± standard deviation		Standardized difference	t value
	Cases	Controls		
Men (N)	(170)	(176)		
Supine SAD, cm	24.3 ± 3.2	23.3 ± 3.5	+0.32	+2.95**
Waist circumference, cm	96.9 ± 10.8	94.5 ± 11.6	+0.21	+1.97*
MTC, cm	50.9 ± 4.9	52.5 ± 5.0	−0.32	−2.94**
Hip circumference, cm	98.8 ± 8.9	98.2 ± 9.7	+0.06	+0.57
SAD/MTC	0.479 ± 0.053	0.444 ± 0.055	+0.65	+6.09***
WTR	1.911 ± 0.196	1.804 ± 0.179	+0.57	+5.28***
WHR	0.980 ± 0.054	0.961 ± 0.057	+0.34	+3.17**
Women (N)	(47)	(85)		
Supine SAD, cm	23.6 ± 3.7	22.4 ± 3.8	+0.32	+1.79
Waist circumference, cm	93.0 ± 13.1	88.3 ± 13.6	+0.35	+1.91
MTC, cm	51.0 ± 6.3	54.1 ± 7.1	−0.46	−2.51*
Hip circumference, cm	100.1 ± 9.5	101.0 ± 11.6	−0.09	−0.48
SAD/MTC	0.465 ± 0.060	0.414 ± 0.049	+0.95	+5.24***
WTR	1.835 ± 0.243	1.638 ± 0.204	+0.90	+4.95***
WHR	0.928 ± 0.085	0.873 ± 0.078	+0.68	+3.77

*$P < 0.05$; **$P < 0.005$; ***$P < 0.0001$.
Abbreviations: SAD = sagittal abdominal diameter; MTC = mid-thigh circumference; WHR = waist circumference/hip circumference; WTR = waist circumference/mid-thigh circumference.

The most important test of an alternative anthropometric dimension, of course, is its ability to predict the incidence of mortality and major diseases. Among men who were measured before about 55 years of age, subsequent mortality due to all causes or to coronary heart disease was associated with their SAD at baseline[5,6]. A positive association between SAD and mortality due to cancer was also identified, but only after adjusting for subcutaneous fat in multivariable analyses[6]. No study has presented data comparing SAD with waist circumference for the prediction of mortality, but reports using standing SAD (men only)[5] and supine SAD (both sexes)[4] have published mortality predictions that compared SAD with WHR. In both of these studies SAD was the superior predictor.

From Atlanta we have reported a case-control study of incident, *non-fatal* coronary heart disease in which we compared the predictive abilities of supine SAD with supine waist circumference[19]. Case subjects were measured early in their hospitalizations. Control subjects free of clinical heart disease were recruited systematically from the community, for the most part, as sex- and age-matched neighbors of the case subjects. Although the cases and controls had nearly identical mean BMI values, the case subjects had larger abdomens than the controls (Table 1). Among men, the case and control groups were discriminated better by their SAD than by their waist circumference. Among women, however, SAD was a slightly weaker discriminator than waist circumference.

Mid-thigh circumference

The complicated anatomy of the hip region makes it difficult to justify measuring hip circumference for the prediction of chronic disease. In addition to important variations in skeletal muscle and adipose tissue, the hip region also includes bony structures of irregular shape (ilium, femoral trochanters) and the pelvic contents. Various landmarks for identifying the hip include the maximum buttocks girth, the anterior superior iliac spine[15], the trochanter level[24], and the level of the iliac crests[1] (elsewhere considered to be the 'waist'[25]!). These alternative definitions may provide strikingly different values for 'hip' circumference[15].

By contrast, a measurement of the mid-thigh circumference (MTC) encompasses little else besides skeletal muscle, subcutaneous (or intramuscular) fat, and the femoral bony shaft. These three tissues in the thigh arguably are analogous to the three tissues (i.e. skeletal muscle, subcutaneous fat, and vertebrae) that surround the intra-abdominal contents. Since the abdomen's compartment of interest is primarily its intra-abdominal component, MTC could serve well as a dimension against which to compare abdominal size.

Instead of measuring thigh circumference at its midpoint (i.e. half way between the midpoint of the inguinal crease and the proximal border of the patella) some have measured the thigh instead at a proximal level immediately below the gluteal fold[13,24,26]. This proximal thigh measurement, however, requires that the tape measure be placed very near the scrotum or labia majora, a procedure that many subjects may find invasive. Alternatively, others have measured thigh circumference at a distal level near the knee[24].

The mid-thigh, however, is probably the most useful point of measurement because it best incorporates the midmuscle zone that reflects muscle mass and exercise experience. Greater muscle mass in the thigh may reflect the benefits of physical activity and may also be a marker for favourable prenatal growth. Birth weight appears to be correlated more strongly with thigh lean tissue than with thigh adipose tissue. If there is an adult cardiovascular benefit to weighing more at birth (the 'fetal origins hypothesis'), it might be mediated by the muscularity of adults who experienced greater prenatal growth in their lower limbs. As growing fetuses, these individuals did not have to restrict their lower-limb tissue development in the interest of protecting their prenatal brain growth. In their subsequent adulthood, large thigh muscles may serve as a major site of increased energy expenditure that protects them against a positive calorie balance and increasing adiposity. By contrast, individuals who as fetuses developed less muscle tissue in their thighs may thereafter experience reduced muscle responsiveness to a fixed insulin signal. Their reduced lower-limb muscularity might help to explain why small size at birth is associated with systemic insulin resistance.

Greater amounts of *adipose* tissue in the thigh may likewise be associated with reduced cardiovascular risk. In contrast to the abdominal location, greater fat mass in the thigh has been associated with a relatively favourable lipid profile in several cross-sectional studies of adults[27]. In thigh subcutaneous fat the expression of mRNA related to resistin is only one fourth as great as its expression in omental or abdominal subcutaneous fat[28].

For both men and women, we found in Atlanta that MTC was inversely associated with incident coronary heart disease whereas hip circumference was not (Table 1)[19]. Of all the available dimensions we found that the strongest discriminator of cases from controls was MTC (inverse association). The next strongest, single-dimension discriminator was supine SAD (positive association). Our multivariable model included the anthropometric dimensions MTC ($t = -6.82$) and supine SAD ($t = +6.64$) simultaneously, along with age, sex and race. We obtained similar results when the model included MTC ($t = -6.67$) and supine waist circumference ($t = +6.26$).

Prospects for an improved anthropometric ratio

This review has provided reasons why a large supine SAD – at least for males – might identify an adverse tissue distribution better than a large waist circumference. There are also reasons why MTC might perform better than hip circumference as a reference or comparison dimension. It should be no surprise then that anthropometric ratios employing MTC in the denominator (i.e. SAD/MTC and WTR) were better predictors of incident, non-fatal, coronary heart disease than WHR that employed hip circumference in the denominator (Table 1)[19]. SAD/MTC and WTR are similarly better predictors, compared to WHR, of *fatal* coronary heart disease[29].

In the Atlanta case-control study we found that neither SAD/MTC nor WTR was associated with height, but WHR was ($r = -0.12$, $P = 0.01$). BMI was positively correlated with WHR, SAD/MTC and WTR ($r = +0.43$, $+0.29$ and $+0.23$), and so was age ($r = +0.16$, $+0.30$, and $+0.40$). After adjustments for multiple risk factors, the superiority of SAD/MTC over WHR in predicting coronary heart disease was eliminated among women, but not among men[19]. With these same multiple adjustments, WTR became slightly superior to SAD/MTC as an independent predictor of coronary heart disease. These changes in predictive ability after adjustments may suggest that SAD/MTC had slightly more co-linearity with traditional cardiovascular risk factors in this population than did WTR. On the other hand, a cross-sectional study of Italians over 66 years old has reported that SAD/MTC had no clear advantage over WHR, SAD, or waist circumference for the prediction of lipid levels, glucose levels, or blood pressure[21].

Waist and hip circumferences have probably retained their popularity because these measurements are well known to most laypersons who buy clothes. But the layperson's casual familiarity with these *nonstandardized* measurements might contribute to lax anthropometric performance in epidemiological or clinical practice. Unlike waist circumference, supine SAD measurement is still unfamiliar to the public and many researchers[3]. SAD measurement has good precision[30], and it does not require the application of tension on a measuring tape. However, the measurement of SAD may be limited by its need for the supine position and for acquiring a bedside caliper. The MTC measurement is also unfamiliar to the public, although it has been part of the US NHANES-III since 1988[25]. (Since 2000 hip circumference has been eliminated from the dimensions collected in NHANES-III.) The MTC also has good precision[30], and it requires no more equipment than the hip circumference. The very novelty of SAD and MTC measurements could serve to make them more reliable than the too-familiar waist and hip measurements.

As of mid-2002, it appears there are net advantages of supine SAD compared with waist circumference, and these advantages might apply also to SAD obtained in the standing position. Evidence suggests also that MTC measurement might have substantial advantages compared with hip circumference for epidemiological or clinical application. Ratios such as SAD/MTC or WTR could likely replace WHR for predicting disease. The research community should finish the task of comparing the predictive utility of these simple anthropometric indices and standardizing the protocols for their use.

Acknowledgement: The thoughts expressed in this paper do not necessarily represent the views of the US Centers for Disease Control and Prevention. A longer version of this paper, including more complete citations, is available as a manuscript on request from the author.

References

1. Larsson B, Svardsudd K, Welin L *et al.* Abdominal adipose tissue distribution, obesity, and risk of cardiovascular disease and death: 13-year follow-up of participants in the study of men born in 1913. *BMJ* 1984; 288: 1401–4.

2. Lapidus L, Bengtsson C, Larsson B *et al.* Distribution of adipose tissue and risk of cardiovascular disease and death: a 12-year follow-up of participants in the population study of women in Gothenburg, Sweden. *BMJ* 1984; 289: 1257–61.

3. Seidell JC. Are abdominal diameters abominable indicators? In: *Progress in Obesity Research: 7*, Angel A, Anderson H, Bouchard C *et al.* (eds), pp. 305–8. London: John Libbey 1996.

4. Sjostrom L, Lonn L, Chowdhury B *et al.* The sagittal diameter is a valid marker of the visceral adipose tissue volume. In: *Progress in Obesity Research: 7* Angel A, Anderson H, Bouchard C *et al.* (eds), pp. 309–19. London: John Libbey, 1996.

5. Seidell JC, Andres R, Sorkin JD, Muller DC. The sagittal waist diameter and mortality in men: the Baltimore Longitudinal Study on Aging. *Int J Obes Relat Metab Disord* 1994; 18: 61–7.

6. Oppert JM, Charles MA, Thibult N *et al.* Anthropometric estimates of muscle and fat mass in relation to cardiac and cancer mortality in men: the Paris Prospective Study. *Am J Clin Nutr* 2002; 75: 1107–13.

7. Kvist H, Chowdhury B, Grangard U, Tylen U, Sjostrom L. Total and visceral adipose-tissue volumes derived from measurements with computed tomography in adult men and women: predictive equations. *Am J Clin Nutr* 1988; 48: 1351–61.

8. Sjostrom L. A computer-tomography based multicompartment body composition technique and anthropometric predictions of lean body mass, total and subcutaneous adipose tissue. *Int J Obes* 1991; 15 (2): 19–30.

9. Pouliot MC, Despres JP, Lemieux S *et al.* Waist circumference and abdominal sagittal diameter: best simple anthropometric indexes of abdominal visceral adipose tissue accumulation and related cardiovascular risk in men and women. *Am J Cardiol* 1994; 73: 460–8.

10. Hill JO, Sidney S, Lewis CE *et al.* Racial differences in amounts of visceral adipose tissue in young adults: the CARDIA (Coronary Artery Risk Development in Young Adults) study. *Am J Clin Nutr* 1999; 69: 381–7.

11. Van der Kooy K, Leenen R, Seidell J, Deurenberg P, Visser M. Abdominal diameters as indicators of visceral fat: comparison between magnetic resonance imaging and anthropometry. *Br J Nutr* 1993; 70: 47–58.

12. Tornaghi G, Raiteri R, Pozzato C *et al.* Anthropometric or ultrasonic measurements in assessment of visceral fat? A comparative study. *Int J Obes Relat Metab Disord* 1994; 18: 771–5.

13. Sjostrom CD, Hakangard AC, Lissner L, Sjostrom L. Body compartment and subcutaneous adipose tissue distribution – risk factor patterns in obese subjects. *Obes Res* 1995; 3: 9–22.

14. Ohrvall M, Berglund L, Vessby B. Sagittal abdominal diameter compared with other anthropometric measurements in relation to cardiovascular risk. *Int J Obes Relat Metab Disord* 2000; 24: 497–501.

15. Houmard JA, McCulley C, Roy LK *et al.* Effects of exercise training on absolute and relative measurements of regional adiposity. *Int J Obes Relat Metab Disord* 1994; 18: 243–8.

16. Weidner MD, Gavigan KE, Tyndall GL, McCammon MR, Houmard JA. Which anthropometric indices of regional adiposity are related to the insulin resistance of aging? *Int J Obes Relat Metab Disord* 1995; 19: 325–30.

17. Richelsen B, Pedersen SB. Associations between different anthropometric measurements of fatness and metabolic risk parameters in non-obese, healthy, middle-aged men. *Int J Obes Relat Metab Disord* 1995; 19: 169–74.

18. Jensen MD, Kanaley JA, Reed JE, Sheedy PF. Measurement of abdominal and visceral fat with computed tomography and dual-energy x-ray absorptiometry. *Am J Clin Nutr* 1995; 61: 274–8.

19. Kahn HS, Austin H, Williamson DF, Arensberg D. Simple anthropometric indices associated with ischemic heart disease. *J Clin Epidemiol* 1996; 49: 1017–24.

20. Gustat J, Elkasabany A, Srinivasan S, Berenson GS. Relation of abdominal height to cardiovascular risk factors in young adults: the Bogalusa heart study. *Am J Epidemiol* 2000; 151: 885–91.

21. Turcato E, Bosello O, Francesco VD *et al.* Waist circumference and abdominal sagittal diameter as surrogates of body fat distribution in the elderly: their relation with cardiovascular risk factors. *Int J Obes Relat Metab Disord* 2000; 24: 1005–10.

22. Harris TB, Visser M, Everhart J *et al.* Waist circumference and sagittal diameter reflect total body fat better than visceral fat in older men and women. The Health, Aging and Body Composition Study. *Ann NY Acad Sci* 2000; 904: 462–73.

23. Marin P, Holmang S, Jonsson L *et al.* The effects of testosterone treatment on body composition and metabolism in middle-aged obese men. *Int J Obes* 1992; 16: 991–7.

24. Callaway CW, Chumlea WC, Bouchard C. Circumferences. In: *Anthropometric standardization reference manual*, Lohman TG, Roche AF, Martorell R (eds), pp. 39–54. Champaign, Illinois: Human Kinetics Publisher, 1988.

25. National Center for Health Statistics Third National Health and Nutrition Examination Survey, 1988–1994, Reference Manuals and Reports (CD-ROM). Centers for Disease Control and Prevention 1996.

26. Seidell JC, Cigolini M, Charzewska J *et al.* Fat distribution in European men: a comparison of anthropometric measurements in relation to cardiovascular risk factors. *Int J Obes* 1992; 16: 17–22.

27. Williams MJ, Hunter G, Kekes-Szabo T, Snyder S, Treuth MS. Regional fat distribution in women and risk of cardiovascular disease. *Am J Clin Nutr* 1997; 65: 855–60.

28. McTernan CL, McTernan PG, Harte AL *et al.* Resistin, central obesity, and type 2 diabetes. *Lancet* 2002; 359: 46–7.

29. Kahn HS, Simoes EJ, Koponen M, Hanzlick R. The abdominal diameter index and sudden coronary death in men. *Am J Cardiol* 1996; 78: 961–4.

30. Williamson DF, Kahn HS, Worthman CM, Burnette JC, Russell CM. Precision of recumbent anthropometry. *Am J Hum Biol* 1993; 5: 159–67.

Progress in Obesity Research: 9. Edited by *Geraldo Medeiros-Neto, Alfredo Halpern* and *Claude Bouchard*
©2003 John Libbey Eurotext Ltd, pp. 644–648.

CHAPTER 134

Body types and health

Peter T. Katzmarzyk, Jean-Pierre Després and Claude Bouchard

School of Physical and Health Education, Queen's University, Kingston, Ontario, Canada; Lipid Research Center, Laval University, St. Foy, Québec, Canada; Pennington Biomedical Research Center, Baton Rouge, Louisiana, USA
[e-mail: katzmarz@post.queensu.ca]

Introduction

The observation that excess adiposity negatively impacts health status and reduces longevity has prompted a dramatic increase in obesity research in recent decades, particularly in light of the current obesity epidemic. Recently, there has been great interest in determining the health risks associated with excess adiposity in specific body fat depots, and technological advances in imaging techniques have made detailed studies of the relation between body fat and health possible in laboratory settings. Historically, the interest was in determining the relationship between morphological characteristics of an individual and biochemical, immunological and psychological markers of health status[1]. Physique, or the overall configuration of the body, is a morphological characteristic that has traditionally been studied in relation to health[2]. In contrast to modern measures of depot-specific body fatness, physique is a holistic measure of one's body type and may have utility in evaluating an individual's global risk of developing metabolic disorders, beyond their level of adiposity. Thus, the purpose of this paper is to review the evidence for a relationship between physique and health status, and to evaluate the efficacy of using measures of physique (somatotype) as an indicator of health risk.

Measurement of physique

Although several measures of physique have been developed, the most comprehensive and widely used index is the somatotype, a three component index including endomorphy, mesomorphy and ectomorphy. There are several methods of estimating somatotype, including the techniques of Sheldon, Parnell, and Heath-Carter[3]; however, the Heath-Carter anthropometric protocol is currently the most widely used[4]. The three components are estimated as follows:

Endomorphy

Endomorphy = $-0.7182 + 0.1451 (X) - 0.00068(X^2) + 0.0000014(X^3)$
where X = [(triceps (mm) + subscapular (mm) + supraspinale (mm) skinfolds) x (170.18/stature (cm))]

Mesomorphy

Mesomorphy = [0.858 x biepicondylar breadth (cm)] + [0.601 x bicondylar breadth (cm)] + [0.188 x CAG] + [0.161 x CCG] – [stature (cm) x 0.131] + 4.50
where CAG = corrected arm girth = flexed arm circumference (cm) minus triceps skinfolds (cm), and CCG = corrected calf girth = maximal calf circumference (cm) minus medial calf skinfold (cm)

Ectomorphy

If SMR = ≥ 40.75, ectomorphy = SMR x 0.732 – 28.58
If SMR < 40.75 but > 38.25, ectomorphy = SMR x 0.463 – 17.63
If SMR = ≤ 38.25, ectomorphy = 0.1
where SMR = stature (cm)/$\sqrt[3]{}$mass (kg)
If any somatotype rating is zero or negative, a value of 0.1 is assigned, as a rating cannot be zero by definition[4].

Somatotype is a three component index, and as such each component should not be considered in isolation without taking into account the other two components. For example, correlations between endomorphy and a risk factor (fasting glucose, cholesterol, etc.) should statistically control for mesomorphy and ectomorphy using partial correlation. Multivariate statistical methods such as MANOVA and canonical correlation are the preferred methods of analysing relations with somatotype[5,6].

The somatotype is a moderately heritable trait that significantly aggregates within families[7-12]. Heritabilities from the available family studies range from 32-68 per cent for the individual somatotype components[9-12]. Further, analysis of a general somatotype index derived from principal components analysis yielded a significant heritability of 64 per cent[12].

Historical studies of physique and health, 1940–69

The study of relationships between physique and health status has a long history in human biology and medicine. Two extremes of body build, one being thin and narrow-chested, and the other being solid and stocky, were recognized by the earliest medical writers. Hippocrates (ca. 460–377 BC) was apparently the first to establish these two extremes of body build, which he called *habitus apoplecticus* and *habitus phthisicus*[13].

Early studies of somatotype and disease were based on the photoscopic somatotyping techniques of Sheldon and colleagues[14]. A series of studies of living and autopsied subjects demonstrated early on that coronary heart disease is more prevalent in mesomorphic individuals and less prevalent in ectomorphic individuals[15-21]. Two early studies also found that blood lipid values were positively related to endomorphy and negatively related to ectomorphy[22-23].

Recent studies of physique and health, 1970 – present

Several recent studies have examined the relationship between somatotype, chronic diseases such as type 2 diabetes and coronary heart disease, and risk factors for chronic diseases. Fredman[24] reported that Tamil diabetics were characterized by higher mesomorphy than controls, and there was a significant positive correlation between mesomorphy and fasting blood glucose levels. In a sample of adults from the Québec Family Study (QFS), those in the upper tertile of the distribution for fasting glucose levels had significantly different somatotypes than those in the lower tertile of the distribution, based on MANOVA[25]. Those in the upper tertile were characterized by higher levels of endomorphy and mesomorphy and lower levels of ectomorphy.

Two recent studies have confirmed and updated the earlier studies of somatotype and blood lipids. Somatotype and blood lipids were significantly related in males but not in females in a study of young (18–25 years old) South Africans[26]. Endomorphic and mesomorphic males had higher total cholesterol and LDL-cholesterol values than ectomorphic males. Further, the first canonical correlation between the somatotype components and blood lipids was significant in the males ($r = 0.42$, $P < 0.01$) but not in the females ($r = 0.31$, NS)[26]. A study of older adults (30–49 years of age) from the QFS indicated that endomorphy was positively correlated with blood lipids in males, and ectomorphy was negatively correlated with blood lipids in females[25]. In general, both males and females in the upper tertile of each risk factor distribution were more endomorphic and mesomorphic and less ectomorphic than those in the lower tertile of the distribution.

Coronary artery stenosis has also been examined in relation to somatotype. Williams *et al.*[27] reported that none of the somatotype components were significantly related to the degree of angiographically determined coronary artery stenosis in a sample of 58 males suspected of having atherosclerosis. However, the sample as a whole showed a limited range of variability in somatotype, with a mean somatotype of high endomorphy (5.7) and mesomorphy (5.6), and low ectomorphy (1.2).

A significant multivariate relationship between somatotype and coronary heart disease risk factors has also been demonstrated in children and youth 9–18 years of age from the QFS[6]. The first canonical correlation between somatotype (endomorphy, mesomorphy, ectomorphy) and risk factors (plasma triglycerides , HDL-cholesterol, LDL-cholesterol and fasting glucose) was 0.29 ($P < 0.001$) in boys and 0.30 ($P < 0.001$) in girls. The pattern of loadings (correlations) from this study (Fig. 1) indicates that a physique characterized by low levels of endomorphy and mesomorphy and high levels of ectomorphy is related to a favourable risk factor profile characterized by low triglycerides, LDL-cholesterol and plasma glucose, and high HDL-cholesterol[6].

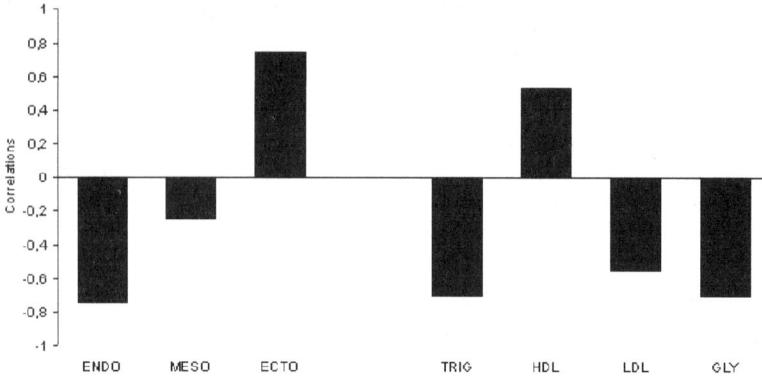

Fig. 1. Correlations between somatotype components, indicators of metabolic fitness and their respective first canonical variates in (a) boys and (b) girls 9–18 years of age from the Québec Family Study. TRIG: triglycerides; HDL: high density lipoprotein cholesterol; LDL: low density lipoprotein cholesterol; GLY: fasting plasma glucose. Adapted from Katzmarzyk *et al. Am J Hum Biol* 1998; 10: 341–350.

Evaluation of physique as a predictor of health risks

Although an association between physique and chronic disease or disease risk factors has been demonstrated in numerous studies as described above, the independence of somatotype from other measures of body composition as a risk factor has yet to be fully delineated. The sum of six subcutaneous skinfolds (SUM) was positively correlated with endomorphy and mesomorphy, and negatively correlated with ectomorphy in youth and adults from the QFS[28]. On the other hand, indicators of subcutaneous adipose tissue (SAT) distribution were largely unrelated to the somatotype components, except in females where a central fat distribution was negatively correlated with mesomorphy. In the same study, SUM, SAT and somatotype components were used to predict coronary heart disease risk factors. All three were significant predictors, together explaining up to 16 per cent of the variance in the risk factors in forward stepwise regression analyses; however, SUM was the best predictor, entering first (most important) in six of 15 significant regressions in males and 14 of 16 significant regressions in females[28].

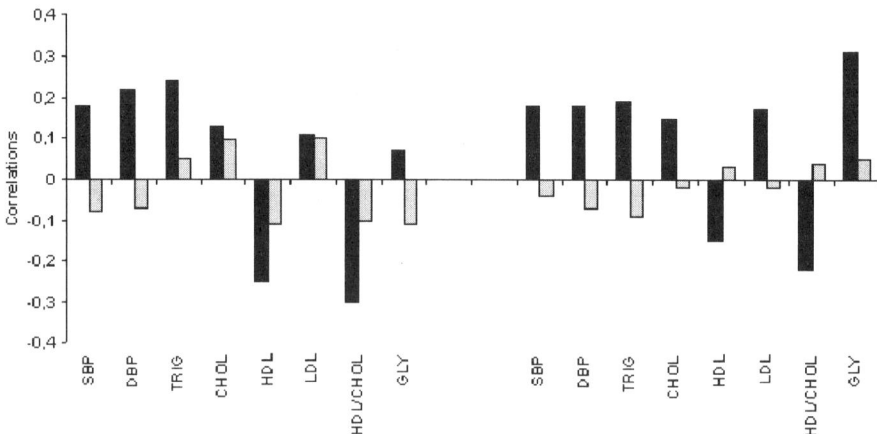

Fig. 2. Correlations between the first principal component of somatotype and risk factors for coronary heart disease in adults from the Québec Family Study. Black bars represent partial correlations controlling for age. Grey bars represent partial correlations adjusted for age and body mass index. SBP: systolic blood pressure; DBP: diastolic blood pressure; TRIG: triglycerides; CHOL: total cholesterol; HDL: high density lipoprotein cholesterol; LDL: low density lipoprotein cholesterol; GLY: fasting plasma glucose.

The body mass index (BMI, kg/m^2) is currently recommended for the identification of overweight and obesity and the associated health risks[29]. In order to examine the influence of BMI on the relationship between somatotype and risk factors for disease in adults (20–60 years of age) from the QFS, principal components analysis was applied to the three somatotype components as described elsewhere[12] and correlations between the first principal component (PC1) and the risk factors were calculated. The correlations were calculated two ways: (1) adjusted for age, and (2) adjusted for age and BMI. PC1 explained 76 per cent of the variance in men and 81 per cent of the variance in women, and was characterized by positive loadings for endomorphy and mesomorphy and a negative loading for ecto-morphy. The correlations between PC1 and the risk factors are presented in Fig. 2. When controlled for age only, PC1 was significantly positively correlated with systolic and diastolic blood pressures, serum triglycerides, total cholesterol and LDL-cholesterol, and negatively correlated with HDL-cholesterol and the ratio of HDL-cholesterol to total cholesterol in both men and women. PC1 was also positively correlated with fasting plasma glucose in women. After further control over BMI, all of the correlations, with the exception of plasma glucose in men, were attenuated, and only the correlations between PC1 and HDL-cholesterol, the HDL-cholesterol to total cholesterol ratio, and plasma glucose were significant in men.

The finding that correlations among somatotype components and risk factors are attenuated after adjustment for BMI is not surprising given that there is considerable covariance among BMI and the individual somatotype components. For example, in the QFS, the correlations with BMI were 0.62 for endomorphy, 0.82 for mesomorphy, –0.87 for ectomorphy and 0.89 for PC1. These results suggest that although somatotype is related to risk factors for heart disease, after control for the BMI, the strength of the relationship is markedly reduced. Thus, the complex measurements and calculations required to derive somatotype may not make it a practical index of CHD risk in comparison with BMI. Further research is required to determine if the holistic approach to examining the relationship between physique and health has clinical implications.

Acknowledgements: The Québec Family Study was supported over the years by the Fonds pour la recherche en santé du Québec (FRSQ), Fonds pour la formation de chercheurs et l'aide à la recherche du Québec (FCAR), Health Canada, and the Medical Research Council of Canada. It is currently supported by the Canadian Institutes for Health Research. Claude Bouchard is funded, in part, by the George A. Bray Chair in Nutrition and Jean-Pierre Després is Chair Professor of Nutrition and Lipidology supported by Parke-Davis/Warner-Lambert and Provigo.

References

1. Damon A. Constitutional medicine. In: *Anthropology and the behavioral health sciences*, Von Mering O, Kasdan L (eds), pp. 179–205. Pittsburgh: University of Pittsburgh Press 1970.

2. Bailey SM. Human physique and susceptibility to noninfectious disease. *Yrbk Phys Anthropol* 1985; 28: 149–73.

3. Malina RM, Bouchard C. Growth, *maturation and physical activity*. Champaign, IL: Human Kinetics 1991.

4. Carter JEL, Heath BH. *Somatotyping – development and applications*. New York: Cambridge University Press, 1990.

5. Cressie NAC, Withers TT, Craig NP. The statistical analysis of somatotype data. *Yrbk Phys. Anthropol* 1986; 29: 197–208.

6. Katzmarzyk PT, Malina RM, Song TMK, Bouchard C. Somatotype and indicators of metabolic fitness in youth. *Am J Hum Biol* 1998; 10(3): 341–50.

7. Song TMK, Malina RM, Bouchard C. Familial resemblance in somatotype. *Am J Hum Biol* 1993; 5: 265–72.

8. Sanchez-Andres A. Genetic and environmental influences on somatotype components: Family study in a Spanish population. *Hum Biol* 1995; 67(5): 727–38.

9. Bouchard C, Demirjian A, Malina RM. Path analysis of family resemblance in physique. *Stud Phys Anthropol* 1980; 6: 61–70.

10. Bouchard C, Demirjian A, Malina RM. Heritability estimates of somatotype components based upon familial data. *Hum Hered* 1980; 30: 112–8.

11. Pérusse L, Leblanc C, Bouchard C. Inter-generation transmission of physical fitness in the Canadian population. *Can J Sport Sci* 1988; 13: 8–14.

12. Katzmarzyk PT, Malina RM, Perusse L, Rice T, Province MA, Rao DC *et al.* Familial resemblance for physique: heritabilities for somatotype components. *Ann Hum Biol* 2000; 27(5): 467–77.

13. Robinson SC, Brucer M. Body build and hypertension. *Arch Intern Med* 1940; 66: 393–417.

14. Sheldon WH, Stevens S, Tucker WB. *The varieties of human physique*. New York: Harper. 1940.

15. Gertler MM, Garn SM, White PD. Young candidates for coronary heart disease. *JAMA* 1951; 147: 621–25.

16. Spain DM, Bradess VA, Huss G. Observations on atherosclerosis of the coronary arteries in males under the age of 46: A necropsy study with special reference to somatotypes. *Ann Intern Med* 1953; 38: 254–77.

17. Gertler MM, White PD. *Coronary heart disease in young adults: a multidisciplinary study.* Cambridge, MA: Harvard University Press. 1954.

18. Spain DM, Bradess VA, Greenblatt IJ. Postmortem studies on coronary atherosclerosis, serum beta lipoproteins and somatotypes. *Am J Med Sci* 1955; 229: 294–301.

19. Spain DM, Nathan DJ, Gellis M. Weight, body type and the prevalence of coronary atherosclerotic heart disease in males. *Am J Med Sci* 1963; 245: 63–8.

20. Damon A. Delineation of the body build variables associated with cardiovascular diseases. *Ann NY Acad Sci* 1965; 126: 711–27.

21. Damon A, Damon ST, Harpending HC, Kannel WB. Predicting coronary heart disease from body measurements of Framingham males. J *Chron Dis* 1969; 21: 781–802.

22. Gertler MM, Garn SM, Sprague HB. Cholesterol, cholesterol esters and phospholipids in health and in coronary artery disease II. Morphology and serum lipids in man. *Circulation* 1950; 2: 380–91.

23. Tanner JM. The relation between serum cholesterol and physique in healthy young men. *J Physiol* 1951; 115: 371–90.

24. Fredman M. Body constitution and blood glucose and serum insulin levels in a group of Tamil Indians. In: *The regulation of the adipose tissue mass*, Vague J, Boyer J (eds), pp. 194–7. New York: American Elsevier; 1974.

25. Malina RM, Katzmarzyk PT, Song TMK, Thériault G, Bouchard C. Somatotype and cardiovascular risk factors in healthy adults. *Am J Hum Biol* 1997; 9: 11–9.

26. Gordon E, Tobias PV, Mendelsohn D, Seftel H, Howson A. The relationship between somatotype and serum lipids in male and female young adults. *Hum Biol* 1987; 59(3): 459–65.

27. Williams SRP, Goodfellow J, Davies B, Bell W, McDowell I, Jones E. Somatotype and angiographically determined athersclerotic coronary artery disease in men. *Am J Hum Biol* 2000; 12(1): 128–38.

28. Katzmarzyk PT, Malina RM, Song TM, Bouchard C. Physique, subcutaneous fat, adipose tissue distribution, and risk factors in the Quebec Family Study. *Int J Obes Relat Metab Disord* 1999; 23(5): 476–84.

29. NIH. Clinical guidelines on the identification, evaluation, and treatment of overweight and obesity in adults – The evidence report. *Obes Res* 1998; 6 (Suppl 2): 51S–209S [published erratum appears in *Obes Res* 1998 Nov; 6(6): 464].

Progress in Obesity Research: 9. Edited by *Geraldo Medeiros-Neto, Alfredo Halpern* and *Claude Bouchard*
©2003 John Libbey Eurotext Ltd, pp. 649–652.

CHAPTER 135

Metabolic syndrome – the role of cytokines

John S. Yudkin

Diabetes and Cardiovascular Risk Academic Unit, University College, London N19 5LW, UK
[e-mail: j.yudkin@ucl.ac.uk]

Type 2 diabetes and impaired glucose tolerance are insulin resistance states, in which skeletal muscle and hepatic actions of insulin show a right shift in the dose response curve[1]. Yet even subjects with normal glucose tolerance demonstrate a wide range of insulin action on glucose metabolism[2]. Moreover, subjects with insulin resistance have been recognized as showing a number of other abnormalities associated with cardiovascular risk, including hypertension and a dyslipidaemia comprising elevated concentrations of triglyceride and low levels of high density lipoprotein (HDL)-cholesterol[3]. The central role of insulin resistance in this syndrome has been proposed[3].

More recently, many other phenotypes, also associated with cardiovascular risk, have been linked to insulin resistance, including impaired fibrinolysis due to elevated levels of plasminogen activator inhibitor-1 (PA1-1)[4], microalbuminuria[5], endothelial dysfunction[6] and hyperfibrinogenaemia[7]. While insulin resistance, or the associated hyperinsulinaemia, might explain the elevated activity of PA1-1, it is more difficult to understand how insulin resistance might explain such phenomena as elevated concentrations of acute phase proteins (fibrinogen), microalbuminuria or endothelial dysfunction.

These observations raise the possibility that the associations described between these phenotypes and insulin resistance is not a consequence, but could represent either cause or the presence of a common antecedent.

Obesity is a powerful determinant of insulin action, and is also associated with many of the metabolic syndrome phenotypes. Thus both endothelial dysfunction[8] and microalbuminuria[9] are linked with obesity, as is hyperfibrinogenaemia[10], in population studies. These observations would suggest that adipose tissue products might play a role in modulating insulin signalling at hepatic, myocyte and adipocyte level, but also might influence other functions in target tissue. Thus endothelial cell nitric oxide synthase in conduit and resistance arteries appears down-regulated in obese subjects[8,11], implying a signalling molecule acting in the systemic circulation. Elevated concentrations of endothelial cell proteins in obese subjects[12] suggest additional capillary actions of such a signal. The elevated concentrations of fibrinogen, as well as of C-reactive protein (CRP)[13] – the archetypal acute phase protein – suggest that in obesity the liver is exposed to high concentrations of circulating pro-inflammatory cytokines.

We have described, in a population study of 107 healthy non-diabetic subjects, associations between composite scores for insulin resistance, endothelial dysfunction and acute phase inflammation[12]. In these subjects, the insulin resistance score and the inflammation score showed a correlation of r = 0.59 (*P* < 0.0001), these associations being little influenced by excluding measures of obesity from the insulin resistance score. More recently, in 32 non-diabetic Pima Indian subjects, we have found powerful associations of both fasting insulin and clamp derived measures of insulin action with concentrations of CRP (Table 1)[14].

More recently, in a case-control study of middle aged men with myocardial infarction, we used factor analysis to explore clustering of insulin resistance and inflammation variables[15]. This technique provided three summary factors, comprising insulin resistance, inflammation and blood pressure. Using a rotation method which permits an exploration of relationships between factors, we found strong and significant correlations between the insulin resistance and the inflammation factor in both cases and controls (Fig. 1), with myocardial infarction cases having higher scores for both insulin resistance and

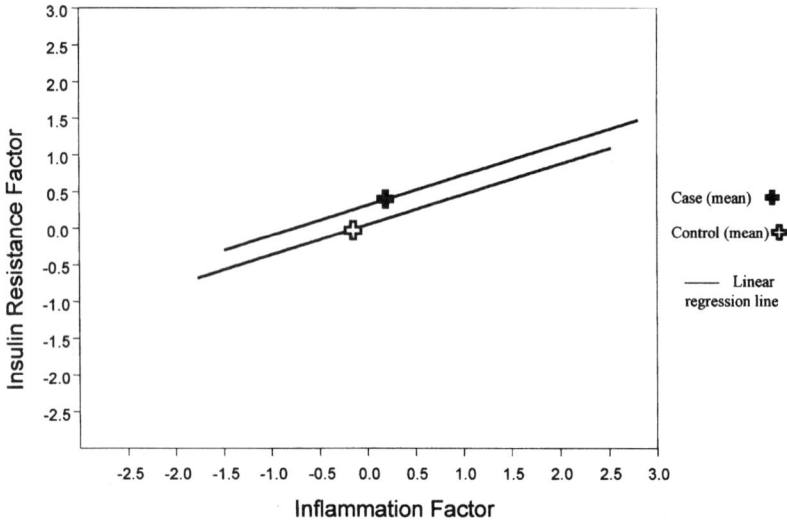

Fig. 1. Scores for obesity/insulin/triglyceride factor and inflammation factor in 364 cases and 331 controls (data from ref.[15]).

inflammation[15]. These observations together suggest that, even in healthy subjects, a state of low grade inflammation exists and is powerfully associated with insulin resistance.

We have explored the possibility that this low grade inflammatory state might be the consequence of asymptomatic infection with a number of agents which have been implicated in the aetiology of coronary heart disease. However when exploring the relationship between circulating inflammatory markers and antibodies to *Chlamydia pneumonie, Helicobacter pylori* and cytomegalvirus, the relationships were weak and inconsistent[12]. Much more powerful were the correlations of levels of these inflammatory markers with measures of body fat (Table 2)[12]. In the Pima Indian Study we found a correlation of 0.85 between levels of CRP and per cent body fat measured by DEXA (Table 1)[14].

Table 1. Correlations of obesity, insulin action and inflammation in 32 Pima Indians (data from ref.[14])

	BMI	% body fat	Fasting insulin	M value	CRP
BMI % body fat	0.83***				
Fasting insulin	0.56**	0.53**			
M value	−0.47**	−0.56**	0.26		
CRP	0.76***	0.85***	0.69***	0.66***	
sPLA$_2$	0.43*	0.41*	0.47**	−0.33	0.54**

Table 2. Relationship of levels of proinflammatory cytokines with antibody titres and obesity (data from ref.[12])

	TNF-α	IL-6	C-reactive protein
Helicobacter pylori titre	0.18	0.28*	0.24*
Chlamydia titre	0.21	0.15	0.25*
Cytomegalovirus titre	0.21	0.17	0.23*
BMI	0.33***	0.19*	0.41***
Waist hip ratio	0.51***	0.41***	0.32**
Subscapular–triceps ratio	0.37***	0.26**	0.21*

We have used the technique of superficial abdominal venous cannulation, combined with arterial sampling, to measure arterio-venous differences of tumour necrosis factor-α (TNF-α) and interleukin 6 (IL-6) across a subcutaneous adipose tissue bed. In 27 subjects we found no evidence of secretion of TNF-α from this adipose bed but abdominal vein concentrations of IL-6 were some 3–4 times higher than arterial concentrations[16]. We estimated, assuming similar IL-6 production in all adipose regions, that up to one third of circulating IL-6 in healthy subjects might derive from adipose tissue. These observations combined suggest that obesity is a low grade inflammatory state.

An important consideration is the distinction between local and systemic actions of cytokines. Tumour necrosis factor-α is powerfully expressed by adipocytes, and influences insulin signalling by inducing serine phosphorylation of the insulin receptor substrate-1, thereby inhibiting insulin action at the adipocyte through autocrine and paracrine mechanisms[17]. However circulating concentrations of TNF-α are unlikely to represent an endocrine signal as these low levels appear to be fully bound to the specific binding proteins[17]. Interleukin 6 is a far more likely candidate for systemic signalling, this being the cytokine, produced in infection and inflammation, which regulates remote hepatic production of CRP and other acute phase proteins. Recent work suggests that IL-6 shares with TNF-α effects on insulin signalling and glucose transport which might also result in insulin resistance at hepatic and skeletal muscle level[18]. Furthermore, as a circulating low grade signal, IL-6 may play a role in endothelial dysfunction and, in turn, in atherogenesis. Weekly injections of interleukin-6 into high fat diet apo-e knockout mice substantially increased plaque formation in these animals[19].

Tissue specific knockout models provide interesting insights into integrative physiology and whole body signalling which can be studied only in intact organisms. Studies from Kahn's group employed adipose tissue-specific GLUT-4 knockouts to induce adipose specific insulin resistance[20]. While isolated hepatocytes and myocytes from these animals showed normal responsiveness to insulin, these tissues were substantially resistant to insulin action *in vivo*[20]. These observations imply that insulin resistance in adipose tissue, even when unrelated to insulin signalling pathways or to inflammation, produces insulin resistance in remote tissues. While dissecting out the particular circulating signal responsible for these changes remains to be completed, the measured concentrations of non-esterified fatty acids (NEFA) in these animals, being lower than in wild type mice, provided no support for the role of NEFA as such signal[20].

In conclusion, obesity appears to be associated with a low grade state of inflammation, probably in consequence of the secretion pro-inflammatory cytokines from adipose tissue beds. These cytokines may well be responsible for inducing many of the components of the insulin resistance syndrome, as well as endothelial dysfunction and, potentially, cardiovascular risk.

References

1. Groop LC, Bonadonna RC, DelPrato S, Ratheiser K, Zyck K, Ferrannini E, DeFronzo RA. Glucose and free fatty acid metabolism in non-insulin-dependent diabetes mellitus. Evidence for multiple sites of insulin resistance. *J Clin Invest* 1989; 84: 205–13.

2. DeFronzo RA, Tobin JD, Andres R. Glucose clamp technique: a method for quantifying insulin secretion and resistance. *Am J Physiol* 1979; 237: E214–E223.

3. Reaven GM. Role of insulin resistance in human disease. Banting Lecture. *Diabetes* 1988; 37: 1595–607.

4. Panahloo A, Yudkin JS. Diminished fibrinolysis in diabetes mellitus and its implication for diabetic vascular disease. *Coronary Artery Disease* 1996; 7: 723–31.

5. Foyle WJ, Carstensen E, Fernandez M, Yudkin JS. A longitudinal study of associations of microalbuminuria with the insulin resistance syndrome and sodium – lithium countertransport in no-diabetic subjects. *Arterioscler Thromb Vasc Biol* 1995; 15: 1330–7.

6. Serne EH, Stehouwer CDA, ter Maaten JC, ter Wee PM, Rauwerda JA, Donker AJM, Gans ROB. Microvascular function relates to insulin sensitivity and blood pressure in normal subjects. *Circulation* 1999; 99: 896–602.

7. Mohamed-Ali V, Gould MM, Gillies S, Goubet S, Yudkin JS, Haines AP. Association of proinsulin-like molecules with lipids and fibrinogen in non-diabetic subjects – evidence against a modulating role for insulin. *Diabetologia* 1995; 38: 1110–6.

8. Steinberg HO, Chaker H, Leaming R, Johnson A, Brechtel G, Baron AD. Obesity/insulin resistance is associated with endothelial dysfunction. Implications for the syndrome of insulin resistance. *J Clin Invest* 1996; 97: 2601–10.

9. Metcalf PA, Scragg RK, Dryson E. Associations between body morphology and microalbuminuria in healthy middle-aged European, Maori and Pacific Island New Zealanders. *Int J Obes Relat Metab Disord* 1997; 21: 203–10.

10. Festa A, D'Agostino R Jr, Williams K, Karter AJ, Mayer-Davis EJ, Tracy RP, Haffner SM. The relation of body fat mass and distribution to markers of chronic inflammation. *Int J Obes Relat Metab Disord* 2001; 25: 1407–15.

11. Arcaro G, Zamboni M, Rossi L, Turcato E, Covi G, Armellini F *et al.* Body fat distribution predicts the degree of endothelial dysfunction in uncomplicated obesity. *Int J Obes Relat Metab Disord* 1999; 23: 936–42.

12. Yudkin JS, Stehouwer CDA, Emeis JJ, Coppack SW. C-reactive protein in healthy subjects: association with obesity, insulin resistance, and endothelial dysfunction. *Arterioscleros Thromb Vasc Biol* 1999; 19: 972–8.

13. Tchernof A, Nolan A, Sites CK, Ades PA, Poehlman ET. Weight loss reduces C-reactive protein levels in obese postmenopausal women. *Circulation* 2002; 105: 564–9.

14. Weyer C, Yudkin JS, Stehouwer CD, Schalkwijk CG, Pratley RE, Tataranni PA. Humoral markers of inflammation and endothelial dysfunction in relation to adiposity and *in vivo* insulin action in Pima Indians. *Atherosclerosis* 2002; 161: 233–42.

15. Yudkin JS, Juhan-Vague I, Hawe E, Humphries SE, di Minno G, Margaglione M, Tremoli E *et al.* on behalf of the HIFMECH Study Group. The insulin resistance syndrome and inflammatory markers in relation to myocardial infarction in the north and south of Europe (HIFMECH Study) (submitted).

16. Mohamed-Ali V, Goodrick S, Rawesh A, Katz D, Miles JM *et al.* Subcutaneous adipose tissue secretes interleukin-6 but not tumour necrosis factor-α *in vivo. J Clin Endo Metab* 1997; 82: 4196–200.

17. Hotamisligil GS, Spiegelman BM. Tumor necrosis factor a: a key component of the obesity-diabetes link. *Diabetes* 1994; 43: 1271–8.

18. Bastard JP, Maachi M, Van Nhieu JT, Jardel C, Bruckert E, Grimaldi A *et al.* Adipose tissue IL-6 content correlates with resistance to insulin activation of glucose uptake both *in vivo* and *in vitro. J Clin Endocrinol Metab* 2002; 87: 2084–9.

19. Huber SA, Sakkinen P, Conze D, Hardin N, Tracy R. Interleukin-6 exacerbates early atherosclerosis in mice. *Arterioscler Thromb Vasc Biol* 1999; 19: 2364–7.

20. Abel ED, Peroni O, Kim JK, Kim YB, Boss O, Hadro E *et al.* Adipose-selective targeting of the GLUT4 gene impairs insulin action in muscle and liver. *Nature* 2001; 409: 729–33.

Progress in Obesity Research: 9. Edited by *Geraldo Medeiros-Neto, Alfredo Halpern and Claude Bouchard*
©2003 John Libbey Eurotext Ltd, pp. 653–656.

CHAPTER 136

Physiological basis of the metabolic syndrome

Richard N. Bergman, Stella P. Kim, Martin Ellmerer, Katrin Huecking, Lisa Getty, Morvarid Kabir, Viorica Ionut, Joyce Richey, Steven Mittelman, Gregg Van Citters and Marilyn Ader

Department of Physiology and Biophysics, Keck School of Medicine, University of Southern California,
Los Angeles 90033, USA
[e-mail: rbergman@usc.edu]

Introduction

There is abundant evidence that adiposity about the visceral organs imparts particular risk for chronic diseases, including not only diabetes, but also hypertension, dyslipidaemia, cardiovascular disease, and colon cancer[1-3]. Yet, the explanation for these associations remains unclear. It appears that insulin resistance may be the link between visceral adiposity and disease, as there is a stronger association between insulin resistance and visceral adiposity than between resistance and adiposity *per se*[4,5].

The mechanism(s) which can account for the relation between visceral fat and insulin resistance are far from clear. It was suggested by Arner and others some years ago that the close physical relationship between the visceral fat depot and the liver might be an important factor[6-8]. The potential exists for delivery of moieties from the adipose tissue stored in the omental circulation directly to the liver, which could induce insulin resistance. While free fatty acids (FFA) are an obvious candidate for inducing insulin resistance, it is now known that a variety of peptides, or 'adipokines' are secreted from the fat cell which could play a role in inducing insulin resistance. Among possible candidates for mediating insulin resistance besides FFA are IL-6, TNF-α, and possibly resistin[9-11]. Alternatively, low levels of the protein adiponectin might play a role[12,13]. Thus, the signaling between the visceral fat depot and insulin sensitive tissues remains to be clarified to explain insulin resistance of the individual with visceral fat.

Canine model

The vast majority of information regarding metabolic syndrome is either associative, or cross sectional. This is true because human subjects generally are studied while the visceral fat depot is extant, and rodent models are difficult to study longitudinally. Therefore, in our laboratory we have exploited the canine model, which enables us to examine metabolic changes while visceral adiposity is developing[14]. In a series of studies we have examined events over 12-week period in which the animals are exposed to a diet elevated in fat. Diets have been either isocaloric, with fat content increased from 36 per cent to 45 per cent (1390–1770 kcal/day) but total calories maintained at the animals 24-h caloric need, or hypercaloric, in which daily fat was ramped up to 2870 kcal/day (54 per cent of daily intake) and total calories in excess of caloric need. Our goal was to follow the development of obesity in these animals, and measure temporally factors which might either cause or be a result of increased adiposity.

Overall, our animals were not obese when first examined (mean per cent adiposity: 16.9 ± 3.3; range: 9.2 to 32.3 per cent). However, increasing the percentage of fat intake to 45 per cent *without* increasing calories (decrease in carbohydrate and protein) had profound effects. Despite little increase in overall body weight (+ 5.5 ± 2.7 per cent; not significant in 6 animals), we found an increase in the intraperitoneal fat depot of 69 per cent, as revealed by magnetic resonance imaging (MRI). We observed a stereotypical metabolic response to increased fat intake: overall insulin sensitivity assessed by hyperinsulinaemic euglycaemic clamp was reduced by 34 per cent. There was an appropriate response which prevented glucose intolerance: a combination of hyperinsulinaemia (basal insulin increased by 68 per cent) as well as a reduction in first-pass hepatic insulin clearance, which reduced from 60 per cent to 44 per cent.

To separate out effects on the liver from systemic effects we performed euglycaemic clamps after 6 or 12 weeks of isocaloric elevated fat intake. The results were dramatic: we observed little change in peripheral insulin resistance; in stark contrast were the effects on liver. Under control conditions during glucose clamps elevated insulin suppressed glucose production to zero, demonstrating the expected exquisite sensitivity of the liver to insulin. Reduction of glucose output was mirrored by suppression of plasma FFA. After 6 week of fat diet, liver was still sensitive to insulin, and during clamps, complete suppression still occurred. More striking was the *total* resistance of the liver to insulin after 12 weeks of elevated but isocaloric diet. Thus, total resistance of the liver to insulin (with respect to glucose metabolism) appears to be a primary defect which can be observed to develop over a 12-week period despite the relative lack of peripheral insulin resistance.

Causes of hepatic resistance

What is the cause of the total resistance of the liver? Several phenomenon were consistent with the 'portal hypothesis', viz. that increased flux of FFA to the liver is responsible for the hepatic resistance. Steven Mittelman in our laboratory has performed insulin dose-response studies and measured net lipolysis of the visceral fat depot compared to total lipolysis[15]. The ED50 of visceral fat was 2.4 times higher than total fat. It can be calculated that during meals suppression of lipolysis in response to insulin would be only 37 per cent whereas suppression of peripheral lipolysis would be much greater ($\sim$ 60–70 per cent). Thus, the liver remains potentially exposed to elevated FFA for 24 h per day due to the particular insulin resistance of the visceral depot. Consistent with this exposure are the deposition of triglyceride in the liver (increased $\sim$ 40 per cent) as well as the expression of rate-limiting proteins in the visceral depot and liver. Dr. Kabir in our laboratory partially cloned (for the first time in the dog) several rate limiting enzymes in visceral depot and liver. Results are consistent with increased visceral fat turnover (increased expression of hormone sensitive lipase, lipoprotein lipase and PPAR-γ) and reduced insulin sensitivity of liver (increased gluconeogenic enzymes glucose-6-phosphatase and PEP carboxykinase). These results are consistent with flux of FFA from visceral depot to liver being responsible for the 'metabolic syndrome' in the dog with moderate increase in dietary fat. We have yet to demonstrate definitively that the actual *flux* of FFA to the liver is increased in this dog model; such a demonstration requires not only measurements of FFA in the portal circulation to the liver, but blood flow measurements as well. Such studies are ongoing.

Role of the sympathetic nervous system

We have recently reported an additional phenomenon which is consistent with the portal hypothesis: direct sympathetic regulation of the visceral fat depot. We recently reported the results obtained by Lisa Getty in our laboratory, who first demonstrated bursts of lipolysis from the visceral adipose depot with approximately one burst every 9–11 min in the fasting state[16]. We showed these bursts to be independent of any cycles of plasma insulin: suppression of the insulin cycles during clamps, if anything increased the magnitude of the FFA pulses. Dr. Getty's results have been extended recently by Katrin Huecking, who has exploited the deconvolution technique to calculate minute-to-minute rates of lipolysis. Dr. Huecking has not only confirmed the existence of the lipolytic bursts, but she has demonstrated that they are mediated via the sympathetic nervous system. The high-affinity blocking agent bupranalol *totally suppressed* the FFA oscillations; yet, basal 'sub-oscillatory' lipolysis continues unabated. These data support the sympathetic nervous system as playing a central role in the presumed increased flux of FFA from the visceral depot to the liver. This sympathetically-driven flux can be expected to further exacerbate the exposure of the liver to elevated FFA when visceral adiposity is increased, and contribute mightily to the metabolic syndrome; i.e. hepatic insulin resistance induced by increased fat in the diet.

But, in human subjects we observe not just hepatic but also substantial peripheral insulin resistance. Do we observe this in the canine model?

Martin Ellmerer has recently completed studies confirming that an *hypercaloric* elevated diet will induce substantial peripheral as well as liver insulin resistance. In fact, with fat intake increased to 54 per cent, and daily calories increased by 33 per cent, insulin sensitivity observed during clamps was reduced 43 per cent.

The results summarized here appear to support the portal hypothesis. Increased fat in the diet – even in the absence of increased calories – generates a syndrome of compensated insulin resistance. Several pathophysiological factors appear to conspire to increase the flux of FFA from the visceral adipose depot to the liver and may induce insulin resistance.

The adipokine hypothesis

Traditionally the adipocyte was considered a relatively benign tissue, which stored fat as triglycerides and released it as FFA. Recently it has become clear that the fat cell can release a plethora of proteins which may well be signals. Thus, the adipocyte can be considered an endocrine organ, in that it releases compounds which flow in the bloodstream and which can be sensed and influenced by distant organs or tissues. It is then important to question whether it may not be lipid itself – FFA – which represent the villain which coverts visceral fat to liver insulin resistance, or whether it is a still underappreciated protein villain secreted by the adipocyte.

There are many candidates for the role of 'villain of the metabolic syndrome'. Among these are the previously stated TNF-α, leptin, resistin, adiponectin (inverse with insulin resistance), and possibly others. It has been estimated that there may be 80–90 different proteins secreted by the adipose cell (B. Corkey, personal communication), most of which remain unidentified. In addition, increases in these adipose cell cytokines have been reported in insulin resistant states, including the metabolic syndrome[17].

Our preliminary data has not supported a separate role of adipokines in the insulin resistance we have observed in the fat-fed dog model. However, it may be that flux of FFA may be a first line of damage which causes insulin resistance, particularly of the liver, and so-called adipokines may mediate either hepatic or peripheral insulin resistance under more chronic conditions of obesity. Further studies of the effects of specific proteins on insulin action in liver and other tissues is clearly warranted.

Last comment

In Westernized countries the increased prevalence of obesity has been associated with endemic increases in disease, including not only diabetes but cardiovascular disease and cancer. Approaches to therapy can include reduction in obesity, which has been a great challenge, treatment of the diseases, or breaking the link between increased fat, insulin resistance and the associated syndrome. Our approach has been to understand not only *if*, but also *why* increased visceral adiposity in particular leads to insulin resistance. We hope that such studies will lead to points of intervention by behavioural or pharmacological approaches which will lessen the burden of adiposity on the health and longevity of the organism.

Reference

1. Vanhala MJ, Pitkajarvi TK, Kumpusalo EA, Takala JK. Obesity type and clustering of insulin resistance-associated cardiovascular risk factors in middle-aged men and women. *Int J Obes Relat Metab Disord* 1998; 22: 369–74.

2. Larsson B, Bengtsson C, Bjorntorp P, Lapidus L, Sjostrom L, Svardsudd K *et al*. Is abdominal body fat distribution a main explanation for the sex difference in the incidence of myocardial infarction? *Am J Epidemiol* 1993; 135: 266–73.

3. Giovannucci E. Insulin, insulin-like growth factors and colon cancer: a review of the evidence. *J Nutr* 2001; 131(11): S3109–S3120.

4. Carey DG, Jenkins AB, Campbell LV, Freund J, Chisholm DJ. Abdominal fat and insulin resistance in normal and overweight women: direct measurements reveal a strong relationship in subjects at both low and high risk of NIDDM. *Diabetes* 1996; 45: 633–8.

5. Lillioja S, Bogardus C. Obesity and insulin resistance: lessons learned from the Pima Indians. *Diab Metab Rev* 1988; 5: 517–40.

6. Vague J. La differenciation sexuelle, facteur determinant des formes de l'obesity. *Presse Méd* 1947; 30: 339–40.

7. Bjorntorp P. Metabolic implications of body fat distribution. *Diab Care* 1991; 14: 1132–43.

8. Arner, P. Role of antilipolytic mechanisms in adipose tissue distribution and function in man. *Acta Med Scand Suppl* 1988; 723: 147–52.

9. Mohamed-Ali V, Goodrick S, Rawesh A, Katz DR, Miles JM, Yudkin JS *et al*. Subcutaneous adipose tissue releases interleukin-6, but not tumor necrosis factor-alpha, *in vivo*. *J Clin Endocrinol Metab* 1997; 82: 4196–200.

10. Hotamisligil GS, Shargill NS, Spiegelman BM. Adipose expression of tumor necrosis factor-α: direct role in obesity-linked insulin resistance. *Science* 1993; 259: 87–91.

11. Steppan CM, Bailey ST, Bhat S, Brown EJ, Banerjee RR, Wright CM *et al.* The hormone resistin links obesity to diabetes. *Nature* 2001; 409: 307–12.

12. Berg AH, Combs TP, Du X, Brownlee M, Scherer PE. The adipocyte-secreted protein Acrp30 enhances hepatic insulin action. *Nature Med* 2001; 7: 947–53.

13. Yamauchi T, Kamon J, Waki H, Terauchi Y, Kubota N, Hara K *et al.* The fat-derived hormone adiponectin reverses insulin resistance associated with both lipoatrophy and obesity. *Nature Med* 2001; 7: 941–6.

14. Mittelman SD, van Citters GW, Kim SP, Davis DA, Dea MK, Bergman RN. The longitudinal compensation for fat induced insulin resistance includes reduced insulin clearance and enhanced B-cell response. *Diabetes* 2000; 49: 2116–25.

15. Mittelman SD, van Citters GW, Kirkman EL, Bergman RN. Extreme insulin resistance of the central adipose depot *in vivo*. *Diabetes* 2002; 51: 755–61.

16. Getty L, Panteleon AE, Mittelman SD, Dea MK, Bergman RN. Rapid oscillations in omental lipolysis are independent of changing insulin levels *in vivo*. *J Clin Invest* 2000; 106: 421–30.

17. Fruhbeck G, Gomez-Ambrosi J, Muruzabal FJ, Burrell MA. The adipocyte: a model for integration of endocrine and metabolic signaling in energy metabolism regulation. *Am J Physiol* 2001; 280: E827–E847.

CHAPTER 137

Impact of obesity on endothelial function and thrombogenic profile

Rainer Rauramaa and Sari B.Väisänen

Kuopio Research Institute of Exercise Medicine, Haapaniementie 16, FIN-70100 Kuopio, Finland
[e-mail: rainer.rauramaa@messi.uku.fi]

Obesity is an independent risk factor for cardiovascular diseases, although the pathophysiologic mechanisms are not yet fully understood. The importance of overweight and obesity have been easily overlooked with the understanding that most, if not all, of the mortality and morbidity were mediated by obesity associated risk factors such as high blood pressure and hyperlipidaemias. The understanding of adipose tissue as a metabolically active tissue rather than merely a passive fat storage has opened a new avenue in research. Obesity is characterized by endothelial dysfunction and the ensuing atherothrombosis. This short review is focused on physical exercise induced changes in endothelial function and the thrombogenecity with regard to body adiposity. Data are still scarce and therefore randomized controlled trials are needed for the identification of optimal exercise programmes to alleviate many obesity associated health problems and morbid consequences. For a more detailed review on endothelial function in obesity, the reader is referred to a recent paper by Williams and coworkers[1].

Obesity, endothelial function and thrombogenesis

Endothelial dysfunction, an early stage in the development of atherosclerosis, is in fact a broad term covering various aspects in vascular pathophysiology. A culminating point is impaired release and function of nitric oxide, secreted by the vascular endothelium. Oxidative stress, due to excessive amounts of superoxide anion, has been considered as a key mechanism for the reduced bioavailability of nitric oxide. Post-prandial hypertriglyceridaemia and hyperglycaemia, both common consequences of obesity associated insulin resistance, induce oxidative stress and ensuing endothelial dysfunction[2]. A major contributor to obesity associated endothelial dysfunction is due to the endocrine role of adipose tissue. Adipocytes secrete a proinflammatory cytokine, tumour necrosis factor alpha (TNF-alpha), circulating levels of which increase up to threefold in obese subjects[3]. Elevated TNF-alpha inhibits the production of endothelial nitric oxide synthase, which may be mediated through an action on insulin metabolism keeping up with oxidative stress. TNF-alpha is also a major inducer of interleukin-6 (IL-6). These cytokines induce hepatic production of acute phase proteins of which high sensitivity C reactive protein (hsCRP), a marker of low-grade systemic inflammation, is a powerful predictor of acute myocardial infarction[4]. TNF-alpha also contributes to the increased circulating levels of insulin and another pro-inflammatory cytokine, transforming growth factor beta (TGF-beta). Chronic elevation of proinflammatory factors and acute phase proteins alone, or in concert with traditional risk factors, lead to endothelial dysfunction.

TNF-alpha, insulin and TGF-beta induce production of plasminogen activator inhibitor type 1 (PAI-1) from endothelium and adipose tissue. Insulin resistance associates with elevated plasminogen activator inhibitor-1 (PAI-1), the primary physiological inhibitor of fibrinolytic system and a powerful thrombogenic risk factor. Furthermore, obesity increases factor VII coagulant activity (FVIIc) and endothelium-derived von Willebrandt factor, thereby interfering with a balance between blood coagulation and fibrinolysis.

Activation of platelets is an early phase in thrombogenesis. Obesity is characterized by increased secretion of leptin, a hormone synthesized primarily in adipocytes and acting on hypothalamic receptors to reduce energy intake and increase energy expenditure. Leptin has a stimulatory effect on platelet aggregation and may thus contribute to acute syndromes in obesity. Recent experimental studies in transgenic mouse provide new insights into the molecular basis of cardiovascular complications in obese subjects. Intraperitoneal injection of leptin into leptin deficient, but not in leptin receptor-deficient mouse shortened the occlusion time after vascular injury, indicating the receptors on platelet mediate the effects of leptin[5]. Weight loss reduces plasma leptin level, while physical exercise without weight decrease does not influence leptin secretion[6].

Effects of physical exercise in postprandial state

Raised level of free fatty acids, a common finding in obese subjects, are harmful to vascular endothelium[7]. Prolonged and frequent postprandial hyperlipaemia and hyperglycaemia cause endothelial dysfunction, and after a long-term exposure lead to atherosclerotic complications. Beneficial effects of physical exercise on blood lipids are well known. However, few data deal with a physiologically more important aspect of postprandial lipaemia.

Hardman and co-workers have studied systematically various determinants of exercise on postprandial lipaemia. Exercise intensity, at constant energy consumption, does not seem to be a key determinant with regard to exercise-induced effects on postprandial lipaemia, at least in young healthy normolipidaemic subjects[8]. To answer the practically valuable question whether exercise needs to be accomplished in one continuous session, or whether several shorter bouts carry similar effects on postprandial lipaemia was investigated[9]. The exercise sessions were either one 90-min session or three separate 30-min sessions at the same moderate intensity level. Both exercise sessions induced approximately 18 per cent lower lipaemic response to a high-fat meal compared with the control study. Moreover, serum insulin response was lower in the intermittent (three exercise bouts) trial compared with the control period. This finding may give some tips as to the frequency of daily exercise sessions. To clarify the issue of fractionation of exercise into a very short periods, sedentary postmenopausal women and in sedentary men walked 30 min briskly, either in one session, or for three separate 10-min exercise bouts. Exercise in either way influenced similarly postprandial lipaemia induced by three meal during the day-long trial[10]. Again, a good message for obese subjects: even short periods of physical activity will bring clear health benefits. Finally, to compare effects of energy consumption with an equivalent energy intake deficit, Gill and Hardman[11] studied postmenopausal women after a control period, after brisk walking for 90 min, and after energy intake restriction. After overnight fasting, the subjects ate a high-fat meal, whereafter blood samples were taken hourly for six hours. As might be expected, exercise reduced postprandial lipaemia significantly, by approximately 20 per cent, while the effect of energy intake restriction did not differ from that of a control period.

Physical exercise improves glucose tolerance and increases insulin sensitivity in healthy subjects[12] as well as in insulin-resistant subjects[13]. This effect has been thought to be due to increased insulin-stimulated glycogen synthesis in skeletal muscle, as well as due to an increase in insulin-stimulated glucose transport-phosphorylation, whereas insulin secretion remains unaffected. During a frequently sampled intravenous glucose tolerance test in healthy non-obese subjects, bicycle exercise at low intensity level decreased blood glucose level below the resting level after 15 min of exercise. Plasma insulin curve followed essentially the glucose curve[12]. High-intensity physical exercise in post-prandial state is accompanied by temporary hyperglycaemia, which however is of smaller magnitude and of shorter duration compared to post-absorptive state[14]. Even if the beneficial effects of physical exercise both in healthy subjects, as well as in those suffering of derangements in glucose metabolism have been known for long time, no such systematic series of studies comparable to the above reports on lipid metabolism seem to be available on postprandial glucose metabolism.

Accumulation of several traits of the metabolic syndrome increases the risk for cardiovascular complications substantially. In this regard the recent study[15] is the most update and important, despite limitations in the study design. Exercise training three times a week for 12 weeks at a relatively high intensity improved endothelial function in subjects with the metabolic syndrome. Obviously, these results need to be replicated in post-prandial conditions in subjects with different degrees of adiposity using variable exercise doses and modes (aerobic exercise, resistance exercise) for optimal exercise prescription to improve endothelial function and prevent thrombogenesis.

Data suggest that regular physical exercise decreases TNF-alpha system activity which may increase insulin sensitivity in obese women with impaired glucose tolerance[16]. However, additional data from randomized controlled trials are needed to confirm the results.

Regular exercise training may decrease PAI-1 level at least in sedentary young men and in elderly men[17], but no corresponding data are available in obese subjects. Strenuous exercise activates platelets acutely, while moderate exercise has a suppressing effect on platelet aggregation in young healthy men. Regular physical activity reduces platelet aggregability in overweight middle-aged men, and in young men and women of normal body weight[17].

References

1. Williams IL, Wheatcroft SB, Shah AM, Kearney MT. Obesity, atherosclerosis and the vascular endothelium: mechanisms of reduced nitric oxide bioavailability in obese humans. *Int J Obes* 2002; 26: 754–64.

2. Ceriello A, Taboga C, Tonutti L, Quagliaro L, Piconi L, Bais B *et al*. Evidence for an Independent and Cumulative Effect of Postprandial Hypertriglyceridemia and Hyperglycemia on Endothelial Dysfunction and Oxidative Stress Generation. *Circulation* 2002; 106: 1211–8.

3. Winkler G, Lakatos P, Salamon F, Nagy Z, Speer G, Kovacs M *et al*. Elevated serum TNF-alpha level as a link between endothelial dysfunction and insulin resistance in normotensive obese patients. *Diabetes Med* 1999; 16: 207–11.

4. Ridker M. High-sensitivity C-reactive Protein. Potential adjunct for global risk assessment in primary prevention of cardiovascular disease. *Circulation* 2001; 103: 1813–18.

5. Konstantinides S, Schäfer K, Koschnick S, Loskutoff DJ. Leptin-dependent platelet aggregation and arterial thrombosis suggests a mechanism for atherothrombotic disease in obesity. *J Clin Invest* 2001; 108: 1533–40.

6. Thong FSL, Hudson R, Ross R, Janssen I, Graham TE. Plasma leptin in moderately obese men: independent effects of weight loss and aerobic exercise. *Am J Physiol Endocrinol Metab* 2000; 279: E307–E313.

7. Steinberg HO, Baron AD. Vascular function, insulin resistance and fatty acids. *Diabetologia* 2002; 45: 623–34.

8. Tsetsonis NV, Hardman AE. Reduction in postprandial lipemia after walking: influence of exercise intensity. *Med Sci Sports Exerc* 1996; 28: 1235–42.

9. Gill JM, Murphy MH, Hardman AE. Postprandial lipemia: effects of intermittent versus continuous exercise. *Med Sci Sports Exerc* 1998; 30: 1515–20.

10. Murphy MH, Nevill AM, Hardman AE. Different patterns of brisk walking are equally effective in decreasing postprandial lipaemia. *Int J Obes Relat Metab Disord* 2000; 24: 1303–9.

11. Gill JM, Hardman AE. Postprandial lipemia: effects of exercise and restriction of energy intake compared. *Am J Clin Nutr* 2000; 71: 465–71.

12. Araujo-Vilar D, Osifo E, Kirk M, Garcia-Estevez DA, Cabezas-Cerrato J, Hockaday TD. Influence of moderate physical exercise on insulin-mediated and non-insulin-mediated glucose uptake in healthy subjects. *Metabolism*. 1997; 46: 203–9.

13. Perseghin G, Price TB, Petersen KF, Roden M, Cline GW *et al*. Increased glucose transport-phosphorylation and muscle glycogen synthesis after exercise training in insulin-resistant subjects. *N Engl J Med* 1996; 335: 1357–62.

14. Kreisman SH, Manzon A, Nessim SJ, Morais JA, Gougeon R *et al*. Glucoregulatory responses to intense exercise performed in the postprandial state. *Am J Physiol* Endocrinol Metab 2000; 278: E786–E793.

15. Lavrencic A, Salobir BG, Keber I. Physical training improves flow-mediated dilation in patients with the polymetabolic syndrome. *Arterioscler Thromb Vasc Biol* 2000; 20: 551–5.

16. Straczkowski M, Kowalska I, Dzienis-Straczkowska S, Stepien A, Skibinska E, Szelachowska M, Kinalska I. Changes in tumor necrosis factor-alpha system and insulin sensitivity during an exercise training programme in obese women with normal and impaired glucose tolerance. *Eur J Endocrinol* 2001; 145: 273–80.

17. Rauramaa R, Väisänen SB. Physical activity in the prevention and treatment of a thrombogenic profile in the obese: current evidence and research issues. *Med Sci Sports Exerc* 1999; (31): S631–S634.

Progress in Obesity Research: 9. Edited by *Geraldo Medeiros-Neto, Alfredo Halpern* and *Claude Bouchard*
©2003 John Libbey Eurotext Ltd, pp. 660–663.

CHAPTER 138

Obesity and lipid cardiovascular risk factors

Benoît Lamarche

Canada Research Chair in Nutrition, Functional Foods and Cardiovascular Health, Institute on Nutraceuticals and Functional Foods, Laval University, Québec, Canada
[e-mail: benoit.lamarche@inaf.ulaval.ca]

Introduction

Obesity has reached epidemic proportions in industrialized countries and medical authorities now worry about the perverse impact that this will have on the population's health as well as societal costs in future years[1]. Obesity may be perceived as a very simple condition attributable to disequilibrium between energy intake and energy expenditure. While this may be fundamentally the case, the scientific community is now more and more recognizing the fact that obesity is very complex in its nature. For example, many obese patients may never develop chronic diseases such as cardiovascular disease or type 2 diabetes. The complex components of obesity make it a rather unique, puzzling and challenging problem to investigate and treat.

The concept that all obesities were not 'created equal' was first put forward by a French investigator, Dr. Jean Vague, in the middle of the 20th-century. Dr. Vague's pioneer work suggested that a preferential accumulation of fat in the abdominal area, the so-called android obesity, was associated with significant health risks that were not observed as frequently among patients accumulating fat in the gluteo-femoral area (gynoid obesity)[2]. It was only 30 years later that investigators followed up on these unique observations and provided supporting evidence to the fact that abdominal obesity was indeed one of the key conditions leading to a series of metabolic alterations predictive of an increased risk of cardiovascular disease and type 2 diabetes[3].

The objective of this short review paper is to summarize some of the evidence indicating that obesity, and in particular abdominal obesity, is a common denominator for a series of metabolic deteriorations related to intravascular lipid metabolism that lead to marked elevations in the risk of cardiovascular disease.

Obesity vs. insulin resistance

It is rather difficult to dissociate abdominal obesity from insulin resistance. The concept of insulin resistance has been recognized for several years when Himsworth and Kerr have documented that patients with diabetes could be categorized into insulin sensitive and insulin resistant subgroups, the latter being more prone to having type 2 diabetes[4]. It was only in the late 1980s that Gerald Reaven proposed that a significant proportion of apparently healthy individuals was characterized by a typical dyslipidaemic state that included high plasma triglyceride (TG) and low HDL cholesterol levels, along with hypertension[5]. His hypothesis was that these metabolic and physiologic alterations were attributable to the presence of a systemic insulin resistance state. This insulin resistance syndrome was first referred to as Syndrome X and has been subsequently extensively investigated over the last 14 years. It has been recently shown that the insulin resistance syndrome may be found in as much as 25 per cent of the American adult population, with numbers rocketing to approximately 45 per cent in men older than 65 years[6]. Interestingly, the initial concept of the insulin resistance syndrome (IRS) did not include obesity as one of its components. In recent years, however, it has been clearly shown that obesity, and particularly abdominal obesity, was one of the key features accompanying insulin resistance and its dysmetabolic state[7]. Whether abdominal obesity precedes the appearance of insulin resistance or *vice versa* remains a matter of much debate and it is beyond the purpose of this short review to comment on this controversy. However, one fact remains virtually beyond debate: abdominal obesity and insulin resistance states are hardly dissociable, with both contributing to increasing the risks of cardiovascular disease through several common metabolic perturbations.

The dyslipidaemic state of obesity

Clinicians have for many years downplayed the importance of TG in managing cardiovascular risk. This was mainly due to the fact that scientists were entangled in a statistical debate on whether plasma TG should be considered as an independent risk factor for CVD, with most of the data suggesting that it should not[8]. This view has changed over the last few years, mainly for two reasons. The first is the publication of a strong and timely meta-analysis of the relationship between plasma TG levels and the risk of CVD indicating that hypertriglyceridaemia (hyperTG) should in fact be considered as an independent risk factor[9]. As indicated above, there is also an increased recognition that hyperTG may be the underlying condition responsible for a series of other highly atherogenic deteriorations in the intravascular metabolism of lipoproteins[10] leading to reduced plasma HDL cholesterol levels and an increased accumulation of small, dense LDL particles.

Several mechanisms have been identified to explain the moderate to marked hyperTG states found among abdominally obese patients. The activity of lipoprotein lipase, the key intravascular enzyme responsible for the hydrolysis and clearance of plasma TG is generally reduced in abdominally obese patients[11]. There is also evidence to suggest that the hepatic output of apoB-containing TG-rich lipoproteins is increased in the presence of chronic hyperinsulinaemia[12]. Interestingly, it has been shown that a reduction in abdominal fat through caloric restriction was associated with an increased (more rapid) catabolism of LDL particles and conversion of VLDL to LDL particles and with a reduced hepatic secretion rate of VLDL particles[13]. These observations point out to the fact that abdominal obesity is an important determinant of the triglyceridaemia.

HyperTG, reduced HDL cholesterol levels and small dense LDL particles

As adequately noted by Reaven when he first described the insulin resistance syndrome, hyperTG and reduced plasma HDL cholesterol levels can hardly be dissociated. Indeed, most of the patients who present increased plasma TG levels generally have reduced plasma HDL cholesterol concentrations as well[14]. The primary mechanisms leading to reduced plasma HDL cholesterol levels in hyperTG states may be due to any one or a combination of the following possibilities[15]:

(1) Small HDL particles, a common feature among hyperTG individuals and which are the product of the intravascular lipolysis of TG-enriched HDL, may be cleared more rapidly from the circulation;

(2) TG-enriched HDL may be intrinsically more unstable in the circulation;

(3) The lipolytic process itself of TG-enriched HDL may lower HDL particle number by causing apo A-I to be shed from the HDL particles and cleared from the circulation;

(4) A reduced LPL activity may contribute to the lowering of HDL levels by reducing the availability of surface constituents of TG-rich lipoproteins that are necessary for the formation of nascent HDL particles. Because abdominal obesity is generally associated with moderate to marked hyperTG and concurrently with TG-enriched HDL, it is therefore not surprising to find reduced plasma HDL cholesterol levels within the abdominally obese population.

Small dense LDL particle is another dyslipidaemic phenotype that is frequently associated with hypertriglyceridaemia[16]. It has been now recognized for more than 20 years that LDL particles were heterogeneous in their composition, size, and density[17]. While there is no doubt that the total cholesterol content of LDL particles, as measured routinely in clinical practice provides a very powerful mean to predict and manage CVD risk, our group and others have provided solid evidence that phenotyping LDL particles beyond their cholesterol content, such as characterizing the particle size and the distribution of cholesterol among large and small particles, may provide valuable and clinically meaningful information on the risk of subsequent cardiovascular disease[18]. For example, we have recently shown that increased concentration of cholesterol found among particles with a diameter < 255 Å was associated with a four–sixfold increase in the risk of ischaemic heart disease in men of the Québec Cardiovascular Study[19]. This relationship was completely independent of concurrent variations in total LDL cholesterol concentrations. While the association between LDL size phenotype and CVD may be also independent of variations in plasma TG levels, the latter is a strong determinant of the former. The mechanisms relating hyperTG to the presence of small dense LDL particles are to some extent similar to those underlying the relationship between hyperTG and reduced HDL cholesterol levels[18]. Indeed, in the presence of high plasma TG levels, there is an increased transfer of TG from TG-rich lipoproteins to LDL particles in exchange of cholesteryl esters. This results in a significant TG enrichment of LDL particles, which become better substrates for HL, thereby promoting the formation of smaller LDL particles. Individuals with completely inactive HL, despite generally showing significant elevations in plasma TG levels as well as massive TG enrichment of LDL particles, have relatively large LDL compared to subjects with normal HL activity[20]. This suggests that while hypertriglyceridaemia may be the primary requirement leading to the formation of small dense LDL particles, HL is probably the limiting factor in this process as evidenced by the unique model of human HL deficiency. Because abdominally obese patients generally have increased plasma TG levels[11], and because it has been shown that intravascular HL activity among abdominally obese patients is elevated[21], it is therefore not surprising to find an increased preponderance of small dense LDL particles among these patients[22].

Finally, the increased output of free fatty acids from the catalytically active intra-abdominal fat is an important factor up regulating the rate at which VLDL particles are secreted from the hepatocytes into the circulation[23]. This not only leads to increased plasma TG levels but also to increased number of VLDL particles, as measured by the concentration of apolipoprotein B-100 (apoB-100). Because VLDL are direct precursors of LDL, and because there is only one apoB-100 per VLDL or LDL particles, the number of plasma atherogenic lipoproteins can be estimated by measuring the concentration of apoB-100[24]. There is accumulating data supporting the fact that apoB-100 is a significant and powerful risk factor for CVD[25,26]. There is also data to suggest that individuals with the IRS and with abdominal obesity have increased number of atherogenic particles as measured by elevated plasma apoB-100 concentration[27].

While abdominal obesity may not be considered as an 'LDL cholesterol' problem (after all, most obese individuals do not display markedly elevated plasma LDL cholesterol concentrations), it should be recognized that abdominally obese patients do indeed have a serious 'LDL problem', mostly in the form of increased number as well as reduced size. This has most certainly a tremendous impact on the risk of CVD in these patients.

Cluster of metabolic abnormalities in abdominal obesity

One concept that has become evident in recent years is that each of the individual metabolic features composing the syndrome of IRS/abdominal obesity rarely occurs as an isolated disorder. For example, we have recently shown that the majority (68.3 per cent) of men with relatively normal plasma TG levels (< 1.6 mmol/l) had none or only one of other metabolic components of the IRS/abdominal obesity syndrome while only 6.4 per cent of these normoTG men had three risk factors simultaneously. On the other hand, the majority (74.2 per cent) of hyperTG men (TG > 1.6 mmol/l) simultaneously accumulated more than one features of the IRS (Pirro *et al.*, unpublished observations). There is also no doubt that accumulating several risk factors of the IRS has a remarkable impact on the risk of CVD. PROCAM was amongst the first studies to suggest that the combination of high plasma TG and reduced HDL cholesterol levels was an important determinant of future CVD[28]. We have also recently observed that the risk of CVD in hyperTG men of the Québec Cardiovascular Study increased in a stepwise fashion according to the number of risk factors, being more than five times greater among men with several risk factors present simultaneously compared to men with no risk factors (Pirro *et al.*, unpublished observations). Finally we have reported that accumulating specific features of the IRS/abdominal obesity syndrome such as increased plasma insulin and apoB-100 levels and small dense LDL particles was associated with a tremendous 20-fold increase in the five-year risk of CVD in men of the Québec Cardiovascular Study[29]. These data clearly emphasize the importance of considering insulin resistance, abdominal obesity as well as their accompanying metabolic disorders in order to assess more adequately the risk of CVD in the population. In that regard, our group has suggested that using a simple measure of waist girth (> 90 cm) combined with a simple measure of plasma TG levels (> 2.0 mmol/) may prove to be an extremely cost-effective and clinically valuable approach to adequately assess the tremendous risk of CVD associated with insulin resistance and abdominal obesity[30].

References

1. Obesity: Preventing and managing the global epidemic. Report on a WHO consultation on obesity. World Health Organization. Geneva 1997.

2. Vague J. Sexual differentiation, a factor affecting the forms of obesity. *Presse Méd* 1947; 30: 339–40.

3. Kissebah AH, Vydelingum N, Murray R, Evans DJ, Hartz AJ, Kalkhoff RK, Adams PW. Relation of body fat distribution to metabolic complications of obesity. *J Clin Endocrinol Metab* 1982; 54: 254–60.

4. Himsworth HP, Kerr RB. Insulin-sensitive and insulin-insensitive types of diabetus mellitus. *Clin Sci* 1939; 4: 119–52.

5. Reaven GM. Role of insulin resistance in human disease. *Diabetes* 1988; 37: 1495–507.

6. Ford ES, Giles WH, Dietz WH. Prevalence of the metabolic syndrome among US adults – Findings from the Third National Health and Nutrition Examination Survey. *JAMA* 2002; 287: 356–9.

7. Després JP. Abdominal obesity as important component of insulin-resistance syndrome. *Nutrition* 1993; 9: 452–9.

8. Gotto AM Jr. Hypertriglyceridemia: risks and perspectives. *Am J Cardiol* 1992; 70, H19-H25.

9. Hokanson JE, Austin MA. Plasma triglyceride level is a risk factor for cardiovascular disease independent of high-density lipoprotein cholesterol level: a meta-analysis of population-based prospective studies. *J Cardiovasc Risk* 1996; 3: 213–9.

10. Lewis GF, Steiner G. Hypertriglyceridemia and its metabolic consequences as a risk factor for atherosclerotic cardiovascular disease in non-insulin- dependent diabetes mellitus. *Diab Metab Rev* 1996; 12: 37–56.

11. Després JP, Moorjani S, Lupien PJ, Tremblay A, Nadeau A, Bouchard C. Regional distribution of body fat, plasma lipoproteins, and cardiovascular disease. *Arterioscler Thromb Vasc Biol* 1990; 10: 497–511.

12. Lewis GF, Uffelman KD, Szeto LW, Steiner G. Effects of acute hyperinsulinemia on VLDL triglyceride and VLDL apo B production in normal weight and obese individuals. *Diabetes* 1993; 42: 833–42.

13. Riches FM, Watts GF, Hua J, Stewart GR, Naoumova RP, Barrett PH. Reduction in visceral adipose tissue is associated with improvement in apolipoprotein B-100 metabolism in obese men. *J Clin Endocrinol Metab* 1999; 84: 2854–61.

14. Lamarche B, Després JP, Moorjani S, Cantin B, Dagenais GR, Lupien PJ. Triglycerides and HDL-cholesterol as risk factors for ischemic heart disease. Results from the Québec Cardiovascular Study. *Atherosclerosis* 1996; 119: 235–45.

15. Lamarche B, Rashid S, Lewis GF. HDL metabolism in hypertriglyceridemic states: an overview. *Clin Chim Acta* 1999; 286: 145–61.

16. Austin MA, Hokanson JE. Epidemiology of triglycerides, small dense low-density lipoprotein, and lipoprotein(a) as risk factors for coronary heart disease. *Med Clin North Am* 1994; 78: 99–115.

17. Shen MM, Krauss RM, Lindgren FT, Forte TM. Heterogeneity of serum low density lipoproteins in normal humans subjects. *J Lipid Res* 1981; 22: 236–44.

18. Lamarche B, Lemieux I, Després JP. The small, dense LDL phenotype and the risk of coronary heart disease. Epidemiology, pathophysiology and therapeutic considerations. *Diabetes Metab* 1999; 25: 199–211.

19. St-Pierre AC, Ruel IL, Cantin B, Dagenais GR, Bernard PM, Després JP, Lamarche B. Comparison of various electrophoretic characteristics of LDL particles and their relationship to the risk of ischemic heart disease. *Circulation* 2001; 104: 2295–9.

20. Connelly PW, Hegele RA. Hepatic lipase deficiency. *Crit Rev Clin Lab Sci* 1998; 35: 547–72.

21. Després JP, Ferland M, Moorjani S, Nadeau A, Tremblay A, Lupien PJ. Role of hepatic-triglyceride lipase activity in the association between intra-abdominal fat and plasma HDL cholesterol in obese women. *Arterioscler Thromb Vasc Biol* 1989; 9: 485–92.

22. Tchernof A, Lamarche B, Nadeau A, Moorjani S, Labrie F, Lupien PJ, Després JP. The dense LDL phenotype: association with plasma lipoprotein levels, visceral obesity and hyperinsulinemia in men. *Diabet Care* 1996; 19: 629–37.

23. Lewis GF. Fatty acid regulation of very low density lipoprotein (VLDL) production. *Curr Opin Lipidol* 1997; 8: 146–53.

24. Sniderman AD, Cianflone K. Lipids and vascular disease: what we do and do not know. *Clin Chim Acta* 1999; 286: 7–22.

25. Lamarche B, Moorjani S, Lupien PJ, Cantin B, Bernard PM, Dagenais GR, Després JP. Apolipoprotein A-I and B levels and the risk of ischemic heart disease during a five-year follow-up of men in the Québec Cardiovascular Study. *Circulation* 1996; 94: 273–8.

26. Walldius G, Jungner I, Holme I, Aastveit AH, Kolar W, Steiner E. High apolipoprotein B, low apolipoprotein A-I, and improvement in the prediction of fatal myocardial infarction (AMORIS study): a prospective study. *Lancet* 2001; 358: 2026–33.

27. Després JP. Dyslipidaemia and obesity. Baillière's *Clin Endocrinol Metab* 1994; 8: 629–60.

28. Assmann G, Schulte H. Relation of high-density lipoprotein cholesterol and triglycerides to incidence of atherosclerotic coronary artery disease (the PROCAM experience). *Am J Cardiol* 1992; 70: 733–7.

29. Lamarche B, Tchernof A, Mauriège P, Cantin B, Dagenais GR, Lupien PJ, Després JP. Fasting insulin and apolipoprotein B levels and low-density lipoprotein particle size as risk factors for ischemic heart disease. *JAMA* 1998; 279: 1955–61.

30. Lemieux I, Pascot A, Couillard C, Lamarche B, Tchernof A *et al.* Hypertriglyceridemic waist: A marker of the atherogenic metabolic triad (hyperinsulinemia; hyperapolipoprotein B; small, dense LDL) in men? *Circulation* 2000; 102: 179–84.

Progress in Obesity Research: 9. Edited by *Geraldo Medeiros-Neto, Alfredo Halpern and Claude Bouchard*
©2003 John Libbey Eurotext Ltd, pp. 664–667.

CHAPTER 139

Managing the obese hypertensive patient

Tobias Pischon and Arya M. Sharma

Franz Volhard Clinic, HELIOS-Klinikum Berlin Buch-Charité, Medical Faculty of the Humboldt University Berlin and Max Delbrück Centre for Molecular Medicine, Berlin, Germany
[e-mail: sharma@fvk berlin.de]

Introduction

In conjunction with the global increase in the prevalence of overweight and obesity, the majority of hypertensive patients are now overweight or obese[1,2]. Obesity substantially increases cardiovascular morbidity and mortality, and the management of obese hypertensive is additionally complicated by the presence of related metabolic co-morbidities including insulin resistance or frank type 2 diabetes, dyslipidaemia, microalbuminuria and left-ventricular hypertrophy[3]. Furthermore, obese patients are less likely to achieve normal blood pressure on treatment than lean patients[4]. As the pathophysiology and hemodynamic alterations found in obese hypertensive patients may substantially differ from those found in non-obese patients, their response to antihypertensive medication may be different. Furthermore, metabolic abnormalities commonly present in obese patients may be be exacerbated by commonly used antihypertensive agents. It therefore appears appropriate to review and discuss the current role of anti-hypertensive treatment options for the obese hypertensive patient.

Weight management

Numerous studies have shown that weight reduction is a very effective measure for lowering blood pressure levels and increasing the response rate to antihypertensive treatment[1,2]. In addition to blood pressure control, obese patients also benefit from weight loss by improvement of other obesity-related risk factors, like insulin resistance and dyslipidaemia. Weight loss can be achieved by reducing energy intake and increasing physical activity, or by pharmacological and surgical interventions. The diet should be moderately calorie reduced, low in saturated and trans fatty acids, and high in polyunsaturated fatty acids and carbohydrates with a low glycaemic index[1,2]. A low sodium diet may further improve blood pressure levels in obese patients[5]. However, because of the limited long-term success of weight loss achieved by behaviour modification, diet, and exercise alone, a large proportion of patients may also benefit from the use of anti-obesity drugs.

Currently, only two substances are widely available for the long-term treatment of obesity. Both result in a 5–10 per cent weight loss that can be largely maintained up to 2 years. Orlistat is a gastrointestinal lipase inhibitor that reduces fat absorption by about 30 per cent. The reductions in blood pressure and heart rate achieved for a given weight loss with orlistat are similar to those expected with weight loss from lifestyle intervention alone[6]. Sibutramine on the other hand, is a serotonin and norepinephrine uptake inhibitor that leads to weight loss by decreasing hunger and enhancing satiety. Its use in hypertensive patients is hampered by its ability to raise blood pressure and heart rate in some patients. However, several studies show that weight loss with sibutramine is associated with modest blood pressure reductions both in normotensive and in treated hypertensive patients, although the fall in blood pressure is only about half of that what may be expected for a given degree of weight loss[7]. Nevertheless, preliminary data suggests that the fall in blood pressure seen in clinical practice with sibutramine may be substantially larger in patients with uncontrolled hypertension[8]. Thus, while orlistat may well be the anti-obesity treatment of choice for the hypertensive high-risk patient, sibutramine can clearly also be used in obese hypertensive patients with controlled hypertension to induce weight loss. Nevertheless, blood pressure and heart rate should be closely monitored in patients treated with sibutramine.

Obesity surgery is currently only recommended for patients with morbid obesity and includes different forms of gastric banding or gastric bypass surgery, liposuction, and abdominoplastic surgery[9]. The potential magnitude of the blood-pressure lowering effects of anti-obesity surgery in morbidly obese patients was recently demonstrated[10], and recent studies have also shown substantial short-term metabolic benefits from large-volume liposuction[11] and omentectomy (visceral fat reduction)[12]. However it should be noted that the long-term effect of surgical weight loss on blood pressure is not clear, as shown by results of the ongoing Swedish Obese Subjects (SOS) study[13], where the prevalence of hypertension was not significantly reduced over an eight-year follow-up period.

Antihypertensive medication

An optimal anti-hypertensive drug for obese patients should effectively lower blood pressure, halt the progression of or even reverse endorgan damage, not impair metabolism, be well tolerated, and significantly reduce morbidity and mortality. These criteria are perhaps best fulfilled by agents that block the renin-angiotensin system. Thus, both ACE-inhibitors and angiotensin receptor blockers have been shown to prevent or reverse endorgan alterations commonly present in obese hypertensives, including left ventricular hypertrophy, heart failure, or microalbuminuria[14,15]. Furthermore, they do not impair metabolism[16] but may in fact substantially reduce the risk of type 2 diabetes[15,17]. Thus, these drugs may be the most appropriate anti-hypertensive agents for obese hypertensive patients[18,19].

Calcium channel blockers have also been considered appropriate for the treatment of obesity hypertension because they do not to impair metabolism[18]. However, the anti-hypertensive effect of calcium channel blockers may be attenuated in obese hypertensives[20], perhaps due to the fact that the peripheral resistance is often decreased in these patients. Because of its negative chronotropic effects, the non-dihydropiridine calcium channel blocker verapamil may be particularly beneficial in obese hypertensives and could perhaps serve as a substitute for β-blockers in these patients[18].

Diuretics reduce blood pressure levels by decreasing cardiac output[2] and should thus be beneficial in obese patients. However, they may also increase sympathetic nerve activity, stimulate the renin angiotensin system, and promote insulin resistance and dyslipidaemia, when used as monotherapy at higher doses. On the other hand, at lower doses, when used as monotherapy, they may be less effective than ACE-inhibitors in obese hypertensives[21]. Thus, diuretics should be preferentially used at lower doses in combination with other agents (such as ACE inhibitors or angiotensin receptor blockers) in the management of obesity-related hypertension.

Alpha-blockers are safe and effective agents for decreasing blood pressure and may be beneficial in patients with dyslipidaemia or glucose intolerance. Prazosin and doxazosin have been associated with reduced glucose levels and improved insulin sensitivity and beneficial effects on insulin sensitivity have also been reported in obese hypertensive patients[22].

Beta-blockers also effectively lower blood pressure levels in obesity hypertension[20]. They are also beneficial for treatment of common obesity-related conditions such as left ventricular hypertrophy and heart failure, and may lower the risk for sudden cardiac death. Thus, β-blockers reduce morbidity and mortality in patients with a number of co-morbidities, including diabetes[23]. On the other hand, however, β-blockers have been shown to interfere with carbohydrate and lipid metabolism, leading to impaired glucose tolerance, increased triglycerides, and reduced HDL-cholesterol levels[24], and may reduce metabolic rate, causing weight gain in some patients[25].

Given the importance of the sympathetic nervous system in the pathogenesis of obesity hypertension, atypical β-blocking agents, including carvedilol or nebivolol, and centrally acting sympatholytic agents, like clonidin or moxonidine, may also be of particular benefit in obese hypertensive patients. Thus, for example, a recent study reported a better metabolic profile beyond blood pressure control, with lower sympathetic activity, in obese hypertensive patients treated with the imidazoline agonist moxonidine compared to the calcium channel blocker amlodipine[26]. These newer compounds, however, remain to be extensively studied in obese hypertensive patients.

Target blood pressure levels in obese patients

Patients at high risk for developing cardiovascular complications require tight blood pressure control and may benefit from blood pressure levels that are sub-normal[1,2]. Obesity is an integral part of the metabolic syndrome with insulin resistance as its key element, and it is tightly linked with type 2 diabetes and hypertension. Obese-hypertensive patients are extremely likely to be insulin resistant and, in turn, are at high risk to develop type 2 diabetes. As shown for type 2 diabetics, tight blood pressure control is one of the most important treatment strategies[27]. Given the high metabolic and hemodynamic risk of obese hypertensive patients, we suggest that these patients should be treated to a blood pressure target level similar to that currently recommended for patients with type 2 diabetes, i.e. 120/80 mmHg[1,2]. The need for optimal blood pressure control in obese patients is further underlined by the fact that the cardiac and renal complications of obesity-hypertension and hypertension in type 2 diabetes are very similar. Thus, as in patients with type 2 diabetes, hypertension markedly increases the risk for the development of microalbuminuria, renal failure, left ventricular hypertrophy, and congestive heart failure in obese patients[28–30].

Conclusions

Weight reduction is by far the most effective strategy in the management of obese hypertensive patients, as it not only improves blood pressure but also obesity-related co-morbidities. The health professional should support the patient's effort to implement this strategy. Anti-obesity drugs may be required when weight reduction or control cannot be achieved by diet and exercise alone. The selection of anti-hypertensive drugs should similarly benefit the patient and support his effort to lose weight and improve metabolic control. ACE-Inhibitors are appropriate first-line drugs in obese patients with uncomplicated hypertension. Calcium channel blockers (preferably non-dihydropyirdine), β-blockers, or low dose diuretics may be added when necessary or alternative medication is needed. Clearly, further research is needed to establish the value of these and newer drugs, like angiotensin receptor blockers, for treatment of obesity-hypertension. Optimal blood pressure levels should be achieved in obese hypertensive patients, particularly those with significant obesity-related comorbidities. However, further research is needed to define the target blood pressure levels for obese individuals.

References

1. The sixth report of the Joint National Committee on prevention, detection, evaluation, and treatment of high blood pressure [published erratum appears in *Arch Intern Med* 1998 Mar 23; 158(6): 573] [see comments]. *Arch Intern Med* 1997; 157: 2413–46.

2. 1999 World Health Organization-International Society of Hypertension Guidelines for the Management of Hypertension. Guidelines Subcommittee. *J Hypertens* 1999; 17: 151–83.

3. Must A, Spadano J, Coakley EH, Field AE, Colditz G, Dietz WH. The disease burden associated with overweight and obesity. *JAMA* 1999; 282: 1523–9.

4. Lloyd-Jones DM, Evans JC, Larson MG, O'Donnell CJ, Roccella EJ, Levy D. Differential control of systolic and diastolic blood pressure: factors associated with lack of blood pressure control in the community. *Hypertension* 2000; 36: 594–9.

5. Sacks FM, Svetkey LP, Vollmer WM, Appel LJ, Bray GA, Harsha D *et al.* Effects on blood pressure of reduced dietary sodium and the Dietary Approaches to Stop Hypertension (DASH) diet. DASH-Sodium Collaborative Research Group. *N Engl J Med* 2001; 344: 3–10.

6. Sharma AM, Golay A. Effect of orlistat-induced weight loss on blood pressure and heart rate in obese patients with hypertension. *J Hypertens* 2002 (in press).

7. Sharma AM. Sibutramine in overweight/obese hypertensive patients. *Int J Obes Relat Metab Disord* 2001; 25(4): S20–S23.

8. Scholze J [Sibutramine in clinical practice – a PMS-study with positive effects on blood pressure and metabolic parameters]. *Dtsch Med Wochenschr* 2002; 127: 606–10.

9. Expert Panel. Executive summary of the clinical guidelines on the identification, evaluation, and treatment of overweight and obesity in adults. *Arch Intern Med* 1998; 158: 1855–67.

10. Haciyanli M, Erkan N, Bora S, Gulay H. Vertical banded gastroplasty in the Aegean Region of Turkey. *Obes Surg* 2001; 11: 482–6.

11. Giese SY, Bulan EJ, Commons GW, Spear SL, Yanovski JA. Improvements in cardiovascular risk profile with large-volume liposuction: a pilot study. *Plast Reconstr Surg* 2001; 108: 510–9 (discussion 520–1).

12. Thorne A, Lonnqvist F, Apelman J, Hellers G, Arner P. A pilot study of long-term effects of a novel obesity treatment: omentectomy in connection with adjustable gastric banding. *Int J Obes Relat Metab Disord* 2002; 26: 193–9.

13. Torgerson JS, Sjostrom L. The Swedish Obese Subjects (SOS) study – rationale and results. *Int J Obes Relat Metab Disord* 2001; 25(1): S2–S4.

14. Garg R, Yusuf S Overview of randomized trials of angiotensin-converting enzyme inhibitors on mortality and morbidity in patients with heart failure. Collaborative Group on ACE Inhibitor Trials. *JAMA* 1995; 273: 1450–6.

15. Dahlof B, Devereux RB, Kjeldsen SE, Julius S, Beevers G, Faire U *et al.* Cardiovascular morbidity and mortality in the Losartan Intervention For Endpoint reduction in hypertension study (LIFE): a randomised trial against atenolol. *Lancet* 2002; 359: 995–1003.

16. Gress TW, Nieto FJ, Shahar E, Wofford MR, Brancati FL. Hypertension and antihypertensive therapy as risk factors for type 2 diabetes mellitus. Atherosclerosis Risk in Communities Study. *N Engl J Med* 2000; 342: 905–12.

17. Yusuf S, Sleight P, Pogue J, Bosch J, Davies R, Dagenais G. Effects of an angiotensin-converting-enzyme inhibitor, ramipril, on cardiovascular events in high-risk patients. The Heart Outcomes Prevention Evaluation Study Investigators. *N Engl J Med* 2000; 342: 145–53.

18. Sharma AM, Pischon T, Engeli S, Scholze J. Choice of drug treatment for obesity-related hypertension: where is the evidence? *J Hypertens* 2001; 19: 667–74.

19. Zanella MT, Kohlmann O Jr, Ribeiro AB. Treatment of obesity hypertension and diabetes syndrome. *Hypertension* 38: 705–8.

20. Schmieder RE, Gatzka C, Schachinger H, Schobel H, Ruddel H. Obesity as a determinant for response to antihypertensive treatment. *BMJ* 1993; 307: 537–40.

21. Reisin E, Weir MR, Falkner B, Hutchinson HG, Anzalone DA, Tuck ML. Lisinopril versus hydrochlorothiazide in obese hypertensive patients: a multicenter placebo-controlled trial. Treatment in Obese Patients With Hypertension (TROPHY) Study Group. *Hypertension* 1997; 30: 140–5.

22. Pollare T, Lithell H, Selinus I, Berne C. Application of prazosin is associated with an increase of insulin sensitivity in obese patients with hypertension. *Diabetologia* 1988; 31: 415–20.

23. UK Prospective Diabetes Study Group. Efficacy of atenolol and captopril in reducing risk of macrovascular and microvascular complications in type 2 diabetes: UKPDS 39. *BMJ* 1998; 317: 713–20.

24. MacMahon SW, Macdonald GJ, Bernstein L, Andrews G, Blacket RB. Comparison of weight reduction with metoprolol in treatment of hypertension in young overweight patients. *Lancet* 1985; 1: 1233–6.

25. Sharma AM, Pischon T, Hardt S, Kunz I, Luft FC. Hypothesis: Beta-adrenergic receptor blockers and weight gain: A systematic analysis. *Hypertension* 2001; 37: 250–4.

26. Sanjuliani AF, Genelhu-Fagunde V, Barroso SG, Duarte AVB, Rodrigues MLG, Castro, RSP *et al.* Effect of a imidazoline agonist on sympathetic activity and components of the insulin resistance syndrome in obese hypertensive brazilian patients. *J Hypertens* 2002; 20 (Suppl 4): S206.

27. Hansson L, Zanchetti A, Carruthers SG, Dahlof B, Elmfeldt D, Julius S *et al.* Effects of intensive blood-pressure lowering and low-dose aspirin in patients with hypertension: principal results of the Hypertension Optimal Treatment (HOT) randomised trial. HOT Study Group. *Lancet* 1998; 351: 1755–62.

28. American Diabetes Association. Diabetic Nephropathy. *Diabetes Care* 2002; 25 (Suppl 1): S85–S89.

29. Hubert HB, Feinleib M, McNamara PM, Castelli WP. Obesity as an independent risk factor for cardiovascular disease: a 26-year follow-up of participants in the Framingham Heart Study. *Circulation* 1983; 67: 968–77.

30. Liese AD, Hense HW, Doring A, Stieber J, Keil U. Microalbuminuria, central adiposity and hypertension in the non-diabetic urban population of the MONICA Augsburg survey 1994/95. *J Hum Hypertens* 2001; 15: 799–804.

©2003 John Libbey Eurotext Ltd, pp. 668–671.

CHAPTER 140

Obesity and cancers of the endometrium and breast

Elizabeth A. Spencer and Timothy J. Key

*Cancer Research UK Epidemiology Unit, University of Oxford, Gibson Building, Radcliffe Infirmary,
Oxford OX2 6HE, UK
[e-mail: elizabeth.spencer@cancer.org.uk]*

Introduction

In 2000, there were an estimated 189,000 cases of and 45,000 deaths from endometrial cancer world-wide, with the highest incidence rates occurring in developed countries[1]. Advancing age, low parity and use of postmenopausal oestrogen replacement therapy (in the absence of a progestagen) are established risk factors whilst use of combined oral contraceptives is protective[2,3].

Breast cancer is the most common cancer among women world-wide, with an estimated 1,050,000 cases and 373,000 deaths in 2000[1]. Western countries have about five times the incidence of less developed countries and Japan, partly due to differences in the reproductive risk factors of age at menarche, parity and age at births and breastfeeding. The only established dietary intake factor is alcohol, which has been convincingly shown to increase risk by about 10 per cent for each alcoholic drink per day[4]. High fat intake has been extensively researched as a risk factor, but currently available data do not support this hypothesis[5]. The evidence on other dietary factors is inconsistent.

Epidemiological evidence on the relationship between obesity and cancers of the endometrium and breast

Endometrial cancer

There is consistent, convincing evidence from both case-control and cohort studies, across a range of populations in Europe, USA, and Asia with a range of ages, to show that obesity is a major, independent risk factor for endometrial cancer, increasing risk by two- to threefold[6]. Most studies have shown the association between body mass index (BMI) and risk to be approximately linear, such that overweight (BMI between 25 and 30 kg/m^2), is also associated with elevated risk, although in some studies the increased risk was only evident in women in the highest category of BMI[6]. Typically the lowest risks have been observed for women with BMI under 22 kg/m^2. Risk estimates have tended to be greater for older than for younger women although there are insufficient data to clarify the relative risks for endometrial cancer among the obese separately for pre- and postmenopausal women.

Adult weight gain, which is likely to represent gain in adipose tissue, is an even better predictor of risk than BMI; most studies have shown that adult weight gain is associated with endometrial cancer risk, in a linear fashion[6].

Premenopausal breast cancer

The relationship between obesity and breast cancer is different for premenopausal women and post-menopausal women. Among premenopausal women, it has been demonstrated in a number of studies in populations with a high incidence of breast cancer, i.e. predominantly developed countries, that obesity is associated with a modest reduction in risk for premenopausal breast cancer[6].

The Pooling Project on Diet and Cancer, a meta-analysis of data from eight prospective cohorts, reported a risk reduction of about 40 per cent among women with BMI of 33 kg/m^2 or greater[7]. It appears that the protective effect may be limited to the obese, with no decreased risk in the overweight. The reduction in risk is largely confined to early stage breast cancer[8], but does not appear to be explicable by detection bias due to delayed diagnosis in obese women[8]. In contrast, studies have demonstrated a positive association of increasing BMI with increasing risk in medium and low-risk countries[9]. This difference between high risk and lower risk countries has not been explained although it was suggested that it may be related to different body fat distribution in these populations[9].

Postmenopausal breast cancer

There is convincing evidence from a large number of studies for a moderate positive association between adult BMI and postmenopausal breast cancer. The recent pooled analysis of eight prospective cohort studies on anthropometric factors and breast cancer found a positive association of BMI with risk, reporting a RR for obese women compared with lean women of about 1.3[7]. The magnitude of this association appears to increase with increasing age[6]. The association remains after controlling for reproductive and lifestyle risk factors[6], and there is some evidence that this relationship is largely independent of physical activity levels[6]. A marked increase in risk has been observed in relation to adult weight gain[10,11] and this increase in breast cancer risk with weight gain is greater among women over 65 years of age[12].

Epidemiology of hormones and cancers of the endometrium and breast

Endometrial cancer risk is determined mainly by exposure of the endometrium to oestrogens in the absence of progestagens[3]. Thus oestrogen replacement therapy increases risk, whereas pregnancy and oral contraceptives are protective[2]. There is some direct evidence that risk for endometrial cancer is related to high circulating levels of oestrogens in postmenopausal women[13,14].

For breast cancer, epidemiological studies have shown that early age at menarche and late age at menopause increase breast cancer risk, indicating that longer exposure of the breasts to ovarian hormones increases risk[15]. There is very little direct evidence on circulating sex hormones and pre-menopausal breast cancer[16]. However, there is evidence that risks for postmenopausal breast cancer are strongly related to circulating serum levels of sex hormones. A pooled analysis of nine prospective studies on endogenous sex hormones and postmenopausal breast cancer showed that women with high levels of oestrogens had two to three times the risk of women with low levels of these hormones; the strongest association was with free oestradiol[17].

Mechanisms by which sex hormones increase cancer risk

The most likely mechanism by which sex hormones affect risk is by determining the mitotic rate of the epithelial cells of the endometrium and breast[18]. High mitotic rates increase risk by increasing the chances of mutations taking place and of these mutations being replicated before the cell can repair the DNA damage, and also increase the growth of early tumours[19].

The 'unopposed oestrogen hypothesis' for endometrial cancer states that risk is increased by exposure to endogenous or exogenous oestrogen which is not opposed by progesterone or a synthetic pro-gestagen[3]. The normal function of oestrogen is to increase the mitotic rate of endometrial epithelium during the first half of the menstrual cycle; if this is not counteracted by a sufficient rise in progester-one, the increased rate of mitosis will continue, leading to increased cancer risk.

Hypotheses for the effect of sex hormones on breast cancer risk are based on the finding that, as opposed to endometrial tissue, mitotic rates in breast epithelium are higher in the luteal phase (second half) of the menstrual cycle than in the follicular phase, possibly because the combination of oestrogen and progesterone causes higher rates of mitosis than oestrogen alone, or because the rise in progester-one during the luteal phase essentially has no effect on mitosis[20].

How obesity increases risks for endometrial and breast cancers via sex hormones

Obesity affects the levels of sex hormones and sex hormone-binding globulin (SHBG), a protein which binds oestradiol and thus reduces its availability to enter cells. The effects of obesity on sex hormones vary by menopausal status (see below), but the effects of obesity on SHBG do not. Numerous studies have all shown that among both pre- and postmenopausal women with high BMI, SHBG is low[21]; how this takes place is not certain but may be largely due to increased insulin levels in heavier people[22].

Premenopausal women

In premenopausal women, the main source of oestradiol is the ovaries. A small amount of oestradiol is produced additionally in the adipose tissue. Serum concentrations of oestrogens are homeostatically controlled by feedback loops involving the hypothalamus and anterior pituitary. The ovaries also synthesise progesterone.

In premenopausal women within the range of BMI 20–30 kg/m^2, as BMI increases, SHBG falls, but there is little variation in bioavailable oestradiol, demonstrating that homeostatic control of free oestradiol is effective[21]. At the level of clinical obesity (BMI over 30 kg/m^2), however, this system appears to be perturbed. One important effect is an increased incidence of anovulatory menstrual cycles. The effect of this on average serum oestradiol levels during a menstrual cycle is unclear; however, on average, oestradiol levels appear to be similar or maybe a little lower in obese women than in normal-weight women, possibly due to faster oestradiol clearance[23,24]. There is little difference in progesterone levels within the range 20–30 kg/m^2, but among obese women, with an increased incidence of anovulatory cycles, there are somewhat lower average progesterone levels in the second half of the menstrual cycle, due to the failure to produce a corpus luteum[25].

In premenopausal women the large increase in risk for endometrial cancer may be explained by the high incidence of anovular menstrual cycles in obese women and the consequent exposure to high levels of oestradiol unopposed by progesterone[3]. The inverse relationship between obesity and premenopausal breast cancer risk found in many studies is as yet unexplained. If oestradiol is the main hormonal factor affecting breast cancer risk, since the level of oestradiol is controlled by feedback mechanisms, obesity premenopausally would not be expected to alter risk. Possibly the decreased risk is partly due to the reduced exposure to progesterone as a result of anovulatory cycles.

Postmenopausal women

After the menopause, the ovaries do not produce oestradiol or progesterone and levels of these hormones fall dramatically. The principal source of oestradiol in postmenopausal women is the adipose tissue: the adrenal glands secrete androgens and an enzyme operating mainly in the adipose tissue aromatizes the precursor androgen, mainly androstenedione, to oestrone; some of this is then converted to oestradiol[26]. This production of oestradiol is not controlled by feedback mechanisms.

Thus obese postmenopausal women, with a large amount of adipose tissue able to convert androgens to oestrogens, have higher levels of serum oestradiol than thin women. As SHBG falls with increasing BMI, the amount of SHBG available to bind the circulating oestrogen falls and therefore the *proportion* of free oestradiol increases. The combination of these effects means the *concentration* of free oestradiol increases by more than double in obese postmenopausal women[27–29].

In postmenopausal obese women the large increase in endometrial cancer risk is due to high levels of free oestradiol together with the normal very low levels of progesterone[3]. The increased levels of free oestradiol in obese women also probably explain the increased risk of postmenopausal breast cancer.

Conclusions

In premenopausal women, obesity causes an increase in the frequency of anovular cycles; this may explain the observed large increase in risk for endometrial cancer and perhaps also the small decrease in risk for breast cancer. In postmenopausal women, obesity causes an increase in serum levels of free oestradiol and this factor causes increased risks for both endometrial and breast cancer. The protective effect of obesity on premenopausal breast cancer incidence does not lead to decreased mortality from breast cancer, and since obesity in young adult life is likely to result in obesity later in life, when risk for breast cancer rises, obesity should be avoided at all ages.

Increases in the prevalence of obesity may contribute to important increases in risk for endometrial cancer and breast cancer. Few risk factors for endometrial cancer and breast cancer are easily modifiable. Whilst obesity is a difficult condition to prevent and treat, reducing obesity does present a possibility for reducing the incidence of cancers of the endometrium and breast. It has been estimated that, in the US, avoidance of overweight and obesity may prevent up to about half of endometrial and up to a fifth of postmenopausal breast cancers[30].

References

1. Ferlay J, Bray P, Pisani P, Partridge DM. Globocan 2000: Cancer incidence, mortality and prevalence worldwide, Version 1.0. IARC CancerBase No. 5. http://www-dep.iarc.fr/globocan/globocan.html [Accessed 2002].

2. Akhmedkhanov A, Zeleniuch-Jacquotte A, Toniolo P. Role of exogenous and endogenous hormones in endometrial cancer: review of the evidence and research perspectives. *Ann NY Acad Sci* 2001; 943: 296–315.

3. Key TJ, Pike MC. The dose-effect relationship between 'unopposed' oestrogens and endometrial mitotic rate: its central role in explaining and predicting endometrial cancer risk. *Br J Cancer* 1988; 57: 205–12.

4. Smith-Warner SA, Spiegelman D, Yaun SS *et al.* Alcohol and breast cancer in women: a pooled analysis of cohort studies. *JAMA* 1998; 279: 535–40.

5. Smith-Warner SA, Spiegelman D, Adami HO *et al.* Types of dietary fat and breast cancer: a pooled analysis of cohort studies. *Int J Cancer* 2001; 92: 767–74.

6. International Agency for Research on Cancer. IARC Handbooks of Cancer Prevention; volume 6: Weight control and physical activity. World Health Organisation, 2002.

7. van den Brandt PA, Spiegelman D,Yaun SS *et al.* Pooled analysis of prospective cohort studies on height, weight, and breast cancer risk. *Am J Epidemiol* 2000; 152: 514–27.

8. Tretli S. Height and weight in relation to breast cancer morbidity and mortality. A prospective study of 570,000 women in Norway. *Int J Cancer* 1989; 44: 23–30.

9. Pathak DR, Whittemore AS. Combined effects of body size, parity, and menstrual events on breast cancer incidence in seven countries. *Am J Epidemiol* 1992; 135: 153–68.

10. Huang Z, Hankinson SE, Colditz GA *et al.* Dual effects of weight and weight gain on breast cancer risk. *JAMA* 1997; 278: 1407–11.

11. Trentham-Dietz A, Newcomb PA, Egan KM *et al.* Weight change and risk of postmenopausal breast cancer (United States). *Cancer Causes Control* 2000; 11: 533–42.

12. Galanis DJ, Kolonel LN, Lee J, Le Marchand L. Anthropometric predictors of breast cancer incidence and survival in a multi-ethnic cohort of female residents of Hawaii. *Cancer Causes Control* 1998; 9: 217–24.

13. Potischman N, Hoover RN, Brinton LA *et al.* Case-control study of endogenous steroid hormones and endometrial cancer. *J Natl Cancer Inst* 1996; 88: 1127–35.

14. Zeleniuch-Jacquotte A, Akhmedkhanov A, Kato I *et al.* Postmenopausal endogenous oestrogens and risk of endometrial cancer: results of a prospective study. *Br J Cancer* 2001; 84: 975–81.

15. Pike MC, Spicer DV, Dahmoush L, Press MF. Estrogens, progestogens, normal breast cell proliferation, and breast cancer risk. *Epidemiol Rev* 1993; 15: 17–35.

16. Key TJ. Serum oestradiol and breast cancer risk. *Endocr Relat Cancer* 1999; 6: 175–80.

17. The Endogenous Hormones and Breast Cancer Collaborative Group. Endogenous sex hormones and breast cancer in postmenopausal women: reanalysis of nine prospective studies. *J Natl Cancer Inst* 2002; 94: 606–16.

18. Albanes D, Winick M. Are cell number and cell proliferation risk factors for cancer? *J Natl Cancer Inst* 1988; 80: 772–4.

19. Preston-Martin S, Pike MC, Ross RK, Jones PA, Henderson BE. Increased cell division as a cause of human cancer. *Cancer Res* 1990; 50: 7415–21.

20. Key TJ, Pike MC. The role of oestrogens and progestagens in the epidemiology and prevention of breast cancer. *Eur J Cancer Clin Oncol* 1988; 24: 29–43.

21. Key TJ, Allen NE, Verkasalo PK, Banks E. Energy balance and cancer: the role of sex hormones. *Proc Nutr Soc* 2001; 60: 81–9.

22. Franks S, Kiddy DS, Hamilton-Fairley D, Bush A, Sharp PS, Reed MJ. The role of nutrition and insulin in the regulation of sex hormone binding globulin. *J Steroid Biochem Mol Biol* 1991; 39: 835–8.

23. Grenman S, Ronnemaa T, Irjala K, Kaihola HL, Gronroos M. Sex steroid, gonadotropin, cortisol, and prolactin levels in healthy, massively obese women: correlation with abdominal fat cell size and effect of weight reduction. *J Clin Endocrinol Metab* 1986; 63: 1257–61.

24. Zhang YW, Stern B, Rebar RW. Endocrine comparison of obese menstruating and amenorrheic women. *J Clin Endocrinol Metab* 1984; 58: 1077–83.

25. Sherman BM, Korenman SG. Measurement of serum LH, FSH, estradiol and progesterone in disorders of the human menstrual cycle: the inadequate luteal phase. *J Clin Endocrinol Metab* 1974; 39: 145–9.

26. Judd HL, Shamonki IM, Frumar AM, Lagasse LD. Origin of serum estradiol in postmenopausal women. *Obstet Gynecol* 1982; 59: 680–6.

27. Potischman N, Swanson CA, Siiteri P, Hoover RN. Reversal of relation between body mass and endogenous estrogen concentrations with menopausal status. *J Natl Cancer Inst* 1996; 88: 756–8.

28. Cauley JA, Gutai JP, Kuller LH, LeDonne D, Powell JG. The epidemiology of serum sex hormones in postmenopausal women. *Am J Epidemiol* 1989; 129: 1120–31.

29. Hankinson SE, Willett WC, Manson JE *et al.* Alcohol, height, and adiposity in relation to estrogen and prolactin levels in postmenopausal women. *J Natl Cancer Inst* 1995; 87: 1297–302.

30. Ballard-Barbash R, Swanson CA. Body weight: estimation of risk for breast and endometrial cancers. *Am J Clin Nutr* 1996; 63: S437–S441.

Progress in Obesity Research: 9. Edited by *Geraldo Medeiros-Neto, Alfredo Halpern and Claude Bouchard*
©2003 John Libbey Eurotext Ltd, pp. 672–675.

CHAPTER 141

Obesity and colorectal cancer

Tim Byers

University of Colorado School of Medicine, 4200 East Ninth Avenue, Denver, Colorado 80262, USA
[e-mail: Tim.Byers@uchsc.edu]

Background

Colorectal cancer is a leading cause of cancer death worldwide. Several nutritional and behavioural factors are known to be associated with a modest increase in risk for colorectal cancer, including dietary factors of low intake of fruits and vegetables, high glycaemic and/or high fat diets, low levels of physical activity, and obesity[1]. This review will briefly summarize what is known about the relationships between body weight and the risk for colorectal neoplasia. The evidence for an overall association will be examined, as well as the patterns by gender, by colorectal subsite, and by stage of carcinogenesis; and the possible biological mechanisms for the associations will be discussed. Colorectal cancers arise predominantly from adenomas, a process that in most people takes at least 10–15 years[2]. Small adenomas first develop from mutated normal colonic epithelium, then some of these grow to become more histologically abnormal as a result of successive mutations, leading eventually to invasive cancer. The relevance of this natural history to weight and weight history is that body weight may have effects on colorectal cancer risk at any of several stages, including initiation, promotion, and progression, over a time period spanning years or decades.

Methods

The epidemiologic literature on the relationship between body weight and colorectal neoplasia comes from case-control and cohort studies. Case-control studies of the association between measures of body fatness and colorectal cancer have appeared frequently in the epidemiologic literature over the past 40 years, but only in the past decade have data become available from several large cohort studies. This brief review is not intended to include all previous studies, as a more comprehensive review of this topic has been recently conducted by the WHO[3]. Only the larger studies are included in this review, and only those that have presented evidence regarding the dose-response relationship between BMI and colorectal neoplasia. Studies that presented only average BMI levels by case and comparison groups were not included. For studies with multiple reports, the report presenting the greatest detail on body weight, or the most recent update (e.g. from ongoing cohort studies) was selected. Because there are many published studies relating body weight to colorectal cancer, this review of cancer studies selected only the larger studies, those with more than 200 cases for each gender. Details of studies of adenomas, colorectal subsite, body fat distribution, and lifetime weight history are included in the recent IARC review on this topic[3].

Findings

The selected epidemiologic studies of the association between BMI and colorectal cancer are summarized in Table 1. The various quantile cutpoints presented in each paper are indicated in Table 1 by the varying cell boundaries for the relative risk estimates in each row. The approximate BMI cut-points used to define each group are indicated in the column headings. For those studies not specifying the BMI cut points, equal-sized categories for quartiles or quintiles were used. Although there is variability across studies, the studies tend to show positive associations between BMI and the risk of colorectal. Across the studies there is about a 50 per cent to 100 per cent higher risk for the upper quartile or quintile of BMI, as compared to the lower quartile or quintile. The specific BMI cutpoints vary across the studies, but the strength of the association corresponds in most studies to about a doubling of risk for those with BMI levels of 30 or over compared to those with BMI of under 23. There is no clear evidence for a threshold effect of BMI, with the overall pattern suggesting a linear dose-response relationship.

Table 1. Findings from epidemiological studies of the relationship between obesity, as estimated by body mass index (BMI) and the risk of colorectal cancer*

Investigator (reference)	Study design	Study dates	Sex	Number of subjects (cases:controls or cases:cohort)	Odds ratio or relative risk by BMI level												
					<20	20	21	22	23	24	25	26	27	28	29	30	>30
LeMarchand (4)	C:C	1987-91	M	698:698			1.0		1.2		1.5			2.2			
			F	494:494			1.0		0.8		0.4			1.2			
Giovannucci (5)	cohort	1986-92	M	203:31,055				1.0		0.84		1.33	1.62			1.82	
Martinez (6)	cohort	1980-92	F	393:89,448		1.0		1.32		1.21			1.35			1.58	
Caan (7)	C:C	1991-94	M	1095:1286		1.0		1.22			1.31		1.79			1.96	
			F	888:1114		1.0		1.20			1.28		1.30			1.45	
Graham (8)	C:C	1975-84	M	205:205			1.0			1.72		1.41			2.20		
			F	223:223			1.0			1.32		1.28			1.84		
Dietz (9)	C:C	1990-91	F	779:2315			1.0			1.1		1.2			1.3		
Kune (10)	C:C	1980-81	M	388:398	0.49			1.0					1.43			1.78	
			F	327:329	0.43			1.0					0.67			0.67	
Chyou (11)	cohort	1965-92	M	289:7840			1.0			0.92		1.22			1.21		
Bostick (12)	cohort	1986-90	F	212:35,215			1.0			0.96		1.68		1.51		1.40	
Russo (13)	C:C	1992-96	M	1124:2067				1.0		1.32	1.19		1.45		1.68		
			F	819:2069				1.0		0.91	0.84		1.16		0.87		
Thun (14)	cohort	1982-88	M	611:5746	0.93		1.0					1.07		1.14		1.36	
			F	539:5746	1.2		1.0					0.98		1.31		1.10	
Ford (15)	cohort	1971-92	Both	222:13,198				1.0		1.79		1.86		2.47		3.72	2.79
Lee (16)	cohort	1964-88	M	302:17,595				1.0		1.30		1.10		1.34		1.52	

The association between BMI and colorectal cancer risk is generally seen more consistently and is generally of higher strength for men than for women (Table 1). The contrast between the genders in this association is quite consistent. The strength of the association is about twice that for males as for females among those studies that have presented results for both genders using the same study methods. The differences in associations between BMI and neoplasia at different colorectal subsites have been examined in several studies. In general, the association is stronger and more consistently observed in the distal colon than in the proximal colon, both among men and women[3]. The few studies of rectal neoplasia have shown little evidence for an association with BMI. The reasons for this greater specificity the BMI association with distal colon neoplasia is unknown.

The association between colorectal neoplasia and body fat distribution, as indicated by the waist/hip ratio has been examined in several studies. In general, the association between WHR and colorectal neoplasia is no stronger than for BMI[3]. It is unlikely, therefore, that the BMI association is only a proxy for a body fat distribution phenotype as indicated by the WHR.

There are fewer studies of BMI and colorectal adenomas[3]. Among the adenoma studies, there is a similar pattern of a positive association as seen for colorectal cancers. For those studies that assessed the BMI association separately for larger as compared to smaller adenomas, there is a pattern suggesting that the BMI association is stronger for larger adenomas. This suggests that obesity-related factors might be acting at a later stage in the development of cancer, perhaps by contributing to the promotion and progression of adenomas toward cancer.

The differences in associations between colorectal neoplasia and reports of weight at different times in life have been examined in a few studies[3], In general, there is not consistent evidence to point to a stronger association between BMI earlier in life and colorectal neoplasia than later in life in those analyses. The association observed between adult obesity and colorectal neoplasia is therefore not likely due simply to a residual effect from a stronger association earlier in life, nearer to the time of adenoma initiation. BMI-associated factors related to adenoma growth and cancer promotion are therefore suggested.

Discussion

In brief, epidemiologic studies have shown that BMI and WHR are positively associated with risk in a dose-dependent way, those associations are seen for both cancer and adenomas (but stronger for advanced adenomas), weight earlier in life is not more associated with risk than weight later in life, and the BMI association is weaker among women.

Adiposity may be only a common sign of the true colorectal cancer risk factor(s), and not truly independently related to colorectal cancer risk. Adiposity may be a correlate of colorectal neoplasia simply because both conditions have a common cause. Caloric imbalance (taking in more calories than one expends on a chronic basis) causes adoposity, and caloric imbalance has also been hypothesized to cause colorectal cancer[1]. The accurate ascertainment of both physical expenditure and caloric intake in epidemiologic studies is problematic. It is not possible, therefore, to measure with certainty the marginal differences between caloric intake and expenditure that constitute the chronic caloric imbalances that lead to obesity. In contrast, however, body weight is relatively easy to measure with accuracy. If physical activity and caloric intake, together or in combination, act to affect colorectal cancer risk independently of adiposity, the limitations of our measurement methods will not allow epidemiologic studies to sort out those relationships with certainty.

Adiposity might be both the cause and the consequence of a metabolic state of increased availability of insulin and insulin-like growth factors that can promote colorectal cancer. Several of the nutritional and behavioural factors known to be associated with a modest increase in risk for colorectal cancer, including dietary factors of low intake of fruits and vegetables, high glycaemic and/or high fat diets, low levels of physical activity, and abdominal obesity, are also risk factors for diabetes and the insulin resistance syndrome. McKeown-Eyssen and Giovannucci proposed a unifying hypothesis linking these observations to findings from the experimental biology of insulin and insulin-like growth factors (IGFs)[17,18]. They hypothesized that insulin and/or IGFs were major factors in human colorectal neoplasia. Specifically, they proposed that the colorectal neoplasia risk factors of high fat or high glycaemic diets, sedentary activity levels, hyper-triglyceridaemia, and obesity are related to colorectal neoplasia via their effects on increasing insulin resistance. Whether the insulin resistance effects are mediated by insulin *per se*, by IGF-1 levels, by IGF-1 binding protein levels, or other mechanisms, is unknown. Recent prospective studies have shown associations between single point-in-time serum markers of insulin resistance and colorectal cancer (2-h insulin levels and IGF-1 levels)[19–21]. Both insulin and IGF are important trophic factors for a variety of tissue types including cells from the colon[22]. By activating the type 1 IGF Receptor they can induce a remarkable series of biologic effects, including cellular proliferation, inhibition of apoptotic cell death, and promotion of neoplastic transformation and angiogenesis. Obesity might also increase colorectal cancer risk via increased production of other factors thought to affect neoplasia, such as cytokines or VEGF.

The observation of a weaker association between BMI and colorectal neoplasia for women than for men is unexplained. It is plausible, however, that this difference might be related to differences in the effects of adiposity on estrogen metabolism in postmenopausal women. It has been shown in observational studies, and now confirmed in the recently-published Womens' Health Initiative trial, that post-menopausal estrogen supplements can decrease the risk of colorectal cancer[23–25]. The mechanisms for this association are not well-understood, but estrogen receptors are expressed by colonocytes. If obesity is a risk factor among both men and women that obesity risk could be partially offset by increased estrogen levels among postmenopausal women who are overweight because overweight leads to higher circulating estrogen levels due to the conversion of estrogen precursors to estrogen in adipose tissues.

In conclusion, it is clear that obesity increases risk for colorectal cancer and colorectal adenomas among both men and women. More advanced adenomas are more associated with obesity that smaller adenomas, and obesity later in life appears to be more strongly associated with risk than obesity earlier in life. Among women, the risk increase from obesity appears to be blunted, perhaps by beneficial effects of obesity on circulating estrogens. The mechanism for risk enhancement by obesity remain only hypothetical. Insulin trophic effects, or the effects of other factors such as insulin-like growth factors, their binding proteins, cytokines, or VEGF, may also play a role, singly or in combination. The needed efforts to reverse the epidemic of obesity in order to reduce risk of cardiovascular diseases, diabetes, and other cancers presents an important additional opportunity to also reduce the risk of colorectal cancer in the future

References

1. Potter J. Nutrition and colorectal cancer. *Cancer Causes Control* 1996; 7: 127–46.

2. Vogelstein B, Fearon ER, Hamilton SR, Kern SE, Preisinger AC, Leppert M *et al*. Genetic alterations during colorectal-tumor development. *N Engl J Med* 1998; 319: 525–32.

3. International Agency for Research on Cancer (IARC) IARC. Handbooks of Cancer Prevention. Weight Control and Physical Activity. Lyon: IARC publications. 2002 (volume 6).

4. Le Marchand L, Wilkens LR, Kolonel LN, Hankin JH, Lyu LC. Associations of sedentary lifestyle, obesity, smoking, alcohol use, and diabetes with the risk of colorectal cancer. *Cancer Res* 1997; 57: 4787–94.

5. Giovannucci E, Ascherio A, Rimm EB, Colditz GA, Stampfer M J, Willett WC. Physical activity, obesity, and risk for colon cancer and adenoma in men. *Ann Intern Med* 1995; 122: 327–334.

6. Martinez ME, Giovannucci E, Spiegelman D, Hunter DJ, Willett WC, Colditz G A. Leisure-time physical activity, body size, and colon cancer in women. Nurses' Health Study Research Group. *J Natl Cancer Inst* 1997; 89: 948–55.

7. Caan B, Coates A, Slattery M, Potter J, Quesenberry C, Edwards S. Body size and the risk of colon cancer in a large case-control study. *Int J Obes* 1998; 22: 178–84.

8. Graham S, Marshall J, Haughey B, Mittelman A, Swanson M, Zielezny M *et al*. Dietary epidemiology of cancer of the colon in western New York. *Am J Epidemiol* 1988; 128: 490–503.

9. Dietz AT, Newcomb PA, Marcus PM, Storer BE. The association of body size and large bowel cancer risk in Wisconsin (United States) women. *Cancer Causes Control* 1995; 6: 30–36.

10. Kune GA, Kune S, Watson LF. Body weight and physical activity as predictors of colorectal cancer risk. *Nutr Cancer* 1990; 13: 9–17.

11. Chyou PH, Nomura AM, Stemmermann GN. A prospective study of weight, body mass index and other anthropometric measurements in relation to site-specific cancers. *Int J Cancer* 1994; 57: 313–7.

12. Bostick R, Potter J, Kushi L, Sellers T, Steinmetz K, McKenzie D *et al*. Sugar, meat, and fat intake, and non-dietary risk factors for colon cancer in Iowa (United States). *Cancer Causes Control* 1994; 5: 38–52.

13. Russo A, Franceschi S, La Vecchia C, Dal Maso L, Montella M, Conti E *et al*. Body size and colorectal-cancer risk. *Int J Cancer* 1998; 78: 161–5.

14. Thun MJ, Calle EE, Namboodiri MM, Flanders WD, Coates RJ, Byers T *et al*. Risk factors for fatal colon cancer in a large prospective study. *J Natl Cancer Inst* 1992; 84: 1491–500.

15. Ford ES. Body mass index and colon cancer in a national sample of adult US men and women. *Am J Epidemiol* 1999; 150: 390–8.

16. Lee IM, Paffenbarger RSJ. Quetelet's index and risk of colon cancer in college alumni. *J Natl Cancer Inst* 1992; 84: 1326–31.

17. McKeown-Eyssen G. Epidemiology of colorectal cancer revisited: are serum triglycerides and/or plasma glucose associated with risk? *Cancer Epidemiol Biomarkers Prev* 1994; 3: 687–95.

18. Giovannucci E. Insulin and colon cancer. *Cancer Causes Control* 1995; 6: 164–79.

19. Renehan AG, O'Dwyer ST, Shalet SMRe: Prospective study of colorectal cancer risk in men and plasma levels of insulin-like growth factor (IGF)-I and IGF-binding protein-3. *J Natl Cancer Inst* 1999; 91: 2051–2.

20. Ma J, Pollak M, Giovannucci E *et al*. Prospective study of colorectal cancer risk in men and plasma levels of insulin-like growth factor (IGF)-I and IGF-binding protein-3. *J Natl Cancer Inst* 1999; 91: 620–5.

21. Giovannucci E, Pollak M, Platz E *et al*. A prospective study of plasma insulin-like growth factor-1 and binding protein-3 and risk of colorectal neoplasia in women. *Cancer Epidemiol Biomarkers Prev* 2000; 9: 345–9.

22. Burroughs KD, Dunn SE, Barrett JC, Taylor JA. Insulin-like growth factor-I: a key regulator of human cancer risk? *J Natl Cancer Inst* 1999; 91: 579–81.

23. Calle E, Miracle-McMahill H, Thun M, Heath C. Estrogen replacement therapy and risk of fatal colon cancer. *J Natl Cancer Inst* 1995; 87: 517–23.

24. Kampman E, Potter J, Slattery M, Caan B, Edwards S. Hormone replacement therapy, reproductive history, and colon cancer: a multicenter, case-control study in the United States. *Cancer Causes Control* 1997; 8: 146–58.

25. Womens' Health Initiative Writing Group. Effects of combined estrogen and progesterone supplementation on morbidity and mortality among postmenopausal women: Results of the Womens' Health Initiative Trial. *J Am Med Assoc* 2002; 288: 321–33.

Progress in Obesity Research: 9. Edited by *Geraldo Medeiros-Neto, Alfredo Halpern and Claude Bouchard*
©2003 John Libbey Eurotext Ltd, pp. 676–679.

CHAPTER 142

Obesity and cancer of the prostate, kidney, gallbladder, and oesophagus

Alicja Wolk

Division of Nutritional Epidemiology, Institute of Environmental Medicine, Karolinska Institutet, Box 210, SE-171 77 Stockholm, Sweden
[e-mail: Alicja.Wolk@imm.ki.se]

Introduction

The first evidence – based on a large prospective study of 750,000 subjects – that overweight and obesity increase risk of mortality from certain cancers was presented over 20 years ago[1]. Since that time the growing number of studies has further linked excess body weight to increased incidence of cancer at several sites[2,3].

In this review the accumulated scientific evidence regarding the association between excess body weight and increased risk of development of cancer in prostate, kidney, gallbladder, and oesophagus is summarized. Possible biological mechanisms behind the observed positive associations are discussed and furthermore, needs for future research are indicated.

Incidence and trends

Incidence and mortality of prostate cancer have systematically increased during the last 30 years[4]. The most striking epidemiologic observation about prostate cancer is the very large, 40-fold difference in the reported age-adjusted incidence between the populations with the highest (US blacks, 130 per 100,000 man-years) and the lowest (China, 3 per 100,000 man-years) risk. Renal cell cancer – the most common malignancy in kidney that accounts for 80–90 per cent of this cancer – is relatively common in western countries, with high incidence rates in Scandinavia[5]. There is a 10-fold variation in the incidence of renal cell cancer over the world. An increasing trend in incidence had been observed in men and women from most areas in the world. Cancer of the oesophagus is the eighth most common form of cancer in the world[5]. The dominating histopathological type is squamous cell carcinoma, which accounts for about 90 per cent of the cases, and its incidence has remained stable during the last few decades[6]. A striking feature in most parts of the industrialized world in recent decades is the rapidly increasing incidence of oesophageal adenocarcinoma. Cancer of the gallbladder is uncommon and there are no recent reliable estimates of incidence available.

Excess adult body weight and risk of prostate, kidney, gallbladder, and oesophagus cancer

Epidemiological investigations of the relation between body size and cancer have focused mainly on weight and measurement of obesity as the body mass index (BMI). The BMI – defined as body weight in kilograms (kg), divided by the square of the height in meters (m^2) – was used as a surrogate for body fat content. In spite of its popularity, there are limitations of BMI as an objective measure of obesity[7]. In recent years, the distribution of body fat has received more attention as an important dimension in studying the relation between obesity and health. The ratio of waist to hip circumferences or waist circumference has been used to estimate upper body fat and abdominal visceral fat.

A number of studies have been done to assess the relation of excess adult body mass to prostate cancer. Out of 11 case-control studies, 10 reported no significant associations between prostate cancer and various measurements including weight, BMI, waist/hip ratio waist, waist circumference, and triceps skinfold thickness[8]. In the majority of these case-control studies the analysis depended upon self-reported anthropometric measures, which might have limitations. What is important to point out in case-control design is that some patients may have lost weight because of their disease. Therefore prospective cohort studies, in which the participants were examined for their weight before they were subsequently diagnosed with prostate cancer, have an obvious advantage over case-control studies in this regard. Results from 12 prospective cohort studies (including one case-control nested within a cohort)[9], are mixed[8]. Seven suggested that there was a positive association of prostate cancer with either BMI, weight, or percentage of desirable weight (relative risk, RR = 1.2–2.4). Two of the 12 studies had death, instead of incident prostate cancer cases, as outcome[10,11]. Both studies found positive associations (RR = 1.4 and 2.4, respectively), which suggests that severity of disease may be an important factor, since the majority of cases with prostate cancer do not die from their disease. The summary relative risk estimate, based upon meta-analysis from six studies, is 1.01 (95 per cent CI 1.00–1.02) per 1 kg/m^2 increment in BMI[12]. There are two additional prospective studies of obesity and prostate cancer with another study design, namely comparing incidence of prostate cancer in a cohort of obese men (BMI >30 kg/m^2) with incidence in the general population[2,3]. In both studies an age-dependent effect of obesity was observed. In the Swedish study there was no association overall, but a positive relation was seen in cases diagnosed before age 60 years (standardized incidence ratio, SIR = 1.5), and a negative relation after age 80 years (SIR = 0.4), with a significant trend through age groups (*P*-value for trend = 0.04)[2]. In the Danish study there was an overall significant positive association (SIR = 1.3). However, obese men, diagnosed with prostate cancer before age of 60 years, had a significant relative risk of 2.5, which decreased to 1.1 among those above 80 years at diagnosis; trend *P*-value through age subgroups was < 0.0013.

Data are sparse in assessing whether birth weight, childhood, adolescence, and young adulthood obesity are more important than mid-life or older age obesity in relation to prostate cancer development. One study indicated that high birth weight is associated with increased risk[13]. In another report, obesity at age 10 years was found to be inversely related to the risk of advanced and metastatic cancer[14]. A recent meta-analysis of results regarding BMI and risk of renal cell cancer has shown that the association is equally strong among women and men, and the summary relative risk (based upon analyses of 14 studies of men and 14 studies of women) is 1.07 (95 per cent CI 1.05–1.09) per 1 kg/m^2 increment in BMI[15]. In our large, population-based case-control study we have observed an increased risk of renal cell cancer among men with a birth weight higher than 3.5 kg (RR = 1.3, 95 per cent CI 1.1–1.8) compared to men with a birth weight 3.0–3.5 kg, especially in the subgroup with hypertension (RR = 1.8, 95 per cent CI 1.2–2.6)[16]. We have reported previously a positive association between number of weight changes (weight loss > 5 kg) and increased risk for renal cell carcinoma[17].

There are very few epidemiological studies of gallbladder cancer. From the six published studies, only two could be included in dose-response meta-analysis, and the summary risk estimate was 1.06 (95 per cent CI 1.00–1.12) per 1 kg/m^2 increment in BMI[12]. In the most recent study, where the incidence of gallbladder cancer in a cohort of 28,129 obese subjects (BMI > 30 kg/m^2) was compared to the incidence in the general population (Sweden), we observed a significantly increased risk (SIR = 1.6, 95 CI 1.1–2.3)[2].

Obesity was found to be associated with an increased risk for oesophagus carcinoma in four of six case-control studies[18]. In the two most recent studies of two specific histological subtypes, there was no association with squamous cell carcinoma, but risk estimates for oesophageal adenocarcinoma cancer were very high[18,19]. In the US study subjects in the highest decile of BMI ($\geq$ 29.5 for men, $\geq$ 31.3 for women) compared to the lowest decile (< 21.7 for men, < 20.2 for women) had over fivefold increased risk (RR = 5.4, 95 per cent CI 2.4–12.0)[19]. In the Swedish study subjects with BMI > 30, compared to those < 22 kg/m^2, had 16-fold increased risk (RR = 16.2, 95 per cent CI 6.3–41.4)[18]. The strongest risk factor for an oesophageal adenocarcinoma is gastro-oesophageal reflux. Among persons with both long-lasting symptoms (duration more than 20 years) and severe symptoms, the adjusted risk estimate was 43.5 (95 per cent CI 18.3–103.5)[20]. It might be speculated that obesity is associated with increased risk of reflux, however, in the Swedish study there was no association between BMI and severity or duration of reflux symptoms[21].

Biological mechanisms

Obesity might be associated with increased risk of various cancers through several hormonal mechanisms[2]. In particular, obesity is associated with insulin resistance, compensatory insulinaemia, and increased growth factor production, which in turn may stimulate carcinogenesis. Obese men have lower levels of sex-hormone binding globulin (SHBG), as well as testosterone. The observed age-dependent effect of obesity on prostate cancer is compatible with findings suggesting that low levels of

SHBG are a risk factor for prostate cancer in younger men, while low levels of testosterone are protective in older men. Obese individuals tend to have lower blood levels of antioxidants[22], perhaps due to lower consumption of fruit and vegetables that are considered protective for several cancer sites[23]. In general, obese consume more calories, which may contribute to increased risk of cancer[24]. Energy restriction in animals has been related to smaller tumours and increased apoptosis. These effects were associated with reduced circulating insulin-like growth factor-I and reduced vascular endothelial growth factor expression, which supports the hypothesis that energy restriction reduces tumour growth by inhibiting tumour angiogenesis[25].

Overweight as avoidable cause of prostate, kidney, gallbladder, and oesophageal cancer

We have recently estimated the proportion of site-specific cases, attributable to excess weight in countries of the European Union[12]. To make these calculations, we used summary risk estimates from the meta-analyses, and we have estimated the prevalence of overweight (BMI = 25.1–30 kg/m^2) and obesity (BMI > 30 kg/m^2) among men and women in 15 European countries. Overweight is prevalent in 50 per cent of adult European men and 35 per cent of women, and obesity in 13 per cent of men and 19 per cent of women. Estimated attributable risk for prostate cancer due to overweight and obesity was 2.9 per cent and 1.6 per cent respectively. Corresponding estimates for kidney cancer were 15.2 per cent and 10.3 per cent in men and 11.1 per cent and 13.4 per cent in women; for gall bladder cancer 14.7 per cent and 10.1 per cent in men and 10.7 per cent and 13.0 per cent in women[12]. The attributable risk for esophageal adenocarcinoma, based on risk estimates from the US study only[19] (relative risk for those with BMI above 25 kg/m^2 in comparison to those below, might be roughly estimated as twofold increase) give us a rough estimate of 38.7 per cent in men and 35.1 per cent in women (Table 1).

Fig. 1. Risk of cancer in relation to excess body weight per unit of BMI increment (from meta-analysis). Comparison of cancer incidence in the cohort of obese subjects (BMI >30 kg/m^2) to incidence in a general population.

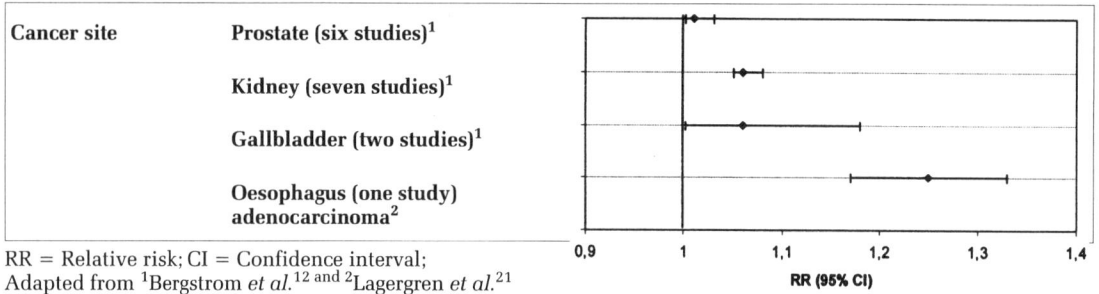

Cancer site		
Prostate (six studies)[1]		
Kidney (seven studies)[1]		
Gallbladder (two studies)[1]		
Oesophagus (one study) adenocarcinoma[2]		

RR = Relative risk; CI = Confidence interval;
Adapted from [1]Bergstrom *et al.*[12 and 2]Lagergren *et al.*[21]

Table 1. Proportion of cancer cases in Europe attributable to BMI > 25 kg/m²

Cancer site	Men	Women
Prostate[1]	4.5%	
Kidney[1]	25.5%	24.5%
Gallbladder[1]	24.8%	23.7%
Oesophagus[2] (adenocarcinoma)	38.7%	35.1%

[1]Adapted from Bergstrom *et al.*[12]; [2]Calculation based on Chow *et al.*[19]

Future research

To advance our knowledge on the association of obesity with cancer, we need inexpensive and uninvasive methods to assess adiposity more accurately than by using BMI or waist/hip ratio. There is a need for more studies of age-dependent aspects of the association between body size and the risk of cancer, e.g. little attention has been paid to the association with birth weight and body size during childhood, adolescence, and early adulthood, as well as potential differences in risk depending on age at diagnosis. Studies should be preferably with a prospective cohort design instead of case-control studies, unless the case-control studies have valid data on anthropometric measurements, pre-dating the diagnosis of cancer. Preferably, blood samples should be collected at the time of anthropometric measurements in cohort studies to enable investigators to measure biomarkers that could be helpful in determining how obesity or related factors are associated with cancer risk. Family history and relevant gene markers should be included in the study in order to enable the investigators to assess gene-environment interactions in relation to body size and cancer of the prostate, kidney, gall bladder, and oesophagus. The association between weight changes and the above mentioned cancer forms also should be studied, especially risk of renal cell cancer. Specific cancer subtypes should be studied separately.

Acknowledgements: The work has been supported by grants from the Swedish Cancer Society.

References

1. Lew EA, Garfinkel L. Variations in mortality by weight among 750,000 men and women. *J Chronic Dis* 1979; 32: 563–76.

2. Wolk A, Gridley G, Svensson M, Nyren O, McLaughlin JK, Fraumeni JF, Adam HO. A prospective study of obesity and cancer risk (Sweden). *Cancer Causes Control* 2001; 12: 13–21.

3. Moller H, Mellemgaard A, Lindvig K, Olsen JH. Obesity and cancer risk: a Danish record-linkage study. *Eur J Cancer* 1994; A30: 344–50.

4. Hsing AW, Devesa SS. Trends and patterns of prostate cancer: what do they suggest? *Epidemiol Rev* 2001; 23: 3–13.

5. Parkin DM. The global burden of cancer. *Semin Cancer Biol* 1998; 8: 219–35.

6. Thomas RM, Sobin LH. Gastrointestinal cancer. *Cancer* 1995; 75: 154–70.

7. Garn SM, Leonard WR and Hawthorne VM Three limitations of the body mass index. *Am J Clin Nutr* 1986; 44: 996–7.

8. Nomura AM. Body size and prostate cancer. *Epidemiol Rev* 2001; 23: 126–31.

9. Gronberg H, Damber L, Damber JE. Total food consumption and body mass index in relation to prostate cancer risk: a case-control study in Sweden with prospectively collected exposure data. *J Urol* 1996; 155: 969–74.

10. Andersson SO, Wolk A, Bergstrom R, Adami HO, Engholm G, Englund A, Nyren O. Body size and prostate cancer: a 20-year follow-up study among 135006 Swedish construction workers. *J Natl Cancer Inst* 1997; 89: 385–9.

11. Snowdon DA, Phillips RL, Choi W. Diet, obesity, and risk of fatal prostate cancer. *Am J Epidemiol* 1984; 120: 244–50.

12. Bergstrom A, Pisani P, Tenet V, Wolk A, Adami HO. Overweight as an avoidable cause of cancer in Europe. *Int J Cancer* 2001; 91: 421–30.

13. Ekbom A, Hsieh CC, Lipworth L, Wolk A, Ponten J, Adami HO, Trichopoulos D. Perinatal characteristics in relation to incidence of and mortality from prostate cancer. *BMJ* 1996; 313: 337–41.

14. Giovannucci E, Rimm EB, Stampfer MJ, Colditz GA, Willett WC. Height, body weight, and risk of prostate cancer. *Cancer Epidemiol Biomarkers Prev* 1997; 6: 557–63.

15. Bergstrom A, Hsieh CC, Lindblad P, Lu CM, Cook NR, Wolk A. Obesity and renal cell cancer – a quantitative review. *Br J Cancer* 2001; 85: 984–90.

16. Bergstrom A, Lindblad P, Wolk A. Birth weight and risk of renal cell cancer. *Kidney Int* 2001; 59: 1110–3.

17. Lindblad P, Wolk A, Bergstrom R, Persson I, Adami HO. The role of obesity and weight fluctuations in the etiology of renal cell cancer: a population-based case-control study. *Cancer Epidemiol Biomarkers Prev* 1994; 3: 631–9.

18. Lagergren J, Bergstrom R, Nyren O. Association between body mass and adenocarcinoma of the esophagus and gastric cardia. *Ann Intern Med* 1999; 130: 883–90.

19. Chow WH, Blot WJ, Vaughan TL, Risch HA, Gammon MD, Stanford JL *et al.* Body mass index and risk of adenocarcinomas of the esophagus and gastric cardia. *J Natl Cancer Inst* 1998; 90: 150–5.

20. Lagergren J, Bergstrom R, Lindgren A, Nyren O. Symptomatic gastroesophageal reflux as a risk factor for esophageal adenocarcinoma. *N Engl J Med* 1999; 340: 825–31.

21. Lagergren J, Bergstrom R, Nyren O. No relation between body mass and gastro-oesophageal reflux symptoms in a Swedish population based study. *Gut* 2000; 47: 26–9.

22. Moor de Burgos A, Wartanowicz M, Ziemlanski S. Blood vitamin and lipid levels in overweight and obese women. *Eur J Clin Nutr* 1992; 46: 803–8.

23. Terry P, Terry JB, Wolk A. Fruit and vegetable consumption in the prevention of cancer: an update. *J Intern Med* 2001; 250: 280–90.

24. Andersson SO, Wolk A, Bergstrom R, Giovannucci E, Lindgren C, Baron J, Adami HO. Energy, nutrient intake and prostate cancer risk: a population-based case-control study in Sweden. *Int J Cancer* 1996; 68: 716–22.

25. Mukherjee P, Sotnikov AV, Mangian HJ, Zhou JR, Visek WJ, Clinton SK. Energy intake and prostate tumour growth, angiogenesis, and vascular endothelial growth factor expression. *J Natl Cancer Inst* 1999; 91: 512–23.

Progress in Obesity Research: 9. Edited by *Geraldo Medeiros-Neto, Alfredo Halpern and Claude Bouchard*
©2003 John Libbey Eurotext Ltd, pp. 680–683.

CHAPTER 143

Intra-uterine and childhood growth and future health outcomes

Johan G. Eriksson

National Public Health Institute, Department of Epidemiology and Health Promotion, Diabetes and Genetic Epidemiology Unit, Mannerheimintie 166, FIN-00300 Helsinki, Finland
[e-mail: bi]

Introduction

The importance of events before birth regarding lifetime health has been observed and confirmed in several epidemiological studies[1-5]. Findings point towards the importance of events during critical periods of growth and development in the pathogenesis of many non-communicable diseases, e.g. cardiovascular disease and type 2 diabetes. In the past when infectious diseases were even more common than nowadays it was self-evident that a non-optimal early growth affected later health. The original 'fetal origins hypothesis' postulates that impaired fetal growth may predispose individuals to heart disease in later life[6]. According to the original observations from Hertfordshire, UK, by Barker and co-workers, deaths from coronary heart disease were more common in men who had been small at birth and who were small at one year of age[1]. Obviously a small body size at birth increases the risk for later coronary heart disease and type 2 diabetes. However, a question of major importance is whether the increased risk for these diseases – associated with a small body size at birth – is modified by childhood growth? Our Helsinki birth cohorts have made it possible to simultaneously assess the importance of body size at birth and growth in childhood with regard to adult health outcomes.

Helsinki birth cohorts

Two birth cohorts born at Helsinki University Central Hospital – consisting of 15,846 men and women – have been followed from 1964 to present date using primarily register linkage[4,5]. The older cohort consists of 7086 individuals born 1924–33 with data on body size at birth as well as data on growth between 7 and 15 years of age. The younger cohort ($n = 8760$) born 1934–44 has more detailed information on growth from birth up to 12 years of age. In both cohorts information on growth was collected from birth records, child welfare records and school records. These records include, in addition to information on growth, information on socio-economic factors. An ongoing clinical examination on 2000 individuals from the younger cohort will further enable more detailed metabolic and genetic studies on the associations between early growth and adult health in the near future.

Early growth and coronary heart disease in adult life

The original study reporting an association between body size at birth and weight in infancy and later coronary heart disease was performed Hertfordshire, UK. Standardized mortality ratios (SMR) fell from 111 in men who weighed ≤ 18 pounds (≤ 8.2 kg) at one year to 42 in those who weighed ≥ 27 pounds (12.3 kg)[1]. There is now convincing evidence from over 100 studies that individuals who had low birth weight, or were thin or short at birth have increased rates of coronary heart disease as well as its risk factors. In the Helsinki Birth Cohorts the importance of body size at birth and growth during childhood has been assessed simultaneously. Deaths from CHD were associated with both a small body size at birth, and an above average body mass index during childhood[4,5,7]. In a simultaneous regression the hazard ratio for CHD mortality increased by 14 per cent for each unit decrease in ponderal index at birth and by 22 per cent for each unit (kg/m^2) increase in body mass index at 11 years of age. In other words, the men who were thin at birth, but whose weight 'caught up' during childhood, had the highest death rates from CHD. These findings show that the consequences of 'catching-up' in body size – are conditioned and modified by growth in utero. Therefore, disease risk does not solely depend on the absolute level of body weight attained. The most unfavourable growth pattern seems to be small body size or thinness at birth, continued slow growth in infancy and thereafter acceleration in growth[7]. The present findings add to the evidence that protection of fetal and infant growth is a key area in strategies for the prevention of many non-communicable adult diseases.

Early growth and type 2 diabetes in adult life

Low birth weight and a small body size at birth are associated with increased rates of type 2 diabetes in adult life[8–10]. This is thought to reflect persistence of changes in glucose and insulin metabolism, which accompany slow growth *in utero*. Type 2 diabetes is also strongly associated with obesity in adult life. Therefore one could speculate that a higher body mass index in childhood would be associated with an increased risk of type 2 diabetes. The cumulative incidence of type 2 diabetes is strongly and positively related to body mass index during childhood. Children, who later developed type 2 diabetes, had a small body size at birth and at one year, after which their weights and body mass indices rose progressively to exceed the average. An early adiposity rebound also seemed to be associated with an increased risk of type 2 diabetes in adult life especially among those born small and thin. The underlying mechanisms explaining these findings are unknown but could be due to alterations in body composition. Babies that are small and thin at birth have a lower muscle mass compared to babies not born small[11]. If these children develop a higher body mass index during childhood they may have a disproportionately high fat mass in relation to lean body mass, which will lead to insulin resistance and subsequently to type 2 diabetes[12].

Early growth and the PPAR γ2 gene

There is a well-established association between the PPAR γ2 gene and type 2 diabetes. We therefore assessed whether the effects of the Pro12Ala polymorphism of the PPARγ gene on insulin sensitivity and insulin metabolism in adult life are modified by size at birth[13]. The effects of the Pro12Pro and Pro12Ala polymorphisms of the PPAR γ2 gene depended on the body size at birth. The well-known association between a small body size at birth and insulin resistance was seen only in individuals with the high risk Pro12Pro allele. In those who had low birth weight, the Pro12Pro polymorphism of the PPAR γ2 gene was associated with increased insulin resistance and elevated insulin concentrations. These findings reflect gene-environment interaction.

Early growth and adult obesity

There is considerable evidence that impaired fetal growth and rapid childhood weight gain is associated with an increased risk of type 2 diabetes and cardiovascular disease. Obesity is closely associated with these disorders but interestingly adult obesity is associated with a large body size at birth[14–16]. Individuals who became obese in adult life had above average body weights and BMIs at all ages from birth to 12 years. Table 1 shows that childhood BMI predicted adult obesity, already from early childhood. Childhood BMI was a stronger predictor of adult obesity than body size at birth. The association with body size at birth points to a role of the early environment in the development of adult obesity. The positive relationship between body size at birth and obesity in adult life has received great attention. Increased muscularity may partly explain the cardiovascular benefits in later life associated with a higher birth weight[11,17]. Therefore individuals with a larger body size at birth may have a larger muscle mass potentially partly protecting them from metabolic disorders in adult life.

Conclusion

The thrifty phenotype hypothesis suggests that the early nutritional environment has a programming effect on metabolism and consequently on health in adult life. The mismatch between a relatively poor intrauterine environment and a nutritionally rich environment in later life is supposed to increase the risk of type 2 diabetes and many other related non-communicable diseases. Adaptation to undernutrition in utero may limit the extent of dietary change to which a generation can be exposed without adverse effects. In other words tendency towards diseases seems to be programmed. This is a very complex area and one must always bear in mind that fetal growth is regulated by genes, hormones, growth factors and placental function – not only by availability of food. Future studies are needed in order to explore the underlying mechanisms between early growth and adult health.

Table 1. Cumulative incidence of obesity according to ponderal index at birth, body mass index at 6 months and 11 years of age in men and women in the Helsinki Birth Cohort born 1934–44

	Men	Women
Ponderal index at birth (kg/m³)		
−25	30.5	29.3
−26	37.8	31.2
−27	31.6	31.1
−28	31.0	34.2
>28	37.8	35.2
P values	0.04	0.008
BMI at 6 months (kg/m²)		
<16.3	28.6	27.5
−16.8	24.2	31.1
−17.3	36.3	33.7
−18.0	32.2	34.5
>18.0	44.1	36.8
P values	<0.0001	0.001
BMI at 11 years (kg/m²)		
−15.8	16.2	19.1
−16.6	23.2	23.9
−17.4	31.3	33.5
−18.5	40.2	28.9
>18.5	63.6	51.8
P values	<0.001	<0.001

Reference

1. Barker DJP, Osmond C, Winter PD, Margetts B, Simmonds SJ. Weight in infancy and death from ischaemic heart disease. *Lancet* 1989; 2: 577–80.

2. Osmond C, Barker DJ, Winter PD, Fall CHD, Simmonds SJ. Early growth and death from cardiovascular disease in women. *BMJ* 1993; 307: 1519–24.

3. Rich-Edwards JW, Stampfer MJ, Manson JE, Rosner B, Hankinson SE, Colditz GA. Birth weight and risk of cardiovascular disease in a cohort of women followed up since 1976. *BMJ* 1997; 315: 396–400.

4. Forsén T, Eriksson JG, Tuomilehto J, Teramo K, Osmond C, Barker DJ. Mother's weight in pregnancy and coronary heart disease in a cohort of Finnish men: follow up study. *BMJ* 1997; 315: 837–40.

5. Eriksson JG, Forsén T, Tuomilehto J, Osmond C, Barker DJ. Early growth and coronary heart disease in later life: longitudinal study. *BMJ* 2001; 322: 949–53.

6. Barker DJ. *Mothers, babies and health in later life* (2nd edn). London: Churchill Livingstone; 1998.

7. Eriksson JG, Forsén T, Tuomilehto J, Winter PD, Osmond C, Barker DJ. Catch-up growth in childhood and death from coronary heart disease longitudinal study. *BMJ* 1999; 318: 427–31.

8. Hales CN, Barker DJP, Clark PMS, Cox LJ, Fall C, Osmond C, Winter PD. Fetal and infant growth and impaired glucose tolerance at age 64. *BMJ* 1991; 303: 1019–22.

9. Rich-Edwards JW, Colditz GA, Stampfer MJ, Willett WC, Gillman MW *et al*. Birthweight and the risk for type 2 diabetes mellitus in adult women. *Ann Intern Med* 1999; 130: 278–84.

10. Forsen T, Eriksson J, Tuomilehto J, Reunanen A, Osmond C, Barker D. The fetal and childhood growth of persons who develop type 2 diabetes. *Ann Intern Med* 2000; 133: 176–82.

11. Eriksson J, Forsen T, Tuomilehto J, Osmond C, Barker D. Size at birth, fat-free mass and resting metabolic rate in adult life. *Horm Metab Res* 2002; 34: 72–6.

12. Eriksson JG, Forsén T, Tuomilehto J, Jaddoe VWV, Osmond C, Barker DJP. Effects of size at birth and childhood growth on the insulin resistance syndrome in elderly individuals. *Diabetologia*. 2002; 45: 342–8.

13. Eriksson JG, Lindi V, Uusitupa M, Forsén TJ, Laakso M, Osmond C, Barker DJP. The effects of the Pro12Ala polymorphism of the peroxisome proliferator-activated receptor-α2 gene on insulin sensitivity and insulin metabolism interact with size at birth. *Diabetes* 2002; 51: 2321–24.

14. Rolland-Cachera MF, Deheeger M, Guilloud-Bataille M, Avons P, Patois E, Sempe M. Tracking the development of adiposity from one month of age to adulthood. *Ann Hum Biol* 1987; 14: 219–29.

15. Sorensen HT, Sabroe S, Rothman KJ, Gillman M, Fischer P, Sorensen TI. Relation between weight and length at birth and body mass index in young adulthood: cohort study. *BMJ* 1997; 315: 1137.

16. Eriksson J, Forsen T, Tuomilehto J,Osmond C, Barker D. Size at birth, childhood growth and obesity in adult life. *Int J Obes* 2001; 25: 735–40.

17. Kahn HS, Narayan KMV, Williamson DF, Valdez R. Relation of birth weight to lean and fat thigh tissue in young men. *Int J Obes* 2000; 24: 1–6.

Progress in Obesity Research: 9. Edited by *Geraldo Medeiros-Neto, Alfredo Halpern and Claude Bouchard*
©2003 John Libbey Eurotext Ltd, pp. 684–692.

CHAPTER 144

Effects of obesity on morbidity in children and adolescents: emerging issues

Aviva Must and Sarah E. Anderson

*Department of Family Medicine and Community Health, School of Medicine, Tufts University, 136 Harrison Avenue,
Boston, MA 02111, USA; Gerald J. and Dorothy R. Friedman School of Nutritional Science and Policy, Tufts
University, 150 Harrison Avenue, Boston, MA 02111, USA*
[e-mail: aviva.must@tufts.edu; sarah.anderson@tufts.edu]

Introduction

The epidemic of childhood obesity might be more aptly termed a pandemic. The rise of obesity in youth has been documented in many countries in both the developed and developing world[1]. Ironically, it co-exists with undernutrition in parts of the world where poverty is common[2]. Warnings regarding the epidemic of obesity and its associated health consequences are not new. In the late 1980s, when Gortmaker and Dietz[3] first identified a trend towards increased obesity prevalence in children across national surveys conducted in the US, they cautioned '... the implications of these increases for the morbidity and mortality of the US population suggest that we can no longer afford to ignore obesity as a medical problem' (p. 539). More recently, the obesity epidemic has been called a failure of primary and secondary prevention. Pinhas-Hamiel[4] asserts 'life-style-related diseases are no longer the exclusive domain of adult medicine' (p. 704).

The health effects of the secular trend towards increasing prevalence of overweight are made more serious by the increased severity of the condition. The population distribution of relative weight (as reflected in BMI z-score) has both shifted upward and become more positively skewed[5]. This means that, not only are more youth overweight, but those youth are *more* overweight. With this increase in severity has come the increased burden on physical and psychosocial health. Heretofore rare medical conditions seen in association with childhood obesity are becoming common enough to be identified in population based, rather than clinical studies. The disturbing secular trends seen in the United States and globally also have important implications for the likelihood of persistence of childhood obesity into adulthood, where substantial additional health consequences accrue. These latter consequences have been recently reviewed[6,7] and will not be considered further here.

Physical health consequences

Historically, disease complications of childhood obesity did not become clinically apparent for decades; immediate consequences of obesity during childhood were thought to be rare. Clinical studies of obese children have identified a wide array of medical conditions for which obese children are at increased risk[8]. As catalogued in table 1, there are few organ systems that severe obesity in childhood does not affect (Table 1).

For the last several decades, the health effects of paediatric obesity documented in population-based studies have been largely limited to intermediate metabolic consequences, such as elevated levels of blood glucose, blood pressure, and cholesterol. Estimates suggest that obesity accounts for approximately 50 per cent of cases of adolescent hypertension[9]. Increased triceps skinfold thickness during adolescence is highly correlated with increased levels of LDL-cholesterol and triglycerides, and significantly decreased levels of serum HDL[10]. These risk factors, which together comprise the metabolic syndrome in adults, also cluster in children. More than half of overweight schoolchildren have at least one other cardiovascular risk factor[11]. Adolescent obesity, particularly in males, is associated with deleterious effects on total cholesterol and LDL-cholesterol in adulthood[12]. In addition, hypertensive children who continue to have high blood pressure into adulthood are more likely to have greater body weight, BMI, skinfold thickness, and substantially greater waist and hip circumferences[13]. The Bogalusa Heart Study has provided a wealth of information on cardiovascular risk factors in childhood as well as their persistence into adulthood[14]. In Bogalusa, overweight during adolescence (BMI > 75th percentile) was associated with a 8.5-fold increase in hypertension, a 2.4-fold increase in the prevalence of total cholesterol values above 240 mg/dl, a threefold increase in LDL values above 160 mg/dl, and an eightfold increase in HDL levels below 35 mg/dl in adults aged 27 to 31 years[15].

Table 1. Physical health conditions associated with childhood and adolescent obesity by system

Orthopaedic:	*Endocrine:*
Slipped capital epiphyses	Insulin resistance/impaired glucose tolerance
Blount's disease (tibia vara)	Type 2 diabetes
Tibial tortion	Menstrual abnormalities
	Polycystic ovary syndrome
Neurological:	
Idiopathic increased intracranial hypertension (e.g. *pseudotumor cerebri*)	*Pulmonary:*
	Sleep apnea
Gastroenterological:	Asthma
Cholelithiasis	Pickwickian syndrome
Liver steatosis	

Emerging physical health consequences

The epidemic of obesity in the paediatric age group has been accompanied by identification of 'new' or proposed associated health conditions. We consider three such conditions in this section: type 2 diabetes, asthma and sleep-disordered breathing; and menstrual abnormalities. The evidence for these conditions as obesity-related diseases in childhood is variable, with the strongest evidence for type 2 diabetes. The three conditions are important because they are prevalent, potentially serious, and carry lifelong consequences to overall health and well-being.

Type 2 diabetes

In addition to metabolic consequences likely to track into adulthood and give rise to substantial adult disease, type 2 diabetes is now a significant health condition in childhood. The emergence of type 2 diabetes in youth, a condition that historically has been seen only in adults, represents a particularly concerning consequence of the obesity epidemic in youth.

The strong upward trend of diabetes prevalence in adulthood, from 4.9 per cent in 1990 to 7.3 per cent in 2000, has been attributed to the epidemic of obesity in adults[16]. Likewise, the increased prevalence and severity of overweight in childhood is likely responsible for the occurrence of diabetes during the first and second decade of life.

As a relatively 'new' disease, the epidemiology and natural history of early type 2 diabetes is in its infancy. Recent findings indicate among newly diagnosed diabetic children, 8–50 per cent have type 2. In a multiethnic cohort of 167 obese children and adolescents recruited from an obesity clinic, impaired glucose tolerance was present in one quarter of obese children and in 21 per cent of obese adolescents by 2-h glucose tolerance test[17]. Undiagnosed diabetes was detected in 4 per cent of adolescents; no diabetes was seen in the younger children. This study, as well as several published case series, identifies minority youth as being at particular risk for type 2 diabetes[18–22].

Because type 2 diabetes has been rare in the paediatric population, relatively little is known about treatment. In the absence of clinical experience in youth, current treatment is modeled on adult treatment protocols. As a progressive condition for which treatment relies heavily on self-management, type 2 diabetes in youth will represent a challenge to caregivers and health care providers. In addition, diagnosis of type 2 diabetes is difficult. At diagnosis, the majority of patients often are either asymptomatic or present with unrelated symptoms such as vaginal monilial infection, rather than the classic triad of polyuria, polydipsia, and weight loss[18].

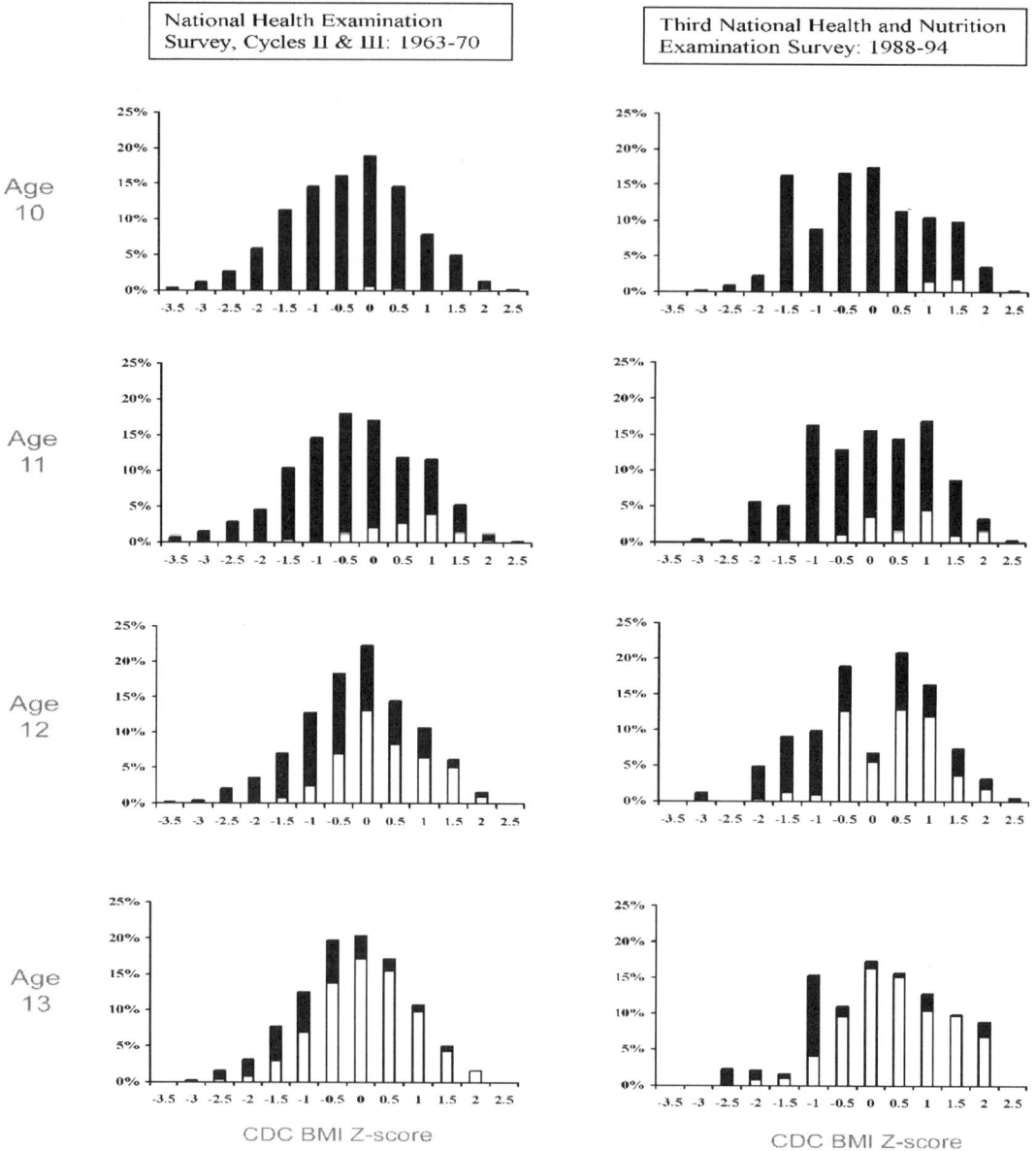

National Health Examination
Survey, Cycles II & III: 1963-70

Third National Health and Nutrition
Examination Survey: 1988-94

Age 10

Age 11

Age 12

Age 13

CDC BMI Z-score

CDC BMI Z-score

Fig. 1. Shift in the distribution of relative weight and menarcheal status between the National Health Examination Survey, Cycles II & III and the Third National Health and Nutrition Examination Survey in girls aged 10–13 years. The percentage of girls with a BMI z-score above the 85th percentile-for-age based on the CDC BMI growth reference increased significantly during the ~25 years between the surveys, and the population BMI z-score distribution shifted toward the right with more girls at higher relative weights. The shaded portion of each bar indicates girls who have not yet reached menarche; the open portions indicate girls who have reached menarche. Higher relative weights are associated with increased likelihood of having reached menarche at a given age.

The population of children with type 2 diabetes is expected to grow and to mirror the current obesity epidemic. Onset of diabetes in youth likely portends advanced complications – cardiovascular disease, kidney failure and amputations – at an early age. Clearly, research into the optimal secondary and tertiary prevention strategies will be crucial to managing this new wave of paediatric disease.

Menstrual problems/early menarche

Menstrual abnormalities and early menarche represent other endocrine responses to excess body fat in girls. Previous studies have established a relationship between obesity and subfertility[23,24]. The impact of high levels of overweight on menstrual problems in adolescents is less well established, however. Oligomenorrhea or amenorrhea associated with obesity, insulin resistance, hirsuitism, acne, and acanthosis nigricans comprise the 'polycystic ovary syndrome'. The appearance of insulin resistance in youth in association with overweight[17] may foreshadow increased prevalence of polycystic ovary disease during adolescence. The prevalence of polycystic ovary syndrome in youth is unknown. It is often not diagnosed in adolescents because they rarely have the characteristic ultrasonic ovarian morphology or because altered menstrual patterns or late menstruation may go unrecognized. However, hormonal patterns typical of polycystic ovary syndrome are increasingly described in obese children[25,26]. In a nested case-control study, increased BMI at age 18, based on recalled height and weight was associated with elevated risk for ovulatory-related infertility in young women[27]. Analyses in the entire Nurses II cohort indicated a positive association between BMI at age 18 and irregular menstrual cycling[27]. In a population-based nationally representative longitudinal study in the United Kingdom, menstrual abnormalities at age 7 increased the risk of later menstrual problems, as well as the risk of hypertension during pregnancy[28].

Menarcheal timing is influenced by weight status, with higher relative weights associated with earlier menarche. Some have suggested that the rise in paediatric obesity will further depress the population age at menarche. In an analysis of data from cycles II and III of the National Health Examination Survey (1963–70) and the Third National Health and Nutrition Examination Survey (1988–94), we observed that the shift upward in the distribution of BMI z-score was paralleled by more girls reaching menarche at a younger age (Fig. 1)[28a].

The putative health consequences of early menarche are both immediate and delayed. Early menarche is an established risk factor for breast cancer and has been linked to other cancers of the female reproductive system[29,30]. Early menarche has also been proposed as a risk factor for the most common psychiatric problems experienced by adolescent girls: depression, disordered eating, and substance abuse, with some supporting research[31,32]. The mechanism for these effects may be affiliation with an older peer group. In addition, early menarche has been linked to increased risk of spontaneous abortion in adulthood[33].

Asthma, asthma symptoms, and sleep disordered breathing

Several cross-sectional studies have identified an association between childhood overweight and asthma[34–37]. In a 2002 report of nationally representative US data on children aged 2 months to 18 years, BMI > 85th percentile was associated with asthma prevalence, independent of age, sex and ethnicity. Socioeconomic status and passive smoking were not independent predictors. Nonetheless, the directionality of any causal relationship is not obvious, because children with asthma are often restricted from vigorous activities and some of the medications used to treat asthma cause weight gain[37]. In nationally representative data from the UK, obesity and asthma were related only in girls in the inner city sample[38]. The coincidence of the increased prevalence of both of these conditions led to a recent paper that explored whether the rise in childhood overweight might explain the rise in childhood asthma[36]. Based on their analysis of National Study of Growth and Health data (1982–94), the authors concluded that the relationship between BMI and asthma outcomes has changed over time, with elevated BMI–asthma associations occurring late in the observation period. The cross-sectional relationship was significant at both time periods, however. In addition, in a 4-year prospective analysis included in the same report, the authors observed relative risks of 4 or more for asthma, or asthma symptoms in the highest weight group compared to the normal weight reference group. A positive association was also reported (in abstract form) for the prospectively studied Growing Up Today cohort of 9–14 year-old offspring of nurses in the Nurses Health Study; after controlling for developmental stage, BMI was significantly associated with 1-year incidence of asthma in boys, with a suggestion of a positive relationship among girls[39]. Asthma and its symptoms are difficult to study. The observation that weight loss improves lung function in obese adults[40] suggests that obesity prevention could decrease the impact of asthma, if not its occurrence.

A more established pulmonary effect of childhood obesity is sleep-associated breathing disorder, seen in association with severe obesity. Sleep disordered breathing refers to a wide spectrum of sleep-related conditions including increased resistance to airflow through the upper airway, heavy snoring, marked reduction in airflow (hypopnea), and complete cessation of breathing (apnea). Obesity-hypoventilation syndrome, also called Pickwickian syndrome (named for Joe in Charles Dickens' *Pickwick Papers*), is a serious condition associated with pulmonary embolism and sudden death in children[41]. In one small study, one-third of subjects with severe obesity had symptoms consistent with sleep apnea, and 5 per cent had severe obstructive sleep apnea[42]. Another report documented abnormal sleep studies in 94 per cent of obese children[43]. Children whose weight was greater than 200 per cent above ideal had markedly abnormal sleep studies; oxygen saturation was below 90 per cent for approximately half of the total sleep time and 40 per cent of the severely obese children demonstrated central hypoventilation. Secondary metabolic correlates of obstructive sleep apnea include insulin resistance, after accounting for obesity severity. Clinically significant effects on learning and memory function in obese children with obstructive sleep apnea represent a particularly troubling consequence of severe obesity[44]. Thus, sleep apnea represents a serious condition that was seen only infrequently when paediatric severe obesity was a rare disease. The changes in the distribution of BMI in children with the elongation of the 'upper tail' translates to a substantial increase in children and adolescents in the 'severely' obese category[45]. In obese adults with sleep apnea, increases in the size of the soft tissue structures that surround the upper airway, including the tongue, soft palate, and lateral pharangeal walls have been noted[46–48]. Presumably, these structural changes occur in obese children as well.

Emerging mental health consequences

The mind-body dualism conceptualized by Descartes in the seventeenth century influenced the distinction that Western medicine has historically drawn between mental and physical health. That such separation is artificial is no longer an unconventional view[49]. Obesity in children and adolescents may have its most immediate effects in the realm of psychological and social consequences.

Stigmatization of obese children and adolescents has long been recognized and is convincingly documented. A classic 1967 study found that young boys (ages 6–10) frequently stereotyped obese body types as being indicative of negative personality characteristics (cheats, lazy, lies, sloppy, naughty, mean, ugly, dirty, stupid)[50]. Similar results have been seen in Australian boys and girls (ages 8–12)[51] and in boys and girls (kindergarten through fourth grade) in the Midwest of the United States with the degree of negative stereotyping increasing with age[52]. Providing children with a medical explanation for obesity did not appreciably affect their negative characterizations of a hypothetical obese peer (especially in older children) and did not influence their lack of desire to share activities with an obese peer[53]. In another classic study, boys and girls (ages 10–11) were asked to rank order a series of drawings of children with various handicaps (crutches, wheelchair, missing a hand, facial disfigurement, obesity) based on which child they would 'like best'; the obese child was *ranked last* irrespective of the ranking child's sex, race, socioeconomic status, living environment, and own disability[54]; these results have recently been replicated[55]. Thus, although childhood obesity has become far more common, the societal reaction to it does not appear to have softened.

The social and economic consequences of obesity in childhood and adolescence are pervasive. In a nationally representative (US) prospective sample, compared to thinner women, we found that obese adolescent women had lower educational attainment, earned less money, had higher rates of poverty, and were less likely to have married[56]. Similar results have been observed in a British cohort[57]. Discrimination towards obese adolescents has been documented in apartment rentals[58], as well as in college admissions, although obesity, at least in the 1960s, does not appear to be related to high-school performance or desire to attend college[59,60].

Given the degree of stereotyping and stigmatization obese children and adolescents face from their peers it might seem obvious that obese youth have fewer friends. An intriguing analysis of social networks in a nationally representative sample of adolescents provides evidence that this may indeed be true; overweight adolescents were 'less popular' than their non-overweight peers as assessed by modeling reported and reciprocated 'friendship nominations' (R.S. Strauss, written communication, 2002). However, a study of 9-year-old girls in the UK did not find that obese or overweight girls were 'less popular'[61]. Peer rejection and lack of friends in childhood has been associated prospectively with reduced psychological functioning in adulthood[62].

As reviewed by French et al., many studies have looked at the association of obesity during childhood and adolescence with self-esteem[63]. The definition of self-esteem is variable, and in some studies comprised of multiple domains (school/intellect, body/appearance, athletic, social, behaviour/conduct, global)[63,64]. In cross-sectional studies of school-age children, results have generally indicated either a weak association between lower self-esteem and obesity or no association[63,65], although reductions in self-esteem associated with obesity appear to differ by race[64] and there is evidence to suggest that athletic and appearance domains of self-esteem are most likely to diminish with obesity[61]. Body dissatisfaction and desire to lose weight have been found to be prevalent even in young children[66], but this desire is not limited to children who are overweight and appears to represent a separate construct. In a prospective analysis of children initially 9–10 years followed for 4 years, obese children did not differ in self-esteem from normal weight children at ages 9–10, but were more likely to decline in self-esteem over the following 4 years; these effects were strongest for white and Hispanic girls but were not absent in boys or in black girls[65]. In cross-sectional studies of adolescents, findings have mainly indicated decreased self-esteem in obese compared to non-obese youth[63,65,67,68], however this effect has not been universally observed[56,69]. In a seven-year follow-up of youth initially aged 16–24, those youth with a BMI above the 95th percentile were not more likely to evidence decreased self-esteem, as assessed by a simple instrument[56].

Few studies have assessed associations of childhood and adolescent obesity with concurrent or subsequent psychopathology, such as depression or anxiety. Braet et al., compared obese children from a clinical and non-clinical setting with normal weight controls and found that while self-esteem was reduced in both obese groups, increased psychopathology was only present in the obese children from the clinical group implying that the factors that caused parents to bring their child for obesity treatment may be more responsible for the effect than the obesity *per se*[70]. A recent study of obesity, depressive symptoms, and weight concerns in California third-graders found a modest and statistically significant association between increasing depressive symptomatology and higher BMI; overweight concerns were also associated with depressive symptoms and girls with higher relative weights reported more overweight concerns[71]. Being teased and feeling unhappy with one's appearance, too often correlates of obesity in children and adolescents, may mediate the psychological consequences of obesity[72]. In a one-year prospective analysis of a nationally representative sample of US adolescents, Goodman and Whitaker, found no evidence for obesity increasing the risk for depression[73]; although depression was dichotomized to depressed or not-depressed based on a screening questionnaire which would have made seeing an effect less likely.

Some of the negative consequences of adolescent obesity result from unhealthy eating behaviours that accompany elevated weight. In a large survey of high-school students in Minnesota, overweight adolescents were more likely to report dissatisfaction with their weight, and there was some evidence for unhealthy eating behaviours (binge eating and chronic dieting); after controlling for age, ethnicity and SES, there was a weak association between obesity and emotional health in boys and a similarly weak association between obesity and suicidal ideation in girls[74]. In a similar survey of Connecticut youth, obese adolescent girls were more likely to report hopelessness, having problems during the prior year, and having attempted suicide than normal weight girls; results were attenuated for boys and did not reach statistical significance[75].

The delineation of the full range of health consequences linked to obesity in the paediatric population may help direct resources to its primary, secondary and even tertiary prevention. Although much remains to be understood, the existence of substantial somatic health consequences of child and adolescent obesity (immediate and longer term) is well established. The evidence regarding the psychological consequences of child and adolescent obesity is more equivocal. Research on the psychological consequences of obesity in childhood and adolescence has been limited, with more information available on psychological correlates such as stigma, self-esteem, and friendship than on identifiable psychopathology. Two recent review articles in adults[76,77] provide useful organizing frameworks for future studies in youth.

References

1. Wang Y, Ge K, Popkin BM. Tracking of body mass index from childhood to adolescence a 6-year follow-up study in China. *Am J Clin Nutr* 2000; 72: 1018–24.

2. Florencio TM, Ferreira HS, De Franca AP, Cavalcante JC, Sawaya AL. Obesity and undernutrition in a very-low-income population in the city of Maceio, northeastern Brazil. *Br J Nutr* 2001; 86: 277–84.

3. Gortmaker SL, Dietz WH, Jr, Sobol AM, Wehler CA. Increasing pediatric obesity in the United States. *Am J Dis Child* 1987; 141: 535–40.

4. Pinhas-Hamiel O, Zeitler P. 'Who is the wise man? – The one who foresees consequences': childhood obesity, new associated comorbidity and prevention. *Preventive Medicine* 2000; 31: 702–5.

5. Flegal KM, Kusczmarski RJ, Johnson CL. Overweight and obesity in the United States: prevalence and trends, 1960–1994. *Int J Obes* 1998; 22: 39–47.

6. Parsons TJ, Power C, Logan S, Summerbell CD. Childhood predictors of adult obesity: a systematic review. *Int J Obes* 1999; 23: S1–S106.

7. NHLBI Obesity Education Initiative Expert Panel. Clinical guidelines on the identification, evaluation, and treatment of overweight and obesity in adults: the evidence report. *Obes Res* 1998; 6: S51–S209.

8. Must A, Strauss RS. Risks and consequences of childhood and adolescent obesity. *Int J Obes* 1999; 23: S2–S11.

9. Rames LK, Clarke WR, Connor WE, Reiter MA, Lauer RM. Normal blood pressure and the evaluation of sustained blood pressure elevation in childhood: the Muscatine study. *Pediatrics* 1978; 61: 245–51.

10. Freedman DS, Burke GL, Harsha DW, Srinivasan SR, Cresanta JL, Webber LS, Berenson GS. Relationship of changes in obesity to serum lipid and lipoprotein changes in childhood and adolescence. *JAMA* 1985; 254: 515–20.

11. Freedman DS, Dietz WH, Srinivasan SR, Berenson GS. The relation of overweight to cardiovascular risk factors among children and adolescents: the Bogalusa Heart Study. *Pediatrics* 1999; 103: 175–1182.

12. Lauer RM, Lee J, Clarke WR. Factors affecting the relationship between childhood and adult cholesterol levels: the Muscatine Study. *Pediatrics* 1988; 82: 309–18.

13. Lauer RM, Clarke WR, Beaglehole R. Level, trend, and variability of blood pressure during childhood: the Muscatine study. *Circulation* 1984; 69: 242–9.

14. Freedman DJ, Serdula MK, Khan LK. The adult health consequences of childhood obesity; In: *Obesity in childhood and adolescence*, Chen C, Dietz Wh (eds), pp. 63–82. Lippincott Williams & Wilkins; 2002.

15. Srinivasan SR, Bao W, Wattigney WA, Berenson GS. Adolescent overweight is associated with adult overweight and related multiple cardiovascular risk factors: the Bogalusa Heart Study. *Metabolism* 1996; 45: 235–40.

16. Mokdad AH, Serdula MK, Dietz WH, Bowman BA, Marks JS, Koplan JP. The continuing epidemic of obesity in the United States. *JAMA* 2000; 284: 1650–1.

17. Sinha R, Fisch G, Teague B, Tamborlane WV, Banyas B *et al.* Prevalence of impaired glucose tolerance among children and adolescents with marked obesity. *N Engl J Med* 2002; 346: 802–10.

18. Scott CR, Smith JM, Cradock MM, Pihoker C. Characteristics of youth-onset non-insulin-dependent diabetes mellitus and insulin-dependent diabetes mellitus at diagnosis. *Pediatrics* 1997; 100: 84–91.

19. Neufeld ND, Raffel LJ, Landon C, Chen Y, Vadheim CM. Early presentation of Type-2 Diabetes in Mexican-American youth. *Diabetes Care* 1998; 21: 80–6.

20. Dabelea RL, Hanson RL, Bennett PH, Roumain J, Knowler WC, Pettitt DJ. Increasing prevalence of Type II diabetes in American Indian children. *Diabetologia* 1998; 41: 904–10.

21. Fagot-Campagna A, Burrows NR, Williamson DF. The public health epidemiology of type 2 diabetes in children and adolescents: a case study of American Indian adolescents in the Southwestern United States. *Clin Chim Acta* 1999; 286: 81–95.

22. Fagot-Campagna A, Pettitt DJ, Engelgau MM, Burrows NR, Geiss LS *et al.* Type 2 diabetes among North American children and adolescents: an epidemiologic review and public health perspective 2000.

23. Zaadstra BM, Seidell JC, Van Noord PA, Te Velde ER, Habbema JD, Vrieswijk B, Karbaat J. Fat and female fecundity: prospective study of effect of body fat distribution on conception rates. *BMJ* 1993; 306: 484–7.

24. Rogers J, Mitchell GW. The relation of obesity to menstrual disturbances. *N Engl J Med* 1956; 247; 53–5.

25. Richards GE, Cavallo A, Meyer WJD, Prince MJ, Peters EJ, Stuart CA, Smith ER. Obesity, acanthosis nigricans, insulin resistance, and hyperandrogenemia: pediatric perspective and natural history. *J Pediatr* 1985; 107: 893–7.

26. Lazar L, Kauli R, Bruchis C, Nordenberg J, Galatzer A, Pertzelan A. Early polycystic ovary-like syndrome in girls with central precocious puberty and exaggerated adrenal response. *Eur J Endocrinol* 1995; 133: 403–6.

27. Rich-Edwards JW, Goldman MB, Willett WC, Hunter DJ, Stampfer MJ, Colditz GA, Manson JE. Adolescent body mass index and infertility caused by ovulatory disorder. *Am J Obstet Gynecol* 1994; 171: 171–7.

28. Lake JK, Power C, Cole TJ. Women's reproductive health: the role of body mass index in early and adult life. *Int J Obes* 1997; 21: 432–8.

28a. Anderson SE, Dallal GE, Must A. Relative weight and race influence average age at menarche: results from two nationally representative surveys of US girls studied 25 years apart. *Pediatrics* 2003; 111: 844–50.

29. Marshall L, Spiegelman D, Goldman M, Manson J, Colditz G, Barbieri R *et al.* A prospective study of reproductive factors and oral contraceptive use in relation to the risk of uterine leiomyomata. *Fertil Steril* 1998; 70: 432–9.

30. McPherson CP, Sellers TA, Potter JD, Bostick RM, Folsom AR. Reproductive factors and risk of endometrial cancer: the Iowa Women's Health Study. *Am J Epidemiol* 1996; 143: 1195–202.

31. Stice E, Presnell K, Bearman SK. Relation of early menarche to depression, eating disorders, substance abuse, and comorbid psychopathology among adolescent girls. *Dev Psychol* 2001; 37: 608–19.

32. Graber JA, Lewinsohn PM, Seeley JR, Brooks-Gunn J. Is psychopathology associated with the timing of pubertal development? *J Am Acad Child Adolesc Psychiat* 1997; 36: 1768–76.

33. Liestol K. Menarcheal age and spontaneous abortion: a causal connection? *Am J Epidemiol* 1980; 111: 753–8.

34. Gennuso J, Epstein LH, Paluch RA, Cerny F. The relationship between asthma and obesity in urban minority children and adolescents. *Arch Pediatr Adolesc Med* 1998; 152: 1197–200.

35. Luder E, Melnik TA, Dimaio M. Association of being overweight with greater asthma symptoms in inner city black and Hispanic children. *J Pediatr* 1998; 132: 699–703.

36. Chinn S, Rona RJ. Prevalence and trends in overweight and obesity in three cross sectional studies of British children, 1974–94. *BMJ* 2001; 322: 24–6.

37. Rodriguez MA, Winkleby MA, Ahn D, Sundquist J, Kraemer HC. Identification of population subgroups of children and adolescents with high asthma prevalence: findings from the Third National Health and Nutrition Examination Survey. *Arch Pediat Adolesc Med* 2002; 156: 269–75.

38. Figueroa-Munoz JI, Chinn S, Rona RJ. Association between obesity and asthma in 4–11 year old children in the UK. *Thorax* 2001; 56: 133–7.

39. Camargo CJ, Field AE, Colditz GA, Speizer FE. Body mass index and asthma in children ages 9–14. *Am J Respir Crit Care Med* 1999; 159: A150.

40. Stenius-Aarniala B, Poussa T, Kvarnstrom J, Gronlund EL, Ylikahri M, Mustajoki P. Immediate and long term effects of weight reduction in obese people with asthma: randomised controlled study. *BMJ* 2000; 320: 827–32.

41. Riley DJ, Santiago T, Edelman NH. Complications of obesity-hypoventilation syndrome in childhood. *Am J Dis Child* 1976; 130: 371–674.

42. Mallory GB, Fiser DH, Jackson R. Sleep-associated breathing disorders in morbidly obese children and adolescents. *J Pediatr* 1989; 115: 892–7.

43. Silvesti JM, Weese-Mayer DE, Bass MT, Kenny AS, Hauptmann SA, Pearsall SM. Polysomnography in obese children with a history of sleep-associated breathing disorders. *Pediatr Pulmonol* 1993; 16: 124–9.

44. Rhodes SK, Shimoda KC, Waid LR, Mahlen P, Oexmann MJ, Collop NA, Willi SM. Neurocognitive deficits in morbidly obese children with obstructive sleep apnea. *J Pediatr* 1995; 127: 741–4.

45. Flegal KM, Troiano RP. Changes in the distribution of body mass index of adults and children in the US population. *Int J Obes* 2000; 24: 807–18.

46. Shelton KE, Woodson H, Gay SB, Suratt PM. Adipose tissue deposition in sleep apnea. *Sleep* 1993; 16, 124–9.

47. Shelton KE, Gay SB, Hollowell DE, Woodson H, Suratt PM. Mandible enclosure of upper airway and weight in obstructive sleep apnea. *Am Rev Respir Dis* 1993; 148: 195–200.

48. Shelton KE, Woodson H, Gay S, Suratt PM. Pharyngeal fat in obstructive sleep apnea. *Am Rev Respir Dis* 1993; 148: 462–6.

49. Rockville MD. Mental Health: a report of the surgeon general; US Department of Health and Human Services. US Department of Health and Human Services, Substance Abuse and Mental Health Services Administration, Center for Mental Health Services, NIH, NIMH; 1999.

50. Staffieri JR. A study of social stereotype of body image in children. *J Pers Soc Psychol* 1967; 7: 101–4.

51. Tiggemann M, Anesbury T. Negative stereotyping of obesity in children: the role of controllability beliefs. *J Appl Soc Psychol* 2000; 30: 1977–93.

52. Brylinsky JA, Moore JC. The identification of body build stereotypes in young children. *J Res Pers* 1994; 28: 170–81.

53. Bell SK, Morgan SB. Children's attitudes and behavioral intentions inward a peer presented as obese: does a medical explanation for the obesity make a difference? *J Pediatr Psychol* 2000; 25: 137–45.

54. Richardson SA, Hastorf AH, Goodman N, Dornsbusch SM. Cultural uniformity in reaction to physical disabilities. *Am Sociol Rev* 1961; 202: 241–7.

55. Latner J, Stunkard A. Getting worse: the stigmatization in sleep apnea. *Obes Res* 2003; 11: 452–6.

56. Gortmaker SL, Must A, Perrin JM, Sobol AM, Dietz W. Social and economic consequences of overweight in adolescence and young adulthood. *N Engl J Med* 1993; 329: 1008–12.

57. Sargent JD, Blanchflower DG. Obesity and stature in adolescence and earnings in young adulthood: analysis of a British birth cohort. *Arch Pediatr Adol Med* 1994; 148: 681–7.

58. Karris L. Prejudice against obese renters. *J Soc Psychol* 1977; 101: 159–60.

59. Canning H, Mayer J. Obesity: its possible effect on college acceptance. *N Engl J Med* 1966; 275: 1172–74.

60. Canning H, Mayer J. Obesity: an influence on high school performance? *Am J Clin Nutr* 1967; 20: 352–4.

61. Phillips RG, Hill AJ. Fat, plain, but not friendless: self-esteem and peer acceptance of obese pre-adolescent girls. *Int J Obes* 1998; 22: 287–93.

62. Bagwell CL, Newcomb AF, Bukowski WM. Preadolescent friendship and peer rejection as predictors of adult adjustment. *Child Dev* 1998; 69: 140–53.

63. French SA, Story M, Perry CL. Self-esteem and obesity in children and adolescents: a literature review. *Obes Res* 1995; 3: 479–90.

64. Kimm SYS, Barton BA, Berhane K, Ross JW, Payne GH, Schreiber GB. Self-esteem and adiposity in black and white girls: the NHLBI growth and health study. *Ann Epidemiol* 1997; 7: 550–60.

65. Strauss RS. Childhood obesity and self-esteem. *Pediatrics* 2000; 105: E15.

66. Robinson TN, Chang JY, Haydel KF, Killen JD. Overweight concerns and body dissatisfaction among third-grade children: the impacts of ethnicity and socioeconomic status. *J Pediatr* 2001; 138: 181–7.

67. French S, Perry C, Leon G, Fulkerson J. Self-esteem and change in body mass index over 3 years in a cohort of adolescents. *Obes Res* 1996; 4: 27–33.

68. Pesa JA, Syre TR, Jones E. Psychosocial differences associated with body weight among female adolescents: the importance of body image. *J Adolesc Health* 2000; 26: 330–7.

69. Renman C, Engstrom I, Silfverdal SA, Aman J. Mental health and psychosocial characteristics in adolescent obesity: a population-based case-control study. *Acta Paediatr* 1999; 88: 998–1003.

70. Braet C, Mervielde I, Vandereycken W. Psychological aspects of childhood obesity: a controlled study in a clinical and nonclinical sample. *J Pediatr Psychol* 1997; 22: 59–71.

71. Erickson SJ, Robinson TN, Haydel KF, Killen JD. Are overweight children unhappy? Body mass index, depressive symptoms, and overweight concerns in elementary school children. *Arch Pediatr Adolesc Med* 2000; 154: 931–5.

72. Thompson JK, Coovert MD, Richards KJ, Johnson S, Cattarin J. Development of body image, eating disturbance, and general psychological functioning in female adolescents: covariance structure modeling and longitudinal investigations. *Int J Eat Disord* 1995; 18: 221–36.

73. Goodman E, Whitaker RC. A prospective study of the role of depression in the development and persistence of adolescent obesity. *Pediatrics* 2002.

74. Neumark-Sztainer D, Story M, French SA, Hannan PJ, Resnick MD, Blum R. Psychosocial concerns and health-compromising behaviors among overweight and non-overweight adolescents. *Obes Res* 1997; 5: 237–49.

75. Falkner NH, Neumark-Sztainer D, Story M, Jeffery R, Beuhring T, Resnick MD. Social, educational, and psychological correlates of weight status in adolescents. *Obes Res* 2001; 9: 32–42.

76. Faith MS, Matz PE, Jorge MA. Obesity-depression associations in the population. *J Psychosom Res* 2002; 52: 1–8.

77. Friedman MA, Brownell KD. Psychological correlates of obesity: moving to the next research generation. *Psychol Bull* 1995; 117: 3–20.

Progress in Obesity Research: 9. Edited by *Geraldo Medeiros-Neto, Alfredo Halpern and Claude Bouchard*
©2003 John Libbey Eurotext Ltd, pp. 693–696.

CHAPTER 145

Regional fat distribution and menopause

André Tchernof

*Molecular Endocrinology and Oncology Research Center, Department of Nutrition, Laval University
Medical Research Center, Canada
[e-mail: andre.tchernof@crchul.ulaval.ca]*

Introduction

According to the World Health Organization, the menopause is defined as the permanent cessation of menstrual cyclicity and reproductive function[1]. Clinically, menopause is defined as the absence of menses for at least 6 months to a year, and the time at which menopause occurs is determined retrospectively as the final menstrual period[1]. Endocrine changes resulting from the menopause transition include reductions of ovarian estrogen, progesterone, androgen and inhibin secretion[1,2], and increased follicle stimulating hormone (FSH) and luteinizing hormone (LH) levels[1]. Peripheral conversion of adrenal steroids such as dehydroepiandrosterone-sulphate and androstenedione remains as the major source of postmenopausal androgens and estrogens in the menopause[2,3], and contributes to increase both the androgen/estrogen and estrone/estradiol ratios.

In recent years, central distribution and accumulation of adipose tissue, and the concomitant insulin resistant-dyslipidaemic state have emerged as important components of a cluster of metabolic abnormalities that are strongly related to coronary heart disease[4]. Therefore, it has been suggested that the menopause may affect body fat distribution, and that postmenopausal hormone replacement therapy could prevent or attenuate these changes[5–7]. The present article is a brief summary of the literature in this area.

The menopause transition and body fat distribution

Results of cross-sectional studies where pre- and postmenopausal women were compared have been equivocal, as some studies found a significant effect of the menopause and others did not. In a recent analysis of these reports[5], we concluded that discrepancies could be attributed to the various methods used for the measurement of body fat distribution, such as circumference measures, dual x-ray absorptiometry, or computed tomography. In studies where anthropometric measurements were used as surrogates of abdominal obesity, no effect of the menopause on body fat distribution was found when statistical adjustment for potential confounding variables such as the degree of obesity or age was performed[5]. Dual X-ray absorptiometry was used in some studies to measure the proportion of fat located in the trunk region. A significant effect of the menopause transition on body fat distribution that was independent of age and total fatness was reported[5]. Studies using the current criterion method for body fat distribution measurement (computed tomography), also found significant effects of the menopause transition on body fat distribution after controlling for BMI[8] or age[9]. Recent results from our laboratory also support an increase in intra-abdominal adipose tissue accumulation with the menopause. In a study by Toth and colleagues[10], early postmenopausal non-obese women were found to have significantly more intra-abdominal adipose tissue compared to premenopausal women, independent of total body fat mass[10]. On the other hand, a few studies using radiologic techniques reported no significant effect of the menopause on abdominal fat accumulation[11,12]. These studies, despite the use of precise methodology, suggested that there is no independent effect of the menopause transition on body fat distribution. However, a very small number of postmenopausal women[11], or no postmenopausal women[12] were examined. Only two studies have examined the effects of the menopause transition on body fat distribution in longitudinal designs[13,14]. In these studies, significant effects of the menopause transition on WHR or waist circumference were noted. Further studies are needed to repeat and confirm these results in other prospective cohorts.

In summary, the discrepancies among previous cross-sectional studies appear to be related to the methodology used for the measurement of body fat distribution[5]. On the other hand, the use of radiologic techniques such as DEXA and computed tomography led to the conclusion that the menopause transition accelerates the selective deposition of intra-abdominal fat. Available longitudinal data also support an increase in central body fatness occurring with menopause, although further investigations using longitudinal designs and more precise methodologies to measure body fat distribution are needed to confirm the effects of the natural menopause transition.

Hormone replacement therapy and body fat distribution

Several cross-sectional comparisons of hormone users and non users were published. Two recent studies using such designs have confirmed that hormone users generally are characterized by reduced abdominal adipose tissue accumulations compared to non-users[15,16]. Although this type of comparison can provide useful information on the effects of hormone replacement therapy, the possibility cannot be excluded that the observed benefits of therapy may be attributable to a study bias where more health conscious and more healthy women have chosen hormone replacement, thereby overestimating the effects of hormone replacement.

The effects of different hormone regimens on body fat distribution have also been examined in several intervention studies. In these studies, treatment times ranged from 1 month to 3 years, and several different regimen were used. The studies that lasted less that 1 year did not find any effect of hormone replacement on body fat distribution[17–19]. Out of the eight studies that lasted from 11 months to 3 years, six found that hormone replacement therapy prevented the increase in abdominal fat accumulation noted in the placebo or control group[20–25], whereas one study found a statistical trend for a protective effect[26]. A recent study also provided evidence that addition of androgens to the preparation may favour trunk fat reductions in postmenopausal women on oral estrogens[27]. However, some of these studies did not include randomization and/or placebo groups. Norman et al.[28], in a systematic review of randomized placebo-controlled studies, concluded that not enough data was available to confirm a significant effect of HRT on body fat distribution.

Recent data on hormone replacement therapy have generated some concern as to the beneficial effects of such treatment on cardiovascular disease outcome in postmenopausal women. Indeed, results from randomized studies have shown that hormone replacement does not seem to provide cardioprotective effects in primary and secondary prevention[29,30]. Moreover, several studies have recently shown a slight increase in the risk of cardiovascular events upon initiation of treatment, which appeared to be related to early proinflammatory and prothrombotic effects of estrogens[29,31]. The possibility remains that hormone replacement through different administration routes provides significant cardioprotective effects. However, these recent results call for caution in the use of hormone replacement therapy. Strategies based on nutritional or lifestyle interventions may represent promising alternatives in this context.

Physiological mechanisms

Abdominal adiposity has been associated with a more androgenic profile, namely increased free testosterone levels and lower sex-hormone binding globulin in both pre- and postmenopausal women. The dramatic modifications in the dynamics of estrogens, free androgens, and SHBG, or the relative androgenicity, have been suggested to be responsible for changes in body fat distribution during this period[5]. Reports by Rebuffé-Scrive and colleagues[32] showed that menopausal women have lower lipoprotein lipase (LPL) activity in femoral adipose tissue compared to premenopausal women, whereas abdominal LPL activity is not different, which is consistent with a shift of adipose tissue accumulation from the gluteal-femoral to the abdominal area[32]. Accordingly, hormonal treatment either with unopposed estrogen or combined estrogen and progestin stimulated LPL activity in the femoral region[32], which suggests that estrogen, or estrogen deficiency, directly influences regional adipose tissue metabolism. More recently, a study by Price and colleagues[33] showed that transdermal estradiol treatment significantly decreased adipose tissue LPL activity, and that this phenomenon was attributable to post-transcriptional modification of protein levels. Taken together, these observations suggest that hormonal changes of the menopause may lead to body fat distribution changes by affecting regional adipose tissue metabolism. Previous findings have also suggested that the energy balance may be affected in postmenopausal women, possibly through estrogen regulation of food intake and energy expenditure[7]. The dual effects of estrogen deficiency on both regional adipose tissue metabolism and energy balance may lead to increased intra-abdominal adipose tissue accumulation in the post-menopausal years.

Conclusions

Careful examination of available studies on body fat distribution and menopause suggests that menopause is associated with an acceleration in the accumulation of abdominal adipose tissue, and most likely, intra-abdominal fat. These results are further supported by hormone replacement studies in which the menopause-induced redistribution of fat was prevented by hormone replacement. However, recent data on proinflammatory and prothrombotic effects of hormone replacement calls for caution in the use of such therapy. Given the central role of body fat distribution in the associations between obesity and risk factors for cardiovascular disease, it is possible that some of the adverse effects of menopause are mediated through increased abdominal (and intra-abdominal) fat accumulation in postmenopausal women. Intervention strategies based on lifestyle modification are likely to provide beneficial health outcomes in the postmenopausal years.

Acknowledgements: Supported by a Grant-in-Aid from the Canadian Diabetes Association and a 'Fonds de la Recherche en Santé du Québec' Scholarship.

References

1. World Health Organization Report of a WHO Scientific Group: Research on the Menopause. Geneva 1981.

2. Couzinet B, Meduri G, Lecce MG, Young J, Brailly S, Loosfelt H *et al.* The postmenopausal ovary is not a major androgen-producing gland. *J Clin Endocrinol Metab* 2001; 86: 5060–6.

3. Labrie F. Intracrinology. *Mol Cell Endo* 1991; 78: C113–C118.

4. Després JP, Marette A. Relation of components of insulin resistance syndrome to coronary disease risk. *Curr Opin Lipidol* 1994; 5: 274–89.

5. Tchernof A, Poehlman ET. Effects of the menopause transition on body fatness and body fat distribution. *Obes Res* 1998; 6: 246–54.

6. Tchernof A, Calles-Escandon J, Sites CK, Poehlman ET. Menopause, central body fatness, and insulin resistance: effects of hormone replacement therapy. *Coron Artery Dis* 1998; 9: 503–11.

7. Tchernof A, Poehlman ET, Després JP. Body fat distribution, the menopause transition, and hormone replacement therapy. *Diabete Metab* 2000; 26: 12–20.

8. Zamboni M, Armellini F, Milani MP, De Marchi M, Todesco T, Robbi R *et al.* Body fat distribution in pre- and post-menopausal women: metabolic and anthropometric variables and their interrelationships. *Int J Obes* 1992; 16: 495–504.

9. Kotani K, Tokunaga K, Fujioka S, Kobatake T, Keno Y, Yoshida S *et al.* Sexual dimorphism of age-related changes in whole-body fat distribution in the obese. *Int J Obes* 18: 207–12.

10. Toth MJ, Tchernof A, Sites CK, Poehlman ET. Effect of menopausal status on body composition and abdominal fat distribution. *Int J Obes* 2000; 24: 226–31.

11. Schreiner PJ, Terry JG, Evans GW, Hinson WH, Crouse JR, Heiss G. Sex-specific associations of magnetic resonance imaging-derived intra-abdominal and subcutaneous fat areas with conventional anthropometric indices. The Atherosclerosis Risk in Communities Study. *Am J Epidemiol* 1996; 144: 335–45.

12. Wang Q, Hassager C, Ravn P, Wang S, Christiansen C. Total and regional body-composition changes in early postmenopausal women: age-related or menopause-related? *Am J Clin Nutr* 1994; 60: 843–8.

13. Björkelund C, Lissner L, Andersson S, Lapidus L, Bengtsson C. Reproductive history in relation to relative weight and fat distribution. *Int J Obes* 1996; 20: 213–9.

14. Poehlman ET, Toth MJ, Gardner AW. Changes in energy balance and body composition at menopause: a controlled longitudinal study. *Ann Intern Med* 1995; 123: 673–5.

15. Sites CK, Brochu M, Tchernof A, Poehlman ET. Relationship between hormone replacement therapy use with body fat distribution and insulin sensitivity in obese postmenopausal women. *Metabolism* 2001; 50: 835–40.

16. Munoz J, Derstine A, Gower BA. Fat distribution and insulin sensitivity in postmenopausal women: influence of hormone replacement. *Obes Res* 2002; 10: 424–31.

17. Anderson EJ, Lavoie HB, Strauss CC, Hubbard JL, Sharpless JL, Hall JE. Body composition and energy balance: lack of effect of short-term hormone replacement in postmenopausal women. *Metabolism* 2001; 50: 265–9.

18. Walker RJ, Lewis-Barned NJ, Sutherland WHF, Goulding A, Edwards EA, de Jong SA *et al.* The effects of sequential combined oral 17beta-estradiol noethisterone acetate on insulin sensitivity and body composition in healthy postmenopausal women: a randomized single blind placebo-controlled study. *Menopause* 2001; 8: 27–32.

19. Münzer T, Harman SM, Hees P, Shapiro E, Christmas C, Bellantoni MF *et al*. Effects of GH and/or sex steroid administration on abdominal subcutaneous and visceral fat in healthy aged women and men. *J Clin Endocrinol Metab* 2002; 86: 3604–10.

20. Espeland MA, Stefanick ML, Kritz-Silverstein D, Finberg SE, Waclawiw MA, James MK *et al*. Effect of postmenopausal hormone therapy on body weight and waist and hip girths. *J Clin Endocrinol Metab* 1997; 82: 1549–56.

21. Reubinoff BE, Wurtman J, Rojansky N, Adler D, Stein P, Schenker JG *et al*. Effects of hormone replacement therapy on weight, body composition, fat distribution, and food intake in early postmenopausal women: a prospective study. *Fertil Steril* 1995; 64: 963–8.

22. Haarbo J, Marslew U, Gotfredsen A, Christiansen C. Postmenopausal hormone replacement therapy prevents central distribution of body fat after menopause. *Metabolism* 1991; 40: 1323–6.

23. Hänggi W, Lippuner K, Jaeger P, Birkhäuser MH, Horber FF. Differential impact of conventional oral or transdermal hormone replacement therapy or tibolone on body composition in postmenopausal women. *Clin Endocrinol* 1998; 48: 691–9.

24. Gambacciani M, Ciaponi M, Cappagli B, Piaggesi L, De Simone L, Orlandi R *et al*. Body weight, body fat distribution, and hormonal replacement therapy in early postmenopausal women. *J Clin Endocrinol Metab* 1997; 82: 414–7.

25. Gambacciani M, Ciaponi M, Cappagli B, De Simone L, Orlandi R, Genazzani AR. Prospective evaluation of body weight and body fat distribution in early postmenopausal women with and without hormonal replacement therapy. *Maturitas* 2001; 39: 125–32.

26. Evans EM, Van Pelt RE, Binder EF, Williams DB, Ehsani AA, Kohrt WM. Effects of HRT and exercise training on insulin action, glucose tolerance, and body composition in older women. *J Appl Physiol* 2001; 90: 2033–40.

27. Dobs AS, Nguyen T, Pace C, Roberts CP. Differential effects of oral estrogen versus oral estrogen-androgen replacement therapy on body composition in postmenopausal women. *J Clin Endocrinol Metab* 2002; 87: 1509–16.

28. Norman, RJ, Flight, IHK, Rees, MCP. Oestrogen and progestogen hormone replacement therapy for peri-menopausal and post-menopausal women: weight and body fat distribution. *Cochrane Library* 3: 2001.

29. Herrington DM, Pouilles JM. Cardiovascular trials of estrogen replacement therapy. *Ann NY Acad Sci* 2001; 949: 153–62.

30. Grady D, Herrington D, Bittner V, Blumenthal R, Davidson M, Hlatky M *et al*. Cardiovascular disease outcomes during 6.8 years of hormone therapy. *JAMA* 2002; 288: 49–57.

31. Cushman M, Legault C, Barrett-Connor E, Stefanick ML, Kessler C, Judd HL *et al*. Effects of postmenopausal hormones on inflammation-sensitive proteins. The postmenopausal estrogen/progestin interventions (PEPI) study. *Circulation* 1999; 100: 717–22.

32. Rebuffé-Scrive M. Steroid hormones and distribution of adipose tissue. *Acta Med Scand* 1988; 723 (Suppl.): 143–146.

33. Price TM, O'Brien SN, Welter BH, George R, Anandjiwala J, Kilgore M. Estrogen regulation of adipose tissue lipoprotein lipase – Possible mechanism of body fat distribution. *Am J Obstet Gynecol* 1998; 178: 101–7.

TRACK V

REGULATION OF ENERGY BALANCE

Progress in Obesity Research: 9. Edited by *Geraldo Medeiros-Neto, Alfredo Halpern and Claude Bouchard*
©2003 John Libbey Eurotext Ltd, pp. 699–702.

CHAPTER 146

Lessons from animal models for the understanding of energy balance regulation

David A. York

Pennington Biomedical Research Center, Louisiana State University, 6400 Perkins Road, Baton Rouge, LA 70808, USA
[e-mail: Yorkda@pbrc.edu]

Introduction

A nimal models have played a major role in developing our understanding of obesity. Initially, this was primarily in relation to the neuroanatomical circuitry of the hypothalamic centres that regulate food intake and energy balance[1,2], and to the physiological, metabolic and behavioural effects of natural gene mutations that caused obesity. However, over the last few years, there has been an explosion in the number of animal models available for studying the development of obesity and its comorbidities. This has resulted from the identification of the human and mouse genomes and the use of transgenic and gene-targeting approaches for proof of function of newly discovered or known genes. Indeed, body weight change on a high fat diet has become a standard phenotype to investigate for all new transgenic and gene knockout studies. These new models have complimented the information that has been gained over several decades from the studies of the spontaneous single gene mutation obesities, the experimental hypothalamic models and from various dietary and endocrine manipulations[3]. This chapter will focus on the rodent models of obesity, but the reader should be aware that there are also many useful models in other animal species including primates[3].

Hypothalamic and CNS control systems

A wide range of methods have been used to damage or activate specific brain sites including selective knife cuts, electrical, and chemical (gold thioglucose, bipiperidyl mustard, monosodium glutamate, ibotenic acid, neurotransmitters, neuropeptides) treatments. More recently a number of viruses have been shown to effect hypothalamic and peripheral tissue functions[4]. The damage or stimulation of hypothalamic sites through these experimental approaches led to the recognition of the different but overlapping functions of specific hypothalamic regions in the control of energy balance. The VMH is recognized as a primary centre regulating the autonomic outflow in response to dietary related signals[5,6]. The lateral hypothalamus has opposing actions to the VMH on the autonomic nervous system normally initiating feeding but causing aphagia after damage or inhibition. In contrast the PVN region has less to do with sympathetic regulation of brown adipose tissue and vagal regulation of insulin secretion but is a powerful site for the regulation of feeding behaviour. It is only in recent years, with the benefit of molecular and genetic studies, that the neurochemical basis for the activities of these centres has been identified. In particular, the two subpopulations of neurons in the arcuate-PVN pathway (NPY/AGRP neurons and POMC/CART neurons) and the identification of MCH and Orexin (hypocretin) in LH neurons has provided neurochemical insight into the function of these sites (Fig. 1).

Integration of feeding behaviour and the autonomic nervous system

All animal obesities appear to be characterized by an imbalance between food intake and specific components of autonomic activity[1]. Extensive literature now documents the close reciprocal integration between food intake and the sympathetic components to brown adipose tissue and heart that regulate thermogenesis and the altered afferent parasympathetic information from the gut together with the efferent parasympathetic drive to the endocrine pancreas seen in many obesities[5–7]. This was concep-

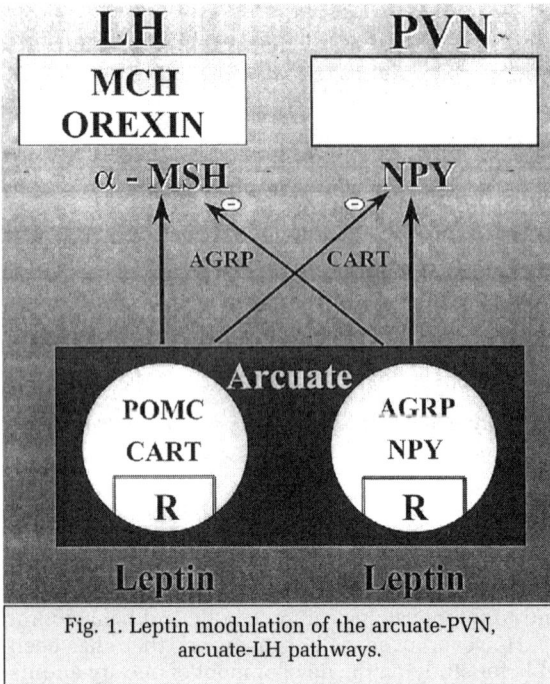

Fig. 1. Leptin modulation of the arcuate-PVN,
arcuate-LH pathways.

tualized in the Autonomic Nervous hypothesis by Bray and York[8]. This relationship holds constant over a wide range of experimental manipulations and pathological changes including the response to hypothalamic damage, various drugs, hormones and neuropeptides, to metabolites and antimetabolites and in comparisons of obese animals with their lean littermates. While there is some evidence for a feedback relationship of a sympathetically induced signal onto food intake, other data would suggest that the parallel controls of feeding behaviour and autonomic activity are a reflection of the CNS effectors independently modulating each arm of the autonomic nervous system as well as feeding behaviour.

Genetic basis of obesity

Initial studies on the genetic basis of obesity focused on five naturally occurring major gene mutations that would cause obesity in mice or rats fed normal chow diets. The identity of each of these genes and their mutations have all been reported[2] (Agouti in the Yellow A^y/a mice, leptin in the obese lep^{ob}/lep^{ob} mouse, the leptin receptor in the diabetes lepr^{db}/lepr^{db} mouse, the fatty lepr^{fa}/lepr^{fa} and Koletsky lepr^{facp}/lepr^{facp} rats, the tub protein in tubby tub/tub mice and carboxypeptidase E in the fat Cpe^{fat}/Cpe^{fat} mouse). The discovery of leptin and the identification of its central actions helped to explain the seminal observations of Coleman[9] and Hervey[10] with parabiosis of lean and obese animals that there was a circulating feedback factor from adipose tissue that could regulate energy balance. The identity of the Agouti gene and protein was also fundamental in the development of insight into the role of the melanocortins within the hypothalamic centres for the regulation of energy balance.

In recent years, the application of transgenic and gene targeting approaches has identified over 80 genes that effect body weight, body composition, energy partitioning or some aspect of feeding behaviour or energy expenditure. These have been reviewed recently[2,11]. The genes include a range of hormones and peptides, receptors, transcriptional regulators, metabolic and structural genes and others that are expressed mainly, but not exclusively in either the CNS or the adipose tissue. The wide range of genes that have been shown to alter the susceptibility to develop obesity emphasize the multicausational nature of this disease. Of particular interest is the recognition that many of the genetic manipulations are without a phenotype until the mice are placed upon a high fat diet (Table 1) illustrating the important interaction between genetic inheritance and environmental influences. This is particularly true of a number of receptor gene manipulations including knock out of neuronal insulin receptors, the NPYY2 receptor, the histamine H1 receptor and the 5HT2c receptor.

Table 1. Gene knockouts that result in obesity on a high fat diet

Gene	Name	Position (Chr, cM)	Knockout (KO)	Comment
Insulin receptor	Insr	8, 1	KO	Neuron specific knockout
aP2	Fabp4	6, 56	KO	Fatty acid binding protein
NPY Y2	Npy2r	3, 36	KO	
MCH	Pmch	10, 47	KO	
Histamine H1	H1r	6, 49	KO	
5HT2C	Htr2c	X, 66.15	KO	
Acyl CoA: diacylglycerol acyl transferase	Dgat		KO	

The important role of glucocorticoids in facilitating the development of obesity has been recognized for many years[12] and this has been substantiated by a number of genetic manipulations of the expression of the glucocorticoid receptor, CRH and CRH binding protein genes. Of particular interest is the development of a mouse model of syndrome X by the transgenic overexpression of 11ß-hydroxysteroid dehydrogenase 1 (11 ßHSD1) in adipose tissue[13]. This enzyme converts cortisone (humans) or 11-dehydrocorticosterone (rodents) into their active glucocorticoid forms of cortisol or corticosterone respectively. The increased adipose tissue production of corticosterone resulted in a visceral form of obesity that was further enhanced by high fat diets. The mice were hyperglycaemic, insulin resistant, hyperlipidaemic and hypertensive, the latter probably resulting from the resultant overexpression of angiotensinogen in the adipose tissue of the transgenic mice. The obesity was associated with a small increase in food intake, decreased BAT thermogenesis and an enhanced partitioning of lipid into adipose tissue through lipoprotein lipase.

Animal models have also illustrated the important effects of background genome on the phenotypic expression of a specific genotype. Early studies had shown that the severity and temporal characteristics of diabetes varied with the background strain on which the lep[ob] was expressed[9]. Similar variations in hyperglycaemia and hypertension have been demonstrated with the Koletzky (fa[cp]) gene that induces a variety of phenotypes of a syndrome X profile on different background strains of rat[14]. Likewise, transgene insertion to prevent the expression of the long form of the leptin receptor in an outbred strain of mice led to wide divergence in the diabetes phenotype and provides another model for studies of the interactions of the leptin system with the background genome[15].

Neural pathways

Animal models have provided new insight into the neurochemical and neuropeptidergic components of the central pathways regulating energy balance. Leptin receptors are expressed in several regions of the brain, but most importantly for energy balance on the POMC/NPY and AgRP/CART neurons in the arcuate nucleus[16]. These neurons project to the paraventricular nucleus and to the lateral hypothalamic melanin concentrating hormone (MCH) and orexin neurons through which the leptin effects in modulating feeding and the autonomic nervous system are modulated[17] (Fig. 1). Several natural mutations and numerous experimental gene manipulations have been used for proof of function of these components. These include the demonstration that knockout of the MCH gene produces a lean phenotype whereas overexpression induces obesity when mice are fed a high fat diet[18,19]. Likewise, POMC null mice become obese[20], as do mice unable to respond to α-MSH through knockout of either the MC3 or MC4 receptors or over expression of Agouti-related protein (AgRP) (see York[2] for review). These and other animal models have helped to identify the important role of the melanocortin and MCH systems in the control of energy balance. In contrast, the application of gene targeting, transgenic and antisense approaches towards identifying the physiological role of the NPY system on energy balance has been less fruitful. Despite the pharmacological and physiological evidence that NPY is the most powerful orexigenic agent, no obvious phenotype presents from many of the genetic manipulations of this system or counterintuitive results, such as the late onset mild obesity in Y2R and Y5R knockout mice, are obtained[2,21]. While it is suggested that counter-regulatory responses within a control system that has probably much redundancy explain these data, it is not clear if this is a valid explanation.

Peripheral signals regulating the CNS control systems for energy balance

While leptin has been the viewed as an important peripheral signal that modulates the central regulatory systems effecting food intake and energy expenditure, work with animal models has shown that it is only one of many such signals. Endocrine manipulations have long been known to influence feeding behaviour and body composition[1-3]. These include peripheral injections of insulin, excessive glucocorticoid activity and ovariectomy. The use of transgenic and gene knockout approaches to manipulate hormone and receptor levels has helped to study the role of insulin, adrenal and gonadal steroids. In addition, these approaches have identified effects of numerous other endocrine influences including pancreatic polypeptide, amylin, IGF-1, CRH, growth hormone and CCK on energy balance. Indeed the gastrointestinal system has been regarded as the major source of inhibitory signals modulating feeding behaviour. Cholecystokinin (CCK) reduces food intake and inhibits gastric emptying through actions on CCKA receptors and afferent vagal information passing to the brain stem regions of the CNS. The physiological role of such receptors is suggested by the obesity seen in rats that have a natural deletion of this gene[22]. In contrast, the growth hormone related peptide ghrelin secreted from the stomach is a powerful stimulator of feeding and can induce excess weight gain and fat deposition when given chronically through its modulation of NPY, AgRP and melanocortin systems in the arcuate-PVN axis[23,24].

References

1. Bray GA, York DA. Obesity. In: *Handbook of physiology*, Sect 7: II(34), pp. 1015–56. Oxford University Press; 2001.

2. York DA. Rodent models of obesity. In: *Handbook of obesity*, GA Bray, C Bouchard, WP James (eds). New York: Marcel Dekker, Inc; 2001 (submitted).

3. York DA, Hansen B. Animal models of obesity. In: *Handbook of obesity*, GA Bray, C Bouchard, WP James (eds), pp. 191–221. New York: Marcel Dekker, Inc; 1997.

4. Dhurandhar NV, Atkinson RL. Viruses and obesity. *Curr Opin Endocrinol Diabetes* 2000; 7: 247–51.

5. Bray GA, York DA, Fisler JS. Experimental obesity: a homeostatic failure due to defective nutrient stimulation of the sympathetic nervous system. *Vitam Horm* 1990; 45: 1–125.

6. Rohner-Jeanrenaud F. A neuroendocrine reappraisal of the dual-centre hypothesis: its implications for obesity and insulin resistance. *Int J Obes* 1995; 19: 517–34.

7. Bray GA, York DA. Reciprocal relation of food intake and sympathetic activity: the Mona Lisa hypothesis. In: *Pennington Center Nutrition Series, nutrition, genetics, and obesity*, pp. 122–43. (vol. 9). Baton Rouge, LA: Louisiana State University Press; 1999.

8. Bray GA, York DA. Hypothalamic and genetic obesity in experimental animals: an autonomica and endocrine hypothesis. *Physiol Rev* 1979; 59: 719–809.

9. Coleman DL. Obesity and diabetes: two mutant genes causing diabetes-obesity syndromes in mice. *Diabetologia* 1978; 14: 141–8.

10. Harris RB, Hervey E, Hervey GR, Tobin G. Body composition of lean and obese Zucker rats in parabiosis. *Int J Obes* 1987; 11: 275–83.

11. York DA. Animal models of obesity. In: *International textbook of diabetes mellitus*, E Ferrannini, P Zimmet, R DeFronzo, H Keen (eds) (3rd edn). United Kingdom: John Wiley, 2002 (submitted).

12. York DA. Lessons from animal models of obesity. *Endocrinol Metab Clin N Am* 1996; 25: 781–800.

13. Masuzaki H, Paterson J, Shinyama H, Morton NM, Mullins JJ, Seckl JR et al. A transgenic model of visceral obesity and the metabolic syndrome. *Science* 2001; 294: 2166–9.

14. Shafrir E. Animal models of non-insulin-dependent diabetes. *Diab Metab Revs* 1992; 8: 179–208.

15. Reichart U, Renner-Muller I, Hoflich A, Muller OJ, Franz WM, Wolf E et al. Contrasting obesity phenotypes uncovered by partial leptin receptor gene deletion in transgenic. *Biochem Biophy Res Commun* 2000; 269: 502–7.

16. Elmquist JK. Hypothalamic pathways underlying the endocrine, autonomic, and behavioral effects of leptin. *Int J Obes Relat Metab Disord* 2001; 25: 878–82.

17. Cowley MA, Smart JL, Rubinstein M, Cerdan MG, Diano S, Horvath TL et al. Leptin activates anorexigenic POMC neurons through a neural network in the arcuate nucleus. *Nature* 2001; 411: 480–4.

18. Shimada M, Tritos NA, Lowell BB, Flier JS, Maratos-Flier E. Mice lacking melanin-concentrating hormone are hypophagic and lean. *Nature* 1998; 396: 670–4.

19. Ludwig DS, Tritos NA, Mastaitis JW, Kulkarni R, Kokkotou E, Elmquist J et al. Melanin-concentrating hormone over expression in transgenic mice leads to obesity and insulin resistance. *J Clin Investigation* 2001; 107: 379–86.

20. Yaswen L, Diehl N, Brennan MB, Hochgeschwender U. Obesity in the mouse model of pro-opiomelanocortin deficiency responds to peripheral melanocortin. *Nature Med* 1999; 5: 1066–117.

21. Bannon AW, Seda J, Carmouche M, Francis JM, Norman MH, Karbon B et al. Behavioral characterization of neuropeptide Y knockout mice. *Brain Res* 2000; 868: 79–87.

22. Fumakoshi A, Miyassaka K, Shinozaki H, Masada M, Kawanami T, Takata Y et al. An animal model of congenital defect of gene expression of cholecystokinin (CCK)-A receptor. *Biochem Biophy Res Commun* 1993; 210: 787–96.

23. Tschop M, Smiley DL, Heiman ML. Ghrelin induces adiposity in rodents. *Nature* 2000; 407: 908–13.

24. Asakawa A, Inui A, Kaga T, Yuzuriha H, Nagata T, Ueno N et al. Ghrelin is an appetite-stimulatory signal from stomach with structural resemblance to motilin. *Gastroenterology* 2001; 120: 337–45.

CHAPTER 147

The viral hypothesis: one new potential pathway to obesity

Nikhil V. Dhurandhar

Department of Nutrition and Food Science, and the Center for Molecular Medicine and Genetics, Wayne State University, Detroit, MI 48202, USA
[e-mail: ndhurand@sun.science.wayne.edu]

Background

The World Health Organization recently declared that we are experiencing an epidemic of obesity. In the past 20 years, the prevalence of obesity has increased by 30 per cent in the United States. The aetiology of obesity is multifactorial and understanding the contribution of various aetiological factors is critical for the successful management of obesity. Sclafani[1] has classified the aetiology of animal obesity in nine different groups, including obesity of neural, endocrine, pharmacological, nutritional, environmental, seasonal, genetic, idiopathic or of viral origin. Although, in the last two decades seven pathogens were reported to cause obesity in animal models, until recently the viral aetiology of obesity had not received significant attention. The relative contribution of these pathogens to human obesity is unknown.

An understanding of the pathogens as aetiological factors is required for better management of obesity. A new perspective about the infectious aetiology of obesity may initiate additional research in the field to assess the contribution of various pathogens in human obesity and possibly to prevent or treat obesity of infectious origin. The following is a review of the role of various pathogens that have been implicated in obesity.

Canine distemper virus (CVD)

Lyons *et al.* published the first report of obesity induced by a virus[2], which showed canine distemper virus (CDV), from the family of paramyxoviruses, induced obesity in Swiss albino mice[2]. Body weight and fat cell size and number increased significantly in mice experimentally infected with CDV. Of the mice surviving CDV infection, hyperplastic and hypertrophic obesity was observed 6 to 20 weeks after the infection in about 26 per cent of the animals infected intracerebrally and in 16 per cent of the animals infected intraperitoneally. The phenomenon of CDV induced obesity in mice was subsequently confirmed and is believed to be due to virus-induced hypothalamic damage[3–6]. Recently, Bernard *et al.*[7] noted down-regulation of expression of the leptin receptor in the hypothalami of CVD infected obese mice and suggested it as the cause of the observed weight gain. Bernard *et al.*[7] feel that the results demonstrate a 'hit and run' type of relationship between CDV and the expression of obesity, i.e. the initial CVD infection of the hypothalamus may set off changes that would continue to promote obesity in animals even after the acute infection has subsided. Additionally, a differential display PCR showed specific down-regulation of melanin-concentrating hormone precursor mRNA (ppMCH) in CVD infected-obese mice[8]. The authors believe that the results show 'the importance of ppMCH in the establishment and maintenance of obesity and the involvement of a virus as an environmental factor'.

CDV is not considered a human pathogen, and the contribution of CVD to human obesity is unknown. However, measles virus is a human virus closely related to CDV and belongs to the paramyxovirus family. Experiments showing the effect of measles virus on adiposity are unavailable.

RAV-7

Experimental infection of chickens with Rous Associated virus 7 causes a syndrome characterized by stunting, hyperlipidaemia, hypercholesterolaemia and obesity[9]. Inoculation of 10-day old chick embryos with RAV-7 via a chorioallantoic route produced fat deposition around crop and abdominal fat pads in the adult birds[9]. The results could be replicated by similar inoculations with the serum obtained from RAV-7 infected adult birds[10]. Interestingly, the RAV-7 induced obesity syndrome and the development of pathology appears to be dependent on the route of inoculation. The intravenous inoculation of 1-day-old chickens with RAV-7 did not produce stunting and obesity. Nevertheless, the infected chickens showed a low incidence of osteoporosis and lymphoid leukosis.

RAV-7 infected chickens developed fatty and yellow colored livers, hepatomegaly, anaemia, and immune suppression. The livers weighed 6.2 per cent and 2.4 per cent of the body weight in the RAV-7 infected and uninfected birds, respectively. These disease manifestations were seen within 3 to 4 weeks after hatching of the eggs. The stunting and hyperlipidaemia was the most striking feature of the syndrome observed in the RAV-7 infected chickens. The mean body weight of 50-day-old RAV-7 infected chickens was 194 g, vs. 515 g of the same age control group. Several chickens from the RAV-7 group had serum triglycerides levels over 2000 mg/dl and one chicken had serum triglycerides over 14,000 mg/dl. Food intake was not different for the RAV-7 infected and the uninfected control groups. Also, dietary fat content did not influence the degree of lipid accumulation in the birds. The reduced thyroid hormone levels observed in RAV-7 infected chickens were a suggested cause of the observed obesity and hyperlipidaemia[9]. Although this work was first reported about 20 years ago, its relevance to human obesity or a detailed mechanism is unknown.

Borna disease virus

Borna Disease virus (BDV) was the third virus to be implicated in obesity. BDV is a single, negative stranded RNA virus which primarily targets the nervous system and also replicates in many other organs[11]. In nature, BDV infections occur in horses and sheep and cause encephalomyelitis, but experimental infection may be produced in birds, rodents and primates. Rats experimentally infected with BDV develop obesity associated with lympho-monocytic inflammation of the hypothalamus, hyperplasia of pancreatic islets, and elevated serum glucose and triglycerides[12].

The expression of BDV-induced obesity syndrome varies with the age of the animals at the time of infection, their genetic background, and the virus strain used[12]. Rats infected as newborns with BDV (passaged and harvested in rabbits) show progressive neurological disease after 12 to 16 months. On the other hand, weanling or adult rats similarly inoculated with BDV develop acute encephalitis and die within 1 to 4 months. Some of these rats survive the infection and develop marked obesity[11]. BDV affects several areas in the brain and the development of obesity perhaps due to a virus-induced hypothalamic damage is a possibility. The exact mechanisms of BDV-induced obesity remain unknown.

Although BDV is not traditionally considered to be a human pathogen, recent studies reported the presence of BDV antigen and antibodies in humans[12]. BDV is associated with schizophrenia and mental depression in humans[13,14] which is responsive to treatment by amantadine, an antiviral[15,16]. Further research is needed to determine if BDV causes depression and/or obesity in humans, and whether the amantadine treatment intended to alleviate BDV-induced depression also reduces body weight.

Scrapie agent

Scrapie is a neurodegenerative disease of a long incubation period, known to occur in sheep and goats. Although the key features of scrapie infections are abnormal behaviour and motor dysfunction, mice[17] and hamsters[18], experimentally infected with scrapie agents also developed obesity. The adipogenic property is a function of scrapie strain but not mouse strain. Regardless of the mouse strain tested, scrapie strain ME7 induced obesity, whereas, scrapie strains 139A or 22L did not induce obesity[19]. The difference in the obesity promoting potential of the strains may be in the pathological lesions produced by the strains. Vacuolation caused by ME7 is in the forebrain of the mouse, whereas, 22L and 139A cause vacuolation in the cerebellum and white matter, respectively[19]. Kim *et al.*[20] demonstrated that adrenalectomy prevents ME7 induced obesity in mice, and suggest that scrapie-induced obesity depends on an effect of scrapie on the hypothalamic-pituitary-adrenal axis. The role of scrapie agents in human obesity is not reported.

SMAM-1 avian adenovirus

SMAM-1, is an avian adenovirus first isolated in India[21], which is serologically similar to Chick Embryo Lethal Orphan (CELO) avian adenovirus present in the United States[21]. Three-week-old chickens experimentally inoculated with SMAM-1 showed 53 per cent greater visceral adiposity but paradoxically lower levels of serum lipids compared to the uninfected controls[22,23]. The effect was noted only three weeks after the inoculation. Subsequently, Dhurandhar *et al.*[24] screened 52 obese humans in Bombay for antibodies to SMAM-1 virus using agar-gel-precipitation test. About 20 per cent of the subjects had antibodies to SMAM-1. The antibody positive subjects had a significantly greater body mass index (35.3 ± 1.5 kg/m^2 vs. 30.7 ± 0.6 kg/m^2, $P < 0.001$) compared to the antibody negative group. Moreover, the SMAM-1 antibody positive subjects had about 15 per cent lower serum cholesterol and 60 per cent lower serum triglycerides. This is the first report of an association of a virus with human obesity.

It is unknown if the SMAM-1 antibodies in humans had developed in response to a past infection with the virus or due to a human adenovirus antigenically similar to SMAM-1. Also, the prevalence of SMAM-1 antibodies in non-obese population is not available. Information about the presence of SMAM-1 in the US is not available.

Human adenovirus Ad-36

Adenoviruses are naked DNA viruses with icosahedral symmetry and a diameter of 65–80 nm. In humans, adenoviruses are frequently associated with acute upper respiratory tract infections, and may cause enteritis and conjunctivitis. There are 50 types of human adenoviruses listed with the American Type Culture Collection. Adenovirus type 36 (Ad-36), the first human virus reported to cause obesity in animal models, does not cross react with most other human adenoviruses[25,26] and therefore, it is antigenically unique. Ad-36 was first isolated in 1978 in Germany in the feces of a 6-year-old girl suffering from diabetes and enteritis[26].

Animal studies: In four separate experiments, chickens and mice were inoculated with human adenovirus Ad-36. These animals developed a syndrome of increased adipose tissue and paradoxically low levels of serum cholesterol and triglycerides[27,28]. This syndrome was not seen in the chickens inoculated with avian adenovirus CELO (Chick Embryo Lethal Orphan virus). Sections of the brain and hypothalamus of Ad-36 inoculated animals did not show any overt histopathological changes. Ad-36 DNA could be detected in adipose tissue, but not in the skeletal muscles of animals for as long as 16 weeks after Ad-36 inoculation[27]. Recent experiments show that Ad-36 upregulates differentiation of preadipocytes[29], which may contribute to the observed increase in adiposity.

Human studies: The prevalence of Ad-36 antibodies in obese (BMI ≥ 27 kg/m^2) and non-obese (BMI $<$ 27 kg/m^2) human serum samples obtained from three sites (Wisconsin, Florida, and New York) pooled together was 5 per cent for the non-obese and significantly greater for the obese subjects (30 per cent)[30]. Also, the antibody positive obese had significantly lower serum cholesterol compared to the antibody negative obese counterparts from the respective site[30], which is similar to the relative hypolipidaemia observed in Ad-36 inoculated animal models.

These data show an association of Ad-36 antibodies with human obesity but do not establish a causation. Due to ethical reasons, the definitive experiment of injecting humans with Ad-36 to determine the role of Ad-36 in human obesity is unlikely to ever be conducted. The relevance of Ad-36 to human obesity would continue to be open to question until perhaps the experiments are conducted in a model more relevant to humans. Recent experiments have suggested the suitability of two non-human primate models, rhesus monkeys and marmosets, to study the adiposity promoting potential of Ad-36[31]. More animal and human research is needed to establish the contribution of Ad-36 in human obesity.

Human adenovirus Ad-37

In an attempt to screen other human adenoviruses for adipogenic potential, Atkinson *et al.*[32] identified the adipogenic potential of yet another virus, Ad-37, which increased adiposity in a chicken model. The adipogenic potential of Ad-36 and Ad-37 is not shared by all human adenoviruses. For instance, Ad-2, another human adenovirus did not increase adiposity in experimentally infected chickens[32]. More information is needed to determine the pathophysiology of Ad-37 induced adiposity.

Discussion

The role of infections in the aetiology of obesity has not been seriously considered until recently. To date, seven pathogens have been implicated in obesity in animal models but their role in human obesity has not been established conclusively. Among the obesity-promoting pathogens, CDV is closely related to human measles virus. Also, humans show evidence of Borna Disease Virus infections. However, avian adenovirus SMAM-1 is the first virus to be implicated in human obesity. Ad-36 is the first human virus to be implicated in obesity. The mechanism responsible for inducing obesity may differ among the pathogens. Apparently, some of the pathogens such as CDV induces obesity via the central mechanism, by affecting the hypothalamus, whereas the action of Ad-36 of upregulating fat cell differentiation is peripheral.

Although four of the seven obesity-promoting pathogens do not have any documented association with human obesity, animal models of pathogen-induced obesity provide remarkable insight in the newly emerging field of 'Infectobesity', obesity of infectious origin. The development of infectobesity depends on factors such as the age of the host, route of infection, and the strain of a pathogen. This selectivity of infection suggests that the resulting obesity is not a non-specific response to just any infection, but results from specific host-pathogen interactions.

More evidence about the role of infections in body weight regulation in humans continues to emerge steadily. Most recently, Dart et al.[33] reported an association between antibodies to chlamydia pneumoniae and increased body mass index. Clearly, the significance of infectobesity depends on determining its relevance to human obesity. Unfortunately, this is not easy. Due to ethical reasons, humans could never be experimentally infected with these pathogens to conclusively determine their role in human obesity and the evidence will have to be indirect. This may include animal experiments, particularly those involving higher animals such as non-human primates. In humans, these experiments could be population based longitudinal studies to show a divergence of body weight or body fat emerging after the development of a marker of infection such as a seroconversion or the presence of an antigen or a pathogen-specific nucleic acid. For instance, in a longitudinal study, an increase in body weight in subjects after the development of antibodies to a particular virus (compared to well matched antibody negative subjects) may strongly implicate the virus infection as the cause of that weight gain. Furthermore, even if infectobesity is present in some humans, its clinical detection and diagnosis is not easy. Unlike some cases of virally induced type 1 diabetes, where the effects of the infection are acutely seen on blood glucose, the onset of obesity is relatively insidious. Therefore, it is difficult to assign the responsibility of weight gain to a particular episode of infection from the past. A detailed understanding of the mechanism of the development of infectobesity and the identification of various markers may be helpful.

If a few types of pathogens can cause obesity, there may be more awaiting discovery. Accepting the concept of infectobesity will add a new perspective about the aetiology of obesity. After the reports published in the past two decades of seven adipogenic pathogens, this acceptance need not be difficult. Evidently, not every case of obesity is of infectious origin. When a relationship between a pathogen and human obesity is well established, vaccines or antimicrobial agents may be employed to prevent or treat obesity induced by that particular pathogen. Such a treatment approach directed specifically to the cause may be a more effective way of managing the multifactorial disease of obesity.

References

1. Sclafani A. Animal models of obesity: classification and characterization. *Int J Obes* 1984; 8: 491–508.

2. Lyons MJ, Faust IM, Hemmes RB, Buskirk DR, Hirsch J, Zabriskie JB. A virally induced obesity syndrome in mice. *Science* 1982; 216: 82–5.

3. Bernard A, Zwingelstein G, Meister R, Fabian Wild T. Hyperinsulinemia induced by canine distemper virus infection of mice and its correlation with the appearance of obesity. *Comp Biochem Physiol* 1988; 91B: 691–6.

4. Bernard A, Fevre-Montange M, Giraudon P, Hardin H, Fabian Wild T and Belin MF. Localization of viral proteins and RNA in hypothalamus of mice infected by canine distemper virus. *Virology* 1991; 313: 545–51.

5. Bernard A, Fevre-Montange M, Bencsik A, Giraudon P, Fabian Wild T et al. Brain structures selectively targeted by canine distemper virus in a mouse model infection. *J Neuropath Exp Neuro* 1993; 52: 471–80.

6. McFerran JB, Adair B, Connor TJ. Adenoviral antigens (CELO, QBV, GAL). *Am J Vet Res* 1975; 36: 527–34.

7. Bernard A, Cohen R, Khuth ST, Vedrine B, Verlaeten O, Akaoka H et al. Alteration of the leptin network in late morbid obesity induced in mice by brain infection with canine distemper virus. *J Virology* 1999; 73(9): 7317–27.

8. Verlaeten O, Griffond B, Khuth ST, Giraudon P, Akaoka H, Belin MF, Fellmann D, Bernard A. Down regulation of melanin concentrating hormone in virally induced obesity. *Mol Cell Endocrinol* 2001; 181(1–2): 207–19.

9. Carter JK, Ow CL, Smith RE. Rous-Associated virus type 7 induces a syndrome in chickens characterized by stunting and obesity. *Infection Immunity* 1983; 39: 410–22.

10. Carter JK, Garlich JD, Donaldson WT, Smith RE. Influence of diet on a Retrovirus induced obesity and stunting syndrome. *Avian Dis* 1983; 27: 317–22.

11. GosztonyiG, Kao M, Bode L, Ludwig H. Obesity syndrome in experimental infection of rats with Borna disease virus. *Clin Neuropathol* 1991; 10: 33–4.

12. Gosztonyi G and Ludwig H. Borna disease: Neuropathology and pathogenesis. *Current Topics in Microbiology and Immunology* 1995; 190: 39–73.

13. Chen CH, Chiu YL, Shaw Ck, Tsai MT, Hwang AL, Hsiao KJ. Detection of Borna disease virus RNA from peripheral blood cells in schizophrenic patients and mental health workers. *Mol Psychiatry* 1999; 4(6): 566–71.

14. Chen CH, Chiu YL, Wei FC, Koong FJ, Liu HC, Shaw CK *et al*. High seroprevalence of Borna virus infection in schizophrenic patients, family members and mental health workers in Taiwan. *Mol Psychiatry* 1999; 4(1): 33–8.

15. Dietrich DE, Bode L, Spannahuth CW, Lau T, Huber TJ, Brodhun B *et al*. Amantadine in depressive patients with Borna disease virus (BDV) infection: an open trial. *Bipolar Disord* 2000; 2(1) 65–70.

16. Ferszt R, Kuhl KP, Bode L, Severus EW, Winzer B, Berghofer A *et al*. Amantadine revisited: an open trial of amantadinesulphate treatment in chronically depressed patients with borna disease virus infection. *Pharmacopsychiatry* 1999; 32(4): 142–7.

17. Kim YS, Carp RI, Callahan SM, Wisniewski HM. Scrapie-induced obesity in mice. *J Infect Dis* 1987 Aug 156(2): 402–5.

18. Carp RL, Kim YS, Callahan SM. Pancreatic lesions and hypoglycemia-hyperinsulinemia in scrapie-injected hamsters. *J Infect Dis* 1990; 161(3): 462–6.

19. Carp RL, Meeker H, Sersen E, Kozlowski P. Analysis of the incubation periods, induction of obesity and histopathological changes in senescence-prone and senescence-resistant mice infected with various scrapie agents. *J Gen Virol* 1998; 79(11): 2863–9.

20. Kim YS, Carp RL, Callahan SM, Wisniewski HM. Adrenal involvement in scrapie-induced obesity. *Proc Soc Exp Biol Med* 1988; 189(1): 21–7.

21. Ajinkya SM. In 'Final Technical Report, ICAR', pp.13–43. Bombay, India: Red and Blue Cross Publishing, 1985.

22. Dhurandhar NV, Kulkarni PR, Ajinkya SM, Sherikar AA. Avian adenovirus leading to pathognomic obesity in chickens. *J Bombay Vet College* 1990; 2: 131–2.

23. Dhurandhar NV, Kulkarni PR, Ajinkya SM, Sherikar AA. Effect of adenovirus infection on adiposity in chickens. *Veterinary Microbiology* 1992; 31: 101–7.

24. Dhurandhar NV, Kulkarni PR, Ajinkya SM, Sherikar AA, Atkinson, RL. Screening of human sera for antibody against avian adenovirus. *Obes Res* 1997; 5: 464–9.

25. Hierholzer JC, Wigand R, Anderson LJ, Adrian T, Gold JWM. Adenoviruses from patients with AIDS: A plethora of serotypes and a description of five new serotypes of subgenus D (Types 43-47). *J Infectious Dis* 1988; 158: 804–13.

26. Wigand R, Gelderblom H, Wadell G. New human adenovirus (candidate adenovirus 36), a novel member of subgroup D. *Arch Virology* 1980; 64: 225–33.

27. Dhurandhar NV, Israel BA, Kolesar JM, Mayhew GF, Cook ME, Atkinson RL. Adiposity in animals due to a human virus. *Int J Obes* 2000; 24(8): 989–96.

28. Dhurandhar NV, Israel BA, Kolesar JM, Mayhew G, Cook ME, Atkinson RL. Transmissibility of adenovirus-induced adiposity in a chicken model. *Int J Obes* 2001; 25: 990–6.

29. Dhurandhar NV, Vangipuram S, Atkinson RL. Human adenovirus that induces adiposity in animals also up-regulates fat cell differentiation. *FASEB J* 2001; 15(4): A300.

30. Atkinson RL, Dhurandhar NV, Allison DB, Bowen R, Israel BA. Evidence for an association of an obesity virus with human obesity at three sites in the United States. *Int J Obes* 1998; 22: S57.

31. Dhurandhar NV, Whigham LD, Abbott DH, Schultz-Darken NJ, Israel BA, Bradley SM *et al*. Human Adenovirus Ad-36 Promotes Weight Gain in Male Rhesus and Marmoset Monkeys. *J Nutr* 2002; 132: 3155–60.

32. Atkinson RL, Whigham LD, Kim YC, Israel BA, Dhurandhar NV, Strasheim A. Evaluation of human adenoviruses as an etiology of obesity in chickens. *Int J Obes* 2001; 25 (Suppl 2): S12.

33. Dart Am, Martin JL, Kay S. Association between past infection with Chlamydia pneumoniae and body mass index, low density lipoprotein particle size and fasting insulin. *Int J Obes* 2002; 26: 464–8.

Progress in Obesity Research: 9. Edited by *Geraldo Medeiros-Neto, Alfredo Halpern and Claude Bouchard*
©2003 John Libbey Eurotext Ltd, pp. 708–712.

CHAPTER 148

Adaptive thermogenesis is important in the aetiology of human obesity: the case for

Abdul G. Dulloo[1] and Jean Jacquet[2]

[1]*Department of Medicine, Division of Physiology, University of Fribourg, Switzerland;*
[2]*Computer Unit, Faculty of Medicine, University of Geneva, Switzerland*
[e-mail: abdul.dulloo@unifr.ch]

Introduction

One of the greatest challenges towards understanding the aetiology of human obesity is to explain how in environments that promote overeating and discourage physical activity, there is always a section of the population who, apparently *without conscious effort*, do not become obese. How do they resist obesity? How is constancy of body weight achieved over decades in these individuals? In addressing the issue of human susceptibility to leanness and fatness, there are three cardinal features of body weight regulation that need to be underlined:

(i)   Humans cannot escape the laws of thermodynamics. Whatever theory is put forward to explain body weight and body composition regulation, it is undeniable that changes in body energy stores (and ultimately body weight) cannot occur unless there is a difference between energy intake and energy expenditure.

(ii)   In individuals maintaining long-term constancy of body weight, the matching between energy intake and energy expenditure must be extremely precise since an error of only 1 per cent between input and output of energy, if persistent, will lead to a gain or loss of 1 kg per year or some 40 kg between the age of 20 to 60 years.

(iii)   Even in individuals that maintain a relatively stable lean body weight over decades, there is no 'absolute' constancy of body weight over days, weeks and years. Instead body weight tends to fluctuate or oscillate around a mean constant value, with deviations from a 'set' or 'preferred' value being triggered by events that are cultural (week-end parties, holiday seasons), psychological (stress, anxiety or emotions) and pathophysiological (ranging from minor health perturbations to more serious disease states). According to Garrow[1], very short-term day-to-day changes in body weight have a standard deviation of about 0.5 per cent of body weight, while longitudinal observations over periods of between 10 and 30 years indicate that individuals experienced slow trends and reversal of body weight amounting to between 7 and 20 per cent of mean weight.

In such a dynamic state within which weight homeostasis occurs, it is likely that long-term constancy of body weight is achieved through a network of regulatory systems and subsystems through which changes in food intake, body composition and energy expenditure are interlinked. In this paper, the case is presented that autoregulatory control systems operating through adjustements in heat production (i.e. in thermogenesis) exists in humans and that they play a crucial role in attenuating and correcting deviations of body weight from its 'set' or 'preferred' value.

Weight regulation through adjustements in energy expenditure

There is in fact a built-in stabilizing mechanism in the overall homeostatic system for body weight[2]. Any imbalance between energy intake and energy requirements would result in a change in body weight which, in turn, will alter the maintenance energy requirements in a direction which will tend to counter the original imbalance and would hence be stabilizing. The system thus exhibits *dynamic equilibrium*. For example, an increase in body weight will increase metabolic rate, which will produce a negative energy balance and hence a subsequent decline in body weight. Similarly, a reduction in body weight would also be automatically corrected since the resulting diminished metabolic rate due to the loss in weight will produce a positive balance and hence a subsequent return towards the 'set' or 'preferred' weight. But in reality, the homeostatic system is much more complex than this simple effect of *mass action*. As demonstrated in the 'weight-clamping' experiments of Leibel *et al.*[3], subjects maintaining body weight at a level 10 per cent above their initial body weight showed an increase in daily energy expenditure even after adjusting for changes in body weight and body composition. Conversely, in subjects maintaining weight at a level 10 per cent below the initial body weight, daily energy expenditure was also lower after adjusting for losses in weight and lean tissues. These compensatory changes in energy expenditure (about 15 per cent above or below predicted values) reflect changes in metabolic efficiency that oppose the maintenance of a body weight that is above or below the 'set' or 'preferred' body weight.

Furthermore, a closer inspection of the data from this study[3] reveals a large inter-individual variability in the ability to readjust energy expenditure, with some individuals showing little or no evidence for altered metabolic efficiency, while others reveal a marked capacity to decrease or increase energy expenditure through alterations in metabolic efficiency. Indeed, the most striking feature of virtually all experiments of human overfeeding is the wide range of individual variability in the amount of weight gain per unit of excess energy consumed. These differences in the efficiency of weight gain are mostly attributed to variability in the ability to covert excess calories to heat, i.e. in the large inter-individual capacity for diet-induced thermogenesis (DIT). In his detailed reanalysis of data from some 150 individuals participating in the various 'Gluttony Experiments' conducted between 1965–99, Stock[4] argues that at least 40 per cent of these overfed subjects must have exhibited an increase in DIT, albeit to varying degrees. Part of this variation in DIT could be explained by differences in the dietary protein content of the diet, with DIT being more pronounced on unbalanced diets which are low or high in per cent protein[4,5]. But we also know from overfeeding experiments of Bouchard *et al.* in identical twins[6] that genes play an important role in variability in metabolism that underlie susceptibility to weight gain and obesity. Conversely a role for genotype in human variability in enhanced metabolic efficiency during weight loss has been suggested from studies of Hainer *et al.*[7] in which identical twins underwent slimming therapy on a very-low-calorie diet.

Taken together, it is therefore evident that in addition to the control of food intake, changes in efficiency of energy utilization (i.e. in adaptive thermogenesis) also play an important role in the regulation of body weight and body composition, and that the magnitude of adaptive changes in thermogenesis is strongly influenced by the genetic make-up of the individual.

What constitutes adaptive changes in thermogenesis?

A main reason for controversies about the importance of adaptive thermogenesis in the aetiology of human obesity reside in difficulties in pin-pointing which component(s) of energy expenditure could be contributing importantly to the changes in metabolic efficiency and hence in adaptive thermogenesis. As depicted in Fig. 1, the energy expenditure measured in the resting state, whether as basal metabolic rate (BMR) or as thermic effect of food (TEF) certainly results in the production of heat (i.e. in thermogenesis), and changes in resting energy expenditure that are unaccounted for changes in body weight and body composition reflect changes in metabolic efficiency, and hence in adaptive changes in thermogenesis. By contrast, the heat production from what is generally clustered under non-resting energy expenditure is more difficult to quantify. The efficiency of muscular contraction during exercise is low ($\sim$ 25 per cent), but that of spontaneous physical activity (SPA) (including fidgeting, muscle tone and posture maintenance, and other low-level physical activities of everyday life) is even lower since these essentially involuntary activities comprise a larger proportion of isometric work which is simply thermogenic. Since actual work done on the environment during SPA is very small compared to the total energy spent on such activities, the energy cost associated with SPA has been referred to as movement-associated thermogenesis or SPA-associated thermogenesis[8]. It can also be argued that since SPA is essentially beyond voluntary control, a change in the *level* or *amount* of such involuntary SPA activity in a direction that defends a 'preferred' body weight also constitute autoregulatory changes in energy expenditure that contribute to the overall changes in metabolic efficiency. In this context, an increase in the amount of SPA in response to overfeeding, or a decrease during starvation, also constitute adaptive changes in thermogenesis. As to whether inter-individual variability in the *amount*

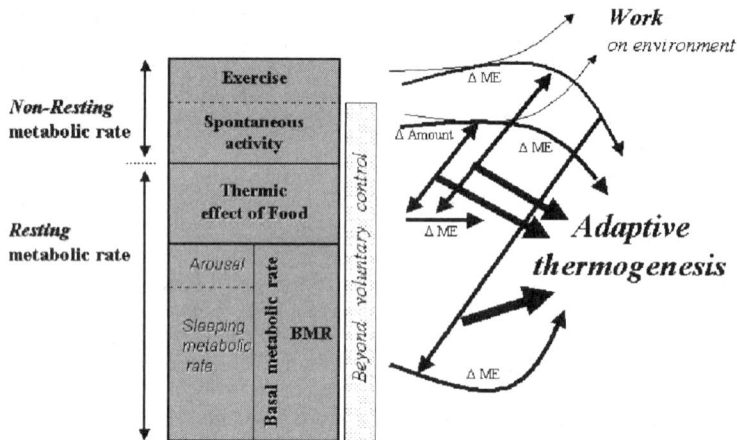

Fig. 1. Schematic diagram showing the various compartements of human energy expenditure, and how changes in metabolic efficiency (ΔME) both within and across these compartments can lead to adaptive changes in thermogenesis.

of SPA during overfeeding contribute to variability in resistance or susceptibility to obesity remains to be demonstrated. By contrast, the marked reduction in the SPA in the men and women who lost 8–25 per cent body weight as a result of chronic food shortage during the Biosphere 2 Experiment[9] could have contributed importantly to their lower daily energy expenditure and enhanced metabolic efficiency.

The importance of SPA-associated thermogenesis in human weight regulation is further underscored by the findings of Ravussin et al.[10] that even under conditions where subjects are confined to a metabolic chamber, the 24 h energy expenditure attributed to SPA (as assessed by radar systems) was found to vary between 100–700 kcal/day, and to be a predictor of subsequent weight gain. In fact, a main conclusion of the early overfeeding experiments of Miller et al.[11] was that most of extra heat dissipation in some of the individuals resisting obesity by increased DIT could not be accounted for an increase in resting metabolic rate but could be due to an increased energy expenditure associated with simple (low-level) activities of everyday life. This notion has recently gained much support from the findings of Levine et al.[12] that more than 60 per cent of the increase in total daily energy expenditure in response to overfeeding was associated with SPA, and that inter-individual variability in energy expenditure associated with SPA – which they referred to as non-exercise-activity thermogenesis (NEAT) – was the most significant predictor of the resistance or susceptibility to obesity. It should however be emphasized that non-resting energy expenditure (Fig. 1) or NEAT could also include heat production resulting from the impact of physical activity on postabsorptive metabolic rate or postprandial thermogenesis. There is in fact some evidence that relatively low-intensity exercise can lead to potentiation of TEF[11,13] and that the effect of physical activity on energy expenditure can persist well after the period of the physical activity (post-exercise or post-SPA stimulation of thermogenesis)[13].

Adaptive thermogenesis as dual-control systems in weight regulation

Thus, any change in metabolic efficiency (ME) in resting or non-resting state that would tend to *attenuate energy imbalance* or to *restore body weight and body composition* towards its 'set' or 'preferred' value constitute adaptive changes in thermogenesis. From a system physiology perspective, the available evidence strongly suggest the existence of two distinct control systems underlying adaptive thermogenesis[14,15]. One control system is a direct function of energy imbalance and responds *rapidly* to attenuate the impact of changes in food intake on changes in body weight; it is suppressed during starvation and increased during overfeeding. By contrast, the other control system has a much *slower* time-constant since it operates as a feedback loop between the size of the fat stores and thermogenesis (i.e. a lipostatic or adipose-specific control of thermogenesis). Whereas its suppression during weight (and fat) losses is to reduce the overall rate of fuel utilization during starvation, its sustained suppression until body fat is recovered during refeeding is to accelerate the replenishment of the fat stores.

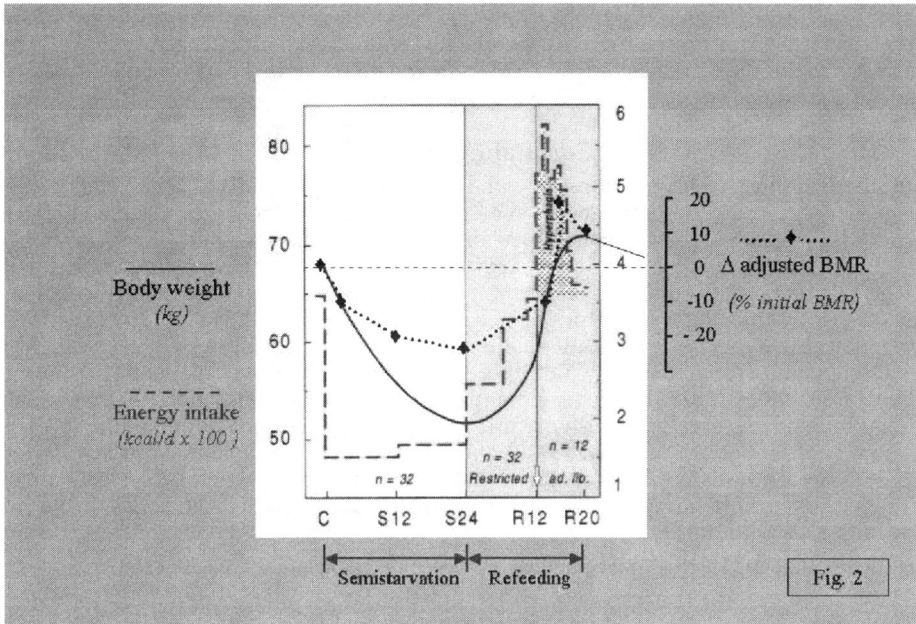

Fig. 2. Pattern of changes in body weight, food intake, and adaptive thermogenesis during the various phases of the longitudinal 'Minnesota Experiment' of human semistarvation and refeeding. The changes in adaptive thermogenesis at the various time-points are assessed as changes in basal metabolic rate (BMR) after adjusting for changes in fat free mass (FFM) and fat mass, and expressed as a percentage of the baseline (control, C) BMR level[17]. C = end of control (baseline) period; S12 and S24 = week 12 and week 24 of semistarvation, respectively; R12 and R20 = week 12 and week 20 after onset of refeeding.

Conversely during periods of excess fat gain, its activation will serve to oppose the maintenance of the excess fat and hence to restore body fat to its 'set' or 'preferred' level.

The operation of this dual control systems for adaptive thermogenesis is consistent with the temporal changes of BMR and body composition during the longitudinal study of semistarvation and refeeding in men from the Minnesota Experiment[16]. The overall pattern of changes in food intake and body weight, together with kinetics of altered thermogenesis (assessed as changes in BMR adjusted for FFM and fat mass, and expressed as a percentage of baseline BMR value) are presented in Fig. 2. During the *phase of weight loss*, the operation of the two control systems for adaptive thermogenesis is suggested by the fact that reduction in thermogenesis is *biphasic* in nature, with an initial reduction in adjusted BMR at week 4 (corresponding to 10 per cent of baseline BMR), followed by a slower reduction in adjusted BMR corresponding to 20 per cent and 25 per cent of baseline BMR at weeks 20 and 24, respectively. At the latter time-points during starvation (at S20 and S24), the magnitude of reduced adjusted BMR was found to be associated with the reduction in fat mass[17] – i.e. the greater the degree of depletion of the fat stores, the greater the suppression of thermogenesis. During the *phase of weight recovery*, the operation of the two control systems for thermogenesis is also suggested by the following:

(a)   The relation between the degree of depletion of fat stores and suppressed thermogenesis persists at week 12 of restricted refeeding[17], at which time-point (R12) the mean adjusted BMR is still about 10 per cent below baseline BMR level (Fig. 2), the body fat is 80 per cent recovered, while body weight and FFM recoveries are less than 50 per cent;

(b)   After withdrawal of the dietary restriction during the subsequent period of *ad libitum* refeeding, the development of hyperphagia is accompanied by a prompt increase in thermogenesis (as judged by increases in adjusted BMR corresponding to about 20 per cent of baseline BMR at week 14 of refeeding); and

(c)   By week 20 after the onset of refeeding (i.e. at R20), when FFM has been almost 100 per cent recovered and body fat had overshot baseline (prestarvation) level by > 70 per cent[18] – a phenomenon that Keys *et al.*[16] referred to as 'post-starvation obesity'– the adjusted BMR remains significantly higher (by about 10 per cent) above baseline BMR despite the fact that hyperphagia is no longer present. This sustained elevation of thermogenesis may well have contributed to the subsequent slow return of body weight towards the baseline level after the phase of fat overshooting.

Concluding remarks

Throughout much of their evolutionary history, the mammalian species have been faced with periodic food shortages, specific nutrient deficiencies and sometimes food abundance. Within such a lifestyle of *famine and feast*, it is conceivable that specialized mechanisms for energy conservation (via enhanced metabolic efficiency), but also for energy wastage (via decreased metabolic efficiency), have evolved to the extent that they constitute key control systems in the regulation of body weight and body composition. These autoregulatory control systems operating through adjustements in heat production or thermogenesis play a crucial role in attenuating and correcting deviations of body weight from its 'set' or 'preferred' value. The extent to which these adjustements through adaptive thermogenesis are brought about is dependent upon the environment (e.g. diet composition), and is highly variable from one individual to another, largely because of variations in the genetic make-up among individuals. In societies where food is plentiful all year round and physical activity demands are low, the resultant subtle variations among individuals in adaptive thermogenesis can, in dynamic systems and over the long-term, be important in determining long-term constancy of body weight in some and in provoking the drift towards obesity in others.

Acknowledgements: Supported by the Swiss National Science Foundation (grant # 3200-061687).

References

1. Garrow J. *Energy balance and obesity in man.* North Holland, Amsterdam: Elsevier; 1974.

2. Payne PR, Dugdale AE. Mechanisms for the control of body weight. *Lancet* 1977; 8011: 583–6.

3. Leibel RL, Rosenbaum M, Hirsch J. Changes in energy expenditure resulting from altered body weight. *N Engl J Med* 1995; 332: 621–8.

4. Stock MJ. Gluttony and thermogenesis revisited. *Int J Obes* 1999; 23: 1105–17.

5. Dulloo AG, Jacquet J. Low-protein overfeeding: a tool to unmask susceptibility to obesity in humans. *Int J Obes* 1999; 23: 1118–21.

6. Bouchard C, Tremblay A, Desprès JP, Nadeau A, Lupien PJ, Thiérault G *et al.* The response to long-term overfeeding in identical twins. *N Engl J Med* 1990; 322: 1477–82.

7. Hainer V, Stunkard AJ, Kunesova M, Parizkova J, Stich V, Allison DB. A twin study of weight loss and metabolic efficiency. *Int J Obes* 2001; 25: 533–7.

8. Girardier L, Clark MG, Seydoux J. Thermogenesis associated with spontaneous activity: an important component of thermoregulatory needs in rats. *J Physiol* 1995; 488: 779–87.

9. Weyer C, Walford RL, Harper IT, Milner M, MacCallum T, Tataranni PA, Ravussin E. Energy metabolism after 2 y of energy restriction: the Biosphere 2 experiment. *Am J Clin Nutr* 2000; 72: 946–53.

10. Ravussin E, Lillioja S, Anderson TE, Christin L, Bogardus C. Determinants of 24-hour energy expenditure in man: Methods and results using a respiratory chamber. *J Clin Invest* 1986; 78: 1568–78.

11. Miller DS, Mumford P, Stock MJ. Gluttony 2. Thermogenesis in overeating man. *Am J Clin Nutr* 1967; 20: 1223–29.

12. Levine JA, Eberhardt NL, Jensen MD. Role of nonexercise activity thermogenesis in resistance to fat gain in humans. *Science* 1999; 283: 212–4.

13. Richard D, Rivest S. The role of exercise in thermogenesis and energy balance. *Can J Physiol Pharmacol* 1989; 67: 402–9.

14. Dulloo AG, Jacquet J. An adipose-specific control of thermogenesis in body weight regulation. *Int J Obes* 2001; 25 (Suppl 5): S22–S29.

15. Dulloo AG, Jacquet J, Montani JP. Pathways from weight fluctuations to metabolic diseases: focus on maladaptive thermogenesis during catch-up fat. *Int J Obes* 2002; 26 (Suppl. 2): S46–S57.

16. Keys A, Brozek J, Henschel A, Mickelson O, Taylor HL. *The biology of human starvation.* Minneapolis: University of Minnesota Press; 1950.

17. Dulloo AG, Jacquet J. Adaptive reduction in basal metabolic rate in response to food deprivation in humans: a role for feedback signals from fat stores. *Am J Clin Nutr* 1998; 68: 599–606.

18. Dulloo AG, Jacquet J, Girardier L. Poststarvation hyperphagia and body fat overshooting in humans: a role for feedback signals from lean and fat tissues. *Am J Clin Nutr* 1997; 65: 717–23.

Progress in Obesity Research: 9. Edited by *Geraldo Medeiros-Neto, Alfredo Halpern* and *Claude Bouchard*
©2003 John Libbey Eurotext Ltd, pp. 713–717.

CHAPTER 149

Adaptive changes in thermogenesis are NOT important in the aetiology of obesity

J.P. Flatt

University of Massachusetts Medical School, Worcester, MA 01605, USA
[e-mail j.p.flatt@umassmed.edu]

Introduction

The metabolic transformations which permit the oxidation of glucose, fatty acids and amino acids in the body generate reducing equivalents (e.g. NADH, FADH2), whose re-oxidation is coupled to the regeneration of ATP from ADP and inorganic phosphate (Pi). About two thirds of the energy liberated can be recovered as high-energy bonds in ATP, while one third appears as heat[1]. ATP is constantly turned over and when used to drive chemical reactions in the body, most of the energy contained in the high-energy bond is also converted into heat, except for the relatively small fraction expended in performing physical work in the environment. Most of the energy liberated by substrate oxidation is thus converted into heat, whose release to the environment is regulated so as to maintain body temperature (Fig. 1). These processes are not usually referred to as 'thermogenesis', a term generally reserved to describe increments in substrate oxidation and heat production in response to cold exposure (i.e. 'cold-induced thermogenesis', which may be shivering or non-shivering), or as an adaptive response to overeating (i.e. 'adaptive thermogenesis') serving to dissipate some of the excess energy consumed (Fig. 2). Because heat is constantly generated (at a rate of some 0.8 to 1.2 kcal/min in resting adults), the use of the word and concept of *thermogenesis* for these additional phenomena only is not logical and therefore apt to promote confusions.

Changes in energy expenditure in response to altered levels of energy intake have long been known and there has been much interest and debate about their significance. Thus, it is well established that during period of food deprivation and starvation, resting energy expenditure declines, and that sustained periods of underfeeding lead to a spontaneous decrease in physical activities as well as to a reduction in work capacity[2]. On the other hand, substantial increases in energy expenditure have been observed in laboratory animals provided with 'cafeteria-diets'[3]. This response is brought about by activation of an un-coupling protein (UCP), which creates a protein leak through the mitochondrial membrane, thereby uncoupling substrate oxidation from ATP regeneration. This process is most active in brown adipose tissue, being induced by cold exposure and during arousal from hibernation, as well as during overfeeding[4]. In the latter case it provides a mechanism limiting fat accumulation during periods of over-consumption[5]. The latter response has been of considerable interest because of its possible influence on body weight regulation. Several forms of UCP have been identified in various tissues, but in spite of considerable research efforts, a significant role for UCPs in body weight regulation in man has not yet been established[6].

In man, changes in resting energy expenditure in response to under- or over-eating are modest and they can merely attenuate their impact on the energy balance. It is important to understand that they are due in part to an increase or a decrease in the 'thermic effect of food' (TEF), which amounts to some 10 per cent of the food energy consumed. The TEF is due mainly to the ATP expended to absorb, transport and store the ingested nutrients[7]. Protein synthesis and gluconeogenesis also involve some ATP expenditure related to the level of nutrient intake. After prolonged periods of negative or positive energy balance, changes in body size account for most of the decreases or increases in resting energy expenditure[2]. Some, but not all studies suggest that changes in energy expenditure are in fact greater

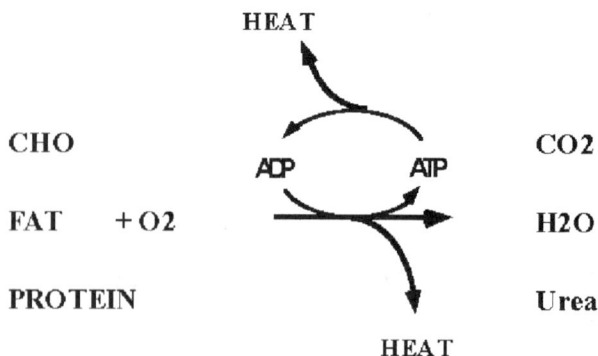

Fig. 1. Heat production during the biological oxidation of substrates.

than what can be attributed to the above mentioned phenomena. While the scope of the unexplained effects is small in comparison to overall energy turnover, one also needs to consider that errors in long-term energy balance are generally small as well, rarely exceeding 1–2 per cent of energy turnover when considered over a one-year period. Indeed, it is still debated whether increments in energy expenditure during overfeeding are important or not for the development of obesity[8-10]. Thus, the issue to be considered here is whether or not lack or weakness of adaptive thermogenesis contributes to the development of obesity.

Discussion

Several facts speak against the view that minor differences in energy expenditure, or in adaptive thermogenesis are important for body weight regulation.

1. Implicit in such a view is the assumption that differences in 'metabolic efficiency' will not be offset by changes in energy intake. This appears as a rather unrealistic assumption, as there is no evidence indicating that average energy intakes in free-living subjects are determined at a given level. By contrast, it is well established that energy density, food quality and diversity influence energy intakes[11,12].

2. Very large daily variations in food intake occur in free-living subjects. This is reflected by the coefficients of variations for intra-individual food intake, which were found to average ± 23 per cent[13]. Physical activities are also susceptible to vary substantially from day to day, and they are not promptly compensated by changes in food intake[14]. This implies that large deviations from daily energy balance occur as a matter of course. The differences in resting

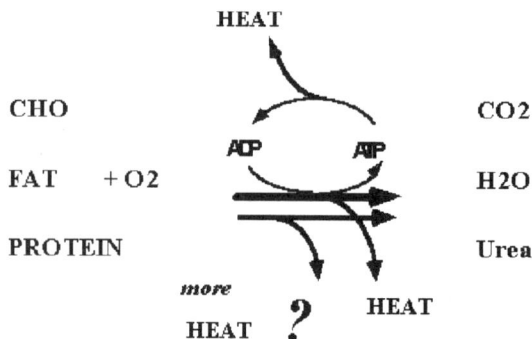

Fig. 2. Adaptive thermogenesis and obesity. The word 'Thermogenesis' is usually reserved to describe either (1) additional heat production by increases in substrate oxidation serving to maintain body temperature during cold exposure, or (2) increased substrate oxidation and heat release serving to dissipate excess energy during period of overfeeding.

Impact of Adaptive Changes in Energy Expenditure
on Energy Deficits and Energy Gains
(other than due to Changes in Body Weight)

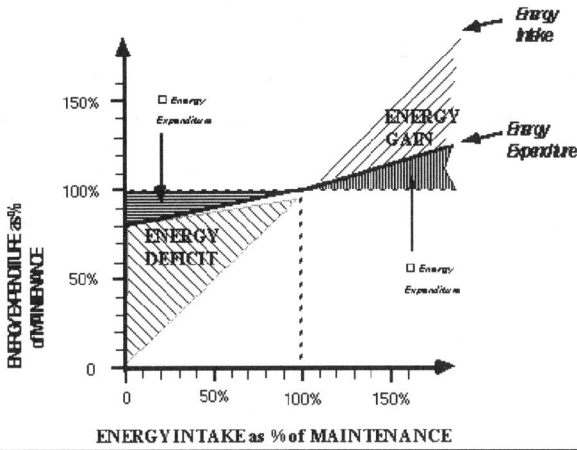

Fig. 3. Impact of changes in energy expenditure during food deprivation or over-consumption on energy balance.

energy expenditure which may be brought about by adaptive changes in thermogenesis are very small and they may not even come into play when days with positive and negative energy balances alternate in quick succession. As shown in Fig. 3, they only modestly attenuate the impact of excessive or insufficient food consumption on the energy balance. Therefore, it is food intake and the phenomena involved in regulating or controlling it, which play the dominant role in the regulation and maintenance of body weight.

Table 1. Impact of height on variance of resting energy expenditure*

Men (n = 6139)				
REE[†] = –328	–9.2 x Age	+22.4x % BodyFat[†]	+1120 x Height	$R^2 = 0.69$
REE = 1637	–10.2 x Age	+24,1x % BodyFat		$R^2 = 0.53$
Women (n = 6103)				
REE = –337	–5.4 x Age	+19.3x % BodyFat	+800 x Height	$R^2 = 0.68$
REE = 993	–5.9 x Age	+19.2x % BodyFat		$R^2 = 0.56$

*Based on NHANES3 data(16).
†Resting energy expenditure (REE) in kcal/day calculated from body weight using Schofield's equations(24); % Body Fat based on bioimpedance data (16); height in m.

Table 2. Impact of age, weight and height on energy expenditure*

Basal energy expenditure†				
Men: BEE = 293	–3.8 x Age	+10.12 x Weight	+456 x Height	$R^2 = 0.64$
Women: BEE = 247	–2.67 x Age	+ 8.60 x Weight	+402 x Height	$R^2 = 0.62$
Total energy expenditure†				
Men: TEE = 864	–9.72 x Age	+PALcoeff x	(14.2 x Weight +503 x Height)	$R^2 = 0.82$
Women: TEE = 387	–7.31 x Age	+PALcoeff x	(10.9 x Weight+661 x Height)	$R^2 = 0.79$

*DRI-Report 2002 (17), based on NHANES3 data;
†Basal Energy Expenditure (BEE) determined by indirect calorimetry, Total Energy Expenditure (TEE) determined by doubly-labeled water (DLW); BEE and TEE in kcal/day; Age in years; weight in kg; height in m; (PAL) = TEE/BEE.

Table 3. Impact of Height on per cent Body Fat*

Men:	% Body Fat† = 21.7+0.16 x Height (N = 7324, P = 0.9)	R^2 = 0
Women:	% Body Fat = 42.4–6.20 x Height (N = 7724, P = 0.0002)	R^2 = 0.0026

*DRI-Report 2002 (17), based on NHANES3 data; †% Body Fat based on bioimpedence data; height in m.

3. Resting energy expenditure (REE) is predominately determined by the size of the lean body mass[15]. Stature has a substantial impact on the lean body mass, yet has no appreciable impact on body fat. In the NHANES3 data, for instance, height was estimated to account for 16 per cent of the variance in lean body mass and REE of adult men and for 12 per cent in women, as judged by the change in R^2 values when height was deleted as a parameter in the regression analysis (Table 1). Yet height had no impact on per cent body fat[16]. In a recently published analysis of daily total energy expenditures (TEE) determined by doubly labeled water measurements[17], height appears as an important factor in predicting TEE (Table 2), but its impact on adiposity, R^2 = 0 in men and R^2 = 0.0026 in women, is biologically insignificant (Table 3). Thus, differences in resting energy expenditure and in total energy expenditure far greater than the small variations in metabolic efficiency or in adaptive thermogenesis have no biologically significant effect on adiposity, as one would have to expect if resting energy expenditure was an important factor for the development of obesity.

4. In many countries, the prevalence of obesity has markedly increased during recent decades[18,19]. It is not plausible to think that this could have been brought about by a sudden failure of adaptive thermogenesis. Rather, it is changes in living conditions, and in particular the increasing ubiquity, availability and promotion of appetizing, energy-dense foods, which have promoted the development of obesity[20], along with further declines in physical activity. Because exercise promotes fat oxidation to a greater extent than carbohydrate oxidation[21], increases in the fat mass are often needed when physical activity is low to raise fat oxidation and make it commensurate with the diet's fat content[20].

In conclusion, analysis of the relationship between stature and adiposity provides data which can be interpreted without the various considerations required to discuss metabolic efficiency. The fact that variations in energy turnover associated with different stature have no appreciable impact on adiposity, demonstrates that differences in resting energy expenditure, as well as adaptive changes in thermogenesis are NOT important in the aetiology of obesity. This finding has several implications.

First, in regard to food regulation. Thus, in spite of the very loose regulation of daily food consumption, underlying phenomena in the regulation of food intake are capable of compensating for the fact that portions served outside of the home are not adjusted for stature. Because these phenomena do not become apparent in studies of food consumption limited to 24 hours, they unfortunately remain poorly understood[22].

Second, in regard to the search for drugs capable of reducing adiposity. Based on the expectation naively derived by consideration of the energy balance equation that increases in energy expenditure are bound to facilitate weight loss[23], considerable efforts have been devoted to find drugs capable of increasing energy expenditure. However, this property does not by itself guarantee weight loss, as made evident by the spontaneous adjustments in food intake which occur in the face of differences in energy turnover. To be effective, a drug must enhance fat oxidation more than carbohydrate oxidation, as is the case with exercise.

Acknowledgement: This publication was made possible by grant number DK 56817 from the National Institute of Health. Its contents are solely the responsibility of the author and do not necessarily represent the official views of the National Institute of Health.

References

1. Pahud P, Ravussin E, Jéquier E. Energy expended during oxygen deficit period of submaximal exercise in man. *J Appl Physiol* 1980; 48: 770–5.

2. Keys A, Brozek J, Henschel A, Mickelsen O, Taylor HL. *The biology of human starvation.* Minneapolis: University of Minnesota Press; 1950.

3. Rothwell NJ, Saville ME, Stock MJ. Effects of feeding a 'cafeteria' diet on energy balance and diet-induced thermogenesis in four strains of rat. *J Nutr* 1982; 112: 1515–24.

4. Himms-Hagen J, Ricquier D. Brown adipose tissue. In: *Handbook of obesity*, GA Bray, C Bouchard, WPT James (eds), pp. 415–41. New York: Marcel Dekker, 1988.

5. Stock MJ. Thermogenesis and energy balance. *Int J Obes* 1992; 16 (Suppl 2): S13–S16.

6. Schrauwen P, Walder K, Ravussin E. Human uncoupling proteins and obesity. *Obes Res* 1998; 7(1): 97–105.

7. Flatt JP. The biochemistry of energy expenditure. *Rec Adv Obesity Res* 1978; 2: 211–28.

8. Leibel RL, Rosenbaum M, Hirsch J. Changes in energy expenditure resulting from altered body weight. *N Engl J Med* 1995; 332: 621–28.

9. Weinsier R, Nelson K, Hensrud D, Darnell B, Hunter G, Schutz Y. Metabolic predictors of obesity: contribution of resting energy expenditure, thermic effect of food, and fuel utilization to four year weight gain of post obese and never obese women. *J Clin Invest* 1995; 95: 980–85.

10. Granata GP, Brandon LJ. The thermic effect of food and obesity: discrepant results and methodological variations. *Nutr Rev* 2002; 60: 223–33.

11. Poppitt SD, Prentice AM. Energy density and its role in the control of food intake: evidence from metabolic and community studies. *Appetite* 1996; 26: 153–74.

12. Rolls BJ. Experimental analysis of the effects of variety in a meal on human feeding. *Am J Clin Nutr* 1985; 42: 932–39.

13. Bingham SA, Gill C, Welch A, Day K, Cassidy A, Khaw KT *et al*. Comparison of dietary assessment methods in nutritional epidemiology: weighed records v. 24h recalls, food-frequency questionnaires and estimated-diet records. *Br J Nutr* 1994; 72: 619–43.

14. Edholm OG, Adam JM, Healey MJ, Wolff HS, Goldsmith R, Best TW. Food Intake and energy expenditure of army recruits. *Br J Nutr* 1970; 24: 1091–107.

15. Ravussin E, Lillioja S, Anderson TE, Christin L, Bogardus C. Determinants of 24-h energy expenditure in man. *J Clin Invest* 1986; 78: 1568–78.

16. Flatt JP, Gupte S. Metabolic efficiency. In: *Nutrition, genetics and obesity*, GA Bray, H Ryan (eds), pp. 73–87. Baton Rouge: Louisiana State Univ Press; 1999.

17. Dietary reference Intakes, Medicine Io, editors. Washington, DC: National Academy of Sciences; 2002.

18. Kuczmarski RJ, Flegal KM, Campbell SM, Johnson CL. Increasing prevalence of overweight among US Adults. *JAMA* 1994; 272: 205–11.

19. Seidell JC. Obesity in Europe: scaling an epidemic. *Int J Obes* 1995; 19: S1–S4.

20. Flatt JP. McCollum Award Lecture, 1995: Diet, lifestyle and weight maintenance. *Am J Clin Nutr* 1995; 62: 820–36.

21. Flatt JP. Integration of the overall effects of exercise. *Int J Obes* 1995; 19: S31–S40.

22. Flatt JP. What do we most need to learn about food intake regulation. *Obes Res* 1998; 6: 307–10.

23. Flatt JP. How NOT to approach the obesity problem. *Obes Res* 1997; 5: 632–3.

24. Schofield WN. Predicting basal metabolic rate, new standards and review of previous work. *Hum Nutr: Clin Nutr* 1985; 39C: 5–41.

Progress in Obesity Research: 9. Edited by *Geraldo Medeiros-Neto, Alfredo Halpern* and *Claude Bouchard*
©2003 John Libbey Eurotext Ltd, pp. 718–723.

CHAPTER 150

Ponderostat: arguments in favour of a set-point

Michel Cabanac

Département de physiologie, Faculté de médecine, Université Laval, Québec, Canada G1K 7P4
[e-mail: michel.cabanac@phs.ulaval.ca]

The tank sketched in Fig. 1A is analog to the processes taking place in animals. In their foods, they receive a flow of energy and matter, and under the form of heat, CO_2, urea, feces, etc., they lose to their environment an equal flow of energy and matter. Living beings are open systems as is the tank. It reaches a steady-state in which the input and output flows of water are equal and the free energy expenditure constant. In the process leading to the steady-state, open systems accumulate free energy and reduce their entropy at the expense of the energy input; e.g. the tank will accumulate water up to a certain level, **h**, which represents a certain amount of potential (free) energy and a reduction of entropy.

The best way to study a system is to perturb it. This is the very nature of the experimental method. A perturbation can be transient or continuous. Systems can be categorized according to the way they respond to transient and continuous perturbations.

When a transient perturbation is applied to an open system in a steady-state, it responds in giving back the perturbation energy to the environment and returns to the original steady-state. If we add a small volume of water to the tank (transient perturbation), the water level will be raised and, in turn, the increased water pressure will increase the outflow until the water level resumes its original value. The same would be true if we scooped some water out of the tank. The lower water level and the decreased pressure would decrease the outflow until the water level resumes its original value. The larger the accumulated energy in an open system, the smaller the change produced by a transient perturbation. The larger the flow through the system, the more quickly it returns to the steady-state.

Steady-state systems have also the property of resisting continuous perturbations within a certain range. If an extra inflow of water (continuous perturbation), or an extra outflow, is added to the water tank, it will change to a new steady-state with a higher, or lower, water level but it will not be destroyed, as would have happened with an closed system. The reason for this is that the rise in the water level caused by an extra inflow, increases the pressure which, in turn, enhances the water outflow. This increased 'response' is the origin of the improvement of stability, but it is not yet regulation. It is only the spontaneous stability of opposing actions of variable energy release and loss to the environment.

In the water tank the stability of the steady-state water level is improved by a float, and a feed back which controls a faucet at the input so as to close it as the level rises (negative feedback) and/or a feed forward to control a faucet in the output so as to open it as the level rises (positive feedforward) (Fig. 1A).

Negative feedback has the same effect as positive feedforward on the water level, which is thus regulated. Regulation, i.e. a regulated system, is therefore a steady-state the stability of which is improved by information loops controlling the inflow and/or outflow of energy.

Examples of physiological regulations show that in most cases the regulation of a given variable is achieved by modulating both inflow and outflow independently, e.g. blood pressure is regulated by the modulation of cardiac output and peripheral resistance. For a biologist, to distinguish whether a regulatory response modulates the inflow (heat production, cardiac output, food-water intake) or the outflow (heat-loss, peripheral resistance, kidney function) is important. The duality of the possible

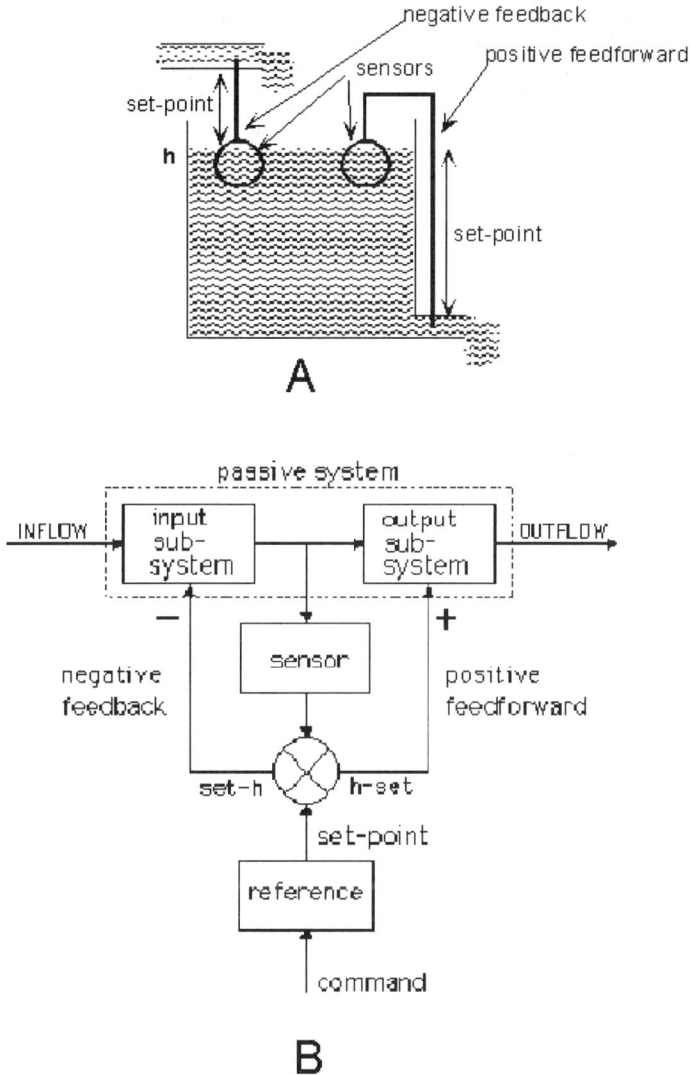

Fig. 1.
A. The steady state becomes a regulation, when equipped with a sensor (float) of the regulated variable (**h**), a negative feedback modulating the input flow, and a positive feed forward modulating the output flow. The set-point of that system is a built-in property incorporated in the length of the shafts between float and input and output faucets.
B. The new diagram proposed for regulation. This underlines the flow of energy and matter through the system, that exists already in the steady state. In addition, it shows that the negative feedback controlling the input is anatomically different from the positive feed forward on the output. Both tend to keep steady the regulated variable **h**. After[45].

response gives one degree of freedom to the system. The block diagram in Fig. 1B pinpoints this duality of functions, inflow vs. outflow. The black boxes are subsystems controlling the inflow and outflow of energy or mass. They represent functions both in the mathematical and physiological sense, e.g. temperature regulation.

The regulatory responses may be interpreted as changes in the parameters of the input and/or output functions resulting from the modulation exerted by the feedback and/or feedforward loops which convey information about the change in the regulated variable, the error signal, elicited by a perturbation, extra inflow or outflow of energy or mass.

The value of the regulated variable in the absence of external perturbation stabilizes at the set-point of the system. This set-point is an information input which may be determined by an external signal to which the regulated variable is compared, or may be determined by the structural characteristics of the system itself. In the regulated water tank, the set-point will depend on the length of the shaft connecting the float to the faucets. Many authors are mistaken when they do not distinguish set-point from reference. The set-point is an information input, e. g. the temperature at which we want our central heating apparatus to regulate the temperature of our house. A reference is a known physical variable to which we can compare an unknown one, e. g. the period of the vibration of a crystal can serve as a reference for time measurement.

The main property of a regulatory system is that a deviation of the regulated variable, triggers a correcting response which opposes the deviation. The minimal deviation tolerated by the system is the error signal.

The set-point may be constant or may be adjustable, cyclically, or unidirectionally during ageing, or under special circumstances (e.g. fever, in the case of temperature regulation). Long term adjustment of the set-point, e.g. increasing arterial pressure with ageing, may be regarded as an adaptation of homeostasis, resulting in an improved adaptation of living organisms to their environment. This phenomenon has been called homeorhesis by Nicolaidis[1] and rheostasis by Mrosovsky[2].

The regulated water tank of Fig. 2A may be used as a model of the ponderostat.

In 1969, Hervey[3] hypothesized that body mass, or a variable closely correlated to body mass, such as body fat content, is constant over the adult life span because it is regulated. This hypothesis has been the object of a debate since, because the concept of set-point appears as a circular explanation to many. As an alternative Wirtshafter and Davis[4] hypothesized that body weight remains constant at, or near, a settling point, the adjustment taking place passively without a regulation and a set-point. Examples from the recent literature show that this point of view is shared by other physiologists who considered the stability of body weight as resulting from the equilibrium between filling and emptying the adipose reservoir. The constancy of body weight in obesity and in *anorexia nervosa* is often described as resulting only from imperfect energy balance, insufficient energy expenditure resulting in elevated body weight, and insufficient food intake resulting in lowered body weight.

If the stability of body weight were produced by a steady state then it would be the simple result of the balance of food intake with energy expenditure, as suggested by the concept of settling point. According to the steady state hypothesis, obesity would be the result of excessive food intake and/or insufficient energy expenditure. Similarly, leanness would be the result of insufficient food intake and/or excessive energy expenditure.

A regulated system is a steady state equipped with regulatory loops. Of course, equal inflow and outflow of energy must also occur, in a regulated system as well as in a steady state, if body weight is to be constant, and transient unequal inflow and outflow of energy must occur if any change in body weight is to be observed. However, the concept of regulation implies that equal flows is not the final cause but rather only a means to achieve the goal of body weight equal to its set-point.

One way to differentiate a regulated system from a simple steady state system consists in measuring how the system responds to a global perturbation. A response opposed to the perturbation indicates that we deal with a regulated system. Thus the fact that food intake increases, after a body weight decrease due to starvation, then returns to control value when body weight has recovered is an indication of a regulated variable closely correlated to body weight.

All the available evidence points to a resistance to body weight changes in health as well as obesity: (1) during hypocaloric diet, the basal metabolism of normal men is depressed. After ending their diet they become hyperphagic and regain their initial body weight; (2) the weight of animals with a circannual cycle is defended by the animals' food intake; (3) after hypothalamic lesions, middle as well as lateral the body weights are defended by the animals' food intake and heat production; (4) periods of limited access to food are followed by compensatory overfeeding when body weight is below set-point but not when body weight is above set-point. Such responses are pathognomonic of regulation. According to the regulation hypothesis, obesity is the result of an elevated set-point (reached through transient increased food intake and/or decreased energy expenditure). Similarly, leanness is the result of a lowered set-point (reached through lowered food intake and/or excessive energy expenditure). All the available evidence shows these to take place.

In open-loop situations, regulatory responses are prevented from rectifying body weight (see review in[5]). The existence of such a response either on the inflow or the outflow is pathognomonic of regulation. Such open loop responses have been used to study the regulation of body weight. The experimental results also point toward a regulated body weight: (1) negative alliesthesia in humans, and disgust mimics in rats tend to disappear when body weight is below set-point, in healthy as well as obese humans and rats; (2) saliva secretion after alimentary stimuli respond similarly; (3) the hoarding of food by rats takes place only when body weight is below set-point in control as well as obese rats; (4) energy expenditure tends to oppose body weight deviations from set-point.

Alliesthesia in humans

Negative alliesthesia with alimentary stimuli contributes to limit quantitatively the amount of ingested food. When subjects are deprived of food for several weeks and lose several kilograms of body weight, negative alliesthesia after a gastric load tends to diminish or to disappear[6–8]. Thus, the size of any meal and total food intake will tend to increase and body weight will tend to return to initial value. In obesity alliesthesia disappears during the period of onset of obesity or 'dynamic obesity', when presumably the patient's body weight is lower than set-point. On the other hand, alliesthesia in patients is similar to that of healthy controls during 'static' obesity, when presumably actual body weight is equal to the elevated set-point[9,10]. This typical pattern of response can be found also with more or less intensity in obese patients under restricted diet, probably in relation with the intensity of the restriction[11–13].

Alliesthesia in rats

The discovery that rats display facial and gestual responses related to the taste stimuli injected into their mouth[14] allows to explore in animals the signals that generate gustatory alliesthesia in humans (among many references see[15–20]). As in humans, the behavioural signal that sweet stimuli arouse pleasure ceases to turn into signs of satiety when rats loose weight; they return when the rats recover[21]. This pattern is, therefore, strictly similar to that of humans.

Saliva secretion

Salivation can be used as an index of appetite[22,23]. The salivary response may, therefore, be used to study the ponderostat. The explicit relation of that response with weight regulation can be found in the measurements made on normal college students[24]. Salivation was stimulated by food odours in dieters (both normal-weight and overweight) and depressed in nondieters (both normal-weight and over-weight). Such a result supports the existence of a ponderostat: the enhanced salivary response shows that dieters were below their body weight set-point and hungry. On the other hand, the inhibited salivary response shows that nondieters were not hungry and presumably at set-point.

Support of the set-point concept was also brought by the study of patients with eating disorders[25]. In response to food odors, bulimic patients salivated more, and anorectic less than controls. This suggests that bulimic patients are below their body weight set-point and anorectic at, or above,set-point.

Hoarding of food by rats

Rats do not hoard pellets when food is continuously available[26,27]. However, when they are placed on schedules in which food is restricted, they start to hoard[28,29]. Yet, the hoarding response is related not to deprivation but rather to body weight decrease: rats hoard food when their body weight is lower than set-point[30]. This behaviour can be considered to be a regulatory response with a magnitude proportional to the decrease of body weight[31]. This method is open loop provided the food hoarded is withdrawn from the rat at the end of the session. The intersept with the x-axis of the regression line of mass hoarded vs. body weight (the threshold of hoarding) provides both the rat's body weight when fed *ad libitum* and the set-point. This set-point in influenced neither by ambient temperature[32], nor by the cost to reach food[33], nor by NPY[34], nor by the size of the pellets to be carried (Charron and Cabanac, in preparation). On the other hand CRH[35], emotion[36], estrogens[37], dexfenfluramine[38] and nicotine (Frankham and Cabanac, submitted) lower it.

Basal metabolism

The outflow of energy from the body is also under control to achieve body weight regulation. The intensity of basal metabolism is adjusted according to the intake and it is possible to manipulate body weight independently from energy metabolism[39]. Thus, energy expenditure does not follow energy intake passively, as would be the case in a steady state. On the contrary, energy expenditure opposes deviations of body weight from set-point. After lateral hypothalamus lesions, the resting metabolic rate of rats supported the hypothesis that their body weight set-point had been lowered by surgery[40,41]. Thus, the rats spent energy at a rate appropriate to the defense of their new body weight set-point.

Another way to manipulate the body weight of rats consists in providing them palatable foods[42]. The obesity produced persists even after the animals have been returned to regular chow[43]. Here again the measurement of energy expenditure of rats rendered and maintained obese with a cafeteria diet showed that they maintained a metabolism lower than would be expected from their mass[44]. In addition when these rats had limited access to food they lost weight but their metabolic rate diminished so as to defend the higher set-point.

In summary, this article focuses on the fact that the set-point for body weight regulation can be discerned from the threshold of responses that oppose body weight drop. Examples of such thresholds can be found with human gustatory pleasure, rats facial responses to sweet stimuli, rat food hoarding behaviour, human saliva secretion, and metabolic responses to changes in body weight. All these responses oppose deviations from body weight set-point. It follows that obesity is likely to result from an elevated, and *anorexia nervosa* from a lowered, body weight set-point.

References

1. Nicolaïdis S. Physiologie du comportement alimentaire. In: *Physiologie humaine*, P. Meyer (ed.), pp. 908–22. Paris: Flammarion; 1977.

2. Mrosovsky, N. *Rheostasis, the physiology of change*. New York: Oxford University Press; 1990.

3. Hervey, G.R. Regulation of energy balance. *Nature* 1969; 223: 629–31.

4. Wirtshafter D, Davis J. Set-points, settling points, and the control of body weight. *Physiol Behav* 1977; 19: 75–8.

5. Cabanac M. Open-loop methods for studying the ponderostat. In: *Appetite and nutrition*, MI Friedman, MG Tordoff, MR Kare (eds), pp. 149–70. New York: Marcel Dekker Inc; 1991.

6. Cabanac M, Duclaux R, Spector NH. Sensory feedbacks in regulation of body weight: is there a ponderostat? *Nature* 1971; 229: 125–7.

7. Herman CP, Polivy J, Esses VM. The illusion of counter-regulation. *Appetite* 1987; 9: 161–9.

8. Cabanac M, Rabe EF. Influence of a monotonous food on body weight regulation in humans. *Physiol Behav* 1976; 17: 675–8.

9. Guy-Grand B, Sitt Y. Alliesthésie gustative dans l'obésité humaine. *Nouv Presse Méd* 1974; 3: 92–3.

10. Guy-Grand B, Sitt Y. Gustative alliesthesia: Evidence supportingthe ponderostat hypothesis for obesity. In: *Recent Advance in Obesity Research: 1*, A. Howard (ed.), pp. 238–41. London: Newman Publishing; 1975.

11. Underwood PJ, Belton E, Hulme P. Aversion to sucrose in obesity. *Proc Nutr Soc* 1973; 32: 93A–94A.

12. Rodin J, Moskowitz HR, Bray G. Relationship between obesity, weight loss, and taste responsiveness. *Physiol Behav* 1976; 17: 591–7.

13. Gilbert DG, Hagen RL. Taste in underweight, overweight and normal-weight subjects before,during and after sucrose ingestion. *Addictive Behav* 1980; 5: 137–42.

14. Grill HJ, Norgren R. Chronically decerebrate rats demonstrate satiation but not bait shyness. *Science* 1978; 201: 267–9.

15. Berridge KC, Flynn FW, Schulkin J, Grill HJ. Sodium depletion enhances salt palatability in rats. *Behav Neurosci* 1984; 98: 652–61.

16. Grill HJ, Roitman MF, Kaplan JM. A new taste reactivity analysis of the integration of taste and physiological state information. *Am J Physiol* 1996; 40: R677–R87.

17. Shulkin J. Hedonic consequences of salt hunger. In: *The hedonics of taste*, RC Bolles (ed.), pp. 89–105. Hillsdale, NJ: Lawrence Earlbaum Associates; 1991.

18. Sclafani A, Clyne AE. Hedonic response of rats to polysaccharide and sugar solutions. *Neurosci Biobehav Rev* 1987; 11: 173–80.

19. Sclafani, A. The hedonics of sugar and starch. In: *The hedonics of taste*, RC Bolles (ed.), pp. 59–87. Hillsdale, NJ: Lawrence Earlbaum Associates; 1991.

20. Cabanac M, Lafrance L. Postingestive alliesthesia: The rat tells the same story. *Physiol Behav* 1990; 47: 539–43.

21. Cabanac M, Lafrance L. Facial consummatory responses in rats support the ponderostat hypothesis. *Physiol Behav* 1991; 50: 179–83.

22. Wooley SC, Wooley OW. Salivation to the sight and thought of food: A new measure of appetite. *Psychosom Med* 1973; 35: 136–42.

23. Booth DA, Fuller J. Salivation as a measure of appetite: A sensitivity issue. *Appetite* 1981; 2: 370–2.

24. Legoff DB, Spigelman MN. Salivary response to olfactory food stimuli as a function of dietary restraint and body weight. *Appetite* 1987; 8: 29–35.

25. Legoff DB, Leichner P, Spigelman MN. Salivary response to olfactory food stimuli in anorexics once bulimics. *Appetite* 19881; 1: 15–25.

26. Wolfe JB. An exploratory study of food storing in rats. *J Comp Psychol* 1939; 28: 97–108.

27. Bindra D. The nature of motivation for hoarding food. *J Comp Physiol Psychol* 1948; 41: 211–8.

28. Morgan CT, Stellar E, Johnson O. Food deprivation and hoarding in rats. *J Comp Psychol* 1943; 35: 275–95.

29. Blundell JE, Herberg LJ. Effectiveness of lateral hypothalamic stimulation, arousal, and food deprivation in the initiation of hoarding behaviour in naive rats. *Physiol Behav* 1973; 10: 763–7.

30. Herberg LJ, Franklin KBJ, Stephens DN. The hypothalamic set-point in experimental obesity. In: *Recent advances in obesity research: 1*, A Howard (ed.), pp. 235–7. Newman Publishing; 1975.

31. Fantino M, Cabanac M. Body weight regulation with a proportional hoarding response in the rat. *Physiol Behav* 1980; 24: 939–42.

32. Fantino M, Cabanac M. Effect of a cold ambient temperature on the rat's food hoarding behavior. *Physiol Behav* 1984; 32: 183–90.

33. Cabanac M, Swiergel AH. Rats eating and hoarding as a function of body weight and cost of foraging. *Am J Physiol* 1989; 257: R952–R957.

34. Cabanac M, Dagnault A, Richard D. The food-hoarding threshold is not raised by acute intraventricular NPY in male rats. *Physiol Behav* 1997; 61: 131–5.

35. Cabanac M, Richard D. Acute intra-ventricular CRF lowers the hoarding threshold in male rats. *Physiol Behav* 1995; 57: 705–10.

36. Michel C, Cabanac M. Opposite effects of gentle handling on body temperature and body weight in rats. *Physiol Behav* 1999; 67: 617–22.

37. Fantino M, Brinnel H. Body weight set-point changes during the ovarian cycle: experimental study of rats during hoarding behavior. *Physiol Behav* 1986; 36: 991–6.

38. Fantino M, Faion F, Rolland Y. Effect of dexfenfluramine on body weight set-point: study in the rat with hoarding behaviour. *Appetite* 1986; 7 (Suppl): S115–S126.

39. Keesey RE. The relation between energy expenditure and the body weight set-point: Its significance to obesity. In: *Handbook of eating disorders*, Part 2, Burrows, Beaumont, and Caspers (eds), pp. 87–102. New York: Elsevier; 1988.

40. Keesey RE, Corbett SW, Hirnoven MD, Kaufman LN. Heat production and body weight changes following lateral hypothalamic lesions. *Physiol Behav* 1984; 32: 309–17.

41. Corbett SW, Wilterdink EJ, Keesey R. Resting oxygen consumption in over- and underfed rats with lateral hypothalamic lesions. *Physiol Behav* 1985; 35: 971–7.

42. Sclafani A, Springer D. Dietary obesity in adult rats: similarities to hypothalamic and human obesity syndromes. *Physiol Behav* 1976; 17: 461–71.

43. Rolls BJ, Rowe EA, Turner RC. Persistent obesity in rats following a period of consumption of a mixed high energy diet. *J Physiol* 1980; 298: 415–27.

44. Corbett SW, Stern JS, Keesey RE. Energy expenditure of rats with diet-induced obesity. *Am J Clin Nutr* 1986; 44: 173–80.

45. Cabanac M, late Russek M. Regulated biological systems. *J Biol Systems* 2000; 8: 141–9.

Progress in Obesity Research: 9. Edited by *Geraldo Medeiros-Neto, Alfredo Halpern and Claude Bouchard*
©2003 John Libbey Eurotext Ltd, pp. 724–728.

CHAPTER 151

The body weight set point – the case against

Ian A. Macdonald

School of Biomedical Sciences, University of Nottingham Medical School, Queen's Medical Centre, Clifton Boulevard, Nottingham NG7 2UH, UK
[e-mail: ian.macdonald@nottingham.ac.uk]

Introduction

The regulation of physiological variables is a fundamental feature of homeostasis. This physiological regulation can be simply described as the control of one or more processes in order to maintain the physiological variable at a set point, or within a set range, in order to achieve optimal function. Such physiological regulation operates for variables such as blood pressure (BP) and body temperature, but it is now clear that for these variables the idea of a set-point is too inflexible, in that the regulated level of the variable is affected by a variety of factors (see below). In order to achieve regulation of a physiological variable, it is necessary to have:

- Sensors (monitoring the level of the variable),

- Afferent signals (between the sensor and the CNS),

- Central integration of the sensed information and comparison of this with the

- Standard level (set point), and

- Effector mechanisms (to bring the regulated variable back towards the 'desired' level).

For variables such as BP and body temperature, a great deal of work has gone into identifying the components of the regulatory systems. This has shown that acute disturbance of BP or temperature leads to compensatory responses designed to restore the original value. However, it is clear for both of these variables that the regulated level (previously termed 'set point') is acutely affected by physiological and external factors. For example, prolonged, sub-maximal exercise leads to a reduction in resting, supine BP in the post-exercise period. Reduced post-exercise BP is seen in both normotensive and hypertensive individuals, and the new BP is maintained during gravitational challenge (i.e. when upright). The latter response to gravitational shifts indicates that the control mechanisms are functioning, but for at least 90 min after the end of exercise these mechanisms do not operate to restore the pre-exercise BP[1]. Hence the BP 'set point' is reset by such exercise.

For complex variables such as BP and body temperature, and also body weight /energy content, one should think more of a range of values within which there is optimal function, rather than a specific set point.

Energy balance

The energy balance equation states that:

Energy intake – Energy expenditure = Change in body energy stores

Whilst this equation is irrefutable (being the application of the Third Law of Thermodynamics to a biological system), its existence does not mean that Body Energy Stores are regulated. It is more helpful to consider that Energy Balance summarizes energy exchange in the body, and to develop the concept of Energy Homeostasis to describe the physiological processes involved (see below).

When one looks at whole-body energy exchanges in human subjects, it is clear that intake and expenditure do not balance over short to medium periods of time (i.e. up to several days). For example, Schutz *et al.*[2] (and many others) have shown a poor matching of 24h energy intake and expenditure in whole body calorimeter studies. Extending these calorimeter studies to 7 days does produce a reasonable balancing of intake and expenditure when subjects consume low fat diets, but not with ad-libitum consumption of normal or high fat diets[3]. Furthermore, the earlier studies of Edholm *et al.*[4] (undertaken in the field) showed reasonable matching of energy intake and expenditure over periods of 28 days, but not from day to day.

Thus, there is somewhat equivocal evidence in support of the idea that energy balance is physiologically regulated. Nevertheless, as many authors have assumed that there is physiological regulation of energy balance, it is worth considering how this system might operate before considering the alternative.

Energy balance – What is the regulated variable?

From the previous description of the components of a regulatory system, it is worth considering what the sensor and afferent signals might be in relation to the regulation of energy balance.

Body weight

If body weight is the regulated variable, how could it be sensed? Presumably, there would need to be either pressure sensors in the lower limbs or feet, or proprioceptors in the joints or muscles. It is well established that proprioceptors are important in determining joint position and monitoring muscle contraction, but there is no evidence that they are affected specifically by body weight. In turn these sensors would need to transmit signals to the brain – presumably via afferent nerves in the way that other proprioceptive information is sent. The major problem with the argument that body weight is the regulated variable is the absence of any evidence of the existence of such weight sensitive sensors, or linking weight with such afferent signals.

Table 1 illustrates the average body composition, by weight and energy content, of a non-obese adult. The most variable component of body weight in such adults is the fat content, and this in turn produces a substantial variation in the total body energy content. Thus, if energy balance was regulated, it is highly unlikely that body weight would be the regulated variable, as the same weight could be associated with marked variations in energy content. Specifically, body weight could remain stable despite an imbalance between energy intake and expenditure if this was combined with a change in body composition.

Table 1. Body energy stores and turnover (mean values for non-obese (60–70 kg), moderately active subjects eating a normal diet)

	Protein	Carbohydrate	Fat
Body pool (kg)	12	0.7	12–18
Energy (MJ)	204	12	460–700
Daily intake (g)	100	300	100
Daily turnover (% stores)	0.8	45	0.5–0.8

Evidence of imprecise regulation of body weight and even poorer control of body energy content comes from the refeeding phase of the Minnesota underfeeding study[5,6]. By the end of 20 weeks of refeeding, after the initial 26 weeks underfeeding, subjects body weight had returned to slightly above the original normally-fed value (Fig. 1). However, the slight excess of regain of body weight was accompanied by a substantial excess storage of body fat. Interestingly, fat free mass was restored much more precisely than body weight. Thus, at the end of the 20 weeks refeeding period, body energy content was greater than the original value. It is clear from this study that fat free mass was the primary variable being restored to the original values, and that this was achieved at the expense of an excessive increase in body energy content.

Other studies have shown that both obese and non-obese, previously weight stable, subjects activate mechanisms to oppose changes in weight and body energy content when experimentally over- or underfed[7]. These studies are interpreted as evidence for the existence of the physiological regulation of

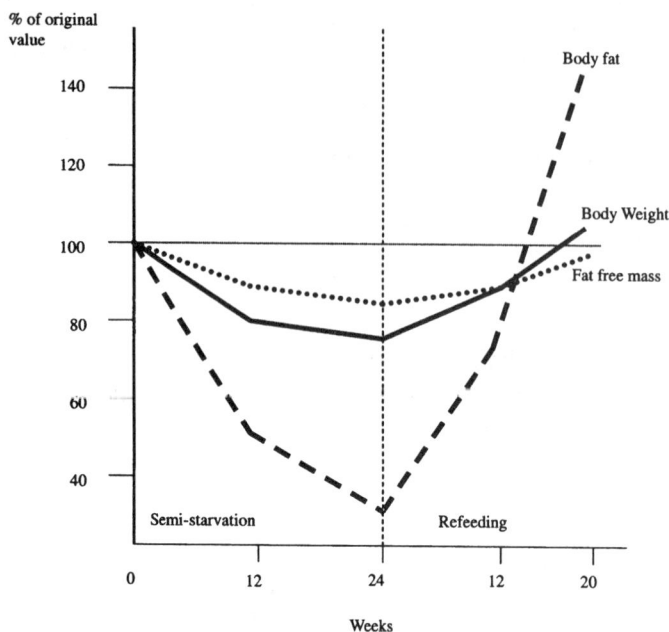

```
% of original
value

140 —

120 —

100 —

80 —

60 —

40 —

        Semi-starvation          Refeeding

    0      12        24       12      20

                Weeks
```

Fig. 1. Changes in body weight and composition during underfeeding and refeeding. The Minnesota study. Adapted from refs.[5,6].

energy balance. However, they do not provide any indication of whether weight, body energy content, or fat free mass is the regulated variable.

In animal studies, the body weight set point has been studied extensively in investigations of feeding behaviour. From studies in obese and lean rats, it is clear that there is a progressive increase in the body weight 'set point' over the first 6 months of life[8]. This 'set point' is the weight threshold for the rat to display food hoarding behaviour if weight falls below this level. However, such growing animals are expanding their fat free mass at this time, and such behavioural responses could equally (and more probably in this author's view) result from physiological mechanisms designed to achieve optimal development of fat free mass during growth. In addition, many strains of rat continuously increase body weight and fat content during adult life,

especially when fed palatable diets. If a set point for body weight exists, it clearly increases as an animal ages. In other animal species there is seasonal variation in body weight and composition[9], so clearly any body weight set point is variable and influenced by a number of external factors.

Body energy/fat

Stock[10] reminded us that 'The ease or difficulty with which one can measure things can often influence the development of scientific ideas'. Body weight is much easier to measure than fat or energy, but that does not mean that weight is the physiologically relevant variable. If energy balance is regulated, it is much more likely that body energy content (or a component of it) is the regulated variable. Kennedy[11] proposed the Lipostatic theory of energy balance regulation over 50 years ago. This theory recognized that fat was the largest, and most variable, energy store in the body, and argued that long-term regulation of energy balance would logically involve this store. The discovery of leptin in the 1990s provided a link between the body fat stores and the hypothalamic control of feeding and metabolism. The demonstration that plasma leptin concentration is proportional to body fat mass was taken as evidence that leptin was the afferent signal indicating the size of the fat stores. Injecting leptin into obese mice or humans with mutations of the *ob* gene, and who are leptin deficient, leads to reductions in food intake and weight loss. This has been used as evidence that body fat is the regulated variable and leptin the feedback signal. However, while significant, the relationship between fat mass and plasma leptin concentration is not sufficiently robust to provide an adequate signal. For example there are gender differences in the relationship between fat mass and plasma leptin (women having higher leptin concentrations at the same fat mass), and the correlation between leptin and subcutaneous fat is much stronger than with intra-abdominal fat[13]. Furthermore, plasma leptin concentration has a circadian pattern[13,14] and is affected by both acute alterations in energy intake and by body fat content[14]. Thus, leptin provides a signal proportional to the size of the fat stores but it does not give an accurate index of total body energy content.

Energy homeostasis

If energy balance is not physiologically regulated, and body weight, energy content or fat content are not regulated variables, what underlying factors do influence the control of energy intake and expenditure?

726

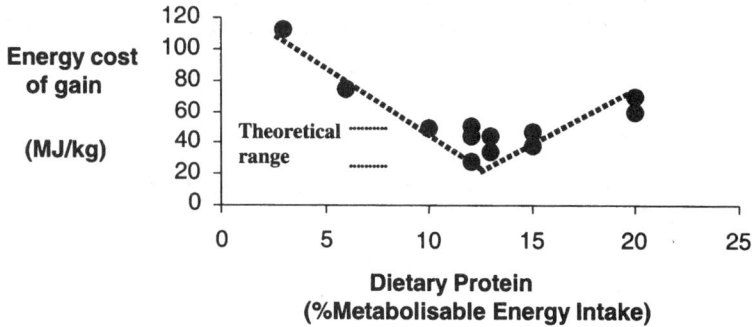

Fig. 2. Energy cost of weight gain in relation to dietary protein content during overfeeding (adapted from ref.[10]).

Three essential metabolic functions are:

- Development and maintenance of optimal fat free mass,
- Maintaining an adequate carbohydrate supply to the CNS[15],
- Maintaining adequate nutritional status for reproduction and growth.

The concept of *Energy homeostasis* encompasses the pathways and mechanisms that underpin these functions. In order to ensure the provision of energy and nutrients to sustain these three functions, macronutrient consumption is needed both to satisfy daily requirements (i.e. growth and energy metabolism) and to support the establishment of adequate energy and nutrient stores. With this approach to the control of energy metabolism, there would be an optimum body weight or energy content, but not a regulated set point. The role of leptin and related signals would be to ensure there were adequate energy stores for reproduction, and to initiate mechanisms to protect against undernutrition and weight loss. Excessive accumulation of body energy does not compromise short-term survival (but obesity clearly reduces life expectancy) and one would not expect elaborate systems to prevent excessive weight gain. However, if dietary quality was poor (i.e. low in protein) an optimal fat free mass could not be achieved with a normal energy intake. In this situation, one might expect more food to be eaten to enable an adequate fat free mass to be achieved, and that some of the excess energy consumed would be expended by protective mechanisms designed to limit fat deposition when fat free mass was compromised.

Support for the idea that energy homeostasis, rather than the regulation of body weight/energy balance, underpins human energy metabolism comes from consideration of human overfeeding studies[10] (Fig. 2). Over a range of protein intakes from 10–15 per cent of dietary energy, overeating leads to weight gain at a predictable rate. However, overfeeding with low protein diets is necessary to satisfy protein requirements and a larger proportion of the excess energy intake is expended rather than stored. Excessive protein contents are also associated with increased energy costs of weight gain, implying activation of mechanisms designed to protect against excessive availability of protein. A final illustration of the importance of energy homeostasis is provided by consideration of Table 1. It can be seen that the daily turnover of the body carbohydrate store amounts to almost 50 per cent of the total store. This store ensures the continued supply of glucose to the CNS, but requires a daily intake of carbohydrate to refill and maintain the store. Thus, a fundamental component of energy homeostasis could be regarded as being related to the original glucostatic theory of food intake control[16]. In this theory, Mayer argued that blood glucose concentration was an important determinant of feeding behaviour. That is likely to be true, but it is also highly probable that liver glycogen content (i.e. the available carbohydrate store) also has an important influence on food intake.

Conclusion

The apparent stability of body weight and existence of behaviours that appear to defend body weight does not mean that it is physiologically regulated around a set point. Any such regulation is more likely to relate to body energy content or a component of it. The increasing prevalence of obesity suggests that any such regulation is failing in large numbers of people, or that the purpose of the regulatory system is directed towards the prevention of undernutrition. Human energy metabolism should be considered in terms of energy homeostasis, with the control systems being directed towards ensuring adequate protein and carbohydrate intake and sufficient nutrient stores to sustain CNS function and support reproduction.

References

1. Bennett T, Wilcox RG, Macdonald IA. Post-exercise reduction in blood pressure in hypertensive man is not due to acute impairment of baroreflex function. *Clin Sci* 1984; 67: 97–103.

2. Schutz Y, Flatt JP, Jequier E. Failure of dietary fat intake to promote fat oxidation: A factor favouring the development of obesity. *Am J Clin Nutr* 1989; 50: 307–14.

3. Stubbs RJ, Harbron CG, Murgatroyd PR, Prentice AM. Covert manipulation of dietary fat and energy density: Effect on substrate flux and food intake in men eating *ad libitum*. *Am J Clin Nutr* 1995; 62: 316–29.

4. Edholm OG. Energy expenditure and food intake. In: *Energy balance in man*, M Apfelbaum (ed.), pp. 51–60. Paris: Masson; 1973.

5. Keys A, Brozek J, Henschel A, Mickelsen D, Taylor HL. *Biology of human starvation*. University of Minnesota Press; 1950.

6. Grande F. Man under caloric deficiency. In: *Handbook of physiology. Adaptation to the Environment*, sect 4, vol 1, chap 59, pp. 911–37. Washington, DC: American Physiological Society; 1964.

7. Hirsch J, Hudgins LC, Leibel R, Rosenbaum M. Diet composition and energy balance in humans. *Am J Clin Nutr* 1998; 67 (Suppl 1): S551–S555.

8. Gosselin C, Cabanac M. Ever higher: Constant rise of body weight set point in growing Zucker rats. *Physiol Behav* 1996; 60: 817–21.

9. Morgan PJ, Mercer JG. The regulation of body weight: lessons from the seasonal animal. *Proc Nutr Soc* 2001; 60: 127–34.

10. Stock MJ. Gluttony and thermogenesis revisited. *Int J Obes* 1999; 23: 1105–17.

11. Kennedy GC. The role of depot fat in the hypothalamic control of food intake in the rat. *Proc Roy Soc* 1953; series B. 140: 578–92.

12. Couillard C, Mauriege P, Prud'homme D, Nadeau A, Tremblay A, Bouchard C *et al.* Plasma leptin concentrations: gender differences and associations with metabolic risk factors for cardiovascular disease. *Diabetologia* 1997; 40: 1178–84.

13. Langendonk JG, Pijl H, Toornvliet AC, Burggraaf J, Frolich M, Schoemaker RC *et al.* Circadian rhythm of plasma leptin levels in upper and lower body obese women: Influence of body fat distribution and weight loss. *J Clin Endocrinol Metab* 1998; 83: 1706–12.

14. Chin-Chance C, Polonsky KS, Schoeller DA. Twenty-four –hour leptin levels respond to cumulative short-term energy imbalance and predict subsequent intake. *J Clin Endocrinol Metab* 2000; 85: 2685–91.

15. Macdonald IA. Assessment of optimal carbohydrate requirements. In: IDECG report, Ed: V.R. Young and B. Schurch, *Eur J Clin Nutr* 1999; 53 (Suppl 1): S101–S106.

16. Mayer J, Arees EA. Ventromedial glucoreceptor system. *Fed Proc* 1968; 27: 1345–8.

Progress in Obesity Research: 9. Edited by *Geraldo Medeiros-Neto, Alfredo Halpern and Claude Bouchard*
©2003 John Libbey Eurotext Ltd, pp. 729–733.

CHAPTER 152

Central insulin in energy balance

Stephen C. Benoit and Stephen C. Woods

University of Cincinnati, Department of Psychiatry, P.O. Box 670559, Cincinnati, OH 45267-0559, USA
[e-mail: Stephen.benoit@uc.edu]

Body weight, or more accurately, adiposity, is a regulated variable. When maintained on an *ad libitum* diet, most animals including humans are able to precisely match caloric intake with caloric expenditure, resulting in relatively stable energy stores as adipose tissue[1,2]. Growing emphasis has been placed on the role of the CNS in controlling this precision of energy homeostasis. However, to balance the energy equation, the brain must receive several kinds of input from the periphery, and some of these should provide information about the status of peripheral energy stores in the form of the adipose mass[3]. At least two peripheral hormones seem to provide key afferent information to the CNS. Leptin, a recently described peptide hormone secreted from adipocytes in proportion to fat mass, has received tremendous attention during recent years, and considerable evidence suggests that leptin acts as one of the body's adiposity signals[4,5]. Leptin levels in the blood are correlated with body fat and administration of leptin reduces food intake and increases energy expenditure. However, leptin levels are better correlated with subcutaneous fat than with visceral fat in humans, such that the reliability of leptin as an adiposity signal varies with the distribution of fat in the body. Because females tend to have more subcutaneous fat than males, on the average, leptin is therefore a better correlate of total adiposity in females than in males. Further, when energy balance is suddenly changed (for example, if an individual is fasted for a day), plasma leptin levels decrease far more than body adiposity in the short term[4,6]. Hence, although much has been written about leptin as an adiposity signal, it is not ideal in and of itself, suggesting that at least one additional signal must exist. The logical candidate is the pancreatic hormone, insulin.

Plasma insulin levels are also highly correlated with adiposity, and they correlate better with visceral than with subcutaneous fat[7,8]. Moreover, when energy balance changes, plasma insulin follows these changes faithfully[9]. Hence, leptin and insulin together provide information to the brain not only about the size of the fat mass, but also about its distribution and important recent changes of metabolic status. The effort of many labs, including in part our own, is concentrated on elucidating how leptin interacts with neural systems controlling energy homeostasis. The focus of this paper is upon insulin.

Insulin as peripheral adiposity signal

Considerable evidence suggests that insulin is a key peripheral regulator of food intake. After Kennedy[2] hypothesized that fat stores produce a hormone that acts as a negative feedback control for adiposity, one early suggestion was that this signal is insulin[10,11]. Data supporting this possibility have been collected over the past two decades and include studies using several species and techniques[7,12,13]. To summarize that literature, levels of plasma insulin correlate directly with body weight, and with body adiposity in particular[14]. Like leptin, insulin is secreted in direct proportion to fat mass. Obese animals and humans have higher basal insulin levels, and secrete more insulin in response to a meal than lean individuals[14,15]. As stated above, plasma insulin levels also reflect more acute changes in energy status. Insulin increases during positive energy balance and decreases during negative energy balance. Obese animals and humans are said to be insulin resistant because more insulin is required to maintain a normal level of blood glucose. This is important because insulin resistance, and visceral fat, correlate with levels of insulin, type 2 diabetes mellitus, and obesity.

The second line of evidence consistent with insulin being a prime candidate as an adiposity signal is the finding that insulin better maps acute changes of energy metabolism and adiposity than its adipocyte cousin, leptin. Insulin secretion faithfully tracks changes of energy balance on the order of minutes to hours, as opposed to days, and these changes are always in direct proportion to the size of the adipose mass. Further, insulin plays a key role in the regulation of glucose and lipid utilization and storage. Without sufficient insulin, most tissues cannot take up much glucose such that glucose accumulates in the blood. At the same time, adipocytes cannot take up and store fat. When insulin resistance occurs in obesity, and more insulin is secreted to regulate glucose, the excess insulin causes increased accumulation of fat in adipocytes. Hence, disruptions of insulin sensitivity are associated with both obesity and diabetes.

Additional support for the hypothesis that insulin acts as an adiposity signal includes the fact that insulin receptors and insulin receptor mRNA are found in CNS regions involved in the regulation of food intake and body weight[5,9,16,17]. In particular, insulin receptors in the ARC are prime candidates for translators of an adiposity signal. Third ventricular (i3vt) administration of insulin decreases expression of the anabolic effector peptide, neuropeptide Y (NPY) in the ARC[18]. ARC NPY fibres project to the PVN, and i3vt insulin also causes increased expression of corticotrophin-releasing hormone mRNA in the PVN[18,19]. These results demonstrate that the insulin signal is tied to the changes in food intake associated with hypothalamic neuropeptides.

One requirement of a humoral adiposity signal is that it should gain access to the brain. Consistent with this, insulin has been found to enter the brain via a saturable transport process that moves it from plasma into brain interstitial fluid[20]. The rate of entry of insulin to CNS is well mapped to normal fluctuations of plasma insulin levels, although higher levels exceed the saturation point[21,22]. With very high plasma levels, the entry of insulin to brain remains relatively constant[9,13]. This is important for regulation of body weight because some types of obesity are known to be associated with disruptions of the insulin transport system.

Finally, and importantly, administration of exogenous insulin into the brain reduces food intake and increases energy expenditure, consistent with its being an adiposity signal. Repeated administration of insulin in small doses, or as a continuous infusion, elicits decreased food intake and increased energy expenditure after several hours and lasts for the duration of the treatment[10,15]. Administration of insulin into the brain also potentiates the anorexic effects of peripherally administered cholecystokinin (CCK)[23]. This suggests that insulin modulates the body's response to short term signals that terminate meals. Importantly, administration of insulin peripherally, in amounts that do not cause hypoglycaemia, also decreases food intake[3,24,25]. In agreement with these data, administration of antibodies to insulin into the brain *increases* food intake and body weight[26,27]. It is important to note that there is no evidence that alterations in food intake after administration of insulin, either systemic or central, produce aversive consequences[28]. That is, administration of exogenous insulin does not appear to make animals ill. Collectively, these data suggest that insulin provides a signal of adiposity to the CNS and that the signal is capable of altering food intake based on the state of energy balance.

In summary, insulin, aside from its important peripheral action for the metabolism of fuels, satisfies all of the criteria for consideration as a general adiposity signal. Indeed, Woods and colleagues[8,29] have suggested that administration of insulin does not simply act to change food intake *per se*, but rather helps determine the level of fat that will be maintained and defended by the animal. That is, levels of circulating plasma insulin help modulate the long-term level of fat stored in the body in any particular environment. It is unclear at present whether, in the obese insulin-resistant state, there are parallel changes of central insulin-sensitive systems.

Central mediation of insulin signaling

Melanocortins (MC) are a family of peptides derived from POMC that have traditionally been associated with skin and hair color. There are now five identified MC receptors, two of which are found in the CNS (MC3 and MC4). MC4 is widely distributed in the CNS. MC3, on the other hand, is found primarily in the hypothalamus[30,31]. Recent work on the melanocortin system has provided evidence that the hypothalamic MC3/4 receptors are involved in the regulation of energy homeostasis[32–35]. This evidence includes behavioural, genetic, and neuroanatomical data.

The first line of evidence that the MC system is important for the regulation of food intake comes from observations that i3vt administration of peptides with affinity for MC3/4 receptors alter food intake[32,35–38]. Several ligands to central MC receptors have been reported to increase or decrease food intake. One of these, a-melanocyte stimulating hormone (α-MSH), is an agonist for both MC3 and 4 receptors[39]. When administered into the third ventricle, α-MSH produces a robust decrease in food intake in rats. Similarly, a synthetic analogue of α-MSH, MTII, that has agonistic properties at both MC3 and MC4 receptors decreases food intake and body weight of both mice and rats[35]. These results suggest that agonists for the MC3/4 receptor may be important mediators for an animal's response to positive energy balance, decreasing both food intake and body weight. The importance of the central melanocortin system is also revealed by the fact that endogenous antagonists, as well as agonists such as α-MSH, are found in the hypothalamus[32,33]. Agouti related protein (AgRP) is an endogenous antagonist for MC3/4 receptors in hypothalamus and is synthesized in NPY neurons in the ARC. I3vt administration of AgRP produces profound and persistent increases in food intake and body weight[40]. In addition, synthetic MC3/4 antagonists such as the AgRP analogue, SHU 9119, also increase food intake and body weight[41].

The second line of evidence implicating the MC system in the control of food intake comes from certain 'knockout' mice. Two strains of these mice lack part of the hypothalamic MC system. One of these, the Agouti mouse, has a mutation resulting in over expression of Agouti signaling protein. The phenotype for this mutation includes a yellow coat to the fur[40]. Interestingly, agouti signaling protein is homologous to AgRP and Agouti mice overeat and become obese[35,40,42,43]. Yet another model with implications for the melanocortin system is the MC4 knockout mouse. As the nomenclature suggests, these mice do not express the MC4 receptor and, as expected, have profound obesity[44]. Collectively, these genetic models also support an important role for the melanocortin system in the control of food intake.

Finally, MC peptides are co-localized with other peptides and receptors in CNS regions important for food intake, particularly in the hypothalamus. The precursor molecule of hypothalamic melanocortins, pro-opiomelanocortin (POMC), is expressed in the ARC, and axons of these neurons project to several other hypothalamic areas including the PVN[34,45]. In addition, administration of MCs can block the effects of other manipulations that alter food intake through hypothalamic systems[41]. Further, neurons which express POMC also have receptors for leptin, indicating that the MC system mediates leptin's anorexic effects[32].

We have recently completed a series of experiments designed to address whether the central melanocortins system mediates the anorexic effects of insulin[46]. First, we observed that POMC neurons in the arcuate nucleus also have receptors for insulin. Second, we found that i3vt insulin infusion stimulated POMC gene expression in fasted rats. These data are consistent with a previous report that when circulating insulin is reduced following streptozotocin, POMC gene expression in the ARC is reduced, and that the administration of insulin systemically restores POMC expression[47]. However, it could not be concluded from that report whether insulin or leptin was the key factor since streptozotocin treatment also results in reduced circulating leptin and since systemic insulin administration leads to an immediate increase in plasma leptin. These findings suggest that insulin may reduce food intake and body weight by acting through the central melanocortin system. Finally, a non-specific melanocortin 3/4 receptor antagonist, SHU-9119, was able to significantly attenuate the reduction in food intake elicited by insulin administration. Hence, like leptin, insulin appears to exert its central catabolic action by acting through melanocortin receptors. Collectively, these recent data demonstrate that the CNS melanocortin system is an important downstream target for the effects of insulin to regulate food intake and body weight[46]. They therefore provide a significant step in delineating the critical pathways that allow for the maintenance of energy balance.

References

1. Keesey RE. *Handbook of eating disorders*, KD Brownell, JP Foreyt (eds), pp. 63–87. Basic Books, 1986.

2. Kennedy GC. The role of depot fat in the hypothalmus control of food intake in the rat. *Proc Roy Soc Lond (Biol)* 1953; 140: 579–92.

3. Chavez M, Kaiyala K, Madden LJ, Schwartz MW, Woods SC. Intraventricular insulin and the level of maintained body weight in rats. *Behav Neurosci* 1995; 109(3): 528–31.

4. Buchanan C, Mahesh V, Zamorano P, Brann D. Central nervous system effects of leptin. *Trends Endocrinol Metab* 1998; 9: 146–50 (Reviews).

5. Matson CA, Wiater MF, Weigle DS. Leptin and the regulation of body adiposity. *Diabetes Rev* 1996; .4: 488–508.

6. Woods SC, Seeley RJ, Schwartz MW. Leptin as an adiposity signal. *Endocrinol Metab* 1997; 4: 77–9.

7. Woods SC *et al.* Insulin: its relationship to the central nervous system and to the control of food intake and body weight. *Am J Clin Nutr* 1985; 42 (Suppl 5): 1063–71.

8. Woods SC, Seeley RJ, Porte DJ, Schwartz MW. Signals that regulate food intake and energy homeostasis. *Science* 1998; 280: 1378–83.

9. Schwartz MW, Figlewicz DP, Baskin DG, Woods SC, Porte D Jr. Insulin in the brain: a hormonal regulator of energy balance. *Endocrine Rev* 1992; 13(3): 387–414.

10. Woods SC *et al.* The evaluation of insulin as a metabolic signal influencing behavior via the brain. *Neurosci Biobehav Rev* 1996; 20(1): 139–44.

11. Baskin DG, Figlewicz DP, Woods SC, Porte DJr, Dorsa DM. Insulin in the brain. *Ann Rev Physiol* 1987; 49: 335–47.

12. Woods SC, Figlewicz DP, Schwartz MW, Porte D Jr. A re-assessment of the regulation of adiposity and appetite by the brain insulin system. *Int J Obes* 1990; 14 (Suppl 3): 69–76.

13. Schwartz MW, Figlewicz DP, Baskin DG, *et al.*: Insulin and the central regulation of energy balance: Update 1994. *Endocrinol Rev* 1994; 2: 109–13.

14. Bagdade JD, Bierman EL, Porte D Jr. The significance of basal insulin levels in the evaluation of the insulin response to glucose in diabetic and nondiabetic subjects. *J Clin Invest* 1967; 46(10): 1549–57.

15. Woods SC, Decke E, Vasselli JR. Metabolic hormones and regulation of body weight. *Psychol Rev* 1974; 81(1): 26–43.

16. Campfield LA, Smith FJ, Burn P. The OB protein (leptin) pathway – a link between adipose tissue mass and central neural networks. *Hormone Metabol Res* 1996; 28(12): 619–32.

17. Schwartz MW *et al.* Inhibition of hypothalamic neuropeptide Y gene expression by insulin. *Endocrinology* 1992; 130(6): 3608–16.

18. Sipols AJ, Baskin DG, Schwartz MW. Effect of intracerebroventricular insulin infusion on diabetic hyperphagia and hypothalamic neuropeptide gene expression. Diabetes. *Diabetes* 1995; 44(2): 147–51.

19. Schwartz MW, Seeley RJ, Campfield LA, Burn P, Baskin DG. Identification of targets of leptin action in rat hypothalamus. *J Clin Invest* 1996; 98(5): 1101–6.

20. Hachiya HL, Halban PA, King GL. Intracellular pathways of insulin transport across vascular endothelial cells. *Am J Physiol* 1988; 255(4 Pt 1): C459–64.

21. Baura G *et al.* Saturable transport of insulin from plasma into the central nervous system of dogs *in vivo*. A mechanism for regulated insulin delivery to the brain. *J Clin Invest* 1993; 92(4): 1824–30.

22. Riedy CA, Chavez M, Figlewicz DP, Woods SC. Central insulin enhances sensitivity to cholecystokinin. *Physiol Behav* 1995; 58(4): 755–60.

23. Brief DJ, Davis JD. Reduction of food intake and body weight by chronic intraventricular insulin infusion. *Brain Res Bull* 1984; 12(5): 571–5.

24. McGowan MK, Andrews KM, Kelly J, Grossman SP. Effects of chronic intrahypothalamic infusion of insulin on food intake and diurnal meal patterning in the rat. *Behav Neurosci* 1990; 104(2): 373–85.

25. McGowan MK, Andrews KM, Grossman SP. Chronic intrahypothalamic infusions of insulin or insulin antibodies alter body weight and food intake in the rat. *Physiol Behav* 1992; 51(4): 753–66.

26. Strubbe JH, Mein CG. Increased feeding in response to bilateral injection of insulin antibodies in the VMH. *Physiol Behav* 1977; 19(2): 309–13.

27. Chavez M, Seeley RJ, Woods SC. A comparison between effects of intraventricular insulin and intraperitoneal lithium chloride on three measures sensitive to emetic agents. *Behav Neurosci* 1995; 109(3): 547–50.

28 .Porte DJ *et al.* Obesity, diabetes and the central nervous system. *Diabetologia* 1998; 41(8): 863–81.

29. Schioth HB, Muceniece R, Wikberg JE. *Pharmacol Toxicol* 1996; 79(3): 161–5.

30. Mountjoy K, Mortrud M, Low M, Simerly R, Cone R. Localization of the melanocortin-4 receptor (MC4-R) in neuroendocrine and autonomic control circuits in the brain. *Molec Endocrinol* 1994; 8(10): 1298–308.

31. Seeley R *et al.* Melanocortin receptors in leptin effects. *Nature* 1997; 390(6658): 349.

32. Thornton JE, Cheung CC, Clifton DK, Steiner RA. Regulation of hypothalamic proopiomelanocortin mrna by leptin in ob/ob mice. *Endocrinology* 1997; 138(11): 5063–6.

33. Mizuno T *et al.* Hypothalamic pro-opiomelanocortin mRNA is reduced by fasting and [corrected] in ob/ob and db/db mice, but is stimulated by leptin. *Diabetes* 1998; 47: 294–7.

34. Fan W, Boston BA, Kesterson RA, Hruby VJ, Cone RD. Role of melanocortinergic neurons in feeding and the agouti obesity syndrome. *Nature* 1997; 385(6612): 165–8.

35. Giraudo SQ, Billington CJ, Levine AS. Feeding effects of hypothalamic injection of melanocortin 4 receptor ligands. *Brain Res* 1998; 809(2): 302–6.

36. Grill HJ, Ginsberg AB, Seeley RJ, Kaplan JM. Brainstem application of melanocortin receptor ligands produces long-lasting effects on feeding and body weight. *J Neurosci* 1998; 18(23): 10128–35.

37. Thiele TE *et al.* Central infusion of melanocortin agonist MTII in rats: assessment of c-Fos expression and taste aversion. *Am J Physiol* 1998; 274(1 Pt 2): R248–54.

38. Cone RD *et al.* The melanocortin receptors: agonists, antagonists, and the hormonal control of pigmentation. *Rec Progr Hormone Res* 1996; 51: 287–320 (discussion 318).

39. Ollmann M *et al.* Antagonism of central melanocortin receptors *in vitro* and *in vivo* by agouti-related protein. *Science* 1997; 278(5335): 135–8.

40. Hagan MM *et al.* Long-term orexigenic effects of AgRP-(83 − −132) involve mechanisms other than melanocortin receptor blockade. *Am J Physiol* 2000; 279(1): R47–R52.

41. Fong TM *et al.* ART (protein product of agouti-related transcript) as an antagonist of MC-3 and MC-4 receptors. *Biochem Biophys Res Commun* 1997; 237(3): 629–31.

42. Yang YK *et al.* Effects of recombinant agouti-signaling protein on melanocortin action. *Molec Endocrinol* 1997; 11(3): 274–80.

43. Huszar D Targeted disruption of the melanocortin-4 receptor results in obesity in mice. *et al. Cell* 1997; 88(1): 131–41.

44. Cheung CC, Clifton DK, Steiner RA. Proopiomelanocortin neurons are direct targets for leptin in the hypothalamus. *Endocrinology* 1997; 138(10): 4489–92.

45. Kim EM, Grace MK, Welch CC, Billington CJ, Levine AS. STZ-induced diabetes decreases and insulin normalizes POMC mRNA in arcuate nucleus and pituitary in rats. *Am J Physiol* 1999; 276(5 Pt 2): R1320–6.

46. Benoit SC, Air EL, Coolen LM, Strauss R, Jackman A, Clegg DJ, Seeley RJ, Woods SC. The catabolic action of insulin in the brain is mediated by melanocortins. *J Neurosci* 2002; 22: 9048–52.

Progress in Obesity Research: 9. Edited by *Geraldo Medeiros-Neto, Alfredo Halpern and Claude Bouchard*
©2003 John Libbey Eurotext Ltd, pp. 734–738.

CHAPTER 153

Cytokines in control of food intake and energy balance

Wolfgang Langhans

*Institute of Animal Sciences, Swiss Federal Institute of Technology (ETH), Schorenstrasse 16, 8603 Schwerzenbach,
Switzerland
[e-mail: wolfgang.langhans@inw.agrl.ethz.ch]*

Introduction

Cytokines are conventionally grouped in families, and act mostly as extracellular messenger molecules. Despite structural differences, several cytokines share the same receptors, which probably accounts for some of their redundant effects. Virtually all cells can produce cytokines in response to a variety of stimuli, with production cycles that typically last from hours to days. A key feature of cytokines is their high potency, which is related to their usually high receptor affinity. Cytokines are known to orchestrate non-specific and specific immune reactions, and they are broadly categorized as being pro-inflammatory or anti-inflammatory. Yet, in addition to their pleiotropic effects in the immune system, cytokines also affect other physiologic functions and cause CNS-mediated effects such as fever, sleep, and an activation of the hypothalamic-pituitary-adrenal axis. Moreover, several cytokines strongly affect energy intake and/or energy expenditure, which is the focus of this review.

Role of cytokines in infection and inflammation

Cytokines are typically produced in response to infections, cancer or local inflammatory stimuli. Several laboratory animal models mimic these situations: Sterile inflammation is modeled by subcutaneous (SC) injection of turpentine[1], inflammatory bowel disease by intrarectal administration of irritants (e.g. trinitrobenzenesulphonic acid [TNB])[2], systemic bacterial infections by peripheral administration of live bacteria or bacterial lipopolysaccharides (LPS)[3], and cancer by experimental tumours[4]. Finally, inoculation of mice with *Toxoplasma gondii* (*T. gondii*) cysts provides an infection model that allows to dissociate the anorexia and hypermetabolism of cachexia[5]. All these models usually produce acute and/or prolonged anorexia, hypermetabolism, an increased expression of cytokine mRNA in various tissues and at least a transient increase in circulating cytokine concentrations. Weight loss is observed with the chronic models. An increased baseline cytokine production and/or cytokine response has also been reported in ageing subjects[6], in which cytokines may be involved in the age-related progressive impairment in insulin action and in geriatric cachexia[6], as well as during high intensity exercise[7]. Finally, adipocytes produce cytokines which may contribute to some of the metabolic and cardiovascular complications associated with obesity[8]. Conversely, the development of obesity may be accompanied by and related to an insensitivity to the actions of cytokines[8]. As it is beyond the scope of this review to deal with all these aspects, I will concentrate on three well characterized models in which a role of cytokines in the accompaning changes in energy intake and energy expenditure has been established.

The peripheral LPS model

LPS are released from Gram-negative bacterial cell walls during bacteriolysis or periods of rapid proliferation. LPS trigger the release of cytokines through the Toll-like receptor[4] (TLR-4)[9]. The cell surface structure CD14 is also involved in this process[9]. We recently found that the feeding suppressive

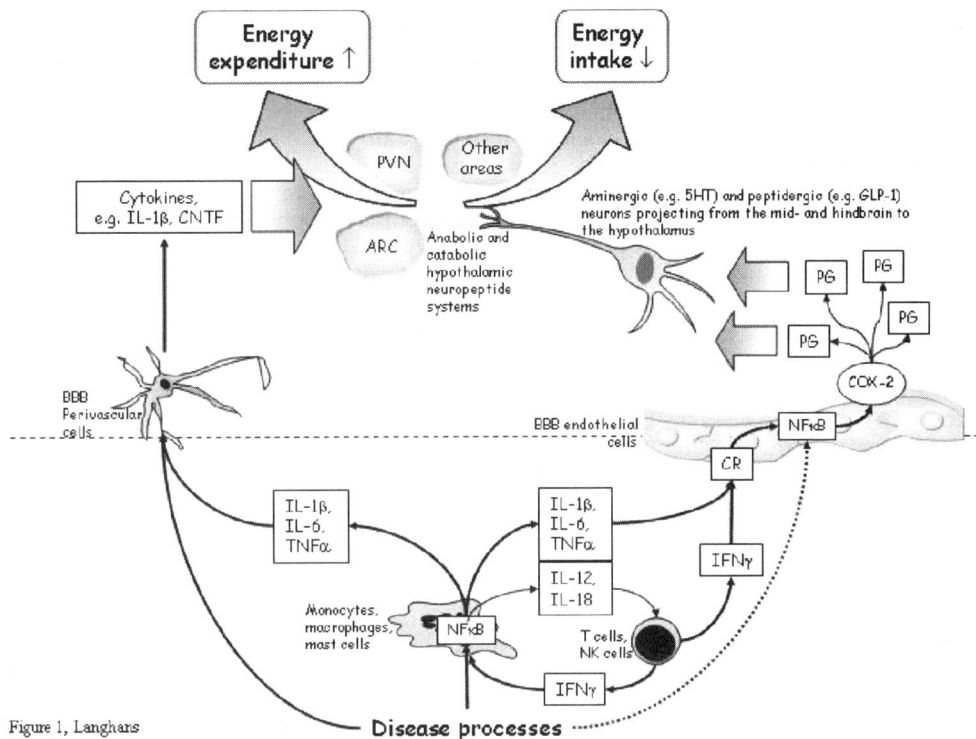

Fig. 1. Possible pathways of cytokine-induced anorexia. 5HT: Serotonin, ARC: Arcuate nucleus, BBB: Blood brain barrier, CNTF: Ciliary neurotrophic factor, COX-2: cyclooxygenase-2, CR: Cytokine receptor, GLP-1: Glucagon-like peptide-1, IFNγ: Interferon-γ, IL-1β (6,12,18): Interleukin-1β (6,12,18), NFκB: Transcription factor nuclear factor κB, PVN: Paraventricular nucleus, TNFα: Tumor necrosis factor-α, NK cells: Natural killer cells.

effect of intraperitoneally (IP) injected LPS is markedly attenuated in mice, genetically deficient of either the TLR4 or the CD14[10], indicating that LPS also induce anorexia through these structures. As expected, IP interleukin-1β (IL-1β) reduced food intake similarly in all genotypes tested. With few exceptions (e.g. 11 for interferon-γ [IFNγ]), studies using knockout (KO) preparations of cytokines and/or cytokine receptors have generally failed to establish a role for a particular cytokine in LPS anorexia (see[12] for review). On the other hand, pharmacological intervention studies suggest that IL-1β and tumour necrosis factor-α (TNFα), in addition to IFNγ, contribute to LPS anorexia (see[12] for review). There is synergism between[13] and the potential for a reciprocal substitution of IL-1β and TNFα in the mediation of LPS anorexia[14]. Thus, several cytokines appear to mediate the feeding suppressive effect of LPS by their combined action. The same probably holds true for the less intensively investigated hypermetabolic effect of LPS, in which a role for IFNγ and TNFα has been established using KO mice[11].

The *T. gondii* model

Intraperitoneal inoculation of Swiss Webster mice with *T. gondii* cysts produces a substantial weight loss within 2–3 weeks[5]. During this time all mice display hypermetabolism (days 1–7) and subsequently (days 7–14 or 7–21) anorexia plus hypermetabolism. In the following chronic phase of infection, the mice show either partial weight recovery (gainers) or no weight regain (non gainers). Gainers are still anorectic but no longer hypermetabolic, whereas non gainers remain anorectic and hypermetabolic. The various periods of infection as well as gainers and non gainers are characterized by different patterns of cytokine expression. This makes experimental *T. gondii* infection in mice a unique model to study phase dependent and individual differences in the mechanisms of infection-induced anorexia and hypermetabolism. The initial hypermetabolic response to *T. gondii* infection was unaffected in TNFα-KO mice, but completely absent in IFNγ-KO mice[15], indicating that the latter but not the former cytokine is indispensable for the acute hypermetabolic response in this infection model.

The turpentine sterile inflammation model

A complete elimination of anorexia and other sickness symptoms in response to SC turpentine injection was observed in IL-6 KO mice[16], which indicates a major role of[16] IL-6 in the responses to sterile localized inflammation. The feeding suppressive effect of SC turpentine administration was also absent in IL-1 receptor-1 KO mice[17], suggesting that IL-1-mediated pathways are also involved. Antagonism of either IL-6 or the IL-1 receptor-1 by monoclonal antibodies also spared body weight and food intake responses to SC turpentine administration[18]. Finally, the hypermetabolic but not the feeding response to SC turpentine was attenuated by pretreatment with TNFα antiserum[19]. Thus, IL-1β, IL-6, and, to a lesser extent, TNFα, all appear to be involved in mediating the responses to sterile inflammation. In sum, several cytokines play a role in the anorectic and hypermetabolic responses in various diseases and/or disease models, and their effects appear to be situationally variable.

Mechanisms of cytokine effects on food intake and energy expenditure

Peripheral LPS administration induces cytokine expression in the periphery and the brain. Cytokines produced in the brain (i.e. within the blood brain barrier [BBB]) can act directly on neural circuitries controlling energy balance. Cytokines produced outside the BBB have local catabolic effects (proteolysis, lipolysis) (see[20] for review) and can affect CNS-mediated functions through afferent nerves or by acting at the blood brain barrier. As an example, I will focus on the effects of the pro-inflammatory cytokines IL-1β and IFNγ.

Feeding suppressive effect of IL-1β

We have shown that afferent autonomic nerves from below the diaphragm are not necessary for the feeding suppressive effect of IP injected IL-1β (see[12,21] for review). Yet, vagal afferents appear to play an important role in the hypermetabolic, i.e. fever response to peripheral IL-1β[22]. Also, leptin does not appear to be a necessary mediator of peripheral IL-1β's anorectic effect because IP injected IL-1β reduces food intake similarly in obese and lean Zucker rats as well as in lean Zucker rats made overweight by cafeteria diet feeding (Lugarini *et al.*, unpublished results). Nevertheless, leptin expression is markedly increased in response to IL-1β[23], and there is evidence for multiple interactions between leptin and IL-1β which may also result in modulation of both peptides' effects on energy balance. Peripheral IL-1β can get direct access to the brain through circumventricular organs and active transport mechanisms[24]. An alternative and not mutually exclusive possibility is that IL-1β triggers the release of downstream mediators by acting through receptors on brain capillary endothelial cells. Peripherally administered IL-1β induces c-fos immunoreactivity in the paraventricular nucleus (PVN) as well as in the arcuate nucleus (ARC) of the hypothalamus[25,26]. The ARC is usually considered to be the major hypothalamic detection site for blood-derived signals. Yet, severing the ARC or its connections to the PVN only slightly attenuates but does not eliminate peripheral IL-1β-induced anorexia[27], indicating that the ARC is involved in but not necessary for peripheral IL-1β-induced anorexia. Several lines of evidence (see[12,21,25]) implicate activation of hindbrain to forebrain aminergic neurons as another major route through which circulating IL-1β affects food intake and metabolism. IL-1β-induced anorexia may in part be mediated through prostaglandin E_2-dependent activation of serotoninergic neurons originating in the raphe nuclei and projecting to the hypothalamus[25]. In line with this idea, systemic administration of a serotonin ($5HT_{2C}$) receptor antagonist and microinjection of the $5HT_{1A}$ autoreceptor agonist 8-OH-DPAT directly into the raphe nucleus both markedly attenuated the feeding suppressive effect of peripherally injected IL-1β (see[21]). Most recent data indicate that activation of serotoninergic neurons ultimately influences the hypothalamic melanocortin pathways of energy balance regulation[28]. The exact mechanisms of this interaction still need to be determined.

Centrally produced IL-1β may contribute to the feeding suppression and hypermetabolism observed in some situations[14,29,30] by affecting the central circuitry of energy balance regulation directly. Also, IL-1β appears to be essential for the production of ciliary neurotrophic factor (CNTF) in response to brain injury or trauma[31]. CNTF was first characterized as a trophic factor for motor neurons in the ciliary ganglion and spinal cord and subsequently found to markedly reduce food intake and body weight (see[32]). Thus, CNTF might be a downstream mediator of IL-1β effects on food intake and energy expenditure. Some data suggest that CNTF ultimately affects energy balance by markedly reducing the expression and action of NPY[33]. A reduction of hypothalamic NPY has also been implicated in the feeding suppressive effect of IL-1β[34]. In sum, several lines of evidence suggest that the pathways of IL-1β-induced suppression of feeding and stimulation of energy expenditure ultimately converge on the well characterized hypothalamic neuropeptide systems that control energy balance.

Hypermetabolic effect of IFNγ

Several cytokines have been shown to stimulate energy expenditure and, hence, induce fever as part of their effects on central nervous system mechanism of energy balance regulation. An alternative pathway of metabolic stimulation has recently been demonstrated for IFNγ. In a whole series of experiments, Arsenijevic et al.[15] demonstrated that IFNγ-dependent hypermetabolism in the initial phase of *T. gondii* infection was mainly due to increased lipid oxidation (based on the observed decrease in respiratory quotient), but that neither a stimulation of uncoupling protein 1 (UCP1) nor of the sympathetic nervous system was involved. The data suggested activation of an extra-mitochondrial mechanism of lipid oxidation, especially in organs rich in macrophage-type cells. Following infection peritoneal macrophages exhibited an enhanced capacity to produce reactive oxygen species, and this capacity was abated in IFNγ-KO mice. In sum these findings suggest that IFNγ-dependent stimulation of the oxidative burst in macrophages can be a major contributor to the hypermetabolic response in some pathological situations[15].

References

1. Wusteman M, Wight DGD, Elia M. Protein-metabolism after injury with turpentine – a rat model for clinical trauma. *Am J Physiol* 1990; 259: E763–E9.

2. Mchugh K, Castonguay TW, Collins SM, Weingarten HP. Characterization of suppression of food intake following acute colon inflammation in the rat. *Am J Physiol* 1993; 265: R1001–R5.

3. Abram M, Vuckovic D, Wraber B, Doric M. Plasma cytokine response in mice with bacterial infection. *Med Inflamm* 2000; 9: 229–34.

4. Cahlin C, Korner A, Axelsson H, Wang WH, Lundholm K, Svanberg E. Experimental cancer cachexia: The role of host-derived cytokines interleukin (IL)-6, IL-12, interferon-gamma, and tumor necrosis factor alpha evaluated in gene knockout, tumor-bearing mice on C57 Bl background and eicosanoid-dependent cachexia. *Cancer Res* 2000; 60: 5488–93.

5. Arsenijevic D, Girardier L, Seydoux J, Chang HR, Dulloo AG. Altered energy balance and cytokine gene expression in a murine model of chronic infection with Toxoplasma gondii. *Am J Physiol* 1997; 272: E908–E17.

6. Yeh S, Schuster MW. Geriatric cachexia: the role of cytokines. *Am J Clin Nutr* 1999; 70: 183–97.

7. Pedersen BK. Exercise and cytokines. *Immunol Cell Biol* 2000; 78: 532–5.

8. Kern PA. Potential role of TNF alpha and lipoprotein lipase as candidate genes for obesity. *J Nutr* 1997; 127: S1917–S22.

9. Tapping RI, Akashi S, Miyake K, Godowski PJ, Tobias PS. Toll-like receptor 4, but not toll-like receptor 2, is a signaling receptor for Escherichia and Salmonella lipopolysaccharides. *J Immunol* 2000; 165: 5780–7.

10. Von Meyenburg C, Hrupka BH, Schwartz GJ, Landmann R, Langhans W. Role for CD14 and TLR2 in bacterial product-induced anorexia. *Appetite* 2002; 39: 105.

11. Arsenijevic D, Garcia I, Vesin C, Vesin D, Arsenijevic Y, Seydoux J et al. Differential roles of tumor necrosis factor-alpha and interferon-gamma in mouse hypermetabolic and anorectic responses induced by LPS. *Eur Cytokine Netw* 2000; 11: 662–8.

12. Langhans W. Anorexia of infection: Current prospects. *Nutrition* 2000; 16: 996–1005.

13. VanderMeer MJM, Sweep CGJF, Pesman GJ, Borm GF, Hermus ARMM. Synergism between IL-1 beta and TNF-alpha on the activity of the pituitary-adrenal axis and on food intake of rats. *Am J Physiol* 1995; 268: E551–E557.

14. Bluthe RM, Laye S, Michaud B, Combe C, Dantzer R, Parnet P. Role of interleukin-1 beta and tumour necrosis factor-alpha in lipopolysaccharide-induced sickness behaviour: a study with interleukin-1 type I receptor-deficient mice. *Eur Neurosci* 2000; 12: 4447–56.

15. Arsenijevic D, de Bilbao F, Giannakopoulos P, Girardier L, Samec S, Richard D. A role for interferon-γ in the hypermetabolic response to murine toxoplasmosis. *Eur Cytokine Netw* 2001; 12: 518–27.

16. Kozak W, Poli V, Soszynski D, Conn CA, Leon LR, Kluger MJ. Sickness behavior in mice deficient in interleukin-6 during turpentine abscess and influenza pneumonitis. *Am J Physiol* 1997; 272: R621–R630.

17. Leon LR, Conn CA, Glaccum M, Kluger MJ. IL-1 type I receptor mediates acute phase response to turpentine, but not lipopolysaccharide, in mice. *Am J Physiol* 1996; 271: R1668–R1675.

18. Oldenburg HSA, Rogy MA, Lazarus DD, Vanzee KJ, Keeler BP, Chizzonite RA et al. Cachexia and the acute-phase protein response in inflammation are regulated by interleukin-6. *Eur J Immunol* 1993; 23: 1889–94.

19. Cooper AL, Brouwer S, Turnbull AV, Luheshi GN, Hopkins SJ, Kunkel S.L et al. Tumor necrosis factor-alpha and fever after peripheral inflammation in the rat. *Am J Physiol* 1994; 269: R1431–R1436.

20. Langhans W. Peripheral mechanisms involved with catabolism. *Curr Opin Clin Nutr Metab Care* 2002; 5: 419–26.

21. Langhans W, Hrupka BJ. Cytokines and appetite. In: *Cytokines and mental health*, Kronfol Z (ed.). Kluwer: Academic Publishers, 2002 (in press).

22. Watkins LR, Goehler LE, Relton JK, Tartaglia N, Silbert L, Martin D, Maier SF. Blockade of interleukin-1 induced hyperthermia by subdiaphragmatic vagotomy: Evidence for vagal mediation of immune brain communication. *Neurosci Letters* 1995; 183: 27–31.

23. Grunfeld C, Zhao C, Fuller J, Pollock A, Moser A, Friedman J, Feingold KR. Endotoxin and cytokines induce expression of leptin, the ob gene product, in hamsters – A role for leptin in the anorexia of infection. *J Clin Invest* 1996; 97: 2152–7.

24. Banks WA, Kastin AJ. Passage of peptides across the blood-brain barrier: Pathophysiological perspectives. *Life Sci* 1996; 59: 1923–43.

25. Ericsson A, Arias C, Sawchenko PE. Evidence for an intramedullary prostaglandin-dependent mechanism in the activation of stress-related neuroendocrine circuitry by intravenous interleukin-1. *J Neurosci* 1997; 17: 7166–79.

26. Herkenham M, Lee HY, Baker RA. Temporal and spatial patterns of c-fos mRNA induced by intravenous interleukin-1: A cascade of non-neuronal cellular activation at the blood-brain barrier. *J Comp Neurol* 1998; 400: 175–96.

27. Reyes TM, Sawchenko PE. Involvement of the arcuate nucleus of the hypothalamus in interleukin-1-induced anorexia. *J Neurosci* 2002; 22: 5091–9.

28. Heisler LK, Cowley MA, Tecott LH, Fan W, Low MJ, Smart JL *et al.* Activation of central melanocortin pathways by fenfluramine. *Science* 2002; 297: 609–11.

29. Mchugh KJ, Collins SM, Weingarten HP. Central interleukin-1 receptors contribute to suppression of feeding after acute colitis in the rat. *Am J Physiol* 1994; 266: R1659–R1663.

30. Plata-Salaman CR, Ilyin SE, Gayle D. Brain cytokine mRNAs in anorectic rats bearing prostate adenocarcinoma tumor cells. *Am J Physiol* 1998; 275: R566–R573.

31. Herx LM, Rivest S, Yong VW. Central nervous system-initiated inflammation and neurotrophism in trauma: IL-1 beta is required for the production of ciliary neurotrophic factor. *J Immunol* 2000; 165: 2232–9.

32. Lambert PD, Anderson KD, Sleeman MW, Wong V, Tan J, Hijarunguru A *et al.* Ciliary neurotrophic factor activates leptin-like pathways and reduces body fat, without cachexia or rebound weight gain, even in leptin-resistant obesity. *Proc Natl Acad Sci USA* 2001; 98: 4652–7.

33. Xu B, Dube MG, Kalra PS, Farmerie WG, Kaibara A, Moldawer LL *et al.* Anorectic effects of the cytokine, ciliary neurotropic factor, are mediated by hypothalamic neuropeptide Y: Comparison with leptin. *Endocrinology* 1998; 139: 466–73.

34. Gayle D, Ilyin SE, Plata-Salamàn CR. Central nervous system IL-1 beta system and neuropeptide Y mRNAs during IL-1 beta-induced anorexia in rats. *Brain Res Bull* 1997; 44: 311–7.

Progress in Obesity Research: 9. Edited by *Geraldo Medeiros-Neto, Alfredo Halpern and Claude Bouchard*
©2003 John Libbey Eurotext Ltd, pp. 739–743.

CHAPTER 154

Leptin: endocrine effects of an adipocyte hormone that promotes homeostasis

Julio Licinio

Interdepartmental Clinical Pharmacology Center, Laboratory for Pharmacogenomics, Neuropsychiatric Institute, David Geffen School of Medicine at UCLA, Los Angeles, CA 90095-1761, USA
[e-mail: licinio@ucla.edu]

Role of clinical investigation

Although translating bench work to clinical practice is an important function for clinical research, translation is not enough. Research in living human beings is necessary and can be safely and ethically conducted to test data-based hypotheses and to generate work that is conceptually novel, as well as medically relevant and that elucidates key points in biology. In addition, there are important ethical and social components to clinical research. Like basic research, successful clinical research requires commitment, luck, and innovation. But because clinical research is closely connected to clinical practice, committed researchers must go beyond discovery and construction of new scientific paradigms to change practice and policy[1]. With this in mind, I will review certain ongoing studies demonstrating that leptin, a peripheral adipocyte hormone[2], regulates key functions of the human central nervous system (CNS), such as the control of neuroendocrine function[3-5].

Leptin and neuroendocrinology

Human life depends on successfully integrating of and responding to a variety of signals that emanate from the environment, from the genome, and from metabolic processes. Neuroendocrinlogy, one of the disciplines that study the integration and transduction of biological signals focuses on the investigation of central and peripheral circuitries that regulate the activity of endocrine glands, related CNS functions and behaviour. Two CNS are key to neuroendocrinology: neuroendocrine transduction and regulation. Neuroendocrine transduction refers to the transformation of neural information mediated by action potentials into informational molecules that can either diffuse from the cell of origin or be secreted; these circulate in the bloodstream and act at distant sites where they regulate the functioning of various systems. The brain integrates information received from the external world and from the internal milieu: Neuroendocrine transduction occurs and molecular signals are sent to various brain regions, as well as to glands localized throughout the body, thereby resulting in neuroendocrine integration, which consists of a complex network of hormones that regulate both the short- and long-term functioning of all organs and systems. The internal milieu sends signals back to the brain; these are integrated with the new information that is constantly arriving from the external world, and the transduction of new neuroendocrine signals results.

Signals from the environment are continuously integrated with feedback received from the internal milieu (both signals that are genetically programmed and others that are the result of metabolic processes) and from external and internal pacemakers. This mechanism causes neuroendocrine transduction and integration to have at the same time elements that control (1) long-term changes, such as those that occur during development and ageing. and (2) rhythms that last for several months (pregnancy), several weeks (the menstrual function), one day (circadian periodicity of hypothalamic-pituitary-adrenal or HPA function), a few hours (insulin response to meals), and a few minutes (short pulses of parathyroid hormone)[6].

Relevance to neuroscience

Data from studies conducted by our group will be reviewed. These were designed to test the hypothesis that the adipocyte hormone leptin modulates neuroendocrine transduction in humans and acts as a key element in neuroendocrine integration by providing a signal of nutritional status to the CNS and peripheral organs. The CNS effects of leptin on neuroendocrine transduction and integration regulate the production of neuropeptides that modulate behaviour and contribute to the pathophysiology of clinical neuroscience disorders, such as major depressive disorder.

Leptin is encoded by a gene located in human chromosome 7q31.3 that spans -20 kb, with three exons and two introns. The promoter region of this gene spans a region of -3 kb, with a TATA box located at −26 to −30, as well as multiple CCAAT/enhancer binding protein and SPA sites, a glucocorticoid response element, and several cAMP response element binding protein sites[7,8]. Transcription and translation of the leptin gene occur in adipose tissue (and during pregnancy in the placenta); the rate of production is directly related to fat mass. Leptin's crystal structure reveals a four-helix bundle similar to that of the long-chain helical cytokine family that also includes interleukin (IL)-6, IL-11, IL-12, leukocyte inhibitory factor, G-CSF, ciliary neurotrophic factor, and oncostatin M[9]. One leptin receptor gene has been cloned: it encodes five or more leptin receptor splice variants including a form predicted to be soluble, several short forms with small intracellular domains, and one long form that is highly homologous to the signaling domain of the type I cytokine receptor family, and uses the JAK/STAT pathway for signal transduction[10]. After it is secreted, principally by white fat cells, leptin circulates in the bloodstream and rapidly enters the brain, where it produces synaptic modulatory effects in the hypothalami[11–12].

Leptin is essential for regulating body weight in humans. Rare genetic mutations in the genes encoding either leptin or its receptor result in normal fetal development and severe postnatal obesity, and in hypogonadism in adults[13–16]. In addition to hypogonadism, individuals with leptin gene mutation have sympathetic system dysfunction, characterized by orthostatic hypotension, inability of blood pressure to rise to cold pressor test and immersion in ice cold water, and the absence of response to median nerve and auditory stimulation in sympathetic skin response test[16]. Thus, intact leptin gene function is required for optimal sympathetic tone. A mutation identified in the human leptin receptor results in a G ? A base substitution in the splice donor site of exon 16. Three sisters who are homozygous for that mutation have been identified; they have a truncated leptin receptor that lacks both the transmembrane and the intracellular domains. These sisters were reported to have early-onset morbid obesity, no pubertal development, and reduced secretion of growth hormone and thyrotropin[15]. The clinical presentation of patients with rare mutations in the genes encoding leptin or its receptor indicates that human leptin bioactivity is required for regulating body weight and neuroendocrine function, as well as for sexual maturation.

Because the vast majority of obese humans present with high levels of leptin, it seems logical to propose that most of cases of obesity could be related to resistance to the effects of leptin, to defective leptin transport into the brain, or to a combination of both[10,17,18]. Conversely, in states of weight loss resulting in low body weight, leptin levels are low[19,20], which in turn results in amenorrhea, indicating that a critical level of leptin is needed to maintain menstrual function. Menstruation ceases when levels are under 1.85 μg/l and leptin levels are a better predictor of amenorrhea than body mass index (BMI), fat mass, and percentage of body fat[21].

To study leptin's role in the neuroendocrine function, it is necessary to develop and validate clinical research protocols that permit a detailed assessment of its function and effects on neuroendocrine regulation. Thus, to test the hypothesis that leptin regulates human endocrine function, we developed a research protocol for rapid sampling of plasma to measure of leptin, as well as pituitary, adrenal, thyroid and ovarian hormones.

The protocol consisted of admission to a dedicated clinical research room at a Clinical Research Center. After two days of acclimatization, blood drawing started at 08: 00, with samples collected through an indwelling intravenous catheter every 7 min for 24 h. During the study, patients received a standardized diet designed to keep them at their admission weight; 20 per cent of calories were consumed at breakfast (08: 30), 35 per cent at lunch (12: 30), 35 per cent at dinner (17: 30) and 10 per cent at an evening snack (21: 00). This rapid-sampling protocol made it possible to determine whether there were rapid fluctuations in circulating leptin levels and to ascertain the impact of fluctuations in the levels of plasma leptin on pituitary-adrenal, pituitary-ovarian, and pituitary-thyroid function[3,4,22,23].

Role in HPA function

Previous studies have showed that leptin contributes to regulating HPA function in experimental animals. In rodents, administration of exogenous leptin suppresses starvation-induced HPA activation and blunts stress-induced elevations in the levels of adrenocorticotrophin hormone (ACTH) and cortisol. *In vitro*, leptin inhibits hypoglycaemia-induced corticotropin releasing hormone (CRH) secretion by perfused rat hypothalami[5]. However, these preclinical studies did not elucidate whether minute-by-minute fluctuations in the plasma levels of leptin affected the dynamics pituitary-adrenal function.

Studying six healthy men under our rapid-sampling protocol, we collected a total of 1242 plasma samples for which we measured the concentrations of leptin, ACTH, and cortisol. A detailed analysis of fluctuations in leptin concentrations revealed statistically significant ultradian and circadian rhythmicity. Total circulating leptin levels exhibited a pattern indicating of pulsatile release, with 32.0 ± 1.5 pulses every 24 h and a pulse duration of 32.8 ± 1.6 min. The finding that circulating human leptin has organized pulsatility opens a new area of investigation aimed at identifying humoral or neural signals that regulate rapid fluctuations in the secretion or clearance of a hormone synthesized by adipocytes dispersed throughout the body, not by an anatomically defined gland.

Also, we showed an inverse relationship between rapid fluctuations in the plasma levels of leptin and those of ACTH (Pearson correlation: $r = 0.651; P < 10^{-9}$) and cortisol ($r = 0.764; P < 10^{-9}$). This highly significant inverse relationship between leptin and pituitary-adrenal hormones raised the following question: Does leptin regulate pituitary-adrenal function or vice versa? To address that question, we studied patients with Cushing's disease before and 10 days after successful surgical removal of ACTH-secreting pituitary adenomas; a 10 to 15-fold reduction in the levels of endogenous HPA function resulted. We showed that leptin levels are the same both at baseline and after CRH stimulation in controls, as well as in patients with Cushing's disease either before or after surgery. The leptin area under the curve during CRH stimulation was 2340 ± 214 ng/m·min in Cushing's patients preoperatively and 2038 ± 185 ng/ml·min postoperatively, a non-significant finding. On the basis of those data, we concluded that endogenous cortisol and ACTH do not seem to acutely affect leptin levels[24]. Although, it should be noted that chronic hypercortisolism causes visceral obesity, and thus results in elevated baseline leptin levels.

In a group of intensively studied men, we found that there was a highly significant inverse correlation between plasma levels of leptin and those of ACTH and cortisol. Preclinical data indicate that leptin acutely regulates CRH secretion; but that endogenous levels of ACTH and cortisol do not seem to affect leptin concentrations. We conclude that leptin acutely regulates human HPA function and propose that leptin, a highly pulsatile signal of nutritional status, can regulate a key function of the CNS, such as the production of CRH, a neuropeptide that modulates HPA function and behaviour and that is abnormally regulated in major depression.

Our data indicate that leptin modulates HPA function. As the HPA axis is essential to life and represents a crucial element in the stress response, it has been proposed that leptin might be a stress hormone with a role in systemic illness. In addition to regulating endogenous levels of cortisol, leptin enhances cytokine production and the phagocytic activity of macrophages. T-cells containing functional leptin receptors. Leptin has a direct and specific effect on T-lymphocyte responses, differentially regulating the proliferation of naive and memory T cells, and increasing Th1 and suppressed Th2 cytokine production[25]. In critically ill patients with acute sepsis, we found that leptin's circadian rhythm was disrupted, with no nocturnal rise in plasma levels and a loss of relationship between plasma leptin and plasma cortisol. Mean leptin levels were three times higher in the patients who survived the septic episode (25.5 ± 6.2 ng/ml, $n = 10$) than in those who did not (8.0 ± 3.7, $n = 6$, $P < 0.01$)[26]. Future studies should test the hypothesis that leptin may be a stress-related hormone whose secretion is important in the pathophysiology of critical illness.

Sex differences: clinical implications

To assess possible sex differences in leptin pulsatility, 14 time series (six women, eight men) containing a total of 2898 measurements were assessed by algorithms that characterize statistically significant pulsatility, spectral (Fourier) analysis, analysis of time intervals and variability, and approximate entropy (ApEn).

ApEn, a statistic that determines the orderliness of a series of values, can differentiate levels of endocrine functioning that are numerically similar but sequentially different[33]. For example, the sequence 'abcabcabcabcabcabcabcabc' has a lower ApEn than the sequence 'abcaabcabcbabcbcabcacabc', which in turn has a lower ApEn than the sequence 'baccaacbbaccbbabcacbacab'. Thus, the last sequence, with the highest ApEn, has less sequential order or structure than the first one, which has a lower ApEn value. Cross-ApEn measures the *relative* pattern orderliness of two data series and quantifies the conditional regularity or synchrony of point-by-point variations across two time series. It is distinct from cross-correlation analysis, because cross-ApEn is lag- and scale-independent. Lower absolute cross-ApEn values denote more conditional regularity or synchronicity. These methods have been elegantly presented by Pincus and have been used to show that older men secrete luteinizing hormone (LH) and testosterone more irregularly and more asynchronously than younger ones[27].

In our comparison study, we found that 24-h profiles of rapidly sampled circulating leptin were over twice as high in young, healthy, normal-weight women as in young, healthy, normal-weight men, with a pulse amplitude that was likewise over twice as high in women[22]. The average 24-h plasma leptin concentrations were 8.49 ± 1.44 ng/ml in women and 3.79 ± 1.24 ng/ml in men; the average heights of leptin pulses were 9.9 ± 1.7 ng/ml in women and 4.6 ± 1.6 ng/ml in men. However, healthy men and women have nearly identical concentration-independent and frequency-related 24-h and ultradian patterns. In other words, the number of leptin pulses/24 h (30 ± 1 in women and 30 ± 2 in men), the duration of each pulse (35.9 ± 1.5 min in women and 34.6 ± 2.0 mins in men), and the interval between pulses (47.4 ± 1.6 min in women and 46.2 ± 2.2 mins in men) were virtually the same. As assessed by ApEn, leptin concentrations have non-random fluctuations over 24 h that are independent of their absolute value and underlying 24-h periodicity and that are similar in men and women. Ultradian periodicities detected by Fourier time series have similar values in men and women. Using several independent methods to analyse endocrine data, we found that the strongest distinction between the sexes in the level of organization of leptin concentrations is *not* at the level of pulse organization or oscillation frequency, but rather in the mass or amount of leptin released per secretory burst, indicating that women might be more resistant to its effects than men.

Leptin is clinically relevant to regulating of body weight and disorders characterized by abnormalities in the regulation of food intake and body weight are more prevalent in women: For example, the female to male ratio for anorexia nervosa is 10 : 1; it is 6 : 1 for bulimia nervosa 5 : 2 for major depression, 3 : 2 for binge eating disorder, and 11.3 : 10 for obesity. Our data may indicate that to maintain normal body weight, women require circulating leptin levels twice as high as men's and that women are therefore relatively more resistant to leptin's effects than men[22]. Future studies should examine whether the relative resistance exhibited by women might contribute to their increased susceptibility to disorders whose pathophysiology involves dysregulation of food intake and body weight.

Clinical protocols

Table 1. Adaptive mechanisms that promote adaptation and survival

FIGHT OR FLIGHT	FEAST
Occurs during confrontation with predators and acute insults	Occurs during weight gain that follows consumption of large amounts of food
ENDOCRINE-IMMUNE MANIFESTATIONS	
Increased HPA responses	Decreased HPA responses
Acute sympathetic discharges	Optimal sympathetic tone
Suppression of immunity	Promotion of immunity
Suppression of reproduction	Promotion of reproductive system function
	↓
	EVOLUTION

Regulation of concentrations of sexual hormones

In addition to its role in regulating body weight, leptin has been shown to affect reproduction: Administering it to immature animals accelerates the onset of puberty[28]. While in adult animals, it corrects the sterility defect in homozygous obese female mice[29]. Leptin corrects hypogonadism in mice starved for forty eight hours, without affecting body weight and in animals fed adlibitum, but not those who are food deprived, it facilitates female sexual behaviour. Those data demonstrate that leptin is a trophic factor necessary for the reproductive system. Because it affects reproduction and because plasma levels of leptin and of hypothalamic-pituitary-ovarian (HPO) hormones are highly pulsatile, we hypothesized that rapidly sampled concentrations of leptin, LH, and estradiol might exhibit pattern coupling or synchronicity. To test this hypothesis, we studied six healthy women whose average age was 25.5 ± 1.6 years and whose average body mass index was 21.6 ± 1.1 kg/m². Plasma was sampled every 7 min for 1442 min (just over 24 h) to measure circulating leptin, LH, and estradiol. Using this protocol we obtained 621 measures per person on a total of 3726 data points in the study[4].

References

1. Sommer A. Albert Lasker Award for Clinical Research. Clinical research and the human condition: moving from observation to practice. *Nature Med* 1997; 3: 1061–3.

2. Zhang Y, Proenca R, Maffei M, Barone M, Leopold L, Friedman JM. Positional cloning of the mouse obese gene and its human homologue. *Nature* 1994; 372: 425–32.

3. Licinio J, Mantzoros C, Negrao AB *et al.* Human leptin levels are pulsatile and inversely related to pituitary-adrenal function. *Nature Med* 1997; 3: 575–9.

4. Licinio J, Negrão AB, Mantzoros C *et al.* Synchronicity of frequently sampled 24-hour concentrations of circulating leptin, luteinizing hormone, and estradiol in healthy women. *Proc Natl Acad Sci* 1998; 95: 2541–6.

5. Ahima RS, Prabakaran D, Mantzoros C *et al.* Role of leptin in the neuroendocrine response to fasting. *Nature* 1996; 382: 250–2.

6. Licinio J, Gold PW. Frontiers in neuroendocrinology. In: *The-Advisory-Committee-on-Health-Research*, pp. 105–28. Neuroscience, Neurology, and Health. Geneva: World Health Organization; 1997.

7. Considine RV, Caro JF. Leptin and the regulation of body weight. *Int J Biochem Cell Biol* 1997; 29: 1255–72.

8. Prolo P, Wong M-L, Licinio J. Molecules in focus: leptin. *Int J Biochem Cell Biol* 1998 (in press).

9. Zhang F, Basinski MB, Beals JM et al. Crystal structure of the obese protein leptin-E100. Nature 1997; 387: 206–9.

10. Flier JS. Leptin expression and action: new experimental paradigms. *Proc Natl Acad Sci* 1997; 94: 4242–5.

11. Glaum SR, Hara M, Bindokas VP *et al.* Leptin, the obese gene product, rapidly modulates synaptic transmission in the hypothalamus. *Mol Pharmacol* 1996; 50: 230–5.

12. Elmquist JK, Ahima RS, Elias CF, Flier JS, Saper CB. Leptin activates distinct projections from the dorsomedial and ventromedial hypothalamic nuclei. *Proc Natl Acad Sci USA* 1998; 95: 741–6.

13. Montague CT, Farooqi IS, Whitehead JP *et al.* Congenital leptin deficiency is associated with severe early-onset obesity in humans. *Nature* 1997; 387: 903–8.

14. Strobel A, Issad T, Camoin L, Ozata M, Strosberg AD. A leptin missense mutation associated with hypogonadism and morbid obesity. *Nature Genet* 1998 ; 18: 213–5.

15. Clément K, Vaisse C, Lahlou N *et al.* A mutation in the human leptin receptor gene causes obesity and pituitary dysfunction. *Nature* 1998; 392: 398–401.

16. Ozata M, Ozdemir IC, Licinio J. Human leptin deficiency caused by a missense mutation: Multiple endocrine defects, decreased sympathetic tone, and immune system dysfunction indicate new targets for leptin action, greater central than peripheral resistance to the effects of leptin, and spontaneous correction of leptin-mediated defects. *J Clinical Endocrinol Metab* 1999; 84: 3686–95.

17. Considine RV, Sinha MK, Heiman ML *et al.* Serum immunoreactive leptin concentrations in normal-weight and obese humans. *N Engl J Med* 1996; 334: 292–5.

18. Caro JF, Kolaczynski JW, Nyce MR *et al.* Decreased cerebrospinal-fluid/serum leptin ratio in obesity: a possible mechanism for leptin resistance. *Lancet* 1996; 348: 159–61.

19. Hebebrand J, Blum WF, Barth N *et al.* Leptin levels in patients with anorexia nervosa are reduced in the acute stage and elevated upon short-term weight restoration. *Mol Psychiatry* 1997; 2: 330–4.

20. Mantzoros C, Flier JS, Lesem MD, Brewerton TD, Jimerson DC. Cerebrospinal fluid leptin in anorexia nervosa: correlation with nutritional status and potential role in resistance to weight gain. *J Clin Endocrinol Metab* 1997; 82: 1845–51.

21. Köpp W, Blum W, von Prittwitz S *et al.* Low leptin levels predict amenorrhea in underweight and eating disordered females. *Mol Psychiatry* 1997; 2: 335–40.

22. Licinio J, Negrão AB, Mantzoros C. *et al.* Sex differences in circulating human leptin pulse amplitude: clinical implications. *J Clin Endocrinol Metab* 1998; 83: 4140–7.

23. Mantzoros CS, Ozata M, Negrao AB, Ziotopoulou M, Caglayan S, Suchard M *et al.* Synchronicity of frequently sampled TSH and leptin concentrations in healthy adults and leptin deficient subjects: evidence for possible partial TSH regulation by leptin in humans. *J Clin Endocrinol Metab* 2001; 86: 3284–91.

24. Cizza G, Lotsikas AJ, Licinio J, Gold PW, Chrousos GP. Plasma leptin levels do not change in patients with Cushing's disease shortly after correction of hypercortisolism. *J Clin Endocrinol Metab* 1997; 82: 2747–50.

25. Lord GM, Matarese G, Howard JK, Baker RJ, Bloom SR, Lechler RI. Leptin modulates the T-cell immune response and reverses starvation-induced immunosuppression. *Nature* 1998; 394: 897–901.

26. Bornstein SR, Licinio J, Tauchnitz R *et al.* Plasma leptin levels are increased in survivors of acute sepsis: associated loss of diurnal rhythm in cortisol and leptin secretion. *J Clin Endocrinol Metab* 1998; 83: 280–3.

27. Pincus SM, Mulligan T, Iranmanesh A, Gheorghiu S, Godschalk M, Veldhuis JD. Older males secrete luteinizing hormone and testosterone more irregularly, and jointly more asynchronously, than younger males: dual novel facets. *Proc Natl Acad Sci USA* 1996; 93: 14100–5.

28. Chehab FF, Mounzih K, Lu R, Lim ME. Early onset of reproductive function in normal female mice treated with leptin. *Science* 1997; 275: 88–90.

29. Chehab FF, Lim ME, Lu R. Correction of the sterility defect in homozygous obese female mice by treatment with the human recombinant leptin. *Nature Genet* 1996; 12: 318–20.

30. Selye H. A syndrome produced by diverse nocuous agents. *Nature* 936; 138: 32.

31. Licinio J. The neurobiology of stress. In: Stress and the nervous system, Bolis CL, Licinio J (eds), pp. 3–13. Geneva: The Advisory Committee on Health Research – World Health Organization; 1998.

©2003 John Libbey Eurotext Ltd, pp. 744–748.

CHAPTER 155

Hormonal modulation of energy intake and expenditure: the multiple contributions of thyroid hormones

Geraldo Medeiros-Neto

Professor of the Department of Clinical Medicine, Division of Endocrinology, University of Sao Paulo Medical School, Sao Paulo 05403-900, Brazil
[e-mail: medneto@uol.com.br]

Introduction

About 100 years ago, Magnus-Levy described the stimulatory effects of thyroid hormones on metabolic rate in humans, leading to the widespread use of basal metabolic rate (BMR) as an index of thyroid function[1]. This method was the standard for many years, the BMR being well above normal in patients with hyperthyroidism and below the expected normal values in patients with decreased thyroid function. Little progress was made during the next 60 years of the past century in determining *HOW* thyroid hormones functioned to produce such effects on oxygen consumption. In the early fifties investigators began to understand mitochondrial structure and function, and a suggestion was put forward that thyroid stimulation of metabolic rate resulted from the uncoupling of oxidative phosphorylation, demonstrated in isolated mitochondria[2]. Few years later it was observed that alterations in nuclear RNA synthesis preceded biochemical changes found in mitochondria[3].

Those findings raised the possibility that nuclear events mediate thyroid hormone-stimulated mitochondrial metabolism. Subsequent studies have supported this hypothesis and have indicated that thyroid hormones exert multiple independent effects via specific receptors located in the nuclei of target tissues[4].

Although the biological and clinical importance of thyroid hormone stimulation of thermogenesis has been recognized, the quantitative contributions of specific energy-consuming processes to total oxygen consumption in absence or excess of thyroid hormones remain relatively unclear. In this chapter it is described the component elements in the thyroid hormones system and it is discussed the current thinking with regard to the mechanism of action of thyroid hormones, in respect to thermogenesis.

The thyroid hormone system

Following absorption in the gut, iodine is efficiently concentrated in the thyroid gland through a sodium-iodide-symporter (NIS) system. The iodide is transported rapidly to the apical membrane where it is transported through this membrane to the colloid space by Pendrin (and possibly other apical membrane proteins). In this new space iodide is oxidatively coupled to tyrosine residues in the thyroglobulin to produce the iodothyronines, L-thyroxine (T4) and triiodothyronine (T3). Although both products are secreted by the thyroid gland, the tetraiodo form predominates. T3 is the most biologically active form of thyroid hormones. It is mostly obtained from peripheral T4 by the action of the deiodinase enzymes. There are two main, quite different forms of these enzymes. Type I is found in liver and kidneys and type II is located in brain and brown adipose tissue. The deiodinase enzymes also convert T3 to diiodothyronines (T2) that are considered inactive metabolites but may have some action in calorigenesis[3].

Thyroid hormones (TH) control of thermogenesis and energy balance

One of the most widely recognized effects of TH in mammals is the regulation of energy metabolism and thermogenesis. Despite there being a substantial literature on this topic, the mechanisms by which TH actually regulate energy and thermogenesis are far from clear. A multitude of biochemical and molecular mechanisms are involved in the control of energy metabolism, with the participation of several cellular compartments.

Both nuclear-mediated and extranuclear action may underline the control exerted by TH on energy metabolism[5]. The nuclear-mediated pathway involves the gene transcription as induced by several T3-binding transcription factors belonging to the nuclear receptor. While the nuclear signaling pathway is universally accepted the extranuclear actions of TH are matter of debate[6].

Mitochondria are considered to be likely subcellular targets for thyroid hormones because of their central role in cellular energy transduction. Both the *activity* and the *number* of these organelles are influenced by the thyroid state of the animal. In skeletal muscle, heart, kidney and liver T3 plans a pivotal role in the mitochondrial function. It is accepted that TH administration increases oxygen consumption and heat production[7]. Two kinds of thyroid hormone action have been reported:

(a) A *short-term influence* occurring within minutes of thyroid hormone treatment;

(b) A more *delayed influence* recorded after a few hours.

Short-term influence

Increased oxygen consumption and oxidative phosphorylation can be detected in isolated liver mitochondria in less than 30 min after TH administration[2]. These effects are not blocked by protein synthesis administration. Moreover when T3 is added *in vitro* to isolated mitochondria from hypothyroid animals, increased oxygen consumption is detected within 2 min of the T3 being present.

Also stimulation of the mitochondrial carrier adenine nucleotide translocase (ANT) has been also confirmed within minutes of T3 administration. Thus, *rapidity*, *refractoriness* to inhibitors of protein synthesis and occurrence in the *absence of nuclei* (isolated mitochondrial preparations) will rule out the involvement of T3 nuclear genomic pathway[2,3].

(a) Mitochondria are a major site for T3 accumulation

Several studies have indicated that the mitochondria is a major compartment of T3 accumulation in the cell[4]. Also ANT (adenine nucleotide translocase) is a major T3 target involved in the short-term influence of this hormone and probably has a high-affinity binding site for T3. Other investigators, however, were unable to find significant binding to purified ANT or protein in the mitochondria[2].

(b) A specific binding site for T3 in mitochondria

The short-term hormonal influence of T3 may be mediated by specificT3 binding sites in mitochondria. A 28 kDa T3 binding protein was localized in the mitochondrial membrane. More recently it was identified a truncated form of T3 nuclear receptor e-Erb Aα1 displaying a similar molecular mass and localization (Fig. 1). This p28 protein is synthetized by alternative translational initiation in the messenger encoding the full-length nuclear receptor[2,3]. As a conclusion p28 could act as a receptor involved in the early mitochondrial T3 influence, as it is localized with components of the respiratory chain, uncoupling proteins (UCPs) and ANT. A second truncated form of the c-Erb Aα1 TH nuclear receptor (p43) was detected in mitochondria and binds T3 with an affinity unsurprisingly similar to that reported for nuclear c-Erb Aα1. Moreover, in contrast to p28, this protein harbors the DNA binding domain of the T3 nuclear receptor[2]. These findings raise the possibility that other members of the TH nuclear receptor superfamily could be imported into the mitochondria.

In the last few years it has become apparent that 3,5 T2, a putative product of the deiodination pathway, could be of biological significance[3]. A rapid stimulation of oxygen consumption, an enhancement of mitochondrial respiratory rate, and stimulation of the COX complex have been demonstrated in mitochondria[3]. These studies gave further support to the notion of a physiological role of 3,5 T2 in mitochondria (Fig. 1).

Delayed actions of T3 are probably induced at nuclear level

Many studies were performed in order to identify the sites of action of T3 involved in increased oxygen consumption. It was concluded that the *proton leak* across the inner membrane of isolated mitochon-

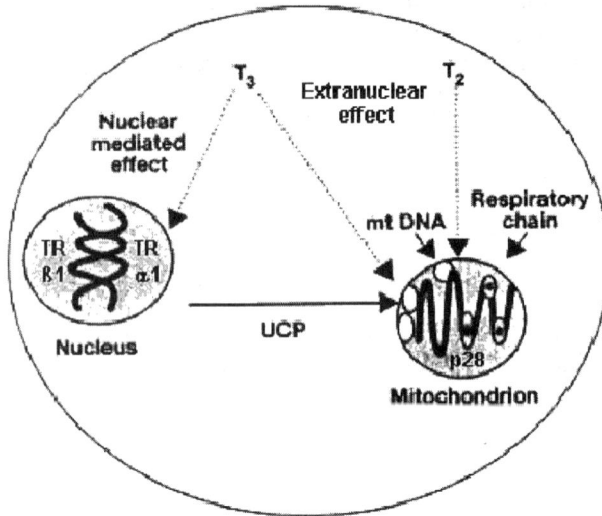

Fig. 1. For a long time it was assumed that TH stimulated only *obligatory* thermogenesis. It is also accepted that it also plays an essential role in *facultative* thermogenesis (in response to cold or feeding). The *nuclear-mediated* pathway involves a control of gene transcription mediated by T3-binding to nuclear receptor superfamily. Mitochondria are considered to be linked to the *extranuclear effect* of T3 because of their central role in cellular energy-transduction. The *proton leak* across the inner membrane of mitochondria is an important target of T3. More recently it has been shown that the α1-TR isoform is indispensable for T3 stimulated-thermogenesis in BAT by an action in elements of the nor-epinephrine signaling pathway. Also other iodothyrosines such as 3,5-T2 seems to act directly on the energy-transduction apparatus by binding withcomponents of the respiratory chain (modified from Lanni *et al.*, *J Endocrinol Invest* 24, 897–913, 2001).

dria is an important target of thyroid hormone. The proton leak represents about 20 per cent of the multifactorial control of mitochondrial respiration[8].

Thyroid hormone increases the proton leak by altering the phospholipid composition of the inner membrane while also increases its area. This will result in increased permeability to protons, recorded 9–12 h after T3 administration. Moreover recent work have indicated that control of mitochondrial UCPs (uncoupling proteins) expression is involved in the T3 regulation of the proton leak. Increased stimulation of *cardiolipin* synthesis activity by T3 will result in substantial increase in cardiolipin that, in turn, stimulated several mitochondrial carriers and enzymes activities[3,8].

Although delayed influence of thyroid hormone on mitochondrial oxygen consumption, involving alterations in phospholipids synthesis, appears to be mainly initiated at *nuclear level*, a direct mito-chondrial effect pathway could also be involved.

Control of energy metabolism by thyroid hormones

Maintenance of transmembrane ionic gradients

(a) Na$^+$/K$^+$ ATPase and thermogenesis

Cells must spend a substantial amount of energy to maintain the gradient of Na$^+$ and K$^+$ with the extracellular fluid[1,4]. This is essential to cell function and they create a transmembrane voltage and provide energy for the transport of a variety of substances. Thyroid hormone increases the activity of the Na/K-ATPase and it was postulated that this effect could account for a significant fraction of the thermogenic effect of T3. About 40 per cent of the increase in oxygen consumption by liver cells treated with T3 may be mediated by direct stimulation of the Na/K ATPase. Moreover the activation of this enzyme may be secondary to gradient perturbations, initiated by a forced influx of Na into the cells[4]. Thus TH could promote a reduction of the gradients of K$^+$ or Na$^+$ by altering the permeability to ions of the cell membrane, possibly by modifying the phospholipid composition. On the other hand, T3 stimulates the synthesis of selective isoforms of the α and β subunits of the enzyme largely by stabilizing the respective mRNAs[4].

(b) Intracellular Ca^{2+} and energy expenditure

It has been estimated that about 10 per cent of the cell energy expenditure is needed simply for cytosolic Ca^{2+} homeostasis, although it depends on the cell type. Studies conducted in skeletal muscle have suggested that TH apparently influence Ca^{2+} turnover by producing increases in both the volume and the density of Ca^{2+}-pumps within the sarcoplasmic reticulum (SR). TH can directly stimulate plasma membrane Ca^{2+}-ATPase activity at physiological concentrations[2,4]. From a *mechanical standpoint*, the increased capacity to pump Ca^{2+} into the SR explains the faster relaxation of the hyperthyroid muscle. In relation to *energy expenditure* the energetic cost of muscle contraction is increased by TH.

(c) Other mechanisms leading to increased thermogenesis

TH stimulates the turnover of *substrates* through metabolic pathways (substrate cycles). This may add little to obligatory thermogenesis, estimated to represent only 3 per cent of the overall thermogenic effect of T3. The substrate cycle that has received most attention is the lipogenesis-lipolysis cycle, stimulated by TH[4]. Thyroid hormone stimulates fatty acid synthesis particularly in the liver through the coordinate induction of the expression of genes encoding the enzymes involved. Also TH stimulates fatty acid chain elongation and desaturation as well as esterification into phospholipids and triglycerides. *Lipolisis* is also positively correlated with thyroid state. T3 enhances lipolysis by increasing the sensitivity of the process to catecholamines, which results in the activation of hormone-sensitive lipase and thereby lipolysis. In addition to promoting lipolysis, T3 also stimulates the oxidation of fatty acids by increasing the activity of the enzyme CPT (carnitine palmitoyl transferase) responsible for transporting fatty acid into the mitochondria[2].

Thyroid hormone stimulates the mitochondrial α-glycerol phosphate dehydrogenase (αGPD) and the increased activity of this enzyme correlates well with the degree of oxygen consumption[4]. The increased activity of the αGPD allows a faster rate of gluconeogenesis from glycerol and may contribute to increased heat production.

Thyroid hormone and uncoupling proteins

Uncoupling protein 1 (UCP-1) is an inner mitochondrial membrane protein expressed exclusively in the brown adipose tissue (BAT). It dissipates the mitochondrial protein gradient generated by the respiratory chain, producing heat instead of ATP[9]. The presence of UCP-1 in BAT together with the finding of a high density of nuclear T3 receptors in BAT have focused attention on a possible role for TH in modifying the function of UCP-1. In fact UCP-1 gene transcription is stimulated by T3, which acts via its receptor in synergy with nor-epinephrine (NE). Local production of T3 by deiodination of T4 is essential for the induction of UCP-1 gene transcription[10].

Other UCPs have been identified in mammals. Briefly UCP3 mRNA is found in skeletal muscle in heart and also in BAT, while UCP-2 is expressed widely in various tissues[11]. Other UCP (UCP-4 and UCP-5) are predominantly expressed in brain.

While UCP-1 is known to play an important role in regulating heat production during cold exposure (increasing whole-body energy expenditure) the biological functions of UCP-2 and UCP-3 are controversial[12]. Possible functions include:

(a)   Control of adaptative thermogenesis in response to cold exposure and diet;

(b)   Control of reactive oxygen species (ROS) production by mitochondria;

(c)   Regulation of ATP synthesis;

(d)   Regulation of fatty acid oxidation.

As T3 increases the expression of both UCP-2 and UCP-3 in heart and skeletal muscle, it may well increase energy expenditure through the functions mentioned above[13,14]. Moreover the UCP-3 gene contains response elements for both thyroid hormone and peroxisome-proliferatior activated receptor (PPAR). Thus UCP-3 has the potential to be the molecular determinant for the regulation of resting metabolic rate by T3[15].

The general conclusion is that UCP-2 and UCP-3 may have distinct primary functions, with UCP-3 implicated in regulating the flux of lipid substrates across the mitochondria and UCP-2 in the control of mitochondrial generation of reactive oxygen species (ROS).

More recently[16] it was confirmed that thyroid hormone contributes to BAT thermogenesis in two ways:

(a)   Stimulating the expression of elements in the signaling pathway of nor-epinephrine (NE);

(b)   Inducing the UCPs directly.

The same group of authors[16] further demonstrated that TH action on the NE signaling pathway is mediated by the α1 TH receptor isoform while the βTR is sufficient to stimulate UCPs. Therefore the α1 TR isoform is indispensable for the NE signaling in the BAT and in other tissues (such as heart) as well. This bring us to an emerging concept of TR isoform-selective response to TR. It might be possible to induce the effects of TH selectively, activating thermogenesis, for example, without concomitant stimulating appetite and lipogenesis, which would counteract the energy dissipation by TH[17]. This may have multiple potential clinical implications in the treatment of obesity.

References

1. Freake HC, Oppenheimer JH. Thermogenesis and thyroid function. *Annu Rev Nutr* 1995; 15: 263–91.

2. Wrutniak-Cabello C, Casas F, Cabello G. Thyroid hormone action in mitochondria. *Mol Endocrinol* 2001; 26: 66–7.

3. Lanni A, Moreno M, Lombardi A, de Lange P, Goglia F. Control of energy metabolism by iodothyronines. *J Endocrinol Invest* 2001; 24: 897–913.

4. Silva JE Thyroid hormone control of thermogenesis and energy balance. *Thyroid* 1995; 5: 481–92.

5. Dauncey MJ Thyroid hormone and thermogenesis. *Proc Nutr Soc* 1990; 49: 203–15.

6. Sestoft L. Metabolic aspects of calorigenic effect of thyroid hormone in mammals. *Clin Endocrinol* 1980; 13: 263–92.

7. Zhang J, Lazar MA. The mechanism of action of thyroid hormones. *Annu Rev Physiol* 2000; 62: 439–66.

8. Brand MD, Steverding D, Kadenbach B, Stivenson PM, Hafiser RP. The mechanism of the increase mitochondrial proton permeability by thyroid hormones. *Eur J Biochem* 1992; 206: 775–81.

9. Ricquier D, Boullaud F. The uncoupling proteins homologues: UCP1, UCP2, UCP3, StUCP and AtUCP. *Biochem J* 2000; 345; 161–79.

10. Bianco AC, Silva JE. Intracellular conversion of thyroxine to triiodothyronine is required for optimal thermogenic function of BAT. *J Clin Invest* 1987; 79: 295–300.

11. Echtay KS, Winkler E, Fuschimuth K, Klingeberg M Uncoupling proteins 2 and 3 are highly active H+ transporters and highly nucleotide sensitive when activated by coenzyme Q *Proc Natl Acad Sci USA* 2001; 98: 1416–21.

12. DeLange P, Lanni A, Beneduce L, Moreno M, Lombardi A, Silvestr E, Goglia F. Uncoupling protein 3 is a molecular determinant for the regulation of resting metabolic rate by thyroid hormone. *Endocrinology* 2001; 142: 340–3.

13. Lombardi A, LanniA, Moreno M, Brand MD, GogliaF. Effect of 3,5 diiodothyronine on the mitochondrial energy-transduction apparatus. *Biochem J* 1998; 330: 51–526.

14. Dulloo A, Samec S. Uncoupling proteins: their role in adaptive thermogenesis and substrate metabolism reconsidered. *Br J Nutr* 2001; 80: 123–39.

15. Boss O, Hagen T, Lowell BB. Uncoupling proteins 2 and 3: potentials regulators of mitochondrial energy metabolism. *Diabetes* 2000; 49: 143–156.

16. Silva JE. The multiple contributions of thyroid hormone to heat production. *J Clin Invest* 2001; 108: 35–7.

17. Ribeiro MO, Carvalho SD, Schultz JJ, Chiellin G, Scanlan TS, Bianco AC, et al. Thyroid hormone-sympathetic interaction and adaptive thermogenesis are thyroid hormone isoforms-specific. *J Clin Invest* 2001; 108: 97–105.

Progress in Obesity Research: 9. Edited by *Geraldo Medeiros-Neto, Alfredo Halpern and Claude Bouchard*
©2003 John Libbey Eurotext Ltd, pp. 749–752.

CHAPTER 156

Ghrelin in the regulation of energy balance

Tamas L. Horvath[1,2], Sabrina Diano[1] and Matthias Tschöp[3]

[1]*Reproductive Neuroscience Unit, Department of Obstetrics and Gynecology; and*
[2]*Department of Neurobiology, Yale Medical School, New Haven, Connecticut, 06520, USA;*
[3]*Department of Pharmacology, German Institute of Human Nutrition, 14558 Bergholz-Rehbrücke, Germany*
[e-mail: tamas.horvath@yale.edu]

The discovery of ghrelin[7,25,29,30] and its influence on appetite, fuel utilization, body weight and body composition that is complementary to ghrelin's growth hormone-releasing effect[49], introduced yet another component to the complexity in the central regulation of energy balance. Ghrelin is predominantly produced by the stomach[12,15,26,29], while substantially lower amounts are expressed in the bowel[12,26], the pituitary[31], the kidney[33], the placenta[19], the testicles[45] and the hypothalamus[24,26,29]. Because circulating ghrelin is predominantly derived from the stomach and intestine and is binding at hypothalamic target neurons, its putative transfer across the blood brain barrier becomes an important factor. Circulating peripheral factors can influence central circuits regulating energy homeostasis, in part, via the so called circumventricular organs that are not protected by the blood brain barrier. These include the median eminence and ventromedial parts of the arcuate nucleus. However, ghrelin receptor expression and ghrelin binding also occurs in central areas that are clearly protected by the blood brain barrier such as the paraventricular nucleus (PVN) or the lateral hypothalamus (LH). In accordance with our own ongoing investigations, recent pilot studies have shown that ghrelin is present in several regions of the hypothalamus[24,26,29]. Ghrelin-positive cells have been identified in varying hypothalamic areas. Detection of hypothalamic ghrelin mRNA expression by use of polymerase-chain reaction (PCR) has also been accomplished[29], however, this issue needs to be further investigated by the detection and regional distribution of ghrelin mRNA by *in situ* hybridization.

Exogenous ghrelin induces adiposity in rodents by stimulating an acute increase in food intake, as well as triggering a reduction in fat utilization[2,22,28,36,40,49,54]. Adipogenic as well as orexigenic effects of ghrelin are independent from its ability to stimulate growth hormone secretion[36,49] and are most likely mediated by a specific central network of neurons that is also modulated by leptin[2,7,16,18,22,27,28,36,38,40,48,49,54]. Regulation of ghrelin secretion, as well as its biological effects, appear to be opposite those of leptin. In addition, a specific role for ghrelin might be to ensure the provision of calories that the pituitary axis require for growth, repair, reproduction and metabolic balance[22,48].

In humans, circulating ghrelin levels are decreased in chronic (obesity)[6,10,21,34,39,50] and acute caloric intake[1,5,8,9,10,17,46,50] states of positive energy balance, while plasma levels of ghrelin are increased by fasting[1,9,10,49] and in cachectic patients with anorexia nervosa, bulimia, cancer cachexia or cardiac cachexia[1,35,43,52]. A recent study shows a pre-meal rise of human plasma ghrelin, suggesting a possible role of ghrelin as a hunger signal triggering meal initiation[9]. Intriguing data in patients with Prader Willi syndrome who suffer from severe hyperorexia and morbid adiposity indicate a possible role for ghrelin in the pathogenesis of this disease: these patients have about three- to fourfold increased levels of circulating ghrelin[10], therefore impressively differing from other obese populations, where ghrelin secretion is significantly decreased[50]. The most promising results to date indicating a physiological role for ghrelin in human energy balance regulation were provided recently by Wren *et al.*, who demonstrated that ghrelin administration in humans caused enhanced appetite and increased food intake[53]. In rodents, fasting and hypoglycaemia increase ghrelin levels, while intake of food, especially carbohydrates (dextrose), decreases ghrelin secretion[3,22,47,49]. We speculate that this obvious connection between glucose levels, ghrelin secretion and GH secretion is likely to be involved in the physiological mechanism of diagnostic procedures such as oral glucose tolerance testing (for acromegaly) and insulin tolerance testing (for growth hormone deficiency).

In the brain, receptors for ghrelin were detected in multiple hypothalamic nuclei as well as in the hippocampus, substantia nigra, ventral tegmental area, and dorsal and median raphe nuclei[20,29,41,42,44] [Willesen et al., 1999]. Dickson and co-workers, first using synthetic GHS-R agonist, and then ghrelin, provided evidence that this novel metabolic hormone, in fact, interacts with hypothalamic peptidergic systems in the central regulation of metabolism[4,13,14,23,32]. For example, they found that following central ghrelin administration, c-fos, an early proto-oncogen that reflects cellular activity, is induced in the medial arcuate nucleus where NPY/AGRP cells are located[23]. It is also known, that Y1-receptor antagonists as well as melanocortin agonists and antisera to both NPY and AGRP may interfere with ghrelin's feeding-inducing effect[1,36,40]. However, absence of NPY in genetically engineered NPY-ko mice does not diminish ghrelin-induced feeding or adiposity suggesting a key-role for AGRP in the mediation of ghrelin's effects on energy balance[49]. The effect of ghrelin on metabolism seems to be the exact opposite to that of leptin[7,16,18,27,30,38,49]. In obesity, when plasma leptin levels are elevated, ghrelin plasma levels are decreased indicating physiological adaptations to the positive energy balance rather than an involvement in the aetiology of obesity[37,50]. Of course, it is important to note that while ghrelin is regulated acutely indicating a role for ghrelin as a meal initiating factor, leptin levels are not regulated by meals, but rather by actual increase of fat mass.

For the insightful and rapid understanding of ghrelin's role in energy homeostasis a broad intetrdisciplinary approach should be followed. This should incorporate the 'leptin experience' with its successes but more importantly with its shortcomings rather then simply replicating the studies conducted for the study of leptin. In fact, it is with the combination of electrophysiological and anatomical techniques with conventional physiological and molecular biological approaches that will most likely accomplish the most in gaining insightful understanding of ghrelin's action in the regulation of energy balance. Failure to do this will likely generate mass amount of data as was accomplished in relation to other promising aspects of energy metabolism rather than delivering cure for metabolism-related disorders, including obesity.

Acknowledgement: Supported by NIH grants MH-59847, RR-14451 and DK-060711.

References

1. Shirakami Ariyasu H, Takaya K, Tagami T, Ogawa Y, Hosoda K, Akamizu T, Suda M et al. Stomach is a major source of circulating ghrelin, and feeding state determines plasma ghrelin-like immunore activity levels in humans. *J Clin Endocrinol Metab* 2001; 86: 4753–8.

2. Asakawa A, Inui A, Kaga T, Yuzuriha H, Nagata T, Ueno N at al. Ghrelin is an appetite-stimulatory signal from stomach with structural resemblance to motilin. *Gastroenterology* 2001; 120: 337–45.

3. Bagnasco M, Kalra PS, Kalra SP. Ghrelin and leptin pulse discharge in fed and fasted rats. *Endocrinology* 2002; 143: 726–9.

4. Bailey AR, von Englehardt N, Leng G, Smith RG, Dickson SL. Growth hormone secretagogue activation of the arcuate nucleus and brainstem occurs via a non-noradrenergic pathway. *J Neuroendocrinol* 2000; 12: 191–7.

5. Beck B, Musse N, Stricker-Krongrad A. Ghrelin macronutrient intake and dietary preferences in long-evans rats. *Biochem Biophys Res Commun* 2002; 292: 1031–5.

6. Bellone S, Rapa A, Vivenza D, Castellino N, Petri A, Bellone J et al. (Circulating ghrelin levels as function of gender, pubertal status and adiposity in childhood. *J Endocrinol Invest* 2002; 25: RC13–15.

7. Bowers CY. Unnatural growth hormone-releasing peptide begets natural ghrelin. *J Clin Endocrinol Metab* 2001; 86: 1464–9.

8. Caixas A, Bashore C, Nash W, Pi-Sunyer F, Laferrere B. Insulin, unlike food intake, does not suppress ghrelin in human subjects. *J Clin Endocrinol Metab* 2002; 87: 1902.

9. Cummings E, Purnell JQ, Frayo SR, Schmidova K, Wisse BE, Weigle DS. A preprandial rise in plasma ghrelin levels suggests a role in meal initiation in humans. *Diabetes* 2001; 50: 1714–9.

10. Cummings DE, Weigle, DS, Frayo RS, Breen PA, Ma MK, Dellinger EP, Purnell JQ. Plasma ghrelin levels after diet-induced weight loss or gastric bypass surgery. *N Engl J Med* 2002; 346: 1623–30.

11. Cummings DE et al. *Nature Med* 2002 (in press).

12. Date Y, Kojima M, Hosoda H, Sawaguchi A, Mondal MS, Suganuma T et al. Ghrelin a novel growth hormone-releasing acylated peptide, is synthesized in a distinct endocrine cell type in the gastrointestinal tracts of rats and humans. *Endocrinology* 2000; 141: 4255–61.

13. Dickson SL, Leng G, Robinson IC. Systemic administration of growth hormone-releasing peptide activates hypothalamic arcuate neurons. *Neuroscience* 1993; 52: 303–6.

14. Dickson SL, Luckman SM. Induction of c-fos messenger ribonucleic acid in neuropeptide Y and growth hormone (GH)-releasing factor neurons in the rat arcuate nucleus following systemic injection of the GH secretagogue, GH-releasing peptide-6. *Endocrinology* 1997; 138: 771–7.

15. Dornonville de la Cour C, Bjorkqvist M, Sandvik AK, Bakke I, Zhao C, Chen D, Hakanson RA. Like cells in the rat stomach contain ghrelin and do not operate under gastrin control. *Regul Pept* 2001; 99: 141–50.

16. Elmquist JK, Maratos-Flier E, Saper CB, Flier JS. Unraveling the central nervous system pathways underlying responses to leptin. *Nature Neurosci* 1998; 6: 445–50.

17. English PJ, Ghatei MA, Malik IA, Bloom SR, Wilding JP. Food fails to suppress ghrelin levels in obese humans. *J Clin Endocrinol Metab* 2002; 87: 2984.

18. Friedman JM, Halaas JL. Leptin and the regulation of body weight in mammals. *Nature* 1998; 395: 763–70.

19. Gualillo O, Caminos J, Blanco M, Garcia-Caballero T, Kojima M, Kangawa K *et al.* Ghrelin a novel placental-derived hormone. *Endocrinology* 2001; 142: 788–94.

20. Guan XM, Yu H, Palyha OC, McKee KK, Feighner SD, Sirinathsinghji DJ *et al.* Distribution of mRNA encoding the growth hormone secretagogue receptor in brain and peripheral tissues. *Brain Res Mol Brain Res* 1997; 48: 23–9.

21. Hansen TK, Dall R, Hosoda H, Kojima M, Kangawa K, Christiansen JS, Jorgensen JO. Weight loss increases circulating levels of ghrelin in human obesity. *Clin Endocrinol* 2002; 56: 203–6.

22. Heiman ML, Tschöp M. Ghrelin acts to provide the calories that growth hormone requires for growth and repair. Denver, CO: Proc 83th Meeting of The Endocrine Society; 2001. p.33.

23. Hewson AK, Dickson SL. Systemic administration of ghrelin induces Fos and Egr-1 proteins in the hypothalamic arcuate nucleus of fasted and fed rats. *J Neuroendocrinol* 2000; 12: 1047–9.

24. Horvath TL, Tschop M, Smith RG, Cowley M, Cone R, Diano S. Ghrelin: a novel hypothalamic neuropeptide with unique anatomical distribution. San Diego, CA: 31st Annual Meeting of the Society for Neuroscience; 2001.

25. Hosoda H, Kojima M, Matsuo H, Kangawa K. Purification and characterization of rat des-Gln14-Ghrelin, a second endogenous ligand for the growth hormone secretagogue receptor. *J Biol Chem* 2000; 275: 21995–2000.

26. Kagotani Y, Sakata I, Yamazaki M, Nakamura K, Hayashi Y, Kangawa K. Localization of ghrelin-immunopositive cells in the rat hypothalamus and intestinal tract. Denver, CO: Proc 83th Meeting of The Endocrine Society; 2001. p. 337.

27. Kalra SP, Dube MG, Pu S, Xu B, Horvath TL, Kalra PS. Interacting appetite-regulating pathways in the hypothalamic regulation of body weight. *Endocr Rev* 1999; 20: 68–100.

28. Kamegai J, Tamura H, Shimizu T, Ishii S, Sugihara H, Wakabayashi I. Central effect of ghrelin, an endogenous growth hormone secretagogue, on hypothalamic peptide gene expression. *Endocrinology* 2000; 141: 4797–800.

29. Kojima M, Hosoda H, Date Y, Nakazato M, Matsuo H, Kangawa K. Ghrelin is a growth-hormone-releasing acylated peptide from stomach. *Nature* 1999; 402: 656–60.

30. Kojima M, Hosoda H, Matsuo H, Kangawa K. Ghrelin: discovery of the natural endogenous ligand for the growth hormone secretagogue receptor. *Trends Endocrinol Metab* 2001; 12: 118–22.

31. Korbonits M Kojima M Kangawa K Grossman AB. Presence of ghrelin in normal and adenomatous human pituitary. *Endocrine* 2001; 14: 101–4.

32. Luckman SM Rosenzweig I Dickson SL. Activation of arcuate nucleus neurons by systemic administration of leptin and growth hormone-releasing peptide-6 in normal and fasted rats. *Neuroendocrinology* 1999; 70: 93–100.

33. Mori K, Yoshimoto A, Takaya K, Hosoda K, Ariyasu H, Yahata K. Kidney produces a novel acylated peptide, ghrelin. *FEBS Letters* 2000; 486: 213–6.

34. Muccioli G, Tschop M, Papotti M, Deghenghi R, Heiman M, Ghigo E. Neuroendocrine and peripheral activities of ghrelin: implications in metabolism and obesity. *Eur J Pharmacol* 2002; 440: 235–54.

35. Nagaya N, Uematsu M, Kojima M, Date Y, Nakazato M, Okumura H *et al.* Elevated circulating level of ghrelin in cachexia associated with chronic heart failure: relationships between ghrelin and anabolic/catabolic factors. *Circulation* 2001; 104: 2034–8.

36. Nakazato M, Murakami N, Date Y, Kojima M, Matsuo H, Kangawa K, Matsukura S. A role for ghrelin in the central regulation of feeding. *Nature* 2001; 409: 194–8.

37. Ravussin E, Tschöp M, Heiman ML, Bouchard C. Plasma ghrelin concentration and energy balance: overfeeding and negative energy balance studies in twins. *J Clin Endocrinol Metab* 2001; 86: 4547–51.

38. Schwartz M, Woods S, Porte D Jr, Seeley RJ, Baskin DG. Central nervous system control of food intake. *Nature* 2000; 404: 661–71.

39. Shiiya T, Nakazato, Mizuta M, Date Y, Mondal MS, Tanaka M *et al.* Plasma ghrelin levels in lean and obese humans and the effect of glucose on ghrelin secretion. *J Clin Endocrinol Metab* 2002; 87: 240–4.

40. Shintani M, Ogawa Y, Ebihara K, Megumi A, Miyanaga F, Takaya K *et al.* Ghrelin, an endogenous growth hormone secretagogue, is a novel orexigenic peptide that antagonizes leptin action through the activation of hypothalamic neuropeptide Y/Y1 receptor pathway. *Diabetes* 2001; 50: 227–32.

41. Shuto Y, Shibasaki T, Wada K, Parhar I, Kamegai J, Sugihara H, *et al.* Generation of polyclonal antiserum against the growth hormone secretagogue receptor (GHS-R): evidence that the GHS-R exists in the hypothalamus, pituitary and stomach of rats. *Life Sci* 2001; 68: 991–6.

42. Smith RG, Leonard R, Bailey AR, Palyha O, Feighner S, Tan C *et al.* Growth hormone secretagogue receptor family members and ligands. *Endocrine* 2001; 14: 9–14.

43. Tanaka M, Naruo T, Muranaga T, Yasuhara D, Shiiya T, Nakazato M *et al.* Increased fasting plasma ghrelin levels in patients with bulimia nervosa. *Eur J Endocrinol* 2002; 146: R1–3.

44. Tannenbaum GS, Lapointe M, Beaudet A, Howard AD. Expression of growth hormone secretagogue-receptors by growth hormone-releasing hormone neurons in the mediobasal hypothalamus. *Endocrinology* 1998, 139; 4420–3.

45. Tena-Sempere M, Barreiro ML, Gonzalez LC, Gaytan F, Zhang FP, Caminos JE *et al.* Novel expression and functional role of ghrelin in rat testis. *Endocrinology* 2002; 143: 717–25.

46. Tolle V, Bassant MH, Zizzari P, Poindessous-Jazat F, Tomasetto C, Epelbaum J, Bluet-Pajot MT. Ultradian rhythmicity of ghrelin secretion in relation with GH, feeding behavior, and sleep-wake patterns in rats. *Endocrinology* 2002; 143: 1353–61.

47. Toshinai K, Mondal MS, Nakazato M, Date Y, Murakami N, Kojima M *et al.* Upregulation of Ghrelin expression in the stomach upon fasting, insulin-induced hypoglycaemia, and leptin administration. *Biochem Biophys Res Commun* 2001; 281: 1220–5.

48. Tschop M, Mayer JP, Heiman ML. Hypophysectomy prevents ghrelin-induced adiposity and increases gastric ghrelin secretion in rats. *Obes Res* 2002 (in press).

49. Tschöp M, Smiley D, Heiman ML. Ghrelin induces adiposity in rodents. *Nature* 2000; 407: 908–13.

50. Tschöp M, Wawarta R, Riepl RL, Friedrich S, Bidlingmaier M, Landgraf R, Folwaczny C. Post-prandial decrease of circulating human ghrelin levels. *J Endocrinol Invest* 2001; 24: RC19–21.

51. Tschöp M, Weyer C, Tataranni PA, Devanarayan V, Ravussin E, Heiman ML. Circulating ghrelin levels are decreased in human obesity. *Diabetes* 2001; 50: 707–9.

52. Wisse BE, Frayo RS, Schwartz MW, Cummings DE. Reversal of cancer anorexia by blockade of central melanocortin receptors in rats. *Endocrinology* 2001; 142: 3292–301.

53. Wren AM, Seal LJ, Cohen MA, Brynes AE, Frost GS, Murphy KG *et al.* Ghrelin enhances appetite and increases food intake in humans. *J Clin Endocrinol Metab* 2001; 86: 5992.

54. Wren AM, Small CJ, Ward HL, Murphy KG, Dakin CL, Taheri S *et al.* The novel hypothalamic peptide ghrelin stimulates food intake and growth hormone secretion. *Endocrinology* 2000; 141: 4325–4328.

Progress in Obesity Research: 9. Edited by *Geraldo Medeiros-Neto, Alfredo Halpern* and *Claude Bouchard*
©2003 John Libbey Eurotext Ltd, pp. 753–756.

CHAPTER 157

Active promoter elements in the human agouti related protein gene

Fulu Bai and George Argyropoulos

Pennington Biomedical Research Center, 6400 Perkins Road, Baton Rouge, LA 70808, USA
[e-mail: argyrog@pbrc.edu]

Introduction

AgRP is a potent anabolic effector of food intake[1]. It is expressed in the arcuate nucleus of the hypothalamus, the testes and the adrenal gland, and is upregulated in obese and diabetic mice[2,3] and by fasting[4]. AgRP exerts its anabolic effects on food intake by antagonizing the alpha-Melanocyte Stimulating Hormone (α-MSH) at its receptors, melanocortin receptors 3 and 4 (MC3R and MC4R)[5]. The murine (mAgRP) and human (hAgRP) orthologs stimulate hyperphagia when administered intracerebroventricularly (i.c.v.)[6,7] or when overexpressed in transgenic mice[8]. In addition, elevated plasma levels of hAgRP have been reported in obese men[9] while a 2-h fast resulted in 73 per cent increase of plasma hAgRP concentration[10].

We have determined the complete genomic structure of hAgRP and identified upstream sequences with significant promoter activities[11,12]. The 5' untranslated exon had significant promoter activity in a periphery cell line only, 24 h following transfection[12], suggesting a role for this exon in the peripheral expression of hAgRP. Here, we present data that show significant activity by the 5' non-coding exon in a mouse hypothalamus cell line 48 h after transfection (the 5' non-coding exon had no activity in this cell line at the shorter interval of 24 h after transfection)[12]. The effects of hormones on hAgRP promoter activity were also examined. Leptin downregulates AgRP expression[13] while ghrelin has opposite effects[14]. We now report regions in the promoter of hAgRP that respond to leptin and ghrelin treatments.

Methods

Constructs to examine promoter activity were directionally cloned (with Sac I and Xho I restriction recognition sites incorporated into the primers) into the pGL3-basic luciferase reporter vector (Promega, Madison, WI). cell culture was carried out under standard conditions in a humidified incubator at 37 °C and 5 per cent CO_2. the GT1-7 cells[15] were grown in DMEM, l-glutamine, and 10 per cent fetal calf serum (FCS) supplemented with the antibiotics penicillin-streptomycin-gentamycin. cells were serum starved for 24 h prior to transfection. Transient co-transfections with promoter/pgl3 constructs and β-gal plasmids were carried out for 24 h in the absence of serum using the geneporter2 transfection reagent as prescribed by the manufacturer (Gene Therapy Systems, San Diego, CA). Subsequently, the media were supplemented with 20 per cent FCS for another 24 h. Cells were harvested using 1x Geneporter2 lysis buffer and the lysates were assayed for luciferase and β-galactosidase activities, as prescribed by the assay manufacturer (Promega, Madison, wi) in a luminometer (Zylux Corporation, Pforzheim, Germany). All luciferase activity measurements were normalized to β-galactosidase values. the data are presented as fold-increase of luciferase activity over the empty vector control (pGL3-basic). In the case of basal promoter activity, a series of four duplicate, independent, transfection experiments were conducted per construct. In the case of the hormone treatments, a series of three duplicate experiments were performed. Leptin (1 nM) and ghrelin (50 nM) were provided in the media for 8 h prior to harvesting the cells.

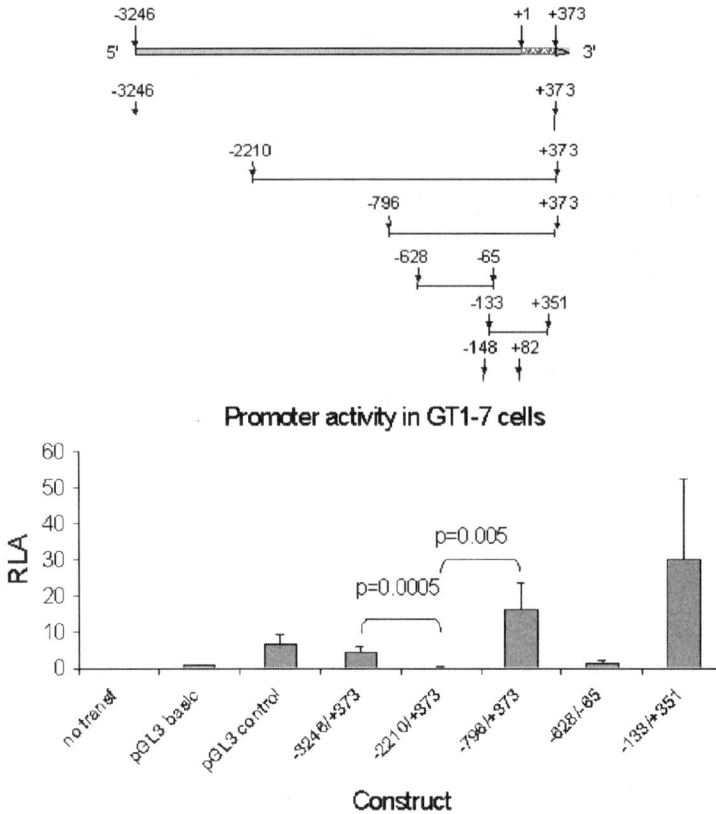

Fig. 1. Transfection constructs and hAgRP promoter activity. (a, top) Schematic representation of transfection constructs in the pGL-3 basic vector and their relative position with respect to the hAgRP gene structure. (b, below) Relative Luciferase Activity (RLA) for promoter constructs in transiently transfected GT1-7 hypothalamus cells is shown as a fold-increase over the pGL-3 basic vector.

Results and discussion

Luciferase reporter constructs of the hAgRP promoter were made in an effort to identify active regions and cis-acting elements that respond to hormonal stimuli. Based on DNA sequences available from the Bacterial Artificial Chromosome (BAC) with GenBank accession number AC027682, we made several overlapping constructs (Fig. 1a). Activity of constructs was examined in the mouse hypothalamus cell line, GT1-7, 48 h after transfection. Suitability of this cell line was confirmed by Real time RT-PCR that showed robust expression of mAgRP (data not shown). Consistent with our previous data for promoter activity in the periphery[12], two constructs that contained the 5' non-coding exon (−796/+373 and −133/+351) had the highest promoter activities but the longer construct that also contained the 5' non-coding exon (−2210/+373) had no promoter activity (Fig. 1b). Given that construct −628/−65, that did not contain the 5' non-coding exon had no activity, we hypothesize that region −2210/−65 might contain binding sites for silencer(s) that are active at basal conditions in this cell line. Promoter activity recovered, however, in the longer −3246/+373 construct, despite the fact that it contained section −2210/−65, which suggests that region −3246/−2210 might be necessary for the transcriptional activation of the gene and it might contain binding sites for transcription co-activators or enhancers.

Leptin downregulates AgRP expression[13], while ghrelin has opposite effects[14]. We therefore treated transiently transfected GT1-7 cells (with promoter constructs) with the two hormones to examine their effects on promoter activity. There were significant effects by leptin on promoter activities of the three constructs we examined ($P = 0.005$) (Fig. 2a). Specifically, two of the three constructs containing the 5' non-coding exon were downregulated by leptin suggesting that the region −769/+373 may contain response elements for leptin's action on AgRP. This is not surprising given that we have identified

Effects of leptin on hAgRP promoter in GT1-7

Effects of ghrelin on AgRP promoter in GT1-7

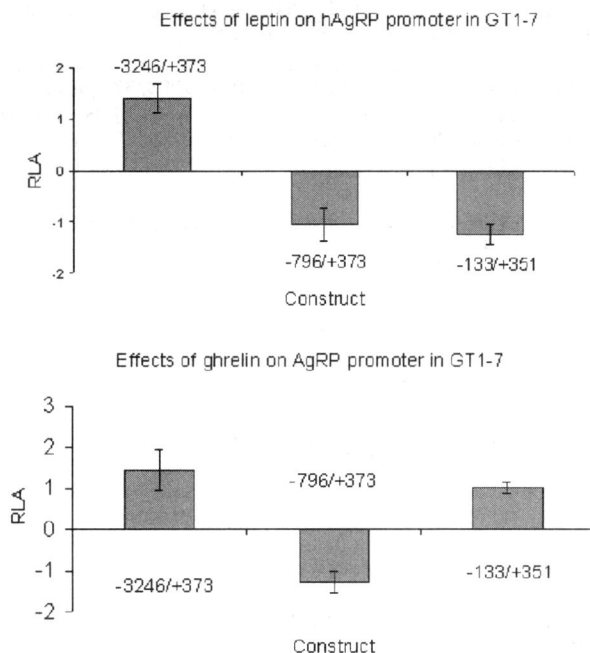

Fig. 2. Hormonal effects on hAgRP promoter activity in GT1-7 hypothalamus cells. Cells were transiently transfected with various promoter constructs and treated with 1 nM of Leptin (a) or 50 nM of Ghrelin (b).

algorithmically two putative binding sites for the Signal Transducers and Activators of Transcription (STATs) in regions −362/−353 and −122/−114. STAT transactivators have docking sites for the long isoform of the leptin receptor and are potential mediators of the anti-obesity effects of leptin[19]. Construct −3246/+373, however, was upregulated by leptin, which may be due to the presence of region −3246/−2210 in the construct, which may have binding sites for transcriptional activators or enhancers (Fig.1b). Ghrelin also had significant effects on the promoter activity of the constructs ($P = 0.0004$) (Fig. 2b). Specifically, constructs −3246/+373 and −133/+351 were upregulated but construct −796/+373 was unexpectedly downregulated. This could be due to the presence of the −628/−65 region in this construct that may have binding sites for silencers (Fig. 1b).

We conclude that regions −3246/−2210 and −65/+351 might be involved in the transcriptional activation while region −2210/−65 might be involved in silencing hAgRP. The promoter activity of region −628/−65 was not only the lowest at basal conditions but was consistently downregulated by both leptin and ghrelin which further suggests a functional role for this region in silencing hAgRP. Additional pull-down and footprinting experiments are required to identify the transcriptional components (i.e. transcription factors, hormone receptors, activators, co-activators, silencers) that bind to these regions in the hAgRP promoter.

Acknowledgements: This project was supported in part by a US Army grant (DAMD 17-97-2-7013).

References

1. Schwartz MW, Woods SC, Porte D Jr, Seeley RI, Baskin DG. Central nervous system control of food intake. *Nature* 2000; 404; 661–71.

2. Ollmann MM, Wilson BD, Yang YK *et al.* Antagonism of central melanocortin receptors *in vitro* and *in vivo* by agouti-related protein. *Science* 1997; 278: 135–8.

3. Shutter JR, Graham M, Kinsey AC, Scully S, Luthy R, Stark KL. Hypothalamic expression of ART, a novel gene related to agouti, is up- regulated in obese and diabetic mutant mice. *Genes Dev* 1997; 11: 593–602.

4. Adam CL, Archer ZA, Findlay PA, Thomas L, Marie M. Hypothalamic gene expression in sheep for cocaine- and amphetamine-regulated transcript, pro-opiomelanocortin, neuropeptide y, agouti-related Peptide and leptin receptor and responses to negative energy balance. *Neuroendocrinology* 2002; 75: 250–6.

5. Ste Marie L, Miura GI, Marsh DJ, Yagaloff K, Palmiter RD. A metabolic defect promotes obesity in mice lacking melanocortin-4 receptors. *Proc Nat Acad Sci USA* 2000; 97: 12339–44.

6. Rosenfeld RD, Zeni L, Welcher AA *et al*. Biochemical, biophysical, and pharmacological characterization of bacterially expressed human agouti-related protein. *Biochemistry* 1998; 37: 16041–52.

7. Rossi M, Kim MS, Morgan DG *et al*. A C-terminal fragment of Agouti-related protein increases feeding and antagonizes the effect of alpha-melanocyte stimulating hormone *in vivo*. *Endocrinology* 1998; 139: 4428–31.

8. Graham M, Shutter JR, Sarmiento U, Sarosi L, Stark KL. Overexpression of Agrt leads to obesity in transgenic mice. *Nature Genet* 1997; 17273–4.

9. Katsuki A, Sumida Y, Gabazza EC *et al*. Plasma levels of agouti-related protein are increased in obese men. *J Clin Endocrinol Metab* 2001; 86: 1921–4.

10. Shen CP, Wu KK, Shearman LP *et al*. Plasma agouti-related protein level: a possible correlation with fasted and fed States in humans and rats. *J Neuroendocrinol* 2002; 14: 607–10.

11. Mayfield DK, Brown AM, Page GP, Garvey WT, Shriver MD, Argyropoulos G. A role for the agouti related protein promoter in obesity and type 2 diabetes. *Biochem Biophys Res Commun* 2001; 287: 568–73.

12. Brown AM, Mayfield DK, Volaufova J, Argyropoulos G. The gene structure and minimal promoter of the human agouti related protein. *Gene* 2001; 277: 231–8.

13. Korner J, Savontaus E, Chua SC Jr, Leibel RL, Wardlaw SL. Leptin regulation of Agrp and Npy mRNA in the rat hypothalamus. *J Neuroendocrinol* 2001; 13: 959–66.

14. Kamegai J, Tamura H, Shimizu T, Ishii S, Sugihara H, Wakabayashi I. Central effect of ghrelin, an endogenous growth hormone secretagogue, on hypothalamic peptide gene expression. *Endocrinology* 2000; 141: 4797–800.

15. Wetsel WC, Eraly SA, Whyte DB, Mellon PL. Regulation of gonadotropin-releasing hormone by protein kinase-A and -C in immortalized hypothalamic neurons. *Endocrinology* 1993; 132: 2360–70.

16. Ahima RS, Hileman SM. Postnatal regulation of hypothalamic neuropeptide expression by leptin: implications for energy balance and body weight regulation. *Regul Pept* 2000; 92: 1–7.

17. Schwartz MW, Baskin DG, Bukowski TR *et al*. Specificity of leptin action on elevated blood glucose levels and hypothalamic neuropeptide Y gene expression in ob/ob mice. *Diabetes* 1996; 45: 531–5.

18. Arvaniti K, Huang Q, Richard D. Effects of leptin and corticosterone on the expression of corticotropin-releasing hormone, agouti-related protein, and proopiomelanocortin in the brain of ob/ob mouse. *Neuroendocrinology* 2001; 73: 227–36.

19. Ghilardi N, Ziegler S, Wiestner A, Stoffel R, Helm MH, Skoda RC. Defective STAT signaling by the leptin receptor in diabetic mice. *Proc Natl Acad Sci USA* 1996; 93: 6231–5.

Progress in Obesity Research: 9. Edited by *Geraldo Medeiros-Neto, Alfredo Halpern and Claude Bouchard*
©2003 John Libbey Eurotext Ltd, pp. 757–759.

CHAPTER 158

CNS melanocortins and the control of food intake

Randy J. Seeley

Department of Psychiatry, University of Cincinnati, Cincinnati OH 45267-0559, USA
[e-mail: Randy.Seeley@uc.edu]

An enormous body of evidence links melanocortin activity in the CNS to the maintained level of body fat stores in the body. The CNS melanocortin system encompasses several peptides and receptors. There are currently five cloned melanocortin (MC) receptors of which both MC3 and MC4 receptor have substantial expression in the CNS. Of these, the stronger case can be made for MC4 receptors being involved in the control of food intake. When administered into the 3rd ventricle of the rat, selective MC4 receptor agonists inhibit and selective MC4 antagonists stimulate food intake[1]. Consistent with this, MC4 receptor 'knockout' mice have increased food intake and frank obesity[2], and they are insensitive to the actions of non-selective MC4 receptor agonists to reduce food intake[3]. MC3 receptor knockouts do have elevated levels of body adiposity but do not have increased food intake or decreased energy expenditure and thus its exact role remains controversial[4].

The precursor molecule of hypothalamic melanocortins is proopiomelanocortin or POMC. In addition to several other important neuropeptides, POMC encodes α-melanocyte stimulating hormone (α-MSH), a melanocortin that is an agonist at both MC3 and MC4 receptors. When given into the 3rd ventricle, α-MSH and other non-selective melanocortin receptor agonists (including the synthetic analogue, MTII) reduce food intake and body weight, whereas administration of melanocortin receptor antagonists (such as SHU-9119) increases food intake and body weight[5,6].

The activity of this melanocortin system appears to be carefully regulated by energy balance. Fasting reduces POMC expression in the ARC[7]. POMC activity is regulated by leptin since there are leptin receptors on POMC neurons[8] and *ob/ob* and *db/db* mice both have dramatically reduced POMC expression levels in the ARC[9,10]. Central leptin replacement reverses the fasting-induced reduction of POMC expression in normal animals[9]. Moreover, direct evidence links leptin effects to changes in melanocortin signaling. Blockade of central melanocortin receptors can completely eliminate the effect of leptin to induce Fos-like immunoreactivity (FLI) in the PVN and to reduce food intake[11]. Preliminary data indicate that in addition to leptin, insulin receptors are also found on POMC neurons and that central melanocortin receptor blockade can also block the anorexic effect of insulin[12]. Involuntary overfeeding that results in increased body weight and circulating levels of leptin and insulin increases POMC gene expression in the ARC and that the hypophagia that follows this regimen can be blocked by central melanocortin receptor blockade[13]. All of this evidence points to the endogenous POMC/α-MSH/MC4 hypothalamic system as being a key effector pathway capable of eliciting robust decreases of food intake and body weight.

One of the unique features of the CNS melanocortin system is the existence of an endogenous antagonist termed Agouti-Related Protein (AgRP). AgRP is a potent antagonist of both MC3 and MC4 receptors[14-16] and is synthesized in a discrete population of neurons only in the ARC nucleus[14]. Interestingly, AgRP is not co-localized with POMC-producing cells but is heavily co-localized with NPY-producing cells[17]. AgRP cells also express long-form leptin receptors[18] and AgRP expression is inhibited by leptin[16]. A biologically active fragment of AgRP administered i3vt potently increases short-term food intake at doses as low as 0.01 nmole[19-20]. Moreover, these low doses produce a robust increase in food intake 24 h after AgRP administration. Even more surprising was that a single administration of AgRP could produce increases in food intake for up to 6 days. When compared at short intervals, AgRP is not as potent as NPY. However, at intervals greater than a few hours, AgRP is far more potent. So whereas

NPY has received considerable attention as a particularly potent orexigenic peptide, the effects of AgRP deserve at least as much attention.

The mechanism by which a single administration of a peptide could exert such long-lasting effects on food intake is unclear. One possibility is that AgRP simply has a very long-half life and exerts its prolonged effect on intake by continuing to act as an antagonist for melanocortin receptors. We tested this hypothesis by administering AgRP and then probing animals with a dose of a melanocortin agonist (MTII) either immediately after the AgRP administration or 24 h later when food intake following a single injection of AgRP is still elevated. As anticipated, when MTII is administered immediately after AgRP, MTII's effect to suppress food intake is completely blocked by AgRP. This implies that the initial orexigenic action of AgRP occurs through antagonism of melanocortin receptors. In contrast, when MTII is administered 24 h after AgRP, it suppresses food intake as potently as if no AgRP had been administered, implying that AgRP is no longer inhibiting melanocortin receptors[19]. The conclusion from these studies is that continued melanocortin receptor antagonism is not the mechanism by which AgRP exerts its long-term effect on food intake. A more likely possibility is that the initial interaction of AgRP with melanocortin receptors produces a cascade of events that involves genomic effects and new protein synthesis that result in an animal that is biased to consume more food over the next several days.

In an attempt to identify the neural circuits that are recruited to mediate these long-term effects of AgRP, we compared the Fos response in a number of brain regions following a single injection of either AgRP or NPY at 2 and 24 h after i3vt administration. Fos-like-immunoreactivity (FLI) measured after 2 h was increased comparably by both AgRP and NPY in several regions of the CNS including the paraventricular nucleus of the hypothalamus (PVN). Hence it would appear that the acute orexigenic effects of these two peptides are mediated by potentially overlapping neuronal circuits[21]. Consistent with its relatively brief stimulation of food intake, NPY did not increase FLI in any brain region 24 h after administration. In contrast, and consistent with its long-lasting effect on food intake, AgRP induced an increase in FLI in several brain regions 24 h after administration. Of particular interest, there was no increase in FLI in the PVN as there had been at 2 h. At 24 h, FLI was dramatically increased in the LH, a site that did not exhibit FLI 2 h after AgRP administration. The LH has long been associated with stimulatory effects on food intake and two peptide systems have been identified in the LH that can increase food intake: melanin concentrating hormone (MCH) and the orexins/hypocretins. MCH and the orexins are not co-localized to the same neurons within the LH. Interestingly, the fos induced by AgRP in the LH is distributed in many of the orexin but not MCH containing neurons indicating that one potential downstream target of AgRP's actions may be the orexins.

Levine, Billington and their colleagues reported that many of the critical effects of NPY, including its stimulatory effect on food intake, depend on downstream activation of opioid receptors[22]. Therefore a reasonable hypothesis is that AgRP-induced food intake also depends on opioid receptors. Consistent with this hypothesis, rats treated with a sub-threshold dose of the non-specific opioid receptor antagonist, naloxone immediately after AgRP, showed no AgRP-induced increase in food intake. However, when given 24 h after AgRP administration, naloxone did not reverse the continued hyperphagia that occurs long after AgRP administration. The conclusion is that whereas the acute effects of AgRP engage opioid receptors, the long-term effects do not[23]. Recently, we have used antagonists specific for one of the three opioid receptor sub-types. While neither a kappa nor mu-specific antagonist could inhibit AgRP-induced food intake, combined kappa and mu receptor blockade blocks AgRP-induced food intake. Future research will need to address the neuroanatomical locations of the critical opioid receptors that are activated by AgRP.

Despite the impressive effects of AgRP to increase food intake when either overexpressed in transgenic mice or administered into the CNS, mice with targeted disruption of the AgRP gene have normal food intake and body weight[24]. Thus, unlike mutations of either the MC4 receptor or POMC that result in increased food intake and obesity[2,25], AgRP would appear to not be essential to normal body weight regulation. This is similar to mice with targeted deletion of NPY who also show no gross differences in total food consumption under *ad libitum* conditions[26]. While a complete discussion of this issue is outside the scope of this review, the gross discrepancy between the pharmacological and the genetic loss-of-function experiments has yet to be sufficiently addressed and deserves further attention using genetic strategies that allow for targeting of these genes at later stages in neural development.

The picture that emerges concerning the CNS melanocortin system is one that provides an essential inhibitory tone to restrain food intake and body weight. That system, however, has multiple mechanisms for regulating its signaling. In addition to having levels of the agonist influenced by a number of important peripheral factors related to energy balance, signaling can be potently regulated by levels of the endogenous antagonist. Thus while the central importance of the melanocortin system to body weight regulation makes it an attractive target as a therapeutic strategy for obesity, the existence of an endogenous antagonist that should be upregulated by weight loss represents a potentially powerful compensatory mechanism that may limit efficacy of MC4 agonists for the treatment of obesity.

Acknowledgements: This work was supported by funds from NIH (DK54080, DK17844, DK56863) and funds from the Procter & Gamble Co.

References

1. Benoit SC *et al.* A novel selective melanocortin-4 receptor agonist reduces food intake in rats and mice without producing aversive consequences. *J Neurosci* 2000; 20(9): 3442–8.

2. Huszar D *et al.* Targeted disruption of the melanocortin-4 receptor results in obesity in mice. *Cell* 1997; 88(Jan 10): 131–41.

3. Marsh D *et al.* Response of melanocortin-4 receptor-deficient mice to anorectic and orexigenic peptides. *Nature Genet* 1999; 21: 19–22.

4. Chen AS *et al.* Inactivation of the mouse melanocortin-3 receptor results in increased fat mass and reduced lean body mass [In: Process Citation]. *Nature Genet* 2000; 26(1): 97–102.

5. Fan W *et al.* Role of melanocortinergic neurons in feeding and the agouti obesity syndrome. *Nature* 1997; 385: 165–8.

6. Thiele T *et al.* Central infusion of melanocortin agonist MTII in rats: assessment of c-Fos expression and taste aversion. *Am J Physiol* 1998; 274: R248–54.

7. Bergendahl M *et al.* Short-term starvation decreases POMC mRNA but does not alter GnRH mRNA in the brain of adult male rats. *Neuroendocrinology* 1992; 56: 913–20.

8. Cheung CC, Clifton DK, Steiner RA. Proopiomelanocortin neurons are direct targets for leptin in the hypothalamus. *Endocrinology* 1997; 138: 4489–92.

9. Schwartz MW *et al.* Leptin increases hypothalamic proopiomelanocoritin (POMC) mRNA expression in the rostral arcuate nucleus. *Diabetes* 1997; 46: 2119–23.

10. Mizuno T *et al.* Hypothalamic pro-opiomelanocortin mRNA is reduced by fasting and in ob/ob and db/db mice, but is stimulated by leptin. *Diabetes* 1998; 47: 294–7.

11. Seeley R *et al.* Melanocortin receptors in leptin effects. *Nature* 1997; 390: 349.

12. Benoit SC *et al.* The catabolic action of insulin in the brain is mediated by melanocortins. *J Neurosci* (in press).

13. Hagan M *et al.* Role of the CNS melanocortin system in the response to overfeeding. *J Neurosci* 1999; 19: 2362–2367.

14. Fong T *et al.* ART (protein product of agouti-related transcript) as an antagonist of MC-3 and MC-4 receptors. *Biochem Biophys Res Commun* 1997; 237: 629–31.

15. Ollmann M *et al.* Antagonism of central melanocortin receptors *in vitro* and *in vivo* by agouti-related protein. *Science* 1997; 278: 135–8.

16. Shutter J *et al.* Hypothalamic expression of ART, a novel gene related to agouti, is up-regulated in obese and diabetic mutant mice. *Genes Dev* 1997; 11: 593–602.

17. Hahn TM *et al.* Coexpression of Agrp and NPY in fasting-activated hypothalamic neurons. *Nature Neurosci* 1998; 1: 271–2.

18. Baskin DG *et al.* Leptin receptor long form splice variant protein expression in neuron cell bodies of the brain and colocalization with neuropeptide Y mRNA in the arcuate nucleus. *J Histochem Cytochem* 1999; 47: 353–62.

19. Hagan MM *et al.* Long-term orexigenic effects of AgRP-(83-132) involve mechanisms other than melanocortin receptor blockade. *Am J Physiol* 2000; 279: R47–R52.

20. Rossi M *et al.* A C-terminal fragment of Agouti-related protein increases feeding and antagonizes the effect of alpha-melanocyte stimulating hormone *in vivo*. *Endocrinology* 1998; 139: 4428–31.

21. Hagan MM *et al.* Immediate and Prolonged Patterns of Agouti-Related Peptide-(83-132)- Induced c-Fos Activation in Hypothalamic and Extrahypothalamic Sites. *Endocrinology* 2001; 142(3): 1050–6.

22. Kotz CM *et al.* Effects of opioid antagonists naloxone and naltrexone on neuropeptide Y-induced feeding and brown fat thermogenesis in the rat. Neural site of action. *J Clin Invest* 1995; 96(1): 163–70.

23. Hagan MM *et al.* Opioid receptor involvement in the effect of AgRP- (83-132) on food intake and food selection. *Am J Physiol Regul Integr Comp Physiol* 2001; 280(3): R814–R821.

24. Qian S *et al.* Neither agouti-related protein nor neuropeptide Y is critically required for the regulation of energy homeostasis in mice. *Mol Cell Biol* 2002; 22(14): 5027–35.

25. Yaswen L *et al.* Obesity in the mouse model of pro-opiomelanocortin deficiency responds to peripheral melanocortin. *Nature Med* 1999; 5(9): 1066–70.

26. Erickson JC, Clegg KE, Palmiter RD. Sensitivity to leptin and susceptibility to seizures of mice lacking neuropeptide Y. *Nature* 1996; 381: 415–8.

Progress in Obesity Research: 9. Edited by *Geraldo Medeiros-Neto, Alfredo Halpern and Claude Bouchard*
©2003 John Libbey Eurotext Ltd, pp. 760–765.

CHAPTER 159

Overview of the central pathways involved in the control of food intake and energy expenditure

Bernard Beck

Centre de Recherches UHP-EA 3453/IFR 111, Systèmes Neuromodulateurs des Comportements Ingestifs, 38 rue Lionnois, Nancy, France
[e-mail: Bernard.Beck@nancy.inserm.fr]

Researchers have focused their interest on central mechanisms that regulate feeding behaviour for over more than sixty years now. An important step was the discovery in the early 1940s of two specific brain areas that could control food intake either positively or negatively[1,2]. These areas are located in the hypothalamus. The ventromedian nucleus (VMN) was considered as 'the' satiety centre as when it is electrolytically destroyed in the rat, the animal becomes hyperphagic and obese. On the other hand, the lateral hypothalamus (LH) was considered as 'the' feeding centre as its electrolytic lesion induces anorexia and weight loss. The discovery of these two areas has led to the dual centre hypothesis for the regulation of food intake. This convincing hypothesis however did not resist to the progress in neuroanatomy and physiology. Several other hypothalamic areas were also involved in the regulation of feeding behaviour. The most important are the paraventricular nucleus (PVN), the dorsomedian nucleus (DMN) and the suprachiasmatic nucleus (SCN)[3–5]. The latter is the biological clock that regulate the different physiological rhythms including the feeding rhythm. The arcuate nucleus (ARC) located on the base of the brain constitute an important interface between these upper centres and periphery.

Progress in tracing techniques has allowed to show that neurons in these areas are closely interconnected through specific axonal projections and therefore constitute complex regulatory networks. These intra-hypothalamic networks receive different inputs from the fore brain (sensory, gustatory, learning, memory). They also receive inputs from the hindbrain and more particularly from the nucleus of the tractus solitarius in the brainstem. This area constitutes an essential link for the integration of peripheral information provided more particularly by the postprandial hormones secreted by the gastrointestinal tract and partly conveyed to the brain by the vagus nerve. The best examples of these hormones are cholecystokinin (CCK) and glucagon-like peptides[6,7]. They are involved in meal termination and constitute satiety signals. This connection with the periphery is not limited to the gut. Organs such as the pancreas and adipose tissue which contribute to the metabolism and storage of the ingested energy also provide information to the brain. The main mediators of this information at the hypothalamic level are leptin[8] and insulin[9]. They are secreted in direct proportion to the quantity of food ingested and the levels of energy stores. These adiposity signals convey their information to the hypothalamus through specific receptors located on different populations of neurons present in the arcuate nucleus. All these signals are integrated in the hypothalamus to produce the adequate feeding response adapted to the need of energy of the entire organism.

Two important pathways in energy homeostasis: the neuropeptide Y (NPY) and pro-opiomelanocortin (POMC) systems

From the discovery of one of the most potent orexigenic peptide, neuropeptide Y in the early 1980s, much attention has been focused on the arcuate and paraventricular nuclei. These areas not only contain NPY but also numerous neuromediators of feeding (Table 1). In the ARC, two separate popu-

Table 1. Peptides with stimulatory or inhibitory effects on food intake

Stimulatory	Inhibitory
Neuropeptide Y*	Leptin*
Melanin-concentrating hormone*	Cholecystokinin*
Orexins A and B*[1]	Corticotropin-releasing hormone*
β-endorphin	Glucagon-like peptides 1 and 2*
Galanin*	Neurotensin*
Ghrelin*	α-MSH*
Agouti-related peptide*	CART*
Growth hormone-releasing factor	Gastrin-releasing peptide
Motilin	Somatostatin
Nociceptin/Orphanin FQ	Thyrotropin-releasing hormone
β-casomorphin	CNTF
Insulin (I.V. infusion)	BDNF
	CGRP
	Bombesin
	Neuromedin
	Urocortin
	Neuropeptide FF
	Xenin
	Enterostatin
	Amylin
	PACAP
	Interleukins
	TNFα
	Apolipoprotein AIV
	Insulin (I.C.V. infusion)
	Glucagon

Asterisks indicate peptides described in the present paper with references in the bibliography.
[1]also named hypocretins 1 and 2.
Abbreviations: MSH: melanocyte-stimulating hormone; CART: cocaine and amphetamine related transcript; CNTF: ciliary neurotrophic factor; BDNF: brain-derived neurotrophic factor; CGRP: calcitonin gene-related peptide; PACAP: pituitary adenylate cyclase-activated peptide. I.V.: intravenous; I.C.V.: intracerebroventricular.

lations of neurons that contain active peptides are particularly well-described[10,11]. The first one co-synthesizes POMC and cocaine-amphetamine related transcript (CART) whereas the second one co-synthesizes NPY and agouti-related protein (AGRP). The two systems exert opposite effects on feeding and metabolism as the first one has a global inhibitory action on food intake whereas the second one has a clear orexigenic action. There is a cross-talk between the two systems. AGRP and alpha melanocyte-stimulating hormone α-MSH), a product of POMC cleavage bind to the type 3 and type 4 melanocortin receptors[10]. NPY is expressed in nerve terminals near POMC neurons and vice-versa[12]. Leptin affect neuronal activity of both populations of neurons by activating the POMC neurons and inhibiting the NPY neurons in order to produce a diminution in food intake. NPY, AGRP and melanocortins signals are integrated in the paraventricular nucleus[13]. In the absence of leptin signaling[14] as in ob/ob mice (default at the level of the protein) and in Zucker fa/fa rats (default at the level of the Ob receptor), NPY is overexpressed in the arcuate nucleus, its synthesis is augmented and its release in the PVN is increased and uncontrolled. The regulation of its levels by the feeding state does not occur. These variations are associated with a profound hyperphagia, a diminished energy expenditure and a massive weight gain. This feeding behaviour and modification in body weight and composition can be reproduced in normal Long-Evans or Sprague-Dawley rats by a chronic and/or continuous infusion of NPY in brain ventricles. Recent data have shown that in the mediobasal hypothalamus, the POMC neurons might be under the influence of an other orexigenic peptide, galanin[15]. Type 1 and 2 galanin receptors are indeed expressed in POMC neurons in the arcuate nucleus. In that case, galanin influences the production of an other product of the POMC cleavage, beta-endorphin. For galanin, the hypothalamic distribution of its perikarya is different from that of NPY. A population of neurons synthesizing galanin exists in the PVN in addition to that found in the arcuate nucleus. Galanin concentration in the PVN is largely augmented in the obese Zucker rat and participate to the general peptidergic dysregulation observed in this model of obesity[14]. A peptide structurally related to galanin (Galanin-like peptide GALP-1-60) has been recently isolated from porcine hypothalamus. It is produced in discrete ARC neurons that express leptin receptors and send projections to the PVN[16]. Through these projections, this new peptide might participate in the integrative processing of the information necessary for establishing a coherent feeding behaviour.

An other important peptide present in the PVN is the corticotropin-releasing hormone (CRH). It inhibits food intake and when infused in Zucker rats, it could prevent their excessive weight gain. It is a link between stress events and energy metabolism[17]. Besides its interaction with leptin, it is possibly linked to some newly detected hypothalamic peptides, the orexins (see below).

Despite of the mass of data already published about these ARC-PVN pathways with NPY as a central point of interest, the importance of these systems in feeding behaviour regulation has been discussed. This is probably related to the creation of knockout and transgenic mouse models[18]. Mice lacking either neuropeptide Y, AGRP or both peptides have a normal food intake and grow normally[18,19]. The same situation is observed for corticotropin-releasing hormone or galanin[18]. There is also a lack of body weight/obesity phenotype in galanin transgenic mouse strains[16]. It was concluded that NPY at least is not necessary for the progressive development of obesity in murine models. However, this opinion must be modulated for several reasons. First, it could be noted that mice deficient in both leptin and NPY (ob/ob NPY −/−) are less obese than ob/ob mice. Second, weight gain progressively augments in POMC null mutant mice or in mice with the deletion of NPY receptors. Sensitivity of the knockout animals to injection of other peptides is changed suggesting that receptiveness of these other neuroregulatory systems of energy homeostasis can be adapted to compensate for the loss of a peptide. It should therefore rather be concluded that each peptide of ARC-PVN axis with its receptors can contribute to the regulation of feeding with an importance depending on the metabolic and environmental conditions.

A renewed interest for 'old' pathways

Since about half a decade now, the discovery of new peptides have reoriented research towards ancient sites implicated in feeding regulation. One is in the periphery and involves the gastrointestinal (GI) tract whereas a second is in the central nervous system and involves the lateral hypothalamus.

In the periphery, research had more or less focused for several decades on satiety factors released after food ingestion and playing a role in meal termination. The best example is cholecystokinin (CCK) for which the circuitry from the GI tract to the brain for its anorexigenic action is well-established[6].

Recent findings have completed this organization and now CCK belongs to the list of peptides that interact with leptin[20]. The activation of neurons as evaluated by the measurement of C-fos expression is enhanced in the brainstem (NTS, area postrema ...) when both peptides are co-injected. This indicates that leptin can influence these hindbrain areas but the mechanism and circuitry of this activation remain to be established.

Since the discovery of a new peptide named ghrelin, a new and different light was shed on the peripheral regulation of feeding by GI peptides. Contrary to all other known GI active peptides which inhibit food intake, ghrelin has orexigenic effects[21]. Ghrelin is indeed primarily produced by the stomach and released in the circulation. As a ligand of the growth hormone (GH) secretagogue (GHS) receptor, it stimulates GH secretion in rats and humans but its stimulation of food intake is GH-independent. It is released just before the beginning of a meal concomitantly with a decrease of blood glucose. These signals could trigger feeding behaviour. After meal ingestion, it progressively decreases. Its circulating levels are dependent on feeding status. It is up-regulated by fasting and decreases after refeeding. After chronic administration, its orexigenic effects led to excess weight gain and adiposity. All these effects are likely due to an interaction with the hypothalamic neuromodulatory pathways. Recent studies have indeed shown that one of its brain target is the hypothalamus and more precisely the arcuate nucleus where it induces Fos and Egr 1 expression. Ghrelin acts on arcuate neurons by increasing the expression of some important orexigenic neuropeptides such as NPY and AgRP. Its orexigenic effect is abolished by co-injection of NPY Y1 and Y5 receptor antagonists. Ghrelin also strongly interacts with the leptin regulatory pathway at the level of the arcuate nucleus[22]. Its changes with feeding status are opposite to those of leptin. Its mRNA expression in the stomach is increased after administration of leptin. When it is co-injected with leptin, it abolishes the leptin induced

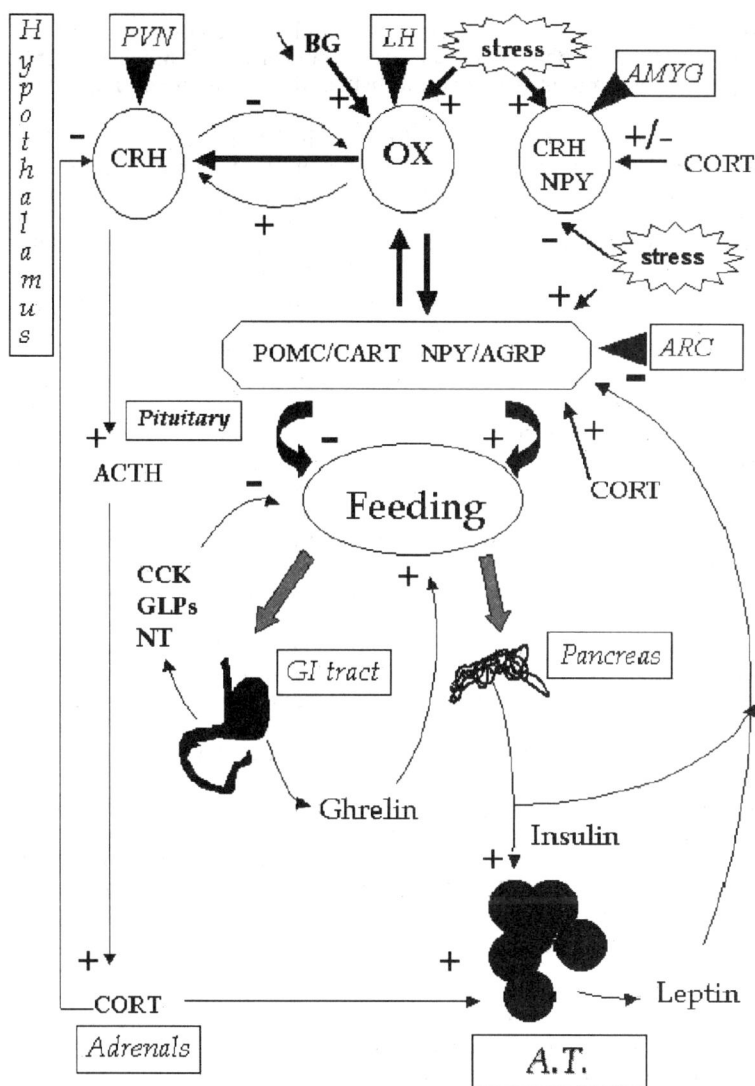

Fig.1. Schematic representation of some recent pathways involved in the regulation of feeding behaviour.
Names of brain areas or peripheral organs are indicated in italics: ARC: arcuate nucleus; PVN: paraventricular nucleus; LH: lateral hypothalamus; AMYG: amygdala; GI tract: gastro-intestinal tract; A.T.: adipose tissue. OX: orexins; CORT: corticosterone; BG: blood glucose; For other peptide abbreviations, see text.

inhibition of food intake in a dose of dependent manner. In the absence of leptin signaling, it is overexpressed in the stomach in the obese Zucker rat (paper in preparation) and in the ob/ob mouse.

As for NPY or galanin in the brain[23], circulating levels of ghrelin are strongly influenced to the type of macronutrients present in the ingested diet[24]. Its plasma concentration are low when a high-fat diet is ingested for a long period of time and it increases when the amount of carbohydrates in the diet increases. Fat-preferring rats have plasma ghrelin levels lower than the carbohydrate-preferring rats. The down-regulation by fat ingestion might serve as a counterregulatory mechanism to limit the development of dietary-induced adiposity. Ghrelin is therefore a new and significant factor mediating food intake. It constitutes a potential target for the drug treatment of obesity.

In the central nervous system, once again, it is the discovery of a new class of neuropeptides, the orexins A and B (also named hypocretins 1 and 2) and the determination of a role in feeding of an already 'old' peptide, the melanin-concentrating hormone (MCH) that put the attention on the lateral hypothalamus[25,26]. The two peptides are synthesized in two distinct populations of neurons in the LH. Both stimulate food intake when they are injected in brains ventricles or in the hypothalamus but in a less intense manner than NPY.

The melanin-concentrating hormone differs from NPY as contrary to NPY, there are clear phenotypes associated with the manipulation of the MCH gene. MCH-overexpressing transgenic mice are obese and hyperphagic when fed on a high fat diet and MCH-knockout mice are lean and hypophagic[18,26]. The MCH neurons are in close relation with the NPY system as NPY neurons in the ARC send some projections towards the MCH population in the LH and vice-versa. They also interact with leptin through receptors located on the neurons. Central injection of leptin inhibits therefore the feeding response elicited by MCH and induces a decrease in MCH mRNA levels. In the obese Zucker rat, the hypothalamic status of MCH looks like that of NPY as its mRNA is overexpressed in the LH with an associated decrease in the expression of at least its type 1 receptor[27,28]. It therefore contributes to the general peptidergic dysregulation leading to hyperphagia and obesity in Zucker rats. It however represents an interesting target for therapeutic compounds as its central distribution is much less large than that of NPY.

The distribution of orexins neurons is also very restricted and confined to the lateral hypothalamus[26,29]. These neurons project widely to different brain areas including the olfactory bulb, the brainstem, the hypothalamus and neurohypophysis in accordance with the variety of biological actions of the peptides. In the hypothalamus, orexin nerve terminals have been mainly located in the arcuate and paraventricular nuclei. On a functional point of view, the orexins system is closely linked to the NPY pathway. Orexin immunoreactive terminals originating in the LH make direct synaptic contact with NPY neurons in the arcuate nucleus and orexin neurons receive innervation from NPY-, AGRP- and alpha-MSH-immunoreactive fibres. The early gene C-Fos is also expressed in NPY neurons of the arcuate nucleus after orexin injection. The regulation of the orexin pathway is slightly different of the NPY system. A small diminution in food intake induced by a chronic leptin treatment induces a large decrease in orexin concentration in the LH whereas in the same animals, the NPY levels remain unchanged[30]. In addition, whereas the NPY mRNA expression is up-regulated in the ob/ob mice and in the Zucker fatty rat, we and others have shown that the entire orexin pathway (peptide content and mRNA expression) is down-regulated in these animal models of obesity. This down-regulation of orexin synthesis might constitute a compensatory mechanism to diminish food intake in the obese rat. The interaction with leptin is possible through leptin receptors located on orexin neurons. Leptin however, is not the sole factor for orexin regulation. The orexins neurons contrary to the MCH neurons are glucose-sensitive and different manipulations of blood glucose levels (insulin-induced hypoglycaemia, injection of 2-deoxyglucose ...) can modify the orexin system in the LH. Besides metabolic factors, other hypothalamic neuropeptides might be potential candidates. Melanocortins and AGRP can be discarded as orexin gene expression is not altered either by interruption of signaling at the MC4 receptor level or in the agouti mice. Corticotropin-releasing hormone (CRH) is a more plausible candidate. Blockade of CRH through an antagonist or an antiserum favours the orexigenic effects of orexin. Physical stressors such as immobilization or cold which stimulates PVN CRH neurons and activates the hypothalamo-pituitary-adrenal axis also induces increase in prepro-orexin mRNA levels in rats. Accordingly, we have recently shown that orexin expression in the LH is dependent on the glucocorticoid status. It is diminished in adrenalectomized rats and restored by a dexamethasone treatment[31]. In addition, CRH neurons in the amygdala are sending projections to the lateral hypothalamus and might modulate orexin action through a separate pathway. It is therefore plausible that the orexin system might integrate through this way some environmental or psychological cues that can influence feeding behaviour.

Conclusion

Knowledge of the different pathways influencing feeding behaviour has considerably progressed over the last twenty years. Their organization for producing an adequate response to the needs of an individual is more and more finely determined. It is very complex and one its characteristic feature is the redundancy of the different circuits. The 'black box' is a little bit open. Brain mechanisms are closely linked to peripheral signals either involved in the digestion or in the storage of the ingested food (Fig. 1).

New targets for drug treatment of feeding and body weight disorders can be explored. Due to the large interaction existing between all these systems, it seems necessary to use several approaches simultaneously to fight these disorders and multitherapy will not remain the apanage of AIDS. In the case of obesity at least, for a complete effectiveness, these pharmacological treatments will have to be associated with strong and voluntary changes in the management of food availability and of activity. These changes have to be done for all the periods of life and for better results as early as possible since all these pathways can already be influenced at prenatal stages[32].

References

1. Anand B K, Brobeck J R. Hypothalamic control of food intake in rats and cats. *Yale J Biol Med* 1940; 24: 123–40.

2. Hetherington AW, Ranson SW. Hypothalamic lesions and adiposity in the rat. *Anat Record* 1940; 78: 149–72.

3. Leibowitz SF, Hammer NJ, Chang K. Hypothalamic paraventricular lesions produce overeating and obesity in the rat. *Physiol Behav* 1981; 27: 1031–40.

4. Bernardis LL, Bellinger LL. The dorsomedial hypothalamic nucleus revisited: 1998 update. *Proc Soc Exp Biol Med* 1998; 218: 284–306.

5. Stoynev AG, Ikonomov OC. Circadian regulation of feeding in rats: suprachiasmatic versus ventromedial hypothalamic nuclei. *Appetite* 1987; 9: 217–29.

6. Beck B. Cholecystokinin, neurotensin and corticotropin-releasing factor - 3 important anorexic peptides. *Ann Endocrinol* 1992; 53: 44–56.

7. Larsen P J, Vrang N, Tang Christensen M, Jensen PB, HaySchmidt A, Romer J et al. Ups and downs for neuropeptides in body weight homeostasis: pharmacological potential of cocaine amphetamine regulated transcript and pre-proglucagon-derived peptides. *Eur J Pharmacol* 2002; 440: 159–72.

8. Ahima RS, Saper CB, Flier JS, Elmquist J K. Leptin regulation of neuroendocrine systems. *Front Neuroendocrinol* 2000; 21: 263–307.

9. Baskin DG, Lattemann DF, Seeley RJ, Woods SC, Porte D, Schwartz MW. Insulin and leptin: dual adiposity signals to the brain for the regulation of food intake and body weight. *Brain Res* 1999; 848: 114–23.

10. Cone RD. The central melanocortin system and energy homeostasis. *Trends Endocrinol Metab* 1999; 10: 211–6.

11. Kalra SP, Dube MG, Pu SY, Xu B, Horvath TL, Kalra PS. Interacting appetite-regulating pathways in the hypothalamic regulation of body weight. *Endocr Rev* 1999; 20: 68–100.

12. Cowley MA, Smart J L, Rubinstein M, Cordan MG, Diano S, Horvath TL et al. Leptin activates anorexigenic POMC neurons through a neural network in the arcuate nucleus. *Nature* 2001; 411: 480–4.

13. Cowley MA, Pronchuk N, Fan W, Dinulescu DM, Colmers WF, Cone R D. Integration of NPY, AGRP, and melanocortin signals in the hypothalamic paraventricular nucleus: Evidence of a cellular basis for the adipostat. *Neuron* 1999; 24: 155–63.

14. Beck B. Neuropeptides and obesity. *Nutrition* 2000; 16: 916–23.

15. Bouret S, Croix D, Mariot M, Loyens A, Prevot V, Jegou S et al. Galanin modulates the activity of proopiomelanocortin neurons in the isolated mediobasal hypothalamus of the male rat. *Neuroscience* 2002; 112: 475–85.

16. Gundlach AL. Galanin/GALP and galanin receptors: role in central control of feeding, body weight/obesity and reproduction? *Eur J Pharmacol* 2002; 440: 255–68.

17. Richard D, Lin Q, Timofeeva E. The corticotropin-releasing factor family of peptides and CRF receptors: their roles in the regulation of energy balance. *Eur J Pharmacol* 2002; 440: 189–197.

18. Beck B. KO's and organisation of peptidergic feeding behavior mechanisms. *Neurosci Biobehav Rev* 2001; 25: 143–58.

19. Qian S, Chen H, Weingarth D, Trumbauer ME, Novi DE, Guan XM et al. Neither agouti-related protein nor neuropeptide Y is critically required for the regulation of energy homeostasis in mice. *Mol Cell Biol* 2002; 22: 5027–35.

20. Emond M, Schwartz GJ, Ladenheim EE, Moran TH. Central leptin modulates behavioral and neural responsivity to CCK. *Am J Physiol* 1999; 45: R1545–R1549.

21. Horvath TL, Diano S, Sotonyi P, Heiman M, Tschop M. Minireview: Ghrelin and the regulation of energy balance – A hypothalamic perspective. *Endocrinology* 2001; 142: 4163–9.

22. Traebert M, Riediger T, Whitebread S, Scharrer E, Schmid HA. Ghrelin acts on leptin-responsive neurones in the rat arcuate nucleus. *J Neuroendocrinol* 2002; 14: 580–6.

23. Beck B. Quantitative and macronutrient-related regulation of hypothalamic neuropeptide Y, galanin and neurotensin. In: *Neural and metabolic control of macronutrient intake*, HR Berthoud, RJ Seeley (eds), pp. 461–70. Boca Raton, CRC Press 1999.

24. Beck B, Musse N, StrickerKrongrad A. Ghrelin, macronutrient intake and dietary preferences in Long-Evans rats. *Biochem Biophys Res Commun* 2002; 292: 1031–5.

25. Sutcliffe JG, deLecea L. The hypocretins: Setting the arousal threshold. *Nature Rev Neurosci* 2002; 3: 339–49.

26. Boutin JA, Suply T, Audinot V, Rodriguez M, Beauverger P, Nicolas JP et al. Melanin-concentrating hormone and its receptors: state of the art. *Can J Physiol Pharmacol* 2002; 80: 388–95.

27. Stricker-Krongrad A, Dimitrov T, Beck B. Central and peripheral dysregulation of melanin-concentrating hormone in obese Zucker rats. *Mol Brain Res* 2001; 92: 43–8.

28. Beck B, Richy S, Dimitrov T, StrickerKrongrad A. Opposite regulation of hypothalamic orexin and neuropeptide Y receptors and peptide expressions in obese Zucker rats. *Biochem Biophys Res Commun* 2001; 286: 518–23.

29. Stricker-Krongrad A, Richy S, Beck B. Orexins/hypocretins in the ob/ob mouse: hypothalamic gene expression, peptide content and metabolic effects. *Regulat Pept* 2002; 104: 11–20.

30. Beck B, Richy S. Hypothalamic hypocretin/orexin and neuropeptide Y: Divergent interaction with energy depletion and leptin. *Biochem Biophys Res Commun* 1999; 258: 119–22.

31. Stricker-Krongrad A, Beck B. Modulation of hypothalamic hypocretin/orexin mRNA expression by glucocorticoids. *Biochem Biophys Res Commun* 2002; 296: 129–33.

32. Kozak R, Burlet A, Burlet C, Beck B. Dietary composition during fetal and neonatal life affects neuropeptide Y functioning in adult offspring. Develop *Brain Res* 2000; 125: 75–82.

Progress in Obesity Research: 9. Edited by *Geraldo Medeiros-Neto, Alfredo Halpern* and *Claude Bouchard*
©2003 John Libbey Eurotext Ltd, pp. 766–769.

CHAPTER 160

Glucosensing neurons

Vanessa H. Routh

*Departments of Pharmacology & Physiology and Neurosciences, New Jersey Medical School (UMDNJ),
Newark, NJ 07103, USA
[e-mail: routhvh@umdnj.edu]*

Glucose homeostasis is of critical concern to the brain, since glucose is its primary fuel. Either a large rise or fall in plasma glucose level cause the brain to activate the sympathetic nervous system[1,2]. Thus, the brain responds to changes in plasma glucose, and initiates compensatory responses to maintain glucose homeostasis. Both central and peripheral glucose sensors may serve to inform the brain that plasma glucose levels are falling to dangerous levels. Much less is known about the mechanisms which sense an increase of plasma glucose. The ventromedial region of the hypothalamus (VMH), which contains both the arcuate nucleus (ARC) and the ventromedial hypothalamic nucleus (VMN), plays an important role in the response to hypoglycaemia[3]. Recent evidence indicates that the brainstem may also play a role[4]. In addition, glucose sensors exist in the portal vein[5] and carotid body[6]. While the efferent mechanisms maintaining glucose homeostasis are fairly well characterized[7], little is known about if and how the brain actually senses and responds to changes in plasma glucose levels.

For many years we have known that glucose regulates neuronal activity. For example, in 1964 two separate laboratories described neurons within the hypothalamus which change their action potential frequency in response to changes in plasma glucose[8,9]. Later studies showed that direct application of glucose increased the action potential frequency of 'glucose responsive' or GR neurons, while decreasing the action potential frequency of 'glucose sensitive' or GS neurons[10]. GR neurons utilize the ATP-sensitive K^+ (KATP) channel to sense glucose[11]. That is, similar to the pancreatic β-cell, rising glucose levels increase the intracellular ATP to ADP ratio and close the KATP channel. This depolarizes the β-cell and activates voltage sensitive calcium channels that mediate insulin secretion[12]. However, glucose initiated depolarization of GR neurons increases action potential frequency. Less is known about the mechanism by which GS neurons sense glucose, although decreased activity of the Na^+/K^+ ATPase with decreased ATP has been suggested[10].

While it is attractive to hypothesize that GR and GS neurons play a role in glucose homeostasis, it is important to note that the majority of studies of these neurons used glucose levels outside the physiologic range (0 to 10 or 20 mM)[10,11,13,14,15]. A cerebrospinal fluid level of 0 mM glucose would be incompatible with life. Moreover, virtually all studies of the central nervous system use 10 mM glucose in the solutions which bathe neurons. However, recent evidence demonstrates that brain glucose concentrations are significantly lower than 10 mM[16]. For example, at 7.6 mM plasma glucose in a fed rat, extracellular brain glucose was only 2.5 mM. Decreasing plasma glucose to 2–3 mM (~40 mg/dl) or increasing to 15.2 mM (~270 mg/dl), caused brain glucose levels of 0.16 mM and 4.5 mM, respectively[16]. One caveat must be mentioned. If the neurons under investigation are in or near a region lacking a blood brain barrier, brain glucose levels may approximate plasma levels. Neurons in these regions may be normally exposed to higher levels of extracellular glucose. However, under physiologic conditions the majority of neurons are unlikely to be exposed to extracellular glucose levels above 5 mM.

Using patch clamp recording in brain slices, our lab has recently characterized glucosensing neurons in the VMN[17], ARC and brainstem (unpublished observations) whose action potential frequency changes in response to changes of extracellular brain glucose from a steady state level of 2.5 mM. We found that glucosensing neurons do respond to physiologically relevant changes in extracellular glucose. VMN glucosensing neurons will be described herein as prototypes of brain glucosensing neurons since we have characterized them extensively[17]. Glucose sensing in the VMN involves a complex convergence of pre- and postsynaptic mechanisms[17]. There are two subtypes of VMN glucosensing neurons which respond directly to a decrease in extracellular glucose. Glucose-excited (GE) neurons increase their action potential frequency as extracellular glucose increases from 0.1 mM to 2.5 mM[17]. Our preliminary data indicate that GE neurons respond to changes in extracellular glucose from 0.1 to 2.5 mM at which point the response to glucose plateaus; their EC_{50} for glucose is 0.64 mM (unpublished observation). Finally, GE neurons are sensitive to changes in extracellular glucose as small as 100 μM (unpublished observation). These GE neurons are similar to the GR neurons described earlier in that they respond to glucose via the KATP channel[17].

On the other hand, glucose-inhibited (GI) neurons decrease their action potential frequency as glucose levels increase from 0.1 mM to 2.5 mM, where the neurons are completely silent. Although these neurons appear to respond in a similar fashion as GS neurons, we do not believe that these are the same class of neuron. It has been suggested that GS neurons sense glucose *via* changes in the Na^+K^+ ATPase pump[10]. However the response to decreased extracellular glucose for GI neurons reversed at the chloride equilibrium potential[17]. This suggests that a chloride channel is involved in their glucose sensing mechanism.

Three other subtypes of physiologically relevant VMN glucosensing neurons are presynaptically modulated by glucose[17]. Although these VMN neurons are not intrinsically glucose sensing but rather modulated by glucose controlled synaptic input, we consider them in the overall category of VMN glucosensing neurons. Of these, 1 subtype is presynaptically excited as extracellular glucose levels fall below 2.5 mM. We refer to these as **p**resynaptically **e**xcited by **d**ecreased glucose or PED neurons. The other two subtypes of presynaptically modulated glucosensing neurons respond to an increase in extracellular glucose from 2.5 to 5 or 10 mM[17]. PER neurons are **p**resynaptically **e**xcited as glucose levels are **r**aised to 5 mM while PIR neurons are **i**nhibited. The presynaptic mechanisms by which PED and PER neurons sense glucose are unclear. However, PIR neurons appear to receive glucose controlled inhibitory input from γ-aminobutyric acid (GABA)-ergic neurons. Moreover, tolbutamide mimics the effect of increased glucose on PIR neurons suggesting the involvement of a KATP channel. We hypothesize that this KATP channel is located on the terminal of the presynaptic GABAergic neuron. Such presynaptic channels have been described in the substantia nigra where glucose has been shown to regulate GABA release[18].

The interactions between pre- and postsynaptic influences are quite interesting. Some directly glucosensing VMN neurons are also presynaptically modulated by other glucosensing neurons. We have often observed a GE neuron receiving inhibitory glucose controlled presynaptic input in response to increased extracellular glucose[17]. This leads to a biphasic response to changes in extracellular glucose in which the GE neuron is inhibited by a deviation in either direction from 2.5 mM. Biphasic responses have also been observed for GI neurons. Finally, VMN neurons receiving glucose controlled presynaptic input in response to decreased glucose also receive glucose controlled presynaptic input in response to increased glucose[17]. Thus, both GI neurons and these latter neurons (PED-PER) are quiescent at steady state levels of 2.5 mM extracellular glucose and excited when glucose levels either increase or decrease. This further supports our hypothesis that GI neurons are not the same class of neurons as GS neurons which are stimulated as glucose levels decrease from 10 or 20 mM to 0 mM. That is, while the GS neurons studied by Oomura were relatively quiescent at 10 or 20 mM[9], ours are active due to presynaptic excitation.

An important issue regarding glucosensing neurons involves the mechanism by which they sense small physiologically relevant changes in extracellular glucose. In this regard, they may be similar to the pancreatic β-cell. Beta cells sense small changes in extracellular glucose with a special hexokinase known as glucokinase (GK, hexokinase IV) whose K_m is in the physiologic range for extracellular glucose[19]. Most neurons possess hexokinase I which is saturated at physiologic glucose levels[20]. In these neurons, small changes in extracellular glucose would not be translated into changes in intracellular metabolism. However, GK is located in brain regions which contain glucosensing neurons[21,22]. Inhibitors of GK block the ability of most GE and GI neurons to sense glucose[23]. Moreover, our preliminary data reveals the presence of mRNA coding for GK in single GE and GI neurons whose ability to sense glucose is blocked by the GK inhibitor, alloxan[24]. Thus, VMN glucosensing neurons may use GK to sense small changes in extracellular glucose.

Finally, regulation of overall energy balance entails more than just the regulation of plasma glucose. Energy balance involves energy intake, energy storage and energy utilization. All of these components are under the regulation of the autonomic nervous system[7,25]. As mentioned above, when plasma glucose levels fall to 2–3 mM, a sympathetically mediated increase in epinephrine release from the adrenal medulla occurs in order to increase liver glucose production and raise plasma glucose[2]. On the other hand, during hyperglycaemia, sympathetic drive to skeletal muscle increases in order to increase peripheral glucose utilization and decrease plasma glucose[1]. Increased plasma glucose also increases insulin levels which promotes glucose entry into tissues such as muscle and adipose; the latter promoting glucose storage as fat[7]. Thus, shifts in plasma glucose affect the energetic status of the body. Glucosensing neurons are located in regions of the brain associated with energy balance[25]. They are also dysfunctional under conditions where energy balance is disturbed. The obese (fa/fa) Zucker rat has dysfunctional K^+ channels and GR neurons[13,26]. Moreover, we have demonstrated that all subtypes of physiologically relevant glucosensing neurons are both dysfunctional and fewer in number in rats that are prone to develop diet-induced obesity and insulin resistance[17]. This is associated with a 50 per cent reduction in the sensitivity of the KATP channel to ATP and sulphonylureas[27].

These data suggest an important interaction between the regulation of glucose homeostasis and overall energy balance. Thus, it is likely that glucosensing neurons also act as metabolic integrators. A number of observations support this hypothesis. Spanswick et al. have shown that VMN GR neurons are inhibited by both insulin and leptin via activation of KATP channels[13,15]. In contrast, Oomura and colleagues have shown that orexin as well as low levels of leptin increase the action potential frequency of medial hypothalamic GR neurons[14]. Similarly, we have found that leptin stimulates both VMN GE and PED neurons[28]. Finally, preliminary data from our lab shows that NE inhibits GE neurons (unpublished observation). Thus, glucosensing neurons respond to other important peptides and transmitters involved in the regulation of energy balance. It is apparent that these glucosensing neurons could serve as integrators of metabolic signals as well as glucose levels and be involved in overall energy homeostasis.

A second question related to the integrative function of glucosensing neurons is whether they specifically sense glucose or whether they respond to any form of energy substrate which produces ATP. Astrocytes sequester glucose and convert it to glycogen for storage. When energy levels drop this glycogen is converted to lactate and transported out of astrocytes and into neurons via monocarboxylate acid transporters. Neurons convert the lactate into pyruvate using lactate dehydrogenase. Pyruvate then fuels mitochondrial oxidative phosphorylation[29]. Whether glucosensing neurons use lactate as a signaling molecule similar to glucose is unclear. In order for glucosensing neurons to act as specific glucose sensors, they should be more sensitive to glucose than lactate under conditions when energy is not limited. The data regarding this are controversial. Yang et al. have shown that VMH glucosensing neurons which increased their action potential frequency in response to increases in glucose over 5 mM were similarly stimulated by early glycolytic intermediates. High levels of lactate (15 mM) also increased the action potential frequency of glucosensing neurons when given in the presence of 5 mM glucose[21]. This would suggest that these glucosensing neurons respond to any metabolic substrate which increases ATP levels. However, steady state lactate levels in the brain are well below 15 mM[29]. Additionally, 15 mM pyruvate did not alter neuronal activity in the presence of 5 mM glucose. Pyruvate did, however, increase action potential frequency when glucose levels were 0 mM[21]. Our preliminary data suggest that 0.5 mM lactate can substitute for glucose in both GE and GI neurons when energy levels are very low (0.1 mM glucose)[30]. We do not know if the same will occur when glucose is not limiting. Thus, it is important to carefully address these issues using physiologic levels of both glucose and lactate.

In conclusion, glucosensing neurons respond to physiologic changes in extracellular glucose. The evidence described above supports the hypothesis that they play a role in the regulation of glucose homeostasis. Finally, it is also likely that glucosensing neurons are not merely glucose sensors. Rather, they function as metabolic integrators to enable the brain to maintain overall energy homeostasis.

References

1. Hoffman RP, Hausberg M, Sinkey CA, Anderson EA. Hyperglycemia without hyperinsulinemia produces both sympathetic neural activation and vasodilation in normal humans. J Diabetes Comp 1999; 13: 17–22.

2. Cryer PE. Glucose counterregulation in man. Diabetes 1981; 30: 261–4.

3. Borg WP, Sherwin RS, During MJ, Borg MA, Shulman GI. Local ventromedial hypothalamus glucopenia triggers counterregulatory hormone release. Diabetes 1995; 44: 180–4.

4. Ritter S, Llewellyn-Smith I, Dinh TT. Subgroups of hindbrain catecholamine neurons are selectively activated by 2-deoxy-D-glucose induced metabolic challenge. Brain Res 1998; 805: 41–54.

5. Niijima A. Glucose-sensitive afferent nerve fibres in the hepatic branch of the vagus nerve in the guinea-pig. J Physiol 1982; 332: 15–323.

6. Alvarez-Buylla R, de Alvarez-Buylla ER. Carotid sinus receptors participate in glucose homeostasis. *Respir Physiol* 1998; 72: 347–60.

7. Nonogaki K. New insights into sympathetic regulation of glucose and fat metabolism. *Diabetologia* 2000; 43: 533–49.

8. Anand BK, China GS, Sharma KN, Dua S, Singh B. Activity of single neurons in the hypothalamus feeding centers: effect of glucose. *Am J Physiol* 1964; 2207: 1146–54.

9. Oomura Y, Kimura K, Ooyama H, Maeo T, Iki M, Kuniyoshi N. Reciprocal activities of the ventromedial and lateral hypothalamic area of cats. *Science* 1964; 143: 484–5.

10. Oomura Y. Glucose as a regulator of neuronal activity. *Adv Metabol Disord* 1983; 10: 31–65.

11. Ashford MLJ, Boden PR, Treherne JM. Glucose-induced excitation of hypothalamic neurones is mediated by ATP-sensitive K+ channels. *Eur J Physiol* 1990; 415: 479–83.

12. Ashcroft FM, Gribble FM. ATP-sensitive K+ channels and insulin secretion: their role in health and disease. *Diabetologia* 1999; 42: 903–19.

13. Spanswick D, Smith MA, Mirshamsi S, Routh VH, Ashford MLJ. Insulin activates ATP-sensitive K+ channels in hypothalamic neurons of lean, but not obese rats. *Nature Neurosci* 2000; 3: 757–8.

14. Shiraishi T, Oomura Y, Sasaki K, Wayner MJ. Effects of leptin and orexin-A on food intake and feeding related hypothalamic neurons. *Physiology & Behavior* 2000; 71: 251–61.

15. Spanswick D, Smith MA, Groppi VE, Logan SD, Ashford MLJ. Leptin inhibits hypothalamic neurons by activation of ATP-sensitive potassium channels. *Nature* 1997; 390: 521–5.

16. Silver IA, Erecinska M. Extracellular glucose concentration in mammalian brain: Continuous monitoring of changes during increased neuronal activity and upon limitation in oxygen supply in normo-, hypo-, and hyperglycemic animals. *J Neurosci* 1994; 14: 5068–76.

17. Song Z, Levin BE, McArdle JJ, Bakhos N, Routh VH. Convergence of pre- and postsynaptic influences on glucosensing neurons in the ventromedial hypothalamic nucleus. *Diabetes* 2001; 50: 2673–81.

18. Levin BE. Glucose-regulated dopamine release from substantia nigra neurons. *Brain Res* 2000; 874: 158–64.

19. Matschinsky FM, Glaser B, Magnuson MA. Pancreatic beta-cell glucokinase: closing the gap between theoretical concepts and experimental realities. *Diabetes* 1998; 47: 307–15.

20. Liu F, Dong Q, Myers AM, Fromm HJ. Expression of human brain hexokinase in Escherichia coli: purification and characterization of the expressed enzyme. *Biochem & Biophys Res Comm* 1991; 177: 305–11.

21. Yang XJ, Kow LM, Funabashi T, Mobbs CV. Hypothalamic glucose sensor: similarities to and differences from pancreatic beta-cell mechanisms. *Diabetes* 1999; 48: 1763–72.

22. Lynch RM, Tompkins LS, Brooks HL, Dunn-Meynell AA, Levin BE. Localization of glucokinase gene expression in the rat brain. *Diabetes* 2000; 49: 693–700.

23. Dunn-Meynell AA, Routh VH, Kang L, Gaspers L, Levin BE. Glucokinase is the likely mediator of glucosensing in both glucose-excited and glucose-inhibited central neurons. *Diabetes* 2002; 51: 2056–65.

24. Kang L, Routh VH, Kuzhikandathil EV, Gaspers LD, Levin BE. Single Cell Reverse Transcription-Polymerase Chain Reaction (SCRT-PCR) Analysis of Glucosensing Neurons in the Ventromedial Hypothalamic Nucleus (VMN). *Soc Neurosci Abstr* 2002 (in press).

25. Levin BE, Dunn-Meynell AA, Routh VH. Brain glucose sensing and body energy homeostasis: role in obesity and diabetes. *Am J Physiol* 1999; 276: R1223–R31.

26. Rowe IC, Boden PR, Ashford MLJ. Potassium channel dysfunction in hypothalamic glucose-receptive neurones of obese Zucker rats. *J Physiol* 1996; 497: 365–77.

27. Routh VH, Levin BE, McArdle JJ. Defective ATP and sulfonylurea sensitivity of the ATP-sensitive K+ (KATP) channel in the ventromedial hypothalamic nucleus (VMN) of obesity-prone (DIO) rats. *FASEB J* 2001; 12: A864

28. Wang W, Routh VH. Leptin excites physiologically relevant glucose sensing neurons in the ventromedial hypothalamic nucleus. *Soc Neurosci Abstr* 2002 (in press).

29. Ames AI. CNS energy metabolism as related to function. *Brain Res Rev* 2000; 34: 42–68.

30. Song Z, Routh VH. Differential effects of lactate on glucosensing neurons in the ventromedial hypothalamic nucleus (VMN). *Soc Neurosci Abstr* 2001; 27: 9472.

Progress in Obesity Research: 9. Edited by *Geraldo Medeiros-Neto, Alfredo Halpern and Claude Bouchard*
©2003 John Libbey Eurotext Ltd, pp. 770–773.

CHAPTER 161

Hypothalamic pathways and energy homeostasis

Joanne A. Harrold, Xue J. Cai, Joanne C. Elliott and Gareth Williams

Diabetes and Endocrinology Research Group, Department of Medicine, University of Liverpool, Liverpool L69 3GA, UK
[e-mail: harrold@liverpool.ac.uk]

Introduction

The regulation of energy homeostasis is extremely complex and is shared between a number of brain regions. During the past decade, our knowledge of CNS-mediated regulation has expanded dramatically. Most interest has focused on the hypothalamus, which has proven to be a key region in the regulation of food intake, energy expenditure and body weight. Consequently, our understanding has moved away from the anatomical concept of feeding and satiety centres towards the presence of specific neurotransmitters that modulate feeding behaviour by acting on discrete neural control pathways. It has become evident that such elaborate regulation involves several neural circuits operating in combination, with each offering a particular function. The relative importance of each contribution varies with the specific conditions of altered energy balance.

Here we shall discuss several of the more recently identified hypothalamic neuropeptides implicated in energy homeostasis. The chosen examples illustrate the functional diversity of regulation and represent some of the most promising potential targets for the development of anti-obesity drugs.

Hypothalamic nutritional signals

Key components of hypothalamic control systems are the nutritional signalling factors which allow the CNS to sense energy requirements. The hypothalamus is widely accessible to a variety of circulating hormones, metabolites and other factors carried by the cerebrospinal fluid. Principal factors include the hormones leptin and insulin and the metabolite glucose.

Leptin

Leptin is encoded by the ob gene, which is expressed by adipose tissue (mainly white) and is secreted into the bloodstream in proportion to body fat mass. Various regions within the CNS express leptin receptors, which are encoded by the *db* gene. Several splice variants of OB-R mRNA have been identified, encoding for at least six leptin receptors. Of these, only the long isoform OB-Rb contains all the sequences required for signal transduction and is the main mediator of leptin's effects[1]. It is abundant within the hypothalamus and is expressed by many of the appetite-regulating neuropeptide systems.

Leptin can readily enter the CNS, where it acts to inhibit feeding, stimulate thermogenesis and reduce body fat and weight. Supporting evidence for this is provided by the genetically obese rodent models: *ob/ob* and *db/db* mice and fa/fa Zucker rat. All demonstrate hyperphagia and severe obesity as a consequence of different mutations in the genes encoding leptin or its receptors[2]. Thus leptin appears to regulate energy balance through a negative feed back loop in which the hormone's antiobesity actions will counteract an increase in body weight.

Insulin

Basal circulating levels of insulin are also broadly proportional to fat mass and concentrations increase after eating. Insulin can readily enter the CNS, where receptors are widely expressed, particularly in the hypothalamic nuclei associated with the control of energy balance, such as the paraventricular

(PVN) and arcuate (ARC) nuclei[3]. Insulin acts on the CNS to affect energy balance and metabolism in a variety of ways; it inhibits food intake following central injection and also stimulates sympathetic outflow to thermogenic tissue, thus enhancing energy expenditure and loss of body fat. Selective knockout of the insulin receptor in the CNS leads to hyperphagia and obesity supporting its participation in a negative feedback loop, comparable to leptin, to keep fat mass constant.

Glucose

Falls in blood glucose powerfully stimulate feeding. Glucose-sensing neurones within the CNS detect these changes in ambient glucose levels and in turn interact with other appetite-regulating neuropeptide systems, e.g. NPY and orexin to induce the appropriate response. The glucose-sensing neurones fall into two classes: glucose-responsive neurones (GRN) that increase their firing rate with rising glucose and glucose-sensitive neurones (GSN) which are stimulated by falling glucose levels[5]. Several hypothalamic nuclei contain glucose-sensing neurones, including the ARC, PVN, ventromedial hypothalamic nucleus (VMH) and the lateral hypothalamic area (LHA), all of which are important to the regulation of energy homeostasis. However, the two populations appear to have a distinct distribution. For example, GRN constitute 40–45 per cent of VMH neurones. Conversely, 30–40 per cent of LHA neurones are GSN, while GRN are rare (5 per cent). This implies that the hypothalamic nuclei serve distinctive functions in terms of altered glucose availability. However, it is not clear how this difference relates to the control of food intake as a whole. Glucose-sensing neurones are also expressed in extrahypothalamic areas, especially the nucleus of the solitary tract (NTS) and their activity is affected by circulating metabolites other than glucose, e.g. insulin and free fatty acids.

Hypothalamic peptides and energy balance

Neuropeptide Y

Neuropeptide Y (NPY) is a 36 amino acid peptide which belongs to the pancreatic polypeptide family. It occurs throughout the central and peripheral nervous system in mammals and is one of the most abundant peptides in rat and human brain[6]. Concentrations are particularly high in the hypothalmus, where the majority is derived from neurones in the ARC. From here, dense NPY-containing projections pass predominantly to the dorsomedial hypothalamic nucleus (DMH) and the PVN.

The anatomical localization of NPY suggests an involvement in the regulation of energy balance. When administered centrally NPY powerfully stimulates food-seeking behaviour and eating (it is one of the most potent central appetite stimulants known). In conjunction with reduced brown adipose tissue thermogenesis and enhanced insulin secretion, which facilitates triglyceride deposition, the overall influence of NPY is the induction of obesity. These effects mimic the key metabolic changes of genetically obese rodents *(ob/ob* and *db/db* mice and fa/fa Zucker rat) and all of these models show increased activity of ARC NPY neurones.

However, NPY does not mediate all forms of obesity. It has been shown that NPY neuronal activity is reduced in animals with dietary-induced obesity. This is illustrated by lowered NPY mRNA concentrations and receptor up-regulation[8]. Thus, the NPY system does not appear to be involved in inducing the hyperphagia associated with palatable diet. In fact, the NPY neurones are inhibited in this situation, potentially in an attempt to limit food intake.

NPY neurones express the 0B-Rb receptor, suggesting that they are modulated by leptin[9]. Overactivity of NPY neurones in genetically obese rodents is apparently due to loss of this leptin regulation, which occurs as a consequence of spontaneously occurring mutations in these animals. Similarly, NPY neurones are stimulated by falling leptin in animals that have lost body weight and fat through starvation, diabetes, lactation and exercise. Like leptin, insulin produces a shift in energy balance by inhibiting feeding, stimulating thermogenesis and inducing weight loss. Such actions are at least partially mediated via inhibition of NPY neurones. However, effects of insulin may be indirectly mediated.

Overall, this data indicates that the physical role of NPY neurones may be to sense energy deficits. Negative energy balance states are characterized by increased hunger and active food-seeking at the expense of other behaviour and by reducing energy expenditure through thermogenesis. These effects mirror NPY's central actions.

Melanocortins

The melanocortin peptides are derived from a common precursor, pro-opiomelanocortin (POMC). Of these, α-melanocyte stimulating hormone (α-MSH) is thought to be the most important in terms of

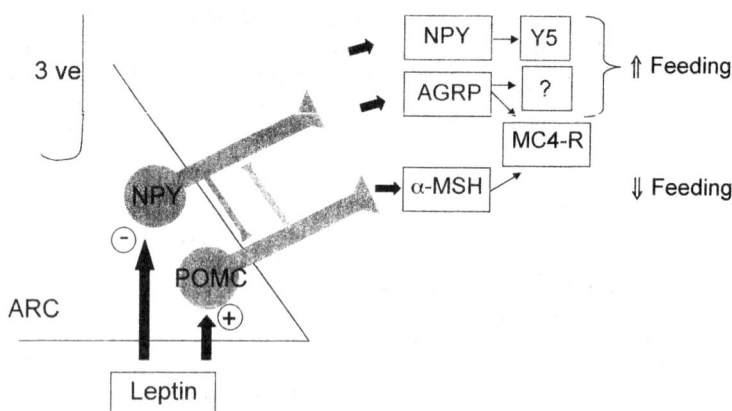

Fig. 1. Reciprocal relationship between neuropeptide Y (NPY)/agouti-related peptide (AGRP) and pro-opiomelancortin neurones of the arcuate nucleus.

feeding. Most POMC neurones lie in the ARC and project to various brain regions, particularly other hypothalamic sites. Three melanocortin receptors are found in the brain (MC3-, MC4- and MC5-R). Of these both MC3- and MC4-R are located in hypothalamic regions concerned with the control of food intake, including the VMH, ARC and DMH. Knockout studies and the use of receptor selective ligands suggests that both MC3- and MC4-R play roles in mediating the appetite-suppressing effects of α-MSH. MC4-R appear to be more important in the response to altered energy balance[11] and it has been suggested that MC3-R act to determine feeding efficiency[12].

The melanocortin system is unique in that it is regulated by both endogenous agonists and antagonists. Two endogenous antagonists are agouti and agouti-related peptide (AGRP). Whilst agouti is only expressed in the hypothalamus of the obese mutant A^Y mouse, AGRP is normally present in the hypothalamus, although its expression is restricted to NPY neurones[13]. Co-injection of α-MSH and AGRP attenuates the melanocortin's anorexigenic effects, whilst injection of AGRP alone produces a prolonged hyperphagia and obesity[14]. AGRP may also stimulate intake independently from the melano-cortin system, possibly via an opioid-dependent pathway.

The melanocortin and NPY systems interact with each other in a reciprocal fashion (Fig. 1). Consequently leptin regulates the melanocortin system in a complementary way to that of NPY. Leptin stimulates melanocortin pathways, consistent with the fact that both factors inhibit feeding and promote weight loss. Approximately 30 per cent of the POMC neurones expressed OB-Rb[15] and pharmacological blockade of MC4-R impairs the ability of leptin to reduce food intake and body weight. Consequently, it has been proposed that the melanocortin system mediates some of the central actions of leptin in the brain.

Orexins

Orexin A and B are homologous 33 and 28 residue peptides respectively, that are derived from the precursor preproorexin. Orexin cell bodies are restricted to the LHA and adjacent zona incerta, from where projections extend to many sites including the PVN, ARC and NTS[16]. Here they interact closely with other appetite-regulating systems, e.g. forming reciprocal connections with ARC NPY/AGRP and POMC/CART neuronal populations. The two classes of orexin receptor (OX1-R and OX2-R) are also widely but differentially distributed within the brain. OX1-R, which is relatively selective for orexin A, is abundant in the VMH. OX2-R, which demonstrates comparable affinity for both orexin peptides, is expressed preferentially in the PVN[17]

Orexin A stimulates feeding when injected centrally, whilst orexin B has a weaker effect (if any) on food intake. However, the actions of orexin A are acute and overall 24 h intake remains unaltered. Consequently, repeated orexin injections do not induce obesity[18]. These short term influences may be partly mediated by NPY and it is reported that they are regulated by plasma leptin. Most orexin neurones carry functional leptin receptors (OB-Rb) and show leptin induced activation of the JACK-STAT pathway. Moreover, central leptin administration is reported to decrease orexin expression[19]. Yet, reductions of plasma leptin, through either food restriction or diabetes, do not alter orexin levels. It appears that increased orexin expression occurs only under very specific conditions of decreased plasma glucose in conjunction with absence of food from the gut[20]. This suggests that orexin pathways are stimulated by hypoglycaemia but rapidly inhibited by neuronal signals from the viscera, such as gastric distension, which are transmitted indirectly to the LHA via the NTS. Orexin neurones are distinct from but intimately related to GSN in the LHA. The two appear to interact functionally to initiate the response to falling glucose and GSN may be partly responsible for mediating the central hyperphagic effects of orexin A.

Overall, orexin neurones may constitute a system for initiating and terminating short-term feeding. At the same time, their widespread distribution indicates a broad range of functions. The orexins are known to play a role in the regulation of the sleepwake cycle and any effects on feeding may simply be related to changes in general arousal.

Conclusion

Energy balance is too vital a function to be regulated by a single control system operating through a single neuropeptide. There can be no doubt that obesity is accompanied by changes in many hypothalamic neuropeptides. Much progress has been made in identifying the neuronal targets for these signals and the ways in which their actions are integrated within the CNS.

References

1. Bjorbaek C. Divergent signaling capacities of the long and short isoforms of the leptin receptor. *J Biol Chem* 1997; 272: 32686–95.

2. Zhang Y. Positional cloning of the mouse obese gene and its human homologue. *Nature* 1994; 372: 425–32.

3. Unger JW. Insulin receptors in the central nervous system: localization, signalling mechanisms and functional aspects. *Prog Neurobiol* 1991; 36: 343–62.

4. Baskin DG. Insulin and leptin: dual adiposity signals to the brain for the regulation of food intake and body weight. *Brain Res* 1999; 848: 114–23.

5. Mizuno Y. Glucose-responding neurons in the nucleus tractus solitarius of the rat, *in vitro* study. *Brain Res* 1984; 307: 109–16.

6. Allen YS. Neuropeptide Y distribution in rat brain. *Science* 1983; 221: 877–9.

7. Billington CJ. Effects of intracerebroventricular injection of neuropeptide Y on energy metabolism. *J Physiol* 1991; 260: R321–R7.

8. Widdowson PS. Reciprocal regional changes in brain NPY receptor density during dietary restriction and dietary-induced obesity in the rat. *Brain Res* 1997; 774: 1–10.

9. Mercer JG. Coexpression of leptin receptor and preproneuropeptide Y mRNA in arcuate nucleus of mouse hypothalamus. *J Neuroendocrinol* 1996; 8: 733–5.

10. Harrold JA. Altered energy balance causes selective changes in melanocortin-4 (MC4-R) but not melancortin-3 (MC3-R) receptors in specific hypothalamic regions: Further evidence that MC4-R activation is a physiological inhibitor of feeding. *Diabetes* 1999; 48: 267–71.

11. Huszar D. Targeted disruption of the melanocortin-4 receptor results in obesity in mice. *Cell* 1997; 88: 131–41.

12. Chen AS. Inactivation of the mouse melanocortin-3 receptor results in increased fat mass and reduced lean body mass. *Nature* 2000; 26: 97–102.

13. Hahn TM. Coexpression of Agrp and NPY in fasting-activated hypothalamic neurons. *Nat Neurosci* 1998; 1: 271–2.

14. Ollmann MM. Antagonism of central melanocortin receptors *in vitro* and *in vivo* by agouti-related protein. *Science* 1997; 278: 1135–8.

15. Cheung CC. Proopiomelanocortin neurons are direct targets for leptin in the hypothalamus. *Endocinology* 1997; 138: 4489–92.

16. Sakurai T. Orexins and orexin receptors: a family of hypothalamic neuropeptides and G protein-coupled receptors that regulate feeding behavior. *Cell* 1998; 92: 573–85.

17. Lu XY. Differential distribution and regulation of OX-1 and OX-2 orexin/hypocretin receptor messanger RNA in the brain upon fasting. *Horm Behav* 2000; 37: 335–44.

18. Haynes A. Effects of single and chronic intracerebroventricular administration of the orexins on feeding in the rat. *Peptides* 1099; 20: 1099–105.

19. Hakansson M. Leptin receptor- and STAT-immunoreactivities in hypocretin/orexin neurones of the lateral hypothalamus. *J Neuroendocrinol* 1999; 11: 653–63.

20. Cai XJ. Hypoglycemia activates orexin neurons and selectively increases hypothalamic orexin B levels. Responses inhibited by feeding and possible mediated by the nucleus of the solitary tract. *Diabetes* 2001; 50: 105–12.

Progress in Obesity Research: 9. Edited by *Geraldo Medeiros-Neto, Alfredo Halpern* and *Claude Bouchard*

©2003 John Libbey Eurotext Ltd, pp. 774–777.

CHAPTER 162

Uncoupling proteins: an overview

Frédéric Bouillaud

CNRS UPR 9078, Meudon, France
[e-mail: bouillau@infobiogen.fr]

Brown adipose tissue and UCP1

Brown adipose is found in mammals, it is exceptionnally well developped in hibernating mammals (of reduced size). It is also found in all newborns. Small mammals retain a functional brown adipose tissue which is recruited for thermogenesis during cold adaptation. In contrast large mammals (such as man) loose most of it. The thermogenic activity of brown adipose tissue is explained by a mitochondrial uncoupling protein called UCP1. Like most of the proteins constituting mitochondria UCP1 is coded by a nuclear gene called *Ucp1*. The proposal was made that brown adipose tissue (and therefore UCP1), could play a role in the control of body weight, independently from the control of body temperature. Unfortunately it became obvious that the occurence of brown adipose tissue and the expression of (UCP1) was almost negligible in adult humans. Genetic studies showed that the influence of *Ucp1* on obesity is not inexistant but of limited importance. Unfortunately no drug able to induce brown adipose tissue activity in man is available yet.

Discovery of UCP2 and UCP3

In 1997 two genes homologous to the *Ucp1* gene were discovered, they were called *Ucp2* and *Ucp3*. These genes are few kilobases apart, and result from the duplication of an ancestral gene. Homologues of (UCP2-UCP3) were found in other organisms than mammals: In birds an homolog of UCP2-UCP3 exists, it is expressed in muscle. Homologues were found also in cold blooded animals and plants. Therefore, although thermogenesis occurs sometimes in these organisms, it suggested that the function of these homologous proteins is distinct from that of UCP1. On the other hand the similarities of the UCP1, UCP2 and UCP3 sequences were high enough to suggest common functional properties. Therefore it was proposed that UCP2 and UCP3 like UCP1 were able to increase energy expenditure by modifying mitochondrial function.

Energy expenditure in mitochondria

Oxidation of substrates leads to reduction of coenzymes (NADH, FADH2). Reoxydation of these coenzymes occurs in the respiratory chain of mitochondria and ends up by the reduction of oxygen to form water. The energy liberated is used by the respiratory chain enzymes to pump protons outside mitochondria. This establishes an electrochemical gradient between the two sides of the mitochondrial inner membrane. When ATP production is not required the respiratory chain builds up a proton gradient high enough to render proton pumping more and more difficult, and this makes respiration much slower. As soon as ADP is made available, its phosphorylation into ATP by the FoF1 ATPase starts using the energy liberated by proton reentry into the mitochondria. This lowers the gradient and authorizes a higher respiratory rate. This ends when the ADP is almost exhausted and consequently when the ATP/ADP ratio becomes the highest, then a steady state is maintained with a high membrane potential 'in equilibrium' with a high phosphorylation potential (ATP/(ADP)) x (Pi)), and a low respiration rate. Therefore respiration is dependent on ATP production, this dependence is called coupling. In fact, most of the ATP is utilized within seconds for cell maintenance. Which means that most of the energy stored into ATP is finally dissipated as a degraded form of energy: heat. Accordingly energy expenditure, and heat production is directly linked to the amount of substrates utilized and therefore to oxygen consumption. In brown adipose tissue UCP1 allows proton reentry without ATP synthesis, therefore it uncouples respiration from ATP synthesis. There is a huge amount of mitochondria in brown adipocytes. The uptake of glucose by these cells could be intense, and their lipidic stores can be mobilized by lipolysis, which is under the control of the adrenergic innervation. UCP1 is provided with a convenient regulatory mechanism since at rest endogenous concentrations of nucleotides maintain UCP1 under inhibition, whereas free fatty acids liberated by lipolysis activate proton transport leading to uncoupling of mitochondria and intense heat production.

UCPs belong to a family of anion carriers present in the mitochondrial inner membrane

There is a need for exchanges between the mitochondria and the cytosol of the cell. For example since mitochondria are ATP providers for the cell, this implies that ADP and phosphate get in and that ATP gets out. This and import of substrates need transporters in the inner membrane. Since the inner membrane should also maintain a high membrane potential these transporters are specific and allow substrate entry/exchange in an energy conservative way (the number of charges exchanged has a fixed stoechiometry). For example the ATP/ADP translocator exchanges one molecule of ATP against one molecule of ADP. These transporters share similarities in their sequences. Based on these simalirities of sequence large sequencing programmes indicated that 30 to 40 genes coding for such proteins are present in the eucaryotic genome. UCP1, UCP2 and UCP3 belong to this family of homologous transporters.

Approaches used to determine the role of UCP2 and UCP3

Many studies showed that the UCP1 produced by a recombinant organism behaves like in brown adipose tissue mitochondria. Therefore this approach was used check whether or not UCP2 or UCP3 are uncoupling proteins. Although in many cases proton transport activity, and therefore an uncoupling activity was observed, the results obtained by different laboratories are not fully consistent. As we said before the inner membrane of mitochondria is submitted to an intense electric field that pushes protons in, and the introduction of a foreign protein, could disturb the membrane and cause a proton leak that is not the result of the normal function of the protein. This could be aggravated by the fact that many recombinant expression systems induce a real overexpression of the protein in comparison with the amount found naturally in mitochondria. There is another point that is neglected: UCP1 is able to transport other ions than protons, for example chloride. Other studies showed that this is the uncoupling activity (proton transport) which is physiologically relevant. Consequently scientists using recombinant expression systems studied the proton transport activity of UCP1. With UCP2 and UCP3 the recombinant expression systems were used the other way around: investigators aimed to demonstrate the existence of a proton transport activity because we suppose that it is the relevant one. Other possible biochemical activities that could be of importance for the cell, have not been looked for. This is aggravated by the fact that according to the conditions used *in vitro*, mitochondrial carriers such as the ATP/ADP translocator are able to uncouple partially mitochondria, although this is not their physiological relevance.

To gain insight on the physiological role of UCP2 and UCP3 investigators aimed to correlate the expression of UCP2 and UCP3 mRNA to various physiological states. This gave some informations, although variations in mRNA expression does not guarantee a similar evolution of protein amount (see below). No correlation could be found between mRNA expression and energy expenditure. For example starvation led to an increase in the mRNA levels whereas it is accompanied by energy sparing. This observation was explained by the fact that UCP2 and UCP3 mRNA expression were induced in presence of increased concentration of fatty acids. This and the existing evidences for the fatty acid cycle catalysed by proteins like UCPs led to the alternative proposal that UCP2 and UCP3 would be fatty acid transporters in charge to remove excess of fatty acids from the mitochondrial matrix.

Inactivation of the *Ucp2* or *Ucp3* gene has been obtained after genetic manipulation of mice. None of these strains of mice developped obesity or overweight, nor they were more sensitive to hyperlipidic diet. These observations made unlikely the role of UCP2 and UCP3 in the control of body weight. *Ucp2* null mice showed an increased insulin secretion and a better response to glucose of the pancreatic beta cells. They showed also a higher resistance to infection due to an overproduction of reactive oxygen species by macrophages. Although no phenotypical alteration could be observed in *Ucp3* null mice it was observed that their muscle mitochondria seem more coupled and submitted to a higher oxidative stress.

Before disregarding Ucps as genes of interest in the control of human overweight, we should consider the association/linkage betwen the *Ucp2-3* locus and several traits relevant to obesity. Indeed genetic studies aimed to decide whether or not, *Ucp2* and *Ucp3* genes are linked to the developpement of (resistance to) obesity and overweight. No systematic association was found between *Ucp2-3* locus and obesity. However two important observations need to be reminded: the first, which was partially at the origin of the discovery of the Ucp2/3 locus is that the chromosomal region containing Ucp2 and Ucp3 genes as well as quite a few others, influences obesity and insulin secretion in mice. This prediction proved to be absolutely right concerning insulin and UCP2 in view of the phenotype of Ucp2 null mice! The second observation was that it exists in man, a statistically significant correlation between genetic variation around the Ucp2-3 locus and the resting metabolic rate. This is exactly what would be predicted if we consider that UCPs operates essentially 'at rest' (see below).

UCPs and oxidative stress.

The level of coupling is dependent upon the permeability of the inner membrane to protons: the lower permeability the higher the coupling/yield. When ATP production is not required the respiration is minimal because the potential accros the inner membrane is maximal. Under these conditions electrons are somehow blocked in the respiratory chain before their normal acceptor (1/2O2) in the cytochrome oxidase. This promotes the combination of one electron with one oxygen molecule to produce super-oxide ion ($O2^{\cdot-}$), this is a reactive molecule which can directly damage cellular components or generate other reactive oxygen species (ROS) potentially dangerous. Long time before the discovery of UCP2/3 it has been proposed that the occurence of a limited proton leak (mild uncoupling) would lower the membrane potential, and therefore allow a slightly higher respiratory rate, which certainly represents a waste of energy but lowers significantly the ROS production. The observations made on *Ucp2* or *Ucp3* null mice reinforced considerably the hypothesis of the existence of a mild uncoupling *in vivo* and of the involvement of UCP2 and UCP3.

Expression level and its regulation

The detection of the protein UCP2 in mitochondria proved to be problematic. This contrasted with UCP1 in brown adipose tissue mitochondria which could be easily detected. The main explanation lies into very different expression levels for the two proteins. UCP1 is abundantly expressed, it reaches per cent of the proteins present in the inner membrane of mitochondria, on the other hand UCP2 is more than two orders of magnitude less expressed in spleen or lung mitochondria (where its expression level is the highest). Such a low level of expression implies that presently available antibodies are used at the limit of their sensitivity and it causes problems because cross hybridization are observed, presumably with other carriers of the mitochondrial inner membrane. This low expression level of UCP2 contrasts with a relatively high mRNA level. Moreover when induction of UCP2 was observed (in lung or gut) after starvation, or injection of lipopolysaccharide (LPS) two situations inducing an oxidative stress, it was observed that the protein level rose whereas there was no change in the mRNA level. This evidenced a translational regulation of UCP2 expression.

No such details are available yet concerning UCP3 expression in muscle. However recent data suggest also dissociation between mRNA and protein levels. It seems that UCP3 expression is highest in glycolytic muscle, since these muscle rely mainly on glycolysis for ATP production, in this place UCP3 would be of little influence on the normal ATP production. Fast glycolytic muscles are usually recruited exceptionnally for intense but short period of exercise, whereas oxidative muscle (fibres) exercise over longer period, for example to counter-balance gravity.

Regulation of UCP activity

A further level of control is brought by the regulation of the protein itself. This is of importance since it is shown experimentally that even a high amount of UCP1 present in the mitochondrial inner membrane can be completely silenced according to the composition of the surrounding medium. Presently the dominant (correct ?) model for UCP activity supposes that all (UCP1/2/3) operate similarly and that fatty acids are obligatory for the UCP activity to take place. Whereas nucleotides are able to inhibit completely this fatty acid induced uncoupling. Therefore efforts concentrated on the description of a fatty acid induced and nucleotide inhibited proton leak in mitochondria. This activity would be present in the wild type mice and and absent in the Ucp2/3 null mice. A recent proposal is that a further activator is required which is the superoxide ion. This explained why in several previous reports no difference was observed between wild type and Ucp2/3 null mice mitochondria. Although there are still uncompletely solved issues concerning this superoxide activation of UCPs, this strengthened considerably the link between UCPs and biochemistry of ROS.

Other studies evidenced differences between the regulation of the different UCPs, most of these reports used the yeast expression system which compares the three proteins in a similar mitochondrial context, however this exotic environment for a mammalian mitochondrial protein has been criticized, in particular since the same expression vectors are used to express similar and fairly high levels of each UCPs in yeast, levels which are fully compatible with the amount of UCP1 in brown adipose tissue, but certainly not with the amount of UCP2 in spleen, lung or white adipose tissue mitochondria. Possible problems linked to overexpression levels have been pointed out.

If the regulation of UC2/3 is similar to that of UCP1 there at least another way of regulating the activity of the protein that is often neglected and has important practical/physiological consequences. The proton transport by the UCP1 is extremely dependent upon the membrane potential that pushes protons through UCP1. When an intense production of ATP occurs the membrane potential is relatively lowered, and therefore UCP1 is a very poor competitor for the phosphorylation by the FoF1ATPase. If a high ATP/ADP ratio is maintained, due either to low ATP usage or to non mitochondrial source of ATP (glycolysis), this result in a higher mitochondrial membrane potential that would greatly stimulate the protonophoric activity of UCP. Therefore the presence of a UCP is not *per se* deleterious for an intense ATP formation, but would lower the maximal value of membrane potential and ATP/ADP ratio that could be attained. It would be easier to understand why UCP2 affects the insulin secretion in the beta cell where the ATP/ADP ration value is used as a signal, and why it, probably as well as UCP3, has little influence on energy expenditure since most of the cells operate with mitochondria permanently recruited for a significant ATP production a condition that would not authorize UCP activity. In other words: in muscle a marginal variation in muscular activity would probably influence much more energy expenditure than UCP3 activity could do. But presence of UCP3 in muscle would avoid that oxidative damage accumulate over time in muscle fibres that are poorly recruited for contraction.

And obesity ...

The situtation is therefore the following: *in vitro* tests failed to give a completely convincing demonstration of the uncoupling activity of UCP2 and UCP3. Experiments made with Ucp2/3 null mice supported indirectly this uncoupling activity, but showed that it has almost no relevance to the control of body weight. This may be explained by the fact that the uncoupling activity operates in cells or conditions which have little influence on energy expenditure. On the other hand overexpression of UCP1 or UCP3 in the muscle of transgenic mice showed that important improvements could be expected if a gain of function of these proteins does occur in muscle or adipose tissue. Therefore it remains possible that recruitment of the uncoupling activity of UCPs, regardless of its physiological significance, would help to increase the overall energy expenditure in man. The interpretation of the effect of the UCP2 on insulin secretion control points to a limitation in the use of UCPs, which if it lowers the maximal ATP/ADP ratio in cells where this is used as a signal, would lead to dysfunction of these cells which are likely to be involved in complex loops of control. This and the exclusive occurence of UCP3 in muscle, an organ responsible for a large part of energy expenditure in man, make UCP3 the best candidate. In this respect the search for specific ligands of the UCP3 showing more specificity than fatty acids, is of interest. Recruitment of the uncoupling activity of UCP1 is still an interesting but challenging objective.

A very short list of reviews is given below.

References

1. Nicholls D. A history of the first uncoupling protein, UCP1. *J Bioenerg Biomemb* 1999; 31: 399–406.

2. Gonzalez Barroso MM, Ricquier D, Cassard-Doulcier AM. The human uncoupling protein-1 gene: present status and perspectives in obesity research. *Obes Rev* 2000; 1: 61–72.

3. Ricquier D, Bouillaud F. The uncoupling protein homologues UCP1, UCP2, UCP3, StUCP, AtUCP. *Biochem J* 2000; 345: 161–79.

4. Boss O, Hagen T, Lowell B. Uncoupling proteins 2 and 3: potential regulators of mitochondrial energy metabolism. *Diabetes* 2000; 49: 143–56.

Progress in Obesity Research: 9. Edited by *Geraldo Medeiros-Neto, Alfredo Halpern and Claude Bouchard*
©2003 John Libbey Eurotext Ltd, pp. 778–780.

CHAPTER 163

The mechanism of mitochondrial proton leak, a major contributor to energy expenditure

Martin D. Brand

MRC Dunn Human Nutrition Unit, Cambridge CB2 2XY, UK
[e-mail: martin.brand@mrc-dunn.cam.ac.uk]

Introduction

Mitochondria couple oxidation of substrates to phosphorylation of ADP by pumping protons from the matrix to the exterior; the electrochemical proton gradient that is generated then drives the protons back to the matrix through the ATP synthase. However, the inner membrane of isolated mitochondria has a finite proton conductance[1–5]. This conductance allows a leak of protons back into the matrix, bypassing the ATP synthase and resulting in oxidative phosphorylation being less than fully coupled *in vitro*. This endogenous uncoupling was originally assumed to be an artefact of mitochondrial isolation, but it is now clear that it is a natural pathway that operates in intact cells and tissues, such as hepatocytes, thymocytes and intact skeletal muscle[6–8].

A high proportion of respiration is used to drive the futile proton cycle across the mitochondrial inner membrane in rat hepatocytes: 20 per cent in active hepatocytes[8] and 25 per cent in resting hepatocytes[6]. In perfused rat muscle the proportion is even greater, 35 per cent in contracting preparations[8] and 50 per cent in resting muscle[7]. The sum of the proton cycling rates in different organs of the rat suggests that 20 per cent of its basal metabolic rate may be devoted entirely to driving this futile cycle[8], making it significant in energy homeostasis and an attractive target for modulation to combat obesity. Indeed, increasing the proton conductance of mitochondria has been shown to be a very effective treatment for obesity. This has been shown using the chemical uncoupler dinitrophenol in clinical practice[9], and in transgenic mice with partial uncoupling of muscle mitochondria caused by overexpression of uncoupling protein 3 (UCP3): the UCP3 overexpressing mice are lean despite significant hyperphagia[10].

The pathway of the basal proton leak has not been established. There is compelling evidence that uncoupling protein 1 (UCP1) in brown adipose tissue mitochondria catalyses an inducible proton conductance that is stimulated by fatty acids and inhibited by purine nucleotides, including ATP and GDP[11,12], although the mechanistic details are under discussion. However, UCP1 does not catalyse the basal uncoupling common to all mitochondria[12]. The UCP1 homologues UCP2 and UCP3 have high sequence similarity to UCP1[13], suggesting the hypothesis that they too may uncouple oxidative phosphorylation.

Results and discussion

Our evidence indicates UCP2 and UCP3 make no significant contribution to basal proton conductance. Although overexpression of UCP3 in mice causes uncoupling and prevents obesity as discussed above[10], physiological manipulation of UCP2 and UCP3 levels by diet has no effect on the basal proton conductance of isolated skeletal muscle mitochondria[14]. Most convincingly, the basal proton conductance of muscle mitochondria from UCP3 knockout mice is the same as that of littermate wild-type controls[15], showing that UCP3 cannot be responsible for the basal proton conductance. Similar observations have recently been made for UCP2 in Bouillaud's group. Reports[16,17] that mitochondria from UCP3 knockout animals have lower proton conductance than controls are probably explained by non-basal assay conditions (so that inducible, not basal proton conductance was changed, see below) or perhaps by effects of genetic background. Other evidence that UCPs are not responsible for basal proton conductance comes from several organisms including the yeast *Saccharomyces cerevisiae*, where basal proton conductance is normal, but UCPs are absent[4,5,18].

Is the basal proton conductance of mitochondria catalysed by any other specific mitochondrial protein, or is it a general background property of the phospholipids and proteins of the mitochondrial membrane? Diffusion of protons through the phospholipid bilayer is one possible mechanism. To examine this possibility, phospholipids from mitochondria with different proton conductance were extracted and reformed into liposomes, and their proton conductance was measured[19,20]. These experiments resolved two issues: the percentage of proton conductance explainable by proton diffusion across the bilayer, and the effect of the phospholipid fatty acyl composition of the bilayer on the conductance. The results showed that passive diffusion in liposomes accounted for only 2.5 to 25 per cent of the proton conductance of mitochondria, implying that some other property of the membrane, such as the presence of proteins, was important in determining the conductance[19]. There was no significant difference in proton conductance between liposomes with very different phospholipid fatty acyl compositions[20], despite a known relationship between the phospholipid fatty acyl composition of intact mitochondria and proton conductance[21]. Perhaps acyl composition is important in mitochondria, but loss of phospholipid asymmetry or of some specific protein causes the effect to be lost in liposomes.

To search for a specific protein catalyst of the basal proton conductance in yeast, we tested whether any member of the mitochondrial carrier family (to which the mammalian UCPs belong) might be an important contributor to basal conductance. There are 35 members of the family in the *S. cerevisiae* genome[4], so we examined the proton conductance of mitochondria isolated from 21 different yeast mutants deleted for each of the carriers that did not have a well-established function and did not give rise to a petite phenotype. None of 21 knockout mutants had decreased proton conductance, showing that none of these mitochondrial carriers is responsible for the basal leak in yeast (or, presumably, mammalian) mitochondria[18].

UCP2 and UCP3 are not responsible for the basal proton leak of mammalian mitochondria, but can they catalyse an inducible proton leak, analogous to the inducible leak catalysed by UCP1? We have expressed UCP2 in *E. coli* inclusion bodies. After refolding, soluble UCP2 binds purine nucleotides with micromolar affinities for ATP and GDP[22]. This corroborates findings in liposomes that UCP2, like UCP1, has high affinity for purine nucleotides. We have recently found that nucleotide-sensitive proton leak can be induced by superoxide in mitochondria that contain UCP1, UCP2 or UCP3, but not in mitochondria that lack any of these proteins[23]. In particular, activation by superoxide is abolished in skeletal muscle mitochondria from UCP3 knockout mice, and appears in mitochondria from yeast expressing mouse UCP1. Thus UCP2 and UCP3, despite their low abundance relative to UCP1, can catalyse a significant inducible proton conductance. The characteristics, mechanism and function of this conductance will not be dealt with here.

The nucleotide-sensitive superoxide-activated uncoupling that is characteristic of native UCPs can be used as a tool to test for native UCP function in the model systems that have been used to examine the putative role of UCPs in basal proton conductance. Previous work has provided evidence for uncoupling by the different UCP1 homologues when they have been overexpressed in yeast, in mammalian cells and in mice[4,5,10,13]. We have tested the yeast[23] and mouse[10,15] UCP expression systems, and find that the uncoupling that occurs is insensitive to superoxide and nucleotides. This confirms our previous contention[4,5,14,24-26] that the uncoupling seen in these expression systems does not reflect a native property of the UCPs, but is an artefact of incorrectly inserted proteins. These expression systems therefore provide no support for the hypothesis that UCPs are involved in the basal proton conductance of mitochondria.

I conclude by stating that UCPs and many other mitochondrial carrier family proteins are not responsible for the basal proton conductance of mitochondria. The pathway for this basal conductance remains to be elucidated.

Acknowledgements: I thank my students and colleagues, past and present, who have contributed enormously to the experiments and ideas outlined in this review.

References

1. Nicholls DG. The influence of respiration and ATP hydrolysis on the proton-electrochemical gradient across the inner membrane of rat-liver mitochondria as determined by ion distribution. *Eur J Biochem* 1974; 50: 305–15.

2. Brand MD. The proton leak across the mitochondrial inner membrane. *Biochim Biophys Acta* 1990; 1018: 128–33.

3. Brand MD, Chien L-F, Ainscow EK, Rolfe DFS, Porter RK. The causes and functions of mitochondrial proton leak. *Biochim Biophys Acta* 1994; 1187: 132–9.

4. Brand MD, Brindle KM, Buckingham JA, Harper JA, Rolfe DFS, Stuart JA. The significance and mechanism of mitochondrial proton conductance. *Int J Obes* 1999; 23 (Suppl 6): S4–S11.

5. Stuart JA, Brindle KM, Harper JA, Brand MD. Mitochondrial proton leak and the uncoupling proteins. *J Bioenerg Biomemb* 1999; 31: 517–25.

6. Nobes CD, Brown GC, Olive PN, Brand MD. Non-ohmic proton conductance of the mitochondrial inner membrane in hepatocytes. *J Biol Chem* 1990; 265: 12903–9.

7. Rolfe DFS, Brand MD. Contribution of mitochondrial proton leak to skeletal muscle respiration and to standard metabolic rate. *Am J Physiol* 1996; 271: C1380–C9.

8. Rolfe DFS, Newman JMB, Buckingham JA, Clark MG, Brand MD. Contribution of mitochondrial proton leak to respiration rate in working skeletal muscle and liver and to SMR. *Am J Physiol* 1999; 276: C692–C9.

9. Harper JA, Dickinson K, Brand MD. Mitochondrial uncoupling as a target for drug development for the treatment of obesity. *Obesity Rev* 2001; 2: 255–265.

10. Clapham JC, Arch JRS, Chapman H, Haynes A, Lister C, Moore GBT *et al.* Mice overexpressing human uncoupling protein-3 in skeletal muscle are hyperphagic and lean. *Nature* 2000; 406: 415–8.

11. Klingenberg M, Huang S-G. Structure and function of the uncoupling protein from brown adipose tissue. *Biochim Biophys Acta* 1999; 1415: 271–96.

12. Nedergaard J, Golozoubova V, Matthias A, Asadi A, Jacobsson A, Cannon B. UCP1: the only protein able to mediate adaptive non-shivering thermogenesis and metabolic inefficiency. *Biochim Biophys Acta* 2001; 1504: 82–106.

13. Ricquier D, Bouillaud F. The uncoupling protein homologues: UCP1, UCP2, UCP3, StUCP and AtUCP. *Biochem J* 2000; 345: 161–79.

14. Cadenas S, Buckingham JA, Samec S, Seydoux J, Din N, Dulloo AG, Brand MD. UCP2 and UCP3 rise in starved rat skeletal muscle but mitochondrial proton conductance is unchanged. *FEBS Letters* 1999; 462: 257–60.

15. Cadenas S, Echtay KS, Harper JA, Jekabsons MB, Buckingham JA, Grau E *et al.* The basal proton conductance of skeletal muscle mitochondria from transgenic mice overexpressing or lacking uncoupling protein-3. *J Biol Chem* 2002; 277: 2773–8.

16. Gong D-W, Monemdjou S, Gavrilova O, Leon LR, Marcus-Samuels B, Chou CJ *et al.* Lack of obesity and normal response to fasting and thyroid hormone in mice lacking uncoupling protein-3. *J Biol Chem* 2000; 275: 16251–7.

17. Vidal-Puig AJ, Grujic D, Zhang C-Y, Hagen T, Boss O, Ido Y *et al.* Energy metabolism in uncoupling protein 3 gene knockout mice. *J Biol Chem* 2000; 275: 16258–66.

18. Roussel D, Harding M, Runswick MJ, Walker JE, Brand MD. Does any yeast mitochondrial carrier have a native uncoupling protein function? *J Bioenerg. Biomemb* 2002; 34: 165–76.

19. Brookes PS, Rolfe DFS, Brand MD. The proton permeability of liposomes made from mitochondrial inner membrane phospholipids: comparison with isolated mitochondria. *J Memb Biol* 1997; 155: 167–74.

20. Brookes PS, Hulbert AJ, Brand MD. The proton permeability of liposomes made from mitochondrial inner membrane phospholipids: no effect of fatty acid composition. *Biochim Biophys Acta* 1997; 1330: 157–64.

21. Hulbert AJ, Else PL, Manolis SC, Brand MD. Proton leak in hepatocytes and liver mitochondria from archosaurs (crocodiles) and allometric relationships for ectotherms. *J Comp Physiol B* 2002; 172: 387–97.

22. Jekabsons MB, Echtay KS, Brand MD. Nucleotide binding to human uncoupling protein-2 refolded from bacterial inclusion bodies. *Biochem J* 2002; 366: 565–71.

23. Echtay KS, Roussel D, St-Pierre J, Jekabsons MB, Cadenas S, Stuart JA *et al.* Superoxide activates mitochondrial uncoupling proteins. *Nature* 2002; 415: 96–9.

24. Harper JA, Stuart JA, Jekabsons MB, Roussel D, Brindle KM, Dickinson K *et al.* Artifactual uncoupling by uncoupling protein 3 in yeast mitochondria at the concentrations found in mouse and rat skeletal muscle mitochondria. *Biochem J* 2002; 361: 49–56.

25. Stuart JA, Harper JA, Brindle KM, Jekabsons MB, Brand MD. A mitochondrial uncoupling artifact can be caused by expression of uncoupling protein 1 in yeast. *Biochem J* 2001; 356: 779–89.

26. Stuart JA, Harper JA, Brindle KM, Jekabsons MB, Brand MD. Physiological levels of mammalian uncoupling protein 2 do not uncouple yeast mitochondria. *J Biol Chem* 2001; 276: 18633–9.

Progress in Obesity Research: 9. Edited by *Geraldo Medeiros-Neto, Alfredo Halpern and Claude Bouchard*
©2003 John Libbey Eurotext Ltd, pp. 781–785.

CHAPTER 164

Uncoupling protein 3 (UCP3) and fatty acid metabolism in muscle

Mary-Ellen Harper, Lisa Bevilacqua, Sheila Costford, Lorenne Doucet, Mahmoud Salkhordeh and Martin Gerrits

Department of Biochemistry, Microbiology and Immunology, Faculty of Medicine, University of Ottawa, 451 Smyth Rd, Ottawa, Ontario, Canada K1H 8M5
[e-mail: mharper@uottawa.ca]

Introduction

The physiological induction and regulation of uncoupling thermogenesis has been of scientific interest for over fifty years, beginning with the identification of brown adipose tissue (BAT). Uncoupling refers to mitochondrial processes that allow protonmotive force (PMF) to be dissipated without the concomitant synthesis of ATP through ATP synthase. Thus the oxidation of energy substrates is uncoupled from ADP phosphorylation, and energy is released as heat. Uncoupling protein-1 (UCP1), expressed exclusively in BAT, allows the return of protons from the intermembrane space into the matrix, bypassing ATP synthase. UCP1 activity is highly regulated. The importance of UCP1 in thermogenesis is reviewed elsewhere in this compendium. The focus here is upon a potential role for UCP3 in muscle fatty acid metabolism.

Identification of UCP 'homologues'

Within the last five years, four genes have been identified as UCP1 homologues, based on their degree of amino acid identity with UCP1 and on initial findings from their heterologous expression in yeast systems. These are referred to as UCP2, UCP3, UCP4, and UCP5 (the latter is also referred to as BMCP1). In particular, UCP2 and UCP3 have been the subject of hundreds of studies into their potential roles in uncoupling thermogenesis, and obesity. UCP4 and BMCP1 are found to a large extent in the central nervous system, and have not been as widely studied as UCP2 and UCP3.

The cloning of the novel UCPs was also met with great interest due to the possibility that they might mediate mitochondrial proton leak, a process that occurs in a wide variety of tissues and that is thought to account for a large proportion (roughly 20 per cent) of basal metabolic rate[1]. We have recently shown an association between rate of proton leak in muscle mitochondria and rate of weight loss in patients in a clinical weight loss programme[2]. The role of proton leak in energy expenditure is also reviewed elsewhere in this compendium. The aim of this brief report is to review recent findings into the possible physiological role(s) of UCP3.

UCP3 and regulation of its expression

UCP3 is expressed in skeletal muscle and BAT, and at low levels in heart; its homology to UCP1 is 57 per cent[3,4]. In human muscle, there are short and long forms of UCP3 mRNA, with the short form lacking the last coding exon[3,5]. The latter results in a truncated protein, lacking the sixth transmembrane domain, but its physiological expression has not been documented. While the relative importance of transcriptional and translational controls is unknown for UCP3, the expression of the long form of the *protein* responds physiologically (e.g. to fasting)[6]. In contrast to the selective tissue expression patterns of UCP1 and UCP3, UCP2 is expressed almost ubiquitously, with high levels in spleen, lung, stomach, and pancreas. However, UCP2 *protein* is found only in tissues having very high levels of mRNA expression and UCP2 protein was undetected in muscle[7].

Transcriptional regulation of UCP3 expression occurs through three putative peroxisome proliferator elements, and one thyroid response element (PPRE and TRE, respectively). Abundant also are recognition motives for muscle-specific factors including E-box sites, and a MEF-2 site[8]. Gong et al.[9] showed that starvation increased expression in muscle and decreased expression in BAT, paralleling starvation-induced changes in fatty acid oxidation in these tissues. Nocturnal norepinephrine (NE) excretion correlated with abundance of UCP2 and UCP3 mRNA in muscle, suggesting that sympathetic tone could be an important factor in the expression, and perhaps function of these genes[10]. As NE stimulates fatty acid oxidation, this indirectly supports the below described role for UCP3 in fatty acid metabolism.

UCP3 and energy expenditure

Support for a role for UCP3 in energy expenditure was initially garnered from reports that UCP3 lowered mitochondrial membrane potential when transfected into yeast (e.g. Gong et al.[9]). However, as described below, the physiological importance of these reports is questionable. Indeed, despite hundreds of publications, there are important controversies and only a very limited understanding of the physiological and biochemical properties of UCP3 has emerged. The following discussion is necessarily brief, but we and others have reviewed the relevant literature elsewhere[11,12]. Because of pronounced differences in the regulation of UCP2 and UCP3 expression in muscle and the apparent absence of significant UCP2 protein in muscle[7], the emphasis in the literature and here is on UCP3.

While some genetic linkage and association studies have supported a relationship between UCP3 and energy expenditure, others have not. Because UCP2 and UCP3 are adjacent on chromosomes 7 and 11 in mice and humans, respectively, linkage markers are in the vicinity of both genes. mRNA expression of UCP3 in muscle was positively correlated with sleeping metabolic rate in obese Pima Indians[13]. Treatment with thyroid hormone, known to stimulate metabolic rate, increased the expression of muscle UCP3 mRNA in lean subjects[14]. However in healthy adults, variability in thyroid hormone, but not UCP2 and UCP3 mRNA, contributed to variability in resting energy expenditure[10]. Thus an important role for UCP3 in energy expenditure is questionnable.

Absence and overexpression of UCP3 in mice

A number of transgenic mouse models for the study of UCPs have been created. The UCP1 −/− mouse is cold-sensitive but is not more predisposed to diet-induced obesity than control mice[15]. Our later studies showed some compensatory energy expenditure through skeletal muscle mitochondrial proton leak that would counter obesity development[16]. Very importantly, however, there were no increases in UCP2 and UCP3 expression in muscle, supporting the idea that the physiological function of UCP2 and UCP3 is distinct from basal mitochondrial proton leak. This supports findings in fasted rats showing that, despite increases in UCP3 protein, muscle mitochondrial proton leak is unchanged[6]. In muscle mitochondria we found higher mitochondrial membrane potential in UCP3 −/− mice than controls, but found that state 4 (non-phosphorylating) respiration was unchanged[17,18]. Vidal Puig et al.[19] observed higher respiratory control ratios in UCP3 −/− muscle mitochondria; they also noted higher levels of serum fatty acids in older UCP3 −/− mice, and increased production of reactive oxygen species in muscle of UCP −/− mice. Cadenas et al.[20] did not detect differences in either membrane potential or respiratory control ratios. Methodological differences and the fact that the groups were using different lines of knockout mice on different and variable genetic backgrounds (e.g. [21]) may explain, in part, discrepancies in findings. Thus results overall support an important role for mitochondrial proton leak in energy expenditure, but do not support a role for UCP3 in muscle mitochondrial proton leak.

Mice that overexpress human UCP3 (hUCP3-tg) in muscle[22] are resistant to obesity, more glucose tolerant and have reduced total plasma cholesterol compared to wild-type mice. mRNA levels of the alpha-skeletal actin-driven expression of the transgene are very high (~66 fold higher than wild-type gene), and the uncoupling observed is thought to reflect an artifact of transgenic expression[20].

What then is the physiological function of UCP3?

Results from UCP3 −/− mice support a role for UCP3 in fatty acid metabolism and in protection from reactive oxygen species. In mitochondria lacking UCP3, production of ROS is increased[19]. In 4–6 month-old mice fed a high fat diet, circulating levels of FFA were higher in knockouts than controls[19]. Our recent studies on the effects of fasting in UCP3 −/− mice have shown lower whole body fat oxidation in knockout vs. control mice[18]. It is important to remember that all of these previous studies were conducted in F1 generation knockouts and control mice – thus, from mouse to mouse, there are variable amounts of the different genetic backgrounds. That genetic background is very important is well acknowledged[21]. Finally, it must be acknowledged that the interpretation of findings from knockout models is often difficult; compensation occurs through unforeseen, and often unknown, mechanisms. Studies are currently underway in our laboratory and other laboratories on mice having identical genetic backgrounds, and different levels of UCP expression (UCP3 –/–, wild type, and UCP3 overexpressors); results from these studies will thus be valuable.

Based on all available findings, it is clear that the physiological function of UCP3 is not proton leak, as originally proposed. The higher mitochondrial membrane potential in UCP3 –/– mitochondria[17,18] could be explained by the absence of the efflux of an anion, or the influx of a cation. Several paradoxes have led to the questioning of the fundamental premise that UCP3 functions primarily as an uncoupling protein. The most important paradox is the increased UCP3 expression that occurs during severe food restriction[23], a condition where *decreased* muscle thermogenesis is well recognized. Moreover, during chronic exposure to cold, UCP3 mRNA expression is not upregulated[23]. Finally, even at thermoneutral temperatures (no need for thermogenesis), fasting causes increased expression[24]. Thus it was not long after its identification that UCP3 that UCP3 was hypothesized to somehow regulate fatty acid metabolism[24].

Hypothesized role for UCP3 in mitochondrial FA export

In 2001 we hypothesized that UCP3 functions as a fatty acid anion exporter to facilitate high rates of fatty acid oxidation[25]. Specifically, we proposed that UCP3 acts in concert with mitochondrial thioesterase-1 (MTE-1) liberating CoASH to support high rates of FA oxidation, and to remove from the matrix the potentially toxic FA anions produced by MTE-1. MTE-1 is a long chain acyl CoA (LCA-CoA) thioesterase in the mitochondrial matrix. LCA-CoA thioesterases are a multigene family having varied intracellular locations, including cytosolic (CTE-1), mitochondrial (MTE-1) and peroxisomal (PTE-1b) compartments. The function of MTE-1 is thought to be the release of CoASH, a metabolite in high demand for matrix reactions involved in FA oxidation. LCA-CoA may sequester CoASH, thus reducing its availability for beta-oxidation and the Krebs cycle. We thus proposed that UCP3 functions with MTE-1 to liberate CoASH, and export potentially detrimental FA anions. Another mechanism, proposed shortly thereafter, posits that UCP3 acts as a FA 'flipase' protein in the mitochondrial inner membrane to remove matrix FA[26]. The latter does not however integrate UCP3 expression with physiological increases in FA oxidation, or with matrix MTE-1 expression, and relies on mitochondrial uptake of fatty acids through a CPT-1 independent mechanism.

While our hypothesis requires further study, support for a role for UCP3 in FA anion export is accruing. In the hUCP3-tg mice, we measured muscle mRNA for many genes important in FA metabolism[27]. The most notable change in gene expression was a threefold increase in MTE-1 expression, both confirming the importance of MTE-1 during increased mitochondrial beta-oxidation, and indirectly supporting the hypothesis that UCP-3 exports fatty acids generated by MTE-1. Lipoprotein lipase mRNA was increased by 50 per cent ($P < 0.05$). UCP2 expression was unchanged. mRNA levels of CPT-1beta and fatty acid binding proteins, and transporters were unchanged, suggesting that increased FA flux through beta-oxidation does not necessarily require marked changes in expression of genes involved in FA metabolism. A recent study in db/db and db/+ mice showed that UCP3 expression in muscle was closely correlated with changes in MTE-1 expression in response to treatment with rosiglitazone or 14,643 (PPAR gamma and delta agonists, respectively)[28]. Findings again support UCP3 and MTE-1 acting in the same pathway, responding to, or regulating, FA oxidation. The inhibition of FA oxidation by etomoxir (inhibits CPT-1, the 'rate-limiting step' for mitochondrial FA uptake) results in decreased UCP3 despite high circulating levels of FFA[29]. Results thus support a direct association between UCP3 and FA oxidation.

Finally, a brief discussion of differences in UCP3 expression between muscle fibre types, and changes induced by fasting is necessary. Muscle is a heterogeneous tissue both structurally and metabolically. Consideration into UCP3 function must take this into account. In non-fasted mice UCP3 mRNA expression is highest in gastrocnemius (mixture of all 3 fibre types, but mainly fast twitch oxidative-glycolytic, and glycolytic fibres; smaller amount of slow twitch oxidative), tibialis anterior (fast twitch oxidative-glycolytic), tensor fascia latae (fast twitch glycolytic), and lower in the soleus (slow twitch oxidative)[3]. The fast and mixed muscle fibre-types account for the bulk of body muscle mass. Fasting increases UCP3 transcription 14-21-fold in white gastrocnemius (glycolytic) and six–eightfold in red gastrocnemius (oxidative) and plantaris (mixed) muscles[30]. No change occurred in soleus muscle. Fasting also increased transcription rate of the lipoprotein lipase (LPL), carnitine palmitoyltransferase I (CPT I), and long-chain acyl-CoA dehydrogenase (LCAD) genes two–fourfold in the fast and mixed fibre-types. Increases in UCP3 with fasting could reflect large relative shifts from glucose to FA oxidation in muscle.

In conclusion, evidence supports a physiological role for UCP3 not in uncoupling thermogenesis, but as a metabolic switch, allowing high rates of fatty acid oxidation. By removing potentially detrimental fatty acid anions from the matrix and thereby lowering mitochondrial protonmotive force, such a mechanism may also underlie the protective role of UCP3 against damage from reactive oxygen species.

Acknowledgements: Supported by NSERC of Canada and the Canadian Institutes for Health Research.

References

1. Rolfe DFS, Brand MD. Contribution of mitochondrial proton leak to skeletal muscle respiration and to standard metabolic rate. *Am J Physiol* 1996; 271: C1380–C9.

2. Harper M-E, Dent R, Monemdjou S, Bezaire V, Van Wyck L, Wells G et al. Decreased mitochondrial proton leak and reduced expression of uncoupling protein 3 in skeletal muscle of obese diet-resistant women. *Diabetes* 2002; 51: 2459–66.

3. Boss O, Samec S, Paoloni-Giacobino A, Rossier C, Dulloo A, Seydoux J et al. Uncoupling protein-3: a new member of the mitochondrial carrier family with tissue-specific expression. *FEBS Letters* 1997; 408: 39–42.

4. Vidal-Puig A, Solanes G, Grujic D, Flier JS, Lowell BB. UCP3: an uncoupling protein homologue expressed preferentially and abundantly in skeletal muscle and brown adipose tissue. *Biochem Biophys Res Commun* 1997; 235: 79–82.

5. Solanes G, Vidal-Puig A, Grujic D, Flier JS, Lowell BB. The human uncoupling protein-3 gene. Genomic structure, chromosomal localization, and genetic basis for short and long form transcripts. *J Biol Chem* 1997; 272, 25433–6.

6. Cadenas S, Buckingham JA, Samec S, Seydoux J, Din N, Dulloo AG, Brand MD. UCP2 and UCP3 rise in starved rat skeletal muscle but mitochondrial proton conductance is unchanged. *FEBS Letters* 1999; 462: 257–60.

7. Pecqueur C, Alves-Guerra M-C, Gelly C, Lévi-Meyrueis C, Couplan E, Collins S et al. Uncoupling protein 2, *in vivo* distribution, induction upon oxidative stress, and evidence for translational regulation. *J Biol Chem* 2001; 276: 8705–12.

8. Acin A, Rodriguez M, Rique H, Canet E, Boutin JA, Galizzi JP. Cloning and characterization of the 5' flanking region of the human uncoupling protein 3 (UCP3) gene. *Biochem Biophys Res Commun* 1999; 258: 278–83.

9. Gong DW, He Y, Karas M, Reitman M. Uncoupling protein-3 is a mediator of thermogenesis regulated by thyroid hormone, beta3-adrenergic agonists, and leptin. *J Biol Chem* 1997; 272: 24129–32.

10. Boivin M, Camirand A, Carli F, Hoffer LJ, Silva JE. Uncoupling protein-2 and -3 messenger ribonucleic acids in adipose tissue and skeletal muscle of healthy males: variability, factors affecting expression, and relation to measures of metabolic rate. *J Clin Endocrinol Metab* 2000; 85: 1975–83.

11. Argyropoulos G, Harper M-E. Uncoupling proteins and thermoregulation. *J Appl Physiol* 2002; 92: 2187–98.

12. Samec S, Dulloo AG. Uncoupling proteins: their roles in adaptive thermogenesis and substrate metabolism reconsidered. *Br J Nutr* 2001; 86: 123–39.

13. Schrauwen P, Xia J, Bogardus C, Pratley RE, Ravussin E. Skeletal muscle uncoupling protein 3 expression is a determinant of energy expenditure in Pima Indians. *Diabetes* 1999; 48: 146–9.

14. Barbe P, Larrouy D, Boulanger C, Chevillotte E, Viguerie N, Thalamas C et al. Triiodothyronine-mediated upregulation of UCP2 and UCP3 mRNA expression in human skeletal muscle without coordinated induction of mitochondrial respiratory chain genes. *FASEB J* 2001; 15: 13–5.

15. Enerback S, Jacobsson A, Simpson EM, Guerra C, Yamashita H, Harper M-E, Kozak LP. Mice lacking mitochondrial uncoupling protein are cold-sensitive but not obese. *Nature* 1997; 387: 90–4.

16. Monemdjou S, Hofmann WE, Kozak LP, Harper M-E. Increased mitochondrial proton leak in skeletal muscle mitochondria of UCP1-deficient mice. *Am J Physiol Endocrinol Metab* 2000; 279: E941–E6.

17. Gong DW, Monemdjou S, Gavrilova O, Leon LR, Marcus-Samuels B, Chou CJ et al. Lack of obesity and normal response to fasting and thyroid hormone in mice lacking uncoupling protein-3. *J Biol Chem* 2000; 275: 16251–7.

18. Bezaire V, Hofmann W, Kramer JK, Kozak LP, Harper M-E. Effects of fasting on muscle mitochondrial energetics and fatty acid metabolism in Ucp3(–/–) and wild-type mice. *Am J Physiol Endocrinol Metab* 2001; 281: E975–E82.

19. Vidal-Puig AJ, Grujic D, Zhang CY, Hagen T, Boss O, Ido Y et al. Energy metabolism in uncoupling protein 3 gene knockout mice. *J Biol Chem* 2000; 275: 16258–66.

20. Cadenas S, Echtay KS, Harper JA, Jekabsons MB, Buckingham JA, Grau E et al. The basal proton conductance of skeletal muscle mitochondria from transgenic mice overexpressing or lacking uncoupling protein-3. *J Biol Chem* 2002; 277: 2773–8.

21. Hofmann WE, Liu X, Bearden CM, Harper M-E, Kozak LP. Effects of genetic background on thermoregulation and fatty acid-induced uncoupling of mitochondria in UCP1-deficient mice. *J Biol Chem* 2001; 276: 12460–5.

22. Clapham JC, Arch JR, Chapman H, Haynes A, Lister C, Moore GB et al. Mice overexpressing human uncoupling protein-3 in skeletal muscle are hyperphagic and lean. *Nature* 2000; 406: 415–8.

23. Boss O, Samec S, Dulloo A, Seydoux J, Muzzin P, Giacobino JP. Tissue-dependent upregulation of rat uncoupling protein-2 expression in response to fasting or cold. *FEBS Letters* 1997; 412: 111–4.

24. Samec S, Seydoux J, Dulloo AG. Role of UCP homologues in skeletal muscles and brown adipose tissue: mediators of thermogenesis or regulators of lipids as fuel substrate? *FASEB J* 1998; 12: 715–24.

25. Himms-Hagen J, Harper M-E. Physiological role of UCP3 may be export of fatty acids from mitochondria when fatty acid oxidation predominates: an hypothesis. *Exp Biol Med* 2001; 226: 78–84.

26. Schrauwen P, Saris WH, Hesselink MK. An alternative function for human uncoupling protein 3: Protection of mitochondria against accumulation of non-esterified fatty acids inside the mitochondrial matrix. *FASEB J* 2001; 15: 2497–502.

27. Moore GB, Himms-Hagen J, Harper M-E, Clapham JC. Overexpression of UCP-3 in skeletal muscle of mice results in increased expression of mitochondrial thioesterase mRNA. *Biochem Biophys Res Commun* 2001; 283: 785–90.

28. Clapham JC, Coulthard VH, Moore GB. Concordant mRNA expression of UCP-3, but not UCP-2, with mitochondrial thioesterase-1 in brown adipose tissue and skeletal muscle in db/db diabetic mice. *Biochem Biophys Res Commun* 2001; 287: 1058–62.

29. Samec S, Seydoux J, Dulloo, AG. Skeletal muscle UCP3 and UCP2 gene expression in response to inhibition of free fatty acid flux through mitochondrial beta-oxidation. *Pflugers Arch* 1999; 438: 452–7.

30. Hildebrandt AL, Neufer PD. Exercise attenuates the fasting-induced transcriptional activation of metabolic genes in skeletal muscle. *Am J Physiol Endocrinol Metab* 2000; 278: E1078–E86.

Progress in Obesity Research: 9. Edited by *Geraldo Medeiros-Neto, Alfredo Halpern* and *Claude Bouchard*
©2003 John Libbey Eurotext Ltd, pp. 786–791.

CHAPTER 165

UCP1 and energy balance

Jan Nedergaard, Valeria Golozoubova, Anita Matthias, Anders Jacobsson and Barbara Cannon

The Wenner-Gren Institute, The Arrhenius Laboratories F3, Stockholm University, SE-106 91 Stockholm, Sweden
[e-mail: jan@metabol.su.se]

The uniqueness of UCP1

When viewed as just one of the mitochondrial carrier proteins, the uniqueness of UCP1 is not evident. It shares with the other members of the mitochondrial carrier family many structural characteristics: all carriers can be envisaged as threefold near-repeats of about 100 amino acids, and many of the amino acid residues occur at the same place in all three repeats in all carriers; this is particularly so for a proline residue found around positions 30/130/230, probably at the end of the ingoing transmembrane α-helices.

Within the family of mitochondrial carriers, a subgroup can be phylogenetically identified; this subgroup can be referred to based on its first identified member, the original uncoupling protein (UCP, thermogenin, now UCP1), and the members may be considered uncoupling-protein-*like* carriers[1]. However, whereas the sequencing of UCP1 occurred after its physiological function was bioenergetically established, all the other members have been identified in the reversed way: first UCP1-like mRNA sequences have been found in EST cDNA libraries, and thereafter a function has been sought for. Based on the early naming of these orphan carriers as UCP2, UCP3 and plant UCPs, it has become implicit that these carriers are also functional uncoupling proteins; it is presently doubtful that this is really the case. However, as these proteins can be subgrouped together within the carrier family, they share certain sequence characteristics, particularly sequences that are probably involved in a nucleotide binding site in the third transmembrane loop (e.g. E190, D209 and H214).

However, within this group of uncoupling-protein-like carriers, the UCP1 group itself is a clearly distinguishable further subgroup. The group consists only of the species variations of UCP1 within different mammals; no UCP1 has been identified in the genome of non-mammalian species. Although there is thus some variation between species in the UCP1 sequences, there are two sequences in UCP1 that attract particular interest: 144SHLHGIKP (facing the matrix) and 299RQTxDCxT (facing the intermembrane space); these sequences are found in all UCP1s but not in any non-UCP1s. Their conservation implies that they endow UCP1 with properties unique and necessary for its function. Correspondingly, experimental analyses of functions of UCPs that fail to observe differences between UCP1 and the other UCPs may be considered to address only those properties that are common within the group and not those that make UCP1 unique.

In the following, we summarise briefly today's knowledge of the significance of UCP1 in energy balance under different physiological conditions. It is not realistic in this short overview to refer to the underlying original studies; instead, with a few exceptions, we refer readers to two of our recent reviews where this information can be identified[1,2]. Original data from our laboratory that are presently not published will be indicated with *.

Concerning the physiological significance of UCP1 for energy balance, the question may be raised with reference to each condition of altered energy balance: is UCP1-dependent thermogenesis essential, optional, additional, coincidental or not at all involved in the phenomenon? After many years of rather indirect approaches to this type of question, the experimental situation was paradigmatically altered when UCP1-ablated mice were developed in L.P. Kozak's laboratory[3]. Most of the present discussion is based on the outcome of studies of these animals.

It is thus evident from the studies of brown-fat mitochondria isolated from these mice that UCP1 is truly an uncoupling protein. Isolated brown-fat *mitochondria* without UCP1 are well coupled, meaning that the exhibit a low rate of oxygen consumption ('thermogenesis'), even in the presence of a surplus of oxidisable substrate, but when an artificial uncoupler is added, respiration is greatly stimulated. In normal brown-fat mitochondria, i.e. with endogenously expressed UCP1, a high rate of thermogenesis is instead observed, which cannot be further increased by an artificial uncoupler. The high rate of respiration can be suppressed to the well-coupled level by addition of GDP, an inhibition that is supposed to reflect the state of UCP1 in the mitochondria of brown-fat cells that are not stimulated (by norepinephrine) to perform thermogenesis.

Correspondingly, isolated brown-fat *cells* without UCP1 have a low respiration and cannot be stimulated by norepinephrine to produce heat (i.e. heat production in brown-fat cells is entirely UCP1-dependent). Brown-fat cells with UCP1 do not have a higher basal rate of respiration (i.e. UCP1 is not leaky) but after addition of norepinephrine, their respiration (thermogenesis) increases about 10-fold.

Thus, there can be no contribution from brown adipose tissue to any thermogenic condition in UCP1-ablated mice. Until recently, UCP1 had only been identified in brown adipose tissue, but there is now evidence that it may be expressed in some cells found within the longitudinal muscle layer in apparently all organs exhibiting peristalsis. The presence of UCP1 within these organs seems to affect their contractile properties*. However, the amounts of UCP1 in these locations are low, and it can therefore not contribute to whole-body thermogenesis. Therefore, based on the UCP1-ablated mice we can analyse the contribution of brown adipose tissue to thermogenesis under different physiological conditions. Based on the apparent 'purpose' of the thermogenesis, we can divide these types of thermogenesis into thermoregulatory and metaboloregulatory thermogenesis.

Thermoregulatory thermogenesis and UCP1

Basal metabolic rate. All animals exhibit a basal metabolic rate, the regulation (and 'purpose') of which is still only partly understood. The basal metabolic rate is by definition circularly defined as the rate observed at thermoneutral temperatures – which are in their term defined as those at which metabolism is at its lowest. The possibility may be discussed that animals possessing brown adipose tissue (UCP1) may constitutively channel some of their metabolism through this tissue, and if this should be the case, the absence of metabolic activity in brown adipose tissue in UCP1-ablated mice should have metabolic consequences: a lowered metabolic rate. This should either result in a correspondingly lower food intake or in the development of obesity. However, the basal metabolic rate is exactly the same in mice possessing UCP1 or not*.

Correspondingly, animals without UCP1, living under normal animal house conditions, do not spontaneously become obese. However, animal house conditions are characterized by ambient temperatures below thermoneutrality, and the mice therefore normally need extra heat production from brown adipose tissue. The absence of this brown-fat-derived heat production is probably the explanation of the markedly reduced life span we have observed of UCP1-ablated mice: their mean life time is only one year*, whereas normal mice live for more than two years.

For this reason, and also because effects of the absence of UCP1 on basal metabolic rate can really only be observed at thermoneutral temperatures, we also followed wild-type and UCP1-ablated mice at 30 °C. Through this, we (re)discovered, in wild-type mice, the phenomenon of 'warmth-induced obesity': the mice became some 20 per cent heavier than wild-type mice living under normal animal house conditions*. However, even at thermoneutrality, no 'extra' obesity was observed in the UCP1-ablated mice*.

Animals in the cold

At all ambient temperatures below thermoneutrality (i.e. below ~30 °C for mice), mammals are required to produce 'extra' heat in order to compensate for the heat lost to the surrounding, otherwise they cannot defend their body temperature. The level of extra heat (and corresponding extra food intake) is for mice in the order of 50 per cent at 24 °C, 100 per cent at 18 °C and 300 per cent at 4 °C. Despite this vast increase in food consumption, the animals do not gain weight; they can thus be said to have become extremely metabolically inefficient. To survive at these temperatures thus puts very high demands on the physical condition of these animals; heart rate, oxygen uptake etc. must incessantly be kept at a fourfold higher level to supply the extra oxygen needed for the combustion to produce the necessary heat. Thus, clear training effects on e.g. heart muscle are observed in cold-acclimated mice*.

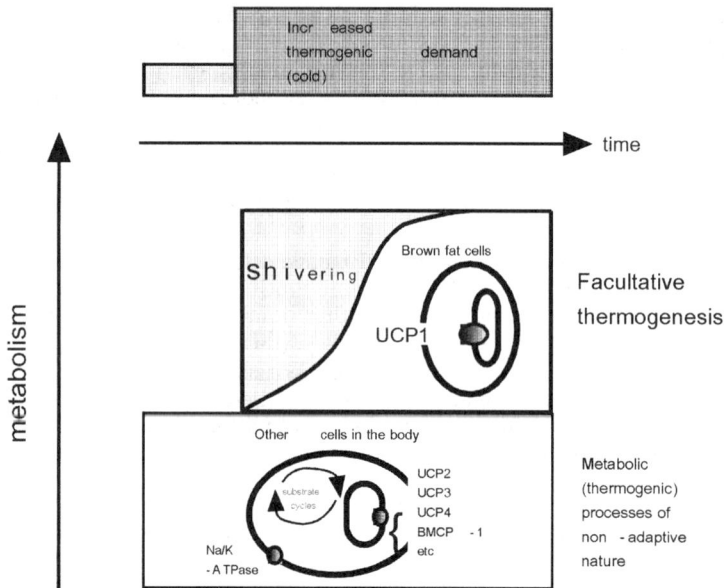

Fig. 1. Thermoregulatory thermogenesis (adapted from Golozoubova et al.[4]).

When animals naive in this respect (i.e. living at thermoneutrality) are exposed to cold, their only possibility to increase heat production is through *shivering* (Fig. 1). Indeed, if shivering is inhibited in acutely cold-exposed animals, they cannot increase their heat production. As shivering occurs through muscular work, and as muscle does not contain UCP1, it is not surprising that shivering is not affected in UCP1-ablated mice.

However, after some weeks in the cold (i.e. really any temperature below thermoneutrality), the phenomenon of *classical nonshivering thermogenesis* develops in normal mice. The animals still exhibit the same high metabolic rate in the cold, but shivering has ceased. Indeed, even if shivering is pharmacologically inhibited, the metabolic rate remains high. Coinciding with the increase in capacity for nonshivering thermogenesis, there is an increase in the amount of UCP1 in brown adipose tissue (the tissue is 'recruited'), and it has been the unconfirmed assumption that this increase in UCP1, and thus in the thermogenic capacity of brown adipose tissue, is the background for the development of nonshivering thermogenesis; however, the existence of alternative means for nonshivering thermogenesis has remained open.

In reality, animals are rarely exposed to a direct transfer from thermoneutral conditions to the cold (4 °C). Animals tested in this type of experiments often come from a partial cold situation (20 °C) to additional cold (4 °C) and they can therefore combine the previously induced, somewhat increased capacity for nonshivering thermogenesis with an acute shivering thermogenesis, allowing them to survive in the cold until their nonshivering thermogenesis capacity is further increased to meet the new requirements. Shivering capacity alone is not sufficient to allow for a direct transfer of mice from thermoneutral temperatures to 4 °C with full control of body temperature.

Similarly, mice without UCP1 that are directly transferred from 24 °C to 4 °C cannot defend their body temperature. However, initially surprisingly, UCP1-ablated mice that are first preacclimated to 18 °C and then transferred to 4 °C can maintain normal body temperatures, even at 4 °C[4]. This observation could indicate that the mice could recruit an alternative form of nonshivering thermogenesis (i.e. not UCP1-dependent). However, this is not the case: even after several weeks at 4 °C, the UCP1-ablated mice shiver as intensely in the cold as they did when directly transferred[4]. No alternative mechanism for nonshivering thermogenesis has thus developed in these mice; UCP1 is thus essential for classical nonshivering thermogenesis. Rather, the improved cold tolerance of these mice preacclimated to 18 °C before transfer to cold must be due to a muscular training process, endowing them with muscles with higher endurance. Indeed, molecular signs of muscular recruitment can be observed in these mice*. That shivering is not an optimal method for producing the heat needed for survival in the cold is witnessed by the fact that these mice, although able to defend their body temperature for many weeks, die after about 100 days in the cold[4]; wild-type mice, to our knowledge, have normal life expectancy in the cold.

As the stimulation of thermogenesis in brown-fat cells *in situ* occurs through the release of nor-epinephrine from the sympathetic nervous system innervating the cells, it is also possible to stimulate the brown-fat cells *in situ* by injection of such high norepinephrine amounts that it mimics synaptic concentrations within the tissue. The thermogenic response to norepinephrine is several-fold aug-mented during acclimation to cold, in parallel with the development of nonshivering thermogenesis and the increase in the amount of UCP1 in brown adipose tissue. It has, however, remained a question as to whether the increase in the thermogenic response to norepinephrine was entirely due to the increase in the amount of UCP1 or whether an alternative mechanism for norepinephrine-induced thermogenesis existed.

Even in UCP1-ablated mice there is a metabolic response to norepinephrine, although only about half that of control mice*. Thus, a thermogenic response to norepinephrine can be mediated via other mechanisms than UCP1. It is, however, unlikely that this UCP1-independent norepinephrine-induced 'thermogenesis' really has thermogenesis as its purpose. This is because it is not possible to increase its magnitude through acclimation to cold*. Thus, there is no cold-acclimation-recruited no-repinephrine-induced thermogenesis without UCP1.

Thus, although UCP1 is essential for the phenomena of classical nonshivering thermogenesis and cold-acclimation-recruited norepinephrine-induced thermogenesis, it is not essential for manifestation of a thermogenic response to cold; rather, UCP1-dependent thermogenesis is optional (and preferred), i.e. the animal will use it as a first source of thermogenesis, to the extent it is available. This also means that the elevated metabolic inefficiency associated with a cold environment is not UCP1-dependent.

Metaboloregulatory thermogenesis and UCP1

A connection between the phenomenon of what is presently referred to as *diet-induced thermogenesis* and brown adipose tissue was established in the 1980s mainly through the work of Rothwell and Stock. In summary, what is found is that animals that are exposed to a diet of palatable human foods overeat (as compared to chow-fed animals) and they do become obese. However, they become less obese than expected, because they display an increased 'basal' metabolic rate, combusting some of the extra energy eaten. These animals also display an increased norepinephrine-induced thermogenesis and signs of a recruited brown adipose tissue (increased amounts of UCP1 etc.). A series or other dietary conditions (high fat diets, high carbohydrate diets, forced ethanol drinking etc.) display similar features.

As brown adipose tissue is recruited in these 'overeating' animals, it is sometimes assumed that it is the hyperphagia itself that leads to recruitment of brown adipose tissue. However, this does not seem to be the case. Thus, conditions such as gestation, lactation and exercise are also characterized by a high food intake – but also by a *decrease* in the amount of UCP1 in brown adipose tissue. Although a cold environment leads to hyperphagia, it is not this hyperphagia that recruits brown adipose tissue in animals in the cold; recruitment takes place even in animals in the cold, pair-fed to animals in the warm. Thus, another explanation for the phenomenon of 'diet-induced thermogenesis' must be sought. A possibility for another explanation can be seen in experiments with so-called post-cafeteria animals[5]. These are animals that have been exposed to a cafeteria diet for several months, have overeaten and have become obese. When these animals are then exposed to a chow diet, they stop overeating, they even undereat, and their body weight starts to decrease but for months remains higher than that of animals that had never been exposed to the cafeteria diet. The remarkable observation is that in such animals (i.e. that are not hyperphagic and not exposed to an unusual diet), brown adipose tissue is still recruited several months after the cessation of the cafeteria diet[5]. As the animals still are obese, it is a likely possibility that it is the obesity that causes the recruitment. Thus, so-called diet-induced thermo-genesis may perhaps more appropriately be referred to as *obesity-induced thermogenesis* (and obesity-induced brown-fat recruitment).

It is perhaps understandable that animals exposed to a tasty diet overeat – but why do animals exposed to a high-fat diet overeat? The answer may be based on the protein-dilution hypothesis formulated by Michael Stock[6]: – consider a chow diet, which has been composed according to best nutritional wisdom and e.g. contains about 18 energy per cent protein. By eating a certain amount of this diet, the animal obtains its daily needs of protein. In most of the classical manipulations of diet, the amount of non-protein in the diet was increased, e.g. by allowing the animals access to Mars bars etc., or by directly adding, for example, fat to the chow mixture. Consequently, the concentration of protein in the diet was diminished. To obtain the same amount of protein per day, the animal must therefore overeat in the question of the total amount of food (calories), and the animal therefore becomes fat.

A possible further scenario is that this increased obesity leads to an increased secretion of leptin from the now overfilled adipose tissue. The leptin in its turn activates brown adipose tissue (via centres in the brain and the normal sympathetic pathway), and we observe the phenomenon of 'diet-induced thermogenesis' (which should thus be called *obesity-induced thermogenesis*). The system of course does not function when the leptin system does not function; indeed, obese animals that do not show brown adipose tissue recruitment invariably also have problems in their leptin pathway.

Again, although it is generally accepted that there is a connection between obesity (diet)-induced thermogenesis and brown adipose tissue, the relative contribution of brown adipose tissue/UCP1 activity to the phenomenon of diet-induced thermogenesis has not been established.

To examine this, we first established that response of wild-type mice to a cafeteria diet. The wild-type mice overate (although not as much as rats) and they gradually responded to the overeating with overt obesity*. This also led to a clear augmentation of the thermogenic response to norepinephrine*, i.e. to a 'diet'-adaptation-recruited norepinephrine-induced thermogenesis. We further observed the expected increase in 'basal' metabolic rate, and that, as expected, after injection of the β-adrenergic inhibitor propranolol there was no longer any difference in the basal metabolic rate between cafeteria-fed and chow-fed mice. It may be noted that the increased 'basal' metabolic rate is in accordance with expectations if the diet-induced thermogenesis is really obesity-induced. That the 'diet-induced' thermogenesis is observable even in short-time starved mice* makes it also less likely that it is secondary to hyperphagia, to specific food components or to processes involved in the processing of the ingested food. The cafeteria-fed mice also maintained a body temperature about 1 °C higher than that of chow-fed mice. This elevated body temperature has sometimes been assumed to be secondary to the diet-induced thermogenesis as such, i.e. it should be a hyperthermia caused by an excessive heat production. Considering that the mice live under conditions below thermoneutrality which thus demands a significant increase in metabolic rate, we find it unlikely that the mice would not be able to dispose of the extra heat; the increased body temperature is thus more probably a defended elevation, i.e. a 'fever' or hyperpyrexia.

UCP1-ablated mice exposed to the cafeteria diet also overate, apparently to the same degree as wild-type mice, and they increased their body weight more on cafeteria diet than on chow diet*. However, in the UCP1-ablated mice, exposure to the cafeteria diet did not lead to any increase in the response to norepinephrine*; thus UCP1 is essential for 'diet'-adaptation-recruited norepinephrine-induced thermogenesis.

Concerning the diet-induced increase in 'basal' metabolic rate, the outcome was less definitive. Even in the UCP1-ablated mice, there was an increased metabolism, but it only amounted to about half the increase in wild-type animals. Similarly, there was an increase in body temperature, but is was only about 0.5 °C *, in contrast to the 1 °C seen in wild-type animals. However, as these clearly occurred in the UCP1-ablated animals, they were UCP1-independent mechanisms. With both norepinephrine-induced thermogenesis and the increase in basal metabolic rate being lower in the UCP1-ablated mice, they should exhibit an increased metabolic efficiency, and with a food intake approximately similar to that of wild-type mice, they should be more obesity-prone. Whether they really do become more obese is presently mainly a question of definition: the body weight of the cafeteria-fed UCP1-ablated mice was not higher than that of cafeteria-fed wild-type mice, but the excess body weight caused by the cafeteria diet was actually somewhat higher in the UCP1-ablated mice than in the wild-type mice*.

There thus would seem to be two mechanisms involved in the process of diet-induced thermogenesis. One is UCP1-independent. It may be caused by increased leptin release from the increased lipid depots. The increased leptin may increase the set-point for the body temperature, as has been observed in other systems, and the increased body temperature may in itself (i.e. for simple chemical kinetics reasons, 'Q_{10}-effects') result in an elevated metabolism. (Other yet unidentified mechanisms for increased metabolism may also be involved.) The other mechanism is UCP1-dependent and is clearly additional to the first. This mechanism is probably due to a leptin effect on the centres controlling brown adipose tissue activity and results in a chronically increased metabolic rate (Fig. 2).

Conclusion and perspectives

Mainly from studies of UCP1-ablated mice, some relationships between UCP1 and energy balance have become clearer. The present interpretation would be as follows:

- UCP1 is *not involved* in (or is optional for, experiments cannot discriminate) for basal metabolic rate (i.e. the rate observed with a standard diet);

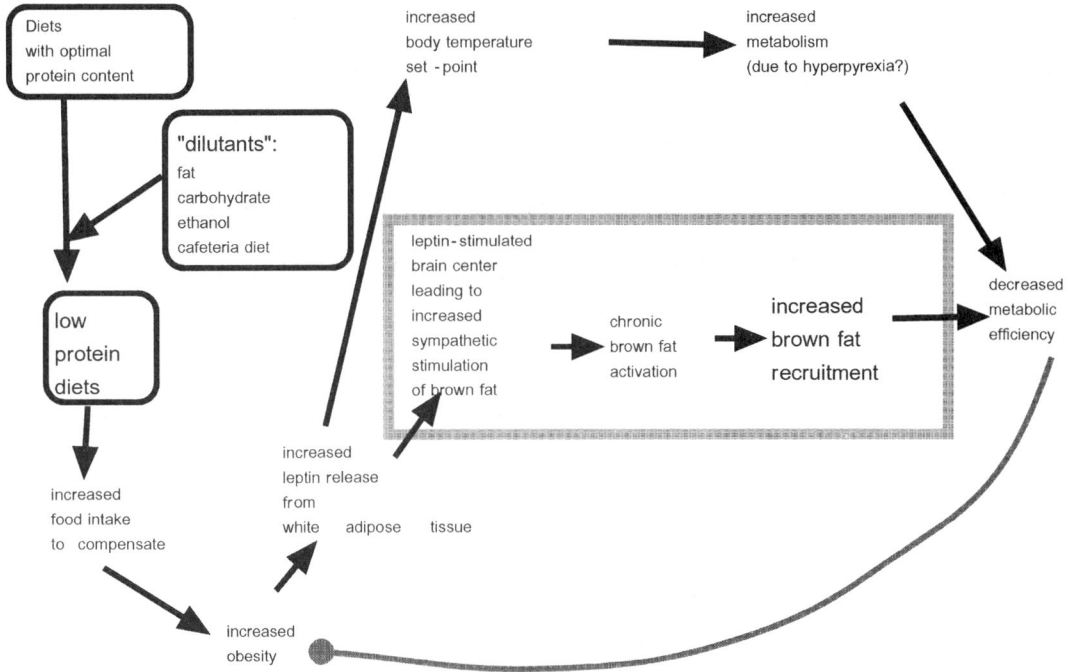

Fig. 2. Metaboregulatory thermogenesis (the grey line with filled circle indicates an inhibitory signal).

- UCP1 is *optional* for cold-induced thermogenesis and the ensuing metabolic inefficiency (i.e. it is – preferentially – utilized to the extent it is present, but its presence only influences the means of thermogenesis (i.e. otherwise shivering);

- UCP1 is an *additional* component to obesity(diet)-induced thermogenesis (i.e. some thermogenesis exists even in the absence of UCP1 but its magnitude is increased when UCP1 is present; in discussions concerning obesity this means that an augmented amount of UCP1 may lead to a proportional increase in thermogenesis and it may thus help to combat obesity);

- UCP1 is *essential* for classical nonshivering thermogenesis (i.e. cold-acclimation-recruited, cold-induced nonshivering thermogenesis) and for cold-acclimation-recruited, norepinephrine-induced thermogenesis, as well as for obesity(diet)-recruited, norepinephrine-induced thermogenesis.

As UCP1 is not found in any nonmammalian species, it is perhaps a surprising realization that a protein that has as its function to alter energy balance so as to make us more metabolically inefficient has probably been of major significance for the evolutionary success of the mammals.

References

1. Nedergaard J, Golozoubova V, Matthias A, Asadi A, Jacobsson A, Cannon B. UCP1: the only protein able to mediate adaptive non-shivering thermogenesis and metabolic inefficiency. *Biochim Biophys Acta* 2001; 1504: 82–106.

2. Cannon B, Nedergaard J. Brown adipose tissue: function and physiological significance. *Physiol Rev* 2003 (in press).

3. Enerbäck S, Jacobsson A, Simpson EM, Guerra C, Yamashita H, Harper M-E, Kozak LP. Mice lacking mitochondrial uncoupling protein are cold-sensitive but not obese. *Nature* 1997; 387: 90–94.

4. Golozoubova V, Hohtola E, Matthias A, Jacobsson A, Cannon B, Nedergaard J. Only UCPI can mediate adaptive nonshivering thermogenesis in the cold. *FASEB J* 2001; 15: 2048–50.

5. Rodriguez AM, Roca P, Palou A. Synergic effect of overweight and cold on uncoupling proteins expression, a role of α2/β3 adrenergic receptor balance? *Pflugers Arch* 2002; 444: 484–90.

6. Stock MJ. Gluttony and thermogenesis revisited. *Int J Obes Relat Metab Disord* 1999; 23: 1105–17.

Progress in Obesity Research: 9. Edited by *Geraldo Medeiros-Neto, Alfredo Halpern and Claude Bouchard*
©2003 John Libbey Eurotext Ltd, pp. 792–796.

CHAPTER 166

Stress, corticotropin-releasing factor (CRF) and the regulation of energy balance in obesity

Denis Richard

D.B. Brown Chair on Obesity Research and Laval Hospital Research Center, Laval University, Québec (Que), G1K 7P4, Canada
[e-mail: denis.richard@phs.ulaval.ca]

The prevalence of obesity has taken epidemic proportions dunng the past twenty years[1]. Obesity is now so widespread that, for the first time in the history of humanity, it is more prevalent than undernutrition or infectious disease. In Canada, the proportion of obese individuals [body mass index (weight in kg/height in cm[2]) above 30] currently exceeds 15 per cent. Alarmingly, the epidemic of obesity has now spread to children, in which the prevalence of the condition has tripled over the past 15 years. Conservative estimates demonstrate that the burden of obesity in industrialized countries now varies between 2 and 7 per cent of the total health costs. Visceral obesity[2], in particular, is associated with the development of costly diseases such as type 2 diabetes, hypertension and atherosclerosis.

Similar to obesity, stress-related disorders are also highly prevalent[3]. The World Health Organization (WHO) Global Burden of Disease Survey has estimated that mental disease, including stress-related disorders, will be the second to ischaemic heart disease as the leading cause of disabilities by the year 2020. Stress (work-related stress, home stress, post-traumatic stress disorders) is now estimated to cost United-States more than $42 billion per year[3].

That the prevalence of obesity and stress-related disorders follows similar trends is not unexpected in the light of the links existing between stress and obesity. Given the positive association between stress and obesity it can be argued that obesity represents a stress-related disorder. Indeed, stress leads to the activation of the hypothalamicpituitary-adrenal (HPA) axis and the secretion of glucocorticoids, which promote the development of visceral (intra-abdominal fat deposition) obesity and its adverse effects[4]. Likewise, there is evidence that stress hampers the control of type 2 diabetes, a known adverse effect of visceral obesity, which currently costs Canadians in cardiovascular complications more than $637 million per year[5].

Alternatively, the positive association between obesity and stress could be interpreted as obesity being the source of stress. Visceral fat releases cytokines capable of stimulating the HPA axis[6]. In addition, the neuropeptidergic/neurochemical and hormonal alterations that preceded or accompanied the development of obesity create a milieu facilitating a stress response. The intolerance to food deprivation, which generates a neurogenic stress in morbidly obese Zucker rats[7,8] is certainly indicative that obesity can generate stress. The general goal of this review is to further speculate on the relationship existing between stress, the corticotropin-releasing factor (CRF) system and the regulation of energy balance in obesity.

Stress

Throughout this short review, the term stress will used as a disruption of the homeostasis associated with the activation of the HPA axis and corticotropin-releasing factor (CRF) system[9]. Stress, which is caused by a myriad of homeostatic challenges or 'stressors' (haemorrhage, infections, exhaustive exercise, sleep deprivation, emotional distress, etc.), is obviously also associated with the stimulation of the sympathetic nervous system (SNS). Despite its importance in the effects of energy metabolism, activation of the SNS should not however be seen as an ultimate marker of stress.

The HPA axis and CRF system

The HPA axis is composed of the hypothalamus, the anterior pituitary and adrenal cortex, three structures functionally united through the interplay of CRF, adrenocorticotropin hormone (ACTH) and species-specific glucocorticoid (either cortisol in human, non-human primates, pigs and dogs or corticosterone in rodents). CRF is released from selective PVH neurons that project to the external layer of the median eminence into the portal blood before attaining the pituitary corticotrophs. These cells release ACTH, a 39 amino-acid residue produced from the proteolytic cleavage of proopiomelanocortin. ACTH via the general circulation activates the adrenal secretion of glucocorticoids, which in turn are capable of a negative control of the pituitary corticotrophs and PVH CRF neurons through a direct or hippocampus-mediated action[10,11].

The mammalian CRF system is not restricted to PVH CRF neurons. The system also includes two CRF-receptor types, a CRF-binding protein, and endogenous CRF-receptor ligands, which comprise the mammalian peptides CRF[12], urocortin (UCN)[13], UCN II[14,15] and UCN III[15,16]. The broad brain distributions of the CRFergic cells, the UCNergic neurons and the CRF receptors conform to the many functions attributed to the CRF system[17]. When injected centrally, CRF evokes autonomic responses[18,19], a widespread arousal[20] and anxiety-like behaviours[19,21]. It respectively activates and inhibits the sympathetic and parasympathetic branches of the autonomic nervous system and thereby stimulates cardiorespiratory functions[22] and inhibits the digestive activity[23]. Because of their selectivity for the CRF type-2 receptor (CRF-R2), UCN II and UCN III[16] (also referred to in humans as stresscopin[15]) have been described as 'stress-coping' peptides[15] capable of exerting anxiolytic effects.

The HPA axis, the CRF system and the regulation of body weight

The role of the HPA axis in the regulation of body weight has been demonstrated in animal models of obesity, which exhibit hyperactivated HPA axis and in which adrenalectomy-induced disruption of the HPA axis prevents or cures obesity via a corticosterone-mediated mechanism. In laboratory rodents, there is also evidence that corticosteroids could promote fat retention (anabolic effects) by eliciting strong inhibitory effects on thermogenesis[24–26] and by stimulating energy intake[27]. In humans, an enhanced HPA axis activity leads to an increase in circulating levels of corticosteroids, which promote visceral fat deposition and the associated adverse health consequences of visceral obesity[2,28]. Resolution of excessive cortisol production normalized fat distribution among patients with Cushing's syndrome, which is well characterized by intra-abdominal fat accretion.

In contrast to corticosteroids, CRF and CRF-related peptides reduce the rate of fat deposition (catabolic effects) due to potent anorectic and thermogenic effects. The sites of the anorectic and thermogenic actions of CRF-related peptides have yet to be fully delineated. There is evidence that CRF and the UCNs can act either centrally[29] or peripherally[30] to elicit anorectic effects. In the brain, PVN has been reported as one among the potential sites for the anorectic effect of CRF[31] and the UCNs[32,33]. There is also evidence that the UCNs evoke anorexia when injected in the lateral septum[34] and that the parabrachial nucleus is the locus of the anorectic action of CRF induced by dehydration[35,36]. The medial preoptic area has been reported as a site for the thermogenic action of CRF[37].

The VMH markedly expresses CRF-R2 and evidence keeps accumulating to emphasize the significance of CRF-R2 in mediating the anorectic effects of CRF-related peptides[38–40]. Recent studies have in fact demonstrated the ability of newly developed CRF-R2 antagonists, such as antisauvagine-30[40] and compound 338-08615[30], to block the effects of CRF and the UCNs on food intake. These results are consistent with the anorectic potential of UCN II[14,15] and UCN III[15,16], which represent specific agonists for CRF-R2. They also are in agreement with studies conducted in CRF-R2-ablated mice[41], which recover a normal food intake more rapidly than do wild-type mice in response to UCN. The involvement of the CRF-R2 in the control of food intake is also in consonance with the changes in the CRF-R2 mRNA levels, which inversely vary with appetite. The expression of the VMH CRF-R2 mRNA is reduced in obese diabetic (unpublished results) and food-deprived[7] rats. It is induced in rats after and intracerebroventricular infusion with leptin (Huang, Q. and Richard, D., unpublished results).

Stress and obesity

In laboratory rodents, stressful events generate intense stress responses, which are generally catabolic. This suggests that the catabolic effects of the CRF system stimulation predominate over the anabolic effects of the HPA axis activation. The importance of the CRF system in the catabolic effects of stress has been particularly emphasized in studies using CRF antagonists, which have been shown to block the anorectic effects of treadmill running[44], restraint stress[45] and emotional stress[46]. Stress-induced activation of the HPA axis and the suppressing effect of stress on the activity of the growth hormone/insulin-like growth factor axis, the hypothalamic-pituitary-gonadal axis, and the thyrotropin-triiodothyronine axis create a hormonal milieu highly favourable to the deposition of intra-abdominal fat[4]. There is indeed strong evidence that stress generates visceral obesity in humans[47–49]. That stress can simultaneously be catabolic and promote visceral obesity is not exclusive, the net predicted effect of concomitant and long lasting activation of the HPA axis and the CRF system being a reduction in total fat deposition and a redistribution of the actual fat stores favoring a visceral deposition.

Recent literature suggests that stress increases food intake in humans only when it is followed with increased cortisol concentrations[48–50], which is consistent with the reported positive associations between stress and obesity [51–53]. In humans, increases in food intake have been reported to occur before and following stress[48]. The intake during stress is probably reduced in the light of the anorectic effect of CRF. There are also studies demonstrating that stress (depending on its strength) can induce weight loss in humans.

It is also worthy of mention that the development of obesity is preceded and accompanied by neuropeptidergic/neurochemical and hormonal alterations creating an environment facilitating stress responses. Obese rodents are characterized by high levels of neuropeptides/neurochemicals such as neuropeptide Y[54], orexins[55] and endocannabinoids[56], which facilitate the stimulation of the HPA axis and the CRF system. In addition, evidence is accumulating to suggest that the CRF-R2-mediated activities could be reduced in obese rats [7,42,43], reducing their ability to cope with stress. The CRF-R2 mediates 'stress-coping' responses such as anxiolysis, 'dearousal' and hypotension[19,38]. Obesity is also associated with leptin resistance, which prevents the antistress effects of leptin[57–59]. The intolerance to food deprivation, which generates a stress response in morbidly obese Zucker rats [7,8] is certainly indicative that obesity can generate stress. Recent observations (Richard, D., unpublished data) suggest that morbidly obese subjects also badly tolerate food deprivation.

References

1. Kopelman PG. Obesity as a medical problem. *Nature* 2000; 404(6778): 635–43.

2. Despres JP. Drug treatment for obesity. We need more studies in men at higher risk of coronary events. *BMJ* 2001; 322(7299): 1379–80.

3. Kalia M. Assessing the economic impact of stress – the modern day hidden epidemic. *Metabolism* 2002; 51(6 Suppl l): 49–53.

4. Van ltallie TB. Stress: a risk factor for serious illness. *Metabolism* 2002; 51(6 Suppl 1): 40–5.

5. Dawson KG, Gornes D, Gerstein H, Blanchard JF, Kahler KH. The economic cost of diabetes in Canada, 1998. *Diabetes Care* 2002; 25(8): 1303–7.

6. Yudkin JS, Kumari M, Humphries SE, Mohamed-Ali V. Inflammation, obesity, stress and coronary heart disease: is interleukin-6 the link? *Atherosclerosis* 2000; 148(2): 209–14.

7. Timofeeva E, Richard D. Functional activation of CRH neurons and expression of the genes encoding CRH and its receptors in food-deprived lean (Fa/?) and obese (fa/fa) Zucker rats. *Neuroendocrinology* 1997; 66: 327–340.

8. Timofeeva E, Richard D. Activation of the central nervous system in obese Zucker rats during food deprivation. *J Comp Neurol* 2001; 441: 71–89.

9. Miller DB, JP OC. Neuroendocrine aspects of the response to stress. *Metabolism* 2002; 51(6): 5–10.

10. De Kloet ER, Vreugdenhil E, Oitzl MS, Joels M. Brain corticosteroid receptor balance in health and disease. *Endocrine Rev* 1998; 19: 269–301.

11. Jacobson L, Sapolsky R. The role of the hippocampus in feedback regulation of the hypothalamic-pitaitary-adrenocortical axis. *Endocrine Rev* 1991; 12: 118–34.

12. Vale W, Spiess J, Rivier C, Rivier J. Characterization of a 41-residue ovine hypothalamic peptide that stimulates secretion of corticotropin and beta-endorphin. *Science* 1981; 213: 1394–7.

13. Vaughan J, Donaldson C, Bittencourt J, Perrin MH, Lewis K, Sutton S *et al.* Urocortin, a mammalian neuropeptide related to fish urotensin I and to corticotropin-releasing factor. *Nature* 1995; 378: 287–92.

14. Reyes TM, Lewis K, Perrin MH, Kunitake KS, Vaughan J, Arias CA *et al.* Urocortin II: A member of the corticotropin-releasing factor (CRF) neuropeptide family that is selectively bound by type 2 CRF receptors. *Proc Nat Acad Sei USA* 2001; 98(5): 2843–8.

15. Hsu SY, Hsueh AJW. Human stresscopin and stresscopin-related peptide are selective ligands for the type 2 corticotropin-releasing hormone receptor. *Nature Med* 2001: 7(5): 605–611.

16. Lewis K, Li C, Perrin MH, Blount A, Kunitake K, Donaldson C et al. Idenfification of urocortin III, an additional member of the corticotropin-releasing factor (CRF) family with high affinty for the CRF2 receptor. *Proc Nat Acad Sci USA* 2001; 98(13): 7570–5.

17. Tumbull AV, Rivier C. Corticotropin-releasing factor (CRF) and endocrine responses to stress: CRF receptors, binding protein, and related peptides. *Proc Soc Exp Biol Med* 1997; 215: 1–10.

18. Brown MR, Fisher LA. Regulation of the autonomic nervous system by corticotropin-releasing factor. In: De Souza EB, Nemeroff CB (eds), *Corticotropin-releasing factor: Basic and clinical studies of a neuropeptide*, pp. 291–8. Boca Raton: CRC; 1990.

19. Heinrichs SC, Tache Y. Therapeutic potential of CRF receptor antagonists: a gutbrain perspective. *Expert Opin Investig Drugs* 2001; 10(4): 647–59.

20. Koob GF, Cole BJ, Swerdlow NR, Le Moal M, Britton KT. Stress, performance, and arousal: focus on CRF. *NIDA Res Monogr* 1990; 97: 163–76.

21. Krysiak R, Obuchowicz E, Herman ZS. Role of corticotropin-releasing factor (CRF) in anxiety. *Pol J Pharmacol* 2000; 52(1): 15–25.

22. Fisher LA, Rivier J, Rivier C, Spiess J, Vale W, Brown MR. Corticotropin-releasing factor (CRF): Central effects on mean arterial pressure and heart rate in rats. *Endocrinology* 1982; 110: 2222–4.

23. Taché Y, Gunion MM, Stephens R. CRF: Central nervous system action to influence gastrointestinal function and role in the gastrointestinal response to stress. In: De Souza EB, Nemeroff CB (eds), *Corticotropin-releasing factor: Basic and clinical studies of a neuropeptide*, pp. 299–307. Boca Raton: CRC, 1990.

24. Strack AM, Bradbury MJ, Dallman MF. Corticosterone decreases nonshivering thermogenesis and increases lipid storage in brown adipose tissue. *Am J Physiol Regul Integr* 1995; 37: R183–R191.

25. Galpin KS, Henderson RG, James WPT, Trayhum P. GDP binding to brown-adipose-tissue mitochondria of mice treated chronically with corticosterone. *Biochem J* 1983; 214: 265–268.

26. Arvaniti K, Ricquier D, Champigny 0, Richard D. Leptin and corticosterone have opposite effects on food intake and the expression of UCP1 mRNA in brown adipose tissue of lepob /lepob mice. *Endocrinology* 1998,139: 4000–4004.

27. Strack AM, Sebastian RJ, Schwartz MW, Dallman MF. Glucocorticoids and insulin: Reciprocal signals for energy balance. *Am J Physiol-Regul Integr* C 1995; 37: R142–R149.

28. Pasquali R, Vicennati V. The abdominal obesity phenotype and insulin resistance are associated with abnormalities of the hypothalamic- pituitary-adrenal axis in humans. *Hormone Metab Res* 2000; 32(11–12): 521–5.

29. Spina M, Merlo-Pich E, Chan RKW, Basso AM, Rivier J, Vale W et al. Appetite-suppressing effects of urocortin, a CRF-related neuropeptide. *Science* 1996; 273: 1561–4.

30. Million M, Saunders P, Rivier J, Vale W, Tache Y. Compound 338-86-15, a novel peptide CRF-R2 antagonist, selectively blocks CRF and stress-induced delayed gastric emptying in rats. *Soc Nurosci Abstr* 2001; 27: 839–17.

31. Krahn DD, Gosnell BA, Levine AS, Morley JE. Behavioral effects of corticotropin-releasing factor: localization and characterization of central effects. *Brain Res* 1988; 443: 63–9.

32. Currie PJ, Coscina DV, Bishop C, Coiro CD, Koob GF, Rivier J et al. Hypothalamic paraventricular nucleus injections of urocortin alter food intake and respiratory quotient. *Brain Res* 2001; 916(1–2): 222–8.

33. Wang C, Mullet MA, Glass MJ, Billington CJ, Levine AS, Kotz CM. Feeding inhibition by urocortin in the rat hypothalamic paraventricular nucleus. *Am J Physiol Regul Integr Comp Physiol* 2001; 280(2): R473–80.

34. Bakshi VP, Newman HC, Weinberg LE, Smith-Roe SL, Kahn NH. Urocortin infusion into lateral septum increases grooming and decreases ingestive behaviors. *Soc Nurosci Abstr* 2001; 27: 414.

35. Kelly AB, Watts AG. The region of the pontine parabrachial nucleus is a major target of dehydration-sensitive CRH neurons in the rat lateral hypothlamic area. *J Comp.Neurol* 1998; 394: 48–63.

36. Watts AG, Sanchez-Watts G, Kelly AB. Distinct patterns of neuropeptide gene expression in the lateral hypothalamic area and arcuate nucleus are associated with dehydration-induced anorexia. *J Neurosci* 1999; 19(14): 6111–21.

37. Egawa M, Yoshimatsu H, Bray GA. Preoptic area injection of corticotropin-releasing hormone stimulates sympathetic activity. *Am J Physiol* 1990; 259: R799–R806.

38. Hashimoto K, Makino S, Asaba K, Nishiyama M. Physiological roles of corticotropin-releasing hormone receptor type 2. *Endocr J* 2001; 48(1): 1–9.

39. Katner JS, Li DL, Grigoriadis DE, Ling N, Iyengar S. Urocortin modulates food consumption and body weight via CRF2á receptor. *Soc Neurosci Abstr* 2001; 27: 477.

40. Cullen MJ, Ling N, Foster AC, Pelleymounter MA. Urocortin, corticotropin releasing factor-2 receptors and energy balance. *Endocrinology* 2001; 142(3): 992–9.

41. Contarino A, Heinrichs SC, Gold LH. Understanding corticotropin releasing factor neurobiology: contributions from mutant mice. *Neuropeptides* 1999; 33(1): 1–12.

42. Richard D, Rivest R, Naïmi N, Timofeeva E, Rivest S. Expression of corticotropin-releasing factor and its receptors in the brain of lean and obese Zucker rats. *Endocrinology* 1996; 137: 4786–95.

43. Makino S, Nishiyama M, Asaba K, Gold PW, Hashimoto K. Altered expression of type 2 CRH receptor mRNA in the VMH by glucocorticolds and starvation. *Am J Physiol Regul Integr* C 1998; 44: R1138–R1145.

44. Rivest S, Richard D. Involvement of corticotropin-releasing factor in the anorexia induced by exercise. *Brain Res Bull* 1990; 25: 169–172.

45. Shibasaki T, Yamauchi N, Kato Y, Masuda A, Imaki T, Hotta M *et al.* Involvement of corticotropin-releasing factor in restraint stress-induced anorexia and reversion of the anorexia by somatostatin in the rat. *Life Sci* 1988; 43: 1103–10.

46. Hotta M, Shibasaki T, Arai K, Demura H. Corticotropin-releasing factor receptor type I mediates emotional stress-induced inhibition of food intake and behavioral changes in rats. *Brain Res* 1999; 823(1–2): 221–5.

47. Bjomtorp P. Do stress reactions cause abdominal obesity and comorbidities? *Obes Rev* 2001; 2(2): 73–86.

48. Epel E, Lapidus R, McEwen B, Brownell K. Stress may add bite to appetite in women: a laboratory study of stress-induced cortisol and eating behavior. *Psychoneuroendocrinology* 2001; 26(1): 37–49.

49. Gohil BC, Rosenblum LA, Coplan JD, Kral JG. Hypothalamic-pituitary-adrenal axis function and the metabolic syndrome X of obesity. *CNS Spectrums* 2001; 6: 581–9.

50. Bjomtorp P, Rossner S, Udden J. 'Consolatory eating' is not a myth. Stress-induced increased cortisol levels result in leptin-resistant obesity. *Lakartidningen* 2001; 98(48): 5458–61.

51. Bradley PJ. Conditions recalled to have been associated with weight gain in adulthood. *Appetite* 1985; 6(3): 235–41.

52. Mellbin T, Vuille JC. Rapidly developing overweight in school children as an indicator of psychosocial stress. *Acta Paediatr Scand* 1989; 78(4): 568–75.

53. Laitinen J, Ek E, Sovio U. Stress-related eating and drinking behavior and body mass index and predictors of this behavior. *Prev Med* 2002; 34(1): 29–39.

54. Jaszberenyi M, Bujdoso E, Telegdy G. The role of neuropeptide Y in orexin-induced hypothalamic-pituitary-adrenal activation. *J Neuroendocrinol* 2001; 13(5): 438–41.

55. Samson WK, Taylor MM, Follwell M, Ferguson AV. Orexin actions in hypothalamic paraventricular nucleus: physiological consequences and cellular correlates. *Regul Pept* 2002; 104(1–3): 97–103.

56. Wenger T, Jamali KA, Juaneda C, Leonardelli J, Tramu G. Arachidonyl ethanolamide (anandamide) activates the parvocellular part of hypothalamic paraventricular nucleus. *Biochem Biophys Res Commun* 1997; 237(3): 724–8.

57. Huang Q, Rivest R, Richard D. Effects of leptin on corticotropin-releasing factor (CRF) synthesis and CRF neuron activation in the paraventricular hypothalamic nucleus of obese (ob/ob) mice. *Endocrinology* 1998; 139: 1524–1532.

Progress in Obesity Research: 9. Edited by *Geraldo Medeiros-Neto, Alfredo Halpern and Claude Bouchard*
©2003 John Libbey Eurotext Ltd, pp. 797–800.

CHAPTER 167

The hypothalamic-pituitary-adrenal axis in obesity

R. Pasquali, V. Vicennati and A. Gambineri

Endocrinology Unit, Department of Internal Medicine, S. Orsola-Malpighi Hospital, University of Bologna, Italy
[e-mail: rpasqual@almadns.unibo.it]

Introduction

Glucocorticoid treatment in experimental animals and humans leads to the development of the abdominal obesity phenotype[1]. Moreover, animal models of obesity have invariably increased levels of corticosterone, the equivalent of cortisol in humans, and in these models adrenalectomy results in the reversal of obesity[1]. The hypothetical role of glucocorticoids in human obesity has been suggested since the abdominal obesity phenotype and syndromes of exogenous or endogenous hypercortisolism share various similarities, including clinical features and different metabolic and endocrine alterations[2]. All pseudo-Cushing syndromes, such as atypical or melancholic depression, alcoholism and the alcohol-withdrawal syndrome, poorly controlled diabetes and some drug-induced conditions (i.e. antiretroviral drugs) are characterized by an abundance of visceral fat tissue[3]. We therefore questioned whether the abdominal obesity phenotype may be considered as another pseudo-Cushing syndrome, as a consequence of inappropriate signals to the different tissues of borderline increased cortisol secretion and/or increased cortisol sensitivity and effectiveness at the level of principal target tissues, specifically the visceral adipose tissue. The recent finding of slightly enlarged adrenal glands in abdominally obese patients[4] may be consistent with this hypothesis. After extensive investigation for many years, however, there are many questions still unanswered: (i) do we have non-controversial evidence that the hypothalamic-pituitary-adrenocortical (HPA) axis is really disrupted in abdominal obesity?; (ii) can we measure these alterations by using simple and reliable methods? This chapter will briefly review all major experimental evidences in humans supporting the hypothesis that the activity and/or the regulation of the HPA axis is altered in the abdominal obesity phenotype, together with some of the suggested pathophysiological mechanisms and aetiologic factors. We will also briefly review the existing evidence for a relationship between alterations of the HPA axis and major features of the metabolic syndrome, such as insulin resistance and hyperinsulinaemia.

Experimental evidence in support of the HPA axis being altered and dysregulated in abdominal obesity

Available evidence indicates that the major abnormalities of the HPA axis described so far include (i) altered basal hormone secretory pattern; (ii) altered response to different neuropeptides and stress stimuli; (iii) altered suppressibility dexamethasone and other substances, at least in women; (iv) altered response to very high carbohydrate ingestion; (v) alteration in the control of tissue cortisol metabolism; and, finally, (vi) alterations in the function of the glucocorticoid receptors.

Most studies found normal or slightly reduced morning cortisol levels in subjects with abdominal obesity[5,6] in whom, however, the ACTH secretory pattern may be disturbed. In fact, despite similar mean ACTH basal concentrations, higher ACTH pulse frequency and lower ACTH pulse amplitude, particularly in the morning, have been found in these subjects with respect to those with peripheral obesity and normal weight controls[7]. Evaluation of 24-h urinary excretion rates of free cortisol (24hFCU) yielded conflicting results, since normal[5], or increased[8] values have been described in subjects with abdominal obesity of both sexes. At variance, even lower 24hFCU values have been reported when obese subjects with obesity but without depressive traits were excluded from the analysis[9]. Finally, increased FCU values in urine samples collected during the nighttime only have been described[10], suggesting that the nighttime, during which the HPA axis drive physiologically increases, could represent a crucial period for detecting alterations of cortisol production and excretion rates in obesity. These findings, on the other hand, are in agreement with those related to alterations of ACTH pulsatile activity cited above.

In general, however, the dysregulation of the HPA axis in abdominal obesity has been more convincingly demonstrated by many dynamic studies, showing both a high secretion of cortisol after laboratory stress test and over-responsiveness after stimulation with various neuropeptides and secretagogues, including CRH and AVP, given alone or in combination, and ACTH[6,11]. Taken together, these studies indicate that hyper-responsive hypothalamic centres, pituitary as well as adrenal regulatory mechanisms, may result in slightly but inappropriately elevated net cortisol production, either continuous or episodic. Studies investigating the appropriateness of HPA axis suppressibility by low-dose dexamethasone have, however, yielded conflicting results, since a lower[12] or normal[13] suppression of circulating cortisol has been reported, although these studies suffer from a limitation since the access of dexamethasone to brain glucocorticoid receptors may be negligible. In fact, rat studies have clearly demonstrated that xenobiotics such as dexamethasone do not cross the brain barrier, unless very high doses are administered[14]. Nonetheless, in a recent study[13] performed in a large number of normal weight and obese subjects of both sexes, we have demonstrated a highly significant effect of dexamethasone blood level concentrations on cortisol and ACTH suppression to different low-dose dexamethasone tests and a significant effect of gender on post-dexamethasone cortisol concentrations, suppression of the HPA axis, and dexamethasone levels, which may be dependent on differences in both cortisol and dexamethasone metabolism. In addition, we demonstrated that pituitary (to which dexamethasone has direct access) sensitivity to feedback inhibition by dexamethasone is preserved in obesity in both sexes even at low dosage, but that, at least in women, abdominal fat distribution may partially counteract the progressively greater suppressibility of the HPA axis that would be expected according to increasing BMI, as conversely occurs in men. These findings partially agree with recent data showing that human obese individuals may present with a relative insensitivity to hydrocortisone inhibition, particularly during the night[15], which cannot exclude a decreased glucocorticoid receptor (GCR) response in the neuroendocrine hypothalamic centres to circulating corticosteroids. Whether this concerns only the abdominal obesity phenotype rather than all obese individuals still needs to be further clarified.

Altered HPA axis activity in obesity may derive from a disruption of the catecholaminergic regulation in the central nervous system, particularly during acute and chronic stress challenges[6,9]. In fact, animal studies have clearly demonstrated that chronic stress exposure is associated with a hyperactivated state of both the HPA and the cathecolaminergic system[16]. Longitudinal studies performed by Shively's group in primates[17] have also shown that, after being exposed for a long time to stressful adverse environmental conditions, all animals developed the abdominal obesity phenotype and all features of the metabolic syndrome, which was associated with hypertrophic adrenal glands and functional hypercortisolemic state. These findings have been somewhat confirmed in humans. In fact, cross-sectional epidemiological studies performed by Bjorntorp's group[12] in adult men have documented a significant relationship of stress-related salivary cortisol concentrations with the abdominal pattern fat distribution and associated metabolic and hemodynamic disturbances. In one study we administered yohimbine, an α2-adrenoreceptor antagonist, in order to achieve steady state norepinephrine plasma levels near to those observed during acute stress, and we found that the ACTH response to combined CRH + AVP challenge was slightly but significantly reduced in normal weight controls, in comparison with that observed during the control test, whereas in obese women, particularly the abdominal phenotype, the response of ACTH was significantly increased[18]. These disparate effects after α2-adrenoreceptor inhibition between normal weight controls and abdominally obese women suggest different sensitivity central noradrenergic tone of the HPA axis activity, and that obese women with abdominal obesity phenotype may escape physiological α2-adrenoreceptor control, thus favouring inappropriate HPA axis excitation in stressed conditions. Taken together, all these findings strongly support the concept that poor coping with long-term exposure to different environmental stressors could favour both the onset and the development of human abdominal obesity through dysregulated endocrine systems, involving both HPA and the sympathetic nervous system, possibly acting at the levels of neuroendocrine centres. This hypothesis, however, needs many more physiopathological and longitudinal studies to be definitely confirmed.

Meals are important synchronizers of the HPA activity during the daytime but contradicting data have been reported after mixed meals in obesity, since normal as well as increased cortisol response have been found[18]. However, recent data of ours indicate that when high carbohydrate meals are administered, ACTH and cortisol surge tend to be significantly higher in women with the abdominal than in those with the peripheral obesity phenotype[19]. We examined two well-defined groups of women with abdominal or peripheral obesity and a group of normal weight controls, to whom high lipid-protein (HLP) or high carbohydrate (HCHO) meals were randomly administered. After the HLP-meal, ACTH tended to similarly but insignificantly increase in all groups, whereas cortisol significantly increased in the peripheral obese group and insignificantly in the other groups. Conversely, both ACTH and cortisol significantly increased only in the abdominal obese group, without any significant changes in either controls or peripheral obese women. The analysis of the interaction between meals and groups clearly indicated that the cortisol response to the HLP-meal and the HCHO-meal was significantly different ($P < 0.025$) between the two obese groups, the abdominal obese group being characterized by a significantly lower response to the HLP-meal and a significantly higher response to the HCHO-meal compared to the peripheral group. Therefore, the response of the HPA axis to meals containing different macronutrient proportions may depend on the pattern of body fat distribution. We suggested that the higher response of the HPA axis to a large CHO meal may be attributable to an increased tone of the noradrenergic drive control of meal digestion and nutrient absorption[19].

Alterations of cortisol metabolism: the role of 11ß-hydroxysteroid dehydrogenase type 1

Obesity is also characterized by increased cortisol metabolic clearance rate (MCR)[21], probably due to multiple factors, including subtle abnormalities of cortisol transport, function and metabolism. In particular, higher numbers of glucocorticoid receptors (GCRs) have been demonstrated in abdominal than in subcutaneous adipocytes, which results in increased intracellular cortisol action and metabolism in the abdominal fat[22]. In addition, alterations of the activity of two enzyme systems, such as impaired activity of the 11β-hydroxysteroid dehydrogenase type 1 (11βHSD-1), which reactivates (acting as a reductase) cortisol from inactive cortisone in the liver and the adipose tissue, and enhanced activity of the 5α-reductase, which metabolizes cortisol to its tetrahydroderivates, have been described in patients with increased central adiposity[23,24]. The importance of the role of excess glucocorticoids produced within the adipose tissue to determine abdominal obesity has been demonstrated by several recent studies. Rask *et al.* found that adipose tissue from obese subjects had increased 11βHSD-1 activity[25]. Using a deuterated cortisol infusion technique, by which whole body cortisol activity of 11βHSD-1 can be adequately measured, it was found that the net conversion of cortisone to cortisol in obesity may be increased by approximately twofold[26]. The importance of 11βHSD-1 activity in the adipose tissue is highly emphasized by recent studies[27] demonstrating that transgenic mice overexpressing 11βHSD-1 selectively in the adipose tissue to an extent similar to that found in adipose tissue from obese humans had increased levels of corticosterone and developed visceral obesity and all features of the metabolic syndrome, particularly insulin resistant diabetes and hyperlipidemia. On the contrary, 11βHSD-1 knock-out mice are protected from the development of obesity and the metabolic syndrome[28]. These findings may have an important impact on systemic biology, since they demonstrate that even a modest increase in the activity of the 11βHSD-1 may play a dominant role in the pathophysiology of abdominal obesity and related metabolic alterations. Moreover, they indicate the 11βHSD-1 system as a target for potential therapeutic intervention.

New insights into adipose tissue biology

We recently demonstrated that the adipose tissue may express CRH receptors and that CRH may have several important metabolic and endocrine functions at the cellular level[29]. In fact we found that both preadipocytes and adipocytes expressed both CRH and its receptors, whose pattern was modified during the differentiation (~40 per cent reduction of CRH receptor density in adipocytes vs preadipocytes). Moreover, we found that CRH in the medium had a dose-response stimulatory effect of lipolysis, as demonstrated by a stimulated glycerol release by mature adipocytes. Finally, we demonstrated that CRH had significant stimulatory effect on both IL-6 and leptin production, even at low concentrations. This finding led us to hypothesize a paracrine/autocrine role of CRH in the adipose tissue, and that both the adipose tissue and the central systems are in close communication, being involved in a regulatory feedback loop.

References

1. Smith SR. The endocrinology of obesity. *Endocr Metab Clin North Am* 1996; 25: 921–42.

2. Bjorntorp P. Centralization of body fat. In: *International textbook of obesity*, Bjorntorp P (ed.), pp. 213–24. Chichester, UK: John Wiley, 2001.

3. Ceroni L, Cota D, Pasquali R. Pseudo-Cushing syndrome. Physiopathologic aspects and differential diagnosis. *Min Endocrinol* 2000; 25: 47–54.

4. De Godoy Matos A. Adrenals and visceral fat. 9th Int Congress of Obesity, Sao Paulo, Brasil, *Int J Obes* 2002; 26 (Suppl 1): S230.

5. Chalew S, Nagel H, Shore S. The hypothalamic-pituitary-adrenal axis in obesity. *Obes Res* 1995; 3: 371–82.

6. Pasquali R, Vicennati V. The abdominal obesity phenotype and insulin resistance are associated with abnormalities of the hypothalamic-pituitary-adrenal axis in humans. *Horm Metab Res* 2000; 32: 521–5.

7. Pasquali R, Biscotti D, Spinucci G, Vicennati V, Genazzani AD, Sgarbi L, Casimirri F. Pulsatile secretion of ACTH and cortisol in premenopausal women: effect of obesity and body fat distribution. *Clin Endocrinol (Oxf)* 1998; 48: 603–12.

8. Marin P, Darin N, Anemiya T, Andersson B, Jern S, Bjorntorp P. Cortisol secretion in relation to body fat distribution in obese premenopausal women. *Metabolism* 1992; 41: 882–6.

9. Vicennati V, Pasquali R. Abnormalities of the hypothalamic-pituitary-adrenal axis in women with the abdominal obesity and relationship with insulin resistance: evidence for a central and peripheral alteration. *J Clin Endocrinol Metab* 2000; 24: 416–22.

10. Duclos M, Corcuff J-B, Etcheverry N, Rashedi M, Tabarin A, Roger P. Abdominal obesity increases overnight cortisol excretion. *J Endocrinol Invest* 1999; 22: 465–71.

11. Vicennati V, Ceroni L, Ragazzini G, Hasanaj R, Gagliardi L, Pasquali R. The role of GABA-system in the regulation of the hypothalamic-pituitary-adrenal (HPA) axis in women with different obesity phenotypes. *J Endocrinol Invest* 2001; 24 (Suppl.7): 78.

12. Rosmond R, Dallman MF, Bjorntorp P. Stress-related cortisol secretion in men: relationships with abdominal obesity and endocrine, metabolic and hemodynamic abnormalities. *J Clin Endocrinol Metab* 1998; 83: 1853–9.

13. Pasquali R, Ambrosi B, Armanini D, Cavagnini F, Degli Uberti E, Del Rio G *et al.* Cortisol and ACTH response to oral dexamethasone in obesity and effects of sex, body fat distribution and dexamethasone concetrations: a dose-response study. *J Clin Endocrinol Metab* 2002; 87: 166–75.

14. De Kloet ER, Vreugdenhil E, Oitzl MS, Joels M. Brain corticosteroid receptor balance in health and disease. *Endocr Rev* 1998; 19: 269–301.

15. Jessop Ds, Dallman MF, Fleming D, Lightman SL. Resistance to glucocorticoid feedback in obesity. *J Clin Endocrinol Metab* 2001; 86: 4109–14.

16. Dallman MF, Bhatnagar S. Chronic stress and energy balance: role of the hypothalamic-pituitary-adrenal axis. In: McEwen BS (ed.) *Handbook of physiology, the environment.* American Physiology Society, Washington, 1998.

17. Shively C, Clarkson T. Regional obesity and coronary atherosclerosis in females: a non-human primate model. *Acta Med Scand* 1989; 723 (Suppl): 71–8.

18. Pasquali R, Vicennati V, Calzoni F, Gnudi U, Gambineri A, Ceroni L *et al.* α2-adrenoreceptor regulation of the hypothalamic-pituitary-adrenocortical axis in obesity. *Clin Endocrinol (Oxf)* 2000; 52: 413–21.

19. Leal AM, Moreira AC. Food and the circadian activity of the hypothalamic-pituitary-adrenal axis. *Braz J Med Biol Res* 1997; 30: 1391–405

20. Vicennati V, Ceroni L, Gagliardi L, Gambineri A, Pasquali R. Response of the hypothalamic-pituitary-adrenocortical axis to high protein-fat and high carbohydrate meals in women with different obesity phenotypes. *J Clin Endocrinol Metab* 2002; 87: 3984–8.

21. Strain GW, Zumoff B, Kream J, Stain JJ, Levin J, Fukushima D. Sex differences in the influence of obesity on the 24h mean plasma concentration of cortisol. *Metabolism* 1982; 31: 209–12.

22. Rebuffé-Scrive M, Lundholm K, Bjorntorp P. Glucocorticoid hormone binding to human adipose tissue. *Eur J Clin Invest* 1985; 15: 267–71.

23. Sandeep TC and Walker BR. Pathophysiology of modulation of local glucocorticoid levels by 11α-hydroxysteroid dehydrogenase. *Trends Endocrinol Metab* 2001; 12: 446–53.

24. Bujalska IJ, Kumar S, Stewart PM. Does central obesity reflect 'Cushing's disease of the omentum'? *Lancet* 1997; 349: 1210–3.

25. Rask E, Olsson T, Doderberg S, Andrew R, Livingstone DE, Johnson O, Walker B. Tissue-specific dysregulation of cortisol metabolism in human obesity. *J Clin Endocrinol Metab* 2001; 86: 1418.

26. Andrew R, Smith K, Jones GC, Walker BR. Use of multideuterated cortisol to distinguish activity of 11α-hydroxysteroid dehydrogenases *in vivo* in man. *J Clin Endocrinol Metab* 2002; 87: 227–85.

27. Masuzaki H, Paterson J, Shinyama H, Morton NM, Mullins JJ, Seckl JR, Flier JS. A transgenic model of visceral obesity and the metabolic syndrome. *Science* 2001; 294: 2166–70.

28. Kotelevtsev Y, Holmes MC, Burchell A, Houston PM, Schmoll D, Jamieson P *et al.* 11α-hydroxysteroid dehydrogenase type I knockout mice show attenuated glucocorticoid-inducible response and resist hyperglycemia on obesity and stress. *Proc Natl Acad Sci USA* 1997; 954: 14924–9.

29. Vicennati V, Vottero A, Zoumakis E, Hiroi N, Pagotto U, Pasquali, Papanicolaou D. Human adipose tissue as a target of corticotropin releasing factor (submitted for publication).

Progress in Obesity Research: 9. Edited by *Geraldo Medeiros-Neto, Alfredo Halpern and Claude Bouchard*
©2003 John Libbey Eurotext Ltd, pp. 801–805.

CHAPTER 168

Adrenal gland and visceral fat

Amelio F. de Godoy Matos, Andrea R. Vieira, Walmir Coutinho, Denise Madeira, Lúcia M. Carraro, Rosa Rodrigues, Gláucia Bastos, Mônica Cabral, André Pantaleão, Jucinéia Oliveira and Ricardo M.R. Meirelles

Department of Nutrology and Metabolism, State Institute of Diabetes and Endocrinology and Catholic University, Rua Visconde Silva 52/704. Botafogo 22271-090 Rio de Janeiro, Brazil
[e-mail: godoymatos@openlink.com.br]

Introduction

There are many clinical similarities between Cushing syndrome and the central type of obesity, what lead to suspicion that a dysfunction in the hypothalamus-pituitary-adrenal axis (HPA) plays a role in the pathophysiology of this type of obesity[1,4]. Indeed, urinary cortisol concentration[6] and higher cortisol response to physical and mental stress factors[2,7,8] have been related to clinical measurements of central obesity as sagital abdominal diameter or waist to hip circumference ratio (WHR). Moreover, a blunted inhibition of cortisol to dexamethasone in obese people with elevated WHR has been observed[9]. Pasquali *et al.*[2] found a higher cortisol and ACTH responses to CRF in patients with upper body fat deposition as compared to patients with lower body fat deposition. Taken together, these findings suggest a disturbed, hypersensitive HPA axis in central obesity.

Major depressive disorder, where the hyperactivity of the HPA axis is one of the most prominent neuroendocrine findings[10,11], have been associated with adrenal gland hyperplasia, as measured by computed tomographic scan (CT)[3,12]. Remarkable in this later study, a 70 per cent increase in the volume of the adrenal glands was significantly reduced after successful therapy of the psychiatric disorder[12].

Despite clear evidence that connecting HPA axis with central and/or visceral obesity and the finding of increased adrenal volume in patients with major depressive disorder, there does not exist, to the best of our knowledge, any study that focus on anatomic evaluation of adrenal gland size in obesity. Our hypothesis was that, if a hyperactivity of HPA axis is present in obesity this might be associated with increased volume of these glands. The aim of this study henceforth, was to demonstrate, through CT scanning of abdominal fat and of adrenal glands, an anatomic association to the malfunction of this axis.

Methods

Subjects

Fifty-two women in recruitment to an anti-obesity drug trial from the obesity clinic of the State Institute of Diabetes and Endocrinology of Rio de Janeiro were invited to participate. Forty-seven patients were obese and five were considered lean. Mean age was 37.53 ± 9.43 years. Informed consent was obtained from the patients at baseline, after the objectives and procedures of the study were fully explained. All patients were free of serious diseases, such as diabetes mellitus, coronary, liver, kidney and endocrine diseases, with special attention paid to signals of hypercortisolism. All volunteers had stable weight (no gain or loss of more than 2.0 kg) over the preceding six months and during this period no one have used any medication with the objective of losing weight.

Recruited volunteers were evaluated by means of clinical and anthropometrical examination, i.e. weight, BMI, height, waistline and hip assessment. All participants were submitted to a CT scan of the abdomen, focusing on the measurement of adrenal gland and visceral and subcutaneous fat at the level of L4-L5. The entire tomographic study was performed by the same radiologist. The tomographic study was carried out in a helicoidal system, without contrast, using the equipment General Electric Model PRO-SPEED. To study adrenal gland, protocol included a helicoidal acquisition in inspiratory apnea with cuts of 5 mm in thickness, 5 mm of spacing between the cuts, a pitch equal to 1 and FOV equal to 50 cm. For evaluation of total abdominal, visceral and subcutaneous fat, a small fan of four cuts, with 10 mm of thickness and 10 mm of spacing, maintaining the same pitch and FOV.

For statistical analysis left plus right adrenal volume were added. Distribution of several variables present in the study were studied, objecting verify the type of distribution, as well as the measurements and their central tendency. Comparison between these variables was carried out through the partial correlation of Pearson, which varied from -1 (negative or inverse correlation) to $+1$ (positive or direct correlation), subsequently testing the statistical significance of the correlated variables, through the transformation Z of Fischer. A comparison of the means between two categories of visceral fat (visceral fat $<$ or > 120 cm^2) was carried out through the Student's t-test, since equality of the variances between the groups tested (the Levene test) was proved. If not proved, non-parametrical forms of this test were carried out (the Scheffe test). Level of significance was of $P < 0.05$.

Results

Correlation between anthropometrical and tomographic data is depicted in Table 1. A positive correlation emerged between weight and waistline measurement ($r = 0.817$; $P < 0.001$), VF ($r = 0.396$; $P = 0.002$) and SCF ($r = 0.813$; $P < 0.001$). Similarly, a positive correlation was found between BMI and waistline measurement ($r = 0.879$; $P < 0.001$), VF ($r = 0.497$; $P < 0.001$) and SCF ($r = 0.795$; $P < 0.001$). BMI also positively correlated with WHR, although weakly ($r = 0.262$, $P = 0.03$).

Table 1. Correlation between anthropometric and tomographic data

	Weight (kg)	BMI (kg/m^2)	Waist (cm)	WHR	VF (cm^2)	SCF (cm^2)	AV L+R (cm^3)
Weight	–	0.930*	0.817*	0.168	0.396***	0.813*	–0.790
BMI	0.930*	–	0.879*	0.262**	0.497*	0.795*	–0.700
Waist	0.817*	0.879*	–	0.627*	0.584*	0.710*	0.060
WHR	0.168	0.262**	0.627*	–	0.471*	0.106	0.272**
VF	0.396***	0.497*	0.584*	0.471*	–	0.297**	0.228#
SCF	0.813*	0.795*	0.710*	0.106	0.297**	–	0.005
AV L+R	–0.790	–0.700	0.060	0.272**	0.228#	0.005	–

Note: * P < 0.001, **P < 0.05 e > 0.01, ***P < 0.005, #P = 0.05. Abbreviations: BMI = Body Mass Index, WHR = Waistline/Hip Ratio, VF = Visceral Fat Area, SCF = Subcutaneous fat area, AV L+R = Adrenal Volume Left+Right.

Measurements of central fat distribution (Table 1) showed that waistline correlated positively with VF ($r = 0.584$) and with SCF ($r = 0.710$), with level of significance being $P < 0.001$ for both. However, another marker of central deposition, WRH, did related to VF ($r = 0.471$; $P < 0.001$) but not to SCF. First evidence of the main objective appeared when WHR was shown to be positively correlated with adrenal volume ($r = 0,272$, $P = 0.02$) (Fig. 1). Moreover, VF showed a direct correlation with the adrenal volume, although at the significance limit ($r = 0.228$, $P = 0.05$).

To evaluate if there was any difference in adrenal volume with different patterns of VF, patients were arbitrarily divided in two groups: those with VF < 120 cm^2 and those with VF ≥ 120 cm^2. Patients with VF ≥ 120 cm^2 have an adrenal volume of 3.56 ± 1.51cm^3 against 2.62 ± 1.37cm^3 of those with VF < 120 cm^2, what was also at the significance limit ($P = 0.05$).

Discussion

Poulliot et al.[5] demonstrated that a simple measurement of the waistline was a better indicator of accumulated VF than was the WHR. Results obtained in the present study even though concordant in general with these and other authors present some peculiarities. Measurement of the waistline evaluated positively VF as well as SCF, but the coefficient was greater with SCF than with VF. What calls more attention is that WHR correlated with VF, but not with SCF, suggesting that WHR predicts intra-abdominal better than subcutaneous fat. On the other hand, when we analysed directly VF and

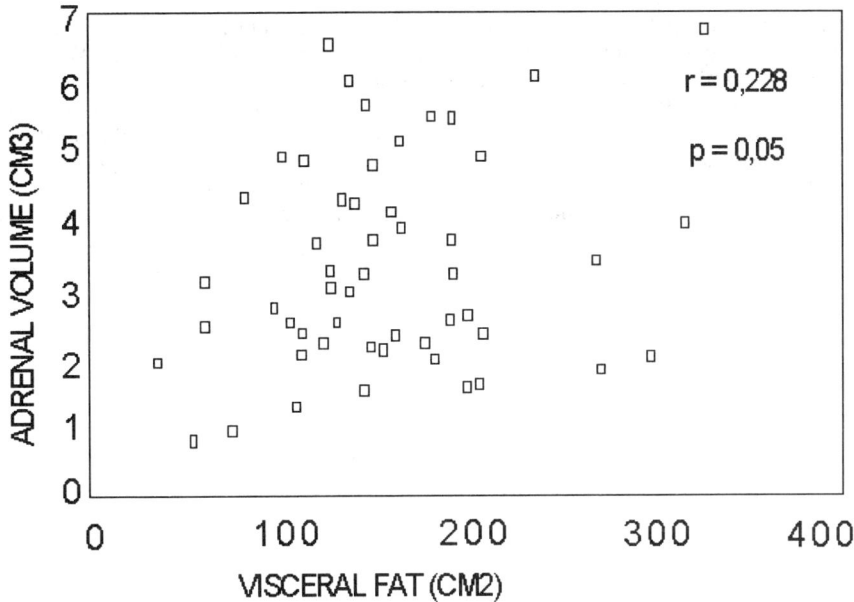

Fig. 1. Relationship between adrenal volume and visceral fat in women.

it's correlation to anthropometric measurements we observed that, indeed, there was a larger correlation with waistline (r = 0.584) than with WHR (r = 0.471). In other words, Waist measured both, VF and SCF and WHR measured essentially VF.

The main proposal of this study, in truth, was to search for an anatomic correlation for the possible functional modifications of the HPA axis in central obesity. We believe that our initial hypothesis was confirmed: WHR in this study evaluated more adequately visceral than subcutaneous fat and was significantly correlated with adrenal volume (r = 0.272, P = 0.02). It was expected also that there would be a direct relationship between visceral fat and adrenal volume and the fact is that this correlation reached borderline significance (r = 0.228, P = 0.05, Table 1, Fig. 1). It is possible that choice of the patients has interfered in these results, reducing the relation coefficient, since central obesity is more commonly associated to median levels of corpulence and our group had in average a very high level of BMI. Apart from this, in an attempt to study a large variation of corpulence, the number of normal volunteers was reduced (only five) and no one patient was located in the intermediary BMI band (between 25 and 30 kg/m^2).

It is noteworthy that adrenal volume did not correlate with any other parameter studied, such as weight and the BMI, suggesting, therefore, that it is not obesity, but the centralization of fat that keeps relationship to HPA axis activity. Further, there was no relationship of adrenal gland volume to SCF, which suggests that HPA axis hyperactivity is not associated with the subcutaneous deposition of fat, but rather with visceral deposition.

Patients with VF ≥ 120 cm^2 presented a bigger adrenal volume (3.56 ± 1.51 cm^3) (P = 0.05) as compared to patients with VF < 120 cm^2 (2.62 ± 1.37 cm^3), confirming that larger areas of VF are associated with the increased volumes of adrenal gland.

Adrenal gland and type 2 diabetes

HPA axis hyperactivity has been related not only to abdominal-visceral fat but also to features of the metabolic syndrome[13]. As type 2 diabetes is a major component of the metabolic syndrome and is related to VF, we hypothesized that there could be differences in adrenal volume of obese diabetic (D) and non-diabetic (ND) women. So we went further and studied 22 obese women, 11 D and 11 ND, utilizing the same protocol as above. In this group we also evaluated plasma cortisol after overnight 1 mg dexametasone suppression (ODS) and 24 h urinary cortisol (UC). Statistical analysis of the sum of the volumes of both adrenal glands was performed with Student ^{t}-test and Spearman correlation.

Results

Tomographic and urinary cortisol data are shown in Table 2. No patient had both, UC and ODS out of reference values. Diabetic were older than non-diabetic ($P = 0.002$). Weight, BMI, WHR and waist circumference were not significantly different between groups. In the same way, VF and SC area were not different between groups, but visceral to subcutaneous ratio (VF/SC) was significantly higher in D as compared to ND (0.818 ± 0.605 vs. 0.401 ± 0.278 $P = 0.004$). Urinary cortisol did not differ between groups (Table 2). Interestingly, AV was significantly bigger in D ($P = 0.001$) as compared to ND (Mean ± SD: AV-D = 4.243 ± 1.514 cm^3; AV-ND = 2.077 ± 1.224 cm^3). There was no association between UC and VF or AV. So, we can conclude that diabetic obese women have enlarged adrenal glands when compared to non-diabetic obese women. Pathophysiologic implications of these findings could be related to hyperactivity of HPA axis, once VF/SC ratio was increased in D patients and type 2 diabetes might be considered as an end stage of this kind of fat deposition. More studies are clearly necessary in this area.

Table 2. Tomographic data and urinary cortisol in diabetic and non-diabetic women

	ND	D	P
Adrenal vol. (AV) cm^3	2.0 ± 1.22	4.24 ± 1.51	0.001
VF (cm^2)	163 ± 61	206 ± 97	0.236
SC (cm^2)	459 ± 121	335 ± 168	0.061
VF/SC ratio	0.401 ± 0.278	0.818 ± 0.605	0.004
UC (μg/24 h)	107 ± 56	86 ± 42	0.351

D = diabetic, ND = non-diabetic.

Omental Cushing hypothesis

Apart from the hyperactivity contribution of the HPA stimulating the adrenal glands, it is possible that other factors can be involved (and coexist) in the pathophysiology of visceral fat accumulation. Re-inckle et al.[14], demonstrated an enhanced mitotic activity of adrenal cells of the lineage NCIh295 incubated with different concentrations of insulin. This suggests that hyperinsulinaemia of patients with larger accumulation of visceral fat could work together with the hyperactivity of the HPA axis to further stimulate enlargement of adrenal gland. Even though this is a workable model to explain this relationship, there are suggestions that omental adipose tissue has a greater activity of oxo redutase enzyme which contributes to an enhanced cortisone to cortisol conversion[15,16,18,19]. Recently, transgenic animals overexpressing 11β-hydroxysteroid dehydrogenase type 1 (11β-HSD1) gene demonstrated increased central fat accumulation and many features of the metabolic syndrome[17]. Therefore, cortisol generated in this tissue can promote accumulation of fat at the visceral level ('Cushing omental'). In fact, in humans 11β-HSD1 predominates in abdominal adipose tissue, being greater in omental[16], increased in obesity[15] and increases with increasing BMI in adipose tissue[18]. By other hand, 5α reductase activity is increased in obesity, augmenting cortisol metabolism[15] and Lottemberg et al.[20] demonstrated that cortisol metabolism is increased in patients with increased amount of visceral fat. Furthermore, 11β-HSD1 is decreased in liver, what suggests an impaired regeneration of cortisol from cortisone in obesity[18,19]. So, this increased inactivation combined with an impaired hepatic regeneration of cortisol may well lead to a compensatory activation of the HPA axis via hypothalamic feed back[18],. This would not exclude a primary HPA hyperactivity, however, and both models can coexist or even work in separated individual type of central fat deposition. In conclusion, our studies suggest that is not obesity itself but fat centralization, or more specifically visceral fat deposition that maintains association to a proposed hyperactivity of HPA axis. Our demonstration of increased adrenal volume related to WHR and to visceral fat deposition can be interpreted as an anatomical correlate of such hyperactivity. Moreover, a good model of the complex visceral fat deposition-insulin resistance is type 2 DM, which exhibited a clear increased adrenal volume. More studies are clearly needed in this area.

References

1. Björntörp P. Endocrine abnormalities in obesity. *Diabetes Rev* 1997; 5: 52–68.
2. Pasquali R, Cantobelli S, Casimiri F et al. The hypothalamic-pituitary-adrenal axis in obese women with different patterns of body fat distribution. *J Clin Endocr Metab* 1993; 77: 341–6.

3. Amsterdam JD, Marinelli DL, Arger P *et al.* Assessment of adrenal gland volume by computed tomography in depressed patients and healthy volunteers: a pilot study. *Psychiatry Res* 1997; 21: 189–97.

4. Björntörp P. Metabolic implications of body fat distribution. *Diabetes Care* 1991; 14: 1132–43.

5. Pouliot M, Després J, Lemieux S *et al.* Waist circunference and abdominal sagital diameter: best simple anthropometric indexes of abdominal visceral adipose tissue accumulation and related cardiovascular risk in men and women. *Am J Cardiology* 1994; v. 73: pp. 460–8.

6. Marin P, Darin N, Amemiya T *et al.* Cortisol secretion in relation to body fat distribution in obese premenopausal women. *Metabolism* 1992; 41: 882–6.

7. Moyer AE, Rodin J, Grilo CH *et al.* Stress-induced cortisol response and fat distribution in women. *Obes Res* 1994; 2: 255–62.

8. Pasquali R, Anconetani B, Chattat R *et al.* Hypothalamic-pituitary-adrenal axis activity and its relationship to the autonomic nervous system in women with visceral and subcutaneous obesity: effects of the corticotropin-releasing factor/arginine-vasopressin test and of stress. *Metabolism* 1996; 45: 351–6.

9. Ljung T, Anderson B, Björntörp P *et al.* Inhibition of cortisol secretion by dexamethasona in relation to body fat distribution: a dose-response-study. *Obes Res* 1996; 4: 277–82.

10. Linkowski P, Mendlewicz J, Leclercq R *et al.* The 24-hour profile of adrenocorticotropin and cortisol in major depressive illness. *J Clin Endocrinol Metab* 1985; 61: 429–38.

11. Tsigos C, Chrousos GP. Physiology of the hipothalamic-pituitary-adrenal axis in health and dysregulation in psychiatric and autoimmune disorders. *End Metab Clin North Am* 1994; 23: 451–66.

12. Rubbin RT, Phillips JJ, Sadow TF *et al.* Adrenal gland volume in major depression. Increase during the depressive episode and decrease with successful treatment. *Arch Gen Psychiatry* 1995; 52: 213–8.

13. Rosmond R, Dallman MF, Björntörp P. Stress-related cortisol secretion in men: relationships with abdominal obesity and endocrine,metabolic and hemodynamic abnormalities. *J Clin Endocrinol Metab* 1988; 83: 1853–9.

14. Reinckle M, Fabnacht S, Väth S *et al.* Adrenal incidentalomas: a manifestation of the metabolic syndrome. *Endocrin Res* 1996; 22: 757–61.

15. Andrew R, Phillips A, Walker BR. Obesity and gender influence cortisol secretion and metabolism in man. *J Clin Endocrin Metab* 1998; 83: 1806–9.

16. Bujalska IJ, Kurnar S, Stewart PM. Does central obesity reflect 'Cushing's disease of the omentum'? *Lancet* 1997; 349: 1210–3.

17. Masuzaki H, Paterson J, Shinyama H *et al.* A transgenic model of visceral obesity and the metabolic syndrome. *Science* 2001; 294: 2166–70.

18. Rask E, Olssom T, Södeberg S *et al.* Tissue-specific dysregulation of cortisol metabolism in human obesity. *J Clin Endocrin Metab* 2001; 86: 1414–21.

19. Rask E, Walker B, Södeberg S *et al.* Tissue-specific changes in Peripheral cortisol metabolism in obese women: increased adipose 11β hydroxysteroid dehydrogenase type 1 activity. *J Clin Endocrin Metab* 2002; 87: 3330–6.

20. Lottemberg AS, Giannella-Neto D, Derendorf H *et al.* Effect of fat distribution on the pharmacokinetics of cortisol in obesity. *Int J Clin Pharm Ther* 1998; 36: 501–6.

Progress in Obesity Research: 9. Edited by *Geraldo Medeiros-Neto, Alfredo Halpern and Claude Bouchard*

CHAPTER 169

Novel mechanism of feeding regulation by ghrelin

Masamitsu Nakazato

Third Department of Medicine, Miyazaki Medical College, Miyazaki 889-1692, Japan
[e-mail: nakazato@post.miyazaki-med.ac.jp]

Introduction

The molecular mechanisms to regulate energy balance are coming to light by the recent robust progresses in the molecular biology and neuroscience. Ghrelin is a novel anabolic peptide that we discovered from the stomach in humans and rats two years ago[1,2]. We describe the molecular mechanism of ghrelin in the regulation of feeding.

Discovery of ghrelin

Growth hormone (GH) secretion from the pituitary has been known to be stimulated by two different pathways: one is the GHRH (growth hormone releasing hormone)/cAMP pathway and the other is the GHS (growth hormone secretagogues)/IP3-calcium pathway. In 1996, the GHS receptor, a G-protein coupled transmembrance receptor and now called the ghrelin receptor, was cloned, but its natural ligand had been unknown until we purified its endogenous ligand peptide, ghrelin. We isolated ghrelin from the human and rat stomach by monitoring an increase in intracellular calcium level in CHO cells that had been designed to express the ghrelin receptor[1]. Ghrelin consists of 28 amino acids in which the Ser-3 is post-translationally modified by the addition of middle-chain fatty acid, octanoyl acid. This acyl modification is indispensable for ghrelin's biological activity. At present, ghrelin is found in the fish, amphibians, birds, and many mammals. In naming the peptide, we associated it with a growth hormone release by naming it a variation of the Proto-Indo-European root, 'ghre'.

Hypothalamic ghrelin

Ghrelin-producing neurons are located in the lateral part of the arcuate nucleus and their nerve fibres are widely distributed in the hypothalamic regions of primary importance in the regulation of feeding[1,3]. Intracerebroventricular (ICV) administration of ghrelin above a minimally active dose of 10 pmol to free-feeding rats during the light phase increased food intake in a dose-dependent manner[2]. Ghrelin-27 that is an alternative splicing product and devoid of a glutamine at position 14, has a same orexigenic potency as ghrelin 28. Ghrelin did not produce unusual behaviour. When we compared doses less than 500 pmol, ghrelin was more potent than neuropeptide Y (NPY) the most powerful orexigenic peptide identified so far. Ghrelin also increased food intake in feeding conditions, such as dark-phase feeding and starvation-induced feeding. A chronic ICV infusion of ghrelin, as few as 250 pmol/day, for 12 days using an osmotic minipump increased food intake and body weight gain over the infusion period. The ghrelin infusion did not affect general activity. At the end of experiment, the plasma concentrations of glucose, insulin, triglycerides, and total cholesterol in the ghrelin-infused group did not differ from those in the control group.

To determine whether an endogenous tone of ghrelin signalling is present in the hypothalamus, we investigated the effect of an antibody against ghrelin on feeding behaviour[2]. Compared with the preimmune serum IgG, anti-ghrelin IgG remarkably suppressed starvation-induced feeding in a dose-dependent manner. Anti-ghrelin IgG also suppressed dark-phase food intake by 36 per cent in free-feeding rats. These findings indicate that ghrelin is a powerful, endogenous orexigenic peptide.

Growth hormone is known to stimulate feeding. To investigate whether ghrelin's orexigenic activity depends on the GH system, we studied the effect of ICV-injected ghrelin in spontaneous growth hormone deficient rats[2]. Ghrelin also stimulated food intake in them. Ghrelin stimulates feeding by the GH-independent mechanism.

Feeding is finely and redundantly regulated by the complicated interaction of many orexigenic and anorectic signals produced in the brain and peripheral tissues. We studied the downstream signalling of the ghrelin system[2]. Ghrelin axon terminals directly contact NPY-containing neurons in double immunohistochemistry. Ghrelin axons make direct synaptic contacts with NPY neurons in electron microscopic immunohistochemistry. To establish the activation of NPY neurons by ghrelin, c-*fos* expression which is a marker of neuronal activation was mapped following an ICV administration of ghrelin. Ghrelin administration induced Fos in 39 per cent of NPY neurons in the arcuate nucleus by double immunohistochemistry. The hypothalamic NPY mRNA level in quantitative *in situ* hybridization increased following ghrelin administration. Ghrelin anatomically lies upstream NPY. To investigate the functional relationship between ghrelin and NPY, the consequence of blocking NPY in ghrelin-induced feeding was observed. ICV administration of anti-NPY IgG 4 h before ghrelin administration abolished ghrelin-induced feeding. An NPY receptor antagonist also abolished ghrelin-induced feeding. NPY neurons are shown to express the ghrelin receptor. These findings indicate that ghrelin lies upstream NPY at both anatomical and functional levels to stimulate food intake.

AgRP (agouti related protein) is another orexigenic peptide produced in the arcuate nucleus. AgRP and NPY co-localize in neurons; however, they exert their activities via different pathways. NPY inhibits an anorectic peptide, corticotropin-releasing hormone (CRH), and AgRP competes with another anorectic peptide, α-melanocyte-stimulating hormone (α-MSH). We studied the functional relationship between ghrelin and AgRP in feeding regulation[2]. Ghrelin-induced feeding was suppressed upon treatment with α-MSH, and blocking of AgRP, with anti-AgRP IgG. These findings indicate that inhibition of endogenous NPY and AgRP can modulate ghrelin-induced feeding. Ghrelin is thought to interact anatomically and functionally with the pathways of these two orexigenic peptides produced in the arcuate nucleus.

The ghrelin receptor is also expressed in the lateral hypothalamus that has been known to be a feeding centre and was recently found to produce two orexigenic neuropeptides, orexin and melanin-concentrating hormone (MCH). Ghrelin may interact with these peptides. Ghrelin fibres are appositioned to orexin neurons. Orexin-producing neurons and their dendritic processes often receive synapses from ghrelin axon terminals[4]. Icv administration of ghrelin induced Fos expression in 23 per cent of orexin-producing neurons. The electrical activity of orexin neurons was activated by ghrelin administration. Orexin is a down stream signal of ghrelin. We further studied the functional relationship between ghrelin and orexin. Pretreatment with anti-orexin IgG reduced ghrelin-induced food intake to one half of the level seen in rats given control IgG + ghrelin. Ghrelin-induced food intake in orexin knockout mice was significantly reduced in comparison with wild-type littermates. Ghrelin-induced feeding is therefore concluded to be mediated in part by the orexin pathway[4]. Ghrelin injection did not induce Fos in any MCH neurons. Pretreatment with anti-MCH IgG did not affect ghrelin-induced feeding, indicating no interaction between ghrelin and MCH[4].

In summary, central ghrelin is verified to act on NPY/AgRP neurons and orexin neurons to stimulate feeding. These neurons are also found to have the leptin receptor. There is a competitive interaction between ghrelin and leptin in these neurons in feeding regulation. Ghrelin nerve fibres project to the median eminence to stimulate GH secretion from the pituitary[5].

Gastric ghrelin

Ghrelin cells are abundant in the oxyntic gland of the stomach in humans and rats in *in situ* hybridization[6]. In immunoelectron microscopy, ghrelin staining is localized on round, compact, electron-dense granules. Until now, three types of endocrine cells: histamine and uroguanylin-producing enterochromaffin-like cells, somatostatin-producing D cells, and serotonin-producing enterochromaffin cells have been identified. Ghrelin cells are a new member of endocrine cells in the gastric body. They make up about 20 per cent of the endocrine cell population in the gastric body of both rats and humans. Ghrelin cells are positioned close to the capillary, and immunoreactive ghrelin is circulating in human plasma at as much as 150 fmol/ml. Ghrelin mRNA expression in the gastric fundus increased after fast, and returned to the control level after refeeding[7]. Ghrelin plasma concentration in the gastric vein increased after fast. The ghrelin mRNA level in the stomach also increased after administration of leptin and insulin. Biosynthesis and secretion of ghrelin is up-regulated under conditions of negative energy balance, which appear to be consistent with ghrelin's anabolic role in the regulation of energy homeostasis[7].

Intravenous administration of ghrelin increased dose-dependently food intake in free-feeding rats. In contrast, intravenous administration of anti-ghrelin IgG reduced feeding in fasted rats. Many anorectic peptides are produced in the gut; however, ghrelin is the first orexigenic peptide present in the periphery[8]. The ghrelin's appetite-stimulating effect was also shown in humans by a double-blind cross-over study[9]. Intravenous infusion of ghrelin significantly increased energy intake from a free-choice buffet lunch compared with saline infusion.

To investigate a possible involvement of ghrelin in the pathogenesis of human obesity, we measured plasma ghrelin concentration in lean and obese non-diabetic individuals[10]. Obese subjects have lower plasma ghrelin concentration than lean subjects. The fasting plasma ghrelin concentration was negatively correlated with body mass index. Ghrelin is downregulated in human obesity, which may represent a physiological adaptation to the positive energy balance. On the other hand, ghrelin is upregulated in anorectic patients, which also is a physiological adaptation to the negative energy balance. Plasma ghrelin concentration of normol subjects decreased after 75 g oral glucose and 10 g intravenous glucose loads[10]. Also in diabetic patients, plasma ghrelin decreased after meal. Plasma ghrelin decreased after insulin injection. Hyperinsulinaemia in glucose load and insulin administration may reduce ghrelin secretion.

The circulating plasma ghrelin level showed a diurnal pattern with preprandial increases and postprandial decreases during the daytime and a maximum peak at 2 a.m.. Ghrelin may be a potent starvation signal and the stomach may apprise the brain of hunger information through the ghrelin system.

Vagus-mediated signalling by ghrelin

How does the stomach-derived ghrelin exert its stimulative action on feeding? We expected two possibilities; one is via the vagus nerve, and the other is via the bloodstream. Some meal-related metabolites, monoamines and peptides as well as mechanical and chemical stimuli transmit their satiety signals to the hindbrain via the vagus nerve. The vagus nerve is a cranial nerve that contains both efferent and afferent fibres. It conveys information to and from viscera as well as to and from brain. Afferent information from the alimentary tract is conveyed to the nucleus of the solitary tract, NTS. Efferent fibres originate from the dorsal motor nuclues, DMN. These two nuclei are located close in the medulla. Approximately 90 per cent of vagus nerve fibres are afferent and composed of unmyelinated, thin, capsaicin-sensitive fibres. There are some afferent endings within the gastrointestinal mucosa and submucosa that are more optimally positioned to monitor bioactive substances released from enteroendocrine cells. Vagal afferent neurons are present within the nodose ganglion located near the jugular foramen. These neurons produce a variety of receptor proteins, and transport them to the vagal afferent terminals in the gastrointestinal tract, for example the receptor protein for cholecystokinin (CCK), an anorectic gut peptide.

Ghrelin's orexigenic activity may depend upon the vagus nerve. Furthermore, it has not been known whether the vagus nerve is involved in the regulation of GH secretion. In order to investigate these possibilities, we examined the effect of ghrelin on feeding using rats with vagotomy or perivagal application of a specific afferent neurotoxin, capsaicin. IV ghrelin (1.5 nmol) stimulated food intake in sham-operated rats[8]. IV ghrelin administered to rats with vagotomy did not induce feeding. And in rats with capsaicin application, ghrelin did not induce feeding. In contrast, feeding induced by ICV ghrelin is not affected by neither vagotomy nor capsaicin treatment[8]. Central ghrelin directly acts on the neuronal circuits in the hypothalamus to increase food intake, and this mechanism is distint from that of gastric ghrelin.

We next studied whether the GH-releasing activity of peripheral ghrelin is also mediated by vagal sensory function. The GH response to ghrelin was profoundly attenuated by both capsaicin treatment and gastric branch vagotomy, but the GH response to GHRH was not affected by these two procedures. The GH-releasing activity of ghrelin is mostly mediated by the vagal afferent nerve, and in part by direct entry into the pituitary via the blood circulation.

Ghrelin IV administered to sham-operated rats induced Fos expression in the arcuate nucleus. In double immunohistochemistry, ghrelin induced Fos expression in 43 per cent of NPY neurons and 15 per cent of GHRH neurons. Neither in capsaicin-treated nor in vagotomized rats, ghrelin did not induce Fos in any neurons of the arcuate nucleus. Stomach-derived ghrelin stimulates NPY and GHRH neurons via the vagal afferent[8]. In order to investigate whether or not the ghrelin receptor is actually synthesized in the vagal afferent neurons, we examined the expression of the ghrelin receptor mRNA[8]. A ghrelin mRNA was found by RT-PCR. Rat nodose ganglion has about 6,000 neuronal cell bodies. *In situ* hybridization showed that the ghrelin receptor mRNA signals were found in 40 per cent of neurons in the nodose ganglion.

We examined the effect of vagal ligation on the accumulation of binding sites detected using ^{125}I-ghrelin in order to study the transport of the ghrelin receptor in the vagus nerve. Binding sites of ^{125}I-ghrelin accumulated in the segments proximal to the ligature. Taken together, stomach-derived ghrelin binds to its receptors synthesized in the vagal afferent neurons then is transported to the vagal afferent terminals. We conclude that ghrelin's starvation signals transmit to the brain through the vagal afferent[8]. To study the influence of ghrelin on vagal afferent, we recorded gastric vagal afferent activity using the electrophysiological method. IV administered ghrelin significantly decreased gastric vagal afferent activity. Des-acyl ghrelin, which lacks the n-octanoylation essential for ghrelin's binding activity to the receptor, did not affect the afferent activity. In contrast, CCK increased vagal afferent activity. The gastric vagal afferent is the major pathway conveying ghrelin's signal for starvation and CCK's signal for satiation.

The ghrelin receptor is expressed in various tissues, and ghrelin has multifaceted roles in systemic organs. For example, ghrelin-immunoreactive cells were colocalized exclusively with glucagon in α-cells of pancreatic islets in both humans anbd rats[11]. The ghrelin receptor is present in pancreatic islets. Ghrelin increased the cytosolic free Ca^{2+} concentration in β-cells and stimulated insulin secretion when it was added to isolated rat pancreatic islets. These findings indicate that ghrelin may regulate islet function in an endocrine and/or paracrine fashion[11]. The next few years will bring answers to questions on the clinical potential for ghrelin, a novel anabolic peptide.

References

1. Kojima M, Hosoda H, Date Y, Nakazato M, Matsuo H, Kangawa K. Ghrelin is a novel growth hormone releasing acylated peptide from stomach. *Nature* 1999; 402: 656–60.

2. Nakazato M, Murakami N, Date Y, Kojima M, Matsuo H, Kangawa K, Matsukura S. A role for ghrelin in the central regulation of feeding. *Nature* 2001; 409: 194–8.

3. Lu S, Guan JL, Wand QP, Uehara K, Yamada S, Goto N *et al.* Immunocytochemical observation of ghrelin-containing neurons in the rat arcuate nucleus. *Neurosci Lett* 2002; 321: 157–60.

4. Toshinai K, Date Y, Murakami N, Shimada M, Guan JL, Wang QP *et al.* Ghrelin-induced food intake is mediated via the orexin pathway. *Endocrinology* 2003; 144: 1506–12.

5. Date Y, Murakami N, Kojima M, Kuroiwa T, Matsukura S, Kangawa K *et al.* Central effects of a novel acylated peptide, ghrelin, on growth hormone release in rats. *Biochem Biophys Res Commun* 2000; 275: 477–80.

6. Date Y, Kojima M, Hosoda H, Sawaguchi A, Mondal MS, Suganuma T *et al.* Ghrelin, a novel growth-hormone-releasing acylated peptide, is synthesized in a distinct endocrine cell type in the gastrointestinal tracts of rats and humans. *Endocrinology* 2000; 141: 4255–61.

7. Toshinai K, Mondal MS, Nakazato M, Date Y, Murakami N, Kojima M *et al.* Upregulation of ghrelin expression in the stomach upon fasting, insulin-induced hypoglycemia, and leptin administration. *Biochem Biophys Res Commun* 2001; 281: 1220–5.

8. Date Y, Murakami N, Toshinai K, Matsukura S, Nijima A, Matsuo H *et al.* The role of the gastric afferent vagal nerve in ghrelin-induced feeding and growth hormone secretion. *Gastroenterology* 2002; 123: 1120–8.

9. Wren AM, Seal LJ, Cohen MA, Brynes AE, Frost GS, Murphy KG *et al.* Ghrelin enhances appetite and increases food intake in humans. *J Clin Endocrinol Metab* 2001; 86: 5992–5.

10. Shiiya T, Nakazato M, Mizuta M, Date Y, Mondal MS, Tanaka M *et al.* Plasma ghrelin levels in lean and obese humans and the effect of glucose on ghrelin secretion. *J Clin Endocrinol Metab* 2002; 87: 240–4.

11. Date Y, Nakazato M, Hashiguchi S, Dezaki K, Mondal MS, Hosoda H *et al.* Ghrelin is present in pancreatic α-cells of humans and rats and stimulates insulin secretion. *Diabetes* 2002; 51: 124–9.

Progress in Obesity Research: 9. Edited by *Geraldo Medeiros-Neto, Alfredo Halpern and Claude Bouchard*
©2003 John Libbey Eurotext Ltd, pp. 810–813.

CHAPTER 170

Pharmacological potential of pre-proglucagon derived peptides as treatment of obesity

Philip J. Larsen, Niels Vrang and Mads Tang-Christensen

Rheoscience, Glerupvej 2, 2610 Rødovre, Denmark
[e-mail: pjl@Rheoscience.com]

In the central nervous system, pre-proglucagon derived peptides, glucagon-like peptide-1 (GLP-1) and glucagon-like peptide-2 (GLP-2) are catabolic neurotransmitters synthesized in neurones of the nucleus of the solitary tract (NTS). In the NTS, pre-proglucagon expression is confined to a subset of non-catecholaminergic neurones[1]. These neurones of the NTS give rise to widespread ascending projections targeting numerous forebrain structures including hypothalamic nuclei involved in regulation of body weight homeostasis. Involvement of the NTS in long-term regulation of energy homeostasis is further emphasized by expression of the long form of the leptin receptor (Ob-Rb) in this nucleus[2,3], although the functional relevance of this is far from fully understood. Dual *in situ* hybridization histochemical experiments have verified that pre-proglucagon expressing neurones also express Ob-Rb suggesting a direct impact of leptin upon intracerebral GLP-1/GLP-2 release[4]. Local administration of leptin into the fourth ventricle as well as systemic injections of leptin induce expression of cFos in ascending catecholaminergic/cholecystokinin (NA/CCK) as well as ascending GLP-1/GLP-2 neurones[5] (own unpublished). However, also local application of leptin at gastric vagal afferents induces neuronal activity of neurones of the nucleus of the solitary tract[6]. These observations imply that brainstem neurones are affected by circulating leptin both via the neurohaemal zone of the area postrema and adjacent subpostreme area as well as via vagal afferents from the gastrointestinal tract. Despite ambiguous results obtained in clinical trials using recombinant human leptin[7], it is possible that activity of satiety inducing neurones is augmented by the concomitant stimulation by leptin. Thus, intracerebroventricular administration of leptin prior to gastric distension of systemic cholecystokinin administration causes much more pronounced satiety than either of the stimuli alone[8,9]. The structural basis for such interaction is likely to be aforementioned ascending neurones of the nucleus of the solitary tract, because postprandial signals of systemic cholecystokinin, GLP-1, and gastric distension as well as leptin converge on these neurones.

Anorectic properties of central GLP-1 are well recognized although the physiological context of endogenous GLP-1 is still subject to debate[10] (Fig. 1). In a recent study, we have shown that the hypothalamic content of GLP-1 and GLP-2 is inversely correlated to the energy balance reflecting that synaptic release of GLP-1/GLP-2 is increased during states of voluntary overfeeding[11]. This observation supports that central pre-proglucagon derived peptides serve roles as satiety factors. Repetitive injection of the GLP-1 antagonist Exendin(9-39) enhance daily food intake in rodents suggesting the existence of a continuous endogenous tone of GLP-1 on neurones involved in the regulation of feeding[12]. Given the wide spread distribution of GLP-1 receptors in the central nervous system[13], it is hardly surprising that several targets is influenced by intracerebroventricular administration of GLP-1 and analogues hereof. In a pharmacological context the relevant question to address is whether centrally acting GLP-1 agonists are candidate anorectic agents with none or only few tolerable side effects. Generally, induction of aversive behaviour is considered an indicator of drug-induced anhedonia and consequently an indicator of potential drug induced malaise. As many other neuropeptides involved in regulation of energy homeostasis, central administration of high doses (10 µg) of GLP-1 induces taste aversion.

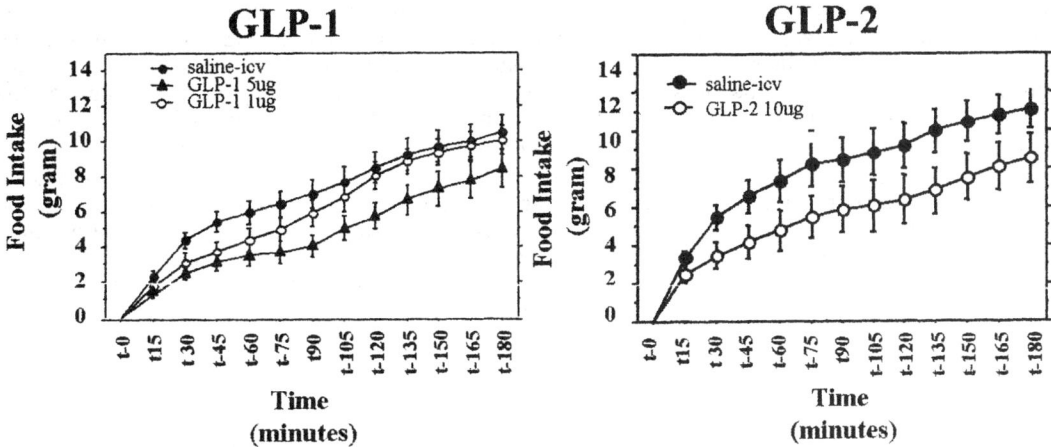

Fig. 1. Food intake in adult male free living rats. Rats were individually housed under a 12 : 12 h light: dark cycle, and immediately prior to the onset of darkness, they received one of several intracerebroventricular doses of GLP-1 or GLP-2. Peptides were dissolved in phosphate buffered saline to which 0.1 per cent (w/v) bovine serum albumin was added. A volume of 10 μl was slowly injected into the right lateral ventricle. Food intake was monitored automatically in a computerized continuous behavioural monitoring system assessing food and water intake as well as locomototion. It is clearly seen that both GLP-1 and GLP-2 abolish food intake normally occurring in rats at the onset of darkness.

However, site directed micro-injections of GLP-1 into the hypothalamic paraventricular nucleus induces pharmacologically specific inhibition of feeding without induction of taste aversive behaviour[14]. In animals having their arcuate nucleus lesioned by neonatal monosodium glutamate treatment, central administration of 10 μg GLP-1 has lost its anorectic potential but is still inducing taste aversion[15] (own unpublished). Further support of dissociated specific satiety inducing central targets of GLP-1 and non-specific taste aversion inducing central targets come from lesion studies by van Dijk and Thiele showing that the hypothalamic paraventricular nucleus constitutes a target where GLP-1 elicits satiety whereas the central amygdala and the parabrachial nuclei constitute areas involved in mediating GLP-1 induced taste aversion[16].

Because GLP-1 and GLP-2 co-exist in ascending neurones of the NTS we speculated that GLP-2 may also constitute a central mediator of satiety. In a recent study we have shown that GLP-2 exerts central actions as a specific transmitter inhibiting feeding behaviour[17] (Fig. 1). The anorexia induced by GLP-2 is not accompanied by taste aversion, and neuroanatomical localization of central GLP-2 receptor expression has shown that GLP-2 receptors are strictly confined to the central compact portion of the dorsomedial hypothalamic nucleus. This region of the dorsomedial nucleus contains a substantial number of neuropeptide Y mRNA expressing neurones, but so far immunohistochemical analyses have failed to reliably demonstrate presence of neuropeptide Y in perikarya and neurites originating from these neurones. Thus, the neurochemical phenotype of GLP-2 receptor expressing neurones is still uncertain but given their localization they are likely to constitute part of the dorsomedial nucleus gain setting entity involved in body weight homeostasis. Central administration of GLP-2 induces premature satiety to freely fed rats as well as inhibition of both starvation and neuropeptide Y induced feeding[17]. Glucagon-like peptide-2 actions on feeding are dependent on intact central GLP-1 receptors because pharmacological antagonism of GLP-1 receptors by prior administration of exendin9-39 abolishes GLP-2 induced anorexia[17]. The most likely interpretation of this finding is that GLP-1 and GLP-2 receptors act in parallel requiring both to be fully operational in order to induce anorexia. Observations from mice have given somewhat different results, because prior central administration of exendin9-39 potentiates the anorectic actions of central GLP-2. The reason for this discrepancy is at present unknown, but our own *in vitro* experiments on transfected cell systems expressing human GLP-2 receptors clearly show that exendin9-39 has virtually no affinity to the GLP-2 receptor[18]. Because of topographically very limited expression of central GLP-2 receptors, they constitute a pharmacologically very interesting target. Ideally, centrally acting GLP-2 agonists could induce satiety via interference with components of the body weight set point generating neuronal circuit. The dorsomedial hypothalamic nucleus constitutes a possible anatomical site for an organismic body weight set point generating device. Lesions of the dorsomedial hypothalamic nucleus render rats hypophagic and with resulting smaller body mass and size, but sham-lesioned animals pair-fed to the dorsomedial nucleus-lesioned become even smaller and display poorer feed efficiency than dorsomedial nucleus-lesioned animals supporting that neurones of the dorsomedial nucleus contribute positively to set the gain of the adipostat[19]. In other words, the neurones of the dorsomedial nucleus render animals less capable of coping with situations characterized by reduced caloric intake.

Experience from both human and animal studies emphasise that GLP-1 also targets peripheral sites with profound impact on feeding and appetite. We and others have shown that chronic GLP-1 infusion confer lasting anorexia in rodent models and the organization of the intricate circuit mediating these actions most likely involve vagal afferents and the adjacent dorsal vagal complex including nucleus of the solitary tract[20]. Pre-proglucagon-like expressing neurones of the nucleus of the solitary tract express leptin receptors and these neurones may constitute part of neurones a central leptin responsive system with negative impact on feeding behaviour.

In the periphery, GLP-1 released from the L-cells is an incretin that stimulate insulin secretion and has a wide spectrum of other effects on pancreatic β-cells, and also inhibits glucagon secretion. However, most importantly GLP-1 also acts as an ileal brake reducing gastric emptying thereby reducing nutrient delivery rate to absorptive portions of the GI tract. Promises of pharmacological use of GLP-1 and analogues hereof as anorectic agents have come from human and rodent studies. Using the long-acting GLP-1 derivative, gamma-L-glutamoyl (N-epsilon-hexadecanoyl)-Lys26, Arg34-GLP-1(7-37), also known as NN2211 (liraglutide), we have shown that acute as well as twice daily administration for 10 days reduces food intake in rats with resultant decrease in body weight and fat content[20]. In a recent human study, continuous infusion of GLP-1 (4.8 pmol/kg/min) to type 2 diabetic patients gave rise to marked improvement of glycaemic control and caused moderate yet non-significant weight loss[21]. There is reason to believe that future studies employing slightly higher doses, larger patient populations, and longer administration periods will prove GLP-1 analogues as efficient weight reducing agents, because subjective sensations of hunger and satiety remained affected even after several weeks of administration[21]. The site of the anorectic action of peripherally administered GLP-1 is unknown but involvement of both central and peripheral sites in GLP-1 are likely, because a recent study has shown that radiolabelled GLP-1 readily gains access to the central nervous system[22]. The nucleus of the solitary tract is situated adjacent to the blood brain barrier free area postrema, and other studies using radiolabelled neuropeptides have shown that peripheral administration of neuropeptides gain access both to the area postrema as well as the adjacent subpostreme regions including the dorsal vagal complex[23]. Thus, it is likely that peripherally administered GLP-1 enters the nucleus of the solitary tract with resulting impact on ascending neurones involved in regulation of food intake. Interaction of GLP-1 with vagal afferents from the gastrointestional tract should also be considered as mediator of its anorectic actions because transection of the vagus nerve renders the stomach of anaesthetized pigs insensitive to the akinetic actions of intravenously administered GLP-1[24]. Probably both vagal afferents and GLP-1 receptors accessible from the periphery are responsible for the anorexia induced by GLP-1, because we have seen that bilateral subdiaphragmatic vagotomy on rats carrying the anorectic GLP-1 producing tumour has no impact on the development of anorexia[25]. Experience from human studies show that the therapeutic window of GLP-1 infusions is limited because infusion doses above 5–6 pmol/kg/min induces nausea and vomiting, probably due to prolonged effects on gastric emptying and activation of emesis mediating pathways having their sensory components in the area postrema[26]. Considering the favourable effects on both glucose homeostasis and appetite, GLP-1 agonists seem obvious candidates for pharmacological treatment of the overweight type 2 diabetes patient improving both glycaemic control and body weight with minimal risk of inducing reactive hypoglycaemia.

References

1. Larsen PJ, Tang-Christensen M, Holst JJ, Orskov C. Distribution of glucagon-like peptide-1 and other preproglucagon- derived peptides in the rat hypothalamus and brainstem. *Neuroscience* 1997; 77: 257–70.

2. Hay-Schmidt A, Helboe L, Larsen PJ. Leptin receptor immunoreactivity is present in ascending serotonergic and catecholaminergic neurons of the rat. *Neuroendocrinology* 2001; 73: 215–26.

3. Mercer JG, Hoggard N, Williams LM, Lawrence B, Hannah LT, Trayhurn P. Localization of leptin receptor mRNA and the long form splice variant (Ob-Rb) in mouse hypothalamus and adjacent brain regions by *in situ* hybridization. *FEBS Letters* 1996; 387: 113–6.

4. Goldstone AP, Mercer JG, Gunn I, Moar KM, Mark C, Edwards B *et al.* Leptin interacts with glucagon-like peptide-1 neurons to reduce food intake and body weight in rodents. *FEBS Letters* 1997; 415: 134–8.

5. Elias CF, Kelly JF, Lee CE, Ahima RS, Drucker DJ, Saper CB, Elmquist JK. Chemical characterization of leptin-activated neurons in the rat brain. *J Comp Neurol* 2000; 423: 261–81.

6. Yuan CS, Attele AS, Wu JA, Zhang L, Shi ZQ. Peripheral gastric leptin modulates brain stem neuronal activity in neonates. *Am J Physiol* 1999; 277: 626–30.

7. Heymsfield SB, Greenberg AS, Fujioka K, Dixon RM, Kushner R, Hunt T *et al.* Recombinant leptin for weight loss in obese and lean adults: a randomized, controlled, dose-escalation trial. *JAMA* 1999; 282: 1568–75.

8. Emond M, Schwartz GJ, Ladenheim EE, Moran TH. Central leptin modulates behavioral and neural responsivity to CCK. *Am J Physiol* 1999; 276: R1545–R1549.

9. Matson CA, Ritter RC. Long-term CCK-leptin synergy suggests a role for CCK in the regulation of body weight. *Am J Physiol* 1999; 276: 1038–45.

10. Tang-Christensen M, Larsen PJ, Göke R, Fink-Jensen A, Jessop DS, Moller M, Sheikh SP. Central administration of GLP-1 (7-36) amide inhibits food and water intake in rats. *Am J Physiol* 1996; 271: R848–R856.

11. Tang-Christensen M, Vrang N, Hartmann B, Larsen LK, Orskov C, Holst JJ, Larsen PJ. The correlation between feeding status and the amount of proglucagon, GLP-1 and GLP-2 in the central nervous system of the rat. *Diabetes* 2001; 50: A373-A1559-P.

12. Meeran K, O'Shea D, Edwards CM, Turton MD, Heath MM, Gunn I *et al.* Repeated intracerebroventricular administration of glucagon-like peptide-1-(7-36) amide or exendin-(9-39) alters body weight in the rat. *Endocrinology* 1999; 140: 244–250.

13. Göke R, Larsen PJ, Mikkelsen JD, Sheikh SP. Distribution of GLP-1 binding sites in the rat brain: evidence that exendin-4 is a ligand of brain GLP-1 binding sites. *Eur J Neurosci* 1995; 7: 2294–2300.

14. McMahon LR, Wellman PJ. PVN infusion of GLP-1(7-36) amide supresses feeding but does not induce aversion or alter locomotion in rats. *Am J Physiol* 1998; 274: R23–R29.

15. Tang-Christensen M, Vrang N, Larsen PJ. Glucagon-like peptide 1(7-36) amides's central inhibition of feeding and peripheral inhibition of drinking are abolished by neonatal monosodium glutamate treatment. *Diabetes* 1998; 47: 530–537.

16. van Dijk G, Thiele TE. Glucagon-like peptide-1 (7-36) amide: a central regulator of satiety and interoceptive stress. *Neuropeptides* 1999; 33: 406–414.

17. Tang-Christensen M, Larsen PJ, Thulesen J, Romer J, Vrang N. The proglucagon-derived peptide, glucagon-like peptide-2, is a neurotransmitter involved in the regulation of food intake. *Nature Med* 2000; 6: 802–807.

18. Larsen PJ, Vrang N, Tang-Christensen M, Jensen PB, Hay-Schmidt A *et al.* Ups and downs for neuropeptides in body weight homeostasis: pharmacological potential of cocaine amphetamine regulated transcript and pre-proglucagon-derived peptides. *Eur J Pharmacol* 2002; 440: 159–172.

19. Bernardis LL, Bellinger LL, McEwen G, Kodis M, Feldman MJ. Further evidence for the existence of an 'organismic' set point in rats with dorsomedial hypothalamic nucleus lesions (DMNL rats): normal catch-up growth. *Physiol Behav* 1988; 44: 561–568.

20. Larsen PJ, Fledelius C, Knudsen LB, Tang-Christensen M. Systemic administration of the long-acting GLP-1 derivative NN2211 induces lasting and reversible weight loss in both normal and obese rats. *Diabetes* 2001; 50: 2530–2539.

21. Zander M, Madsbad S, Madsen JL, Holst JJ. Effect of 6-week course of glucagon-like peptide 1 on glycaemic control, insulin sensitivity, and beta-cell function in type 2 diabetes: a parallel-group study. *Lancet* 2002; 359: 824–830.

22. Hassan M, Eskilsson A, Nilsson C, Jonsson C, Jacobsson H, Refai E *et al.* In vivo dynamic distribution of 131I-glucagon-like peptide-1 (7-36) amide in the rat studied by gamma camera. *Nucl Med Biol* 1999; 26: 413–420.

23. Whitcomb DC, Taylor IL. A new twist in the brain-gut axis. *Am J Med Sci* 1992; 304: 334-338.

24. Wettergren A, Wojdemann M, Holst JJ. Glucagon-like peptide-1 inhibits gastropancreatic function by inhibiting central parasympathetic outflow. *Am J Physiol* 1998; 275: 984–992.

25. Jensen PB, Blume N, Mikkelsen JD, Larsen PJ, Jensen HI, Holst JJ, Madsen OD. Transplantable rat glucagonomas cause acute onset of severe anorexia and adipsia despite highly elevated NPY mRNA levels in the hypothalamic arcuate nucleus. *J Clin Invest* 1998; 101: 503–510.

26. Larsen J, Jallad N, Damsbo P. One-week continuous infusion of GLP-1(7-37) improves the glycemic control in NIDDM. *Diabetes* 1996; 45: A233.

CHAPTER 171

Regulation of thyoasing hormone (TRH) gene expression by hypothalamic signaling pathways involved in energy expenditure

Marisol E. Lopez and Anthony N. Hollenberg

Division of Endocrinology, Beth Israel Deaconess Medical Center and Harvard Medical School, Boston MA 02215, USA
[e-mail: thollenb@caregroup.harvard.edu]

Introduction

The production of thyroid hormones (thyroxine (T4) and triiodothyronine (T3) by the thyroid gland is essential for normal human development after birth. In addition to its critical role in development thyroid hormone is also a major regulator of energy expenditure in man principally through its effects on metabolic rate which may in part be related to mitochondrial energy uncoupling[1]. The regulation of thyroid hormone synthesis is mediated by an endocrine system which originates in the hypothalamus with the production of thyrotropin-releasing hormone (TRH), a tripeptide, which acts on the thyrotroph in the pituitary to produce thyroid-stimulating hormone (TSH) which then binds to its cognate receptor on follicular cells in the thyroid to allow for thyroid hormone synthesis[2]. This system is kept in check by a feedback system such that thyroid hormones (principally T3) inhibit the synthesis of TRH and TSH.

However, it has also long been known that other systemic processes, such as nutritional stress, can effect the thyroid axis at multiple levels in order to decrease energy expenditure. Indeed, in order to survive a prolonged fast rodents rapidly decrease thyroid hormone levels. This process is mediated by the rapid suppression of TRH gene expression in the paraventricular nucleus of the hypothalamus[3]. Thus, TRH gene expression is governed by pathways important in energy expenditure. Confirmation of this was provided for in experiments where administration of the adipocyte-derived hormone leptin (which also falls during a fast) prevented the fall of thyroid hormone levels by stimulating TRH gene expression[4]. More recent experiments have confirmed that this system is operative in humans by demonstrating that mutations in the leptin signaling system leads to central hypothyroidism[5] and in addition leptin can regulate thyroid hormone levels in humans[6]. Furthermore, other hypothalamic peptides that are important in regulating both food intake and energy expenditure also appear to regulate TRH gene expression. Thus, the regulation of TRH expression in the hypothalamus provides an ideal model system in which to explore the mechanisms by which pathways important in energy expenditure mediate their effects on physiologically relevant targets.

The TRH neuron

TRH is expressed widely in the brain and in other tissues. The essential role of TRH in the regulation of the thyroid axis has been demonstrated in TRH knockout mice which develop central hypothyroidism[7]. While other roles for the central expression of TRH have been postulated, none has been phenotypically confirmed in this genetic model. Within the hypothalamus TRH is expressed in multiple areas including the lateral hypothalamus and PVH. However, it is the TRH neurons within the PVH which project to the median-eminence (hyophysiotropic neurons) which regulate the function of the thyrotroph in the pituitary and are thus critical in the regulation of thyroid function[8]. Indeed these neurons within the parvocellular division of the PVH also co-express the cocacaine and amphetmeine related transcript (CART) while other TRH neurons within the hypothalamus do not[9]. It has become

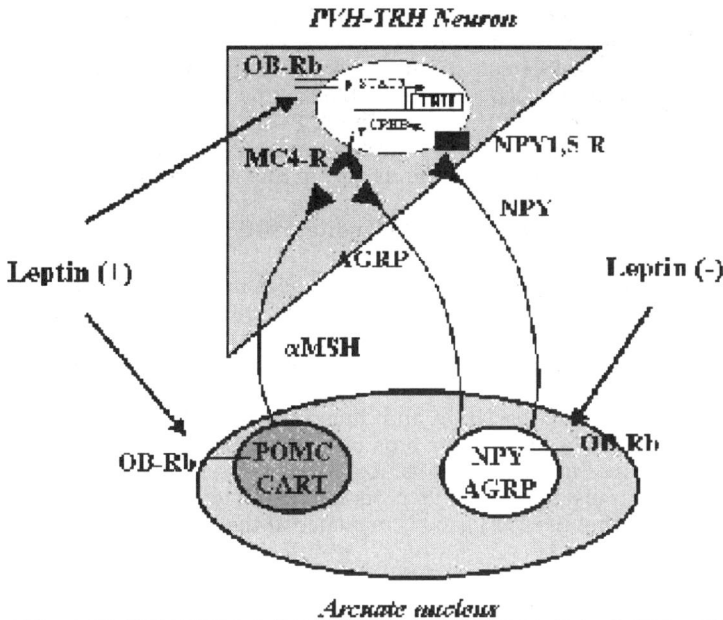

Fig. 1. Leptin signaling pathways which engage the TRH neuron in the brain. Shown are the direct and indirect pathways which are potentially engaged by leptin. Leptin could either cross the blood brain barrier and act on the TRH neuron in the PVH via the arcuate nucleus or directly contact the TRH neuron in the PVH. In the absence of leptin, AgRP and NPY expression is increased in the arcuate nucleus and these peptides can then directly target the TRH neuron in the PVH. The TRH promoter integrates all of these signals at the level of transcription.

clear that the hypophysiotropic TRH neurons are specifically-regulated by thyroid hormone and pathways important in energy expenditure. However, TRH expression in other regions of the brain could also be regulated by such pathways.

The TRH neuron in the PVH is regulated by peripheral signals (ie leptin and thyroid hormone) and as well by central connections from catecholamine neurons in the brainstem and also from the arcuate nucleus in the hyothalamus. As shown in Fig. 1, the arcuate nucleus possesses two principal classes of neurons both of which project to the TRH neuron in the PVH. The first group of neurons termed pro-opiomelanocortin (POMC)/CART neurons are stimulated by leptin and produce the POMC derived peptide α-MSH as well as the peptide CART[10,11]. The second group of arcuate neurons co-express both Agouti-related protein (AgRP), an α-MSH antagonist[12,13], and neuropeptide Y (NPY). AgRP and NPY are both are potent orexigenic peptides and their expression is inhibited by leptin[14]. The TRH neuron in the PVH expresses the centrally expressed melanocrtin 4-receptor (MC4-R)[15,16] which binds its agonist, α-MSH, and antagonist, AgRP, and the NPY-receptor isoforms 1 and 5[17,18]. In addition, a small percentage of TRH neurons also express leptin receptors indicating that they may be able to respond both directly to leptin and indirectly via the arcuate nucleus[9,16]. Thus, the TRH neuron is the PVH is poised to integrate signal from multiple pathways which play a role in the regulation of body weight.

The regulation of TRH gene expression

T3 is a potent inhibitor of TRH gene expression. Its actions are mediated specifically in the PVH only[19], by the thyroid hormone receptor α2 (TRα2) isoform which in the presence of T3 binds to a target binding sequence in the proximal TRH promoter termed Site 4[20,21]. *In vivo* proof that this regulation is occurring at the level of transcription is provided for by our recent studies showing that T3 can directly suppress TRH heteronuclear RNA expression (Lopez and Hollenberg, unpublished data). However, much remains to be deciphered in this process as it remains unclear by what mechanism TRα2 is mediating its effects.

As described previously, TRH gene expression is rapidly suppressed by a fast and this repression can be reversed by the administration of leptin. Indeed, leptin may act both indirectly through the arcuate nucleus and directly to stimulate TRH gene expression. An indirect pathway is supported by data demonstrating that lesions to the arcuate nucleus block the effects of leptin on TRH expression and in addition centrally administered α-MSH can stimulate TRH expression[22,23]. Furthermore, in hypothalamic explants the effect of leptin on TRH release are blocked by the MC4-R antagonist AgRP[24]. Our laboratory has demonstrated that most TRH neurons in the PVH express the MC4-R and that stimulation of the MC4-R in heterologous cells leads to activation of the TRH promoter through the phosphorylation of the transcription factor CREB which binds also to Site 4[16]. Phosphorylation of CREB in the PVH by α-MSH has also been recently demonstrated *in vivo*[25]. However, thyroid hormone levels are normal in MC4-R knockout mice suggesting that this indirect pathway is not required for the maintenance of normal thyroid function[26].

In contrast, mutations in the leptin receptor in both mice and humans cause central hypothyroidism which suggests that direct actions of leptin on the TRH neuron are possible[5]. This is supported by the fact that both 10–15 per cent of both TRH neurons in the PVH and primary hypothalamic neurons in culture appear to co-express the long form of the leptin receptor and TRH[16,27]. Furthermore, activation of the leptin receptor by its ligand leads to the activation of the TRH promoter in heterologous cells. This effect is mediated by the phosphorylation and dimerization of the transcription factor STAT-3 which binds just upstream of Site 4 in the TRH promoter. Mutation of this site or a nearby SP-1 site significantly impairs the response to leptin[16]. Thus, like α-MSH signaling, leptin signaling can lead to direct activation of TRH gene transcription via its promoter. However, it is important to point out that it has not been proven *in vivo*, that the TRH gene is regulated at the level of transcription by the leptin and melanocortin signaling pathways.

The activation of STAT-3 and CREB by leptin and α-MSH respectively provides a paradigm in which to understand the input of other signaling pathways on the TRH promoter and TRH gene expression. Indeed, down regulation of either transcription factor would lead to the inhibition of TRH gene expression. This is supported by the demonstration that CREB and TRα2 both bind competitively to Site 4 suggesting that this competition may mediate negative regulation by T3. In addition, it has recently been demonstrated that the central infusion of NPY can suppress TRH mRNA expression in the PVH[18]. Indeed, in our heterologous system both the NPY-Y1 and Y5 receptor isoforms inhibit CREB phosphorylation in the presence of NPY and down regulate the TRH promoter. Similarly, AgRP also inhibits CREB phosphorylation both in the presence of α-MSH indicating that it to would be a potent inhibitor of TRH gene expression. Cross-talk between these pathways also occurs such that co-stimulation of cells with both leptin and α-MSH leads to synergisitc activation of the TRH promoter suggesting that activation of both pathways may lead to the enhanced recruitment of a necessary cofactor such as CBP/p300[28]. However, this hyothesis remains to be proven *in vivo*.

Conclusions

The regulation of TRH gene expression in the PVH is essential for the maintenance of thyroid hormone levels in rodents and man. Such regulation allows for adaptations to nutritional stress which may require a rapid reduction in energy expenditure. It is clear that the TRH neuron within the PVH has adapted to integrate signals from multiple pathways important in the regulation of body weight. This integration appears to occur at the transcriptional level such the TRH promoter across species contains conserved TR,CREB and STAT binding sites which allow it to respond to T3, melanocortin and leptin pathways respectively. However, much work remains to be done in understanding the pathways activated at the transcriptional level *in vivo* and to definitively show that they target the TRH promoter. Further investigations using the TRH neuron as a model system are likely to yield important new insights into the molecular mechanisms by which nutritional pathways regulate gene expression.

Acknowledgements: This work was supported by grants DK57658 and DK56123 from the NIH.

References

1. Lebon V, Dufour S, Petersen KF, Ren J, Jucker BM, Slezak LA *et al*. Effect of triiodothyronine on mitochondrial energy coupling in human skeletal muscle. *J Clin Invest* 2001; 108(5): 733–737.

2. Nillni EA, Sevarino KA. The biology of pro-thyrotropin-releasing hormone-derived peptides. *Endocr Rev* 1999; 20(5): 599–648.

3. Blake NG, Eckland DJ, Foster OJ, Lightman SL. Inhibition of hypothalamic thyrotropin-releasing hormone messenger ribonucleic acid during food deprivation. *Endocrinology* 1991; 129(5): 2714–2618.

4. Ahima RS, Prabakaran D, Mantzoros C, Qu D, Lowell B, Maratos-Flier E *et al*. Role of leptin in the neuroendocrine response to fasting. *Nature* 1996; 382(6588): 250–252.

5. Clement K, Vaisse C, Lahlou N, Cabrol S, Pelloux V, Cassuto D *et al.* A mutation in the human leptin receptor gene causes obesity and pituitary dysfunction [see comments]. *Nature* 1998; 392(6674): 398–401.

6. Rosenbaum M, Murphy EM, Heymsfield SB, Matthews DE, Leibel RL. Low dose leptin administration reverses effects of sustained weight-reduction on energy expenditure and circulating concentrations of thyroid hormones. *J Clin Endocrinol Metab* 2002; 87(5): 2391–2394.

7. Yamada M, Saga Y, Shibusawa N, Hirato J, Murakami M, Iwasaki T *et al.* Tertiary hypothyroidism and hyperglycemia in mice with targeted disruption of the thyrotropin-releasing hormone gene. *Proc Natl Acad Sci USA* 1997; 94(20): 10862–7.

8. Jackson IMD, Wu P, Lechan RM. Immunohistochemical localisation in the rat brain of the precursor for thyrotropin-releasing hormone. *Science* 1985; 229: 1097–1100.

9. Elias CF, Lee C, Kelly J, Aschkenasi C, Ahima RS, Couceyro PR *et al.* Leptin activates hypothalamic CART neurons projecting to the spinal cord. *Neuron* 1998; 21(6): 1375–85.

10. Cheung CC, Clifton DK, Steiner RA. Proopiomelanocortin neurons are direct targets for leptin in the hypothalamus. *Endocrinology* 1997; 138(10): 4489–92.

11. Elias CF, Aschkenasi C, Lee C, Kelly J, Ahima RS, Bjorbaek C *et al.* Leptin differentially regulates NPY and POMC neurons projecting to the lateral hypothalamic area. *Neuron* 1999; 23(4): 775–86.

12. Ollmann MM, Wilson BD, Yang YK, Kerns JA, Chen Y, Gantz I *et al.* Antagonism of central melanocortin receptors *in vitro* and *in vivo* by agouti-related protein [published erratum appears in Science 1998 Sep 11; 281(5383): 1615]. *Science* 1997; 278(5335): 135–8.

13. Shutter JR, Graham M, Kinsey AC, Scully S, Luthy R, Stark KL. Hypothalamic expression of ART, a novel gene related to agouti, is up-regulated in obese and diabetic mutant mice. *Genes Dev* 1997; 11(5): 593–602.

14. Hahn TM, Breininger JF, Baskin DG, Schwartz MW. Coexpression of Agrp and NPY in fasting-activated hypothalamic neurons. *Nat Neurosci* 1998; 1(4): 271–2.

15. Mountjoy KG, Mortrud MT, Low MJ, Simerly RB, Cone RD. Localization of the melanocortin-4 receptor (MC4-R) in neuroendocrine and autonomic control circuits in the brain. *Mol Endocrinol* 1994; 8(10): 1298–308.

16. Harris M, Aschkenasi C, Elias CF, Chandrankunnel A, Nillni EA, Bjorbaek C *et al.* Transcriptional regulation of the thyrotropin-releasing hormone gene by leptin and melanocortin signaling. *J Clin Invest* 2001; 107: 1–11.

17. Broberger C, Visser TJ, Kuhar MJ, Hokfelt T. Neuropeptide Y innervation and neuropeptide-Y-Y1-receptor-expressing neurons in the paraventricular hypothalamic nucleus of the mouse. *Neuroendocrinology* 1999; 70: 295–305.

18. Fekete C, Kelly J, Mihaly E, Sarkar S, Rand WM, Legradi G *et al.* Neuropeptide Y has a central inhibitory action on the hypothalamic-pituitary-thyroid axis. *Endocrinology* 2001; 142(6): 2606–13.

19. Segerson TP, Kauer J, Wolfe HC, Mobtaker H, Wu P, Jackson IM *et al.* Thyroid hormone regulates TRH biosynthesis in the paraventricular nucleus of the rat hypothalamus. *Science* 1987; 238(4823): 78–80.

20. Hollenberg AN, Monden T, Flynn TR, Boers ME, Cohen O, Wondisford FE. The human thyrotropin-releasing hormone gene is regulated by thyroid hormone through two distinct classes of negative thyroid hormone response elements. *Mol Endocrinol* 1995; 9(5): 540–50.

21. Abel ED, Ahima RS, Boers ME, Elmquist JK, Wondisford FE. Critical role for thyroid hormone receptor beta2 in the regulation of paraventricular thyrotropin-releasing hormone neurons. *J Clin Invest* 2001; 107(8): 1017–23.

22. Legradi G, Emerson CH, Ahima RS, Rand WM, Flier JS, Lechan RM. Arcuate nucleus ablation prevents fasting-induced suppression of ProTRH mRNA in the hypothalamic paraventricular nucleus. *Neuroendocrinology* 1998; 68(2): 89–97.

23. Fekete C, Legradi G, Mihaly E, Huang Q-H, Tatro JB, Rand WM *et al.* (alpha)-Melanocyte-stimulating-hormone is contained in nerve terminals innervating thyrotropin-releasing hormone synthesizing neurons in the hypothalamic paraventricular nucleus and prevents fasting induced suppression of Prothyrotropin-releasing hormone gene expression. *J Neurosci* 2000; 20: 1550–8.

24. Kim MS, Small CJ, Stanley SA, Morgan DGA, Seal LJ, Kong WM *et al.* The central melanocortin system affects the hypothalamo-pituitary thyroid axis and may mediate the effect of leptin. *J Clin Invest* 2000; 105: 1005–11.

25. Sarkar S, Legradi G, Lechan RM. Intracerebroventricular administration of alpha-melanocyte stimulating hormone increases phosphorylation of CREB in TRH- and CRH-producing neurons of the hypothalamic paraventricular nucleus. *Brain Res* 2002; 945(1): 50–9.

26. Huszar D, Lynch CA, Fairchild-Huntress V, Dunmore JH, Fang Q, Berkemeier LR *et al.* Targeted disruption of the melanocortin-4 receptor results in obesity in mice. *Cell* 1997; 88(1): 131–41.

27. Nillni EA, Vaslet C, Harris M, Hollenberg A, Bjorbak C, Flier JS. Leptin Regulates Prothyrotropin-releasing Hormone Biosynthesis. Evidence for direct and indirect pathways. *J Biol Chem* 2000; 275(46): 36124–33.

28. Hollenberg AN. Thyroid hormone receptor isoforms, nuclear corepressors and coactivators and their role in thyroid hormone action. *Current Opinions in Endocrinology and Diabetes* 1998; 5: 314–20

Progress in Obesity Research: 9. Edited by *Geraldo Medeiros-Neto, Alfredo Halpern and Claude Bouchard*
©2003 John Libbey Eurotext Ltd, pp. 818–821.

CHAPTER 172

Energy balance and reward

Stephanie Fulton, Barbara Woodside and Peter Shizgal

Center for Studies in Behavioral Neurobiology, Concordia University, 1455 de Maisonneuve, H-1013, Montreal, Quebec, Canada. [e-mail: shizgal@csbn.concordia.ca]

Introduction

Behaviour is an integral component of the energy-balance equation, both on the input and output sides. Appetitive and consummatory behaviours are the means through which energy inputs are obtained, and all behaviour entails energy expenditure. In turn, the metabolic state of the organism is a potent influence on the type and amount of behaviour that it will exhibit. The tendency to engage in or maintain a particular behaviour is also influenced by the rewarding properties of goal objects and goal-oriented activities. Thus, one way in which energy balance signals could modify behaviour is by modulating brain reward circuitry. If so, identifying and characterizing the neural circuitry responsible for the rewarding properties of stimuli and behaviours has implications for understanding energy balance and imbalance. This paper reviews selected findings concerning (1) the reward efficacy of food; (2) the modulation of brain reward circuitry by long-term regulatory signals; and (3) neurochemical components of brain reward circuitry.

Reward efficacy of food

A meaningful index of reward effectiveness can be obtained by measuring the willingness of the subject to work for the goal object. In the progressive ratio (PR) schedule of reinforcement, the subject is required to emit an increasing number of operant responses (e.g. lever presses) for each successive reward. Eventually performance falls below a preset criterion. The number of responses emitted to obtain the last reward (the 'break point') serves as the index of willingness to work.

The break point derived from the PR schedule is a well-validated measure of reward magnitude and the motivational state of the animal[1]. For example, the break point declines when the nutritional value of the food reward is reduced and increases as a function of body weight loss[1]. Not all factors that influence food intake alter the reward efficacy of food. Jewett and colleagues[2] found that while 2-deoxyglucose administration, a manipulation that induces intracellular glucoprivation, can substantially increase food intake, it fails to increase break points derived from the PR schedule. Thus, determining the amount of freely available food consumed is not equivalent to measuring willingness to work for food. Interestingly, recent evidence suggests that PR performance for grain is enhanced in the genetically obese Zucker rat relative to lean rats, suggesting that neural mechanisms underlying food reward may contribute to the development of obesity in this model[3]. These findings illustrate how willingness-to-work measures can track changes in both the quality of a food reward and the internal state of the animal while differentiating obese subjects from normals.

Brain stimulation reward and energy balance

A parallel approach to measuring reward effectiveness is to determine the strength of a rewarding stimulus that is required to entice the subject to perform at a criterion level. The strongest control over reward strength is achieved through the use of direct electrical brain stimulation. Vertebrates, from goldfish to humans, will work vigorously to initiate electrical stimulation of certain brain regions. The effect that maintains instrumental responding is called brain stimulation reward (BSR). BSR represents a valuable tool for investigating neural systems mediating reward because of (1) the strength of the rewarding effect; (2) the lack of satiation; (3) the lack of sensory adaptation; and (4) the ability to focally activate discrete brain regions.

The medial forebrain bundle (MFB) supports robust self-stimulation behaviour in rats. Many structures implicated in energy balance are interconnected with MFB neurons. The strength of BSR at MFB sites is demonstrated by the finding that rats will choose the stimulation over food even under conditions of severe food deprivation. In spite of its unique features and artificial basis, BSR can compete with, summate with, and substitute for the rewarding effect of natural stimuli such as food [4].

In a subset of rats with electrodes in the perifornical region of the lateral hypothalamus (LH) the rewarding effect of the stimulation is enhanced by chronic food restriction and body weight loss, whereas in rats with electrodes in neighboring LH sites BSR is unaffected by food restriction[5-7]. We have recently shown that the influence of food restriction on BSR depends on the placement of the stimulating electrode[8]. In some rats with multiple stimulating electrodes, the rewarding impact of the stimulation was potentiated by weight loss at one stimulation site and not the other. This evidence implies that functionally different subpopulations of reward neurons can be activated by LH stimulation.

In contrast to the influence of chronic food restriction, manipulation of short-term energy reserves by means of a 48 hour period of food deprivation failed to alter BSR at restriction-sensitive sites suggesting that the potentiation of BSR is contingent upon the reduction of long-term energy reserves[7]. This finding is consistent with the demonstration that other factors that affect short-term energy stores, such as glucoprivation or lipoprivation do not alter restriction-sensitive reward circuitry[9]. Thus, manipulation of long-term energy stores appears to exert a modulatory influence on signals arising in a sub-population of reward-related neurons.

The discovery of circulating molecules that link adiposity stores to central mechanisms controlling energy balance opened exciting new avenues for investigating the modulation of BSR by food restriction. Leptin and insulin serve as adiposity hormones informing the brain about the status of the fat mass to regulate food intake and energy expenditure[10]. Central leptin administration can oppose the reward-enhancing effects of food restriction on BSR, but only at restriction-sensitive stimulation sites[7,11]. Similarly, it has been shown that central insulin administration can attenuate the rewarding effect of stimulating restriction-sensitive sites[12]. These findings suggest that leptin and insulin may couple the state of long-term energy stores to restriction-sensitive reward circuitry.

Several neuropeptides act downstream of leptin and insulin to influence energy balance, such as neuropeptide Y (NPY), α-melanocyte-stimulating hormone, agouti-related peptide (AgRP), melanin-concentrating hormone (MCH) and corticotropin-releasing hormone (CRH)[13,14]. We found that the influence of CRH, like the influence of leptin, depends on the sensitivity of BSR to food restriction[15]. Nonetheless, CRH generally had no impact on BSR obtained at restriction-sensitive sites, suggesting that it is not involved in the process whereby food restriction facilitates BSR. In a similar manner, central administration of NPY[16] failed to alter BSR at restriction-sensitive sites, despite the significant elevations in food intake produced by these agents. Taken together, the data suggest that the modulation of restriction-sensitive reward circuitry is not mediated by these neuropeptidergic signaling systems.

What is the nature of the rewarding signal produced by stimulating restriction-sensitive sites? In consideration of the evidence that food deprivation, a manipulation that dramatically increases the value of food, does not augment BSR obtained from restriction-sensitive sites[7,11], it is difficult to characterize these neurons as encoding information about the rewarding impact of food or the motivation to eat. Nonetheless, it should be noted that feeding can be elicited by stimulation ('stimulation-induced feeding') via electrodes in the perifornical region of the LH and at perifornical sites where self-stimulation is increased by food restriction[5,17]. Alternatively, the potentiating effect of weight loss on perifornical self-stimulation may be tied to the influence of long-term energy stores on non-ingestive behaviours that defend body weight, such as food hoarding[18]. In this respect, it is worth mentioning that electrical stimulation of sites in the LH that elicit feeding also produces food hoarding behaviour[19]. Additional work is required to determine the precise function of this circuitry and the manner in which it contributes to energy balance.

Some neurochemical components of brain reward circuitry

Several brain areas have been implicated in the processing of rewarding stimuli including the nucleus accumbens (NAc), prefrontal cortex (PFCX), amygdala, sub-lenticular extended amygdala, hypothalamus, pedunculopontine and laterodorsal tegmental regions. Many neurotransmitter systems are represented in these brain regions. Among those implicated in reward and energy balance are the dopamine (DA) projections from midbrain ventral tegmentum (VTA) to forebrain structures including the NAc, striatum and PFCX that comprise the mesocorticolimbic dopamine system. Changing dopaminergic tone influences the behavioural effectiveness of rewards such as food, sex, BSR and drugs of abuse. Nonetheless, it is not yet clear how or where the dopaminergic neurons contribute to the circuitry underlying such rewarding effects. This question is receiving intense attention on both the empirical and theoretical levels[20-22]. A recent report shows that the response of DA neurotransmission to rewarding and aversive stimuli varies among different DA terminal areas in the forebrain[23]. This promising result suggests that finer-grain analysis may succeed in reconciling apparently conflicting results from prior studies.

Investigations of the influence of NAc DA depletions on food-motivated behaviour have produced inconsistent results. This may be due, at least in part, to difference between behavioural testing paradigms. For example, it has been shown that NAc DA depletions are more effective in reducing the procurement and consumption of food when the work requirement is high[24]. In studies of BSR, it is well documented that dopaminergic manipulations can alter the rewarding impact of MFB stimulation. However, non-dopaminergic cells may predominate among the MFB neurons directly activated by BSR[25]. In addition, DA levels in the NAc fall to unmeasurable value during a prolonged BSR session, while the vigor of the behaviour is maintained[26]. It would be of considerable interest to determine whether the DA modulation of BSR differs at restriction-sensitive and restriction-insensitive sites.

A large body of evidence ties the influence of another set of neurochemicals found in the NAc to the rewarding effects of food: the opioids. The opioid family comprises multiple peptides including the endorphins, enkephalins, dynorphins and orphanin. These peptides as well as their receptors subtypes (μ, δ, κ, ORL1) are distributed throughout many regions of the brain and play a role in emotional regulation, responses to pain and stress, and energy balance. It was shown in early studies that increased opioid neurotransmission, elicited by non-selective opioid agonists such as morphine, can increase preference for sweet solutions. Such findings gave rise to the hypothesis that opioid peptides modulate the palatability of food. Subsequent studies found that the NAc is particularly sensitive to the influence of opioids on feeding and palatability, and that stimulation of the μ opioid receptor produces particularly robust increases in food intake[27]. More germane to issues of motivation and reward, Kelley and coworkers recently found that DAMGO infusion into the NAc increases break points in a PR paradigm, suggesting that opioidergic stimulation via μ receptors in the NAc augments the rewarding effects of food[28]. These findings are consistent with earlier evidence from Glass et al.[29] showing that peripheral administration of naloxone, a non-selective opioid antagonist, can decrease break points for food reward in a PR schedule of reinforcement. Together, this evidence points to a role for NAc μ opioid receptors in the rewarding properties of food and feeding.

Recent studies have begun to elucidate the neural pathways affected by μ opioid receptor stimulation in the NAc. The expression of Fos (a marker of neuronal activation) was detected in several output regions of the NAc such as the LH, dorsomedial hypothalamus (DMH), VTA and gustatory relay nuclei in the hindbrain following NAc DAMGO infusion and fat consumption[27]. A role for the LH, DMH and VTA in these opioidergic effects on feeding is further supported by demonstrations that food intake can be blocked by injection of the GABA$_A$ agonist muscimol in these nuclei[27].

In addition to the data tying opioidergic stimulation to the rewarding and palatable effects of food, other studies have linked opioid modulation to rewarding brain stimulation in the LH. Carr and coworkers found that the magnitude of increase in the rewarding effect of the stimulation grows as a function of the severity of the weight loss and that the opioid antagonist, naltrexone, reverses the weight-loss induced potentiation of BSR[6]. In a later study, Carr and Papadouka[30] examined the effect of selective opioid receptor antagonists and found that μ and κ antagonists could selectively reverse the enhancement of BSR by food restriction. It would be of interest in future studies to track down which nuclei are responsible for these effects by assessing the ability of microinjections of μ and κ antagonists into distinct brain regions, such as the NAc, to enhance the rewarding effect of restriction-sensitive stimulation.

Summary: Behavioural analyses that measure the willingness of an animal to work for goal objects, such as food and BSR, have shown that fluctuations in energy balance can lead to changes in reward effectiveness. Investigations of BSR at discrete regions in the LH point to a subset of reward neurons that respond to changes in body weight and circulating hormones such as leptin. These studies illustrate how BSR can be used to tease apart functionally different subsets of neurons. It stands to reason that BSR sites will be found where the rewarding effect is tied to additional signals involved in motivated behaviour such as those contributing to short-term energy balance, hydromineral balance, reproductive behaviour and exploration. Identifying the neurons and signaling molecules responsible for the modulation of BSR by long-term energy stores and by leptin is a challenge for future research. Several neuropeptides known to mediate the actions of leptin on food intake have been examined as potential mediators, and none of them has yet been shown to contribute. Research addressing the role of neurotransmitter systems in energy balance may help identify the neurochemical components of the restriction-sensitive reward circuitry. Of particular interest are findings linking opioid modulation to changes in the rewarding properties of food and BSR. These discoveries and the flood of recent findings concerning the neurochemical basis of energy balance offer exciting opportunities for achieving a better understanding of the role of brain reward circuitry in foraging, ingestion and other behaviours that contribute to regulation and its disorders.

Acknowledgements: The authors thank the 'Fonds pour la Formation de Chercheurs et l'Aide à la Recherche du Québec' (grant #00ER0124) and the Natural Science and Engineering Research Council of Canada (grant #OGP0000308) for research support

References

1. Hodos W. Progressive ratio as a measure of reward strength. *Science* 1961; 134: 943–4.

2. Jewett DC, Cleary J, Levine AS, Schaal DW, Thompson T. Effects of neuropeptide Y, insulin, 2-deoxyglucose, and food deprivation on food-motivated behavior. *Psychopharmacology (Berl)* 1995; 120: 267–71.

3. Glass MJ, O'Hare E, Cleary JP, Billington CJ, Levine AS. The effect of naloxone on food-motivated behavior in the obese Zucker rat. *Psychopharmacology (Berl)* 1999 ; 141(4): 378–84.

4. Shizgal P. Neural basis of utility estimation. *Curr Opin Neurobiol* 1997; 7: 198–208.

5. Blundell JE, Herberg LJ. Relative effects of nutritional deficit and deprivation period on rate of electrical self-stimulation of lateral hypothalamus. *Nature* 1968; 219: 627–8.

6. Carr KD, Wolinsky TD. Chronic food restriction and weight loss produce opioid facilitation of perifornical hypothalamic self-stimulation. *Brain Res* 1993; 607: 141–8.

7. Fulton S, Woodside B, Shizgal P. Modulation of brain reward circuitry by leptin. *Science* 2000; 287: 125–8.

8. Fulton S, Woodside B, Shizgal P. Restriction-sensitivity of brain stimulation reward: Individual or electrode placement differences? *Society for Neuroscience Abstracts* 2002.

9. Cabeza De Vaca S, Holiman S, Carr KD. A search for the metabolic signal that sensitizes lateral hypothalamic self-stimulation in food-restricted rats. *Physiol Behav* 1998; 64: 251–60.

10. Woods SC, Seeley RJ. Adiposity signals and the control of energy homeostasis. *Nutrition* 2000; 16: 894–902.

11. Fulton S, Richard D, Woodside B, Shizgal P. Modulation of brain stimulation reward by food restriction and leptin in lean and obese Zucker rats. *Society for Neuroscience Abstracts* 2001; 635–2.

12. Carr KD, Kim G, Cabeza de Vaca S. Hypoinsulinemia may mediate the lowering of self-stimulation thresholds by food restriction and streptozotocin-induced diabetes. *Brain Res* 2000; 863: 160–8.

13. Spiegelman BM, Flier JS. Obesity and the regulation of energy balance. *Cell* 2001; 104: 531–43.

14. Grill HJ, Kaplan JM. The neuroanatomical axis for control of energy balance. *Front Neuroendocrinol* 2002; 23: 2–40.

15. Fulton S, Richard D, Woodside B, Shizgal P. Interaction of CRH and energy balance in the modulation of brain stimulation reward. *Behav Neurosci* 2002; 116: 651–9.

16. Fulton S, Woodside B, Shizgal P. Does neuropeptide Y contribute to the modulation of brain stimulation reward by chronic food restriction? *Behav Brain Res* 2002; 134: 157–64.

17. Hernandez L, Hoebel BG. Food intake and lateral hypothalamic self-stimulation covary after medial hypothalamic lesions or ventral midbrain 6-hydroxydopamine injections that cause obesity. *Behav Neurosci* 1989; 103: 412–22.

18. Shizgal P, Fulton S, Woodside B. Brain reward circuitry and the regulation of energy balance. *Int J Obes Relat Metab Disord* 2001; 25 (Suppl 5): S17–S21.

19. Herberg LJ, Blundell JE. Lateral hypothalamus: hoarding behavior elicited by electrical stimulation. *Science* 1967; 155: 349–50.

20. Berridge KC, Robinson TE. What is the role of dopamine in reward: hedonic impact, reward learning, or incentive salience? *Brain Res Brain Res Rev* 1998; 28: 309–69.

21. Salamone JD, Cousins MS, Snyder BJ. Behavioral functions of nucleus accumbens dopamine: empirical and conceptual problems with the anhedonia hypothesis. *Neurosci Biobehav Rev* 1997; 21: 341–59.

22. Schultz W. Reward signaling by dopamine neurons. *Neuroscientist* 2001; 7: 293–302.

23. Bassareo V, De Luca MA, Di Chiara G. Differential expression of motivational stimulus properties by dopamine in nucleus accumbens shell versus core and prefrontal cortex. *J Neurosci* 2002; 22: 4709–19.

24. Salamone JD, Cousins MS, Snyder BJ. Behavioral functions of nucleus accumbens dopamine: empirical and conceptual problems with the anhedonia hypothesis. *Neurosci Biobehav Rev* 1997; 21: 341–59.

25. Shizgal P, Murray B. Neuronal basis of intracranial self-stimulation; In: *The neuropharmacological basis of reward*, Liebman JM, Cooper SJ (eds), pp.106–63. Oxford; Oxford University Press 1989.

26. Garris PA, Kilpatrick M, Bunin MA, Michael D, Walker QD, Wightman RM. Dissociation of dopamine release in the nucleus accumbens from intracranial self-stimulation. *Nature* 1999; 398: 67–9.

27. Kelley AE, Bakshi VP, Haber SN, Steininger TL, Will MJ, Zhang M. Opioid modulation of taste hedonics within the ventral striatum. *Physiol Behav* 2002; 76: 365–77.

28. Zhang M, Balmadrid C, Kelley A. Nucleus accumbens opioid, GABAergic, and dopaminergic modulation of palatable food motivation: contrasting effects revealed by a progressive ratio study in the rat. *Behav Neurosci* 2002 (in press).

29. Carr KD, Papadouka V. The role of multiple opioid receptors in the potentiation of reward by food restriction. *Brain Res* 1994; 639: 253–60.

Progress in Obesity Research: 9. Edited by *Geraldo Medeiros-Neto, Alfredo Halpern and Claude Bouchard*
©2003 John Libbey Eurotext Ltd, pp. 822–825.

CHAPTER 173

Appetite control and palatability of food in humans: does the pleasure of eating lead to obesity?

John E. Blundell and Joanna Le Noury

PsychoBiology Research Group, University of Leeds, Leeds LS2 9JT, UK
[e-mail: J.E.Blundell@leeds.ac.uk]

Pleasure of eating: a risk factor for weight gain?

At the outset it is useful to pose some questions in order to focus attention on certain key issues. Firstly, do people who gain weight and become obese have a different response to the palatability of food compared with people who remain lean? If the answer to this question is yes, then do obese people perceive food as being *more* or *less* pleasant than lean people? Put another way, do obese people have a suppressed or a super-sensitive response to the palatability of food? These questions are theoretically important since both possibilities could account for over eating among obese people. If food is perceived as being low in pleasantness then it could be argued that people would need to eat *more* food in order to gain an adequate level of pleasure. Conversely, if food is perceived as being very pleasant then this would stimulate *more* eating in order to gain maximal pleasure. The attraction of foods probably involves motives of 'liking' (reward) and 'wanting' (incentive salience)[1], qualities that are difficult to dissect in humans.

Secondly, how can the biological purpose of eating be reconciled with the strong social, cultural and psychological aspects? As noted in the recent National Nutrition-Health Programme (2001–2005) in France, an individual's food choice is a 'free act' and eating is recognized as a moment of pure pleasure. 'Must we from now on sacrifice the gentle principle of pleasure to the all powerful precautionary principle?'

A key proposal is that the palatability of foods constitutes a behavioural risk factor that promotes overconsumption. Although sedentariness is widespread, there is also much evidence that weight gaining individuals consume excessive amounts of food[2] and that weight gain is associated with specific food habits including the consumption of fatty foods, eating outside of the home and the availability of fast foods. Physiological satiety signals can be overwhelmed by the potency of high energy dense highly palatable foods[3], and preferences for these foods are expressed as behavioural traits or risk factors (e.g. Blundell[4]). Do these particular food habits stimulate eating either wholly or in part via the high palatability that forms an important part of their appeal?

Homeostasis and hedonics: separate identities?

In the homeostatic approach to energy balance, drives (such as hunger) that arise in part from biological needs, are balanced by physiological satiety signaling systems. The substrate comprises a network of neuropeptides and biogenic aminergic neurotransmitters which links peripheral and central components (e.g. Schwartz *et al.*[5]). There is also a biological substrate that mediates hedonic processes. Are these circuits for energy homeostasis and hedonic mediation independent of each other? Pharmacological evidence suggests that the circuits are rather separate. For example, in obese subjects administration of the serotonin drug d-fenfluramine[6] suppressed the sensation of hunger but had no effect on the appreciation of the pleasantness of food. Conversely, nalmafene, an opioid antagonist, reduced the rated pleasantness of palatable foods but had no effect on hunger[7]. This double dissociation concept indicates that appreciation of palatability is associated with a specific biological substrate that can be pharmacologically dissected from the substrate mediating hunger[8].

Hunger and pleasure – do they interact?

A recent survey of a sample of French subjects has confirmed the effect of palatability of foods on total food intake. High palatability ratings were associated with larger meal sizes of longer duration resulting in a greater amount of food consumed[9]. As anticipated the variability in the pleasantness ratings among these self selected foods was low (all foods eaten tended to be highly acceptable and tasty). This outcome confirms the expectation that people eat more food when the taste is good. However, the study could not examine the mechanism.

The possibility of an interaction between palatability and hunger was specifically investigated almost 20 years ago. On separate occasions subjects consumed a fixed energy meal composed of either highly preferred foods or less preferred equivalent food items[10]. Hunger was increased when subjects first saw and then began to eat the highly preferred food. Hunger remained high during the meal. However, this fixed meal design did not allow the disclosure of any effect on energy intake. In a more sophisticated series of experiments Yeomans has manipulated the palatability of foods by the use of flavours of varying strength. Compared with bland food, a flavouring of 4 per cent oregano increased hunger and prolonged eating leading to an increased energy intake (Yeomans[11,12]. In contrast an 8 per cent addition of oregano was too strong and hunger was reduced along with the amount eaten. The use of temporal ratings of hunger during the meal (as in the Hill *et al.* study[10]) together with the continuous measurement of intake by means of a universal eating monitor, allowed the experimenters to mathematically model the interactions between hunger and food consumption for foods of different degrees of palatability[13]. In subsequent studies, this team has investigated the effect of food palatability on the degree of energy compensation following preloads[14]. The presence of more palatable food prevented compensation. Taken together these studies indicate that the palatability of food does exert an effect on energy intake, and this appears to be mediated via a modulation of hunger. This means that when the homeostatic and hedonic systems are stimulated simultaneously (by food) a synergy occurs that modulates the control of appetite. This process appears to constitute one way through which palatability of foods could lead to weight gain. However, the system does appear to operate asymmetrically; although high palatability foods can augment hunger (and therefore food intake), the presence of strong satiety (large preload) does not down regulate palatability. Indeed it has been documented that subjects in a state of satiety can be induced to prolong their eating by offering highly palatable foods. It is also noticeable that the reasons people give for stopping eating emphasise fullness and loss of hunger rather than a decline in the pleasantness of the food[15].

Food choice, palatability and obesity

In addition to an interaction between palatability and hunger, the perceived pleasantness of foods could also modulate appetite control indirectly by influencing the choice of foods. There is considerable evidence that this is the case. In an experiment in which subjects sampled a range of foods containing varying amounts of fat and rated their sensory preferences, there was a positive relationship between the rated pleasantness of the fat content of the foods and measures of the adiposity of the subjects[16]. The fatter the subjects the greater was their rated pleasantness of the fatty foods. More recently, the food choices of monozygotic twins discordant for body weight have been assessed[17]. The twins with the highest degree of fatness displayed a significantly higher preference for fatty foods. If it is assumed that the expression of food preferences is influenced at least in part by the pleasure yielded by the foods, then these studies have demonstrated that levels of body fat are associated with greater rating of pleasantness of fat containing foods. In addition female obese subjects have demonstrated a significantly higher preference for sweet high fat foods than lean subjects [18]. Also, using the database from a national food survey in the UK, it has been shown that obese subjects (BMI 30 plus) reported a greater consumption of sweet fat foods than subjects with lower BMIs[19]. However, this relationship only emerged after the suspected under-reporters had been removed from the database, leaving only subjects whose reports were likely to be more valid. Taken together these findings indicate that palatability of foods promotes the choice of foods (high in fat) that are known to favour the attainment of a positive energy balance. Obese individuals appear to be particularly vulnerable to display this maladaptive food choice process.

These studies indicate that palatability can influence appetite control (and therefore food intake) via effects on food choice or on energy intake (via hunger). Recent investigations of behavioural phenotypes characterized by habitual food choices suggests that these phenomena can co-exist. Groups of obese and lean young males matched for age and the habituahabitual high consumption of fat (high fat phenotypes) were compared[20]. Although both groups were eating a diet known to favour a positive energy balance, the obese phenotypes consumed greater amounts of the high fat foods in a test meal and reported greater feelings of pleasantness, satisfaction and tastiness for the foods consumed. One interpretation of these data is that, for a least one group of obese people, they habitually self select (fatty) foods with a high probability of generating a positive energy balance (on the basis of their energy density), consume these foods in greater amounts and derive greater pleasure from this eating. This outcome also demonstrates that obese people have a disposition to perceive foods as being more pleasant than their lean counterparts. This may indicate a super sensitivity in components of the neural circuitry forming the substrate for hedonic properties of foods. Given this capacity to obtain a high level of pleasure from foods (and eating), it is not surprising that obese people show a tendency to self-select high palatability foods. There is evidence that dopamine D2 receptors – implicated in hedonic processes – are altered in obese individuals[21] although the interpretation of these data may be complicated[1]. The evidence indicating a role for palatability in appetite control creates a problem for nutritional strategies to deal with obesity. Within the field of functional foods (or nutriceuticals) there is a strong movement to produce foods that will enhance satiety. However, the food industry is also committed to producing foods which are highly palatable; this will have the intended effect of promoting acceptability and consumption (see data above). Palatability increases the willingness of people to consume (and carries the potential to over consume). This means that within a particular food, different components may enhance and diminish the disposition to eat. Is this achievable? Is it possible to design foods with enhanced palatability (to promote and ensure consumption) and at the same time to improve satiety (which implies a reduction in the desire to eat)?

Pharmaceutical strategies

Although low levels of physical activity contribute to body weight gain, there is no doubt that many weight gaining and obese individuals display behavioural risk factors such as patterns of eating, food selection, weak satiety and a recurring drive to eat that favour the attainment of a positive energy balance[22]. To these risk factors should be added a super sensitive hedonic capacity. Currently pharmaceutical strategies for the treatment of obesity are concerned with the reduction of energy assimilated – by improving satiety (sibutramine) or by reducing fat intake and fat digestion (Orlistat). Given the evidence cited above, some consideration should be given to the concept of diminishing the hedonic response to foods, particularly in the light of the ever-increasing palatability of foods entering the market place. The strategy would counter one significant risk factor that predisposes people to gain weight. The identification of a neural substrate that mediates aspects of the hedonic response, reward value of foods or their incentive salience, identifies pharmacological targets. Of particular interest are the endocannabinoids which are known to be involved in food consumption and especially the intake of highly palatable foods[23]. CB1 receptor antagonists such as SR141716A (Rimonabant) may be effective in helping people to diminish consumption of high-risk foods, adapt to more appropriate food choices and resist cravings. This type of approach would add a useful dimension to pharmaceutical treatments and may be especially helpful for a subset of obese people who overconsume because of a potent hedonic response to food.

References

1. Berridge KC, Robinson TE. What is the role of dopamine in reward: hedonic impact, reward learning, or incentive salience? *Brain Res Rev* 1998; 28: 309–69.

2. Pearcey SM, de Castro JM. Food intake and meal patterns of weight-stable and weight-gaining persons. *Am J Clin Nutr* 2002; 76: 107–12.

3. Blundell JE, Lawton C, Cotton JR, Macdiarmid JI. Control of human appetite: implications for the intake of dietary fat. *Ann Rev Nutr* 1996; 16: 285–319.

4. Blundell JE. Food choice phenotypes: biology or environment. *Euro J Clin Nutr* 2001; 54 (Suppl 4): S4–S5.

5. Schwartz MW, Woods SC, Porte D, Seeley RJ, Baskin DG. Central nervous system control of food intake. *Nature* 2000; 404(6778): 661–71.

6. Blundell JE, Hill AJ. Serotoninergic modulation of the pattern of eating and the profile of hunger-satiety in humans. *Int J Obes* 1987; 11: 141–53.

7. Yeomans MR, Wright P. Lower pleasantness of palatable foods in nalmefene-treated human volunteers. *Appetite* 1991; 16(3): 249–59.

8. Blundell JE, Rogers PJ. Hunger, hedonics and the control of satiation and satiety. In: *Chemical senses*, vol. 4, *Appetite and Nutrition*, Friedman M, Tordoff M, Kare M (eds), pp.127–48. New York: Dekker; 1991.

9. de Castro JM, Bellisle F, Dalix AM. Palatability and intake relationships in free-living humans: measurement and characterization in the French. *Physiol & Behav* 2000; 68(3): 271–2770.

10. Hill AJ, Magson LD, Blundell JE. Hunger and palatability: Tracking ratings of subjective experience before, during and after the consumption of preferred and less preferred food. *Appetite* 1984; 5(4): 361–71.

11. Yeomans MR. Palatability and the microstructure of eating in humans: the appetizer effect. *Appetite* 1996; 26: 119–33.

12. Yeomans MR, Symes T. Individual differences in the use of pleasantness and palatability ratings. *Appetite* 1999; 32: 383–94.

13. Yeomans MR. Rating changes over the course of meals: what do they tell us about motivation to eat? *Neurosci Biobehav Rev* 2000; 24: 249–59.

14. Yeomans MR, Lee MD, Gray RW, French SJ. Effects of test-meal palatability on compensatory eating following disguised fat and carbohydrate preloads. *Int J Obes & Related Metab Disord* 2001; 25(8): 1215–24.

15. Mook DG, Votaw MC. How important is hedonism? Reasons given by college students for ending a meal. *Appetite* 1992; 18: 69–75.

16. Mela DJ, Sacchetti DA. Sensory preferences for fats: relationship with diet and body composition. *Am J Clin Nutr* 1991; 53: 908–15.

17. Rissanen A, Hakala P, Lissner J, Mattlar C-E, Koskenvuo M, Ronnemaa T. Acquired preference especially for dietary fat and obesity: a study of weight-discordant monozygotic twin pairs. *Int J Obes* 2002; 26: 973–7.

18. Drewnowski A, Krahn DD, Demitrack MA, Nairn K, Gosnell BA. Taste responses and preferences for sweet high-fat foods: evidence for opioid involvement. *Physiol & Behav* 1992; 51: 371–9.

19. Macdiarmid JI, Cade JE, Blundell JE. High and low fat consumers, their macronutrient intake and body mass index: further analysis of the national diet and nutrition survey of British adults. *Euro J Clin Nutr* 1996; 50: 505–12.

20. Le Noury JC, Lawton C, Blundell JE. Food choice and hedonic responses: difference between overweight and lean high fat phenotypes. *Int J Obes* 2002; 26 (Suppl 1): S125.

21. Wang GJ, Volkow ND, Logan J, Pappas NR, Wong CT, Zhu W *et al.* Brain dopamine and obesity. *Lancet* 2001; 357: 354–7.

22. Blundell JE, Cooling J. Routes to obesity: phenotypes, food choices and activity. *Br J Nutr* 2000; 83 (Suppl): 33–8.

23. Kirkham TC, Williams CM. Endogenous cannabinoids and appetite. *Nutr Res Rev* 14: 65–86.

Progress in Obesity Research: 9. Edited by *Geraldo Medeiros-Neto, Alfredo Halpern and Claude Bouchard*
©2003 John Libbey Eurotext Ltd, pp. 826–828.

CHAPTER 174

Endocannabinoids: novel lipid mediators involved in the neural control of appetite

George Kunos, Douglas Osei-Hyiaman, Lei Wang, Jie Liu and Sandor Batkai

National Institute on Alcohol Abuse & Alcoholism, National Institutes of Health, Bethesda, MD 20892-8115, USA
[e-mail: gkunos@mail.nih.gov]

Endogenous cannabinoids are lipid-like molecules produced by neurons in the brain as well as some peripheral tissues that bind to cannabinoid receptors and elicit effects similar to those produced by plant-derived cannabinoids. The two substances that received most of the attention to date are anandamide or arachidonoyl ethanolamide discovered in 1992 by Mechoulam and coworkers[1] and 2-arachidonoyl glycerol or 2-AG discovered 3 years later[2,3]. There are also two subtypes of cannabinoid receptors discovered to date, the brain type or CB 1 receptor that mediates the neurobehavioural as well as some other effects of cannabinoids[4], and the CB2 receptor, which is expressed exclusively on cells of the immune system[5], and is involved in immunemodulation.

In addition to its well-known psychoactive properties, marijuana and its active principle, delta-9-tetrahydrocannabinol, affects many other physiological variables, including blood pressure and heart rate, intraocular pressure, motor functions and appetite. It is well known that smoking marijuana causes the 'munchies' increases appetite, particularly for palatable foods. Recent studies have also indicated that in some rodent models of food intake, treatment with the CB1 receptor antagonist rimonabant (SR141716A) reduces appetite and food intake[6–9], which could suggest that endocannabinoids are tonically active in maintaining normal levels of food intake. However, this antagonist is known to possess inverse agonist properties[10] (i.e. direct effects opposite to those of cannabinoids), which makes it difficult to unequivocally attribute its effect to antagonism of endogenous ligands. We therefore took advantage of genetically altered mice lacking the CB 1 receptor to examine the involvement of endocannabinoids in the physiological control of appetite and food intake. Furthermore, because of the central role of the adipocyte-derived hormone leptin in regulating appetite at the hypothalamic level, we examined the possibility that the endocannabinoid system may be part of the leptin-regulated neural circuitry in the brain that is involved in the control of appetite and food intake.

Methods

CB 1 knockout mice and their wild-type littermates were obtained from heterozygote breeding pairs, developed by Andreas Zimmer[11]. Obese *db/db* and *ob/ob* mice and their lean controls were purchased from Jackson Laboratories.

Food intake was measured during the first 3 h of the dark cycle in free feeding or 24 h food-restricted animals, as indicated. Animals received an i.p. injection of vehicle or 3 mg/kg SR141716A 10 min prior to the test period. In the chronic treatment paradigm, food intake was measured daily for one week, and animals received daily injections of the same dose of the antagonist or vehicle.

Endocannabinoid levels in the brain were measured by HPLC-APCI-MS as described elsewhere[12] and expressed as pmol (for anandamide) or nmol (for 2-AG) per g of wet brain tissue.

Plasma leptin levels were measured by radioimmunoassay from trunk blood obtained by decapitation.

Results and discussion

As illustrated in Fig. 1, the low level food intake of free-feeding mice was similar in wild-type (CB 1$^{+/+}$) and CB1 knockout (CB 1$^{-/-}$) animals. However, when animals were made hungry by 24 h food restric-

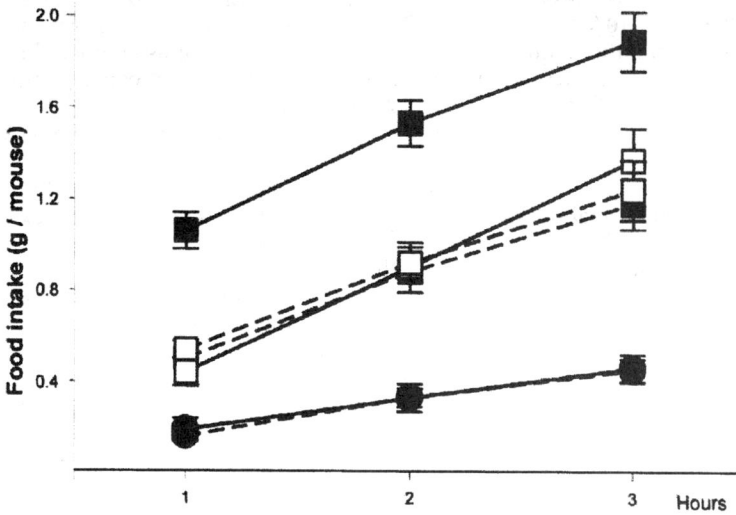

Fig. 1. Food intake in CB1$^{+/+}$ (solid lines) and CB1$^{-/-}$ mice (dashed lines) was tested in free-feeding animals (circles) or in 24-h food-restricted animals pretreated with vehicle (solid squares) or 3 mg/kg SR141716A 10 min prior to testing (open squares). Points and vertical bars are means ± SE from 5–9 animals. In the food-restricted state, food intake was significantly greater in vehicle-treated CB1$^{+/+}$ mice than in SR-treated CB1$^{+/+}$ mice.

tion before the test, the observed increase in food intake was much greater in the wild-type than in the knockout mice.

Leptin is known to produce its anorexigenic effects by downregulating orexigenic peptides, such as NPY, and upregualating anorexigenic peptides, such as α-MSH, in the hypothalamus[13]. To test whether endocannabinoids in the hypothalamus are also under the regulatory influence of leptin, we measured endocannabinoid levels in the hypothalamus of genetically obese mice which do not produce leptin *(ob/ob* mice) or have defective leptin signaling due to a mutation in their leptin receptor *(db/db* mice). The level of 2-AG was significantly higher in the hypothalamus of both *db/db* and *ob/ob* mice than in their respective lean controls, whereas anandamide levels were slightly higher[12]. These findings could suggest that hypothalamic endocannabinoids, particularly 2-AG, are under the negative regulatory influence of leptin.

The elevated hypothalamic level of endocannabinoids suggested that they may contribute to the hyperphagia that leads to the development of obesity in these animals. We therefore tested the effect of acute teatment with SR141716A (3 mg/kg i.p.) on food intake in free-feeding *ob/ob* and *db/db* mice. In both strains, SR141716A caused a significant reductuion in food intake, as measured during the first

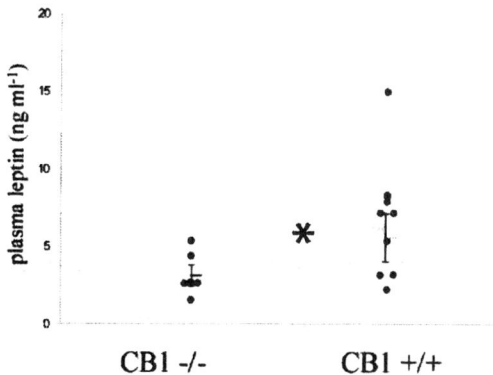

Fig. 2. Plasma leptin levels are significantly lower (*$P < 0.05$) in CB1 knockout mice than in their wild-type littermates. Plasma leptin was measured by radioimmunoassay in trunk blood, as described in Methods.

3 h of the dark period. We then tested whether chronic treatment of *db/db* mice with daily injections of the same dose of SR141716A for one week affects their weight gain. Such treatment resulted in a significant decrease in weight gain during the first 4 days of treatment as compared to vehicle-treated control *db/db* mice, after which catch-up growth in the SR 141716A-treated group eliminated the difference. These results therefore indicate that endocannabinoids contribute to the hunger-induced increase in food intake, whether hunger is elicited by food restriction in normal animals or by a genetic defect in leptin signaling in obese mice.

Genetic defects in leptin or melanocortin signaling are known to result in obesity[14,15], suggesting that these pathways are critical for maintaining the balance between orexigenic and anorexigenic pathways. In contrast, mice lacking NPY[16] or CB1 receptors[1,17] have normal levels of food intake and body weight, suggesting that compensatory changes may offset the loss of some orexigenic signals. As indicated by the data in Fig. 2, plasma leptin levels are significantly lower in CB $1^{-/-}$ mice than in their wild-type littermates. This could suggest that the loss of orexigenic signaling by endocannabinoids is compensated in the knockouts by reduced anorexigenic signaling by leptin.

In summary, endocannabinoids are orexigenic factors that are not tonically active in free-feeding animals, but are activated by hunger. They appear to be part of the leptin-regulated neural circuitry involved in the control of food intake and energy homeostasis. The relative role of the two endocannabinoids as orexigenic regulators, their exact site of action in the brain and the downstream mediators of their effect on food intake are subjects of ongoing investigations

References

1. Devane WA, Hanus L, Breuer A, pertwee RG, Stevenson LA, Griff C *et al.* Isolation and structure of a brain constituent that binds to the cannabinoid receptor. *Science* 1992; 258: 1946–9.

2. Sugiura T, Kodaka T, Nakane S, Kishimoto S, Kondo S, Waku K. 2-Arachidonoylglycerol: a possible endogenous cannabinoid ligand in brain. *Biochem Biophys Res Commun* 1995; 215: 89–97.

3. Mechoulam R, Ben-Shabat S, Hanus L, Ligumski L, Kaminski NE, Schatz AR *et al.* Identification of an endogenous 2-monoglyceride, present in the gut, that binds to cannabinoid receptors. *Biochem Pharmacol* 1995; 50: 83–90.

4. Matsuda LA, Lolait SJ, Brownstein MJ, Young AC, Bonner TI. Structure of a cannabinoid receptor and functional expression of the cloned cDNA. *Nature* 1990; 346: 561–4.

5. Munro S, Thomas KL, Abu-Shaar M. Molecular characterization of a peripheral receptor for cannabinoids. *Nature* 1993; 365: 61–5.

6. Colombo G, Agabio R, Diaz G, Lobina C, Reali R, Gessa GL. Appetite suppression and weight loss after the cannabinoid antagonist sR 141716. *Life Sci* 1998; 63: PL113-PL117.

7. Freedland CS, Poston JS, Porrino LJ. Effects of SR141716A, a central cannabinoid receptor antagonist, on food-maintained responding. *Pharmacol Biochem Behav* 2000; 67: 265–70.

8. Kirkham TC, Williams CM. Synergystic effects of opioid and cannabinoid antagonists on food intake. *Psychopharmacology* 2001; 153: 267–70.

9. Rowland NE, Mukherjee M, Robertson K. Effects of the cannabinoid receptor antagonist SR 141716, alone and in combination with dexfenfluramine or naloxone, on food intake in rats. *Psychopharmacology* 2001; 159: 111–6.

10. Shire D, Calandra B, Bouaboula M, Barth F, Rinaldi-Carmona M, Casellas P, Ferrara P. Cannabinoid receptor interactions with the antagonists SR141716A and SR144528. *Life Sci* 1999; 65: 627–35.

11. Zimmer A, Zimmer AM, Hohmann AG, Herkenham M, Bonner TI. Increased mortality, hypoactivity, and hypoalgesia in cannabinoid CB1 receptor knockout mice. *Proc Natl Acad Sci USA* 1999; 96: 5780–5.

12. Di Marzo V, Goparaju SK, Wang L, Liu J, Batkai S, Jarai Z *et al.* Leptin-regulated endocannabinoids are involved in maintaining food intake. *Nature* 2001; 410: 822–5.

13. Friedman JM, Halaas JL. Leptin and the regulation of body weight in mammals. *Nature* 1998; 395: 763–70.

14. Huszar D, Lynch CA, Fairchild-Huntress V, Dunmore JH, Fang Q, Berkemeier LR *et al.* Targeted disruption of the melanocortin-4 receptor results in obesity in mice. *Cell* 1997; 88: 131–41.

15. Chen H, Charlat O, Tartaglia LA, Woolf EA, Weng X, Ellis SJ *et al.* Synergystic effects of opioid and cannabinoid antagonists on food intake. *Psychopharmacology* 2001; 153: 267–70.

16. Erickson JC, Clegg KE, Palmiter RD. Sensitivity to leptin and susceptibility to seizures in mice lacking neuropeptide Y. *Nature* 1996; 381, 415–421.

17. Ledent C, Valverde O, Cossu G, Petitet F, Aubert J-F, Beslot F *et al.* Unresponsiveness to cannabinoids and reduced addictive effects of opiates in CB1 receptor knockout mice. *Science* 1999; 283: 401–4.

CHAPTER 175

Organochlorine pollutants and energy balance

A. Tremblay and C. Pelletier

Division of Kinesiology, PEPS, Laval University, Ste-Foy (Québec), G1K 7P4, Canada
[e-mail: angelo.tremblay@kin.msp.ulaval.ca]

Introduction

In the last century, we have seen numerous scientific innovations susceptible to improve quality of life. However, some of them, first very effective and useful, were then found to represent environment, wildlife and/or human health threats. Organochlorine compounds (OC), characterized by their chemical structure containing carbon, chlorine and hydrogen atoms, carbon-chlorine bonds and cyclic carbon chains, are part of these man-made products. These compounds regroup two main classes of products. First, polychlorinated biphenyls (PCBs) which began to be used in 1929, were employed in industries as plasticizers in inks, plastic and rubber and as lubricants and coolants in electrical appliances. The second class is organochlorine insecticides, which appeared on the market after the Second World War. They were used in agriculture as well as in public health programmes to control vectors of diseases such as malaria. Organochlorines were banished in most countries in the 1970s when reports documented their adverse effects on environment, wildlife and human health, but insecticides are still used in countries where malaria is endemic.

Although their use is restraint since about 30 years, organochlorines are still found in every organism on the planet, due to the characteristics of these compounds. First, organochlorines degrade very slowly. Half-lives of the order of months to 6–12 years have been reported for these compounds[1,2]. Moreover, organochlorines are fat-soluble, so they accumulate in fatty tissues. Thus, an organism that is high in the food chain will accumulate a greater quantity of organochlorines with its ingested food, a phenomenon called biomagnification. For humans, the principal exposure to organochlorines occurs via fish, meat and dairy products intake. Since organochlorines are stored in fat and could have adverse health effects, we explored the association between fat mass and contamination by organochlorines and the impact of these compounds on components of energy metabolism during weight loss.

Organochlorine concentration in lean and obese individuals

As fat mass is the storage depot for organochlorines, adiposity could influence the organochlorine concentration between individuals. It could be suspected that obese persons have a low concentration of organochlorines (when expressed on a lipid basis), since they have a high fat mass to dilute these compounds. However, obese individuals have a greater caloric intake than lean persons, thus their contamination by organochlorine could be higher since these compounds are ingested with food. Plasma organochlorine concentration was compared between endurance athletes, lean sedentary persons and obese individuals, who differ by their fat mass and caloric intake. In this study, athletes had the lowest plasma organochlorine concentration whereas obese individuals had the highest[3]. As the results for fat mass followed the same trend, the possible relationship between fat mass and plasma organochlorine concentration was investigated. Athletes were not included in this analysis, since physical activity could modify the relationship. In the sedentary group (lean + obese individuals), a positive correlation was found between fat mass and plasma organochlorine concentration[3]. These results are in accordance with the pharmacokinetic model suggested by Wolff and Anderson[4]. In this model, the difference in organochlorine concentration between lean and obese persons depends on the phase of exposure. When exposure is occurring, it is similar between obese and lean persons, so organochlorine concentration is higher in lean individuals since obese individuals have a higher fat mass to dilute the compounds. However, when exposure ceased, as it is the case in industrialized countries, clearance rate seems to be greater in lean persons and after about 15 years, obese individuals display a higher organochlorine concentration than lean persons. A higher clearance rate of organochlorine in leaner persons was also reported in individuals occupationally exposed to β-HCH. In these persons, the half-life of β-HCH was positively correlated to the percentage of body fat[5].

Table 1. Relative organochlorine body burden in athletes and in lean and obese sedentary individuals

	Lean	Athletes	Obese
Total plasma OC concentration (u./kg lipids)	1	0.70	1.33
Fat mass (kg)	1	0.78	2.34
Body burden (u.)	1	0.55	3.11

OC, organochlorine; u., units. Adapted from Pelletier *et al.*[3]

Obese persons having a higher organochlorine concentration expressed on a lipid basis and a higher fat mass than lean persons, their total body burden of organochlorines is expected to be much more elevated than that of lean individuals. Results from Pelletier *et al.*[3] were used to extrapolate the total organochlorine body burden of lean and obese persons. Means of total plasma organochlorine concentration and fat mass for the lean sedentary group were equalized to 1, whereas means for the athlete and obese groups were adjusted relatively to the reference value of the lean sedentary group (Table 1). Since variations in plasma organochlorine concentrations are highly representative of those observed for adipose tissue[6], organochlorine body burden was calculated as the product of total plasma organochlorine concentration (u./kg lipids) and fat mass (kg). Results shown in Table 1 suggest that, in this study, organochlorine body burden is about two times lower in athletes and three times higher in obese individuals than in lean persons.

Impact of organochlorine pollutants on energy metabolism

Organochlorine compounds may exert many adverse effects on health. They have been associated with alteration of the immune system[7] and with increased breast cancer risk[8–11]. They have also been associated with alteration of thyroid function. Negative correlations were found between plasma organochlorine and triiodothyronine (T3) or thyroxine (T4) concentrations[12,13]. Since thyroid hormones are implicated in the control of energy metabolism, it could be hypothesized that organochlorines could have a negative impact on metabolic rate.

Plasma organochlorine concentration increases during body weight loss as a result of fat mobilization[14,15]. This increase in plasma organochlorine concentration has also been positively associated to the increase in basal lipolysis of subcutaneous adipocytes[16]. When circulating, organochlorines may reach their target organs and exert their effects. Since T3 concentration and resting metabolic rate (RMR) decrease during weight loss, relationships between the changes in these variables and the organochlorine increase was investigated. Thus, plasma organochlorine concentration, T3 concentration and RMR were measured before and after a 15-week weight loss programme. Even after adjustment for body weight loss, the increase in plasma organochlorine concentration was negatively correlated with the decreases in T3 concentration and in RMR[17]. Furthermore, when fat mass, fat free mass, leptin concentration, T3 concentration and plasma organochlorine concentration were entered as predicting variables in a stepwise multiple regression analysis with RMR as dependent variable, changes in organochlorine concentration were the best predictor of changes in RMR during weight loss[17]. These results suggest that organochlorine release could affect T3 concentration and RMR during weight loss, but other studies are needed to explore the causality of the relationships obtained.

Another component of energy balance that may be affected by organochlorines is the capacity for fatty acid oxidation. Capacity for lipid oxidation in skeletal muscle cells is altered in obese persons, and this impairment is not improved with weight loss[18]. Markers of the oxidative capacity are mitochondrial enzymes such as beta-hydroxyacyl CoA dehydrogenase (HADH), citrate synthase (CS) and cytochrome *c* oxidase (COX), which may be inhibited by organochlorines[19]. The possible effect of organochlorine on lipid oxidative capacity was thus explored during a weight loss programme. In men, the increase in plasma organochlorine concentration was correlated with the decrease in skeletal muscle HADH, CS

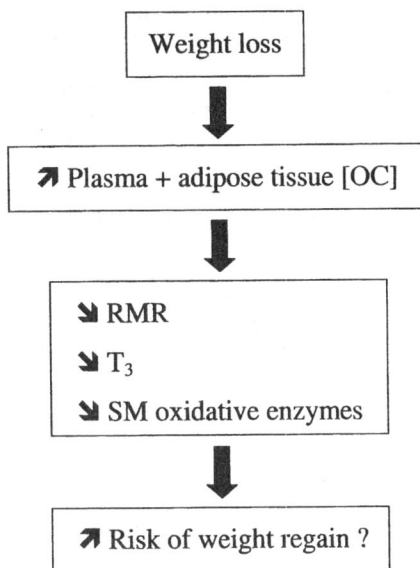

Fig. 1. Illustration of the impact of organochlorine pollutants on energy metabolism during weight loss. OC, organochlorine compounds. Adapted from Pelletier *et al.*[6].

and COX activities[20]. Thus, organochlorine release may play a role in the impairment of the capacity for lipid oxidation in reduced-obese individuals.

Conclusion

The subtle effects of organochlorine release during weight loss on energy balance which are reported in this paper may be considered as 'adverse effects' of weight loss. Indeed, as summarized in Fig. 1, decreases in T_3 concentration, RMR[17], and skeletal muscle oxidative capacity[20] associated to the increase in plasma organochlorine concentration may favour weight regain or increase the difficulty to further weight loss. These physiological changes might be perceived as protection mechanisms to avoid a substantial release of organochlorine compounds into blood, which could increase risk to develop health problems associated to organochlorines.

Obese persons, who are the most susceptible to lose weight, present higher organochlorine body burden than lean individuals, and so may be at greater risk for an important increase in plasma organochlorine concentration during weight loss. Thus, for the obese person who wants to lose weight, the release of organochlorines into blood during weight loss may be alarming since these compounds may have adverse effects such as increasing cancer risk. However, it is not certain if the change in the concentration of organochlorines during an usual weight loss of about 10 per cent of the initial body weight is high enough to cause health problems. Up to now, health benefits of weight loss as decreased risk for cardiovascular diseases, hypertension or diabetes surpass health risks associated to the increase in plasma organochlorine concentration. Body weight loss in obese individuals should thus not be discouraged on the basis that it would increase the plasma organochlorine concentration. Nevertheless, a moderate weight loss could be privileged as long as we know that it could normalise metabolic profile[21]. Thus, risks for diseases associated to obesity would be decreased whereas a substantial release of organochlorines, and so risks of health problems due to these compounds, could be avoided.

References

1. Wolff MS. Half-lives of organochlorines (OCs) in humans. *Arch Environ Contam Toxicol* 1999; 36: 504.

2. Morgan DP, Roan CC. Absorption, storage, and metabolic conversion of ingested DDT and DDT metabolites in man. *Arch Environ Health* 1971; 22: 301–8.

3. Pelletier C, Després JP, Tremblay A. Plasma organochlorine concentrations in endurance athletes and obese individuals. *Med Sci Sports Exerc* 2002; 34: 1971–5.

4. Wolff MS, Anderson HA. Correspondence re: J. M. Schildkraut *et al.*, Environmental contaminants and body fat distribution. Cancer Epidemiol Biomark Prev 1999; 8: 179–83. *Cancer Epidemiol Biomarkers Prev* 1999; 8: 951–2.

5. Jung D, Becher H, Edler L, Flesch-Janys D, Gurn P, Konietzko J *et al*. Elimination of beta-hexachlorocyclohexane in occupationally exposed persons. *J Toxicol Environ Health* 1997; 51: 23–34.

6. Pelletier C, Imbeault P, Tremblay A. Energy balance and pollution by organochlorines and polychlorinated biphenyls *Obes Rev* 2003; 4: 17–24.

7. Svensson BG, Hallberg T, Nilsson A, Schutz A, Hagmar L. Parameters of immunological competence in subjects with high consumption of fish contaminated with persistent organochlorine compounds. *Int Arch Occup Environ Health* 1994; 65: 351–8.

8. Demers A, Ayotte P, Brisson J, Dodin S, Robert J, Dewailly E. Plasma concentrations of polychlorinated biphenyls and the risk of breast cancer: a congener-specific analysis. *Am J Epidemiol* 2002; 155: 629–35.

9. Aronson KJ, Miller AB, Woolcott CG, Sterns EE, McCready DR, Lickley LA *et al*. Breast adipose tissue concentrations of polychlorinated biphenyls and other organochlorines and breast cancer risk. *Cancer Epidemiol Biomark Prev* 2000; 9: 55–63.

10. Romieu I, Hernandez-Avila M, Lazcano-Ponce E, Weber JP, Dewailly E. Breast cancer, lactation history, and serum organochlorines. *Am J Epidemiol* 2000; 152: 363–70.

11. Güttes S, Failing K, Neumann K, Kleinstein J, Georgii S, Brunn H. Chlororganic pesticides and polychlorinated biphenyls in breast tissue of women with benign and malignant breast disease. *Arch Environ Contam Toxicol* 1998; 35: 140–7.

12. Hagmar L, Rylander L, Dyremark E, Klasson-Wehler E, Erfurth EM. Plasma concentrations of persistent organochlorines in relation to thyrotropin and thyroid hormone levels in women. *Int Arch Occup Environ Health* 2001; 74: 184–8.

13. Sala M, Sunyer J, Herrero C, To-Figueras J, Grimalt J. Association between serum concentrations of hexachlorobenzene and polychlorobiphenyls with thyroid hormone and liver enzymes in a sample of the general population. *Occup Environ Med* 2001; 58: 172–7.

14. Backman L, Kolmodin-Hedman B. Concentration of DDT and DDE in plasma and subcutaneous adipose tissue before and after intestinal bypass operation for treatment of obesity. *Toxicol Appl Pharmacol* 1978; 46: 663–9.

15. Chevrier J, Dewailly E, Ayotte P, P, M, Després JP, Tremblay A. Body weight loss increases plasma and adipose tissue concentrations of potentially toxic pollutants in obese individuals. *Int J Obes* 2000; 24: 1272–8.

16. Imbeault P, Chevrier J, Dewailly E, Ayotte P, Després JP, Tremblay A, Mauriège P. Increase in plasma pollutant levels in response to weight loss in humans is related to *in vitro* subcutaneous adipocyte basal lipolysis. *Int J Obes* 2001; 25: 1–7.

17. Pelletier C, Doucet E, Imbeault P, Tremblay A. Associations between weight-loss induced changes in plasma organochlorine concentrations, serum T3 concentration and resting metabolic rate. *Toxicol Sci* 2002; 67: 46–51.

18. Kelley DE, Goodpaster B, Wing RR, Simoneau JA. Skeletal muscle fatty acid metabolism in association with insulin resistance, obesity, and weight loss. *Am J Physiol* 1999; 277: E1130–E41.

19. Pardini RS. Polychlorinated biphenyls (PCB): effect on mitochondrial enzyme systems. *Bull Environ Contam Toxicol* 1971; 6: 539–45.

20. Imbeault P, Tremblay A, Simoneau JA, Joanisse DR. Weight loss-induced rise in plasma pollutant is associated with reduced skeletal muscle oxidative capacity. *Am J Physiol Endocrinol Metab* 2002; 282: E574–E9.

21. Tremblay A, Doucet E, Imbeault P, Mauriege P, Despres JP, Richard D. Metabolic fitness in active reduced-obese individuals. *Obes Res* 1999; 7: 556–63.

Progress in Obesity Research: 9. Edited by *Geraldo Medeiros-Neto, Alfredo Halpern and Claude Bouchard*
©2003 John Libbey Eurotext Ltd, pp. 833–836.

CHAPTER 176

Ageing and energy balance

John E. Morley

*Division of Geriatric Medicine, Saint Louis University School of Medicine, and GRECC, St. Louis VA Medical Center,
St. Louis, Missouri, USA*
[e-mail: morley@slu.edu]

Introduction

In persons over the age of 70 years weight loss is an excellent predictor of mortality and morbidity. Weight loss occurs both physiologically and pathologically in older persons. Physiological weight loss is a combination of decreased food intake and a loss of muscle mass. When an older person becomes ill, there is an acceleration of weight loss with severe muscle wasting, i.e. cachexia, that is due to a combination of worsening anorexia and cytokine release resulting in muscle catabolism and a rapid decrease in circulating albumin and prealbumin. Recently it has been suggested that cytokines produce cachexia by activating the coactivator of PPAR$_\delta$, PGC-1, which leads to an uncoupling of cellular respiration leading to energy imbalance in the cell. Sarcopenia is analogous to osteoporosis and occurs when an older person develops muscle loss two standard deviations below that of a younger person. Persons with excess muscle loss who maintain excess adiposity become the 'fat frail' and have worse outcomes than those who lose both muscle and fat.

Physiological anorexia of ageing

Animal studies

Rodents decrease food intake and lose weight. This is associated with a decline in lean mass and an increase in leptin levels[1]. The increase in leptin levels is associated with an increase in peripheral but not visceral fat. There is also a decline in testosterone levels with ageing.

Our early studies demonstrated that older Fisher-344 rats were 10 to 100 times more sensitive than younger animals to the suppressive effects of naloxone on feeding[2]. In addition, older rats were less responsive to the feeding enhancement of the Kappa opiate agonist, butorphanol tartrate. In addition, we found that mice were more sensitive to the satiating effects of cholecystokinin (CCK), but not to bombesin and gastrin releasing peptide[3].

In addition, the orexigenic neuropeptide, NPY, has been shown to have decreased hypothalamic gene expression in older animals[4]. Testosterone replacement increases NPY mRNA and reduces cocaine-amphetamine-regulated transcript mRNA in older animals[5]. Troglitazone, a PPAR$_\delta$ activator, increased food intake and decreased leptin in older rats[6].

Our previous studies have suggested that nitric oxide places an integral effect in activating food intake[7]. Both leptin and NPY produce their effects on feeding through nitric oxide[8] and orexin A fails to increase food intake in nitric oxide synthase (brain) knockout mice (unpublished data). Both pharmacological studies and measurement of nitric oxide synthase suggest a role for nitric oxide in the anorexia of aging[9].

Human studies

It is well established that with ageing there is a decline in food intake. In 1988, we termed this condition the anorexia of ageing[10]. The reasons for this decline in food intake are multifactorial. It includes an alteration in the perception of the hedonic qualities of food, due to a decrease in olfaction and an increase in taste threshold.

A major reason for the anorexia of ageing is the development of early satiation. This is related to delayed gastric emptying when large volume meals are ingested[11]. There is evidence that with ageing there is a decline in fundal adaptive relaxation[12]. This is not probably due to a decrease in nitric oxide synthase activity. The reduction in adaptive compliance leads to more rapid antral filling and early satiation[13].

CCK is a classic satiating hormone. In older individuals basal levels of CCK are increased as well as the levels obtained after intraduodenal lipid[14]. Glucagon-like peptide-1 and Peptide YY did not differ between young and older persons. CCK-8 was twice as potent at suppressing food intake in older compared to younger persons[15]. This increased satiating apprea to be related to the higher serum levels of CCK-8 in older persons due to delayed plasma clearance. These findings strongly suggest a role for CCK in the anorexia of ageing.

Wilson *et al.*[16] showed that older persons ingested less fat and carbohydrate. Satiety was more prolonged in old compared to young individuals. When a caloric preload was given 60 min before a meal the older person ate more than when it was administered immediately before meals. These studies suggest that caloric supplements should be given at least 60 min before a meal.

Leptin levels increase with the increasing fat mass at middle age[17]. The high leptin levels are less anorexia than expected because of leptin resistance that occurs in part because of a reduction in blood barrier transport of leptin[18]. The elevated leptin levels are related to peripheral, rather than visceral, obesity[19]. In older men leptin levels increase despite a decline of total fat mass[20]. This is predominantly due to declining testosterone levels[21] and the increased leptin levels are decreased with testosterone treatment in older males[22]. Testosterone also reverses the sarcopenia of aging[23]. It would appear that the increased anorexia that occurs in men compared to women with ageing is due to the decline in testosterone.

While there is evidence that in humans the hypodipsia of ageing is related to a failure of the opioid drinking drive[24], older males seem to retain their sensitivity to the opioid feeding drive[25]. The possibility of gender differences in opioid sensitivity deserve further investigation.

Pathological anorexia

There is not good evidence that multiple cytokines cause anorexia[26]. Older persons develop multiple conditions from cancer to infections that result in elevated cytokine levels. Megestrol acetate increases food intake in older persons[27]. It decreases cytokine levels and is more effective in older persons with elevated cytokine levels[28].

The most common cause of weight loss in older persons is depression[29,30]. Antidepressants that increase food intake, e.g. mirtazapine, are preferable to selective serotonin receptor uptake inhibitors in depressed older persons who are losing weight. A psychosocial intervention also improves nutritional status and decrease dysphoria in older persons[31].

There are numerous treatable causes of anorexia and weight loss that are easily remembered by the mneumonic – MEALS-ON-WHEELS (Table 1).

Table 1. MEALS-ON-WHEELS menmonic for treatable causes of weight loss

Medications (e.g. digoxin, theophylline, cemetidene)
Emotional (e.g. depression)
Alcoholism, elder abuse, anorexia tardive
Late life paranoia
Swallowing problems
Oral factors
Nasocomial infections (e.g. tuberculosis)
Wandering and other dementia related factors
Hyperthyroidism, hypercalcaemia, hypoadrenalism
Enteral problems (e.g. gluten enteropathy)
Eating problems
Low salt, low cholesterol and other therapeutic diets
Stones (cholecystitis)

Dronabinol, a purified tetrahydrocannibinol, has been shown to increase food intake in older persons[32]. It also decreases behaviour disturbances. It can be used to decrease nausea. There is a need for further studies on the role of dronabinol in reversing the anorexia of ageing.

Conclusion

Anorexia and weight loss are deleterious conditions in older persons. In many situations, these conditions can be effectively treated if recognized early and an appropriate diagnosis made.

References

1. Wolden-Hanson T, Marck BT, Smith L, Matsumoto AM. Cross-sectional and longitudinal analysis of age-associated changes in body composition of male Brown Norway rats: association of serum leptin levels with peripheral adiposity. *J Gerontol Biol Sci* 1999; 54(3): B99–B107.

2. Gosnell BA, Levine AS, Morley JE. The effects of aging on opioid modulatio of feeding in rats. *Life Sci* 1983; 32(24): 2793–9.

3. Silver AJ, Flood JF, Morley JE. Effect of gastrointestinal peptides on ingestion in old and young mice. *Peptides* 1988; 9(2): 221–5.

4. Matsumoto AM, Marck BT, Gruenewald DA, Wolden-Hanson T, Naai MA. Aging and the neuroendocrine regulation of reproduction and body weight. *Experiment Gerontol* 2000; 35(9–10): 1251–65.

5. Sohn EH, Wolden-Hanson T, Matsumoto AM. Testosterone (T)-induced changes in arcuate nucleus cocain-amphetamine-regulated transcript and NPY mRNA are attenuated in old compared to young male brown Norway rats: contribution of T to age-related changes in cocaine-amphetamine-regulated transcript and NPY gene expression. *Endocrinology* 2002; 143(3): 954–63.

6. Wolden-Hanson T, Marck BT, Matsumoto AM. Troglitazone treatment of aging Brown Norway rats improves food intake and weight gain after fasting without increasing hypothalamic HPY gene expression. *Experiment Gerontol* 2002; 37(5): 679–91.

7. Morley JE, Flood JF. Competitive antagonism of nitric oxide synthetase causes weight loss in mice. *Life Sci* 1992; 51(16): 1283–9.

8. Morley JE, Alshaher MM, Farr SA, Flood JF, Kumar VB. Leptin and neuropeptide Y (NPY) modulate nitric oxide synthase: Further evidence for a role of nitric oxide in feeding. *Peptides* 1999; 20(5): 595–600.

9. Morley JE, Kumar VB, Mattammal MB, Farr S, Morley PM, Flood JF. Inhibition of feeding by a nitric oxide synthase inhibitor: effects of aging. *Eur J Pharmacol* 1996; 311(1): 15–9.

10. Morley JE, Silver AJ. Anorexia in the elderly. *Neurobiol Aging* 1988; 9(1): 9–16.

11. Clarkston WK, Pantano MM, Morley JE, Horowitz M, Littlefield JM, Burton FR. Evidence for the anorexia of aging: gastrointestinal transit and hunger in healthy elderly vs. young adults. *Am J Physiol* 1997; 272(1 Pt 2): R243–R8.

12. Rayner Ck, MacIntosh CG, Chapman IM, Morley JE, Horowitz M. Effects of age on proximal gastric motor and sensory function. *Scand J Gastro* 2000; 35(10): 1041–7.

13. Jones KL, Doran SM, Hveem K, Bartholomeusz FD, Morley JE, Sun WM *et al*. Relation between postprandial satiation and antral area in normal subjects. *Am J Clin Nutr* 1997; 66(1): 127–32.

14. MacIntosh CG, Andrews JM, Jones KL, Wishart JM, Morris hA, Jansen JB *et al*. Effects of age on concentrations of plasma cholecystokinin, glucagons-like peptide 1, and peptide YY and their relation to appetite and pyloric motility. *Am J Clin Nutr* 1999; 69(5): 999–1006.

15. MacIntosh CG, Morley JE, Wishart J, Morris H, Jansen JB, Horowitz M *et al*. Effect of exogenous cholecystokinin (CCK)-8 on food intake and plasma CCK, leptin, and insulin concentrations in older and young adults: evidence for increased CCK activity as a cause of the anorexia of aging. *J Clin Endocrinol Metab* 2001; 86(12): 5830–7.

16. Wilson MM, Purushothaman R, Morley JE. Effect of liquid dietary supplements on energy intake in the elderly. *Am J Clin Nutr* 2001; 75(5): 944–7.

17. Perry HM III, Morley JE, Horowitz M, Kaiser FE, Miller DK, Wittert G. Body composition and age in African-American and Caucasian women: relationship to plasma leptin levels. *Metabolism: Clin Exper* 1997; 46(12): 1399–405.

18. Banks WA, DiPalma CR, Farrell CL. Impaired transport of leptin across the blood-brain barrier in obesity. *Peptides* 1999; 20(11): 1341–5.

19. Baumgartner RN, Ross RR, Waters DL, Brooks WM, Morley JE, Montoya GD, Garry PJ. Serum leptin in elderly people: associations with sex hormones, insulin, and adipose tissue volumes. *Obes Res* 1999; 7(2): 141–9.

20. Baumgartner RN, Waters DL, Morley JE, Patrick P, Montoya GD, Garry PJ. Age-related changes in sex hormones affect the sex difference in serum leptin independently of changes in body fat. *Metabolism* 1999; 48(3): 378–84.

21. Morley JE, Kaiser FE, Perry HM 3rd, Patrick P, Morley PM, Stauber PM *et al*. Longitudinal changes in testosterone, luteinizing hormone, and follicle-stimulating hormone in healthy older men. *Metab: Clin Exper* 1997; 46(4): 410–3.

22. Sih R, Morley JE, Kaiser Fe, Perry HM 3rd, Patrick P, Ross C. Testosterone replacement in older hypogonadal men: a 12-month randomized controlled trial. *J Clin Endocrinol Metab* 1997; 82(6): 1661–7.

23. Morley JE. Anorexia, sarcopenia, and aging. *Nutrition* 2001; 17(7–8): 660–3.

24. Silver AJ, Morley JE. Role of the opioid system in the hypodipsia associated with aging. *J Am Geriatr Soc* 1992; 40(6): 556–60.

25. MacIntosh CG, Sheehan J, Davani N, Morley JE, Horowitz M, Chapman IM. Effects of aging on the opioid modulation of feeding in humans. *J Am Geriat Soc* 2001; 49(11): 1518–24.

26. Baez-Franceschi D, Morley JE. Pathophysiology of catabolism in undernourished elderly patients. *Zeitschrift fur Gerontologie und Geriatrie* 1999; 32 (Suppl 1): I12–19.

27. Karcic E, Philpot C, Morley JE. Treating malnutrition with egestrol acetate: Literature review and review of our experience. *J Nutr Hlth & Aging* 2002; 6(3): 191–200.

28. Yeh SS, Wu SY, Levine DM, Parker TS, Olson JS, Stevens MR, Schuster MW. The correlation of cytokine levels with body weight after megestrol acetate treatment in geriatric patients. *J Gerontol Med Sci* 2001; 56(1): M48-M54.

29. Wilson MM, Vaswani S, Liu D, Morley JE, Miller DK. Prevalence and causes of undernutrition in medical outpatients. *Am J Med* 1998; 104(1): 56–63.

30. Morley JE, Kraenzle D. Causes of weight loss in a community nursing home. *J Am Geriatr Soc* 1994; 42(6): 583–5.

31. Suda Y, Marske CE, Flaherty JH, Zdrodowski K, Morley JE. Examining the effect of intervention to nutritional problems of the elderly living in an inner city area: a pilot project. *J Nutr, Hlth & Aging* 2001; 5(2): 118–23.

32. Volicer L, Stelly M, Morris J, McLaughlin J, Volicer BJ. Effects of dronabinol on anorexia and disturbed behaviour in patients with Alzheimer's disease. *Int J Geriatr Psych* 1997; 12(9): 913–9.

Progress in Obesity Research: 9. Edited by *Geraldo Medeiros-Neto, Alfredo Halpern and Claude Bouchard*
©2003 John Libbey Eurotext Ltd, pp. 837–841.

CHAPTER 177

Energy density of food and energy balance

Catherine M. Champagne, Silvia Morales, Ray Allen and Michael Lefevre

Pennington Biomedical Research Center, Louisiana State University, 6400 Perkins Road, Baton Rouge, LA 70808 USA
[e-mail: ChampaCM@pbrc.edu]

Introduction

Ecological studies usually associate low fat, and thus low energy dense, diets with low rates of obesity[1]. However, despite the decrease in dietary fat content and the abundance of lower fat foods in the marketplace, Astrup[2] noted that the US has rapidly increasing obesity rates, giving rise to the term, 'the American paradox'. The relationship between energy density of the food supply and energy balance or regulation has received renewed interest as an area for further study. Decades of research in metabolic wards using formula fed diets showed that the carbohydrate-to-fat ratio could vary widely with little or no impact on energy requirements for weight maintenance[3]. However changes in dietary energy density as fat, carbohydrate, or mixtures can result in profound effects on energy intake and body weight[4–7]. These findings were obtained under strictly controlled conditions and the authors point out that in real life situations subjects can alter the food eaten in the context of amount, type, and composition resulting in perhaps different compensatory responses.

Energy density clearly has an effect on the human appetite and subsequent energy intake, thereby affecting energy balance or regulation[8]. Additionally, the response to energy density and fat content in the diets of lean compared to obese individuals has been studied, with evidence indicating differences between the two groups in food intake and taste preference[9,10].

Energy density in the context of sugar content has also been explored, with results suggesting that the use of sweeteners to reduce energy density may provide short-term reduction in energy intake[11]. Few data are available to evaluate the effects of sweeteners for long-term weight control[11,12].

There are data to suggest that some populations consume diets of similar food volumes independent of food energy. One such study by Bell[13] indicated that energy density influenced energy intake when diets were similar in volume but when diets containing different energy densities were provided to normal weight women, significantly different energy intakes resulted. The implication of this study is that overconsumption of high fat foods may be due to their high energy density as opposed to just their fat content.

However, if the volume of food is energy dense, it may in fact be imposing health risks because of its potential adverse energy, simple sugar and fat profiles. Regardless, diets with extremely high energy density or extremely low energy density pose challenges to healthy nutritional status[14].

Most of the available information on the influence of macronutrient composition and energy density on energy balance has been derived from controlled feeding experiments. This paper will attempt to illustrate the roles of energy density, macronutrient intake, and their subsequent effects on weight through evaluation of subjects participating in intervention counseling studies which were designed to investigate dietary fat effects on blood lipids and cardiovascular risk.

Methods

Subjects participating in two intervention studies form the basis of this manuscript. Study 1 will be referred to as MedStep and study 2 will be referred to as PBS (peanut butter sterol). MedStep was designed to be a comparison of the Mediterranean diet vs. the American Heart Association Step 1. One hundred thirteen subjects between the ages of 35 and 65 years of age participated in the study. Total cholesterol was required to be above 200 mg/dl and LDL-cholesterol greater than 130 but less than 200 mg/dl. Subjects were excluded if they had hypertension or diabetes or were using lipid lowering drugs or foods. Primary endpoints were blood lipids, including total cholesterol, HDL cholesterol, LDL cholesterol and triglycerides. We recruited five cohorts to reach the final numbers needed and to achieve adequate subject management. Subjects were randomized to either a Step 1 diet therapy plan (30 per cent of calories from total fat, less than 10 per cent of calories from saturated fat, and less than 300 mg of dietary cholesterol per day) or a Mediterranean diet therapy plan (37 per cent of calories from total fat, less than 10 per cent of calories from saturated fat, less than 300 mg of dietary cholesterol per day, and approximately 21 per cent of calories from monounsaturated fat). Participants were counseled for 6 months using both group and individual sessions to follow their prescribed diets. Increased fruit, vegetable, and grain consumption was advocated on both dietary regimes. Seven day food records were used to derive endpoint dietary information.

The 15-week PBS study consisted of an initial 3 week run-in period on control treatment followed by a three period cross-over phase – each period lasting 4 weeks. Subjects were instructed prior to the run-in period on an American Heart Association Step 1 diet and followed the diet plus incorporating four tablespoons (64 g) of control peanut butter during the 3 week period. The treatment levels were 'control peanut butter', 'peanut butter with 1.5 g sterol per day' and 'peanut butter with 3.0 g sterol per day'. Measurements were taken at the end of each period. The primary endpoints were blood lipids, including total cholesterol, HDL cholesterol, LDL cholesterol and triglycerides. Each of 30 subjects was randomized to one of six three-treatment sequences with the goal to obtain balanced residual effects. However, it was assumed that any carry-over effects would wash out rapidly. Twenty-eight subjects were used in the statistical analysis, as two subjects dropped out before any baseline measurements were taken. Four day food records were collected at baseline (3 weeks following instruction on the Step 1 diet and addition of 4 tablespoons, 64 g, of test peanut butter per day), 7, 11 and 15 weeks.

Dietary intakes from both studies were analysed utilizing a Food Diary application which was developed from the MENu (Moore's Extended Nutrient) Database (Pennington Biomedical Research Foundation, Baton Rouge, LA).

Statistical analysis

The response variables of the MedStep data were analysed by Repeated Measures Analysis of Variance. Diet, week, gender, and their interactions were the fixed effects of interest. The baseline measurement of the response variable was included as a covariate. Week was used as a within subject factor to take into account that observations had been taken repeatedly on the same subject, i.e. at week 12 and week 24. The comparison of energy density between the two weight change groups (subjects who had lost at least 1 kg of weight by week 24 and subjects who had not) was done by one-way Analysis of Covariance. Baseline energy density was the covariate.

The statistical analysis of the PBS data proceeded in a similar manner, however without the diet information in the fixed effects list. No particular structure was imposed upon the covariance among the repeated observations at weeks 7, 11 and 15 of this study. Weight change was analysed by one-way ANCOVA, with gender defining the two populations and baseline weight serving as the covariate.

All tests were non-directional and established through adjusted means predicted by the model (Least Squares Means). Statements concerning the significance of tests were based on a type I error rate of 0.05 without adjustment for multiple comparisons. The statistical analyses were performed using SAS, version 8.2.

Results and discussion

Table 1. Baseline demographic data for the MedStep (Step 1 and Mediterranean diet arms) and the PBS (Peanut Butter Sterol) studies

Diet	Step 1	Mediterranean	PBS
n	56	57	28
Male/females	21/35	22/37	12/16
Age, y	50 ± 8	49 ± 9	49 ± 2
Weight, kg	81 ± 12	77 ± 13	80 ± 3
Total cholesterol, mg/dl	240 ± 28	234 ± 26	233 ± 6
LDL cholesterol, mg/dl	154 ± 17	154 ± 15	160 ± 4
BMI, kg/m^2	28.8 ± 0.5	27.1 ± 0.5	28.1 ± 0.9

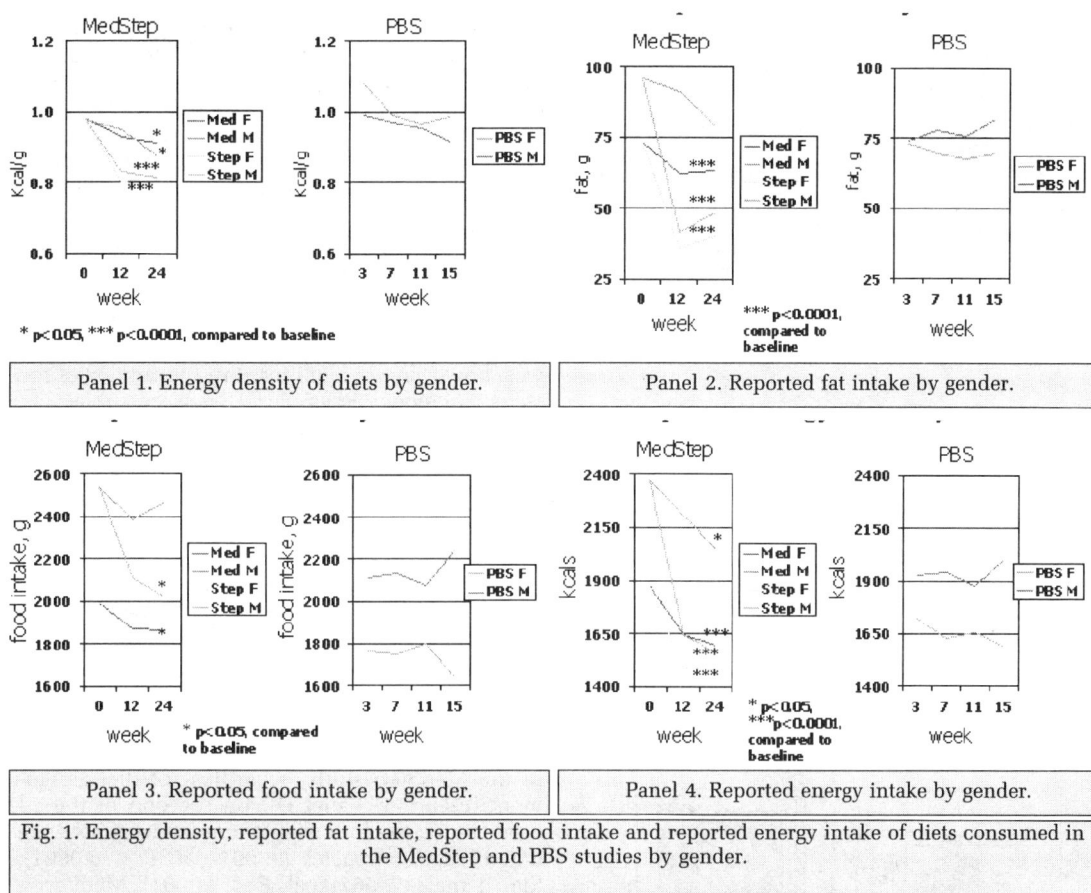

Panel 1. Energy density of diets by gender.

Panel 2. Reported fat intake by gender.

Panel 3. Reported food intake by gender.

Panel 4. Reported energy intake by gender.

Fig. 1. Energy density, reported fat intake, reported food intake and reported energy intake of diets consumed in the MedStep and PBS studies by gender.

The demographic information for the subjects at baseline from both studies is contained in Table 1. Even though these were two different studies, the inclusion and exclusion criteria were the same and the subjects therefore were very similar. Fewer subjects were in the PBS study. Approximately 60 per cent of the subjects were female in both studies. Subjects were middle aged and body weights were similar. All subjects had elevated serum cholesterol and LDL-cholesterol levels and were classified as overweight (body mass index > 25).

Subjects in the MedStep study were successfully able to comply with the dietary regimens they were instructed to follow. At baseline the mean fat consumption was between 35.0–35.7 per cent of calories. The subjects on the Mediterranean diet continued to consume approximately 35 per cent of calories from fat for the remainder of the study, though shy of the initial goal of 37 per cent of calories from fat. Those subjects on the Step 1 diet were able to lower their fat intakes to approximately 23 per cent by 12 weeks and 25 per cent by 24 weeks. In response to the successful compliance to the Step 1 diet, those subjects lost 2.6 ± 0.3 kg ($P < 0.0001$) by 12 weeks and completed the study at 24 weeks with a weight loss of 3.0 ± 0.5 kg ($P < 0.0001$). It is worthy of note that the Mediterranean group also lost weight, 1.4 ± 0.3 kg ($P < 0.0001$) by 12 weeks and 1.1 ± 0.4 kg ($P = 0.0064$) by 24 weeks. Subjects in the PBS study remained essentially weight stable throughout the 15 week trial. A significant diet effect ($P = 0.0056$) and diet by week interaction ($P = 0.0150$) were noted in MedStep.

Energy density, food intake, fat intake and energy intake for the subjects in both studies are contained in Fig. 1. The most striking observation from Panel A of Fig. 1 is that the diets of subjects participating in both studies is the low energy density of the diets of these free-living individuals, even at baseline. Bell[13] classified a low energy dense diet as having 1.02 kcal/g of food, medium density 1.17 kcal/g of food, and high density 1.34 kcal/g of food. Additionally, in the MedStep study, the subjects reduced the energy density of their diets even further, dramatically so for those in the Step 1 treatment arm (change from baseline at 24 weeks, $P < 0.0001$). Male and female subjects in the Mediterranean

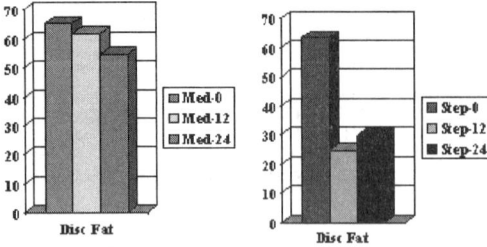

Panel 1. Discretionary fat consumption (g/day) by week in MedStep.

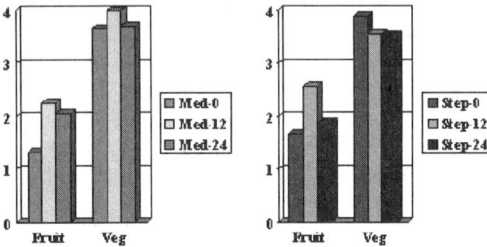

Panel 1. Fruit and vegetable consumption (servings/day) by week in MedStep.

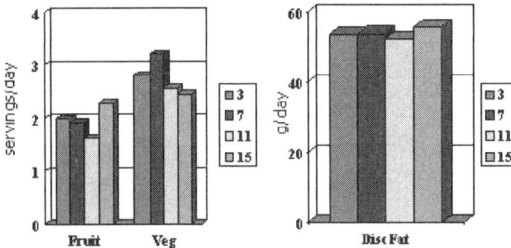

Panel 1. Fruit, vegetable and discretionary fat consumption by week in MedStep.

Fig. 2. Discretionary fat intake and fruit and vegetable consumption reported in the MedStep and PBS studies.

treatment arm each reduced energy density of their diets (change from baseline at 24 weeks, $P < 0.05$). There were also differences between diet treatments, both at 12 ($P < 0.0001$) and 24 weeks ($P < 0.01$). Subjects participating in the PBS study, while consuming low energy dense diets, did not lower the energy density of their diets.

Panel B of Fig. 1 contains the reported fat intake of subjects by gender in MedStep and PBS. Step 1 subjects and female Mediterranean subjects reduced reported fat intake both at 12 and 24 weeks ($P < 0.0001$). Males following the Mediterranean diet reported a trend to lower fat intake which was, however, not significant in the context of the statistical model. Regardless of gender, subjects in the Mediterranean arm reduced fat intake ($P < 0.0001$). Subjects in PBS did not significantly change their fat intake.

Reported total food intake in grams (Figure 1, Panel C) was lower at both 12 and 24 weeks for those MedStep males following the Step 1 diet ($P < 0.05$) and females following the Mediterranean diet ($P < 0.05$). Decreases in total food intake in Step 1 females and Mediterranean males were not significant at either 12 or 24 weeks. There were no differences in reported total food intake in subjects in the PBS study.

Reported energy intake decreased for all subjects in the MedStep study, regardless of diet assignment (Figure 1, Panel D). By the end of the 24 week study, the following energy reductions were noted: Step 1 females (–509 kcal, $P < 0.0001$), Step 1 males (–567 kcal, $P < 0.0001$), Mediterranean females (–366 kcal, $P < 0.0001$), and Mediterranean males (–197 kcal, $P = 0.0163$). For subjects in the PBS study, reported energy intakes changes were not significant at 15 weeks (females, $P = 0.18$; males, $P = 0.45$).

In an effort to determine the specific dietary pattern changes that may have occurred over the course of the two studies, we examined changes in discretionary fat consumption and in servings of fruits and vegetables. Figure 2 contains information on discretionary fat and fruit and vegetable consumption by the subjects in both studies. In the MedStep study, discretionary fat usage tended to decrease slightly in the Mediterranean treatment arm but the trend was more noticeable in the Step 1 treatment arm. Concerning changes in fruit and vegetable consumption in the MedStep study, no changes were noted that could explain the decrease in energy density. The PBS study subjects showed no measurable changes in either discretionary fat use or servings of fruits and vegetables.

Because of the interest in weight loss, we addressed the specific question of energy density of the diet in relation to weight loss for those subjects participating in the MedStep study. Individuals were divided into one of two categories: (1) weight stable, defined as individuals who lost less than 1 kg, or either maintained or gained weight (weight gain in this study was negligible); or (2) weight losers, defined as individuals who lost more than 1 kg. When we compared these individuals, the energy density of the diet was lower in the weight losers (0.82) when compared to the weight stable individuals (0.91) ($P = 0.0207$).

Summary

While the studies reported here were not designed to address energy density, clearly all groups reported low energy dense diets at baseline. Energy density further decreased over time in the MedStep study to levels less than 1.02, the low category reported by Bell[13]. Energy density was correlated with weight loss in MedStep, with lowest density diets consumed by those losing more than 1 kg body weight. There appears to be an important relationship between energy density of food and energy balance, certainly in the context of weight loss and maintenance.

References

1. Tataranni PA, Ravussin E. Effect of fat intake on energy balance. *Ann NY Acad Sci* 1997; 819: 37–43.

2. Astrup A. The American paradox: the role of energy-dense fat-reduced food in the increasing prevalence of obesity. *Curr Opin Clin Nutr Metab Care* 1998; 1: 573–7.

3. Hirsch J, Hudgins LC, Leibel RL, Rosenbaum M. Diet composition and energy balance in humans. *Am J Clin Nutr* 1998; 67 (Suppl.): S551–S555.

4. Stubbs RJ, Harbron CG, Murgatroyd PR, Prentice AM. Covert manipulation of dietary fat and energy density: effect on substrate flux and food intake in men feeding *ad libitum*. *Am J Clin Nutr* 1995; 62: 316–30.

5. Stubbs RJ, Ritz P, Coward WA, Prentice AM. Covert manipulation of the ratio of dietary fat to energy density: effect on food intake and energy balance in free-living men feeding *ad libitum*. *Am J Clin Nutr* 1995; 62: 330–8.

6. Stubbs RJ, Johnstone AM, O'Reilly LM, Barton K, Reid C. The effect of covertly manipulating the energy density of mixed diets on *ad libitum* food intake in 'pseudo free-living' humans. *Int J Obes* 1998; 22,(10): 980–987.

7. Prentice AM. Manipulation of dietary fat and energy density and subsequent effects on substrate flux and food intake. *Am J Clin Nutr* 1998; 67 (Suppl.): S535–S541.

8. Blundell JE, Stubbs RJ. High and low carbohydrate and fat intakes: limits imposed by appetite and palatability and their implications for energy balance. *Eur J Clin Nutr* 1999; 53 (Suppl. 1): S148–S165.

9. Bell EA, Rolls BJ. Energy density of foods affects energy intake across multiple levels of fat content in lean and obese women. *Am J Clin Nutr* 2001; 73: 1010–8.

10. Levine AS. Energy density of foods: building a case for food intake management. *Am J Clin Nutr* 2001; 73: 999–1000.

11. Drewnowski A. Intense sweeteners and energy density of foods: implications for weight control. *Eur J Clin Nutr* 1999; 53: 757–63.

12. Yao M, Roberts SB. Dietary energy density and weight regulation. *Nut Rev* 2001; 59: 247–58.

13. Bell EA, Castellanos VH, Pelkman CL, Thorwart ML, Rolls BJ. Energy density of foods affects energy intake in normal-weight women. *Am J Clin Nutr* 1998; 67: 412–20.

14. Rolls BJ. The role of energy density in the overconsumption of fat. *J Nutr* 2000; 130: S268–S271.

Progress in Obesity Research: 9. Edited by *Geraldo Medeiros-Neto, Alfredo Halpern and Claude Bouchard*
©2003 John Libbey Eurotext Ltd, pp. 842–847.

CHAPTER 178

The obesity phenotype and ageing connection in genetically altered FORKO mice

M. Ram Sairam, Min Wang, Natalia Danilovich and Weirong Xing

Molecular Reproduction Research Laboratory, Clinical Research Institute of Montreal, 110 Pine Avenue West, Montreal, Quebec, Canada H2W 1R7
[e-mail: sairamm@ircm.qc.ca]

Introduction

Obesity is one of the most serious nutritional disorders that has become a national problem in many industrialized countries and rapidly gaining ground in a growing number of developing countries. In addition to changes in food habits, physical activity and metabolic factors, gender and hormonal status including ageing play a significant role in the appearance as well as the severity of obesity. Ovarian steroid hormones for example exert significant modulating influence on the metabolism of adipose tissue[1–4] in the female. In addition, estrogen plays an important role in determining the regional specificity of distribution of adipose tissue localization and metabolism[5–7]. Disorders such as polycystic ovarian disease that afflict many women of reproductive age is a condition of steroid imbalance and androgen excess causing infertility and inducing obesity in approximately 50 per cent of the cases. In many of these overweight and obese individuals, obesity is predominantly abdominal[8]. Abdominal obesity occurring in many postmenopausal women is considered to be major risk factor for the higher incidence of cardiovascular complications and disease[6]. There is cross talk between steroid hormones and adipose tissue because the latter is known to impact on the metabolism of sex hormones[9] particularly after menopause when ovarian hormone production declines very steeply. Adipose tissue is the major site of peripheral aromatization of androgens to estrogens after menopause[10,11]. Thus, understanding the effects of ovarian function on adipose tissue is of major importance in tackling the problem of obesity and its associated ill effects on health during ageing such as type 2 diabetes and heart disease.

In this report we highlight the obesity phenotype that appears in genetically modified female and male mice in which the receptor for the glycoprotein hormone FSH (follitropin) has been deleted by homologous recombination. The null females are sterile due to failure of ovulation[12]. Due to estrogen deficiency, they develop various disorders that typify the postmenopausal state in women including obesity, kyphosis[13] ovarian tumours[14] as well as changes in the central and peripheral nervous systems[15]. The FSH receptor (FSH-R) is a major signaling system in the ovary that is expressed exclusively in granulosa cells of the follicle that contribute to estrogen production during each reproductive cycle. Our investigations reveal that major changes occur in the adipose tissue in null females and show how the lipid abnormalities may be corrected by estrogen replacement therapy[16].

Materials and methods

The single gene that codes for a variety of FSH-R's was deleted by homologous recombination techniques and mice of all three genotypes were obtained breeding the heterozygous mice in the SV129 background. Mice of different ages were used in our investigations as noted in the text or figure legends. The animals were fed normal diet chow without accounting for any phytoestrogen contribution that might be present in commercial formulations. Serum hormone levels and tissue estrogen receptor isoform determinations were performed by radioimmunoassay and western blotting respectively using specific antibodies[13]. Histological examination of different tissues at various months was performed to monitor the progression of age related changes. Plasma lipid profiles including Apo E content was performed by appropriate techniques as recently described[16]. Glucose intolerance was monitored by feeding the overnight fasted mice with glucose (1 mg/g body weight) and measuring serum glucose levels with the aid of Abbott diagnostics glucometer. Evaluations for statistical significance were performed by ANOVA or the *t*-test.

Results and discussion

Hormonal profiles (Figs. 1A, B)

The gene knockout studies in mice confirm that the FSH-R is a critical player in determining ovarian development and function. These include the two vital tasks of gametogenesis and steroidogenesis that are essential for species propagation. Consequently, abrogation of this gene results in complete sterility in the female and reduced fertility in the mutant male mutant[13]. In terms of key hormonal profiles we may note that estrogen is virtually absent from circulation in null females and the hormone FSH rises markedly as in postmenopausal women due to lack of negative steroid feedback. A notable difference

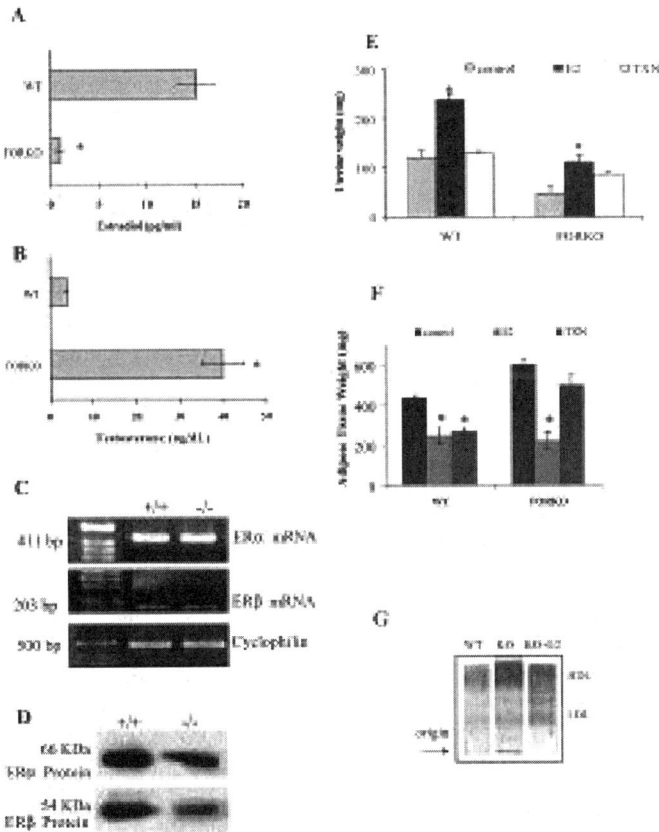

Fig. 1. Estrogen deficiency, nuclear receptors and hormone replacement in FORKO mice. (A and B) Estradiol-17ß and testosterone levels in 3–5 month old wild-type (WT) and FORKO females; (C) Expression (RT-PCR) of estrogen receptors α and ß mRNA's in uterus. The sizes of the amplified fragment and Mr ladder are shown; (D) Western blots of uterine extract using monoclonal antibody to ER α and ER ß peptide antibody; (E) Uterine weights in wild type and FORKO before and after estrogen treatment. *Signifies statistical difference (P < 0.01); (F) Adipose tissue weights and the effect of estrogen treatment; (G) Gel electrophoresis of plasma lipoproteins in female mice. Lane 1 – wild type, 2 – FORKO 3. Profile corrected by estrogen treatment.

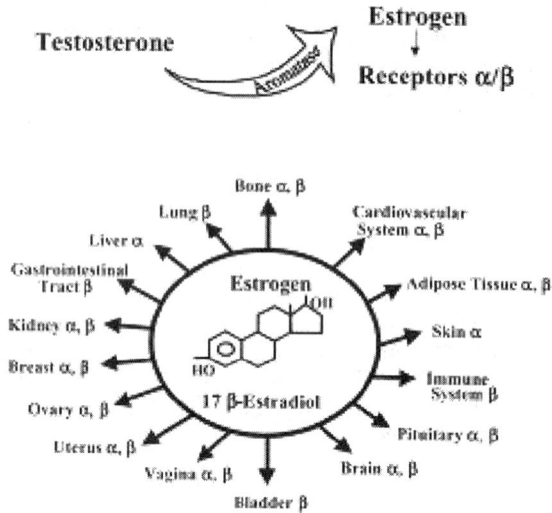

Fig. 2. Estrogen is a versatile hormone affecting many tissues in the female. It is formed from ovarian androgen by aromatase action and exerts its effects via at least two nuclear receptors ER α and ß whose distribution might vary. The diagram depicts a summary inferred from different studies. In the FORKO female estrogen is not formed despite high testosterone.

however, is the early elevation of serum testosterone that persists at different ages. In the mutant male the production of androgen is reduced by about 50 per cent[12] due to imbalances in the intracellular communication among testicular compartments. This induces a state equivalent to andropause that continues for the rest of the life in null males. Events that occur in the haploinsufficient females are of great interest because this represents a model of accelerated biological aging[17]. These +/– females that initially show reduced fertility undergo early reproductive senescence and become infertile similar to middle aged women. Consequently their hormonal profiles upon early ageing are altered to a form that resembles the null mouse. Despite the chronic loss of estrogen, the null females continue to express the ER α and ß receptors in target tissues as seen by the example of their evaluation in the atrophic uterus (Figs. 1C, D).

Body weight and obesity phenotype

At 3–4 months of age, the mutant females housed and fed under identical conditions were larger and heavier. A comparison of their body weights revealed a definite tendency towards obesity in proportion to disruption of the FSH-R gene. There was no evidence of hyperphagia in the genetically altered mice. The body weights of the FORKO and heterozygous animals were 20 per cent (23.5 g, $P < 0.03$) and 9.6 per cent (21.5 g) higher than age matched wild-type mice (19.6 g). These effects are also seen after ovariectomy[18], a surgical procedure that creates a loss of ovarian steroids as well as other secretions. Virtually all FORKO females revealed an increased deposition of abdominal adipose tissue (Fig. 1E). The total weight of adipose tissue in the abdominal area increased two fold in FORKO mice over the values in wild-type animals (600.2 ± 21.9 mg vs. 335.3 ± 15.5 mg, $P < 0.004$). Interestingly, although the body weight of 3–4 month-old heterozygotes is not yet significantly different from the wild-type littermates, around 10–12 months of age, all heterozygous females become obese (not shown). This age dependent phenomenon in heterozygous mice is related to the alteration of ovarian dynamics and accelerated loss of reproductive function induced by partial FSH-R gene disruption[17].

Estradiol 17 ß the principal estrogen in the female is a versatile hormone exerting positive and negative effects on many tissues in the body (see Fig. 2) including the adipose tissue. Its genomic actions are mediated by at least two nuclear receptors ER α and ß that may be differentially distributed in various targets. Estrogen is formed from the androgen (testosterone or androstenedione) in a reaction mediated by aromatase expressed in several tissues. In the null FORKO female the enzyme remains inactive and despite high substrate levels in the cell (Fig. 1B) no estrogen is produced. Among other effects[13] the lack of estrogen induces obesity in the FORKO females (both null and +/– but at different ages). The

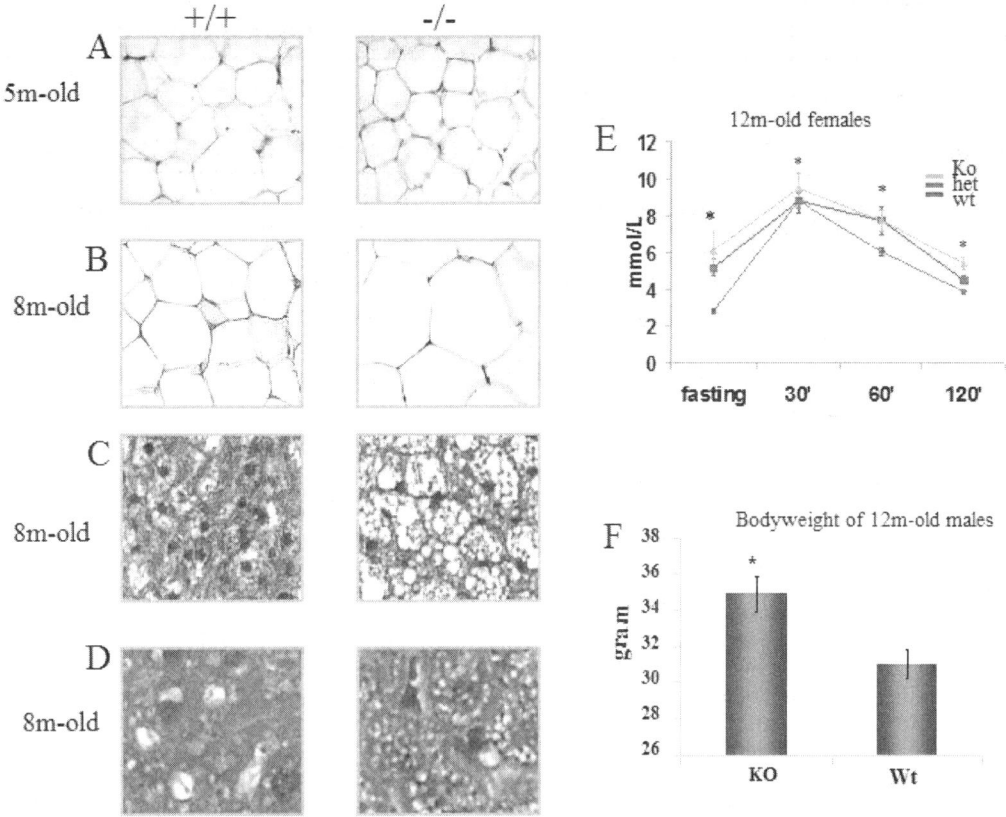

Fig. 3. Histology of adipose tissue and liver in females. (A) note more cells /area in –/– the adipose tissue indicating proliferation; (B) adipose tissue at 8 months indicates hypertrophy in –/– mice; (C) Brown adipose tissue; (D) Liver; (E) Higher basal glucose as well as glucose intolerance in aged –/– and +/– females; (F) Ageing and androgen deficient FORKO males show increased body weight.

appearance of obesity in ERα [19] and aromatase knockout mice[20] also confirms that lack of estrogen is an important contributor to the induction of obesity in the female.

Based on our histological and cellular examinations (Figs. 3A and B) we have concluded that lack of estrogen in FORKO females produces a proliferation of the adipocyte because cells appear to be smaller but numbers increase. With age these cells become bigger and accumulate more lipid stores. The brown adipocytes of FORKO's are also loaded with lipid at 8 months of age (Fig. 3C). The structures of hepatocytes are also different suggesting probable signs of steatosis (Fig. 3D), a condition that needs to be studied in greater detail. Ageing null females and heterozygotes develop glucose intolerance and by 1 year of age, their basal fasting glucose levels are significantly elevated. Clearance is also different from the wild type females. These data are reminiscent of those postmenopausal or PCO patients who develop type 2 diabetes under conditions of estrogen deficiency or androgen excess. Although we have not studied the null males in detail it is interesting to note that significant body weight difference occur in older mutants indicating signs of apparent obesity (Fig 3F).

Estrogen effects

In mice the major cholesterol carrier is HDL, an entity that is elevated in FORKO females (Fig. 1F, lane 2). These data are also supported by quantitative FPLC profiles of plasma lipoproteins[16]. Estrogen treatment of 5-month-old obese FORKO's completely reverses not only the amount of adipose tissue (Fig. 1G) but also corrects the plasma lipoproteins (Fig. 1F, lane 3) and increases Apo E levels[16]. Whether chronic estrogen deficiency contributes to the induction of atherogenesis is a question that needs to be addressed in future studies.

	Putative ERE	Putative PRE (GRE, ARE)
consensus binding site	**_GGTC_ACTGTGACC**	**T_GTAC_AGGAT_GTT_CT**
mFABP (GI: 507169)	2666—GGTAGATGTGACC--2678	2000...TGAGAACAGTGTGGT--2014
mUCP-1 (GI: 1519064)	900– GGTGAATGGGGCC–912	1222–TAGTTAAATTGTTCT--1236
mAcrp30 (GI: 13160934)	2007...GGTCAGAGAGATC..2020	595...AGTCTGGAGTGTTCT...609
mLeptin (GI: 1845603)	1943...AGCCTGGGTGACC..1955	5170...AGAGGGCTCTGTTCT..5184
mPPAR (GI: 20832062)	1777...GGTTAATCTGACC..1789	11150...TATTCAAACTGTTCT..11164
mResistin (GI: 20860492)	1748...GGTCATCCTGGTG..1760	2418...GAACCACATTGTACA...2432
hPTP1B (GI: 13919644)	19......AGGCAACCTGACC....31	436...TTTCTCTCTTGTTCT..422

Table 1. Potential steroid hormone response elements in adipocyte and related target genes

Based on a preliminary survey of the data in the gene bank we have highlighted a few genes that might impact on the adipose tissue and contain putative hormone responsive elements in their promoter regions (Table 1). Although this is not an exhaustive compilation, the list includes several adipocyte-derived proteins. A positive or negative regulation of these and other genes would affect significantly on the metabolic activity of the adipose tissue. With the recent recognition of the adipose tissue as an endocrine organ, we are currently exploring some of the novel adipocyte derived factors that could be altered in the estrogen deficient state. Using the FORKO model there is an excellent opportunity for exploring the genomic and proteomic profiles of adipose tissue at different stages of obesity aiding the discovery of novel therapeutic measures including non-hormonal agents that are selectively targeted to the adipocyte.

References

1. Hansjen. FM, Fahmy N, Nielsen JH. The influence of sexual hormones on lipogenesis and lipolysis in rat fat cells. *Acta Endocrinol* 1980; 95: 566–70.

2. Pedersen SD, Borglum JD, Moller-Pedersen T, Richelsen B. Effects of *in vitro* estrogen treatment on adipose tissue metabolism and nuclear estrogen binding in isolated rat adipocytes. *Mol Cell Endocrinol* 1992; 85: 13–9.

3. Krakower GR, James RG, Arnaud C, Etienne J, Keller RH, Kissebah AH. Regional adipocyte precursors in the female rat. Influence of ovarian factors. *J Clin Invest* 1988; 81: 41–648.

4. Rebuffé-Scrive M, Lonnroth P, Wesslau MC, Bjorntorp P. Regional adipose tissue metabolism in men and post menopausal women. *Int J Obes* 1987; 11: 347–55.

5. Lacasa D, Agli B, Mur, Dausse JP, Giudicelli Y. Influence of ovarian status and regional fat distribution on protein kinase C in rat fat cells. *J Endocrinol* 1994; 140: 257–82.

6. Larsson B, Bengtsson C, Bjorntorp P, Lapidus L, Sjostrom L, Svardsudd K *et al.* Is abdominal body fat distribution a major explanation for the sex difference in the incidence of myocardial infarction? The study of men born in 1913 and the study of women in Goteborg, Sweden. *Am J Epidemiol* 1992; 135: 266–73.

7. Gambacciani M, Ciaponi M, Cappagli B, Piaggesi L, De Simone L, Orlandi R, Gemazzani AR. Body weight, body fat distribution and hormonal replacement therapy in early postmenopausal women. *J Clin Endocrinol Metab* 1997; 82: 414–7.

8. Gambineri A, Pelusi C, Vicennati V, Pagotto U, Pasquali R. Obesity and the polycystic ovary syndrome. *Int J Obes* 2002; 26: 883–96.

9. Desypere JP, Verdonk L, Vermulen A. Fat tissue: a steroid reservoir and site of steroid metabolism. *J Clin Endocrinol Metab* 1985; 61: 564–70.

10. Simpson ER, Merril JC, Hollub AJ, Graham-Lorence S, Mendelson CR (Regulation of estrogen biosynthesis by human adipose cells. *Endocr Rev* 1989; 10: 136–48.

11. Szymczak J, Milewicz A, Thijssen JHH, Blankenstein MA, Daroszewski J. Concentration of sex steroids in adipose tissue after menopause. *Steroids* 1998; 63: 319–21.

12. Sairam MR, Dierich A, Monaco L, Fimia GM, Gansmuller A, LeMeur M, Sassone-Corsi P. Impairing follicle-stimulating hormone (FSH) signaling *in vivo*. Targeted disruption of the FSH receptor leads to aberrant gametogenesis and hormonal imbalance. *Proc Natl Acad Sci* 1998; 95: 13612–7.

13. Danilovich N, Babu PS, Xing W, Gerdes M, Krishnamurthy H, Sairam MR. Estrogen deficiency, obesity and skeletal abnormalities in follicle-stimulating hormone receptor knockout (FORKO) female mice. *Endocrinology* 2000; 141: 4295–308.

14. Danilovich N, Roy I, Sairam MR. Ovarian pathology and high incidence of sex cord tumors in follitropin receptor knockout (FORKO) mice. *Endocrinology* 2001; 142: 3673–84.

15. Tam J, Danilovich N, Nilsson K, Sairam MR, Maysinger D. Chronic estrogen deficiency leads to molecular aberrations related to neurodegenerative changes in follitropin receptor knockout female mice. *Neuroscience* 2002; 114: 493–506.

16. Sairam MR, Danilovich N, Lussier-Cacan S. The FORKO mouse as a genetic model for exploring estrogen replacement therapy. *J Reprod Med* 2002; 47: 412–8.

17. Danilovich N, Sairam MR. Haploinsufficiency of the Follicle-Stimulating Hormone Receptor Accelerates Oocyte Loss Inducing Early Reproductive Senescence and Biological Aging in Mice. *Biol Reprod* 2002; 67: 361–9.

18. Ke HZ, Paralkar VM, Grasser WA, Crawford DT, Qi H, Simmons HA, Pirie CM *et al*. Effects of CP-336,156, a new, nonsteroidal estrogen agonist/antagonist, on bone, serum cholesterol, uterus and body composition in rat models. *Endocrinology* 1998; 139: 2068–76.

19. Heine PA, Taylor JA, Iwamoto GA, Lubahn DB, Cooke PS. Increased adipose tissue in male estrogen receptor á knockout mice. *Proc Natl Acad Sci* 2000; 97: 12729–34.

20. Jones MEE, Thorburn AW, Britt KL, Hewitt KN, Wreford NG, Proietto J *et al*. Aromatase-deficient (ArKO) mice have a phenotype of increased adiposity. *Proc Natl Acad Sci* 2000; 97: 12735–40.

Progress in Obesity Research: 9. Edited by *Geraldo Medeiros-Neto, Alfredo Halpern and Claude Bouchard*
©2003 John Libbey Eurotext Ltd, pp. 848–851.

CHAPTER 179

Effects of estrogen and phytoestrogen signaling through estrogen receptor α (ERα) and ERβ on adipose tissue in males and females

Paul S. Cooke[1,2], Afia Naaz[1], Patricia A. Heine[1], Melissa A. Zakroczymski[1], Philippa T.K. Saunders[3], Julia A. Taylor[4], Robert H. Eckel[5], Dalan R. Jensen[5], William G. Helferich[2,6] and Dennis B. Lubahn[4]

Departments of [1]Veterinary Biosciences and [6]Food Science and Nutrition and [2]Division of Nutritional Sciences, University of Illinois, Urbana, IL 61802, USA; [3]MRC Human Reproductive Sciences Unit, Centre for Reproductive Biology, The University of Edinburgh Academic Centre, Edinburgh EH16 4SB, Scotland, UK; [4]Departments of Biochemistry and Child, University of Missouri-Columbia, Columbia, MO 65211, USA; [5]Department of Medicine, University of Colorado Health Sciences Center, Denver, CO 80262, USA
[email: p-cooke@uiuc.edu]

Introduction

The high and increasing incidence of obesity in human populations worldwide, and the associated impact on human morbidity and mortality, have made understanding the factors that regulate adipose tissue an important research priority. Estrogens such as 17β-estradiol (E2) regulate the growth, development and function of female reproductive organs, but it has become increasingly clear in recent years that estrogens have critical actions in a variety of non-reproductive targets such as the cardiovascular system, bone, immune system and adipose tissue, and that estrogens also have important functions in males[1–3]. This review will focus on recent studies related to understanding how estrogens act to regulate the amount and activity of adipose tissue, and will also discuss effects on adipose tissue of phytoestrogens, plant-derived estrogens that are consumed by humans as well as companion, food and laboratory animals.

Results and discussion

Lack of estrogen receptor alpha (ERα) induces obesity in both male and female mice

It has been know for many years that estrogen is a major regulator of adipose tissue in females, based on the increase seen in adipose tissue in laboratory animals following ovariectomy and in women following menopause, and the ability of estrogen replacement to reverse this increase. However, the specific role of individual estrogen receptors in adipose tissue deposition and function, as well as the possible role of estrogen in male adipose tissue, has been unclear. In mammals, E2 acts through two nuclear receptors, the classical ERα and the more recently discovered ERβ, though there is evidence that membrane estrogen receptors may also be important for some aspects of E2 signaling. ERα and ERβ are widely distributed in reproductive and non-reproductive tissues in both males and females, and human adipose tissue expresses both ERα and ERβ[4].

The recent availability of knockout animals, in which a particular gene is inactivated and the resulting phenotypic and functional changes can be studied, has provided a powerful tool to assess the role of both ERα and ERβ in adipose tissue. We have used the ERα knockout (αERKO) mouse to gain insight into the role of E2/ER signaling in both male and female adipose tissue.

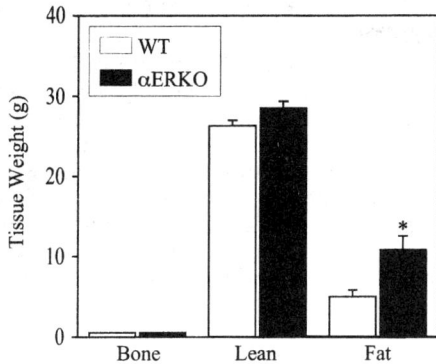

Fig. 1. Dual energy X-ray absorptiometry (DEXA) analysis of body composition in WT and αERKO mice (120–150 days old). A significant* increase was observed in adipose tissue in the αERKO compared to the WT mice ($P < 0.01$).

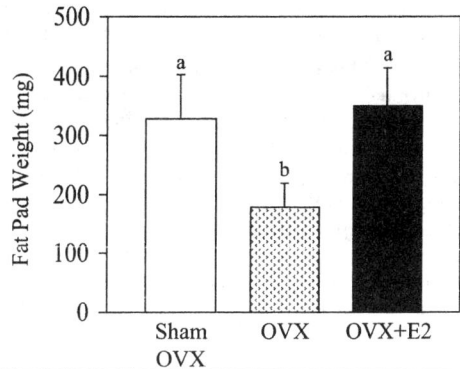

Fig. 2. Inguinal fat pad weights 28 days after surgery in αERKO mice that were either sham ovariectomized (Sham OVX) or ovariectomized with (OVX-E2) or without (OVX) E2 replacement (5 μg/kg/day). Values with different superscripts are significantly different from each other at $P < 0.05$. The $n = 7$, 5 and 9 for the Sham OVX, OVX-E2 and OVX groups respectively. Data are shown as mean ± SEM.

Male and female αERKO mice both have increased adult body weight compared to wild-type (WT) mice. Utilizing dual energy X-ray absorptiometry, we were able to show that this increase in weight resulted from an increase in adipose tissue (Fig. 1). Individual fat pad weights were increased in αERKO vs. WT mice, and this increase was age-related; for example, fat pads in αERKO males weigh 140–185 per cent more than those in WT mice at days 270–360. Morphometric examination indicated that the increase in adipose tissue in αERKO males was due to both adipocyte hypertrophy and hyperplasia[5].

The obesity observed in αERKO mice is not associated with an increase in food intake. Indirect calorimetry studies show that αERKO mice have a lower energy expenditure that is attributable primarily to a decreased resting metabolic rates but also appears to be due to a reduction in voluntary activity (Heine *et al.*, unpublished).

The obese phenotype in αERKO mice is associated with glucose intolerance and insulin resistance in both male and females. Humans with genetic mutations that result in either a non-functional ERα gene or a lack of endogenous estrogen production also show alterations in glucose tolerance and insulin sensitivity and have a tendency toward obesity[6], indicating that the αERKO mouse model appears highly relevant to humans.

The obese phenotype and many of the adipocyte and metabolic changes seen in the αERKO mouse are also seen in the aromatase knockout (ArKO) mouse[7]. ArKO mice cannot produce endogenous estrogens and are therefore deficient in E2 signaling through both ERα and ERβ. The similar obese phenotypes in both αERKO and ArKO mice, despite the loss of both ERα and ERβ signaling in the latter, indicates that ERα is the major signaling pathway through which E2 or other compounds such as dietary phytoestrogens act to regulate adipose tissue.

Effects of E2/ER signaling in adipose tissue

Circulating E2 is increased 10-fold in αERK0 females, and some metabolic and/or phenotypic changes seen in obese αERKO mice could involve ER signaling. To analyse this, we ovariectomized αERKO mice to determine if the loss of E2/ERβ signaling in an endocrine environment where E2/ERα signaling had already been eliminated resulted in phenotypic or functional changes in adipose tissue.

Age-matched female WT or αERKO (12–13 weeks old) mice were ovariectomized or sham ovariectomized and maintained on a phytoestrogen-free diet. Mice were treated with vehicle or E2, and body weights were measured. After 28 days, WT mice showed an increase in body weight, but αERK0 mice showed a 6 per cent decrease[8]. Inguinal and parametrial fat pads of ovariectomized αERKO mice showed about a 45 per cent decrease in weight compared to sham or E2-replaced ovariectomized αERKO mice (Fig. 2). There was a 16 per cent decrease in adipocyte circumference in ovariectomized αERKO mice compared to sham ovariectomized αERKO mice, and this decrease was reversed by E2 replacement (circumference = 250 ± 5 μm, 191 ± 2 μm and 270 ± 4 μm for sham ovariectomized, ovariectomized and E2-replaced ovariectomized αERKO mice respectively).

Blood glucose levels were lower both before and after a bolus injection of glucose in ovariectomized αERKO mice compared to sham ovariectomized αERKO mice, and E2 treatment partially reversed these effects[8]. Immunohistochemical analysis revealed strong staining for ERβ in adipose tissue. These observations suggest that estrogen might affect adipose tissue even in the absence of ERα, possibly through ERβ. ERβ signaling may have a stimulatory effect on adipose deposition, and removing E2/ERβ signaling by ovariectomy of mice lacking ERα appears to concomitantly decrease body weight, fat pad weight and adipocyte size, and improve glucose metabolism. Though E2 effects on adipose tissue appear to be predominately mediated by ERα, these results suggest ERβ can have effects on adipose tissue that are opposite those mediated by ERα, and the opposing effects of these two ERs in adipose tissue are similar to those in organs such as uterus[9].

The phytoestrogen genistein can have effects on adipose tissue

Phytoestrogens are plant-derived estrogens, which can bind to ER and mimic the actions of E2 on target tissues. The isoflavone genistein is a phytoestrogen found in high concentrations in soy and soy products, and is a major source of phytoestrogen exposure for both humans and animals. Genistein acts as an estrogen *in vivo* and causes uterine growth, both in intact and ovariectomized animals. Genistein binds to both ERα and ERβ. Binding affinity is greater for ERβ than ERα, but genistein is a complete agonist through ERα, and only a partial agonist through ERβ.

Although genistein is a weaker estrogen than E2, humans and animals can be exposed to high levels of this isoflavone. For example, genistein and other soy isoflavones are consumed by Oriental populations at a level of up to 1 mg/kg/day, and human infants fed soy formula consume even higher quantities of isoflavones on a per weight basis[11]. Humans consuming soy/isoflavone supplements are exposed to isoflavone levels that exceed those obtained with even a high-soy diet[12]. Soy is an economical source of high-quality protein, and soy is used extensively in feed for animals such as swine, dogs and cats[13]. Most commercial rodent chows used for laboratory rodents are also soy-based[14]. Thus, different segments of the human population, as well as some food, companion and laboratory animals, are exposed to high amounts of genistein and other isoflavones.

Based on its known estrogenicity, we hypothesized that genistein could induce anti-lipogenic effects in mice, and to test this we recently analysed the ability of injected and dietary genistein to inhibit the increase in adipose tissue which normally occurs after ovariectomy[15]. Daily subcutaneous injections of genistein (80 or 200 mg/kg/day) into juvenile or adult (30- or 100-day-old) ovariectomized C57/BL6 mice for 28 days produced significant decreases in fat pad weight compared to vehicle-treated controls. These doses of genistein produce peak serum genistein concentrations greater than those reported in humans or animals consuming genistein. In addition, injection produces differences in pharmacokinetics and metabolism compared to dietary ingestion. Despite the effects of injected genistein, it was therefore unclear whether dietary genistein at levels that produce serum genistein concentrations in the range of those reported in humans and animals under different nutritional conditions would produce demonstrable effects on adipose tissue. To test the effects of dietary genistein, mice (32- to 34-day old) were fed for 12 days with a semi-purified phytoestrogen-free diet (AIN-93G) to which 0, 300, 500, 1000 or 1500 parts per million (ppm) of genistein were added. Mice fed 500, 1000 or 1500 ppm of dietary genistein had significant dose-responsive decreases in parametrial fat pad weights of 37 per cent, 40 per cent and 57 per cent, respectively, compared to controls[15]. Parametrial fat pad weights in mice fed 300 ppm genistein were not different from controls. Average serum genistein concentrations in the mice fed 500–1500 ppm dietary genistein were between 1.79 and 3.81 μM[15], less than the concentrations reported in humans under certain nutritional conditions[11].

Previous work has indicated that rats or mice fed soy-based diets weighed less than those fed similar diets without soy[16], and the saponins have been implicated as one component in soy that can have effects on adipose tissue[17]. The adipose effects seen with serum genistein concentrations in the physiological range for both humans and animals indicates that dietary isoflavones can induce clear effects on adipose tissue and may do so at serum concentrations that humans and animals could realistically be exposed to.

Acknowledgements: This work supported by grants from the United Soybean Board, the Illinois Council on Food and Agricultural Research (CFAR), and Animal and Health and Disease Research Funds from the University of Illinois.

References

1. Yellayi S, Naaz A, Szewczykowski MA, Sato T, Woods JA, Chang J *et al.* The phytoestrogen genistein induces thymic and immune changes: A human health concern? *Proc Natl Acad Sci* 2002; 99: 7616–21.

2. Yellayi S, Teuscher C, Woods JA, Welsh THJ, Tung KS, Nakai M *et al.* Normal development of thymus in male and female mice requires estrogen/estrogen receptor-alpha signaling pathway. *Endocrine* 2000; 12: 207–13.

3. Hess RA, Bunick D, Lee KH, Bahr J, Taylor JA, Korach KS, Lubahn DB. A role for estrogens in the male reproductive system. *Nature* 1997; 390: 509–12.

4. Pedersen SB, Bruun JM, Hube F, Kristensen K, Hauner H, Richelsen B. Demonstration of estrogen receptor subtypes alpha and beta in human adipose tissue: influences of adipose cell differentiation and fat depot localization. *Mol Cell Endocrinol* 2001; 182: 27–37.

5. Heine PA, Taylor JA, Iwamoto GA, Lubahn DB, Cooke PS. Increased adipose tissue in male and female estrogen receptor-alpha knockout mice. *Proc Natl Acad Sci* 2000; 97: 12729–34.

6. Morishima A, Grumbach MM, Simpson ER, Fisher C, Qin K. Aromatase deficiency in male and female siblings caused by a novel mutation and the physiological role of estrogens. *J Clin Endocrinol Metab* 1995; 80: 3689–98.

7. Jones ME, Thorburn AW, Britt KL, Hewitt KN, Wreford NG, Proietto J, Oz OK, Leury BJ, Robertson KM, Yao S, Simpson ER. Aromatase-deficient (ArKO) mice have a phenotype of increased adiposity. *Proc Natl Acad Sci* 2000; 97:12735–40.

8. Naaz A, Zakroczymski MA, Heine P, Bunick D, Saunders P, Lubahn DB, Taylor JA, Cooke PS. Effect of ovariectomy on adipose tissue of mice in the absence of estrogen receptor α (ERα): a potential role for estrogen receptor β (ERβ). *Endocrinology* 2002; 34:758–63.

9. Weihua Z, Saji S, Makinen S, Cheng G, Jensen EV, Warner M, Gustafsson JA. Estrogen receptor (ER) beta, a modulator of ER alpha in the uterus. *Proc Natl Acad Sci* 2000; 97: 5936–41.

10. Kuiper GG, Carlsson B, Grandien K, Enmark E, Haggblad J, Nilsson S, Gustafsson JA. Comparison of the ligand binding specificity and transcript tissue distribution of estrogen receptors alpha and beta. *Endocrinology* 1997; 138: 863–70.

11. Setchell KD, Zimmer-Nechemias L, Cai J, Heubi JE. Exposure of infants to phyto-oestrogens from soy-based infant formula. *Lancet* 1997; 350: 23–7.

12. Busby MG, Jeffcoat AR, Bloedon LT, Koch MA, Black T, Dix KJ *et al.* Clinical characteristics and pharmacokinetics of purified soy isoflavones: single-dose administration to healthy men. *Am J Clin Nutr* 2002; 75: 126–36.

13. Court MH, Freeman LM. Identification and concentration of soy isoflavones in commercial cat foods. *Am J Vet Res* 2002; 63: 181–5.

14. Brown NM, Setchell KD. Animal models impacted by phytoestrogens in commercial chow: implications for pathways influenced by hormones. *Lab Invest* 2001; 81: 735–47.

15. Naaz A, Yellayi S, Szewczykowski MA, Bunick D, Lubahn DB, Helferich WG, Cooke PS. The soy isoflavone genistein decreases adipose deposition in mice. *Endocrinology* (in press).

16. Aoyama T, Fukui K, Takamatsu K, Hashimoto Y, Yamamoto T. Soy protein isolate and its hydrolysate reduce body fat of dietary obese rats and genetically obese mice (yellow KK). *Nutrition* 2000; 16: 349–54.

17. Kawano-Takahashi Y, Ohminami H, Okuda H, Kitagawa I, Yoshikawa M, Arichi S, Hayashi T. Effect of soya saponins on gold thioglucose (GTG)-induced obesity in mice. *Int J Obes* 1986; 10: 293–302.

Progress in Obesity Research: 9. Edited by *Geraldo Medeiros-Neto, Alfredo Halpern and Claude Bouchard*

©2003 John Libbey Eurotext Ltd, pp. 852–856.

CHAPTER 180

Aromatase deficient (ArKO) mice have a phenotype of increased adiposity

Margaret E.E. Jones[1], Anne W. Thorburn[2], Kara L. Britt[1], Kylie N. Hewitt[1], Marie L. Misso[1], Nigel G. Wreford[3], Joseph Proietto[2], Orhan K. Oz[4], Brian J. Leury[5], Kirsten M. Robertson[1], Shenggen Yao[6] and Evan R. Simpson[1]

[1]*Prince Henry's Institute of Medical Research, Clayton, Victoria, Australia;* [2]*Department of Medicine, Royal Melbourne Hospital, Victoria, Australia;* [3]*Department of Anatomy, Monash University, Clayton, Victoria, Australia;* [4]*University of Texas, Southwestern Medical Center, Dallas, Texas, USA;* [5]*Department of Animal Production, University of Melbourne, Victoria, Australia;* [6]*Howard Florey Institute, Parkville, Victoria, Australia*
[e-mail: Margaret.Jones@med.monash.edu.au]

Introduction

Estrogen plays an integral role in lipid homeostasis and adipose tissue deposition and distribution. The sexually dimorphic distribution of adipose tissue in humans has implicated sex steroids in the regulation of adiposity and distribution of fat depots[1,2]. Estrogen insufficiency is thought to be largely responsible for the increase in adiposity during menopause since postmenopausal women who receive estrogen replacement therapy do not display the characteristic abdominal weight gain pattern usually associated with menopause[3,4]. The role that estrogens play in lipid metabolism in the body is also highlighted by the fact that individuals of both sexes with natural mutations of the gene encoding aromatase, the enzyme responsible for estrogen biosynthesis, develop truncal obesity, insulin resistance, hypercholesterolaemia and hypertriglyceridaemia[5–8].

We have developed a mouse model of estrogen insufficiency by targeted disruption of the aromatase gene (the ArKO mouse)[9]. Aromatase is encoded by the *Cyp*19 gene and catalyses the final step in the biosynthesis of C_{18} estrogens from C_{19} steroids. Hence we have further investigated the relationship between estrogen and fat by exploring the phenotype of our estrogen-deficient mouse model. This review summarizes our observations and presents evidence for the role of estrogens in lipid homeostasis.

ArKO mice accumulate excess adipose tissue

Previous studies by this group[9,10] have reported that female ArKO mice are significantly heavier and have significantly larger fat deposits than WT littermates from 3 months onwards (Fig. 1). Male ArKO mice also have significantly heavier fat pads than WT males (Fig. 1). In agreement with this data, both MRI and body composition analyses have shown that ArKO mice have a significantly greater percentage of adipose tissue than their WT litter mates from as early as 10 weeks, through to 1 year. Body composition analyses confirmed that the increase in fat mass was accompanied by a significant decrease in lean mass in the ArKO mice[10].

Administration of exogenous 17β-estradiol to female and male ArKO mice restored their fat depots to masses comparable to, or less than, those of WT littermates[10], indicating a significant role between the action of estrogen and the accumulation of fat. Stereological analyses of sectioned fat depots revealed that this increase in fat mass resulted from an increase in both adipocyte volume and number which also was reversed with 17β-estradiol treatment (Table 1)[10].

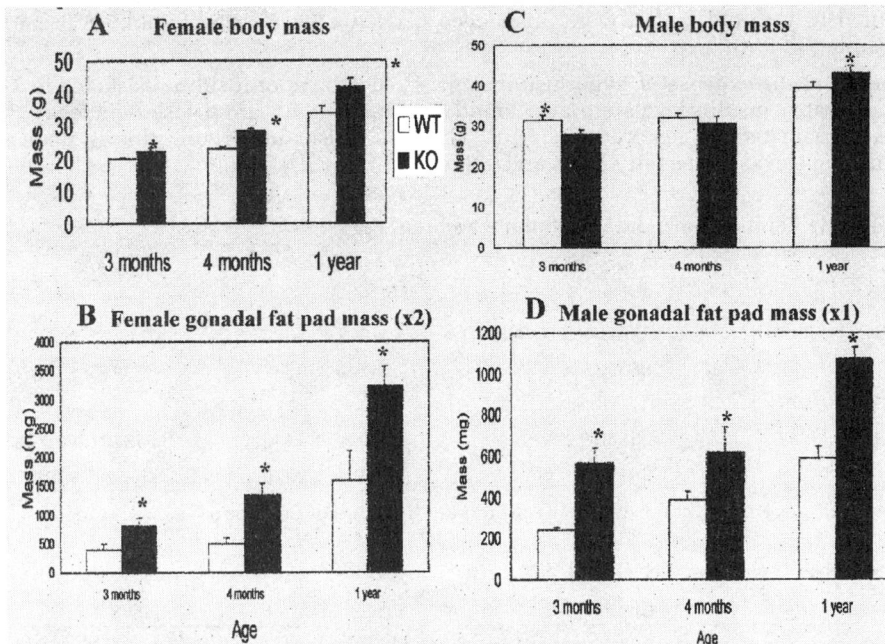

Fig. 1. (A) Body mass (g) for ArKO vs. wildtype female mice; (B) Gonadal fat pad (x2) mass (g) for ArKO vs. wildtype female mice; (C) Body mass (g) for ArKO vs. wildtype male mice; (D) Gonadal fat pad (x1) mass (g)for ArKO vs. wildtype male mice. *$P \leq 0.05$.

ArKO mice are not hyperphagic

Increased adiposity in the ArKO mice has not been associated with hyperphagia. In fact, there has been reported a strong trend for food intake to be lower in ArKO mice compared to WT mice (15.7 ± 0.8 vs. 19.1 ± 1.1 kcal/day, $P = 0.06$)[10]. Adiposity in the older female ArKO mice, however, has been related to reduced spontaneous physical activity with ArKO mice half as active as WT mice (43,285 ± 4205 vs. 93,839 ±15,925 ambulatory movements/d, $P < 0.01$). A similar trend was observed in the younger mice although this was not significant. Resting energy expenditure was not significantly lower in ArKO mice compared to WT mice (5.99 ± 0.33 vs. 6.68 ± 0.56 kcal/day) and fat oxidation rates were not significantly higher in the ArKO mice compared to WT mice (0.34 ± 0.02 vs. 0.32 ± 0.03 mg/min). Glucose oxidation rates, however, were 59 per cent lower in the ArKO mice (0.11 ± 0.03 vs. 0.26 ± 0.05 mg/min, $P < 0.02$).

The reduced spontaneous physical activity found in the ArKO mice may be partly responsible for the increase in fat pad mass. It is of interest that reduced physical activity is also reported to be a feature of estrogen deficiency in both ovariectomized animals[11] and postmenopausal women[12]. Reduced physical activity in the ArKO mice may be secondary to the increase in fat mass and decrease in lean body mass seen in these mice, however, it is also possible that this inactivity is caused by an effect of estrogen insufficiency on the function of the central nervous system in these mice.

Circulating cholesterol, triglycerides and HDL

Although there are no differences in serum cholesterol, triglycerides and HDL between knockout and WT young (3–4 months) ArKO male and female mice, differences are observed by one year of age in both genders. One year old female and male ArKO mice had significantly elevated circulating cholesterol and HDL levels compared to gender-matched WT control littermates. At 1 year there was no difference in circulating triglyceride levels between ArKO and WT females. However, triglyceride levels were significantly elevated in 1-year-old ArKO vs. WT males (Table 2).

ArKO mice may be insulin resistant

By 1 year ArKO males have a fourfold increase in the levels of insulin compared to WT mice (47.14 ± 12.46 mU/l (6) vs. 12.42 ± 3.27 mU/l,[5] mean ± SEM (n), $P = 0.02$). Glucose levels on the other hand, when measured in year old males, were unchanged (ArKO: 8.52 ± 1.56 mmol/l;[3] WT: 8.61 ± 2.02 mmol/l,[3] mean ± SEM (n))[10].

Normoglycaemia at the expense of hyperinsulinaemia is suggestive of insulin resistance in 1-year-old ArKO mice. Elevated insulin levels are also found in humans with aromatase deficiency[5–7]. Insulin resistance is a characteristic feature of obesity. The mechanism underlying this is unclear, but it appears to involve elevated free fatty acids and TNFα[13,14].

Table 1. Adipocyte volume (μm³) data for female and male mice

		3 months	4 months	1 year
Females				
	ArKO	293280 ± 42383	509872 ± 36947*	458277 ± 53401*
	WT	288534 ± 51976	253296 ± 59477	319955 ± 24510
Males				
	ArKO	259504 ± 47184	531090 ± 44499*	652191 ± 67285*
	WT	264197 ± 60913	236304 ± 25756	254998 ± 50774

Mean ± SEM; *indicates $P \leq 0.05$ compared to WT. Minimum five animals per group.

Table 2. Serum lipid profile of ArKO and WT mice

	Cholesterol	Triglycerides	HDL
Females 1 year			
ArKO	4.34 ± 0.63 (5)*	2.28 ± 0.57 (5)	2.92 ± 0.33 (5)*
WT	2.74 ± 0.28 (5)	2.23 ± 0.49 (5)	1.77 ± 0.18 (5)
Males 1 year			
ArKO	4.79 ± 0.73 (7)*	3.27 ± 0.39 (7)*	2.84 ± 0.33 (7)*
WT	3.39 ± 0.29 (8)	2.08 ± 0.43 (8)	2.10 ± 0.26 (8)

All measurements reported in mmol/l. Mean ± SEM (n); * indicates at least $P < 0.05$ compared to WT.

Table 3. Serum leptin levels in ArKO and WT mice

	Females	Males
4 months		
ArKO	8.18 ± 0.78 (5)*	8.79 ± 1.83 (6)*
Wildtype	2.92 ± 0.68 (5)	3.81 ± 1.00 (7)
1 year		
ArKO	19.86 ± 4.90 (6)*†	8.47 ± 1.85 (7)*
Wildtype	6.19 ± 2.33 (4)†	4.89 ± 0.72 (8)

All measurements reported in ng/ml; Mean ± SEM (n).
* indicates at least $P < 0.05$ compared to age-matched WT mice;
† indicates at least $P < 0.05$ compared to 4-month old, genotype- and sex-matched mice.

Serum leptin levels are elevated

Circulating leptin levels were elevated two–threefold in 4 month old and 1 year old male and female ArKO mice compared to their WT littermates (Table 3). An age-related increase in leptin concentration is evident in both ArKO and WT female mice.

Elevated levels of circulating leptin in ArKO mice is not surprising, given the established association between obesity and increased production of leptin in most human subjects[15] and most animal models of obesity[16–19]. Leptin regulates body fat predominantly by decreasing food intake[20]. The fact that food intake is reduced in our ArKO mice suggests that these mice are responding normally to leptin.

Hepatic steatosis

General inspection of internal organs at necropsy revealed that in 1-year-old ArKO animals the liver was often larger and paler in colour than that of WT littermates. Following fixation, sectioning and staining, the livers of 3 month old and 1 year old ArKO animals were observed to have a greater accumulation of lipid droplets than WT control animals.

The observation that ArKO mice develop a fatty liver phenotype may be related to the observed hypercholesterolaemia. One of the ways in which estrogen is believed to lower circulating cholesterol is by increasing the level of LDL receptor expression in the liver and thus enhancing LDL uptake [21]. Moreover, mice deficient in the oxysterol receptor LXR (LXR–/–) fail to induce transcription of cholesterol 7β-hydroxylase (*Cyp* 7a), the rate-limiting enzyme in bile acid synthesis, and accumulate cholesterol in the liver and have marked hypercholesterolaemia [22]. It has been reported that estrogen and progesterone increase the activity of cholesterol 7α-hydroxylase[23], so it is conceivable that both the fatty liver and hypercholestrolaemia in the ArKO mice are due to a reduction in bile acid synthesis secondary to estrogen deficiency. Concomitant with a possible perturbation in this pathway, Nemoto *et al.* report impairment in hepatocellular fatty acid β-oxidation in an aromatase-deficient mouse model they have independently generated[24]. Analyses revealed a decrease in both mRNA expression and activities of specific enzymes required in fatty acid β-oxidation. Evidently estrogens play multiple roles in lipid homeostasis, crucially involved not only in adipose depot accretion, but also lipid turnover in the liver.

Conclusions

Studies on the Aromatase knockout (ArKO) mouse reinforce and extend the concept that estrogens play an important role in the regulation of adiposity as a function of age in both males and females[25]. ArKO mice of both sexes with estrogen insufficiency develop a progressive increase in adiposity, primarily as an accumulation of intra-abdominal fat. This excess fat accretion was associated with an increase in adipocyte volume and number, hyperleptinaemia, hyperinsulinaemia, and hypercholesterolaemia. However, unlike many other rodent models of obesity, excess body fat in the estrogen-insufficent ArKO mice was not due to hyperphagia or reduced resting energy expenditure, but was associated with decreased lean mass and reduced spontaneous physical activity. The obese phenotype is likely to be due to estrogen insufficiency rather than testosterone excess since 17β-estradiol treatment normalized body fat content in the ArKO mice, and the obese phenotype is similar in both male and female ArKO mice despite their greatly different testosterone levels. Furthermore, a similar phenotype of fat accumulation is observed in estrogen-deficient ovariectomized rats, which cannot synthesise androgens[11].

Evidence that estrogen action plays an important role in body fat deposition is provided not only by these studies on the ArKO mouse, but also by other rodent models of estrogen deprivation. Ovariectomized rats show an increase in body mass and fat deposition[11], as do follicle-stimulating hormone receptor (FORKO)[26] and estrogen receptor-α (αERKO) knockout mice[27]. Estrogen receptor-β (βERKO) mice, on the contrary, do not accumulate excess adipose tissue[28]. This observation suggests that estrogen action in terms of accumulation of fat is mediated via ERα rather than ERβ, consistent with reports by ourselves and others that ERα, but not ERβ, is present in adipose tissue[27–29].

At present it is not known whether the increase in abdominal adiposity resulting from estrogen deficiency reflects direct actions of estrogens on the adipose depots or central actions or both. Estrogen is known to have direct effects on adipose tissue, for example, oophorectomy decreases lipolysis in adipose tissue[30] of rats, and estradiol treatment lowers fatty acid synthesis and increases lipolysis in fat cells[31]. However, estrogen may also be involved in the central regulation of body weight. The fact that estrogen receptors are expressed within the central nervous system makes it possible that obesity in the ArKO and αERKO mice[27] is due, at least in part, to impaired signaling of estrogen through the α-estrogen receptor found in the hypothalamus of the brain. Investigations are currently underway to unravel the cellular and biochemical mechanisms underlying the physiological phenomena reported here.

Acknowledgements: This work is supported by USPHS grant #R37-AG 08174, grant # 169010 from the NHMRC, and by the Victorian Breast Cancer Research Consortium.

Abbreviations: ArKO, aromatase knockout; WT, wildtype.

References

1. De Ridder CM, Brunung PF, Zonderland ML, Thijssen JH, Bonfrer JM, Blankenstein MA *et al. J Clin Endocrinol Metab* 1990; 70: 888–93.

2. Elbers JMH, Asscheman H, Seidell JC, Gooren LJG. *Am J Physiol* 1999; 276: E317–E25.

3. Gambacciani M, Ciaponi M, Cappagli B, Piaggesi L, De Simone L, Orlandi R et al. *J Clin Endocrinol Metab* 1997; 82: 414–7.

4. Haarbo J, Marslew U, Gotfredsen A, Christiansen C. *Metab: Clin Experiment* 1991; 40: 1323–6.

5. Morishima A, Grumbach MM, Simpson ER, Fisher C, Qin K. *J Clin Endocrinol Metab* 1995; 80: 3689–98.

6. Carani C, Kenan K, Simoni M, Faustini-Fustini M, Serpente S, Boyd J et al. *New Engl J Med* 1997; 337: 91–5.

7. Bilezikian JP, Morishima A, Bell J, Grumbach MM. *New Engl J Med* 1998; 339: 599–603.

8. Conte FA, Grumbach MM, Ito Y, Fisher CR, Simpson ER. *J Clin Endocrinol Metab* 1994; 78: 1287–92.

9. Fisher CR, Graves KH, Parlow AF, Simpson ER. *Proc Natl Acad Sci* 1998; 95: 6965–70.

10. Jones MEE, Thorburn AW, Britt KL, Hewitt KN, Wreford NG, Proietto J et al. *Proc Natl Acad Sci* 2000; 97: 12735–40.

11. Wade GN. Gonadal hormones and behavioral regulation of body weight. *Physiol Behav* 1972; 8(3): 523–34.

12. Poehlman ET, Tchernof A. Traversing the menopause: changes in energy expenditure and body composition. *Coronary Artery Dis* 1998; 9(12): 799–803.

13. Unger RH. Lipotoxicity in the pathogenesis of obesity-dependent NIDDM. Genetic and clinical implications. *Diabetes* 1995; 44(8): 863–70.

14. Hotamisligil GS, Spiegelman BM. Tumor necrosis factor alpha: a key component of the obesity-diabetes link. *Diabetes* 1994; 43: 1271–8.

15. Hamilton BS, Paglia D, Kwan AY, Deitel M. Increased obese mRNA expression in omental fat cells from massively obese humans. *Nature Med* 1995; 1(9): 953–6.

16. Zhang Y, Proenca R, Maffei M, Barone M, Leopold L, Friedman JM. Positional cloning of the mouse obese gene and its human homologue. *Nature* 1994; 372(6505): 425–32.

17. Ogawa Y, Masuzaki H, Isse N, Okazaki T, Mori K, Shigemoto M et al. Molecular cloning of rat obese cDNA and augmented gene expression in genetically obese Zucker fatty (fa/fa) rats. *J Clin Invest* 1995; 96(3): 1647–52.

18. Collins S, Surwit RS. Pharmacologic manipulation of ob expression in a dietary model of obesity. *J Biol Chem* 1996; 271(16): 9437–40.

19. Funahashi T, Shimomura I, Hiraoka H, Arai T, Takahashi M, Nakamura T et al. Enhanced expression of rat obese (ob) gene in adipose tissues of ventromedial hypothalamus (VMH)-lesioned rats. *Biochem Biophys Res Commun* 1995; 211(2): 469–75.

20. Farooqi IS, Jebb SA, Langmack G, Lawrence E, Cheetham CH, Prentice AM et al. Effects of recombinant leptin therapy in a child with congenital leptin deficiency. *New Engl J Med* 1999; 341(12): 879–915.

21. Kovanen PT. Regulation of plasma cholesterol by hepatic low-density lipoprotein receptors. *Am Heart J* 1987; 113(2 Pt 2): 464–9.

22. Peet DJ, Turley SD, Ma W, Janowski BA, Lobaccaro JA, Hammer RE, Mangelsdorf DJ. Cholesterol and bile acid metabolism are impaired in mice lacking the nuclear oxysterol receptor LXR alpha. *Cell* 1998; 93(5): 693–704.

23. Chico Y, Fresnedo O, Botham K, Lacort M, Ochoa B. Regulation of bile acid synthesis by estradiol and progesterone in primary cultures of rat hepatocytes. Exp Clin Endocrinol. *Diabetes* 1996; 104(2): 137–44.

24. Nemoto Y, Toda K, Ono M, Fujikawa-Adachi K, Saibara T, Onishi S et al. J Altered expression of fatty acid-metabolizing enzymes in aromatase-deficient mice. *Clin Invest* 2000; 105(12): 1819–25.

25. Simpson ER, Rubin G, Clyne C, Robertson K, O'Donnell L, Jones M, Davis S. Natural (human) and experimental (mouse) models of estrogen insufficiency have revealed hitherto unexpected roles for estrogens in both males and females. In postmenopausal women, and in men, estrogen no longer. *Trends Endocrinol Metab* 2000, 11: 5: 184–188.

26. Danilovich N, Babu PS, Xing W, Gerdes M, Krishnamurthy H, Sairam MR. Estrogen deficiency, obesity, and skeletal abnormalities in follicle-stimulating hormone receptor knockout (FORKO) female mice. *Endocrinology* 2000; 141(141): 4295–308.

27. Heine PA, Taylor JA, Lubahn DB, Cooke PS. Increased adipose tissue in male and female estrogen receptor-alpha knockout mice. *Proc Natl Acad Sci* 2000; 97(23): 12729–34.

28. Couse JF, Korach KS. Estrogen receptor null mice: what have we learned and where will they lead us? *Endocrine Reviews* 1999; 20(3): 358–417.

29. Murata Y, Boon WC, Cox V, Oz OK, Thorburn A, Proietto J et al. US Endocrine Society 81st Annual Meeting. 1999; P2–198

30. Darimont C, Delansorne R, Paris J, Ailhaud G, Negrel R. Influence of estrogenic status on the lipolytic activity of parametrial adipose tissue *in vivo*: an *in situ* microdialysis study. *Endocrinology* 1997; 138(3): 1092–6.

31. Hansen FM, Fahmy N, Nielsen JH. The influence of sexual hormones on lipogenesis and lipolysis in rat fat cells. *Acta Endocrinol* 1980; 95(4): 566–70.

TRACK VI

MANAGEMENT AND TREATMENT

Progress in Obesity Research: 9. Edited by *Geraldo Medeiros-Neto, Alfredo Halpern and Claude Bouchard*
©2003 John Libbey Eurotext Ltd, pp. 859–865.

CHAPTER 181

Quality of life in the management of obesity

M.E.J. Lean and Jose Lara

Human Nutrition at Glasgow, University of Glasgow, Queen Elizabeth Building, Royal Infirmary, Glasgow G31 2ER, UK
[e-mail: lean@clinmed.gla.ac.uk]

Introduction

Why do people seek and undergo treatment for a medical problem? A simple enough question, but one which doctors, and other health professionals have too frequently failed to ask. Thus treatments have been developed for cancers which clinical trials can prove effective for limiting tumours growth, but which patients reject for the simple reason that they do not feel better. Patients commonly stop taking effective drugs for epilepsy (e.g. sodium valproate) or schizophrenia (atypical anti-psychotics) or diabetes (insulin, sulphonylureas) if they gain weight as a side effect. They do not, on balance, feel better, despite control of seizures or psychosis, or diabetes, if they gain weight, ie they perceive a decline in overall satisfaction or quality of life.

On the face of it, it might seem self-evident that being overweight or obese will make people feel unwell or unhappy, and weight loss can reasonably be expected to make them feel better. The surprise is that people who seek, and embark on, weight management so often stop treatment after very little weight loss, and put the weight back on.

There is evidence from a variety of sources that 'quality of life' is seriously impaired in overweight and obese people, compared to normal weight individuals. Obesity is the disease process of excess fat accumulation, which leads to a huge range of physical symptoms, organ-specific and systemic patholo- gies, and to psycho-social dysfunctions (Table 1). Because body weight increases over time, and so many of the medical and psycho-social consequences of weight gain are also functions of age. What is seen for many is an accelerated development of age-related medical problems in people who are overweight. This means that any analyses need to adjust for age. There are also associations between weight-gain and gender, socio-economic status, etc which need to be adjusted for analyses. Whether comparisons should be adjusted for level of physical activity, or for diet composition, are more difficult questions, because these two factors are aetiologically linked to weight gain, directly affected on a consequence of weight gain and also have weight-independent effects on symptoms and quality of life.

Choosing measures

It is important to choose appropriate measures for both overweight and for quality of life. The first issue should always be to establish exactly why they are to be measured – i.e. the purpose of the study or survey.

To measure overweight, we usually seek a measure of body fat. This is difficult to measure directly. The best indirect method is probably from deuterium dilution (to measure water space). If this rather expensive method is not availabie, the field methods include BMI, anthropometry by skinfolds orwaist circumference. The evidence is that waist, or skinfolds give reasonable estimates of total body fat in population (using underwater weighing as the reference method), with coefficients of determination about $R^2 = 0.8$. BMI is more influenced by variations in muscle mass and other tissues, so correlates a little less well with body fat ($R^2 = 0.7$)'. More indirect methods such as bio-electrical impedance h ave not been shown to be better measures of body fat than a simple waist circumference[2].

Although these methods give reasonable estimates of body fatness in groups, they are generally less precise than ideal for estimation in individuais. When changes in body composition and quality of life are under study, body weight often has to be taken as the independent variable – recognizing that although it will generaly give a good index of change in body fat during weight loss, there may be other influences on body weight change and the relationship between body weight change and fat change may vary between individuals.

Table 1. Medical and psychosocial consequences of overweight and obesity

Physical symptoms	Metabolic problems	Social problems
Tiredness	Hypertension	Isolation
Breathlessness	NIDDM	Agoraphobia
Varicose veins	Hepatic steatosis	Unemployment
Back pain	Hyperlipidaemia	Family/marital stress
Arthritis	Hypercoagulation	Discrimination
Oedema/cellulitis	IHD and stroke	Financial
Sweating/ intertrigo		
Stress incontinence		
Anaesthetic/surgical	**Endocrine problems**	**Psychological problems**
Sleep apnea	Hirsutism	Low self-esteem
Chest infections	Oligomenorrhea/infertility	Self-deception
Wound dehiscence	Metromenorrhea	Cognitive disturbance
Hernia	Oestrogen dependent	Distorted body image
Venous thrombosis	Cancers: breast, uterus, prostate	Depression

For these methods to measure body fat, to indicate 'overweight' or 'obesity' there is no true 'goldstandard' or correct answer, but they have ali been developed in terms of their ability to predict a reliable laboratory-based method – the reference method. The position is rather different in that there is no reference method for measuring quality of life. Instead, there are large numbers of questionnaires which address a range of issues which reflect some aspect of well-being, satisfaction, happiness or health. The emphasis given to different components varies between questionnaires. Many do not incorporate subject-specific weighting, to take account of individuais' personal evaluations of the impact of problems.

At a very simple level, quality of life may be influenced by factors in the external environment, in factors related to lifestyle and activities, factors related to interpersonal relationships, and to factors stemming from within the individual. The distinction between assessment of quality of life and of health should be a very fine one if the WHO[3] definition of health is taken, to include evaluation of all components of physical, mental and social well-being. However, for practical uses, questionnaire assessment of health status is usually, restricted to a small number of key concepts or domains, as a *generic* measure of health status, which is likely to give a reasonably close approximation to overall quality of life for most people or for groups.

Some generic questionnaires have been more commonly used, e.g. SF-36, however other questionnaires falling in this category are also available. They share many similarities, but some hold particular characteristics. For example the physical domain as assessed by the Nottingham Health Profile[4] emphasizes mobility, while the SF-36 has a broader approach to overall physical functioning. Thus although the Nottingham Health Profile[4] is considered as a generic instrument, it may be more appropriate for particular purposes, i.e. as 'disease-related quality of life' measure, such as the impact of hip replacement surgery, it is important to recognise that it has been found to reflect other diseases usefully. It is possible that some 'generic' questionnaires could be complementary to each other as well as to the disease-specific ones, however it is also true that some sections will not apply to the subjects under study.

More generic symptom questionnaires are available, but symptoms form only one aspect of the impact of disease on health, and disease forms only one of many influences on an individual's perceived

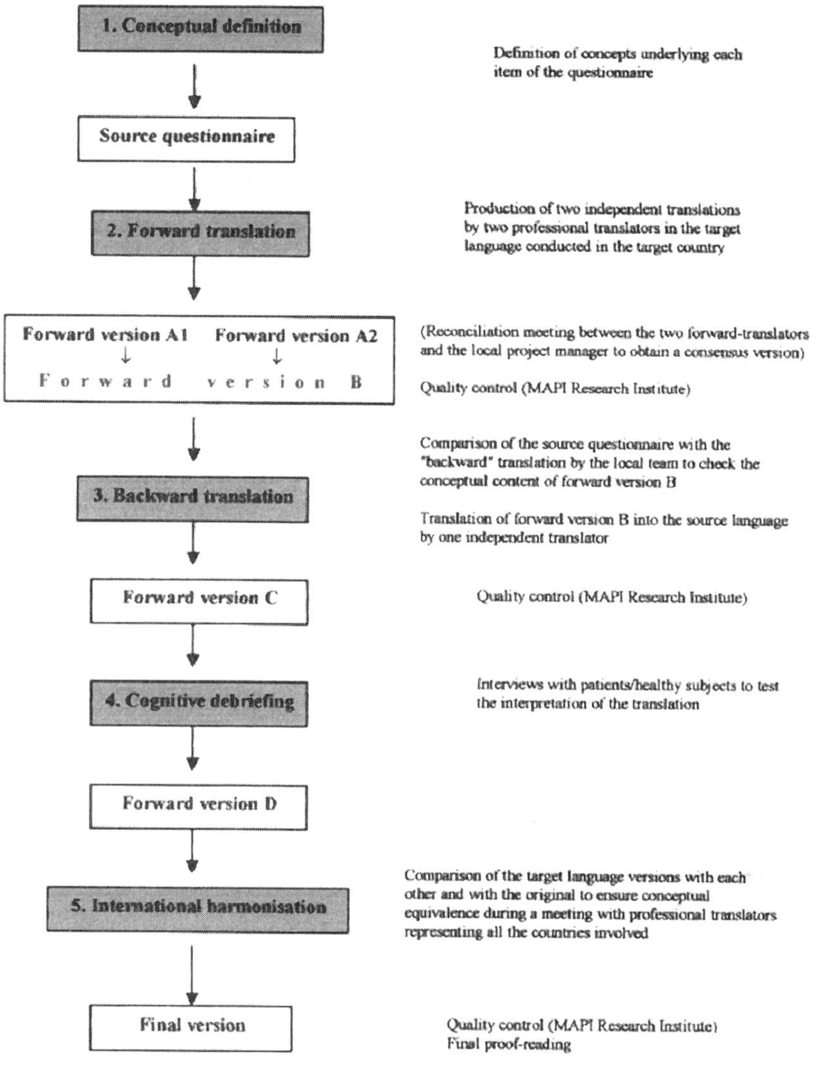

Fig. 1. MAPI Research Institute's linguistic validation process[6].

well-being or quality of life. Moreover, it is not possible simply to add up numbers of symptoms and produce a score which has any useful meaning. Perceived symptom severity needs to be incorporated, but also an evaluation of the impact of each symptom on that individual subject. Symptoms can be physical or mental of course, but subjects' evaluations are likely to reflect some of their own attribution and interpretation of symptoms.

Disease specific measures (often confusingly referred to as health-related!) often focus heavily on symptoms and functional consequences of disease which are likely to respond to treatment, and this may lead to misleading results when trying to predict overall well-being or satisfaction with treatment. For example, cancer treatment historically focussed heavily on pain. It came as a surprise to most doctors that the impact of pain for cancer patients is much less than that of fatigue[5].

Evidence for improved quality of life is increasingly used by pharmaceutical companies to persuade doctors to prescribe. This may be misleading if it is based on very specific or restricted disease-related ('health-related') topics. A further important issue is that mood or affect of subjects may affect how they respond to quality of life questionnaires, as well as affecting perceived quality of life. Patients may seek treatment when relatively depressed for other reasons. When other problems recede, and mood lifts, their disease or symptoms become less of a burden.

Values and norms differ between cultures, thus the fact that an original instrument has undergone a proper and comprehensive validation process does not guarantee that a translation into another language or to another population will possess satisfactory properties. The MAPI Research Institute[6] in France recommends a linguistic validation process summarized in Fig. 1. In addition, the Medical Outcome Trust has also established a minimal translation criteria required before endorsing any new translation[7]. To facilitate the search for relevant instruments, QOLID the 'Quality of Life Instruments Database'[6] developed by MAPI, and the Medical Outcomes Trust[7], offer a list of instruments validated and translated to other languages.

SF-36 Health Profile

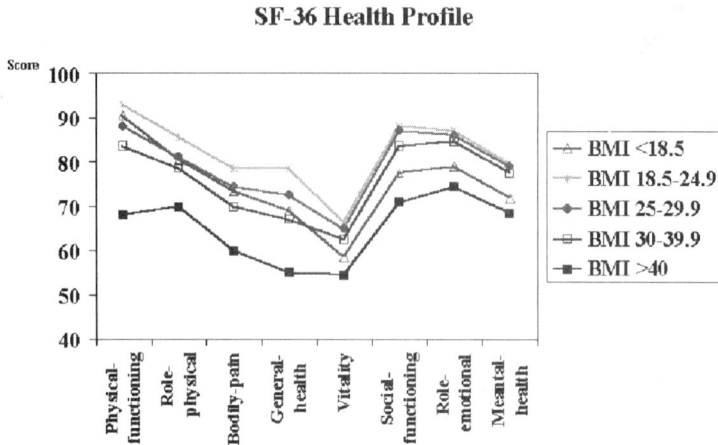

Fig. 2. SF-36 Health profiles in relation to body mass index in a Swedish population study[14].

Quality of life and obesity

Health status

The plethora of organ specific pathologies, and of body systems affected by obesity, coupled with its complicated 'vicious cycle' relationship with life circumstances lifestyle, personal relationships, self-esteem etc, underlines the need to include a generic measure of health status. The SF-36 is a simple, short, well validated tool, available in many languages, which addresses eight functional domains – physical functioning, measures the ability to perform of daily living and strenuous activities (10 items); role-physical, reflects the extent that physical health has a limiting effect on work or other activities (four items); bodily pain, concerns the amount of pain felt and whether it interferes with normal activities (two items); general health, measures perceived general health status (five items); vitality, includes items on energy, tiredness, etc (four items); social functioning, concerns how social activities are affected by physical health or emotional problems (two items); role-emotional, reflects the extent that work or other activities are limited by emotional problems (three items); and mental health, measures emotional well-being (five items) – which are influenced by a variety of health problems[8]. It consistently identifies impaired physical and mental function in obese people[9,10]. Its use provides the opportunity to relate scores for different domains and for overall score, obtained in the overweight and obese, with scores obtained in other patient and population groups.

In cross-sectional general population surveys, SF-36 has shown consistently that higher BMI or waist impairs physical functioning and increases bodily pains, but will little impact on mental health[11,12]. These surveys are generally dominated by large numbers in a relatively narrow BMI range. When subjects with more extreme obesity are studied – e.g. BMI > 40, all components including mental health are affected dramatically[13]. People who are seeking obesity treatment, who often are heavier and have experienced repeated failure, commonly report poorer quality of life and score worse on SF-36[14,15]. Sullivan *et al.*[16] showed worse scores for every domain of SF-36 in obese subjects (Fig. 2).

The SF-36 cannot be assumed to measure global quality of life in obesity or any other disease, although it may be a reasonable generic index. For example, inability to carry shopping or walk upstairs can be considered disabilities, but would not impair quality of life (or even perceived health) for people with no need for these activities.

Global well-being

A second type of measure which might be considered, therefore, in assessing quality of life is obesity or weight management as an instrument which measures global well-being. These are not so well described or widely used, but a well-designed and simple instrument is SEIQOL method[17]. This has the advantage of incorporating individual weightings of the issues included for each domain. SEIQOL was originally developed for use in patients with diabetes, a disease whose symptomatology overlaps substantially with overweight[18], and it is available in several languages.

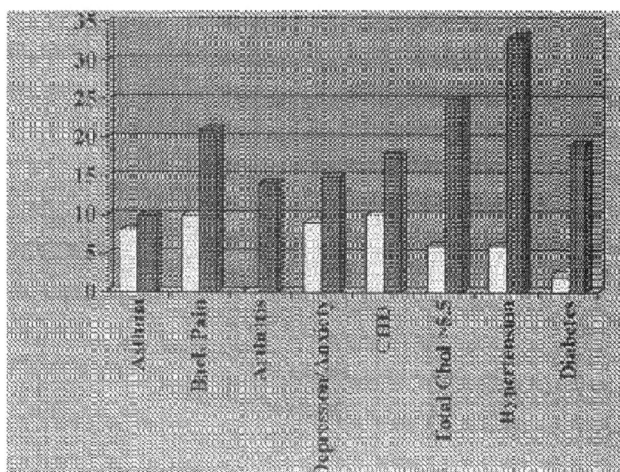

Fig. 3. Co-morbidities in subjects with BMI = 30 (red columns) and subjects with BMI in the range 18.5–24.9 (yellow columns) (McCombie and Lean, unpublished).

Global quality of life aims to assess the general sense of happiness and satisfaction with our lives and our environment. It therefore needs to encompass all aspects of life – e.g. health, recreation, culture, rights, values, beliefs, aspirations, housing and neighbourhood, job satisfaction, family and personal relationships and many more. Inevitably, any practical instrument can touch on only a few of these areas. The aim is to address those which are most frequently important influences on the overall balance of global quality of life. Individually weighted scales, taking variation in topic impact into account, aim to be more discriminating, but even they cannot be used unthinkingly. The best questionnaire in the world cannot be expected to assess quality of life accurately in Manchester the day after a victory (or loss) for Manchester United. To some extent, this increase in quality of life is mediated by mood (elated after a victory, depressed after a loss). However, mood of the individual is only one aspect. A victory will raise the spirits of everybody in town, and thereby also impact those who have not heard the football results.

Mood

Since mood can modify perceived quality of life, and also influence how questionnaires are completed,

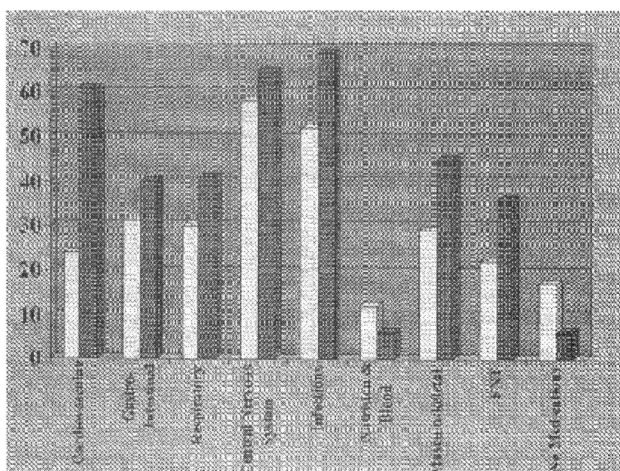

Fig. 4. Drugs prescription by BNF Category in Glasgow (McCombie and Lean, unpublished).

it is valuable to have an independent measure of mood. Two scales are in wide use – the Profile of Mood States (POMS)[19], and the Hospital Anxiety and Depression Scale (HADS)[20]. POMS gives measures of six mood states – tension, depression, anger, vigour, fatigue and confusion. Its design is slanted towards detecting central side effects of drugs, but these components will be affected by a variety of external factors. Perhaps more widely used is the HAD scale[20], a 14-item self-report questionnaire sensitive to mild forms of anxiety (seven items) and depression (seven items), and translated to at least 33 different languages. All items are scored on a 4-point scale from 0 to 3, thus giving a range of possible scores from 0 to 21 for each sub-scale, with higher values indicating higher anxiety or depression. Neither severe psychological symptoms, less common in non-psychiatric clinical-patients, nor physical indicators of psychological distress, which could give false positive results if they are due to an underlying medical illness, are included in the scale thus making it suitable for use in subjects with different medical conditions. Different studies support the validity of HADS. Factor analysis has generally shown two relatively independent dimensions of anxiety and depression. In addition a good internal consistency for the HADS subscale (mean Cronbach's alpha coefficient 0f 0.83 for anxiety (range 0.68 to 0.93), and 0.82 for depression (0.67 to 0.90)). Finally the sensitivity and specificity of the anxiety and depression sub-scales, with a cut-off point score, were most often found to be approximately 0.80 (range of 0.70 to 0.90)[21].

Obesity-related quality of life

The aim of disease-related (or 'health-related') quality of life measures is not to assess global quality of life, but to estimate the impact of the disease and its treatment on known consequences which will impact quality of life. It may be valuable to establish the pattern of effects on quality of life through the time-course of obesity – and to dissect the effects of weight gain from those of ageing, or to examine the effects of treatment on consequences of obesity. These questionnaires are therefore correctly measuring aspects of health status, not necessarily quality of life[22]. They have value for clinical use, for public health surveys to guide resource planning, and for pharmaceutical companies to evaluate impacts of interventions.

Tools to assess health-related quality of life for, say, rheumatoid arthritis can reasonably be limited to mobility, pain, stiffness, fatigue and specific side-effects of treatment. Obesity, on the other hand, is a much more diffuse, multi-system disease, with a huge range of common medical and psycho-social consequences (Table 1). There is also a mis-match between the symptomatic impact of obesity on individuals and the relatively small and distant impact of cardiovascular and metabolic risk factors which dominate the thinking of health planners.

Figure 3 shows the excess of a number of medical problems in people with BMI > 30 from the records of a general practice in Glasgow (Scotland), and the excess in drug prescribing in every BNF category except 'nutrition'! (Fig. 4). The impact of obesity on health status, or quality of life, is therefore impacted by a whole range of specific disease-related fields, and by a colossal number of drugs with a bewildering array of potential side effects.

It is difficult at this stage to make any firm recommendation to use one specific obesity-related quality of life questionnaire. It seems likely that some kind of large 'bank' of questions will emerge, from the large number of tools under development. It will not be possible to assume equal impact of specific obesity consequences in different cultures, and it will be up to clinicians, researchers, and public health planners to choose questions appropriate to these needs, whilst recognizing the limitations of the approach used.

It does seem clear though, that non-experts cannot simply pick an 'off-the-shelf' quality of life measure and expect simple or meaningful results.

Comparative and longitudinal assessment

A number of studies have attempted to compare health status or quality of life of obese subjects in comparisons with people with other medical conditions. Sullivan et al.[16] used the Sickness Impact Profile Score to suggest that health status of people with severe obesity (BMI >35 kg/m^2) was worse that that of cancer survivors. Others have offered hypothetical choices (obesity or amputation) to suggest that people would prefer amputation or stroke (check reference) to obesity. Studies of this kind catch headlines, but should not be used to suggest impact on quality of life or to guide policy.

Almost whatever instrument is used, weight loss in obese subjects leads to improved scores for health status, and for apparent quality of life. Thus Karlsson et al.[23] importantly showed improvements in mood, vitality and mental health. Worryingly, however, these improvements occurred acutely but were usually only maintained if weight loss (with surgery) was over 30 kg. There were improvements in mental well-being, but clearly factors other than adiposity are more dominant during the sort of weight loss which can be achieved in routine clinical settings.

When longitudinal or intervention studies are undertaken it is vital to include control groups because quality of life is affected by many external factors. There may also be a component of regression towards the mean if people enter trials when relatively depressed for other reasons. Consideration must be given to standardizing the conditions under which quality of life questionnaires are completed. Time of day, day of the week, relationship to most recent meal, coffee or alcohol could all affect results. Such factors are likely to be less for administered questionnaires than for postal surveys, but reported quality of life may be different when subjects are in unusual clinical or research environments.

It should go without saying that all measures chosen should be rigorously validated, including pilot work to ensure reliability in the specific subject group under study[24].

References

1. Lean MEJ, Han T, Deurenberg P. Predicting body composition by densitometry from simple anthropometric measurements. *Am J Clin Nutr* 1996; 63: 4–14.

2. Han TS, Lean ME. Bioelectrical impedance analysis in nutritional research. *Nutrition* 1998; 14: 707–8.

3. World Health Organization. Preamble to the Constitution of the World Health Organization as adopted by the International Health Conference, 19–22 June 1946; New York, p.100.

4. Hunt SM, McEwen J, McKenna SP. Measuring health status: A new tool for clinicians and epidemiologists. *J Roy Coll Gen Pract* 1985; 35: 185–8.

5. Stone P, Richardson A, Ream E, Smith AG, Kerr DJ, Kearney N. On behalf of the Cancer Fatigue Forum: Cancer-related fatigue: Inevitable, unimportant and untreatable? Results of a multi-centre patient survey. *Ann Oncol* 2000; 11: 971–75.

6. MAPI Research Institute Website: Available from: URL: http://www.mapi-research-inst.com/index02.htm.

7. Medical Outcomes Trust Website: Available from: URL: http://www.outcomes-trust.org/instruments.htm.

8. Ware JE Jr, Snow KK, Kosinski M, Gandek B. SF-36 *Health survey manual and interpretation guide.* Boston: Nimrod Press; 1993.

9. Lean ME, Han TS, Seidell JC. Impairment of health and quality of life in people with large waist circumference. *Lancet* 1998; 351: 853–6.

10. Doll HA, Petersen SE, Stewart-Brown SL. Obesity and physical and emotional well-being: associations between body mass index, chronic illness, and the physical and mental components of the SF-36 questionnaire. *Obes Res* 2000; 8: 160–70.

11. Han TS, Tijhuis MA, Lean ME, Seidell JC. Quality of life in relation to overweight and body fat distribution. *Am J Public Health* 1998; 88: 1814–20.

12. Lean ME, Han TS, Seidell JC. Impairment of health and quality of life using new US federal guidelines for the identification of obesity. *Arch Intern Med* 1999; 159: 837–43.

13. Larsson U, Karlsson J, Sullivan M. Impact of overweight and obesity on health-related quality of life – a Swedish population study. *Int J Obes Relat Metab Disord* 2002; 26: 417–24.

14. Fontaine KR, Cheskin LJ, Barofsky I. Health-related quality of life in obese persons seeking treatment. *J Fam Pract* 1996; 43: 265–70.

15. Fontaine KR, Bartlett SJ, Barofsky I. Health-related quality of life among obese persons seeking and not currently seeking treatment. *Int J Eat Disord* 2000; 27: 101–5.

16. Sullivan M, Karlsson J, Sjöström L, Taft L. Why quality of life measures should be used in the treatment of patients with obesity. In: *International textbook of obesity*; Bjorntorp P (ed.), pp. 485–510. Chichester: John Wiley, 2002.

17. Bradley C. Achieving accessibility with quality: questionnaire measurement of condition-specific individualised quality of life. *Proc Br Psychol Soc* 1999; 7 (Suppl 2): 143.

18. UKPDS Group. UK Prospective Diabetes Study 7: response of fasting plasma glucose to diet therapy in newly presenting type II diabetic patients. *Metabolism* 1990; 39: 905–12.

19. McNair DM, Lorr M, Droppleman LF. Profile of Mood States (POMS) Manual, Educational and Industrial Testing Service. San Diego; 1992.

20. Zigmond AS, Snaith RP. The Hospital Anxiety and Depression Scale. *Acta Psychiatr Scand* 1983; 67: 361–70.

21. Bjelland I, Dahl AA, Haug TT, Neckelmann D. The validity of the Hospital Anxiety and Depression Scale. An updated literature review. *J Psychosom Res* 2002; 52: 69–77.

22. Bradley C. Importance of differentiating health status from quality of life. *Lancet* 2001; 357: 7–8.

23. Karlsson J, Sjostrom L, Sullivan M. Swedish obese subjects (SOS) – an intervention study of obesity. Two-year follow-up of health-related quality of life (HRQL) and eating behavior after gastric surgery for severe obesity. *Int J Obes Relat Metab Disord* 1998; 22: 113–26.

24. MOT (1995) SAC Instrument Review Criteria. Medical Outcome Trust Bulletin. 3, 4. Available from: URL: http://195.101.204.50: 443/public/34sacrev.htm.

Progress in Obesity Research: 9. Edited by *Geraldo Medeiros-Neto, Alfredo Halpern* and *Claude Bouchard*
©2003 John Libbey Eurotext Ltd, pp. 866–869.

CHAPTER 182

Behavioural approaches to the management of obesity

Donald A. Williamson

Pennington Biomedical Research Center, 6400 Perkins Road, Baton Rouge, LA, USA
[e-mail: williada@pbrc.edu]

Theoretical basis of behavioural treatment

There is a significant genetic component to the development of obesity, and it is generally believed that some interaction of genetics and environment may predispose selected persons to gain weight[1]. The focus of a behavioural intervention incorporates modification of eating behaviours and physical activity to yield energy imbalance. Behavioural theory postulates that eating and exercise habits are conditioned[2]. Classical conditioning refers to the set of circumstances by which cues in an individual's environment become associated with a particular behaviour. When an environmental stimulus is repeatedly paired with a behaviour, the stimulus itself becomes a 'trigger' to elicit a behavioural reaction. In the case of eating behaviour, many aspects of the environment may become associated with hunger sensations and with eating. The smell or sight of food may become conditioned stimuli to eating and therefore trigger hunger sensations. This association is conditioned because the smell and sight of food are repeatedly paired with eating behaviour. However, additional stimuli, when paired with eating, may become associated with feelings of hunger. For example, if an individual habitually eats while watching television, then hunger sensations can be elicited by watching television (independently of physiological hunger). Operant conditioning refers to the influence of reinforcement contingencies upon the learning of behavioural habits. The natural consequences of eating, e.g. the good taste of food and reduction of hunger, promote the development of overeating habits; whereas, the natural consequences of exercise, e.g. fatigue and muscle soreness, promote the development of a sedentary lifestyle. Furthermore, as a person gains weight, the natural consequences of exercise become even more aversive, resulting in less physical activity as obesity increases.

Behavioural treatment methods

Components of behavioural weight loss interventions

Self-monitoring. A central feature of behavioural weight loss interventions is self-monitoring of eating and exercise habits[2]. Self-monitoring involves recording food intake and intentional efforts to increase physical activity. This monitoring should occur at the time of each behavioural event, i.e. at each meal or snack or immediately after a bout of exercise. Self-monitoring also generally involves recording (1) environmental events associated with eating and exercise, e.g. place and time of day, (2) cognitive and emotional reactions, e.g. eating in response to stress, and (3) hunger ratings before and after eating. Self-monitoring serves several purposes: (1) enhanced awareness of habits, patterns of behaviour, and amount of food eaten at meals and snacks, (2) record of behaviour that can be used to evaluate progress and to set goals for reinforcement, and (3) dietary record that can be analysed for the adequacy of the person's nutritional intake across time.

Stimulus control. Stimulus control procedures are designed to alter the relationship between antecedent stimuli and eating and exercise habits[2]. Commonly used stimulus control procedures are: (1) eating at the same time and place at each meal, (2) slowing eating by putting utensils down between bites, (3) eating on small plates, (4) resisting the urge to have second portions, (5) eating while seated, (6) leaving a small amount of food on one's plate, (7) serving small portions of food, and (8) exercising at the same time each day. These procedures serve several functions: (1) extinction of the conditioned association between certain environmental events and unhealthy eating or exercise habits, (2) conditioning of a three meal/day eating pattern that is associated with specific environmental cues, (3) slowing the pace of eating, and (4) developing a consistent pattern of physical activity that becomes habitual.

Reinforcement/shaping/goal setting. Unfortunately, alteration of the natural consequences of eating is difficult without pharmacological or surgical intervention, but fortunately, the development of healthy physical activity habits makes some of the natural consequences of exercise less aversive over time. Behavioural weight control programmes are very 'goal oriented'. Typically, the person will set a weight goal, a calorie goal, and an exercise goal. Individualized goals are usually established. These goals might include such things as: cessation of eating certain types of foods, e.g. soft drinks, walking up stairs instead of using elevators, or modification of snacks, e.g. eating fruit instead of ice cream. The principle of shaping is generally employed when reinforcement contingencies to modify behaviour are formulated. Shaping refers to setting small, but reasonable goals at first, and then gradually making them more challenging over the course of treatment.

Behavioural contracting. To enhance the person's motivation for achieving these goals, a procedure called behavioural contracting is often used. Behavioural contracting involves clearly specifying behavioural goals in terms of frequency, duration, or intensity, e.g. 'I agree to walk at least 30 min per day for at least five days per week'. A behavioural contract generally includes some type of reinforcement contingency for successful attainment of the goal, e.g. 'if I meet my exercise goal for this week, I will reward myself by purchasing a copy of my favorite magazine'.

Meal planning. Goals related to nutrient intake may take many forms, e.g. calories, fat grams, or dietary exchanges. In general, research has shown that explicit meal plans are most effective for compliance. An explicit meal plan might include an actual menu to be followed each day. The use of portion-controlled foods that are prepackaged for use in diets can be quite useful for persons who have difficulty following a self-selected meal plan. A dietitian should manage this aspect of the programme.

Modification of physical activity. Programmes to increase physical activity generally include increasing exercise and decreasing sedentary behaviour. Research has found that aerobic exercise is the most effective form of exercise prescription and that compliance is best when the exercise programme is incorporated into their normal lifestyle.

Problem-solving. Formal training in problem-solving is a common component of most behavioural weight control programmes. This type of training involves assisting the person to: (1) identify problems that are obstacles to successful weight management, (2) define the problem in objective behavioural terms, (3) brainstorm about potential solutions to the problem, (4) conduct a cost/benefit analysis for each solution, (5) select a solution and develop a plan of action, and (6) evaluate the success or failure of the plan of action and revise it, based upon this evaluation. This component of treatment is often useful in modifying obstacles that negatively impact compliance with the basic behavioural weight management programme.

Social support. Enhancement of social support for behaviour change has been found to be a very important factor in successful weight management. Social support may be derived from a spouse, family members, or friends. In the treatment of childhood or adolescent obesity, involvement of the parents in the therapy programme has been found to be very useful. Enhancement of social support is best accomplished by inviting family members and friends to attend some of the therapy sessions. In these sessions, support persons learn to reinforce healthy behaviour change and are discouraged from engaging in actions that sabotage progress toward behaviour change.

Components of behavioural weight maintenance programmes

Relapse prevention. Returning to old, unhealthy habits is a primary cause of relapse and regain of weight that has been lost[3]. Relapse prevention programmes generally assist in the identification of situations that place the person at risk for returning to old, unhealthy habits and to develop specific plans to manage these high-risk situations. For example, parties might be a high-risk situation for overeating. The person might develop a plan of action that involves healthy eating before going to the party to reduce hunger and standing/sitting in areas that are away from tempting foods. Relapse prevention programmes also often include a discussion of the distinction between lapses and relapse. People often engage in 'all-or-nothing' thinking so that when they deviate from the behavioural prescriptions of the programme, they feel as though they have failed, resulting in loss of motivation and returning to old habits.

Booster treatment. Booster treatment generally involves periodic therapeutic contact during the period of weight maintenance. This therapeutic contact may take many forms, including face-to-face sessions, scheduled telephone calls, or Internet exchanges. Since obesity is now viewed as a chronic illness, most experts believe that some type of booster treatment may be needed over the course of an entire lifetime, if weight loss is to be successfully maintained.

Tests of efficacy

Early studies (1967–1990)

Behavioural methods for the treatment of obesity were first applied over thirty years ago. In 1967, Richard B. Stuart[4] was among the first to describe the application of learning principles to the treatment of obesity. His first behavioural programme successfully treated eight overweight women, who attained an average weight loss of 17 kg over a 12-month period. It was Stuart's early success story that sparked researchers' interest in this approach to the treatment of obesity.

The research studies that followed in the 1970s were modeled on Stuart's behavioural weight control programme; however, there were some notable differences in the application of the treatment protocol. In Stuart's programme, he used an individualized approach, tailoring the programme to fit the needs of the individual patient. Treatment sessions took place three times per week for the first 4 to 5 weeks, then less frequently as treatment progressed. The studies of the 1970s, that followed Stuart's early studies, moved in a different direction. These studies delivered treatment to small groups of six to ten persons and usually met for once per week for 12 to 16 weeks. As noted by Williamson and Perrin[2], this approach to behavioural weight loss treatment resulted in less impressive results (average weight loss of about 4 to 5 kg).

Since the 1970s behavioural treatment programmes for obesity have been intensified in terms of length and aggressiveness, yielding average weight losses of about 8.5 kg. However these weight losses usually occur in the short-term and are not maintained in the long-term, after treatment ends. Most people who receive behavioural weight control regain much of the weight that was lost, though the regain of weight usually takes about 5 years.

Intensive lifestyle behaviour modification (1990–2000)

Increased duration of treatment. After the trend of regaining weight was frequently observed, behavioural researchers in the 1990s tried to identify more effective long-term strategies. One strategy was to increase the length of treatment[5]. Treatment length increased from an average of 8 weeks in 1974 to an average of 21 weeks by the 1990s[2]. Comparable increases in weight loss have occurred with increases in treatment duration. In 1974 the average weight loss associated with the 8-week treatment protocol was 3.8 kg, and in 1990, the average weight loss associated with a 21-week treatment protocol was 8.5 kg. Average weight losses in behavioural treatment studies have increased by approximately 75 per cent in studies conducted over the past 30 years and this improved weight loss has occurred in conjunction with the approximate doubling of treatment duration over the last 30 years. In his review in 1998, Perri[3] concluded that longer duration of treatment has been consistently associated with greater weight loss.

Very low calorie diets and meal planning. One way of improving weight loss is to incorporate a very low calorie diet (VLCD), defined as less than 800 kcal/day, into the treatment protocol. Most behavioural weight control programmes have used low calorie diets (LCD), which usually consist of approximately 1200 to 1500 kcal/day. The initial studies of combining behaviour therapy with VLCDs found that a VLCD combined with behaviour therapy was more successful, than a LCD combined with behaviour therapy, in producing more initial weight loss (in the short-term); however, this initial weight loss did not improve long-term outcome. Williamson and Perrin[2] concluded that the addition of behaviour therapy to a VLCD, in the active treatment phase, did not yield weight loss above that usually associated with VLCDs alone; however, the addition of behaviour therapy did seem to slow the rate of weight regain.

In addition to VLCD's, diets that are more structured have also been incorporated into behavioural treatment protocols. Food provision (actually providing the persons with the appropriate food) was effective in improving the amount of initial weight loss in one study, but was no more effective in the long-term than was a condition that had a standard calorie goal of 1000–1500 kcal/day[6]. Subsequent studies have found that the most important component of food provision is the provision of structured meal plans and grocery lists (not the provision of food, *per se*), which appear to exert their effects by assisting people in selecting healthy foods, and by creating a regular meal pattern (i.e. breakfast, lunch, dinner)[6].

Exercise. Unlike the dietary approaches mentioned above, increased attention to exercise has been related not only to enhanced short-term weight loss, but also long-term weight loss. In fact, the benefit of exercise has been particularly effective in the long-term. Recent research has focused on the types and amount of exercise that produce the best weight losses and best weight maintenance. These studies have generally found no differences in treatment programmes using aerobic exercise, resistance training (weight lifting), or the combination of aerobic exercise and resistance training, although all yielded significant weight losses[6]. It is clear, however, that ultimately, the person should incorporate lifestyle exercise with a goal of 2,000 to 2,500 kcal/week, into their daily routine[5,6]. It is possible that exercise is effective in the long-term because it increases lean body mass, elevates metabolic rates, and/or decreases appetite.

Social support. Enhancement of social support has been tested as a means of improving long-term weight loss. The most common way to enhance social support has been to include spouses, or friends in the treatment process. Wing[6] concluded that there are both short-term and long-term benefits to including spouses in obesity treatment. Wing and Jeffery[7] found similar results with the inclusion of friends in the treatment process, revealing that persons who entered treatment with friends had better success at maintaining weight losses 6 months after a 4-month behavioural treatment programme.

Increased therapist contact during the maintenance phase. Obesity researchers have tested the impact of increasing therapist contact during the weight maintenance phase, as a means of facilitating long-term success. Perri and colleagues[3] found that the addition of therapist contact via the telephone and mail, significantly enhanced maintenance of weight loss for a group that received behaviour therapy plus relapse prevention training. Similar results have been obtained with the use of booster sessions to enhance maintenance of weight loss[5]. Perri and colleagues reported that women in a behavioural weight control programme that received one year of additional contact (biweekly treatment contacts of various sorts) maintained their weight losses better than the group of women who received no contact during the maintenance phase[3]. In recent years the Internet has been employed as a means of increasing therapist contact to improve long-term weight maintenance, and preliminary results of this approach are encouraging[8].

Relapse prevention. Relapse prevention training has been used to help people learn to 'nip lapses in the bud' in order to obtain better long-term weight maintenance. There is general consensus[2,5] that development of skills to respond immediately to overeating, periods of inactivity, or to small weight gains, is useful for long-term management of obesity, though the effects of this intervention are relatively small in comparison to the effects of exercise, structured meal plans, and social support[5].

References

1. Bouchard C, Perusse L, Rice T, Rao DC. The genetics of human obesity. In: *Handbook of obesity*, Bray G, Bouchard C, James P (eds), p.157. New York: Marcel Decker, 1999.

2. Williamson DA, Perrin LA. Behavior therapy for obesity. Endocrinology and Metabolism *Clinics of North America* 1996; 25: 943–54.

3. Perri MG. The maintenance of treatment effects in the long-term management of obesity. *Clin Psychol Science Pract* 1998; 5: 526–43.

4. Stuart R. Behavioral control of overeating. *Behav Res Ther* 1967; 5: 357–65.

5. Perri MG, Corsica JA. Improving the maintenance of weight loss in behavioral treatment of obesity. In: *Handbook of obesity treatment*, Wadden T, Stunkard A (eds), p. 357. New York: Guilford Press; 2002.

6. Wing RR. Behavioral weight control. In: *Handbook of obesity treatment*, Wadden T, Stunkard A (eds), p. 301. New York: Guilford Press; 2002.

7. Wing RR, Jeffery RW. Benefits of recruiting participants with friends and increasing social support for weight loss maintenance. *J Consult Clin Psychol* 1999; 67: 132–38.

8. Tate D, Wing RR, Winett R. Development and evaluation of an Internet behavior therapy program for weight loss. *JAMA* 2001; 285: 1172–7.

Progress in Obesity Research: 9. Edited by *Geraldo Medeiros-Neto, Alfredo Halpern and Claude Bouchard*
©2003 John Libbey Eurotext Ltd, pp. 870–880.

CHAPTER 183

The 'Agita São Paulo' model in promoting physical activity

**Victor Matsudo, Sandra Matsudo, Douglas Andrade, Timoteo Araujo,
Erinaldo Andrade, Luis Carlos de Oliveira, Glaucia Braggion and Marcos Ausenka**

*Centre of Studies of the Physical Fitness Research Laboratory, from São Caetano do Sul - CELAFISCS,
Agita São Paulo Program, Brazil*
[e-mail: celafiscs@celafiscs.com.br]

Introduction

Promoting an active-life style in the general population as an important tool to prevent or control consequences of obesity or overweight has been difficult in the past. The purpose of this paper is to present some of the experiences of the Agita São Paulo programme, a multi-level, community-wide, physical activity intervention programme that was created in Brazil[1,2]. The programme was especially addressed to the people in the state of São Paulo, but because its positive impact, it serves as basis for Agita Brasil and Agita America (Physical Activity Network for the Americas). More recently, WHO decided to celebrate World Health Day 2002 on the topic of Physical Activity, taken the slogan Agita Mundo: Move Health. Brasil is a country in the epidemiologic transition, as shown by an increase in deaths from cardiovascular diseases[3,4], and obesity prevalence[5], while experiencing a decrease in infectious and parasitic diseases. Cardio-vascular diseases (CVD) are responsible for the deaths of about 300,000 Brazilians a year, representing one death every 2 min[6]. The rate in the São Paulo state (30.8 per cent) is higher than the national average[7]. This can, in part, be explained by several survey results that have indicated a large proportion of Brazilians are not meeting physical activity guidelines. In the São Paulo metropolitan region, a survey estimated that in the early 1990s[8], 69.3 per cent of the adults were not sufficiently active, and was more true of women (80.2 per cent) than men (57.3 per cent). A national survey in 1997 ($n = 2,504$) showed 60 per cent of adults were insufficiently active[9]. That prevalence was higher than any other risk factor, i.e. diabetes (6.9 per cent), obesity (18 per cent), hypertension (22.3 per cent), or smoking (37.9 per cent).

It is interesting to note that recent epidemiological studies based upon 25,341 men[10] have demonstrated that the cardiovascular death risk was lower among active, fat men than leaner, sedentary ones; and lower among active, hypertensive men than among nonhypertensive men; and in a similar manner was lower among active, diabetic men than among non-diabetic men[11]. Moreover, another recent epidemiological study demonstrated that the risk is still lower when highly fit men with three risk-factors were compared to non-active men with no risk-factors[12].

Physical activity has been considered the 'best buy' in public health, since two million deaths/year may be attributed to the consequences of sedentariness. In 1995, the United States spent US\$24billion (9.4 per cent of total health expenditures) to deal with that problem (CDC[13]). It is estimated that sedentariness costs about US\$330/person/year.

A comprehensive analysis of the preceding data shows that even in developing countries there is a need for population-wide interventions to increase physical activity and reduce risks of chronic diseases. However, the greatest challenge is to create population-modification programmes for physical activity that consider the economic, political, social, and cultural realities of a developing country. Moreover, if a programme is successful in Brazil, it can serve as a model for other developing countries.

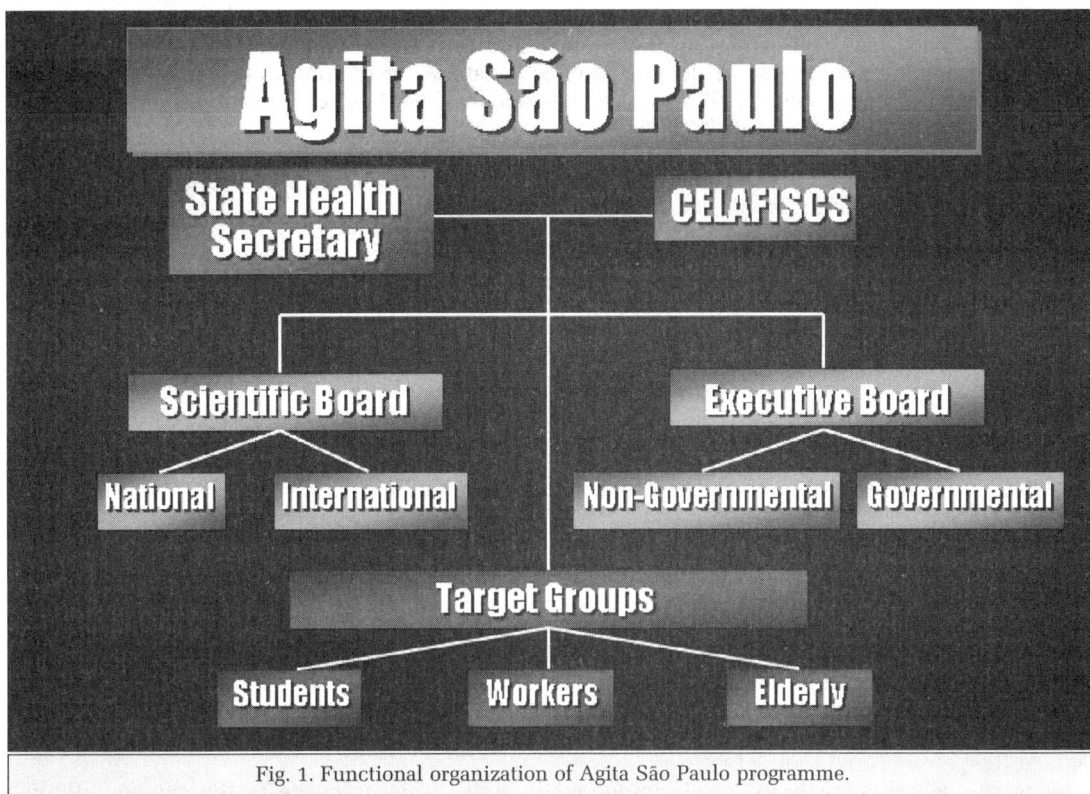

Fig. 1. Functional organization of Agita São Paulo programme.

CELAFISCS background

Research centres do not usually conduct intervention programmes; therefore it is of interest to realize that the Physical Fitness Research Centre in São Caetano do Sul (CELAFISCS) in São Paulo, Brazil is an independent, non-profit, scientific institution founded in 1974 for the purpose of conducting research on sports sciences in a developing country and to train professionals to conduct such research. During the last 29 years the Centre trained more than 189 professionals of different fields (physicians, physical education teachers, nutritionists, physical therapists, psychologists) from Brazil and other South America countries. CELAFISCS has conducted research on the growth and development of fitness variables throughout a person's life span, assessing the impact of biological maturation, malnutrition, socioeconomic level, and participation in sports. One line of research determined talent profiles for different sports, and another, that began in 1977, included an ongoing longitudinal study of fitness, physical activity, and chronic disease risk factors in young people[14].

Establishment of Agita São Paulo

In 1995, CELAFISCS started to consider how it could make a contribution to the promotion of physical activity. Emerging data on the high prevalence of physical inactivity in the state's population, particularly among the low socioeconomic and undernourished groups, indicated that a physical activity promotion effort was needed. The State Secretary for Health in São Paulo requested CELAFISCS to develop a state-wide programme.

Two major challenges had to be faced in creating the programme. First, there was meager scientific literature on promoting physical activity in developing countries. Second, the São Paulo state comprised a population of about 37 million inhabitants in a 248,808 km^2 area with 645 municipalities. The city and metropolitan region of São Paulo was the second largest in the world, with 16,446,000 inhabitants.

A 2-year planning process included consultation with the Pan American Health Organization, the US's Centres for Disease Control and Prevention (CDC), the United Kingdom's Health Education Authority, the Institute for Aerobics Research in Dallas, Texas, and advisors from Brazil, the US, Finland, England,

and Australia. CELAFISCS developed a programme document delineating the scientific basis for the necessity to promote physical activity in the population, goals, target populations, strategies, actions, and desired results of the programme for the São Paulo state. After the preparation phase, 'Agita São Paulo' was launched in December 1996 with support from multiple state governments, non-governmental organizations, and the private sector (Fig. 1).

The name Agita was selected after two years consideration with the assistance of professional marketing consultants; it is a special word that represents not only the desire for physical activity, but also includes considerations of the mind, social health, and citizenship.

The scientific basis

Multiple models were used to guide the design of the programme because a variety of intervention strategies were needed. The Transtheoretical Model[15] was applied to the assessment of changes in the readiness of various subgroups and the selection of change methods relevant to people in each stage. The 'one-step-ahead model' expressed the aim to help people at each stage and progress to the next stage. Other methods used were:

(a)   The Social Cognitive Theory[16];

(b)   The community planning for partnership and health promotion[17,18];

(c)   Social marketing[19,20];

The preceding models were useful to conceptualize particular intervention components, but most of the models addressed the education of individuals or groups; the reliance on educational approaches may be one reason for the disappointing results of previous change efforts in communities[21]. Consequently, ecological models were used to plan and coordinate changes on multiple levels[21–23]. Mass communications and community organizations were used to enhance social influences for physical activity. Community organization partnerships were used to create sustainable changes in institutions. Government partnerships led to policy changes that supported physical activity, including improvements in the physical environment.

Target group segmentation is extremely important in Agita São Paulo due to the extreme ethnic, economic, geographic, and cultural diversity of the population. Literature on mass media and health promotion was consulted for guidance because mass media was expected to be included in the mix of interventions[24].

The goal of Agita

The goals of the Agita programme were to increase the population's knowledge of the benefits of physical activity for health (biological, psychological, social) and to increase participation in moderate physical activity, upgrading each person's stage of physical activity by at least one level – a principle of the Transtheoretical Model[15]. The programme aims for the sedentary to be at least irregularly active, the irregularly active to be regularly active, the regularly active to be very active, and the very active to maintain that level while reducing the risk of injuries. The goal of the programme is to increase the level of knowledge by 50 per cent and the level of physical activity over 20 per cent in 10 years (2 per cent per year).

The Agita message and target groups

Traditional health promotion guidelines for physical activity do not usually obtain population adherence because of the suggested duration time of 50–60 min, the high intensity of effort (70 per cent of maximal heart rate or over), and requests for a medical screening.

The Agita São Paulo programme adopted the current public health recommendation for adults on new evidence of the accumulative benefits of moderate intensity physical activity. This recommendation is to accumulate at least 30 min of moderate-intensity physical activity on most, and preferably all, days of the week[25]. The activity can be performed continuously or accumulated in sessions of 10 to 15 min. This recommendation is endorsed by different international organizations such as the World Health Organization (WHO), CDC, ACSM, AHA among others[26], and adopted in national campaigns in Canada, England and Australia.

The recommendation emphasizing the accumulation of moderate intensity physical activity is particularly relevant for the São Paulo culture. In the São Paulo metropolitan area, lack of time is perceived as a major barrier to being active[27,28]), so accumulating activity in brief sessions may be perceived as more feasible. Similarly, moderate intensity is more likely to be accepted in a hot, tropical country than a vigorous activity programme.

Three main target groups were identified: students (children and adolescents), elderly, and workers (blue and white collar). Programmes and materials were developed for each target group.

Agita structure

Partnership

To face the programme development challenge, partnerships were adopted as a key strategy. Intellectual partnerships were instrumental in obtaining experiences from other national and international programmes. Thus, several professionals with well-established expertise in intervention were invited to visit the Agita Centre, and to compose a national and international scientific board.

The Governmental and Non-Governmental Organizations Partnership represents the key factor of the Agita success. More than 250 strong institutions comprise its Executive Board, which discusses main Agita actions at its monthly meeting. Different society sectors are represented on that board, such as education, sports, health, industry, commerce, and services[29]).

Scientific and Executive Board

The structure of Agita São Paulo shows the relationship between the Scientific Board and the Executive Board; inter-sectorial, but mainly intra-sectorial balance seemed to be of utmost importance. For example, when support of the Industry Federation was obtained, the Chamber of Commerce was solicited; when the Lions Club support was obtained, the Rotary Club was solicited. In academic circles, the same trend was used; federal, state, and private universities were also encouraged to join.

Empowerment

Another important approach was to empower existing programmes instead of preparing a new agenda for them. This gave a common flag to all groups; the combined programme developed a strong identity in cause and a diversity in action.

Agita programme details

Inclusion

Agita reflects the inclusion and diversity concerns with its 'inclusion principle'; this is also clear when the main messages were selected, i.e. 'active living' and 'physical activity for health' substituting for the traditional and ineffective 'sport' and 'fitness' jargons.

One-step-ahead

The 'one-step-ahead model' is another example of the inclusion process allied to the Transtheoretical Model. In that approach, instead of a general message, targeting messages were developed asking the sedentary to become more active; the somewhat active to be regularly active; and those who were already active or very active, to remain active without injuries[1].

Culture links

The 'half-hour man' became the mascot of the campaign, reflecting the attention to culture aspects, since fun is a crucial factor for Brazilians. A 'half-hour woman' and a 'half-hour cowboy' were created, attempting to adapt to regional cultures and genders; a 'half-hour seashoreman' was also selected from an inter-school contest.

Agita settings

Three settings were selected: home, transport, and leisure time. Everyday home activities were the most reinforced, concentrating on the importance of walking (even while walking a dog), gardening, home-chores, avoidance of sedentary behaviours (sitting, watching TV); endeavours were made to give meaning to home activities while using humor to attract the Brazilians' attention. Walking and stair climbing were stimulated in the transport setting. Dance became the most important inclusion message among leisure activities because children, adolescents, adults, and elderly can dance, and Brazilians love to dance.

Educational materials

The biological benefits of active living were listed in the guideline materials (Governo do Estado de São Paulo[30,31]; however, these are long-term benefits not easily perceived by the normal population. The benefits of mental and social health were stressed since they seemed to be more effective in changing behaviour as people could 'feel' and observe them in a shorter time! In other words, it is easier to feel changes in mood or self-esteem, than to notice changes in body plasma, cholesterol, or glucose.

Medical Committee

Medical groups deserve special attention[32]. The Medical Committee activities determined medical doctors had a low knowledge level for prescribing exercise. Because the traditional culture to 'prescribe a medicine for each health problem', the 'Agitol', or the 'formula for active living' was developed which could be taken in doses of 30, 15 or 10 min – presented in a typical pharmaceutical format. A good sense of humor made Agitol quite popular among health professionals, and a good example to encourage the shifting from the traditional 'treatment disease' to a 'health promotion' approach.

Physical activity among teenagers

Data from the Agita Lab showed that physical activity is declining among the lower socio-economic boys, where classes C, D and E (lower, poorer) were less active than classes A and B (higher, richer). This is understandable because urban changes have decreased safety on the streets and availability of appropriate activity space[33]. Brazilian boys are less involved in sports activities than US boys, and watching TV is their first option for use of free time[34]. The problem is important because they watch TV for about four hours/day; and even more among girls and low socioeconomic groups. This behaviour impairs all fitness indices as adiposity, lower limb strength, anaerobic power, and mainly aerobic power[35].

Moreover, physical education is in crisis all around the world, and more marked in Latin America where the number of weeks of classes is decreasing; is not implemented in 50 per cent of the schools; and is conducted under inadequate conditions in 100 per cent of the cases[36].

This research provided information to be applied in the target message approach and educational materials were developed – like the physical activity pyramid. In the pyramid, TV watching was listed as the least desirable behaviour – at the top, while everyday physical activity was placed at the bottom, being the most recommended. The nutrition pyramid was printed with a physical activity pyramid (Agita message), permitting the two to reach the population together; it was sent to more than 6 million students.

Andrade and other colleagues from our Centre observed that girls from low socio-economic region were more involved in vigorous physical activity than boys at the same age[37]. This is a surprise because literature systematically reported a superiority of boys regarding levels of physical activity. However, this information was mostly based on samples from well-developed countries. Our case sample consisted of girls from Ilhabela, an ocean island between Rio de Janeiro and São Paulo, where local culture probably played an important role. When we analysed the data further, it was observed that the main difference for this was explained by the girl's involvement in strenuous housekeeping, which was much more evident in girls (41.7 per cent), than boys (5.9 per cent). In fact, 70.5 per cent of the boys answered that they were 'not at all' involved in strenuous housekeeping activities! However, when transportation to/from school was analysed, 100 per cent of the boys utilized active transportation, compared to only 57.1 per cent of the girls.

Agita mega-events

Realizing that knowledge cannot change behaviour *per se*, creative and radical interventions are necessary. Therefore, three mega-events are usually organized each year, one for each target group: the Agita Galera Day – that means agitate the crowd or the Active Community Day – dedicated to the school communities; the Active Worker Day, for the laborers; and the Active Elderly Day.

Agita Galera Day. The Agita Galera Day was held the last five years on the last Friday of August, when over 6,000 public and private school students discussed the positive effects of active living; they later walked through the streets. They also discussed methods to establish permanent actions promoting active school setting environments. It has involved more than 6 million students and their communities; the preparation requires war-like logistics efforts, including training hundreds of educational and health care professionals in the 640 state cities. A special educational manual was prepared, and sent to all school systems, to sensitive teachers, health providers, and the media, in an approach to encourage active living that even includes a cable TV teleconference.

A concerted effort has been made to show that an active-living culture cannot be the responsibility of physical education teachers only, but it is a responsibility of all teacher disciplines, and examples were given to the other teachers. Although many activities were scheduled for Agita Galera Day, the central theme was to discuss the benefits of active living for 15 to 20 min during regular school classes, and then have a community walk or other physical activity. The outcome was fantastic with crowds of students occupying the streets and main squares from the very small to the large cities of São Paulo. A helicopter brought the State Secretary of Health to the so-called mega-focus of Agita, to recognize the efforts of the different communities.

Active Worker Day. In order to promote physical activity in the workplace, a tailored set of education material, involving manual, folders, banners, booklets, and stickers were made. Information in the materials included short explanations focusing on the healthy benefits of physical activity offering suggested durations, frequencies and intensities. Beyond the Agita São Paulo suggestions, an important point to attain success for intervention strategies is to consider the institutional perspectives in preparing information according to the different groups needs. Several interesting experiences have occurred, since lectures are given at the beginning of the workday journey, until stopping the assembly line, as in the General Motors-Brazil, to read and discuss about the benefits of active-living. Another important point has been the direct participation of labour unions through their communication system to the employees trying to promote the importance of active daily living. In the last several years, we have estimated that over 5 million employees from different industries have participated in the Active Worker Day.

Active Elderly Day. The Agita São Paulo programme has developed specific material to distribute and spread the message to the elderly population. The programme produced a brochure and a poster for this specific group in which the programme calls attention to how people can get and maintain their functional independence by being physically active. A mega-event is organized every year on the occasion of the national and international elderly day at the end of September. It has been a walking event in order to promote the joining of generations to celebrate the special fact of being alive. In this event, sun-hats, a special bag with the brochures, hand-fans, and some sweets are provided because the people love to get gifts and to take something home. The walking day includes a short walk (no more than 30 minutes) in the cities' green parks and is combined with some recreational and leisure activities, including dances, games, and assistance for other elderly groups.

Agita media exposure

Mega-events like Agita Galera are crucial in bringing media attention to the programme. There is a special section in Agita headquarters to follow-up on the impacts of these activities. The media impact might be recognized by a potential TV audience of 21 million people/year, representing the impressive amount of almost 13 million dollars savings/year (non-paid media approach). Strong supportive reports were published in 28 state and 42 regional newspapers, two national and 8 international magazines, and broadcast on seven state and four national TV programmes. These reports have a special significance since Agita does not spend any financial resources for media exposure – the so called 'non-paid media approach'. Agita developed a media surveillance service that tracks how many newspaper columns were published, their seasonal variation, and in what regions. The media coverage areas per year includes over $39,399.80$ cm^2, which represented an average of 237.6 cm^2 per article of media coverage[38].

Special Agita promotional activities

As mentioned earlier, culture and social manifestations are essential elements in the Agita Programme. Special intervention promotions were developed for Carnival; a special hand-fan was distributed during the samba-school parade and a 'half-hour woman' and a 'half-hour seashoreman' were developed to attract gender and regional attention.

Agita has used several marketing materials. Red sticker marketing materials became popular national-wide. Most of those did not require any Agita funding, e.g. electricity company bills with our message imprinted reached 7 million families, our message was displayed in the largest, private soccer stadium and at the metro stations (over 2 million people/day); and messages were broadcast on truck driver's radio-station programmes.

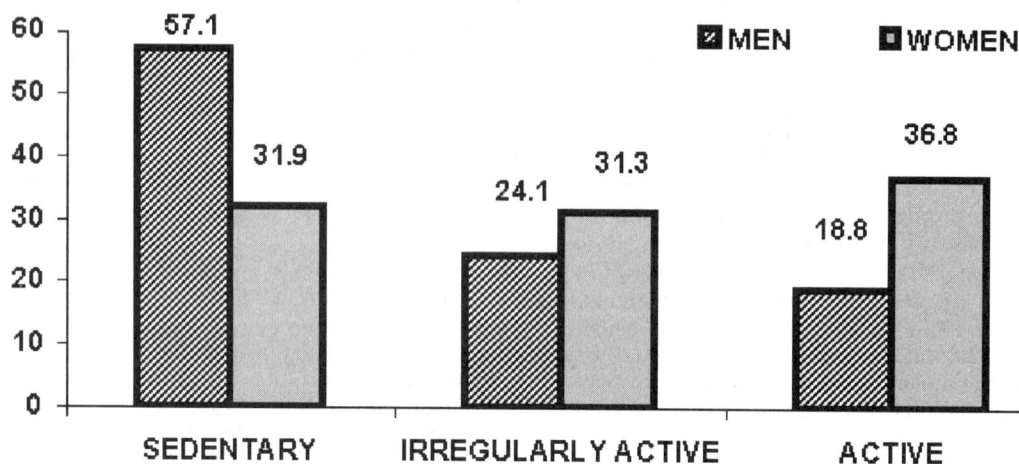

Fig. 2. Physical activity prevalence among men and woman (645) in São Paulo Metropolitan Area.

Nutritional issues in the Agita model

Special attention is dedicated to nutritional issues and to the consequences of the metabolic syndrome. In the Agita programme, e.g. the combination of the nutritional and physical activity pyramid. Joint efforts were developed with other advocacy groups, such as nutrition (Brazilian Multi-professional Society for Infancy and Maternal Nutrition); obesity (The Brazilian Association of the Studies on Obesity – ABESO), diabetes (The National Association for Assistance of Diabetics – ANAD and The Juvenile Diabetes – ADJ); and hypertension (The Association of Protection and Friends of Hypertension). Presentations were conducted at their major conferences, and invitations were received to publish editorial articles[39] in their journals and Agita may review research projects that were developed[40,41].

A good example of the transitional phase, represented by a decline in physical activity and probable increase in calorie intake, is given by two studies developed in Ilhabela, the ocean island between Rio and São Paulo. Teodosio[42] verified adiposity and weight secular trends (1980–2000) among boys and girls from a low socioeconomic region, and found an increase of 10.7 per cent in weight, 12.2 per cent in total adiposity, and 21.6 per cent in central adiposity. Meanwhile, a negative secular trend was observed in physical fitness variables for upper limb strength (–35.5 per cent in boys and –28.9 per cent in girls); no changes were found in lower limb strength or cardio-respiratory variables[43].

Nutrition and physical activity profiles were analysed in an elderly target group of the Agita programme, comprising 71 women over 50 years of age[44]. A significant increase in frequency (48 per cent) as consequence of Agita message, involvement in moderate physical activity (123 per cent), and walking duration (150 per cent) was reported; no changes in body composition were observed, probably because of the short time intervention. However, it was noted that women who received physical activity advice presented a positive change in nutrition intake, even without any nutritional orientation. Those women spontaneously decreased total calories (from 1,581.4 kcal/day to 1,316.6 kcal/day) and fat intake (from 65.4 g/day to 48.2 g/day), suggesting that an active life-style promotion may enhance other healthy behaviours, including nutritional habits.

In another study within the Agita programme, the relationships among nutrition behaviour, physical activity, and mental well-being were explored through measures of self-image. It was shown that among adolescents under a restricted diet, those who were regularly active (1,734 kcal/day total intake) presented higher values of self-image satisfaction than those who were more sedentary (1,565 kcal/day total intake) although they reported similar total calories intake[45].

Another interesting feature developed by the Agita São Paulo team[46] is that among 41 elderly women (aged 50 to 69 years), body image seems to be more related ($P < 0.05$) to body weight (r: 0.52 to 0.67), body mass index (r: 0.57 to 0.74), and adiposity (r: 0.45 to 0.59), than to calorie intake (r: 0.11 to 0.41).

Agita São Paulo outcomes

The evaluation process included surveillance by central office and out-side groups and included measurements of physical activity levels, physical activity knowledge, barriers, attitudes, behaviour stage, and knowledge about the programme.

Data was obtained from a home visiting survey of 645 randomly selected homes. These data, stratified by sex, age, education, and socio-economic level, revealed that 55.7 per cent have heard about Agita; among those, 23.1 per cent knew the main message, over 60 per cent of the best educated had heard about Agita, and 37 per cent knew about the Agita purpose. Recall of Agita and knowledge of its purpose were well distributed among different socioeconomic levels and was known by 67 per cent of the most educated.

Figure 2 shows that 18 per cent of the men and about 36 per cent of women were already reaching the CDC/ACSM recommendation after four years of the programme. Because walking is an important strategy of Agita, it would be of interest to analyse the influence of that behaviour on physical activity levels. When walking was included, 54.8 per cent of the total sample have reached the CDC/ACSM recommendation, 48.7 per cent among men and 61 per cent among women (Table 1).

Table 1. Participation in recommended physical activity, including walking, among men and women from São Paulo Metropolitan area

Gender	Participation (%)	95 % CI
Overall	54.8	50.6–59.0
Male	48.7	42.8–54.6
Female	61.0	55.1–66.8

CI: Interval of confidence.

The prevalence of those who reached the CDC/ACSM recommendation, as related to Agita message knowledge were analysed in an attempt to verify the impact of the programme on physical activity levels more specifically. Table 2 clearly shows that the chances to reach adequate levels of physical activity were higher among those who knew the Agita purpose and objectives (43.0 per cent) than among those did not (35.3 per cent). The influence became more marked when walking was included (Table 3); overall inactivity declined to 10.9 per cent, but the risk of being inactive was almost double among whose did not know the Agita purpose (13.1 per cent) when compared to whose that knew the programme objectives (7.1 per cent).

Table 2. Participation in recommended physical activity as related to Agita purpose knowledge, excluding walking, in São Paulo Metropolitan area

Gender	Participation (%)	95 % CI
Overall	38.1	32.5–43.7
Yes	35.3	28.4–42.2
No	43.0	33.5–52.5

CI: Interval of confidence.

Table 3. Participation in recommended physical activity as related to Agita São Paulo purpose knowledge, including walking, in São Paulo Metropolitan area

Gender	Participation (%)	95 % CI
Overall	10.9	7.2–14.5
Yes	13.1	8.1–18.0
No	7.1	2.0–12.1

CI: Interval of confidence.

These are remarkably lower than the index of 69 per cent of sedentariness obtained 10 years ago, supported by recent findings of Andrade[47], suggesting that Agita played some role in the change because inactivity was more prevalent among those who did not know the programme. The level of physical activity declined, as in other countries, as age increased, although moderate walking messages were more popular among middle-age adults and elderly groups, than among young adults[48].

A school setting intervention revealed a marked increase ($P < 0.05$ per cent) in the time involved in vigorous physical activity among girls and boys, 11–14 years of age[49]. Those results are consistent with the increased physical activity knowledge in those groups in that time period[50].

Table 4 shows some of the factors the programme coordinators considered the most important to emerge from the Agita experience.

Table 4. Lessons from the past for guidance in the future: key-factors emerged from Agita São Paulo experience

a.	The inclusion principle
b.	Intellectual and institutional partnership principle
c.	Inter and intra-sectorial partnership balance
d.	Empowering the partner institution agenda
e.	Similar in cause; and diverse in action
f.	Scientific sound
g.	Non-paid media approach
h.	Clear, simple and feasible message
i.	Cultural adaptation
j.	One-step ahead model
k.	Surveillance
l.	Links with other risk-factor advocacy groups

National and international impact

The Agita São Paulo programme has diffused to other states, developing the Brazilian Networking and launching the Agita Bahia and the Mexe Campina among others, which caused the Ministry for Health to request the Agita Centre to organize the Agita Brazil. The research centre, CELAFISCS, was also requested to support other countries, e.g. Colombia (Muevete Bogota, Risaralda Activa), Argentina (A moverse), and Uruguay (Movete Uruguay) to launch their programmes!

Panamerican Health Organization in conjunction with the CDC are supporting the creation of the network to promote physical activity in the Americas. The Physical Activity Network for the Americas (Agita America) now includes about 20 countries in the Continent! WHO considered Agita as a model, and published it in the World Health Report[1]. Morover, WHO decided to dedicate World Health Day 2002 to promote Physical Activity, using the slogan 'Agita Mundo – Move for Health'. Dra. Gro Brundtland, Director General of WHO, came to São Paulo to officially start the celebration, comprising 1644 events in 125 countries.

Conclusions

In conclusion, based upon the Agita São Paulo experience, it appears that a multi-level community-wide intervention to promote physical activity may obtain a good impact if it is considers in the model: (a) inclusion principles; (b) intellectual and institutional partnerships; (c) inter and intra-sectorial partnership balance; (d) empowerment of the partner institution agenda; (e) similarity in cause; and diverse in action; (f) scientific soundness; (g) non-paid media approach; (h) clear, simple and feasible messages; (i) cultural adaptation; (j) one-step ahead model; (k) surveillance; and (l) links with other risk-factor advocacy groups.

References

1. Matsudo VKR. Passaport for health. World Health Organization Report 1997; 3: 16–7.
2. Matsudo VKR, Andrade DR, Matsudo SMM, Araujo TL, Andrade E, Figueira Jr AJ *et al.* Physical education, health and well-being. Proceedings of the World Summit on Physical Education 2001; 2: 85–94.

3. Ministério da Sáude Programas e Projetos Doenças Cardiovasculares.[on line] Available from: URL: http//: www.saude.gov.br/programas/cardio/cardio.htm [Accessed 6 July 2000].

4. Barreto ML e Carmo EH. Determinantes das condições de saúde e problemas prioritários no país. In: XI Conferência Nacional de Saúde; Brasília. 2000. pp. 1–13.

5. Monteiro C, Benificio M, Conde W. Shifting obesity trends in Brazil. *Eur J Clin Nutr* 2000; 54: 342–6.

6. Lotufo PA. Mortalidade precoce por doenças do coração no Brasil. Comparação com outros países. *Arquivos Brasileiros de Cardiologia* 1998; 70: 321–5.

7. Ministério da Saúde. Datasus. [on line] Available from: URL: http//: www.datasus.gov.br/cgi/tabcgi.exercício [Accessed 23 February 2001].

8. Rego A, Berardo F, Rodrigues S. Fatores de risco para doenças crônico não transmissíveis: Inquérito domiciliar no município de São Paulo, SP (Brasil). Metodologia e resultados preliminares. *Revista Brasileira de Saúde Pública* 1990; 24: 277–85.

9. Data Folha Jornal Folha de São Paulo. Levantamento Nacional de Atividade Física. 1997.

10. Farrell SW, Kampert JB, Kohl III HW, Barlow CE, Macera CA, Paffenbarger Jr RS *et al.* Influences of cardiorespiratory fitness levels and other predictors on cardiovascular disease mortality in men. *Med Sci Sports Exerc* 1998; 30: 889–905.

11. Kohl H. What is the magnitude of risk for cardiovascular disease associated with sedentary living habits? In: *Physical activity and cardiovascular health – A National Consensus*, Arthur L (ed.), pp. 26–33. Champaing: Human Kinetics; 1997.

12. Blair S, Kampert JB, Kohl HW, Barlow CE, Macera CA, Paffenbarger RS, Gibbons LW Influences of cardiorespiratory fitness and other precursors on cardiovascular disease and all-cause mortality in men and women. *JAMA* 1996; 276: 205–10.

13. Centers for Disease Control and Prevention. Promoting physical activity: a best buy in public health. A Report from the CDC; 2000.

14. Oliveira LC, Matsudo V, Matsudo S. CELAFISCS – XX years of history in sports sciences. XIX International Symposium on Sports Sciences. São Paulo; 1994. p. 5–18.

15. Prochaska JO, Marcus BH. The transtheoretical model: Applications to exercise. In: *Advances in exercise adherence*, Dishman RK (ed.), pp.161–80. Champaign, Illinois: Human Kinetics, 1994.

16. Bandura A. *Social foundations of thought and action: A social cognitive theory*, pp. 1–386. Englewood Cliffs, NJ: Prentice-Hall; 1986.

17. Bracht N, Kingsbury L, Rissel C. *A five-stage community organization model for health promotion: Empowerment and partnership strategies. Health promotion at the community level 2: New advances*, Bracht N (ed.) (2nd edn), pp. 83–104. Thousand Oaks, CA: Sage Publications; 1999.

18. Minkler M, Wallerstein N. Improving health through community organization and community building. In: *Health behavior and health education: Theory, research and practice* (2nd edn), Glanz K, Lewis FM, Rimer BK (eds). San Francisco: Jossey-Bass; 1997.

19. Donovan RJ, Owen N. *Social marketing and population interventions. Advances in exercise adherence*, Dishman RK (ed.), pp. 249–90. Champaign, IL: Human Kinetics; 1994.

20. Lefebvre R, Rochlin I. Social marketing. In: *Health behavior and health education: Theory, research and practice*, Glanz K, Lewis FM, Rimer BK (eds) (2nd edn), pp. 384–402. San Francisco: Jossey-Bass; 1997.

21. Sallis J, Bauman A, Pratt M. Environmental and policy interventions to promote physical activity. *Am J Prevent Med* 1998; 415: 379–97.

22. Mcleroy KR, Bibeau D, Steckler A. An ecological perspective on health promotion programs. *Health Educ Qtly* 1998; 15: 355–77.

23. Sallis J, Owen N. Ecologic models. In: *Health behavior and health education: Theory, research and practice*, Glanz K, Lewis FM, Rimer BK (eds) (2nd edn), p. 4. San Francisco: Jossey-Bass; 1997.

24. Finnegan J, Viswanath K. Mass media and health promotion: lessons learned, with implications for public health campaigns. In: *Health promotion at the community level 2: New advances*, pp. 119–34. Newbury Park, California: Sage; 1999.

25. Pate R, Pratt M, Blair SN, Haskell W, Macera CA, Bouchard C *et al.* Physical activity and public health: a recommendation from the Centers for Disease Control and Prevention and the American College of Sports Medicine. *JAMA* 1995; 273: 402–7.

26. Blair S, Booth M, Gyarfas I. XDevelopment of public policy and physical activity initiatives internationally. *Sports Medicine* 1995; 321: 157–63.

27. Andrade DR, Matsudo SMM, Matsudo VKR, Figueira Jr A, Araújo T, Andrade E, Oliveira L. Barriers to exercise adherence among activity young adults. *Medicine and Science in Sports and Exercise Supplement* 1998; 30: S182.

28. Oliveira LC, Andrade DR, Figueira Jr A, Araújo T, Matsudo VKR, Matsudo SMM, Andrade E. Physical activity barrier as related to behavior stage in white collar workers. *Medicine and Science in Sports and Exercise Supplement* 1998; 30: S121.

29. Maresman S, Matsudo VKR, Nieves C, Araújo TL, Matsudo SMM, Andrade DR, Andrade EL, Oliveira LC. *Coaliciones multisectoriales en salud – La experiencia de Agita São Paulo PAHO.* In press, 2003.

30. Governo do Estado de São Paulo – Secretaria de Estado da Saúde. Programa Agita São Paulo Manual de orientação. São Paulo; 1998.

31. Governo do Estado de São Paulo – Secretaria de Estado da Saúde. Programa Agita São Paulo. The São Paulo manifesto: promoting physical activity in the Americas. *ICSSPE Bulletin* 2000; 28–37.

32. Matsudo V, Matsudo S, Araújo T, Andrade DR, Andrade EL, Oliveira LC *et al.* Agitando o médico e os agentes de saúde. In: *Agita São Paulo: proposta de intervenção em grupos de profissionais de saúde.* Anais do XXII Simpósio Internacional de Ciências do Esporte. São Paulo, Brasil; 1999. p.162.

33. Gonçalves LG, Figueira Jr A, Oliva M, Matsudo VKR. Atividade física espontânea relacionada com o nível sócio – econômico. Anais do XVIII Simpósio Internacional de Ciências do Esporte. São Paulo, Brasil; 1992; S22.

34. Paschoal V, Andrade D, Matsudo S, Matsudo VKR. Nutrition knowledge and physical activities habits in Ilhabela (Brazil) and the United States. The International Pre-Olympic Scientific Congress. Dallas, Texas: USA; 1996. S1047.

35. Matsudo SMM, Matsudo VKR, Andrade DR, Rocha JR. Physical fitness and time spent watching T.V. in children from low socioeconomic region. *Medicine and Science in Sports and Exercise* 1997; (Suppl 29): 237.

36. Hardman K, Marshall J. World-wide survey on the state and status of physical education in schools. Proceedings of the World Summit on Physical Education. Berlin: ICSSPE; 2001. pp. 15–36.

37. Andrade DR, Matsudo SMM, Matsudo VK, Araújo T, Andrade EL, Rocha A *et al.* Physical activity patterns in girls and boys from low socioeconomic region physical activity level in adolescents. In: XIXth International Seminar on Pediatric Work Physiology Heavitree Road; 1997.

38. Figueira Jr A, Oliveira LC, Araújo TL, Matsudo SMM, Andrade DR, Andrade EL, Matsudo VKR. Impacto do programa de promoção de atividade física na mídia não paga: experiência do programa Agita São Paulo. *Revista Brasileira de Atividade Física e Saúde* 2000; 5: 38–47.

39. Bracco M, Araújo T, Matsudo VKR, Matsudo S, Andrade D, Andrade E *et al.* Atividade Física: Quanto e como fazer para a prevenção e controle do Diabetes Mellitus tipo 2. *Revista Diabetes Clínica* 2000; 4: 368–370.

40. Costa HD, Matsudo VKR, Matsudo SMM, Andrade EL. Effect of walking program on physical fitness and glycemic control in patients with diabetes type II (NIDDM). *Medicine Science Sports Exercise* 1998; 30: S361.

41. Pereira MHN. Mudança na adiposidade de mulheres adultas após um programa de exercícios enriquecidos das técnicas de modificação do comportamento. *Revista Brasileira de Ciência e Movimento* 1990; 4: 18–27.

42. Teodosio JP, Araújo TL, Figueira Jr A, Raso V, Matsudo VKR. Tendência secular da adiposidade de escolares residentes em região de baixo nível sócio-econômico. XXIII Simpósio internacional de ciências do esporte, p.149. São Paulo: Brasil; 2000.

43. Marques AC, Araújo TL, Figueira Jr A, Raso V, Matsudo VKR. Tendência secular das variáveis de aptidão física relacionadas à saúde em adolescentes de uma região de baixo nível sócio-econômico. XXIII Simpósio Internacional de Ciências do Esporte. São Paulo: Brasil; 2000. p. 125.

44. Ferreira M, Matsudo S, Andrade E, Braggion G, Matsudo V. Relação entre a adequação alimentar e variáveis antropométricas de mulheres de 55 a 75 anos fisicamente ativas. XXIII Simpósio Internacional de Ciências do Esporte. São Paulo: Brasil; 2000. p. 99.

45. Braggion GF, Matsudo SMM, Matsudo VKR. Consumo alimentar, atividade física e percepção da aparência corporal em adolescentes. *Revista Brasileira de Ciência e Movimento* 2000; 8: 15–21.

46. Braggion GF, Matsudo SMM, Matsudo VKR, Andrade EL. Energy intake, anthropometric variables and body image in active elderly women as related to age. *Medicine Science Sports Exercise* 2000; 32(5): S219.

47. Andrade EL, Matsudo VKR, Matsudo SMM, Andrade DR, Araújo TL, Oliveira LC *et al.* Level of physical activity in adults, including and excluding walking, according to the knowledge of Agita São Paulo Program. *Medicine Science in Sports Exercise* 2001; 33: S179.

48. Matsudo V, Matsudo S, Araújo T, Andrade DR, Andrade EL, Oliveira LC *et al.* XModerate, vigorous, and walking messages adopting in a physical activity intervention program, as related to chronological age. *Medicine and Science in Sports and Exercise Supplement* 2001; 33: S1192.

49. Matsudo VKR, Andrade DR, Matsudo SMM, Araujo T, Andrade E, Figueira Jr A, Oliveira LC. Impact of a community – school intervention program on physical activity behavior of male and female adolescents. *Medicine and Science in Sports and Exercise Supplement* 1999; 31: S1327.

50. Andrade D, Matsudo S, Matsudo V, Araújo T, Andrade E, Figueira Jr A *et al.* Changes in physical activity knowledge level as related to health promotion among students after one year intervention program. *Medicine and Science in Sports and Exercise* 2000; 32: S94.

Progress in Obesity Research: 9. Edited by *Geraldo Medeiros-Neto, Alfredo Halpern* and *Claude Bouchard*
©2003 John Libbey Eurotext Ltd, pp. 881–886.

CHAPTER 184

Practical prescribing

Peter G. Kopelman

Barts & The London, Queen Mary's School of Medicine & Dentistry, Turner Street, London E1 2AD, UK
[e-mail: p.g.kopelman@qmul.ac.uk]

Background

Obesity causes or exacerbates many health problems, both independently and in association with other diseases. Overweight and obesity must be considered as a disease in which an excess of body fat has accumulated such that health may be adversely affected. Life-insurance and epidemiological studies confirm that increasing degrees of overweight and obesity are important predictors of decreased longevity. In spite of this evidence, some clinicians still consider obesity to be a self-inflicted condition of little medical significance that does not warrant medical intervention nor consideration of drug therapy.

Rationale for prescribing for overweight and obesity

Obesity is not a single disorder but a heterogeneous group of conditions with multiple causes. Although genetic differences are of undoubted importance, the marked rise in the prevalence of obesity is best explained by behavioural and environmental changes that have resulted from technological advances. The most variable component of energy expenditure is physical activity, representing 20–50 per cent of total energy expenditure – an analysis of physical activity of an individual should be a critical element of any therapeutic assessment. Cross-cultural studies of physical activity and BMI demonstrate a sevenfold increased risk of overweight (BMI > 25) in those with a low physical activity ratio (total energy expenditure/RMR). Thus the primary intervention for overweight and obesity should address an increase in regular physical activity.

The understanding of the role of energy intake in the aetiology of obesity is confounded by failure to report food intake accurately. Under-reporting is widely recognized as a feature of obesity, with comparisons of energy intake and expenditure showing a consistent shortfall in self-reported food intake of approximately 30 per cent of energy requirements. An initial assessment of any patient with a weight problem must include a dietary review and considered dietary advice.

Current drug treatment of obesity is directed at reducing energy/food intake either by an action on the gastrointestinal system or via an action through the central nervous system control of appetite and feeding. In prescribing a drug, a clinician must assess firstly whether the type of drug action is appropriate for a particular patient (i.e. the evidence that the patient is currently eating in excess of calorie needs) and, secondly, the likelihood of a favourable weight loss response. This requires a detailed clinical assessment of the patient.

Clinical assessment

An outline of a scheme for the clinical assessment of an overweight or obese patient is given in Table 1. Height should be measured accurately using a stadiometer and weight measured by accurate scales calibrated against known weights. Fat distribution is assessed by measurement of the waist circumference and used to refine an assessment of risk for patients with a BMI of 25 to 34.9. Waist circumference is taken as the mid-point between the lower rib margin and the iliac crest.

An examination of the resting pulse rate and blood pressure are important as is the measurement of the neck circumference – a neck circumference of 43cm (17 inches) or greater indicates a likelihood of obstructive sleep apnoea. An examination of the skin is important – acanthosis nigricans (pigmented, 'velvety', skin creases especially in the axillae) suggests insulin resistance. Moderate hirsutism in women may indicate the polycystic ovary syndrome. Gastrointestinal reflux is a common cause of persistent cough in an obese patient.

Table 1. Examination

1.	Height, weight – calculate BMI
2.	Waist circumference
3.	Neck circumference
4.	Blood pressure and resting pulse rate
5.	Any evidence for cardiac valvular disease
6.	Any evidence for pulmonary hypertension, cor pulmonale or congestive cardiac failure
7.	Signs of dyslipidaemia
8.	Signs of thyroid disease
9.	Ophthalmic evidence for diabetes or sustained hypertension

Assessment of risk

An assessment of an obese patient's absolute risk status requires an assessment of associated disease conditions (established CHD, other atherosclerotic disease, type 2 diabetes and sleep apnoea), other obesity-associated diseases such as gynaecological abnormalities, osteoarthritis, gallstones and stress incontinence and cardiovascular risk factors. These will include cigarette smoking, hypertension, high-risk LDL cholesterol (>4 mmol/l), low HDL cholesterol (<1 mmol/), impaired fasting blood glucose and a family history of premature CHD.

Patients are classified as being of high absolute risk if they have three of these risk factors. Such patients usually require specific management of the risk factors.

Assessment of motivation to lose weight

Not all patients are prepared for weight reduction despite a referral to a medical practitioner. Indeed, many see the prescription of an anti-obesity drug as an alternative to lifestyle change that includes dietary restriction. As a consequence, it is often useful to apply the stages of change model to assess the 'readiness to change' to confirm that a patient understands the need for weight loss, and is prepared to follow medical advice to achieve and maintain an agreed weight goal.

Goals of weight loss

The success or failure of a treatment programme may be judged by an arbitrarily chosen target weight loss. After an initial period of relatively rapid weight reduction, an average continuing weight loss of anything up to 1 kg per week should be considered as acceptable. Assessment of success must take account of the age of the patient, the initial degree of overweight and obesity, the presence of indicators of associated risk or complications and previous attempts at weight control.

Weight loss goals for overweight and obese patients should be tailored to the individual. A weight loss of 5 per cent of the initial body weight will result in some improvement, while a loss of 10 per cent is of major benefit, with clinically useful changes such as lowered blood pressure, reduction in plasma total cholesterol and triglycerides, an increase in HDL cholesterol and a significant improvement in diabetic control.

The primary goal of treatment for patients treated with an anti-obesity drug should be a 10 per cent reduction from the initial weight with consequential amelioration of many of the associated risk factors. Nevertheless, weight loss should be approached incrementally with new weight loss goals negotiated with the patient once the original target is achieved.

Selection of patients suitable for anti-obesity drug therapy

It is important that doctors who use such drugs are fully familiar with either the primary literature or an authoritative summary.

The accepted first line strategy for weight reduction and weight maintenance is a combination of diet, exercise and behaviour modification. The first line of management should be at least 3 months of managed care that includes dietary control and changes in lifestyle. Exceptionally, this period may be shortened when the clinician judges that drug treatment is justified at an earlier stage due to over-riding medical circumstances. Table 2 lists the criteria that should be applied to judge the suitability of a patient for drug treatment.

Table 2

1.	Drug treatment may be appropriate where diet and exercise have not achieved acceptable weight loss relative to associated medical risk.
2.	Weight lowering drugs should be targeted at those at high risk from obesity, not obesity alone.
	The following priorities for drug treatment are applicable:
1.	Patients with established co-morbidities such as type 2 diabetes, hypertension, dyslipidaemia.
2.	Patients who are physically restricted by their weight either as a consequence of breathlessness or arthritis.
3.	Patients considered to be at high risk – for example, those with family histories of overweight or obese parents who died prematurely from CHD or developed type 2 diabetes with complications.

Appropriate prescribing – therapeutic 'responsiveness'

The criteria applied to the use of an anti-obesity drug are similar to those applied to the treatment of other relapsing disorders. It is important to avoid offering anti-obesity drug therapy to patients who are seeking a 'quick fix' for their weight problem. The initiation of drug treatment will depend on the clinician's judgement about the risks to an individual from continuing obesity. It may be appropriate after at least 3 months of supervised diet, exercise and behavioural management, or at a subsequent review, if a patient's BMI is equal or greater than 30 kg/m^2 and weight loss is less than 10 per cent of the presenting weight. In certain clinical circumstances it may also be appropriate to consider anti-obesity drug treatment for those patients with established co-morbidities whose BMI is 27 kg/m^2 or greater if this is permitted by the drug's licence. An anti-obesity drug should never be prescribed for a patient whose BMI is less than that specified in the product licence for the drug.

It would appear pointless to prescribe a drug if a patient continues to gain weight after initial dietary and non-drug management have been initiated, because the chance of relapse on cessation of drug therapy (which of itself is for a relatively limited time) is extremely likely.

The experience from the use of anti-obesity drugs during 12–24 month randomized controlled trials indicate that approximately 50 per cent of the actively treated patients respond as judged by 5–10 per cent reduction in body weight maintained over 12 months. The weight loss occurs in the 'responder' group within 12 weeks. This indicates a suitable time period when a response to drug treatment can be identified and a decision taken to continue the medication. Continuing assessment of drug therapy for efficacy and safety is essential. If the drug is efficacious in helping a patient to lose and/or maintain weight loss, and there are no serious side effects, it may be continued. If not, it should be discontinued. Once a weight loss target has been achieved, there should be an opportunity for re-negotiation of a new target, if indicated, and/or long term monitoring with reinforcement.

Monitoring and longer term follow up

Patients prescribed anti-obesity drugs require the following:

- An individualized weight loss management programme;
- Concomitant advice about diet, physical activity and lifestyle change;
- Monitoring of weight (ideally monthly – no greater than two monthly);
- Monitoring of pulse rate and blood pressure;
- The treatment plan should be recorded for each patient and incorporated into local audit data recording systems;

- As weight loss progresses adjustments of medications taken by the patient may be necessary. For example, the dose of an oral hypoglycaemic agent may need to be reduced as insulin sensitivity increases with weight loss.

The duration of treatment should be considered in the light of the clinical circumstance but should never exceed the period indicated by the product licence.

Once the drug is discontinued patients should be monitored for at least a further 6 months in order to discourage weight regain. Weight loss during treatment with an anti-obesity drug is usually regained over time following cessation of treatment but typically at a slower rate than that experienced during weight loss. On average it appears to take about three additional years to regain the weight that has been lost over a year on the drug.

Appropriate setting for anti-obesity drug treatment

Any centre that claims to specifically provide expertise in weight management should incorporate the essential elements outlined in Table 3.

Table 3

1.	Trained staff directly involved in the running of the weight loss programme. These staff [medical, nursing and other healthcare professionals] should have attended courses on the management of obesity and must be provided with an opportunity to continue their education.
2.	A printed programme for weight management that includes clearly outlined dietary advice, behavioural modification techniques, physical exercise and strategies for long term life style change. Such a programme may include a family and/or group approach.
3.	Suitable equipment, in particular accurate and regularly calibrated weighing scales and stadiometer.
4.	Specified weight loss goals with energy deficits being achieved through moderating food intake and increasing physical expenditure.
5.	Documentation of individual patients' health risks. This will include BMI, waist circumference, blood pressure, blood lipids, cigarette smoking and other co-morbid conditions.
6.	A clearly defined follow up procedure which involves collaboration between the different settings of care, and provides regular monitoring and documentation of progress and includes details of criteria for judging the success of weight loss. This will allow a weight loss programme to be properly supported, medical conditions to be monitored and problems or issues to be addressed at the earliest opportunity. It is wise to have available a checklist of possible adverse drug effects e.g. anxiety, disturbances of sleep, breathlessness, depression and diarrhoea.

Types of drug treatment for overweight and obesity

There are currently two categories of anti-obesity drugs – those that act on the gastrointestinal system (pancreatic lipase inhibitors) and those which act on the central nervous system to suppress appetite.

Drugs acting on the gastrointestinal system – pancreatic lipase inhibitors

Orlistat inhibits pancreatic and gastric lipase thereby decreasing ingested triglyceride hydrolysis. It produces a dose-dependent reduction in dietary fat absorption thereby leading to weight loss in obese subjects.

Centrally acting anti-obesity drugs

Sibutramine promotes a sense of satiety through its central action as a serotonin and norepinephrine re-uptake inhibitor. In addition, it may have enhancing effect on thermogenesis through stimulation of peripheral norepinephrine receptors although this has not been proven in clinical practice.

Indications for a particular type of anti-obesity drug in clinical practice

There are no good clinical studies that have directly evaluated sibutramine against orlistat nor explored which particular patient may better benefit from one or other of the two drugs. Nevertheless, there are some simple pointers:

Patients who may be suitable for sibutramine:

- Uncontrollable appetite and eating;

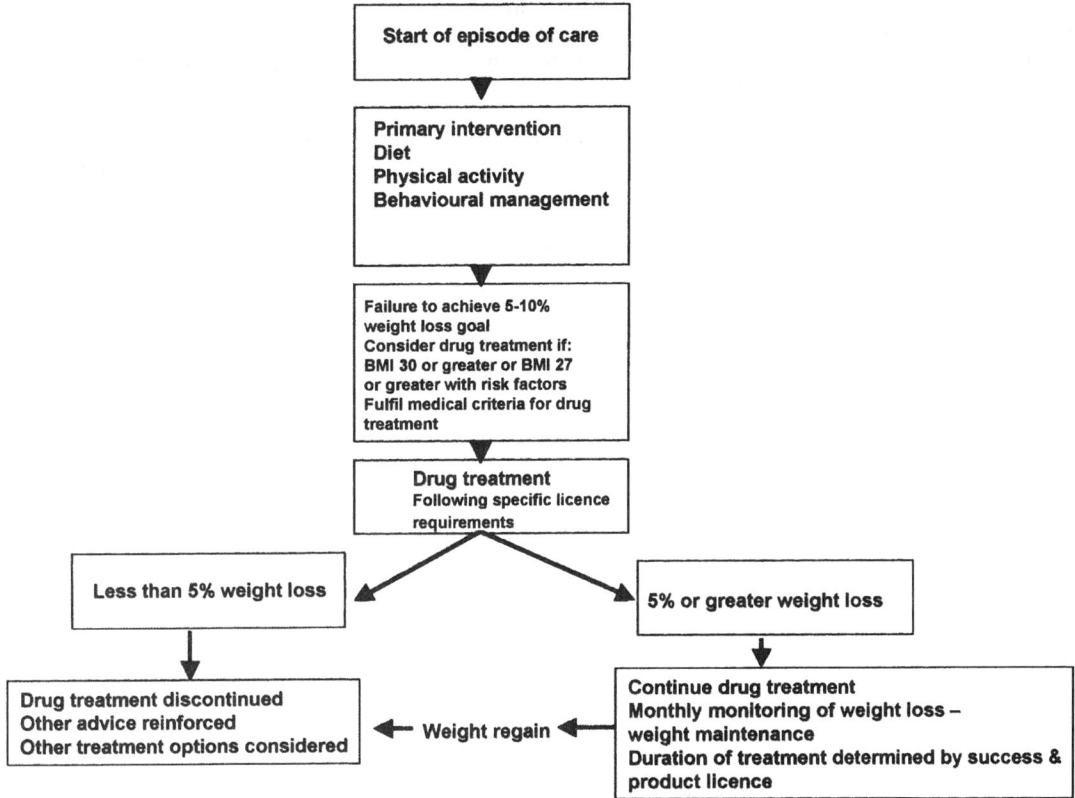

Fig. 1.

- Frequent snacking;

- Nocturnal eaters;

- Need for immediate weight loss for medical reasons;

- No contraindications to use of sibutramine (specifically cardiac abnormalities or an elevated blood pressure –>140/90 mm Hg).

Sibutramine should be discontinued if the resting pulse rate is increased >10 beats per minute and the blood pressure exceeds 145/95 mm Hg.
Patients who may be suitable for orlistat:

- Those who have lost at least 2.5 kg in weight prior to consideration of drug treatment;

- Patients requiring longer term behavioural change;

- Patients in whom a dietary assessment suggests high fat intake;

- Previous repeated short term weight loss followed by rapid weight regain;

- Ability to adhere to a low fat diet for the longer term.

The product licence for sibutramine advises that treatment should only be continued beyond 4 weeks if the patient has lost 2 kg or greater.
The prescription for both sibutramine and orlistat may be continued beyond three months if a patient has lost at least 5 per cent of their body weight from the start of drug treatment. The drug should be stopped thereafter if weight regain occurs despite continuation of the treatment.

Combination therapy with anti-obesity drugs is contraindicated because of the absence of evidence for synergy between the two drugs, and lack of information about safety. Logic would suggest no additional benefit from taking the two drugs together given their specific actions on suppressing eating and reducing fat absorption – if a patient does not eat there seems little point in prescribing a drug to reduce fat absorption.

There is limited information about the use of anti-obesity drugs in patients over the age of 75 years – in such a circumstance, the accepted practice is to aim for weight maintenance rather than weight loss. Neither drug is licensed for use in children.

Longer term anti-obesity drug treatment (beyond 2 years)

A calculation of cost effectiveness for current anti-obesity drugs suggest a figure of £15,000–30000 ($/Euro22,500–45,000) per QUALY gained.

At the present time, the benefits from longer term drug therapy are merely expectations derived from epidemiological data and observed changes in surrogate end-points such as lipids, blood pressure and diabetic status. There is no hard data related to defined outcomes, including a reduction in early mortality, because of the absence of clinical trials that extend beyond two years. This is important to bear in mind when considering drug therapy for a patient.

Selected Bibliography – from which the evidence base for the text is drawn

1. Kopelman PG. Obesity as a medical problem. *Nature* 2000; 404: 635–643.

2. US Department of Health and Health Sciences (PHS). Physical activity and health: a report of the Surgeon General (Executive Summary). Superintendent of Documents, Pittsburgh; 1996.

3. National Institutes of Health (NIH), National Heart, Lung & Blood Institute (NLLBI). *Clinical guidelines on the identification, evaluation and treatment of overweight and obesity: the evidence report.* US Government Press, Washington; 1998.

4. Committee on Nutrition, Massachusetts Medical Society. Obesity treatment using drug therapy, White Paper. The Massachusetts Medical Society: Waltham MA; 1998.

5. National Task Force on the prevention and treatment of obesity. Long-term pharmacotherapy in the management of obesity. J Am Med Soc 1996; 276: 1907–1915.

6. Scottish Intercollegiate Guidelines Network (SIGN). *Integrating prevention with weight management.* SIGN: Edinburgh; 1996.

7. Royal College of Physicians of London. Clinical management of overweight and obese patients with particular reference to the use of drugs; 1998.

8. National Institute for Clinical Excellence (NICE). Guidance on the use of orlistat for the treatment of obesity in adults (March 2001) – Available from: URL:

9. http: // www.nice.org.uk.

10. National Institute for Clinical Excellence (NICE). Guidance on the use of sibutramine for the treatment of obesity in adults; 2001 oct. Available from: URL: http: //www.nice.org.uk

11. Haddock CK, Poston WSC, Dill PL, Foreyt JP, Ericsson M. Pharmacotherapy for obesity: a quantitative analysis of four decades of published randomised clinical trials. *Int J Obes* 2002; 26: 262–73.

Progress in Obesity Research: 9. Edited by *Geraldo Medeiros-Neto, Alfredo Halpern* and *Claude Bouchard*

CHAPTER 185

Is there still a place for catecholaminergic drugs in the treatment for obesity? The contrary view

P.A. Tataranni

Clinical Diabetes and Nutrition Section, NIH-NIDDK-DHHS, 4212 N. 16th Street, Phoenix, AZ 85016, USA
[e-mail: antoniot@mail.nih.gov]

Introduction

O besity is a chronic relapsing disease resulting from a positive energy balance. With the exception of rare congenital forms, the exact aetiologic cause(s) for the majority of cases is unknown. Because of its chronic nature and undefined aetiology, cure of obesity is rare[1,2], but palliation is a realistic clinical goal.

While it is generally recognized that the best public health approach is to concentrate on measures to prevent obesity, pharmacological treatment of obesity represents one of the major unmet clinical needs of our time. Similar to the treatment of other chronic diseases (hypertension, dyslipidaemias, etc.), drugs to treat obesity may have to be used for life. In contrast to lipid lowering and antihypertensive drugs, however, any effective weight loss drug carries the risk of being widely used for cosmetic purposes because of the social stigma attached to obesity. Therefore, it is not unreasonable to require that weight loss drugs be judged against very high safety and efficacy standards.

As a result of a history tarnished by a host of therapeutic disasters[3] and the limited success of currently available weight loss drugs, treatment of obesity is still the subject of much debate[4,5]. However, in 1998 a panel of experts appointed by the NIH critically reviewed the evidence linking obesity to increased morbidity and mortality and recommended that safe and effective therapeutics be employed to treat overweight and obese patients to reduce their risk of type 2 diabetes, hypertension and dyslipidaemias[6]. Several studies indicate that this can be achieved only when weight loss is greater than 5–10 per cent of the initial body weight.

Is treatment of obesity by any pharmacological mean justified as long as a clinically meaningful weight loss is achieved? Hirsch has proposed that the clinical desirability (DE) of an antiobesity therapy is directly proportional to the drug induced weight loss leading to reduction in mortality and morbidity (M) and indirectly proportional to the hazard of the drug (H). He argued that if one subscribes to the simple expression of this equation (DE = [1+M]/[1+H]), DE is not likely to be high when therapeutics are not specific for the abnormalities that characterize obesity. This is because the non-specific mechanism of action of the drug will also carry an increased risk of untoward effects, ultimately inflating the denominator of the above equation[7].

Recognizing that the pharmacological alternatives for the treatment of obesity are extremely limited (Orlistat, Metformin), the aim of this manuscript is to criticize the use of catecholaminergic drugs based on two main arguments: (1) catecholaminergic drugs are not very specific for the abnormalities that characterize obesity; and (2) catecholaminergic drugs have a safety/efficacy profile that is only marginally acceptable, even in the absence of pharmacological alternatives.

Physiological and pharmacological influences of the catecholaminergic system on energy metabolism

Food intake

Experimental evidence in animals suggests that central-acting catecholamines (norepinephrine [NE] and dopamine [DA]) are involved in the modulation of non-specific aspects of eating behaviour, such as behavioural arousal[8]. Stimulation of specific receptor subtypes can result in behaviourally opposite responses. NE is the endogenous ligand for all adrenoceptors including $\alpha_{1,2}$ and $\beta_{1,2,3}$ receptor subtypes. In rodents, changes in brain NE can either increase or decrease food intake. The stimulatory effect of NE on eating has been linked to stimulation of α_2 adrenoceptors in the hypothalamus and the number of these receptors increases sharply before the onset of feeding. Conversely α_1 and β_2 receptor agonists inhibit eating[9]. Administration of NE, NE-releasing drugs and NE-reuptake inhibitors is associated with suppression of eating in rodents, but it is unclear which areas of the brain and/or neuronal pathways are ultimately responsible for mediating this response. Specifically, it is unknown how central-acting catecholamines interact with neuropeptide Y (NPY) and pro-opio-melanocortin (POMC) producing neurons that play a central role in the control food intake in the hypothalamus[10]. The central effects of dopamine are mediated by five subclasses of dopamine receptors (D1-5) which are primarily involved in the control of movement, pleasure/reward and neuroendocrine regulation of the pituitary gland. Drugs acting on dopamine receptors can also alter eating behaviour. However, this effect is complex, as indicated by the inverted U shape of the relationship between food intake and brain dopaminergic activity[8].

Thermogenesis

Administration of NE causes increased thermogenesis and weight loss in experimental animals. The main site of action for this response is the brown adipose tissue (BAT). This is a special form of adipose tissue which is well suited to produce heat under catecholaminergic stimulation primarily by upregulation of UCP-1 and uncoupling of oxidative phosphorylation. BAT is abundant in small mammals and infants, but not in adult humans. Thermogenesis in animals can be induced by either central stimulation of the SNS (cold, leptin, insulin) or peripheral stimulation of β-adrenoceptors. However, chronic stimulation of thermogenesis via peripheral administration of catecholamines results in tachyphylaxis due to down regulation of these receptors[11].

Role of catecholamines in the pathophysiology of human obesity

Very little is known about the neurophysiology of the catecholaminergic system and its adaptive changes in response to weight gain in humans. Abnormalities of the dopamine receptor-2-subtype may be present in the striatum of obese individuals[12]. There is no knowledge as to whether NE tone is increased or decreased in the brain of obese individuals, but a higher concentration of NE has been observed in the CSF of people at high risk for the development of the disease (PAT, unpublished observation).

Norepinephrine is the main neurotransmitter by which peripheral terminals of the sympathetic nervous system (SNS) control metabolism and the vasculature. In humans, SNS activity seems to affect all aspects of energy metabolism, including resting energy expenditure, energy expenditure due to physical activity, and diet-induced thermogenesis. Fasting suppresses, whereas feeding stimulates, the SNS which in turn increases or decreases energy expenditure, thus buffering energy surfeits or deficits.

Low sympathetic nervous system (SNS) activity and a low resting metabolic rate have been shown to be risk factors for the development of obesity in Pima Indians[13,14], but not in other populations. Whether a pharmacological increase of the catecholaminergic tone would prevent the onset of the disease in these individuals remains unknown.

In experimental animals, a low catecholaminergic tone precedes the development of and is associated with obesity[15]. Unlike animals, accumulation of total and central fat is associated with increased catecholaminergic activity in humans. The higher catecholaminergic tone in obese individuals has been interpreted as a compensatory mechanism to limit further weight gain via its stimulatory effects on energy expenditure and fat oxidation. A drawback of the weight-limiting effects of increased catecholaminergic activity in response to weight gain is its effect on the cardiovascular system. The pathophysiological mechanisms predisposing obese individuals to hypertension are not completely understood, but the increase in SNS plays an important role[16].

Use of catecholaminergic drugs for the treatment of obesity

Catecholaminergic drugs have been available to physicians worldwide for over 30 years. They fall under four main categories: a1-agonists, NE-releasers, NE-reuptake inhibitors and NE/DA/5HT-reuptake inhibitors (Table 1). NE-releasers and reuptake inhibitors are thought to have minimal dopaminergic effects as well. The main mechanism of action of all these drugs is suppression of food intake. Mazindol and sibutramine have been shown to induce thermogenesis in animals, but a sustained thermogenic effect in humans has not been observed.

Table 1. Catecholaminergic drugs

Generic name	FDA approval	DEA schedule	No. of studies[a]	Length of any study ≥ 6 months[a]
Benzphetamine	Few weeks	III	3	No
Diethylpropion	Few weeks	IV	13	Yes
Mazindol	Few weeks	IV	28	No
Phendimetrazine	Few weeks	III	–	No
Phentermine	Few weeks	IV	9	Yes
Phenylpropanolamine	No	OTC	9	No
Sibutramine	Long term	IV	5	Yes

[a]Published, randomized and controlled clinical trials (adapted from [17]).

Efficacy

The efficacy of an antiobesity drug is established by demonstrating that in double-blind randomized clinical trials it produces greater weight loss than a placebo drug, that the weight loss induced is clinically relevant (i.e. sufficient to induce improvement of comorbidities) and that the weight loss is chronically maintained while the drugs is used. An in-depth review of all published clinical trials using catecholaminergic drugs is beyond the scope of this manuscript and the reader is referred to the excellent review by Bray & Greenway[3]. In general, efficacy data for this class of drugs are based on short-term trials often lacking adequate control groups. In some of these trials, catecholaminergic drugs produced a larger weight loss compared to placebo. A meta-analysis of all published, randomized, and controlled trials revealed that the placebo-subtracted weight loss induced by all catecholaminergic drugs never exceeds 4.0 kg[17]. Table 1 lists the catecholaminergic drugs that are approved by the FDA for the short-term treatment of obesity, which is widely interpreted as up to 12 weeks.

Sibutramine is the only drug in its class that has been extensively evaluated in several clinical trials lasting up to two years; it has been approved for the long-term treatment of obesity (Table 1). Sibutramine was found to produce dose dependent weight loss, with maximum weight loss achieved at 6 months and maintained for over 1 year. The amount of weight loss varied among individuals but on average it was very modest, i.e. 5–7 kg compared to 1–3 kg in the placebo treated group (for a more comprehensive review see[18]).

None of the catecholaminergic drugs, including sibutramine, has been shown to reduce comorbidities above and beyond the effect expected from the loss of body weight.

Safety

Because amphetamine is addictive, the potential for abuse of the catecholaminergic drugs that share a similar chemical structure (phentermine, phenylpropanolamine, diethylpropion) has been the subject of significant controversy[3]. Notwithstanding the debate, all FDA approved catecholaminergic drugs, are currently designated by the DEA in the US as schedule III and IV drugs, a regulatory classification indicating the potential for abuse (Table 1).

All catecholaminergic drugs share a side effect profile that is consistent with their sympathomimetic mechanism of action. Insomnia, dry mouth, asthenia, and constipation are the most commonly reported side effects. Most important, all catecholaminergic drugs have the potential to increase blood pressure. For some drugs in this class, this seems to be offset by the blood pressure lowering effect of weight loss[3].

The use of phenylpropanolamine (PPA) at high doses has been associated with increased risk of hypertension. Based on a report linking the use of PPA (an ingredient in OTC products for the treatment of either nasal congestion or obesity) to hemorrhagic stroke, in the year 2000 the FDA aanounced the intention to remove PPA from the US market (http: //www.fda.gov/bbs/topics/ANSWERS/ANS01051. html). This led to similar action by numerous regulatory agencies around the world.

The use of sibutramine in placebo-controlled trials was associated with significant increases in systolic/diastolic blood pressure and heart rate[19]. Sibutramine is, therefore, contraindicated in obese patients with a history of CVD. However, it is difficult to identify all patients at risk since many obese patients may have occult cardiac disease. In March 2002, Italian authorities temporarily suspended the marketing of sibutramine after the use of the drug was associated with seven serious adverse reactions including arrhythmias and cardiac arrests resulting in two deaths. Since then, several other European Countries and Canada have announced plans to conduct a safety review of this prescription drug[20]. However, these actions have not resulted in a permanent withdrawal of sibutramine in any country.

Conclusion

The use of catecholaminergic drugs does not seem to be very specific for the abnormalities that characterize obesity, a disease associated with increased peripheral catecholaminergic tone. The side effect profile of these drugs, especially their potential for inducing hypertension, is highly undesirable in individuals who are already at increased risk for cardiovascular complications. Finally, detailed information on long-term efficacy and safety for most of these drugs is not available, but on balance their effect on weight loss seems to be small. Based on the above considerations, the use of most catecholaminergic drugs for the treatment of obesity is unwarranted. Sibutramine, the only catecholaminergic drug approved for long-term use, represents a sub-optimal therapeutical option at best.

Thus, in answer to the question of whether there is still a place for catecholaminergic drugs in the treatment of obesity, it seems fair to conclude that a place for this class of drugs in the pharmacopoeia for the treatment of obesity is only justified by the near absence of pharmacological alternatives.

References

1. Oral EA, Simha V, Ruiz E, Andewelt A, Premkumar A, Snell P *et al.* Leptin-replacement therapy for lipodystrophy. *N Engl J Med* 2002; 346: 570–578.

2. Farooqi IS, Jebb SA, Langmack G, Lawrence E, Cheetham CH, Prentice AM *et al.* Effects of recombinant leptin therapy in a child with congenital leptin deficiency. *N Engl J Med* 1999; 341: 879–84.

3. Bray GA, Greenway FL. Current and potential drugs for treatment of obesity. *Endocr Rev* 1999; 20: 805–75.

4. Kassirer JP, Angell M. Losing weight – an ill-fated New Year's resolution. *N Engl J Med* 1998; 338: 52–54.

5. Halsted CH. Should drugs be used in the treatment of obesity. *Am J Clin Nutr* 1998; 67: 1–4.

6. NIH-NHLBI Obesity Initiative Task Force. Clinical guidelines on the identification, evaluation, and treatment of overweight and obesity in adults –The Evidence Report *Obes Res* 1998; 6: 1–209.

7. Hirsch J. The treatment of obesity with drugs. *Am J Clin Nutr* 1998; 67: 2–4.

8. Stricker EM, Zigmond MJ. Brain catecholamines and the central control of food intake. *Int J Obes* 1984; 8 (Suppl 1): 39–50.

9. Gedeon Y, Ramesh GT, Wellman PJ, Jadhav AL. Changes in mesocorticolimbic dopamine and D1/D2 receptor levels after low level lead exposure: a time course study. *Toxicol Lett* 2001; 123: 217–226.

10. Schwartz MW, Woods SC, Porte DJ, Seeley RJ, Baskin DG. Central nervous system control of food intake. *Nature* 2000; 404(6778): 661–71.

11. Dulloo AG. Biomedicine. A sympathetic defense against obesity. *Science* 2002; 297: 780–1.

12. Wang GJ, Volkow ND, Logan J, Pappas NR, Wong CT, Zhu W *et al.* Brain dopamine and obesity. *Lancet* 2001; 357: 354–7.

13. Tataranni PA, Young JB, Bogardus C, Ravussin E. A low sympathoadrenal activity is associated with body weight gain and development of central adiposity in Pima Indian men *Obes Res* 1997; 5: 341–347.

14. Ravussin E, Lillioja S, Knowler WC, Christin L, Freymond D, Abbott WG *et al.* Reduced rate of energy expenditure as a risk factor for body-weight gain. *N Engl J Med* 1988; 318: 467–72.

15. Bray,GA. Obesity, a disorder of nutrient partitioning: the MONA LISA hypothesis. 1991; *J Nutr* 121: 1146–62.

16. Ravussin E, Tataranni PA. The role of altered sympathetic nervous system activity in the pathogenesis of obesity. *Proc Nutr Soc* 1996; 55: 793–802.

17. Haddock CK,Poston WS, Dill PL, Foreyt JP, Ericsson M. Pharmacotherapy for obesity: a quantitative analysis of four decades of published randomized clinical trials. *Int J Obes Relat Metab Disord* 2002; 26: 262–73.

18. Astrup A, Toubro S. When, for whom and how to use sibutramine? *Int J Obes Relat Metab Disord* 2001; 25 (Suppl 4): S2–S7.

19. Bray GA. Sibutramine and blood pressure: a therapeutic dilemma. *J Hum Hypertens* 2002; 16: 1–3.

20. Woolterton E. Obesity drug sibutramine (Meridia): hypertension and cardiac arrhythmias. *CMAJ* 2002; 166: 1307–8.

Progress in Obesity Research: 9. Edited by *Geraldo Medeiros-Neto, Alfredo Halpern and Claude Bouchard*
©2003 John Libbey Eurotext Ltd, pp. 891–892.

CHAPTER 186

There still is a place for catecholaminergic drugs on the treatment of obesity

Alfredo Halpern

Hospital das Clíncas da Faculdade de Medicina, University of São Paulo, Brazil
[e-mail: halpern@netpoint.com.br]

It is undoubtfully confirmed that many cases of obesity require pharmacologic treatment. Pharmaceutical companies are exerting themselves, trying to discover new drugs, aiming at obesity. Nevertheless, nowadays there are only a few of these drugs that are really approved for the treatment of obesity. These are: (1) orlistat; (2) sibutramine; and (3) catecholaminergic drugs.

Among these drugs there is a quite clear tendency to choose orlistat and sibutramine, due to many clinical researches that were held using both drugs and showing good results with regard to efficacy, tolerability and which included safety. Furthermore, there were several studies with these drugs, with 3 or more years of duration, that also evidenced efficacy, tolerability and safety in the long run.

Unfortunately, there are not such extended studies with catecholaminergic drugs.

In other words, the efficacy, safety and tolerability of such drugs have not been tested during a significant period of time.

Why has this happened?

It is my opinion this took place for several reasons, among them the devaluation of obesity as a real, factual disease, some years ago; the general existing fear with regard to amphetamines, and the lack of interest of pharmaceutical industry regarding obesity at the time catecholaminergic drugs were launched.

Today things have changed dramatically in a positive sense: obesity is being considered a very important disease, with many morbid associated conditions, and its treatment constitutes a real challenge. Pharmaceutical industries are largely interested in this field, among other reasons due to the number of affected patients very high constantly increasing, what constitutes a fantastic market in the field of drugs.

On the other hand, there unfortunately is no interest in investing on long studies with catecholaminergic drugs, particularly due to their cheap cost and to the fact they are manufactured by many industries. In spite of this, several studies have been made in the past with such drugs. The most studied ones were diethylpropine, phentermine and mazindol.

With regard to the fear concerning amphetamines, it must be said that these compouds (such as phentermine, and diethylpropion) share with amphetamines only the phenetylamine nucleus, which is the exact responsible for the anorectic action of same. Nevertheless, their profile of collateral events (including the potential for addiction) is much lower than amphetamine. The only catecholaminergic drug that is a precursor of amphetamine is fenproporex, but even it has a lower incidence of side effects than amphetamine.

The main reason for the withdrawal of amphetamine from the market was its potential power for addiction. Such potential is provided by dopamine and is not related to the phenetilamine nucleus. Mazindol, another catecholaminergic drug, does not have such a nucleus.

The most comprehensive study ever published with catecholaminergic drugs was held during 52 weeks (the phen-fen study was longer but it included phentermine and phenfludamine) and was made with diethylpropion.

Practically all studies, including a revision made by Scoville for the FDA evidenced that:

(1)   Catecholaminergic drugs are effective in producing weight loss;

(2)   Efficacy is similar with any of the catecholaminergic drugs;

(3)   Tolerability and safety profiles are considerably accetable.

I, particularly, have been using catecholaminergic drugs for more than 30 years and am each time more convinced that they still hold an efficient place in the treatment of obesity.

Although studies have not been held for more than one year, I am convinced that, once obesity is a chronic disease, it requires chronic treatment. That is why several patients in my clinic have been treated for more than 20 years with catecholaminergic drugs, with no apparent adverse effects. Furthermore, when the administration of drugs was interrupted, the tendency was to regain weight in most of them.

I sometimes have good results changing catecholaminergic drugs for sibutramine, but not always. It has been observed that there are good and bad responders to sibutramine and that there are good and bad responders to catecholaminergic drugs. Sometimes good results have been observed when catecholaminergic drugs were introduced in patients that did not show good results with sibutramine.

It is my firm opinion that catecholaminergic drugs still have a significant place in the treatment of obesity for the following reasons:

(1)   They are effective in many cases, with an acceptable profile of adverse effects (but in general worse than sibutramine or orlistat);

(2)   They can sometimes be effective when sibutramine does not work;

(3)   Mainly, due to the fact that they are much cheaper than sibutramine and orlistat, what heavily accounts for their use, particularly in obese people of lower economic classes, as it happens in developing countries such as Brazil.

In our Ambulatory of Obesity at the Hospital das Clínicas of the University of São Paulo, at least 60 per cent of our prescription of antiobesity drugs are composed of catecholaminergic drugs and our results seem to be similar to those of studies held elsewhere.

Bibliography

Bray GA, Greenway FL. Current and potential drugs for treatment of obesity. *Endocr Rev* 1999; 20: 805.

Cession-Fossio NA. Sur quelques propriétés pharmacologiques du fenproporex Chez le rat. *Arch Int Pharmacodyn Ther* 1970; 87: 192.

Connolly HM, McGoon MD. Obesity drugs and the heart. *Curr Probl Cardiol* 1999; 24: 745.

Enzi G, Baritussio A, Marchiori E, Crepaldi G. Short-term and long-term clinical evaluation of a non-amphetaminic anorexiant (mazindol) in the treatment of obesity. *J Int Med Res* 1976; 4: 305.

Inoue S. Clinical studies with Mazindol. *Obes Res* 1995; 3 (Suppl 4): 549S.

Matos AFG. Tratamento da Obesidade: – anorexígenos. In: *Obesidade*, Halpern, Matos, Suplicy, Mancini, Zanella (eds), p. 281, 1998.

McKay RH. Long-term use of diethylpropion in obesity. *Curr Med Res Opin* 1973; 1: 489.

Munro JF, MacCuish AC, Wilson EM, Duncan LPJ. Comparison of continuous and intermittent anorectic therapy in obesity. *BMJ* 1968; 1: 352.

National Task Force on the Prevention and Treatment of Obesity. Long-term pharmacotherapy in the management of obesity. *JAMA* 1996; 276: 1907.

Scoville BA. Review of Amphetamine – like drugs by the FDA: Clinical data and value judgements in Bray, editor. Obesity in Perspective. Proceedings of the Fogarty Conference 1975. p. 441.

Silverstone JT, Solomon T. The long-term management of obesity in general practice. *Br J Clin Pract* 1965; 19: 395.

Sullivan AC, Triscar J, Cheng L. Appetite regulation by drugs and endogenous substances. *Fed Proc* 1982; 44: 139.

Weintraub M, Taves DR, Mushlin DI, Locwood DH. Determinants of responses to anorexiants. *Clin Pharmacol Ther* 1981; 30: 528.

Weintraub M, Sundaresan PR, Madan M *et al.* Long-term weight control study.I (weeks 0 to 34). The enhancement of behaviour modification, caloric restriction, and exercise by fenfluramine plus phentermine versus placebo. *Clin Pharmacol Ther* 1992; 51: 586.

Progress in Obesity Research: 9. Edited by *Geraldo Medeiros-Neto, Alfredo Halpern and Claude Bouchard*
©2003 John Libbey Eurotext Ltd, pp. 893–897.

CHAPTER 187

Novel peptides

Len Storlien, David G.A. Morgan, John C. Clapham, Sven Sjögren, Stephan Hjorth, Andrew V. Turnbull and Björn C.L. Carlsson

AstraZeneca R & D, Mölndal, Sweden and Alderley Park, UK
[e-mail: leonard.storlien@astrazeneca.com]

Introduction

The last 8 years have been exciting ones for obesity research. The discovery of leptin paved the way for revelations about the endocrine role of white adipose tissue and the complex peptide machinery of energy homeostasis. The convergence of this knowledge explosion and the growing recognition of the world-wide medical implications of the obesity epidemic has galvanized the field. Unfortunately, this enthusiasm has to be balanced against the reality that the promise of simple drug intervention in the leptin/neuropeptide signalling axes has been, thus far, somewhat illusory. Is it just too soon? Are the best targets already there in the literature and just waiting for the magic bullets to be made, or will they, like some already prominent examples, yield one by one not joy to the obese and to the pharmaceutical industry, but disappointment to both?

The 'new order' of energy balance

There is little utility in listing the novel peptides of energy balance as they have been reviewed extensively and with great insight very recently[1-3]. Suffice it to say that they broadly fall into 3 (overlapping) categories: adipose tissue secreted; brain (hypothalamic and forebrain), and gut derived. Leptin of course is the landmark adipose-derived peptide which began the recasting of the fat cell from passive pantry of our gluttonous excess to master control organ of energy flux. It was the key to making sense of, and uncovering new elements in, the network of neuropeptides downstream of its brain effects. Extensive evidence has amassed on the neuropeptide Y/Agouti related peptide (NPY/AgRP) orexigenic/energy conserving systems, and the balancing proopiomelanocortin/cocaine amphetamine regulated transcript (POMC/CART) anorexigenic/catabolic systems both linked to leptin function[1-3]. It is now also becoming clear that even the endocannabinoid system with its notable links to nutritional state and appetite control (e.g.[3]) is at least under partial regulation of leptin[5].

Equally, the implications that the discovery of leptin had for the adipocyte as endocrine organ spawned a successful search for other adipocyte-secreted peptides. Whilst the role of some, eg resistin, is controversial, adiponectin (aka, ACRP30 or AdipoQ) has been shown to have important effects across a range of aspects of both glucose and lipid metabolism[6-7].

Just as for insulin resistance, leptin resistance has meant that simple elevation of leptin levels does not provide any longterm solution. The issue with leptin is therefore not its importance as an entity, and/or its interaction with a range of regulatory systems. It is the fact that it circulates in great abundance in the bloodstream of obese individuals, the vast majority who have genetically normal leptin receptors, but it does not function to limit weight increase. That is a condition which we might not unreasonably call 'leptin resistance'. Recent research with long-term diet induced obesity adds weight to the concept of leptin resistance[8-9]. These data show that expression of orexigenic peptides, including NPY and AgRP, which are normally downregulated by leptin, increase in rodents made obese by long-term feeding of high fat diets, suggesting that the increased levels of leptin are no longer effective. This concept may add further support to the idea that blocking the action of such orexigenic hypothalamic peptides, downstream of the leptin receptor, may have good treatment potential for obesity.

The hypothalamic neuropeptide control of feeding is complicated not only by the number of peptides that have been implicated in this process, but also by the fact that the majority of these peptides appear to have multiple receptor subtypes as potential candidate targets. Moreover, from a perspective of drug intervention most of the peptide receptors subserve multiple potential functions, raising the possibility of significant side-effects. Of the NPY receptors implicating in feeding, the NPY Y5 receptor appeared an attractive target as a result of pharmacological, antisense and early antagonist food intake/body weight data in rodents, while at the same time appearing to be a receptor that had involvement in few other physiological processes[10–11]. Indeed many NPY Y5 antagonists have been developed by a number of groups and a significant proportion of these have been claimed to have inhibitory effects on feeding (see[12] for references). However, one of the best studied of these, CGP 71683A has been demonstrated to be equally as efficacious at reducing food intake in either NPY or NPY Y5-deficient mice as in their wild-type controls[13], indicating that antagonism of the NPY Y5 receptor is not its principal mechanism of action. Others[12] have similarly reported hypophagic effects of NPY Y5 antagonists in NPY Y5 knockouts, but the lack of correlation between Y5 antagonism and *in vivo* activity suggests that NPY Y5 antagonism and inhibition of feeding do not necessarily share a cause–effect relationship. In support, two groups have reported that antagonists that clearly antagonize the NPY Y5 receptor in brain do not affect NPY-induced feeding[12–14], and recent studies have now gone on to show that selective antagonism of the NPY Y5 receptor in brain does not have a major effect on feeding or body weight in rats[12]. Whether NPY Y1 or NPY Y2 approaches to influencing NPY's contribution to body weight regulation deliver greater success in the long term remains to be seen.

Equally, of course, obesity research does not just concentrate on a single neuropeptide and recently melanocortin concentrating hormone (MCH) antagonists have been shown to persistently and substantially reduce food intake and body weight in rodent models[15–16]. If such effects are lacking in MCH receptor knockout mice, then it may be that this is an outstanding possible therapeutic target. Only time will tell, but along with the melanocortin system, MCH seems one of the most promising 'hypothalamic' targets. It can be hoped that these mediators of leptin action will yield to the intensive efforts being exerted by the pharmaceutical industry, and provide useful therapeutic agents in the future. However, even if successful, such research will not deliver a drug to the market within at least the better part of a decade.

The current pipeline

So what is in the pipeline? It may reflect the youth of the discoveries of the new peptide regulators of energy balance that of the new types of potential pharmaceutical treatments for obesity at least into phase II trials (studies in affected humans, ie, obese – short-term, dose-ranging), none are from the classes of novel peptides thought to be of the direct, energy-balance type. Instead they are: (1) more specific 5HT2c receptor agonist follow-ups of the classic enhancers of the serotonin (5-HT) neurotransmission, exemplified initially by fenfluramine and more currently by sibutramine (a dual serotonin-noradrenaline reuptake inhibitor). Interestingly, there are data to suggest that the anorexigenic effect of fenfluramine is mediated indirectly via enhanced 5-HT2c receptor activation[17]); (2) a cannabinoid receptor 1 antagonist (likely affecting 'reward'/motivation and appetite systems in the forebrain as well as hypothalamus – see[4]); (3) adrenergic beta-3 receptor agonists which reduce visceral fat mass[18]; (4) a neurotrophic factor; and (5) a growth hormone fragment that does not apparently operate via the growth hormone receptor[19]. The fourth of these, axokine (Regeneron), is a modified truncated form of the human ciliary neurotrophic factor (CNTF) and is therefore an injectable peptide. CNTF is a cytokine which was originally identified as a survival factor for isolated neurons, promoting differentiation, maturation and survival of oligodendrocytes The interesting thing about this possible pharmaceutical approach is that while a 12-week trial at what was described as an 'optimal' dose produced only approximately a 5 per cent weight loss below control in massively obese individuals (e.g. for an individual with a BMI of 40, this would be approximately a reduction to a BMI of 38), this weight loss was maintained for almost a year after cessation of treatment[20]. This is an important and intriguing finding as weight maintenance is much, much more difficult than initial weight loss. The question is whether this is a genuine 'resetting' of the brain's ponderostat (that old term which indicated that somehow the brain sensed the totality of body fatness, and acted, like a thermostat to maintain some optimal level). This possible resetting is, in many ways, an extraordinary concept but if this indeed were true, the question would have to arise as to whether such an effect is open to substantial abuse by segments of the population driven by the desire to be pathologically thin? Developments using this approach are awaited with great interest.

So where do we go now – the 'drivers' of the obesity epidemic

On what road do we travel in the quest for truly effective anti-obesity agents? One approach could be by viewing targets within the concept 'thrifty genotype rendered detrimental by progress'[21]. As Andrew Prentice has noted in the recent article based on his British Nutrition Foundation Annual Lecture[22], this thrifty gene hypothesis is a 'nebulous and ill-defined concept entirely lacking in any proof'. However in the context of his analysis it has, and we agree, 'become a very intriguing one'. 'Progress' in the Neel sense give us an understanding of the 'drivers' of the modern epidemic of obesity. 'Drivers' can be described as environmental factors which have changed and exposed genetic predispositions to obesity. These include reduced physical activity and the consequences for muscle morphology, altered dietary habits, and increased stress and immune challenges. What is difficult for our true understanding of these drivers is that energy balance is just that, a fine balance where as little as a 1–2 per cent excess of intake over expenditure, prolonged over the course of a single year, will theoretically lead to body fat gain of 1–2 kg to 10–20 kg in a decade. We have no way on a population basis of measuring either energy intake or expenditure with anywhere near the precision to even say whether an increase in intake or a decrease in expenditure really has driven the obesity pandemic. The published data do not support an increase in total caloric intake or of fat as a percentage of calories (e.g.[23–24]). However, under-reporting has been shown at least in some studies to increase with increasing overweight, and are these data then biased by that confounder? On the energy expenditure side of the equation Professor Frank Booth has, in particular, passionately argued that an increasing proportion of our time spent in sedentary activities is the key element[25] and certainly the data showing the rise in obesity and incidence of diabetes with the parallel rise in television watching deserve at least close scrutiny for causality. This sedentary behaviour may not only dispose obesity by reducing energy expenditure but also lead to an actual decrement in whole-body capacity to burn fat for energy which is reversible, at least to some extent, by exercise[26]. Finally, in the drivers category it needs to be emphasized that acute phase markers of inflammation are chronically elevated in individuals with the metabolic syndrome and may reflect a specially potent role of omental fat as not only a triglyceride storage depot but also an immune organ driving, in some way, metabolic abnormalities via cytokine or other inflammatory peptide delivery directly to the liver, causing both steatosis and insulin resistance. It is interesting here that work from Arner's laboratory[27] has recently shown that surgical removal of a small amount of omental fat during a gastric banding operation to alleviate morbid obesity, had a powerful, early, potentiating effect on insulin senstivity which persisted and increased along with much greater rate of weight loss over the two years following surgery.

Coming back to the sedentary behaviours angle, it is worth a few moments discussing weight maintenance. When we think of possible novel peptides for obesity therapy we must think of the disease as we know it. Weight loss of 10, even 15, kg is quite achieveable over periods of 3–6 months in a surprisingly high proportion of overweight and obese individuals who want to lose weight. Success rates in excess of 80 per cent of subjects are not unusual in weight loss studies[28]. What is much, much more difficult, and psychologically devastating with failure, is maintenance of the reduced weight (note the weight regain in the control group and the dropout rate of > 50 per cent in both groups of this last referenced study[28]). We already know that reduced capacity for fat utilization (or at least reduced propensity for fat to be used under standardized conditions) is strongly related to propensity for weight regain (e.g.[29]). Understanding the metabolic mechanisms predisposing weight regain should be a fruitful approach and the lean phenotype of mice with a knockout in an enzyme of the 'fat burning' pathway, ACC2, is interesting[30]. Equally, the fact that physical activity shifts fibre type mixture and enzymatic activities towards increased oxidative capacity and hence increased capacity for using fat as fuel may then be important in the corollary; physical inactivity and reduced fat-utilizing capacity as a driver of obesity.

Obesity is not a single entity

One final point that should be made in the search for novel peptides of energy balance is that obesity is not a single entity. We know that central/visceral fat is more deleterious than lower body adiposity. Also, impairments in insulin action are markedly different between individuals at the same whole-body level of adiposity with intramyocellular and intrahepatic fat accounting for a great deal of that variability. Therefore targets which modulate fat distribution without necessarily impacting on total body fatness may have equal, or even potentially more important, beneficial consequences in relation to the comorbidities of obesity. Here it is worth a reminder about the results of Arner and coworkers and the fact that certain fat pads may also play particular, and particularly nasty, roles in the metabolic dysfunction of obesity. Lastly in this section it should again be emphasized that leptin, when it is functioning well, is a potent mobiliser of intramyocellular lipid. Looking for pathways in skeletal muscle downstream of the leptin receptor may provide interesting new ways to attack obesity. Equally, effective mobilization of fat by leptin from pancreatic β-cells should improve insulin secreting capacity. Since maintained weight loss has recently been shown to prevent some 80 per cent of new cases of diabetes which would have occurred in an obese population[31], it may be that weight-loss induced improvement in leptin sensitivity at the pancreatic level plays a role in that exceptionally important outcomes finding.

Obesity and the complexity of metabolism

While it is now agreed that the genetic component of obesity is high – 60–70 per cent of the variance in body weight – it is a polygenic disease and we must think in terms of a predisposing collusion in a number of metabolic pathways. Therefore an overriding consideration that must be always borne in mind is that energy balance involves the entire complex, interconnected range of metabolic pathways and that metabolism is a fine balance. Completely disabling an element in a pathway with a sledge hammer and ascribing function to the resulting perturbation is often disilluminating. Thus, major changes in body adiposity, be it fatness or leanness which develop, for example, from a single gene knockout, may be misleading – a sledgehammer taken to one part of a car's engine may stop the engine from functioning but it is not illuminating about the normal function of the parts concerned. A finer grained analysis is needed. For the best illustration of this point, the reader is referred to an excellent article in relation to type 2 diabetes, another polygenic disease[32]. In this publication it was shown that individuals with a frameshift/premature stop mutation (i.e. reduction of function) in *either* PPARγ (which is highly expressed in adipose tissue and the target of the well-known thiazolodinediones used for treatment of diabetes) or in PPP1R3A (a muscle specific regulatory subunit of protein phosphatase 1 which is thought to play an important role in the insulin-induced signalling cascade leading to glycogen storage) were metabolically fairly normal – no severe insulin resistance, modest changes in blood lipids. However, individuals with *both* mutations were severely insulin resistant and had major blood lipid abnormalities. As the authors conclude 'These findings provide evidence that mutations that, when present alone, have at most subtle effects on different, metabolically relevant tissues can combine to result in extreme disturbances of human insulin action'[32]. This conclusion should be kept firmly in mind for obesity. The disease has many genetic and environmental determinants. Treatment will need to be aimed at modulating metabolism in multiple pathways.

Equally, the systems which defend the body so effectively against weight loss, may not be at all designed to defend against weight gain. Teleologically this makes sense as survival of the organism depends on its ability to withstand energy deficit, but this is not nearly so obvious for energy excess, a point to which we will return. Second, energy balance may be too important to leave to the mercy of single higher brain systems. There may be effective metabolic pathways functioning to cap obesity but simplistic mesencephalicocentric approaches targeted at individual hypothalamic peptides may not deliver what seemed recent promise. As Grill and Kaplan have argued, the current knowledge base may suggest 'a distributionist (as opposed to hierarchical) model for the control of energy balance'[3]. Finally, modulation of cellular processes of signal transduction subsequent to peptide-receptor interactions may prove more productive, particularly if we understand the metabolic systems that we need to modulate and recognise that we may need to 'tweak' more than one system, given the likely redundancy in systems controlling such fundamental homeostatic functions.

Summary and concluding thoughts

The explosion of knowledge in the past 8 years is still a long way from being translated into the clinic. Novel peptides, and the small synthetic molecule pharmaceuticals which will be developed out of their discovery, are still a long way from the clinic. One of them may turn out to be the magic bullet. However, it is much more likely that in a complex disease like obesity more than one target, more than one pathway, will need to be modulated and this combination therapy will come from both within, and outside, the direct pathways of energy balance. Firm data are needed to understand whether the current 'explosion' of obesity really is driven somewhat more by sloth than gluttony. Successful interventions will then be more likely to come from our understanding of what this means for metabolism. Thus, novel therapeutics will need to drive systems rendered dysfunctional by 'progress' and they will need to be developed with a view to restoring the metabolic flexibility that humans developed to cope with major discontinuties of both supply of, and demand for, energy.

References

1. Beck B. Neuropeptides and obesity. *Nutrition* 2000; 16: 916–923.

2. Clapham JC, Arch JRS, Tadayyon M. Anti-obesity drugs: a critical review of current therapies and future opportunities. *Pharmacol Therapeutics* 2001; 89: 81–121.

3. Grill HJ, Kaplan JM. The neuroanatomical axis for control of energy balance. *Frontiers Neuroendocrinol* 2002; 23: 2–40.

4. Kirkham TC, Williams CM, Fezza F, di Marzo V. Endocannabinoid levels in rat limbic forebrain and hypothalamus in relation to fasting, feeding and satiation: stimulation of eating by 2-arachidonyl glycerol.. *Br J Pharmacol* 2002; 136: 550–57.

5. di Marzo V, Goparaju SK, Wang L, Liu J, Bátkai S, Járai Z *et al*. Leptin-regulated endocannabinoids are involved in maintaining food intake. *Nature* 2002; 410: 822–25.

6. Tsao T-S, Lodish HF, Fruebis J. ACRP30, a new hormone controlling fat and glucose metabolism. *Eur J Pharmacol* 2002; 440: 213–21.

7. Berg AH. Combs TP, Scherer PE. ACRP30/adiponectin: an adipokine regulating glucose and lipid metabolism. *Trends Endocrinol Metab* 2002; 13: 84–90.

8. Gao J, Ghibaudi L, van Heek M, Hwa JJ. Characterization of diet-induced obese rats that develop persistent obesity after 6 months of high-fat followed by 1 month of low-fat diet. *Brain Res* 2002; 936: 87–90.

9. Lin S, Thomas TC, Storlien LH, Huang XF. Development of high fat diet-induced obesity and leptin resistance in C57B1/6J mice. *Int J Obes* 2000; 24: 1–8.

10. Zimanyi IA. Poindexter GS. NPY-ergic agents for the treatment of obesity. *Drug Dev Res* 2000; 51: 94–111.

11. Tang-Christensen M, Kristensen P, Stidsen CE, Brand CL, Larsen PJ. Central administration of Y5 receptor antisense decreases spontaneous food intake and attenuates feeling in response to exogenous neuropeptide Y. *J Endocrinol* 1998; 159: 307–12.

12. Turnbull AV, Ellershaw L, Masters DJ, Birtles S, Boyer S, Carroll D *et al*. Selective antagonism of the NPY5 receptor does not have a major effect on feeding in rats. *Diabetes* 2002; 51: 2441–49.

13. Bannon AW, Seda J, Carmouche M, Francis JM, Norman MH, Karbon B, McCaleb ML. Behavioral characterization of neuropeptide Y knockout mice. *Brain Res* 2000; 868: 79–87.

14. Kanatani A, Ishihara A, Iwaasa H, Nakamura K, Okamoto O, Hidaka M *et al*. L-152,804: orally active and selective neuropeptide Y Y5 receptor antagonist. *Biochem Biophys Res Com* 2000; 272: 169–173.

15. Borowsky B, Drukin MM, Ogozalek K, Marzabadi MR, DeLeon J, Heurich R *et al*. Antidepressant, anxiolytic and anorectic effects of a melanin-concentrating hormone-1 receptor antagonist. *Nature Med* 2002; 8: 825–30.

16. Takekawa S, Asami A, Ishihara Y, Terauchi J, Kato K, Shimomura Y *et al*. T-226296: a novel, orally active and selective melanin-concentrating hormone receptor antagonist. *Eur J Pharmacol* 2002; 438: 129–35.

17. Vickers SP, Dourish CT, Kennett GA. Evidence that hypophagia induced by d-fenfluramine and d-norfenfluramine in the rat is mediated by 5-HT2c receptors. *Neuropharmacol* 2001; 41, 200–9.

18. Borst SE, Hennessy M. β-3 adrenergic agonist restores skeletal muscle insulin responsiveness in Sprague-Dawley rats. *Biochem Biophys Res Commun* 2001; 289,1188–91.

19. Heffernan MA, Jiang WJ, Thorburn AW, Ng FM. Effects of oral administration of a synthetic fragment of human growth hormone on lipid metabolism. *Am J Physiol* 2000; 279, E501–7.

20. Weinstein S, Vicary C, Elttinger M, Littlejohn T, Schwartz S, Weiss S *et al*. Maintenance of weight loss 48 weeks after treatment with axokine®. *Int J Obes* 2002; 26 (Suppl 1): S136.

21. Neel JV. Diabetes mellitus: a 'thrifty' genotype rendered detrimental by 'progress'. *Am J Human Genetics* 1962; 14: 3–362.

22. Prentice AM. Fires of life: the struggles of an ancient metabolism in a modern world. *Nutr Bull* 2002; 26: 13–27.

23. Arnett DK, Xiong B, McGovern PG, Blackburn H, Luepker RV. Secular trends in dietary macronutrient intake in Minneapolis-St. Paul, Minnesota, 1980–1992. *Am J Epidemiol* 2002; 152: 868–73.

24. Prentice AM, Jebb SA. Obesity in Britain: gluttony or sloth? *Br Med J* 1995; 311(7002): 437–39.

25. Booth FW, Gordon SE, Carlson CH, Hamilton MT. Waging war on modern chronic diseases: primary prevention through exercise biology. *J Applied Physiol* 2000; 88: 774–87.

26. Schrauwen P, van Aggel-Leijssen DPC, Hul G, Wagenmakers AJM, Vidal H, Saris WHM, van Baak MA. The effect of a 3-month low-intensity endurance training program on fat oxidation and acetyl-CoA carboxylase-2 expression. *Diabetes* 2002; 51: 2220–26.

27. Thörne A, Lönnqvist F, Apelman J, Hellers G, Arner P. A pilot study of long-term effects of a novel obesity treatment: omentectomy in connection with adjustable gastric banding. *Int J Obes* 2002; 26: 193–99.

28. James WPT, Astrup A, Finer N, Hilsted J, Kopelman, Rössner S, Saris WHM, van Gaal LF. Effect of sibutramine on weight maintenance after weight loss: a randomised trial. *Lancet* 2000; 356: 2119–25.

29. Valtuena S, Salas-Salvado J, Lorda PG. The respiratory quotient as a prognostic factor in weight-loss rebound. *Int J Obes* 1997; 21: 811–17.

30. Abu-Elheiga L, Matzuk MM, Abo-Hashema KAH, Wakil SJ. Continuous fatty acid oxidation in mice lacking acetyl-CoA carboxylase 2. *Science* 2001; 291: 2613–17.

31. Torgerson JS, Sjöström L. The Swedish Obese Subjects (SOS) study – rationale and results. *Int J Obes* 2001; 25 (Suppl 1): S2–S4.

32. Savage DB, Agostini M, Barroso I, Gurnell M, Luan J, Meirhaeghe A *et al*. (2002): Digenic inheritance of severe insulin resistance in a human pedigree. *Nature Genet* 31: 379–84.

Progress in Obesity Research: 9. Edited by *Geraldo Medeiros-Neto, Alfredo Halpern and Claude Bouchard*
©2003 John Libbey Eurotext Ltd, pp. 898–902.

CHAPTER 188

Pharmacotherapy of obesity: historical perspective

Bernard Guy-Grand

Service de Medecine et Nutrition, Hotel-Dieu, 1 Place du Parvis Notre-Dame, Paris, France
[e-mail: bernard.guy-grand@htd.ap-hop-paris.fr]

The history of pharmacotherapy of obesity – i.e. that of drugs designed for helping patients to lose weight – is a long one, starting at the end of the 19th century – for restricting us to the so called modern era of medicine – with the introduction of thyroid extracts, later on thyroid hormones, based on the belief that obese patients had hypothyroidism. At the beginning of the 21st century, drug therapy has still difficulties in being fully accepted, unequivocally recommended, commonly and properly prescribed and few drugs are available. This is a major difference with other chronic metabolic diseases – hypertension, type 2 diabetes, hyperlipidaemia – which treatment has been shifted over the last fifty to thirty years from very poorly efficient dietary prescriptions to a number of powerful drugs. Among the different ways that such an history can be told, the most fruitful is probably to place it in the general context of the evolution of the understanding of the physiological and pathophysiological mechanisms at work in energy balance and obesity itself and, more importantly, of the purposes of obesity treatment and of the needs of their attainments. Of course this evolution have strongly influenced the nature of the drugs, the expectations from them, the evaluation processes, the regulations and the practices.

Figure 1 provides a list of the major drugs that have been widely used in the second half of the 20th century; many of them have been withdrawn for safety reasons either obvious (dinitrophenol, amphetamine, aminorex) or more or less alleged (fenfluramines – when widely associated with phentermine) or abandoned in many countries for poorly demonstrated effectiveness (many amphetamines derivatives developed between the 1940s and the 1960s).

However the most illustrating perspective of the history of pharmacotherapy of obesity is perhaps to try following the evolution of what was expected from drugs by the professionals (doctors and pharmaceutical companies) not the public nor the quacks, and accordingly from the authorities licensing them. We can easily recognize several steps in the different ways of thinking, corresponding broadly to the last three decades, even if this classification is somewhat artificial and schematic.

Until the mid-1970s

Until the mid seventies, drugs were commonly expected to induce rapid and large weight losses and used as starters with the naive hope that these 'magic bullets' could be able to restore a more normal weight that the patients were kindly (not always!) asked to maintain. Implicit to this attitude was the belief that they must be cured from their guilty gluttony.

As a consequence, trials were of short-term duration, mostly lasting 12 weeks, sometimes less, rarely 24 weeks. Cross over designs were quite popular. They included, usually in one centre, some tens of poorly characterized patients who received the placebo or the drug frequently without any additional advice. Dropouts were mostly not accounted for even if it was clear that in many studies they were more than 60 per cent (for examples and references, see ref.[1,2]).

Weight loss was usually evaluated by comparing the mean decrease in weight expressed in absolute terms between placebo and drug-treated patients completing the studies; the placebo group typically achieved only a trivial weight loss. However in late 1950s Stunkard and McLaren Hume[3] had proposed the first categorical analysis of the data: the criterion for success was a comparison of the proportion

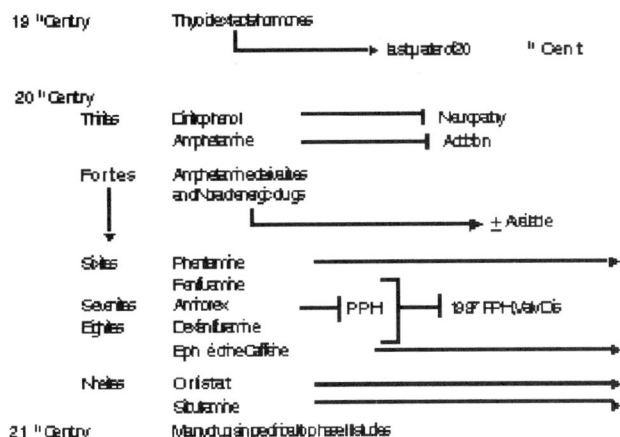

Fig. 1. Major anti-obesity drugs that have been licensed.

of patients losing more than 9 kg or more than 18 kg in drug treated and control groups. Cut of points of such a magnitude are clearly indicating that the expected weight loss was quite large and that reverting bodyweight to the 'normal' range was at hope. In addition, since absolute weight loss is dependent on starting weight, comparing different trials including patients differing in weight was impossible.

In 1975, in his FDA review of drugs, Scoville[4] used the rate of weight loss to evaluate efficacy: losing more than 0.125 kg/week in excess of placebo or how many patients lost more than 0.45 kg/week or more than 1.4 kg/week were the criteria. Since the rate of weight loss slows down with time, these criteria are only adapted to trials lasting three months or less. The major expectation was to assess the pharmacological potency of drugs and not their clinical usefulness.

Due to the fear of the addictive properties of almost all the drugs available during this period, that were derivatives of amphetamine, often classified under schedule III and inducing self administration in animals (with the exception of fenfluramine), their administration was restricted to short periods of time, usually three months. These restrictions lasted until late nineties.

The 1980s

At the turn of the eighties it was progressively understood that short-term treatment of obesity could be mostly a non-sense because relapse almost invariably occurs when the treatment is stopped. Therefore the need for long-term strategies to control body weight came into view[5,6] as the concept of obesity as a chronic status progressively emerged. It was realized that the treatments, including drugs, were only palliative and not curative in nature whereas maintenance over time of a reduced body weight was the goal (Fig. 2)[7,8].

Also a shift from weight loss in itself towards a long-term medically useful improvement in comorbidities started off, that will be officially and universally recognized ten years later in the WHO report[9]. The question of long-term (eventually lifelong) drug therapy was raised[10,11]. Thus, drugs that were considered ineffective because weight regain occurred after withdrawal – an issue however hardly surprising and the admitted rule for other chronic diseases – began to be viewed differently, even if some 10 years were needed for such an obviousness to be accepted by the many.

In accordance with this line, the characteristics that a useful drug must meet were precised[12]: (1) demonstrated effect on body weight and weight dependant diseases, (2) bearable and/or transient side effects, (3) no addictive properties, (4) few escapes when continued long-term, (5) rare hazards after years of administration, (6) known mechanisms of action. New standards for reporting results were proposed[13].

Soon after appeared the first multicentre long-term (1 year) controlled trial, the Index study with dexfenfluramine[14] which served as a model for many subsequent studies. Dexfenfluramine and placebo were associated with a calorie deficit diet. Many lessons were derived from that study:

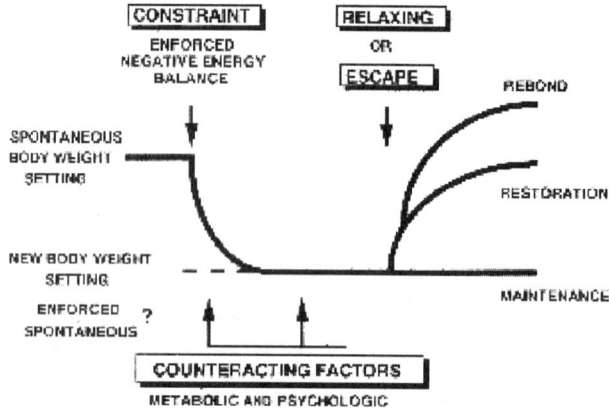

Fig. 2. Schematic evolution in body weight in treated obese patients (adapted from[7]).

(1)   Evidence that medium term drug administration was able to help maintaining a lower body weight, a feature that needs to be shown: the failure of fluoxetine was an example of the contrary[15];

(2)   Weight loss is restricted to the first 6–8 months and body weight is then plateauing whereas regain in weight is observed in the placebo group. This weight stability is therefore not indicative of a 'tolerance' to the drug which would have become ineffective but the witness of its limits of action;

(3)   Weight loss expressed relatively to starting weight is a better end point than absolute number of kilograms lost, allowing comparisons of subjects with different BMI;

(4)   Not only mean weight loss on the drug – treated group compared with that of placebo – that is biased by default when there is an excess of drop outs over that of placebo – should be assessed, but percentage of patients entered in the study and losing more than a given end point (categorical analysis with LOCF) provides a more relevant estimate of the clinical usefulness of the drug. In INDEX study a cut off point of 10 per cent weight loss was shown to be achieved by twice as many drug-treated patients than placebo receiving patients; a target of the same order of magnitude was found later on with orlistat[16] and sibutramine[17]. It was mostly on the grounds of that study and on those confirming it that FDA approved a new drug (dexfenfluramine) for the first time in 25 year.

The 1990s

Several important issues occurred during the nineties. First it was shown that modest (5–10 per cent) intentional weight loss were able to improve mortality from several diseases clearly linked to obesity[18]. This was important because many epidemiological studies had reported that weight changes, including weight loss, could be positively linked to overall mortality. Also Goldstein[19] in his review of the literature of drug induced weight loss pointed out the improvement – at least in the short to medium term – of most of the obesity associated risk factors with modest weight loss. Guidelines from NAASO reflected the consensus for such targets[20]. Second, maintenance of body weight and improvement in comorbidities tended to take the preference over weight loss per se, as stressed in 1997 by the IOTF/WHO report[9]. Therefore the designs of the trials lasted 1 to 4 years with phentermine/fenfluramine[21], sibutramine[17] and orlistat[16] and were aimed at demonstrating a lasting effect. Many trials in obese patients suffering from type 2 diabetes, hypertension and hypercholesterolaemia were specifically designed in order to assess the improvement of drug induced weight loss in the control of these diseases[22] or to substantiate drug related effect in addition to the action of weight loss/maintenance per se[23]. Furthermore a study designed to assess the potential preventive effect of weight loss and maintenance on the appearance of type 2 diabetes in obese patients with impaired glucose tolerance started in 1998; the positive results of XENDOS study have been presented at the 9th ICO (Sjöström, unpublished data). Third: during the1990s, when body fat became routinely available and the importance of visceral fat was unanimously recognized as a major feature of the metabolic syndrome (in fact a story that started long time ago), fat loss and fat distribution were considered as secondary end points. Also the need for a global management of obese patients put improvement of quality of life into consideration. The current regulatory criteria for establishing efficacy of anti obesity drugs adopted in the late nineties both by FDA and CPMP, and discussed in another chapter of this book by F. Kelly reflects this evolution.

Safety concerns

Safety of anti obesity drugs has been a matter of concerns from the very beginning of their use and many drama occurred (see Fig. 1), feeding the prejudice they have suffered. Apart from the symptomatic side effects, often temporary, and rarely leading to withdrawal, that are systematically recorded, very harmful consequences of some drugs have strewn suspicion and led to prudent withdrawal of many. The cardiovascular side effects of sibutramine[17] have led to the recommendation of precise medical monitoring. The fact that primitive pulmonary hypertension was attributed to the fenfluramines only after years of administration in many millions of patients and particularly after long-term administration, is justifying precise pharmacovigilance and more research on the potential predictors (possibly via pharmacogenetics) of very harmful drawbacks. The concept of long term treatment, however, remains realistic.

Beginning of the 21st century

The future of pharmacotherapy remains, by definition conjectural. We can however guess that history is not over. Several questions are still open.

One of the most important is to bring evidence that anti-obesity drugs can significantly help preventing associated morbidity and mortality on a quite long time frame. Full acceptance of pharmacotherapy of obesity is relying on such outcome studies that have to demonstrate that its benefit/risk ratio is acceptable. The same has been true in the past for the use of lipid lowering drugs in hyperlipidaemia.

When new drugs will appear on the market? Theoretically an anti-obesity drug can reduce food intake, increase energy expenditure, limit intestinal absorption or modify nutrient partitioning.

Today, with the exception of orlistat, acting peripherally for limiting fat absorption, the other available drugs act merely by modifying the monoaminergic control of food intake; as such they are derived from the discoveries of the neurosciences that were already known thirty years ago. The explosion of knowledge in the past 20 years has shown the complexity of the system regulating energy balance, from the role of GI Tract to that of adipose tissue itself and including the roles of autonomic nervous system, of the peptidergic control of food intake and of several genetic mutations located in several points of this complex network. So far a lot of new drugs are in development: the history tells us that many of them will fail to appear on the market but we can hope that obesity will benefit of as many drugs as hypertension.

Many other questions will need answers and more research. Some examples are: advantages/disadvantages of associating behaviour modification with drugs risks/benefits of association of drugs with different mechanisms of action as is currently the case in hypertension and type 2 diabetes. How to limit misuse? Are anti obesity drugs worth refunding by social organization in specific comorbidities?

Guessing that answers will be brought in some of the future international congresses on obesity is probably no too optimistic.

References

1. Munro JF. *Clinical use of antiobesity agents in the treatment of obesity*, pp. 85–123. Lancaster, England: MTP Press Limited; 1979.

2. Bray GA. *The obese patients.* W.B. Saunders Comp Philadelphia, 1976.

3. Stunkard AJ, McLaren Hume. The results of treatment for obesity. *Arch Int Med* 1959; 103: 79–85.

4. Scoville BA. Review of amphetamine like drugs by the FDA. In: *Obesity in perspective DHEW* 75-108 Bethesda 1975; pp. 441–43.

5. Bray GA. To treat or not to treat. That is the question. In: *Recent advances in obesity research II.* Proceedings 2nd ICO, Bray G (ed.), pp. 248–65. London: Newman Publishing, 1978.

6. Stunkard AF, Pennick SP. Behavior modification in the treatment of obesity, the problem of maintaining weight loss. *Arch Gen Psychiatry* 1979; 36: 801–6.

7. Guy-Grand B, Waysfeld B. Pharmacology of obesity. In: *Traité de pharmacologie clinique*, pp. 924–936. Exp. Scientifique Française. Girond JP, editor; Paris; 1978.

8. Munro JF, Ford MJ. Drug treatment of obesity. In: *Drugs and appetite*, Silverstone T (ed.), pp.125–157. London: Academic Press; 1982.

9. Preventing and managing the global epidemic. Report of a WHO consultation on obesity. WHO/NUT/NCD/98.1

10. Guy-Grand B. A new approach to the treatment of obesity. *Ann NY Acad Sci* 1987; 499: 313–17.

11. Munro JF. Drug treatment: an overwiew. *Int J Obes* 1987; 11(Supp 3): 13–5.

12. Guy-Grand B. Long-term pharmacotherapy in the management of obesity. From theory to practice. In: *Obesity in Europe 1988*. Proceedings of 2nd ECO. Björntorp P, Rössner S (eds), pp. 311–318. London: John Libbey; 1989.

13. Apfelbaum M, Björntorp P, Garrow J *et al.* Standards for reporting the results of treatment of obesity. *Am J Clin Nutr* 1987; 45: 1035–36.

14. Guy-Grand B, Apfelbaum M, Crepaldi G *et al.* International trial of long-term dexfenfluramine in the management of obesity. *Lancet* 1989, II: 1142–44.

15. Darga L, Caroll-Michels L, Botsford, Lucas C. Floxetine's effect on weight loss in obese patients. *Am J Clin Nutr* 1991; 54: 321–25.

16. Sjöström L, Rissanen A, Andersen T *et al.* For the European Multicentre Orlistat Study Group. Randomized placebo-controlled trial of orlistat for weight loss and prevention of weight regain in obese patients. *Lancet* 1998; 352: 167–73.

17. James WPT, Astrup A, Finer N *et al.* For the STORM Study Group. Effect of Sibutramine on weight maintenance after weight loss: a randomized trial. *Lancet* 2000; 356: 2119–25.

18. Williamson DF, Pamuck E, Thurn M *et al.* Prospective study of international weight loss and mortality in never smoking overweight US white women aged 40–64 years. *Am J Epidemiol* 1995; 141(12): 1128–41.

19. Goldstein DJ. Beneficial health effects of modest weight lost. *Int J Obes* 1992; 16: 397–415.

20. North American Association for the Study of Obesity. Guidelines for the approval and use of drugs to treat obesity. *Obes Res* 1995; 3: 473–78.

21. Weintraub M, Sundaresan PR, Schuster B *et al.* Long term weight control: the National Heart, Lung and Blood Institute funded multimodal intervention study. I-VII. *Clin Pharmacol Ther* 1992; 51: 581–646.

22. Hollander PA, Elbein SC, Hirsh IB *et al.* Role of orlistat in the treatment of obese patients with type 2 diabetes. A 1-year randomized double-blinded study. *Diabetes Care* 1998; 21: 1288–94.

23. Muls E, Kolanowski J, Scheen A, Van Gaal L. For the ObelHyx Study Group. The effects of orlistat on weight and on serum lipids in obese patients with hypercholesterolemia: a randomized, double-blind, placebo-controlled, multicentre study. *Int J Obes* 2001; 25: 1713–21.

Progress in Obesity Research: 9. Edited by *Geraldo Medeiros-Neto, Alfredo Halpern and Claude Bouchard*
©2003 John Libbey Eurotext Ltd, pp. 903–905.

CHAPTER 189

International perspective of drug therapy

Stephan Rössner

Obesity Unit, Huddinge University Hospital, S-141 86 Stockholm, Sweden
[e-mail: Stephan.Rossner@medhs.ki.se]

Background

George Bray has summarized the development of pharmaco-therapy for obesity in the following, remarkably drastic way: Almost all drug treatments for obesity have generated undesirable outcomes that resulted in their termination (Table 1)[1]. Bray particularly points out that the previous use of amphetamine created a negative halo, spread by the addictive property of this drug[2]. Because amphetamine is addictive, other derivatives were presumed addictive and considered guilty by association, which lead to restrictions on the entire class of these drugs in several countries. Although some of these compounds would have appetite-depressing effects with little potential for abuse, many of them were lumped together and banned.

Table 1. Disasters with drug treatments for obesity (from G. Bray with permission, ref[1])

Date	Drug	Outcome
1893	Thyroid	Hyperthyroidism
1933	Dinitrophenol	Cataracts, neuropathy
1937	Amphetamine	Addiction
1967	Rainbow pills (digitalis, diuretics)	Death
1971	Aminorex	Pulmonary hypertension
1997	Fenfluramine + phentermine Dexfenfluramin+ phentermine	Valvular insufficency
2000	Phenylpropanolamine	Haemorrhagic stroke

Associated with the early and understandably negative attitudes to pharmaco-therapy of obesity was the primitive understanding that anti-obesity drugs did not work, since patients relapsed, when they stopped taking the medication. As Bray and others have pointed out, the truth is quite the contrary, since obesity is a chronic disease which like other chronic diseases, such as asthma, rheumatism, schizophrenia, psoriasis will require chronic treatment.

In spite of meticulous pre-registration research, unexpected negative side effects of anti-obesity drugs may still be experienced. The Fen-Phen drug combination with two well documented drugs, the combination of which had however never been formally accepted, resulted in valvulopathy, initially reported to affect up to 35 per cent of the patients[3]. Obviously, with this historical background, it is understandable that international health authorities, physicians and patients, however hopeful they are that a drug be delivered which will help to combat the obesity epidemic, remain sceptical.

National attitudes to antiobesity drugs and financial aspects

In most national health care systems, treatment of obesity is not reimbursed by society. Reimbursement has been made possible when treatment of obesity has been shown to directly improve serious comorbidities, but not even that has always been the case.

The presently available drugs which can be found almost over the world (sibutramine and orlistat) are costly in all countries, and the price varies surprisingly little in developed and developing countries. The time frame for acceptance and registration of new drugs for the treatment of obesity are markedly variable in different countries. Whereas orlistat brandnamed as Xenical (Roche) has been available in the United States and in Europe already during the previous millennium, the drug was not launched in China until 2001 and has not yet been registered in Japan in 2002.

Sibutramine, registered as Meridia/Reductil in many countries (Abbott) is available in China under several various other brand names. The development of sibutramine was hampered for a few months after an Italian report in early 2002 to the health authorities after two deaths, presumed to be associated with this product, but careful scrutinty of these records did not reveal any reason to alter present clinical routines. The event illustrates a certain vulnerability of the international control system, in that it seems that the temporary restriction that followed these reports was not evidence based. Patients benefiting from this treatment in many countries outside Italy were obviously concerned, when these reports reached wide publicity and some stopped using the medication.

It is interesting to note that dexfenfluramine, which was removed from almost all markets in 1997 is still easily available as an OTC product in China.

Reimbursement strategies may reflect attitudes to obesity rather than being based on proper scientific analyses. In Sweden, a country with a tax level up to 60 per cent for a sizeable proportion of the population, the national health care system is basically free, with only minor costs to be covered by the individual and only up to a certain level. The arrival of orlistat led to massive prescriptions of this drug, to which the government reacted by removing some drugs, such as those for impotency treatment and obesity from the reimbursement list. This manoeuvre was obviously intended to control drug costs and performed with political and not a scientific backup. It is ironic that at the same time, the British NICE (National Institute for Clinical Excellence) recommended that orlistat treatment be reimbursed in the United Kingdom if prescribed as a way to control obesity induced comorbidities[4].

Pharmacotherapy of obesity obviously has followed different courses in different countries. In some parts of world, access to such drugs has always been and remains liberal, whereas in other countries the access has been restricted. The ephedrine-caffeine combination, which was scientifically well documented through studies, in particular from Denmark[5], has been popular in the United States as an OTC product, whereas this product is not available in the neighbouring country Sweden and is not much used in other countries.

Alternative medicine

It is obvious that a huge number of overweight and obese patients are using alternative medication, completely outside the control of the medicine health care system. Allison has recently reviewed these products and identified 18 treatment strategies for which at least some scientific documentation could be found[6]. The overall impression is that these compounds are not well researched, have never been systematically tested in clinical trials and also may have potential serious side effects, which have never been properly addressed. The use of Ma Huang, which is a herbal natural source of ephedrine has raised concerns because of serious side effects. The Ma Huang reports illustrate the fact that herbal compounds cannot always be relied upon for safety, since the amount of the pharmacologically active compound may vary dramatically from batch to batch, resulting in either lack of efficacy or serious side effects.

New indications

With the present international trend that anti-obesity drugs are not reimbursed, it is but natural that several pharmaceutical companies are identifying avenues to achieve reimbursement status by looking at the effects of the drugs on the obesity associated comorbidities. Orlistat has been shown to have several beneficial effects in the prevention and management of diabetes mellitus, possibly also outside the effects achieved by weight loss in itself[7,8]. Orlistat has also been found to lower LDL cholesterol in overweight hypercholesterolaemic patients.

Likewise, the preliminary studies with sibutramine, such as the STORM study, indicate that sibutramine has a pronounced capacity to increase HDL cholesterol[9]. This effect actually exceeds that of many compounds, such as the fibrates, which are indicated in many countries for the treatment of the low HDL cholesterol levels, associated with atherosclerosis.

Prescription practices

No doubt, further studies will elucidate the potential role of these compounds in treating the obesity-associated complications in addition to inducing weight loss.

The concern that in the future problems may arise, as in the past, with anti-obesity drugs has lead to a discussion concerning methods to prevent future pharmaco-therapeutical disasters. As one way to increase security it has been suggested that restrictions in prescription rights of currently available drugs might prevent abuse. However, in reality it is not realistic to restrict prescription of these drugs to 'obesity specialists', since in every country the number of such specialists is extremely small and the proportion of the population, theoretically qualifying for treatment according to internationally accepted standards, is certainly at least around 10 per cent of the adult population. Thus it is obvious that drug treatment for obesity, also in the future, needs to be given by clinicians with a wide range of specialties: family physicians, general practitioners, endocrinologists, diabetologists, cardiologists, gynecologists etc.

The educational consequence of this pragmatic reality is that since restriction of prescription rights is no constructive way forwards, training of physicians in the management of obesity, which then also includes appropriate prescription competence, will become a priority of opinion leaders and policy makers.

So far, systematic training in management of obesity is rare. The Czech republic is one of the few countries where there is an attempt to develop a subspecialty, built on a network of dedicated teachers in a nummers of clinical units throughout the country. The CORE programme, initially developed in the United States but spreading also to other parts of the world, is an interesting attempt to provide a standardized programme, which can easily be used in various settings

References

1. Bray GA. *Contemporary diagnosis and management of obesity.* Pennsylvania: Handbooks in Health Care Co., 1998.

2. Bray GA. Use and abuse of appetite-suppressant drugs in the treatment of obesity. *Ann Intern Med* 1993; 119: 707–13.

3. Conolly HM, Crary JL, McGoon MD *et al.* Valvular heart disease associated with fenfluramine-phentermine. *N Engl J Med* 1997; 337: 581–8.

4. Foxcroft D, Luddens J. Orlistat for the treatment of obesity. Southampton: Wessex Institute for Health Research and development. Development and Evaluation Committee Report; 1999. Report 101.

5. Astrup A, Breum L, Toubro S *et al.* The effect and satiety of an ephedrine/caffeine compound compared to ephedrine, caffeine and placebo in obese subjects on an energy restricted diet. A double blind trial. *Int J Obes Relat Metab Disord* 1992; 16: 269–77.

6. Allison DB, Fontaine KR, Heshka S, Mentorer JL, Heimsfield SB. Alternative treatment for weight loss. A critical review. *Critical Reviews in Food Science and Nutrition* 2001; 41(1): 1–28.

7. Kelley DE, Jnedi M. Orlistat in the treatment of type 2 diabetes mellitus. *Expert Opin Pharmacother* 2002; 3(5): 599–605.

8. Keating GM, Jarvis B. Orlistat in the prevention and treatment of type 2 diabetes mellitus. *Drugs* 2001; 61(14): 2107–19.

9. James WPT, Astrup A, Finer N, Hilsted J, Kopelman P, Rössner S *et al.* Effect of sibutramine on weight maintenance after weight loss: a randomised trial. *Lancet* 2000; 356: 2119–25.

CHAPTER 190

Long-term therapy with drugs for the treatment of obesity – regulatory issues

Finian Kelly

84 Waterloo Place, Dublin 4, Ireland
[e-mail: finiankelly@ireland.com]

Introduction

The treatment of obesity with drugs remains controversial despite the licensing in recent years of two new treatments, sibutramine and orlistat. Underlying this unease with drug treatment are negative experiences with earlier drugs used in weight control, and negative attitudes to obesity as a condition that can be treated medically.

History of drug treatment of overweight and obesity

In order to understand these negative attitudes, a review of the history of drug treatment of obesity, and its accompanying pharmacological disasters, is useful in providing context. Historically, overweight was long a sign of prosperity and therefore desirable. It was not until the early nineteenth century that fashion dictated that less weight might be more aesthetically desirable. As now, reducing weight was no easy task and medical or chemical means of weight loss were sought. Thus the experimentation with extracts of thyroid gland that proved successful in reducing weight though only at the expense of inducing symptoms and signs of hyperthyroidism. The use of thyroid extracts for weight control, although medically unacceptable, continued until the latter quarter of the twentieth century.

In the early twentieth century, dinitrophenol was observed to induce weight loss, but its use was halted by the induction of severe neuropathies and cardiac complications. Amphetamines, powerful anorectic drugs, became widely used for weight control in the 1930s. The abuse potential of amphetamines lead to problems of addiction. As important was their central nervous system and cardiovascular stimulation, which lead to increased mortality from strokes and myocardial infarctions. 'Rainbow pills', so called for their many colours, were a compound mixture of amphetamines, digitalis and diuretics. This particularly lethal concoction, ignoring the narrow therapeutic index of digitalis, lead to many fatalities.

In 1971, aminorex was widely used in Europe for weight control. An epidemic of primary pulmonary hypertension (PPH), a rare and fatal respiratory disorder, was linked to the use of aminorex.

Fenfluramine, a serotonin-releasing agent, was the first of the newer generation of drugs used for weight control. Its anorectic effect was postulated to be due to an enhancement of satiety. It was later succeeded by its dextro-isomer, dexfenfluramine[1]. A landmark study published in 1992 demonstrated clinically significant weight loss with long term maintenance in obese patients treated by a combination of fenfluramine and phentermine, a sympathomimetic agent. Both drugs were then licensed in the United States only for short-term use. This lead to widespread use of this drug combination.

In the early 1990s both fenfluramine and dexfenfluramine were associated with cases of primary pulmonary hypertension in Europe. Despite this, in April 1997 dexfenfluramine became the first drug licensed by the Food and Drugs Administration of the United States for long-term (12 months) weight management. High expectations were fuelled by intense media coverage of the introduction of this supposed 'wonder diet drug', and prescription volumes were very high. In May 1998, reports associating the use of fenfluramine or dexfenfluramine with unexplained left-sided cardiac valve dysfunction emerged. Both drugs were withdrawn from all markets internationally in September 1998.

Phenylpropanolamine, a sympathomimetic, had been available as a non-prescription weight loss medication in the United States since the 1950s. A review of its safety profile revealed an increased risk of haemorrhagic stroke and it was withdrawn from the market in 1999. In Europe, in the wake of the withdrawal of the fenfluramines, the Committee for Proprietary Medicinal Products (CPMP) of the European Agency for the Evaluation of Medicinal Products (EMEA) undertook a scientific review of anorectic agents licensed in European Union countries. Marketing authorizations for eleven agents, including phentermine, mazindol and amfepramone, were withdrawn, based on an unfavourable risk/benefit ratio.

Thus the historical perspective of drugs used to control weight is coloured by the occurrence of a series of pharmacological disasters, many of which resulted in fatal illnesses.

Current drug treatments for obesity

Only two drugs are licensed for long-term treatment of obesity, sibutramine and orlistat. In this context, long-term means for a period of 12 months. Sibutramine is an inhibitor of the reuptake of serotonin, noradrenaline and dopamine, which acts to increase satiety; very limited evidence suggests a possible effect to increase metabolism[2]. Efficacy trials demonstrate weight loss that is active to 5–6 months of treatment, followed by maintenance to a further 18 months of continuous treatment[3]. This weight loss is accompanied by improvements in parameters of glucose metabolism, and in lipid profiles. Blood pressure does not show decreases, in fact the contrary, likely due to its noradrenergic enhancement.

Orlistat, an inhibitor of gastric lipase activity, decreases absorption of ingested fat by approximately 30 per cent[4]. Weight loss has been shown to continue for six months with demonstration of maintenance of that weight loss to two years. Improvement of obesity related risk factors including glucose, lipids and blood pressure have been demonstrated. Preliminary evidence suggests a lowering of the risk of progression from impaired glucose tolerance (IGT) to type 2 diabetes[5]. In the United States and some other countries (but not the European Union), some drugs are available for short-term treatment of obesity. These include phentermine, diethylpropion, mazindol and some sympathomimetcs. Data on both efficacy and safety of these drugs collected from controlled trials is lacking.

In addition to drugs licensed directly for the treatment of obesity, several drugs are used 'off-label' in this condition. Serotonin reuptake inhibitors are used, based on early data that demonstrated short-term weight loss with fluoxetine. A 12-month trial, however, demonstrated that the early weight loss was followed by weight regain with no difference between drug and placebo at the end of one year of treatment. Bupropion, an inhibitor of dopamine reuptake, licensed as an antidepressant in the United States, and globally as an aid to smoking cessation, has been shown to produce moderate weight loss. Topiramate, licensed as adjunctive therapy in epilepsy, produces profound, and unexplained weight loss in some patients. This has lead to its use in obesity. Other drugs used off-label include naltrexone and diazoxide.

Despite the safety and tolerability issues experienced in the use of the fenfluramine/phentermine combination, clinicians continue to experiment with combinations of drugs for obesity treatment. This practice is hazardous, since a combination drug therapy requires just as careful evaluation as each single therapy required. No systematic efficacy and tolerability data has been collected for these combinations.

Regulatory guidance for anti-obesity drug development

Both the US FDA and the European EMEA have published notes for guidance for development of drugs for 'weight control'[6,7]. These guidelines are not prescriptive. Both sets of guidelines set out primary and secondary efficacy criteria that should be attained. Both agencies mandate trials of at least one year duration, and FDA also seek data in 200–500 patients treated for two years. In the experience of this author, these guidelines represent the minimum requirements. Drug development programmes should improve on the last licensed drug in the field, and should be conducted in very large numbers of patients, probably 6,000 to 10,000 patients.

Attitudes to drug treatment of obesity

Despite educational initiatives of medical and allied organizations to educate the general public and healthcare professionals, there remain attitudes to obesity as a medical condition that requires medical treatment. Even at the level of regulatory agencies the attitudes expressed are not in consort with prevailing medical opinion. Obesity is still regarded by many medical practitioners as a lifestyle condition, which requires exercise of self-control rather than medical treatment to obtain a positive therapeutic outcome. The use of drugs in obesity is tainted by historical events: anorectic drugs are construed as inevitably having abuse potential; drug-induced weight loss is regarded as always accompanied by negative tolerability issues; weight control drugs are regarded as inherently unsafe. This skewed thinking insists on a unique test of efficacy for anti-obesity drugs: weight regain on cessation of treatment is interpreted as evidence of lack of efficacy. Thus, anti-obesity drugs are the only drugs expected to work when they are not taken.

The attitudes of regulatory agency assessors are, in the experience of the author, changing; the standards of efficacy data are now far beyond those laid down in the guidances for weight-control drugs. They will argue that the duration of drug trials have not been sufficiently long to show real long-term benefit; and further they will argue that weight loss and improvement in risk factors (for example, fasting glucose, blood pressure, fibrinogen, lipids) are simply surrogates for long-term mortal and morbid outcomes.

Thus the real questions for anti-obesity drug development have to be:

(1)   Is intentional weight loss beneficial in the long term?

(2)   Will drug-induced weight loss be as beneficial as non-drug induced weight loss?

These are the real issues for regulatory agencies.

Intentional weight loss

Data on intentional weight loss is lacking. Most data derive from studies not primarily intended to examine the effect of intentional weight loss. Singh *et al.* (1992) published results from a 1-year randomized controlled trial of a 'cardioprotective diet' in East Indian patients hospitalized with recent myocardial infarction (mean age 50 years, mean BMI about 24 kg/m^2)[8]. Although this study was not designed to specifically test the efficacy of intentional weight loss on lower mortality, the authors found that those who lost at least 0.5 kg had a 50 per cent lower incidence of cardiac events and a 54 per cent lower risk of overall mortality compared with counterparts who lost < 0.5 kg.

In a prospective observational study, Williamson *et al.* assessed weight loss intention and its relationship to mortality and morbidity[9]. Data from 43,457 overweight (BMI > 27), never-smoking women ages 40 to 64 years were analysed. In women with obesity-related co-morbidities, intentional weight loss of any amount was associated with a statistically significant 20 per cent reduction in all-cause mortality, mainly due to a significant reduction in mortality from obesity-related cancers. Diabetes-related mortality was also significantly reduced in those who intentionally lost weight. In women with no co-morbidities, intentional weight loss was generally unrelated to mortality.

Three studies provide evidence of an association between weight loss and delay in progression to type 2 diabetes in subjects with impaired glucose tolerance (IGT). The Da Qing study demonstrated that diet and exercise interventions reduced the relative risk of developing type 2 diabetes by 31 to 46 per cent[10]. In the Finland Diabetes Prevention Study, the effect of lifestyle interventions on the progression from IGT to type 2 diabetes was evaluated[11]. Mean weight loss at the end of year 2 in the intervention group was 3.4 kg compared to 0.8 kg in the control group. The cumulative incidence of type 2 diabetes after 4 years was 11 per cent in the intervention group compared to 23 per cent in the control group. Thus, the risk of diabetes was reduced by 58 per cent in the intervention group.

The Diabetes Prevention Program (DPP) is the first major clinical trial to show that lifestyle intervention (diet and exercise) delays the development of type 2 diabetes in a cohort of non-diabetic overweight patients with IGT[12]. The trial was halted 1 year ahead of schedule because interim data indicated that lifestyle intervention and treatment with metformin delayed the onset of type 2 diabetes. Compared with placebo, subjects in the intensive-lifestyle intervention group showed a 58 per cent reduction in the incidence of type 2 diabetes, associated with a 7 per cent weight loss.

In the ongoing Swedish Obese Subjects (SOS) intervention study, severely obese subjects treated by surgery are compared to a matched cohort group treated with standard care[13]. At eight years, mean weight reduction was 16.6 per cent in the surgically treated group compared to a mean gain of 0.9 per cent in the control group[14]. This weight reduction was associated with a diabetes incidence of 3.6 per cent compared to 18.5 per cent in the controls. However, no advantage of weight loss was apparent for hypertension, with no difference between the groups; incidence was 25.8 per cent in the treated group compared to 26.4 per cent in the controls.

Achieving acceptance of long-term drug treatment of obesity

To achieve acceptance of long-term drug treatment of obesity several stakeholders must play a role. Opinion leaders, experts and clinical investigators must ensure that a process of education of physicians, healthcare professionals and regulators is continuous. This education should aim to convince that obesity is a serious disorder with appalling health consequences; that moderate weight loss is beneficial; and that pharmcotherapy is often appropriate in treating obesity. Additionally, opinion leaders, experts and clinical investigators must ensure that drugs for obesity are developed to the highest standards. These stakeholders should further provide support to patient advocacy groups.

Prescribers must use licensed anti-obesity drugs within their labeling, respecting contra-indications and precautions. Patients most likely to benefit should be targeted and therapy should not continue in patients who do not respond. If drugs are used off-label for treatment of obesity, great care should be taken to monitor the patients' response; the patient should understand and agree to the use of medication in this manner. Clinicians should be aware that combination drug therapies are potentially hazardous, keeping in mind the 'fen-phen' problems. Such combination therapies need just as rigorous evaluation as the use of single drugs.

The pharmaceutical industry contributes by ensuring that drugs are developed in comprehensive programmes, with sufficient trials of sufficient length to show benefits on a wide range of surrogate endpoints. Guideline must be complied with and improvement on best previous practice is desirable. Non-pharmacological weight loss therapies should be standardized within trials so that data from different centres are comparable. Safety issues should be proactively addressed, including the historical safety concerns, primarily abuse potential, valvulopathy and pulmonary hypertension. Relevant animal models should be use and the mechanism of action of a drug should be demonstrated since unexplained weight loss is often medically associated with serious illness.

To the future

Improved drug development guidelines are desirable. The professional obesity bodies have a major role to persuade regulatory agencies to enter into dialogue on guidelines, with appropriate contributions from the pharmaceutical industry. Improved guidelines will help in ensuring high quality development programmes. Prediction of efficacy responders should be attempted. Safety issues will remain paramount; therefore determination of predictors of poor tolerability would greatly improve the risk-benefit ratio for drugs.

Pharmaceutical companies will have to commit to long-term evaluation of their drugs after licensing authorization is granted. This will entail commitment to performing outcome studies examining mortality and morbidity. There are lessons to be learned from the outcome studies with statins which proved their long-term benefits and lead to the acceptance of these drugs in routine medical practice[15,16]. Primary endpoints for outcome studies include total mortality and cardiovascular mortality. Secondary endpoints would include major coronary events, carotid intimal wall thickness, and progression to diabetes and to diabetes complications.

Conclusion

If long-term treatment of obesity with pharmacological agents is to become acceptable, a continuing process of education on the validity of obesity as a serious medical condition must be undertaken. More valid data on the benefits of intentional weight loss by any method are needed. The challenge for the pharmaceutical industry is to prove that drug-induced weight loss has long-term benefits that outweigh any tolerability and safety issues.

References

1. Guy-Grand B, Apfelbaum M, Crepaldi G *et al.* International trial of long-term dexfenfluramine in obesity. *Lancet* 1989; 2: 1142–45.

2. Connoley IP, Heal DJ, Stock MJ. A study in rats of the effects of sibutramine on food intake and thermogenesis. *Br J Pharmacol* 1995; 114–388.

3. James WPT, Astrup A, Finer N *et al.* Effect of sibutramine on weight maintenance after weight loss: a randomized trial. *Lancet* 2000; 356: 2119–25.

4. Hvizdos KM, Markham A. Orlistat: a review of its use in the management of obesity. *Drugs* 1999; 58: 743–60.

5. Heymsfield SB, Segal KR, Hauptman J *et al. Arch Intern Med* 2000; 160: 1321–26.

6. Guidance for the clinical evaluation of weight-control drugs. Food and Drug Administration, Rockville: Maryland; 1996.

7. Note for guidance on clinical investigationof drugs used inweight control Committee for Proprietary Medicinal Products, EMEA, London: UK; 1997.

8. Singh RB. Randomised controlled trial of cardioprotective diet in patients with recent acute myocardial infarction: resultsof one year follow-up. *BMJ* 1992; 304: 1015–19.

9. Williamson DF, Pamuk E, Thun M, Flanders D, Byers T, Heath C. Prospective study of intentional weight loss and mortality in never-smoking overweight US white women aged 40–64 years. *Am J Epidemiol* 1996; 141: 1128–41.

10. Pan XR, Li GW, Hu YH *et al.* Effects of diet and exercise in preventing NIDDM in people with impired'glucose tolerance. The Da Qing and diabetes study. *Diabetes Care* 1997; 20: 537–44.

11. Tuomilehto J, Lindstrom J, Eriksson JG *et al.* Preventionof type 2 diabetes mellitus by changes in lifestyle among subjects with impaired glucose tolerance. *N Engl J Med* 2001; 344: 1343–50.

12. Knowler WC, Barrett-Connor E, Fowler SE *et al.* Reduction in the incidence of type 2 diabeteswith lifestyle intervention or metformin. *N Engl J Med* 2002; 346: 393–403.

13. Sjostrom L, Larsson B, Backman L, Bengtsson C, Bouchard C, Dahlgren S *et al.* Swedish Obese Subjects (SOS): recruitment for an intervention study and a selected description of the obese state. *Int J Obes Relat Metab Disord* 1992; 16: 465–79.

14. Sjostrom CD, Peltonen M, Wedel H, Sjostrom L. Differentiated long-term effects of intentional weight loss on diabetes and hypertension. *Hypertension* 2000; 36: 20–5.

15. Scandinavian Simvastatin Survival Study Group. Randomised trial of cholesterol lowering in 4444 patients with coronary heart disease: the Scandinavian Simvastatin Survival Study (4S). *Lancet* 1994; 344: 1383–89.

16. Shepherd J. Prevention of coronary heart disease with pravastatin in men with hypercholesterolemia.West of Scotland coronary prevention study. *N Engl J Med* 1995; 24: 1839–48.

Progress in Obesity Research: 9. Edited by *Geraldo Medeiros-Neto, Alfredo Halpern and Claude Bouchard*
©2003 John Libbey Eurotext Ltd, pp. 911–916.

CHAPTER 191

Which diet or dietary approach – a consumer's approach?

Sonia Nigro Rosso

Department of Clinical Nutrition, School of Nutrition, State University, Uruguay
[e-mail: nigro@adinet.com.uy]

Dietary management is one of the well-established and evaluated therapies for the treatment of overweight. It is a basic strategy but as difficult as any other lifestyle changes. The aim of this paper is to discuss the best dietary approach to promote healthy weight. It analyses different options to identify the most effective methods to obtain acceptable weight loss benefits with fewer negative consequences.

The problem

Obesity is a chronic disease that affects groups of all ages, both in developed and under developing countries. It can be observed as an iceberg of a defined cluster of noncommunicable diseases, being a major risk factor for the most important health problems[1]. It is a serious disease that requires long term treatment to involve the development and maintenance of life-long healthy patterns. This chronic condition and its consequent difficult management, explain the frequent therapeutic failure.

It is a serious disease that requires long term treatment to involve the development and maintenance of life-long healthy patterns. This chronic condition and its consequent difficult management, explain the frequent therapeutic failure.

In 1958, Stunkard concluded his review of the past 30 years: 'Most obese persons will not stay in treatment for obesity. Of those who stay in treatment, most will not lose weight, and of those who do lose weight, most will regain it'[2]. Almost half a century later, this reality had changed only a little: maybe 80 per cent of patients will stay in treatment for 5 weeks and will lose more than 10 per cent of the initial weight but most of them will still regain it[3].

Data on behaviour therapy, very-low-calorie diet interventions and pharmacotherapy reveal that the majority of people who lose weight, regain it within 3 to 5 years after lifestyle intervention and within 1 year after leaving use of drugs[4].

The weight loss maintainers appear to be lighter, to be older and have dieted for longer, to have tried healthy eating more frequently, to be motivated for psychological reasons and are those who believe in the importance of weight for health[5].

The diet compliance is difficult because of problems associated with the consumer and the professional. The obese people modify food consumption waiting for weight reduction. At first it may seem a moderate effort if they can see good results. But the professional can make it harder if he/she does not consider individual aspects like eating patterns, appetite, previous diets and results, behaviour and motivation, social conditions, use of drugs and special clinical situations.

There is a weak basis in our knowledge about long-term effect of dietary treatment. Diet itself or diet combined with behaviour modification appears to show a success rate of 15 per cent of cases, three or more years later. Diet combined with group therapy lead to better long-term outcome (median 27 per cent)[6]. Great restrictions do not make it better for maintenance; very low calorie diets (VLCD) are as ineffective as conventional diets when we evaluate them in the long term[7].

That is why traditional weight loss treatments have been recently questioned in addition to the unsuccessful results, for the psychological costs: eating disorders because of restriction and deprivation, reduction of self-esteem because of cyclic failure, body unsatisfaction, irritability, increased anxiety and depression[8].

These observations lead us to question our professional function and the objective of the traditional weight loss treatments. The 'Health at any size philosophical foundation' (H@AS) supporters and other non official groups are recommending programmes based on psychological changes, not on diet focused as an alternative approach[9]. At the same time, some medical positions propose light diet recommendations. With those strategies, patients change the range of physical activities and adhere to a stable diet with liberal eating, aiming at health and obtaining modest weight loss.

The consumers point of view

Body unsatisfaction is a general feeling, specially in women and it is increasing in all communities. The desire to be slender is so strong and so widespread that it is difficult to persuade somebody to only maintain his/her weight, even when it is within a normal range. Patients spend economic and material resources to lose sizes, with significant differences between the obese that had made previous treatments and other obese and non-obese persons[10]. These people would not accept general recommendations, they expect solutions.

Without stereotyping, patients can be classified in two groups when they are derived for dietary management:

- People who are not interested in dietary guidelines because they ask for pharmacological treatment, or they do not want to be on a diet because they have never associated their health problem with overweight or with dietetic effectiveness.

Perhaps the first ones might have had numerous and difficult experiences trying all kinds of diets, they know the main basis of a caloric restriction and drug therapy is the key to accept lifestyle changes. The other members of this group need to understand and consent to be treated; maybe specific indications can change their food intake and could achieve the initial aim of the treatment.

- On the other hand there are patients looking for answers, anxious to change the dietary intake and be controlled.

Probably they have never been on a diet at least under professional supervision, or they are attempting to initiate a new stage. They require special attention to learn food selection, meal size, meal timing and energy restriction. Obviously the non-dietary focused strategy can not be the approach, they do not come for recommendations looking for a lifestyle change. They expect special indications to have a real treatment context.

Men are more likely to practice physical activity and to adhere to diet. Those with more attempts to lose weight (probably the majority), accept dietetic indications and recommendations to attend slimming groups[11].

The most obese are more likely to have negative views on treatments developed by health professionals and they regard themselves as second class clients[11]. Maybe they are right because there has been evidence that the patient's weight affects physician attitudes such as the time that they would spend for attention, the number of tests prescribed and different prejudices around obese capacities and responses[12]. Fortunately, this happens outside of specialized healthcare teams and particularly between health workers who have not understood obesity as a disease yet.

The youngest prefer vigorous forms of exercising and those without medical problems are more likely to engage in physical activity. Women are the most demanding: they want to have instant results, prefer slimming products, to swim and keep fit but are less likely to see dieticians and generally ask for medication[11].

To sum up, the preferences and usefulness of different methods for losing weight varies according to the number of attempts, gender, age, obesity stage and medical condition. Anyway, we need to define strategies; the challenge is to find which is the best approach.

Looking for answers

The education in food intake and eating habits is basically aimed at facilitating weight control. Dietary management is the most conventional treatment for overweight and obesity in spite of its poor long-term effectiveness, especially when used in isolation.

Traditionally we have modified the total energy intake, reducing amounts according to scientific data and aiming at weight changes. In the last years the epidemiological and experimental observations, showed beneficial effects by modifying diets' nutrient composition of diets. Low-fat diets had appeared to have better long-term outcome and to prevent or treat risky factors. In spite of that evidence, the rate of weight loss can be generally greater when low-fat dieting is coupled with a reduction in energy intake[13].

The WHO at this moment recognizes four modalities for dietary management:

- Individualized modest energy deficit diets: usually well tolerated, they promote a deficit of 500–600 kcal/day of the energy requirement with approximately 20–30 per cent or less energy fat, 15 per cent as protein and 55–60 per cent or higher as complex carbohydrate. The prescribed energy level should not be lower than 1200 kcal/day. Correctly used, this approach can lead in larger weight losses, educating the patient on a dietary plan looking for better dietary patterns. We have adapted this modality, reducing 20–40 per cent of the initial energy intake, to be sure that we are making gradual changes and at the same time the reduction is enough to have a negative energy balance. This methodology requires time and experience to estimate the habitual food intake.

- Low-fat high-carbohydrate diets: based on the beneficial effect on cardiovascular risk factors, proposes a fat level next to 10 per cent of total energy diet. Reduction of dietary fat is an easier way to have a low energy density. At the same time high carbohydrates consumption increases satiety and prevents the passive overconsumption of palatable high fat food. In addition to this advantage, rich complex carbohydrate diets promote energy expenditure to be stored like fat. This means that an *ad libitum* low-fat high carbohydrate diet programme has a great role in prevention and maintenance and may be useful to promote a modest but significant decrease of body kilograms, proportional to pre-treatment weight. It is a great strategy as initial counselling. We do not use it during treatment because of our eating patterns and the reduced industry availability of low-fat food in our country.

- Severe/moderate energy deficit diets: usually used in commercial systems for slimming, because of the quick weight reduction. Providing 1000–1200 kcal/day induce 15 per cent weight loss over 10–20 weeks, but they need a maintenance programme to keep the initial success. We use it only in certain patients or for a short time, because of the difficulty in compliance and the risk in basal metabolic rate reduction. Data shows good results when they are combined with behaviour modification, but this strategy is rare in our health care systems.

- Very-low-calorie diets: they are able to induce rapid weight loss with an energy level of less than 800 kcal/day. They are reserved for special conditions, they need medical supervision and should not be recommended as a common prescription. We do not have experience with them, except as an alternative diet used for few days within a conventional hypocaloric plan.

Comparing results of different diets, there are two ways to classify the success rate: in the short-term the greatest energy restrictions induce major weight loss, but in the long-term there are no major differences between different dietary approaches.

With hypocaloric balanced diets (individualized modest energy deficit diets), patients can lose nearly 0.5–1 kg per week, depending on the initial weight and the treatment stage. They do not have detrimental side effects, they are able to warrant optimal nutrient composition, they may control appetite through their physicochemical characteristics, and with them we may take into consideration the prevention or treatment of the frequent associated diseases[1]. But many patients do not accept them without any other added strategies. Anyway this is the conventional and basic therapy to promote nutritional changes.

Low-fat high-carbohydrate diets induce a weight loss of 3 kg in 6 months (20–30 g per week). Although exceptions, they are not accepted as an initial diet plan[14].

Low energy diets or VLCD induce rapid weight loss, nearly 1–2.5 kg per week, but they are used for specific applications, as part of a great weight loss programme, because of clinical and nutritional detrimental effects and the problems associated with compliance and psychological effects[7].

There are no data about weight loss over general diet recommendations; surely they can not induce countable results without other additional therapies.

All this indicates that it is necessary a long-term dietary programme, based on education about food and eating habits. It may be useful to promote a great initial weight loss as the first step of a management programme, attending to the evidence that it improves a sustained weight maintenance[15]. But this is still controversial in relation with the patient situation and with the therapies to cause the

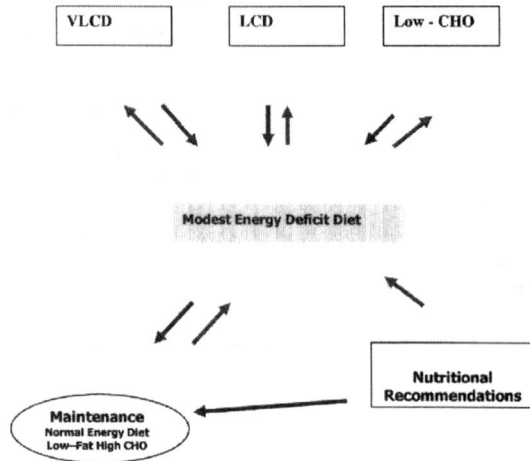

Fig. 1. The dietary treatment process. The green arrows mark good response to the strategy and define the next stage. The red arrows announce no evolution with that approach and suggest a new kind of diet. VLCD = Very Low Calorie Diets. LCD = Low Calorie Diets. Low-CHO = Low carbohydrate.

large weight loss as well as its greater maintenance. To accomplish that great initial weight loss, a drug therapy may be needed at an early stage and/or severe restrictions and strong changes should be recommended in a short time. That can not be suitable for all patients.

The ideal strategy

The best way of achieving healthy weight is by adopting a healthy diet with an energy level that does not exceed expenditure, low in fat, providing adequate amounts of all food groups attending the Dietary Guidelines of each country. At the same time, people will complete their lifestyle change through physical activity. These changes in behaviour should be tailored for each patient in order to ensure an optimal and well tolerated treatment, to produce gradual weight loss preventing negative psychological consequences[4]. In the same way, it is necessary to reduce the patient's focus on weight loss, trying to motivate self size-acceptance[16]

This theory proposal, is limited for different reasons:

- Not every patient loses enough weight due to global lifestyle changes, and even less with a healthy diet alone.

- Not every obese patient is able to reduce weight maintaining the ingestion of adequate amounts of all food groups because sometimes the solution is the restriction of a specific macronutrient.

- We have to prevent psychological consequences of restrictive diets, and at the same time the frustration for the unsuccessful weight loss because of insufficient restrictions.

- We can not probably suggest forgetting weight loss as the main objective because as professionals we are extremely focused on weight, too[17]. On the contrary, in some cases we are responsible to advise and improve weight loss because the clinical situation requires it and the patient has not noticed it.

We think the solution is to moderate dietary restrictions according to the health status. We have to communicate the indications in easy ways, looking for plans that do not make obese feel they are on a diet. We need to forget the weight as the main goal wherever there are no medical reasons to focus on it. In other words, our proposal is to change the professional point of view trying to be as flexible as we can, promoting the minimum weight loss to attend the clinical and psychological demands to prevent cycling failure or eating disorders.

Possible solutions

It is necessary to understand the obese patient treatment as a process, centred in the management of a possible and stable weight. According to the stage of treatment and attending to individual aspects, the clients may receive advice of healthy diet as general recommendations or may need a specific dietary management, presented as conventional hypocaloric diet or as greater restrictions. These diets can develop a circuit to travel aiming at the targets and the effectiveness.

An individualized approach

The prognosis and evolution are associated with the clinical situation and the diet compliance, and it is conditioned by multiple aspects to consider.

The dietary approach needs to take into account particular variables such as gender, age, degree of overweight, personal weight history, genetic susceptibility, physical activity, motivation, number of weight-loss attempts and type of previous treatments and responses, mood disturbances or eating disorders, co-morbidity or risk factors, drug therapy, nourishing behaviour, previous food intake and preferences.

At the same time, it is important to analyse the patient's context: government health policies, care service support, food industry, nutritional education, social situation, economic resources and family involvement.

In order to address these factors it is very important to have an interview to investigate and to register those details. At the same time it facilitates the patient – professional rapport to warrant the first compliance.

In spite of the difficulty of reporting the previous dietary intake, we prefer to approach it, using combined methods to define qualitative and quantitative diet characteristics. It is necessary to know, at least, the meal frequency, food selection and cooking methods, diet composition and an estimate of energy intake. It may project an energy deficit that the patient can sustain, translated into a dietary plan based on healthy eating principles suitable to his/her circumstances. It should educate patients to facilitate better long-term weight loss/control.

Using a guideline to choose the best diet strategy

This proposal is based on our observation and experience, which unfortunately is not yet documented. So it is presented as a hypothesis open to discussion. Frequent situations of obese patients were matched with possible best dietary approaches to begin treatment.

Situations Type A:

- Both gender, little weight gain, BMI < 25 (probable increased waist circumference), associated with physical activity reduction or quitting smoking.

- Both gender, first weight loss attempt with previous high energy diet and without co-morbidity.

Dietary strategy: nutritional recommendations emphasizing lower fat, high fibre and moderate meal size, known as qualitative diet.

Situation Type B:

- Situation A but with co-morbidity or genetic susceptibility.

- Female BMI < 25, first weight loss attempt, previous physical activity and acceptable eating habits.

Dietary strategy: dietary plans to promote minimum energy deficit or at least to define clear changes in diet composition. They need or demand more accuracy. Food exchange system is a good method; it can be used to express all food groups or only the ones that have high energy density.

- Situation Type C:

- Males, multiple weight loss attempts.

- Females, multiple weight loss attempts, sedentary behaviour, previous free food intake.

- Obese with important eating disorders.

Dietary strategy: conventional hypocaloric diet, modest energy deficit tailored to individual characteristics. Pharmacological treatment may be considered accounting BMI, co-morbidity and causes of previous failure.
Situation Type D:

- Female, multiple weight loss attempts, habitually restrained eater.

Dietary strategy: severe/moderate energy deficit. Drug therapy may be the central choice, depending on the clinical situation.

The nutrient energy distribution in all situations is done according to appetite, associated diseases, eating patterns and eating disorders. People who overeat need high protein diets; metabolic disease can be treated with carbohydrates or lipids modifications and when there is carbohydrate appetite it is useful to maintain complex carbohydrates evenly distributed. Sometimes pharmacological treatment makes the difference, too.

In all cases, an integral approach will be considered, including physical activity and additional therapies, maintaining basic criteria such as: re-education from the previous intake, considering co-morbidities and seeking agreement. Patients motivation or economic resources, may change the strategy or at least the way to communicate the indications being as flexible as possible to prevent failure.

References

1. World Health Organisation. Obesity: Preventing and managing the global epidemic. Report Geneva; 1997.
2. Ogden J. The correlates of long term weight loss: a group comparison study of obesity. *Int J Obes* 2000; 24: 1018–25.
3. Wadden TA. Treatment of obesity by moderate and severe calorie restriction: results of clinical research trials. *Ann Intern Med* 1993; 119: 688–93.
4. American Dietetic Association. Position of the American Dietetic Association: Weight management. *J Am Diet Assoc* 1997; 97: 71–4.
5. Latner JD, Stunkard AJ, Wilson G.T, Jackson M, Zelitch DS, Labouvie E. Effective long-term treatment of obesity: a continuing care model. *Int J Obes* 2000; 24: 893–8.
6. Ayyad C, Andersen T. Long-term efficacy of dietary treatment if Obesity: a systematic review of studies published between 1931 and 1999. The International Association for the Study of Obesity. *Obesity Rev* 2000; 1: 113–19.
7. Mustajoki P, Pekkarinen T. Very low energy diets in the treatment of obesity. *Obes Rev* 2001; 2: 61–72.
8. Ikeda JP *et al.* A commentary on the new obesity guidelines from NIH. *J Am Diet Assoc* 1999; 99: 918–19.
9. Miller WC, Jacob AV. The health at any size paradigm for obesity treatment: the scientific evidence. *Obes Rev* 2001; 2: 37–45.
10. Sherwood NE *et al.*: Predictors of weight gain in the Pound of Prevention study. *Int J Obes* 2000; 24: 395–403.
11. Thompson RL, Thomas DE. A cross-sectional survey of the opinions on weight loss treatments of adult obese patients attending a dietetic clinic. *Int J Obes* 2000; 24: 164–70.
12. Hebl MR, Xu J. Weighing the care: physicians' reactions to the size of a patient. *Int J Obes* 2001; 25: 1246–52.
13. Bray GA, Popkin BM. Dietary fat intake does affect obesity! *Am J Clin Nutr* 1998; 68: 1157–1173.
14. Saris WHM *et al.* Randomized controlled trial of changes in dietary carbohydrate/fat ratio and simple vs. complex carbohydrates on body weight and blood lipids: the CARMEN study. *Int J Obes* 2000; 24: 1310–18.
15. Asturp A, Rössner S. Lessons from obesity management programmes: greater initial weight loss improve long-term maintenance. *Obes Rev* 2000; 1: 17–9.
16. Parham ES. Promoting body size acceptance in weight management counseling. *J Am Diet Assoc* 1999; 99: 920–5.
17. McArthur LH., Ross JK. Attitudes of registered dietitians toward personal overweight and overweight clients. *J Am Diet Assoc* 1997; 97: 63–6.

Progress in Obesity Research: 9. Edited by *Geraldo Medeiros-Neto, Alfredo Halpern and Claude Bouchard*
©2003 John Libbey Eurotext Ltd, pp. 917–921.

CHAPTER 192

The roles of behaviour modification in the management of obesity

Patrick Mahlen O'Neil

*Weight Management Center, Department of Psychiatry and Behavioral Sciences,
Medical University of South Carolina, Charleston, SC 29425, USA
[e-mail: oneilp@musc.edu]*

Definition and purposes of behaviour modification

Behaviour modification is the application of principles of learning to produce a change in target behaviours. It includes the analysis and modification of relationships among stimuli, behaviour, and consequences. Specific behaviours most germane to the overall presenting problem are identified, the stimuli or cues that are probabilistically related to those behaviours are isolated, and the results of the behaviour under those conditions are identified and assessed as either increasing or decreasing the future probability of the behaviour. These relationships are then altered to attempt to produce a change in the target behaviours.

The realm of behaviour modification is often currently taken to include 'cognitions' (thoughts) and emotions as stimuli, behaviours, and consequences. Therapeutic approaches that attend to the patient's reported thought and emotional patterns as well as overt behaviours are referred to broadly as cognitive behavioural therapy. To acknowledge another less precise use of the word 'behavioural' in the obesity literature, as an adjective it is sometimes used to mean 'psychological'.

Behaviour modification has a foundation in the experimental psychology areas of classical (Pavlovian) and operant (Skinnerian) conditioning. Beginning in the 1960s, it quickly became the subject of extensive research and clinical application in clinical psychology and, to a lesser extent, other mental health disciplines, as it was applied to the treatment of a variety of psychological disorders and behavioural problems.

The concept of using behaviour modification principles to assist obese patients was first proposed by Ferster in a 1962 paper[1]. Shortly thereafter, in another landmark paper, Stuart in 1967[2] described the successful application of behavioural techniques to weight loss efforts of a series of obese patients. This prompted scores of clinical and research projects by psychologists on ways to evaluate and extend the effectiveness of behaviour modification as a weight loss intervention. Some of the most productive and long-standing clinical researchers in this area are Albert Stunkard, John Foreyt, Thomas Wadden, Kelly Brownell and Michael Perri.

Although Stuart reported the results of individual treatment of a series of individual patients, rather quickly the norm for treatment became protocol-based structured treatments conducted in group settings by one or two behavioural specialists, usually psychologists or psychology trainees. This remains the most frequent structure for the behavioural treatments of obesity that are reported in the clinical outcomes literature. Indeed, comprehensive behavioural treatment also includes substantial education and counseling regarding nutrition and exercise, and is increasingly referred to as 'lifestyle change'. However, it must be emphasized that behavioural techniques may also be applied in work with individual patients by non-behavioural providers, in limited interventions focusing on a very few behaviours at any one time.

Although obesity is neither a behaviour nor a psychiatric diagnosis, the importance of behaviour change in weight loss and maintenance is apparent. Weight loss requires negative energy balance in the near term, and weight loss maintenance requires long-term energy balance. Both require changes in the amount, type and pattern of caloric intake and the amount of energy expended in daily activities and exercise.

These dietary, exercise and activity changes are frequently difficult to achieve for a variety of reasons. Genetic factors and physiological and biological processes, both normative and aberrant, may predispose the individual to excess intake, preference for certain calorically dense items, and energy conservation via inactivity. The individual's longstanding behavioural, cognitive, and emotional patterns may present a compelling baseline of competing, undesired behaviours. Various aspects of the environment may pose obstacles to desired behaviours and facilitate the undesired behaviours; this includes physical, social, cultural and nutritional features of the environment.

Consideration of the naturally occuring consequences of weight-related behaviours provides further understanding of how weight-increasing behaviour patterns are established and maintained in the natural environment. Behaviours may have both immediate and delayed consequences, and the two may be quite different in type and valence. From an operant point of view, the immediate consequences have the greatest influence on the behaviour. The immediate consequences of many unhealthful behaviours (e.g. consumption of a high-calorie dessert or watching television rather than exercising) tend to be immediate and rewarding (e.g. pleasant taste and post-ingestive physical state; avoidance of physical discomfort). These consequences are also relatively certain and known to the individual. Although the likely long-term consequences of the unhealthful behaviours are accepted as undesirable (e.g. obesity, poor fitness), they are remote, only probable, and perhaps not within the person's experience. Therefore the naturally occurring consequences oppose the behaviour patterns necessary for weight control.

Behaviour modification techniques

A variety of behaviour modification techniques are used to support the introduction and continuation of desired behaviours despite the numerous obstacles just discussed.

Goal-setting

Attainment of a weight loss objective requires a number of behavioural changes that must be established and maintained over weeks and months, and weight maintenance requires longer-term behaviour change. Translating the desired weight outcome to the specific behaviours required to achieve it is necessary to provide a plan for behaviour change. The focus is on immediate behaviour changes. For example, a patient who wishes to lose 20 kg may be counseled to plan for a 0.5 kg loss per week. That weekly loss may require following a specific food and exercise plan which should be stated in behavioural terms. Thus, 'lose 20 kg' is transformed to 'lose one half kilo this week' which is translated to 'follow the 1200 kcal diet and walk 45 minutes five times'.

Behavioural goals should be *specific* and *observable*, that is, they should be clearly and unambiguously defined, and confined to a reasonably short time frame. While requiring meaningful change, they should also be *attainable* given the patient's current status. For example, the currently sedentary patient should not attempt to walk 10 km daily the first week of exercise. Finally, in clinical practice, it is often useful to use goals that are somewhat *forgiving*, i.e. that do not require perfect performance every day of the targeted time period. This allows the patient to succeed at attaining meaningful goals despite an occasional 'off' day.

Shaping

Shaping is the use of successive approximations to an ultimate behavioural target which may be quite remote from current behavioural patterns in extent and time. For example, a sedentary individual may have to develop a programme of moderately intensive exercise for 45 min, 5 days a week, and maintain that programme for months. Achieving that benchmark in the first week is unlikely and may be undesirable. This objective is best met by breaking down the ultimate goal to a series of smaller, less ambitious units, each closer to the ultimate goal. Goals should be set so that success is likely at each step.

Rewards

As noted earlier, the naturally occurring consequences of undesired behaviours are often rewarding, certain and familiar. The healthier alternative behavioural goals may not be immediately rewarding and may involve discomfort or deprivation. Therefore, patients who have difficulty meeting goals may be counseled to implement a system of rewards for achieving the goal. The specific reward should be designated at the time of goal-setting, and may be tangible (e.g. purchase of some desired item) or intangible (e.g. time to oneself).

Self-monitoring

Self-monitoring refers to the systematic observation and recording of one or more aspects of one's behaviour. When applied to dietary assessment, the patient is asked to record all (caloric) food and drink intake over a specified period of time, often with forms that are provided. Data to be recorded may include types and amounts of foods and drinks consumed, methods of preparation, the time, duration and place of consumption, and the social, emotional and physical conditions. Self-monitoring is also useful for other behaviours, particularly exercise. Regular recording of bodyweight is another long-term application of self-monitoring.

Self-monitoring often changes the monitored behaviour in the desired direction. Studies by Kirschenbaum and associates demonstrate convincingly the contribution that self-monitoring can play in enhancing weight loss. Baker and Kirschenbaum[3] followed 56 patients during 12 weeks after an initial treatment period (average of 40 weeks) during which they had lost an average of 9.5 kg (21 lb). The authors assessed the consistency of subjects' self-monitoring on a weekly basis during the 12 weeks and found a strong relation of self-monitoring consistency to weight loss during this time (r = 0.41–0.44, P < 0.01). When subjects were divided into quartiles based on extent of monitoring, the top quartile lost far more weight during the 12-week period (10.0 kg; 22.1 lb) than did the bottom quartile, which gained 0.7 kg (1.6 lb). Further, subjects lost significantly more weight in their best week of monitoring than in their worst week of monitoring. A later study by Boutelle and Kirschenbaum[4] closely replicated the above findings, and two other studies showed that self-monitoring improved weight control during the end-of-the-year holiday season[5,6].

Stimulus control

Many habitual behaviours are elicited much more reliably in the presence of certain cues or stimuli, such as visible food, place, time, activity, or even mood. For example, watching television at certain times, or driving, or boredom may be triggers for unplanned eating. Restricting eating to a smaller number of stimuli may make it easier to control eating. For example, the patient may be encouraged to limit eating to one location in the home, or to avoid pairing eating with certain other stimuli, or to keep most food items out of sight. The power of stimuli in eliciting behaviours may also be employed to promote desirable behaviours by, for example, encouraging exercise by making it a regular occurrence at certain times, or by changing to walking shoes before returning home from work.

Eating behaviour changes

Sometimes the manner in which food is consumed contributes to excessive consumption, as when, for example, the patient eats so rapidly that the planned portion of the meal is completed before satiety signals have had a chance to develop. Various methods may be used to slow eating rate so that satiety has begun before the meal has ended, for example, monitoring the time required to consume a meal, building in pauses during the meal, or placing utensils down before bites. These and other eating behaviour changes (e.g. not engaging in other activities while eating) may also increase awareness of what is eaten to reduce excess consumption.

Cognitive restructuring and relapse avoidance skills

The patient's expectations about and interpretations of the course of weight loss may influence the success of behavioural change efforts in both the short and long term. For example, unrealistically perfectionistic standards may prove self-defeating, and overly harsh assessments of setbacks may promote an expectation of failure. Similarly, failure to assume responsibility for successes may encourage the patient to see them as random and unlikely. It can be useful to encourage the patient to examine cognitive patterns related to weight control efforts and to attempt to replace maladaptive patterns with more productive alternatives.

Weight loss maintenance requires life-long change, and relapse to older patterns with consequent weight regain is common. Behavioural treatment tries to prepare the patient for this long-term challenge, especially when preparing the patient to deal with slips and setbacks. It is important for both the provider and the patient to maintain a non-judgmental approach that recognizes the innate difficulty and environmental obstacles that can provoke occasional lapses. Patients should be encouraged to try to quantify the degree to which they have strayed from their goals and should be taught problem-solving skills to regain control by analysing the determinants of the setback and revising goals.

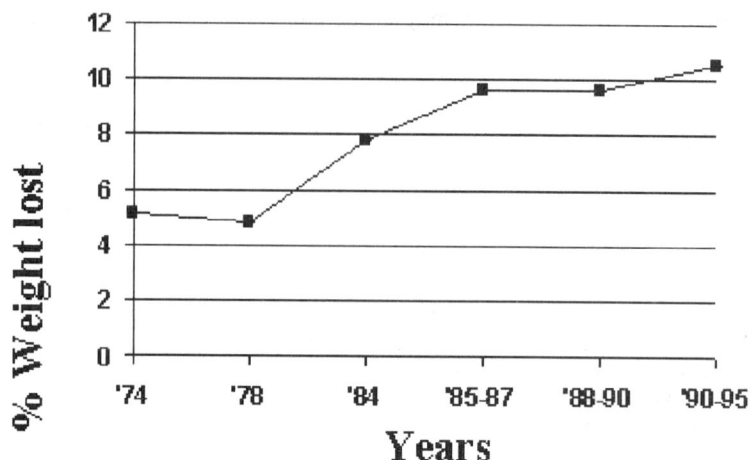

Fig. 1. Mean weight loss results of behaviour modification trials. Each data point reflects mean loss of studies in designated time period in trials using moderate caloric restriction (based on summaries by Wadden[7] and Wing[8]).

Targets of behaviour modification that do not directly involve the energy balance equation

Other behaviour modification approaches can play a role in obesity treatment beyond simple alteration of the energy balance equation. Cognitive-behavioural programmes to improve body image may be important when problems in this area either exist initially or become manifest with weight loss. Frequently, patients who report difficulty enacting weight control techniques because of competing demands may be helped with stress management and time management training. Assessment and enhancement of lifestyle balance may be useful for patients for whom eating may represent the only reward and/or relaxation that they permit themselves.

Results of behavioural weight control programmes

As mentioned earlier, most of the studies examining the results of behaviourally based programmes have involved protocol-driven treatments usually conducted in group settings by behavioural or nutritional professionals, with some components addressing dietary and exercise changes. Figure 1 summarizes the results of several scores of such trials (all entailing moderately calorically restrictive diets) conducted over more than 20 years. It is noteworthy that the more recent trials show that behaviourally based treatment produces a weight loss approximating 10 per cent of initial bodyweight, an amount often adequate to improve co-morbidities. This amount of loss is also commensurate with that seen in most trials of weight loss medications. It should be noted that over the years the duration of treatment has also increased, to an average of 27 weeks in the last time period shown[7,8].

Methods of enhancing utility of behavioural methods

Figure 1 suggests that comprehensive behavioural treatments, while achieving a clinically significant weight loss, may have reached a ceiling of effectiveness as commonly studied. There are numerous promising methods of increasing the usefulness of the behavioural approach, in terms of both average weight loss to participants and number of eligible participants. Several studies have shown that improved weight loss can be achieved when behavioural programmes are combined with other modalities such as meal replacements, other means of structuring dietary intake, and weight loss medications(e.g.[9-11]). The maintenance of weight loss has been shown to be improved by various types of post-treatment contact[12].

As noted earlier, the trials of behavioural treatments have typically examined group-based programmes in university or hospital settings requiring weekly attendance for a half-year or more. Such programmes are unavailable to most obese persons because of cost or geographic proximity. Accessibility to behaviourally based programmes can be increased by greater insurance coverage of fee-for-service programmes, by provision of such programmes at no or little cost by health maintenance programmes or government health programmes, and by designing programmes that can be delivered by persons other than behavioural or nutritional specialists. In particular, means should be developed to incorporate the most effective behavioural techniques into primary care medical settings (e.g.[13]). The internet offers a promising means of vastly increasing access to the elements of behavioural treatment, although the in-person contact is necessarily diminished or lost[14].

The time required of patients and providers in the research behavioural programmes is an obstacle to both widespread implementation and widespread acceptance. Obviously, the necessary staff time greatly increases the expense of delivering such programmes. Even when available, most people attempting to lose weight do not use such programmes, whether because of cost, time or personal preference[15–16]. A challenge is to distill the lessons of behavioural trials to develop interventions that employ the most effective techniques in formats that are more acceptable and accessible to the majority of obese persons. In a related vein, it is important to note that nearly all of the behavioural trials have been conducted in the US. Future studies should attempt to demonstrate how best to modify these programmes for use in other countries with different cultural features.

References

1. Ferster CB. Nurnberger JI, Levitt EB. The control of eating. *J Mathetics* 1962; 1: 87–107.

2. Stuart RB. Behavioral control of overeating. *Behav Res Ther* 1967; 5: 357–65.

3. Baker RC, Kirschenbaum DS. Self-monitoring may be necessary for successful weight control. *Behav Ther* 1993; 24: 377–94.

4. Boutelle KN, Kirschenbaum DS. Further support for consistent self-monitoring as a vital component of successful weight control. *Obes Res* 1998; 6: 219–24.

5. Baker RC, Kirschenbaum DS. Weight control during the holidays: Highly consistent self-monitoring as a potentially useful coping mechanism. *Health Psychol* 1998; 17: 367–70.

6. Boutelle KN, Kirschenbaum DS, Baker RC, Mitchell ME. How can obese weight controllers minimize weight gain during the high risk holiday season? By self-monitoring very consistently. *Health Psychol* 1999; 18: 364–68.

7. Wadden TA. Treatment of obesity by moderate and severe caloric restriction. Results of clinical research trials. *Ann Int Med* 1993; 119: 688–93.

8. Wing R. Behavioral approaches to the treatment of obesity. In: *Handbook of obesity*, GA Bray, Bouchard C, James WPT (eds), pp. 855–73. New York: Marcel Dekker; 1998.

9. Ashley JM, St. Jeor ST, Perumean-Chaney S, Schrage J, Bovee V. Meal replacements in weight intervention. *Obes Res* 2001; 9: S312–20.

10. Wing RR, Jeffery RW, Burton LR, Thorson C, Nissinoff KS, Baxter JE. Food provision vs. structured meal plans in the behavioral treatment of obesity. *Int J Obes Relat Metab Disord* 1996; 20: 56–62.

11. Wadden TA, Berkowitz RI, Sarwer DB, Prus-Wisniewski R, Steinberg C. Benefits of lifestyle modification in the pharmacologic treatment of obesity: a randomized trial. *Arch Intern Med* 2001; 161: 218–27.

12. Perri, MG. Improving the maintenance of weight lost in behavioral treatment of obesity. In: *Handbook of obesity treatment*, Wadden TA, Stunkard AJ (eds), pp. 357–82. New York: The Guilford Press, 2002.

13. Wadden TA, Berkowitz RI, Vogt RA, Steen SN, Stunkard AJ, Foster GD. Lifestyle modification in the pharmacologic treatment of obesity: a pilot investigation of a potential primary care approach. *Obes Res* 1997; 5: 218–26.

14. Tate DF, Wing RR, Winett RA. Using Internet technology to deliver a behavioral weight loss programme. *JAMA* 2001; 285: 1172–77.

15. Binks, M, O'Neil PM. Referral sources to a weight management programme: Relationship to outcome. *J Gen Int Med* 2002; 17: 596–603.

16. Levy AS, Heaton AW. Weight control practices of US adults trying to lose weight. *Ann Int Med* 1993; 119: 661–6.

©2003 John Libbey Eurotext Ltd, pp. 922–926.

CHAPTER 193

Alternative treatments for weight loss: range, rationale, and effectiveness

Garry Egger[1], Rosemary Stanton[2] and David Cameron-Smith[3]

[1]*Centre for Health Promotion and Research, PO Box 313, Balgowlah, NSW, Australia & School of Health Sciences, Deakin University, Burwood Hwy., Melbourne, Australia;* [2]*Consultant Dietitian; University of New South Wales, Sydney, Australia;* [3]*School of Health Sciences, Deakin University; Burwood Hwy., Melbourne, Australia* [e-mail: eggergj@ozemail.com.au]

Introduction

Up to 72 per cent of men and 85 per cent of women in some countries are currently trying to lose, or at least not gain, weight[1]. However, less than 30 per cent of those trying to lose and 20 per cent of those trying not to gain, report using 'traditional' treatments to do so[2]. 'Alternative' treatments seem to be more popular, although their effectiveness has not been established.

In this paper we used appropriate electronic searches to add to the findings from three earlier reviews of 'alternative' treatments in weight loss[3–5]. 'Alternative' here is defined as those treatments not involving modifications of energy balance through traditional means, as shown in Table 1. The report is narrative and we do not claim to cover all treatments, or use quantitative standards of assessment. Also, for brevity, only new data since the earlier reviews are reported. We consider alternative treatments in three categories; ingestible substances, non-ingestible treatments and alternative forms of delivery.

Table 1. Traditional treatment approaches for obesity

Target population	Interventions
Overweight/obese (with co-morbidities)	Medical/surgery/VLEDs
Overweight/obese (with disordered eating patterns or cognitions)	Psychology/behaviour modification
Overweight/obese	Individual education and skills training
General population	Population education and awareness raising

Ingestible substances

As many as 7 per cent of the US population[2], and up to 28 per cent of young, obese women[6], regularly use non-prescription, over-the-counter (OTC) substances for weight loss. In previous reviews, no evidence of long-term beneficial results for any of the ingredients commonly contained in these preparations has been found. We concurred with other authors that while several products do have a reasonable physiological rationale, claims of effectiveness are usually not based on well controlled studies published in reliable peer-reviewed literature. The effectiveness of substances that may interact is also difficult to assess.

Since our last report[3] we have identified a number of newly promoted compounds including: bissey nut extract, citrus aurantium, coleus forskolin, ephedra alkaloids, ginseng, green tea extract, guarana, L-tyrosine, magnesium stearate, gymnema sylvestre and pyruvate. We have been unable to find acceptable evidence supporting any of these for long-term weight loss in humans. Rat studies which claim hydroxycitric acid (HCA) may reduce food intake were partly supported by a 2 week single-blind crossover trial in humans in the Netherlands which reported a 5–30 per cent decrease in 24-h energy intake, although without changes in appetite profile or dietary restraint[7]. However, another study of 89 mildly obese women found no effects of HCA on appetite variables and no satiety effect[8].

Several recent trials confirm the earlier short-term successes reported for caffeine and ephedra in various forms. The Chinese herb ma-huang has featured in many of these. However, widespread side effects and some deaths have lead the US Food and Drug Administration (FDA) to take action against marketers of this product and their continued availability and long-term safety is currently under question

In summary, there have been no good recent data produced to change the conclusions of earlier reviews showing that while some alternative substances have a reasonable theoretical rationale, none can be recommended for use on the basis of current evidence or long-term safety.

Non-ingestible treatments

As well as ingestibles, there is a wide, and rapidly changing range of alternative non-ingestible treatments claiming benefits for weight loss. We have chosen some of the most common and enduring for inclusion.

Skin applications

Most skin creams claiming weight loss properties are focused primarily on 'cellulite' reduction[9]. Cellulite creams are diverse with 32 products surveyed containing 263 ingredients[10]. Commonly reported as an active ingredient is caffeine although no published evidence supports a role for topically applied caffeine in cellulite reduction. In their review of thigh creams, Alison *et al.*[5] conclude that any changes resulting from these are at most, cosmetic, and there is no evidence for medical/health benefits of these treatments. There has been no evidence since this review to change this conclusion. Slimming soaps which contain seaweed extract as the active ingredient have also been claimed to have weight loss effects[11], but again, there is no published supporting evidence, or physiological basis for these claims.

Acupuncture and acupressure

Acupuncture and related oriental techniques are frequently cited as strategies to curb appetite and lower body weight. At least four controlled studies have found no such effect[12], although improved psychological status has been observed in a recent randomized, placebo-controlled trial[13]. In one controlled study, combined acupressure and transcutaneous electrical stimulation of the auricular branch of the vagal nerve using an AcuSlim device suppressed appetite and body weight (−3.0 ± 1.4 kg) when applied twice weekly for four weeks[14]. However, auricular acupressure without electrical stimulation has not been found to have any effect[15]. Further studies are required to provide data on the longer term effectiveness of acupressure techniques in weight loss.

Muscle electrostimulation (transcutaneous electrical nerve stimulation)

Electronic muscle stimulation (EMS) or transcutaneous electrical nerve stimulation (TENS) apparati are used as a supplementary treatment option in the management of selected muscular rehabilitation and conditioning. At least one study has shown significant weight loss with TENS compared to a control group[14] prompting a suggestion for further independent research on this process. However no impact of EMS on bodyweight has been demonstrated[16].

Hypnosis

Hypnotherapy is often used as an adjunct treatment in weight loss, although few controlled studies exist on its effectiveness. A meta-analysis of five controlled studies using hypnosis for weight loss demonstrated a small non-significant effect, but a further review of the same data set, with the inclusion of one additional study, suggested a small significant effect (2.6 kg)[17]. In more recent studies, a slight benefit (mean loss of 2 kg) occurred with hypnosis plus overt aversion (electric shock, disgusting tastes and smells) compared with hypnosis alone[18] although a similar study did not confirm this[19]. In another study, 60 obese patients with obstructive sleep apnoea were randomized to receive two forms of hypnosis (directed at stress reduction or reducing energy intake reduction) compared to standard dietary advice alone. After initial weight loss in all groups, the hypnotherapy for stress reduction was the only intervention to achieve persistent weight loss (mean 3.8 kg)[20].

Other techniques

Several other alternative treatment approaches including massage, body wrapping and strapping, eastern stress management techniques such as Yoga and Tai Chi, and a range of passive exercise devices have been proposed for weight loss, but none currently have any reliable evidence supporting their use for weight loss.

In summary therefore, minor weight loss benefits have been reported with hypnosis, and possibly acupressure with electrical stimulation in some situations, suggesting a possible justification for further research.

Alternative methods of delivery

Perhaps more interesting than alternative therapeutic treatments, are alternative forms of delivery of otherwise traditional treatments. Standard weight loss treatments are usually delivered through clinical or educational services in a one-on-one, or group situation in line with the steps approach shown in Table 1. Alternative methods of delivery are considered here under four main headings, with discussion of a fifth example encompassing a combination of these approaches. Only those approaches with the potential for a high penetration in the population have been considered.

Correspondence

Correspondence programmes offer a cost-effective means of delivering weight control programmes to a large number of people. Consumer preferences indicate that this approach may also be more desirable for many than face-to-face formats, particularly in higher education and income level groups[21]. Programmes can range from being totally self-help with minimal contact to adding a component to a shared-care programme. They have also been offered at no cost, at commercial rates, or with different forms of cost incentives. Reported success rates are generally higher with some level of payment, perhaps indicating a level of self selection through commitment. Telephone based interventions have also been found to have reasonable success in some cases. Correspondence may be more effective in some groups than others and may depend on the type of intervention required. King et al.[22] found exercise is easier to maintain in men using minimal contact strategies than dietary approaches focusing on modification of energy intake.

Internet

The development of the Internet provides unique opportunities for alternative delivery of weight loss programmes. However there is currently a huge variation in relevance and quality of sites, with probably less than 5 per cent providing sound weight loss advice[23]. Also, despite the wide proliferation of services, there is almost a complete lack of evidence of the effects of the Internet on health care outcomes[24]. One study comparing passive web-site education with more intensive Internet behaviour therapy did find positive short-term (6 month) effects on weight loss, with bigger effects in the more intensive group[25]. This suggests a greater role in future for Internet based programmes or combining the Internet with other approaches such as shared care or correspondence.

Mass media and multi-media

Mass media programmes in lifestyle change were initially tested in the 1970s with limited success. More recently, mass media in community interventions have been found to increase awareness, but have limited impact on weight loss at the population level[26,27].

The development of multi-media systems presents a new and expanded opportunity for programme delivery. Some existing correspondence programmes have used elements of this such as videos, audio-tapes and print. However, the current availability of computer-based audio and video CDs and e-mail, and Internet delivery of these provides promising new opportunities to satisfy the requirements of many people for minimal contact, interactive services. Currently however there is no evidence of the benefits of such systems.

Shared care

Shared-care has been used as an effective delivery option for many health-related programmes ranging from asthma to pregnancy. Because weight control ideally calls for multi-disciplinary input, the idea of shared care between disciplines is a logical approach to service delivery. This is often referred to in principle, although surprisingly few evaluative studies have been reported. However, there is some evidence of better weight loss than in conventional single disciplinary interventions[28]. Options that optimise use of the practitioner's time by combining with developed programmes and correspondence courses may be a logical direction for the future.

Combined delivery services

While each of the delivery services discussed here has potential for improving outcomes in weight control, a combination of these approaches would seem to have logical advantages over any single approach. This has been attempted over the last decade in a programme developed for men in Australia[29]. GutBusters was developed as a shared care, correspondence course carried out in conjunction with trained General Practitioners (GPs). Participating GPs were required to complete at least part of a Post Graduate Medical Certificate in Weight Control Management.

A random survey was carried out with 266 participating doctors and 607 overweight patients in 1998. The results showed that after the training programme, 96 per cent said they felt more confident in helping patients lose weight, and 28 per cent claimed to have lost weight themselves. In addition, 23 per cent of patients claimed to have lost weight on the programme. A further 50 per cent had not yet taken the programme up, but intended to in the future, while 27 per cent had discontinued the programme. Patient satisfaction with GPs being involved in shared-care was high, with 96 per cent expressing a positive reaction.

As a result of the appeal of the programme, and the availability of new technology, the GutBuster programme has now been modified and expanded to include a range of weight loss programmes at different levels of intervention, using multi-media materials in a correspondence pack connecting participants to an interactive Internet site (www.professortrim.com) and shared care with over 1,000 GPs and 100 specially trained 'Personal Weight Coaches'. Prospective evaluation is being established to monitor the ongoing effectiveness of the programme.

References

1. Kottke TE, Clark MM, Aase LA, Brandel CL, Brekke MJ, Brekke LN *et al*. Self-reported weight, weight goals, and weight control strategies of a midwestern population. *Mayo Clin Proc* 2002; 77(2): 114–21.

2. Khan LK, Serdula MK, Bowman BA, Williamson DF. Use of prescription weight loss pills among US adults in 1996–1998. *Ann Intern Med* 2001; 20: 134(4): 282–6.

3. Egger G, Cameron-Smith D, Stanton R. The effectiveness of popular, non-prescription weight loss supplements. *Med J Aust* 1999; 171: 604–8.

4. Dyck DJ. Dietary fat intake, supplements, and weight loss. *Can J Appl Physiol* 2002; 25(6): 495–523

5. Allison DB, Fonatine KR, Heshka S, Mentore J, Heymsfield SB. Alternative treatments for weight loss: A critical review. *Cr Rev Food Sc Nut* 2001; 41(1): 1–28.

6. Blanck HM, Khan LK, Serdula MK. Use of nonprescription weight loss products: results from a multistate survey. *JAMA* 2001; 22–29; 286(8): 930–5.

7. Westerterp-Plantenga MS, Kovacs EM. The effect of (-)-hydroxycitrate on energy intake and satiety in overweight humans. *Int J Obes Relat Metab Disord* 2002; 26(6): 870–2.

8. Mattes RD, Bormann L. Effects of (-)-hydroxycitric acid on appetitive variables. *Physiol Behav* 2002; 71(1–2): 87–94.

9. Rosenbaum M, Prieto V, Hellmer J, Boschmann M, Krueger J, Leibel RL, Ship AG. An exploratory investigation of the morphology and biochemistry of cellulite. *Plast Reconstr Surg* 1998; 101(7): 1934–9.

10. Sainio EL, Rantanen T, Kanerva L. Ingredients and safety of cellulite creams. *Eur J Dermatol* 2000; 10(8): 596–603.

11. Marshall S. It's so simple: Just lather up, watch the fat go down the drain. *Wall Street J* 1995; 226(87): B1.

12. Ernst E. Acupuncture/acupressure for weight reduction? A systematic review. *Wien Klin Wochenschr* 1997; 31: 109(2): 60–2.

13. Mazzoni R, Mannucci E, Rizzello SM, Ricca V, Rotella. Failure of acupuncture in the treatment of obesity: a pilot study. *Eat Weight Disord* 1999; 4(4): 198–202.

14. Richard D, Marley J. Stimulation of auricular acupuncture points in weight loss. *Aust Fam Phys* 1998; 27 (Suppl 2): S73–77.

15. Allison DB, Kreibich K, Heshka S, Heymsfield SB. A randomised placebo-controlled clinical trial of an acupressure device for weight loss. *Int J Obes Relat Metab Disord* 1995; 19(9): 653–8.

16. Porcari JP, McLean KP, Foster C, Kernozek T, Crenshaw B, Swenson C. Effects of electrical muscle stimulation on body composition, muscle strength, and physical appearance. *J Strength Cond Res* 2002; 16(2): 165–72.

17. Kirsh I. Hypnotic enhancement of cognitive-behavioral weight loss treatments another meta-reanalysis. *J Consult Clin Psychol* 1996; 64(3): 517–9.

18. Johnson DL. Weight loss for women: studies of smokers and nonsmokers using hypnosis and multicomponent treatments with and without overt aversion. *Psychol Rep* 1997; 30(3 pt 1): 931–3.

19. Johnson DL, Karkut RT. Participation in multicomponent hypnosis treatment programs for women's weight loss with and without overt aversion. *Psychol Rep* 1996; 79(2): 659–68.

20. Sreadling J, Roberts D, Wilson A, Lovelock F.Controlled trial of hypnotherapy for weight loss in patients with obstructive sleep apnoea. *Int J Obes* 1998; 28: 278–81.

21. Sherwood NE, Morton N, Jeffery RW, French SA, Neumark-Sztainer D, Falkner NH. Consumer preferences in format and type of community-based weight control programs. *Am J Health Promot* 1998; 13(1): 12–8.

22. King AC, Frey-Hewitt B, Dreon DM, Wood PD. Diet vs. exercise in weight maintenance. The effects of minimal intervention strategies on long-term outcomes in men. *Arch Intern Med* 1989; 149(12): 2741–6.

23. Miles J, Petrie C, Steel M. Slimming on the Internet. *J Roy Soc Med* 2000; 93(5): 254–7.

24. Bessell TL, McDonald S, Silagy CA, Anderson JN, Hiller JE, Sansom LN. Do Internet interventions for consumers cause more harm than good? A systematic review. *Health Expect* 2002; 5(1): 28–37.

25. Tate DF, Wing RR, Winett RA. Using Internet technology to deliver a behavioral weight loss program. *JAMA* 2001; 7: 285(9): 1172–7.

26. Jeffery RW. Community programs for obesity prevention: the Minnesota Heart Health Program. *Obes Res* 1995; 3 (Suppl 2): 283–88.

27. Miles A, Rapoport L, Wardle J, Afuape T, Duman M. Using the mass-media to target obesity: an analysis of the characteristics and reported behaviour change of participants in the BBC's 'Fighting Fat, Fighting Fit' campaign. *Health Educ Res* 2001; 16(3): 357–72.

28. Richman RM, Webster P, Salgo AR, Mira M, Steinbeck KS, Caterson ID. A shared care approach in obesity management: the general practitioner and a hospital based service. *Int J Obes Relat Metab Disord* 1996; 20(5): 413–9.

29. Egger G, Bolton A, O'Neill, Freeman D. Effectiveness of an abdominal obesity reduction programme in men: the GutBuster 'waist loss' programme. *Int J Obes* 1996; 23(6): 564–69.

Progress in Obesity Research: 9. Edited by *Geraldo Medeiros-Neto, Alfredo Halpern and Claude Bouchard*
©2003 John Libbey Eurotext Ltd, pp. 927–930.

CHAPTER 194

Obesity, sleep apnea and cardiovascular disease

Ronald R. Grunstein

Associate Professor and Head, Centre for Respiratory Failure and Sleep Disorders, Royal Prince Alfred Hospital and Sleep Research Group, Woolcock Institute of Medical Research, Sydney, Australia
[e-mail: rrg@mail.med.usyd.edu.au]

Introduction

Sleep-disordered breathing is defined by the loss of a normal pattern of breathing during sleep and encompasses a spectrum of abnormality from snoring to obstructive sleep apnea (OSA) through to profound nocturnal hypoventilation and respiratory failure during sleep (when associated with severe obesity, called obesity-hypoventilation syndrome, OHS)[1]. Significant upper airway obstruction can occur in the absence of complete collapse of the upper airway. Increased airway resistance can produce a measurable reduction in airflow (hypopnoea) with the same consequences (hypoxaemia and arousal) as an apnoea. Even very minor increases in airway resistance (without detectable reductions in airflow) can produce recurrent arousals and excessive daytime sleepiness. The usual measure of OSA is the apnea –hypopnea index (apneas, hypopneas per hour of sleep, AHI) or respiratory disturbance index[1].

Patients with OHS develop prolonged episodes of sleep-related hypercapnic hypoxaemia with 'resetting' of chemoreceptors with subsequent blunted daytime chemosensitivity and the development or worsening of daytime hypercapnic respiratory failure. In addition, the prolonged exposure to hypoxaemia and hypercapnia leads to pulmonary hypertension and right-sided heart failure. This is reversible with non-invasive ventilation during sleep. The reason why only some severely obese patients develop OHS may be explained by the observation that this disorder is more strongly associated with leptin resistance than the actual degree of obesity[2].

Central apnoea refers to cessation of airflow with no detectable respiratory effort (in contrast to obstructive apnoeas where breathing efforts are often vigorous). These classically occur as part of the periodic breathing seen in patients as a consequence of congestive cardiac failure (also called Cheyne-Stokes breathing)[3]. In the remaining text, the focus will be on the cardiovascular risk of OSA which is the most common breathing disorder during sleep.

Epidemiology – OSA and obesity

The Wisconsin Sleep Cohort Study is the largest reported prevalence study where sleep studies were performed. This group found an AHI of > 5 events/h in 9 per cent of female and 24 per cent of male middle-aged public servants. An AHI of > 15 events/h was found in 4 per cent of women and 9 per cent of men[4]. Our group has found a similar prevalence of OSA in an Australian rural community using home monitoring of breathing[5]. Obesity is one of the strongest risk factors for OSA and there are a number of ways in which obesity can reduce upper airway size and therefore predispose the upper airway to collapse causing repeated airway obstruction during sleep. A BMI of > 30 is associated with up to 18 times the risk of OSA compared with a BMI of < 25[5]. Anthropometry indicates that OSA is associated with a central pattern of obesity[6].

There are limited data on the prevalence of sleep apnoea in the obese population. The Swedish Obese Subjects study, which examined 3034 subjects with BMI > 35, found that over 50 per cent of obese men reported habitual loud snoring[7] as compared to 15 per cent in age-matched non-obese subjects.

Similarly, 33 per cent of men and 12 per cent of women in this study reported a history of frequent witnessed apnoeas. Given that questionnaires tend to underestimate the prevalence of OSA, it is clear that OSA and related conditions occur in a very high proportion of obese subjects. More recent longitudinal studies have demonstrated a strong association between weight gain and the development of sleep-disordered breathing. Even relatively small changes in weight may have a powerful impact on the degree of sleep-disordered breathing. Other important risk factors for OSA are facio-maxillary status (brachycepahlic face), menopausal status and upper airway masses (tonsillar hypertrophy in children and adults, acromegaly)[1].

Excessive daytime sleepiness (EDS) is characteristic of sleep apnoea predominantly related to repetitive arousal and sleep fragmentation, but a direct effect of hypoxaemia is possible.

OSA is characterized by a range of EDS and there is a relatively poor correlation between markers of severity of OSA, such as AHI, and daytime sleepiness[1]. It seems likely that people vary in their susceptibility to the effects of sleep fragmentation and sleep deprivation. Sleepiness may lead to both impaired work performance and driving. Patients with untreated OSA form an important risk group for motor vehicle accidents. Driving performance on various simulators is impaired in patients with OSA. The detrimental effects of OSA have other social implications, with data from the Swedish Obese Subjects study showing that, in equally obese men and women, OSA is associated with impaired work performance, increased sick leave and a higher divorce rate[8].

Treatment

Nasal continuous positive airway pressure (CPAP) is the most effective commonly used treatment in OSA. Randomized controlled trials demonstrate that CPAP dramatically improves daytime sleepiness, quality of life and driving simulator performance[9]. CPAP is also a useful research tool to separate the effects of OSA and obesity. CPAP compliance can be measured effectively and also can be controlled by oral placebo or even sham or sub-therapeutic CPAP. Weight loss, either by caloric restriction or bariatric surgery significantly reduces the severity of OSA but long term data on the relationship of weight reduction treatment and OSA is lacking.

Impact of OSA on cardiovascular health

The acute cardiovascular effects seen during obstructive events have been well characterized with marked changes in both systemic and pulmonary arterial blood pressure[3]. As an obstructive apnoea progresses, there are increasing swings in pleural pressure, worsening hypoxaemia, bradycardia (vagally mediated) and increased sympathetic nerve activity. As the apnoea is terminated by arousal, with increased ventilation, heart rate increases and both systolic and diastolic blood pressure increase markedly, often by more than 100 mmHg. These profound haemodynamic fluctuations are largely due to surges in muscle sympathetic nerve activity (MSNA) resulting from the combination of blood gas derangement, large swings in intrathoracic pressure and arousals[3]. Patients with OSA have increased MSNA through the night, with persistence into wakefulness. Importantly, it has been shown that OSA is a crucial determinant of awake MSNA in obesity. Reduction in awake MSNA is closely related to hours of nightly CPAP use[3]. Studies using an elegant canine model of OSA have shown that sustained hypertension develops after one to three months of OSA[10]. Studies in rats have found that intermittent hypoxia induces a persistent increase in diurnal blood pressure, mediated through renal sympathetic nerve activity and the renin-angiotensin system[3].

Patients have a potent pressor response to hypoxia compared to normal subjects, indicating endothelial dysfunction attenuating arterial vasodilation[11]. This has been confirmed by direct measurement of endothelial function. Nasal CPAP use appears to improve endothelial function[12]. There is also increasing evidence that OSA leads to a chronic inflammatory state potentially promoting atherogenesis[3,13–14]. OSA is associated with higher levels of fibrinogen, measures of thrombotic tendency and platelet aggregation, vascular endothelial growth factor, leptin, highly selective C-reactive protein and adhesion molecules[3,13–14]. Promoters of atherogenesis including superoxide radicals and monocyte adension are also higher in OSA. Nasal CPAP normalizes the levels of many of these vascular mediators or markers of a pro-atherogenic state independent of weight change[3,13–14]. Other data has shown that OSA is associated with insulin resistance and CPAP can improve insulin sensitivity[3,15]. Other features of the metabolic syndrome of obesity common to OSA include low growth hormone and testosterone levels. These endocrine parameters are also normalized with CPAP independent of weight change[16].

OSA and cardiovascular disorders

Sleep apnoea is a common finding among patients in hypertension clinics and similarly, many patients with OSA have hypertension[3]. Data from the Sleep Heart Health Study, a large cross-sectional community based study with more than 6000 subjects, found that AHI and percentage of sleep time with an oxygen saturation below 90 per cent were significantly associated with systemic hypertension, independent of anthropomorphic variables such as BMI, waist-hip ratio and neck circumference[17]. Prospective data from the Wisconsin Sleep Cohort Study, which followed more than 700 subjects for over 4–8 years, have found a dose-response association between sleep-disordered breathing and hypertension, independent of measures of obesity. In this study, compared with no OSA, an AHI < 4.9 events/h had an odds ratio for hypertension at follow-up of 1.42, with an odds ratio of 2.03 and 2.89 for an AHI of 5.0–14.9 and >15 respectively[18]. A recent randomized trial comparing the effects of therapeutic and sub-therapeutic CPAP has shown a powerful blood pressure lowering effect of effective treatment in patients with more severe OSA or those with currently treated hypertension[19].

Coronary artery disease and stroke

A number of groups have reported an increased risk of myocardial infarction and stroke in sleep apnoea[3]. Recent data, again from the Sleep Heart Health Study, have demonstrated a relationship between AHI and prevalent cardiovascular disease (as defined by various manifestations of ischaemic heart disease, heart failure and stroke). The odds ratios were fairly modest and surprisingly there did not appear to be a dose-response ratio above an AHI of 10[20]. However, a criticism of this study is the mean age of the group (65 years)[13]. Data from prospective follow up may establish the exact role of OSA in hard cardiovascular endpoints but this may be complicated by the increasing use of CPAP in the community to prevent sleepiness. Small long term follow studies strongly suggest the adverse impact of OSA on these endpoints in the presence or absence of baseline cardiovascular disease[3,13].

Implication for obesity research

OSA can no longer be considered 'an innocent bystander' in the relationship between obesity and health outcomes. This is well established for psycho-social factors and accumulated data over the past 10 years has now shown this for cardiovascular risk factos and diseases. This has implications for screening for OSA in obese populations and a strong argument can be mounted for measuring OSA as an outcome variable for weight loss treatments in the same way we already investigate diabetes, hyperlipidaemia and hypertension.

References

1. Redline S, Strohl KP. Recognition and consequences of obstructive sleep apnea hypopnea syndrome. *Clin Chest Med* 1998; 19: 1–19.

2. Phipps P, Staritt E, Caterson ID, Grunstein RR. Association of serum leptin with hypoventilation in obesity. *Thorax* 2002; 57: 75–6.

3. Leung R, Bradley D. Sleep apnea and cardiovascular disease. *Am J Respir Crit Care Med* 2001; 164: 2147–65.

4. Young T, Palta M, Dempsey J *et al*. The occurrence of sleep-disordered breathing among middle-aged adults. *N Engl J Med* 1993; 328: 1230–5.

5. Bearpark H, Elliott L, Grunstein R *et al*. Snoring and sleep apnea. A population study in Australian men. *Am J Respir Crit Care Med* 1995; 151: 1459–65.

6. Grunstein R, Wilcox I, Yang TS *et al*. Snoring and sleep apnoea in men: association with central obesity and hypertension. *Int J Obes Relat Metab Disord* 1993; 17: 533–40.

7. Grunstein RR, Stenlof K, Hedner J, Sjostrom L. Impact of obstructive sleep apnea and sleepiness on metabolic and cardiovascular risk factors in the Swedish Obese Subjects (SOS) Study. *Int J Obes Relat Metab Disord* 1995; 19: 410–8.

8. Grunstein RR, Stenlof K, Hedner J, Sjostrom L. Impact of self-reported sleep-breathing disturbances on psychosocial performance in the Swedish Obese Subjects (SOS) Study. *Sleep* 1995; 18: 635–43.

9. Jenkinson C, Davies RJ, Mullins R *et al*. Comparison of therapeutic and subtherapeutic nasal continuous positive airway pressure for obstructive sleep apnoea: a randomised prospective parallel trial. *Lancet* 1999; 353: 2100–5.

10. Brooks D, Horner RL, Kozar LF *et al*. Obstructive sleep apnea as a cause of systemic hypertension. Evidence from a canine model. *J Clin Invest* 1997; 99: 106–9.

11. Hedner JA, Wilcox I, Laks L *et al*. A specific and potent pressor effect of hypoxia in patients with sleep apnea. *Am Rev Respir Dis* 1992; 146: 1240–5.

12. Imadojemu V, Gleeson K, Quraishi S *et al.* Impaired vasodilator responses in obstructive sleep apnea are improved with continuous positive airway pressure therapy. *Am J Respir Crit Care Med* 2002; 165: 950–3.

13. Peker Y, Hedner J, Norum J, Kraiczi H, Carlson J. Increased incidence of cardiovascular disease in middle-aged men with obstructive sleep apnea. A 7-year follow-up. *Am J Respir Crit Care Med* 2002; 166: 159–165.

14. Dyugovskaya, Lavie P, Lavie L. Increased adhesion molecules expression and production of reactive oxygen species in leukocytes of sleep apnea patients. *Am J Respir Crit Care Med* 2002; 165: 934–39.

15. Brooks B, Cistulli PA, Borkman M *et al.* Obstructive sleep apnea in obese noninsulin-dependent diabetic patients: effect of continuous positive airway pressure treatment on insulin responsiveness. *J Clin Endocrinol Metab* 1994; 79: 1681–5.

16. Grunstein RR, Handelsman DJ, Lawrence SJ *et al.* Neuroendocrine dysfunction in sleep apnea: reversal by continuous positive airways pressure therapy. *J Clin Endocrinol Metab* 1989; 68: 352–8.

17. Nieto FJ, Young TB, Lind BK *et al.* Association of sleep-disordered breathing, sleep apnea, and hypertension in a large community-based study. Sleep Heart Health Study. *JAMA* 2000; 283: 1829–36.

18. Peppard PE, Young T, Palta M *et al.* Prospective study of the association between sleep-disordered breathing and hypertension. *N Engl J Med* 2000; 342: 1378–84.

19. Pepperell JCT, Ramdassingh-Dow S, Crosthwaite N *et al.* Ambulatory blood pressure after therapeutic and subtherapeutic nasal continuous positive airway pressure for obstructive sleep apnoea: a randomised parallel trial *Lancet* 2002; 359: 204–10.

20. Shahar E, Redline S, Lee ET *et al.* Sleep-disordered breathing and cardiovascular disease cross sectional results of the sleep heart health study. *Am J Respir Crit Care Med* 2001; 163: 19–25.

Progress in Obesity Research: 9. Edited by *Geraldo Medeiros-Neto, Alfredo Halpern and Claude Bouchard*
©2003 John Libbey Eurotext Ltd, pp. 931–935.

CHAPTER 195

Obesity, type 2 diabetes and dyslipidaemia

André J. Scheen

*Division of Diabetes, Nutrition and Metabolic Disorders, Department of Medicine, CHU Sart Tilman,
B-4000 Liège, Belgium*
[e-mail: andre.scheen@chu.ulg.ac.be]

Introduction

The concept of syndrome X or metabolic syndrome was introduced by Reaven to explain the clustering of cardiovascular risk factors such as obesity, insulin resistance, impaired glucose tolerance or type 2 diabetes mellitus, dyslipidaemia and hypertension[1]. Numerous studies have clearly demonstrated that obesity is a major risk factor for abnormal glucose and lipid metabolism[2-4], and that insulin resistance is the link between fat excess, essentially abdominal adiposity, and such metabolic complications[5-7]. A net positive energy balance and disordered fat storage and mobilization appear to be central factors in the pathogenesis of many of the metabolic features of the insulin resistance syndrome, especially type 2 diabetes and dyslipidaemia[8]. This theory in no way precludes an important role for peptides and hormones that are secreted by adipocytes and may link adiposity to insulin resistance and type 2 diabetes[9,10]. Thus, excessive circulating free fatty acid levels, ectopic intracellular triglyceride deposition, and abnormal production of molecules by large adipocytes probably play a crucial role in the intimate relationship between obesity, insulin resistance, type 2 diabetes and dyslipidaemia. Conversely, weight loss improves insulin sensitivity, glucose metabolism and lipid profile in obese patients, and, interestingly enough, significant metabolic improvements have already been reported after modest weight reduction, especially among obese diabetic individuals[11,12].

The present concise review aims at describing some epidemiological observations and pathophysiological mechanisms linking obesity, type 2 diabetes and dyslipidaemia. We will also analyse results of various intervention trials demonstrating the potential reversibility of this strong association after weight reduction, using lifestyle modifications, antiobesity agents and/or bariatric surgery.

Epidemiological observations

Obesity and type 2 diabetes

Besides genetic predisposition, obesity is considered as the most important risk factor for type 2 diabetes. The strong exponential relationship between the risk of developing diabetes mellitus, on the one hand, body mass index or weight gain, on the other hand, has been demonstrated in several studies including both men and women[2,3,13]. Besides the degree of obesity *per se*, several other factors obviously play a crucial role such as the abdominal distribution of adiposity[6,7] and the duration of overweight[3]. Conversely, numerous studies have demonstrated that, among obese subjects, successful weight loss results in a reduction in both the incidence and the severity of type 2 diabetes, whatever the therapeutic means used[14-16]. The respective beneficial effects of negative energy balance and weight reduction per se have been extensively analysed in well-designed short-term and long-term clinical studies[11].

Obesity and dyslipidaemia

Dyslipidaemia is part of the metabolic syndrome and contributes to worsen cardiovascular prognosis of obese subjects with syndrome X[1,5,7,17]. Lipid disturbances associated with obesity typically consists of high triglyceride and low HDL levels, particularly if type 2 diabetes mellitus is also present. In most cases, total and LDL cholesterol concentrations are only mildly elevated, but small dense LDL, oxidized

LDL and postprandial hyperlipidaemia are frequently increased in presence of abdominal obesity[6,7,17]. Dyslipidaemia augments the risk of cardiovascular complications of obese subjects, especially coronary heart disease[1,2,7,17].

Pathophysiological mechanisms

Obesity and type 2 diabetes

Type 2 diabetes results from a defect in both insulin action and insulin secretion[18]. It occurs when obese subjects are not able to maintain hyperinsulinaemia to compensate for decreased insulin sensitivity, and progression of the disease is best explained by an exhaustion of insulin secretion in face of persistent insulin resistance[19]. These two defects are perpetuated and exaggerated by both lipotoxicity and glucotoxicity in a vicious circle which may explain the progressive metabolic deterioration generally seen in obese patients with type 2 diabetes[19].

Insulin resistance plays a key-role in the intimate relationship between obesity and diabetes[18]. Metabolic, hormonal and haemodynamic abnormalities could contribute to decreased insulin sensitivity in obese individuals[3]. Obesity, especially visceral adiposity, is associated with increased release and higher plasma levels of free fatty acids (FFA) which may trigger a reduction in insulin sensitivity at both the hepatic and the muscular levels[5–7]. In the liver, high FFA supply results in an increased glucose output (essentially due to enhanced gluconeogenesis) and a decreased insulin extraction while in the skeletal muscle such metabolic abnormality results in a reduction in glucose uptake, oxidation and storage as glycogen.

Besides this classical paradigm, known as the 'portal/visceral metabolic hypothesis' or Randle's effect, to explain the link between obesity and type 2 diabetes, two new paradigms have emerged recently, i.e. the 'ectopic fat storage' paradigm and the 'adipocyte as an endocrine organ' paradigm[10]. Most obese subjects shunt lipid into skeletal muscle and liver: the degree of triglyceride infiltration into skeletal muscle is highly correlated with insulin resistance[8] and non alcoholic fatty liver is now considered as being part of the insulin resistance syndrome[20]. The endocrine paradigm results from the observation that adipocytes secrete a variety of peptides and endocrine hormones such as TNF-α, interkeukin-6, leptin, resistin, adiponectin. Several studies have demonstrated a positive association between insulin resistance and all these adipocyte products, except adiponectin. Adiponectin concentrations are decreased in obese subjects, and a significant negative relationship has been consistently reported between adiponectin levels and insulin resistance. The role of these peptides/hormones in the relationship between obesity, insulin resistance and type 2 diabetes has been clearly demonstrated in various animal models. However, even if several human studies supporting such an hypothesis have been published recently, much work remains to be done to understand the precise contribution of these adipocyte secretory products to the pathophysiology of insulin resistance and type 2 diabetes in human obesity[10].

Obesity and dyslipidaemia

Hypertriglyceridaemia, the most common lipid disturbance in obesity, insulin resistance and type 2 diabetes, is primarily due to VLDL overproduction, with reduced VLDL clearance playing a significant role only in some instances. Some of the other prominent features of the dyslipidaemia characterizing these patients, such as low HDL and excessive small, dense LDL particles, may be secondary to VLDL overproduction[17]. Because of expanded VLDL pool and cholesterol ester protein (CETP) overactivity, there is increased neutral lipid exchange resulting in triglyceride enrichment of both HDL and LDL. Furthermore, triglyceride rich HDL and LDL particles undergo increased lipolysis due to overactivity of hepatic lipase, especially in overweight type 2 diabetic patients. This results in the generation of smaller, more dense lipoprotein particles with altered physiological function. On the one hand, small dense HDL particles have diminished reverse cholesterol transfer capacity and reduced antioxidant properties, hence reducing the anti-atherogenic potential of HDL. On the other hand, small dense LDL particles exhibit increased toxicity to endothelial cells, increased tendency to absorption by macrophages to form foam cells, increased susceptibility to oxidative and glycative modification, and increased tendency to induce free radical release, all factors contributing to increased atherogenic potential[17]. Dyslipidaemia associated to overweight and visceral adiposity is exacerbated in the obese patient with poorly controlled type 2 diabetes, who presents both insulin resistance and relative insulinopenia[21].

Hepatic VLDL production is primarily substrate driven, with the most important regulatory substrates FFAs being increased in obesity. Nevertheless, increased FFA availability per se is not sufficient to explain the high VLDL production rates seen in obese patients with insulin resistance syndrome and/or diabetes mellitus[8,17,21]. VLDL overproduction occurs as a result of a composite set of factors, which includes flux of fatty acids from extrahepatic tissues to the liver and directly from lipoprotein remnant uptake, increased hepatic *de novo* fatty acid synthesis, preferential esterification vs. oxidation of fatty acids etc. While the increased flux of FFAs to the liver arises from adipose tissue resistance to insulin action, we do not definitely know whether the hepatic effects arise as a result of insulin resistance or hyperinsulinaemia per se. It is possible that the changes in liver metabolism may be due to both increased and reduced insulin action, with some biochemical pathways in the liver remaining responsive to insulin, whereas others are downregulated[8].

Therapeutic approaches

Intervention trials in obesity essentially include lifestyle changes (diet, physical exercise), new antiobesity agents (orlistat, sibutramine), and obesity surgery (gastroplasty, gastric bypass)[14,16].

Obesity and type 2 diabetes

Lifestyle changes, including hypocaloric low-fat diet and regular physical exercise, generally induce a modest weight reduction that is, however, sufficient to significantly delay or prevent the progression from impaired glucose tolerance to overt diabetes[22]. In addition, the same therapeutic approaches are able to markedly improve blood glucose control of obese diabetic patients, although long-term success rate may be somewhat disappointing, essentially because of patients' poor compliance to such intervention programmes[14-16]. The role of dietary fat in the promotion of obesity and type 2 diabetes is a topic of considerable debate[23]. Simply reducing dietary fat seems unlikely to be an effective treatment for most obese patients. Furthermore, while dietary fat type is recognized as a contributing factor in dyslipidaemia, linkage to obesity, insulin resistance and type 2 diabetes remains uncertain.

The two recently marketed anti-obesity agents, sibutramine and orlistat, showed a potential role in the management of the obese diabetic patient[24]. Sibutramine, a new noradrenaline and 5-hydroxytryptamine reuptake inhibitor, has been shown to regulate appetite and produce a dose-related weight loss in obese subjects, with optimal doses of 10–20 mg/day[4]. Favourable results were reported with sibutramine in three 6-month and two one-year randomized clinical trials in obese type 2 diabetic patients[16,24]. All studies demonstrated that, when compared to placebo, an average 3–5 kg further weight loss resulting from the prescription of sibutramine is sufficient to improve fasting blood glucose and glycated haemoglobin levels, especially in patients losing ≥ 10 per cent of their baseline body weight. The observation that changes in plasma glucose levels observed on sibutramine and placebo were similar for the same degree of weight loss suggests an indirect rather a direct action of the drug on glucose metabolism. Orlistat, a semisynthetic derivative of lipstatin, is a potent and selective inhibitor of gastric and pancreatic lipases that reduces lipid intestinal absorption and induces a dose-dependent reduction in body weight, with an optimal dosage regimen of 120 mg tid[4]. Interestingly enough, orlistat-associated moderate weight loss was shown to have beneficial effects on insulin sensitivity and beta-cell function and to significantly reduce the relative risk of developing overt type 2 diabetes in obese patients with impaired glucose tolerance[24]. Orlistat may also be used in the treatment of obese patients with type 2 diabetes. Four one-year prospective randomized placebo-controlled multicentre clinical trials demonstrated that orlistat promotes weight loss, decreases fasting plasma glucose and glycated haemoglobin levels and/or allows to decrease the doses of other antidiabetic agents in obese patients with type 2 diabetes treated with sulphonylureas, metformin or insulin[16,24]. Furthermore, the cardiovascular risk profile was also improved in patients treated with orlistat as compared to those receiving placebo. Although no direct comparative studies are available, indirect comparison of sibutramine and orlistat trials suggests that orlistat 120 mg tid may be slightly less effective than sibutramine 15–20 mg od in reducing body weight, but that it may be more effective in improving blood glucose control and lipid profile in obese type 2 diabetic patients.

The crucial contribution of weight excess to hyperglycaemia in the obese diabetic patient justifies that aggressive weight reduction strategies may be considered in well-selected individuals with refractory severe obesity and persistent hyperglycaemia despite classical medical approaches[14-16]. Our group demonstrated that the recovery of ideal body weight in severely obese non-diabetic patients submitted to a gastroplasty resulted in a complete normalization of insulin secretion, action and metabolism, as compared to lean controls[15]. Several studies have reported that bariatric surgery is able to markedly improve blood glucose control in most obese diabetic patients, with drastic reduction or even normalization of fasting plasma glucose and glycated haemoglobin levels after gastroplasty, gastric bypass or biliopancreatic diversion. The metabolic improvement following weight loss allows the suppression or at least marked reduction of antidiabetic drugs, especially insulin and sulphonylureas, in most patients[14–16]. The 8-year follow-up preliminary results of the large prospective Swedish Obese Subjects (SOS) study[26] showed a remarkable reduction in the incidence of type 2 diabetes after a major and sustained weight loss of 20–40 kg resulting from bariatric surgery (either gastroplasty or gastric bypass).

Obesity and dyslipidaemia

Significant improvement of dyslipidaemia has been reported after weight reduction, whatever the treatment applied, i.e. lifestyle modifications, drugs and surgery[27]. However, although weight loss is associated with improvements in the plasma lipid prolfile, factors other than weight loss per se are involved[28]. Furthermore, whether the lipid changes that are observed in the short term are sustained in the long term and whether the manner of weight loss has any impact on long-term outcomes remains to be determined. Lifestyle modifications may profoundly alter lipid profile. High intake of fat, especially saturated fatty acids, increases total and LDL cholesterol concentrations while diet rich in sucrose and/or alcholol may increase triglyceride levels; thus, restriction in these food components should be recommended to improve lipid profile, especially in obese individuals. Regular endurance exercise contributes to increase HDL concentrations, probably by improving insulin sensitivity. While the improvement of lipid profile with sibutramine strictly depends on its positive effect on weight reduction, the best results being observed in individuals with weight loss above 10 per cent of initial body weight, orlistat exerts a specific cholesterol lowering effect beyond its action resulting from weight Loss per se, due to its selective intestinal lipase inhibitor activity[29]. Finally, gastroplasty resulted in marked and sustained weight reduction and concomitantly was associated with significant improvement of biological abnormalities related to the metabolic syndrome. While only a mild reduction of total cholesterol concentration was observed, a clear-cut diminution of triglyceride levels and a significant increase of HDL cholesterol concentration were reported[26,30]. An even greater change in lipid parameters may be observed after surgical procedures leading to partial intestinal malabsorption such as gastric bypass and, especially, biliopancreatic bypass, but with a higher risk of complications.

Conclusions

Obesity is strongly associated with type 2 diabetes mellitus and lipid disturbances, a well-known metabolic syndrome associated with poor cardiovascular prognosis. Insulin resistance obviously plays a major role in the intimate relationship between obesity and abdominal adiposity on the one hand, type 2 diabetes and dyslipidaemia on the other hand. The crucial role of excessive circulating free fatty acid levels has been clearly evidenced during the last decade, and the deleterious effect of ectopic intracellular triglyceride deposition, both in the skeletal muscles and in the liver, has been recently emphasized. Whereas numerous observations are available in rodents supporting the paracrine/endocrine role of adipocytes, controversies still persist regarding the contributing roles of increased TNF-α, interleukin-6, leptin and resistin concentrations in human obesities. Recently, a crucial role has been devoted to adiponectin whose levels are decreased in obesity which may contribute to increase insulin resistance and favour type 2 diabetes. Thus, new emerging paradigms, i.e. the ectopic fat storage syndrome and the adipocyte as an endocrine organ, constitute the framework for the study of the links between our obesogenic environment and diabetes risk in the next decade. They may also trigger the search for new pharmacological interventions aiming at reducing the metabolic risk related to weight excess.

Weight loss prevents the development of type 2 diabetes and significantly improves insulin sensitivity, glucose metabolism and lipid profile in obese diabetic patients. Undoubtedly, diet and physical exercise remain the cornerstones of prevention and treatment of obesity and type 2 diabetes. When those fail (and they do frequently), pharmacological approaches may be considered. Anti-obesity drugs, such as sibutramine and orlistat, can be used in addition to diet since the resulting greater weight loss, even modest on average, can improve blood glucose control and other risk factors, especially dyslipidaemia in patients receiving orlistat. Overall metabolic improvement is already observed after a rather modest weight loss of 5–10 per cent of initial body weight. Aggressive weight reduction programmes may be used in severely obese individuals with type 2 diabetes, refractory to conventional diet and drug treatment. Surgical approaches, such as gastroplasty and gastric bypass, may be helpful in diabetic subjects with morbid obesity, provided that they are performed by a well-trained multidisciplinary team in well-selected and carefully supervised patients. Long-term prospective studies, such the Swedish Obese Subjects trial, should demonstrate that sustained improvements in glucose and lipid metabolism associated with weight loss will be able to ameliorate the poor cardiovascular prognosis of obese subjects having the metabolic syndrome related to insulin resistance.

References

1. Reaven GM. Role of insulin resistance in human disease. *Diabetes* 1988; 37: 1595–1607.

2. National Task Force on the Prevention and Treatment of Obesity. Overweight, obesity and health risk. *Arch Intern Med* 2000; 160: 898–904.

3. Scheen AJ. Obesity and diabetes. In: *The management of obesity and related disorders*, pp. 11–44. Kopelman PG (eds). London, UK: Martin Dunitz, 2001.

4. Yanovski SZ, Yanovski JA. Obesity. *N Engl J Med* 2002; 346: 591–602.

5. DeFronzo RA, Ferrannini E. Insulin resistance: a multifaceted syndrome responsible for NIDDM, obesity, hypertension, dyslipidemia, and atherosclerotic cardiovascular disease. *Diabetes Care* 1991; 14: 173–94.

6. Wajchenberg BJ. Subcutaneous and visceral adipose tissue: their relation to the metabolic syndrome. *Endocr Rev* 2000; 21: 697–738.

7. Després J-P. The insulin resistance-dyslipidemic syndrome of visceral obesity: effects on patients' risk. *Obes Res* 1998; 6 (Suppl 1): S8–17.

8. Lewis GF, Carpentier A, Adeli K, Giacca A. Disordered fat storage and mobilization in the pathogenesis of insulin resistance and type 2 diabetes. *Endocr Rev* 2002; 23: 201–29.

9. Kahn BB, Flier JS. Obesity and insulin resistance. *J Clin Invest* 2000; 106: 473–81.

10. Ravussin E, Smith SR. Increased fat intake, impaired fat oxidation, and failure of fat cell proliferation result in ectopic storage, insulin resistance, and type 2 diabetes mellitus. *Ann NY Acad Sci* 2002; 967: 363–78.

11. Williams KV, Kelley DE. Metabolic consequences of weight loss on glucose metabolism and insulin action in type 2 diabetes. *Diabetes Obes Metab* 2000; 2: 121–9.

12. Maggio CA, Pi-Sunyer FX. The prevention and treatment of obesity. Application to type 2 diabetes. *Diabetes Care* 1997; 20: 1744–66.

13. Willett WC, Dietz WH, Colditz GA. Guidelines for healthy weight. *N Engl J Med* 1999; 341: 427–34.

14. Scheen AJ, Lefèbvre PJ. Management of the obese diabetic patient. *Diabetes Rev* 1999; 7: 77–93.

15. Scheen AJ. Aggressive weight reduction treatment in the management of type 2 diabetes. *Diabetes Metab* 1998; 23: 116–23.

16. Scheen AJ. Current management strategies for coexisting diabetes mellitus and obesity. *Drugs* 2003; 63: 1165–84.

17. Després JP. Dyslipidaemia and obesity. *Baillière's Clin Endocrinol Metab* 1994; 8: 629–60.

18. Scheen AJ, Paquot N, Letiexhe MR *et al*. Glucose metabolism in obese subjects: lessons from OGTT, IVGTT and clamp studies. *Int J Obes* 1995; 19 (Suppl 3): S14–20.

19. Scheen AJ. From obesity to diabetes. Why, when and who? *Acta Clin Belg* 2000; 55: 9–15.

20. Luyckx FH, Lefèbvre PJ, Scheen AJ. Non-alcoholic steatohepatitis: association with obesity and insulin resistance, and influence of weight loss. *Diabetes Metab* 2000; 26: 98–106.

21. Garg A, Grundy SM. Diabetic dyslipidemia and its therapy. *Diabetes Rev* 1997; 5: 425–33.

22. Diabetes Prevention Program Research Group. Reduction in the incidence of type 2 diabetes with lifestyle intervention or metformin. *N Engl J Med* 2002; 346: 393–403.

23. Hajduk CL, Roberts SB, Saltzman E. Dietary treatment of obesity. *Curr Opin Endocrinol Diabetes* 2001; 8: 240–6.

24. Scheen AJ, Ernest PH. New antiobesity agents in type 2 diabetes: overview of clinical trials with sibutramine and orlistat. *Diabetes Metab* 2002; 28: 437–45.

25. Heymsfield SB, Segal KR, Hauptman J *et al*. Effects of weight loss with orlistat on glucose tolerance and progression to type 2 diabetes in obese adults. *Arch Intern Med* 2000; 160: 1321–26.

26. Sjöström CD, Lissner L, Wedel H, Sjöström L. Reduction in incidence of diabetes, hypertension and lipid disturbances after intentional weight loss induced by bariatric surgery: the SOS Intervention Study. *Obes Res* 1999; 7: 477–84.

27. Datillo AM, Kris-Etherton PM. Effects of weight reduction on blood lipids and lipoproteins: a meta-analysis. *Am J Clin Nutr* 1992; 56: 320–28.

28. Noakes M, Clifton PM. Weight loss and plasma lipids. *Curr Opin Lipidol* 2000; 11: 65–70.

29. Muls E, Kolanowski J, Scheen A, Van Gaal L. For the Obelhyx Study Group The effects of orlistat on weight and on serum lipids in obese patients with hypercholesterolemia: a randomized, double-blind, placebo-controlled, multicentre study. *Int J Obes* 2001; 25: 1713–21.

30. Luyckx FH, Scheen AJ, Desaive C *et al*. Effects of gastroplasty on body weight and related biological abnormalities in morbid obesity. *Diabetes Metab* 1998; 24: 355–61.

©2003 John Libbey Eurotext Ltd, pp. 936–941.

CHAPTER 196

Obesity in the elderly – a growing dilemma

Gary A. Wittert

Associate Professor, Department of Medicine, Royal Adelaide Hospital, North Terrace, Adelaide SA 5064, Australia
[e-mail: gary.wittert@adelaide.edu.au]

Age related changes in body composition

By 2030, demographers estimate that one in five Americans will be age 65 or older. Body weight increases until approximately the age 60 to 65 and decreases in over 60 per cent of the population thereafter. Muscle mass peaks in the third to fourth decade, followed by a steady decline of about 1.2 kg per decade in men and by about 0.1 kg per decade in women. Overall there is an approximately 15 per cent decrease in muscle mass and 30 per cent decline in muscle strength and activity between 2nd and 7th decades[1]. The age related changes that occur in muscle include a disproportionate atrophy of type 2 a (fast twitch) muscle fibres, a decrease in muscle protein synthesis, an approximately 25 per cent decrease in mitochondrial oxidative enzyme activity and muscle capillarization, a decrease in myosin heavy chain synthesis and a decrease in the number of functional motor units accompanied by irregularity of motor unit firing. Factors which may be responsible for, or are at least associated, with these changes are decreased physical activity, inadequate nutrition, vascular disease, increased activity of the cytokines IL1, IL6, and TNF-α and decreased levels of the anabolic hormones testosterone, DHEA, GH, and IGF-1[2].

The contribution of fat mass to the weight loss that occurs in the elderly is small and seen predominantly in women over the age of 70 years[3,4]. Fat mass has also been reported to increase with increasing age in both men and women[1]. More importantly fat tends to be redistributed toward the abdomen, particularly viscerally, in both genders[5]. Longitudinal changes that occurred between the ages of 65–70 and 80–85 have been reported in elderly Europeans from nine towns that were included in the SENECA study. Stature decreased by 1.5–2 cm, mean weight decreased by 2.6 kg to 4.2 kg in three towns, but on average body weight increased by 5 kg in 13 per cent of men and women whereas baseline weight decreased by 5 kg in 23 per cent of men and 27 per cent women. Small decreases in arm circumference occurred. Waist circumference increased by 3–4 cm[6].

After age 60 in a group of men and women followed longitudinally between 1986 and 1994 although overall body weight in men did not change significantly fat mass increased by approximately 1.2 kg and total appendicular skeletal muscle decreased by approximately 0.8 kg. In women both body weight and fat mass were reduced by about 0.8 kg and appendicular skeletal muscle mass decreased by about 0.4 kg[7]. In one study the oldest subjects had a thinner body frame and malnutrition was present in 5 per cent of both genders. Waist circumference and waist: hip ratio values were higher for the youngest men than for the oldest men, whereas in women the waist: hip ratio values were higher in the oldest women, suggesting that visceral redistribution in old age predominantly affects females[47].

Assessment of obesity in the elderly

The body mass index (BMI) calculated as kg/m^2, is used as an approximation of adiposity. BMI reaches a maximum in the 5th decade in both males and females. The 75th year of age is a turning point for BMI[8]. At different ages, however, the same levels of BMI correspond to different amounts of fat and fat-free mass. Some individuals with low BMI have as much fat as those with high BMI[9]. Therefore the increases with age in the prevalence of overweight and obesity and in the risks for chronic disease may be underestimated using BMI[10]. Low lean body mass is probably better reflected by low BMI, whereas increased (abdominal) fatness is better reflected by increased waist circumference[9,10]. The accurate identification of sarcopenic obesity requires precise methods of simultaneously measuring fat and lean components, such as dual-energy X-ray absorptiometry[10].

Prevalence of obesity in the elderly

Studies of the prevalence of obesity in the elderly are all based on standard BMI criteria. The prevalence of obesity has been reported to be 28 per cent and 16 per cent in elderly Italian women and men respectively[11]. In a representative sample of elderly Mexicans from five Southwestern states in the USA, 23 per cent of men and 35 per cent of women were obese[12]. In elderly Taiwanese subjects the prevalence of overweight was 27.3 per cent in men and 34.9 per cent in women, and that of obesity was 3.2 per cent in men and 6.4 per cent in women[13]. The Dutch nutrition survey of 539 apparently healthy, independently living elderly aged 65–79 years, found an overall prevalence of obesity of 13 per cent[14]. In urban Mexican women, mean age 71.6, the proportion of overweight and obese women was 60.7 per cent, 36.2 per cent and 76.5 per cent in urban, rural and marginal areas respectively[15].

Among residents aged over 50 in a defined area in Jerusalem the prevalence of obesity standardized by age and sex was 21 per cent in 1970 and 25 per cent in 1986, although the increase was statistically significant only in men[16]. In elderly Italians age 65–95 the prevalence of obesity in 1985 was 28 per cent women and 13 per cent men and increased to 16 per cent in men in a little over a decade, while remaining unchanged in the women[11]. Analysis of data from the Longitudinal Study of Aging and the Assets and Health Dynamics of the Oldest Old Survey showed that the prevalence of obesity, over time, increased among those 70 and older[17]. Data from male participants of the Normative Aging Study showed that new cases of obesity, defined on the basis of BMI, increased over time while the numbers of subjects classified as lean and intermediate decreased. Among oldest subjects both the lean and obese had slight but significant decreases in mean BMI. Among the lean, only the young showed consistent increments[18].

Mechanisms responsible for the changes in body composition with ageing

Energy expenditure decreases by around 165 kcal/decade in men and 103 kcal/decade in women, primarily due to changes in voluntary physical activity and to a lesser extent a decrease in RMR[19]. In a population-based cohort of 33,466 men aged 45–79 years in central Sweden total daily physical activity was found to decrease by approximately 4 per cent between age 45 and 79. Obese men reported 2.6 per cent lower physical activity than normal weight men. Men with self-rated poor health had –11.3 per cent lower levels of physical activity than those reporting very good health[20]. Data from cross section studies show that after the age of 40 there is a progressive decline is resting metabolic rate which is explained both by a loss of fat free mass and a decrease in physical activity. Resting metabolic rate is around 6 per cent higher in physically active older men than in untrained older men independent of differences in fat free mass[21].

Energy intake decreases with advancing age, but probably to a lesser extent than energy expenditure[21]. Up to 30 per cent community dwelling older persons have diets deficient in at least one major nutrient[22]. In a recent cross-sectional study of 15,266 healthy men aged 55–79 years, total energy and energy from fat, but not from other nutrients, increased linearly with increasing BMI. BMI increased by 0.53 and 0.14 kg/m^2 for every 500 kcal of fat and total energy consumed, respectively[23].

Other changes that occur with ageing that increase the propensity to the accumulation of fat include, a decrease in whole body fat oxidation (0.5 g/year from age 30–70) associated with the decrease in fat-free mass[24], a diminished ability to use fat as a fuel during exercise[25], reduced adipose tissue lipoprotein lipase activity[26], catecholamine[25] and leptin[26] resistance.

The consequences of obesity in the elderly

Overall mortality

The relative contribution of increased fat mass to mortality may be less pronounced in elderly people. There is some variability between studies. In 2,032 subjects (999 men, 1,033 women), mean age 80 years, recruited by random sampling of the Old Age and Disability Allowance Schemes in Hong Kong, stratified by sex and 5-year age groups from 70 years onwards, overall mortality was negatively associated with body mass index and participation in physical activity, after adjusting for age and sex[27]. In a another study, older men and women at a BMI range of 25 to less than 32 kg/m^2 were shown to have no excess mortality[28]. The BMI range of 25 to 27 has also been reported not to be risk factor for all-cause and cardiovascular mortality among elderly persons, whereas overweight (BMI > 27) was a significant prognostic factor for all-cause and cardiovascular mortality among 65 to 74 year olds, and there was also a significant positive association between overweight and all-cause mortality among those 75 years or older[29]. Overall it is clear that higher BMI values are associated with a smaller relative mortality risk in elderly persons compared with young and middle-aged populations[29]. The standardized mortality rate increases with increasing BMI but, within each BMI group, the standardized mortality rate decreases with age.

A high waist circumference (in non-smoking men) may be a better predictor of all-cause mortality than high BMI[9]. In a prospective cohort study of 31,702 healthy Iowa women aged 55–69 years, waist-hip ratio was the best anthropometric predictor of total mortality[31]. In men and women age 67–78 waist circumference and supine sagittal abdominal diameter are most closely related to CVD risk factors[32]. The elderly at greatest risk are those who are simultaneously sarcopenic and obese[2]. Low BMI and weight loss in the elderly are both strong and independent predictors of subsequent mortality, and low BMI better predicts mortality than low waist circumference[9]. Prior weight history has also been shown to be important in predicting risk. Older heavier people who gained more than 10 per cent of midlife body weight or thinner older people who had lost 10 per cent or more of body weight show high risk compared with thinner people with stable weight[33].

Disease-specific risks

Mobility related disability

Among 2714 women and 2095 men, 65–100 years, there was a positive association between fat mass and disability at baseline. Moreover fat mass was predictive of disability 3 years later, independent of low fat free mass, age, physical activity or chronic disease[34]. Data from the USA National Health and Nutrition Examination Survey (NHANES) I (1971 through 1987) showed that high BMI is a strong predictor of long-term risk for mobility disability in older women and that this risk persists even to very old age. There was a paradoxical increase in risk associated with weight loss in very elderly women[35].

Impaired glucose tolerance and type 2 diabetes mellitus

The prevalence of type 2 diabetes increases progressively with age, peaking at 16.5 per cent in men and 12.8 per cent in women at the age of 75–84 years. Over age 65, diabetes or glucose intolerance was present in 30–40 per cent of Framingham Study subjects[36]. Among 1972 male participants in the Department of Veterans Affairs Normative Aging Study cohort – prospective relation between abdominal adiposity and the risk of diabetes[37]. An age associated increase in total adiposity is a major contributor to impaired glucose tolerance in middle-aged and older men. Increased body fatness and increased abdominal obesity, rather than ageing per se are thought to be directly linked to the greatly increased incidence of type 2 diabetes mellitus among the elderly[38]. Nevertheless, there is evidence that insulin secretion decreases with age even after adjustments for differences in adiposity, fat distribution, and physical activity[39].

Hypertension

Data from the Honolulu Heart Program show that obesity and high blood pressure continue to be highly correlated even in old age[40]. Furthermore the Veterans Administration Normative Aging Study showed that abdominal accumulation of body fat, apart from overall level of adiposity, was associated with both increased blood pressure and an increased risk of hypertension[41].

Fatty liver

The prevalence of fatty liver has been reported to be 3.3 per cent in male and 3.8 per cent in female non-obese and 21.6 per cent in male and 18.8 per cent in female obese elderly individuals, and was shown to be an independent correlate of coronary risk[42].

Pulmonary function

Among 1094 men and 540 women from the Baltimore Longitudinal Study of Aging there was a strong inverse association of WHR with FEV^1 and FVC in men but not women[43]. Weight loss has been shown improves static lung volumes, not dynamic pulmonary function, in moderately obese, sedentary men[44].

The management of obesity in the elderly

Modification of behavioural factors (physical activity, smoking, and obesity) and other cardiovascular risk factors (diabetes, HDL cholesterol and blood pressure) are associated with maintenance of good health in older adults[45]. Many obesity-related health conditions (e.g. hypertension, dyslipidaemia, insulin resistance, glucose intolerance) can be ameliorated independently of weight loss[46]. It is appropriate to advise a reduction in fat intake, to increase fibre and to ensure that the diet contains sufficient micronutrients.

Calorie restriction

Thinness and weight loss (regardless of initial BMI) are associated with increased mortality rates in humans, independent of smoking or weight loss resulting from sub-clinical disease. For overweight individuals in good health, there is no good evidence to show that mortality rates are reduced with weight loss. Even among overweight persons with one or more obesity-related health conditions, specific weight loss recommendations may be unnecessary[46].

Physical activity

Regular exercise is the best predictor of successful weight maintenance. An increase in physical activity leads to an improved insulin sensitivity and glucose tolerance, and a reduction in all cause and cardiovascular mortality[46]. Endurance training increases fatty acid oxidation, leads to a reduction in visceral fat, and increases, or attenuates the decline in RMR[24]. Beginning moderately vigorous sports activity, quitting cigarette smoking, maintaining normal blood pressure, and avoiding obesity were separately associated with lower rates of death from all causes and from coronary heart disease among middle-aged and older men[49]. Resistive training has particular benefits and improves quality and function of skeletal muscle, decreases total and intraabdominal fat, improves insulin action and lowers blood pressure[50,51]. Improvements in fitness have been shown to attenuate age-related increases in adiposity. People who exercise regularly have a lower risk of cardiovascular disease[52], and appear to accumulate less adipose tissue in upper, central body regions as they get older, potentially reducing the risk for the metabolic disorders associated with upper body obesity[30].

Drugs and surgery

Most clinical trials exclude older patients and little is known about benefits of diets or drugs inducing weight loss in these age groups. Bariatric surgery can be safely performed in patients above age 70 with the same benefits as for younger subjects.

References

1. Hughes VA, Frontera WR, Roubenoff R, Evans WJ, Fiatarone Singh MA. Longitudinal changes in body composition. *Am J Clin Nutr* 2002; 76: 473–81.

2. Morley JE, Baumgartner RN, Roubenoff R, Mayer J, Nair KS. Sarcopenia. *J Lab Clin Med* 2001; 137: 231–43.

3. Mott JW, Wang J, Thornton JC, Allison DB, Heymsfield SB, Pierson RN Jr. Relation between body fat and age in 4 ethnic groups. *Am J Clin Nutr* 1999; 69: 1007–13.

4. Perry III HM, Morley JE, Horowitz MH, Kaiser FE, Miller DK, Wittert GA. Leptin, Body composition and Age in African American Women. *Metabolism* 1997; 46: 1399–1405.

5. Beaufrere B, Morio B. Fat and protein redistribution with aging: metabolic considerations. *Eur J Clin Nutr* 2000; 54 (Suppl 3): S48–53.

6. de Groot CP, Enzi G, Matthys C, Moreiras O, Roszkowski W, Schroll M. Ten-year changes in anthropometric characteristics of elderly Europeans. *J Nutr Health Aging* 2002; 6: 4–8.

7. Gallagher D, Ruts E, Visser M, Heshka S, Baumgartner RN, Wang J et al. *Am J Physiol Endocrinol Metab* 2000; 279: E366–75.

8. Perissinotto E, Pisent C, Sergi G, Grigoletto F. Anthropometric measurements in the elderly: age and gender differences. *Br J Nutr* 2002; 87: 177–86.

9. Seidell JC, Visscher TL. Body weight and weight change and their health implications for the elderly. *Eur J Clin Nutr* 2000; 54 (Suppl 3): S33–9.

10. Baumgartner RN, Heymsfield SB, Roche AF. Human body composition and the epidemiology of chronic disease. *Obes Res* 1995; 3: 73–95.

11. Perissinotto E, Pisent C, Sergi G, Grigoletto F. Anthropometric measurements in the elderly: age and gender differences. *Br J Nutr* 2002; 87: 177–86.

12. Ostir GV, Markides KS, Freeman DHJ, Goodwin JS. Obesity and health conditions in elderly Mexican Americans: the Hispanic EPESE. Established Population for Epidemiologic Studies of the Elderly. *Ethn Dis* 2000; 10: 31–38.

13. Chiu HC, Chang HY, Mau LW, Lee TK, Liu HW. Height, weight, and body mass index of elderly persons in Taiwan. *J Gerontol A Biol Sci Med Sci* 2000; 55: M684–90.

14. Lowik MR, Schrijver J, Odink J, van den Berg H, Wedel M, Hermus RJ. nutrition and aging: nutritional status of 'apparently healthy' elderly (Dutch nutrition surveillance system). *J Am Coll Nutr* 1990; 9: 18–27.

15. Gutierrez LM, Llaca MC, Cervantes L, Velasquez AM, Irigoyen ME, Zepeda M. Overweight in elderly Mexican women of a marginal community. *J Nutr Health Aging* 2001; 5: 256–58.

16. Gofin J, Abramson JH, Kark JD, Epstein L. The prevalence of obesity and its changes over time in middle-aged and elderly men and women in Jerusalem. *Int J Obes Relat Metab Disord* 1996; 20: 260–66.

17. Himes CL. Obesity, disease, and functional limitation in later life. *Demography* 2000; 37: 73- 82.

18. Grinker JA, Tucker K, Vokonas PS, Rush D. Overweight and leanness in adulthood: prospective study of male participants in the Normative Aging Study. *Int J Obes Relat Metab Disord* 1996; 20: 561–69.

19. Elia M. Obesity in the elderly. *Obes Res* 2001; 9 (Suppl 4): S244–S248.

20. Norman A, Bellocco R, Vaida F, Wolk A. Total physical activity in relation to age, body mass, health and other factors in a cohort of Swedish men. *Int J Obes Relat Metab Disord* 2002; 26: 670–75.

21. Poehlman ET. Energy expenditure and requirements in aging humans. *J Nutr* 1992; 122: 2057–65.

22. Morley JE. Nutritional status of the elderly. *Am J Med* 1986; 81: 679–95.

23. Satia-Abouta J, Patterson RE, Schiller RN, Kristal AR. Energy from fat is associated with obesity in US men: results from the Prostate Cancer Prevention Trial. *Prev Med* 2002; 34: 493–501.

24. Poehlman ET, Toth MJ, Fonong T. Exercise, substrate utilization and energy requirements in the elderly. *Int J Obes Relat Metab Disord* 1995; 19: S93–96.

25. Blaak EE. Adrenergically stimulated fat utilization and ageing. *Ann Med* 2000; 32: 380–82.

26. Berman DM, Rogus EM, Busby-Whitehead MJ, Katzel LI, Goldberg AP. Predictors of adipose tissue lipoprotein lipase in middle-aged and older men: relationship to leptin and obesity, but not cardiovascular fitness. *Metabolism* 1999; 48: 183–89.

27. Woo J, Ho SC, Yuen YK, Yu LM, Lau J. Cardiovascular risk factors and 18-month mortality and morbidity in an elderly Chinese population aged 70 years and over. *Gerontology* 1998; 44: 51–5.

28. Bender R, Jockel KH, Trautner C, Spraul M, Berger M. Effect of age on excess mortality in obesity. *JAMA* 1999; 281: 1498–1504.

29. Heiat A, Vaccarino V, Krumholz HM. An evidence-based assessment of federal guidelines for overweight and obesity as they apply to elderly persons. *Arch Intern Med* 2001; 161: 1194–1203.

30. Kohrt WM, Malley MT, Dalsky GP, Holloszy JO. Body composition of healthy sedentary and trained, young and older men and women. *Med Sci Sports* 1992; 24: 832–37.

31. Folsom AR, Kushi LH, Anderson KE, Mink PJ, Olson JE, Hong CP et al. Associations of general and abdominal obesity with multiple health outcomes in older women: the Iowa Women's Health Study. *Arch Int Med* 2001; 160: 2117–128.

32. Turcato E, Bosello O, Francesco VD, Harris TB, Zoico E, Bissoli L et al. Waist circumference and abdominal sagittal diameter as surrogates of body fat distribution in the elderly: their relation with cardiovascular risk factors. *Int J Obes* 2000; 24: 1005–10.

33. Harris TB, Launer LJ, Madans J, Feldman JJ. Cohort study of effect of being overweight and change in weight on risk of coronary heart disease in old age. *BMJ* 1997; 314: 1791.

34. Visser M, Langlois J, Guralnik JM, Cauley JA, Kronmal RA, Robbins J, Williamson JD, Harris TB. High body fatness, but not low fat-free mass, predicts disability in older men and women: the Cardiovascular Health Study. *Am J Clin Nutr* 1998; 68: 584–90.

35. Launer LJ, Harris T, Rumpel C, Madans J. Body mass index, weight change, and risk of mobility disability in middle-aged and older women. The epidemiologic follow-up study of NHANES I. *JAMA.* 1994; 271: 1093–98.

36. Wilson PW, Kannel WB. Obesity, diabetes, and risk of cardiovascular disease in the elderly. *Am J Geriatr Cardiol* 2002; 11: 119–25.

37. Cassano PA, Rosner B, Vokonas PS, Weiss ST. Obesity and body fat distribution in relation to the incidence of non-insulin-dependent diabetes mellitus. A prospective cohort study of men in the normative aging study. *Am J Epidemiol* 1992; 136: 1474–86.

38. Colman E, Katzel LI, Sorkin J, Coon PJ, Engelhardt S, Rogus E, Goldberg AP. The role of obesity and cardiovascular fitness in the impaired glucose tolerance of aging. *Exp Gerontol* 1995; 30: 571–80.

39. Muller DC, Elahi D, Tobin JD, Andres R. The effect of age on insulin resistance and secretion: a review. *Semin Nephrol* 1996; 16: 289–98.

40. Masaki KH, Curb JD, Chiu D, Petrovitch H, Rodriguez BL. Association of body mass index with blood pressure in elderly Japanese American men. The Honolulu Heart Program. *Hypertension* 1997; 29: 673–77.

41. Cassano PA, Segal MR, Vokonas PS, Weiss ST. Body fat distribution, blood pressure, and hypertension. A prospective cohort study of men in the normative aging study. *Ann Epidemiol* 1990; 1: 33–48.

42. Akahoshi M, Amasaki Y, Soda M, Tominaga T, Ichimaru S, Nakashima E *et al.* Correlation between fatty liver and coronary risk factors: a population study of elderly men and women in Nagasaki, Japan. *Hypertens Res* 2001; 24: 337–43.

43. Harik-Khan RI, Wise RA, Fleg JL. The effect of gender on the relationship between body fat distribution and lung function. *J Clin Epidemiol* 2001; 54: 399–406.

44. Womack CJ. Womack CJ, Harris DL, Katzel LI, Hagberg JM, Bleecker ER *et al.* Weight loss, not aerobic exercise, improves pulmonary function in older obese men. *Gerontol A Biol Sci Med Sci* 2000; 55: M453–7.

45. Burke GL, Arnold AM, Bild DE, Cushman M, Fried LP, Newman A *et al.* Factors associated with healthy aging: the cardiovascular health study. *J Am Geriatr Soc* 2001; 49: 254–62.

46. Gaesser GA. Thinness and weight loss: beneficial or detrimental to longevity? *Med Sci Sports Exerc* 1999; 31: 1118–28.

47. Perissinotto E, Pisent C, Sergi G, Grigoletto F. Anthropometric measurements in the elderly: age and gender differences. *Br J Nutr* 2002; 87: 177–86.

48. Laws A, Reaven GM. Effect of physical activity on age-related glucose intolerance. *Clin Geriatr Med* 1990; 6: 849–63.

49. Paffenbarger RSJ, Hyde RT, Wing AL, Lee IM, Jung DL, Kampert JB. The association of changes in physical-activity level and other lifestyle characteristics with mortality among men. *N Engl J Med* 1993; 328: 538–45.

50. Ryan AS, Hurlbut DE, Lott ME, Ivey FM, Fleg J, Hurley BF, Goldberg AP. Insulin action after resistive training in insulin resistant older men and women. *J Am Geriatr Soc* 2001; 49: 247–53.

51. Hurley BF, Roth SM. Strength training in the elderly: effects on risk factors for age-related diseases. *Sports Med* 2000; 30: 249–68.

52. Paffenbarger RSJ, Hyde RT, Hsieh CC, Wing AL. Physical activity, other life-style patterns, cardiovascular disease and longevity. *Acta Med Scand* 1986; 711: 85–91.

©2003 John Libbey Eurotext Ltd, pp. 942–950.

CHAPTER 197

Management of morbid obesity

Richard L. Atkinson

Departments of Medicine and Nutritional Sciences University of Wisconsin Madison, Wisconsin 53706, USA
[e-mail: rla@medicine.wisc.edu]

Introduction

As the prevalence of obesity has increased across the world in the last approximately 20 years, the number of individuals with massive amounts of excess adipose tissue has also increased[1-2]. This condition, known as morbid obesity, appears to differ from lesser degrees of obesity, perhaps in aetiology, but certainly in the requirements for management. This review will examine the definitions of morbid obesity, complications particularly important in the morbidly obese, and the elements of management ranging from diet and exercise programs to obesity surgery.

Definitions and frequency of morbid obesity

Morbid obesity has been defined by cutpoints of body mass index (kg/m^2). Unfortunately, there has not been sufficient research to define morbid obesity by body fat content, which would be the most logical. The most accepted definition of morbid obesity is a body mass index of 40 kg/m^2.[1,3,4] In 1991 a Consensus Development Conference sponsored by the National Institutes of Health in the United States proposed an additional definition based on the presence of major complications of obesity that would be expected to have a significant impact on morbidity or mortality[5]. The consensus from the conference agreed upon a cut-point BMI of 35 kg/m^2 along with a major complication, as a second definition of morbid obesity[5]. Some of the more important complications of obesity are listed in Table 1.

In the United States, the prevalence of obesity meeting the definition for morbid obesity is approximately 5 per cent of the total population[1,2,6]. The prevalence of morbid obesity in other countries of the world is difficult to document, but for most countries certainly is lower than in the United States[1].

Complications of morbid obesity

All of the complications of morbid obesity listed in Table 1 occur at lesser degrees of obesity, but several of them deserve special mention in relation to morbid obesity. Insulin resistance, with or without diabetes mellitus, increases with increasing BMI level[7-9]. This is also true for blood pressure. Hypertension occurs in more than 25 per cent of obese patients[9], and in our experience, morbidly obese people have a prevalence of hypertension of about 50 per cent. Serum cholesterol and triglycerides, which are accepted as major risk factors for cardiovascular disease, have an interesting pattern. There is a strong positive correlation of these serum lipids with increasing BMI level up to a BMI of about[45], then the curve flattens out and may even decline slightly. The mechanisms and implications of this pattern in morbid obesity are not clear.

Pulmonary disease merits special attention because it is predominantly a disease of massive obesity. The two major manifestations of pulmonary disease in morbidly obese people are sleep apnea and obesity-hypoventilation syndrome[8,11-14]. The estimates of the prevalence of sleep apnea with obesity range from about 25 to 50 per cent, and patients with morbid obesity have a higher prevalence[12-14]. Peppard *et al.*[13] reported that weight gain increases the risk of developing sleep apnea sixfold over a 4-year period. The end stage of sleep apnea and obesity-hypoventilation syndrome is Pickwickian syndrome, characterized by congestive heart failure, severe hypersomnolence, and a 5-year mortality rate of 70 per cent if left untreated[15]. Fortunately, sleep apnea is highly responsive to weight loss and more than 90 per cent of cases respond to obesity surgery[16,17].

Table 1. Complications of obesity

1. Metabolic complications

    a. Non-insulin-dependent diabetes
    b. Insulin resistance, hyperinsulinaemia
    c. Dyslipidaemia
    d. Gout
    e. Abnormalities of growth hormone secretion

2. Diseases of organ systems

    a. Atherosclerotic and arteriosclerotic vascular diseases
        (1) Coronary heart disease
        (2) Hypertension
        (3) Congestive heart failure
        (4) Cerebrovascular disease

    b. Respiratory system abnormalities
        (1) Obesity-hypoventilation syndrome
        (2) Sleep apnea

    c. Digestive system abnormalities
        (1) Gall bladder disease
        (2) Hepatic disease
        (3) Gastro-esophageal reflux disease

    d. Renal system
        (1) Proteinuria
        (2) Obesity-related glomerulopathy
        (3) Urinary incontinence

    e. Reproductive system abnormalities

    f. Nervous system
        (1) Pseudotumour cerebri
        (2) Adiposis dolorosa

    g. Immune system dysfunction

    h. Skin diseases

    i. Cancers

        (1) Breast   (5) Prostate
        (2) Uterus   (6) Pancreas
        (3) Gallbladder (7) Renal
        (4) Colon

3. Mechanical complications of obesity

    a. Arthritis
    b. Increased intra-abdominal pressure

4. Surgical complications

    a. Perioperative risks: anesthesia, wound comlications, thrombophlebitis, infections
    b. Incisional hernias

5. Psycho-social complications

    a. Social stigma: job and career discrimination, marriageability
    b. Poor self esteem
    c. Poor body image

Sugerman and colleagues[18–23] in a series of papers have described a syndrome of increased intra-abdominal pressure, associated with multiple complications that are normally attributed to excess weight. These investigators postulate that the increased visceral fat contributes to raising the pressure within the abdominal cavity to levels that would constitute a surgical emergency if seen in a trauma ward[18–23]. Using animal models with an inflatable intra-abdominal balloon to increase pressure, they have shown that systemic hypertension and increased cerebrospinal fluid pressure (CSF) occur. One of the serious complications of increased CSF pressure is pseudotumour cerebri, with intractable headaches[18,23]. In humans, an apparatus designed to lower intra-abdominal pressure results in reducing headaches, tinnitus, and CSF pressure[23]. Obesity surgery, with its attendant rapid weight loss, reduces or eliminates the increased intra-abdominal pressure syndrome in more than 80 per cent of cases.

Morbidly obese individuals have a high prevalence of perioperative complications such as wound infections, wound dehiscence, thrombophlebitis and pulmonary emboli, and postoperative pneumonia[8,24]. Also, patients with sleep apnea are prone to suppression of respiration in the immediate postoperative period, perhaps due to sequestration of anaesthetic agents in adipose tissue. These individuals may awaken after surgery, then drift off to sleep, undergo an apneic episode, and the level of anesthaesia may be sufficient to suppress the arousal response. It is recommneded that morbidly obese patients with sleep apnea be kept longer in the surgical intensive care unit after surgery to monitor respiration.

Morbid obesity is associated with several complications that usually do not threaten life, but that dramatically lower the quality of life. These include degenerative arthritis, urinary incontinence, and gastro-esophageal reflux disease (GERD). Obesity is the most common precipitating factor for degenerative joint disease (DJD)[25–27], and a high percentage of morbidly obese patients have DJD. The presence of DJD limits the ability to perform physical activity and may result in a downward spiral of decreasing activity, increasing body weight, and further deterioration of joints. Because many surgeons will not replace hips or knees in morbidly obese patients due to a high postoperative failure rate, morbidly obese patients may end up disabled and confined to a wheelchair.

Urinary incontinence occurs in a high percentage of morbidly obese patients[8,16,20–30], particularly women, but few patients will volunteer the information on a routine history and physical examination without being asked. GERD also may not be mentioned during the history and many patients do not realize the relationship of morbid obesity to GERD and urinary incontinence. Fortunately, with significant weight loss, particularly after obesity surgery, urinary incontinence and GERD usually improve dramatically and may disappear[16,28].

Treatments of morbid obesity

There is a logical progression of treatments of morbid obesity starting with prescription of a diet, exercise, and behaviour modification programme and proceeding through obesity surgery (Table 1). Since the vast majority of patients have previously been on a weight reduction programme, simply prescribing diet and exercise rarely is effective. An option that may be presented to patients is very low calorie dieting (VLCD). Anderson et al.[32] performed a metaanalysis of studies evaluating long term weight maintenance. When standard diets were compared to VLCD, whatever the outcome measure and whenever the follow-up period, VLCD gave superior results. However, the long term success rate is very low, and additional measures are almost always needed. The next step for most patients is obesity drugs. Major weight loss and long term success are rare, but if a patient has not been treated with drugs previously, a trial of one or more drugs is warranted to determine if the individual will be a 'superresponder' who loses large amounts of weight. The usual outcome of treatment with obesity drugs is moderate weight loss, but morbid obesity persists. The only option left in these cases is obesity surgery. A brief discussion of each of these treatments is presented below.

Diet and exercise: The standard diet used for many years for the treatnent of obesity is low in fats (less than 30 per cent of kcal), high in carbohydrates (CHO) (more than 50 per cent of kcal), and containing about 15 per cent of kcal as protein[33,34]. Recently, this conventional wisdom has been challenged by investigators giving higher protein in the diet[35]. Higher protein diets, containing about 25–35 per cent of kcal/day, produce decreased hunger and somewhat better weight loss, fat loss, and compliance than do lower protein, higher CHO diets[35]. Although recently there have been a few studies of high protein, high fat diets, most authorities do not recommend them because the longest follow-up period has been one year[35]. High protein diets are associated with increased kidney size, but no evidence of damage to kidneys during the follow-up period[36].

VLCDs provide approximately 10–12 kcal per kg of 'desirable' body weight, which may be defined as the body weight at a BMI of 22. VLCDs may consist of liquid formulas or predominantly high protein foods. Protein intakes of about 1.0–1.5 g per kg minimize loss of lean body mass. VLCDs usually do not provide sufficient vitamins and minerals, so they need to be supplemented. VLCDs produce very rapid weight loss and dramatic improvement in complications of obesity such as hyperinsulinaemia, hyperglycaemia, hypertriglyceridaemia, and hypertension[39]. Wadden et al.[40] reported that VLCDs of up to 16 weeks were well tolerated. Anderson et al.[32] reported in a metaanalysis that patients on a VLCD have a better outcome, no matter what the outcome measure, than patients on a conventional diet.

As discussed above, exercise may be difficult for many morbidly obese patients because of pain from DJD. Also, morbidly obese people usually are extremely physically unfit and may be able to walk only very short distances before getting short of breath. An activity programme must be carefully tailored to the individual and take into account the person's physical limitations. For most morbidly obese people, walking is a good initial exercise programme. For those with severe DJD who cannot walk for an extended period, deep water exercise provides a good workout. Length of the exercise session may have to be limited to 5–10 min initially until the patient builds endurance. Strength training twice weekly helps build muscle mass, which may increase fatty acid oxidation. Because the early stages of weight loss are associated with the greatest changes in fluid and electrolyte balance and changes in substrate utilization, the potential for arrhythmias is greatest during this time. Exercise programmes for morbidly obese patients should be delayed until there is an initial weight loss of 5–10 kg by dieting, or for the first 4–6 weeks after starting weight loss.

Table 2. Progression of treatment of morbid obesity

1. Energy deficient diet
2. Increased actiyity
3. Increased exercise
4. Very low calorie diet
5. Pharmacotherapy
6. Obesity surgery

Table 3. Drugs for the treatment of morbid obesity

1. Adrenergic agonists	Generic name	Trade names	DEA schedule
	Benzphetamine	Didrex	III
	Dextroamphetamine[a]	Dexidrine	II
	Diethylpropion	Tenuate	IV
	Mazindol[b]	Mazanor, Sanorex	IV
	Methamphetamine[a]	Desoxyn	II
	Phendimetrazine	Bontril, Plegine, Prelu-2	III
	Phentermine	Adipex, Fastin, Ionamin	IV
	Phenylpropanolamine[b]	Dexatrim, Acutrim	OTC
2. Serotonin agonists: DEA IV: d,l-fenfluramine[b], d-fenfluramine[b]			
3. Combined adrenergic and serotonergic agonist: DEA IV: Sibutramine			
4. Drug affecting absorption: Orlistat			

[a]Amphetamine compounds not recommended for clinical use for obesity;
[b]These drugs have been removed from the US market by the manufacturer or the MA, but some may be available in other countries.

Table 4. Drugs used 'off label' for morbid obesity

Acarbose
Bupropion
Metformin
Topiramate
Fluoxetine
Sertraline
Citalopram

Obesity drugs: The selection of drugs approved for obesity is quite limited (Table 3). With the exception of orlistat, all obesity drugs act on the central nervous system (CNS). Adrenergic drugs increase concentrations of norepinephrine in critical areas in the CNS that are involved in regulating food intake or energy expenditure. Phendimetrazine and benzphetamine are rated as Schedule III by the US Food and Drug Adminstration (FDA), signifying a supposedly greater addictive potential. Phentermine and diethylpropion are in Schedule IV, but animal studies suggest that diethylpropion has somewhat greater reinforcement activity than phentermine[42]. One head-to-head study suggested that phentermine produced significantly greater weight loss than diethylpropion[43]. All of the above adrenergic drugs were approved many years ago and were evaluated for only brief periods of time. Phentermine was evaluated for 36 weeks in two studies[44,45] and found to produce weight losses of about 13 per cent of initial body weight. The most common side effects of the central adrenergic drugs is dry mouth. Pulse rate may increase slightly, and increases in blood pressure are reported, although the overall effect is a reduction in blood pressure due to weight loss.

Sibutramine is the only drug approved for obesity that increases both norepinephrine and serotonin in the CNS[46]. Weight loss averages about 6–8 per cent of initial body weight at 1 year[46]. Sibutramine produces improvements in diabetes control, lowers serum lipids, and on average reduces blood pressure, but these effects appear to be due to the effects of weight loss, and are not independent effects of the drug[46,47]. Side effects include slight increases in blood pressure and pulse rate in some patients, and in about 5 per cent of patients, a paradoxical increase in appetite[46,47].

Orlistat acts entirely in the gastrointestinal tract by binding intestinal lipases and resulting in loss of about one third of ingested fat[48,49]. Weight losses are reported to be about 10 per cent of initial body weight at 1 year and about 8 per cent after 2 years[48,49]. Orlistat reduces serum cholesterol and LDL levels, partially due to the effects of weight loss, but there is an additional independent effect of orlistat on the serum lipids[49]. Reductions in serum glucose and insulin are due to the weight loss effect[50,51]. Side effects include diarrhoea and rare instances of fecal incontinence[48,51]. Serum fat soluble vitamin levels decrease slightly, so vitamin replacement is recommended.

All of the drugs mentioned above have only modest effects on patients with morbid obesity and there is a high failure rate in maintaining weight loss. The limited response to current drugs approved for the treatment of obesity has led some physicians to use combinations of drugs or drugs not approved for treating obesity, so called 'off label' use. Some of the drugs used off label are listed in Table 4.

When orlistat is added to a regimen of either phentermine or sibutranine, there is minimal or no additional weight loss[52,53]. Anecdotal or preliminary reports of the combination of phentermine with fluoxetine suggests that there may be some additive effects[54,55], but more research is needed to determine if this combination will be useful for morbid obesity. The combination of phentermine and fluoxetine does not appear to cause damage to heart valves.

Bupropion and topiramate are drugs approved for other purposes, depression and seizures, respectively, but not for treating obesity. Bupropion has been studied for up to 1 year and produces weight losses of about 8 per cent of initial body weight[56,57]. Topiramate was reported to produce weight losses of up to 17 per cent of initial body weight in obese epileptic patients[58] (personal communication, M. Fitchet). A recent clinical trial on subjects with uncomplicated obesity showed a loss of up to 6.3 per cent at 6 months[58a]. Metformin has been shown to cause modest weight losses in obese people[59,60]. Individual physicians are using bupropion, topiramate and metformin in combination with phentermine or other obesity drugs, but there are minimal or no published data on these combinations.

Surgery for obesity: Several types of surgery have been used for morbid obesity, including gastric bypass, vertical banded gastroplasty (VBG), biliopancreatic bypass, and duodenal switch. Gastric bypass appears to be the most effective with tolerable side effects[16,61–66]. Sugerman et al.[62] performed a randomized trial of gastric bypass compared to VBG. Gastric bypass produced a greater weight loss that was better maintained. Biliopancreatic bypass and duodenal switch produce malabsorption[16,61], and some investigators believe that the risks of these operations does not outweigh the benefits. Biliopancreatic bypass and duodenal switch produce weight losses of up to 75 per cent of excess body weight, compared to about 65 per cent for gastric bypass and about 50 per cent for VBG[67,68].

It has not been possible to identify predictors of success with obesity surgery, although one study noted that Blacks have a lower weight loss than do Caucasians[16]. Many surgeons insist on psychological evaluation preoperatively, but this has limited utility in predicting weight loss or outcome of surgery[69].

The complications of surgery include perioperative problems such as wound dehiscence, wound infections, anastomotic leaks, pneumonia and pulmonary emboli[5,16,61]. Super-obese patients (BMI > 50) lose more mass, but less percentage of body weight and have more complications, particularly pulmonary emboli, wound infections and death[70]. VBG is associated with increased nausea and vomiting, particularly after meals, presumably due to the small residual gastric pouch and gastric outflow obstruction fixed by the gastric band. Gastric bypass produces a high prevalence of the dumping syndrome and in some patients is associated with reduced absorption of vitamin B_{12}, calcium and iron[16]. Supplements of these nutrients must be given indefinitely after surgery. Biliopancreatic bypass and duodenal switch produce diarrhea, malabsorption of vitamins, macrominerals and trace minerals[16,67,68]. Supplements of vitamins and minerals must be given indefinitely after surgery. Unfortunately, a number of surgeons who perform obesity surgery do not insist on long term follow-up and they refer patients back to their primary care physicians, who may not be familiar with the myriad of chronic problems that may be produced by the surgery. Surgeons who undertake obesity surgery should have a defined follow-up programme or refer patients to physicians who have expertise in the area.

Special considerations in treating morbidly obese patients

There are a number of special considerations that must be kept in mind when treating morbidly obese patients. Medications such as certain antibiotics, pain medications, and anaesthetic agents are fat soluble, or are diluted in the increased blood volume seen in morbidly obese patients, so dosages of drugs must always be considered when treating these patients[71,72]. Obese patients do poorly after trauma. Choban et al.[73] noted that as compared to lean patients, obese patients have a remarkably higher mortality rate despite similar degrees of injury. Many of the deaths were due to adult respiratory distress syndrome. Morbidly obese people are susceptible to dehydration because of their increased surface area and the fact that the subcutaneous fat layer provides greater insulation. Particular attention must be paid by the patient and the physician to ensure adequate fluid intake.

Summary and conclusions

Morbidly obese patients are at increased risk of multiple complications of obesity and have a poorer quality of life than do lean and moderately obese people. Standard medical treatment of obesity usually meets with limited or no success in producing long term weight loss. Occasional patients respond to obesity drugs with long term, large scale weight loss, so a trial of obesity drugs is indicated to identify these 'super-responders'. For most morbidly obese patients, obesity surgery offers the best hope of long term, large scale weight loss. A wide variety of perioperative risks and the occurrence of long term problems with absorption of vitamins and minerals may be seen with gastric bypass, biliopancreatic bypass, and duodenal switch. These problems mandate very careful selection of candidates for obesity, surgery and careful long term follow-up. Morbidly obese people may be more fragile during acute illness and have a higher mortality rate. They may require higher doses of certain medications and careful attention to hydration status. Additional research is needed to identify the aetiology of morbid obesity and the special considerations that must be given to their care.

Acknowledgement: Supported in part by funds from the Beers-Murphy Clinical Nutrition Center, University of Winsconsin, Madison.

References

1. World Health Organisation. Preventing and managing the global epidemic of obesity: report of a WHO Consultation on Obesity. Geneva, 3–5 June 1997. WHO/NUT/NCD98.1, Geneva, 1998.

2. Flegal KM, Carroll MD, Ogden CL, Johnson CL. Prevalence and trends in obesity among US adults, 1999–2000. *JAMA* 2002 Oct 9;288(14):1723-7.

3. Foster WR, Burton BT. Health Implications of obesity, National Institutes of Health Consensus Development Conference. *Ann Intern Med* 1985; 103 (6 pt 2): 981–1077.

4. Clinical Guidelines on the identification, evaluation, and treatment of overweight and obesity in adults – The Evidence Report. *Obes Res* 1998; 6 (Suppl 2): S51–S209.

5. Gastrointestinal surgery for severe obesity. Proceedings of a Nacional Institutes of Health Consensus Development Conference. March 25–27, 1991, Bethesda, MD. *Am J Clin Nutr.* 1992; 55(2 Suppl): S487–S619.

6. Centers for Disease Control and Prevention, National Center for Health Statistics avaiable from: http//www.cdc.gov/nchs/hus.htm

7. Hunt SC, Williams RR, Adams TD. Biochemical and anthropometric characterization of morbid obesity in a large Utah pedigree. *Obes Res* 1995; 3 (Suppl 2): S165–S172.

8. Grundy SM, Barnett JP. Metabolic and health complications of obesity. *Dis Mon* 1990; 36(12): 641–731.

9. Wilson PW, D'Agostino RB, Sullivan L, Parise H, Kannel WB. Overweight and obesity as determinants of cardiovascular risk: the Framingham experience. *Arch Intern Med* 2002; 9: 162(16): 1867–72.

10. Vierhapper H, Nardï A, Grosser P. Prevalence of paradoxically normal serem cholesterol in morbidly obese women. *Metabolism* 2000; 49: (5) 607–610.

11. Suratt PM, Dee P, Atkinson RL, Armstrong P, Wilhoit SC. Fluoroscopic and computed tomographic features of the pharyngeal airway in obstructive sleep apnea. *Am Rev Resp Dis* 1983; 127: 487–92.

12. Young T, Palta M, Dempsey J, Skatrud J, Weber S, Badr S. The occurrence of sleep disordered breathing among middle-aged adults. *N Engl J Med* 1993; 29: 328(17): 1230–5.

13. Peppard PE, Young T, Palta M, Skatrud J. Prospective study of the association between sleep-disordered breathing and hypertension. *N Engl J Med* 2000; 11; 342(19): 1378–84.

14. Resta O, Foschino-Barbaro MP, Legari G, Talamo S, Bonfitto P, Palumbo A *et al.* Sleep-related breathing disorders, loud snoring and excessive daytime sleepiness in obese subjects. *Int J Obes Relat Metab Disord* 2001; 25(5): 669–75.

15. Miller A, Granada M. In-hospital mortality in the Pickwickian syndrome. *Am J Med* 1974; 56: 144–7

16. Sugerman HJ. Bariatric surgery for severe obesity. *J Assoc Acad Minor Phys* 2001; 12(3): 129–36.

17. Dixon JB, Schachter LM, O'Brien PE. Sleep disturbance and obesity: changes following surgically induced weight loss. *Arch Intern Med* 2001; 161(1): 102–6.

18. Sugerman HJ, DeMaria EJ, Felton WL 3rd, Nakatsuka M, Sismanis A. Increased intra-abdominal pressure and cardiac filling pressures in obesity-associated pseudotumor cerebri. *Neurology* 1997; 49(2): 507–11.

19. Sugerman HJ, Bloomfield GL, Saggi BW. Multisystem organ failure secondary to increased intra-abdominal pressure. *Infection* 1999; 27(1): 61–6.

20. Bloomfield GL, Ridings PC, Blocher GR, Marmarou A, Sugerman HJ. A proposed relationship between increased intra-abdominal, intrathoracic, and intracranial pressure. *Critical Care Med* 1997; 25(3): 496–503.

21. Bloomfield GL, Blocher CR, Fakhry IF, Sica DA, Sugermann HJ. Elevated intra-abdominal pressure increases plasma renin activity and aldosterone levels. *J Trauma-Injury Infection Critical Care* 1997; 42(6): 997–1004 (discussion 1004–5).

22. Sugerman HJ, Felton WL 3rd, Salvant JB Jr, Sismanis A, Kellum JM. Effects of surgically induced weight loss on idiopathic intracranial hypertension in morbid obesity. *Neurology* 1995; 45: 1655–59.

23. Sugerman HJ, Felton III WL 3rd, Sismanis A, Saggi BH, Doty JM, Blocher C, Marmarou A, Makhoul RG. Continuous negative abdominal pressure device to treat pseudotumor cerebri. *Int J Obes Relat Metab Disord* 2001; 25(4): 486–90.

24. Forse RA, Karam B, MacLean LD, Christou NV. Antibiotic prophylaxis for surgery in morbidly obese patients. *Surgery* 1989; 106(4): 750–6.

25. Anderson JJ, Felton DT. Factors associated with osteoarthritis of the knee in the first National Health and Nutrition Examination Survey. *Am J Epidemiol* 1988; 128: 179–89.

26. Carman WJ, Sowers M, Hawthorne VM, Weissfeld LA. Obesity as a risk factor for osteoarthritis of the hand and wrist: a prospective study. *Am J Epidemiol.* 1994; 15: 139(2): 119–29.

27. Cooper C, Inskip H, Croft P, Campbell L, Smith G, McLaren M, Coggon D. Individual risk factors for hip osteoarthritis: obesity, hip injury, and physical activity. *Am J Epidemiol* 1998; 15: 147(6): 516–22.

28. Deitel M, Stone E, Kassam HA, Wilk EJ, Sutherland DJ. Gynecologic-obstetric changes after loss of massive excess weight following bariatric surgery. *J Am Coll Nutr* 1988; 7(2): 147–53.

29. Mommsen S, Foldspang A. Body mass index and adult female urinary incontinence. *World J Urol* 1994; 12(6): 319–22.

30. Chiarelli P, Brown WJ. Leaking urine in Australian women: prevalence and associated conditions. *Women Health* 1999; 29(1): 1–13.

31. Choban PS, Atkinson RL, Moore BJ *et al. Guidance for treatment of adult obesity.* Shape Up America! Bethesda, 1996.

32. Anderson JW, Konz EC, Frederich RC, Wood CL. Long-term weight-loss maintenance: a meta-analysis of US studies. *Am J Clin Nutr* 2001; 74(5): 579–84.

33. Astrup A, Ryan L, Grunwald GK, Storgaard M, Saris W, Melanson E, Hill JO. The role of dietary fat in body fatness: evidence from a preliminary meta-analysis of *ad libitum* low-fat dietary intervention studies. *Br J Nutr* 2000; 83 (Suppl 1): S25–S32.

34. Astrup A, Astrup A, Buemann B, Flint A, Raben A. Low-fat diets and energy balance: how does the evidence stand in 2002 *Proc Nutr Soc.* 2002; 61(2): 299–309.

35. Skov AR, Toubro S, Ronn B, Holm L, Astrup A. Randomized trial on protein vs. carbohydrate in *ad libitum* fat reduced diet for the treatment of obesity. *Int J Obes Relat Metab Disord* 1999; 23(5}: 528–36.

36. Skov AR, Toubro S, Bulow J, Krabbe K, Parving HH, Astrup A. Changes in renal function during weight loss induced by high vs. low-protein low-fat diets in overweight subjects. *Int J Obes Relat Metab Disord* 1999; 23(11): 1170–7.

37. Fisler JS; Drenick EJ. Starvation and semistarvation diets in the management of obesity. *Ann Rev Nutr* 1987; 7: 465–84.

38. Pasquali R, Casimirri F, Melchionda N. Protein metabolism in obese patients during very low-calorie mixed diets containing different amounts of proteins and carbohydrates. *Metabolism* 1987; 36(12.): 1141–8.

39. Atkinson, R.L. Usefulness and limits of VLCD in the treatment of obesity. In: *Progress in Obesity Research: 1990*, Y Oomura, S Tarui, S Inoue, T Shimazu (eds), pp. 473–80. London, John Libbey, 1991.

40. Wadden TA, Foster GD, Letizia KA. One-year behavioral treatment of obesity: comparison of moderate and severe caloric restriction and the effects of weight maintenance therapy. *J Consult Clin Psychol* 1994; 62(1): 165–171.

41. Fisler JS. Cardiac effects of starvation and semistarvation diets: safety and mechanisms of action. *Am J Clin Nutr.* 1992; 56(1 Suppl): S230–S234.

42. Griffiths RR, Brady JV, Bradford LD. Predicting the abuse liability of drugs with animal drug self-administration procedures: psychomotor stimulants and hallucinogens. *Adv Behav Pharm* 1979; 2: 163–208.

43. Valle-Jones JC, Brodie NH, O'Hara H, O'Hara J, McGhie RL. A comparative study of phentermine and diethylpropion in the treatment of obese patients in general practice. *Pharmatherapeutica* 1983; 3(5): 300–4.

44. Munro JF, MacCuish AC, Wilson EM, Duncan LJP. Comparison of continuous and intermittent anorectic therapy in obesity. *BMJ* 1968; 1: 352–4.

45. Steel AL Munro JF, Duncan LJ. A comparativo trial of different regimens of fenfluramine and phentermine in obesity. *Practitioner* 1973; 211(262): 232–6.

46. Heal DL Aspley S, Prow MR, Jackson HC, Martin KF, Cheetham SC. Sibutramine: a novel anti-obesity drug. A review of the pharmacological evidence to differentiate it from d-amphetamine and d-fenfluramine. *Int J Obes Relat Metab Disord* 1998; 22 (Suppl 1): S18–S28.

47. Weintraub M, Rubio A, Golik A, Byrne L, Scheinbaum ML. Sibutramine in weight control: a dose-ranging, efficacy study. *Clin Pharmacol Ther* 1991; 50(3): 330–7.

48. James WP, Avenell A, Broom J, Whitehead J. A one year trial to asses the valise of orlistat in the management of obesity. *Int J Obes* 1997; 21 (Suppl 3): S24–S30.

49. Davidson MH, Hauptman J, DiGirolamo M, Foreyt JP, Halsted CH, Heber D. Weight control and risk factor reduction in obese subjects treated for 2 years with orlistat: a randomized controlled trial. *JAMA* 1999; 281(3): 235–42.

50. Greenway F. Obesity medications and the treatment of type 2 diabetes. *Diabetes Technol Ther* Fall 1999; 1(3): 277–87.

51. Kelley DE, Jneidi M. Orlistat in the treatment of Type 2 diabetes mellitus. *Expert Opin Pharmacother* 2000; 3(5): 599–605.

52. Bowen RL, Atkinson RL. Addition of orlistat to long term phentermine treatment for obesity. *Obes Res* 2000; 8: 118.

53. Wadden TA, Berkowitz RI, Womble LG, Sarwer DB, Arnold ME, Steinberg CM. Effects of sibutramine plus orlistat in obese women following 1 year of treatment by sibutramine alone: a placebo controlled trial. *Obes Res* 2000; 8(6): 431–37.

54. Dhurandhar NV, Atkinson RL. Comparison of serotonin agonists in combination with phentermine for treatment of obesity. *FASEB J* 1996; 10: 561.

55. Griffen L, Anchors, M. The 'phen-pro' diet drug combination is not associated with valvular heart disease. *Arch Intern Med* 1998; 158: 1278–9.

56. Gadde KM, Parker CB, Maner LG, Wagner HR 2nd, Logue EJ, Drezner MK, Krishnan KR. Bupropion for weight loss: an investigation of efficacy and tolerability in overweight and obese women. *Obes Res* 2001; 9(9): 544–51.

57. Anderson JW, Greenway FL, Fujioka K, Gadde KM, McKenney J, O'Neil PM. Bupropion SR enhances weight loss: a 48-week double-blind, placebo- controlled trial. *Obes Res.* 2002 10(7): 633–41.

58. Reife R, Pledger G, Wu SC. Topiramate as add-on therapy: pooled analysis of randomized controlled trials in adults. *Epilepsia* 2001; 41 (Suppl 1): S66–S71.

58a. Bray GA, Hollander P, Klein S, Kushner R, Levy B, Fitchet M, Perry BH. A 6-month randomized, placebo-controlled, dose-ranging trial of topiramate for weight loss in obesity. *Obes Res* 2003; 11(6): 722-33.

59. Lee A Morley JE. Metformin decreases food consumption and induces weight loss in subjects with obesity with type II non-insulin-dependent diabetes. *Obes Res* 1998; 6(1): 47–53.

60. Kay JP, Alemzadeh R, Langley G, D'Angelo L, Smith P, Holshouser S. Beneficiai effects o metformin in normoglycemic morbidly obese adolescents. *Metabolism* 2001; 50(12): 1457–61.

61. Kral JG. Surgical treatment of obesity. In: *Handbook of obesity*, Bray GA, Bouchard C, James WPT (eds), pp. 977–93. New York: Marcel Dekker, 1997.

62. Pories WJ, Flickinger EG, Meelheim D *et al*. The effectiveness of gastric bypass over gastric partition in morbid obesity. *Ann Surg* 1982; 196: 389–99.

63. Sugerman HJ, Londrey GL, Kellum JM, Wolf L, Liszka T, Engle KM, Birkenhauer R, Starkey JV. Weight loss with vertical banded gastroplasty and roux-y gastric bypass for morbid obesity with selective versus random assignment. *Am J Surg* 1989; 157: 93–102.

64. Gjorup IE, Gotzsche PC, Baden H, Andersen B. Surgical treatment of morbid obesity. A survey of overall outcome 1968–1989. *Dan Med Bull* 1991; 38(5): 405–7.

65. MacLean LD, Rhode BM, Sampalis J, Forse RA. Results of the surgical treatment of obesity. *Am J Surg* 1993; 165(1): 155–60.

66. DeMaria EJ, Sugerman HJ, Kellum JM, Meador JG, Wolfe LG. Results of 281 consecutive total laparoscopic Roux-en-Y gastric bypasses to treat morbid obesity. *Ann Surg* 2002; 235(5): 640–5.

67. Bajardi G, Ricevuto G, Mastrandrea G, Branca M, Rinaudo G, Cali F, *et al.* Surgical treatment of morbid obesity with biliopancreatic diversion and gastric banding: report on an 8-year experience involving 235 cases. *Ann Chir* (2000); 125(2): 155–62.

68. Baltasar A, Bou R, Bengochea M, Arlandis F, Escriva C., Miro J *et al.* Duodenal switch: an effective therapy for morbid obesity – intermediate results. *Obes Surg* 2001; 11(1): 54–8.

69. Grana. AS, Coolidge FL, Merwin MM. Personality profiles of the morbidly obese. *J Clin Psychol* 1989; 45(5): 762–5.

70. Bloomston M, Zervos EE, Camps MA, Goode SE, Rosemurgy AS. Outcome following bariatric surgery in super versus morbidly obese patients: does weight matter? *Obes Surg* 1997; 71.7{5}: 414–9.

71. Forse RA, Karam B, MacLean LD, Christou NV. Antibiotic prophylaxis for surgery in morbidly obese patients. *Surgery* 1989; 106(4): 750–6 (discussion 756–7).

72. Graves DA Batenhorst RL, Bennett RL, Wettstein JG, Griffen WO, Wright BD, Foster TS. Morphine requirements using patient-controlled analgesia: influence of diurnal variation and morbid obesity. *Clin Pharm* 1983; 2(1): 49–53.

73. Choban PS, Weireter LJ Jr, Maynes C. Obesity and increased mortality in blunt trauma. *J Trauma* 1991; 31(9): 1253–7.

Progress in Obesity Research: 9. Edited by *Geraldo Medeiros-Neto, Alfredo Halpern* and *Claude Bouchard*
©2003 John Libbey Eurotext Ltd, pp. 951–955.

CHAPTER 198

The effects of surgically induced weight loss on obesity co-morbidity: results from the SOS-study

Ingmar Naslund

The SOS-study group, University of Gothenburg and University Hospital of Orebro, Sweden
[e-mail: ingmar.naslund@orebroll.se]

Introduction

The aim of any kind of treatment of obesity is to achieve weight loss, but the reason for this treatment varies. Most patients seek help because they want relief from their psychosocial burden and the impairment of quality of life caused by obesity. The political and the health care systems are hoping weight loss to be efficient from an economic point of view. On the other hand, the medical profession prefers to focus on the effects upon cardiovascular risk factors, co-morbidity and mortality. This paper has the latter perspective.

Surgery offers the possibility to study effects of weight loss on co-morbidity and quality of life of obesity. Drug and other conservative treatment methods have hitherto not been effective and long-lasting enough for this purpose. This means that surgery is the foundation for the present knowledge of the effects of weight loss upon body and mind.

Method

The SOS-study (Swedish Obese Subjects) is an ongoing nationwide intervention trial of obesity that began 1987. The primary aim is to determine whether mortality and morbidity rates in obese persons can be reduced by surgical treatment and weight reduction. The study consists of two parts, a cross-sectional registry study, which also serves as a recruitment base for the other part that is a controlled, prospective intervention study. A cross-sectional population study of randomly selected individuals from the general population is also affiliated with the project.

In the intervention study, 2010 surgically treated, severely obese patients will be compared to 2038 controls. The controls were selected and recruited from the register study with the help of a computerized matching procedure taking 18 different matching variables such as age, weight, height, sex, anthropometrics, biochemistry, smoking, four different psychological variables related to mortality, and two personality traits related to treatment preferences into account. The two groups are followed in the same way with a planned follow-up of 20 years[1,2]. The study is ongoing and several analyses of subgroups of varying sizes with a follow-up to 10 years have been published.

The treatment was restrictive surgery, mainly gastroplasty. About two thirds were operated upon with vertical banded gastroplasty, a fifth with gastric banding and 13 per cent with gastric bypass. Ten per cent of the operations were laparoscopic procedures. Twenty-five different surgical departments all over Sweden are involved in surgery and follow-up. 3220 intervention and control subjects have so far (October 2001) been followed up for 2 years (follow up rate 86.3 per cent) and 724 for 10 years (77.8 per cent). The average weight loss in the surgical group was after 2 years 23 per cent and after 10 years 16 per cent. The control group with conventional treatment at 480 primary health care centres had at two years a weight reduction of 0.1 per cent and a weight increase at 10 years of 1.4 per cent.

Results and discussion

Mortality

The increased mortality associated with severe obesity is well known, but we do not know if intentional weight loss will reduce this mortality. So far, hard endpoints (total mortality, myocardial infarction and stroke) have been collected over 32,000 person-years (August 2002) in the SOS-study. In the study protocol the first publication of such endpoint results is planned after 40,000 person years of observation. The circumstance that the Safety Monitoring Committee of the study not yet has given us permission to publish such data could indicate that a weight loss of 17 per cent over 10 years is not enough to decrease mortality. But on the other hand we know for sure that surgically treatment of obesity dose not increase the risk (including a peroperativ mortality of 0.25 per cent).

Cardiovascular risk factors

The effects of weight loss upon cardiovascular co-morbidity and risk factors as compared to findings in controls 2 and 10 years after intervention are summarized in Table 1. These results can be expressed in at least three different ways: recovery from the co-morbidity or risk factor, reduction of the incidence, i.e. protection from developing a risk factor, and change of the mean value of the risk factor (The SOS research group: Impact of interventional weight loss over 10 years on life style and cardiovascular risk factors: The SOS experience. In manuscript).

Table 1. Summary of results. Favourable effects upon cardiovascular risk factors of surgically induced weight loss as compared to findings in controls two and ten years after intervention

	Incidence of risk		Recovery from risk		Mean change of risk factor	
	2 yr	10 yr	2 yr	10 yr	2 yr	10 yr
Diabetes	+	+	+	+		
Glucose					++	++
Insulin					++	++
Hypertension	0	0	+	+		
Systolic BP					++	(+)
Diastolic BP					++	0
Triglycerides	++	(+)	++	++	++	++
HDL cholesterol	++	0	++	+	++	++
Total cholesterol	0	0	0	0	+	(+)
Uric acid	+	+	+	+	+	+

0 = no effect of weight loss; $+$ = $P < 0.05$; $++$ = $P < 0.001$. In no case surgically induced weight loss caused non-favourable effects on risk factors.

Recovery from diabetes among patients with diabetes at baseline was higher in the surgical group compared to the controls. Incidences were lower, i.e. the proportions of subjects that were euglucaemic at baseline and later developed diabetes were much smaller in the surgical group than in the control group. This difference means that about one out of twenty developed diabetes over 10 years in the surgical group, whereas the corresponding number in the weight stable control group was about one out of four. Surgically induced weight loss has a strong effect upon recovery as well as protection from developing diabetes among severe obese. Significant decreases of mean blood-glucose and plasma-insulin values at 2 and 10 years were observed.

Weight loss induced recovery from hypertension, but the effect was not as profound as in diabetes. Although weight loss improved systolic (at 2 and 10 years) and diastolic values (at 2, but not 10 years) the incidences were not significantly different between the two groups.

Surgically induced weight loss caused recovery in a significantly higher proportion as compared to the controls regarding hypertriglyceridaemia, hypo-HDL and hyper-urecaemi, but not hyper-cholesterolaemi. Reductions of incidence and mean values of these risk factors followed a similar pattern (Table 1). In no case surgically induced weight loss caused non-favourable effects on these cardiovascular risk factors.

Weight loss also caused favourable structural and functional changes in the cardiovascular system. In subsamples of the SOS study and a lean reference group Karason[3,4] examined cardiac anatomy and function with two dimensional and Doppler echocardiography. At base line the systolic and diastolic blood pressure, left ventricular mass, and relative wall thickness were increased in the obese whereas the systolic function measured as left ventricular ejection fraction and the diastolic function measures as E: A fraction were decreased. After one year all these variables had improved in the surgically treated group but not in the obese control group. When pooling the two obese groups and plotting left ventricular mass or E: A ratio as a function of quintiles of weight change, a 'dose' dependency was revealed; that is the larger the weight reduction the larger the reduction of left ventricular mass and the more pronounced the improvement in the diastolic function. Unchanged weight was in fact associated with a measurable deterioration in diastolic function over 1 year.

The speed of the atherosclerotic process in obese was shown to be slowed down by surgical treatment[5]. Intima-media thickness of the carotid bulb was measured by ultrasonography in surgically treated obese, obese control subjects and lean controls matched for gender, age and height. The two first groups were measured over four years and the lean reference group over three years. The annual progression rate was almost three times higher in the obese control group compared with lean reference subjects. In the surgical treated group, the progression was normalized.

Various cardiopulmonary symptoms and complaints are also improved by weight loss. In a report based on questionnaire data from 1210 surgically treated patients and 1099 obese SOS control subjects examined at base line and after two years it was found that dyspnoea and chest discomfort was reduced in a much larger fraction of the surgically treated patients[6]. In the surgical group 87 per cent reported baseline dyspnea when climbing two flights of stairs, whereas only 19 per cent experienced such dyspnoea at the two years follow-up. Corresponding figures in the obese control group were almost unchanged, 69 and 57 per cent respectively. Further, at baseline a high likelihood for sleep apnoea syndrome was observed in 23 per cent of the surgically treated patients but only in 8 per cent after two years. In the control group the figures were 22 and 20 per cent respectively ($P < 0.001$).

Effects of other organ systems

Pain in joints, especially the legs and the back, are reduced by weight loss. Incontinence of urine among women is reduced. Dermal infections of the groins and sub mammary areas become a less problem, as well as oedema and varicose ulcers of the legs. Infertility can in many cases change to child bearing.

Non-favourable effects

The surgical intervention can cause peroperative complications. During the first 90 days there were 291 patients (14.5 per cent) of the 2010 surgical cases with one or more complications that were regarded to cause at least one extra day of hospital stay or an extra surgical intervention. 2.9 per cent (2.5 per cent during the primary hospital stay) were reoperated upon. There were five deaths (0.25 per cent).

Late complications (> 90 days to 10 years) have not yet been analysed in SOS. But incisional hernias are reported in several series as high as 20 per cent. Bowel obstruction can be seen after any gastrointestinal surgery. The surgical SOS-group had a higher cost for consumption of drugs for miscellaneous gastrointestinal symptoms as compared to the control group over 6 years[10].

There are also non-favourable effects of weight loss *per se*. Biliary tract diseases – gallstone formation with pain, cholecystitis, cholecystectomy and pancreatitis – are more common among obese compared to lean, and increase during weight loss (Torgersson J, Lindroos AK, Naslund I, Peltonen M: Gallstone, gallbladder disease and pancreatitis. Cross-sectional and two year data from the Swedish Obese Subjects (SOS) and SOS-reference studies. In manuscript). The larger the weight loss the higher the proportions of biliary tract diseases.

Iron deficiency anaemia is common especially in women before menopause and is probably related to a low iron intake. B12-deficiency is common after gastric bypass and malabsorptive procedures. Gastric bypass has been proposed to cause osteoporosis, but this has so far not been reported in long-term follow up series over ten years.

Effects related to specific procedure

Some of the effects upon risk factors and co-morbidity are more or less related to the specific surgical procedures rather than to the weight loss *per se*. Procedures, which bypass duodenum and the upper jejunum, have a more profound anti-diabetic effect with a reduced need for insulin medication much faster than what can be explained by loss of body fat.

At a per oral glucose test 1 year after surgery gastric bypass had a significantly lower S-glucose level that gastroplasty which only partly was explained by differences in weight loss. (unpublished data, Naslund)

The amount of weight loss

The improvements of the cardiovascular risk factors mentioned above were proportional to the weight loss[7]. The larger the weight loss the better. When data from 1281 consecutive obese control subjects and surgically treated subjects were pooled together, and this sample was divided into decentiles of percentage of weight change, no subject with a weight loss of at least ten per cent developed diabetes[8]. Among those who had a smaller weight loss or a weight increase a significant number developed diabetes. A weight loss of only 10 per cent seemed to be enough to prevent the development of diabetes over 2 years, whereas other risk factors such as total-cholesterol and diastolic blood pressure seemed to be more resistant to weight loss.

Also regarding quality of life improvements there was a strong relationship to the amount of weight loss, not for the initial first year but for the long-term effects[9].

Life-style effects

Closely related to the effects of weight loss upon co-morbidity are the effects upon life-style of which energy intake and physical activity are the two most important aspects.

The average energy intake was in the range of 2500–2400 kcal during 10 years of observation in the control group. In the surgical group it dropped immediately after surgery from about 3000 kcal/day to 1500 kcal, and later stabilized in the range of 2000–2100 kcal. The differences between the groups were statistically significant. (The SOS research group: Impact of interventional weight loss over 10 years on life style and cardiovascular risk factors: The SOS experience. In manuscript).

The proportions of individuals being physically active during leisure were significantly larger in the surgically treated group compared to the control group over 10 years. A similar although less dramatic pattern, the difference only statistically significant during the first 4 years, was seen for the proportion of individuals who were physically active during work time (The SOS research group: Impact of interventional weight loss over 10 years on life style and cardiovascular risk factors: The SOS experience. In manuscript).

An altered lifestyle with an increased physical activity and a decreased energy intake is not only a prerequisite for a long-term maintained weight loss, it is in it self an important part of an improved quality of life and subsequent beneficial effects upon co-morbidity.

Conclusion

- Surgery is the main basis for the knowledge of the effect of weight loss upon co-morbidity, cardiovascular risk factors (and quality of life).

- It increases the possibility of recovery from diabetes, hypertension and most other cardiovascular risk factors.

- It improves structural and functional changes and symptoms of the heart and it slows down the atherosclerotic process.

- Weight loss decreases the risk to develop diabetes and several other risk factors.

- The required weight loss differs for different co-morbidities and risk factors.

- There are specific effects related to the procedure *per se.*

- Complications of the surgical procedure and non favourable effects of weight loss, e.g. increase of incidence of biliary tract diseases, have to be taken into account.

If total mortality is reduced by weight loss is not yet known.

References

1. Sjostrom L, Larsson B, Backman L, Bengtsson C, Bouchard C, Dahlgren S *et al.* Swedish obese subjects (SOS). Recruitment for an intervention study and a selected description of the obese state. *Int J Obes Relat Metab Disord* 1992; 16: 465–79.

2. Sjostrom L. Surgical intervention as a strategy for treatment of obesity. [Review] [130 refs]. *Endocrin J UK* 2000; 13: 213–30.

3. Karason K, Wallentin I, Larsson B, Sjöström L. Effects of obesity and weight loss on left ventricular mass and relative wall thickness: survey and intervention study. *BMJ* 1997; 315: 912–16.

4. Karason K, Wallentin I, Larsson B, Sjostrom L. Effects of obesity and weight loss on cardiac function and valvular performance. *Obes Res* 1998; 6: 422–9.

5. Karason K, Wikstrand J, Sjostrom L, Wendelhag I. Weight loss and progression of early atherosclerosis in the carotid artery: a four-year controlled study of obese subjects. *Int J Obes Rel Metab Disord* 1999; 23: 948–56.

6. Karason K, Lindroos AK, Stenlof K, Sjostrom L. Relief of cardiorespiratory symptoms and increased physical activity after surgically induced weight loss: results from the Swedish Obese Subjects study. *Arch Intern Med* 2000; 160: 1797–802.

7. Sjostrom CD, Lissner L, Sjostrom L. Relationships between changes in body composition and changes in cardiovascular risk factors: the SOS Intervention Study. Swedish Obese Subjects. *Obes Res* 1997; 5: 519–30.

8. Sjostrom CD, Peltonen M, Wedel H, Sjostrom L. Differentiated long-term effects of intentional weight loss on diabetes and hypertension. *Hypertension* 2000; 36: 20–5.

9. Sullivan M, Karlsson J, Sjostrom L, Taft C. Why quality of life measures should be used in the treatment of patients with obesity. In: *International textbook of obesity*, Bjorntorp B (ed.), pp. 485–510. Chichester: John Wiley and Sons; 2001.

10. Narbro K *et al.* Comparison with a randomly selected population sample and long-term changes after conventional and surgical treatment: The SOS intervention study. *Am J Gastroenterol* 2003; 98: 1032–41.

Progress in Obesity Research: 9. Edited by *Geraldo Medeiros-Neto, Alfredo Halpern and Claude Bouchard*
©2003 John Libbey Eurotext Ltd, pp. 956–964.

CHAPTER 199

Principles for re-operative bariatric surgery problem solving applied to open and minimally invasive approaches

George Cowan, Jr and M. Lloyd Hiler

University of Tennessee, Memphis, USA
[e-mail: owcinc@mindspring.com]

Introduction

The principles for decision-making are, for all intents and purposes, pretty much the same for open versus minimally invasive in re-operative bariatric surgery. The bariatric surgeon's decision-making is the key element rather than whether to use an 'open' or 'closed' approach. The principles elements, and options are many and complex as the patient presentation, with many choices being unique to the individual – the paper will provide guidance, including new operative considerations/procedures/techniques we have developed for additional options. We will first define re-operative bariatric surgery as well as its work-up.

Potential re-operative bariatric surgery candidates have had bariatric surgery at least thirty days previously and experience significant problems which appear related to this earlier surgery. The prior bariatric surgery may have been any of a wide variety of restrictive, malabsorptive or combined, open or laparoscopic, procedures with a stomach cut between staples, stapled *in situ* or partially resected, ante- or retro-colic(-gastric) alimentary limb, limbs of varying lengths, different pouch constructions, anastomoses, and, if present, band or ring characteristics. Some patients may have had prior re-operative bariatric surgery(-ies), up to fourteen in our experience. Additional patient variables include prior complications and surgery, BMI, weight loss/gain/regain, gender, age, race, family history, co-morbidities, dietary habits, medications, presenting complaints, national origin, compliance, and psycho-social status.

From our approximately eight hundred re-operative bariatric surgery patient experience, too few individuals exist with sufficiently matching variables among all these possibilities to develop large, definitive, useful series. The insightful clinician, therefore, will assume the role of a clinical detective and carefully handle each presentation as a case unique in itself, employing experience-derived principles, guidelines, options, and precautions as presented in this chapter.

With the general principles in Table 1 in mind, consider the not uncommon circumstances of a patient presenting with chief complaints of nausea, vomiting, dysphagia, abdominal pain and a history of prior bariatric surgery.

General principle: be sceptical

Initial presentations of patients, particularly opinionated, knowledgeable, ones may make their diagnosis seem obvious and avoid re-operative surgery for a potentially non-surgical problem. This may lead to taking shortcuts, skipping a full work-up or less than full history-taking. 'Rush' patients who come from a long distance and claim to have little time to spend prior to re-operative surgery deserve to complete a full work-up without compromise (Table 2).

An adequately detailed history and physical examination, in conjunction with basic studies is valuable for documentation and to direct further work-up as required. While the basic work-ups are similar to primary bariatric surgical work-ups, additional GI tract and malnutrition evaluations are important considerations. Also of note, we have found a surprisingly large number of re-operative candidates, among whom are the nicest, most respectable-appearing patients, who have positive alcohol-drug screens.

Table 1. General principles for re-operative bariatric surgery are the same whether performed open or laparoscopically

Be sceptical
Defer surgery if any doubt
Inexperience dangerous
Expect the unexpected
Making 'psych' diagnosis is by exclusion
Get old operative note(s) if possible

Table 2. Basic pre-op re-operative bariatric surgery work-up

H and P with detailed 'detective work'
CBC, SMAC, Mg, lipids, PT, PTT
Thyroid function tests
Amylase, lipase
Vitamins, zinc
HIV if nutritional problem
Chest X-ray
Electrocardiogram
Pulmonary function tests (if indicated)
Echocardiogram (if indicated)
Anaemia and other work-up (if indicated)
Drug and alcohol screen in all

General principle: inexperience dangerous

Reoperative bariatric surgery can provide challenges as great as the general surgeon will encounter. Therefore, consulting about re-operative cases with experienced colleagues can prove valuable. When in doubt, refer. The bariatric surgeon is wise to delay any re-operative bariatric surgery until completing at least thirty, and preferably more, primary bariatric surgeries to a well-experienced re-operative bariatric surgeon or have one assist.

The International Federation for the Surgery of Obesity recommends considerable prior experience with primary bariatric surgery and encourages discussion of problems with more experienced colleagues or referral to them[1].

General principle: expect the unexpected

In the vast majority of our 800 re-operative bariatric surgical procedures, we have found more than one problem to address for nausea, vomiting, abdominal pain and dysphagia. It has included, but not exclusively, large diverticula at a stapled enteroenterostomy or a gastroenterostomy, internal hernia, redundant partially obstructing alimentary limb above the mesocolon, kinked gastric pouch due to liver adhesion, surgery not described in prior surgical operative note(s), fistula, incarcerated ventral hernia, tumour, gall bladder or other pathology.

General principle: 'psych problem' is a diagnosis of exclusion

It can be far too easy to explain a patient's complaints on the basis of 'it is all in his/her mind', or, worse, 'she's/he's crazy'. Patients may have co-existent or pre-existing psychopathology or it may have arisen in response to the patient's inability to cope with organic problems. Each deserves a complete work-up before excluding every other possibility prior to attributing the patient's complaints as essentially psychiatric in origin.

General principle: get old operative note if possible

Where prior operative notes have not been available, it is possible to 'figure out' the prior operative procedure. However, this effort may lead to extended anesthesia and surgical time required for additional dissection and exploration. The uncertainty increases chances of unexpected findings during surgery with, sometimes, additional or modified procedure(s) as a result.

Upper GI endoscopy and radionuclide scanning

The basic work-up (Table 2) is usually followed by upper GI endoscopy (EGD) which may demonstrate the source of the basic problem as listed in Table 3. Most of these entities, such as peptic ulcer, stomal stenosis, bezoar and pouch gastritis are potentially amenable to non-surgical treatment. Others, such as fistula, stenosis not remediable with intra-luminal dilatation, short alimentary limb or loop gastric bypass with reflux esophagitis and gastritis, diverticula are objective indications for surgery.

Where an EGD is not diagnostically productive, liquid and solid phase radionuclide scanning is indicated. It has the ability to clearly identify quantitatively the presence (or absence) of incomplete emptying and slow transit times. It is sometimes the strongest objective indication to proceed with re-operative bariatric surgery.

Table 3. Some possible endoscopic findings by direct visualization

Ulcer
Stenosis stoma or gastric pouch
Foreign body erosion
Gastric pouch bezoar
Gastric pouch inflammation
Fistula
Loop gastric bypass
Gastric or jejunal diverticulum
Jejunitis
Bile or bile staining

Other diagnostic possibilities

Detailed history-taking concerning nausea and vomiting may uncover a history of dizziness, vertigo, hearing changes or car-sickness. A trial of medication may alleviate much of the problem. Additionally, chronic draining sinusitis material may be the source of pouch gastritis, vomit or regurgitation and abdominal pain. Although patients are warned to avoid aspirin and NSAIDS, their arthritic or other pain problems may 'demand' their use with subsequent gastritis, ulceration, stenosis, GI bleeding and even perforation. Malnutrition may be elicited by history or physical findings such as cheilosis, magenta tongue, oro-pharyngeal or esophagel (by EGD) moniliasis. Other infections such as actinomycosis and *H. pylori* may also be responsible for symptomatology.

When reactive hypoglycaemia is documented, we have recommended frequent, smaller meals and acarbose 25 mg tid po with benefit. Dumping syndrome symptomatology may also be controlled by dietary modifications and medications.

Diarrhea, with or without malnutrition, may be associated with short bowel syndrome, gastro-colic fistula (barium enema may be the only way to demonstrate due to pressure differentials between the stomach and colon), *C. difficile* or other GI infection, medication side-effects, low serum zinc, low serum calcium or patient non-compliance. Diarrhoea may be effectively treated with *per os* lactobacillus, donnatal, metamucil, a BRATT (bananas, rice, apple sauce, tea and toast) diet, but the patient may require hospital admission for re-hydration, as well as TPN.

Once treated medically, surgery may sometimes become unnecessary or, at least, deferred for further observation longer-term. The surgical treatment of a purely medical condition has limited chance for success.

Psychosocial pathology

Considerable psychosocial pathology exists in the bariatric surgical population, much secondary to their condition. For example, eighty-nine per cent of patients presenting to our clinic for consideration for primary bariatric surgery tested positive for depression, which appeared largely centred around their inability to achieve a sustained weight loss[2]. This presentation is often exacerbated in patients presenting with significant problems following earlier bariatric surgery. In many, their abdominal pain and other symptoms were considerably magnified by depression. We have documented Von Munchhausen's syndrome associated with incredible histories and clinical course[3].

Substance abuse

Many re-operative candidates receive chronic narcotic prescriptions for headaches, low back pain, abdominal pain and other complaints. A few others test positive for alcohol, marihuana and non-prescribed medications. It is important to know one's patient sufficiently in order to balance re-operative risks where surgically-remediable problems exist versus benefits in a known addict, substance abuser or chronic pain patient. When we have performed surgery in these patients, they soon taught us the wisdom of deferring substance abuse treatment until full post-operative recovery.

Patient requests surgical reversal of bariatric surgery

Very rarely is bariatric surgical reversal justified. Following reversal, patient weight increases to earlier, pre-op levels often plus a bonus for the weight gain that would have occurred during the post-bariatric surgical period. Ultimately, the reversed patient has had two major surgical procedures without any long-term benefit. Patients often present with anger, at themselves or others, for having undergone this surgery which they find themselves unable to tolerate. They may be almost hysterical, anxious or unreasonable. A counseling session by an experienced bariatric surgeon followed by a 'cooling off' period may allow the patient to become more reasonable and permit constructive counseling and further work-up. As a result, more than half of patients may accept alternatives such as pouch or enteral limb modification in lieu of complete reversal. Some patients seek general surgeons who may be all-too-willing to reverse them. It seems irresponsible for a general surgeon, lacking qualifications and experience in bariatric surgery, to reverse a bariatric surgery.

Pre-op principle: have complete bowel prep and antibiotic cover

The unexpected needs to be covered since re-operative bariatric surgery can result in different procedures than planned pre-operatively. Dense adhesions may also result in inadvertent spillage of gastric or intestinal content. Prophylactic antibiotics are known to reduce risk of post-operative infection. The contents of the bypassed stomach have about a two-thirds chance of containing microorganisms[4]. Therefore, we regularly use propylene glycol bowel prep and quadruple antibiotics, usually gentamycin, clindamycin, flucanazole and Cipro and recommend them for use by others.

Pre-op principle: documented, complete informed consent is important

Informed consent is a process which begins with the patient first becoming aware of bariatric surgery. The experience of prior bariatric surgery and its sequellae also informs the patient in addition to information learned from other patients, the bariatric surgeon and staff. The patient has a responsibility to not sign the final stage of the informed consent process until he/she is satisfied that he/she understands the nature of the proposed procedure(s), options, risks, benefits, possible complications, implications and has had the opportunity to have questions answered satisfactorily.

The informed consent process is usually concluded by the patient signing a document certifying, among other things, that he/she is adequately informed about the proposed operative procedure(s). This process is meant to assure that the patient understands the procedure(s) and alternative options as well the risks, benefits, possible complications and implications of the surgery to be performed by the named surgeon(s). Most bariatric surgeons do an excellent job of informed consent for primary bariatric surgery[5]. From a risk management perspective, it would seem extremely difficult for a patient to claim not to have understood the informed consent material when he/she has, signed and witnessed, correctly answered questions concerning it.

Re-operative bariatric surgery, however, is more unpredictable than primary bariatric surgery. Unforeseen findings during laparotomy are considerably more frequent, necessitating change(s) to the originally planned re-operative bariatric surgical or other procedure. By signing, the patient indicates that he/she knows of this possibility as well as the possibility of a future re-operation being required.

Table 4. The pre-operative principles for re-operative bariatric surgery are the same whether performed open or laparoscopically

Pre-operative principles
Full bowel prep and antibiotics begun
Careful, complete informed consent documented
Use the 'fifty percent rule' to counsel
Defer surgery if any doubt
Re-review work-up and old op note
Gastric X-rays hanging in OR

Table 5. Dissection and resection basic principles for re-operative bariatric surgery are the same whether performed open or laparoscopically

Remove old hardware if not too burdensome
Resect or modify large diverticuli

If operating that area,
    Be flexible with gastric dissection
    (but, keep pouch orientation)
    Mark old gastric staple-lines
    Measure all intestinal limbs
    Dissect from the edges

Table 6. Principles to minimize post-operative problems following re-operative bariatric surgery

Place omentum or other barrier between gastric pouch and liver
Use oro-gastric tube, not naso-gastric tube
Make your most recent re-op procedure your best

Pre-operative principle: use the 'fifty percent rule' to counsel

Some time during the patient-surgeon encounter for possible re-operative bariatric surgery, we have found it useful to ask the patient 'If we were to improve your problems 50 per cent, would that be satisfactory for you?' At later post-operative office visits, we ask whether we have achieved this goal and usually the answer is 'Yes, you have exceeded it'. and indicate 90 per cent or better. This helps prevents patient dissatisfaction with even a 95 per cent or 99 per cent good outcome expectation. It is wise to have this understanding in writing to later refer to if needed.

General principle: defer surgery when in any doubt

It takes 'courage' to re-schedule surgery where the easiest course is to proceed as initially scheduled. However, patients with marginal or poor nutrition, actual or potential infection, questionable behaviour (also by their significant others), inadequate documentation, concernworthy work-up findings and even the surgeon having 'an uneasy feeling' are valid bases for canceling surgery even as late as the immediate pre-operative period.

Pre-op principle: re-review work-up and old op note and gastric x-rays on view box in OR

When available, prior operative note(s) may be valuable. Well-performed upper GI studies provide useful 'road-maps', augmenting endoscopic study; we insist on having them displayed in the OR during surgery. They are often a good guide to dissection or its prudent limitation.

The following are discussions of dissection/resection principles of re-operative bariatric surgery that apply to the surgery itself (Table 5).

Dissection/resection principle: remove old hardware if not burdensome

During re-operative surgery, we prefer, as a general principle, to remove pre-existing, bypassed, foreign bodies, such as Marlex mesh vertical banded gastroplasty bands or rings. However, bands that erode through the mucosa are a necessity to remove due to their septic potential; we have seen them in association with pylephlebitis, hepatic abscess and septicaemia. Since the foreign bodies are often located in the bypassed stomach, they are not easily visualized for direct evaluation, and possible endoscopic management, at some later time.

Dissection/resection principle: resect or modify large diverticuli

The dynamically motile stomach may migrate under the band to enlarge the pouch, sometimes producing a Zenker's-like diverticulum hanging over the band. Band replacement or removal is necessary.

The end-to-side gastroenteric anastomosis can result in the small intestine hanging from the gastric pouch like the crook of a cane. The blind end may preferentially fill and, over time, become enlarged, producing symptoms of nausea, vomiting abdominal pain, regurgitation and dysphagia. Moderate or large diverticula, are sometimes found unexpectedly at surgery, and may be considered a potential source of pre-op complaints. Alternatively, the surgeon may elect to elevate the enteric diverticulum, suturing it to the lateral aspect of the gastric pouch, sometimes to reinforce a fresh pouch staple or suture line.

A stapled, functional end-to-side enterostomy not uncommonly produces, long-term, two blind end diverticula. When sufficiently large, particularly when they are being moved to the biliopancreatic limb, resection as prophylaxis for subsequent stasis with blind limb syndrome is wise.

Dissection/resection principle: if operating in the region of the stomach, be flexible with dissection (and, keep pouch orientation to avoid excessive bleeding)

Dense adhesions often make it difficult to dissect around different parts of the gastric pouch. However, at least one of the multiple different approaches inevitably works. This includes dissecting: (1) across and caudal to the Angle of His; (2) high lesser curvature gastro-hepatic omentum; (3) lower lesser curvature gastro-hepatic omentum; (4) lesser sac via opening the gastro-colic ligament; (5) craniad along the proximal small intestine, starting with the most visible part and continuing to the gastric pouch; (6) as a continuation of peri-esophageal dissection but in a caudad direction.

When anterior gastric dissection becomes tedious and bloody, pack the area and dissect posteriorly through one of the other approaches listed. It helps to avoid injuring short gastric or lesser curvature vessels by periodically pausing and re-orienting dissection towards the bougie or other tube passed into the gastric pouch. With prior horizontal gastric stapling, cautiously approach and handle the staple line near the greater curvature as it is often adherent in the region of the splenic hilar vessels.

Dissection/resection principle: if operating upon the stomach, mark old gastric staple-lines

Identify staples and mark them with through-and-through #3-0 silk sutures two to three centimeters apart. An intra-gastric naso-gastric tube or bougie may be manipulated against, or through, staple lines to identify the location of staple line gaps by palpation. Occasionally, a gastrotomy is required to determine exact staple location or absence visually or by internal palpation. Traction on the sutures guides precise stapler placement on either side.

Dissection/resection principle: if altering small intestinal length, measure all intestinal limbs

Decisions regarding limb length adjustments are best made with a knowledge of the length of each intestinal Roux-en-Y limb. Following surgery, even years later, recorded limb lengths may be valuable information regarding potential for re-operative obesity surgery or its avoidance. Measurement of the stretched intestine along the anti-mesenteric border is the generally performed measurement.

Dissection/resection principle: dissect from the edges

It is easy for the surgeon to persist in dissection until reaching his/her goal and wind up 'digging in a hole' which may produce more problems than benefits. The wise surgeon is alert to reaching this point and moves his/her attention to either side, i.e. towards the 'edges' away from the prior dissection. Later, the dissections along this 'broad front' unite promoting further, deeper dissection.

Principles to minimize post-op problems: place omentum or other barrier between gastric pouch and liver

Adhesions between the liver and gastric pouch can cause pouch kinking with partial or complete obstruction. Omental interposition removes this possibility. When omentum is inadequate for this purpose, material such as Seprafilm may be used satisfactorily in its place.

961

Principles to minimize post-op problems: use oro-gastric tube, not naso-gastric tube

Post-op fever of unknown origin may arise from the nasal sinuses due to tube trauma, inflammation and partial obstruction in conjunction with use of a nasogastric tube. The alternative use of an oro-gastric tube placed after anesthetic induction works well and appears to lower post-operative complications from this source. Post-operatively, the old habit of leaving in an NGT is rarely useful and it is best removed (or, better still, not inserted) in most instances.

Principles to minimize post-op problems: make your most recent re-op procedure your best

Nowhere else in bariatric surgery is it more important than to learn from one's operative experience. The goal is to do better each operative case than the one preceding.

Some specific guidance points are offered in addition to the more generalized principles.

Guidance: handling small bowel obstruction (partial or total, recurrent)

Severe, intractable peri-umbilical, colicky pain, poorly responsive to narcotics, often with nausea and without a recent bowel movement or flatus, is a small bowel obstruction until proven otherwise. Patients with distal obstruction may not vomit early in the course of the obstruction. This is no reason for surgical delay. The old adage 'Never let the sun set on a small bowel obstruction' remains relevant and wise.

We have had a 2 per cent incidence of small bowel obstruction following bariatric surgery, with 2.5 per cent of these patients developing recurrent obstruction. The majority of obstructions are due to an obstructing band in the ileum around which small intestine may form a volvulus or a severe angulation. Massive weight loss lengthens and thins out the intestinal mesentery making it capable of volvulus around adhesions which shift with massive weight loss. We have seen only two cases of intussusception in over 4000 bariatric surgical patients; other experienced bariatric surgeons personally communicated similar incidences. During surgery for possible obstruction, it is important to explore further for internal herniation, particularly following laparoscopy. Potential sites include the enteroenterostomy mesenteric junction and the mesocolic opening for retro-colic alimentary limb passage.

Guidance: handling bilio-pancreatic (afferent) limb obstruction

Bilio-pancreatic (afferent) limb obstruction or partial obstruction is a potentially lethal condition, particularly because it may be overlooked by the inexperienced clinician. The afferent limb represents the bypassed small intestine and, therefore, orally-ingested contrast material does not reach it. The back pressure of a complete or partial bilio-pancreatic limb obstruction on the common bile duct, pancreatic duct, native (distal, bypassed) stomach increases with time, usually causing elevations in serum amylase, lipase and liver function tests as well as tachycardia and hypotension. Ante-colic alimentary limb blood supply may be interrupted by marked distention of the native (by-passed) stomach that over-stretches the limb anteriorly and may result in limb gangrene or stomal disruption. CT scan of the abdomen will usually detect a distended C-loop, native stomach and, sometimes, an overstretched alimentary limb; it is best to review the films with the radiologist who may not be completely familiar with this potentially-lethal presentation.

Operative guidance: mesenteric imbrication for recurrent volvulus

Following massive weight loss, the intestinal mesentery lengthens up to about 30 cm. as measured from the mesenteric root to the intestine. In the rare instances of recurrent large or small intestinal volvulus, we have imbricated all of the lengthened mesenteric visceral peritoneum to 10 cm or less so that it no longer can twist upon itself to re-form a volvulus. We employ #3-0 silks held with snaps, taking care to angle them in towards the root of the mesentery. The visceral peritoneum lies quite loosely over its contained vessels following the mesenteric fat loss and is readily sutured without damage taking five or so small bites per suture. We have experienced no post-operative problems related to this technique[6].

Operative guidance: gastric pouch re-modeling and 'Bermuda triangles'

Exceptionally enlarged gastric pouches may be reduced in size by stapling off a new pouch within the old. Edward E. Mason first named this pouch-in-a-pouch 'Faberge' technique.

Straight gastric staple lines do not always remain straight. Over time, they can become irregular, often S-shaped. During re-operative surgery, firing a straight stapler over an incompletely-defined S-shaped staple line can unintentionally entrap one or more gastric segments, appropriately named 'Bermuda triangles'. They may become cystic due to gastric mucosal secretion, enlarge further and disrupt, sometimes disastrously. To prevent Bermuda triangles, we carefully mark prior gastric staple lines with sutures, as described earlier, before gastric re-stapling or resection.

Operative guidance: pouch banding/re-banding

Gastric bands added to, or removed from, gastric bypass procedures appear responsible for 15 to 40 pounds additional weight loss or gain. Following band removal, repair of gastrogastric fistula or pouch re-sizing, a gastric band may be placed. Location ideally is as a proximal 'sling' around the Angle of His and across the lesser curvature about 2 to 3 cm from its uppermost end. The band circumference is usually 6.5 cm, sometimes larger. The only band which has not eroded in our series is the composite band.

Operative guidance: composite band. composite banding

For about 15 years, we have been placing a 'composite band' around selected re-operative gastric pouches to maintain the pouch diameter long-term. The band consists of a 1½ x 9 cm midline fascial strip obtained while opening the abdomen. The central 6½ cm is measured and marked at its extremes with metal clips. Multiple bites with a #5 Ethibond suture are taken in the outer side side of the band along the 6½ cm marked length. The band is placed through a previously-channeled posterior gastric pouch track with the #5 suture on the outside and then sutured to its opposite end at the 6½ cm clip marker level. The suture is tied with a #34F or #36F bougie in place. We have had no recorded erosions of any composite band, experience supporting theory that the fascial band buffers the suture from eroding the gastric pouch. This 'belt and suspenders' construction provides the suture to maintain the desired diameter in case the fascia weakens.

Operative guidance: limb lengths

The average small bowel length in the morbidly obese patient is twenty feet. If the patient with prior gastric bypass is not having frequent or diarrhea stools, he/she has demonstrated the likely ability to handle half of the total enteric length being bypassed – unlike the non-operated bariatric population, this person has passed the 'bariatric surgery intestinal tolerance test'. For weight re-gain or refractoriness to weight loss, we have frequently bypassed at least half of the enteric length. This involves fashioning a three foot alimentary limb and a seven foot common limb, with the remainder constituting the biliopancreatic limb. Where the total of alimentary limb and common limb lengths exceed twelve feet, little additional weight is lost beyond the weight loss experienced with a regular gastric bypass. It is wise to document small bowel limb lengths particularly when altering them. We use a known length of umbilical tape along the well-stretched anti-mesenteric border, moving the tape proximally from the ileo-cecal valve. Other patients 'flunk' the 'gastric bypass tolerance test' and develop dumping syndrome.

Controlling dumping

Remedial surgery was required on five patients referred with uncontrollable dumping following gastric bypass Roux-en-Y. In each case, we divided and re-anastomosed the two ends of a ninety centimeter segment of the common limb *in situ*. We also divided the intestinal mesentery down to its root at both intestinal division points. This effectively interrupted intestinal hyperperistalsis sufficient to control the patients' dumping.

Operative guidance: thal-type patches

On occasion, the surgeon may become concerned about the integrity of a gastric pouch suture or staple line. To buttress it, we have rotated the native (bypassed) stomach sufficiently to place a tension-free row of interrupted #3-0 silk sutures between the sero-muscularis of the posterior by-passed stomach wall and the pouch posterior to the staple or suture line. We then complete encirclement of the gastric pouch reinforcement site with an anterior row of sutures between the two stomach segments, tying them when completed.

This variation of a Thal patch has also functioned as a buttress over closure of a fistula or acute gastric leak. It is important to avoid tension between the structures and not use the gastrostomy tube for enteral feeding since the distended bypassed stomach may damage the repair.

Operative guidance: proximal jejunal diverticuli resected and as reinforcement patches

The end-to-side anastomosis of gastric pouch to small intestine leaves a stapled end of small intestine protruding laterally. With time, the intestine may enlarge and become dependent, overlapping the gastroenterostomy like a Zenker's diverticulum. This may be accompanied by intermittent nausea, vomiting and dysphagia. At upper GI endoscopy, the scope may advance directly into the diverticulum rather than pass through the gastroenterostomy stoma; an upper GI radiography may show the diverticulum filled with contrast material that may not readily empty. To minimize this occurrence during primary bariatric surgery, we advance the jejunum craniad and suture it with three #3-0 silks to the lateral distal one-half of the gastric pouch.

When a jejunal diverticulum at the stoma is present, we have either resected it or tacked it to the lateral aspect of the gastric pouch, sometimes surrounding a stapled and divided gastrogastric fistula as a reinforcement. When present, it is a convenient alternative to the Thal-type gastric patch.

Operative guidance: gastrostomy tube

Patients who have had pre-operative nausea, vomiting, dysphagia may need time to readjust to adequate oral intake. Post-operative native stomach decompression as well as possible post-operative gastrostomy feedings and medications are indications for tube placement where a residual, bypassed stomach exists.

Operative guidance: drains

Post-operative leakage rarely occurs but, when it does, early warning is important. A drain can serve this function and also potentially channel drainage externally as a 'controlled leak'. Our preferred drain is a large triple-lumen Davol surrounded on either side with a wide Penrose drain that buffers the intermittent low Gomco drainage suction from causing harm to adjacent tissues; in addition, we make sure that no part of any drain comes within 2 to 3 cm of any suture or stapling site. We suture the Penrose drains as well as the Gomco collar to the skin with #0 Silk and also place a suture through the collar edge and one of the Gomco sump channels to prevent drain migration due to traction. Any questionable drainage can be sent to the lab for an amylase analysis which, if elevated, indicates probable leakage.

Conclusion

The logic and principles for performing re-operative bariatric surgery open or laparoscopically as described herein are essentially the same. This surgery involves an integration of this complex information into practice. The surgeon also requires knowledge of options to detect and handle different, unique or unexpected situations, sometimes causing the original operative plan to be altered. In complex cases or early in the re-operative bariatric surgeon's experience, discussion of the optimal use of these options is ideally carried out before surgery with a well-experienced bariatric surgeon. This will help optimize decision-making which is the key to successful re-operative bariatric surgery.

References

1. The Cancun IFSO statement on bariatric surgeon qualifications. *Obes Surg* 1998; 8: 36.

2. Cowan GSM, III, Buffington CK, Vickerstaff S, Cowan GSM, Jr. Psychological status of the morbidly obese. *Obes Surg* 6: 107, 1996.

3. Cowan GSM Jr, Battle AO, Buffington C *et al*. Munchausen's syndrome in post-operative bariatric surgical patients. *Obes Surg* 1997: 98–9.

4. Uramatsu S, Cowan GSM Jr, Hiler ML *et al*. Infectious potential of the bypassed stomach in gastric bypass patients. *Obes Surg* 1996; 6: 307 (Abstract).

5. Cowan, G.S.M., Jr. Informed Consent in Bariatric Surgery, Chapter 27 in *Obesity surgery*, M. Deitel (ed.), pp. 327–337. Lea & Febiger, 1989.

6. Cowan GSM, Hiler ML. A new anti-volvulus imbrication technique to correct mesenteric lengthening which occurs following massive weight loss. *Obes Surg* 3: 2002 (in press).

Progress in Obesity Research: 9. Edited by *Geraldo Medeiros-Neto, Alfredo Halpern* and *Claude Bouchard*
©2003 John Libbey Eurotext Ltd, pp. 965–968.

CHAPTER 200

Cost-effectiveness of surgery

Kristina Narbro

Department of Body Composition and Metabolism, The Sahlgrenska Academy at Göteborg University, Sahlgrenska University Hospital, SE-413 45 Göteborg, Sweden
[e-mail: kristina.narbro@medfak.gu.se]

Introduction

Obesity-related chronic diseases and poor psychosocial functioning impose a sizeable economic burden on both society and the individual in terms of health care expenditures and losses in productivity[1]. Obesity-related costs due to productivity losses, i.e. indirect costs, in the US are similar to those due to diseases attributable to cigarette smoking[2]. In Sweden, an estimated 7 to 10 per cent of the total indirect cost of sick leave and disability pension is related to obesity[3]. Direct health care expenditures attributable to obesity are estimated at 1 to 6 per cent in affluent countries[1]. Although these cost-of-illness estimates give a picture of the economic consequences of the natural course of obesity and stress the importance of the disease, they provide no indication of whether or not the money spent on obesity and obesity-related disorders is used in an efficient way. Thus, economic evaluations, e.g. cost-effectiveness analysis, that take into account both costs and effects of alternative strategies for treating obesity are needed.

Effect of surgery on health care utilization and costs

Although the effect of weight loss on *total* health service utilization is sparsely studied, some studies have reported a reduced use of medication following surgically-induced weight loss. MacDonald *et al.*[4] studied 232 obese patients with non-insulin dependent diabetes mellitus (NIDDM), and found that the proportion of surgically treated patients on diabetes medication decreased from 32 per cent before treatment to 9 per cent after 9 years, while in the weight-stable, obese control group the corresponding figures were 56 per cent at baseline and 87 per cent after 6 years. A recent report from the ongoing nation-wide intervention study of obesity, the Swedish Obese Subjects study (SOS) showed that nearly a third of the surgically treated patients with an average weight loss of 16 per cent were able to discontinue their diabetes medication after 6 years, while none of the conventionally treated obese controls with a relative weight increase of 1 per cent were[5].

Weight loss has also been associated with a decreased use of other medications. Surgical studies with average weight losses of 30–35 per cent have reported a 30–50 per cent reduction in the number of patients requiring medication for hypertension 4 to 6 years after surgery[6,7]. In the SOS study, 38 per cent of the surgically treated and 9 per cent of the conventionally treated patients were able to discontinue medication for cardiovascular disease (CVD) after 2 years. The corresponding figures at the 6-year follow-up were 35 per cent and 14 per cent, respectively[5].

Few studies have estimated changes in the direct *costs* of health care in relation to weight reduction. Collins and Anderson[8] analysed medication costs among 32 obese persons with NIDDM, who partici-pated in a hypocaloric programme. An average weight loss of 9 per cent over 1 year was associated with a 50 per cent reduction per person in the out-of-pocket cost for diabetes and hypertension medications. Greenway *et al.*[9] analysed pharmaceutical costs in 73 patients treated with weight loss medications. After 2 to 3 months of treatment and weight losses of 6–10 per cent of the initial body weight, a net pharmaceutical cost saving was observed. In contrast, Ågren *et al.*[5], who have analysed pooled data from 965 surgically and conventionally treated patients in the SOS study, report that a weight reduction of ≥ 15 per cent of initial body weight is required to reduce the average cost for diabetes and CVD medication over 6 years among patients initially taking these medications.

Unpublished SOS data show that the cost for diabetes and cardiovascular disease medication was markedly lower in the surgically treated group compared with the conventionally treated group during 6 years of follow-up. However, these cost reductions were counter-balanced by higher costs for other types of medication, resulting in similar total cost for prescribed medications among surgically and conventionally treated patients over 6 years. Data from the SOS study also show an increased hospitalization and higher costs for in-patient care over 6 years among the surgically treated patients compared with the conventionally treated patients.

Effect of surgery on working ability

Several studies have reported a decrease in sick leave and an increase in employment rates after surgical treatment of obesity. For example, in a study of 240 surgically treated patients, Hawke et al.[10] found that employment rates improved from 38 per cent before surgery to 60 per cent after 3 years. Similarly, a smaller study by van Gemert et al.[11] of vertical banded gastroplasty (VBG) patients reported improved employment rates from 19 per cent before treatment to 48 per cent 2 years after surgery. They also reported that sick leave decreased from 38 per cent to 10 per cent among these patients. In the SOS study[12], the surgically treated patients averaged 35 per cent more days of sick leave plus disability pension than the weight stable control group during the first postoperative year, but they had 10–14 per cent fewer days during years 2 to 3 after inclusion. However, during the fourth year of follow-up the difference between the groups decreased. It is noteworthy that the differences between the surgical group and the control group 2 to 4 years after inclusion were greatest among the older patients.

Cost-effectiveness analysis

In cost-effectiveness analysis (CEA), all relevant costs arising from a treatment are related to one or several measures of outcome[13]. However, there is no available golden standard for what might be a cost-effective alternative. This is a question of relative cost-effectiveness, i.e. how cost-effective a certain treatment is in relation to existing alternative treatments.

Costs are expressed in monetary terms and the outcomes are expressed in natural units, such as cost per patient treated, cost per kg weight loss, cost per life saved, or cost per year of life saved. Costs included in cost-effectiveness analysis vary depending on the perspective of the analysis, e.g. the patient's, the payer's, the government's or the society's[13].

If the elements included in the economic evaluation are uncertain, a sensitivity analysis may be performed to supplement ordinary statistical analysis[13]. Sensitivity analysis varies estimates of uncertain factors (e.g. the effectiveness of the treatment) within some plausible range to determine how sensitive the conclusions of the economic evaluation are to these variations.

A special form of CEA, sometimes called cost-utility analysis (CUA), takes into account the effects of a treatment on the quality and the length of life[13]. The health outcomes of a treatment are then valued, combined and reported in quality-adjusted years of life saved, so-called QALYs. The number of QALYs are calculated as the product of the time spent in a specific health state and a quality weight assigned to that particular health state. The quality weights are derived either from population-based or research-based assessments of the value of not having or not getting a certain disease. CUA is useful when the evaluated treatment influences morbidity more than mortality. CUA can also be used to compare treatments for different diseases, but the lack of standard methods to value health outcomes makes comparisons somewhat problematic.

Cost-effectiveness analysis of surgery

Several studies have estimated how much it would cost to achieve a 1 per cent-unit reduction in the rate of overweight. Estimates in the United States average less than US$35 for behavioural therapy and very low calorie diet programmes[14]. In Denmark, the cost was about US$12 per person for a diet programme[15]. Although conventional treatment may be cost-effective in the short-term as shown in these studies, weight loss is seldom maintained over a longer period[1,14]. Therefore, in the long run, more expensive treatments with large and sustained weight losses could be more cost-effective than conventional treatment. This is illustrated in a study by Martin et al.[16], in which they compared the cost per pound of weight loss for gastric bypass with the costs for a medical programme that consisted of a very-low-calorie diet in combination with behaviour modification. The direct cost per patient in the medical programme over 1.5 years was US$3000, while surgery (including pre-operative testing) was estimated to cost eight times that. However, estimates of the cost per pound lost showed that after 2 years the cost of surgery was only two and a half times that of the medical programme (US$100). Notably, after 6 years the cost of surgery was actually less than that of the medical programme, US$750 vs. US$1600. In these estimates, all patients who were lost to follow-up were assumed to have no weight loss. When these patients were excluded from the analysis the cost per pound lost was decreased markedly but was still higher in the medically treated group compared to the surgically treated group at 6-year follow-up.

Cost-utility analysis of surgery

To date, few published studies have reported on cost-utility analysis of obesity treatment. In a literature-based analysis of obesity surgery from the United Kingdom[17] the cost per QALY was calculated for VBG in the treatment of morbid (BMI $\geq$ 40 kg/m^2) obesity. The success rate of VBG treatment was derived from the literature, and it was estimated that among 100 patients treated, 24 to 44 QALYs could be gained over a 5-year period. It was assumed that no QALYs were gained after 5 years. The direct health care cost of VBG and 5 years of follow-up totalled UK£5800 per patient. Depending on the assumptions of revision and reoperation, the cost of treating 100 patients with VBG ranged from UK£635,000–727,000 and the cost per QALY gained ranged from UK£14,500–30,300.

Another recent literature review from the United Kingdom[18] compared different types of surgery with non-surgical treatment. Costs (including pre-operative treatment, surgery, management of complications/revisions and annual follow-up), cost savings from avoiding diabetes, and QALYs were calculated over 20 years. The direct treatment costs for 100 patients ranged from UK£696,400 for non-surgical treatment to UK£1,079,500 for silicone adjustable gastric banding (SAGB). For 100 patients treated, it was estimated that VBG yielded 26 more QALYs than non-surgical treatment and the cost-utility was calculated to be UK£10,237 per QALY gained. SAGB yielded 45 more QALYs than non-surgical treatment and the cost per QALY gained was UK£8527. The corresponding figures for Roux-en-Y gastric bypass were 45 QALYs and UK£6289. In a sensitivity analysis the assumptions about the length of hospital stay, costs for pre- and post-operative care, costs for treating comorbidities, weight loss, and utility gain were altered, and the cost per QALY gained for surgical compared to non-surgical treatment was then estimated to be UK£20,000–30,000.

In an individually based study from the Netherlands[11], vanGemert *et al.* calculated the 2-year direct cost of VBG (including management of complications, out-patient visits and hospitalizations) in a group of 21 morbidly obese patients. Compared to the pre-operative status, the quality of life improved markedly 2 years after the intervention. The authors assumed that this improvement would persist over the remaining lifetime and estimated that 12 QALYs could be gained in a life-long scenario. Surgical intervention was assumed to save direct health care costs for obesity-related co-morbidities. Compared to a 'do nothing' alternative (estimated as the lifetime direct cost-of-illness), the intervention was estimated to save about US$100–180 per QALY gained. When savings in indirect costs were included in the analysis, surgical treatment was reported to save about US$4000 per QALY gained.

The study by vanGemert *et al.*[11] reported on savings in direct health care costs per QALY gained, while the literature-based studies[17,18] estimated a relative large direct health care cost per QALY gained. This discrepancy could owe to differences in treatment costs in the different countries, different time perspectives for the analyses, and different assumptions about the possible gain in quality of life after treatment.

The results from the studies of surgical treatment can be compared with literature-based studies of the drugs orlistat[19] and sibutramine[20]. Compared to placebo, orlistat had a direct treatment cost per QALY gained of UK£45,000 (range in sensitivity analysis: UK£19,450–55,400)[19]. In a comparison of sibutramine with placebo over 5 years, the net direct cost (including cost savings for coronary heart disease and diabetes) per QALY gained was estimated to be UK£10,500 (range in sensitivity analysis: UK£5700–35,200)[20].

Although the cost per person for surgical treatment is higher than for pharmaceutical treatment, the cost per QALY gained seems to be similar or even lower. However, all studies are based on several assumptions about costs and the possible gain in quality of life after treatment. The time perspective and the type of costs included differed between the studies and some studies included cost savings while other studies did not. Hence, the results from these CUA must be interpreted with some caution.

Conclusions

Sick leave and disability pension rates might be decreased with surgically induced weight loss. Surgical obesity treatment also reduces some of the increased health care expenditures that have been observed among the obese. On the other hand, other health care costs are increased by bariatric surgery and, so far, there is no evidence that surgical treatment of obesity reduces total health care expenditures over the first 6 years. However, this does not rule out the possibility that health care costs can be reduced in a longer perspective.

When both costs and consequences of surgical treatment are taken into account it seems that surgical treatment of obesity compared to life style changes produces extra QALYs at an incremental cost. Surgery might be cost-effective compared to pharmaceutical treatment, but long-term controlled intervention studies with data on both costs and consequences of different treatments are needed before really valid estimates can be obtained.

Acknowledgements: This study was supported by grants from The Swedish Medical Research Council (grant no. 05239), Stockholm, and The Centre for Public Sector Research, Göteborg University, Göteborg, Sweden.

References

1. World Health Organization. Obesity: Preventing and managing the global epidemic. Report of a WHO consultation, Geneva: WHO. 2000.

2. Wolf AM, Colditz GA. Current estimates of the economic cost of obesity in the United States. *Obes Res* 1998; 6: 97–106.

3. Narbro K, Jonsson E, Larsson B, Waaler H, Wedel H, Sjöström L. Economic consequences of sick-leave and early retirement in obese Swedish women. *Int J Obes Relat Metab Disord* 1996; 20: 895–903.

4. MacDonald KG, Long SD, Swanson MS, Brown BM., Morris P, Dohm GL, Pories WJ. The gastric bypass operation reduces the progression and mortality of non-insulin-dependent diabetes mellitus. *J Gastrointest Surg* 1997; 1: 213–20.

5. Ågren G, Narbro K, Näslund I, Sjöström L, Peltonen M. Long-term effects of weight loss on pharmaceutical costs in obese subjects. A report from the SOS intervention study. *Int J Obes Relat Metab Disord* 2002; 26: 184–92.

6. Carson JL, Ruddy ME, Duff AE, Holmes NJ, Cody RP, Brolin RE. The effect of gastric bypass surgery on hypertension in morbidly obese patients. *Arch Intern Med* 1994; 154: 193–200.

7. MacGregor AM, Rand CS. Gastric surgery in morbid obesity. Outcome in patients aged 55 years and older. *Arch Surg* 1993; 128: 1153–7.

8. Collins RW, Anderson JW. Medication cost savings associated with weight loss for obese non-insulin-dependent diabetic men and women. *Prev Med* 1995; 24: 369–74.

9. Greenway FL, Ryan DH, Bray GA, Rood JC, Tucker EW, Smith SR. Pharmaceutical cost savings of treating obesity with weight loss medications. *Obes Res* 1999; 7: 523–31.

10. Hawke A, O'Brien P, Watts JM, Hall J, Dunstan RE, Walsh JF et al. Psychosocial and physical activity changes after gastric restrictive procedures for morbid obesity. *Aust NZ J Surg* 1990; 60: 755–8.

11. van Gemert WG, Adang EM, Kop M, Vos G, Greve JW, Soeters PB. A prospective cost-effectiveness analysis of vertical banded gastroplasty for the treatment of morbid obesity. *Obes Surg* 1999; 9: 484–91.

12. Narbro K, Ågren G, Jonsson E, Larsson B, Näslund I, Wedel H, Sjöström L. Sick leave and disability pension before and after treatment of obesity. *Int J Obes Relat Metab Disord* 1999; 23: 619–24.

13. Drummond MF, O'Brien BJ, Stoddart GL, Torrance GW. *Methods for the economic evaluation of health care programmes* (2nd edn). Oxford: Oxford University Press; 1997.

14. Stunkard AJ, Cohen RY, Felix MR. Weight loss competitions at the worksite: how they work and how well. *Prev Med* 1989; 18: 460–74.

15. Siggaard R, Raben A, Astrup A. Weight loss during 12 weeks' *ad libitum* carbohydrate-rich diet in overweight and normal-weight subjects at a Danish work site. *Obes Res* 1996; 4: 347–56.

16. Martin LF, Tan TL, Horn JR, Bixler EO, Kauffman GL, Becker DA, Hunter SM. Comparison of the costs associated with medical and surgical treatment of obesity. *Surgery* 1995; 118: 599–607.

17. Bryant J, Best L, Milne R. Gastroplasty for severe obesity. Southampton: Wessex Insitute for Health Research and Development. DEC Report No. 68; 1997.

18. Clegg AJ, Colquitt J, Sidhu MK, Royle P, Loveman E, Walker A. The clinical effectiveness and cost-effectiveness of surgery for people with morbid obesity: a systematic review and economic evaluation. *Health Technol Assess* 2002; 6(12): 1–153.

19. Foxcroft D, Ludders J. Orlistat for the treatment of obesity. Southampton: Wessex Institute for Health Research and Development. Development and Evaluation Committee Report No.101; 1999.

20. O'Meara S, Riemsma R, Shirran L, Mather L, ter Riet G. The clinical effectiveness and cost-effectiveness of sibutramine in the management of obesity: a technology assessment. *Health Technol Assess* 2002; 6(6): 1–97.

Progress in Obesity Research: 9. Edited by *Geraldo Medeiros-Neto, Alfredo Halpern and Claude Bouchard*

CHAPTER 201

Baseline description of the SOS study group and nutritional changes over 10 years

Anna Karin Lindroos

*Department of Body Composition and Metabolism, The Sahlgrenska Academy at Göteborg University,
Sahlgrenska University Hospital, SE-413 45 Göteborg, Sweden
[e-mail: anna.karin.lindroos@medfak.gu.se]*

Introduction

The SOS study is an on-going intervention trial designed to determine whether the mortality and morbidity rates among obese individuals who lose weight by surgical means differ from rates associated with conventional treatment. The SOS study started in 1987 and the last participants were recruited to the study in December 2000. The design of the SOS Registry and Intervention studies have previously been describes in great detail[1]. Over the years several interim reports have been published from the on-going SOS study. A summary of results until year 2000 have been published by Sjöström[2]. The aim of the following presentation is to give an outline of the SOS study, to describe the study groups in the SOS Intervention study and nutritional changes after intervention.

Study design

The SOS study is made up of three different parts: a registry study, a reference study and an intervention study (Fig. 1). The SOS study is a collaboration between the primary health care, medical departments and surgical clinics in Sweden and the study is administered by a steering committee. A safety monitoring committee consisting of three members continuously supervises the mortality and the two hard end points cardiovascular events and stroke. All data collection is computerized and managed centrally from the SOS-secretariat in Gothenburg.

The SOS Registry study

The aim of the SOS Registry study was to find and offer obese subjects treatment, describe the obese patient with respect to body composition, metabolic aberrations, dietary habits, psychological and socio-economic variables. Furthermore to investigate the dependency of obesity on genetics and cultural factors and to serve as a recruitment base for the SOS Intervention study. Obese volunteers were recruited to the SOS registry study through advertisements in the mass media. Before the subjects were offered a health examination extensive questionnaires were mailed to them[1]. The questionnaires had to be completed and returned before the health examination. The health examination included anthropometry, systolic and diastolic blood pressure, ECG and blood sampling. Inclusion criteria for the registry study were age between 37 and 57 years, completed questionnaires, weight according to a weight-for-height-table giving BMIs for the shortest in each interval of 34 kg/m² for men and 38 kg/m² for women. A total of 6328 obese subjects (2460 men and 3868 women) are health examined in the SOS Registry study.

The SOS Intervention study

In the on-going SOS Intervention study surgically treated obese patients are compared with conventionally treated, obese controls. The primary aim of the SOS Intervention study is to study the influence of weight change on total mortality. Secondary aims are to study effects of weight change on risk factors and mortality and morbidity of specific diseases. Additional secondary aims are to study genetics, quality of life, economy and dietary habits in relation to obesity and weight reduction. The inclusion criteria for the SOS Intervention study were 37–60 years and BMI ≥ 34 kg/m² for men and ≥ 38 kg/m²

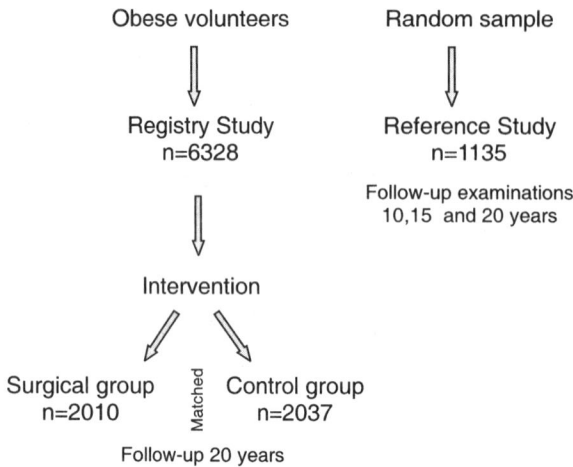

SOS
Swedish Obese Subjects

Obese volunteers   Random sample

Registry Study   Reference Study
n=6328   n=1135

Follow-up examinations
10,15 and 20 years

Intervention

Surgical group Matched Control group
n=2010   n=2037

Follow-up 20 years

Fig. 1. Schematic description of the SOS study design.

for women. Surgical methods used in the study are gastric banding, variable gastric banding, vertical banded gastroplasty and gastric bypass. The conventionally treated control patients are treated according to existing routines for obesity management at their respective primary health care centre. The patients undergo health examinations and complete extensive questionnaires at certain intervals. These are year: 0, 0.5, 1, 2, 3, 4, 6, 8, 10, 15 and 20. Blood samples are collected for centralised analysis at 0, 2, 10, 15 and 20 years.

The intervention study is not randomized as the Ethic committees did not approve of such design considering the high postoperative mortality in the early 1980s (1–5 per cent). Therefore a matched controlled design was chosen. A computerized matching program was used to select controls from potential controls in the registry. The matching procedure, that is carried out on group level, takes gender and the following 18 variables into account: age, weight, height, waist circumference, hip circumference, waist/hip ratio, systolic blood pressure, s-cholesterol, s-triglycerides, smoking, diabetes, pre/post menopausal state among women, four psychological variables known to be associated with mortality (current health, availability of social interaction, availability of attachment,

Table 1. Comparison of variables used for matching in the SOS Intervention study. Values presented as means and standard deviations or proportions.

	Surgery group		Control group		P^1
Number of subjects	2010		2037		
Sex, % men	29.4		28.9		0.782
Age, years	46.0	5.8	47.4	6.1	<0.001
Height, m	168.9	9.1	169.1	9.2	0.644
Weight, kg	119.2	16.1	116.9	15.4	<0.001
Waist, cm	124.1	10.6	122.2	10.1	<0.001
Hip, cm	125.9	9.7	124.4	9.3	<0.001
Waist-hip ratio	0.9871	0.007	0.984	0.07	0.195
Systolic blood pressure, mmHg	140.6	18.7	139.9	18.2	0.206
Total serum cholesterol, mmol/l	5.8	1.1	5.7	1.1	0.005
S-Triglycerides, mmol/l	2.2	1.4	2.1	1.5	0.088
Diabetes, %[2]	7.4		6.1		0.132
Daily smoking, %[2]	27.9		20.2		<0.001
Postmenopausal women, %[3]	37.2		41.3		0.026
1 – Current health scale	21.4	6.1	22.7	6.2	<0.001
2 – Monotony avoidance	22.5	5.1	22.6	5.0	0.447
3 – Psychastenia	23.9	5.2	23.1	5.3	<0.001
4 – Availability of social interaction	6.0	2.4	6.1	2.5	0.387
5 – Availability of attachment	4.3	1.3	4.3	1.3	0.479
6 – Stressful life events	2.5	1.3	2.4	1.3	0.092

[1]Test of equality of the surgery and control groups, t-test for continuous variables, Fisher's exact test for proportions and Mann-Whitney test for psychological scores; [2]From self-administered questionnaire; [3]Proportion of women.

stressful life events) and two personality traits related to treatment preferences (psychastenia, monotony avoidance).

When recruitment to the study ended in December 2000, the surgical group consisted of 2010 subjects (591 men and 1419 women) and the conventionally treated control group of 2037 subjects (589 men and 1448 women).

The SOS Reference study

In order to get comparable reference data to the SOS Registry and Intervention studies the SOS Reference study was initiated. Subjects living in the two communities Mölndal and Örebro in Sweden have been randomly selected from the population registry by means of a computer program to participate in the reference study. Between August 1994 to December 1999, 816 men and 936 women from Mölndal and 160 men and 125 women from Örebro were invited to participate in the study. Nine hundred and fifty eight (426 men and 532 women) in Mölndal and 179 (98 men and 79 women) in Örebro accepted to participate in the study. The overall participation rate was thus 53.7 per cent for men and 57.6 per cent for women. All participants have been health examined and completed the same questionnaires as in the SOS Registry study. Re-examinations of the reference population are planned after 10, 15 and 20 years.

The SOS dietary questionnaire

The SOS dietary questionnaire was developed with particular attention to capture dietary intake in obese subjects[3]. The questionnaire includes 49 questions and food items believed to be problematic for obese subjects such as for example sandwiches, candies and chocolates are described in great detail. Furthermore portion sizes of prepared main meals are described separately for potatoes/rice/pasta, meat/fish and vegetables with the help of coloured photographs. In other respects this questionnaire is fairly typical of the food frequency approach. An English translation of the questionnaire is published as an appendix to Lindroos *et al.*[3]. The validity of the dietary questionnaire has been evaluated in obese and non-obese subjects and reported mean intake showed good agreement with estimated energy expenditure in both the obese and nonobese groups, based on measured BMR and reported physical activity level[3]. Furthermore the between method correlation was 0.34 ($P < 0.01$) in the total group and 0.32 ($P < 0.05$) in the obese group. Based on the results from the validation study it was concluded that it is possible to obtain energy intake values from obese subjects that are at least as valid as those from normal weight subjects. Furthermore the SOS dietary questionnaire may be a useful dietary assessment tool in studies of diet and obesity-related diseases.

SOS Registry study versus SOS Reference study

The obese men from the SOS Registry study had a mean BMI ± SD of 38 ± 4.4 compared to 25.8 ± 3.4 among the randomly selected reference men. Among women mean BMI ± SD was 41.3 ± 4.4 and 24.7 ± 4.1, respectively. Severely obese men in the SOS Registry study were more often smokers than reference men, had a lower educational level and were less likely to have a partner. The obese women were less educated than the reference women, but smoking and cohabitation did not differ between the women. The prevalence of cardiovascular risk factors was much higher among obese men and women than among reference men and women. For example, diabetes was five times as common among obese men compared to reference men and hypertension twice as common. Corresponding figures for women were six times for diabetes and three times for hypertension.

Results from the SOS Intervention study

Baseline description of the study groups

The variables used for matching in the SOS Intervention study are presented in Table 1. On average surgical cases were younger, heavier, had a larger waist and hip circumference, higher total cholesterol level and were more likely to be smokers than controls. Since women in the surgical group were younger they were also less likely to be menopausal than the control women. Two of the six psychological scores also differed. Gender distribution, height, waist/hip ratio, systolic blood pressure, proportion having diabetes and four of the psychological variables did not differ significantly between the two groups.

Weight change

357 conventionally treated controls and 367 surgical cases have so far been followed for 10 years. Drop-out rate in the surgical group is 21.1 per cent versus 23.4 per cent in the control group. The

conventionally treated control group has essentially been weight stable over the 10 year period. The surgical groups reached minimum weights at 1 year. After 1 year they slowly started to relapse. Weight loss after 10 years is on average 16 per cent in the three surgical groups.

Changes in physical activity

The rapid weight loss in the surgical groups resulted in an increased physical activity level. When controlling for age, sex, initial weight and physical activity level at baseline a significantly higher proportion of the subjects in the surgical group report being physically active at leisure time compared to the weight stable control group.

Changes in dietary intake

Energy intake decreased rapidly after surgery and reported energy intake was significantly lower in the surgical group over the entire 10 year period, when age, sex, baseline weight and reported energy intake at baseline was controlled for. Large differences in macronutrient intake were also noted after surgery. In the surgical group the proportion of energy intake coming from protein was significantly lower than in the control group. Furthermore type of carbohydrates consumed differed between the groups. The proportion of energy intake coming from simple carbohydrates was significantly higher and the proportion from complex carbohydrates significantly lower in the surgical group compared to the control group during the entire 10 year period. Furthermore surgical cases with large weight losses after 10 years had a higher proportion of their total energy intake coming from simple carbohydrates than surgical cases with a more moderate weight loss.

Conclusion

The large sample of obese subjects in the SOS Registry study provides a unique opportunity to describe obesity with respect to weight development, morbidity, genetics, economy, and life style factors such as diet and physical activity. Furthermore the information obtained from the SOS Reference population also makes it possible to compare obese subjects with a normal population. Comparing the SOS Registry subjects with the SOS Reference subjects confirm previously published results showing a much higher morbidity among obese subjects than a normal population, when the first 1006 subjects in the SOS Registry were compared with participants in two Swedish population studies[1].

Recruitment to the SOS Intervention study has now stopped. In the 367 surgical cases followed for 10 years surgery resulted in more than 15 per cent weight loss. In contrast the conventionally treated control group was on average weight stable. The effects of weight change on cardiovascular risk factors, cardiovascular structure and function as well as health related quality of life and direct and indirect costs are further discussed elsewhere[4-6]. In the surgical group, where large weight losses were seen, physical inactivity after two years is decreased[7]. After 10 years the physical activity level was still higher in the surgical group. Another report from the SOS study have suggested that among subjects treated with Gastric banding and Vertical banded gastroplasty, the largest weight losses were seen in those who were able to reduce their total energy intake by eating less sandwiches, rice, pasta, potatoes and meat but who continued to eat sweet foods[8]. This was also true after 10 years. This result high lights the need for nutritional supplementation after Gastric banding and Vertical banded gastroplasty and stresses the need for nutritional education before and after obesity surgery.

References

1. Sjöström L. *et al.* Swedish obese subjects (SOS). Recruitment for an intervention study and a selected description of the obese state. *Int J Obes* 1992; 16: 465–79.

2. Sjöström L. Surgical intervention as a strategy for treatment of obesity. *Endocrine* 2000; 13: 213–30.

3. Lindroos AK, Sjöström L, Lissner L. Validity and reproducibility of a self-administered dietary questionnaire in obese and nonobese subjects. *Eur J Clin Nutr* 1993; 47: 461–81.

4. Sjöström D. Effects of 10 year weight loss retension on cardiovascular risk factors. In: *Progress in Obesity Research: 9*. Proceedings of Sao Paulo Congress 2002, pp. 973–6. Paris: John Libbey Eurotext, 2003.

5. Karason K. Cardiovascular effects of surgically induced weight loss: results from the SOS study. In: *Progress in Obesity Research: 9*. Proceedings of Sao Paulo Congress, 2002: pp. 977–82. Paris: John Libbey Eurotext, 2003.

6. Torgerson J. Effects of long-term weight loss maintenance on health-related quality of life and obesity related costs. In: *Progress in Obesity Research: 9*. Proceeding of Sao Paulo Congress 2002: pp. 983–6. Paris: John Libbey Eurotext, 2003.

7. Karason K *et al.* Relief of cardiorespiratory symptoms and increased physical activity after surgically induced weight loss: results from the Swedish Obese Subjects study. *Arch Intern Med* 2000; 160(12): 1797–802.

8. Lindroos A-K, Lissner L, Sjöström L. Weight change in relation to intake of sugar and sweet foods before and after weight reducing gastric surgery. *Int J Obes* 1996; 20: 634–43.

Progress in Obesity Research: 9. Edited by *Geraldo Medeiros-Neto, Alfredo Halpern and Claude Bouchard*
©2003 John Libbey Eurotext Ltd, pp. 973–976.

CHAPTER 202

Effects of 10 year weight loss retention on cardiovascular risk factors: results from the Swedish Obese Subjects study

C.D. Sjöström

Department of Anaesthesiology and Intensive Care and Dept. of Body Composition and Metabolism,
Sahlgrenska University Hospital, Göteborg, Sweden
[e-mail: david.sjostrom@medfak.gu.se]

Study group

The first 724 patients included in the SOS intervention study have now been followed for 10 years. The dropout rates are only 23 per cent for controls and 21 per cent for the surgically treated patients. Mean matching variables (SD) for 357 controls and 367 surgically treated patients who have been followed for 10 years are: age 46.9 (5.9), 45.9 (5.7) years, weight 116.3 (15.8), 118.3 (15.5) kg, BMI 40.7 (4.3), 41.2 (3.8) kg/m^2, respectively.

Results

Weight changes

After a 10-year follow up the controls had gained 1.1 (13.7) kg, which corresponds to a 1.4 per cent weight increase. The surgically treated patients had reduced their body weight 19.5 (13.7) kg or 16 per cent. There were large differences depending on surgical technique, banding (100 patients) −13 per cent, vertical banded gastroplasty (240 patients) −16 per cent and gastric by-pass (27 patients) −23 per cent of their initial body weight. Maximum weight losses in the surgically treated patients were seen after 1 year, banding −20 per cent, vertical banded gastroplasty −25 per cent and gastric by-pass −37 per cent of initial body weight. After the 1-year examination a slow but steady weight increase was observed until the 10-year examination. Figure 1 shows the weight changes during an 8 year observation period.

Risk factor changes

At 10 years the differences in relative risk factor changes between controls and surgically treated patients were large and highly significant ($P < 0.001$) for glucose, insulin, uric acid, triglycerides and HDL-cholesterol. There were no significant differences in relative changes for systolic and diastolic blood pressures or for total cholesterol.

Blood pressure

From 3 years and onwards, despite an initially large drop, systolic blood pressure in the surgically treated patients followed the same track as in the control group. The absolute level of diastolic blood pressure in the surgically treated group was significantly higher than among the controls from 6 years and onwards. In the control group the diastolic blood pressure decreased all through the study period. After 10 years the pulse pressure was significantly higher in the control group. Figure 2 shows blood pressure changes over 8 years.

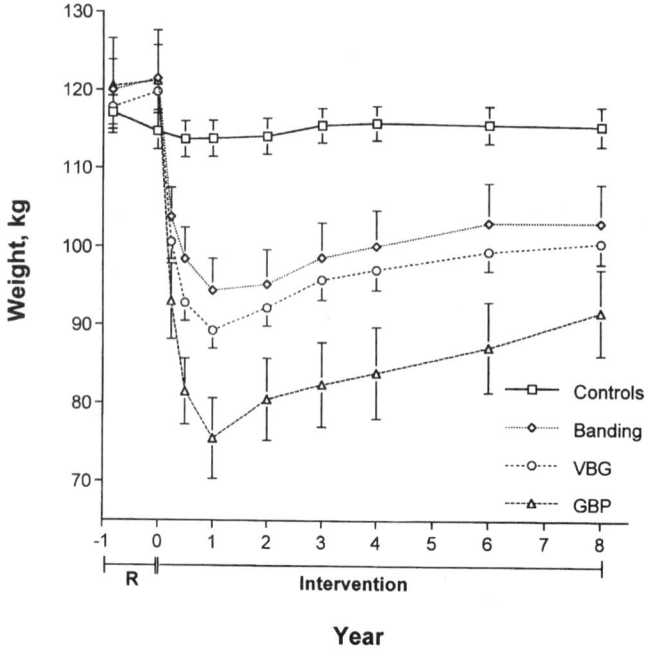

Fig. 1. Weight change (95 per cent CI) in 232 obese controls and 251 surgically treated obese patients from matching until end of year 8 in the SOS intervention study. Analysis based on completer population. Each one of the three surgical groups had a significantly ($P < 0.01$) larger weight reduction than the controls. R = Registry study with collection of matching variables, VBG = Vertical banded gastroplasty, GBP = Gastric bypass (from ref.[10], by permission of the publisher Lippincott, Williams & Wilkins).

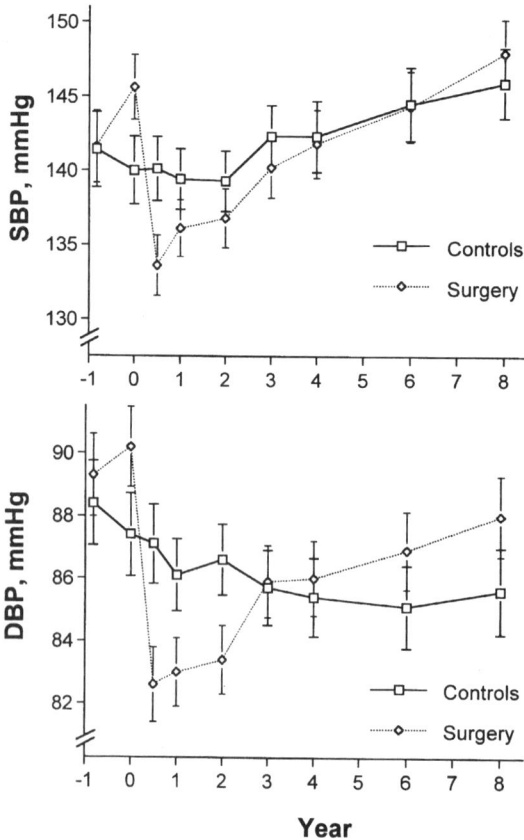

Fig. 2. Development of SBP and DBP (95 per cent CI) over 8 years in 232 obese controls and 251 surgically treated obese patients. Analysis based on completer population. Blood pressures during the intervention period are adjusted for sex, age, inclusion weight, inclusion blood pressure and at each measuring point for current: blood pressure medication (y/n), smoking (y/n), alcohol intake (g/day), energy intake (J/day), physical activity during work and leisure time (four levels) (from ref.[10], by permission of the publisher Lippincott, Williams & Wilkins).

Incidence calculations

The risk factor improvements at 10-years were only sufficient to reduce the incidence of diabetes and hyper-uricaemia among the surgically treated patients as compared to the controls. The odds ratio (95 per cent CI) for the incidence of diabetes was 0.16 (0.09–0.27) at 2 years and 0.24 (0.14–0.41) at 10 years ($P < 0.001$ for both). At two years there were also reduced incidences of hyper-triglyceridaemia, OR 0.31 (0.22–0.44), and hypo-HDL cholesterolaemia, OR 0.22 (0.14–0.34) in the surgically treated group. The incidences of hypertension and hyper-cholesterolaemia were not affected at 2 or 10 years.

Effect of weight loss and ageing in the pooled study group

In the pooled study group the adjusted effect of weight loss was evaluated using a weight stable reference group. In order to achieve any significant changes in risk factor levels over 10 years very large weight losses were required. For insulin a weight loss of more than 10 kg was needed, for systolic blood pressure > 15 kg, for diastolic blood pressure, glucose, HDL-cholesterol and uric acid > 20 kg, for triglycerides > 30 kg. No significant weight loss dependent change was observed for total cholesterol. The effect of a 10 kg weight loss, adjusted for sex, inclusion weight, height and age, was calculated by multiple regression. After 10 years a 10 kg weight loss corresponded to an average change in systolic blood pressure of –2.4 mmHg, diastolic blood pressure –1.5 mmHg, uric acid –19 µmol/l, HDL-cholesterol +0.06 mmol/l, triglycerides –0.19 mmol/l, blood glucose –0.37 mmol/l, insulin –3.9 mU/l and no significant change for total cholesterol.

The unadjusted effect of 10 years ageing assuming no weight change was also estimated. In the obese SOS patients systolic blood pressure changed +4 per cent, diastolic blood pressure –1 per cent, pulse pressure +16 per cent, blood glucose +15 per cent, insulin +11 per cent, total cholesterol –6 per cent, HDL-cholesterol +12 per cent. Uric acid and triglycerides showed no significant spontaneous variations independent of weight change.

Discussion

Weight and risk factor changes

By using weight reducing gastric surgery we have to a large extent overcome one large problem in weight reduction studies, namely the regain of lost weight. The 10-year results on weight reduction in the SOS study are far better than any two-year result from pharmacological or lifestyle modification studies[1]. Despite showing large weight losses, after 10 years the surgically treated patients are still obese, mean BMI 35 kg/m^2.

As compared to our earlier published two-year data[2,3] the effects of weight loss on risk factor levels had diminished. After 10 years we only saw an effect on the incidences of diabetes and hyper-uricaemia. Also, much larger weight losses were needed in order to achieve any improvements in risk factor levels than reported in more short-term studies[2,4]. Still the effects on diabetes are most convincing[5].

Reports from the literature are often very optimistic concerning the response of risk factors to weight loss. The following figures are used by WHO in the resent report on obesity[6]. For a 10 kg weigh loss systolic blood pressure will fall10 mmHg, diastolic blood pressure 20 mmHg, triglycerides 30 per cent, total cholesterol 10 per cent and HDL-cholesterol increase 8 per cent. Our results are much more modest. Some reports support our more moderate calculations of the effects of weight loss. Dattilo *et al.*[7] quantified the effect of weight loss on plasma lipids in a meta-analysis of 70 trials. The results were very similar to ours regarding triglycerides and HDL-cholesterol but not for total cholesterol where we saw no effect of weight loss. However, relapse of cholesterol after treatment but with retained weight loss has also been observed by others[8].

A lot of the discrepancies in results concerning the effect of weight loss are due to timing of the analysis, as risk factor levels vary depending on whether the body is in an anabolic or catabolic state. This is not only true concerning lipids[8], but also regarding blood pressure[9]. For a given body weight the blood pressure is significantly higher if weight is currently gained than lost. In the SOS study the surgical group was in a moderate positive energy balance at the 2-year examination and virtually weight-stable over the last two years preceding the 10-year examination. However, the picture is further complicated as risk factor levels change over time independently of weight change. Assuming no weight change, different risk factors changed between –6 per cent and +16 per cent during our 10-year follow-up.

Weight change and blood pressure development

We have thoroughly analysed the blood pressure response to weight loss induced by gastric surgery in previously published papers[10,11]. A regain of blood pressure after weight loss has been shown also in other studies. Due to short follow-up the relapse usually did not have time to be completed[9,12]. The relapse of systolic blood pressure to control levels after a few years (Fig. 2) might partly be explained by on-going weight increases. Data from the SOS study[10] as well as from others[13] indicate that ongoing weight change is more closely related to blood pressure than the initial body weight. An often over-looked aspect is the effect of time. We have shown how one elapsed year has 2.5 to 4 times larger impact on blood pressure than one regained kilogram[11].

The analysis of weight change on blood pressure is further complicated by the natural development of blood pressure. In normal weight populations diastolic blood pressure starts to decline after an age of approximately 60 years[14]. This decrease is due to a reduced arterial compliance. In the severely obese this decline starts more than 10 years earlier than normal[11] (Fig. 2). The combination of a continuously increasing systolic blood pressure and a decreasing diastolic blood pressure inevitably leads to a rapidly increasing pulse pressure, which has been associated with an increased intima-media thickness[15]. The SOS study has shown that large retained weight losses can slow down the rapid increase in pulse pressure seen in weight stable obese. This observation is in accordance with the reduced progression rate of the intima-media thickness seen in weight reduced obese patients after 4 years[16].

Larger weight losses are required to improve risk factors after 10 years than in short term studies. Gastric surgery improves some but not all risk factors after 10 years. It is still uncertain whether these risk factor changes will be sufficient to reduce hard end points.

Acknowledgements: Major sponsors of this study were The Swedish Medical Research Council (grant no 05239), Stockholm, Sweden and Hoffmann-La Roche Ltd., Basel, Switzerland. Support was also obtained from The Volvo Research Foundation, Göteborg, CEFOS, Göteborg, The Swedish Social Welfare Board, Stockholm, Ministry of Education, Stockholm, and Skandia Insurance, Stockholm, all in Sweden.

References

1. Phelan S, Wadden TA. Combining behavioral and pharmacological treatments for obesity. *Obes Res* 2002; 10: 560–74.

2. Sjöström CD, Lissner L, Sjöström L. Relationships between changes in body composition and changes in cardiovascular risk factors: the SOS Intervention Study. Swedish Obese Subjects. *Obes Res* 1997; 5: 519–30.

3. Sjöström CD, Lissner L, Wedel H, Sjöström L. Reduction in incidence of diabetes, hypertension and lipid disturbances after intentional weight loss induced by bariatric surgery: the SOS Intervention Study. *Obes Res* 1999; 7: 477–84.

4. Blackburn G. Effect of degree of weight loss on health benefits. *Obes Res* 1995; 3 (Suppl 2): 211–216.

5. Pinkney JH, Sjöström CD, Gale EA. Should surgeons treat diabetes in severely obese people? *Lancet* 2001; 357: 1357–9.

6. WHO. Obesity: Preventing and Managing the Global Epidemic – Report of a WHO Consultatin on Obesity. Geneva: World Health Organization, 2000.

7. Dattilo AM, Kris-Etherton PM. Effects of weight reduction on blood lipids and lipoproteins: a meta-analysis. *Am J Clin Nutr* 1992; 56: 320–8.

8. Wadden TA, Anderson DA, Foster GD. Two-year changes in lipids and lipoproteins associated with the maintenance of a 5 per cent to 10 per cent reduction in initial weight: some findings and some questions. *Obes Res* 1999; 7: 170–8.

9. Dornfeld LP, Maxwell MH, Waks AU, Schroth P, Tuck ML. Obesity and hypertension: long-term effects of weight reduction on blood pressure. *Int J Obes* 1985; 9: 381–9.

10. Sjöström CD, Peltonen M, Wedel H, Sjöström L. Differentiated long-term effects of intentional weight loss on diabetes and hypertension. *Hypertension* 2000; 36: 20–5.

11. Sjöström CD, Peltonen M, Sjöström L. Blood pressure and pulse pressure during long-term weight loss in the obese: the Swedish Obese Subjects (SOS) Intervention Study. *Obes Res* 2001; 9: 188–95.

12. Carson JL, Ruddy ME, Duff AE, Holmes NJ, Cody RP, Brolin RE. The effect of gastric bypass surgery on hypertension in morbidly obese patients. *Arch Intern Med* 1994; 154: 193–200.

13. Sonne-Holm S, Sørensen TI, Jensen G, Schnohr P. Independent effects of weight change and attained body weight on prevalence of arterial hypertension in obese and non-obese men. *BMJ* 1989; 299: 767–70.

14. Franklin SS, Gustin Wt, Wong ND et al. Hemodynamic patterns of age-related changes in blood pressure. The Framingham Heart Study. *Circulation* 1997; 96: 308–15.

15. Boutouyrie P, Bussy C, Lacolley P, Girerd X, Laloux B, Laurent S. Association between local pulse pressure, mean blood pressure, and large-artery remodeling. *Circulation* 1999; 100: 1387–93.

16. Karason K, Wikstrand J, Sjöström L, Wendelhag I. Weight loss and progression of early atherosclerosis in the carotid artery: a four-year controlled study of obese subjects. *Int J Obes Relat Metab Disord* 1999; 23: 948–56.

Progress in Obesity Research: 9. Edited by *Geraldo Medeiros-Neto, Alfredo Halpern and Claude Bouchard*
©2003 John Libbey Eurotext Ltd, pp. 977–982.

CHAPTER 203

Cardiovascular effects of surgically induced weight loss: results from the SOS study

Kristjan Karason

Department of Cardiology, Sahlgrenska University Hospital, Göteborg University, Göteborg, Sweden
[e-mail: kristjan.karason@medfak.gu.se]

Introduction

One major cause of premature morbidity and mortality in obesity is cardiovascular disease[1]. Body fat accumulation is associated with the development of hypertension, dyslipidaemia and diabetes mellitus and has been shown to be an important determinant of coronary heart disease. Furthermore, obesity is related to left ventricular hypertrophy and cardiac failure and contributes to an increased risk of arrhythmia and sudden death. A heightened awareness of the cardiovascular complications of the obese state, together with the increasing prevalence of obesity, has stimulated increasing research into the interactions between obesity and the cardiovascular system.

Although it appears reasonable to assume that sustained weight reduction would favour cardiovascular improvements, no data are available to support such a belief. Analyses of the balance between the benefits and risks of obesity treatment are further complicated by epidemiological studies showing associations between weight loss and increased mortality, as well as case reports describing serious cardiovascular complications following rapid weight reduction.

Results from numerous observational studies and controlled clinical trials have clearly demonstrated that weight loss is associated with improvements hemodynamic and metabolic risk factors. Weight reduction induces a fall in blood volume and cardiac output[2] and results in reduced blood pressure[3]. Moreover, weight loss produces favourable changes in glucose tolerance, plasma insulin and lipoprotein-lipid levels.[4] Although these beneficial effects of weight loss appear to outweigh possible risks, important aspects still need to be resolved. The extent to which disturbances in cardiovascular structure and function can be reversed by weight reduction is not yet clear and the crucial question of whether weight loss reduces the risks for major morbidity, such as heart attack, stroke and death, remains unanswered.

The overall aim of this study is to investigate the effects of large, sustained weight losses on the cardiovascular system in patients with severe obesity.

Methods

Obese patients included in this study were recruited from the SOS (Swedish Obese Subjects) study. SOS is an ongoing nationwide project designed to determine whether the morbidity and mortality rates among obese people who lose weight by surgical means differ from those in a matched obese reference group[5]. Briefly, SOS consists of a registry study and an intervention study. The aim of the registry study is to describe the obese state with respect to physical health and psychosocial well-being and to serve as a recruitment base from which eligible patients are enrolled into the intervention study. The criteria of inclusion for the intervention study are age between 37 and 60 years and BMI ≥ 38 kg/m^2 for women and BMI ≥ 34 kg/m^2 for men.

The intervention study consists of one surgically treated group and one conventionally treated control group. The study is not randomized since a procedure of this kind was not approved by the ethics committees in Sweden due to high perioperative mortality (2–5 per cent) in studies available in 1987. Instead, the groups are matched to one another with respect to sex and 18 other clinical variables.The treatments offered to the surgical group consist of gastric bypass, vertical banded gastroplasty and gastric banding[6]. These operations, as well as follow-ups of surgically treated patients, are conducted at 25 different surgical departments in Sweden. Control subjects receive conventional dietary recommendations and are followed up at 480 primary health care centres located throughout the country. Each group will contain 2000 subjects and the follow-up period is 10 years.

In the present study forty one patients treated with gastric surgery, 31 obese patients receiving conventional dietary recommendations and 43 normal weight subjects were included. Body weight and blood pressure measurements were obtained and metabolic risk factors, as well as urinary norepinephrine excretion, were analysed. Two-dimensional and Doppler echocardiography were performed to evaluate cardiac structure and function and 24-h Holtrer recordings used to assess heart rate variability. Carotid ultrasonography was performed to determine intima-media thickens, an estimate of atherosclerosis. All study groups were investigated at baseline and the two obese groups were re-examined after 1–4 years of follow-up. In addition, 1290 obese surgical cases and 1099 matched obese control subjects, followed for two years, were compared with respect to symptoms of breathlessness and chest pain and levels of leisure-time physical activity.

Results

Patients with obesity had higher blood pressure, larger left ventricular mass and increased relative wall thickness compared with lean subjects. They also had impaired left ventricular filling and reduced left ventricular ejection fraction. Heart rate variability was lower and norepinephrine excretion was higher in obese subjects than in lean subjects. An adverse metabolic risk factor profile was noted in patients with obesity, who also had increased intima-media thickness in the carotid artery bulb, compared with lean controls.

Obese patients treated with surgery displayed substantial weight losses, whereas the average weight in the obese control group remained essentially unchanged. Following weight loss, blood pressure, left ventricular mass and relative wall thickness diminished and left ventricular filling patterns, as well as ejection fraction, were favourably influenced. Heart rate variability increased and norepinephrine excretion decreased. The weight loss group also showed improvements in metabolic risk factors and appeared to have a lower progression rate of carotid bulb intima-media thickness than the group with persistent obesity. Finally, weight loss was associated with a marked relief in symptoms of dyspnea and chest pain and increased levels of leisure-time physical activity.

Discussion

This controlled intervention study of subjects with severe obesity demonstrates that large intentional weight losses are associated with improvements in several aspects of cardiovascular structure and function. Moreover, weight reduction is associated with a marked relief of symptoms of breathlessness and chest discomfort and promotes increased leisure-time physical activity. In most cases, the cardiovascular improvements occurring in connection with weight loss showed a dose-response pattern. These findings are in line with accumulating evidence that intentional weight reduction in obese subjects is associated with improvements in physical health[7] and mental well-being[8].

Cardiac structure

Several autopsy[9] and echocardiographic[10] studies have demonstrated that obesity, as well as hypertension, is associated with left ventricular hypertrophy. The development of increased left ventricular mass in obese patients is related to an augmented hemodynamic load, but is most probably also influenced by various humoral factors. Left ventricular hypertrophy has been shown to be a major risk indicator of cardiovascular disease[11] and its recognition and treatment is therefore of importance. Previous trials have observed the regression of left ventricular hypertrophy after pharmacological treatment of hypertension[12], whereas studies investigating the effects of weight loss on cardiac mass are limited and have produced inconsistent results.

To explain the discrepancy in previous studies, it has been suggested that beneficial effects of weight loss on cardiac structure may occur only if the obesity is mild or of short duration. In the present study, however, a mean weight loss of 33 kg (28 per cent) in subjects with long-term morbid obesity resulted in a 15 per cent reduction in left ventricular mass, clearly supporting the reversibility of left ventricular hypertrophy in obese patients. The degree of reversal was related to weight reduction in a dose-response manner and the average improvement was comparable with that seen after antihypertensive therapy[12].

The increments in left ventricular chamber size and wall thickness observed in obese subjects are in accordance with previous studies[13]. Furthermore, the ratio of wall thickness to chamber radius, or relative wall thickness, was higher in obese subjects compared with lean ones, indicating a concentric left ventricular pattern. Whereas changes in left ventricular volumes and dimensions at follow-up did not differ significantly between the obese surgical and control groups, left ventricular wall thickness showed definite reductions with weight loss. As a result, relative wall thickness also decreased. This is an important finding since a concentric left ventricular pattern has been shown to be associated with increased cardiovascular risk[14].

Cardiac function

Although the development of left ventricular hypertrophy in obesity is initially an adaptive response to augmented hemodynamic load, it commonly leads to disturbances in left ventricular filling and diastolic dysfunction. In agreement with previous reports[15,16], obese patients in the present study had several echocardiographic findings characteristic of impaired ventricular relaxation, including increased atrial size, prolonged isovolumetric relaxation time and a lower E/A ratio. However, it should be noted that these echocardiographic measurements of diastolic function can also be influenced by other factors such as age, heart rate and loading conditions.

In the present study, weight loss was followed by an increase in E/A ratio and a tendency towards decreased isovolumetric relaxation time and reduced left atrial size, supporting improvements in diastolic function. Furthermore, pulmonary venous inflow patterns were normal after weight reduction which excludes any form of 'pseudonormalization' of transmitral flow due to elevated atrial pressures. Increases in E/A ratio were correlated with reductions in left ventricular mass and heart rate, suggesting that improved filling patterns could be due to enhanced ventricular relaxation and prolonged diastole. On the other hand, changes in left ventricular volumes and blood pressure, which are crude indicators of preload and afterload, were not related to changes in E/A ratio.

Cardiac autonomic control

In the present study we used an index of long-term heart rate variability, the standard deviation of all RR intervals in the 24 h period (SDANN), as a measurement of sympathetic activity. A main contributor to SDANN is the shift in the mean RR level from daytime to night-time. This basic biological rhythm is severely reduced in conditions such as heart failure[17] and post-myocardial infarction[18] where heightened levels of sympathetic activation spread into night-time and limit the shift in the RR level. In the present study, the SDANN was reduced in subjects with obesity, but it improved after weight loss. Moreover, the urinary excretion of norepinephrine, which is a crude marker of global sympathetic activity, was elevated in obese patients and decreased with weight reduction. Taken together, these findings suggest that obese subjects have generally increased levels of sympathetic neural and neurohumoral activity and that this increment in adrenergic activity may be reversed following weight loss.

The high frequency (HF) component of heart rate variability is widely accepted as a measurement of pure vagal activity. Several cross-sectional studies have reported decreased HF power in obese subjects, reflecting vagal withdrawal[19]. Nevertheless, it is still unclear whether vagal tone varies along with weight changes. In the present study, the weight loss group displayed a significant increase in both the standard deviation of all RR intervals in the 24-h period (SDNN) index and HF amplitude, strongly suggesting a reversal of vagal withdrawal following weight reduction.

Atherosclerosis

The relationship between obesity and atherosclerotic disease remains somewhat controversial. Although excess body fat promotes multiple cardiovascular risk factors[20,21] and epidemiological evidence demonstrates an association between body weight and cardiovascular disease[22], studies based on angiography and autopsy have not been able to demonstrate a consistent relationship between obesity and the degree of atherosclerosis.

In accordance with previous studies, obese patients in this study had an adverse risk factor profile with increments in blood pressure, total cholesterol, triglycerides, glucose and insulin. One novel finding was that obese patients had a thicker intima-media complex in the carotid artery bulb compared with lean subjects and a higher intima-media thickness progression rate during four years of follow-up. These observations strongly suggest that obesity predisposes subjects to the development of atherosclerosis and that the disease process is likely to be mediated by hemodynamic and metabolic risk factors.

As expected, weight loss in our obese subjects was associated with improvements in several risk factors, including reductions in blood pressure, triglycerides and insulin and an increase in HDL-cholesterol. One important observation was that the obese control group displayed a significant increase in carotid bulb intima-media thickness at follow-up, while the weight loss group did not. The progression rate of intima-media thickness in the weight loss group was only about one-third that found in the obese control group and was similar to that observed in lean subjects. However, the difference between the weight loss group and the obese control group did not reach statistical significance, but this could be due to small sample sizes. Taken together, our findings suggest that weight loss, along with concomitant risk factor improvements, may reduce the progression rate of atherosclerosis.

Symptoms and physical activity

Apart from the increased work of ambulation, exertional dyspnea in obesity may be related to disturbances in both circulation and respiration. Left ventricular hypertrophy and associated disturbances in diastolic filling may contribute to the elevation in pulmonary venous pressures and cause dyspnea, particularly on exertion, and impairments in respiratory mechanics and gas exchange may further exacerbate breathlessness. The regression of left ventricular hypertrophy and improved diastolic filling after weight loss, as well as weight loss-related improvements in pulmonary function and arterial blood gases[23], are likely to contribute to the marked improvement in dyspnea observed after weight loss in the present study.

Although obesity is associated with signs of premature atherosclerosis, it is unlikely that the high frequency of effort-related chest pain reported by obese patients in the present study is entirely due to underlying coronary heart disease. Chest pain may arise from left ventricular hypertrophy as a result of an imbalance between oxygen supply and demand[24], and an elevation in intra-abdominal pressure associated with visceral adiposity predisposes subjects to gastroesophageal reflux and symptoms of heartburn[25]. Finally, obstructive sleep apnea, has been reported to simulate angina pectoris even in the absence of coronary atherosclerosis[26]. Since these conditions improve following surgically-induced weight loss, they are likely to contribute to the relief in chest pain also observed after weight reduction in our patients.

The relationship between body weight and physical activity is complex and the directionality of this relationship has not been fully determined. Several investigators have emphasized the primary role of a sedentary lifestyle in the development of obesity[27,28], while the opposite possibility, that effort-related symptoms in obese subjects might limit exercise performance, has received less attention. In the present study, weight loss was associated with an increase in physical activity, possibly encouraged by the concomitant relief in effort-related symptoms. Our findings thus suggest that sedentary behaviour may be secondary to obesity to some extent and support the hypothesis that physical inactivity and the accumulation of body fat reinforce one another in the process of developing and maintaining the obese state. The breaking of this vicious circle with surgical intervention, thereby permitting enhanced leisure-time activity, should be regarded as favourable, not only because it promotes general well-being, but also because improved physical fitness has been shown to reduce cardiovascular morbidity and mortality[29,30].

Clinical implications

Left ventricular hypertrophy has assumed an important clinical role as a major risk indicator of cardiovascular disease[11]. Although not yet known, it is reasonable to believe that the regression of left ventricular mass will lead to a reduction in cardiovascular risk. Both obesity and hypertension are associated with left ventricular hypertrophy[31], but in the present study, improvements in left ventricular structure correlated more closely with the degree of weight loss than with the accompanying reduction in blood pressure. It can therefore be concluded that, in order to prevent or improve abnormal heart structure in obese subjects weight control should be a primary goal and should be regarded as being at least as important as regulating blood pressure.

From a clinical point of view, it is important to recognize that diastolic heart failure has distinct pathophysiological features which differ from the properties of systolic dysfunction and requires specific treatment measures[32]. It has been reported that diastolic dysfunction can be reversed by the medical treatment of hypertension[33] and the present study shows that improvements in diastolic filling can also be obtained by weight reduction. These results useful, since it can be concluded that weight loss is beneficial for obese subjects with diastolic heart dysfunction.

In view of the increased risk of arrhythmia and sudden death in the obese population, the correction of autonomic balance following weight loss should be regarded as favourable and an indication of improved health. Furthermore, the observations that obese subjects who lose weight appear to have a reduced progression rate in carotid intima-media thickness compared with subjects with persistent obesity are valuable, not only because intima-media thicness measurements are an estimate of carotid atherosclerosis, but also because they are a surrogate measurement of coronary heart disease[34].

Shortness of breath and chest discomfort on exertion are common complaints of obese patients. These are debilitating symptoms that limit exercise performance and contribute to sedentary behaviour as well as to poor well-being. In addition, chest pain is an alarming symptom, that may lead to frequent hospital admissions. The marked relief of these symptoms following weight loss is an important finding since it is likely to allow enhanced physical activity, reduce utilization of health care services and improve quality of life.

The overall findings of the present thesis aid to the accumulating evidence that weight loss offers considerable health benefits to patients with severe obesity. The widespread cardiovascular improvements observed are likely to have favourable effects on long-term prognosis and support that obesity should be treated. As today, surgical treatment is the only available method resulting in large sustained weight losses and is reserved for the morbidly obese. However, the advancing understanding energy balance, will probably lead to the development of more effective pharmacological therapy in the near future. Nevertheless, it is of crucial importance that lifestyle modification, including healthful diet and regular exercise, will continue to play a central role in all forms of prevention and treatment.

References

1. Eckel RH. Obesity and heart disease: a statement for healthcare professionals from the Nutrition Committee, American Heart Association. *Circulation* 1997; 96: 3248–50.

2. Alexander JK, Peterson KL. Cardiovascular effects of weight reduction. *Circulation* 1972; 45: 310–8.

3. Chiang BN, Perlman LV, Epstein FH. Overweight and hypertension. A review. *Circulation* 1969; 39: 403–21.

4. Sjöström CD, Lissner L, Sjöstrom L. Relationships between changes in body composition and changes in cardiovascular risk factors: the SOS Intervention Study. Swedish Obese Subjects. *Obes Res* 1997; 5: 519–30.

5. Sjöström L, Larsson B, Backman L *et al.* Swedish obese subjects (SOS). Recruitment for an intervention study and a selected description of the obese state. *Int J Obes Relat Metab Disord.* 1992; 16: 465–79.

6. Sagar PM. Surgical treatment of morbid obesity. *Br J Surg* 1995; 82: 732–9.

7. Van Gaal LF, Wauters MA, De Leeuw IH. The beneficial effects of modest weight loss on cardiovascular risk factors. *Int J Obes Relat Metab Disord* 1997; 21 (Suppl 1): S5–9.

8. Karlsson J, Sjöstrom L, Sullivan M. Swedish obese subjects (SOS)-an intervention study of obesity. Two-year follow-up of health-related quality of life (HRQL) and eating behavior after gastric surgery for severe obesity. *Int J Obes Relat Metab Disord* 1998; 22: 113–26.

9. Amad KH, Brennan JC, Alexander JK. The cardiac pathology of chronic exogenous obesity. *Circulation* 1965; 32: 740–5.

10. Messerli FH, Sundgaard-Riise K, Reisin ED *et al.* Dimorphic cardiac adaptation to obesity and arterial hypertension. *Ann Intern Med* 1983; 99: 757–61.

11. Levy D, Garrison RJ, Savage DD *et al.* Prognostic implications of echocardiographically determined left ventricular mass in the Framingham Heart Study. *N Engl J Med* 1990; 322: 1561–6.

12. Dahlöf B, Pennert K, Hansson L. Reversal of left ventricular hypertrophy in hypertensive patients. A metaanalysis of 109 treatment studies. *Am J Hypertens* 1992; 5: 95–110.

13. Lauer MS, Anderson KM, Kannel WB *et al.* The impact of obesity on left ventricular mass and geometry. The Framingham Heart Study. *JAMA* 1991; 266: 31–6.

14. Koren MJ, Devereux RB, Casale PN *et al.* Relation of left ventricular mass and geometry to morbidity and mortality in uncomplicated essential hypertension. *Ann Intern Med* 1991; 114: 345–52.

15. Ku CS, Lin SL, Wang DJ *et al.* Left ventricular filling in young normotensive obese adults. *Am J Cardiol* 1994; 73: 613–5.

16. Alpert MA, Lambert CR, Terry BE *et al.* Influence of left ventricular mass on left ventricular diastolic filling in normotensive morbid obesity. *Am Heart J* 1995; 130: 1068–73.

17. Casolo G, Balli E, Taddei T *et al.* Decreased spontaneous heart rate variability in congestive heart failure. *Am J Cardiol* 1989; 64: 1162–7.

18. Bigger Jr. JT, Kleiger RE, Fleiss JL *et al.* Components of heart rate variability measured during healing of acute myocardial infarction. *Am J Cardiol* 1988; 61: 208–15.

19. Peterson HR, Rothschild M, Weinberg CR *et al.* Body fat and the activity of the autonomic nervous system. *N Engl J Med* 1988; 318: 1077–83.

20. Kannel WB, Gordon T, Castelli WP. Obesity, lipids, and glucose intolerance. The Framingham Study. *Am J Clin Nutr* 1979; 32: 1238–45.

21. Sjöström CD, Hakangard AC, Lissner L *et al.* Body compartment and subcutaneous adipose tissue distribution-risk factor patterns in obese subjects. *Obes Res* 1995; 3: 9–22.

22. Manson JE, Willett WC, Stampfer MJ *et al.* Body weight and mortality among women. *N Engl J Med* 1995; 333: 677–85.

23. Weiner P, Waizman J, Weiner M *et al.* Influence of excessive weight loss after gastroplasty for morbid obesity on respiratory muscle performance. *Thorax* 1998; 53: 39–42.

24. Marcus ML, Harrison DG, Chilian WM *et al.* Alterations in the coronary circulation in hypertrophied ventricles. *Circulation* 1987; 75: 119–25.

25. Sugerman H, Windsor A, Bessos M *et al.* Intra-abdominal pressure, sagittal abdominal diameter and obesity comorbidity. *J Intern Med* 1997; 241: 71–9.

26. Loui WS, Blackshear JL, Fredrickson PA *et al.* Obstructive sleep apnea manifesting as suspected angina: report of three cases. *Mayo Clin Proc* 1994; 69: 244–8.

27. Rissanen AM, Heliovaara M, Knekt P *et al.* Determinants of weight gain and overweight in adult Finns. *Eur J Clin Nutr* 1991; 45: 419–30.

28. Prentice AM, Jebb SA. Obesity in Britain: gluttony or sloth? *BMJ* 1995; 311: 437–9.

29. Blair SN, Kohl HW 3rd, Barlow CE *et al.* Changes in physical fitness and all-cause mortality. A prospective study of healthy and unhealthy men. *JAMA* 1995; 273: 1093–8.

30. Wannamethee SG, Shaper AG, Walker M. Changes in physical activity, mortality, and incidence of coronary heart disease in older men. *Lancet* 1998; 351: 1603–8.

31. Levy D, Anderson KM, Savage DD *et al.* Echocardiographically detected left ventricular hypertrophy: prevalence and risk factors. The Framingham Heart Study. *Ann Intern Med* 1988; 108: 7–13.

32. Wheeldon NM, Clarkson P, MacDonald TM. Diastolic heart failure. *Eur Heart J* 1994; 15: 1689–97.

33. White WB, Schulman P, Karimeddini MK *et al.* Regression of left ventricular mass is accompanied by improvement in rapid left ventricular filling following antihypertensive therapy with metoprolol. *Am Heart J* 1989; 117: 145–50.

34. Hulthe J, Wikstrand J, Emanuelsson H *et al.* Atherosclerotic changes in the carotid artery bulb as measured by B-mode ultrasound are associated with the extent of coronary atherosclerosis. *Stroke* 1997; 28: 1189–94.

Progress in Obesity Research: 9. Edited by *Geraldo Medeiros-Neto, Alfredo Halpern and Claude Bouchard*

CHAPTER 204

Effects of long-term weight loss maintenance on health-related quality of life and obesity related costs

Jarl S. Torgerson

SOS secretariat, Department of Body Composition and Metabolism, Sahlgrenska University Hospital, Göteborg, Sweden
[e-mail: jarl.torgerson@medfak.gu.se]

Introduction

Physicians, patients and politicians/decision makers tend to have slightly different views on treatment effectiveness. The medical focus is mainly on measures of signs and symptoms, survival time, side effects et cetera. Paradoxically, better health according to such traditional indicators is not automatically accompanied by improved well being or perceived health gain. This is especially true in chronic disorders such as obesity[1]. Politicians and decision makers are facing a relative scarcity in health care resources and have to give priority to different treatment options. Consequently, their focus is more on optimal allocation and use of available resources. This chapter will outline results from the Swedish Obese Subjects (SOS) study[2] on the effects of long-term weight loss maintenance on health-related quality of life and direct as well as indirect costs of obesity.

Health-related quality of life

The SOS survey on health-related quality of life (HRQL) includes both generic and disease specific questionnaires. Generic measures capture HRQL dimensions that are not specific to obesity, thereby allowing comparisons with other patient groups, while disease specific questionnaires are designed to be sensitive to treatment induced changes[1].

HRQL at baseline

Obese SOS patients, irrespective of gender, rated their health status and mental well being worse than a healthy reference population. Furthermore, anxiety and depression was more common in the obese[3]. Compared to other groups of chronically diseased patients (e.g. rheumatoid arthritis and disease free cancer survival) the obese had worse mental well being. In fact, only subjects with cancer recurrence or non-responders to treatment for chronic pain had similar or slightly poorer well being. The obese also had more symptoms of anxiety and depression than almost all other examined patient groups[3]. Finally, patients in SOS operated group generally had lower HRQL levels at baseline than the conventionally treated controls[4].

General remarks on HRQL following weight loss

A very consistent pattern of improvements in all HRQL dimensions emerged after intervention. All measures differed significantly between operated and conventionally treated patients after 24 months. Generally, peak values appeared after six to twelve months, followed by a small to moderate decline after 2 to 4 years. Only minor changes were found in the conventionally treated group[1,4]. There was a dose dependent relation between two-year improvements in HRQL and weight loss, while the association between weight reduction and early change in HRQL was generally weak[4]. After four years HRQL ratings remained stable in subjects that had lost more than 30 kg, while a regression was seen in patients losing less weight. Subjects with less than 10 kg weight loss tended to return towards baseline levels[1].

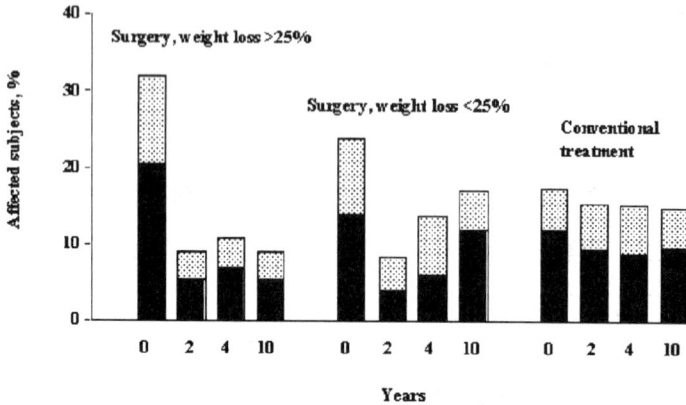

Fig. 1. Prevalence of depression in operated and conventionally treated obese patients. Operated patients are divided by magnitude of the ten-year weight loss. Data from baseline and 2-, 4- and 10-year examinations are shown. The Hospital Anxiety and Depression (HAD) scale was used. The scale range is 0–21. Scores below eight are in the normal range, while scores between eight and ten indicate a possible (black bars) and above ten a probable (dotted bars) clinical depression (Karlsson J et al., unpublished data).

Specific examples of HRQL following weight loss

Figure 1 shows the prevalence of clinical depression at baseline and two, four and ten years after surgery or conventional obesity treatment. The generic Hospital Anxiety and Depression (HAD) scale was used. The operated patients were more frequently depressed at baseline. Following intervention the prevalence of depression was reduced in operated patients, especially in those who lost more than 25 per cent in weight, while ratings remained stable in the conventionally treated control group (Karlsson J et al., unpublished data).

The OP scale is a specific module measuring the proportion of patients being bothered by common situations such as going to a restaurant, trying on and buying clothes or having intimate relation with partner. The fraction of bothered subjects was dramatically reduced two and four years after bariatric surgery. Generally, the number of bothered individuals was two to five times smaller than at baseline[1]. Improvements in OP scale scores were related to weight loss in a dose dependent fashion even after ten years (Karlsson J et al., unpublished data).

Concluding remarks on HRQL

A general conclusion from SOS is that all measures of HRQL are dramatically improved following surgically induced weight loss. Long-term improvements are related to the amount of weight loss. Since short-term changes in HRQL and body weight are only weakly related there is a definite need for

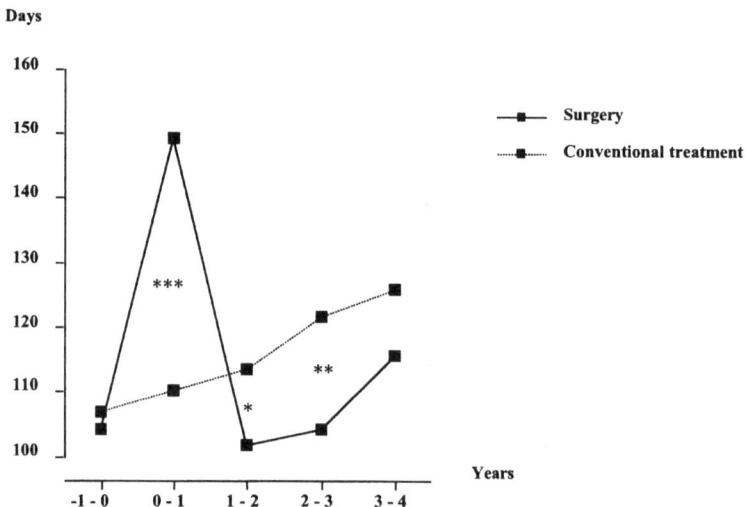

Fig. 2. Number of days per year of sick leave and disability pension in operated (solid line) and conventionally treated (dotted line) obese subjects. *P < 0.05, ** P < 0.01, *** P < 0.001. Adapted from ref.[7] with permission.

long-term intervention and follow-up in obese patients. The improvement in HRQL was maintained in patients that lost more than 30 kg, while a deterioration was seen in patients losing less. This implies that the profound improvements in HRQL seen after successful obesity surgery cannot be directly extrapolated to pharmacological obesity treatment since weight reduction achieved with drugs is generally much smaller.

Health economics

Direct (health care expenditures) and indirect (productivity losses) costs of obesity have been analysed in the SOS study.

The baseline situation

Obese women had about twice as many days per year of sick leave and disability pension as the general Swedish population. The incremental annual indirect cost in obese women was 3.6 billion Swedish crowns (1994 prices and wages)[5]. Obese SOS patients were more frequently prescribed medication than a reference population (52 and 36 per cent, respectively). The obese were more often on medication against diabetes, cardiovascular disease (CVD), asthma and pain, while there was no difference in medication against psychiatric and gastrointestinal disorders. The total annual cost for drug treatment was 77 per cent higher in the obese[6]. There was no baseline difference in sick leave or disability pension when operated patients and the conventionally treated controls were compared [7]. The annual cost for diabetes medication was significantly higher in the operated group, while there was no difference in the costs for other types of medication[6].

Indirect costs following weight loss

Figure 2 indicates that sick leave and disability pension was reduced in the operated group[7]. The first year after inclusion the operated had a 50 per cent increase in sick leave, mainly due to normal post-operative convalescence. All operations were performed in the pre-laparoscopic era. Year two and three, but not year four, there were significantly fewer days of sick leave and disability pension in the operated group. When sick leave and disability pension were analysed separately there was a significant reduction in disability pension (but not in sick leave) among the operated also year four. This latter finding might be due to partial weight relapse, late complications or additional surgery resulting in increased sick leave in operated patients[8]. The initial increase in post-operative sick leave was thus counterbalanced during subsequent years. It is noteworthy that the long-term difference between surgery and conventional treatment was mainly driven by patients above median age (46.7 years)[7].

Direct costs following weight loss

Two and six years after inclusion in SOS there were fewer patients on medication against diabetes and CVD in the operated group than in the control group. This was the case both in subjects who were, or who were not, on medication at baseline. A weight loss greater than ten per cent significantly reduced the long-term risk of having CVD medication, while an effect on diabetes medication was observed only after two years[9]. Although the operated patients had a significant reduction in the cost for medication against diabetes (69 per cent) and CVD (31 per cent), this was counterbalanced by increased costs for drugs against other diseases e.g. gastrointestinal disorders and anaemia. In spite of a huge weight loss difference the average annual drug costs during six years were similar in operated and conventionally treated patients[6]. Furthermore, the six-year costs for hospitalization were higher in the operated group than among the conventionally treated patients (Narbro K *et al.*, unpublished data).

Concluding remarks on health economy

Obesity surgery seemed to decrease the number of days of sick leave and disability pension and also the cost of medication against common obesity-related comorbidities such as diabetes and CVD. However, there was no decrease in total drug treatment costs and the in-patient costs were increased. So far the SOS study does not provide evidence for reduced costs following obesity surgery. However, we need still longer observation time to get a clearer picture. Furthermore, health economic studies of different obese subgroups e.g. subjects with type 2 diabetes will be important.

References

1. Sullivan M, Karlsson J, Sjöström S, Taft C. Why quality of life measures should be used in the treatment of patients with obesity. In: *International textbook of obesity*, Björntorp P (ed.), pp. 485–510. Chichester: John Wiley & Sons, Ltd., 2001.

2. Sjöström L, Larsson B, Backman L, Bengtsson C, Bouchard C, Dahlgren S, Hallgren P *et al.* Swedish obese subjects (SOS). Recruitment for an intervention study and a selected description of the obese state. *Int J Obes* 1992; 16: 465–79.

3. Sullivan M, Karlsson J, Sjöström L, Backman L, Bengtsson C, Bouchard C *et al.* Swedish obese subjects (SOS) – an intervention study of obesity. Baseline evaluation of health and psychosocial functioning in the first 1743 subjects examined. *Int J Obes* 1993; 17: 503–12.

4. Karlsson J, Sjöström L, Sullivan M. Swedish obese subjects (SOS) – an intervention study of obesity. Two-year follow-up of health-related quality of life (HRQL) and eating behavior after gastric surgery for severe obesity. *Int J Obes* 1998; 22: 113–26.

5. Narbro K, Jonsson E, Larsson B, Waaler H, Wedel H, Sjöström L. Economic consequences of sick-leave and early retirement in obese Swedish women. *Int J Obes* 1996; 20: 895–903.

6. Narbro K, Ågren G, Jonsson E, Näslund I, Sjöström L, Peltonen M. Pharmaceutical costs in obese individuals: comparison with a randomly selected population sample, and long-term changes after conventional and surgical treatment: the SOS intervention study. *Arch Inter Med* 2002; 162: 2061–69.

7. Narbro K, Ågren G, Jonsson E, Larsson B, Näslund I, Wedel H, Sjöström L. Sick leave and disability pension before and after treatment for obesity: A report from the Swedish obese subjects (SOS) study. *Int J Obes* 1999; 23: 619–24.

8. Sjöström L. Surgical intervention as a strategy for treatment of obesity. *Endocrine* 2000; 13: 213–30.

9. Ågren G, Narbro K, Näslund I, Sjöström L, Peltonen M. Long-term effects of weight loss on pharmaceutical costs in obese subjects. A report from the SOS intervention study. *Int J Obes* 2002; 26: 184–92.

TRACK VII

CONTINUING MEDICAL EDUCATION

Progress in Obesity Research: 9. Edited by *Geraldo Medeiros-Neto, Alfredo Halpern and Claude Bouchard*
©2003 John Libbey Eurotext Ltd, pp. 989–993.

CHAPTER 205

Overview of the genetic susceptibility to obesity

Claude Bouchard

Pennington Biomedical Research Center, Baton Rouge, LA 70808, USA
[e-mail: Bouchac@pbrc.edu]

Introduction

There has been a dramatic increase in the prevalence of obesity in this century, and current trends suggest that the problem will get worse in the coming decades (WHO[1]). How many of the obese individuals have developed their condition as a result of a major deficiency in one gene? How many are obese as a consequence of a strong genetic predisposition determined by DNA sequence variation at several genes? How many have only a slight genetic predisposition but have gained large amounts of body weight because they had poor nutritional habits and a sedentary lifestyle? How many do not have any genetic susceptibility but nonetheless became overweight or obese? Obviously we cannot yet answer these questions. However, in recent years, genetic epidemiology and molecular genetic studies have begun to generate data which allow us to formulate these questions in more relevant terms and to sketch some response elements. This chapter will examine the genetic epidemiology aspect of the obesity epidemic.

Variation in body fat is caused by a complex network of genetic, nutritional, metabolic, energy expenditure, psychological, and social variables, all playing a role in the regulation of body weight with age. Figure 1 displays the key determinants and suggests that the impact of genetic differences on food intake, energy expenditure, energy partitioning, and adipogenesis can lead to obesity over time.

Heritability level

C.B. Davenport described in 1923 the first comprehensive attempt to understand the role of inheritance in human body mass for stature (Davenport[2]). Among his findings, normal weight parents sometimes have obese adult offspring and the converse: obese parents frequently have normal weight adult descendants. In the aggregate, however, his study demonstrated convincingly that BMI values were more similar among family members than among unrelated persons.

Except for some rare Mendelian disorders, the vast majority of obese patients do not exhibit a clear pattern of Mendelian inheritance. Despite the large number of studies on the familial aggregation and heritability of the obesity phenotypes, there is no unanimity among researchers regarding the quantitative importance of genetic factors. Only a brief summary of the main findings is presented here. A more detailed exposé of these studies can be found in Maes *et al.*[3] and Bouchard *et al.*[4].

The level of heritability is simply the fraction of the population variation in a trait (e.g. BMI) that can be explained by genetic transmission. The level of heritability has been considered in a large number of twin, adoption, and family studies. Overall the results depend on the sampling strategy, the sample size, and the kinds of relatives upon which they are based. For instance, studies conducted with identical twins and fraternal twins or identical twins reared apart have yielded the highest heritability levels with values clustering around 70 per cent of the variation in BMI[5]. In contrast, the adoption studies have generated the lowest heritability estimates, that is about 30 per cent and less[4]. The family studies have generally found levels of heritability intermediate between the twin and the adoption study reports.

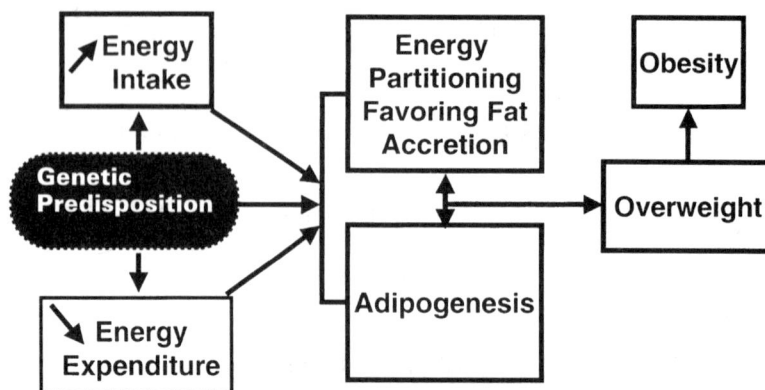

Fig. 1. Diagram of the determinants of positive energy balance and fat deposition with indication about the sites of action of a genetic predisposition.

It is fair to say that there are divergent views on the interpretation of these statistical genetic studies. Some see them as evidence for a strong genetic role in obesity. The most vocal claim that the heritability of the disease is of the order of 70 to 90 per cent of the total population variance. Among the implications of such high heritability levels, one finds a good number of predisposing genes or a few predisposing alleles at key genes present at high frequencies in human populations. In contrast, other scientists conclude that the heritability level reaches a much more modest fraction of the population variance. One implication of this position is that the changes in lifestyle experienced in this century have played a dominant role in the current overweight and obesity epidemic. At present, it is not possible to establish whether one school of thought is closer to the truth than the other.

Familial risk of obesity

The risk of becoming obese when a first-degree biological relative is overweight or obese can be quantified using the lambda coefficient, defined as the ratio of the risk of being obese when a biological relative is obese compared to the risk in the population at large, i.e. the prevalence of obesity in the same population. Estimates of lambda for obesity based on BMI data were recently reported[6-8]. Age and gender risk ratios obtained from 2349 first degree relatives of 840 obese probands and 5851 participants of the National Health and Nutrition Examination Survey III revealed that the prevalence of obesity is twice as high in families of obese individuals than in the population at large[8]. Moreover, the risk increases with the severity of obesity in the proband. Thus, the risk of extreme obesity (BMI of 45 and above) is about seven to eight times higher in families of extremely obese subjects. Other large studies report similar trends.

These lambda values are accepted as evidence for a strong genetic effect for obesity, particularly severe obesity. However, the picture is more complex than originally suggested. For instance, Katzmarzyk and collaborators, using data from 15,245 participants, aged from 7 to 69 years, from the 1981 Canada Fitness Survey, showed that the familial risk of obesity was five times higher for relatives in the upper 1 per cent of the distribution of BMI values than in the general Canadian population[7]. But the study suggested that the familial risk was not due entirely to genetic factors as the risk was also markedly elevated in the spouse of the proband. Future replication studies need to consider not only a genetic hypothesis, i.e. assessing the familial risk in a first-degree relative of the proband, but also a mixed-model in which the familial risk is assessed in a non-biological but cohabitating relative of the same proband.

Genotype-environment interactions

A genotype-environment interaction (GxE) effect arises when the response of a phenotype to environmental changes depends on the genotype of the individual. From a reasonable body of data, it is known that there are interindividual differences in the responses to various dietary interventions or to exercise programmes. However, few attempts have been made to verify whether these differences are genotype-dependent, particularly for obesity-related phenotypes.

Overfeeding

Twin A

Negative Energy Balance

Twin A

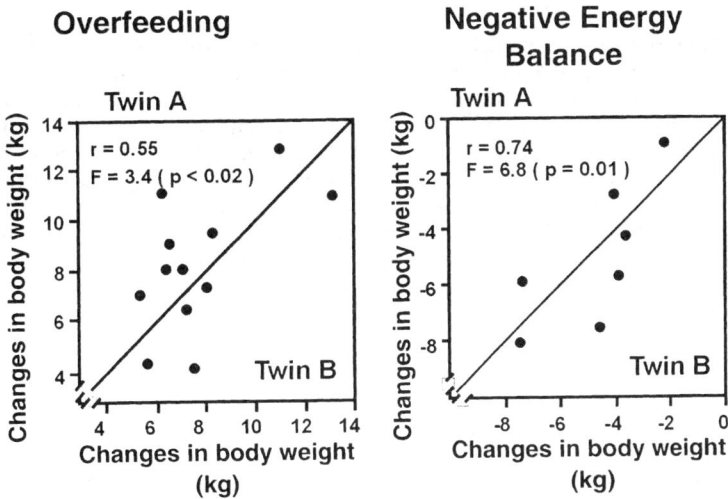

Fig. 2. Intrapair resemblance in the response of identical twins to long-term changes in energy balance. (*left*) Twelve pairs of identical twins were submitted to an 84,000 kcal energy intake surplus over 100 days; (*right*) Seven pairs were subjected to a negative energy balance protocol caused by exercise. The energy deficit was 58,000 kcal over 93 days (reproduced by permission from Bouchard[9,10]).

Studies conducted with identical twins strongly suggest that undetermined genetic characteristics may play an important role in the responsiveness to standardized alterations in energy balance conditions. Experiments performed with monozygotic twins revealed that the response to a positive or negative energy balance protocol is very heterogeneous among twin individuals but quite homogeneous within members of the same twin pair.

In one study, 12 pairs of male MZ twins ate a 4.2 MJ (1000 kcal) per day caloric surplus, six days a week, during a period of 100 days for a total caloric surplus of 353 MJ (84,000 kcal) over the energy cost of weight maintenance[9]. Significant increases in body weight and fat mass were observed after the period of overfeeding. Data showed that there were considerable interindividual differences in the adaptation to excess calories and that the variation observed was not randomly distributed, as indicated by the significant within-pair resemblance in response. There was at least three times more variance in response between pairs than in response within pairs for the gains in body weight (Fig. 2, left panel) and body fat. These data demonstrate that some individuals are more at risk than others to gain fat when energy intake surplus is clamped at the same level for everyone and when all subjects are confined to a sedentary lifestyle and that the amount of weight gained is likely influenced by the genotype.

In another experiment, seven pairs of young adult male identical twins completed a negative energy balance protocol during which they exercised on cycle ergometers twice a day, nine out of ten days, over a period of 93 days, while being kept on a constant daily energy and nutrient intake[10]. The mean total energy deficit caused by exercise above the estimated energy cost of body weight maintenance reached 244 MJ (58,000 kcal). Mean body weight loss was 5.0 kg. Intrapair resemblance was observed for changes in body weight (Fig. 2, right panel) and body fat content. Even though there were large individual differences in response to the negative energy balance and exercise protocol, subjects with the same genotype were more alike in responses than subjects with different genotypes.

The results of both experiments are remarkably similar. They demonstrate that the response to positive or negative energy balance is heterogeneous. A two to three fold range in response to the protocols was typically observed for body mass, body composition, and other obesity-related phenotypes.

The experiments also reveal that being genetically identical translates into a similar pattern of adaptation[11]. Overall these studies provide highly suggestive evidence for the presence of genotype-environment interaction effects that are of critical importance for the understanding of the predisposition to obesity and of the response to a variety of obesity treatments. Ultimately, we would like to know the genes and DNA sequence variants that are at the origin of this individuality in adaptation.

Assortative mating

Dozens of studies have reported a spousal correlation for BMI or adiposity phenotypes[12,13]. In general, the correlation is low at about 0.2 or less, although there are exceptions. Assortative mating may, however, be stronger at the upper end of the distribution of BMI values. This is exactly what has been found in some recent studies. This has led to the speculation that adiposity genes are present at a higher frequency among heavy or obese parents and that such genes are passed along to their offspring resulting over time in an increase in the genetic risk for obesity in this segment of the population. Two recent studies have provided data that are compatible with this scenario[12,13]. Childhood overweight and obesity were in both cases more frequent in families in which both parents were themselves obese. However, since obese parents may have reduced fertility, the true contribution of this phenomenon to the evolution of the genetic risk in large populations remains unknown. Note that opposite forces may be acting at the other end of the distribution although it is not yet clear from the existing studies. If this was the case, the effect would be to increase the frequency of the leanness genes in another segment of the population.

Other considerations

Several investigators have attempted to establish whether there was a maternal effect in the risk for obesity[4]. In the aggregate, the evidence is negative. Both parents seem to contribute more or less equally to the genetic risk. Moreover, there is no clear evidence for a role of non Mendelian maternal inheritance as would be the case if mitochondrial DNA was a major contributor to the risk level. Whether obese parents have more frequently obese boys or girls has been considered in several studies and the results were generally negative. Thus the transmission of risk from parents to offspring does not appear to be sex-specific.

In the Swedish Obese Subjects (SOS) study, the severely or morbidly obese proband is typically ten to 15 BMI units heavier than his or her siblings[14-16]. The same observation has been made in other studies of severely obese men and women. There is at present no good explanation for such a difference. However, the ratio of severely obese to other offspring in such families is around one out of three or four siblings. This is compatible with the ratio expected if a single recessive gene with a large effect was contributing to the risk. Under this scenario, the homozygotes for the recessive allele would be severely affected. Such a gene (and there may be several of them) has not been identified yet but candidates have emerged recently.

Finally, if current societal trends are maintained for generations, almost every individual living in a knowledge-based economy and well developed society will eventually be living in an obesogenic environment. One consequence of such a trend will be that the genetic component of the resistance to or the protection against positive energy balance will increase. Another implication will be that those with some genetic predisposition to the disease will naturally evolve towards obesity.

Conclusion

Excessive adiposity is a complex multifactorial trait evolving under the interactive influences of dozens of affectors from the social, behavioural, physiological, metabolic, cellular, and molecular domains. Segregation of the genes is not easily detected in familial or pedigree studies and whatever the influence of the genotype on the aetiology, it is generally attenuated or exacerbated by nongenetic factors, particularly in the present obesogenic environment of the Western world.

The distinction between the genes causing obesity and those predisposing to obesity is particularly relevant. We have begun to make progress in the first category perhaps because the effect of a major disruption in a gene is more evident. Progress in the identification of the predisposing genes is much slower. However, in the interim, populations of informative patients have been assembled. Geneticists and gene hunters are expected to move forward faster in the coming years and should be able to isolate many of these genes. It will nonetheless be a daunting task to define how genetic individuality interacts with factors in our environment to make some people resistant to obesity and others very much at risk of becoming obese.

The task can be seen as even more complex when the phenomenon of gene-gene interactions is considered. We will need all the power of genetics and molecular biology to unravel the genetic basis of the predisposition to obesity.

References

1. World Health Organization. Obesity – preventing and managing the global epidemic. Report of a WHO consultation on obesity. World Health Organization. Obesity; 1998.

2. Davenport CB. Build, Its Definition and Its Ontogeny. Body-Build and Its Inheritance. Washington: The Carnegie Institution of Washington; 1923. pp. 3–169.

3. Maes HH, Neale MC, Eaves LJ. Genetic and environmental factors in relative body weight and human adiposity. *Behav Genet* 1997; 27: 325–51.

4. Bouchard C, Perusse L, Rice T, Rao DC. The genetics of human obesity. In: Bray G, Bouchard C, James WPT (eds) *Handbook of obesity*, pp. 157–90. New York: Dekker Inc; 1998.

5. Stunkard AJ, Harris JR, Pedersen NL, McClearn GE. The body-mass index of twins who have been reared apart. *N Engl J Med* 1990; 322: 1483–7.

6. Allison DB, Neale MC, Kezis MI, Alfonso VC, Heshka S, Heymsfield SB. Assortative mating for relative weight: genetic implications. *Behav Genet* 1996; 26: 103–11.

7. Katzmarzyk PT, Perusse L, Rao DC, Bouchard C. Familial risk of obesity and central adipose tissue distribution in the general Canadian population. *Am J Epidemiol* 1999; 149: 933–42.

8. Lee JH, Reed DR, Price RA. Familial risk ratios for extreme obesity: implications for mapping human obesity genes. *Int J Obes Relat Metab Disord* 1997; 21: 935–40.

9. Bouchard C, Tremblay A, Despres JP, Nadeau A, Lupien PJ, Theriault G *et al.* The response to long-term overfeeding in identical twins. *N Engl J Med* 1990; 322: 1477–82.

10. Bouchard C, Tremblay A, Despres JP, Theriault G, Nadeau A, Lupien PJ *et al.* The Response to Exercise with constant energy intake in identical twins. *Obes Res* 1994; 2: 400–10.

11. Bouchard C. *Genetic and energy balance interactions in humans.* In: Carolyn D. Berdanier (ed.) Nutrients and gene expression: clinical aspects, pp. 83–100. Boca Raton: CRC Press; 1996.

12. Hebebrand J, Wulftange H, Goerg T, Ziegler A, Hinney A, Barth N *et al.* Epidemic obesity: are genetic factors involved via increased rates of assortative mating? *Int J Obes Relat Metab Disord* 2000; 24: 345–53.

13. Katzmarzyk PT, Hebebrand J, Bouchard C. Spousal resemblance in the Canadian population: implications for the obesity epidemic. *Int J Obes Relat Metab Disord* 2002; 26: 241–6.

14. Lissner L, Sjostrom L, Bengtsson C, Bouchard C, Larsson B. The natural history of obesity in an obese population and associations with metabolic aberrations. *Int J Obes Relat Metab Disord* 1994; 18: 441–7.

15. Perusse L, Chagnon YC, Bouchard C. Etiology of massive obesity: role of genetic factors. *World J Surg* 1998; 22: 907–12.

16. Reed DR, Bradley EC, Price RA. Obesity in families of extremely obese women. *Obes Res* 1993; 1: 167–72.

Progress in Obesity Research: 9. Edited by *Geraldo Medeiros-Neto, Alfredo Halpern* and *Claude Bouchard*

©2003 John Libbey Eurotext Ltd, pp. 994–998.

CHAPTER 206

Lipodystrophy-lipoatrophy

Steven R. Smith

Endocrinology Laboratory, 6400 Perkins Road, Pennington Biomedical Research Center, Baton Rouge, LA 70808, USA
[e-mail: smithsr@pbrc.edu]

Classification schema

The Online Mendeliam Inheritance in Man (OMIM) serves to coordinate the classification and diagnostic criteria of most inherited monogenic disorders[1]. The OMIM can be accessed on-line: http: //www.ncbi.nlm.nih.gov/Entrez. Recently, Premkumar, *et al.* suggested diagnostic criteria for the lipodystrophies that are listed in Table 1[2]. The reader is referred to the excellent review by Garg[3] for a more detailed discussion and the finer points of the diagnosis of the lipodystrophic syndromes. The purpose of this review is to provide a broad stroke/review of these diseases and recent progress. Lipodystrophy can be defined as an absolute or relative decrease in adipose tissue mass that leads to the ectopic fat storage in liver, muscle and the pancreatic beta cell. This ectopic fat causes increased triglycerides, insulin resistance, and diabetes. Lipodystrophy can be due to either genetic or acquired causes.

Familial partial lipodystrophy

(FPL, OMIM # 151660) Familial partial lipodystrophy, also known as Köbberling–Dunnigan syndrome is an autosomal dominant disorder that manifests during or after puberty and results in the near absence of fat in the extremities. A hallmark of this syndrome is an increase in fat around the neck, face and/or viscera.

FPL is most apparent in women due to the muscular appearance of the extremities and the greater amount of body fat of women in general. Most patients are severely insulin resistant, have dyslipidaemia with elevated triglycerides, low HDL-cholesterol and often develop overt diabetes at an early age. Köbberling–Dunnigan syndrome should not be confused with Madelung's disease (multiple symmetric lipomatosis, which also results in excess growth of adipose tissue in the upper torso, neck, and/or arms. Madelung's disease is not associated with decreased fat in the extremities, and develops in the middle years rather than at adolescence[4].

In 2000, mutations in lamin A/C were identified in patients with FPLD (Köbberling–Dunnigan syndrome)[5,6]. The lamins are structural components of the nuclear pore that are thought to be involved in the trafficking of molecules between the cytoplasm and nucleus[7]. Lamin A and C differ only in their differentially spliced C-terminal domains. Many different diseases are caused by mutations this one protein:

- Emery-Dreifuss muscular dystrophy[8];

- Limb girdle muscular dystrophy 1B[9];

- Autosomal dominant dilated cardiomyopathy and conduction system disease[10];

- Autosomal recessive Charcot-Marie Tooth disease;

- Dunnigan type FPLD

Recent evidence suggests that Lamin A interacts with SREBP 1a and 1c[11]. Given the role of SREBP/ADD in adipocyte differentiation, it is possible that mutations in LMNA block SREBP mediated adipocyte differentiation. Dhe-Paganon, S, *et al.* solved the structure of the globular tail of nuclear lamin and

---

Table 1. Proposed criteria for the diagnosis of well-characterized genetic syndromes of lipoatrophy

congenital generalized lipoatrophy

(Presence of two of the three major criteria and at least three supportive criteria needed for diagnosis)

Major criteria

Autosomal recessive inheritance

Paucity of fat apparent at birth or within the first year of life

Emergence of at least one of the following metabolic abnormalities within the first decade of life:

Fasting insulin levels of more than 30mU/ml

Fasting triglycerides levels of 200 mg/dl

Presence of diabetes as defined by American Diabetes Association criteria (fasting blood sugar > 126 mg/dl on two consecutive tests or 2-h oral glucose tolerance test glucose level >200 mg/dl on two consecutive tests)

Enlarged liver with evidence of fatty infiltration and no other genetic disease present

Supporting criteria

Acromegalic features

Cardiomegaly

Increased body hair during childhood

Evidence of hyperandrogenism in girls

Preservation of supportive fat in temporal fossa, palms, and soles of the feet; presence of glandular breast tissue in girls

Evidence of hypogonadotrophic hypogonadism

Long bones with multiple sclerotic and lytic lesions

MR images that reveal complete absence of fat in abdomen and extremities as well as absence of bone marrow fat

Early heavy proteinuria with no other features of nephrotic syndrome

Leptin levels of less than 2 ng/ml

Decreased IQ or attention deficit, particularly in boys

Familial partial lipodystrophy or Dunnigan-Kobberling syndrome

(Presence of two major criteria or of one major and two supporting criteria needed for diagnosis)

Major criteria

Autosomal dominant inheritance in pedigree (male patients are easy to miss; therefore, at least one affected first-degree female relative required to substantiate the diagnosis)

Change in body habitus at or after puberty (clear increase of fat deposits around face and neck)

Presence of mutations on lamin A gene (if the test is available)

Clear absence of subcutaneous fat in the extremities and trunk with increased fat around face and neck or viscera (suspected on basis of physical examination and supported by MR imaging findings)

At least one of the following metabolic abnormalities

Fasting insulin level of more than 30 mU/ml

Fasting triglycerides level of more than 200 mg/ml

Presence of diabetes as defined by American Diabetes Association criteria

Evidence of fatty infiltration of the liver

Supporting criteria

Presence of 'buffalo hump'

High-density lipoprotein level of less than 35 mg/dl

Evidence of premature coronary artery disease

Evidence of hyperandrogenism or menstrual abnormalities in female patients

---

identified a region of mutations that were specific for FPLD which were similar to the SREBP binding sites identified by Lloyd[12]. These discoveries generate hypotheses and hopefully the exact mechanism by which these mutations result in impaired adipocyte differentiation will be uncovered. This is especially important given the role of adipocyte differentiation in the development of diabetes[13,14].

As an alternate mechanism, several authors have identified defects in nuclear envelope structure. Lamin A and C are expressed in adipose tissue, with higher ratios of Lamin A to Lamin C in subcutaneous vs. omental AT. Whether this is related to the relative sparing of visceral/omental adipose tissue in this disorder is uncertain[15].

Mandibuloacral dysplasia

(MAD; OMIM # 248370) Once thought to be a separate disease genetic studies clearly demonstrate MAD is a LMNA mutation[16]. MAD is characterized by FPL-like fat loss and other congenital defects: hypoplastic mandible w/ dental crowding, persistently wide cranial sutures and multiple Wormian bones, postnatal growth retardation, skeletal malformations (hypoplastic scapulae), mottled cutaneous pigmentation and acroosteolysis[17].

Congenital generalized lipodystrophy

(CGL; OMIM # 269700) Congenital generalized lipodystrophy, also known as Berardinelli-Seip syndrome, is an autosomal recessive disorder that manifests at birth as a complete absence of adipose tissue, hepatomegaly, and severe nonketotic insulin resistant diabetes. Additional features include acanthosis nigricans and an elevated metabolic rate. Mechanical fat in the hands, feet, orbit, scalp and peri-articular fat is usually preserved[18]. Recent genetic studies revealed that Congenital generalized lipodystrophy is the result of mutations in guanine nucleotide-binding protein (G protein), gamma 3-linked gene (Gng3lg) a.k.a Seipin[19]. The exact function of Seipin is unknown. There is probably another gene that causes CGL. For example, Heathcote et al. describe two distinct phenotypes of CGL in Oman[20]. CGL- Type A is similar to previous reports of CGL. CGL- Type B is distinguished by: a lack of acanthosis nigricans, normal insulin, hypertrophic pyloric stenosis, muscle abnormalities (increased CPK), phlebomegaly, bone abnormalities and cardiac disturbances. Importantly, these phenotypic differences are consistent with the finding that the CGL-Type B do not harbor mutations in the Seipin gene[21].

Other mutations in patients without LMNA mutations

Recently, several pedigrees were described with severe insulin resistance, diabetes, and peripheral fat wasting without CGL or FPL. The manifestation of this inherited partial lipodystrophy syndrome is quite similar to the metabolic syndrome-X, with the exception that these patients do not respond to the anti-diabetic thiazolidinediones (TZD's). These families were found to have mutations in the PPAR-γ nuclear transcription factor gene at the ligand binding pocket. This results in impaired activation of gene transcription by the TZD's. Newer PPAR-γ ligands with a different structural backbone have been shown to bypass CGL mutations in vitro. Although rare, these mutations are instructive in the sense that the metabolic sequelae are almost identical to the 'garden-variety' obesity/syndrome-X. Agarwal and Garg describe a C to T heterozygous mutation at nucleotide 1273 in exon 6 of the PPAR-γ gene with a phenotype of lipodystrophy[22]. Other familial syndromes are also likely to exist. For example, the NIH group has identified a 'new' autosomal dominant FPL syndrome[2] that does not fit any of the existing classification schemas.

Acquired generalized lipodystrophy (AGL) (also known as Lawrence-Seip syndrome)

AGL is a disease of childhood and adolescence with progressive loss of adipose tissue across the entire body. Girls are affected at a rate three times greater than boys AGL is most likely an autoimmune disease. It is characterized by a generalized progressive loss of adipose tissue and loss of fat from the soles of the feet and palms of the hands may occur.

Acquired partial lipodystrophy (APL) (also known as Barraquer-Simons syndrome)

APL affects mainly young women. The progressive loss usually affects the face and neck and spreads downward with sparing of the pelvic girdle and lower extremities. Many of these patients exhibit altered complement activation and develop glumerulonephritis with subsequent renal failure[23]. Metabolic complications, such as insulin resistance and dyslipidaemia, are less common (~50 per cent) than in CGL, which is compatible with the relatively normal blood levels of leptin and adiponectin[24].

Juvenile dermatomyositis associated lipodystrophy

Juvenile dermatomyositis associated lipodystrophy begins as a partial lipodystrophy and progresses to generalized lipodystrophy. Intraabdominal adipose tissue is usually preserved.

'Other' types of acquired lipodystrophy

HIV associated lipodystrophy

HIV and HIV therapy are associated with alterations in body composition; lipoatropy, lipid storage as abdominal adipose tissue or buffalo hump, and a mixed syndrome[25]. The aetiology of this finding is unclear, however, in-vitro studies demonstrate a variety of direct effects of HIV drugs on adipocytes and insulin sensitivity in animals and humans. Several studies suggest that activation and rebound of the immune system during HAART are associated with lipodystrophy[26,27]. Recent molecular studies demonstrate multiple alterations in adipose tissue transcription factors (PPAR-γ and SREBP1/ADD) and an increase in mRNA for TNF-β; in addition, the metabolic alterations are highly correlated with the blood levels of the soluble TNF receptor (sTNF-RII)[27].

Therapy

PPAR-γ agonists

Given that (a) lipodystrophy is a disorder of inadequate adipocyte growth, (b) the anti-diabetic thiazolidenediones promote the differentiation of adipose tissue, and (c) *in vitro* studies demonstrate TZDs activate differentiation in cells from lipodystrophic patients[28], TZD therapy is a logical treatment for lipodystrophy. Arioglu *et al.* demonstrate a good response in patients treated with a first generation TZD: troglitazone[29]. As a cautionary note, one of these patients developed liver complications during therapy with troglitazone and liver enzyme testing at regular intervals may be more important than in the routine diabetic patient. Given this caveat, the newer TZD's, which are less likely to cause liver toxicity, are likely to become a first line therapy for lipodystrophic metabolic syndromes.

Leptin

Given that leptin levels are low in lipodystrophy patients and that leptin plays an important role to regulate fat oxidation and neuroendocrine function, and positive results in lipodystrophic mice, leptin is an obvious therapeutic choice for patients with lipodystrophy. Recent reports demonstrte a stunning decrease in hepatomegaly–steatosis, reversal of insulin resistance and an improvement in glucose control in patients treated with recombinant leptin. Similarly, disordered neuroendocrine function is reversed by the same treatment[30]. Additional studies are needed to determine the efficacy of this therapy in patients with milder forms of lipodystrophy and those with higher leptin levels[30,31].

Energy balance

Older temporarily effective therapies include plasmapheresis to remove triglycerides. A prudent diet is indicated in individuals with any of the lipodystrophy syndromes. For example, Montenegro *et al.* carefully controlled fat intake and diet in a child with CGL and were able to reverse the elevated blood sugar levels[32].

Conclusion

The lipodystrophies represent a variety of underlying genetic and acquired disorders with a common metabolic phenotype: ectopic fat, insulin resistance and diabetes. The recent discoveries of the genetic basis of these diseases will assist in their care and the care of millions of others with garden-variety metabolic syndrome and diabetes. The nuance of the diseases and the familial cases that do no have mutations in known genes highlight that we still have much to learn.

Acknowledgements: I would like to acknowledge the support of the Bristol-Myers-Squibb Lipodystrophy initiative and the USDA that provide support for this work. I also acknowledge the contributions of Dr. George Bray through his lively and enlightening discussions.

References

1. Hamosh A, Scott AF, Amberger J, Valle D, McKusick VA. Online Mendelian Inheritance in Man (OMIM). *Hum Mutat* 2000; 15(1): 57–61.

2. Premkumar A, Chow C, Bhandarkar P, Wright V, Koshy N, Taylor S *et al.* Lipoatrophic-lipodystrophic syndromes: the spectrum of findings on MR imaging. *AJR Am J Roentgenol* 2002; 178(2): 311–8.

3. Garg A. Lipodystrophies. *Am J Med* 2000; 108(2): 143–52.

4. Zancanaro C, Sbarbati A, Morroni M, Carraro R, Cigolini M, Enzi G *et al.* Multiple symmetric lipomatosis. Ultrastructural investigation of the tissue and preadipocytes in primary culture. *Lab Invest* 1990; 63(2): 253–8.

5. Speckman RA, Garg A, Du F, Bennett L, Veile R, Arioglu E *et al.* Mutational and haplotype analyses of families with familial partial lipodystrophy (Dunnigan variety) reveal recurrent missense mutations in the globular C-terminal domain of lamin A/C. *Am J Hum Genet* 2000; 66(4): 1192–8.

6. Cao H, Hegele RA. Nuclear lamin A/C R482Q mutation in canadian kindreds with Dunnigan-type familial partial lipodystrophy. *Hum Mol Genet* 2000; 9(1): 109–12.

7. Genschel J, Schmidt HH. Mutations in the LMNA gene encoding lamin A/C. Hum Mutat 2000; 16(6): 451–9.Emery AE. Emery-Dreifuss muscular dystrophy – a 40 year retrospective. *Neuromuscul Disord* 2000; 10(4–5): 228–32.

8. Kitaguchi T, Matsubara S, Sato M, Miyamoto K, Hirai S, Schwartz K *et al.* A missense mutation in the exon 8 of lamin A/C gene in a Japanese case of autosomal dominant limb-girdle muscular dystrophy and cardiac conduction block. *Neuromuscul Disord* 2001; 11(6–7): 542–6.

9. Jakobs PM, Hanson EL, Crispell KA, Toy W, Keegan H, Schilling K *et al.* Novel lamin A/C mutations in two families with dilated cardiomyopathy and conduction system disease. *J Card Fail* 2001; 7(3): 249–56.

10. Lloyd DJ, Trembath RC, Shackleton S. A novel interaction between lamin A and SREBP1: implications for partial lipodystrophy and other laminopathies. *Hum Mol Genet* 2002; 1(7): 769–77.

11. Dhe-Paganon S, Werner ED, Chi YI, Shoelson SE. Structure of the globular tail of nuclear lamin. *J Biol Chem* 2002; 277(20): 17381–4.

12. Weyer C, Foley JE, Bogardus C, Tataranni PA, Pratley RE. Enlarged subcutaneous abdominal adipocyte size, but not obesity itself, predicts type II diabetes independent of insulin resistance. *Diabetologia* 2000; 43(12): 1498–506.

13. Danforth E Jr. Failure of adipocyte differentiation causes type II diabetes mellitus? *Nature Genet* 2000; 26(1): 13.

14. Lelliott CJ, Logie L, Sewter CP, Berger D, Jani P, Blows F *et al.* Lamin expression in human adipose cells in relation to anatomical site and differentiation state. *J Clin Endocrinol Metab* 2002; 87(2): 728–34.

15. Novelli G, Muchir A, Sangiuolo F, Helbling-Leclerc A, D'Apice MR, Massart C *et al.* Mandibuloacral Dysplasia Is Caused by a Mutation in LMNA-Encoding Lamin A/C. *Am J Hum Genet* 2002; 71(2): 426–31.

16. Simha V, Garg A. Body fat distribution and metabolic derangements in patients with familial partial lipodystrophy associated with mandibuloacral dysplasia. *J Clin Endocrinol Metab* 2002; 87(2): 776–85.

17. Seip M, Trygstad O. Generalized lipodystrophy, congenital and acquired (lipoatrophy). *Acta Paediatr Suppl* 1996; 413: 2–28.

18. Magre J, Delepine M, Khallouf E, Gedde-Dahl T Jr, van Maldergem L, Sobel E *et al.* Identification of the gene altered in Berardinelli-Seip congenital lipodystrophy on chromosome 11q13. *Nature Genet* 2001; 28(4): 365–70.

19. Heathcote K, Rajab A, Magre J, Syrris P, Besti M, Patton M *et al.* Molecular analysis of Berardinelli-Seip congenital lipodystrophy in Oman: evidence for multiple loci. *Diabetes* 2002; 51(4): 1291–3.

20. Rajab A, Heathcote K, Joshi S, Jeffery S, Patton M. Heterogeneity for congenital generalized lipodystrophy in seventeen patients from Oman. *Am J Med Genet* 2002; 110(3): 219–25.

21. Agarwal AK, Garg A. A novel heterozygous mutation in peroxisome proliferator-activated receptor-gamma gene in a patient with familial partial lipodystrophy. *J Clin Endocrinol Metab* 2002; 87(1): 408–11.

22. Levy Y, George J, Yona E, Shoenfeld Y. Partial lipodystrophy, mesangiocapillary glomerulonephritis, and complement dysregulation. An autoimmune phenomenon. *Immunol Res* 1998; 18(1): 55–60.

23. Haque WA, Shimomura I, Matsuzawa Y, Garg A. Serum adiponectin and leptin levels in patients with lipodystrophies. *J Clin Endocrinol Metab* 2002; 87(5): 2395.

24. Carr A, Samaras K, Thorisdottir A, Kaufmann GR, Chisholm DJ, Cooper DA. Diagnosis, prediction, and natural course of HIV–1 protease-inhibitor- associated lipodystrophy, hyperlipidaemia, and diabetes mellitus: a cohort study [see comments]. *Lancet* 1999; 353(9170): 2093–9.

25. Ledru E, Christeff N, Patey O, de Truchis P, Melchior JC, Gougeon ML. Alteration of tumor necrosis factor-alpha T-cell homeostasis following potent antiretroviral therapy: contribution to the development of human immunodeficiency virus-associated lipodystrophy syndrome [In Process Citation]. *Blood* 2000; 95(10): 3191–8.

26. Mynarcik DC, McNurlan MA, Steigbigel RT, Fuhrer J, Gelato MC. Association of severe insulin resistance with both loss of limb fat and elevated serum tumor necrosis factor receptor levels in HIV lipodystrophy [In Process Citation]. *J Acquir Immune Defic Syndr* 2000; 25(4): 312–21.

27. Fischer P, Moller P, Bindl L, Melzner I, Tornqvist H, Debatin KM *et al.* Induction of adipocyte differentiation by a thiazolidinedione in cultured, subepidermal, fibroblast-like cells of an infant with congenital generalized lipodystrophy. *J Clin Endocrinol Metab* 2002; 87(5): 2384–90.

28. Arioglu E, Duncan-Morin J, Sebring N, Rother KI, Gottlieb N, Lieberman J *et al.* Efficacy and safety of troglitazone in the treatment of lipodystrophy syndromes [see comments]. *Ann Intern Med* 2000; 133(4): 263–74.

29. Oral EA, Ruiz E, Andewelt A, Sebring N, Wagner AJ, Depaoli AM *et al.* Effect of leptin replacement on pituitary hormone regulation in patients with severe lipodystrophy. *J Clin Endocrinol Metab* 2002; 87(7): 3110–7.

30. Petersen KF, Oral EA, Dufour S, Befroy D, Ariyan C, Yu C *et al.* Leptin reverses insulin resistance and hepatic steatosis in patients with severe lipodystrophy. *J Clin Invest* 2002; 109(10): 1345–50.

31. Montenegro RM Jr, Montenegro AP, Fernandes MI, de Moraes RR, Elias J Jr, Gouveia LM *et al.* Triglyceride-induced diabetes mellitus in congenital generalized lipodystrophy. *J Pediatr Endocrinol Metab* 2002; 15(4): 441–7.

Progress in Obesity Research: 9. Edited by *Geraldo Medeiros-Neto, Alfredo Halpern and Claude Bouchard*

©2003 John Libbey Eurotext Ltd, pp. 999–1003.

CHAPTER 207

Body composition: an overview

Steven B. Heymsfield

New York Obesity Research Center, St. Luke's-Roosevelt Hospital, Columbia University, Institute of Human Nutrition, College of Physicians and Surgeons, New York, NY 10025, USA
[e-mail: SBH2@Columbia.edu]

Introduction

Quantifying the amount and distribution of adipose tissue and its related components is important to the study and treatment of human obesity and other nutritional disorders. Body composition research is a field devoted to the development and extension of methods for the *in vivo* quantification of adipose tissue and other related components[1,2].

The human body consists of multiple components distributed across four main organizational levels: atomic, molecular, cellular, and tissue system (Fig. 1)[3,4]. The sum of all components at each level of body composition is equivalent to total body mass.

An understanding of the theoretical basis of these levels and of the inter-relationships among the components at different levels is important in properly applying body composition methods. In the section that follows I review the main characteristics of each body composition level. Some general references are listed at the end[1–9].

Body composition levels

The human body is comprised of 11 elements that account for > 99 per cent of total body mass[1]. Three elements, C, H and O are found in storage triglycerides. The average proportion of triglyceride as C, H an O are stable at approximately 76.7 per cent, 12.0 per cent, and 11.3 per cent, respectively. These stable elemental triglyceride proportions permit development of methods for deducing total body fat from total body carbon and other elements[8].

The above elements, including essential trace elements that are found in small quantities, combine to form chemical compounds that may be grouped into broad classes that define the molecular level of body composition. The main molecular level components include lipids, water, proteins, minerals and carbohydrates[1–3].

Three main components are included in the cellular level: cell mass, extracellular fluid, and extracellular solids. Connective, epithelial, nervous, and muscular cells are specific cell types. Adipocytes or fat cells serve as the primary storage site for triglycerides. Storage triglycerides are usually excluded in the estimation of 'body cell mass', a term which refers to the active protoplasmic portion of cells. Accordingly the cellular level can be considered as fat, body cell mass, extracellular fluid, and extracellular solids.

The main components at the tissue-system level are adipose tissue, skeletal muscle, bone, and visceral organs (e.g. liver, kidneys, heart, etc.). Magnetic resonance imaging (MRI) methods are now replacing CT as a means of quantifying VAT and other tissue-system level body composition components. In addition to adipose tissue, all major organs and tissues can now be quantified *in vivo* by MRI and other related methods.

The whole body level, not shown in Figure 1, includes characteristics such as body mass, stature, body density, resistance, skinfold thicknesses, and circumferences. Most clinical methods for estimating the main body composition components are at the whole-body level of body composition. These measurements, such as skinfold thicknesses, are often used with prediction equations to estimate components (e.g. fat and skeletal muscle) at the other four-body composition levels[1–3].

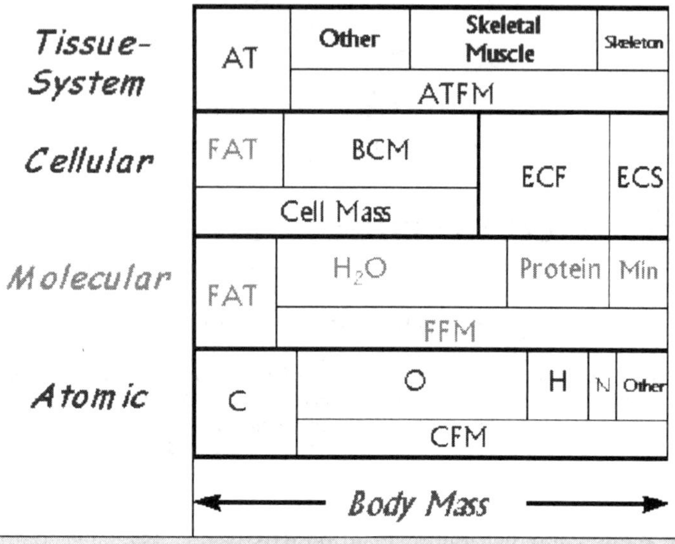
Tissue-System
AT
Other
Skeletal Muscle
Skeleton
ATFM
Cellular
FAT
BCM
ECF
ECS
Cell Mass
Molecular
FAT
H2O
Protein
Min
FFM
Atomic
C
O
H
N
Other
CFM
Body Mass

Fig. 1. The first four body composition levels and their respective main components. The fifth body composition level, whole-body, is not shown in the figure. Abbreviations: AT, adipose tissue; ATFM, adipose tissue-free body mass; BCM, body cell mass; CFM, carbon-free body mass; ECF, extracellular fluid; ECS, extracellular solids; FFM, fat-free body mass; and Min, mineral mass. From[2] with permission.

Body composition methods

The following sections provide an overview of whole-body and regional measurement methods.

Anthropometry

Anthropometry is the least expensive and most widely used method of assessing human body composition. Anthropometric measurements are used in clinical and epidemiological studies to grade the degree of malnutrition or obesity in populations[7]. Anthropometric measurements useful in the clinical and research setting include body weight, stature, skinfold thicknesses, circumferences of the trunk and limbs, and sagittal diameter.

The most widely used weight-stature index is Quetelet's body-mass index (BMI), $BMI = W/S^2$ where weight (W) is measured in kilograms and stature (S) is measured in meters. This index has the advantage of being inexpensive, safe and easy to obtain. It only requires a standard scale and stadiometer.

Skinfold thickness and circumference measurements are widely applied and can be used alone in evaluating nutritional status. As the cost of anthropometric methods is low and they are easily applied, they are useful in field and clinical studies of subject populations at baseline and over time. The main disadvantages of anthropometry are that technical skill is required for proper application and accuracy/reproducibility even with correct application are lower than for research-based methods.

Bioimpedance analysis

Over the past decade bioimpedance analysis (BIA) was introduced as a simple, safe, and relatively inexpensive means of quantifying body composition components. The main concept upon which BIA is based is that tissues rich in water and electrolytes are less resistant to the passage of an electrical current than lipid-rich adipose tissue. In concept a subject with no adipose tissue would have minimum impedance, and impedance would increase to a maximum when all lean tissue was replaced by lipid-filled adipose tissue. Impedance methods include an estimate of height to adjust for between-individual differences in electrical path length. The path length typically evaluated is arm-to-leg, although the measurement of an isolated limb or trunk impedance is increasing in popularity.

Impedance methods are often single frequency systems, mainly 50 kHz, although multiple frequency systems are widely available. Measured impedance is associated mainly with tissue fluid content and therefore single-frequency BIA methods are usually calibrated for estimating total body water or fat-free mass. Once fat-free mass is known total body fat can be calculated as the difference between body weight and fat-free mass[1,2].

With BIA a critical issue is that subject measurement conditions must be standardized. Subject and room temperature, body position, electrode lead placement, and other controllable factors such as eating or drinking and proximity of aerobic exercise to time of evaluation should all be considered and standardized if possible.

Practically all BIA body composition methods are based on 'empirical' prediction models. This is important because developed prediction formulas should only be applied to populations for whom the regression model was developed. Inaccurate results can be anticipated when, for example, BIA is applied in obese subjects and component prediction formulas are used which were developed in normal weight individuals.

Isotope dilution

The most important isotope dilution method is dilution of labeled water (^3H_2O, D_2O and $H_2^{18}O$). Total body water estimates also allow evaluation of fat-free mass and fat. The classic method of estimating fat and fat-free body mass is based on the assumed stable hydration of fat-free mass (i.e. total body water/fat-free mass = 0.73)[3]. Fat-free mass can be calculated using this ratio once total body water is known from isotope dilution. Fat can then be calculated as the difference between body weight and fat-free mass.

The widespread applicability of total body water methods is based on their simplicity, low cost, and overall safety, particularly of stable water isotopes. The main limitation of this useful method is the model error introduced when hydration is rendered abnormal (i.e. = 0.73) by various diseases and with other states such as normal ageing.

Dual-energy X-ray absorptiometry (DXA)

Although DXA was originally introduced for measuring the amount of mineral within bone, this important method can also be used to estimate soft-tissue fat and lean.

DXA is based on the differential attenuation of a collimated photon beam at two effective energy levels as it passes through the body. The ratio of the mass attenuation coefficients, the so-called R-value, at the two energy levels is used to estimate soft tissue and bone mineral and the fraction of fat in the soft-tissue on a pixel-by-pixel basis. The pixel composition estimates are summed to provide total body estimates. For pixels that contain both soft and bone tissues, the fat content of the soft tissue component is interpolated from the nearest pixels that do not contain bone. DXA estimates bone mineral, fat, and lean soft-tissue masses for the whole body and separately for the arms, legs, and trunk.

Now there are many validation studies comparing DXA with those derived by other research methods[1-3]. The limitation of DXA in obesity research surrounds calibration issues in the obese population and the limited capacity of most commercial scanners to accommodate subjects with BMI in excess of about 35 kg/m^2. Half-body scans are proposed as a means of overcoming the body-size problem encountered when evaluating morbidly obese subjects.

In vivo neutron activation analysis (IVNA) and whole body counting

Four elements – O, C, H and N– account for over 95 per cent of body mass and with an additional seven – Na, K, P, Cl, Ca, Ma and S – comprise 99.5 per cent of body mass[1,3]. Elements maintain stable or relatively stable associations with the other major elements. Several of these well-recognized associations are (kg/kg): S/N = 0.062; N/protein = 0.16; C/triglyceride = 0.77; K/intracellular water = 150 mmol/l; and H/body weight = 0.10.[1] These are important 'constants' applied in body composition research[3].

Neutron activation analysis methods can quantify the major elements *in vivo*, including total body H, C, N, O, Na, Ca, P and Cl. Total body potassium (TBK) can be measured with ^{40}K whole-body counting alone or as part of some IVNA protocols. Potassium is mainly found as non-radioactive ^{39}K, although a small portion (0.0118 per cent) consists of radioactive ^{40}K. This natural mixture of K isotopes also occurs in human tissues, and ^{40}K can be estimated by whole-body counting. Once the subject's ^{40}K content is known, TBK (mmol) can be estimated as TBK = ^{40}K/0.0118. The estimated TBK can then be used to derive body cell mass (BCM) as, BCM (kg) = TBK (mmol) x 0.0083. Total body K can also be used to estimate total body skeletal muscle mass and intracellular fluid[1-3]. Neutron activation systems expose patients to ionizing radiation and therefore pregnant women and children are not usually studied. Whole-body counting for potassium is without known hazard.

1001

Imaging

Both computerized axial tomography (CT) and magnetic resonance imaging (MRI) afford the opportunity to evaluate tissue-system level components *in vivo*. High-resolution cross-sectional images can be produced by CT and MRI and software then used to estimate various pixel areas. Multiple cross-sectional images can then be used to reconstruct tissue volumes including: total, subcutaneous, and visceral adipose tissue; skeletal muscle; brain; visceral organs such as liver, spleen, kidneys, and heart; skin; bone; and other smaller organs and tissues. Mass can then be calculated as the product of organ/tissue volume and assumed density.

The CT/MRI multicomponent approach represents a major advance in the study of human body composition. The entire tissue-system level of body composition can be analysed *in vivo* with high accuracy and reproducibility. While CT exposes subjects to radiation, MRI is without any known hazard.

Imaging techniques are revolutionizing body composition research. New insights into energy exchange, metabolic processes, and functional properties of tissues are provided by nuclear magnetic spectroscopy and other concurrently applied methods such as positron emission tomography. The recognition of these exciting areas is supported by the recent addition of a biomedical imaging institute at the National Institutes of Health.

Method selection

The available instruments, specific question posed, and evaluated subject group collectively determine the appropriate measurement method. Evaluation of large subject populations in field surveys requires simple, practical, and safe portable methods. Small-scale studies examining limited numbers of subjects or a single individual at one or more time points require reliable adiposity measurement methods. Methods applied in children, women of child bearing potential, or women who are pregnant must meet different safety criteria from methods applied in the elderly or ill patients. A summary of some of these considerations is provided for the various methods in Table 1. Methods in this qualitative survey tend to group among these characteristics: accurate methods tend to be more costly to purchase and operate, are less practical to apply, and are usually associated with some risk. In contrast, the field methods tend to be less expensive to purchase and operate, simple to apply, and are safe for application in most populations. These various considerations determine method selection.

Table 1. Qualitative characteristics of body composition methods

Method	Research	Clinical	Cost	Safety	Accessibility
Neutron activation	****	*	****	*	*
WBC	****	*	***	****	*
DXA	***	***	***	***	***
Hydrometry+	***	**	**	****	**
UWW-AP	***	**	**	****	**
BIA	**	****	*	****	****
Anthropometry	*	****	*	****	****

Scores range from low (*) too high (****). +assumes stable isotope;
Abbreviations: WBC, whole body ^{40}K counting; DXA, dual-energy x-ray absorptiometry; UWW-AP, underwater weighing and air plethysmography; BIA, bioimpedance analysis.
Accessibility refers to availability of measurement systems. From[3] with permission.

Conclusions

There are many methods of estimating body composition components, particularly in the context of evaluating human obesity and its associated risks. The method selection depends on the specific purpose of the measurements: questions posed will dictate the requirement for method accuracy and precision and turn will relate to method cost, safety, practicality, and availability. These are important considerations as most research centres now have multiple available methods ranging from CT and MRI to DXA, BIA, and anthropometry. Few centres today have whole-body counters and IVNA systems.

These modern body composition methods should aid in establishing pathogenesis and quantifying risk and treatment response of a serious nutritional disorder human obesity.

References

1. Wang ZM, Pierson RN Jr, Heymsfield SB. The five level models: a new approach to organizing body composition research. *Am J Clin Nutr* 1992; 56: 19–28.

2. Pietrobelli A, Heymsfield SB, Wang ZM, Gallagher D. Multi-component body composition models: recent advances and future directions. *Eur J Clin Nutr* 2001; 55: 69–75.

3. Hoffman D, Humber RK, Allison DB, Wang Z, Shen W, Heymsfield SB. *Human body composition* (in press).

4. Wang ZM, Heshka S, Pierson RN Jr, Heymsfield SB. Systematic organization of body composition methodology: overview with emphasis on component-based methods. *Am J Clin Nutr* 1995; 61: 457–65.

5. Moore FD, Oleson KH, McCurray JD, Parker HV, Ball MR, Boyden CM. *Body cell mass and its supporting environment: body composition in health and disease.* Philadelphia: WB Saunders; 1963.

6. Behnke AR. Role of fat in gross body composition and configuration. In: *Fat as a tissue,* Rodahl K (ed.), pp. 285–313. New York: McGraw Hill, 1964.

7. Heymsfield SB. Anthropometric assessment. In: Wright RA, Heymsfield SB (eds) *Nutritional assessment of the hospitalized patient,* pp. 27–82. Boston: Blackwell Scientific; 1984.

8. Heymsfield SB, Wang ZM, Baumgartner RN, Ross R. Human body composition: advances in models and methods. *Annu Rev Nutr* 1997; 17: 527–58.

9. Forbes GB. *Human body composition.* New York: Springer-Verlag; 1987.

Progress in Obesity Research: 9. Edited by *Geraldo Medeiros-Neto, Alfredo Halpern and Claude Bouchard*

CHAPTER 208

Race differences in body composition

Dympna Gallagher and Stanley Heshka

New York Obesity Research Center, St. Luke's/Roosevelt Hospital and Columbia University, Institute of Human Nutrition, New York, New York, USA
[e-mail: sh311@columbia.edu]

T he study of body composition differences among race/ethnic groups is pursued for several reasons – some immediately practical, some more theoretical. There are known biological differences among race/ethnic groups in some important dimensions, for example, bone mineral density, and differences in prevalence of certain disorders such as diabetes and coronary vascular disease (CVD) in African Americans compared to Caucasians. Differences in body composition may mediate or play an explanatory or causal role in the prevalence of disease rates or risk factors. In the more exploratory and investigative sense newly identified differences in body composition may lead to the discovery of important health correlates or consequences of which we are not yet aware.

The literature on ethnic differences in body composition is large and an integrative overview is not possible in this limited space. A sample of findings indicating the range of investigations that have been conducted is presented here.

In studies of populations of different race/ethnic groups, whether living in the US or in their native countries, it should be borne in mind that phenotypic differences are likely to be influenced by the environment and lifestyle characteristic of the local culture as well as by expression of genetic endowment.

Studies in adults

Soon after the adoption of the body mass index (kg/m^2, BMI) as a universal index for the definition of overweight and obesity by the WHO[1], it became apparent that race differences in the amount of fat existed at the threshold percentiles of overweight and obesity (25th and 30th BMI). If the deleterious effects of obesity are a function of fat mass rather than body mass then the manner in which fat mass varies as a function of race for a given BMI may be important.

An investigation of this question was reported by Gallagher *et al.*[2]. Using dual energy x-ray absorptiometry (DXA) and a 4-compartment model for determination of fat mass, three samples of race/ethnic groups (Caucasian, African American and Asian) from the UK, USA and Japan were compared. The results indicated that African Americans tended to have less percent body fat and Asians tended to have more percent body fat at most age/sex groups compared to Caucasian subjects (Table 1).

Hispanics in the USA are a difficult ethnic group to study because of the range of racial genetic admixture, reflecting the mixed racial heritage of their country of origin and their own particular genetic inheritance. Methods using genetic markers based on known frequency of occurrence of certain alleles within race groups are required for more definitive genotyping[3]. Nevertheless, a study by Fernandez *et al.*[4] using a sample of Puerto Rican Hispanics showed that the women tended to have greater percent body fat at low BMI (< 30) and smaller percent body fat at higher BMI (> 35) than European American women.

Race differences in the distribution of fat, especially along the central versus peripheral, or the intra-abdominal versus subcutaneous dimensions[5], are of interest since evidence suggests that central and visceral deposits are associated with more adverse health conditions than peripheral/subcutaneous deposits[6,7]. Mexican Americans have been shown to have greater trunk fat deposits as measured by skinfold thickness compared to Caucasians[8,9]. In a sample of Asians (mainly of Chinese and Korean descent) living in New York city, Park *et al.*[10] found larger visceral adipose tissue (VAT) deposits with increasing age, compared to those of Caucasian women. VAT deposits in Pima Indians, an ethnic group with high insulin resistance and hyperinsulinaemia, have been compared with those of equally obese Caucasians, and found to be not significantly different[11]. Several studies have reported relatively less VAT in African Americans compared to Caucasians[12,13].

Table 1. Percentage body fat by sex, age and race

BMI	Caucasian	African-American	Asian	Caucasian	African-American	Asian
kg/m²	F	F	F	M	M	M
			Age 20–39			
18.5	21	20	25	8	8	13
25.0	33	32	34	21	20	23
30.0	39	38	40	26	26	28
			Age 40–59			
18.5	23	21	25	11	9	13
25.0	35	34	36	23	22	24
30.0	41	39	41	29	27	29
			Age 60–79			
18.5	25	23	26	13	11	14
25.0	38	55	36	25	23	24
30.0	43	41	41	31	29	29

F = female; M = male; age in years.

The studies mentioned above were concerned with fat mass and its distribution. There are also studies investigating quantity and quality of skeletal muscle and other tissues and organs. Amount of skeletal muscle, for instance, is correlated with bone mineral density (BMD), which is an important factor in bone fractures, and to measures of physical functioning. Race differences in BMD are well known[14], however the role of skeletal muscle in contributing to the development and maintenance of BMD has not been clearly delineated. Nevertheless, race differences have been observed in appendicular skeletal muscle such that after adjusting for age, weight and stature, African Americans had more than Caucasians[15].

Total body potassium (TBK) measurement, carried out by counting the gamma particles given off by a naturally-occurring isotope of potassium, ^{40}K, has been used to measure lean body mass as the body's potassium is located almost entirely in lean tissue[16]. Because skeletal muscle makes up approximately 60 per cent of lean body mass, TBK measurement may be used to track changes in lean tissue and skeletal muscle[17]. Consistent with findings reported earlier, research in our laboratory shows race differences in peak values of TBK and in rate of decline with ageing in women and men.

The quality as well as quantity of skeletal muscle is also of interest. As persons age and/or gain weight, adipose tissue deposits increase within the muscle area. Inter- and intra-muscular adipose tissue (IMAT) is a depot measured by MRI in our laboratory, where inter-muscular adipose tissue is the adipose tissue visible between named muscles and intra-muscular adipose tissue is visible within a specific muscle, between fascicles. There is preliminary evidence that these deposits may affect insulin sensitivity and glucose disposal, as strongly as, and perhaps even more than VAT. Preliminary results from our laboratory (unpublished) show that there are race/ethnic differences in IMAT deposits that do not track the size of deposits in other adipose compartments. These observations may provide an insight into the development or correlates of diabetes and CVD.

Another type of tissue/organ study has investigated possible differences in the mass of certain 'high metabolic rate' organs (liver, brain, kidney, heart) as an explanation for observed resting energy expenditure (REE) differences of 200–400 kJ/day between African American and Caucasian women matched for age, height, weight and fat-free mass. The mass of the relevant organ/tissues was quantified using MRI scans and algorithms for volume rendering of these organs. Regression analyses showed that

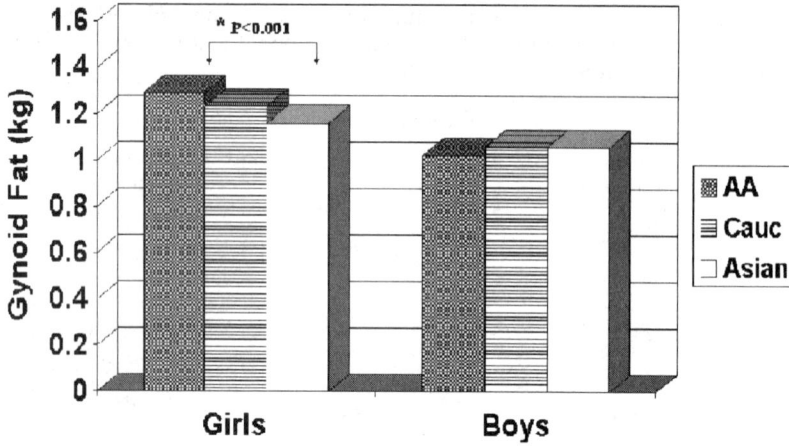

Fig. 1a. Log-transformed values for DXA-derived gynoid fat. *Adjusted multiple *post-hoc* comparisons ($P <$ 0.01) were used to compare the adjusted means for Asians to those for African-Americans and Caucasians. Boys and girls were analysed separately.

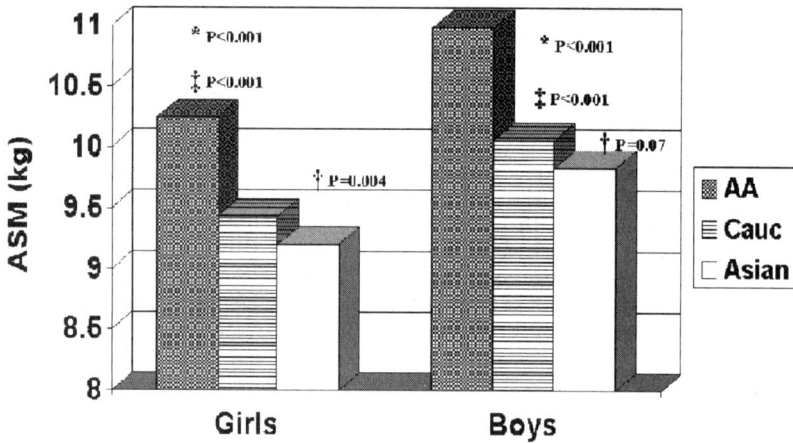

Fig. 1b. Appendicular skeletal muscle mass in Asian (left), Caucasian (middle), and African-American (right) females and males. Mean values adjusted for height, weight, and age are presented; P values are: *Asian vs. African-American; †Asian vs. Caucasian; ‡Caucasian vs. African-American.

race is a statistically significant factor in accounting for the total mass of high metabolic rate organs. The regression of organ mass on height, weight, and age yielded a multiple correlation coefficient of 0.56; the addition of race to the regression model significantly increased the correlation to 0.66 indicating that African American females had less 'high metabolic rate' tissue then Caucasians of equivalent weight, height and age. Thus, if metabolic coefficients (energy requirement per unit weight per unit time) of organs are equivalent across races, this difference in mass may explain observed REE differences.

Studies in children

Although most work has been carried out in adults, recently there have been investigations to determine whether race/ethnic differences already exist in early childhood, and to identify correlates of such differences.

A series of studies by He *et al.*[18] investigated race differences in fat distribution in African American, Asian, and Caucasian children at prepuberty, early puberty and late puberty. Findings show that the amount of extremity and gynoid fat and the pattern of sexual dimorphism of fat distribution in prepuberty (Fig. 1a) and with advance in pubertal age differed in Asians compared to African-Americans and Caucasians. Boys had less extremity and gynoid fat in late puberty compared to prepuberty. Trunk fat deposits have been associated with increased blood pressure at all pubertal stages in boys[19]. Greater limb lean tissue mass has been found in African American compared to Caucasian children through all Tanner stages[20]. Song *et al.*[21], using a sample of African American, Asian and Caucasian prepubertal children confirmed previously reported race differences in appendicular skeletal muscle between African American and Caucasians, and reported that Asian girls and boys had less skeletal muscle than African Americans and Caucasians (Fig. 1b).

Differences in bone mineral content are already present at pre-puberty. Horlick *et al.*[22], investigated total body bone mineral content (TBBMC) adjusted for total body bone area, age, height, and weight in prepubertal African American and Caucasian females ($n = 172$) and males ($n = 164$). TBBMC was greater in males than in females ($P = 0.01$), and this sex difference was independent of race. African American children had greater TBBMC than Asian and Caucasian children ($P = 0.001$). No differences were found between Asian and Caucasian children.

Race differences in REE of approximately 200 kJ/day have been noted between African American and Caucasian children. Although it is unclear whether REE differences play a role in the development of obesity, these differences are of interest for basic biological understanding of organ growth and the underlying causes of these race differences in REE are being investigated.

References

1. Obesity: preventing and managing the global epidemic. Report of a WHO Consultation on Obesity, Geneva, 3–5 June 1997.

2. Gallagher D, Heymsfield SB, Heo M, Jebb SA, Murgatroyd PR, Sakamoto Y. Healthy percentage body fat ranges: an approach for developing guidelines based on body mass index. *Am J Clin Nutr* 2000; 72: 694–701.

3. Shriver MD. Ethnic variation as a key to the biology of human disease. *Ann Intern Med* 1997; 127: 401–403.

4. Fernández J, Heo M, Heymsfield SB, Pierson RN, Pi-Sunyer FX, Wang ZM, Wang J, Hayes M, Allison DB, Gallagher D. Is per cent body fat differentially related to BMI in Hispanic- African- and European-Americans? *Am J Clin Nutr* 2003; 77(1): 71–5.

5. Fujimoto WY, Bergstrom RW, Boyko EJ, Leonetti DL, Newell-Morris LL, Wahl PW. Susceptibility to development of central adiposity among populations. *Obes Res* 1995; 3 (Suppl 2): 179S–186S.

6. Seidell JC, Bjorntorp P, Sjostrom L, Kvist H, Sannerstedt R. Visceral fat accumulation in men is positively associated with insulin, glucose, and C-peptide levels, but negatively with testosterone levels. *Metabolism* 1990; 39: 897–901.

7. Larsson B, Svardsudd K, Welin L, Wilhelmsen L, Bjorntorp P, Tibblin G. Abdominal adipose tissue distribution, obesity, and risk of cardiovascular disease and death: 13 year follow up of participants in the study of men born in 1913. *BMJ (Clin Res Ed)* 1984; 288: 1401–4.

8. Greaves KA, Puhl J, Baranowski T, Gruben D, Seale D. Ethnic differences in anthropometric characteristics of young children and their parents. *Hum Biol* 1989; 61: 459–477.

9. Casas YG, Schiller BC, DeSouza CA, Seals DR. Total and regional body composition across age in healthy Hispanic and white women of similar socioeconomic status. *Am J Clin Nutr* 2002; 73: 13–18.

10. Park YW, Allison DB, Heymsfield SB, Gallagher D Larger amounts of visceral adipose tissue in Asian Americans. *Obes Res* 2001; 9: 381–7.

11. Gautier JF, Milner MR, Elam E, Chen K, Ravussin E, Pratley RE . Visceral adipose tissue is not increased in Pima Indians compared with equally obese Caucasians and is not related to insulin action or secretion. *Diabetologia* 1999; 42: 28–34.

12. Hill JO, Sidney S, Lewis CE, Tolan K, Scherzinger AL, Stamm ER Racial differences in amounts of visceral adipose tissue in young adults: the CARDIA (Coronary Artery Risk Development in Young Adults) study. *Am J Clin Nutr* 1999; 69: 381–7.

13. Perry AC, Applegate EB, Jackson ML, Deprima S, Goldberg RB, Ross R, Kempner L, Feldman BB. Racial differences in visceral adipose tissue but not anthropometric markers of health-related variables. *J Appl Physiol* 2000; 89: 636–43.

14. Bachrach LK, Hastie T, Wang MC, Narasimhan B, Marcus R Bone mineral acquisition in healthy Asian, Hispanic, black, and Caucasian youth: a longitudinal study. *J Clin Endocrinol Metab* 1999; 84: 4702–12.

15. Gallagher D, Visser M, De Meersman RE, Sepúlveda D, Baumgartner RN, Pierson RN, Harris T, Heymsfield SB. Appendicular skeletal muscle mass: effects of age, gender, and ethnicity. *J Appl Physiol* 1997; 82: 229–39.

16. Moore FD, Olesen KH, McMurrey JD, Parker JHV, Ball M. *The body cell mass and its supporting environment: body composition in health and disease.* Philadelphia: WB Saunders, 1963.

17. Cohn SH, Vaswani A, Zanzi I, Aloia JF, Roginsky MS, Ellis KJ Changes in body chemical composition with age measured by total-body neutron activation. *Metabolism* 1976; 25: 85–95.

18. He Q, Horlick M, Thornton J, Wang J, Pierson RN, Heshka S, Gallagher D Sex and race differences in fat distribution among Asian, African-American, and Caucasian prepubertal children. *J Clin Endocrinol Metab* 2002; 87: 2164–70.

19. He Q, Horlick M, Fedun B, Wang J, Pierson RN, Heshka S, Gallagher D Trunk fat and blood pressure in children through puberty. *Circulation* 2002; 105: 1093–8.

20. Sun M, Gower BA, Bartolucci AA, Hunter GR, Figueroa-Colon R, Goran MI. A longitudinal study of resting energy expenditure relative to body composition during puberty in African-American and white children. *Am J Clin Nutr* 2001; 73: 308–15.

21. Song M, Kim J, Horlick M, Wang J, Pierson RN, Heo M, Gallagher D Prepubertal Asians have less limb skeletal muscle. *J Appl Physiol* 2002; 92: 2285–91.

22. Horlick M, Thornton J, Wang J, Levine LS, Fedun B, Pierson RN Bone mineral in prepubertal children: gender and ethnicity. *J Bone Miner Res* 2000; 15: 1393–7.

Progress in Obesity Research: 9. Edited by *Geraldo Medeiros-Neto, Alfredo Halpern and Claude Bouchard*
©2003 John Libbey Eurotext Ltd, pp. 1009–1014.

CHAPTER 209

Obesity and diabetes

H. Hauner

German Diabetes Research Institute, Auf'm Hennekamp 65, 40225 Düsseldorf, Germany
[e-mail: hauner@ddfi.uni-duesseldorf.de]

Numerous reports have clearly established that obesity has become a global epidemic during the last decades and there is little doubt that this unfavourable trend is still unchanged or has even accelerated[1]. At present, between 15 and 25 per cent of the total population in the industrialized countries are obese with a BMI ≥ 30 kg/m^2 and another 40 per cent are moderately overweight with a BMI ranging from 25 to 29.9 kg/m^2. There has also been an even more dramatic rise in overweight and obesity in most developing countries. According to present calculations the number of over-weight/obese people in the world is currently surpassing the number of people suffering from under-nutrition.

As a consequence of the obesity epidemic between 5 and 8 per cent of the total population in the Western countries are now suffering from type 2 diabetes mellitus. It is particularly alarming in this context that type 2 diabetes is more frequently diagnosed in young people and there is a growing number of type 2 diabetic subjects among obese children and adolescents[2]. Likewise, there is an even stronger trend for a rise in the prevalence of type 2 diabetes in developing countries. Therefore, it is projected that the number of subjects with diabetes will have more than doubled to approximately 300 million by the year 2025[3].

Obesity – the most important risk factor for type 2 diabetes

There is now overwhelming evidence from a variety of prospective studies that obesity is by far the most important modifiable risk factor for the development of type 2 diabetes. This is particularly true for women in whom already a body weight in the upper normal range is associated with an increased incidence of type 2 diabetes[4], but similar data have been reported for men[5]. This is in contrast to other cardiovascular risk factors, where the incidence starts to increase at clearly higher body weight levels. Consistent with this observation, changes in body weight throughout adult life have a direct impact on the risk of diabetes. A weight increase between 11 and 19.9 kg since the age of 18 in middle-aged women was associated with a 5.5-fold increase in the risk of diabetes compared to weight-stable women. This degree of weight gain represents the average change in body weight in the industrialized countries. Thus, preventing weight gain during adult life would be sufficient to prevent up to 80 per cent of all cases of type 2 diabetes. In contrast, those participants in the two above quoted studies who were able to reduce their body weight were found to reduce their risk of diabetes considerably[4,5]. The detrimental role of obesity is also suggested by data showing that the mean BMI of men and women with type 2 diabetes under the age of 70 is between 29 and 30 kg/m^2. However, it should be noted that only between 30 and 50 per cent of all obese subjects will develop diabetes in future life, whereas the majority of patients will remain free of this disease due to differences in genetic susceptability. It is also important to note that the risk of metabolic complications is particularly elevated if there is an abdominal pattern of fat distribution as indicated by a waist circumference > 85 cm in females and > 100 cm in men. The independent contribution of an abdominal fat distribution for the development of type 2 diabetes had first been described in a prospective study from Gothenburg[6] and was confirmed by many subsequent studies.

Pathophysiology of obesity-associated type 2 diabetes

Although the molecular mechanisms that underly the development of type 2 diabetes are still far from being understood, there is compelling evidence that obesity induces a state of insulin resistance, however to a highly variable extent. Those individuals with marked insulin resistance are particularly prone to develop clinical diabetes. The currently prevailing hypothesis indicates that there is an additional defect of the β-cells. As long as insulin resistance is compensated by an increased production and secretion of insulin blood glucose concentrations will remain in the normal range. Only when the secretory capacity of the β-cells fails to maintain hyperinsulinaemia type 2 diabetes will develop[7]. The later stages of type 2 diabetes are characterized by further continuous deterioration of β-cell function which may finally lead to insulin deficiency and the requirement of insulin supplementation, independent of the degree of body weight[8]. In addition, there are recent data indicating that obesity also promotes disturbances in insulin secretion via the high turnover of fatty acids and the elevated production of leptin which was found to inhibit insulin release. Finally, obesity is characterized by an increased hepatic glucose production which is also a feature of the diabetic state.

In this context, it is also important to mention that obesity is not only a promoter of type 2 diabetes but also the common soil for the simultaneous development of dyslipidaemia and hypertension. Thus, the development of type 2 diabetes is frequently accompanied or even preceded by other metabolic disturbances, which may explain the elevated risk for cardiovascular complications. Therefore, it is not surprising that type 2 diabetes and atherosclerosis are developing in parallel and result from long-standing more or less pronounced metabolic disturbances which may also involve a chronic inflammatory process.

Indication for the treatment of obesity and treatment goals

There is agreement among obesity experts that overweight in subjects with type 2 diabetes should be treated if the BMI exceeds 27 kg/m^2. Weight reduction is the more urgent the more associated risk factors are detectable. Unfortunately, the enormous impact of obesity on the development and course of diabetes is not adequately addressed by current recommendations for the treatment of diabetes. These guidelines promote a strict control of blood glucose, blood pressure and blood lipids, but are rather diffuse and inconcrete with respect to the management of overweight or obesity. Usually, an adequate body weight by appropriate caloric intake is recommended which does not fully reflect the clinical importance of elevated body weight.

The treatment strategies for obese subjects with type 2 diabetes are in principle the same as those for subjects without diabetes. Generally, a modest to moderate weight loss is strived for, but weight goals should always take the individual situation into account. Most guidelines recommend a weight loss of 5 to 10 per cent which is a rather realistic goal and can be achieved by the majority of patients if adequate obesity programmes are applied. In addition, as type 2 diabetes and its accompanying risk factors are chronic conditions, long-term maintenance of the reduced body weight is an essential target.

The first step in any weight management programme is the establishment of a healthy life-style which consists of a moderately energy-reduced balanced diet, an increase in physical activity and behaviour modification. There are now several randomized controlled trials demonstrating that this approach is at least partially successful and can induce weight loss for limited time periods[9]. Other evidence-based treatment components that may be also applied are summarized in Table 1. It has been convincingly shown by clinical studies that there exists a dose-response relationship between the extent of weight loss and improvement in metabolic variables including blood pressure[10]. It is currently unclear for how long subjects may benefit from weight loss programmes. Unfortunately, in most studies there was a rapid and at least partial weight regain which was associated with a deterioration in metabolic control[11], pointing to the importance of weight maintenance. Long-term follow-up data from the ACS Cancer Prevention Study I also indicate that intentional weight loss in subjects with diabetes is associated with a decrease in overall mortality by up to one third[12]. Similar supportive data on the effect of weight loss on life expectancy have previously been published in a retrospective study of diabetic subjects in Scotland[13].

The potential of weight-lowering drugs in obese subjects with type 2 diabetes

To date, all studies on the long-term outcome of weight loss are more or less disappointing. Most participants usually regain most or all of the body weight they had lost. Therefore, a lot of efforts were made in the past to improve long-term results. One approach to solve this problem is to develop drugs which may help to control body weight.

Table 1. Components for the treatment of overweight/obese patients with type 2 diabetes

Nutrition

Moderately energy-reduced healthy diets (energy deficit 500–800 kcal/day)
       Low-fat, carbohydrate *ad libitum* diets
       Very-low-calorie diets (VLCD)
              for a limited period of time (max. 3 months)
              intermittent (e.g. one day per week)
       Meal-replacement strategy (one main meal/day by formula diet)

Increase in physical activity
Regular physical activity in daily life   Additional leisure time activity, e.g. sports (low-to-moderate intensity)
Behaviour modification
Weight-lowering drugs

Orlistat
       Sibutramine
       (Metformin)

Bariatric surgery

Gastric bypass
       Vertical banded gastroplasty (VBG)
       Laparoscopic gastric banding

At present, there is only limited information on the use and efficacy of weight lowering drugs for the treatment of obese individuals with type 2 diabetes. There is wide agreement that these drugs should only be taken if a weight loss ≥ 5 per cent is not achieved by conventional methods within a period of 3 months at minimum. In addition, weight-lowering drugs should be used only above a threshold BMI of 27 kg/m^2. Two drugs, which have been recently approved in most countries, may be used for adjunct treatment of obese subjects.

Orlistat is a pancreatic lipase inhibitor which was found to reduce body weight by reducing fat absorption in the small intestine. There are currently two clinical studies available on the effect of orlistat on body weight and metabolic control in obese subjects with type 2 diabetes treated with either oral anti-diabetic agents or insulin[14,15]. The average additional weight loss in both studies was 1.9 kg and 2.6 kg, respectively. At the end of the 1-year treatment period there was an additional decrease in mean HbA$_{1c}$ by 0.5 per cent and 0.3 per cent, respectively, compared to the control groups despite a greater reduction in anti-diabetic medication[14,15]. Furthermore, a modest improvement in other risk factors, particularly total and LDL-cholesterol, was observed. Drug treatment was well tolerated, but the drop-out rates under orlistat were substantial, although not different from the respective control group.

Sibutramine is a selective serotonine and noradrenaline reuptake-inhibitor which reduces energy uptake and modestly increases energy expenditure. Two studies have been published so far that prove the weight lowering potential of this drug also in type 2 diabetic subjects (16)(17). In the first study, addition of sibutramine for 3 months led to an additional weight loss of 2.3 kg which was associated with a reduction of HbA$_{1c}$ by 0.3 per cent[16]. In a more recent study from Turkey, treatment with sibutramine for 6 months resulted in additional weight loss by 8.7 kg and a decrease in HbA$_{1c}$ by 2.7 per cent[17]. Administration of sibutramine was well tolerated but there remains some concern as to whether the sympathomimetic action of the drug may cause undesired blood pressure elevation in a population prone to the development of hypertension.

Thus, there is only limited data available concerning the benefit and safety of weight lowering drugs in this particular patient group. Therefore, the database is not sufficient to give general recommendations for the optimal use of these drugs in the management of obese subjects with type 2 diabetes, although this option could become a helpful treatment component in the future. Moreover, there is an urgent need for clinical outcome studies, before a firm and reliable conclusion can be drawn concerning the clinical benefit of both drugs. So far, these drugs should only be used with caution and only for limited periods of time.

Anti-diabetic agents and body weight

Weight control in subjects with type 2 diabetes may be complicated by the concomitant administration of anti-diabetic agents. There is now a substantial amount of data from clinical trials indicating that the effect of the single glucose-lowering agents on body weight is highly variable. In a recent meta-analysis of randomized controlled trials in lean and obese patients with type 2 diabetes it turned out that the use of sulphonylureas is associated with an average weight gain of 1.7 kg, while treatment with metformin results in a mean average weight loss of 1.2 kg at the same degree of amelioration of HbA_{1c} levels, suggesting that replacing sulphonylureas with metformin goes along with a weight advantage of roughly 3 kg which is equivalent to the weight-lowering potential of an anti-obesity drug[18]. For this and other reasons, e.g. reduction in cardiovascular morbidity and mortality[19], metformin is currently considered as the drug of first choice in overweight/obese subjects with type 2 diabetes.

Among the other anti-diabetic agents α-glucosidase inhibitors were found to have a modest weight lowering potential, while all other novel drugs including thiazolidinediones and glinides increase body weight[20]. Average weight increase is greatest under insulin treatment which may be accompanied by a deterioration in associated cardiovascular risk factors[21], thereby diminishing or even abolishing the beneficial effect of improved glycaemic control.

Are more aggressive weight reduction strategies required?
The role of very-low-calorie diets

Apart from the use of weight-lowering agents there are two other promising strategies to reduce body weight more effectively. The first is the use of very-low-calorie diets (VLCD). There is considerable evidence from a variety of studies showing that application of VLCD not only results in a greater initial weight reduction but may also promote an acute amelioration of insulin resistance. Some studies also suggest that VLCD treatment may improve long-term metabolic control in obese diabetic patients even if weight is regained[22]. There is also recent indication that the long-term results of VLCDs may be better than those of moderately hypocaloric diets, at least in subjects without diabetes[23]. Therefore, it appears that VLCDs could represent a more efficient strategy to better maintain weight loss than conventional strategies. Clinical experience suggests that intermittent VLCD for 1–2 days a week or similar concepts may serve this purpose with particular efficacy, but clinical data supporting this clearly are missing. On the other hand, it must not be neglected that VLCDs have a much greater risk of adverse effects and require much tighter medical supervision[22].

Obesity surgery

Bariatric surgery is another means of reducing body weight, but its application is restricted to those with a BMI over 40 or at least over 35 kg/m² and in whom conventional strategies have failed to achieve treatment goals. There is now a number of studies available, mostly in small samples of morbidly obese subjects, showing that the substantial weight loss usually achieved by such surgical techniques results in a dramatic improvement in glucose metabolism and insulin resistance. This improvement is usually observed despite the fact that body weight is not normalized and despite a marked reduction in anti-diabetic medication[24]. A retrospective study of 154 extremely obese individuals with type 2 diabetes undergoing gastric bypass surgery reported not only an improvement in glycaemic control and a reduced requirement for anti-diabetic agents but also a reduction in the overall mortality rate (1.0 per cent per year vs. 4.5 per cent per year in a group of 78 control subjects) over an observation period of up to nine years[25]. In addition, a recent analysis of the Swedish Obese Subjects (SOS) study demonstrated that substantial weight loss by bariatric surgery dramatically reduces the incidence of type 2 diabetes mellitus over up to 8 years[26]. Therefore, bariatric surgery appears to be an extremely effective and beneficial therapeutic approach in well selected severely obese patients with diabetes mellitus. Nevertheless, a careful selection of the patients, special training of the surgeon and continuous medical care are required to obtain excellent results and minimize the risk of serious complications.

Is it more difficult for obese subjects with diabetes to lose weight?

There is some evidence from clinical studies that weight loss is more difficult to achieve in subjects with diabetes, but not all studies confirm this finding. However, there are several aspects which may be considered in this context and which may explain why the effects of weight loss strategies may be smaller in individuals with type 2 diabetes than in non-diabetic subjects. Firstly, obese patients with type 2 diabetes are usually older and have more health problems than obese subjects without diabetes. Higher age is known to be associated with smaller weight reduction[9]. Secondly, depression is more frequent in diabetic as compared to non-diabetic subjects and may reduce the compliance to weight loss measures. Thirdly, many obese subjects with type 2 diabetes focus more on blood glucose control than on body weight management. Finally, the majority of patients takes anti-diabetic drugs that promote weight increase or make weight loss more difficult.

How can long-term weight reduction and maintenance be achieved in subjects with type 2 diabetes?

Long-term weight stabilization is still a target that is not sufficiently achieved by current strategies and remains the greatest challenge in obesity treatment. However, the following components were found to support long-term weight maintenance at least in younger obese subjects without diabetes: a permanently moderate caloric intake, in particular a low-fat diet, regular physical activity in daily life and additional sports, regular contact with the treatment team, and social and emotional support by family members, friends or self-help groups. A particular risk factor for weight increase in subjects with diabetes is the introduction of insulin treatment. Therefore, when patients are put on insulin treatment attention should be directed to this potential adverse effect and advice should be given to prevent weight gain. It is currently a matter of debate as to whether a strategy that contains preprandial administration of small amounts of rapid-acting insulin is superior to a more conventional scheme of two daily injections of premixed insulin.

In conclusion, the management of overweight/obesity plays a central and still underestimated role in the treatment of subjects with type 2 diabetes. The treatment principles are the same as those for individuals without diabetes. As several anti-diabetic drugs including insulin and sulphonylureas are known to increase body weight, concomitant management of body weight has to be a mandatory component of any diabetes treatment strategy. For several reasons including a weak anorectic effect metformin is the anti-diabetic agent of choice in overweight/obese individuals with type 2 diabetes. Due to the elevated risk of subjects with diabetes for cardiovascular complications, a more strict and aggressive weight management is advocated to reduce this risk by greater and more sustained weight loss.

References

1. World Health Organization. Obesity: preventing and managing the global epidemic. Report of a WHO Consultation. WHO Technical Report Series 894. Geneva: World Health Organization; 2000.

2. Sinha R, Fisch G, Teague B, Tamborlane WV, Banyas B, Allen K *et al.* Prevalence of impaired glucose tolerance among children and adolescents with marked obesity. *N Engl J Med* 2002; 346: 802–10.

3. King H, Aubert RE, Herman WH. Global burdens of diabetes, 1995–2025: prevalence, numerical estimates and projections. *Diabetes Care* 1999; 21: 1414–31.

4. Colditz GA, Willett WC, Rotnitzky A, Manson JE. Weight gain as a risk factor for clinical diabetes in women. *Ann Intern Med* 1995; 122: 481–6.

5. Chan JM, Rimm EB, Colditz GA, Stampfer MJ, Willett WC. Obesity, fat distribution, and weight gain as risk factors for clinical diabetes in men. *Diabetes Care* 1994; 17: 961–9.

6. Ohlson LO, Larsson B, Svärdsudd K *et al.* The influence of body fat distribution on the incidence of diabetes mellitus. 13,5 years of follow-up of the participants in the study of men born in 1913. *Diabetes* 1985; 34: 1055–8.

7. Polonsky KS, Sturis SJ, Bell GI. Non-insulin-dependent diabetes mellitus – a genetically programmed failure of the beta cell to compensate for insulin resistance. *N Engl J Med* 1996; 334: 777–83.

8. Kahn BB, Flier JS. Obesity and insulin resistance. *J Clin Invest* 2000; 106: 473–81.

9. Brown SA, Upchurch S, Anding R *et al.* Promoting weight loss in type II diabetes. *Diabetes Care* 1996; 19: 613–24.

10. Wing RR, Koeske R, Epstein LH *et al.* Long-term effects of modest weight loss in type II diabetic patients. *Arch Intern Med* 1987; 147: 1749–53.

11. Wing RR, Marcus MD, Salata R *et al.* Effects of a very-low-calorie diet on long-term glycemic control in obese type 2 diabetic subjects. *Arch Int Med* 1991; 151: 1334–40.

12. Williamson DF, Thompson TJ, Thun M *et al.* Intentional weight loss and mortality among overweight individuals with diabetes. *Diabetes Care* 2000; 23: 1499–51.

13. Lean ME, Powrie JK, Anderson AS, Garthwaite PH. Obesity, weight loss, and prognosis in type 2 diabetes. *Diab Med* 1990; 7: 228–33.

14. Hollander PA, Elbein SC, Hirsch IB *et al.* Role of orlistat in the treatment of obese patients with type 2 diabetes. *Diabetes Care* 1998; 21: 1288–98.

15. Kelley DE, Bray GA, Pi-Sunyer FX *et al.* Clinical efficacy of orlistat therapy in overweight and obese patients with insulin-treated type 2 diabetes. *Diabetes Care* 2002; 25: 1033–9.

16. Finer N, Bloom SR, Frost GS, Banks LM, Griffiths J. Sibutramine is effective for weight loss and diabetic control in obesity with type 2 diabetes: a randomised, double-blind, placebo-controlled study. *Diab Obes Metab* 2000; 2: 105–12.

17. Gokcel A, Karakose H, Ertorer EM *et al.* Effects of sibutramine in obese female subjects with type 2 diabetes and poor blood glucose control. *Diabetes Care* 2001; 24: 1957–60.

18. Johansen K. Efficacy of metformin in the treatment of NIDDM. *Diabetes Care* 1999; 22: 33–7.

19. UKPDS. Effect of intensive blood-glucose control with metformin on complications in overweight patients with type 2 diabetes. *Lancet* 1998; 352: 854–65.

20. Hauner H. Current pharmacological approaches to the treatment of obesity. *Int J Obes* 2001; 25 (Suppl 1): S102–S106.

21. Yki-Järvinen H, Ryysy L, Kauppila M *et al.* Effect of obesity on the response to insulin therapy in non-insulin-dependent diabetes mellitus. *J Clin Endocrinol Metab* 1997; 82: 4037–43.

22. Henry RR, Gumbiner, B. Benefits and limitations of very-low-calorie diet therapy in obese NIDDM. *Diabetes Care* 1991; 14: 802–23.

23. Anderson JW, Konz EC, Frederic RC, Wood CL. Long-term weight loss maintenance: a meta-analysis of US studies. *Am J Clin Nutr* 2001; 74: 579–84.

24. Pories WJ, MacDonald KG, Morgan EJ *et al.* Surgical treatment of obesity and its effects on diabetes: 10-y follow-up. *Am J Clin Nutr* 1992; 55: S582–S585.

25. MacDonald KG, Long SD, Swanson MS *et al.* The gastric bypass operation reduces the progression and mortality of non-insulin-dependent diabetes mellitus. *J Gastrointest Surg* 1997; 1: 213–20.

26. Sjöström CD, Peltonen M, Wedel H, Sjöström L. Differentiated long-term effects of intentional weight loss on diabetes and hypertension. *Hypertension* 2000; 36: 20–5.

CHAPTER 210

The metabolic syndrome

Per Björntorp

Dept. of Heart & Lung Diseases, Sahlgren's Hospital, University of Göteborg, Sweden
[e-mail.: Per.Bjorntorp@hjl.gu.se]

The metabolic syndrome is usually defined as a cluster of risk factors where abdominal obesity, insulin resistance, dyslipidaemia and hypertension are included. These are all powerful risk factors for diabetes mellitus type 2, cardiovascular disease and stroke. Recent research has indicated the possibility of common pathogenetic factor(s) for this syndrome. This will be reviewed in the following. Recent overviews have been published, and several of the references to original work will be found in these summaries[1–5].

In principle two approaches to the understanding of the syndrome have appeared. One is that insulin resistance is the primary event, followed by dyslipidaemia and hypertension by known or suggested mechanisms[6]. The putative primary factor, insulin resistance could be caused by physical inactivity, stress, smoking or other known mediators of this symptom. The problem with this attempt to explanation is, however, that it is difficult to understand how abdominal obesity comes into the picture. Abdominal obesity is one of the cornerstones of the metabolic syndrome and needs to be included in attempts to find a common explanatory mechanism.

The other approach to find an explanation is that central neuroendocrine abnormalities are the primary factor. The main players here are the both stress axes, the hypothalamic-pituitary-adrenal (HPA) axis and the central sympathetic nervous system (SNS). The latter has been established as a major pathogenetic factor in the generation of primary hypertension[7]. The activation of the HPA axis is followed by an increased secretion of cortisol. Subsequently the central gonadal and growth hormone axes are inhibited[8]. This results in on the one hand elevated cortisol and, on the other, low sex steroid and growth hormone concentrations in circulation. These hormonal abnormalities are each alone and, particularly in combination, resulting in accumulation of fat in intra-abdominal, visceral fat depots due to variations in specific receptor density in different adipose tissue regions. Cortisol activates the rate limiting enzyme for lipid uptake, the lipoprotein lipase, while sex steroids in combination with growth hormone have opposite effects[9].

It is thus apparent that these endocrine abnormalities are able to explain the accumulation of fat in central, visceral depots. In addition, the other major part of the metabolic syndrome, the insulin resistance can be explained by these hormonal changes. The ability of cortisol to induce insulin resistance is classical knowledge. This might occur either directly at the cellular level or via permissive effects on the lipolytic process. Since the SNS activity also frequently is elevated in the metabolic syndrome this will result in an excessive fat mobilization and elevated levels of circulating free fatty acids. Free fatty acids are powerful inducers of insulin resistance.

In addition, low sex hormones and, surprisingly, growth hormone deficiency is associated with insulin resistance. The cause-effect relationship here is supported by intervention studies, which improve or diminish the symptoms, and by the known mechanisms by which this is occurring[1–3].

The situation seems to be different in men and women. The cortisol is the predominant active hormone in men. In women adrenal androgens seem to be the major factor. Androgens in women have in essence the same affects as cortisol[9].

The dyslipidaemia is likely to be a consequence of the hyperinsulinaemia created by the insulin resistance, again via mechanisms which are essentially known[6]. It has been argued that the hypertension included in the syndrome might be a consequence of the prevailing hyperinsulinaemia via activation of the central SNS[6]. It seems at least equally likely that the elevated blood pressure is a

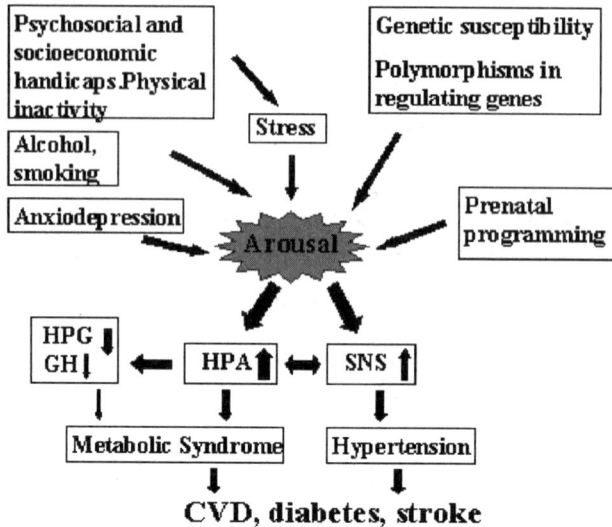

Fig. 1. The pathogenesis of an 'arousal syndrome' as a background to the metabolic syndrome (for details, see text).
Abbreviations: HPG: Hypothalamic-pituitary-gonadal axis. GH: Growth hormone. HPA: Hypothalamic pituitary-adrenal axis. SNS: Sympathetic nervous system. CVD: Cardiovascular disease.

consequence of a parallel activation of the both stress axes, the HPA axis and the SNS. These axes are difficult to activate separately[8], and, as mentioned above primary hypertension is know generally considered to be a consequence of SNS activation[7].

This explanation of the pathogenesis of the metabolic syndrome via central events has the advantage that it takes a holistic view on all the parts of the syndrome and there is strong evidence for the mechanisms involved for each symptom.

Primary pathogenetic factors involved

The brief review above then indicates that frequently repeated or chronic activation of the both stress axis, the HPA axis and the SNS, are followed by the metabolic syndrome. An important question then becomes whether or not these axes are activated in the syndrome, and what the potential factors causing this would be.

There is considerable evidence that such factors are prevalent in the metabolic syndrome. There are several socioeconomic and psychoscial handicaps associated with the syndrome. These include low social class, low education, physical types of comparably poorly paid jobs, low housing standards and a poor social environment[10,11]. Such circumstance would most likely cause frequent situations of stress reactions. In addition, symptoms of depression and anxiety, as well as use of too much alcohol and tobacco smoking are often found in subjects with the syndrome. All these factors are known to activate the HPA axis and the SNS[12]. There are likely more factors involved, not yet determined.

To sum up at this point, it appears that a cluster of factors, alone or more likely, in combinations are activating the both stress axes, the HPA axis and the SNS, to result in a cascade of peripheral and autonomic abnormalities which are able to induce the different components of the Metabolic syndrome. The prevalence of these pathogenetic factors is high in modern society, and therefore it is not surprising that the prevalence of the metabolic syndrome has been estimated to be as high as in the order of 25 per cent in the population[6].

Models

The interpretation of the situation leading to the metabolic syndrome, reviewed above, finds support in a number of other situations. First, Cushing's syndrome, with excess cortisol secretion is associated with a classic metabolic syndrome, which disappears after successful treatment.

In addition, and more to the point are experiments in non-human primates in captivity. Such animals form social hierarchies where the monkeys at the bottom of the social ladder are stressed and depressed. Under these fully controlled, mild forms of social stress these bottom monkeys develop the full metabolic syndrome, including elevated cortisol secretion, seen as enlargements of the adrenals, accumulation of visceral fat, insulin resistance with decreased glucose tolerance, hypertension and early coronary atherosclerosis[13]. This is strong evidence from prospective, controlled studies in these close relatives to man, that the metabolic syndrome can be induced by psychosocial stress.

Other evidence comes from studies of a socioeconomic gradient in the Whitehall studies, where a low socioeconomic status is associated with the metabolic syndrome and vice versa[14]. Furthermore, depression is associated with the metabolic syndrome, and this is a classical example of increased activity of the HPA ans SNS axes.

Additional evidence now also seems to emerge from the 'small baby syndrome'. At adult age subjects born small for gestational age develop the metabolic syndrome. Such subjects have a sensitive HPA axis which might be a consequence of a programming during *in utero*[15].

Genetic aspects

Genetic factors are clearly involved in the pathogenesis of the metabolic syndrome. With the background provided above it would be logical to seek abnormalities in genes regulating the stress axes. Such studies have recently begun and shown associations to potential candidate genes, including for example the glucocorticoid receptor gene and, in women the aromatase gene[16–18]. These studies are ongoing.

References

1. Björntorp P. Etiology of the metabolic syndrome. In: Bray GA, Bouchard C, JamesWPT (eds), *Handbook of obesity*, pp. 573-600. New York: Marcel Dekker; 1998.

2. Björntorp P. Hypothalamic origin of prevalent human disease. In: Pfaff D, Arnold A, Etgen A, Fahrbach S, Rubin R, Hormones *et al.* (eds), vol. 5, pp. 607–35. San Diego: Academic Press; 2000.

3. Björntorp P, Rosmond R. Obesity and cortisol. *Nutrition* 2000; 16: 924–36.

4. Björntorp P, Holm G, Rosmond R. Hypothalamic arousal, insulin resistance and type 2 diabetes mellitus. *Diabetic Med* 1999; 16: 373–401.

5. Björntorp P. Neuroendocrine perturbations as a cause of insulin resistance. *Diab Metab Res Rev* 1999; 15: 427–41.

6. Reaven GM. Role of insulin in human disease. *Diabetes* 1988; 37: 1595–1607.

7. Björntorp P, Holm G, Rosmond R, Folkow B. Primary hypertension and the metabolic syndrome: Closely related central origin? *Blood Press* 2000; 9: 71–82.

8. Chrousos GP, Gold PW. The concept of stress and stress system disorders. Overview of physical and behavioral homeostasis. *JAMA* 1992; 267: 1244–52.

9. Björntorp P. The regulation of adipose tissue distribution in humans *Int J Obes* 1996; 20: 291–302.

10. Rosmond R, Lapidus L, Björntorp P. The influence of occupational status and social factors on obesity and body fat distribution in middle-aged men. *Int J Obes Relat Metab Disord* 1996; 20: 599–607.

11. Björntorp P. Visceral obesity: A 'Civilization Syndrome'. *Obes Res* 1993; 1: 216–22.

12. Björntorp P, Rosmond R. Hypothalamic origin of the metabolic syndrome X. *Ann NY Acad Sci* 1999; 892: 297–307.

13. Shively CA, Laber-Laird K, Anton RF. Behavior and physiology of social stress and depression in female cynomolgus monkeys. *Biol Psychiatry* 1997; 41: 871–882.

14. Brunner E, Marmot MG, Nanchatal K, Shipley MJ, Stansfield SA, Juneja M. Social inequality in coronary risk: central obesity and the metabolic syndrome. Evidence from the Whitehall II study. *Diabetologia* 1997; 40: 1341–1349.

15. Phillips DIW, Barker DJP, Fall CHD, Seckl JR, Whorwood CB, Wood PJ, Walker BR. Elevated cortisol concentrations: A link between low birth weight and the insulin resistance syndrome? *J Clin Endocr Metab* 1998; 83: 757–60.

16. Rosmond R, Chagnon YC, Holm G, Chagnon M, Pérusse L, Lindell K *et al.* A glucocorticoid receptor gene marker is associated with abdominal obesity, leptin and dysregulation of the hypothalamic-pituitary-adrenal axis. *Obes Res* 2000; 8: 211–8.

17. Rosmond R, Chagnon YC, Chagnon M, Pérusse L, Bouchard C, Björntorp P. A polymorphism in the 5'-flanking region of the glucocorticoid receptor gene locus is associated with basal cortisol secretion in men. *Metabolism* 2001 (in press).

18. Baghaei F, Rosmond R, Westberg L, Hellstrand M, Eriksson E, Holm G, Björntorp P. Androgens as disease predictors in women. 2002. (Submitted).

Progress in Obesity Research: 9. Edited by *Geraldo Medeiros-Neto, Alfredo Halpern and Claude Bouchard*
©2003 John Libbey Eurotext Ltd, pp. 1018–1021.

CHAPTER 211

Portion-controlled diets

Marion Flechtner-Mors

Department of Internal Medicine, University of Ulm, Robert-Koch-Str. 8, 89081 Ulm, Germany
[e-mail: marion.mors@medizin.uni-ulm.de]

Introduction

Obesity, often viewed as a 'Western' problem, is rapidly becoming a major health concern worldwide[1]. There are numerous complex and interrelated factors that may cause obesity, including: genetics, neurologic, physiologic, biochemical, cultural and psychosocial factors. However, environmental changes are the main contributors to the global increase in obesity.

The environment has changed dramatically in comparatively recent times. It is only in the past one hundred years or so that many humans have had a surplus of food. Agriculture evolved about ten thousand years ago, and modern Western diets have been in existence for only a few hundred years. 50,000 years ago seeds, roots, tubers, leaves, stalks beans and fruits were the principal source of nutrients. Nowadays we eat refined pasta, flour, cereal, rice chicken, red meat, pizza, ice cream, yogurt, cheese, whole milk and oil. The food we eat is often processed. It is common to add fat or sugar, thereby increasing the energy content. For example, potatoes are very good for a healthy diet, if they are eaten as grown. However, potatoes are usually eaten with added fat. Two-hundred grams of cooked potatoes contain 0.2 g of fat, mashed potatoes 3 g, fries 30 g, potato pancakes 40 g and chips 78 g. Also, the consumption of refined sugar is very high. Often sugar is added as a substitute for fat to enhance taste (for example in cookies, cakes and low fat peanut butter). Water is often replaced by soft drinks with very high glucose content. We eat processed foods that have very high energy density. Processed food is available everywhere and is relatively inexpensive.

Essentials of obesity therapy

Obesity is a chronic disorder with serious consequences, including death, and must be treated in order to reduce the associated morbidity and mortality[2]. Diet remains an essential component of obesity therapy. The challenge that confronts us is to develop effective guidelines for healthy living that obese people can follow for the long-term to reduce body weight and maintain it at a desirable level. It is necessary to have freedom of food choices to form healthy dietary patterns for weight loss and maintenance that take into account the varied needs of individuals, families, communities and populations. There must be an emphasis on sound nutritional planning to meet nutrient intake requirements. Three components are essential for the development of an effective nutrition programme: (1) dietary variety, (2) portion size and (3) long-term outcome of treatment.

Dietary variety plays a key role in energy intake and body fatness in free-living people consuming self-selected diets. It has been shown in many studies that subjects consume more total food when offered a variety of different foods than when only a single food is presented. A study by McCrory *et al.*[3] addressed the question of whether daily energy intake varies according to dietary variety. Within different food groups tested, consumption of a greater variety of foods was associated with a greater energy intake from those foods. These short-term influences on food and energy intake exert a large long-term effect on increased body fatness. For weight reduction it is also important to keep the portion size low. This is very difficult for many people and may partially explain the widespread perception that long-term reduction in body weight is difficult to achieve. Indeed, many studies measuring the long-term impact of dieting, as reported in the literature, are unimpressive[4]. However, there are some long-term studies with low calorie diets and very low calorie diets that show excellent results.

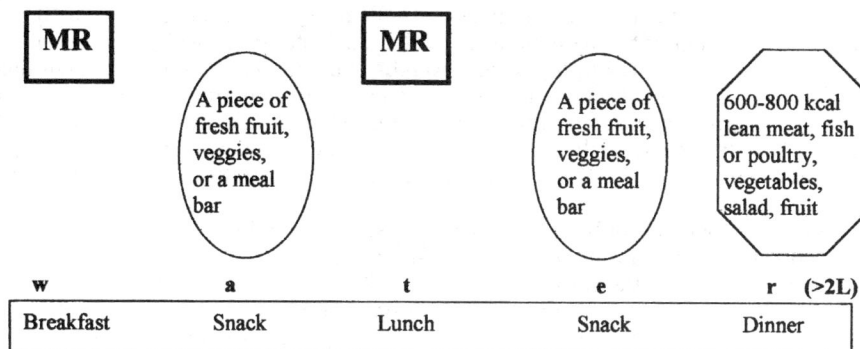

Fig. 1. Structured diet plan.
Meal replacements (MR) can be formula diet drinks, soups, prepackaged foods or frozen low-calorie meals. For weight loss two of three main meals are replaced. For weight maintenance one main meal is replaced.

A meta-analysis of 29 studies by Andersen and coworkers compared the effect of low calorie diets (LCDs) and very low calorie diets (VLCDs) long-term[5]. The weight loss phase ranged from 8 to 30 weeks. After one year of follow-up the VLCD group had lost 17 kg and the LCD group had lost 6.5 kg. This initial weight loss with VLCDs was significantly greater than with LCDs. After 5 years of follow-up, weight loss was 7.0 kg for the VLCD group, and 2.0 kg for the LCD group. Thus, VLCDs showed acceptable results regarding long-term outcome.

However, designing VLCDs using conventional food requires careful selection of food and time for preparation that is often inconvenient. When VLCDs are composed of powdered or liquid formula and used as the only means of nutrition, drop out rate is very high, since patients describe the diet as monotonous and unpalatable[6].

Structured portion controlled-diet plans

Formula diets can be integrated into a conventional diet regimen and used as replacements for a main meal, usually composed of conventional food. This structured diet plan (Fig. 1) consists of meal replacements of breakfast and lunch or breakfast and dinner. One or two main meals remain. They are composed of conventional food with ample vegetables and fruits.

The structured diet using meal replacements conforms to the essentials of obesity therapy: it provides a simple guide for healthy nutrition, since the structured diet is easy to follow. In today's fast food environment fewer meals are prepared at home. The advantage of using meal replacements is that no special food must be bought and cooked. Further, the structured diet plan maintains freedom of food choices. The remaining meals can be composed of individual food preferences. This helps meet the specific needs of individuals, families and communities. People are not isolated with a special diet and can take part in normal social life. The structured diet plan meets the Recommended Dietary Allowances[7] only when meal replacements are used that are nutritionally balanced. Using meal replacements it may be easier to meet the various dietary guidelines recommended by national health organizations.

Clinical evidence for the effectiveness of portion-controlled diets

Few studies have tested the effectiveness of meal replacement as a weight loss strategy long-term. In our 4 year trial at the University Hospital (Obesity Centre at the University Hospital of Ulm, Germany), we performed a study integrating formula diet drinks as meal replacements in a low energy diet regimen[8]. Each meal replacement (SlimFast; [SF] SlimFast Foods Company, West Palm Beach, FL) provided 220 kcal. In the study 100 patients (21 men, 79 women) were treated for 51 months. Phase I was a 3 month weight loss period. Patients were randomly assigned to two diet groups with 1200–1500 kcal/day (20 per cent protein, 50–60 per cent carbohydrate and 20–30 per cent fat). One group of overweight or obese people had a conventional low calorie diet. In the other group, subjects replaced two main meals with a diet shake and had a third regular meal of 600–800 kcal. Phase II was a 4 year weight maintenance period. All patients replaced one main dish with a diet shake and had two conventional main dishes (400 and 700 kcal). All 100 patients completed phase I of the study and body weight was reduced in both groups after 3 months. In patients with a conventional diet (Group A), initial weight loss was 1.5 per cent, whereas patients with meal replacements (Group B) lost 7.8 per cent. After 4 years, 75 per cent of the patients were evaluated. Total mean weight loss was 3.2 per cent for Group A and 8.4 per cent for Group B. During weight maintenance, there was a significant group effect in which Group B had a greater percentage change from baseline for all time points. This change was attributable to the difference in the initial weight loss observed at the completion of the first 3 months. These results demonstrate that a diet plan with meal replacements is more effective in achieving and sustaining weight loss than a traditional healthy diet with the same prescribed caloric value.

Portion-controlled diets work, not only in a university-based setting, but also out in the real world. In a community-based setting with minimal clinical intervention a study was performed in a free-living population in a community in northern rural Wisconsin, USA[9]. One hundred and forty-nine overweight men and women participated in the study. For comparison purposes each participant was matched with three other overweight community members of the same gender and approximately the same age. Overweight people who replaced one or two meals a day for 5 years with a diet shake (SF) were able to lose weight and keep it off. Women lost a mean 4.2 kg and men lost 5.8 kg. In contrast, in the comparison group men gained 6.7 kg and women gained 6.5 kg.

Meal replacements are also effective in traditional lifestyle interventions[10]. In a randomized trial 113 overweight pre-menopausal women were randomly assigned to a traditional dietitian-led intervention group (group A), a traditional dietitian-led intervention group incorporating meal replacements (group B), or a primary care office intervention group incorporating meal replacements with individual physician and nurse consultations (group C). Subjects in groups B and C replaced two main meals per day with a diet shake (SF). After weight loss of 10 per cent of initial body weight, they were instructed to replace only one main meal each day with a meal-replacement shake. Seventy-four subjects completed one year. Retention rates among the three groups were similar. Weight loss was similar in the dietitian-led group and physician led group. However, when patients were instructed by a dietitian and when they incorporated meal replacements daily, weight loss was significantly greater than in the other groups.

Portion-controlled diets have also been shown to be effective in patients with co-morbidities such as type 2 diabetes[11]. Compared to a conventional diet meeting the American Diabetes Association recommendations[12], integration of meal replacements induced greater short term weight loss. Lipid profiles, glycaemia (fasting blood glucose), fasting insulin and hemoglobin A1c were improved. Similar results have been reported using a comprehensive prepackaged meal plan in patients with type 2 diabetes[13].

Why portion-controlled diets improve weight loss

The results of studies performed with meal replacements incorporated in portion-controlled diets seem to be superior to results obtained from studies with conventional food. Thereare several possible explanations for the different results[14]:

(1) It is easier to plan meals. No preparation time is necessary. Meal replacements are readily available and can be stored at home. They are convenient to use and simplify dietary compliance. Furthermore, the diet can be easily tailored to meet individual needs.

(2) Barriers to dietary adherence are reduced. Beginning a diet does not mean turning away from normal social life. Meal replacements can be easily incorporated into contemporary lifestyles. They may be consumed anywhere, including the workplace.

(3) Regular eating patterns are established and reinforced. The structured meal plan, with fixed times for meal replacements, facilitates adherence to the diet. When people have their regular meal pattern the time between meals is not long. People will remember that they did eat something. They are unlikely to assume that they have not eaten for hours and eat an extra large portion to compensate. There is also a reduction in the number of decisions required for food choices and this may help to prevent unintended dietary failures.

(4) There may be an improvement in the accuracy of calorie estimation and the estimation of portion size. A meal replacement strategy is simple and easy to understand. It offers individuals clear and direct control of their energy intake.

(5) The quality and quantity of foods consumed may be improved. Meal replacements must be nutritionally balanced, i.e. vitamin- and mineral-fortified.

(6)   Meal replacements may have positive effects on self-monitoring. Using a meal replacement strategy, food choices are made that guide the development of healthy nutrition lifestyle.

Conclusion

Portion-controlled diets that include meal replacement products induce weight loss and improvement in biomarkers of health. They provide the simplicity and nutrient composition necessary for long-term weight maintenance and healthy nutrition. They offer a promising strategy for treating obesity.

References

1.   World Health Organization. Obesity: Preventing and Managing the Global Epidemic. WHO Obesity Technical Report Series 894. Geneva, Switzerland: World Health Organization, 2000.

2.   Garrow J. Should obesity be treated? Those who consult should be treated. *BMJ* 1994; 29; 309(6962): 1158.

3.   McCory MA, Fuss JP, McCallum JE, Yao M, Vinken AG, Hays NP, Roberts SB. Dietary variety within food groups: association with energy intake and body fatness in men and women. *Am J Clin Nutr* 1999; 69: 440–7.

4.   Garne, DM, Wooley SC. Confronting the failure of behavioural and dietary treatments for obesity. *Clin Psychol Rev* 1991; 11: 729–80.

5.   Andersen JW, Konz EC, Frederich RC, Wood C. Long-term weight-loss maintenance: a meta-analysis of US studies. *Am J Clin Nut* 2001; 74: 579–84.

6.   Howard AN. The historical development of very low calorie diets. *Int J Obes* 1989; 13 (Suppl 2): 1–9.

7.   National Research Council, Subcommittee on the Tenth Edition of the RDAs. Recommended Dietary Allowances, Washington: National Academy Press; 1989.

8.   Flechtner-Mors M, Ditschuneit HH, Johnson TD, Suchard MA, Adler G. Metabolic and weight loss effects of long-term dietary intervention in obese patients: four year results. *Obes Res* 2000; 8: 399–402.

9.   Rothacker DQ. Five-year self-management of weight using meal replacements: Comparison with matched controls in rural Wisconsin. *Nutrition* 2000; 16: 344–8.

10. Ashley JM, St Jeor ST, Schrage JP, Perumean-Chaney SE, Gilbertson MC, McCall NL, Bovee V. Weight control in the physician's office. *Arch Intern Med* 2001 Jul 9; 161(13): 1599–604.

11. Yip I, Go VLW, DeShields S, Saltsman P, Bellman M, Thames G *et al*. Liquid meal replacements and glycemic control in obese type 2 diabetes patients. *Obes Res* 2002; 9 (Suppl 4): S341–S347.

12. American Diabetes Association. Nutrition recommendations and principles for people with diabetes mellitus. *Diabetes Care* 1996; 19 (Suppl 1): 516–519.

13. Pi-Sunyer FX, Maggio CA, McCarron DA, Reusser ME, Stern JS, Haynes RB *et al*. Multicenter randomized trial of a comprehensive prepared meal programme in type 2 diabetes. *Diabetes Care* 1999; 22: 191–7.

14. Wing RR, Jeffery RW. Food Provision as a strategy to promote weight loss. *Obes Res* 2001; 9 (Suppl 4): S271–S275.

Progress in Obesity Research: 9. Edited by *Geraldo Medeiros-Neto, Alfredo Halpern and Claude Bouchard*
©2003 John Libbey Eurotext Ltd, pp. 1022–1025.

CHAPTER 212

Popular diets: low carbohydrate vs. low fat

Wim. H.M. Saris

Nutrition Research Institute NUTRIM, University of Maastricht, P.O. Box 616, 6200 MD Maastricht, The Netherlands
[e-mail: w.saris@hb.unimaas.nl]

Introduction

Consumers are desperately seeking new dietary weight control products which are convenient and which provide an effective solution to weight loss and for the long term weight maintenance. Eighty-six per cent of the US weight-loss market is attributed to low fat, low calorie, sugar free foods or soft drinks. These are all related to the carbohydrate/fat content of the food or the diet.

Apart from genetic factors, it is now commonly accepted that obesity is the result of an imbalance between food intake and daily physical activity. Efforts to reduce the prevalence of obesity have focused on three particular factors, namely to increase levels of physical activity, to reduce total fat intake and to reduce intake of sugars and rapidly digested carbohydrates. There is general acceptance of the urgency to take public action to increase the level of daily physical activity in all sectors of the population. However with respect to the dietary factors, total fat intake and glycaemic carbohydrates, there is much more debate in the literature. Throughout the 1960s and 1970s there was a tendency to consider carbohydrates and especially sugar as an important factor for weight gain. Since then, the attention has been shifted towards fat as the major nutritional component promoting excess energy intake and weight gain[1].

Dietary carbohydrates have been generally viewed as a beneficial macronutrient with references to body weight control[2]. This positive effect was based on the accumulating evidence that energy balance is based on the sum of the independent macronutrient balances[3]. This requires that net oxidation of each nutrient equals the intake of the same nutrient in the diet. Evidence that the regulation of the carbohydrate balance has a much higher priority in the hierarchy compared to fat as well as the knowledge that *de novo* lipogenesis is limited has contributed to the general perception that carbohydrate ingestion is less likely to promote fat storage[4]. Despite the controversy about the particular role of sugar, the message that the role of fat in the diet is determining the excess energy intake became stronger, leading recommendations for reducing fat intake in dietary guidelines all over the world. The low-fat market expanded rapidly but so did the prevalence of obesity in particular in the US. Reason why more recently this concept of low fat diets as a better tool for body weight control has been challenged. For example Katan *et al.* have questioned the importance of low-fat/high carbohydrate diets in the prevention and treatment of obesity[5]. Randomized controlled trials show only limited weight reduction and the so-called 'fat paradox' can be seen in several countries where there is a poor association between dietary fat intake and the percentage of the population that is overweight or obese. Also a direct relation between dietary fat and energy density was questioned on the basis that many low-fat foods currently available are based on sugar or high glycaemic carbohydrates leading to energy density values similar to those of their high-fat counterparts[6]. At the same time the discussion about the glycaemic index of the diet and body weight control was started. High glycaemic food could lead to overfeeding and thus to weight gain compared to low glycaemic food and a low glycaemic diet[7].

In the following, these issues related to the macronutrient content of diet and body weight control are addressed in more detail. No attention will be given to a specific popular diet with a low fat or low carbohydrate content since the focus of this paper is more related to the physiological and energetic aspects of macronutrient selection and body weight control.

Dietary fat and body weight control

It is now generally accepted that protein and carbohydrate balance are regulated more closely than fat balance. There are a number of potential mechanisms to explain this effect. In metabolic terms, fat is more readily absorbed and assimilated into body fat stores and less rapidly oxidized than other macronutrients. In addition the satiety signals arising from fat ingestion are weaker and perhaps most important, the energy density per gram is twice as high than from carbohydrate and protein. This explains why, when subjects are allowed to eat *ad libitum* over a day or longer, they consume and store more energy as the proportion of fat in the diet increases. In Table 1 the hierarchy of the different physiological factors in relation to energy balance is tabulated.

Table 1. Hierarchy of the macronutrients in the different physiological factors leading to expansion of the body fat stores

	Protein	CHO	Fat	Alcohol
Satiety	4	3	2	1
Energy density	3/4	3/4	1	2
Diet induced thermogenesis	4	3	1	2
Faecal energy loss	3	4	2	1
Storage capacity	3	2	1	4
E costs to convert to fat	4	2	1	3
Overall score	4	3	1	2

This phenomenon has been described as 'passive over-consumption'. As demonstrated in the well-controlled study of Stubbs *et al.*[8], a group of male volunteers were allowed to eat *ad libitum* a diet with 20, 40 or 60 per cent fat for one week. On the 20 per cent fat diet they experienced a modest decrease in body fat, whereas on the 60 per cent fat diet, they gained around 0.5 kg body fat in seven days due to a considerable positive energy balance.

Iso-energetic substitution of fat with carbohydrate does not substantially change the energy expenditure although on theoretical grounds it is expected to be lower. A difference in diet induced thermogenesis of only ~120 kJ per day can be calculated between a 20 per cent fat diet or 60 per cent diet in an individual eating 10 MJ per day.

Also the metabolic conversion to store excess energy into the adipose tissue is most favourable for dietary fat. Horton *et al.* demonstrated by overfeeding men for 14 days each with iso-energetic amounts of fat or carbohydrate that fat storage is higher with fat (90–95 per cent) than with carbohydrate overfeeding[9]. This confirms the biochemical findings that the conversion from glucose to fat is energetically a very costly process compared to fat which should lead to a ~ 20 per cent lower fat deposition at an equi-energetic excess intake. Furthermore it can be argued that *de novo* lipogenesis from glucose is very limited and occurs only when oxidation is nearly completely covered by carbohydrate and the glycogen stores are filled.

Also epidemiological observations have found a positive relation between fat intake and prevalence of obesity[10]. Although one should be very cautious regarding the outcome as simple food questionnaires are used in large-scale epidemiological studies. Many studies have shown convincingly that especially obese subjects underreport their food intake up to 50 per cent[11]. Even more problematic is the selective underreporting of macronutrients. With the increasing awareness of the relation between fat intake and disease risk in particular obesity, subjects are more likely to selectively underreport fatty foods. By using the doubly labeled water and water balance technique to check for both underreporting and selective fat underreporting, it was clearly demonstrated that both phenomenon's occurred in obese men[12]. The reported percentage of energy from fat was a function of the level of underreporting energy intake. This selective fat underreporting could also explain the so-called 'American paradox'. With increasing prevalence of obesity, the observed fat intake based on food questionnaires is decreasing. To explain the fat paradox, it is more likely that the combination of the exponential increase in obesity especially in the US and the increasing awareness of the danger of fat in the diet resulted in a grossly selective underreporting of fat by a growing segment of the population.

The physiological considerations as well as the epidemiological results including the bias related to fat and perhaps also to sugar strengthens confidence in the importance of a reduction in fat intake to control body weight as was concluded from the meta-analysis of *ad libitum* low fat dietary intervention studies[13]. Extracted data from 16 trials with 19 intervention groups and 1910 individuals showed 3.2 kg body weight loss at a 10.3 per cent fat reduction in the low-fat diet groups compared to the control groups. Having a body weight 10 kg higher than the average pre-treatment body weight was associated with a 2.6 kg greater difference in weight loss. It was concluded that a decrease in body weight of this magnitude in the general population could reduce the prevalence of obesity from 25 per cent to 15 per cent. Even a few kilograms weight loss on a low-fat diet may, therefore, have an important public health impact. This is especially true considering that the observed 3–4 kg weight loss produced by *ad libitum* low-fat diets is more likely an underestimation of the real effect due to the compliance problem inherent to most dietary interventions. This was elegantly demonstrated by Swinburn *et al.* who showed that the poorly compliant groups lost only 1 kg compared to 6 kg in the more compliant group after 1 year[14]. Furthermore one can argue from evolutionary point of view that the human genome is selected to prevent weight loss and instead to store excess energy intake. Therefore from a theoretical point of view it is expected that the effects of a low fat diet to prevent the gaining of weight most probably is more effective compared to the weight loss results after reduction of fat intake. However so far no intervention trial with such prospective design has been published.

Dietary carbohydrate and body weight control

As shown in Table 1, different carbohydrates influence the thermogenic response. We investigated the impact on energy expenditure and post-prandial substrate utilization for 6 h after oral ingestion of 75 g of glucose, fructose, sucrose or starch in healthy volunteers[15]. The integrated areas under the glucose and insulin response, curves above baseline were highest with glucose and starch, intermediate with sucrose and lowest with fructose. The rise in energy expenditure was lowest for glucose and starch and highest for fructose and especially sucrose. The differences in post-ingestive thermogenesis between these carbohydrates can be attributed to their differences in metabolism. Because fructose uptake is handled by a different transporter compared to glucose. Furthermore fructose avoids the first rate limiting enzymes of glycolysis and is therefore more rapidly metabolized resulting in the accumulation of three-carbon components which are available for gluconeogenesis and glycogen formation. Carbohydrate oxidation, glycogen formation and down regulation of lipid oxidation have been reported after fructose and to a lesser extend after sucrose and glucose ingestion. The finding that fructose and sucrose ingestion results in a higher thermogenic response than glucose ingestion despite the fact that fructose has only a slight effect on insulin secretion, indicates that the thermogenic response after carbohydrate ingestion is not directly related to the plasma insulin concentration. It is difficult to extrapolate the above finding of the effect of acute carbohydrate ingestion on the thermogenic response to a situation of long-term energy balance. The more pronounced suppression of lipid oxidation with ingestion of glucose and starch may result in a larger effect on daily fat oxidation. However, evidence of differences in the effects of various carbohydrates on long-term energy or substrate balance is lacking. The response of different carbohydrate containing foods on glucose/insulin plasma levels is a topic that has attracted renewed attention in recent years[7]. High glycaemic food does give by definition higher excursions of the plasma glucose levels. Long-term monitoring of blood glucose levels indicate that glucose and insulin levels are necessarily related to satiety and food intake but that the dynamic declines in blood glucose levels are of importance to initiate a meal request[16]. Several studies have compared the effects of different classes of carbohydrate on energy balance and rate of weight loss. Animal studies do not show differences among carbohydrate diets in energy expenditure, energy efficiency and energy intake. These data, indicating no effect of the class of carbohydrate on energy balance on energy balance, are consistent with studies in men[2]. In a study on the effects of three hypocaloric diets (3 weeks, 3.4 MJ) with either 45 per cent polysaccharide or 45 per cent sugar, the decrease in fat mass was comparable.

During the past 20 years longer-term intervention trials have shown that an increase in the carbohydrate/fat ratio has a positive effect on body weight control. Most cross-sectional studies linking carbohydrate intake expressed in energy per cent and body fatness expressed as BMI show an inverse relation[4]. This relation is even stronger for the intake of sugars or high glycaemic food and BMI[17]. Recently the first large scale randomized controlled trial addressing the type of carbohydrate and the carbohydrate/fat ratio simultaneously was published. In this CARMEN study the impact of 6 months of *ad libitum* intake of low-fat diets, rich in either simple or complex carbohydrates on energy intake, body weight and health variables was investigated[18], The results showed that both low-fat diets reduced body weight by 1.6 and 2.4 kg respectively compared to the control group. The body fat in the simple and complex carbohydrate low-fat was −1.3 kg and −1.8 kg respectively. The slightly lower weight and body fat loss in the simple carbohydrate group did not reach statistical significance. Furthermore, no detrimental effects on blood lipids were observed in the high carbohydrate groups as was suggested in the past[5,6]. According to this first RCT the type of carbohydrate does not seem to have much effect on body weight regulation and health risk factors, as was previously suggested.

The findings from the CARMEN study underline the importance of public measure to reduce fat intake compared to simple carbohydrates in particular sugar. However we need confirmation of these results in large scale randomized controlled intervention trials using different types of carbohydrates.

References

1. Lissner L, Heitman BL. Dietary fat and obesity – evidence from epidemiology. *Eur J Clin Nutr* 1995; 49: 79–90.

2. Blaak EE, Saris WHM. Health aspects of various digestible carbohydrates. *Nutr Res* 1995; 15: 1547–73.

3. Flatt J. The difference in the storage capacities for carbohydrate and for fat and its implications in the regulation of body weight. *Ann NY Acad Sci* 1987; 499: 104–23.

4. Astrup A, Raben A. Carbohydrate and obesity. *Int J Obes* 1995; 19 (Suppl 5): 527–537.

5. Katan MB, Grundy SM, Willet WC. Beyond low-fat diets. *New Eng J Med* 1997; 337: 563–6.

6. Willet WC. Is dietary fat a major determinant of body fat? *Am J Clin Nutr* 1998; 62: S264–S274.

7. Brand-Miller JC, Holt SHA, Pawlak DB, McMillan J. Glycemic index and obesity. *Am J Clin Nutr* 2002; 76: S285–S291.

8. Stubbs RJ, Ritz P, Coward WA, Prentice AM. Covert manipulation of the ratio dietary fat to energy density: effect on food intake and energy balance in men feeding *ad libitum*. *Am J Clin Nutr* 1995; 62: 330–8.

9. Horton TJ, Drougas H, Brackey A, Reecy W, Peters JC, Hill JO. Fat and carbohydrate overfeeding in humans: different effects on energy storage *Am J Clin Nutr* 1995; 62: 19–29.

10. Bolton-Smits C, Woodward M. Dietary composition and fat sugar ratios in relation to obesity. *Int J Obes* 1994; 8: 820–8.

11. Schoeller DA. How accurate is self-reported dietary energy intake? *Nutr Rev* 1990; 48: 373–9.

12. Goris AHC, Westerterp-Plantenga MS, Westerterp KR. Under-eating and under-recording of habitual food intake in obese men: elective underreporting of fat intake. *Am J Clin Nutr* 2000; 71: 130–4.

13. Astrup A, Grunwals GK, Meanson EL, Saris WHM, Hill JO. The role of low-fat diets in body weight control a meta-analysis of *ad libitum* dietary intervention studies. *Int J Obes* 2000; 24: 1545–52.

14. Swinburn BA, Metcalf PA, Ley S. Long-term (5-year) effect of a reduced-fat diet intervention in individuals with glucose intolerance. *Diabetes Care* 2001; 24: 619–624.

15. Blaak EE, Saris WHM. Post-prandial thermogenesis and substrate utilization after ingestion of different dietary carbohydrates. *Metabolism* 1996; 45: 1235–42.

16. Melanson KJ, Westerterp-Plantenga MS, Campfield H, Saris WHM. Blood glucose patterns and appetite in time-blinded humans: carbohydrate vs. fat. *Am J Physiol* 1999; 27: R227–R345.

17. Hill JO, Prentice AM. Sugar and body weight control. *Am J Clin Nutr* 1995; 62: S264–S274.

18. Saris WHM, Astrup A, Prentice AM *et al.* Randomised controlled trial of changes in dietary carbohydrate/fat ratio and simple vs. complex carbohydrates on body weight and blood lipids: the CARMEN study. *Int J Obes* 2000; 24: 1310–8.

Progress in Obesity Research: 9. Edited by *Geraldo Medeiros-Neto, Alfredo Halpern* and *Claude Bouchard*
©2003 John Libbey Eurotext Ltd, pp. 1026–1029.

CHAPTER 213

Long-term maintenance of weight loss

James O. Hill and Rena R. Wing

*Center for Human Nutrition, University of Colorado Health Sciences Center and Department of Psychiatry, Brown
University School of Medicine, 4200 E. Ninth Avenue, Denver, Colorado 80262, USA
[e-mail: James.Hill@uchsc.edu]*

Introduction

Does anyone succeed in long-term maintenance of weight loss? In reality, we have to define success in weight loss maintenance before we can answer this question. It is common to hear that fewer than 5 per cent of those attempting weight loss succeed over the long-term. This figure comes from a weight loss intervention study conducted in the 1950s[1]. Have things really not improved since the 1950s?

If we ask how many obese individuals (BMI $\geq$ 30 kg/m^2) lose and maintain sufficient weight to return them to a BMI $\leq$ 25 kg/m^2, the success rate may close to 5 per cent (although we do not have sufficient data to determine an exact success rate). In recent years, it has become clear that substantial health benefits can be accrued in obese individuals with weight losses of 5–10 per cent; losses that usually leave them with a BMI well above that considered healthy[2]. Wing and Hill[3] have defined success in weight loss maintenance as achieving and maintaining at least a 10 per cent reduction in body weight for at least 1 year. By this definition, success in long-term weight maintenance is closer to 20 per cent, which means that one in every five obese individual who attempts weight loss achieves success.

Regardless of how success is defined, we need to learn how to improve obesity treatment especially when it comes to helping individuals keep off the weight they lose. One way to learn about effective strategies for weight loss and maintenance of weight loss is to study individuals who have succeeded in long-term weight loss maintenance. The largest study of individuals who have succeeded in long-term weight loss maintenance is the National Weight Control Registry (NWCR), established by Drs. James O. Hill and Rena R. Wing in 1992.

The National Weight Control Registry (NWCR)

The NWCR is a longitudinal research project aimed at identifying characteristics of, and strategies used by individuals who succeed in long-term maintenance of weight loss. The key finding from the NWCR have recently been summarized in a review[3].

To qualify for membership in the NWCR, individuals must have maintained at least a 30 lb weight loss for at least 1 year. An individual who lost 40 lb and kept off 30 lb for one year would be eligible but not an individual who lost 40 lb and only kept off only 20 lb. The intent in developing these criteria was to capture individuals who are clearly successful in long-term weight maintenance without making the criteria so stringent that few would qualify. The NWCR was set up to capture information for these individuals over time, whether or not they continue to be successful in maintaining their weight loss.

NWCR members are recruited in several ways. Most participants learn about the NWCR through the media. The project has been featured in hundreds of newspapers and magazines. It has been the subjects of several television specials. Additionally, many weight management programmes provide information to participants about the NWCR and encourage those who continue to keep their weight off to join.

Potential participants contact NWCR staff via a toll-free telephone number (1-800-606-NWCR) or through a website (http: //www.nwcr.ws). Those who qualify for membership are asked first to complete an informed consent form, followed by completing a set of baseline questionnaires. These questionnaires are designed to provide information about current and past weight. Co-morbid conditions, quality of life measures, and current and past behavioural strategies used for weight management. Some NWCR participants have participated in metabolic studies conducted at the University of Colorado Health Sciences Center.

Who is in the National Weight Control Registry?

Currently there are over 3200 members of the NWCR. These individuals have maintained an average weight loss of 30 kg for about 5.5 years. Over 15 per cent of NWCR participants have maintained their weight loss for over 10 years. NWCR participants reported losing an average of 10 BMI units (from 35 kg/m^2 to 25 kg/m^2).

The NWCR is a non-representative sample, and it has been suggested that these successful individuals may differ substantially from those who are unsuccessful in weight management efforts. In other words, weight loss in these individuals may have been 'less difficult' than for those who fail. This does not seem likely since 60 per cent of NWCR participants have a family history of obesity and 67 per cent reported that their obesity began in childhood. Further, over 90 per cent of registry participants reported that they had failed in previous weight loss attempts before finally losing the weight and keeping it off.

How did NWCR participants lose weight?

Eighty-nine per cent of NWCR subjects reported that they used both diet and exercise to lose weight, 9 per cent did it with diet alone and only 1 per cent did it with exercise alone. This is strong support for ensuring that physical activity is an important part of weight loss plans.

There was surprisingly little similarity in the dietary strategies used for weight loss. While we did not ask about specific branded diets, we did ask about behavioural strategies used for dieting. Some participants countered calories, other counted fat gram and still others used structured meal plans. A large number used diets that few nutritionists would consider as sound ways to lose weight. All in all, we were not able to identify any particular dietary strategy for weight loss that was common among NWCR participants.

One advantage of the NWCR is that it allows entry for individuals who lost weight on their own, without a formal diet programme. About half of NWCR participants reported that they used a formal weight loss programme to lose weight and about half reported that they lost the weight on their own. Women were more likely to use a formal programme while men were more likely to lose weight on their own. There was no difference in amount or duration of weight loss between those who used a formal programme and those who lost weight on their own.

We asked participants to describe any triggering event that facilitated there determination to succeed in weight loss maintenance. The most frequent triggering events were a medical trigger (32 per cent) an emotional trigger (32 per cent) or a lifestyle trigger (26 per cent).

Maintenance of weight loss

When we assessed behavioural strategies being used to keep weight off, we found several common strategies used by NWCR members. We have described four weight maintenance behaviours that are common to this group.

Eating a low fat, high carbohydrate diet

Self-reported food intake was assessed using a food frequency. NWCR participants reported eating a diet containing 24 per cent energy from fat, 20 per cent energy from protein and 56 per cent energy from carbohydrate. It is interesting, given the current high interest in low carbohydrate diets (such as the Atkins diet) in weight management, that few NWCR subjects report using such a diet for weight maintenance. It is important to realize that the type of diet consumed for weight maintenance is not necessarily the type of diet used by these subjects for weight loss. This suggests that the most effective strategies for losing weight may not always be the most effective strategies for keeping the weight off.

Frequent self monitoring

Frequent self-monitoring is a common characteristic of NWCR members. They weigh themselves frequently, with about 75 per cent of them weighing themselves more than once per week and many weighing themselves daily. Further, about half of the NWCR subjects report that they still keep records of food eaten, with many continuing to count calories or fat grams. Self monitoring has consistently

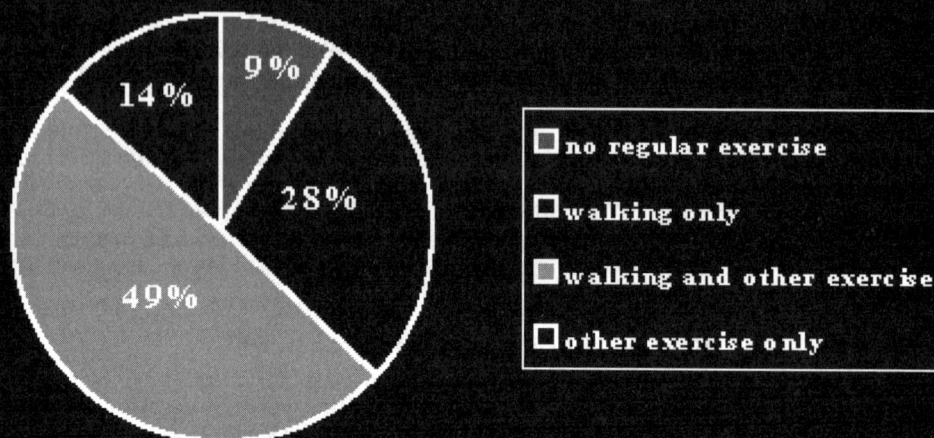

Classification of NWCR members into 4 exercise categories

- 9%
- 14%
- 28%
- 49%

□ no regular exercise

□ walking only

■ walking and other exercise

□ other exercise only

Fig. 1. This figure shows the types of physical activity reported by individuals in the National Weight Control Registry.

been found to predict success in weight management[4]. Frequent self monitoring may provide an 'early warning system' for reduced obese individuals, allowing them to implement predetermined strategies when weight is up.

Eating breakfast

Most (78 per cent) NWCR members eat breakfast every single day[5]. Only 4 per cent report that they never eat breakfast. Eating breakfast seems to be an important weight maintenance strategy for these individual, perhaps because eating breakfast may help with hunger management during the remainder of the day.

High levels of physical activity

NWCR participants report engaging in very high levels of physical activity. Using the Paffenbarger Physical Activity Scale, NWCR subjects report engaging in about 2800 kcal/week of physical activity[3]. This is roughly equivalent to 60–90 min/day of moderate intensity physical activity. Figure 1 shows the breakdown of the types of physical activity reported by NWCR subjects. Walking was the most frequent physical activity reported, but a large number of NWCR participants used walking in conjunction with another type of physical activity. Weight lifting was a common form of physical activity.

Only 9 per cent of NWCR subjects reported maintaining their weight loss with diet alone. While it is possible to keep weight off without making physical activity a priority, it is rare in this group of successful weight loss maintainers.

Regular physical activity has been found by others to be a predictor of success in weight loss maintenance[6,7]. In fact, there is reasonable consistency among studies as to the amount of physical activity required to maintain a substantial weight loss. It appears that 60–90 min/day of moderate intensity physical activity may be required to keep weight off in previously obese subjects. This amount is higher than that recommended by US Public Health officials[8]. Whether less physical activity may be required for primary prevention of weight gain (vs. prevention of weight regain) is not clear.

Discussion

Regardless of how it is defined, success in weight loss maintenance is less than desirable. The National Weight Control Registry consists of over 3200 individuals who have lost an average of 30 kg and kept it off for an average of 5.5 years. While not necessarily representative of the larger population of individuals engaging in weight management, this group of successful weight loss maintainers can provide some indication of the characteristics and behaviours of people who do succeed in long-term weight loss maintenance.

There is surprisingly little similarity in how these individuals lost their weight beyond the fact that they used both diet and physical activity rather than diet alone. To date, we have identified four behaviours that these individuals tend to have in common: (1) eating a low fat, high carbohydrate diet; (2) frequent self-monitoring of weight and food intake; (3) eating breakfast every day; and (4) 60–90 min/day of physical activity. It should be emphasized that while these behaviours are seen frequently among NWCR subjects, there are exceptions to each of these behaviours. While there may be different ways to keep weight off, there is surprising similarity in behaviours of NWCR subjects. It seems reasonable to look closely at these similarities when designing behavioural programmes for weight management.

The National Control Registry shows that many people do succeed in losing weight and keeping it off long-term. Further, we have found that these subjects live 'normal' lives after weight loss and consistently report that life is better after weight loss. Our subjects tell us that their success requires substantial effort but that it is worth it. Finally, our data suggest that it does get easier to maintain weight loss over time. Once you have maintained a weight loss for 2–5 years, the chances of longer-term success greatly increase. While weight loss maintenance may be a lifelong struggle, the struggle may get easier if you can just get through those first 2–5 years.

References

1. Stunkard AJ, McLaren-Hume M. The results of treatment for obesity. *Arch Intern Med* 1959; 103: 79–85.

2. National Institutes of Health, National Heart, Lung and Blood Institute. Clinical guidelines on the identification, evaluation and treatment of overweight and obesity in adults – the evidence report. *Obes Res* 1998; 6: S51–S209.

3. Wing RR, Hill JO. Successful weight loss maintenance. *Annu Rev Nutr* 2001; 21: 323–41.

4. Baker RC, Kirschenbaum DS. Self-monitoring may be necessary for successful weight control. *Behav Ther* 1993; 24: 377–94.

5. Wyatt HR, Grunwald GK, Mosca C, Wing RR, Hill JO. Long-term weight loss and breakfast consumption in reduced-obese subjects in the National Weight Control Registry. *Obes Res* 2002; 10: 2: 78–82.

6. Schoeller DA, Shay K, Kushner RF. How much physical activity is needed to minimize weight gain in previously obese women? *Am J Clin Nutr*1997; 66: 551–6.

7. Weinsier RL, Hunter GR, Desmond RA, Byrne NM, Zuckerman PA, Darnell BE. Free-living activity energy expenditure in women who are successful and unsuccessful in maintaining a normal body weight. *Am J Clin Nutr* 2002; 75: 499–504.

8. US Department of Health and Human Services. Physical Activity and health: A Report of the Surgeon General. Atlanta, GA: US Department of Health and Human Services, Centers for Disease Control and Prevention, National Center for Chronic Disease Prevention and Promotion; 1996.

Progress in Obesity Research: 9. Edited by *Geraldo Medeiros-Neto, Alfredo Halpern* and *Claude Bouchard*
©2003 John Libbey Eurotext Ltd, pp. 1030–1034.

CHAPTER 214

Health benefits associated with weight loss

F. Xavier Pi-Sunyer

New York Obesity Research Center, St. Luke's-Roosevelt Hospital, Columbia University, New York, NY 10025, USA
[e-mail: fxp1@columbia.edu]

Benefits associated with weight loss

Obesity is associated with a number of health hazards. These include the development of insulin resistance leading to impaired glucose tolerance and eventual type 2 diabetes, hypertension, dyslipidaemia, clotting abnormalities, coronary artery disease, stroke, non-alcoholic steato hepatitis, sleep apnea, arthritis, gout, gall bladder disease, and certain cancers (colon and prostate in men and endometrial and breast in women)[1]. Weight loss has been reported in various studies to decrease the presence of there conditions. Most of the studies of the effect of weight loss on the co-morbidities of obesity have been short-term[2], but there are a significant number of long-term studies that show a sustained effect over time[3]. Intentional weight loss in a 12-year follow-up of more than 15,000 middle-aged, overweight women (BMI 1.27) with obesity-related conditions at baseline was associated with dramatic reductions in mortality[4].

Insulin resistance

Obese persons develop insulin resistance. This is manifested by an elevation of their circulating insulin both fasting and post-prandially[5]. Also, there is a diminished ability to oxidize and store glucose[6–8]. The insulin resistance, in individuals whose pancreatic beta cells cannot keep up with the secretory demand, leads to diabetes mellitus[9]. The effect of weight loss on insulin resistance is well known. With even moderate decrease in caloric intake and a drop of between 5 and 10 per cent of body weight, insulin resistance improves. Weight loss in patients with impaired glucose tolerance, who have insulin resistance, prevents the progression to diabetes and, in some, actually reverts their glucose metabolism back to normal. In both the Finnish diabetes prevention study[10] and the American DPP[11], there was a 58 per cent greater prevention of progression to diabetes with a 7 lb weight loss and increased physical activity over a period of 3 years of follow-up. Insulin resistance is known to cause other health risks besides glucose tolerance. Included are hypertension, dyslipidaemia, coronary heart disease, and stroke. A longitudinal study by Haffner *et al.*[12] has reported that reducing insulin resistance through weight loss will reduce cardiovascular risk in patients who are 'prediabetic'. The effect of weight loss on all of these is positive and will be discussed below.

Diabetes mellitus

In patients who are already diabetic, weight loss has a positive effect on increasing glucose control and decreasing the need for medications. Short-term studies initially showed this[13,14]. A 1-year study by Wing *et al.*[15] showed that the greater the weight loss the greater the positive effect on HgAlc. Other studies of at least a year[16,17] have shown a similar positive effect. Since the onset and progression of diabetic complications are strongly associated with poor glycaemic control[18], better glycaemic control has now become a standard of care for type 2 diabetes patients. Thus, weight loss has been re-emphasized as the first line of therapy in patients who develop type 2 diabetes[17].

Hypertension

There is an increased prevalence of high blood pressure in individuals who are obese[19]. The JNC VII has recommended non-pharmacologic therapy as the initial treatment of 'mild' hypertension[20]. A study of recent myocardial infarction patients who were placed on a weight loss diet and lost an average of 6.3 kg lowered both their systolic and diastolic blood pressure[21]. In the TOHMS study[22], comparing six antihypertensive intervention for the treatment of high blood pressure, a weight loss initially of 4–5 kg which averaged 2.6 kg after 4 years of intervention showed a decrease of 8.6 mmHg systolic and 9.1 mm diastolic for the diet non-drug group[22]. Other studies have also shown a positive effect of weight loss on lowering blood pressure[2-5] hypertension levels. The TAIM study[26] (showed that a mean net reduction of 4.7 kg reduced systolic pressure by 2.8 mm and diastolic by 2.5 mm[26].

Dyslipidaemia

It is well known that risk of coronary artery disease is associated with high levels of LDL cholesterol, low levels of HDL cholesterol, and elevated triglycerides. These all occur in obese patients. Some obese patients do not have a rise in LDL, but their LDL particles are small and very atherogenic[27]. Low levels of HDL have been correlated to premature cardiovascular disease mortality[28]. A number of randomized controlled trials have shown that weight loss is associated with improvement of lipid parameters[29-33]. Examples are the studies of Hellenius[30], Karvetti[31], Marniemi[32] and Svensen[33], among others. As weight loss occurs, there is a decrease in FFA flux and in hyperinsulinaemia, leading to a decreased production of VLDL lipids. The effect of weight losses of 5 to 10 per cent from baseline will elevate low HDL levels[34,35] is clear. A study in women reported that the capacity for *in vitro* oxidation of non-HDL lipoprotein particles was greater in the obese subjects than in normal weight ones[36]. A weight reduction of 7 per cent in 6 months resulted in a significant reduction in *in vitro* oxidation[36].

Thrombosis

Obesity has recently been related to changes in blood clotting factors that make it easier for thrombosis to occur and to be cleared more slowly. This is particularly true if central fat distribution is present. Plasminogen activator one (PAI-I) has been reported to be elevated in obese persons[37]. Also, fibrinogen is elevated and fibrinolytic activity is decreased[38,39]. With weight loss, clotting activity improves[40].

Pulmonary function and sleep apnea

Obesity, particularly as it gets more severe, is often associated with respiratory impairment. This is manifested by a decreasing oxygen saturation and hypercarbia, with a loss of ventilatory drive[41]. An increase in one standard deviation in BMI is accompanied with a fourfold increase in hypoventilation[42]. There is a marked increase in sleep apnea as the obesity increases[43].

Weight loss is associated with an improvement of both sleep apnea and pulmonary function. In morbidly obese patients who undergo bariatric surgery, the benefits can be very great. Two long-term studies, the SOS[44] and one by Sugerman *et al.*[45] have reported marked improvement. More modest weight loss of 10 kg or so by very low calorie diet can also greatly improve pulmonary function and sleep apnea[46-48].

Cardiovascular disease

Obesity is an independent risk factor for cardiovascular disease[1]. Whether weight loss improves risk for cardiovascular events has not been studied. There was an observational study by Higgins *et al.* (1993)[49] that found an association between weight loss and cardiovascular disease, although this finding almost certainly results from the fact that the study does not distinguish disease-related involuntary weight loss from voluntary weight reduction.

In a longitudinal study of individuals who had had a myocardial infarction, a mean weight loss of 6.3 kg was associated with a reduction in cardiac events and total mortality[21]. Ornish *et al.*[50] reported a regression of coronary atherosclerosis in patients adopting his diet, which targets both weight and lipids. Williamson *et al.*[4] found a 20 per cent reduction in all-cause mortality in women with obesity-related health conditions reporting an intentional weight loss of 1–19 lb, while the reduction in mortality rate from cardiovascular disease was 9 per cent. Future trials need to investigate further the effect of lifestyle change (diet and exercise) on cardiovascular events. Presently, the LookAhead Trial supported by the NIH is investigating this in diabetic patients.

Heart failure

With obesity, there is an increase in blood volume, an increase in blood pressure, and an increased cardiac output. This can lead to left ventricular hypertrophy and eventual heart failure. Weight loss generally improves the impaired cardiac function[47]. A study by McMahon *et al.*[51] showed a decrease in left ventricular mass in a group of obese persons who lost an average of 8.3 kg.

Gallstones

Obese persons produce bile which tends to be supersaturated with cholesterol. As a result, they are prone to the development of cholesterol gallstones[52,53]. The gallbladder in obese persons also has poor contractility, so that the bile is not optimally ejected and pools in a stagnant fashion also promoting the crystallization of the cholesterol to form sludge and stones[54]. The Nurses' Health Study has reported that weight loss is associated with the formation of gallstones and risk for cholecystectomy. The risk increases for those losing 4.0 to 9.9 kg and is even greater for those losing 10 kg or more[55]. It is important to add that during the period of active weight loss, lithogenicity of the bile increases[56], but after a new, lower weight plateau has been reached, the lithogenicity is less than it was at the initial baseline weight.

Arthritis

In cross-sectional studies, increasing weight is associated with increasing prevalence of osteoarthritis[1]. Small reductions in weight are associated with decreased pain and improved walking time in patients with arthritis'[57].

Conclusion

Obesity is associated with a number of health risks. These health risks tend to be improved with weight loss[2,3,58]. Even a small weight loss of 5 to 10 per cent of baseline weight has an important effect on reducing risk. It seems incumbent on physicians to treat this widespread condition, which is increasing in prevalence around the world.

References

1. Pi-Sunyer FX, Health hazards of obesity. *Ann Int Med* 1993; 119: 665.

2. Pi-Sunyer FX. Short-term medical benefits and adverse effects of weight loss. *Ann Int Med* 1993; 119: 722–6.

3. Pi-Sunyer FX A review of long-term studies evaluating the efficacy of weight loss in ameliorating disorders associated with obesity. *Clin Therap* 1996; 18: 1006–35.

4. Williamson DF, Pamuk E, Thun M *et al.* Prospective study of intentional weight loss and mortality in never-smoking overweight US white women aged 40–64 years. *Am J Epidemiol* 1995; 141: 1128–41.

5. Polonsky KS, Given BD, Hirsh LJ *et al.* Abnormal patterns of insulin secretion in non-insulin dependent diabetes mellitus. *N Engl J Med* 1988; 318: 1231–9.

6. Reaven GM. Role of insulin resistance in human disease. *Diabetes* 1988; 37: 1595–607.

7. Bogardus C, Lillioja S, Mott D, Reaven GR, Kashiwagi A, Foley JE. Relationship between obesity and maximal insulin stimulated glucose uptake *in vivo* and *in vitro* in Pima indians. *J Clin Invest* 1984; 73; 800–5.

8. Olefsky JM, Kolterman OG, Scarlett JA. Insulin action and resistance in obesity and noninsulin-dependent type II diabetes mellitus. *Am J Physiol* 1982; 243: E15–30.

9. Ward WK, Beard JC, Porte D Jr. Clinical aspects of islet B-cell function in noninsulin-dependent diabetes mellitus. *Diabet Metab Rev* 1986; 2: 297–313.

10. Tuomilehto J, Lindstrom J, Eriksson JG, Valle TT, Hamalainen H *et al.* Prevention of type 2 diabetes mellitus by changes in lifestyle among subjects with impaired glucose tolerance. *N Engl J Med* 2001; 344: 1343–50.

11. Diabetes Prevention Program. Reduction in the incidence of type 2 diabetes with lifestyle intervention or metformin. *N Engl J Med* 2002; 346: 393–403.

12. Haffner SM, Stern MP, Hazuda HP, Mitchell BD, Patterson JK. Cardiovascular risk factors in confirmed prediabetic individuals. Does the clock for coronary disease start ticking before the onset of clinical diabetes? *J Am Med Assoc* 1990; 262: 2893–8.

13. Liu GC, Coulston AM, Lardinois CK, Hollenbeck CB, Moore JG, Reaven GM. Moderate weight loss and sulfonylurea treatment of non-insulin-dependent diabetes mellitus. *Arch Int Med* 1985; 145: 665–9.

14. Henry RR, Wiest-Kent TA, Scheaffer L, Koltennan OG, Olefsky JM.. Metabolic consequences of very-low-calorie diet therapy in obese non-insulin-dependent diabetic and nondiabetic subjects. *Diabetes* 1986; 35: 155–64.

15. Wing RR, Loeske R, Epstein LH *et al.* Long-term effects of modest weight loss in type II diabetic patients. *Arch Int Med* 1987; 47: 1749–53.

16. Hanefield M, Fischer S, Schinechel H *et al.* Diabetes intervention study. *Diabetes Care* 1991; 14: 308–17.

17. UK Prospective Diabetes Study 7. Response of fasting plasma glucose to diet therapy in newly presenting type II diabetic patients. *Metabolism* 1990; 39: 905–12

18. Diabetes Control and Complications Trial Research Group. The effect of intensive treatment of diabetes on the development and progression of long-term complications in insulin dependent diabetes mellitus. *N Engl J Med* 1993; 329: 977–86.

19. Stamler R, Stamler J, Riedlinger WF *et al.* Findings in hypertension screening of 1 million Americans. *J Am Med Assoc* 1978; 240: 1607–10.

20. JNC VII. The seventh report on the joint national committee on prevention, detection, evaluation, and treatment of high blood pressure. Executive summary. *J Am Med Assoc* 2002.

21. Singh RB, Rastogi SS, Verma R *et al.* Randomized controlled trial of cardioprotective diet in patients with recent acute myocardial infarction: results of one-year follow-up. *BMJ* 1992; 304: 1015–9.

22. Neaton JD, Grimm RH, Prineas RJ, Stamler J, Grandits GA *et al.* Treatment of mild hypertension study. *J Am Med Assoc* 1993; 270: 713–24.

23. Stamler R, Stamler J, Gosch FC *et al.* Primary prevention of hypertension by nutritional-hygienic means: final report of a randomized, controlled trial. *J Am Med Assoc* 1989; 262: 1801–7.

24. Sugennan HJ, Fairman RP, Sood RK *et al.* Long-term effects of gastric surgery for treating respiratory insufficiency of obesity. *Am J Clin Nutr* 1992; 55: S597–S601.

25. Wassertheil-Smoller S, Blaufox MD, Oberman AS, Langford HG, *et al.* The Trial of Antihypertensive Interventions and Management (TAIM) Study: adequate weight loss, alone and combined with drug therapy in the treatment of mild hypertension. *Arch Int Med* 1992; 152: 131–6.

26. Langford HG, Davis BR, Blaufox D *et al.* Effect of drug and diet treatment of mild hypertension on diastolic blood pressure. The TAIM Research Group. *Hypertension* 1991; 17: 210–7.

27. Després JP. Dyslipidaemia and obesity. *Clin Endocr Metab* 1994; 8: 629–260.

28. Kaplan RM, Wilson DK, Hartwell SL *et al.* Prospective evaluation of HDL cholesterol changes after diet and physical conditioning programs for patients with type II diabetes mellitus. *Diabetes Care* 1985; 8: 343–8.

29. NHLBI. Clinical guidelines on the identification, evaluation, and treatment of overweight and obesity in adults. The evidence report. *Obes Res* 1998; 6: S51–S209.

30. Hellenius ML, Defaire U, Berglund B *et al.* Diet and exercise are equally effective in reducing risk for cardiovascular disease. Results of a randomized controlled study in men with slightly to moderately raised cardiovascular risk factors. *Atherosclerosis* 1993; 103: 81–91.

31. Karvetti RL, Hakala P. A 7-year follow-up of a weight reduction programme in Finnish primary health care. *Eur J Clin Nutr* 1992; 46: 743–53.

32. Marniemi J, Seppanen A, Hakala P. Long-term effects on lipid metabolism of weight reduction on lactovegetarian and mixed diet. *Int J Obes* 1990; 14; 113–25.

33. Svensen OL, Hassager C, Christiansen C. Effect of an energy-restrictive diet, with or without exercise, on lean tissue mass, resting metabolic rate, cardiovascular risk factors, and bone in overweight post-menopausal women. *Am J Med* 1993; 95: 131–40.

34. Wolf RN, Grundy SM. Influence of weight reduction on plasma lipoproteins in obese patients. *Arteriosclerosis* 1983; 3; 160–9.

35. Sorbris R, Petersson BG, Nilsson-Ehlem P. Effect of weight reduction on plasma lipoproteins and adipose tissue metabolism in obese subjects. *Eur J Clin Invest* 1981; 11; 491–8.

36. VanGaal LF *et al.* Human obesity: from lipid abnormalities to lipid oxidation. *Int J Obes* 1995; 19: S21–S26.

37. Hamsten A, Walldius G, Szamosi A *et al.* Plasminogen activator in plasma: risk factor for recurrent myocardial infarction. *Lancet* 1987; 2: 3–9.

38. Meade TW, Ruddock V, Stirling Y *et al.* Fibrinolytic activity, clotting factors and long term incidence of ischemic heart disease in the Northwick Park Heart Study. *Lancet* 1993; 11: 342–5.

39. Vague P, Juhan-Vague J, Ailhaud MF *et al.* Correlation between blood fibrinolytic activity, plasminogen activator inhibitor level, plasma insulin level and relative body weight in normal and obese subjects. *Metabolism* 1986; 35: 250–3.

40. Folsom AR, Qamhieh HT, Wing RR, *et al.* Impact of weight loss on plasminogen activator inhibitor (PAI-1), Factor VII and other hemostatic factors in moderately overweight adults. *Arterioscler Thromb* 1993; 13: 162–9.

41. Kopelman, P. Obesity as a medical problem. *Nature* 2000; 404: 635–43.

42. Young T, Palta M, Dempsey J *et al.* (The occurrence of sleep-disordered breathing among middle-aged adults. *N Engl J Med* 1993; 328: 1230–5.

43. Vgontzas AN, Tan TL, Bixler EO *et al.* Sleep apnea and sleep disruption in obese patients. *Arch Int Med* 1994; 154: 1705–11.

44. Karason K, Lindroos AK, Stenlof K, Sjöström L. Relief of cardiorespiratory symtoms and increased physical activity after surgically induced weight loss: results from the Swedish Obese Subjects study. *Arch Int Med* 2000; 160; 1797–802.

45. Sugerman HJ, Fairman RP, Sood RK *et al.* Long-term effects of gastric surgery for treating respiratory insufficiency of obesity. *Am J Clin Nutr* 1992; 55: S597–S601.

46. Kansanen M, Vanninen E, Tuunainen *et al.* The effect of a very low-calorie diet-induced weight loss on the severity of obstructive sleep apnoea and autonomic nervous function in obese patients with obstructive sleep apnoea syndrome. *Clin Physiol* 1998; 18: 377–85.

47. Suratt PM, McTier RF, Findley LJ *et al.* Changes in breathing and the pharynx after weight loss in obstructive sleep apnea. *Chest* 1987; 92: 631–37.

48. Suratt PM, McTier RF, Findley LJ *et al.* Effect of very-low calorie diets with weight loss on obstructive sleep apnea. *Am J Clin Nutr.*1992; 56: S182–S184.

49. Higgins M, D'Agostino RB, Kannel W, Cobb JL. Benefits and adverse effects of weight loss: observations from the Framingham Study. *Ann Int Med* 1993; 119: 758–63.

50. Ornish D, Brown SE, Scherwitz B *et al.* Can lifestyle changes reverse coronary heart disease? *Lancet* 1990; 336; 129–33.

51. McMahon SW, Wilkens DE, MAcDonald GJ. The effect of weight reduction on left ventricular mass: a randomized controlled trial in young overweight hypertensives. *N Engl J Med* 1986; 314: 334–9.

52. Maclure KM, Hayes KC, Colditz GA *et al.* Weight, diet, and the risk of symptomatic gallstones in middle-aged women. *N Engl J Med* 1989; 321: 563–9.

53. Bennion LJ, Grundy SM. Effects of obesity and caloric intake on biliary lipid metabolism in man. *J Clin Invest* 1975; 56: 996–1011.

54. Marzio L, Capone F, Neri M, Mexetti A, DeAngelis C, Cuccurullo F. Gallbladder kinetics in obese patients. Effect of a regular meal and low-calorie meal. *Dig Dis Scl* 1988; 33: 4–9.

55. Stampfer MJ, Maclure KM, Colditz GA *et al.* Risk of symptomatic gallstones in women with severe obesity. *Am J Clin Nutr* 1992; 5: 652–8.

56. Liddle RA, Goldstein RB, Saxton J. Gallstone formation during weight-reduction dieting. *Arch Int Med* 1989; 149: 1750–3.

57. Bradley MH, Golden EL. Powdered meal replacements – can they benefit overweight patients with concomitant conditions exacerbated by obesity? *Curr Ther Res* 1990; 47: 429–36.

58. Goldstein DJ. Beneficial effects of modest weight loss. *Int J Obes* 1992; 16: 397–415.

CHAPTER 215

Non-pharmacologic treatment of obesity: herbal aids to weight loss

Frank Greenway

Medical Director and Professor, Pennington Biomedical Research Center, 6400 Perkins Road, Baton Rouge, Louisiana 70808-4124, USA
[e-mail: greenwfl@pbrc.edu]

Introduction

The use of herbal dietary supplements and alternative treatments increased dramatically in the United States with the passage of the 1994 Dietary Supplements Health Education Act. This act classifies dietary herbal supplements as foods that are generally recognized as safe. This allows the manufacturers to market these products without proving efficacy or safety, relying on the FDA to prove them unsafe in order to remove them from the market. The FDA has limited resources to test these products and relies on adverse event reports to monitor their safety. Adverse event reports cannot establish cause and effect. This puts the medical profession in a difficult position when asked to advise patients on the safety and efficacy of these products. This paper will review the, often inadequate, information on safety and efficacy of dietary herbal supplements sold for the treatment of obesity in an attempt to provide some basis upon which advise the obese patient. Dietary herbal supplements will be reviewed starting with dietary fibres, amino acids and neurotransmitter modulators, agents effecting fat metabolism and nutrient partitioning and ending with agents effecting thermogenesis. This last category includes the bulk of the dietary herbal supplements sold for the treatment of obesity. It is not only the category with the greatest amount of scientific data to support conclusions, but it is also the category that provokes the most controversy.

Fibres

Plant fibre

The decline in the amount of dietary fibre associated with starchy food in the diet of Western countries since 1900 has been postulated to be one of the reasons for an upsurge in the incidence of obesity[1]. Efforts to evaluate the relationship between dietary fibre and weight regulation began in the 1980s. There have been at least a dozen controlled, clinical trials evaluating dietary fibre for the treatment of obesity. One can summarize these studies by saying that the bulk of evidence supports dietary fibre decreasing food intake and decreasing hunger. These studies used dietary fibre supplements between 5 and 40 g/day. This led to weight losses of 1 to 3 kg more than placebo. This difference is less than the 5 per cent of body weight felt to be the threshold for a medically significant weight loss[2]. Nevertheless, since dietary fibre has salutary effects on cardiovascular risk factors and appears to be safe, it should be included in weight loss diets. In fact, the caloric density of food has been inversely related to food intake and to the use of fibre[3].

Chitosan

Chitosan is acetylated chitin. Chitin is dietary fibre from animals and is derived from the exoskeletons of crustaceans like shrimp. It was designed to bind fat within the gut. Mice fed chitosan as 3–15 per cent of their diet for 9 weeks gained less weight, had less hyperlipidaemia, fatty liver and a high excretion of fecal fat than high fat fed controls[4]. Two controlled clinical trials using 2.4–3.6 g/day

1

chitosan gave no more weight loss than a placebo. Although chitosan appears safe at the amounts given in these trials, it does not decrease caloric density sufficiently to give weight loss.

Table 1.

Herbal treatment	Evidence of efficacy	Evidence of safety
Thermogenic		
Caffeine and ephedra	Good – clinical trial	Good
Green tea catechins	Good – metabolic study	Excellent
Synephrine	Modest – clinical trial	Excellent
Capsaicin	Good – clinical trial	Excellent
L-tyrosine	None	Excellent
Fat metabolism and nutrient modulation		
Conjugated linoleic acid	Weak – clinical trial	Questionable
Garcinia cambogia	Poor – clinical trial	Excellent
Dehydroepiandrosterone	Minimal, if any – clinical trial	Questionable
Chromium picolinate	Ineffective	Good
Betahydroxymethylbutyrate	Ineffective for weight loss	Good
Amino acids and neurotransmitter modulation		
5-hyrdoxytryptophan	Modest – clinical trial	Excellent
Fibres		
Dietary fibre	Modest – clinical trial	Excellent
Chitosan	Ineffective – clinical trial	Excellent

Serotonin (5-HT)

Serotonin is well-recognized to play a role in the central regulation of appetite, and the weight loss properties of fenfluramine are mediated through serotonin. Rats infused with serotonin eat less. Osborne-Mendle rats that have reduced activity of tyrosine hydroxylase, the enzyme that converts tryptophan to serotonin, are predisposed to obesity. There have been two clinical trials comparing serotonin 8 mg/kg/day to a placebo over a 5- to 15-week period. Although there was a statistically significant weight loss compared to placebo in both studies, the studies were small and the difference from placebo was 3 kg at 12 weeks. This suggests the efficacy and safety of serotonin for weight loss, but confirmation of these findings is clearly needed.

Fat metabolism and nutrient partitioning

Hydro-beta-methylbuterate (HMB)

HMB is sold as a supplement to burn fat, increase strength and build muscle tissue. It is a metabolite of leucine that, when supplemented at 1.5–3 gm/day, reduces muscle catabolism, and increases fat free mass during a 2–6 week weight lifting programme. HMB appears to be safe, but has not been tested as an obesity treatment.

Chromium

Chromium increases muscle mass and decreases fat mass during the growth phase in swine known as 'finishing'. The most popular salt of chromium for this purpose is chromium picolinate. Chromium, though its incorporation into glucose tolerance factor is thought to increase insulin sensitivity. Increased insulin sensitivity has been postulated to result in weight loss through an anorectic effect of on the brain. At least nine trials have been performed to evaluate the effect of chromium on loss and body composition. Although none of these trials gave greater weight loss than placebo, by Trent and Thieding-Cancel was the largest and most persuasive. Two hundred twelve navy personnel were randomized to chromium picolinate 400 mcg/day or placebo for 16 though there was a small weight and fat loss during the study, there was no effect of the chromium picolinate compared to placebo[5]. Chromium, in the doses used in these studies, appears safe, but gives no weight loss in humans.

Dehydroepiandrosterone (DHEA)

DHEA is an effective weight loss agent in rodents, an animal that makes very little DHEA. DHEA is the most abundant steroid produced in humans, and it declines with age and illness. Studies of DHEA in doses up to 1600 mg/day have generally been without effect on weight. One study using 200 mg/day, however, gave a 1 kg weight loss over 1 month in obese women. In an effort to evaluate this conflicting result, ageing humans were treated with 50 mg DHEA/day for 6 months, a dose that raised their level of DHEA to that seen during youth. There was no change in body fat. The dose was then increased to 100 mg DHEA/day for the next year. Body fat decreased 1 kg in men but not women. The women gained 1.4 kg, but the men did not. DHEA appears safe, but is minimally effective, if effective at all for weight loss[6].

Garcinia cambogia (hydroxycitric acid)

Garcinia cambogia contains hydroxycitric acid. One of the 16 isomers of hydroxycitric acid is an inhibitor of citrate lyase, an enzyme that catalyses the first step in fatty acid synthesis outside the mitochondrion. Roche Pharmaceuticals studied sodium hydroxycitrate in rodents during the 1970s. The rodents lost weight, but, contrary to expectations, the weight loss was due to a decrease in food intake. Pair-feeding experiments were used to demonstrate the importante of a decrement in food intake, rather than an inhibition of fat synthesis in the animal's weight loss. Despite the weight loss with hydroxycitrate in rodents, human clinical trials have been disappointing. Although three trials evaluating garcinia cambogia failed to demonstrate weight loss, the trial with 135 obese participants randomized to 1500 mg/day of calcium hydroxycitric acid derived from garcinia cambogia or placebo was the most convincing. At the end of a 12-week treatment period, the group treated with garcinia cambogia lost 3.2 kg, an amount not different from the 3.1 kg lost by the placebo group[7]. No blood levels of hydroxycitrate were drawn during this study. Therefore, it is not clear whether the sodium salt that was effective for weight loss in rodents was absorbed more efficiently than the calcium salt used in humans, or if humans and rodents are different in their response to hydroxycitrate. Hydroxy-citrate appears to be safe, but the preparations currently on the market are ineffective for weight loss.

Conjugated linoleic acid (CLA)

The cis-9, trans-11 isomer of conjugated linoleic acid is formed in the rumen of cattle, and has anticancer properties. When conjugated linoleic acid is chemically synthesized the trans-10, cis-12 isomer that is responsible for changes in body composition is also formed. CLA retards weight gain without effecting food intake, decreases body fat, increases fat oxidation and increases lipolysis in rodents. Metabolic rate was increased and respiratory quotient decreased in rodents. The trans-10, cis-12 isomer also causes insulin resistance. A clinical trial in humans gave no weight loss compared to placebo. Therefore, CLA is not effective for weight loss in humans, and the increased insulin resistance in rodents raises concerns about its safety.

Thermogenic aids

Herbal caffeine and ephedrine

During the 1970s, ephedrine with theophylline or caffeine was commonly used for the treatment of asthma in adults and children. Theophylline and caffeine are both methylxanthines that inhibit phos-phodiesterase and the adenosine receptor, 1 mg of theophylline being equivalent to 2 mg of caffeine. This ephedrine with methylxanthine combination was noted to give weight loss comparable to diethyl-propion in a 12-week controlled trial[8]. Caffeine 200 mg with ephedrine 20 mg taken three times a day is an approved prescription medication for the treatment of obesity in Denmark, and has a good safety record.

The pivotal 24-week, double-blind, randomized Danish trial used to approve caffeine with ephedrine as an obesity treatment enrolled 180 subjects who were assigned to placebo, ephedrine 20 mg tid, caffeine 200 mg tid or the combination of caffeine and ephedrine. Weight loss in the caffeine and ephedrine group was greater than placebo from the eighth week of the trial, but neither caffeine nor ephedrine alone was different than placebo. Adverse events were not serious and reached placebo levels by week 8 where they remained for the remainder of the trial. The blood pressure and pulse rat in the caffeine with ephedrine group were below baseline by week 8 of the trial, and caffeine protect from the rise in pulse rate seen with ephedrine alone. At the end of 24 weeks, subjects continued caffeine and ephedrine for an additional 6 months, and maintained their weight loss over that period[9]. Caffeine with ephedrine is sold as a dietary herbal supplement in the USA, a category that presumes safety. Due to adverse events reported to the FDA MedWatch system, the presumption of safety has been questioned[10]. Three billion doses of herbal caffeine and ephedrine products were produced in 1999, giving an incidence for serious adverse events (mostly cardiovascular and neurological) of 1 for every 70 million doses[11]. This compares to one serious adverse event (mostly gastrointestinal) per 25 million doses of 200 mg ibuprofen[12]. The incidence of adverse events with low dose aspirin use is one to three times higher than ibuprofen, suggesting that caffeine and ephedrine have a safety profile better than some common non-prescription drugs.

The real measure of safety is derived from clinical trials where a placebo group is available with which to compare. Due to the limited numbers of subjects in clinical trials with caffeine and ephedra, rare serious events with an incidence less than 1 per cent would not be detected. Herbal ephedra is composed of four isomers, the most potent of which is ephedrine[13]. Thus, ephedra would be expected to be safer on a milligram for milligram basis than ephedrine. Nevertheless, many of the herbal products makers may not properly standardize the dose or use good manufacturing practices. Caffeine and ephedra products may also contain herbs capable of causing drug interactions. For example, one commercial product contains forskolin that, like caffeine and ephedrine, result in sympathetic activation.

The longest controlled clinical trial of herbal caffeine and ephedrine compared 192 mg of caffeine per day and 90 mg of ephedrine a day to placebo in a 6-month trial. The 46 subjects (55 per cent) finishing the trial in the caffeine and ephedrine group lost 7.8 per cent of their initial body weight compared to 3.5 per cent in the 36 subjects (43 per cent) completing the trial in the placebo group ($P < 0.001$). No serious adverse events were recorded, the caffeine with ephedrine group lost more fat and had a 4 beat per minute rise in pulse rate[14].

L-tyrosine

Although the conversion of tyrosine to norepinephrine is normally enzyme-limited, drugs like ephedrine that release catecholamines convert this to a substrate-limited reaction in rodents. Thus, tyrosine can increase ephedrine induced suppression of food intake in rodents by 50 per cent through a central effect[14]. Although tyrosine is included in some herbal weight loss supplements along with caffeine and ephedrine, this combination has not been tested in human clinical trials.

Green tea catechins

Green tea contains catechins and caffeine. Epigallocatechin gallate is the most potent of these catechins and inhibits, catachol-o-methyl transferase, an enzyme that degrades norepinephrine. Epigallocatechin gallate synergistically increases oxygen consumption in a brown fat cell assay when combined with caffeine and ephedrine[15]. Green tea (catechin and caffeine) increased oxygen consumption by 4.5 per cent in a metabolic chamber compared to 3.2 per cent with the same dose of caffeine alone[16].

Citrus aurantium

Citrus aurantium (bitter orange) contains small amounts of synephrine and octopamine, direct and indirect sympathetic agonists. Although citrus aurantium is included in some herbal weight loss preparations, it has only given more weight loss compared to baseline rather than to placebo. Citrus aurantium may be milder than caffeine with ephedrine, but a bioequivalence trial has not been reported.

Chili peppers

Capsaicin from chili peppers stimulates fat oxidation and thermogenesis[17]. Reports of modest weight loss also exist in subjects consuming chili peppers regularly.

References

[1]brink MJ. Dietary fiber, plasma insulin, and obesity. *Am J Clin Nutr* 1978; (10 Suppl): S277–S279.

[ ] and Nutrition Board. *Weighing the options*; Paul R. Thomas (ed.), p. 16. Washington: National Academy 1995.

[ ] Hetherington M, Burley VJ. Sensory stimulation an energy density in the development of satiety. *hav* 1988; 6: 727–33.

4. Han LK, Kimura Y, Okuda H. Reduction in fat storage during chitin-chitosan treatment in mice fed a high-fat diet. *Int. J Obes Relat Metab Disord* 1999; 23: 174–9.

5. Trent LK, Thieding-Cancel D. Effects of chromium picolinate on body composition. *J Sports Med Phys Fitness* 1995; 35: 273–80.

6. Morales AJ, Haubrich RH, Hwang JY, Asakura H, Yen SS. The effect of six months treatment with a 100 mg daily dose of dehydroepiandrosterone (DHEA) on circulating sex steroids, body composition and muscle strength in age-advanced men and women. *Clin Endocrinol* 1998; 49: 421–32.

7. Heymsfield SB, Allison DB, Vasselli JR, Pietrobelli A, Greenfield D, Nunez C. Garcinia cambogia (hydroxycitric acid) as a potential antiobesity agent: a randomized controlled trial. *JAMA* 1998; 280: 1596–600.

8. Malchow-Moller A, Larsen S, Hey H, Stokholm KH, Juhl E, Quaade F. Ephedrine as an anorectic: the story of the 'Elsinore pill'. *Int J Obes* 1981; 5183–7.

9. Astrup A, Breum L, Toubro S, Hein P, Quaade F. The effect and safety of an ephedrine/caffeine compound compared to ephedrine, caffeine and placebo in obese subjects on an energy restricted diet. A double blind trial. *Int J Obes Relat Metab Disord* 1992; 16: 269–77.

10. Haller CA, Benowitz NL. Adverse cardiovascular and central nervous system events associated with dietary supplements containing ephedra alkaloids. *N Engl J Med* 2000; 343: 1833–8.

11. Dietary supplement market view. Washington: FDC Reports; 2000.

12. Moore N, Noblet C, Breemeersch C. Focus on the safety of ibuprofen at the analgesic antipyretic dose. *Therapie* 1996; 51: 458–63.

13. Vansal SS, Feller DR. Direct effects of ephedrine isomers on human beta-adrenergic receptor subtypes. *Biochem Pharmacol* 1999; 58: 807–10.

14. Hull KM, Maher TJ. L-tyrosine potentiates the anorexia induced by mixed-acting sympathomimetic drugs in hyperphagic rats. *J Pharmacol Exp Ther* 1990; 255: 403–9.

15. Dulloo AG, Seydoux J, Giradier L. Tealine and thermogenesis: interactions between polyphenols, caffeine and sympathetic activity. *Int J Obes Relat Metab Disord* 1996; 20 (Suppl 4): 71.

16. Dulloo AG, Seydoux J, Girardie L, Chantre P, Vandermander J. Green tea and thermogenesis: interactions between catechin-polyphenols, caffeine and sympathetic activity. *Int J Obes Relat Metab Disord* 2000; 24: 252–8.

17. Henry CJ, Emery B. Effect of spiced food on metabolic rate. *Hum Nutr: Clin Nutr* 1986; 40: 165–8.

CHAPTER 216

Evaluation of obese patient before treatment

Julio C. Montero

J.E. Uriburu 1312. (1114). Pta. Baja 'A'. Buenos Aires, Argentina
[e-mail: jcmontero@cotelnet.com.ar]

Introduction

Adaptative response to the positive energetic balance results in increasing fat in adipose tissue: a situation that could be called: 'physiological overweight'[1] recognized as a change that increases the possibility of survival in starvation conditions. However, if the amount of fat accumulated in the adipose tissue is excessive, if it is deposited in abnormally high amount in upper body or there are triglycerides ectopically accumulated elsewhere (e.g. muscle)[2] for a long time or even chronically, the originally protective condition is slowly progressing towards the morbid status known as 'obesity illness' or simply obesity[3]. It is necessary to keep in mind that even the moderate and mild obese patients suffer a dynamic impact over their metabolism and endocrine system, but morbid obese ones also have an important heart, hemodynamic[4], respiratory and osteoarticular overload[5] and increased prevalence of hormone-dependent and gastrointestinal cancers[3]. On triggering general compensative metabolic mechanisms such as insulin resistance, obesity can have a negative impact on the majority of organs and tissues, inducing confusion between causes and consequences. Obesity can be considered an illness in itself as it causes myocardial dysfunction, mechanical overcharge and psychological burden or 'the mother' of other ones as it stresses chronically metabolic pathways, distorting hormonal systems and pre-existent pathologies.

We must not forget psychological aspects as unhappy feelings related to negative image, physical impairments and social discrimination. Depression and hyperphagic disorders[6] which are frequently associated to obesity, could be seen again as the double condition of cause and consequence of psychological discomfort[7-9]. Related to those multiple confounding aspects, obesity treatment usually generate conflictive points of view and criticism from the general opinion and even from some physicians. These reasons force us to make an accurate diagnosis and prognosis in order to choose a therapeutic prescription considering physiopatological mechanisms, health risks and life expectancies. For all this, it is relevant to evaluate the patient before the treatment.

Evaluation of obese patient requires both clinical and complementary diagnostic techniques.

Anamnesis

Disease at present. Symptomatology. Consultation reason

Interview gives esential information which can be very useful in the evaluation of obese patient. Obesity-related consultation is usually limited to three main aspects: image, morbidities and risks. Real and subjective image can give information about personality, motivation and expectancies, that can be ·lpful in the global management. Sometimes organic or functional morbidities symptomatology (not ·sity) triggered or worsened by obesity can be the reason of consultation. Clinical signs and symp- must be interpreted in their particular context (age, medical antecedents, occupation, etc). In- ¹ risks related to weight gain can be related to morbities above mentioned or by genetic nts. Most frequent health problems and symptomatology associated with obesity are[34]: Greatly 'relative risk > 3): diabetes, gallbladder disease, hypertension, dyslipidaemia, insulin resis- ʰlessness, sleep apnea. Moderately increased (relative risk 2–3): coronary heart disease, (knees), hyperuricaemia and gout. Slightly increases (relative risk 1–2): cancer (breast cancer in postmenopausal women, endometrial cancer, colon cancer), reproductive hormone abnormalities, polycystic ovary syndrome, impaired fertility, low back pain, increased anesthetic risk, fetal defects from maternal obesity.

History of obesity. Personal antecedents. Weight evolution

Maternal nutrition during pregnancy together with anthropometrical fetal measures at delivery time could be suggestive of fetal life influences prone to obesity and its associations[10].

Onset of obesity. The earlier the onset of obesity, the higher the possibility of obesity and associated risks. The precocity of 'rebound' in the early infancy is a negative prognosis factor because of its relationship to obesity afterwards in life[11,12].

Length of obesity. The longer the obesity evolution, the higher the risks of dismetabolic associations[13].

Recent weight change. It is important to know if the weight patient is increasing or is steady. Sustained weight gain suggest present factors operating on energetic balance (smoking cessation, some drugs, depression, suppression of physical activity, change of work, etc). These should be detected by the physician since they could be corrected. Due to the impossibility to know accurately which the regulatory component that is operating in each particular case is, it is only possible to attempt to modify the triggering active circumstance or counteract the most probable physiopathological mechanism. Drugs related to weight gain such as antidopaminergics, tricyclic antidepressants, antiepileptics (valproate), steroids (glucocorticoids, estrogen, progestins, oral contraceptives), sulphonylurea, glitazonas, cyproheptadine, etc. are aetiologic factors potentially reversible[14].

Familiar antecedents. Weight history of parents or siblings could help us predict the possible evolution of the illness related to inheritance, since several studies have shown the powerful influence of the genetic background to developing obesity and its associations(hypertension, dyslipaemias, insulin-resistance, diabetes, etc)[15-20].

Lifestyle

Energy intake. Food habits. A food recall should be asked to the patient because it collects valuable data about: (a) Macronutrients ingested: related to neurohormonal eating regulation and metabolic needs, that are expressed in different ways, such as hunger, appetite, satiety or as non-specific signals such as anxiety, insomnia and other. (b) Bulk of food ingested: connected to gastric compliance, satiation and early digestive signals. Highest gastric capacity seems to be more frequently associated with binge. (c) Frequency of food. Regular time eating is important to improve meals control. Some obese people usually eat once or twice a day[21] while others suffer 'craving' or 'nibbling'. All these eating behaviours make the control of energetic intake difficult.

Eating behaviour. Abnormal eating behaviour has been associated with worse prognosis, psychological problems and treatment complexity[22]. Schematically, undesirable eating behaviour can be: compulsive (e.g. binges, craving) or purgative (e.g. vomits). Macronutrients eaten besides eating behaviour give the necessary information to select the best strategy to modify the energy intake, such as avoiding addictive foods and suggesting the more effective and possible food changes and pharmacological intervention.

Energy expenditure. Physical activity level

Physical activity level of working and leisure activities (sportive or recreative) gives us an idea about the amount of energy usually spent and the possibilities of increasing the energetic expenditure. Regulation of the intensity, frequency and length of programmed physical activities can turn it into a controllable energetic and metabolic therapeutical tool. Exhaustive physical activity is considered as a purgative expenditure behaviour frequently associated with some eating disorders[23].

Psychological profile. Although depression is frequently associated with weight gain and overweight, some antidepressive drugs such as tryciclics can do the same. Antipsychotics(phenotiazinas and butyrophenones) and lithium can induce weight gain[24].

Physical examination

Symptomatology from the interview added to check-up give information about obesity features and some co morbid conditions as:

(1) Early obesity, craniofacial and limb deformation, mental retardation, reproductive alteration[25] suggesting genetic obesity syndromes; (2) Headache, impaired vision, amenorrhea, impotence, convulsions, coma[26] in hypothalamic obesity; (3) Central, truncal, facial obesity, cutaneous striae, thin atrophic skin and hypertension associated to hypercortisolism; (4) Acanthosis nigricans associated to insulin – resistance syndrome; (5) Xanthoma, xhantelasma, corneal arcus, ischaemia, in dyslipidae-

mias; (6) Hirsutism, infertility, abnormal menses, oligoanovulation[27] in polycystic ovary syndrome; (7) Sleep apnea, daytime tiredness, short and wide neck (= 43 cm)[28,29]; (8) Chronic airflow limitation, sleep apnea, cyanosis[30].

Weight and risks. It is important to measure the height and weight to calculate the body mass index (BMI: Weight (kg)/Height (m^2)). It is also required to measure the body circumference at the waist and hip level. Overweight in adults and risks of weight related-comorbilities are classified according to BMI. In spite of the fact of not being specifically fat-sensitive, BMI maintains a good correlation (0.7–0.8) with total fat mass[31]. Cutt-off points of the classification belong to Caucasic people. For Asiatics, Africans and other ethnic groups different values should be used[3] (see Table 1).

Table 1.

Classification	BMI (kg/m^2)	Risk of co-morbidities
Underweight	< 18.5	Low
Normal range	18.5–24.9	Average
Overweight	≥ 25	
Pre-obese	25–29.9	Increased
Obese class I	30–34.9	Moderate
Obese class II	35–39.9	Severe
Obese class III	≥ 40	Very severe

Several studies have shown that mortality increases in accordance with BMI both in males and females, related to cardiovascular disease, cancer and all another causes[32].

Among relative risks of death cardiovascular diseases are the most increased as a consequence of excessive weight[33]. As most people gain weight with advancing age, some of them become overweight (BMI > 25). As long as overweight people do not develop any of the morbid clinical condition related to excessive weight they are called: preclinical overweight group (BMI 25–30). Finally, the group of overweight people (BMI > 30) that develop some of the typical weight-related morbidities belongs to the clinical overweight group[34].

Fat and risks. Upper body fat is another risk predictor recognized since Vague[35] as 'android fat'. This includes the central or abdominal fat (subcutaneous and visceral). The waist to hip ratio value is better to indicate the body shape than to indicate the risks derive from central fat (when > 1 in men and > 0.85 in women)[36]. Nowadays, waist circumference has been proposed as the best indicator of central fat[37–40]. Table 2 shows the WHO cut-off points for central fat-associated metabolic complications[3].

It is said that for BMI = 32 kg/m^2 the waist circumference is a stronger risk predictor than BMI.

Table 2. Risk of obesity-associated metabolic complications

	Increased	Substancially increased
Men	≥ 94 cm (37 inches)	≥ 102 cm (40 inches)
Women	≥ 80 cm (32 inches)	≥ 88 cm (35 inches)

According to The Practical Guide of National Institutes of Health, waist circumference is measured at the top of the right iliac crest level. The tape measure is parallel to the floor. The measurment is made at the end of a normal expiration.

Complementary diagnostic techniques

(a) Routine: fasting glucose. Total, LDL and HDL cholesterol, triglycerides, apoprotein B. Uraemia, uricaemia. Urine determinations. (b) Specific (if necessary): glucose oral test with insulin curve.T3, T4 free, TSH; 24 h urinary cortisol, cortisol production rate, dexametasona suppression test; LH, FSH, testosterone, SHBG, growth hormone. (c) Other (if necessary): ECG.Rx torax.Ovarian ultrasound. Echocardiography. Polysomnography.

Some biochemistry abnormalities can be suspected from physical inspection data as insulin resistance if acanthosis nigricans were present or from clinical manifestations such as amenorrhea in the polycystic ovarian syndrome, though they must be afterwards confirmed and controlled from laboratory data.

Evaluation and prognosis

Overall risks related to BMI can be adjusted taking into consideration some variables such as weight gain; plasmatic triglycerides, HDL cholesterol; fasting glucose, etc. For this objective the method proposed by Bray shown in Table 3[41] can be useful.

Table 3. Risk – Adjusted BMI for metabolic variables

	ADJUSTEMENT SCORES			Adjustment score
SCORE	0	+2	+4	
Weight gain from age of 18	< 5	5–15	> 15	
Ratio TG/HDL	< 5	5–8	> 8	
Blood pressure (mmHg)	< 140/ < 90	140–160/ 90–100	> 160/ > 100	
Fasting glycaemia (mg/dl)	< 95	95–126	> 126	
Waist (cm)	< 94 < 81	94–102 81–89	> 102 > 89	
Sleep apnea	Absent	–	Present	
Physical activity	Regular activity	Sedentary		
RISK – ADJUSTED INDEX				

Conclusions

Evaluation before treatment is a valuable tool. It must be the most complete, rational and comprehensive possible. As the majority of treatments of overweight and obesity imply significant and permanent lifestyle changes, it is very important to make the most suitable prescription, according to the patient possibilities related to biological status, perspectives of weight loss, potential benefits and risks associated with the treatment.

References

1. Garrow JS. *Treat obesity seriously: A clinical manual.* New York: Churchill Livingstone; 1990.

2. Unger RH, Orci L. Lipotoxic diseases of nonadipose tissues in obesity. *Int J Obes Relat Metab Disord.* 2000 Nov; 24 (Suppl 4): S28–32. Review.

3. World Health Organization. Obesity: prevention and management of the global epidemic. The WHO Consultation on Obesity. Clinical guidelines on the identification, evaluation and treatment of overweight and obesity in adults, National Institutes of Health. Geneva: National Heart Lung and Blood Institute 1998.

4. Rillaerts E, van Gaal L, Xiang D *et al.* Blood viscosity in human obesity. Relation to glucose tolerance and insulin status. *Int J Obes* 1989; 13: 739–45.

5. Wirth, A. Cardiac adaptation in obese subjects with and without hypertension -therapeutic implications. *Progress in Obesity Research: 8*, Guy-Grand B, Aillaud G (eds), pp. 593–604. London: John Libbey, 1999.

6. Stunkard, AJ. The dieting depression: Untoward responses to weight reduction. *Am J Med* 1957; 23: 77.

7. Sullivan M *et al.* Swedish Obese Subjects (SOS) – an interventional study of obesity. Baseline evaluation of health and psychosocial functioning in the first 1743 subjects examined. *Int J Obes* 1993; 17: 502–12.

8. Sarlio-Lahteenkorva S, Stunkard A, Rissanen A. Psychological factors and quality of life in obesity. *Int J Obes* 1995; 19 (Suppl 6): S1–S5.

9. Kral JG, Sjostrom LV, Sullivan MBE. Assessment of quality of life before and after surgery for severe obesity. *Am J Clin Nutr* 1992; 55: S611–S614.

10. Pettit DJ, Baird HR, Aleck KA, Bennett PA, Knowler WC. Excessive obesity in offspring of Pima Indian women with diabetes during pregnancy. *N Engl J Med* 1983; 308: 242–5.

11. Rolland-Cachera MF, Deheeger M, Guilloud-Bataille M. Tracking the development of adiposity from one month of age to adulthood. *Ann Hum Biol* 1987; 14: 219–29.

12. Whitaker RC, Pepe MS, Wright JA, Seidel KD, Dietz WH. Early adiposity rebound and the risk of adult obesity. *Pediatrics* 1998 Mar; 101(3): E5.

13. Everhart JE, Pettitt DJ, Bennett PH, Knowler WC. Duration of obesity increases the incidence of NIDDM. *Diabetes* 1992; 41: 236–40.

14. Psychotropic drug-induced obesity. In: *Obesity*, Per Bjorntorp, Bernard Brodoff (eds), pp. 445–53. Philadelphia: JB Lippincott Company; 1992.

15. Ravelli ACJ, van der Muelen JHP, Michels RPJ, Osmond C, Barker DJP *et al.* Glucose tolerance in adults after prenatal exposure to famine. *Lancet* 1998; 351: 173–7.

16. Ravelli ACJ, van der Muelen JHP, Osmond C, Barker DJP, Bleker OP. Obesity at the age of 50 y in men and women exposed to famine prenatally. *Am J Clin Nutr* 1999; 70: 811–6.

17. Larsson B, Svardsudd K, Welin L, Wilhelmsen L, Bjorntorp P, Tibbllin G. Abdominal adipose tissue distribution, obesity, and risk of cardiovascular disease and death: 13 year follow up of participants in the study of men born in 1913. *BMJ* 1984; 288: 1401–4.

18. Bouchard C. Human adaptability may have a genetic bases. In: Landry F (ed.) *Health risk estimation. risk reduction and health promotion*. Ottawa: Canadian Public Health Association; 1983.

19. Poelhman ET, Tremblay A, Després JP *et al.* Genotype-controlled changes in body composition and fat morphology following overfeeding in twins. *Am J Clin Nutr* 1986, 43: 723.

20. Bouchard C, Pérusse L. Heredity and body fat. *Annu Rev Nutr* 1988; 8: 259.

21. Fabry P, Fodor J, Hejl Z *et al.* The frequency of meals: Its relationship to overweight, hypercholesterolaemia, and decreased glucose-tolerance. *Lancet* 1964; 2: 14.

22. Kruger S, Shugar G, Cook RG. Co-morbidity of binge eating disorder and the partial binge eating syndrome with bipolar disorder. *Int J Eating Disorders* 1996; 19: 45–52.

23. Mitchell JE, Hatsukami D, Eckert ED *et al.* Characteristics of 275 patients with bulimia. *Am J Psychiatry* 1985; 142: 482.

24. Bernstein JG. Management of psychotropic drug-induced obesity. In: *Obesity*, Per Bjorntorp, Bernard Brodoff (eds), pp. 445–53. JB Lippincott; 1992.

25. Bray GA. Classification and evaluation of the obesities. *Med Clin North Am* 1989; 73: 161–84.

26. Bray GA. Syndromes of hypothalamic obesity in man. *Pediatr Ann* 1984; 13: 525.

27. Goldzieher JW. Polycystic ovarian disease. *Fertil Steril* 1981; 35(4): 371.

28. Finer N. Clinical assessment, investigation and principles of management: realistic weight goals. In: *Clinical obesity*. Kopelman PG, Michael J Stock (eds), p. 369. Oxford: Blackwell Science; 1998.

29. Strollo PJ Jr, Rogers RM. Current concepts: obstructive sleep apnea. *N Engl J Med* 1996; 334: 99–104.

30. Leech J, Onal E, Baer P, Lopata M. Determinants of hypercapnia in occlusive sleep apnea syndrome. *Chest* 1987; 92: 807–13.

31. Epstein F, Higgins M. Epidemiology of obesity. In: *Obesity*, Per Bjorntorp, Bernard Brodoff (eds), p. 330. Lippincott: JB; 1992.

32. Calle E *et al.* BMI and mortality in a prospective cohort of US adults. *N Engl J Med* 1999; 341: 5.

33. Hubert H, Feinleb M, McNamara P, Castelli W. Obesity as an independent risk factor for cardiovascular disease: a 26-year follow-up of participants in the Framingham study. *Circulation* 1983; 67: 968–77.

34. Bray GA. *Contemporary diagnosis and management of obesity*. Newtown: Handbooks in Health Care Co; National Center for Health Statistics; 1998.

35. Vague J. The degree of masculine differentiation of obesities: a factor determining predisposition to diabetes, arteriosclerosis, gout and uric calculous disease. *Am J Clin Nutr* 1956; 4: 20–34.

36. James WPT. The epidemiology of obesity. In: Chadwick DJ, Cardew GC (eds), *The origins and consequences of obesity*, pp. 1–16. Chichester, Wiley: Ciba Foundation Symposium 201; 1996.

37. Lean MEJ, Hans TS, Morrison CE. Waist circumference as a measure for indicating need for weight management. *BMJ* 1995; 311: 158–61.

38. Lemieux S, Prud'homme D, Tremblay A, Bouchard C, Després JP. Anthropometric correlates to changes in visceral adipose tissue over 7 years in women. *Int J Obes Relat Metab Disord* 1996; 20: 618–24.

39. Lemieux S, Prud'homme D, Bouchard C, Tremblay A, Després JP. A single threshold value of waist girth identifies normal-weight and overweight subjects with excess visceral adipose tissue. *Am J Clin Nutr* 1996; 64: 685–93.

40. Lemieux S, Prud'homme D, Nadeau A, Tremblay A, Bouchard C, Després JP. Seven-year changes in body fat and visceral adipose tissue in women. Association with indexes of plasma glucose-insulin homeostasis. *Diabetes Care* 1996; 19: 983–91.

41. Bray, GA. *Contemporary diagnosis and management of obesity*. Handbooks in Health Care Co. Newtown; 1998.

Progress in Obesity Research: 9. Edited by *Geraldo Medeiros-Neto, Alfredo Halpern and Claude Bouchard*

CHAPTER 217

Orlistat in the treatment of obesity

Alfredo Halpern

University of São Paulo, São Paulo, Brazil
[e-mail: halpern@netpoint.com.br]

O besity prevalence has reached epidemic proportions[1]. Overweight and obesity are associated to health consequences and mortality and represent a serious public health issue[2,3]. In addition, obesity is associated to high economic costs, being responsible for 2–6 per cent of health total cost in some countries[4,5]. Weight loss, even moderate, clearly improves co-morbidities associated to obesity[6,7]. Interventions based on diet and behaviour have had little success at long term[8,9], which indicates the need for long-term effective and safe pharmacological interventions. In-excess fat consumption is recognized as an important factor in obesity genesis[10], and fat absorption inhibition is a useful target for pharmacological intervention. Our aim is to review the use of orlistat, a powerful gastrointestinal lipase inhibitor in the control of overweight and its co-morbidities.

History

From the study of bacteria and fungi isolated from soil samples, a compound with a high gastrointestinal-lipase inhibiting activity, named lipstatin, produced by *Streptomyces toxytricini*[11,12] was identified in 1981. A more stable compound was produced in 1983 from hydrogen reaction and named tetrahydrolipstatin (THL) or orlistat.

Mechanism of action

Orlistat is a highly lipophilic compound; a potent and selective inhibitor of gastrointestinal lipases. Lipases participate in fat digestion process through hydrolysis of dietary triacylglycerol in fatty acids and monoacylglycerol that are subsequently absorbed by intestinal mucosal wall. Orlistat irreversibly inhibits the hydrolysis of dietary triacylglycerol by covalently binding to the active site of lipase, resulting in reduction of dietary fat absorption. Fat absorption reduction is dose-dependent inhibition of 30 per cent of fat absorption with the dose of 120 mg t.i.d.[13]. In contrast with lipase inhibition, orlistat does not inhibits other intestinal enzymes, including hydrolases, trypsin, phospholipase A2 or liver carboxylesterases. Due to its little systemic absorption it has no effect on plasmatic lipases[14].

Pharmacokinetics[14]

Absorption: Orlistat acts exclusively on gastrointestinal tract with negligible systemic absorption.

Distribution: Orlistat distribution volume may not be determined as it is minimally absorbed and has no defined systemic pharmacokinetics.

Metabolism: Orlistat is mostly metabolized within the gastrointestinal wall cells. Two orlistat metabolites have been detected at minimal concentrations in the plasma (M1 and M3) and do not show clinical activity.

Elimination: Almost 97 per cent of an oral dose of orlistat is eliminated by faeces, with 83 per cent eliminated intact in the feces.

Drug interactions: Orlistat do not showed interaction with the most frequently used drugs (anti-hypertensive agents, cardiovascular agents, contraceptives and alcohol) were studied. Drug interaction studies showed that phenytoin, warfarin, digoxin, oral contraceptive, statins, nifedipine and alcohol pharmacokinetics are not affected by concomitant use of orlistat.

Clinical efficacy

Orlistat effect has been extensively studied. Patients amounting to 13.5 million are estimated to have received orlistat since its launching in 1998, and more than 30,000 patients participated in clinical trial programmes with this medication

Weight loss and prevention of weight regain

Multicentre, double-blind, randomized, placebo-controlled studies showed orlistat efficacy in weight loss and maintenance[15-18]. In a European multicentre study[15], a total of 743 obese subjects (BMI 28–47 kg/m^2) were included, and received a hypocaloric diet (deficit of 600 kcal/day with 30 per cent calories from fat) and placebo for a 4-week period. After this period, 683 patients remained and were then randomized to receive hypocaloric diet and orlistat 120 mg t.i.d. ($n = 343$), or placebo ($n = 340$) for 1 year. After 1 year treatment the average body weight reduction was 10.2 per cent (10.3 kg) for the group receiving orlistat compared to 6.1 per cent (6.1 kg) reduction in the placebo group. This weight reduction was 68 per cent higher with orlistat ($P < 0.001$). Compared with placebo, a significantly higher proportion of patients treated with orlistat achieved weight loss higher than 5 per cent (68.5 per cent vs. 49.2 per cent; $P < 0.05$), while twice the patients receiving orlistat lost more than 10 per cent of the initial weight (38.8 per cent vs. 17.6 per cent; $P < 0.05$). During the second year of the study, patients received guidance for an isocaloric diet for weight maintenance and were again randomized to continue with the same treatment regimen (orlistat or placebo t.i.d.) or changing to an alternative regimen. During the second year, those patients who continued with orlistat regained half of the weight in average compared to those who were changed to placebo ($P < 0.001$). Patients who were changed from placebo to Orlistat lost an additional 0.9 kg during the second year, compared with an average regain of 2.5 kg in those patients who continued with placebo ($P < 0.001$).

Another study also carried out in European centres[16], randomized 729 obese patients (BMI 28–43 kg/m^2) to receive placebo ($n = 243$), orlistat 60 mg ($n = 242$) or orlistat 120 mg ($n = 244$) t.i.d. associated to a hypocaloric diet (deficit of 600 kcal with 30 per cent energy from fat). Weight loss with orlistat 120 mg and 60 mg (9.7 per cent and 8.6 per cent) was significantly higher than weight loss with placebo (6.4 per cent) after 1 year treatment ($P < 0.001$). Weight loss higher than 5 per cent or higher than 10 per cent was significantly higher in the group using orlistat ($P < 0.001$). After 1 year, those patients who lost > 3 kg received guidance for an isocaloric diet and those patients that lost less than 3 kg were kept in the usual diet. Medications were kept in the usual doses for one additional year. Those patients who had received orlistat 120 mg or 60 mg showed less weight regain than the placebo group ($P < 0.001; P < 0.05$).

In a multicentre study carried out in the United States[17], 892 patients were randomized to receive orlistat 120 mg t.i.d. ($n = 668$) or placebo ($n = 224$) associated to a hypocaloric diet for 1 year. The average body weight reduction was 8.8 per cent of the initial weight for the group receiving orlistat compared to a 5.8 per cent reduction for the group receiving placebo ($P < 0.001$). Compared with placebo, a significantly proportion of patients treated with orlistat achieved weight loss higher than 5 per cent (65.7 per cent vs. 43.6 per cent; $P < 0.01$), and higher than 10 per cent of the initial weight (38.9 per cent vs. 24.8 per cent; $P < 0.004$). After 1 year treatment, all patients that remained in the study received an isocaloric diet for weight maintenance. The placebo group continued to receive placebo ($n = 133$) while orlistat group was randomized to receive placebo ($n = 138$), orlistat 60 mg ($n = 152$) or 120 mg ($n = 153$) t.i.d. for an additional year. Those patients who received orlistat 120 mg showed lower weight regain (3.2 ± 0.45 kg) than those who received orlistat 60 mg (4.26 ± 0.57 kg) or placebo (5.63 ± 0.42 kg) during the second year ($P < 0.05$). A total of 34.1 per cent of the patients who received orlistat 120 mg for the two years maintained weight loss higher than 10 per cent of the initial weight in relation to only 17.5 per cent of the patients who received placebo for 2 years ($P < 0.02$).

Orlistat efficacy was also investigated in a study carried out in 17 primary care centres of USA[18]. This study differs from the previous ones as the patients were advised by not-expert health staff in obesity management. The patients watched several videos on behaviour modification for weight loss and received material with information on diet and lifestyle modification. A total of 635 patients were randomized to receive placebo ($n = 212$), orlistat 60 mg ($n = 213$) or orlistat 120 mg ($n = 210$) t.i.d. for a year, associated to hypocaloric diet. Those patients treated with orlistat lost significantly more weight (7.1 kg and 7.9 kg for 60 mg and 120 mg orlistat, respectively) than those treated with placebo (4.1 kg) within one year ($P < 0.001$). More patients of orlistat group lost more than 5 per cent of the initial weight (48.8 per cent and 50.5 per cent for 60 and 120 mg, respectively) compared with placebo group (30.7 per cent, ($P < 0.001$). After 1 year, patients were directed to follow weight maintenance diet and maintain medications in use. A small percentage of placebo group patients maintained weight loss higher than 5 per cent (24.1 per cent) compared with 34.3 per cent in the group receiving orlistat 120 mg (($P = 0.02$). In spite of the patients having regained weight in all groups, the lost weight recovery per cent was higher in the placebo group (60 per cent) than in the orlistat group 60 and 120 mg (37 per cent, 38 per cent). The average weight loss in this study for both groups (placebo or orlistat) was slightly lower than that achieved in other clinical trials with orlistat.

Efficacy in reducing waist circumference

Waist circumference measure has been considered as an important indicator of cardiovascular risk[19]. Studies showed that waist above 94 cm in men and above 80 cm in women is associated to a prevalence of 1.5 to 2 times higher cardiovascular risk factors in relation to general population. Those with waist above 102 cm, in the case of men, and above 88 cm in the case of women, show 2.5 to 3 times more risk factors in relation to general population[20].

Meta analysis carried out from five studies evidenced that the patients who received orlistat showed a significant reduction in abdominal circumference measure in relation to the group that received placebo (men: –6.7 vs. –4.9 cm; $P < 0.001$/women: –6.9 vs. –4.5 cm; $P < 0.001$ respectively)[21].

Efficacy in the treatment of diabetes

Several studies have confirmed the strong association between overweight and type 2 diabetes mellitus[22,23]. Around 80 per cent of diabetic people show overweight or obesity. Weight loss, even though moderate, is associated to an improvement in the disease control or progression[24,25].

Heymsfield et al.[26], analysed data from three similar clinical studies with orlistat in order to determine if a small weight reduction had improved glucose tolerance and reduced diabetes onset rate in obese patients. This meta-analysis included only those patients who received orlistat 120 mg t.i.d. or placebo for 2 years. After two years, the patients who received orlistat lost significantly more weight than those who received placebo (6.7 kg vs. 3.8 kg; $P < 0.001$). Intolerance to glucose was present in 18.7 per cent and 15.8 per cent of orlistat group and placebo group patients, respectively. After 2 years, a small percentage of these patients progressed to diabetes in the orlistat group (3.0 per cent) vs. placebo (7.6 per cent; $P = 0.04$) and 71.6 per cent of the patients treated with orlistat normalized glucose intolerance at the end of treatment compared to 49.1 per cent in placebo group ($P = 0.04$). Thus, addition of orlistat to conventional treatment for weight loss significantly improved oral tolerance to glucose and decreased progress rate to the development of type 2 diabetes.

A multicentre, randomized, placebo-controlled study was carried out in five Latin-American countries in order to assess the effect of orlistat on weight loss, glycaemic profile and other risk factors in obese patients with type 2 diabetes[27]. A total of 338 patients were randomized for the treatment with orlistat 120 mg ($n = 164$) or placebo ($n = 174$) t.i.d. associated to hypocaloric diet for 6 months. The orlistat group showed higher weight loss than placebo group (4.7 per cent vs. 3.0 per cent; $P = 0.0003$). More patients from orlistat group showed weight loss higher than 5 per cent of the initial weight in relation to placebo group (30 per cent vs. 17 per cent; $P = 0.003$). Orlistat was associated to a significant improvement in glycaemic control, compared to placebo, as reflected by a higher reduction of HbA1c (–0.6 per cent vs. –0.2 per cent; $P = 0.06$), fasting plasma glucose (–1.00 vs. –0.01 mmol/l; $P = 0.04$) and postprandial glucose (–1.06 vs. + 0.17 mmol/l; $P = 0.05$). There was a significant improvement in relation to total cholesterol and LDL-cholesterol levels. Orlistat associated to diet may be effective in the control of type 2 diabetes.

The treatment with sulphonylureas is frequently associated to weight gain and may negatively affect diabetes control. Hollander et al.[28], studied orlistat efficacy in promoting weight loss in 322 obese and diabetic patients who were receiving sulphonylureas. Patients were randomized for orlistat 120 mg t.i.d. or placebo combined with hypocaloric diet (deficit of 500 kcal/day). Patients treated with orlistat lost more weight (–6.2 per cent) that placebo group (–4.3 per cent; $P < 0.001$). Compared with placebo, twice the patients treated with orlistat achieved weight loss higher than 5 per cent (48.8 per cent vs. 22.6 per cent; $P < 0.001$), and 17.9 per cent of the patients who received orlistat lost more than 10 per cent of the initial weight compared with only 8,8 per cent of placebo group. The treatment with orlistat plus diet compared with placebo plus diet was associated to a significant improvement of glycaemic control, as reflected by HbA1c decreases ($P < 0.001$), by fasting plasma glucose ($P < 0.001$) and by the reductions of oral sulphonylureas ($P < 0.01$).

The insulin therapy is generally started in those patients for whom diet and antidiabetic agents have failed. However, long-term insulin therapy is frequently associated to weight gain, as observed in

UKPDS. Also, there are evidences that obese patients do not respond to insulin therapy as well as non-obese patients[29]. Thus, weight control is a particular issue in overweight diabetic patients receiving insulin. Bray *et al.*[2] evaluated the effect of orlistat in overweight type 2 diabetic patients receiving insulin. Diabetic patients with BMI from 28–43 kg/m^2 and HbA1c of 7.5–12.0 per cent were randomized for treatment with hypocaloric diet (daily deficit of 600 kcal/day) plus orlistat 120 mg t.i.d. ($n = 269$) or placebo ($n = 266$). After 1 year, the orlistat group patients lost significantly more weight (−3.76 ± 0.3 per cent of initial body weight) than those patients receiving placebo (−1.22 ± 0.3 per cent; $P = 0.002$). In addition, more patients from orlistat group achieved weight loss ≥ 5 per cent (33 per cent vs. 13 per cent; $P = 0.000$) or ≥ 10 per cent (10 per cent vs. 4 per cent; $P = 0.001$). The group receiving orlistat also showed significantly higher decreases in HbA1c (−0.62 ± 0.08 per cent vs. +0.27 ± 0.08 per cent; $P = 0.002$), fasting plasma glucose (−1.63 ± 0.3 vs. −1.08 ± 0.3 mmol/l; $P = 0.02$), insulin doses (−8.1 ± 1.5 vs. −1.6 ± 1.7 U/day; $P = 0.007$), and other antidiabetic medications. These results indicate that orlistat plus diet is a useful adjuvant treatment to improve glycaemic control in type 2 diabetes obese patients that are sub-optimally controlled with insulin and other antidiabetic medications.

Metformin results lower weight gain than insulin or sulphonylureas, thus, being preferably used for diabetic obese patients. Miles *et al.*[30] evaluated orlistat effect on body weight, glycaemic control and cardiovascular risk factors in diabetic obese subjects treated with metformin (1000–2500 mg/day) isolated or combined with other oral agents. Patients with BMI of 28–43 kg/m^2 and HbA1c of 7.5–12.0 per cent were randomized for hypocaloric diet plus orlistat ($n = 249$) or placebo ($n = 254$). After 1 year, weight loss was significantly higher than placebo (−4.6 ± 0.3 per cent vs. −1.7 ± 0.3 per cent of initial body weight; $P < 0.001$), and a major proportion of orlistat group achieved weight loss ≥ 5 per cent (39.0 per cent vs. 15.7 per cent; $P < 0.001$), and weight loss ≥ 10 per cent (14.1 per cent vs. 3.9 per cent; $P < 0.001$). Reduction of HbA1c ≥ 0.5 per cent (61 per cent vs. 43 per cent; $P < 0.01$) and ≥ 1.0 per cent (46 per cent vs. 29 per cent; $P < 0.01$) was significant in orlistat group in relation to placebo. More patients treated with orlistat decreased or discontinued at least one antidiabetic medication compared to placebo (17 per cent vs. 8 per cent). This data show that orlistat is useful in weight control and results in improvement of glycaemic control in obese patients that are being treated with metformin for type 2 diabetes mellitus.

Thus, there are currently considerable evidences that the treatment with orlistat associated to diet produces a significant weight loss and has additional favourable effects on glycaemic control of overweight diabetic patients using or not antidiabetic medications (sulphonylureas, metformin or insulin). Orlistat is a useful therapeutic choice for overweight diabetic patients.

Efficacy in dyslipidaemia control

Dyslipidaemia is one of the major risk factors for coronary disease. Overweight is frequently associated with elevated total cholesterol, LDL-cholesterol and triglyceride levels, and with a decrease in HDL-cholesterol[31]. Improvement of lipid profile may be achieved with weight loss[32].

Randomized clinical studies showed that the use of orlistat associated to diet has a positive effect on plasma lipids, especially total cholesterol and LDL-cholesterol reduction[15–17]. In the study by Sjöstrom *et al.*[15], there was a reduction of 0.36 per cent in total cholesterol and 1.15 per cent in LDL-cholesterol after 1 year treatment in the group treated with orlistat compared with an increase of 4.91 per cent and 5.18 per cent in the group that received placebo ($P < 0.001$). Another study showed that after a 2-year treatment with orlistat 120 mg there was a significant reduction of LDL-cholesterol in relation to placebo that was independent of the higher weight loss of orlistat group[17].

Muls *et al.*[33] evaluated the effect of orlistat on lipid levels of hypercholesterolaemic obese patients. This study, carried out in 19 centres in Belgium, was a 24-week randomized, double-blind, placebo-controlled study. Treatment with orlistat was associated with significant reduction in total cholesterol (−11.9 per cent vs. −4.0 per cent; $P < 0.001$) and LDL-cholesterol (−17.6 per cent vs. −7.6 per cent; $P < 0.001$) in relation to placebo. For any weight loss category during treatment, from gain to loss ≥ 10 per cent of the initial weight, the changes in LDL-cholesterol were higher in orlistat group than in placebo, indicating that orlistat has a direct effect on cholesterol reduction independent of the weight reduction.

Mittendorfer *et al.*[34] evaluated the hypothesis that orlistat inhibits cholesterol uptake from diet as a possible mechanism responsible for the orlistat additional effect on the reduction of total cholesterol and LDL-cholesterol. In this study, the treatment with orlistat caused a 25 per cent reduction in cholesterol uptake, from 53 ± 6 per cent for 44 ± 5 per cent ($P < 0.01$).

Effect on blood pressure

A moderate weight loss is associated to major blood pressure reduction in obese patients. A meta-analysis of five randomized, double-blind, placebo-controlled studies showed that the patients presenting increased diastolic blood pressure (DBP ≥ 90 mmHg) had a reduction of 7.9 mmHg in DBP when treated with orlistat compared to a reduction of 5.5 mmHg when treated with placebo after 1-year treatment (P = 0.06). In patients with increased systolic blood pressure at randomization time (SBP ≥ 140 mmHg), treatment with orlistat resulted in a significant reduction in relation to placebo group (−10.9 vs. −5.1 mmHg; $P < 0.05$)[35].

Adverse events

Orlistat is practically not absorbed and systemic adverse events are not expected. The most frequent side effects are the gastrointestinal ones related to the pharmacological action of the medication, and include in frequency order: oily spotting, flatus and discharge, fecal urgency, fatty/oily stool; oily evacuation, increased defecation and fecal incontinence[36]. In a meta-analysis comparing the results of 1740 patients treated with placebo and 2038 patients treated with orlistat, gastrointestinal events were significantly higher in orlistat group, but were considered as slight, occurring in the first weeks of treatment, and reducing frequency after 12-week therapy[37]. In placebo-controlled studies, between 1.1–6 per cent of the patients treated with orlistat and 0.6–1.3 per cent of the patients treated with placebo discontinued the study due to gastrointestinal events[38].

Cholecystokinin is one of the most important mediators of gallbladder emptying and its release depends on the presence of long-chain fatty acids in the intestine. Postprandial cholecystokinin release and gallbladder contraction might be decreased by orlistat, potentially resulting in an increased risk of gallstone formation. However, short-terms studies in healthy volunteers and obese patients do not suggest an increased risk of gallstone formation during the treatment with orlistat[39].

During 2-year clinical studies, plasma concentration of soluble vitamins (A, D, E and beta-carotene) decreased among patients who received orlistat, but remained often within normal range. In the study by Davidson *et al.*[17], vitamin supplement was required in 14.1 per cent of the orlistat group compared with 6.3 per cent of the placebo group.

Special conditions: use in adolescents

Obesity prevalence and severity is increasing in the paediatric population. There are no pharmacological agents currently approved for the treatment of child obesity. However, clinical studies are being developed with the use of orlistat for this population. An open-label pilot study using orlistat in adolescents for a 3-month period showed orlistat to be effective in weight loss, total cholesterol and LDL-cholesterol reduction and a significant improvement of insulin-sensitivity[39]. The true benefit and safety for this population requires further investigation in large controlled clinical studies.

References

1. World Health Organization. Obesity: Preventing and Managing the Global Epidemic. Report of a WHO consultation on obesity. Geneva, 3–5 June 1997: World Health Organization, 1998.

2. Pi-Sunyer FX. Medical hazards of obesity. *Ann Intern Med* 1993; 119: 655–60.

3. Bray GA. Health hazards of obesity. *Endocrinol Metab Clin North Am* 1996; 25: 907–19.

4. Wolf AM, Colditz GA. Current estimates of the economic cost of obesity in the United States. *Obes Res* 1998; 6: 97–106.

5. Seidell J, Deerenberg I. Obesity in Europe-prevalence and consequences for the use of medical care. *Pharmacoeconomics* 1994; 5 (Suppl 1): 38–44.

6. Goldstein DJ. Beneficial health effects of modest weight loss. *Int J Obes* 1992; 6: 397–415.

7. Pi-Sunyer FX. A review of long-term studies evaluating the efficacy of weight loss in ameliorating disorders associated with obesity. *Clin Ther* 1996; 18: 1006–35.

8. Kramer FM, Jeffrey RW, Forster JL *et al.* Long-term follow-up of behavioral treatment for obesity: patterns of weight regain among men and women. *Int J Obes* 1989; 13: 123–36.

9. Sarlio-Lähteenkorva S, Rissanen A, Kaprio J. A descriptive study of weight loss maintenance: 6 and 15-year follow-up of initially overweight adults. *Int J Obes* 2000; 24: 116–25.

10. Golay A, Bobbioni E. The role of dietary fat in obesity. *Int J Obes* 1997; 21 (Suppl3): S2–S11.

11. Weibel EK, Hadvary P, Hochuli E, Kupfer E, Lengsfeld H. Lipstatin, an inhibitor of pancreatic lipase, produced by Streptomyces toxytricini I. Producing organism, fermentation, isolation and biological activity. *J Antibiotics* 1987; 40: 1081–5.

12. Hochuli E, Kupfer E, Maurer R, Meister W, Mercadal Y, Schmidt K. Lipstatin, an inhibitor of pancreatic lipase, produced by Streptomyces toxytricini II. Chemistry and structure elucidation. *J Antibiotics* 1987; 40: 1086–91.

13. Zhi J, Melia AT, Guerciolini R, Chung J, Kinberg J, Hauptman JR. Retrospective population-based analysis of the dose-response (fecal fat excretion) relationship of orlistat in normal and obese volunteers. *Clin Pharmacol Ther* 1994; 56: 82–5.

14. Guerciolini R. Mode of action of orlistat. *Int J Obes* 1997; 21 (Suppl 1): S12–S23 .

15. Sjostrom L, Rissanen A, Andersen T *et al.* Randomised placebo-controlled trial of orlistat for weight loss and prevention of weight regain in obese patients. *Lancet* 1998; 352: 167–72.

16. Rösner S, Sjostrom L, Noack 'R, Meinders AE, Noseda G. Weight loss, weight maintenance and improved cardiovascular risk factors after 2 years treatment with orlistat for obesity. *Obes Res* 2000; 8: 49–61.

17. Davidson MH, Hauptman J, DiGirolamo M *et al.* Weight control and risk factor reduction in obese subjects treated for 2 years with orlistat. *JAMA* 1999; 281: 235–42.

18. Hauptman J, Lucas C, Boldrin MN, Collins H. Orlistat in the long-term treatment of obesity in primary care settings. *Arch Farm Med* 2000; 9: 160–7.

19. Seidell, JC, Cigolini M., Charzewska J, Ellsinger BM, Deslypere JP, Cruz A. Fat distribution in European men: comparison of anthropometric measurements in relation to cardiovascular risk factors. *Int J Obes* 1992; 16: 17–22 .

20. Hans TS, van Leer EM, Seidell JC, Lean ME. Waist circumference in the identification of cardiovascular risk factors: prevalence study in a random sample. *BMJ* 1995; 311: 1401–5.

21. Desprès JP. The impact of orlistat on the multifactorial risk profile of abdominally obese patients. *Diabetes* 1999; 48 (Suppl 1): A1344.

22. Hu FB, Manson JE, Stampfer MJ *et al.* Diet, lifestyle, and the risk of type 2 diabetes mellitus in women. *N Engl J Med* 2001; 345: 790–7.

23. Carey VJ, Walters EE, Colditz GA *et al.* Body fat distribution and risk of non-insulin-dependent diabetes mellitus in women. The Nurse's Health Study. *Am J Epidemiol* 1997; 145: 614–9.

24. Moore LL, Visioni AJ, Wilson PWF. Can sustained weight loss in overweight individuals reduce the risk of diabetes mellitus? *Epidemiology* 2000; 11: 269–73.

25. Wing RR, Koeske R, Epstein Leonard, Nolwalk MP, Gooding W, Becker D. Long-term effects of modest weight loss in type II diabetic patient. *Arch Intern Med* 1987; 147: 1749–53.

26. Heymsfield SB, Segal KR, Hauptman J *et al.* Effects of Weight Loss With Orlistat on Glucose Tolerance and Progression to Type 2 Diabetes in Obese Adults. *Arch Intern Med* 2000; 160: 1321–6.

27. Halpern A. Latin-American multicentric study with orlistat in overweight or obese patients with type 2 diabetes (abstract). *Diabetes* 2001; 50 (Suppl 2): 437.

28. Hollander PA, Elbein SC, Hirsch IB *et al.* (1): Role of orlistat in the treatment of obese patients with 2 diabetes. A 1-year randomized double-blind study. *Diabetes Care* 21, 1288–1294.

29. Yki-Jarvinen H, Ryysy L, Kauppila M *et al.* Effect of obesity on the response to insulin therapy in noninsulin-dependent diabetes mellitus. *J Clin Endocrinol Metab* 1997; 82: 4037–43.

30. Bray GA, Pi-Sunyer FX, Hollander P *et al.* Effect of orlistat in overweight patients with type 2 diabetes receiving insulin therapy. *Diabetes* 2001; 50 (Suppl 2): 433.

31. Miles JM, Aronne LJ, Hollander P, Klein S. Effect of orlistat in overweight and obese type 2 diabetes treated with metformin. *Diabetes* 2001; 50 (Suppl 2): 442–3.

32. Brown CD, Higgins M, Donato KA *et al.* Body mass index and the prevalence of hypertension and dislipidaemia. *Obes Res* 2000; 8: 605–19.

33. Dattilo AM, Kris-Etherton PM. Effects of weight reduction on blood lipids and lipoproteins: a meta-analysis. *Am J Clin Nutr* 1992; 56: 320–8.

34. Muls E, Kolanowski J, Scheen A, van Gaal L. The effects of orlistat on weight and serum lipids in obese patients with hipercholesterolaemia: a randomized, double-blind, placebo-controlled, multicenter study. *Int J Obes* 2001; 25: 1713–21.

35. Mittendorfer B, Ostlund RE, Patterson BW, Klein S. Orlistat inhibits dietary cholesterol absorption. *Obes Res* 2001; 9: 599–604.

36. Zavoral JH. Treatment with orlistat reduces cardiovascular risk in obese patients. *J Hypertension* 1998; 16: 2013–7.

37. Ballinger A . Orlistat in the treatment of obesity. *Expert Opin Pharmacother* 2000; 1: 841–7.

38. McNeely W, Benfield P. Orlistat. *Drugs* 1998; 56: 241–50.

39. Ballinger A, Peikin SR. Orlistat: its current status as an anti-obesity drug. *Eur J Pharmacol* 2002; 440: 109–17 .

40. McCann S, McDuffie J, Nicholson J, Sastry L, Calis K, Yanovski J. A pilot of the efficacy of orlistat in overweight adolescents. *Obes Res* 2002; 8 (Suppl 1): 58.

Progress in Obesity Research: 9. Edited by *Geraldo Medeiros-Neto, Alfredo Halpern and Claude Bouchard*
©2003 John Libbey Eurotext Ltd, pp. 1051–1057.

CHAPTER 218

The role of sibutramine in the clinical management of obesity

Donna H. Ryan

Pennington Biomedical Research Center, 6400 Perkins Road, Baton Rouge, LA 70808, USA
[e-mail: ryandh@pbrc.edu]

Sibutramine – pharmacology and mechanism of action

Sibutramine (marketed as Meridia in the US and Reductil in Europe) is a selective reuptake inhibitor for norepinephrine, serotonin, and dopamine[1]. The drug is rapidly metabolized to two active metabolites, whose half-life is 14–16 h, with the peak concentration at 3 to 4 h and a plateau from 3 to 7 h[2]. This pharmacologic profile allows for once a day dosing, an advantage when appetite regulation is the aim.

In clinical trials with humans, sibutramine decreases food intake in non-dieting men[3] and women[4], by increasing meal-induced satiety[3-5]. Sibutramine also affects energy expenditure in humans on the order of 3–5 per cent increase in metabolic rate beginning 3 h from ingestion and lasting less than 24 h[5]. The expected decline in resting energy expenditure usually observed with weight loss is blunted in sibutramine-treated patients, equivalent to 100 kcal/day[6].

Sibutramine – clinical efficacy

The key clinical efficacy features of sibutramine are illustrated in Table 1[7-20].

A key feature of sibutramine's efficacy is the dose: response relationship. Sibutramine 1, 5, 10, 15, 20 and 30 mg and the effect on weight loss is illustrated by a study reported by Bray et al.[8] and depicted in Table 1, which shows the results of a double-blind, placebo controlled study conducted in seven centres and enrolling 1047 subjects. The recommended dose levels for use in clinical practice are 5–15 mg/day and these doses produced –3.9 per cent, –6.1 per cent and –7.4 per cent loss from baseline at week 24. As can be observed, the behavioural approach used with pharmacotherapy in this study was relatively weak, since the mean weight loss associated with placebo was only 1.2 per cent from baseline at 24 weeks. Mean weight loss is useful information, but another way of analysing results is appropriate. Physicians should find it useful to evaluate the chances of an individual patient achieving significant weight loss. Weight loss of 5 per cent and 10 per cent from baseline are useful benchmarks, because these are associated with significant health benefits. Of persons taking sibutramine 5, 10 and 15 mg doses in this study, 37.4 per cent, 59.5 per cent and 63.7 per cent achieved 5 per cent weight loss from baseline compared to only 19.5 per cent of those taking placebo.

The intensity of the behavioural component of the weight loss programme also influences the amount of weight loss with sibutramine. Since sibutramine enhances satiety, a dietary programme that takes advantage of this mechanism is likely to produce greater weight loss. Wadden[21] illustrates the advantage of a highly structured dietary intervention in combination with sibutramine. In that study 53 women were randomized to receive sibutramine 10–15 mg daily versus the same dosing scheme with a group lifestyle modification programme, versus the same dosing scheme with a highly structured portion-controlled diet included in the first 4 months of the lifestyle modification programme. The group that received an initial 4 months of a highly structured diet (four servings of nutritional supplements and an evening meal of a frozen entrée, fruit and salad) lost the greatest amount (16.5 per cent from baseline) compared to the other two groups who lost 4.1 per cent (drug alone) and 10.8 per cent (drug + lifestyle).

Table 1. Clinical trials with sibutramine of ≥ 24 weeks duration and with placebo control

Author	Year	No. of subjects Started	No. of subjects Completed	Dose (mg/day)	Duration of study (weeks)	Initial weight (kg) Placebo	Initial weight (kg) Drug	Weight loss (kg) Placebo	Weight loss (kg) Drug	Weight loss (%) Placebo	Weight loss (%) Drug	Comments
Bray et al.[7]	1996	24 24 25 25 25 24 26	23 21 24 22 20 22 23	0 1 5 10 15 20 30	24	92.0	95.8 90.9 87.2 89.7 90.9 91.4	−0.75	−2.96 −2.87 −6.19 −6.89 −7.30 −8.24	−0.77	−3.20 −3.07 −6.91 −7.77 −8.06 −9.17	Part of multi-centre study (8), data on completing men and women
Bray et al.[8]	1999	148 149 151 150 152 146 151	87 95 107 99 98 96 101	0 1 5 10 15 20 30	24	95	94 94 91 93 93 95	−1.3	−2.4 −3.7 −5.7 −7.0 −8.2 −9.0	−1.2	−2.7 −3.9 −6.1 −7.4 −8.8 −9.4	Multi-centre phase III trial
Apfelbaum et al.[9]	1999	181 82	48 60	0 10	52	97.7	95.7	+0.2	−6.1	+0.2	−6.4	Multi-centre; those with > 6 kg weight loss after 4 weeks VLCD were randomized
Fanghanel et al.[10]	2000	55 54	44 40	0 10	26	86.4	87.5	−4.6	−8.8	−4.8	−9.9	BMI > 30 kg/m². Diet 30 kcal/kg of ideal body weight
James et al.[11]	2000	115 352	57 204	0 10–20	78	102.1	102.3	−4.7	−10.2	−4.4	−10.0	Multi-centre trial in subjects who lost ≥ 5 per cent on 10 mg sibutramine in 6 months
Cuellar, et al.[12]	2000	9/34 placebo 22/35 sibutramine		0 15	24	90.1	86.0	−1.3	−10.4	−1.4	−10.4	
Smith, et al.[13]	2001	80/163 placebo 94/161 10 mg 82/161 20 mg	163 161 161	80 90 82	87	87	87 87	−1.6	−4.4 −6.4	−1.8	−5.0 −7.3	
Dujovne, et al.[14]	2001	54/160 placebo 48/162 20 mg	160 162	54 48	102.0	99.7		−0.6	−4.9	−0.6	−4.6	Obese subjects with dyslipidaemia

Table 1. Contd.

Author	Year	No. of subjects		Dose (mg/day)	Duration of study (weeks)	Initial weight (kg)		Weight loss (kg)		Weight loss (%)		Comments
		Started	Completed			Placebo	Drug	Placebo	Drug	Placebo	Drug	
Wirth, et al.[15]	2001	146/201 325/405 15 mg 315/395 intermittent *intermittent therapy		201 415 395* *intermittent therapy	146 325 315	98.2	98.6 98.2	-3.9	-7.9 -7.8	-3.9	-8.2 -8.1	After > 2% loss at 4 weeks, subjects randomized to placebo vs. 15 mg sibutramine vs. intermittent sibutramine (weeks 1–12, 19–30.37–48).
Sibutramine trials in obese patients with diabetes												
Fujioka et al.[16]	2000	89 86	61 60	0 5–20	24	98.2	99.3	-0.4	-3.7	-0.5	-4.5	Multi-centre trial in diabetics
Gokcel, et al.[17]	2001	30 30	25 29	0 20	24	95.5	98.6 98.2	-0.9	-9.6	NA	NA	Obese females with poorly controlled diabetes
Serrano-Rios, et al.[18]	2002	65 69	57 53	0 15	24	94.2	92.0	-1.7	-4.5	-1.7	-4.5	Obese patients with diabetes stable on sulphonylurea therapy
Sibutramine trials in obese patients with hypertension												
McMahon et al.[19]	2000	150 142	74 69	0 5–20	52	95.5	97.0	-0.5	-4.4	-0.7	-4.7	Multi-centre trial in hypertensives on calcium channel blockers ± beta blockers, thiazide diuretics
McMahon et al.[20]	2002	74 146	36 84	0 20	52	99.0	96.7	-0.4	-4.5	-0.3	-4.8	Hypertensive patients on ace inhibitor ± diuretic

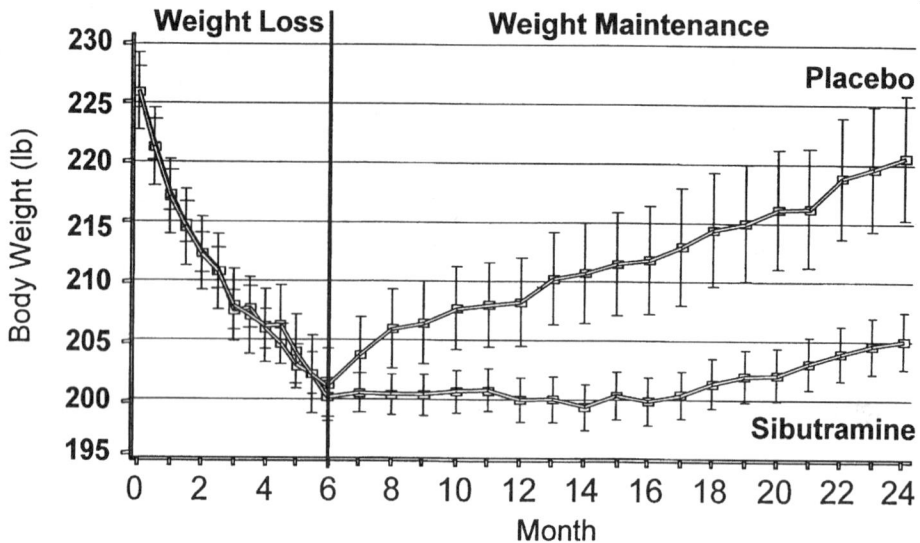

Fig. 1. The STORM trial: a multicentre study enrolling 605 obese patients. For the first 6 months patients received sibutramine 10 mg daily and a calorie deficit diet. At 6 months, patients were randomized to placebo vs. sibutramine for an additional 18 months.
*Same diet, exercise for sibutramine, placebo; $P \leq 0.001$, sibutramine vs. placebo for weight maintenance.
Adapted with permission from James WPT et al., Lancet 2000; 356: 2119.

Perhaps the greatest advantage of sibutramine is its efficacy in weight loss maintenance. Three trials have been designed to address this issue[9,11,15]. After inducing weight loss with very low calorie liquid diet[9] or with sibutramine[11,15], patients were randomized to placebo or sibutramine for maintenance of weight loss for up to 18 months. The STORM trial[11] illustrates that sibutramine is quite effective for inducing and maintaining weight loss for up to 2 years and provides a number of notable lessons, as illustrated in Fig. 1. In this multicentre European study, patients received sibutramine 10 mg and a calorie deficit diet for six months. Of the 605 obese patients who entered the trial, 467 (77 per cent) achieved weight loss of at least 5 per cent from baseline. Those patients were then randomized to receive sibutramine (doses could be titrated from 10 to 20 mg daily) or placebo. Following 24 months of observation, weight loss of the sibutramine treated group averaged 10.2 kg baseline compared to 4.7 kg for placebo. Physicians might infer from this study that about three-quarters of obese patients who are prescribed sibutramine 10 mg/day with a diet programme will achieve meaningful weight loss. If medication is continued, albeit with dose increase as needed, almost half of those will maintain 80 per cent of the weight loss.

Obesity is associated with increased risk for type 2 diabetes and for hypertension and in clinical practice, these comorbidities are frequently encountered. The experience with sibutramine used in controlled clinical trials of > 24 weeks in obese patients with hypertension and with diabetes are presented in Table 1. In all instances the weight loss pattern favours sibutramine.

Three studies of ≥ 24 weeks describe sibutramine use in patients with diabetes. In the study by Gokcel[17] 60 female patients with diabetes who had poorly controlled glucose levels (HbA1c > 8 per cent) on maximal doses of sulphonylureas and metformin were randomly assigned to sibutramine 10 mg twice daily or placebo. The weight loss at 24 weeks was −9.6 kg in sibutramine treated patients and −0.9 kg in those on placebo. The improvements in glycaemic control were equally striking. In the sibutramine treated patients, Hg Alc fell −2.73 per cent compared to −0.53 per cent with the placebo. Insulin levels fell −5.66 µU/ml compared to −0.68 for placebo and fasting glucose fell −124.88 mg/dl compared to −15.76 mg/dl for placebo. While the weight loss in most of the studies of patients with diabetes does not appear as great as in non-diabetic patients, in all of the studies the percentage of patients who achieved weight loss ≥ 5 per cent from baseline was significantly greater than placebo. In all studies the degree of weight loss corresponds to the degree of improvement in glycaemic control.

Two trials have been reported using sibutramine to treat hypertensive patients over one year[19,20] (Table 1). McMahon et al.[29] reported a 52-week trial in hypertensive patients whose blood pressure was latory blood pressure, as well as pharmacokinetics. The study will provide important safety and efficacy data relevant to address the growing epidemic of childhood obesity.

Another trial explores the feasibility of maximizing weight loss through use of meal replacements. 'SLIM-MER' combines meal replacements (Slim-Fast®) with sibutramine for otherwise healthy obese men and women with BMI 30–40 kg/m². This study provides three months of sibutramine 10 mg with a diet of two Slim-Fast® shakes and one regular meal daily in a lifestyle modification programme. At 3 months patients are randomized to placebo and regular meals vs. sibutramine 15 mg/day and one Slim-Fast® shake with two regular meals daily for the remaining nine months of the study.

There is a long-term weight maintenance study underway that has randomized 466 highly motivated adult patients age 20–78 years. Those volunteers documented loss of > 10 kg for 6 months by non-pharmacologic means and had gained back < 50 per cent peak weight loss. They are randomized to receive a behavioural modification program and either placebo or sibutramine 15 mg/day for 5 years. This study will provide valuable information on medicating with sibutramine for the long-term. If obesity is a chronic disease that requires continued medication for control, this data will be quite valuable.

The SCOUT study – Sibutramine Cardiovascular Outcome Study – will address the important issues of sibutramine use in patients at risk for a CV event and may address the issue of sibutramine's mixed effects on cardiovascular risk factors by using cardiovascular events as the study's primary endpoint. This is a double-blind, randomized, placebo-controlled, parallel-group, global, multicentre study with a single-blind sibutramine lead-in period. There will be 12,000 patients enrolled in the lead-in period. Patients will be 55 years or older with BMI $\geq$ 27 kg/m² or $\geq$ 25 kg/m² with waist circumferences $\geq$ 102 cm (males) or $\geq$ 88 cm (females). In addition, patients will have documented cardiovascular disease or type 2 diabetes. The primary endpoint is time from randomization to the first occurrence of nonfatal myocardial infarction, nonfatal stroke, resuscitated cardiac arrest or cardiovascular death. Over 400 clinical sites are expected to participate.

Conclusion

Sibutramine promotes weight loss through a dual mechanism of action. It has demonstrated efficacy in inducing and maintaining weight loss for up to two years. Future studies will expand this experience to five years and explore the safety of sibutramine in patients at risk for cardiovascular events. The SCOUT study is expected to evaluate sibutramine's efficacy in cardiovascular risk reduction.

References

1. Heal DJ, Aspley S, Prow MR, Jackson HC, Martin KF, Cheetham SC. Sibutramine: a novel anti-obesity drug. A review of the pharmacological evidence to differentiate it from d-amphetamine and d-fenfluramine. *Int J Obes Relat Metab Disord* 1998; 22 (Suppl 1): S19–S28.

2. Luque CA, Rey JA. Sibutramine: A serotonin-norepinephrine reuptake-inhibitor for the treatment of obesity. *Ann Pharmacother* 1999; 33: 968–78.

3. Chapelot D, Marmonier C, Thomas F, Hanotin C. Modalities of the food intake-reducing effect of sibutramine in humans. *Physiol Behav* 2000; 68: 299–308.

4. Rolls BJ, Shide DJ, Thorwart ML, Ulbrecht JS. Sibutramine reduces food intake in non-dieting women with obesity. *Obes Res* 1998; 6: 1–11.

5. Hansen DL, Toubro S, Stock MJ, Macdonald IA, Astrup A. Thermogenic effects of sibutramine in humans. *Am J Clin Nutr* 1998; 6; 1180–6.

6. Walsh KM, Leen E, Lean MEJ. The effect of sibutramine on resting energy expenditure and adrenaline-induced thermogenesis in obese females. *Int J Obes Rel Met Dis* 1999; 23(10): 1009–15.

7. Bray GA, Ryan DH, Gordon D, Heidingsfelder S, Cerise F, Wilson K. A double-blind randomized placebo-controlled trial of sibutramine. *Obes Res* 1996; 4: 263–70.

8. Bray GA, Blackburn GL, Ferguson JM, Greenway FL, Jain AK, Mendel CM *et al.* Sibutramine produces dose-related weight loss. *Obes Res* 1999; 7: 189–98.

9. Apfelbaum M, Vague P, Ziegler O, Hanotin C, Thomas F, Leutenegger E. Long-term maintenance of weight loss after a very-low-calorie diet: A randomized blinded trial of the efficacy and tolerability of sibutramine. *Am J Med* 1999; 106: 179–84.

10. Fanghanel G, Cortinas L, Sanchez-Reyes L, Berber A. Second phase of a double-blind study clinical trial on Sibutramine for the treatment of patients suffering essential obesity: 6 months after treatment cross-over. *Int J Obes Relat Metab Disord* 2001; 25(5): 741–7.

11. James WPT, Astrup A, Finer N, Hilsted J, Kopelman P, Rossner S *et al.* for the STORM Study Group. Effect of sibutramine on weight maintenance after weight loss: a randomised trial. *Lancet* 2000; 356: 2119–25.

controlled with calcium channel blockers with or without β-blockers or thiazides. Sibutramine doses were increased from 5 to 20 mg/d during the first 6 weeks. Weight loss was significantly greater in the sibutramine-treated patients, averaging –4.4 kg (4.7 per cent) as compared to –0.5 kg (0.7 per cent) in the placebo-treated group. Diastolic BP decreased –1.3 mmHg in the placebo-treated group and increased by 2.0 mmHg in the sibutramine-treated group. The SBP increased +1.5 mmHg in the placebo-treated group and by +2.7 in the sibutramine-treated group. Heart rate was unchanged in the placebo-treated patients, and increased +4.9 bpm in the sibutramine-treated patients[23].

Weight loss with sibutramine is associated with improvement in lipids, waist circumference, measures of glycaemic control and quality of life. The need for brevity does not allow us to review those benefits here. The cardiostimulatory effects of sibutramine mean that the drug may have mixed effects on cardiovascular risk factors and this shall be discussed in detail later.

Sibutramine safety and tolerability

The side effects of sibutramine (insomnia, asthenia, dry mouth, and constipation) are generally mild and transient. Sibutramine is not associated with valvulopathy[23]. Although the drug is scheduled as a Class IV substance, there is no evidence for abuse potential, as demonstrated in a study of 31 male recreational stimulant users[24]. There is no evidence for a clinically relevant interaction of sibutramine with alcohol in impairment of cognitive function[25].

If sibutramine acts via central nervous system stimulation of norepinephrine and serotonin and through the sympathetic nervous system to increase thermogenesis, then, cardiostimulatory effects are to be expected. The principle concerns with sibutramine safety have been the increase in blood pressure and pulse rate that averages 1–3 mm Hg for BP and a 4–6 beats/min increase in pulse[26,27]. The mean increases do not tell the whole story. Some patients are sensitive to sibutramine and will experience blood pressure and pulse increases to unacceptable levels. In the clinical trials reviewed in this article, that usually represents < 2 per cent of patients exposed to sibutramine. It is recommended in the prescribing information that patients be monitored for blood pressure and pulse changes at 2–4 weeks after initiating the medication. If, after prescribing sibutramine, blood pressure is in the hypertensive range or pulse > 100 beats/min, the drug should be stopped.

The mean increase in blood pressure and pulse are problematic on another level besides just the tendency to cause clinically significant changes in some patients, and represent a therapeutic dilemma when viewed from a population perspective. If sibutramine has mixed effects on risk factors, increasing blood pressure while producing the decreases in cholesterol and improvement in other risk factors associated with weight reduction, how are we to judge the net result?

It has been suggested that the blood pressure effects of sibutramine are mitigated by greater weight loss[27]. That is, with increasing amounts of weight loss the blood pressure change may actually be a net decrease, albeit less than that observed with similar non-pharmacologic weight loss. Thus, for an individual patient who has successfully achieved weight loss with sibutramine, the blood pressure may be reduced from baseline, although the blood pressure reduction may not be as great as that associated with the same degree of weight lost without medications. One strategy for managing the blood pressure is to use guidelines of 135/85 or ≤ 10 mm increase in systolic or diastolic blood pressure as acceptable limits. If a conservative approach to acceptable blood pressure is taken, the clinician cannot be faulted for using sibutramine to induce meaningful weight loss.

Another strategy to deal with the cardiostimulatory effects of sibutramine has been described by Berube-Parent *et al.*[28]. In this intervention, an aerobic exercise programme was added to a weight loss programme that combined diet and sibutramine 10 mg. This small (*n* = 8 men) observational study should not be extrapolated to a larger, more diverse, population. However, the study did show promise in terms of enhanced weight loss (10.7 kg in 12 weeks) and a benefit in mitigating the cardiostimulatory side effects of sibutramine with the aerobic exercise component.

Future directions for sibutramine study

Four clinical trials[29], in progress or in planning, are worthy of note. 'AWESOME', Adolescent Weight Loss Study of Meridia®, addresses pharmacotherapy for obesity in children age 12–16 years. The BMI (body mass index) of enrolled children is 28–48 kg/m^2. There are 498 randomized participants. Patients are randomized 3 : 1 to sibutramine 10 mg vs. placebo for 6 months. The BMI is assessed at 6 months; if < 10 per cent decrease in BMI, sibutramine is increased to 15 mg or if > 10 per cent, it is continued at 10 mg/day. The study gathers data on left ventricular wall thickness by echocardiogram and ambu-

12. Cuellar GEM, Ruiz AM, Monsalve MCR, Berber A. Six-month treatment of obesity with sibutramine 15 mg/ a double-blind, placebo-controlled monocenter clinical trial in a Hispanic population. *Obes Res* 2000; 8(1): 71–82.

13. Smith IG, Goulder MA. Randomized placebo-controlled trial of long-term treatment with sibutramine in mild to moderate obesity. *J Fam Pract* 2001; 50(6): 505–12.

14. Dujovne CA, Zavoral JH, Rowe E, Mendel CM. Effects of sibutramine on body weight and serum lipids: a double-blind, randomized, placebo-controlled study in 322 overweight and obese patients with dyslipidaemia. *Am Heart J* 2001; 142(3): 489–97.

15. Wirth A, Krause J. Long-term weight loss with sibutramine. *JAMA* 2001; 286(11): 1331–9.

16. Fujioka K, Seaton TB, Rowe E, Jelinek CA, Raskin P, Lebovitz HE *et al.* Weight loss with sibutramine improves glycaaemic control and other metabolic parameters in obese patients with type 2 diabetes mellitus. *Diab Obes Metab* 2000; 2: 175–87.

17. Gokcel A, Karakose H, Ertorer EM, Tanaci N, Tutuncu NB, Guvener N. Effects of sibutramine in obese female subjects with type 2 diabetes and poor blood glucose control. *Diabet Care* 2001; 24(11): 1957–60.

18. Serrano-Rios M, Melchionda N, Moreno-Carretero E. (Spanish Investigators). Role of sibutramine in the treatment of obese Type 2 diabetic patients receiving sulphonylurea therapy. *Diabet Med* 2002; 19(2): 119–24.

19. McMahon FG, Fujioka K, Singh BN, Mendel CM, Rowe E, Rolston K *et al.* Efficacy and safety of sibutramine in obese white and African American patients with hypertension. *Arch Intern Med* 2000; 160; 2185–91.

20. McMahon FG, Weinstein SP, Rowe E, Ernst KR, Johnson F, Fujioka K. Sibutramine is safe and effective for weight loss in obese patients whose hypertension is well controlled with angiotensin-converting enzyme inhibitors. *J Hum Hypertens* 2002; 16(1): 5–11.

21. Wadden TA, Berkowitz RI, Sarwer DB, Prus-Wisniewski R, Steinberg C. Benefits of lifestyle modification in the pharmacologic treatment of obesity. *Arch Intern Med* 2001; 161: 218–27.

22. Hazenberg BP. Randomized, double-blind, placebo-controlled, multicenter study of sibutramine in obese hypertensive patients. *Cardiology* 2000; 94: 152–8.

23. Bach DS, Rissanen AM, Mendel CM, Shepherd G, Weinstein S, Kelly F. Absence of cardiac valve dysfunction in obese patients treated with sibutramine. *Obes Res* 1999; 7(4): 363–9.

24. Cole JO, Levin A, Beake B, Kaiser PE, Scheinbaum ML. Sibutramine: a new weight loss agent without evidence of the abuse potential associated with amphetamines. *J Clin Psychopharmacol* 1998; 18(3): 231–6.

25. Wesnes KA, Garratt C, Wickens M, Gudgeon A, Oliver S. Effects of sibutramine alone and with alcohol on cognitive function in healthy volunteers. *Br J Clin Pharmacol* 2000; 49(2): 110–7.

26. Lean ME. Sibutramine – a review of clinical efficacy. *Int J Obes* 1997; 21: S30–S36.

27. Sharma AM. Sibutramine in overweight/obese hypertensive patients. *Int J Obes Relat Metab Disord* 2001; 25 (Suppl 4): S20–S23.

28. Berube-Parent S, Prud-homme D, St-Pierre S, Doucet E, Tremblay A. Obesity treatment with a progressive clinical tri-therapy combining sibutramine and a supervised diet – exercise intervention. *Int J Obes Relat Metab Disord* 2001; 25(8): 1144–53.

29. Renz C. Personal communication. Abbott Laboratories, Inc., North Chicago.

Author Index

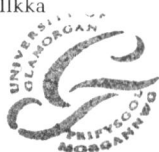

Achevé d'imprimer par Corlet, Imprimeur, S.A.
14110 Condé-sur-Noireau
N° d'Imprimeur : 72626 - Dépôt légal : août 2003

Imprimé en France